Universal Precautions: Prevention of Transmission of Human Immunodeficiency Virus, Hepatitis B Virus, and Other Blood-Borne Pathogens in Health Care Settings

Under universal precautions, blood and certain body fluids of all clients are considered potentially infectious for human immunodeficiency virus (HIV), hepatitis B virus (HBV), and other blood-borne pathogens. Blood is the single most important source of HIV, HBV, and other blood-borne pathogens in health care settings. Infection control efforts for HIV, HBV, and other blood-borne pathogens must focus on preventing exposures to blood as well as delivery of HBV immunization.

Epidemiologic evidence has implicated only blood, semen, vaginal secretions, and possibly breast milk in transmissions. Although the risk is unknown, universal precautions also apply to tissues and to the following fluids: cerebrospinal fluid, synovial fluid, pleural fluid, peritoneal fluid, and amniotic fluid. Universal precautions do not apply to feces, nasal secretions, sputum, saliva (except in a situation in which contamination with blood is likely, such as a dental setting), sweat, tears, urine, and vomitus, unless they contain visible blood. The risk of transmission of HIV and HBV from these materials is extremely low or nonexistent.

Health care workers are at risk for exposure to blood from clients infected with HIV, HBV, and other blood-borne pathogens. Health care workers must consider *all* clients as potentially infected with blood-borne pathogens and must adhere rigorously to infection control precautions for *all* clients.

Precautions to Prevent Transmission of HIV

General Precautions

- Consider *all* clients as potentially infected.
- Wear gloves when touching blood, body fluids containing blood, and body fluids to which universal precautions apply; for handling items or surfaces soiled with blood or applicable fluids; and for performing venipuncture and other vascular access procedures. Change gloves after each contact with a client.
- Use protective barriers (ie, wear masks, protective eyewear or face shields and gowns or aprons) when performing procedures that may produce blood or body fluid droplets or splashes.
- Wash hands and skin surfaces immediately and thoroughly with warm soap and water if contaminated with blood or other body fluids to which universal precautions apply; wash between clients and after removal of gloves even when they are intact.
- Take precautions to prevent injuries from needles, scalpels, and other sharp instruments during procedures, when cleaning instruments, during disposal, or when handling. To prevent needlestick injuries, needles should not be recapped, purposely bent or broken by hand, removed from disposable syringes, or otherwise manipulated. After they are used, disposable syringes and needles, scalpel blades, and other sharp items should be placed in puncture-resistant containers for disposal.
- Use mouthpieces, resuscitation bags, or other ventilation devices when mouth-to-mouth resuscitation is likely to be performed in emergency situations.

Special Considerations

- Health care workers who have exudative lesions or weeping dermatitis should refrain from all direct patient care and from handling patient care equipment until the condition resolves.
- Pregnant health care workers are not known to be at greater risk of contracting HIV infection than health care workers who are not pregnant; however, if a health care worker develops HIV infection during pregnancy, the infant is at risk of infection resulting from perinatal transmission. Because of this risk, pregnant health care workers should be especially familiar with and strictly adhere to precautions to minimize the risk of HIV transmission.

Precautions for Invasive Procedures

(Here an invasive procedure is defined as any surgical entry into tissues, cavities, or organs or repair of major traumatic injuries.) General blood and body fluid precautions listed earlier, combined with the precautions listed here, should be the *minimal precautions for all such invasive procedures*.

- All health care workers who participate in invasive procedures must routinely use appropriate barrier procedures to prevent skin and mucous membrane contact with all patient's blood and other body fluids to which universal precautions apply.
- Gloves and surgical masks must be worn for all invasive procedures.
- Protective eyewear or face shields should be worn for all procedures that commonly result in generation of droplets, splashing of blood, body fluids containing blood, and other applicable body fluids.
- Gowns or aprons made of materials providing an effective barrier should be worn during invasive procedures likely to result in the splashing of blood or other pertinent body fluids.
- All health care workers who perform or assist in vaginal or cesarean delivery should wear gloves and gowns when handling the placenta or the infant until blood and amniotic fluid have been removed from the infant's skin. Gloves should be worn until postdelivery care of the umbilical cord.
- If a glove is torn or a needlestick or other injury occurs, the glove should be removed and a new glove used as promptly as client safety permits; the needle or instrument involved in the incident should also be removed from the sterile field.

(Centers for Disease Control. [1987]. Recommendations for prevention of HIV transmission in health care settings. *Morbidity and Mortality Weekly Report, 36*[Suppl. 25]; Centers for Disease Control. [1988]. Update: Universal precautions for prevention of transmission of human immunodeficiency virus, hepatitis B virus, and other bloodborne pathogens in health-care settings. *Morbidity and Mortality Weekly Report, 37*[24]; and [1989] *Morbidity and Mortality Weekly Report, 38*[Suppl. 6], 9–18.)

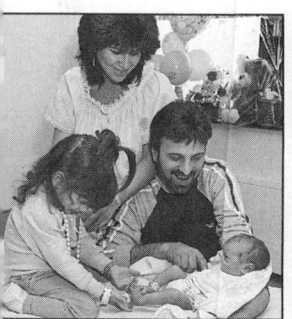
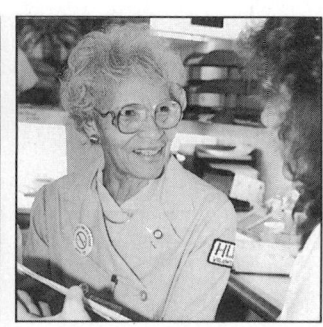
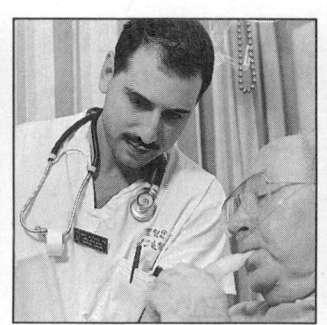
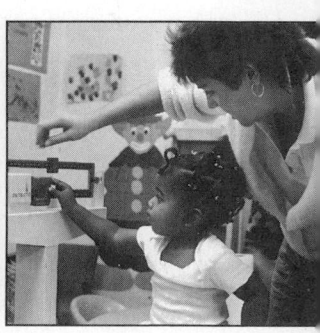

FUNDAMENTALS OF
NURSING

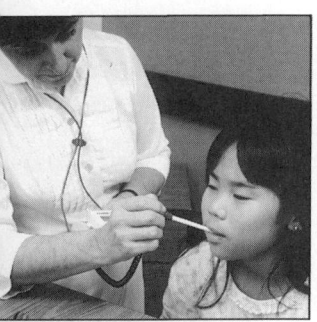

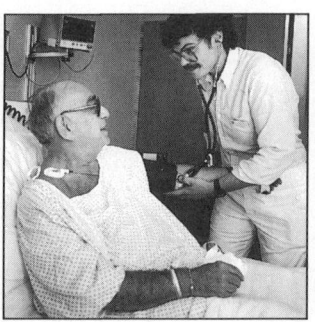

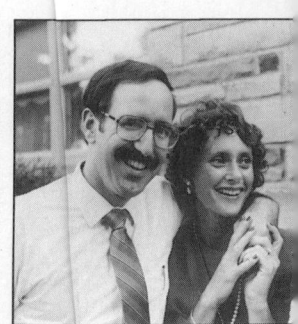

Carol Taylor
CSFN, RN, MSN,
PhD (Candidate)
Assistant Professor,
Nursing
Georgetown University
Washington, DC
Holy Family College
Philadelphia, Pennsylvania

Carol Lillis
RN, MSN
Associate Professor
Department of Nursing
Delaware County
Community College
Media, Pennsylvania

Priscilla LeMone
RNC, DSN
Assistant Professor
University of Missouri—
Columbia
Columbia, Missouri

SECOND EDITION

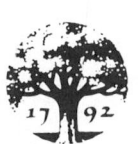

J. B. Lippincott Company   Philadelphia

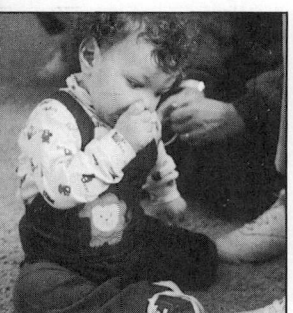
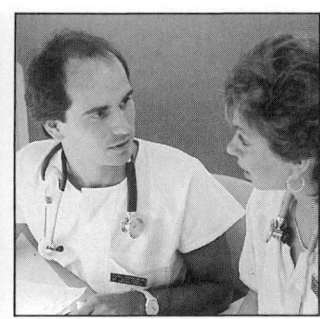

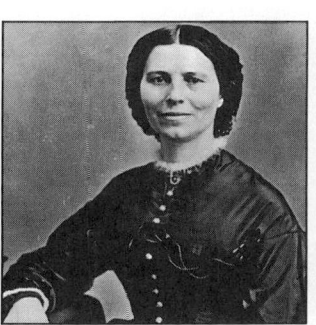

FUNDAMENTALS OF
NURSING

THE ART AND SCIENCE OF NURSING CARE

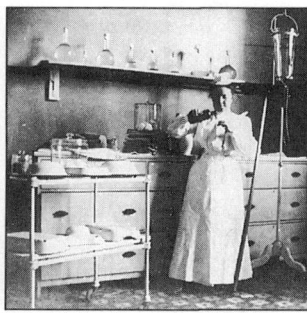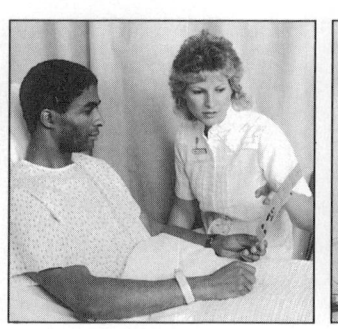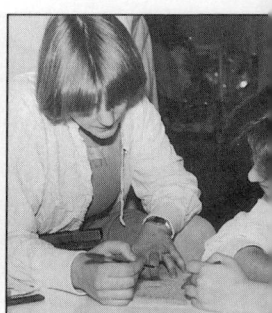

Sponsoring Editor: Donna L. Hilton, RN, BSN
Editorial Assistant: Susan Perry
Project Editors: Grace R. Caputo and Mary Rose Muccie
Indexer: Ann Cassar
Design Coordinator: Kathy Kelley-Luedtke
Designer: Tracy Baldwin
Production Manager: Helen Ewan
Compositor: Circle Graphics
Printer/Binder: R. R. Donnelley & Sons Company

2nd Edition

Copyright © 1993, by J. B. Lippincott Company.

Copyright © 1989, by J. B. Lippincott Company. All rights reserved. No part of this book may be used or reproduced in any manner whatsoever without written permission except for brief quotations embodied in critical articles and reviews. Printed in the United States of America. For information write J. B. Lippincott Company, 227 East Washington Square, Philadelphia, Pennsylvania 19106-3780.

6 5 4 3 2

Library of Congress Cataloging-in-Publication Data

Fundamentals of nursing : the art and science of nursing care /
  [edited by] Carol Taylor, Carol Lillis, Priscilla LeMone.—2nd ed.
    p.   cm.
  Includes bibliographical references and index.
  ISBN 0-397-54917-2
  1. Nursing. I. Taylor, Carol. II. Lillis, Carol. III. LeMone,
Priscilla.
  [DNLM: 1. Health Promotion. 2. Nursing. 3. Nursing Process. WY
16 F981]
RT41.F882   1993
610.73—dc20
DNLM/DLC
for Library of Congress   92-48786
                                    CIP

Any procedure or practice described in this book should be applied by the health-care practitioner under appropriate supervision in accordance with professional standards of care used with regard to the unique circumstances that apply in each practice situation. Care has been taken to confirm the accuracy of information presented and to describe generally accepted practices. However, the authors, editors, and publisher cannot accept any responsibility for errors or omissions or for any consequences from application of the information in this book and make no warranty, express or implied, with respect to the contents of the book.

Every effort has been made to ensure drug selections and dosages are in accordance with current recommendations and practice. Because of ongoing research, changes in government regulations and the constant flow of information on drug therapy, reactions and interactions, the reader is cautioned to check the package insert for each drug for indications, dosages, warnings and precautions, particularly if the drug is new or infrequently used.

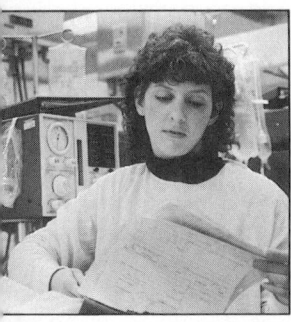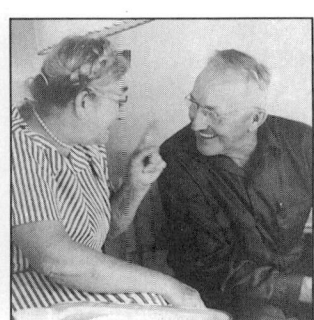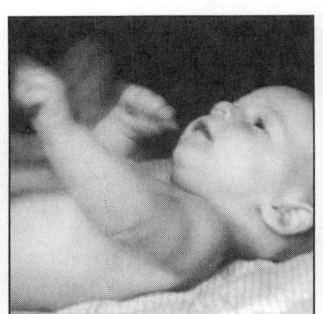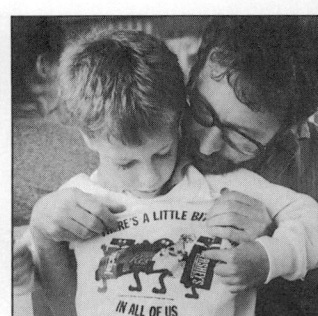

To my family, whose support enables me to
meet each new day with love and courage

Carol Taylor

To Mom and Dad, Cass and John—parents,
counselors, and friends—par excellence!

Carol Lillis

To the special people in my life who made
me truly understand caring: my parents,
Gordon and Sybil, and my husband, Jacque

Priscilla LeMone

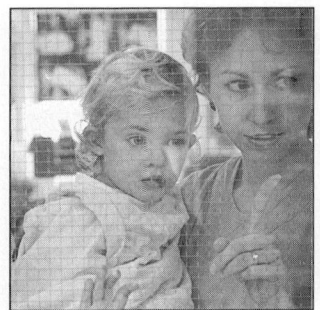
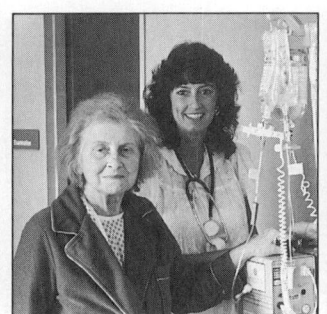
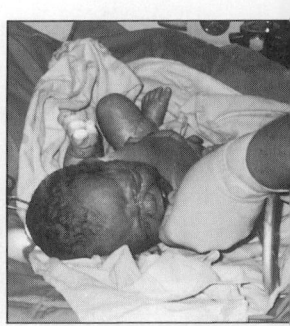

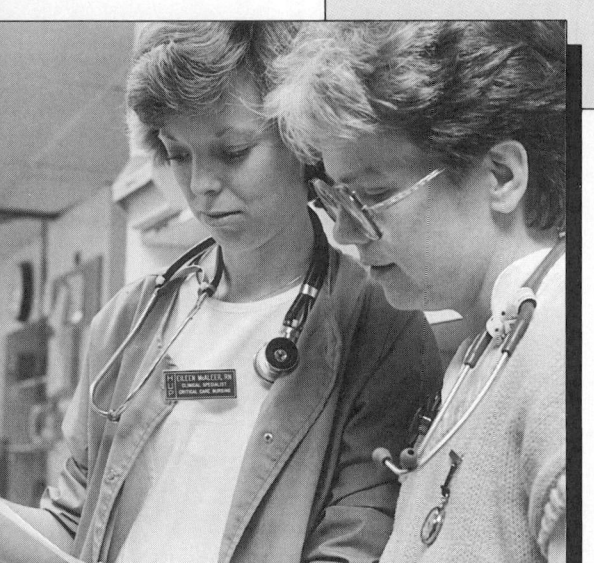

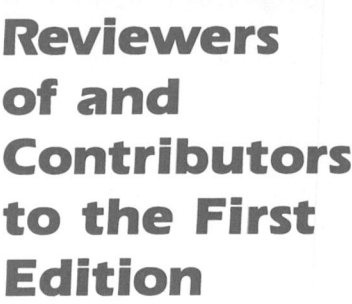

Reviewers of and Contributors to the First Edition

Joan Berends, PhD, RN
Formerly Director, Nursing Program
Grand Rapids Community College
Grand Rapids, MI

Deborah J. Borelli, RN, CCRN, MSN
Instructor
Nursing Department
St. Petersburg Junior College
Pinellas Park, FL

Nancy L. Bradley, RN, BSN, MEd
Formerly Coordinator, Sophomore
   Nursing
Assistant Professor of Nursing
School of Nursing
Kent State
Kent, OH

Anne Carlson, BS, HEc, RD
Health Consultant—Registered Dietician
Women's Health Resources Grace
   Hospital
Calgary, Alberta, Canada

Anne M. Carty, MA, MSN, RN
Formerly Director, Associate Degree
   Nursing Program
Southwest Missouri State University
West Plains, MO

L. Diane Clayton, MA, MEd, RN
Professor
Department of Nursing
Rockland Community College
Suffern, NY

Donita D'Amico, EdM, RN
Assistant Professor
RN Program Coordinator
Department of Nursing
William Paterson College
Wayne, NJ

Dorcas D. Williams Davidson, RN, BSN, MSN, MS, Ed
Assistant Professor
Acting Academic Advisor
College of Nursing
Chicago State University
Chicago, IL

Susan Dudek, RD, BS
Consultant Dietitian
Bertrand Chaffee Hospital
Springville, NY

Vicki V. Earnest, RN, MS
Professor
Nursing Faculty
Community College of Denver
Denver, CO

Blanca Rosa Garcia, RNC, FNP, MSN
Chairperson and Professor
Department of Registered Nurse
   Education
Del Mar College
Corpus Christi, TX

Ellen B. Gloyd, RN, MSN
Professor Emeritus
Nursing Department
Montgomery College
Takoma Park, MD

Ruth E. Gordon, RNC, MSN, CRNP (Doctoral Candidate)
Assistant Professor
Department of Nursing
Millersville University
Millersville, PA

Sharolyn B. Heatwole, RN, MSN
Associate Professor
Nursing Program
Division of Health Technology
J. Sargeant Reynolds Community
   College
Richmond, VA

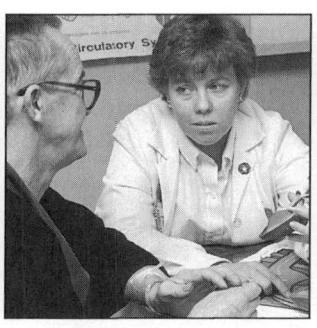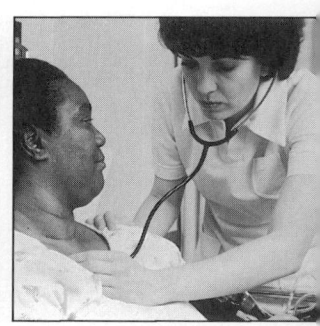

Daisy Hines, RNC, PHN, BSN, MSN
Professor of Nursing
Associate Degree Nursing Program
Long Beach City College
Long Beach, CA

Sylvia Huber, RN, BScN
Formerly Instructor
Department of Nursing and Allied
   Health
Mount Royal College
Calgary, Alberta, Canada

June Johnson, RN, MS
Professor and Curriculum Coordinator
Department of Nursing
Sinclair Community College
Dayton, OH

Cheryl Kleffer, MSN, RN, CS
Instructor
Department of Nursing
Southeast Missouri State University
Cape Girardeau, MO

Jane McCausland Kurz, RN, MSN,
CCRN
Instructor in Nursing
Delaware State College
Dover, DE

Monica Kwong, MS, RN
Clinical Nurse Educator
Medical–Surgical–Hospice Division
Department of Hospital Nursing
Kaiser Permanente—Oakland Medical
   Center
Oakland, CA

Kathleen Sweeney Malic, RN,
BSN, MA
Clinical Instructor
Prairie State College
Chicago Heights, IL

Filomela A. Marshall, RN, MSN
Assistant Professor
Division of Nursing
Holy Family College
Philadelphia, PA

Rosemary Russo Miley, RN, BSN
Formerly Clinical Supervisor
Mercy Catholic Medical Center
Darby, PA

Mary C. Mitchell
Associate Professor of Nursing
School of Nursing, Business and
   Hospitality
SUNY/Morrisville College
Morrisville, NY

Maureen J. Osis, RN, MN
Clinical Nurse Specialist
Adjunct Assistant Professor
Calgary District Hospital Group and
   University of Calgary
Calgary, Alberta, Canada

Paulette LaCava Osterman, RN,
BSN, MSN
Professor of Nursing
Doctoral Student
Community College of Rhode Island
Warwick, RI

Gracie H. Perry, MSN, CRNP
School Nurse Practitioner
School District of Philadelphia
Coadjutant Instructor
Delaware County Community College
Media, PA

Faith M. Reierson, RN, MN
Coordinator, Nursing Programs
Olympic College
Bremerton, WA

Linda Ann Robinson, RN, MSN
Instructor
Department of Nursing
College of Allied Health Sciences
Thomas Jefferson University
Philadelphia, PA

Marylen Robinson, RNC, MSN
Adjunct Professor of Nursing
Bethel College
Mishawaka, IN

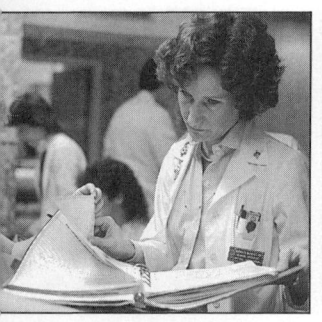  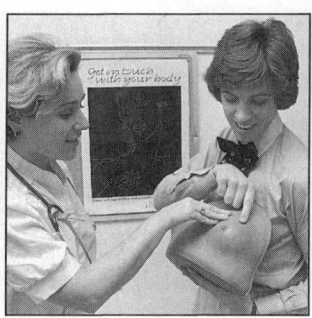  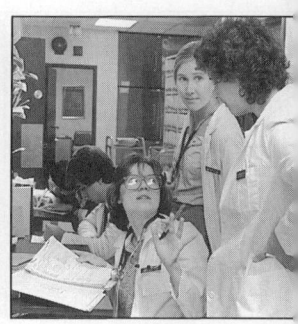

Christine M. Rosner, RN, MSN
Assistant Professor
Division of Nursing
Holy Family College
Philadelphia, PA

Lynn Schneidler, BSN, MOED, RN, C
Professor of Nursing
Nursing and Allied Health
New Hampshire Technical College
Stratham, NH

Joyce Soehnlen, RN, MSN
Assistant Professor
Department of Nursing
Walsh College
North Canton, OH

Shirley M. Solberg, RN, MN
Associate Professor
School of Nursing
Memorial University of Newfoundland
St. Johns, Newfoundland, Canada

Melissa Spezia, RN, DSN
Assistant Professor
University of Tennessee—Memphis
College of Nursing
Memphis, TN

Wanda Stephenson, MS, RN
Department Head, Nursing
Ann Arundel Community College
Arnold, MD

Janet L. Storch, RN, BScN, MHSA, PhD
Dean and Professor
Faculty of Nursing
University of Calgary
Calgary, Alberta, Canada

Barbara Stright, BSN, MSN
Assistant Professor of Nursing
Clarion University of Pennsylvania
Venango Campus
Oil City, PA

Jacqueline Sullivan, RN, MSN, CCRN, CNRN
Clinical Nurse Specialist
Neurosensory Intensive Care Unit
Clinical Assistant Professor
Thomas Jefferson University Hospital
Philadelphia, PA

Barbara Timby, RNC, BSN, MA
Nursing Professor
Glen Oaks Community College
Centreville, MI

Karen L. Wall, BScN
Curriculum Coordinator
Nursing Department
Red River Community College
Winnipeg, Manitoba, Canada

Joyce Welliver, RN, MSN
Assistant Professor
Director of Continuing Education
Division of Nursing
Holy Family College
Philadelphia, PA

Eileen M. Williams, RN, MSN
Professor of Nursing
School of Nursing and Allied Health
Mesa State College
Grand Junction, CO

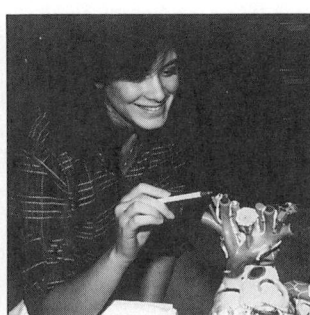
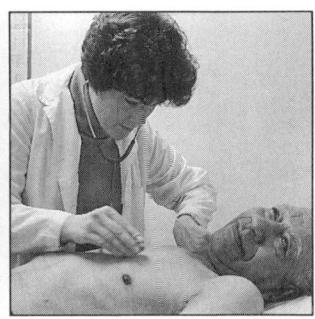

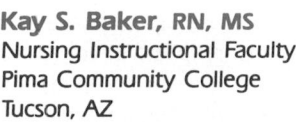

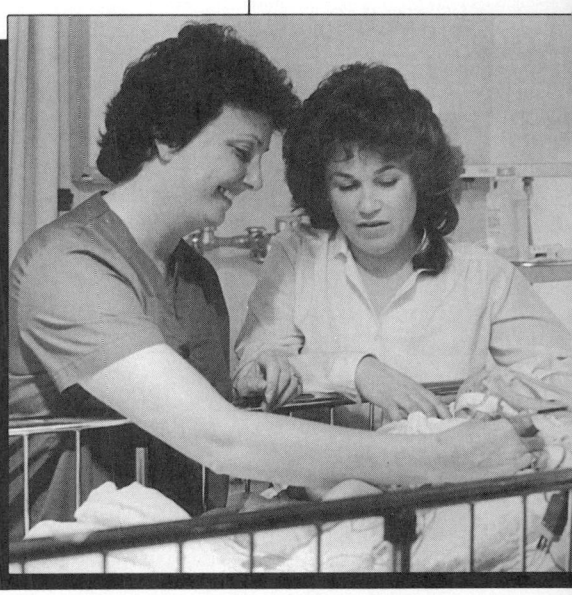

Kay S. Baker, RN, MS
Nursing Instructional Faculty
Pima Community College
Tucson, AZ

Nancy Bradley, RN, BSN, MEd
Formerly Coordinator, Sophomore
 Nursing
Assistant Professor of Nursing
School of Nursing
Kent State University
Kent, OH

L. Diane Clayton, MA, MEd, RN
Professor
Department of Nursing
Rockland Community College
Suffern, NY

Patricia Connors
Instructor
Division Allied Health
Brookdale Community College
Lincroft, NJ

Dauna L. Crooks, MScN, BScN, RN
Assistant Professor
School of Nursing
McMaster University
Hamilton, Ontario, Canada

Norma Hill Freeborn, MSN, RNC
Chairman
Division of Nursing and Health Science
College of the Sequoias
Visalia, CA

Blanca Rosa Garcia, RNC, FNP, MSN
Chairperson and Professor
Department of Registered Nurse
 Education
Del Mar College
Corpus Christi, TX

Mary Elizabeth Haney, RN, BSN, MA, Ed
Instructor
Nursing Department
Asheville Buncombe Technical
 Community College
Asheville, NC

Cathy Michalenko
Instructor
Red Deer College
Red Deer, Alberta, Canada

Barbara L. Ogden, MSN, RN, C
Assistant Professor
Faculty Liaison
University of Florida
College of Nursing
Gainesville UAMC
Gainesville, FL

Faith Reierson, RN, MN
Coordinator, Nursing Programs
Olympic College
Bremerton, WA

Enid A. Schwartz, RN, C, MS
Nursing Instructor
Cochise College
Douglas, AZ

Kathleen Simon, DNSc, RN
Assistant Professor
College of Nursing
Medical University of South Carolina
Charleston, SC

Joyce K. Soehnlen, RN, MSN
Associate Professor
Department of Nursing
Walsh College
North Canton, OH

Maryanne Werner-McCullough, RN, MS, MNP
Instructor
Nursing Department
Contra Costa College
San Pablo, CA

Reviewers of the Second Edition

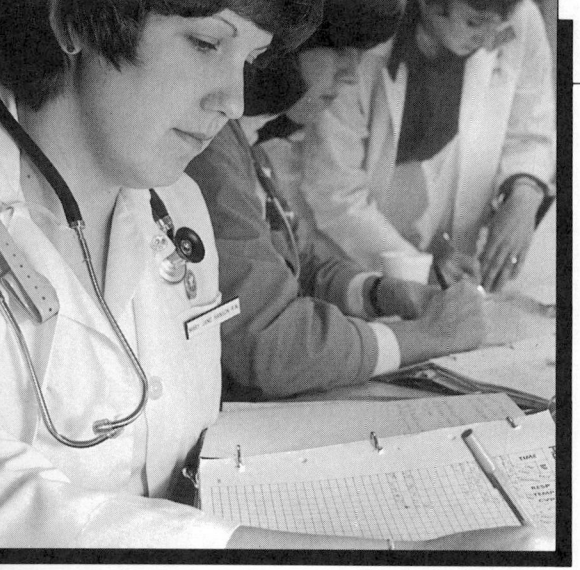

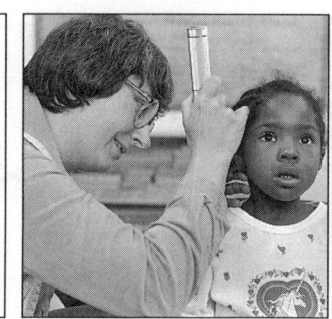

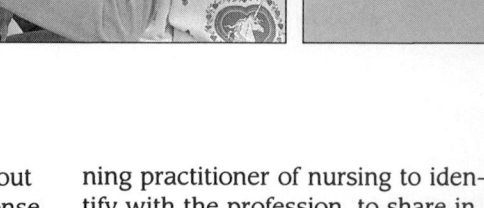

Preface

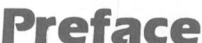

We are very pleased about the enthusiastic response the first edition of *Fundamentals of Nursing: The Art and Science of Nursing Care* generated. Nothing so excites us as meeting students in different parts of the country who express their delight in having a text they actually *enjoy* reading. We are deeply grateful to each educator who affirmed our vision of nursing fundamentals education. To those who have now taught with the text for several years and who have shared with us suggestions for revision we are especially grateful. We hope you will find your suggestions incorporated in this revision.

This second edition aims once again to prepare those beginning the study of nursing to competently and confidently confront the challenges of clinical nursing. Care is taken to present nursing as an exciting and demanding profession that affords its practitioners real opportunities to make a difference in the health and well-being of those they encounter. The authors recognize that those new to nursing can quickly become overwhelmed by the demands placed on the nurse's knowledge, technical competence, interpersonal skills, and commitment. And thus much care has once again gone into the selection of both the content of this edition and the manner of its presentation. Throughout, our aim is to capture the unique essence of both the art and science of nursing, distilling what the person beginning the study of nursing needs to know and presenting this content in a straightforward manner. We consistently focus on the caregiver role of the nurse and invite the begin-

ning practitioner of nursing to identify with the profession, to share in its pride, and to respond to its challenges.

The authors are sensitive to the different meanings nurses attach to the terms "client" versus "patient." We chose to use the term "client" to emphasize respect for the autonomy (self-determination) of the client and to encourage the nurse to actively involve the client and family as much as possible in care decisions. Care has been taken to communicate that both nurses and clients may be male or female and that they come from every racial and ethnic background and socioeconomic group. Whenever possible we have tried to avoid male/female distinctions in personal pronouns.

Realizing that our textbook is used by a variety of people throughout North America, we attempted to generalize many statements and use references to Canada throughout the book. Other Canadian materials appear in the Appendices and the Canadian Instructor's Manual.

Organization

The textbook is organized into nine units. The learner is first introduced to the concepts "nurse," "client," and "nursing process," and then to basic nursing roles and actions common to nursing practice. The remaining units focus specifically on how nurses can work with clients to promote healthy physiologic and psychosocial responses. Although, ideally, the text is followed sequentially, every effort has been made to respect the differing needs of diverse curricula and students. Thus each chapter stands on its own merit and

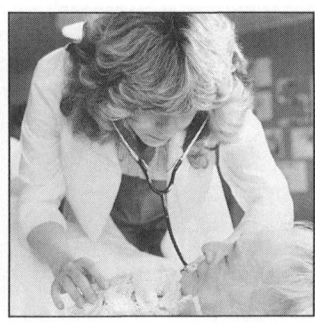

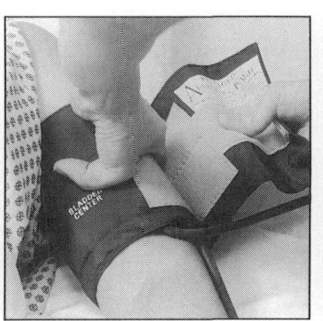
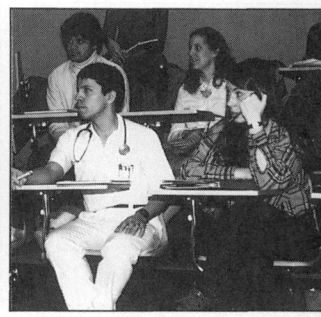

may be read independently of others.

Unit I, The Nurse: Foundations for Nursing Practice, describes contemporary nursing. Chapters focus on the profession of nursing, nursing's role in promoting wellness in health and illness, the changing health care system, nursing theories, and the ethical and legal dimensions of nursing practice.

Unit II, The Client: Concepts for Holistic Care, offers foundational knowledge about clients, essential to accurate nursing assessments and effective nurse–client interactions. Chapters describe the human needs of individuals, families, and communities and explore the concepts of culture and ethnicity, and stress and adaptation.

Unit III, Promoting Wellness Across the Life Span, provides a comprehensive picture of growth and development throughout the life span and acknowledges the differing needs for nursing arising from different developmental stages and abilities to meet developmental tasks. The unit includes chapters on basic developmental concepts, conception to midlife, and the older adult, and the concepts of loss, grief, and death.

Unit IV, The Nursing Process, offers a detailed step-by-step guide to each component of the nursing process. Practical guidelines and examples are included in each chapter. Separate chapters address the nursing process as a whole, assessing, diagnosing, planning, implementing, and evaluating. Documentation guidelines are discussed in the chapter on implementing and are noted wherever appropriate.

Unit V, Roles Basic to Nursing Care, describes major roles in which nurses function as they interact holistically with clients. Chapters focus on the communicator, teacher and counselor, and leader, researcher and advocate roles of the nurse as caregiver.

Unit VI, Actions Basic to Nursing Care, presents the foundational skills used by nurses in most practice settings. Skills are developed in measuring vital signs, performing nursing assessments (physical examination), ensuring client safety, maintaining asepsis, assisting with diagnostic procedures, and promoting continuity of care.

Unit VII, Promoting Healthy Physiologic Responses, explores the nurse's role in helping clients meet basic physiologic needs: hygiene, activity, rest and sleep, comfort, nutrition, bowel elimination, urinary elimination, oxygenation, and fluid, electrolyte, and acid–base balance. In each chapter guidelines are included for assessing and diagnosing unhealthy responses and for planning, implementing, and evaluating appropriate care strategies. Chapters conclude with a case study illustrating the use of the nursing process to resolve selected nursing diagnoses.

Unit VIII, Promoting Healthy Psychosocial Responses, using the same format as Unit VII, focuses on psychosocial needs of clients: self-concept, sensory stimulation, sexuality, and spirituality.

Unit IX, Promoting Optimal Health in Special Situations, includes chapters describing nursing responsibilities related to medication administration, diagnostic procedures, wound care, and perioperative nursing.

Integrated Nursing Process

After the nursing process is introduced in Unit IV, it provides the organizational framework for successive chapters. Chapters in Units VII and VIII, which deal with physiologic and psychosocial responses, begin with a succinct background discussion of the concept followed by an identification of factors that influence how different individuals respond to these needs. Steps in the nursing process are used to describe related nursing responsibilities.

Assessing. Common elements of both a comprehensive and problem-focused nursing assessment are presented; sample interview questions are included, and specific physical assessment techniques described.

Diagnosing. NANDA-approved nursing diagnoses related to the human need being discussed are identified, and tables illustrate the relationship between diagnostic cues, contributing factors, and the problem statement.

Planning. Sample client goals are suggested based on client strengths. Each chapter concludes with a care plan designed for the client described in a case study.

Implementing. Nursing measures are clearly explained and are illustrated when this is deemed helpful. Procedures have been streamlined to facilitate mastery. A sufficient variety of nursing interventions is provided to enable the development of a repertoire of nursing actions that

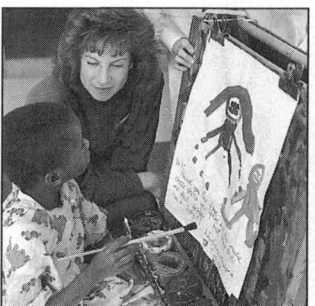

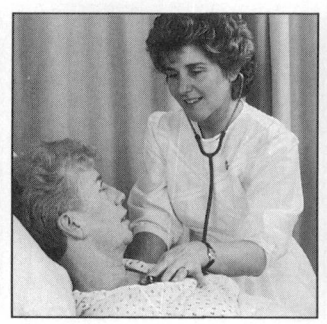

makes practicing the art of nursing possible.

Evaluating. Criteria for evaluating the effectiveness of the plan of care are suggested.

Each chapter in Units VII and VIII concludes with the workup of several diagnoses that demonstrate the comprehensive nursing management of common nursing problems. This section and the concluding case studies with a nursing care plan afford the reader ongoing illustrations of the correct use and documentation of nursing process. As the learner progresses through the text, the nursing process becomes an integral part of nursing care.

Key Features

In preparing this edition we wanted to capitalize on the strengths of the first edition and address new priorities. We chose to further develop or strengthen the following features:

Nursing as an Art and Science. As a science, nursing is characterized by a growing body of knowledge that links technical and interpersonal interventions to desired client outcomes; as an art, nursing demands of its practitioners sufficient competency to creatively design individualized strategies to assist clients to reach personal health goals. Always a unique spirit of caring must prevail.

Wellness Orientation. A wellness rather than an illness orientation provides a framework for presentation of content. Wellness promotion displays highlight assessment check-points for specific components of high-level wellness and include suggestions for designing a self-care prescription. These displays serve a two-fold purpose: a self-care model for the learner and an invaluable aid for the learner who is newly developing the role of client educator.

Nurse as Role Model. Learners are directed to assess their own health behaviors before attempting to help clients; health goals for the nurse are presented in each clinical chapter.

Aims of Nursing. Learners are gradually introduced to the theory, interpersonal skills, and nursing procedures that will enable them to work successfully with clients to promote wellness, prevent illness, restore health, and facilitate coping with altered functioning. Early attention to these broad aims of nursing will prepare learners to meet the needs of clients in diverse health care settings.

Through the Eyes of a Student. Remembering the loneliness and embarrassment that accompanied the execution of many "nursing firsts" in the clinical arena, the authors invited "experienced" nursing students to share their "nursing firsts" with learners attempting these skills for the first time. It is hoped that these accounts will go a long way toward reducing student anxiety and forging the bond that unites practitioners of nursing everywhere.

Basic Human Needs. Common to all people and essential to wellness and survival are basic human needs. The clinical chapters in Units VII and VIII prepare the learner to assist clients and family members in meeting these needs. Learners are encouraged to explore *human responses* to health and illness as indicators of how well an individual is functioning to meet basic human needs.

Holistic Care Across the Life Span. Holistic orientation to basic human needs exists across the life span. Unit III, growth and development factors in Units VII and VIII, age considerations in many procedures, and the diverse ages and needs of clients represented in the case presentations in clinical chapters address the life span continuum. Wherever appropriate, cultural considerations are included.

Attention to the Special Needs of the Elderly. Nurses today confront growing numbers of elderly clients in all practice settings. The chapter on the older adult and the Focus on the Older Adult display that appears in many clinical chapters aim to sensitize learners to the special nursing needs of the elderly.

Continuity of Care. Clients today spend fewer days in the hospital, are frequently transferred both within the hospital and between health care institutions, and need to rely on rapidly proliferating community-based health care resources. The text emphasizes the nurse's role in ensuring continuity of care and in preparing clients and family members through consistent education, early discharge planning, and advocacy strategies, to manage their own care.

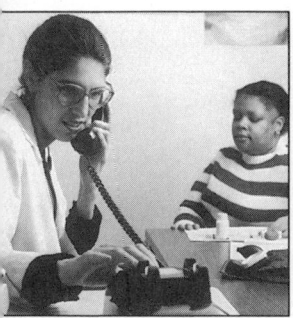
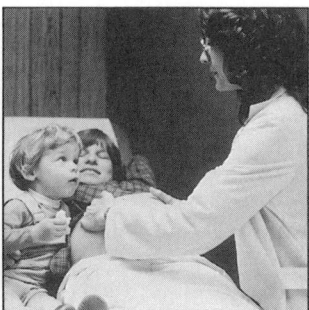
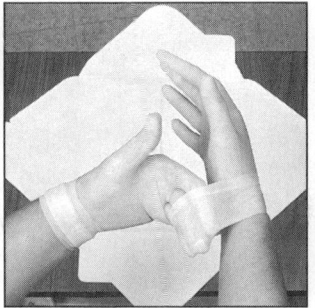

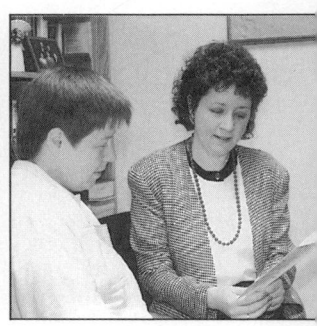

Respect for Client Autonomy.
The learner is consistently reminded to actively involve the client and family (significant others), according to their ability and motivation, in all aspects of care.

Nursing Process. Fundamental to nursing care is the nursing process, discussed earlier in the Preface. Every effort has been made to enhance the nursing process strengths of this text.

Collaborative Dimensions of Care. The client's achievement of health goals is related to the efficient functioning of the health care team. The nurse, who possesses unique knowledge of the client, is encouraged to work collaboratively with the health team, respecting the contributions of different members of the team.

Nursing Procedures. Procedures are presented in a concise, straightforward, and simplified format that is intended to facilitate competent performance of nursing skills. Scientific rationale accompany each nursing action, and the many photographs and illustrations further reinforce mastery. New special considerations (eg, for home care or the elderly) are included where appropriate.

Broad Scope of Nursing. The text has been written to encompass learning fundamental skills in a laboratory as well as in actual clinical settings caring for well or ill clients. Numerous examples are given to illustrate nurses interacting with clients of all ages and backgrounds, in traditional and nontraditional set-

tings, to acquaint learners with the many exciting career options in nursing. The authors draw on their rich experience in multiple practice settings.

Nursing Today: Challenges and Solutions. This recurring feature highlights some of today's most pressing issues: the needs of people with AIDS, the gender gap in research, the special needs of children, and so on. Nursing's creative solutions to these problems are highlighted and learners are encouraged to help nursing make a difference.

Research Highlights. The research displays that appear in many chapters assist learners to value research and to see its relevance to practice. Learners are challenged to become informed participants in or consumers of clinical research.

Computer Highlights. Various computer displays acquaint the learner with innovative computer applications in nursing and health care.

Key Terms/Glossary. Key terms precede the text in each chapter. When these terms are defined in the chapter, they are boldfaced for clarity. A Glossary appears at the back of the book for easy studying of terms used in the book.

Sample Test Questions. Sample test questions appear at the end of each chapter in Units VI through IX to facilitate mastery of chapter content. These exercises will assist students who are attempting to improve their objective test-taking skills.

Teaching/Learning Package

To facilitate mastery of this text's foundational content, a comprehensive teaching/learning package has been developed to assist faculty and students.

Two supplemental books are available for the learner. A Performance Checklists Manual includes a checklist for each procedure to facilitate learner evaluation. Foundations of learning developed in the text are augmented in the Student Study Guide. Chapter-by-chapter exercises enable learners to gain expertise in theory comprehension and application. In addition to developing valuable testing skills, learners using the study guide will find case presentations in each clinical chapter that facilitate their mastery of nursing process skills.

Supplemental materials for the faculty member include an Instructor's Manual, a printed and computerized Test Bank, and Transparency Acetates. The Instructor's Manual provides theoretical and clinical resources. Chapter objectives and learning activities encompass a range of cognitive, affective, and psychomotor domains. Acetate transparencies enable faculty to visually enhance their lectures and presentations. A computerized test bank program assists faculty members in testing knowledge attained by learners during the course. Questions are based on material presented in *Fundamentals of Nursing*.

Carol Taylor, CSFN, RN, MSN,
  PhD (Candidate)
Carol Lillis, RN, MSN
Priscilla LeMone, RNC, DSN

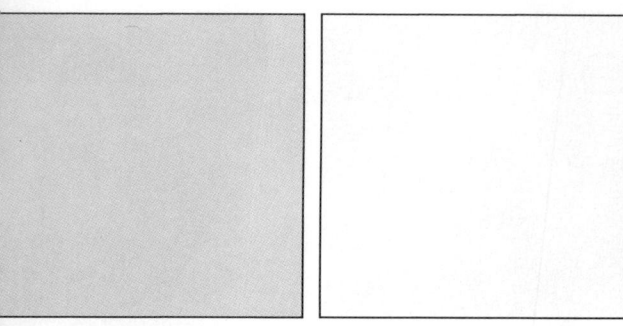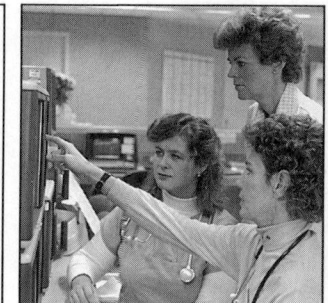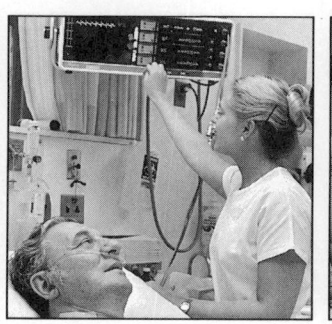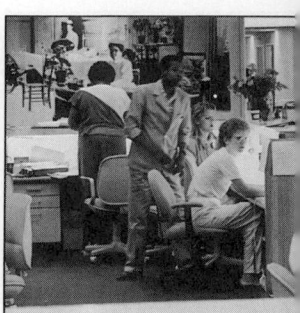

 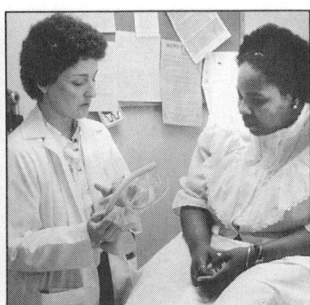 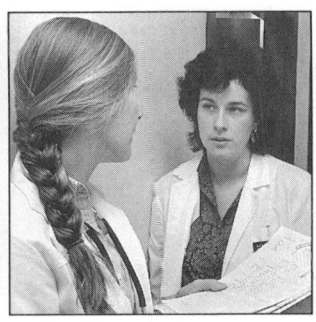

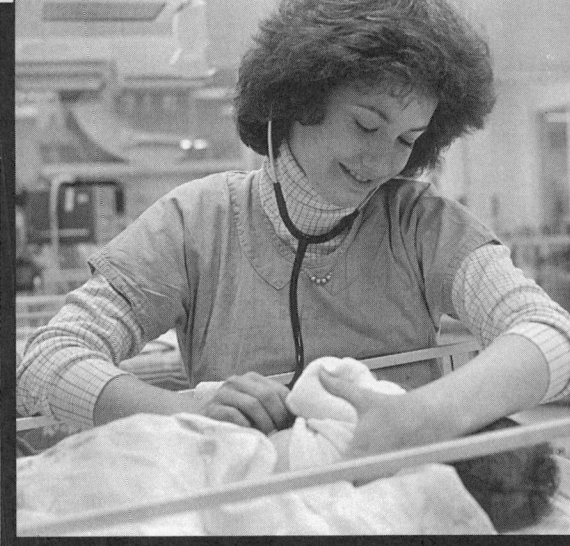

Acknowledgments

This revision is the work of many talented and committed people and we wish to gratefully acknowledge the assistance of all who have contributed in any way to the completion of this project. Our first debt of gratitude is to all the nurse educators and students who have adopted the text and shared with us their experiences in using the teaching and learning package. We are deeply grateful for your revision suggestions and trust they will enhance the learning experiences of others.

Our special thanks to the Nursing Department of J. B. Lippincott: Donna L. Hilton, Senior Editor; Susan Perry, Editorial Assistant; and Diana Intenzo, Vice President and Publisher; to Grace Caputo, Project Editor, who followed through each step of production with patience and determination; and to the sales staff, who worked tirelessly to make the first edition such a success. To Carole Wonsiewicz, our Developmental Editor, whose expert direction brought improved clarity and consistency to this revision, we are grateful.

Since the first edition remains central to this revision we need once again to express our heartfelt gratitude to the friends who made the first edition possible: Eleanor Faven, and our contributors and reviewers.

Tracy Baldwin coordinated the art program and designed the book. Her suggestions and talents give a visual interpretation to the text. She patiently worked through deadlines, shooting schedules, and various drafts of manuscript to perform her craft, for which we express our thanks.

The illustration program seeks to communicate the excitement and spirit of the multi-disciplined and person-centered character of nursing. The energies of many people contributed to that end. We thank all who generously gave their time, ideas, and resources. We gratefully acknowledge the special contributions of the following:

Bob Jackson and
Leslie Foster Roesler, illustrators

Ken Kasper, Barbara Proud,
Don Walker, and Robert Neroni,
photographers

Gates Rhodes and Denise Angelini,
School of Nursing, University of Pennsylvania

Maryanne Lieb, Cheryl Meyer, and Pat Welsh, Delaware County Community College (DCCC) faculty and administrators, and DCCC students who served as models for many of the text s photos.

Patty McBride, coordinator of infection control, and Nancy Stout, infection control practitioner, Bryn Mawr Hospital, Bryn Mawr, PA, for advising and updating us on changing infection control protocols.

Marie Clark, who developed the math problems and solutions in Chapter 42.

Joan E. Lynaugh, RN, PhD, FAAN, Director, the Center for the Study of the History of Nursing

As for the actual writing of the text, we gratefully acknowledge the influence of our mentors and teachers; each person we have been privileged to care for as nurses; our students, who continually challenge us to find more effective means to teach nursing; our professional colleagues; and perhaps most importantly, our friends, whose love sustained us through the lonely hours of research and writing.

Finally we are grateful to our reviewers, whose expertise has broadened both the scope and depth of the text.

Carol Taylor
Carol Lillis
Priscilla LeMone

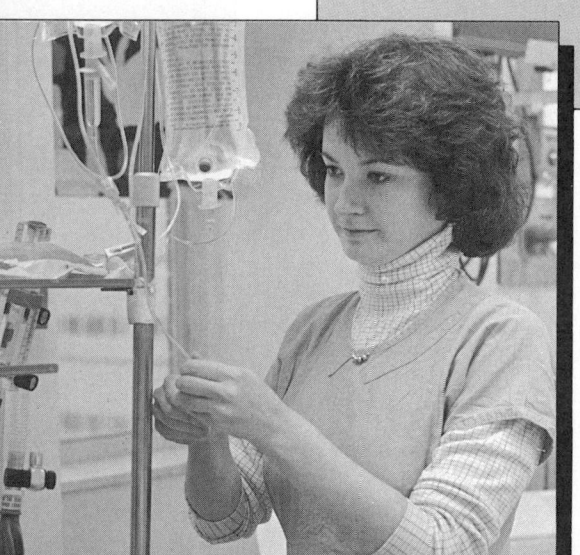
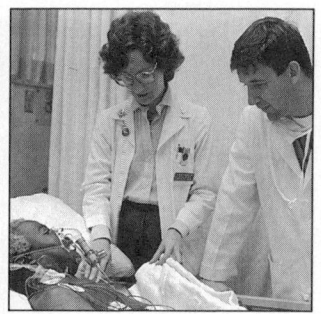

Contents

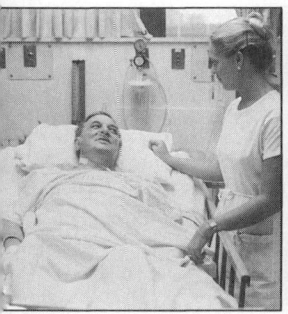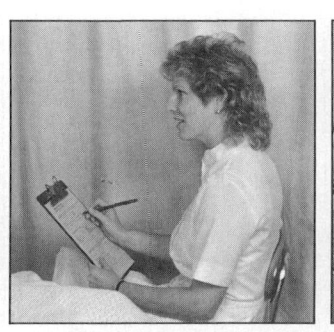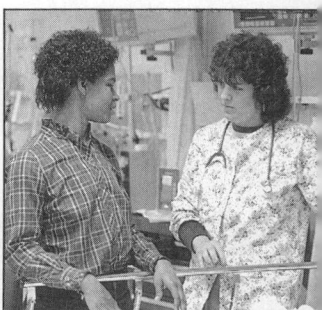

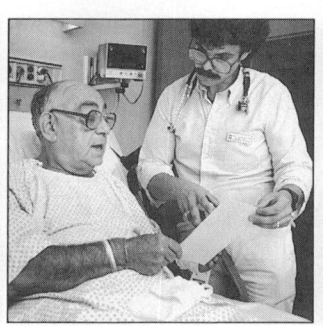
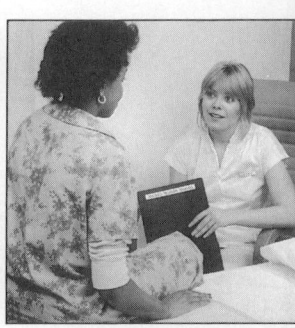
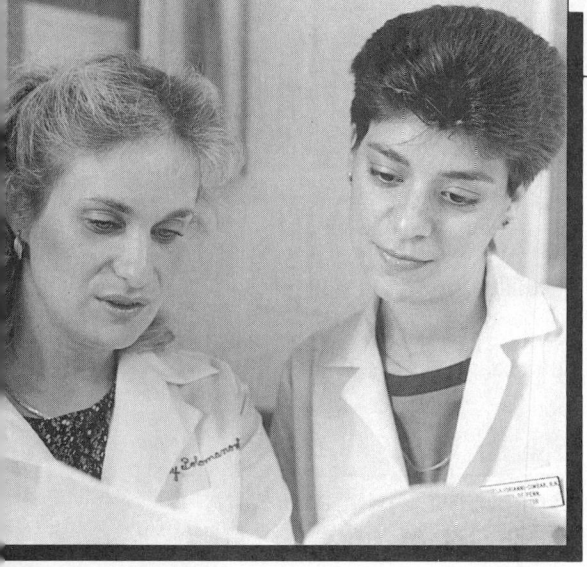

Expanded Contents

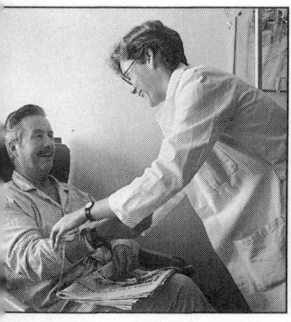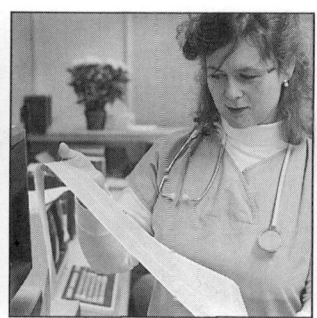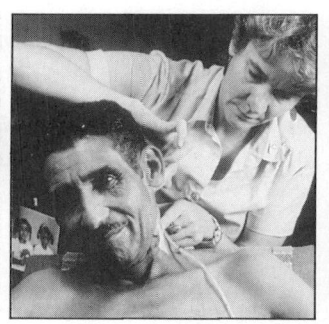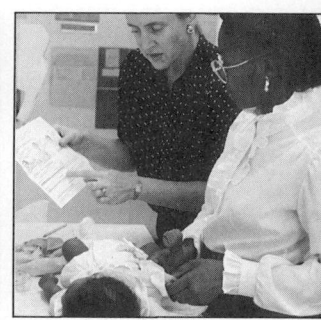

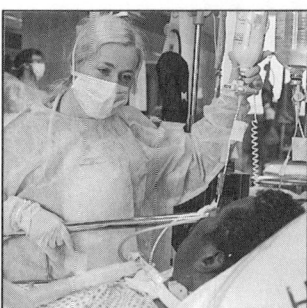
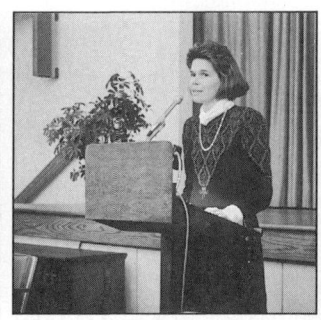
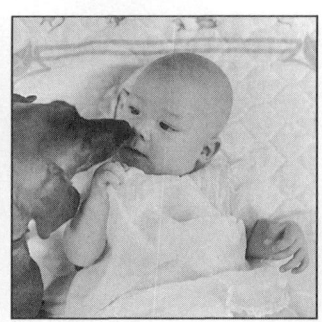

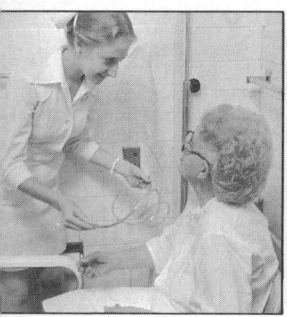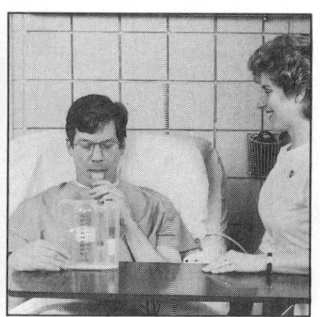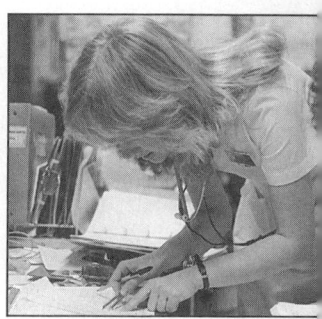

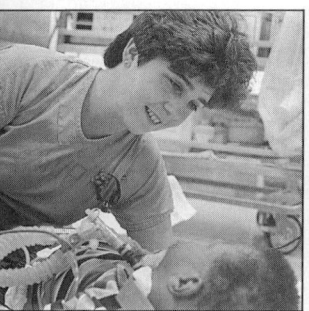
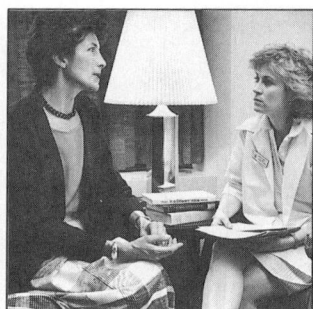

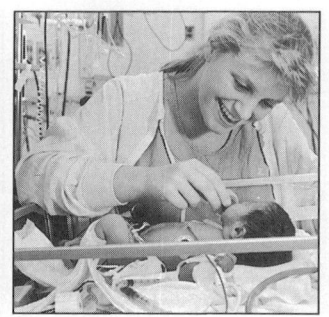

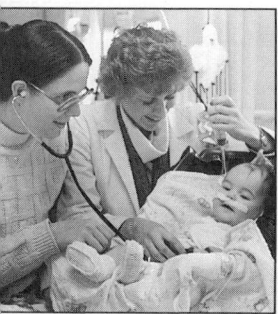

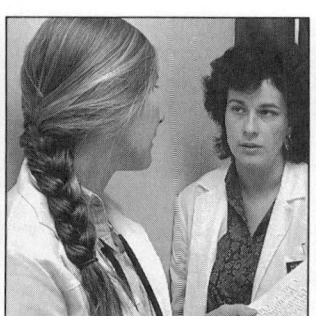
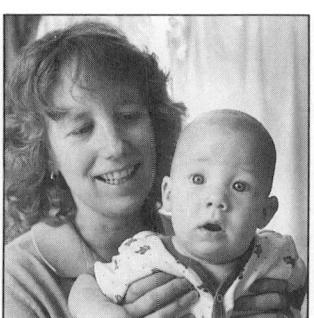

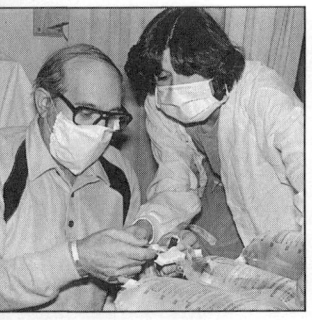

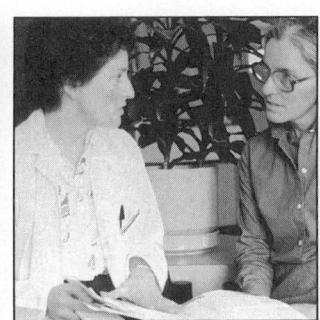
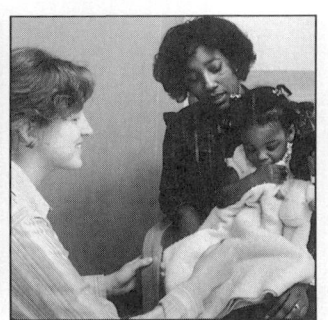
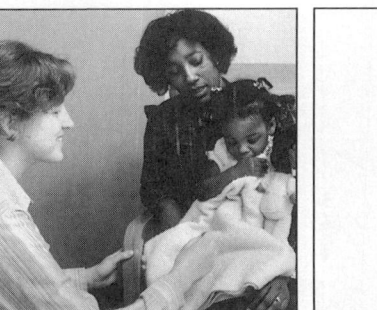

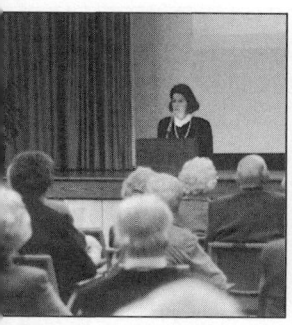

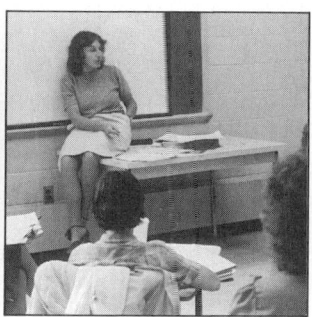
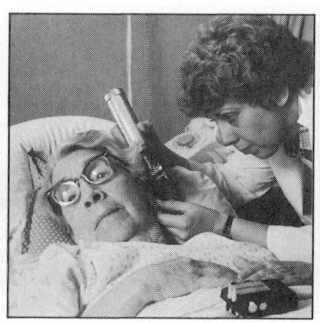

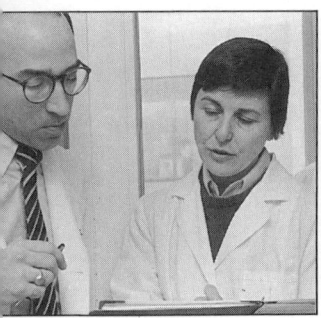

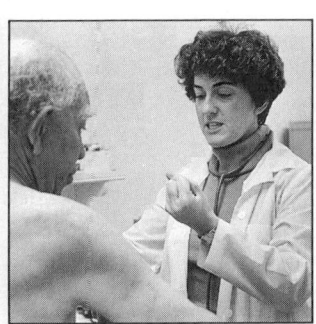
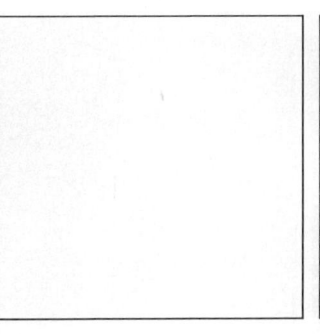
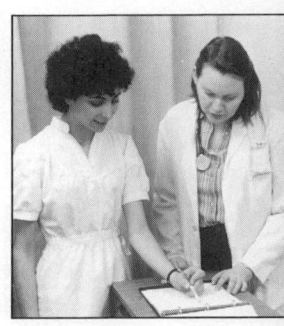

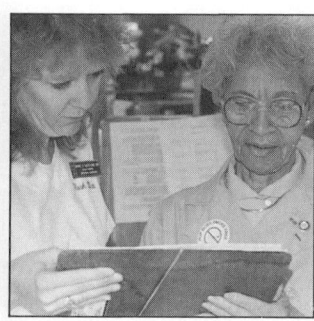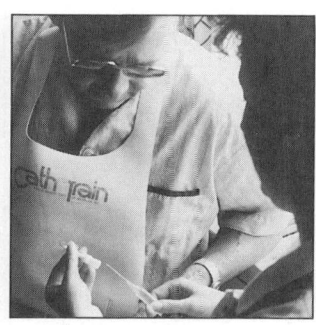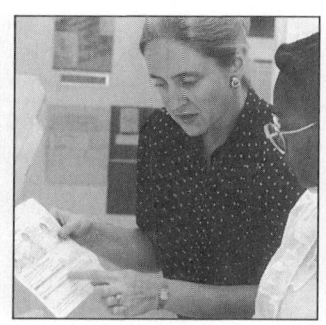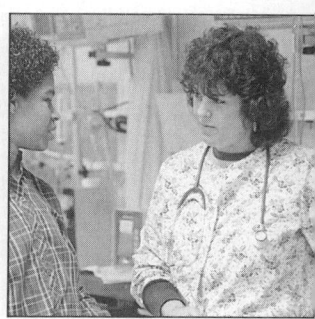

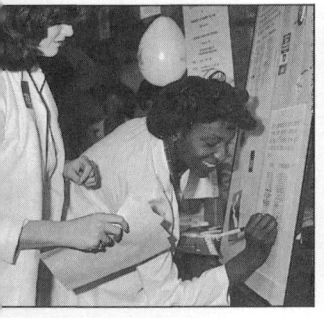  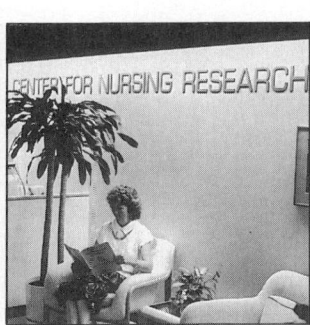 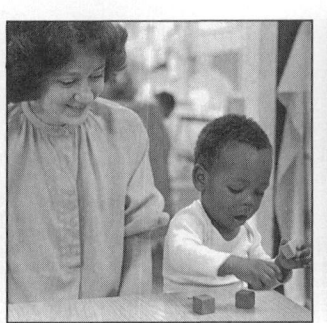 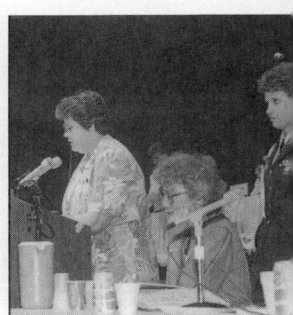

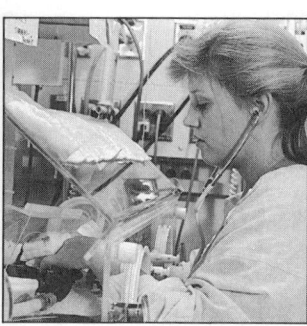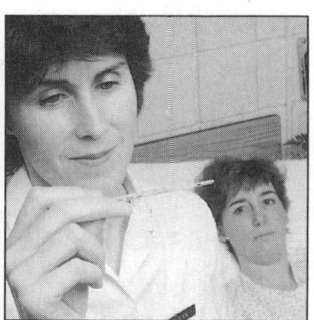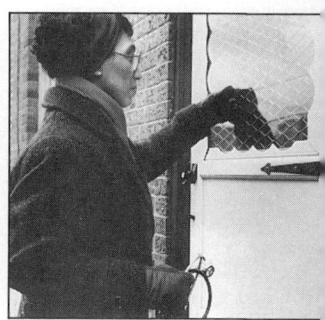

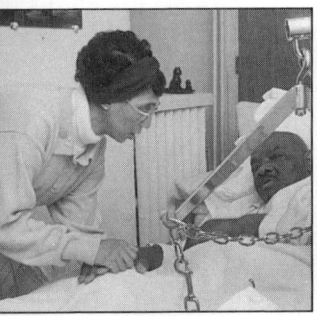
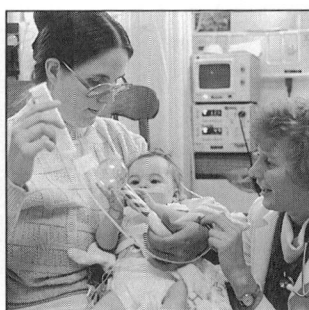
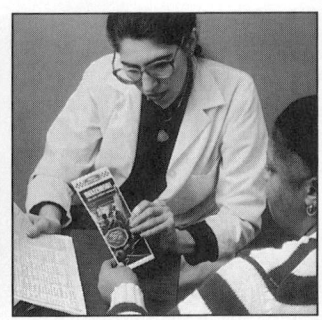
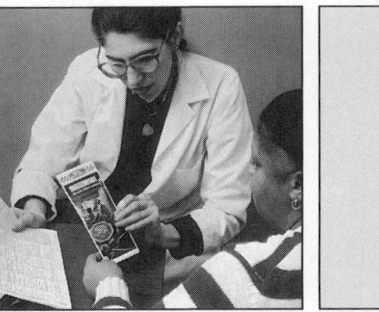

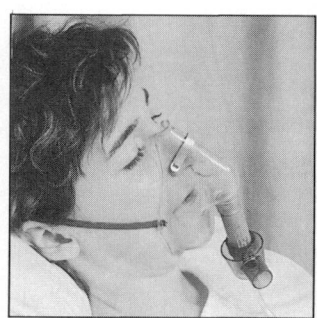
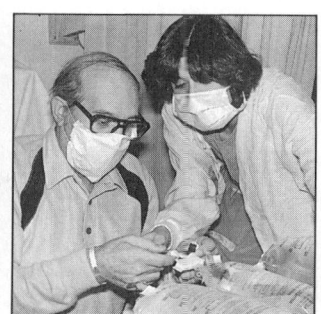

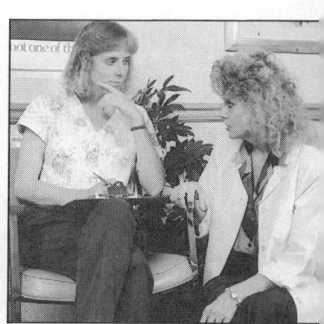

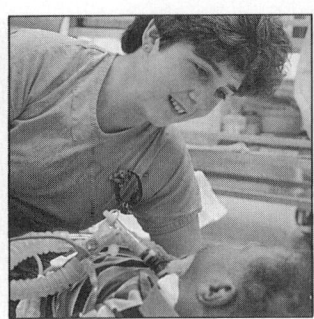
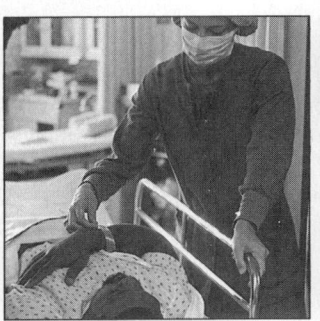
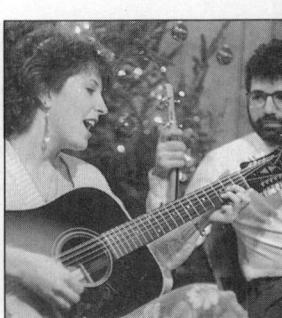

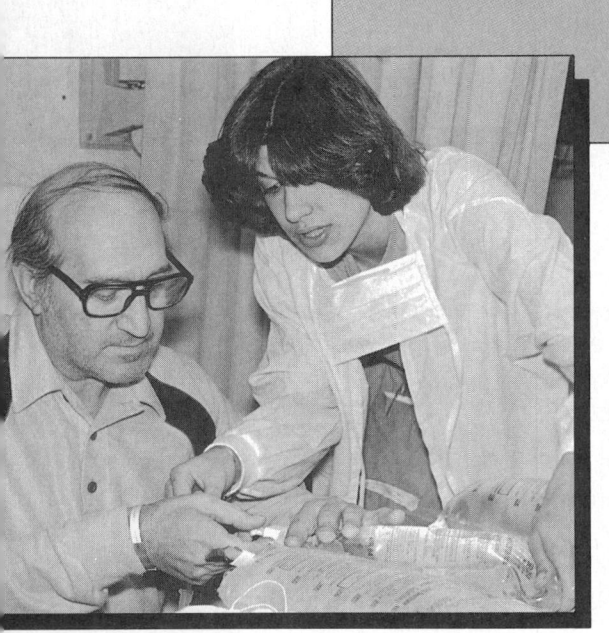

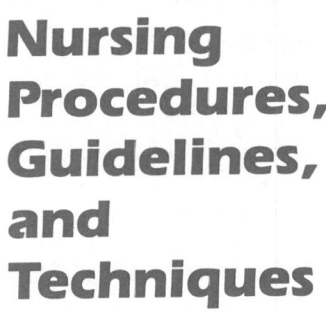

Nursing Procedures, Guidelines, and Techniques

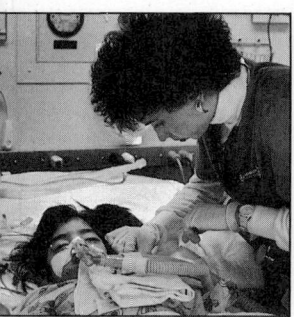

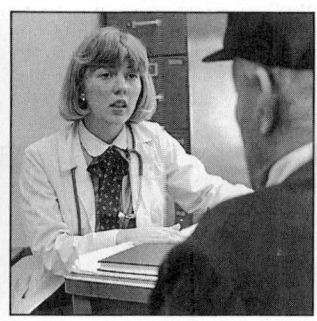

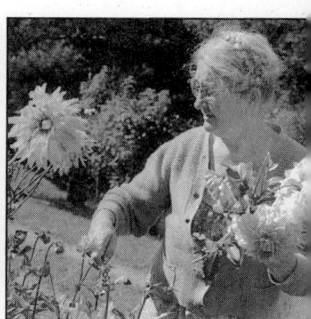

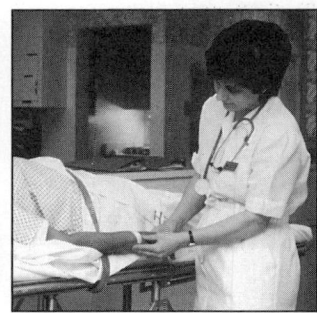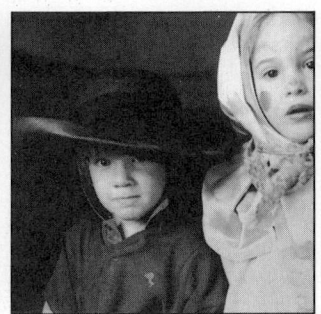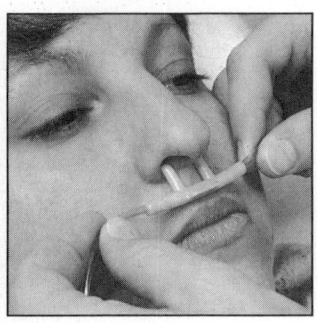

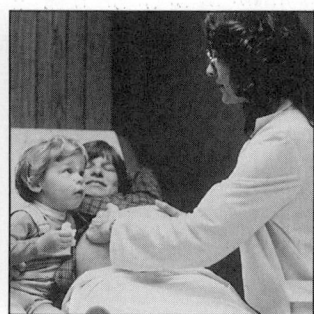
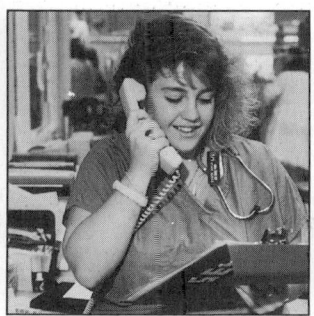
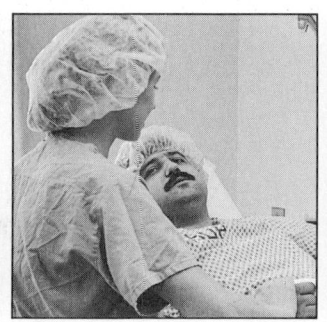
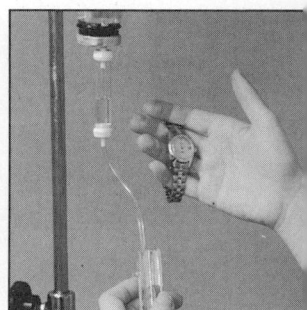

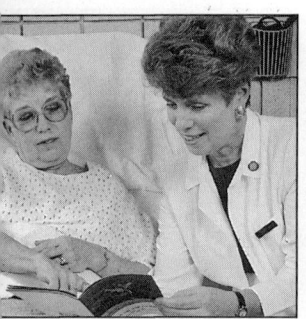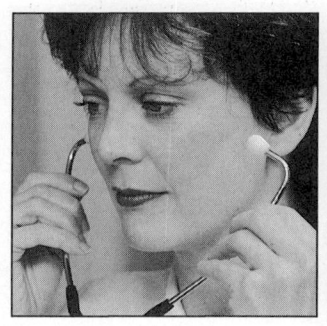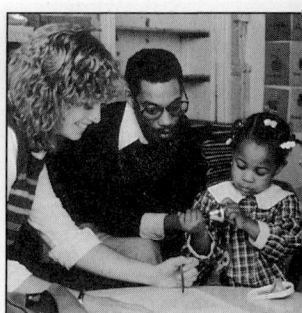

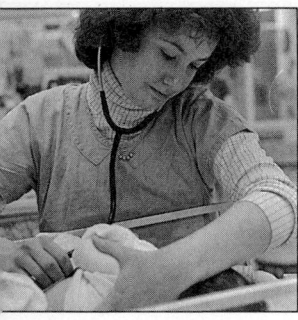

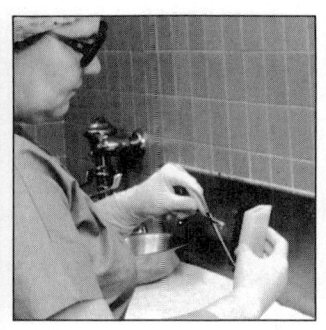
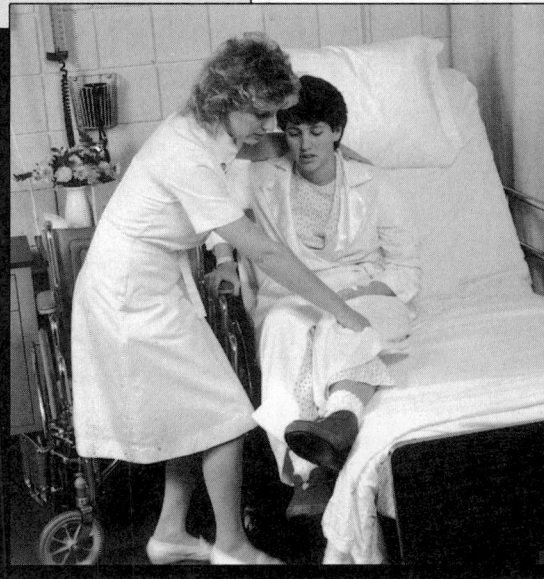

Nursing Process in Clinical Practice

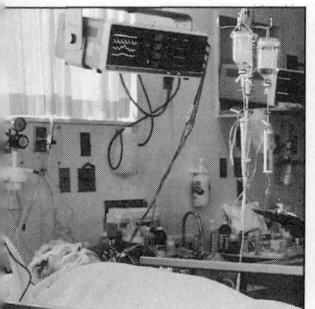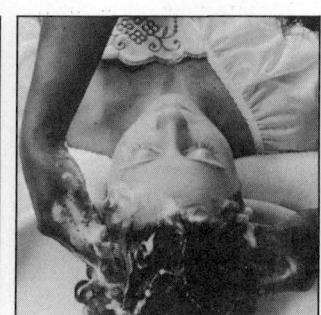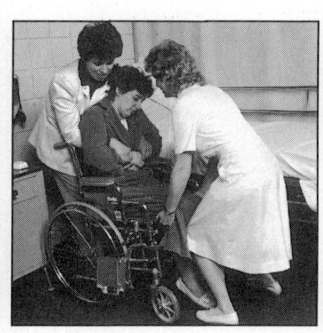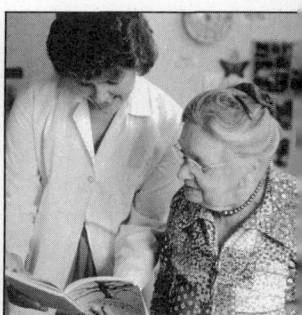

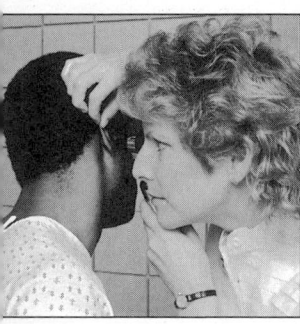

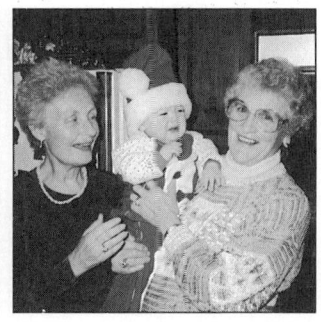
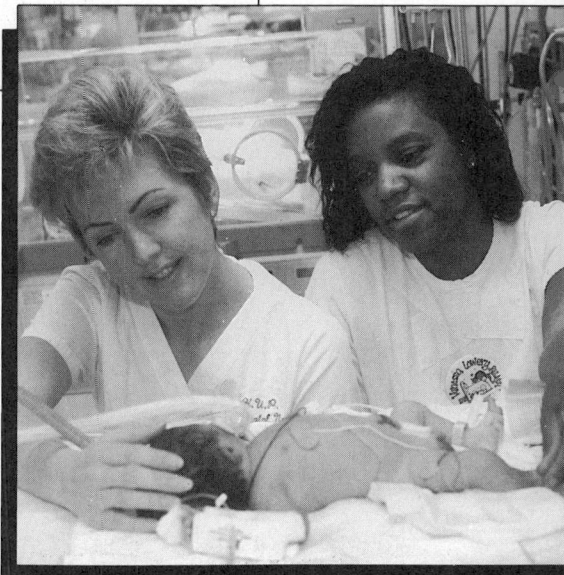

Nursing Care Plans

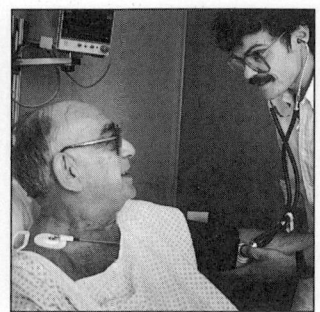
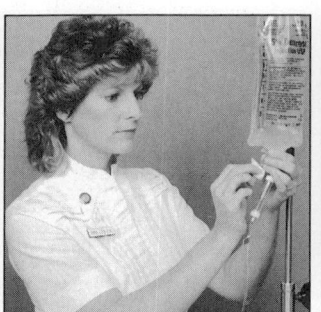
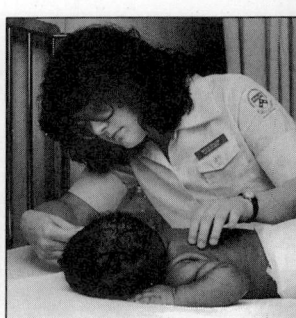

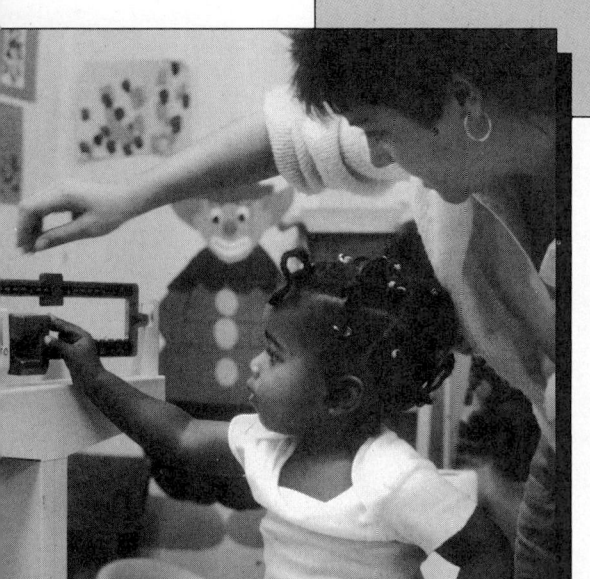

Summary of Recurring Displays

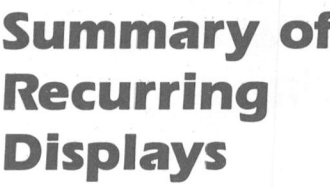

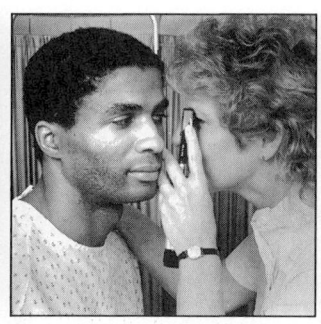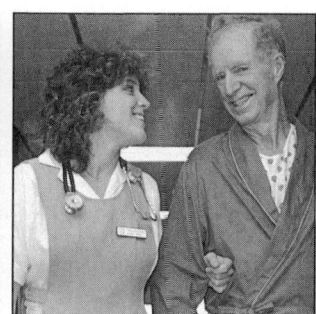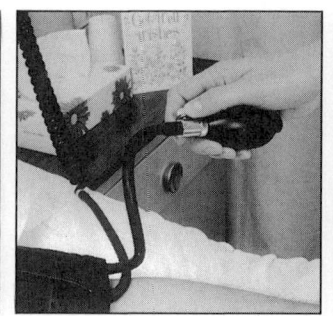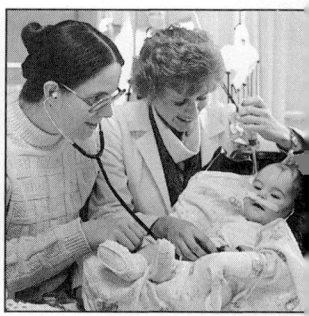

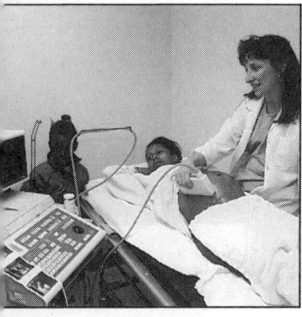

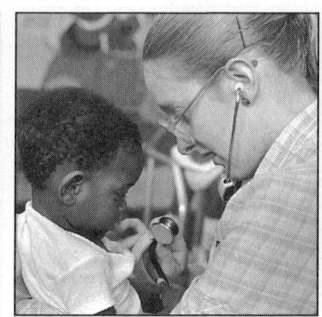
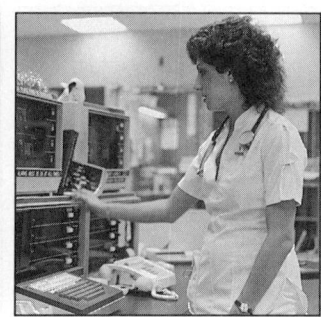

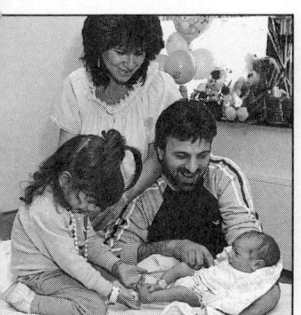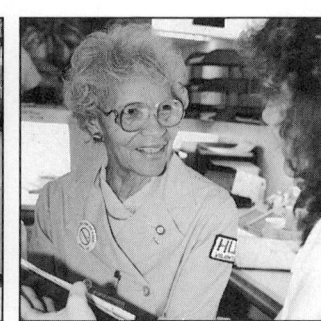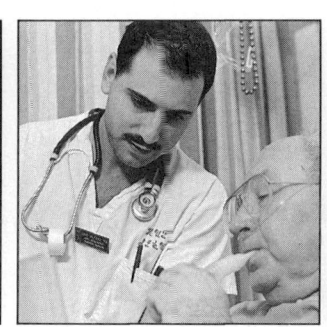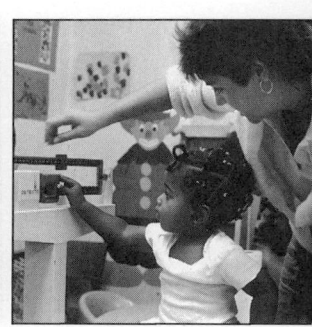

FUNDAMENTALS OF
NURSING

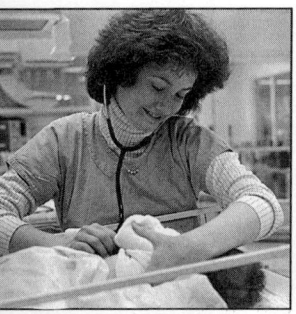  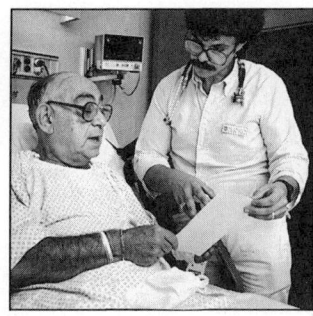 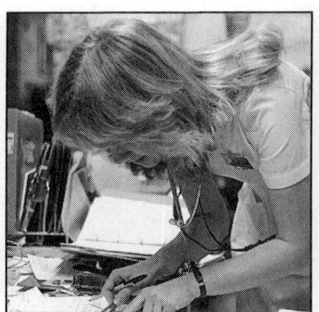 

The Nurse: Foundations for Nursing Practice

Nursing is both an art and a science. It is a profession that uses specialized skills and knowledge to give care to the whole person in both health and illness and in a variety of practice settings. Unit I introduces concepts necessary to provide nurses with the foundations for nursing practice by defining nursing as a whole. Chapters in this unit introduce the profession of nursing, the concepts of health and illness, the health care system, the theoretical base for nursing, and the ethical and legal implications of nursing practice.

Historical perspectives, educational preparation, professional organizations, and guidelines for professional nursing practice serve as a base for understanding what nursing is and how it is organized. An understanding of basic human needs and the individualized definitions of wellness and illness prepare the nurse to integrate the human dimensions—the physical, intellectual, emotional, sociocultural, spiritual, and environmental aspects of each person—into the care given to promote wellness, prevent illness, restore health, and facilitate coping with altered function or death. Knowledge of the varied methods of health delivery is necessary in today's complex health care system.

Nursing theories provide a base for nursing practice, defining the rationale for nursing actions and offering a focus for nursing care. An understanding of the influence of values on human behavior and of the ethical dimensions of nursing practice is essential to responsible and accountable client care. Finally, sensitivity to the legal implications of professional nursing practice is imperative in today's culture.

Unit I explores the foundations for nursing practice from the perspective of the nurse. Initiates are introduced to a challenging and rewarding profession, and are provided with a knowledge base to ground the development of caregiving skills, professional relationships, and professional behaviors.

I

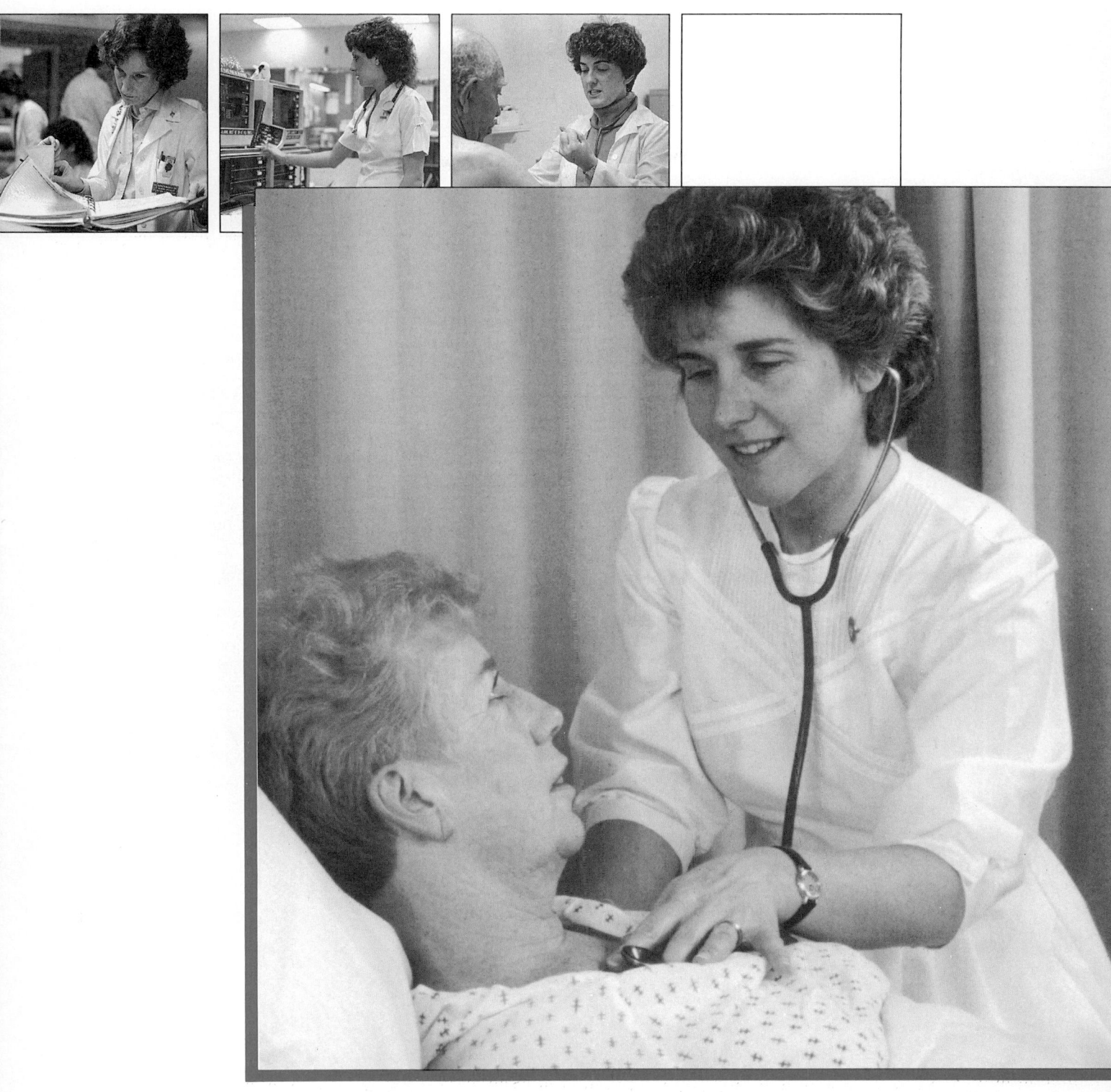

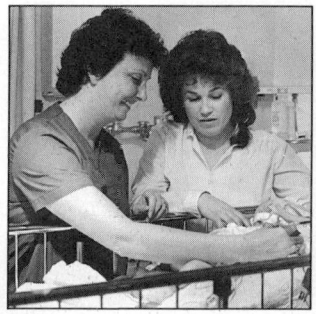
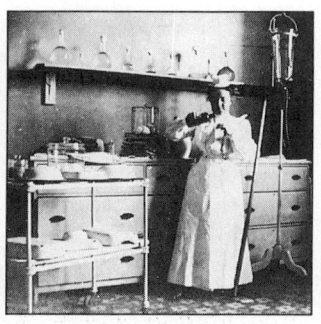

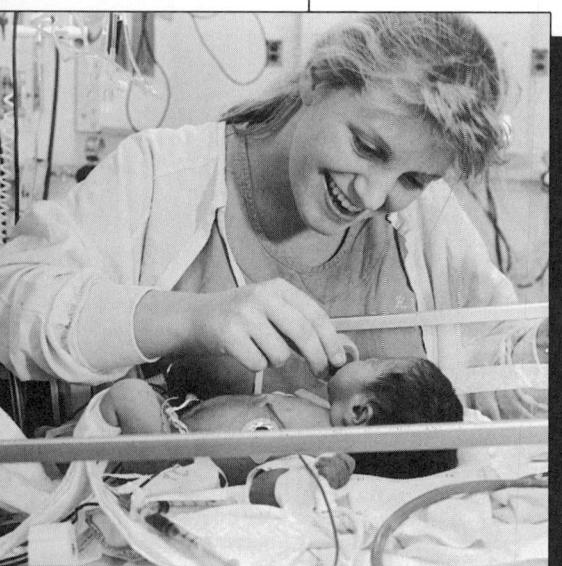

Introduction to Nursing

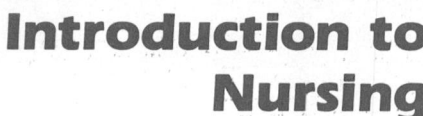

O B J E C T I V E S

After studying this chapter, the learner should be able to:

Define key terms used in the chapter.

Describe the historical background, the definitions of nursing, and the status of nursing as a profession and as a discipline.

Identify the aims of nursing as they interrelate to facilitate maximum function and quality of life for clients.

Describe the various levels of educational preparation in nursing.

Discuss the effect of nursing organizations, standards of nursing practice, nurse practice acts, and the nursing process on the practice of nursing.

Identify current trends in nursing.

K E Y   T E R M S

continuing education
dependent nursing actions
discipline
holistic health care
independent nursing actions
in-service education
interdependent nursing actions
licensure
nurse practice act
nursing
nursing education
nursing process
profession
standards
wellness

1

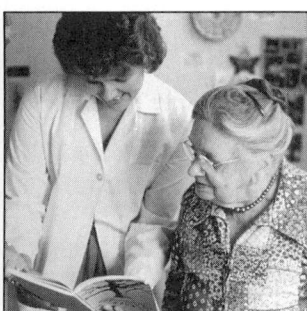

Nursing is a difficult word to define because nurses carry out many different activities in many settings. If your class were asked to complete the sentence, "Nursing is _____," a number of different responses would emerge, because each person would provide an answer based on his or her own personal experience and knowledge of nursing. As you progress toward graduation, those definitions will change, reflecting changes within yourself as you learn about and experience nursing.

Most basically defined, **nursing** is the care of others. That care may involve any number of activities, ranging from carrying out complicated technical procedures to something as seemingly simple as holding a hand. All nursing actions focus on the person receiving care and are a blend of the art and the science of nursing. The *science of nursing* is the knowledge base for what is done, and the *art of nursing* is the skilled application of that knowledge to help others reach maximum function and quality of life.

This chapter introduces you to nursing as a whole, including a brief history of nursing from its beginnings to the present, and to definitions of nursing by different individuals and organizations. Educational preparation, professional organizations, and guidelines for professional nursing practice serve as a base for understanding what nursing is and how it is organized. Because nursing is a part of an ever-changing society, a brief discussion of trends in nursing is also included.

Nursing: An Emerging Profession and Discipline

Historical Background

From the beginning of time, the nurse has been regarded as a caregiver. This role was and is defined by groups, communities, and societies. Health care and nursing as we currently know it is based on what has happened in the past.

In early civilizations, humans believed that illness had supernatural causes. The theory of animism was developed in an attempt to understand the cause of the mysterious changes in bodily functions. This theory was based on the belief that everything in nature was alive with invisible forces and endowed with power. Good spirits brought health, whereas evil spirits brought sickness and death. The roles of the physician and the nurse were separate and distinct. The physician was the medicine man who treated disease by chanting, inspiring fear, or opening the skull to release evil spirits (Dolan, Fitzpatrick, & Herrmann, 1983). The nurse usually was the mother who cared for her family during sickness by providing physical care and herbal remedies. This nurturing and caring role of the nurse has continued to the present.

As tribes became civilizations, temples became the centers of medical care because of the belief that illness was caused by sin and the gods' displeasure (ie, disease meant "dis-ease"). Priests were highly regarded as physicians, but neither human life nor women were valued by society; the nurse was viewed as a slave, carrying out menial tasks based on the orders of the priest–physician. In contrast, during the same period, the ancient Hebrews proposed rules for ethical human relationships, mental health, and disease control through the Ten Commandments and the Mosaic Health Code. Nurses cared for sick people in the home and the community and also practiced as nurse–midwives (Dolan et al., 1983).

With the beginning of Christianity, nursing began to have a formal and more clearly defined role. Led by the belief that love and caring for others were important, women called *deaconesses* led the first organized visit to sick people, and members of male religious orders gave nursing care and buried the dead. During the Crusades, both male and female nursing orders were founded. Hospitals were built to care for the enormous number of pilgrims needing health care, and nursing became a respected vocation. The early Middle Ages ended in chaos, but nursing had developed purpose, direction, and leadership.

At the beginning of the 16th century, society changed from one with a religious orientation to one that emphasized warfare, exploration, and expansion of knowledge. Many monasteries and convents closed, leading to a tremendous shortage of people to care for sick people. To meet this need, women who had committed crimes were recruited into nursing in lieu of serving jail sentences. From this background evolved a long-held view of society that nurses were disreputable and that respectable women did not work outside the home. Along with a poor reputation, nurses received low pay and worked long hours in poor conditions.

From the middle of the 18th century to the 19th century, social reforms changed the roles of nurses and of women in general. It was during this time that nursing, based on many of the beliefs and examples of Florence Nightingale, began as we currently know it. Florence Nightingale was born in 1820 to a wealthy family. She grew up in England and was well educated and traveled extensively. Despite strong opposition from her family, Nightingale received nurse's training at age 31 years. The outbreak of the Crimean War and a request by the British to organize nursing care for a military hospital in Turkey gave Nightingale an opportunity for achievement (Kalish & Kalish, 1986). Because she was able to overcome enormous difficulties successfully, Nightingale challenged prejudices against women and elevated the status of all nurses. After the war, she returned to England, where she established a training school for nurses and wrote books about health care and nursing education.

Florence Nightingale's contributions are numerous and far-reaching:

- Recognizing that nutrition is an important part of nursing care
- Instituting occupational and recreational therapy for sick people
- Identifying personal needs of the client and the role of the nurse in meeting those needs
- Establishing standards for hospital management
- Establishing a respected occupation for women
- Establishing nursing education
- Recognizing the two components of nursing—health and illness
- Believing that nursing is separate and distinct from medicine
- Stressing the need for continuing education for nurses

Florence Nightingale elevated the status of nursing to a respected occupation, improved the quality of nursing care, and founded modern nursing education. Florence Nightingale and other images of nursing care in the 19th century are shown in Figure 1-1.

Nursing in North America

The work of Florence Nightingale and the care provided for battle casualties during the Civil War focused attention on the need for educated nurses in both Canada and the United

Florence Nightingale, initiator of major reforms in health care and nursing training in England

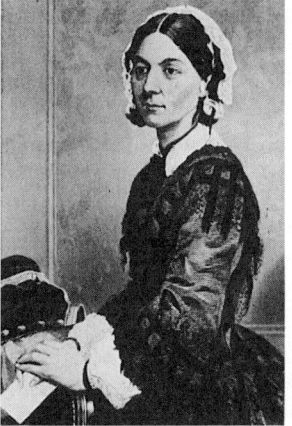

FIGURE 1-1

Images of nurses spanning more than 100 years of service. (Courtesy of The Center for the Study of the History of Nursing, University of Pennsylvania.)

Clara Barton, founder of the American Red Cross in 1882

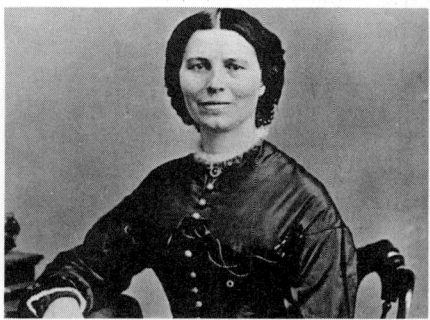

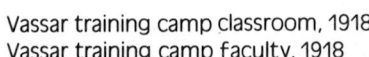
Vassar training camp classroom, 1918
Vassar training camp faculty, 1918

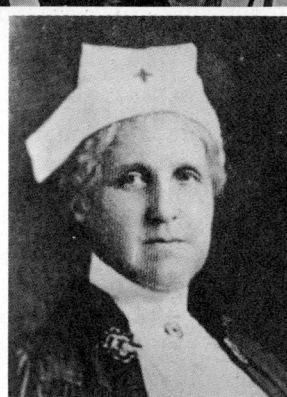

Jane Delano, an Army nurse, instrumental in the organization of the Red Cross Nursing Service in the early 1900 s

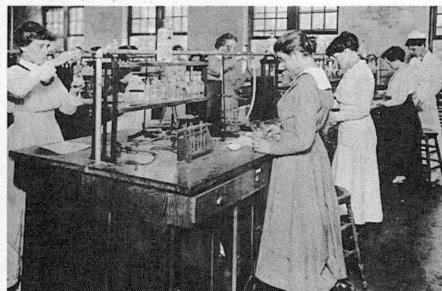

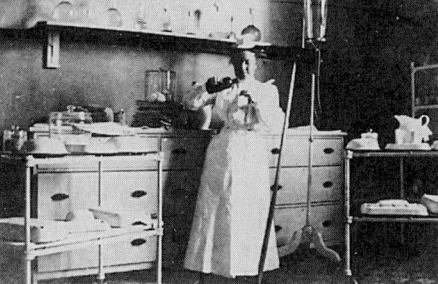

Philadelphia General Hospital nurse, late 1800 s

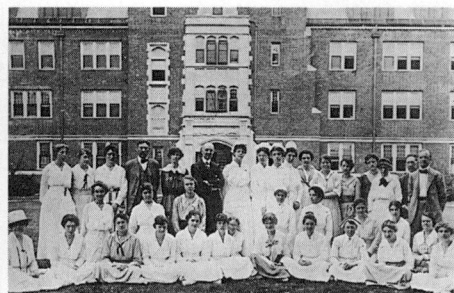

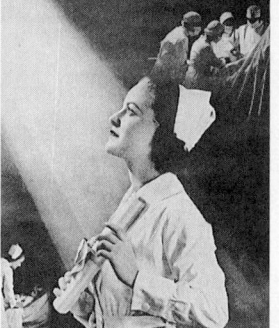

Post-WWII nursing school poster

The Art of Nursing

Nursing is caring: Nurses give care; they also demonstrate non-possessive caring about and for others.

Nursing is sharing: Nurses share themselves with each other, with other members of the health care team, and with clients.

Nursing is laughing: Nurses who laugh with others know that humor is a part of feelings of comfort and belonging.

Nursing is crying: Nurses accept tears from others and themselves as a normal response to both happiness and sadness.

Nursing is touching: Nurses touch to comfort, massage, give care—touching says "I care" and "I know what to do to help you."

Nursing is helping: Nurses help others in two broad areas: understanding and taking action.

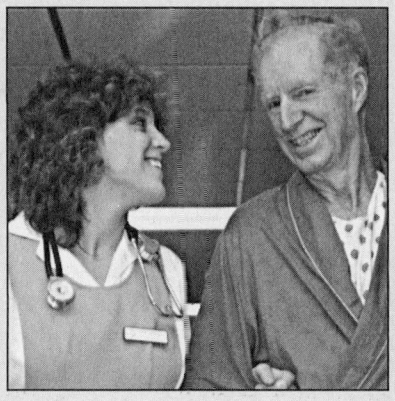

Nursing is believing in others: Nurses believe that others have the desire and ability to reach their individual potential in all areas of human functioning.

Nursing is trusting: Nurses demonstrate trust in others by accepting people as they are and by always expecting positive results from actions.

Nursing is believing in self: Nurses believe they have the knowledge and ability to help others maintain wellness.

Nursing is learning: Nurses learn new or expanded knowledge and skills throughout their career.

Nursing is respecting: Nurses demonstrate respect for others through unconditional acceptance, ensuring privacy, and individualizing care.

Nursing is listening: Nurses listen to what is said verbally but also are equally attentive to what is not said.

Nursing is doing: Nurses carry out assessments and interventions with knowledge and skill to give safe, comprehensive client care.

Nursing is feeling: Nurses share in the sorrows, joys, frustrations, and satisfactions of others.

Nursing is accepting: Nurses must first accept themselves before they can accept others.

States. Schools of nursing were founded in connection with hospitals, but although these schools were established on the works of Nightingale, the training they provided was based more on apprenticeship than on educational programs. Hospitals saw an economic advantage in having their own school, and most hospital schools were organized to provide more easily controlled and less expensive staff for the hospital. This resulted in the loss of clear guidelines separating nursing service and nursing education. As students and as graduates, female nurses were under the control of male hospital administrators and physicians. The lack of educational standards, the male dominance of health care, and the pervading Victorian belief that women depended on men combined to contribute to several decades of slow progress toward professionalism in nursing (Kalish & Kalish, 1986).

World War II had an enormous effect on nursing. For the first time, large numbers of women worked outside the home. In the process, they also became more independent and assertive. These changes in women and in society resulted in an increased emphasis on education. The war itself had identified a need for more nurses and had resulted in a knowledge explosion in medicine and technology, which broadened the role of nurses. After World War II, efforts were directed at upgrading nursing education. Schools of nursing were based on educational objectives and were increasingly developed in university and college settings, leading to degrees in nursing for both men and women.

Since the 1950s, nursing has broadened in all areas, including practice in a wide variety of health care settings, the development of a body of knowledge specific to nursing, the conduct and publication of nursing research, and the recognition of the role of nursing in promoting wellness. Increased emphasis on the importance of nursing knowledge as the base for nursing practice has led to the growth of nursing as a profession and as a discipline.

Definitions of Nursing

The word *nurse* originated from the Latin word *nutrix*, meaning to nourish. Ellis and Hartley (1992) used this word origin in describing the nurse as a person who nourishes, fosters, and protects; a person prepared to take care of sick, injured, and aged people. This definition has general acceptance, but it does not include the expanding roles and functions of the nurse today. This section offers several definitions of nursing that provide a broad perspective of nursing. Chapter 4 provides further definitions of nursing by specific nursing theorists.

International Council of Nurses   The following definition was written by Virginia Henderson and adopted by the International Council of Nurses (ICN) in 1973:

The unique function of the nurse is to assist the individual, sick or well, in the performance of those activities contributing to health or its recovery (or to peaceful death) that he would perform unaided if he had the necessary strength, will, or knowledge. And to do this in such a way as to help him gain independence as rapidly as possible.

American Nurses' Association In 1965, the American Nurses' Association (ANA) Committee on Education issued a position paper that broadly defined nursing as an independent profession. The statement said,

Nursing is a helping profession and, as such, provides services which contribute to the health and well-being of people. Nursing is a vital consequence to the individual receiving services; it fills needs which cannot be met by the person, by the family, or by other persons in the community.

The essential components of professional nursing are care, cure, and coordination. The care aspect is more than "to take care of"; it is "caring for" and "caring about," as well. It is dealing with human beings under stress, frequently over long periods. It is providing comfort and support in time of anxiety, loneliness, and helplessness. It is listening, evaluating, and intervening appropriately.

The promotion of health and healing is the cure aspect of professional nursing. It is assisting clients to understand their health problems and helping them to cope. It is the administration of medication and treatments. And it is the use of clinical nursing judgment in determining, on the basis of clients' reactions, whether the plan for care needs to be maintained or changed. It is knowing when and how to use existing and potential resources to help clients toward recovery and adjustment by mobilizing their own resources.

Professional Nursing Practice is this and more. It is sharing responsibility for the health and welfare of all those in the community, and participating in programs designed to prevent illness and maintain health. It is coordinating and synchronizing medical and other professional and technical services as these affect clients. It is supervising, teaching, and directing all those who give nursing care.

These concepts and beliefs were expanded by ANA in 1980 in *Nursing: A Social Policy Statement,* when the ANA Congress for Nursing Practice (1973) defined *nursing practice* as "the diagnosis and treatment of human responses to actual or potential health problems" (p. 9). This definition further legitimized the assessment and analysis of signs and symptoms and the use of nursing knowledge to implement and evaluate nursing actions taken to meet needs for potential or actual health problems.

Canadian Nurses Association The Canadian Nurses Association (CNA) made the following philosophical statement about nursing:

The nursing professional exists in response to a need of society and holds ideals related to man's

health throughout his life span. Nurses direct their energies toward the promotion, maintenance, and restoration of health, the prevention of illness, the alleviation of suffering and the ensuring of a peaceful death when life can no longer be sustained. Nurses value a holistic view of man and regard him as a biopsychosocial being who has the capacity to set goals and make decisions and who has the right and responsibility to make informed choices congruent with his own beliefs and values. Nursing, a dynamic and supportive profession guided by its code of ethics, is rooted in caring, a concept evident throughout its four fields of activity—practice, education, administration, and research. (1989, p. iii)

In all of the definitions, the central focus is the person receiving care (client), which includes the physical, emotional, social, and spiritual dimensions of that person. Nursing is no longer considered to be primarily concerned with illness; the concepts and definitions have expanded to include the prevention of illness and the maintenance of health for individuals, families, and communities.

Nursing: A Profession and a Discipline?

As definitions of nursing have expanded to more clearly describe the roles and actions of nurses, increased attention has also focused on the question of nursing as a profession and as a discipline. Nursing is gaining recognition as a **profession,** based on the criteria that a profession must have
- A strong scientific base
- A strong service orientation
- Recognized authority by a professional group
- A code of ethics
- A professional organization that sets standards
- Ongoing research
- Autonomy (DeYoung, 1985)

A **discipline** has a specific and unique body of knowledge that uses existing and new knowledge to creatively solve problems and meet human needs within ever-changing boundaries. To be considered a discipline, certain criteria must be met:
- An impressive body of lasting works
- Suitable techniques
- Concerns that are relevant to human activities
- Relevant traditions that inspire future knowledge development
- Considerable scholarly recognition and achievement (Shermis, 1962)

Nursing involves specialized skills and application of knowledge based on education that has both theoretical and clinical components. Nursing upholds standards set forth by professional organizations and follows an established code of ethics. The concerns of nursing focus on human responses to actual or potential health problems and are increasingly focused on wellness, an area of caring that encompasses nursing's unique knowledge and abilities. Nursing is rich in tradition, which is used to develop and redefine both the art and science of nursing. Furthermore, nursing is increasingly being recognized as scholarly, with academic qualifications, research, and publications specific to nursing becoming more widely accepted and respected.

Nursing has evolved through history from a technical service to a person-centered process that affects the lives of others to allow maximizing of potential in all human dimensions. This has been an active process, as the profession and the discipline of nursing has developed by using lessons from the past to gain knowledge for practice in the present and in the future.

Aims of Nursing

Apparently, many definitions of nursing exist. From these definitions, the following four broad aims of nursing practice can be identified:

- To promote wellness
- To prevent illness
- To restore health
- To facilitate coping

To meet these aims, the nurse uses knowledge and skills to give care in a variety of traditional and expanding nursing roles. The primary role of the nurse as caregiver is given shape and substance by the interrelated roles of communicator, teacher, counselor, leader, researcher, and advocate. These roles, as well as expanded career roles and functions of nurses, are defined in Tables 1-1 and 1-2, and fully discussed in Unit V. Activities within the roles are carried out by the nurse in many different settings, ranging from traditional hospital care to innovative home care. These activities are directed toward maximum wellness for the client and his or her family. Health care settings are discussed in Chapter 3.

Promoting Wellness

Wellness is a state of human functioning that may be defined as the achievement of one's maximum attainable potential. The American Hospital Association (1980) further described wellness as follows:

> The objective of wellness is not merely to avoid illness or to prolong life; rather, its objective is to enhance the quality of a person's life through activities that are designed to continually improve the state of his physical, mental, emotional and spiritual well being . . . wellness is as achievable by the aged, the chronically ill, or the handicapped as by anyone else. (p. 1)

Nurses promote wellness by maximizing strengths that are specific and individualized within each person requiring care. Wellness is an essential part of each of the other aims of nursing, with identification and analysis of client strengths a component of preventing illness, restoring health, and facilitating coping with disability or death. Every client, no matter how acutely or chronically ill, has strengths. The nurse must identify and use these strengths to help the client reach maximum function and quality of life or meet death with dignity (Houldin, Saltstein, & Ganley, 1987).

Wellness promotion is the framework for nursing activities. The client's self-awareness, health awareness, wellness skills, and use of resources are all considered as the nurse gives care. Through knowledge and skill, the nurse

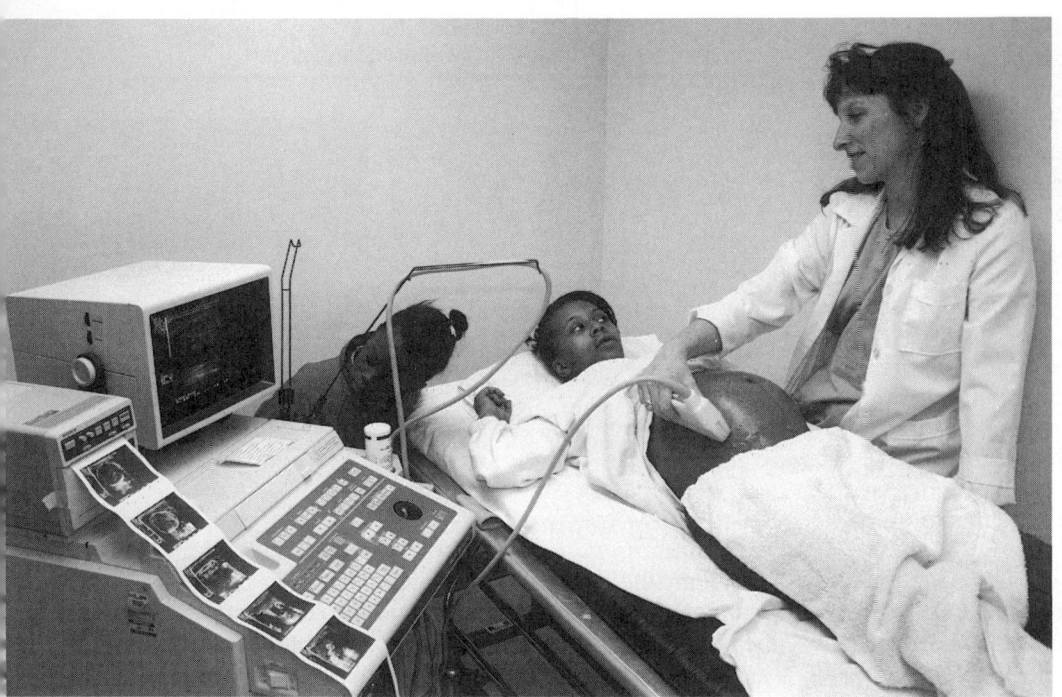

F I G U R E   1 - 2

Growing numbers of women's health centers staffed with certified nurse practitioners and nurse midwives provide affordable health maintenance care. (Photo by Gates Rhodes, courtesy School of Nursing, University of Pennsylvania.)

- Increases self-awareness by facilitating decisions about life-style that enhance the quality of life and by encouraging acceptance of responsibility for one's own health
- Increases health awareness by assisting in the understanding that health is more than just not being ill and by teaching that certain behaviors and factors can contribute to or diminish wellness
- Teaches wellness skills (1) by promoting decision making so that self-care activities maximize achievement of goals that are realistic and attainable, and (2) by serving as a role model
- Encourages the use of wellness resources by providing information about resources that can be used to bring about desired change (Abood & Burkhead, 1938)

Preventing Illness

The objectives of illness-prevention activities are to reduce the risk of illness, to promote good health habits, and to maintain the individual's optimal functioning. Health promotion is carried out by organizations and institutions as well as by nurses. Nurses primarily promote health by teaching and by personal example. Such activities include the following:

- Hospital educational programs in areas such as prenatal care for pregnant women, smoking-cessation programs, and stress-reduction seminars
- Community programs and resources that encourage healthy life-styles, including aerobic exercise classes, swimnastics, and physical fitness programs
- Literature and television information on diet, exercise, and the importance of good health habits
- Health assessments in institutions, clinics, and community settings that identify areas of strength and the potential for illness

Restoring Health

Activities directed to restore health encompass those most traditionally considered to be the nurse's responsibility and probably are an area in which most practicing nurses are employed. This area focuses on the individual with an illness but ranges from early detection of a disease to rehabilitation and teaching during recovery. Activities include

- Providing direct care of the person who is ill, by such measures as physical care, administration of medications, and carrying out procedures and treatments
- Performing diagnostic measurements and examinations (eg, taking blood pressure, measuring blood sugars) that detect an illness
- Referring questions and abnormal findings to other health care providers as appropriate
- Planning, teaching, and carrying out rehabilitation for illnesses such as heart attacks, arthritis, and strokes
- Working in mental health and chemical-dependency programs

TABLE 1-1

Roles and Functions of Nurses

Role	Function
Caregiver	The provision of care to clients that combines both the art and the science of nursing in meeting physical, emotional, intellectual, sociocultural, and spiritual needs. As a caregiver, the nurse integrates the roles of communicator, teacher, counselor, and leader, researcher, advocate to promote wellness through activities that prevent illness, restore health, and facilitate coping with disability or death. The role of caregiver is the primary role of the nurse.
Communicator	The use of effective interpersonal and therapeutic communication skills to establish and maintain helping relationships with clients of all ages in a wide variety of health care settings.
Teacher	The use of communication skills to assess, implement, and evaluate individualized teaching plans to meet learning needs of clients and their families.
Counselor	The use of therapeutic interpersonal communication skills to provide information, make appropriate referrals, and facilitate the client's problem-solving and decision-making skills.
Leader	The assertive, self-confident practice of nursing when providing care, effecting change, and functioning with groups.
Researcher	The participation in or conduct of research to increase knowledge in nursing and improve client care.
Advocate	The protection of human or legal rights and the securing of care for all clients based on the belief that clients have the right to make informed decisions about their own health and lives.

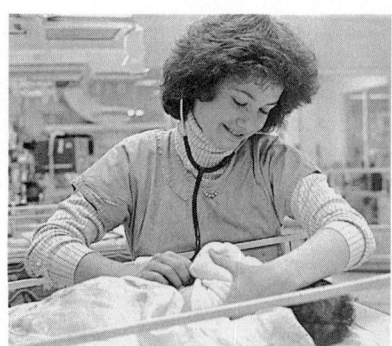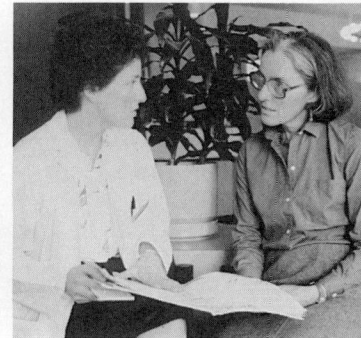

Facilitating Coping

Although the major focus of health care is promoting, maintaining, or restoring health, these goals cannot always be met. Nurses also facilitate client and family coping with altered function, life crisis, and death. *Altered function* re-

TABLE 1-2

Expanded Career Roles and Functions of Nurses

Title	Description
Clinical nurse specialist (eg, enterostomal therapist, geriatrics, infection control, medical–surgical, maternal–child, oncology, quality assurance, nursing process)	A nurse with an advanced degree, education, or experience who is considered to be an expert in a specialized area of nursing; carries out direct client care, consultation, teaching clients, families, and staff, and conducting research
Nurse practitioner	A nurse with an advanced degree, certified for a special area or age of client care; works in a variety of health care settings or in independent practice to make health assessments and deliver primary care
Nurse anesthetist	A nurse who completes a course of study in an anesthesia school; carries out preoperative visits and assessments, administers and monitors anesthesia during surgery, and evaluates postoperative status of clients
Nurse midwife	A nurse who completes a program in midwifery; provides prenatal and postnatal care and delivers babies to women with uncomplicated pregnancies
Nurse educator	A nurse, usually with an advanced degree, who teaches in educational or clinical settings; teaches theoretical knowledge and clinical skills; conducts research
Nurse administrator	A nurse who functions at various levels of management in health care settings; responsible for the management and administration of resources and personnel involved in giving client care
Nurse researcher	A nurse with an advanced degree who conducts research relevant to the definition and improvement of nursing practice and education
Nurse entrepreneur	A nurse, usually with an advanced degree, who may manage a clinic or health-related business, conduct research, provide education, or serve as an adviser or consultant to institutions, political agencies, or businesses

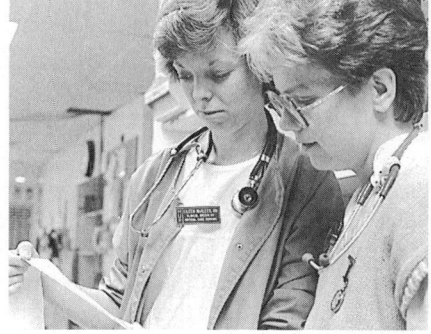
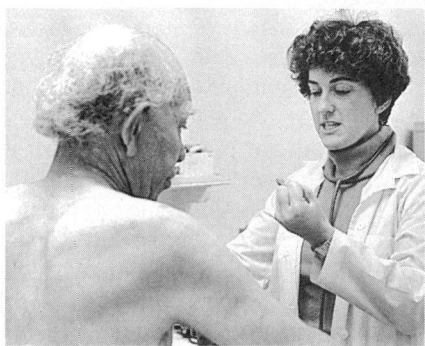
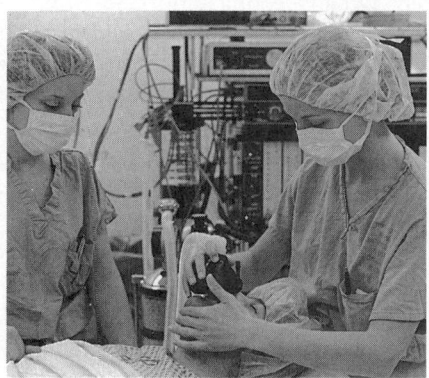
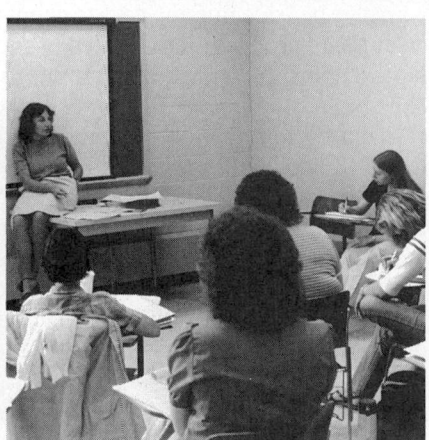

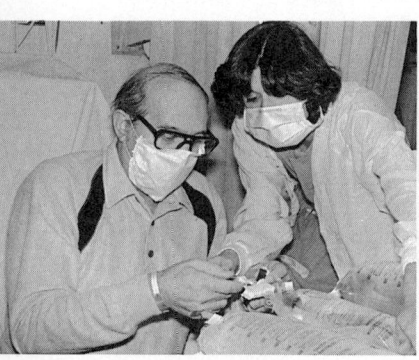
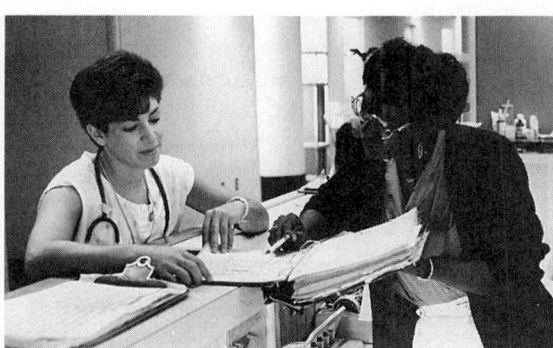

(Photos by Gates Rhodes and Denise Angelini, courtesy of School of Nursing, University of Pennsylvania.)

sults in a decrease in an individual's ability to carry out activities of daily living and expected roles. Nurses can facilitate an optimal level of function through understanding and acceptance of the individual and family, the maximizing of strengths and potentials, teaching, and knowledge and referral to community support systems. Nurses provide care to both clients and families during the terminal illness, and they do so in hospitals, long-term nursing facilities, and homes. Nurses are also becoming more active in hospice programs, which are developed to assist individuals and their families in preparing for death and in living as comfortably as possible until death occurs.

Educational Preparation for Nursing Practice

Levels of Education

Educational preparation for nursing practice currently involves several different types of programs. Students may choose to enter a practical nursing program and be licensed as a licensed practical nurse (LPN) or licensed vocational nurse (LVN), or they may enter a diploma, an associate degree, or a baccalaureate program to be licensed as a registered nurse (RN). State laws in the United States and in some provinces of Canada recognize both the LPN or LVN and RN as having the proper credentials to practice nursing, although the responsibilities are different for the two levels. Graduate programs are also available in nursing, providing master's and doctoral degrees.

One of the major issues in nursing currently involves nursing education. The multiple educational systems are confusing to institutions employing nurses, to consumers of health care services, and to nurses themselves. Nursing organizations are working hard to answer questions such as, "What is technical nursing?" and "What is professional nursing?" as well as, "Should graduates of all programs take the same kind of licensing examination and have the same title?" These questions should be resolved during your nursing career.

This section discusses education for LPNs and RNs, as well as graduate nursing education, continuing education for nurses, and in-service education.

Practical and Vocational Nursing Education

Practical nursing was established to provide graduates who give bedside nursing care to clients. Schools for practical nursing programs are located in such varied settings as high schools, technical or vocational schools, community colleges, or independent agencies. Most programs are 1-year programs divided into one-third classroom and two-thirds clinical laboratory hours. On completion of the program, graduates are eligible to take the National Council Licensure Examination (NCLEX-PN) for licensure as practical nursing. In Canada, some provinces offer a similar program for practitioners called registered nursing assistant.

LPNs work under the direction of a physician or RN to give direct care to clients, focusing on meeting health care needs in hospitals, nursing homes, and home health agencies.

Registered Nursing Education

Three primary types of educational programs lead to **licensure** as an RN. In the United States, these types are (1) diploma, (2) associate degree, and (3) baccalaureate programs; in Canada, (1) 2-year community college, (2) 3-year hospital-based diploma, and (3) university baccalaureate programs. Graduates of all types of programs take the same RN licensing examination. In the United States, grad-

uates take the NCLEX-RN examination, and graduates of Canadian schools take the Canadian Nurses' Association Testing Service examination. Although both are national examinations, they are administered by, and the nurse is licensed in, each state or province. It is illegal to practice nursing unless one has a license verifying completion of an accredited (by the state or province) program in nursing and has passed the licensing examination. Nurses gain legal rights to practice nursing in another state or province by applying to that state's or province's board of nursing and receiving reciprocal licensure.

Diploma in Nursing Most nurses practicing in the United States received their basic nursing education in 3-year, hospital-based diploma schools of nursing (Ellis & Hartley, 1988). The first schools of nursing established to educate nurses were diploma programs, and until the 1960s, they were the major source of graduates. In recent years, as nursing organizations have begun to take a stand on the need for education for nursing in institutions of higher education, the number of diploma programs has decreased.

Current graduates of diploma programs have a sound foundation of the biologic and social sciences, with a strong emphasis on clinical experience in direct client care. Graduates work in acute, long-term, and ambulatory health care facilities (Ellis & Hartley, 1992).

Associate Degree in Nursing Associate degree nursing education is based on a research project carried out by Dr. Mildred Montag from 1952 to 1957. At that time, a shortage of nurses existed, and the project was created to meet the needs of society by preparing nurses in less time than was required in diploma programs. The emphasis of this type of program was education instead of service (Grippando, 1986).

Currently, most associate degree programs are in community junior colleges and universities. These 2-year educational programs attract more men, more minorities, and more nontraditional students than do the other types of programs. Associate degree education prepares nurses to give care to clients in structured settings (acute and long-term facilities). Graduates of these programs are technically skilled and well prepared to carry out nursing roles and functions. Competencies of the associate degree nurse on entry into practice, as defined by the National League for Nursing (NLN), are listed in the accompanying display.

Baccalaureate in Nursing The first baccalaureate nursing programs were established in the United States and Canada in the early 1900s. However, the number of programs and the number of enrolling students did not increase markedly until the 1960s. (Most graduates receive a bachelor of science in nursing [BSN] degree and, hence, are referred to having a BSN throughout this section.)

The increase in number of programs and student enrollment is the result of recommendations made by ANA, NLN, and CNA that the entry level for professional practice be at the baccalaureate level. Although nurses with a BSN practice in a wide variety of settings, the 4-year degree is

Educational Outcomes of Associate Degree Nursing Programs: Competencies at Graduation

On graduation, the associate degree nurse demonstrates the following competencies:

Role as Provider of Care

Assessment

- Obtains data through assessment of the client.
- Collects additional data relative to the client from family, significant others, health records, health care team members, and other resources.
- Identifies changes in health status that affect the client's ability to meet needs.
- Contributes the information to a data base.

Diagnosis

- Identifies actual or potential health care needs on the basis of assessment.
- Selects nursing diagnoses on the basis of analysis and interpretation of data.

Planning

- Participates with the client, family, significant others, and members of the health care team to establish the client-centered goals directed toward promoting and restoring the client's optimal level of health, preventing illness, and providing rehabilitation.
- Establishes priorities for care with recognition of client's diagnoses and needs.
- Develops care plan incorporating data related to the client's cultural and spiritual beliefs and physiologic, psychosocial, and developmental needs and strengths.
- Collaborates with other health care workers in the development of individualized teaching plans that include health counseling, discharge planning, and implementation of a therapeutic regimen.
- Supports client's right to make decisions regarding care.

Implementation

- Implements a care plan according to priority of goals.
- Initiates nursing interventions in response to client's needs.
- Adjusts priorities for nursing interventions in response to client's needs.

- Uses current technology to enhance client care.
- Demonstrates safe performance of nursing skills.
- Provides for physical safety of the client.
- Promotes an environment conducive to maintenance or restoration of the client's ability to carry out activities of daily living.
- Promotes the rehabilitation potential of the client.
- Administers and monitors the prescribed medical regimen for the client undergoing diagnostic tests and/or therapeutic procedures.
- Promotes psychological safety of the client.
- Demonstrates caring behavior in providing nursing care.
- Uses communication techniques that assist the client, family, and significant others to cope with and resolve problems.
- Communicates verbally and in writing client behaviors, responses to nursing interventions, and responses to medical regimen.
- Implements teaching plans that are specific to the client's level of development, knowledge, and learning needs.
- Provides for continuity of care in the management of chronic health care needs.
- Makes referrals on the basis of identified client needs and knowledge of available resources.

Evaluation

- Determines the effects of nursing interventions on the status of the client.
- Participates with the client, family, significant others, and members of the health care team in the evaluation of client's progress toward goals
- Revises care plan as needed.

Role as Manager of Care

- Establishes priorities for nursing care for a group of clients.
- Delegates aspects of nursing care to other health care workers commensurate with their education preparation and experience.
- Is accountable for nursing care delegated to other workers.

- Assists other nursing personnel to develop skills in providing nursing care.
- Interacts with other members of the health care team in a collegial manner.
- Uses appropriate channels of communication to accomplish goals related to delivery of client care.
- Provides for continuity of care within the employing institution.
- Serves as an advocate for clients.
- Seeks assistance from other members of the health care team when the situation encountered is beyond the nurse's knowledge and experience.
- Uses current technology to increase efficiency of management of client care and resources.
- Practices in a cost-effective manner.

Role as Member Within the Discipline of Nursing

- Practices within the ethical and legal framework of nursing.
- Maintains confidentiality of information regarding clients.
- Communicates truthfully in verbal and written form the client's behavior and responses to interventions.
- Reports concerns regarding quality of care to the appropriate person.
- Values nursing as a career and values own practice.
- Supports peers and other workers in the delivery of client care.
- Recognizes and reports ethical dilemmas encountered in practice.
- Serves as a role model to members of the nursing team.
- Uses information from current literature to provide safe nursing care.
- Recognizes the importance of nursing research in advancing nursing practice.
- Uses resources for continuous learning and self-development.
- Uses constructive criticism and suggestions for improving nursing practices.

(National League for Nursing. [1990]. *Educational outcomes of associate degree nursing programs: Roles and competencies* [Pub. No. 23-2348]. New York: Author, Council of Associate Degree Programs.)

required for many administrative and supervisory as well as community health positions.

In BSN programs, the major in nursing is built on a general education base with concentration on nursing at the upper level. Students acquire knowledge of theory and practice related to nursing and other disciplines, provide nursing care to individuals and groups, work with members of the health care team, understand research, and have a foundation for graduate study (Grippando, 1986). The accompanying display describes the characteristics of the graduate of the baccalaureate program in nursing as defined by NLN.

Graduate Education in Nursing

The two levels of graduate education in nursing are the master's and doctoral degrees. A master's degree in nursing prepares the graduate to function in educational settings, in managerial roles, as clinical specialists, and as nurse practitioners. Nurses with doctoral degrees meet requirements for academic advancement or tenure and also are prepared to carry out research necessary to advance nursing theory and practice.

Continuing Education

The ANA (1974) *Standards for Continuing Education in Nursing* defines **continuing education** as "planned learning experiences beyond a basic nursing education program. These experiences are designed to promote the development of knowledge, skills, and attitudes for the enhancement of nursing practice, thus improving health care to the public" (p. 11).

Formal continuing education through courses, seminars, and workshops is offered by colleges, hospitals, voluntary agencies, and private groups. In some states, continuing education is required to maintain licensure.

In-Service Education

Many hospitals and health care agencies provide education and training for employees of their institution or organization. This is called **in-service education** and is designed to increase the knowledge and skills of the nursing staff. Programs might involve learning a nursing skill or how to use new equipment or might update knowledge.

Professional Nursing Organizations

Before a profession can be described as a profession, one of the criteria it must meet is having a professional organization that sets standards for nursing practice and nursing education. Nursing does meet this criterion through its professional organizations. Professional organizations also are concerned with current issues in nursing and health

---

Characteristics of the Graduate of the Baccalaureate Program in Nursing

The graduate of the baccalaureate program in nursing is able to

- provide professional nursing care, which includes health promotion and maintenance, illness, care, restoration, rehabilitation, health counseling, and education based on knowledge derived from theory and research
- synthesize theoretical and empirical knowledge from nursing, scientific, and humanistic disciplines with practice
- use the nursing process to provide nursing care for individuals, families, groups, and communities
- accept responsibility and accountability for the evaluation of the effectiveness of their own nursing practice
- enhance the quality of nursing and health practices within practice settings through the use of leadership skills and a knowledge of the political system
- evaluate research for the applicability of its findings to nursing practice
- participate with other health care providers and members of the general public in promoting the health and well-being of people
- incorporate professional values as well as ethical, moral, and legal aspects of nursing into nursing practice
- participate in the implementation of nursing roles designed to meet emerging health needs of the general public in a changing society

(National League for Nursing. [1987]. *Characteristics of baccalaureate education in nursing* [Pub. No. 15–1758]. New York: Author.)

---

care, and they influence health care legislation. The benefits of belonging to a professional nursing organization include networking with colleagues, having a voice in the legislation affecting nursing, and keeping current with trends and issues in nursing.

National Nursing Organizations

North America has three major professional organizations for nurses: (1) ANA, (2) CNA, and (3) NLN. **ANA** is the professional organization for RNs in the United States. Founded in the late 1800s, its members are state nurses' associations, with individual nurses belonging to the state organization. ANA establishes standards of practice, encourages research to advance nursing practice, represents nursing through legislative actions, and supports the National Student Nurses' Association (NSNA).

CNA is the national nursing association for RNs in Canada. CNA has provincial organizations, supported by local districts. CNA supports the same goals as ANA—to improve standards of health, to foster high standards of nursing, and to promote the professional development and welfare of nurses. CNA has also been active in nursing education, licensing, and registration for nurses.

NLN is an organization open to all people in nursing, including nurses, nonnurses, and agencies. Established in 1952, its objective is to foster the development and improvement of all nursing services and nursing education. The following are the major activities of NLN:

- Conducts one of the largest professional testing services in the United States, including pre-entrance testing for potential students, achievement testing to measure student progress, and state board examinations for licensure
- Sponsors continuing education workshops and seminars nationwide
- Serves as the primary source of research data about nursing education; conducts annual surveys of schools and new RNs
- Provides voluntary accreditation for educational programs in nursing

The national organizations for student nurses are NSNA in the United States and the Canadian University Nursing Student Organization in Canada. These organizations comprise members who are students actively enrolled in nursing education programs. Programs and activities focus on professional development and health care.

International Nursing Organization

ICN was the first international organization of professional women. The organization was founded in 1899, with nurses from both the United States and Canada among the charter members. By sharing a commitment to maintaining high standards of nursing service and nursing education and by promoting ethics, ICN provides a way for national nursing organizations to work together. The ICN *1973 Code for Nurses* states, "The need for nursing is universal. Inherent in nursing is respect for life, dignity and rights of man. It is unrestricted by considerations of nationality, race, creed, color, age, sex, politics, or social status."

Specialty Nursing Organization

A wide variety of nursing organizations currently are available to nurses. These organizations provide information on specific areas of nursing, often have publications directed toward the specialty area of nursing, and may be involved in certification activities. The following examples illustrate the variety of organizations:

American Association of Critical Care Nurses
Association of Operating Room Nurses
American Indian Nurses' Association
Canadian Gerontological Nursing Association
National Black Nurses' Association, Inc.
Nurses' Christian Fellowship

Guidelines for Nursing Practice

As the preceding historical discussion makes evident, nursing is a dynamic process that continues to evolve and change to meet the needs of society. The ANA Congress for Nursing Practice (1973) stated that a profession must control its practice to guarantee the quality of its service to the public and that "a profession that does not maintain the confidence of the public will soon cease to be a social force." Nursing controls and guarantees its practice through standards of practice, nurse practice acts and licensure, and use of the nursing process. Each of these will guide your nursing education as a student and your nursing practice after graduation.

Standards of Nursing Practice

The ANA (1991) *Standards of Clinical Nursing Practice* define the activities of nurses that are specific and unique to nursing. **Standards** allow nurses to carry out professional roles, serving as protection for the nurse, the client, and the institution where health care is given. Each nurse is accountable for his or her own quality of practice and is responsible for the use of these standards to ensure knowledgeable, safe, and comprehensive nursing care. The standards, outlined in the accompanying display, apply to the practice of all RNs and lay the foundation for the practice of professional nursing in all settings. The CNA (1987) publication *A Definition of Nursing Practice: Standards for Nursing Practice* provides a parallel purpose in Canada, although some provinces have opted to write their own standards. These standards are outlined in the accompanying display.

Nurse Practice Acts and Licensure

Nurse practice acts are laws established in each state (United States) and province (Canada) to regulate the practice of nursing. They are broadly worded and vary among jurisdictions, but all of them have certain elements in common. In general, they

- Are designed to protect the public by defining the legal scope of nursing practice, excluding untrained or unlicensed people from practicing nursing
- Create a state board of nursing or regulatory body having the authority to make and enforce rules and regulations concerning the nursing profession
- Define important terms and activities in nursing, including legal requirements and titles for RNs and LPNs
- Establish criteria for the education and licensure of nurses

American Nurses' Association Standards of Clinical Nursing Practice

Standards of Care

Assessment: The nurse collects client health data.

Diagnosis: The nurse analyzes the assessment data in determining diagnoses.

Outcome identification: The nurse identifies expected outcomes individualized to the client.

Planning: The nurse develops a plan of care that prescribes interventions to attain expected outcomes.

Implementation: The nurse implements the interventions identified in the plan of care.

Evaluation: The nurse evaluates the client's progress toward attainment of outcomes.

Standards of Professional Performance

Quality of care: The nurse systematically evaluates the quality and effectiveness of nursing practice.

Performance appraisal: The nurse evaluates his or her nursing practice in relation to professional practice standards and relevant statutes and regulations.

Education: The nurse acquires and maintains current knowledge in nursing practice.

Collegiality: The nurse contributes to the professional development of peers, colleagues, and others.

Ethics: The nurse's decisions and actions on behalf of clients are determined in an ethical manner.

Collaboration: The nurse collaborates with the client, significant others, and health care providers in providing client care.

Research: The nurse uses research findings in practice.

Resource use: The nurse considers factors related to safety, effectiveness, and cost in planning and delivering client care.

(American Nurses' Association. [1991]. *Standards of clinical practice.* Kansas City, MO: Author. Copyright © 1991, ANA.)

The board of nursing for each state or province is given legal authority to administer the licensing examination to graduates of approved schools of nursing. The individual who successfully meets the requirements for **licensure** is then given a license to practice nursing in the state or province. The license, which must be renewed annually, is valid during the life of the holder and is registered (listed with) in the state or province. The license and the right to practice nursing can be denied, revoked, or suspended for professional misconduct (eg, incompetence, negligence, chemical impairment, or criminal actions).

As nursing roles continue to expand, and as issues in nursing are resolved, nurse practice acts will reflect those changes. It is essential that nurses understand and keep abreast of the specific nurse practice act under which they practice.

Nursing Process

Although the nursing process is fully described in Unit IV, it is introduced in this chapter because it is one of the major guidelines for nursing practice. The caregiving role of the nurse is implemented through the **nursing process,** which integrates both the art and the science of nursing. That is, the implementation of the nursing process is nursing made visible. Yura and Walsh (1983) described the nursing process as follows:

> The nursing process is the core and essence of nursing; it is central to all nursing actions; it is applicable in any setting . . . there is a basic theme that underlies the process; it is organized, systematic, and deliberate. (p. 1)

The nursing process allows the nurse to identify health care needs and strengths of the client, to establish and carry out a plan of care to meet those needs, and to evaluate the effectiveness of the plan. The nursing process allows the nurse to focus on the client as an individual and to define those areas of client care that are within the domain of nursing (Carpenito, 1989).

Nursing in Transition

Nursing is constantly changing in response to the needs and resources of society as a whole. Nursing also changes in response to those factors identified in this chapter—definitions of nursing, aims of nursing, educational levels of nursing, and expanded practice roles. Current issues and trends in nursing that are briefly discussed in this section are new directions in nursing, changes in client needs, and increased responsibility. These are complex subjects and the information provided is only intended to serve as an introduction. Many of these trends and issues also are discussed in other chapters.

New Directions in Nursing

Currently, despite increased numbers of students entering schools of nursing and more nurses actively practicing nursing, there is still a shortage of nurses to provide care. Various factors have been identified as responsible for this shortage, including a change in the health care needs of clients, economic conditions affecting the setting in which care is given, and career mobility.

Individuals requiring care are more acutely ill but spend less time within the hospital setting as a result of health care reimbursement plans (see Chapter 3). This has resulted in an increased demand for nursing care both in the hospital and in community and home settings. With advanced education and expanded roles, nurses are taking advantage of career mobility to move into management, educational, and community and home clinical settings. This shift has further depleted the number of nurses available to give traditional hospital care.

In addition, nurses are finding they have increased autonomy (ie, freedom to regulate their work behavior) in making decisions about the care of others and are being better paid for their knowledge and skill. As this trend continues, increased numbers of better qualified nurses should become available.

Changes in Client Needs

Changes such as the growing tendency to discharge clients from the hospital earlier have created new needs for nursing. Client education is an important aspect of care—teaching clients and their families how to care for the clients after dismissal from the hospital literally begins on admission. Consideration of the health care needs of the client and the family in the home setting is a major component of planning client care. It is essential to maintain continuity in care between the nurse in the hospital and the nurse in the home setting. In addition, the complex needs of the client during the acute stage of illness or injury while in the hospital setting requires nursing knowledge and skill that is accurate and kept up to date.

Another aspect of changes in client needs is the increasing population of elderly who require both wellness promotion and health restoration. This issue is discussed in Chapters 3 and 12. Other changes in client needs that require nursing consideration involve the homeless, indigent, and people with acquired immunodeficiency syndrome. These groups, as well as others, require innovative nursing care to meet special needs.

Increased Responsibility

Three issues affect nursing in transition: (1) technological advances, (2) the concept of holistic nursing care, and (3) nursing actions. It is impossible to visit a health setting of almost any type without being aware of the rapid advances that have been made in technology. Diagnostic procedures, inpatient and outpatient surgical procedures, intensive care units and client care units are all heavily based on high-tech concepts and machines. These machines often follow the client into the home, where ventilators, kidney dialysis machines, intravenous fluids, and a wide variety of monitors are becoming more common. The nurse must continually update his or her knowledge and skills to use the technology to give safe, individualized care. In addition, computerization in a wide variety of applications has become commonplace in health care, providing more accurate assessments, monitoring infusion rates, and providing documentation and care plan capabilities (computer applications in nursing are included throughout this text).

Canadian Nurses Association Standards of Nursing Practice

These four standards are necessarily interdependent and interrelated.

Standard I. Nursing practice requires that a conceptual model(s) for nursing be the basis for that practice.

Nurses are required to have a clear idea, conception, or understanding of (1) goal, (2) client, (3) role of the nurse, (4) source of difficulty, (5) focus and modes of intervention, and (6) consequences.

Standard II. Nursing practice requires the effective use of the nursing process.

Nurses are required in any practice setting to do the following: (1) collection of data, (2) analysis of data, (3) planning of the intervention, (4) implementation of the intervention, and (5) evaluation.

Standard III. Nursing practice requires that the helping relationship be the nature of the client–nurse interaction.

Nurses are required to perform the following parts of the helping relationship: (1) initiation, (2) maintenance, and (3) termination.

Standard IV. Nursing practice requires nurses to fulfill professional responsibilities.

Nurses are expected to respect or comply with the following: (1) legislation, (2) ethics, and (3) collaboration.

(Summarized and adapted from the Canadian Nurses Association Standards for Nursing Practice. Prepared and revised by a Task Group to Develop a Definition of Nursing Practice and Standards for Nursing Practice, Ottawa, Canadian Nurses Association, 1987).

The concept of holistic nursing care is a trend that has great implications for nursing. No longer do nurses focus solely on the medical problem or the technical skills needed for client care. Holistic care considers all aspects of the client—the physical, psychosocial, and spiritual dimensions that make each individual unique. This focus allows the nurse to provide care that is person centered and wellness oriented.

Nursing actions, which are the activities (or interventions) nurses carry out as caregivers, are also in transition. Nurses were long considered to have only a dependent role. With changes in nursing, nursing autonomy has increased and the special role of the nurse in providing care has been recognized. It is important to realize that with authority to carry out actions also comes responsibility for one's actions. Even if an action is carried out on the direct order of a physician, the nurse is still responsible. Because this area encompasses terminology that is changing, both traditional and more recent definitions of nursing actions are given.

Traditionally, nursing actions have been divided into three categories:

Dependent nursing actions: Those activities that the nurse does based on physician orders. Even dependent actions (eg, administering prescribed medications) require knowledge and skill, as well as the legal responsibility to question any order that is inappropriate.

Interdependent nursing actions: Those activities that the nurse carries out in collaboration with other members of the health care team. Examples include monitoring the client for the side effects of medications or for changes in the results of diagnostic test, and reporting findings that indicate increased potential for illness to the appropriate person.

Independent nursing actions: Those activities that the nurse orders and carries out based on assessments, knowledge, and judgment. A wide range of activities are included in this area, including health assessments, nursing diagnoses and care plans, teaching, and counseling.

As nursing continues to differentiate itself from medicine, nursing actions are being defined more precisely, with the terminology more clearly reflecting the role of the nurse. Although the independent activities remain as previously described, other definitions may be used that encompass the dependent and interdependent activities of the nurse. Nursing interventions for collaborative problems include making assessments to detect early complications of illness, performing nursing actions that are ordered, and carrying out nursing actions based on standard policy and procedure manuals (Alfaro, 1990). Nursing actions may also be classified as independent or delegated, in which independent interventions are nursing prescribed and delegated interventions are physician prescribed (Bulechek & McCloskey, 1985; Carpenito, 1991). Regardless of the type of intervention, independent nursing judgment is required as the intervention is carried out.

Providing holistic, individualized client care is a combination of both independent and collaborative (or delegated) actions. As nurses become more assertive in defining their own practice, the special and distinctive role of nursing in caring for others will become increasingly recognized.

KEY POINTS

- Nursing has always involved caring; the role of the nurse as caregiver has been present since early civilization.
- Definitions of nursing have changed and expanded through time in response to societal needs and the social and political structure in which nursing has existed.
- The base for nursing practice and nursing education as we currently know it was established by Florence Nightingale, who positively influenced health care standards, nursing practice, nursing education, and women's rights.

- Nursing education in North America has changed from service-oriented hospital training schools to educational programs primarily offered in colleges and universities.
- The roles, functions, and professional status of nursing have been defined and described by ICN, ANA, and CNA. In all definitions, the central focus of nursing is the person receiving care.
- Nursing is an emerging profession and discipline. It is a practice that applies knowledge through specialized skills, upholds standards developed by and for the profession, develops theories and conducts research, and uses the nursing process to give individualized and holistic care.

BIBLIOGRAPHY

Abood, D. A., & Burkhead, E. J. (1988). Wellness: A valuable resource for persons with disabilities. *Health Education,* April/May, 21–26.

Alfaro, R. (1990). *Applying nursing diagnosis and nursing process: A step-by-step process* (2nd ed.). Philadelphia: Lippincott.

American Hospital Association. (1980). Wellness: What is it? *Promoting Health, 1*(1), 1–5.

American Nurses' Association. (1965). American Nurses' Association first position paper on education for nurses. *American Journal of Nursing, 12,* 106–111.

American Nurses' Association. (1974). *Standards for continuing education in nursing.* Kansas City, MO: Author.

American Nurses' Association. (1980). *Nursing: A social policy statement.* Kansas City, MO: Author.

American Nurses' Association. (1991). Standards of clinical nursing practice. Kansas City, MO: Author.

American Nurses' Association, Committee on Education. (1965). *A position paper.* New York: Author.

American Nurses' Association, Congress for Nursing Practice. (1973). *Standards: Nursing practice.* Kansas City, MO: Author.

Bailey, D. R. (1988). Computer applications in nursing: A prototypical model for planning nursing care. *Computers in Nursing, 6*(5), 199–203.

Barnum, B. (1989). Nursing's image and the future. *Nursing and Health Care, 10*(1), 18–21.

Baumgart, A. (1990). Celebrating nursing. *Canadian Nurse, 86*(8), 24–25.

Bulechek, G. M., & McCloskey, J. C. (1985). *Nursing interventions: Treatments for nursing diagnoses.* Philadelphia: Saunders.

Canadian Nurses Association. (1987). *A definition of nursing practice: Standards for nursing practice.* Ottawa, Canada: Author.

Carnevali, F. (1986). Computers in nursing. *Canadian Critical Care Nursing Journal, 3*(4), 22–26.

Carpenito, L. J. (1992). *Nursing diagnosis: Application to clinical practice* (4th ed.). Philadelphia: Lippincott.

Carpenito, L. J. (1991). *Nursing care plans and documentation: Nursing diagnoses and collaborative problems.* Philadelphia: Lippincott.

Competencies of the associate degree nurse on entry into practice. (1978). (Pub. No. 23-1731). New York: National League for Nursing.

Curtin, L. L. (1990). Designing new roles: Nursing in the '90s and beyond. *Nursing Management, 21*(2), 7–8.

Dalton C. (1990). The sleeping giant awakes. *Canadian Nurse, 86*(9), 17–18.

DeYoung, L. (1985). *Dynamics of nursing* (5th ed.). St. Louis: Mosby.

Diers, D. (1990). The art and craft of nursing. *American Journal of Nursing, 90*(1), 65–66.

Dolan, J. A., Fitzpatrick, M. L., & Herrmann, E. K. (1983). *Nursing in society: A historical perspective.* Philadelphia: Saunders.

Drugge S. (1991). The essence of nursing. *Canadian Nurse, 87*(10), 28.

DuBrey, R. J. (1982). *Promoting wellness in nursing practice.* St. Louis: Mosby.

Ellis, J., & Hartley, C. (1992). *Nursing in today's world: Challenges, issues, trends* (4th ed.). Philadelphia: Lippincott.

Grippando, G. (1986). *Nursing perspectives and issues* (3rd ed.). Albany, NY: Delmar.

Hammond, M. (1990). Is nursing a semi-profession? *Canadian Nurse, 86*(2), 21–23.

Hood, G. (1985). At issue: Titling and licensure. *American Journal of Nursing, 5,* 592.

Houldin, A. D., Salstein, S. W., & Ganley, K. M. (1987). *Nursing diagnoses for wellness.* Philadelphia: Lippincott.

International Council of Nurses. (1973). *1973 code for nurses.* Geneva: Impimeries Populaires.

Kalish, P., & Kalish, B. (1986). *The advance of American nursing* (2nd ed.). Boston: Little, Brown.

Kelly, L. Y. (1992). *The nursing experience: Trends, challenges, and transitions.* (2nd ed.). New York: McGraw-Hill.

Lindberg, J. B., Hunter, M. L., & Kruszewski, A. Z. (1990). *Introduction to nursing: Concepts, issues and opportunities.* Philadelphia: Lippincott.

McCann-Flynn, J., & Heffron, P. B. (1988). *Nursing: From concept to practice* (2nd ed.). Norwalk, CT: Appleton & Lange.

McCloskey, J. C., & Bulecheck, G. (1992). *Nursing interventions classification (NIC).* St. Louis: Mosby.

McCloskey, J. C., & Grace, H. K. (1990). *Current issues in nursing* (3rd ed.). St. Louis, MO: Mosby.

Moccia, P. (1992). In 1992: A nurse in every school. *Nursing and Health Care, 13*(1), 14–18.

National League for Nursing. (1978). *Characteristics of baccalaureate education in nursing* (Pub. No. 23-1731). New York: Author.

Parse, R. R. (1989). Essentials for practicing the art of nursing. *Nursing Science Quarterly, 2*(3), 111.

Shermis, S. (1962). On becoming an intellectual discipline. *Phi Delta Kappan, 44*(1), 84–86.

Smith, M. J. (1988). Nursing: What's in a name? *Nursing Science Quarterly, 1*(4), 142.

Westfall, VE. (1987). Standards of practice: Nursing values made visible. *Journal of Nursing Quality Assurance, 1*(2), 21–30.

Yura, H., & Walsh, M. (1988). *The nursing process: Assessing, implementing, evaluating* (5th ed.) Norwalk, CT: Appleton-Century-Crofts.

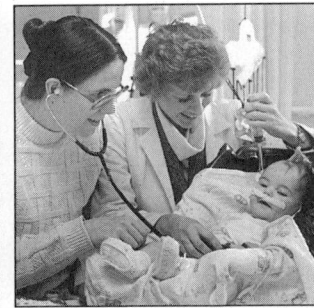
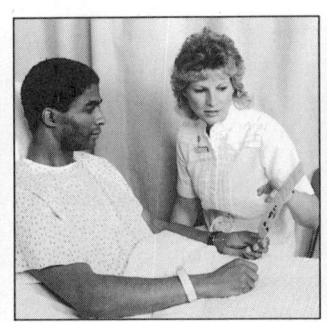
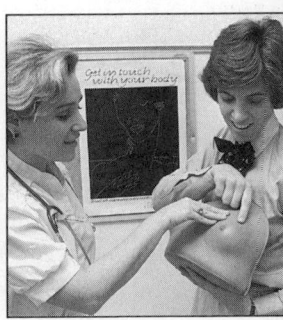

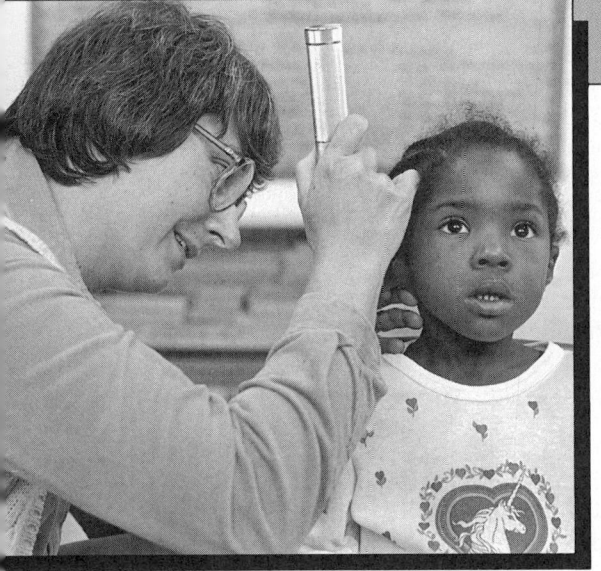

Promoting Wellness in Health and Illness

OBJECTIVES

After studying this chapter, the learner should be able to:

Define key terms used in the chapter.

Describe wellness, health, and illness.

Identify the factors influencing health and illness, including the human dimensions, basic human needs, and self-concept.

Compare and contrast acute illness and chronic illness.

Summarize the role of the nurse in promoting wellness based on knowledge of risk factors for illness, illness behaviors, and the effects of illness on the family.

Describe the levels of preventive care.

KEY TERMS

acute illness
agent–host–environment model
basic human needs
chronic illness
disease
health
health-belief model
health–illness continuum
high-level wellness
illness
primary preventive care
risk factor
secondary preventive care
tertiary preventive care

2

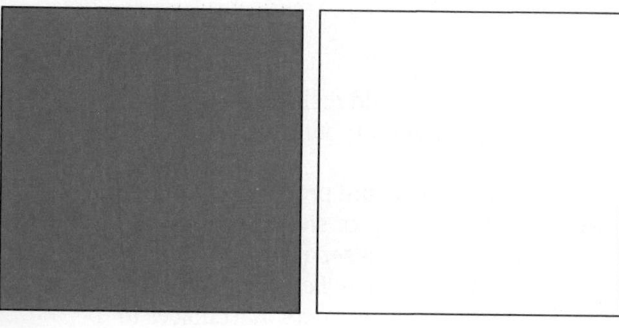

The primary role of the nurse as caregiver is to maximize wellness in clients of all ages, in a variety of settings, and in both health and illness. Chapter 1 focused on the historical background and broad perspectives of nursing. This chapter discusses how the practice of nursing is also influenced by the **client**—the person receiving care. To give holistic care, the nurse must accept and respect each person's definition of wellness and response to illness.

Defining Wellness in Health and Illness

Wellness is defined by each person relative to his or her own values and beliefs. That individualized definition is also influenced by the family, community, and society in which a person lives. Consider the following examples:

- Brian Taft, age 5 years, was born with a heart defect. However, the defect was repaired when Brian was a baby, and he is an active member of his kindergarten class, plays soccer for the community little league, and wants to be a firefighter when he grows up.
- Sara Wall is a 34-year-old mother of two school-age children. She has chronic rheumatoid arthritis and is in a wheelchair. Sara takes care of her house and her family, and uses a specially designed car to get to her part-time job.
- Howard Streete is 78 years old. He had a minor heart attack and takes medications to treat high blood pressure. Howard is retired but spends 3 days weekly as a volunteer in a local hospital as a transport technician.

Would Brian, Sara, and Howard be defined as well? Although they have a physical condition that would allow them to define themselves as ill, they are all productive members of their society and would say they are healthy.

Wellness and health are not just the absence of illness. Health must be defined by each person and must consider the dimensions of that person—the physical, intellectual, emotional, sociocultural, spiritual, and environmental aspects that compose the whole person. Equal consideration of all these interrelated and interdependent components of the whole person serves as the basis for holistic nursing care (Fig. 2-1).

Because health is individualized to each person and is affected by so many factors, definitions are difficult. The most widely accepted definition of **health,** which includes the concept of wellness, was made in 1947 by the World Health Organization: Health is a state of complete physical, mental, and social well-being, not merely the absence of disease or infirmity (p. 1). This definition has been expanded since the 1940s (see Models of Health and Illness). In contrast to definitions from the scientific community, most individuals describe and define health by how they feel ("I feel terrible"); by the absence or presence of symptoms of illness ("My headache was awful, but now it is gone"); or their ability to carry out their normal activities of daily living ("I felt so much better that I got up and cooked supper").

Definitions of illness are also individualized to each person who experiences an alteration in health. Illness is also difficult to define, because the terms *disease* and *illness* are often used to mean the same process. **Disease** is a medical term, meaning that there is a pathologic change in the structure or function of the body or mind. It is a condition that has specific symptoms and boundaries, whereas health and illness are individualized perceptions and definitions of oneself. An **illness** is an abnormal process in which the person's level of functioning is changed compared with a previous level. It is important to remember that a person may have a disease, and consider himself or herself to be ill, but still achieve maximum functioning and quality of life, which is wellness.

Models of Health and Illness

Because definitions of health and illness are not specific, **health models** (examples developed to give a visual impression of something that cannot be observed directly) have been developed to help describe the concepts and

FIGURE 2-1

The human dimensions. All of these interdependent parts compose the whole person.

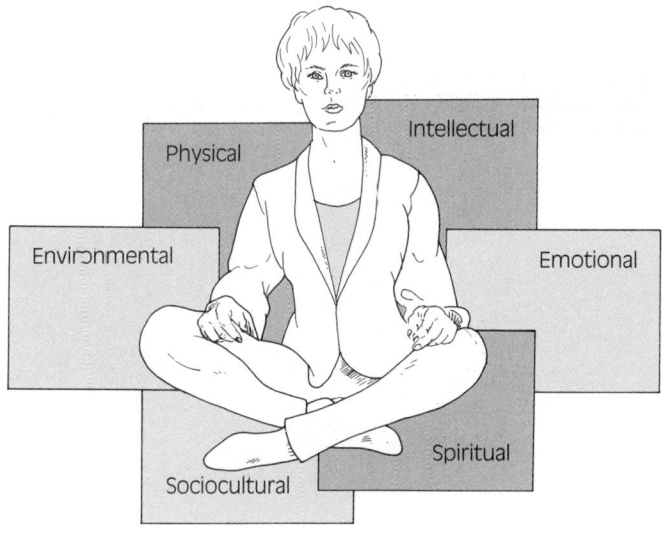

relationships involved in health and illness. The models described in this chapter are the health–illness continuum, the high-level wellness model, the agent–host–environment model, and the health-belief model.

The Health–Illness Continuum

One way to measure a person's level of wellness is to use the **health–illness continuum**. According to this model, health is a constantly changing state, with high-level wellness and death being on opposite ends of a graduated scale, or continuum (Fig. 2-2). The nurse must be aware that a client with a chronic illness may place himself or herself at different points on the continuum at any given time, depending on how well the client believes he or she is functioning for the illness (McCann-Flynn & Heffron, 1988).

High-Level Wellness Model

Halbert Dunn (1961) described his model of **high-level wellness** as functioning to one's maximum potential while maintaining balance and purposeful direction in the environment. The concept of high-level wellness can be applied to the individual, family, community, environment, and society. This discussion focuses on Dunn's model as it applies to the individual.

Dunn differentiates "wellness" from "good health," believing that good health is a passive state wherein the person is not ill. Wellness, on the other hand, is a more complex and active state.

In this model, humans are viewed as having five aspects:

1. Each individual functions as a total personality.
2. Each person possesses dynamic energy.
3. Each person is at peace with inner and outer worlds.
4. Each person has a relationship between energy use and self-integration (the interweaving of all the aspects of life).

F I G U R E   2 - 2

The health–illness continuum.

5. Each person has an inner world (cells making up the organized whole) and an outer world (environment).

Combined with these five aspects are processes that help the person know who and what he or she is. These processes are *being* (recognizing self as separate and individual); *belonging* (being part of a whole); *becoming* (growing and developing); and *befitting* (making personal choices to befit the self for the future).

Dunn's model is holistic, allowing the nurse to care for the total person with regard for all dimensional factors affecting the person's state of being as he or she strives to reach maximum potential. For example, when planning and giving care to a young male college student paralyzed after a diving accident, the nurse would include nursing activities to meet his educational needs (intellectual dimension); incorporate friends and family (sociocultural dimension); provide or refer for counseling (emotional dimension); and ask the hospital chaplain to visit (spiritual dimension).

Agent–Host–Environment Model

The **agent–host–environment model** of health and illness, developed by Leavell and Clark (1965), initially concentrated on community health but is also appropriate when examining the causes of disease in an individual (the "multiple causation" of disease). The model is actually more useful in predicting illness than in promoting wellness, although recognition of risk factors resulting from interaction of agent–host–environment is important in the promotion and maintenance of health.

The three variables involved are defined as follows:

Agent: A factor that must be present or absent for an illness to occur. It may be biologic, chemical, physical, mechanical, or psychosocial.

Host: Living beings (ie, human or animal) capable of being infected or affected by an agent. Host reaction is influenced by family history, age, and health habits.

Environment: Everything external to the host that makes illness more or less likely. Examples of environmental factors are living conditions and sound (noise) levels.

The triangle in Figure 2-3 shows that each of the agent–host–environment factors affects and is affected by the others. The factors are constantly interacting, and a combination of factors increases the possibility of illness. When the variables (agent–host–environment) are balanced, health is maintained; when they are out of balance, disease occurs. Thus, health is an ever-changing state.

Health-Belief Model

In the United States and Canada, free or low-cost screenings and information are available to help in the early detection of disease and to educate about healthy living to prevent illness. Why then don't more people take advantage of these services or change their life-styles? This ques-

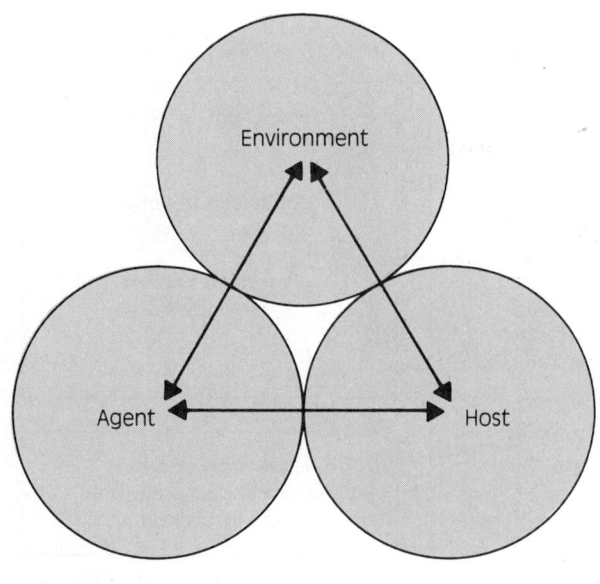

FIGURE 2-3

The agent–host–environment triangle.

tion can be answered through the widely used health-belief model, which describes health behavior.

The **health-belief model** (Rosenstock, 1974) is based on what people perceive, or believe, to be true about themselves in relation to health. This model is based on three components: (1) perceived susceptibility to a disease, (2) perceived seriousness of a disease, and (3) perceived value of action.

Perceived susceptibility to a disease is an individual's belief that he or she either will or will not contract a disease. Perceived susceptibility may range from being afraid of contracting a disease to complete denial that certain behaviors will result in illness. For example, the person who smokes cigarettes may believe he or she is at danger for lung cancer and may stop smoking, or the person may believe smoking will pose no serious threat and, hence, will continue to smoke.

Perceived seriousness of a disease involves two factors: (1) seriousness of the disease and (2) its perceived effect on the person's life-style. This component is based on how much the person knows about the disease and can result in a change in health behavior. If the person who smokes believes that lung cancer could lead to physical disability or death and would affect his or her ability to work and care for the family, the person is more likely to stop smoking. Both perceived susceptibility to a disease and perceived seriousness of a disease are part of beliefs about the threat of disease.

Perceived value of action is concerned with how effective the individual believes preventive measures will be in preventing illness. It is influenced by two factors: (1) conviction that carrying out a recommended action will prevent or modify the disease and (2) the person's perception of the cost and unpleasant effects of performing the health

behavior (compared with not taking any action). Based on this component, the person may believe that stopping smoking will prevent altered respiratory function and that the initial withdrawal symptoms can be overcome, and therefore will stop smoking.

Figure 2-4 illustrates the component health-belief perceptions and modifying factors. This model is useful in teaching individuals about health and illness. The nurse can identify the client's health beliefs and then structure goals to realistically meet client needs. Teaching and wellness-promotion activities are ineffective unless the client believes they are important and necessary.

Factors Affecting Health and Illness

As the preceding models of health and illness illustrate, many factors influence a person's health status. These factors may be internal or external to the individual, and may or may not be under conscious control. However, they do affect client responses to nursing care. To plan and give holistic care, the nurse must understand how these factors influence behavior in both healthy and ill clients.

This section addresses factors that affect health and illness, including factors influencing health–illness status, beliefs, and practices; basic human needs; and self-concept. This section serves only as an introduction to these concepts; other chapters in the book fully discuss each topic.

Factors Influencing Health–Illness Status, Beliefs, and Practices

The factors influencing health–illness status, health beliefs, and health practices are described as they relate to the person in terms of the human dimensions previously discussed (see Fig. 2-1). Each person is a composite of these human dimensions, and each dimension influences the behaviors of the person receiving care. As you assess, plan, give, and evaluate nursing care of clients, consideration of these dimensions is an integral part of the nursing process (Fig. 2-5).

Physical Dimension Genetic makeup, age, developmental level, race, and sex are all part of an individual's physical dimension and strongly influence health status and health practices. Examples are as follows:

- The toddler just learning to walk, who is prone to fall and injure himself
- The young woman who has a family history of breast cancer and diabetes and therefore is at higher risk to develop these conditions
- The middle-aged African-American man who is more prone to develop high blood pressure
- The elderly person with normal aging changes that result in diminished sight and hearing

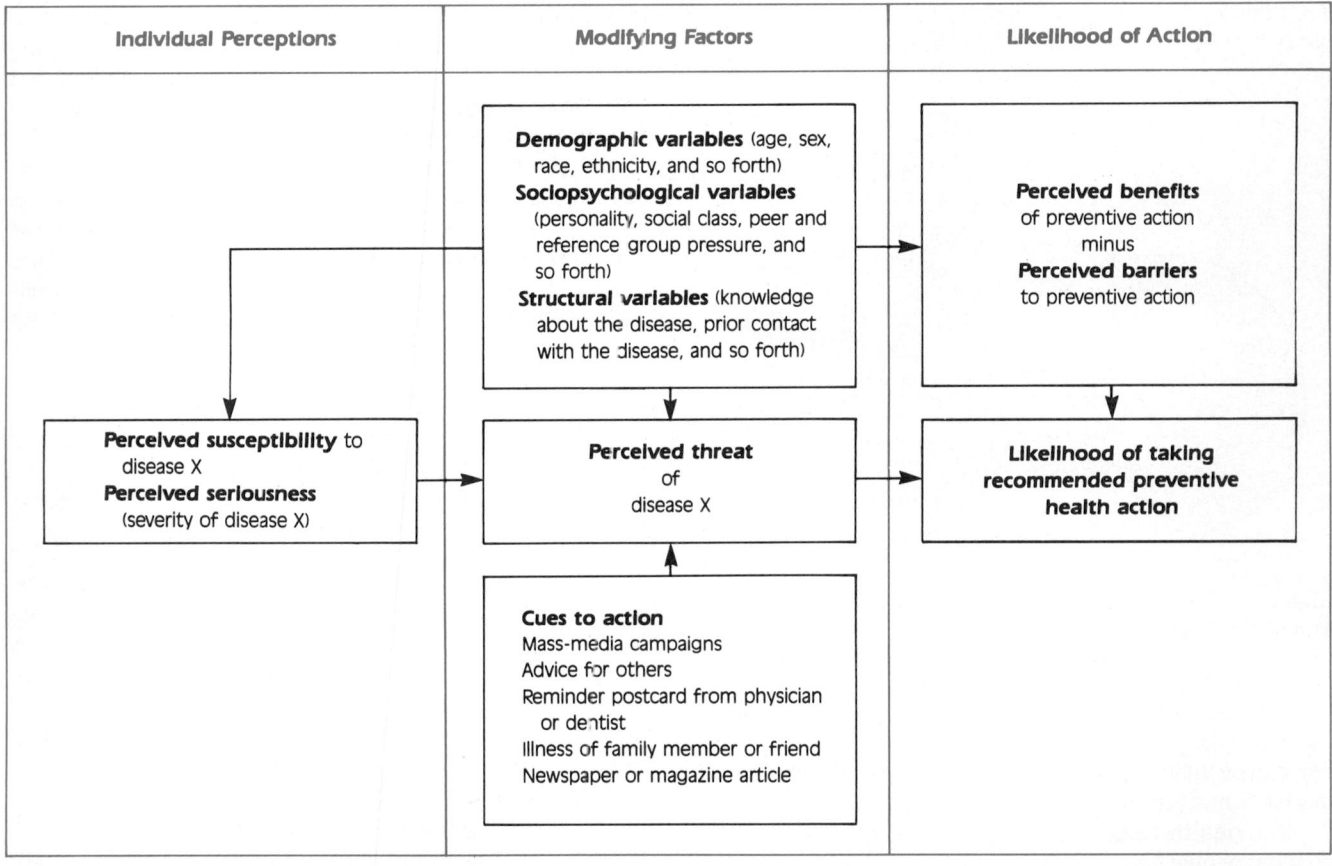

F I G U R E 2 - 4

Health belief model. (Becker, M. [Ed.]. [1974]. *The health belief model and personal health behavior.* Thorofare, NJ: Charles B. Slack.)

Emotional Dimension How the mind and body interact to affect body function and to respond to body conditions also influences health. Long-term stress affects the body systems and anxiety affects health habits; conversely, calm acceptance and relaxation can actually change body responses to illness. Consider the following:
- Before a test, a student always has diarrhea.
- Worried about her teenage son, a mother chain smokes.
- The adolescent who is not socially outgoing begins to experiment with drugs.
- Extremely nervous about surgery, a man experiences severe pain after his operation.
- Using relaxation techniques, a young woman reduces her pain during the delivery of her baby.
- After learning biofeedback skills, a man reduces his previously elevated blood pressure.

Intellectual Dimension The intellectual dimension encompasses cognitive abilities, educational background, and past experiences. These influence a client's responses to teaching about health and reactions to nursing care during illness. They also play a major role in health behaviors.

Examples of situations involving this dimension include the following:
- An elderly woman who has only a third-grade education who needs to be educated about a complicated diagnostic test
- A young college student with diabetes who follows a diabetic diet but continues to drink beer and eat pizza with friends several times a week
- A young woman who quits taking her high blood pressure medication after developing unpleasant side effects

Environmental Dimension The environment has many influences on health and illness. Housing, sanitation, climate, and pollution of air, food, and water are aspects of the environmental dimension. There are many examples of environmental causes of illness, including these selected few:
- Deaths, especially among the elderly, resulting from inadequate heating and cooling
- Increased incidence of asthma and respiratory problems in large cities with smog
- Food poisoning
- Drowning

Sociocultural Dimension Health practices and beliefs are strongly influenced by a person's economic level, life-style, family, and culture. Low-income groups are less likely to seek medical care to prevent or treat illness; high-income groups are more prone to stress-related habits and illness. The family and the culture to which a person belongs determine patterns of living and values about health and illness that are often unalterable. All of these factors are involved in personal care, patterns of eating, life-styles, and emotional stability. For example:

- The adolescent who sees nothing wrong with smoking or drinking because his parents smoke and drink
- The parents of a sick baby who do not seek medical care because they have no money
- The single parent, abused as a child, who in turn physically abuses her own small son
- The person of Asian descent who uses herbal remedies and acupuncture to treat an illness

Spiritual Dimension Spiritual and religious beliefs and values are important components of the way a person behaves in health and illness. It is important that the nurse accept these values and understand their importance to the individual client. Included in this dimension are the following examples:

- Roman Catholics require baptism for both live births and stillborn babies.
- Orthodox and Conservative Jews may observe kosher laws, prohibiting the intake of pork or shellfish.
- Jehovah's Witnesses are opposed to blood transfusions.
- A person with a strong Fundamentalist belief may accept a serious disease as a punishment from God.

FIGURE 2-5

Comprehensive nursing care involves using skills and knowledge effectively to meet a variety of needs. (Photo by Gates Rhodes, courtesy of School of Nursing, University of Pennsylvania.)

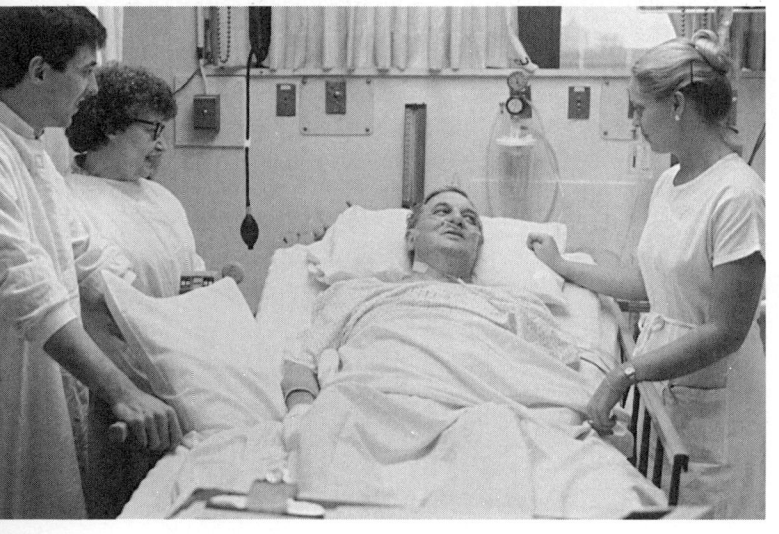

Basic Human Needs

All of us are familiar with the following occurrences:
- A drink of water "goes the wrong way" and you experience a sense of panic until you can take a breath.
- You are too busy to eat breakfast and are "starving to death" by lunch.
- As you start your first college class, your thoughts are filled with questions about how you will react to the new experience.
- You plan to spend a part of each weekend with your family.
- A neighbor has emergency surgery and you volunteer to care for her children.

These actions—and many more like them—are the result of needs. A *need* is something that is *essential* to the emotional and physiologic health and survival of humans. Because needs are essential and are common to all people, they are called **basic human needs.** All people strive to meet basic needs; at any given time, an individual's needs may be met, partially met, or unmet. A person whose needs are met may be considered to be healthy, and a person with one or more unmet needs is at increased risk for illness or health alterations in one or more of the human dimensions.

Needs are an integral part of each person's human dimensions.

Physical needs involve all of the body's physiologic processes, including breathing, the intake and output of food and fluids, temperature, circulation, and movement.

Emotional needs are concerned with the feelings of a person, such as fear, happiness, sadness, and loneliness.

Intellectual needs are focused on processes such as thinking, learning, problem solving, and decision making.

Environmental needs deal with our physical surroundings as they affect safety and security, and include housing, neighborhood, climate, and atmosphere.

Sociocultural needs relate to the relationships and communications a person has with others, such as friends, a sense of belonging to a group or community, and being loved by others.

Spiritual needs concern a person's values and beliefs as they relate to a higher being and to the performance of activities to help others.

The nursing procedures and actions that you will learn as you progress through your education are aimed toward meeting your clients' basic human needs. Chapter 7 describes each level of human needs (called Maslow's hierarchy of needs), and family and community influences on basic human needs (see Fig. 7-1).

Self-Concept

Another variable influencing health and illness is self-concept, which incorporates both how a person feels about self (*self-esteem*) and the way the person perceives his or her physical self (*body image*). Self-concept has both physical and emotional aspects, and is an important factor in the way each individual reacts to stress and illness, follows self-care health practices, and interrelates with others. For example, the teenager who has anorexia nervosa and is dangerously thin may still perceive self as being overweight and refuse to eat. In contrast, the person who is overweight may feel that nothing he or she does will change the way others see him or her or will have an effect on the person's acceptance by others. Thus, the person refuses to follow a diet and exercise program.

A person's self-concept is the product of a variety of past experiences, interpersonal interactions, physical and cultural influences, and education. It includes a person's perceptions of his or her own strengths and weaknesses. Illness can alter self-concept as it affects roles, independence, and relationships with important others. Chapter 38 fully discusses self-concept.

Promoting Wellness and Preventing Illness

This section examines the client at risk for illness and the client who becomes ill. Nurses often work with clients entering the health care system because of an illness (the causes of illness are outlined in the accompanying display). Therefore, illness behavior and the effects of illness on the family are discussed. Acute and chronic illness are defined to serve as a base for learning about different kinds of illnesses. Furthermore, the levels of health care activities carried out by nurses to promote health and prevent illness are included to illustrate the expanded role of nurses in society.

Risk Factors

A **risk factor** is a factor in a person's human dimensions that increases that person's chance for illness or injury. Risk

---

T A B L E 2 - 1

Major Areas of Risk Factors

Risk Factor	Example
Age	School-aged children are at high risk for communicable diseases.
	After menopause, women are more likely to develop cardiovascular disease.
Genetic	A family history of cancer or diabetes predisposes a person to developing the disease.
Physiologic	Obesity increases the possibility of heart disease.
	Pregnancy places increased risk on both the mother and the developing fetus.
Health habits	Smoking increases the probability of lung cancer.
	Poor nutrition can lead to a variety of health problems.
Life-style	Multiple sexual relationships increase the risk of sexually transmitted diseases (eg, gonorrhea or AIDS).
	Events that increase stress (eg, divorce, retirement, work-related pressure) may precipitate accidents or illness.
Environment	Working and living environments (such as hazardous materials and poor sanitation) may contribute to disease.

---

factors can be categorized into six major areas. These areas, with examples, are listed in Table 2-1.

As with other components of health and illness, risk factors are often interrelated; as the number of risk factors increases, so does the possibility of disease. For example, the overweight executive, under pressure to increase sales, smokes and drinks alcohol in excess. These factors, combined with a family history of heart disease, place this person at higher risk for illness. The older adult is also at risk for illness or injury (see the accompanying display).

A health-risk appraisal is an assessment of the total person. The "picture" of the individual that is made from the assessment indicates areas of risk of disease or injury, as well as areas that support health. There are a variety of forms used to perform the assessment, but all of them take a broad approach to health, focusing on life-style and health behaviors. (Such an appraisal appears in the display, Health-Style: A Self-Test.) After the appraisal, the client can be taught to continue healthy living habits and change unhealthy life-styles.

Certain practices are supportive of health:
- Sleeping regularly, 7 to 8 hours per night
- Eating breakfast
- Eating regular meals, with few snacks
- Maintaining ideal body weight
- Using alcohol in moderation
- Discontinuing smoking
- Maintaining positive mental health and self-concept

Causes of Diseases

- Inherited genetic defects
- Developmental defects resulting from exposure to such factors as virus or chemicals during pregnancy
- Biologic agents or toxins
- Physical agents such as temperature, chemicals, radiation
- Generalized tissue responses to injury or irritation
- Physiologic and emotional reactions to stress
- An excessive or insufficient production of body secretions (hormones, enzymes, and so forth)

As the number of health practices increases, so does the level of wellness.

Acute and Chronic Illness

An **illness** is the result of a disease in which a pathophysiologic change in the structure or function of the body or mind causes a resultant change in an individual's level of health functioning. Illnesses are classified in terms of being either acute or chronic. A person may be acutely and chronically ill at the same time—for example, the adult with diabetes who has flu. Each of these broad classifications of illness are discussed in the following section.

Acute Illness

An **acute illness** has a rapid onset of symptoms but lasts only a limited and relatively short time. Although an acute illness may be life threatening, many do not require medical attention. If medical intervention is required, specific treatment with medications (eg, antibiotics for pneumonia) or surgical procedures (eg, an appendectomy for appendicitis) will return the person to normal functioning. With self-treatment and use of over-the-counter (OTC) medications, simple acute illnesses such as the common cold or diarrhea are resolved without problems.

Illness Behaviors   When a person becomes acutely ill, certain illness behaviors are seen in identifiable stages. Although these stages of illness may be seen in the chronically ill person, they are much more typical of acute illness.

Stage 1: Experience of Symptoms   How do people define themselves as "sick"? The first indication of an illness is usually the recognition of symptoms that are incompatible with our personal definition of health. Although pain is the most significant symptom indicating illness, other common symptoms include a rash, fever, chills, or cough.

The person then defines himself or herself as being sick, seeks validation of this experience from others, gives up normal activities, and assumes a "sick role." At this stage, most people center on their symptoms and bodily functions. Depending on individual health beliefs and practices (and on the variables discussed previously), the person may choose to do nothing, buy OTC medications to relieve symptoms, or seek health care for diagnosis and treatment. In this society, an illness becomes truly legitimate when the diagnosis and prescribed treatment are determined by a physician. When these activities occur, the person becomes a client and enters the next stage.

Stage 2: The Dependent Role   A major part of accepting the dependent role is the decision to accept the diagnosis and follow the treatment plan. This stage of illness is complex and involves all of the human dimensions and basic human needs.

In the dependent sick role, a person conforms to the opinions of others, often requires assistance in carrying out activities of daily living, and needs emotional support through acceptance, approval, physical closeness, and protection.

It is at this stage that many clients enter the hospital. To facilitate adherence to treatment plans, the hospitalized client needs effective relationships with caregivers, knowledge about the illness, and an individualized plan of care. The client is expected, by both caregivers and family, to get well and resume normal roles.

Stage 3: Recovery and Rehabilitation   Recovery and rehabilitation may begin in the hospital and conclude at home. As hospitals become increasingly acute-care centered, more and more clients will complete this final stage of illness behavior at a convalescent center or at home.

In this stage, the person is expected to give up the dependent role and resume normal activities and responsibilities. If the plan of care included health education, the individual may return to health at a higher level of functioning (and at a higher level on the health–illness continuum) than was present before the illness.

There are no specific timetables for the stages of illness behaviors. The stages may occur rapidly or slowly and are highly individualized. The nursing roles throughout the stages remain constant. In all stages, the nurse accepts the client as an individual, gives nursing care based on priority of needs, and facilitates recovery through physical care, emotional support, and health education.

FOCUS ON THE OLDER ADULT

Risk Factors for Illness and Injury in Older Adults

- The older adult is at increased risk for illness or injury as a result of changes that occur with aging:
  - Decreased vision can increase the danger of accidents in the home and while driving.
  - Atrophy of taste buds can interfere with nutrition.
  - Decreased response to sensory stimulation can increase the risk of burns, frostbite, and other injury.
- Falls are a major cause of injury and death and may be the result of poor vision, loss of balance, the effects of chronic illness, or the effects of medications.
- Women who are past menopause may be estrogen deficient, resulting in the loss of bone mass and density (osteoporosis). As a result, risk for fractures of the hip and vertebrae is increased.

Health Promotion

Challenges

- In many schools, especially in inner-city areas, students are Hispanic. Many do not speak English. They face problems of gang violence, suicide, drug abuse, depression, pregnancy, AIDS and other sexually transmitted diseases, and depression.
- Nurses must take a good look at their own life-styles first, and then take care of their clients' health promotion. Included are stress management; obesity; use of alcohol, tobacco, and other drugs; nutrition; and exercise.

Nursing Solutions

- Nurses at the school-based clinic at one California high school provide individual health teaching every time they come into the office. In addition, the faculty and staff have received information about problems and make referrals. The clinic is funded through the Robert Wood Johnson Foundation through its School-Based Adolescent Health Care Program.
- A nurse who serves as assistant chief of the US Air Force Health Promotion Program establishes policy and sets programming for health promotion activities at 120 Air Force bases worldwide. The program includes the components of smoking cessation, nutrition, physical fitness, stress management, hypertension, and drug and alcohol abuse prevention.
- A doctorally prepared nurse works for the National Institutes of Health to coordinate research findings with health education programs and educational materials for use by nurses in the workplace. The office coordinates national programs on high blood pressure education, cholesterol education, smoking education, asthma education, and heart attack early action.

(Selby, T. [February, 1990]. Home health care finds new ways of caring. *American Nurse*, 1.)

Chronic Illness

A **chronic illness** is an impairment or a deviation from normal health with one or more of the following characteristics:

- It is a permanent change
- It causes, or is caused by, irreversible alterations in normal anatomy and physiology
- It requires special client education for rehabilitation
- It requires a long period of care or support

Chronic illnesses usually have a slow onset and commonly have periods of *remission* (when the disease is present, but the person does not experience symptoms) and *exacerbation* (the symptoms reappear). With exacerbation, the person is in the acute phase of the chronic illness. Examples of common chronic illnesses are heart problems, diabetes mellitus, lung diseases, and arthritis.

More nursing care of clients with chronic illnesses will be required as we advance into the 21st century. As the population ages, there will also be a corresponding rise in chronic illnesses. The care needed for clients with chronic illnesses will also increase as a result of AIDS, which is an international health crisis. Although not all people with a chronic illness require care, there are certain needs that all people who are chronically ill must meet to be able to live with the illness on a day-to-day basis for the rest of their lives:

- Living as normally as possible, despite the symptoms and treatment that make an individual feel different from others
- Learning to modify activities of daily living, relationships, and self-care activities
- Maintaining a positive self-concept and sense of hope
- Grieving over losses in physical structure and function, financial income, status, role and dignity
- Learning how to live with chronic discomfort
- Following the prescribed medical therapy
- Maintaining a feeling of being in control
- Confronting the inevitability of death (Miller, 1983; Pollock, 1986)

As a nurse, you will care for individuals of all ages who have a chronic illness and you will provide that care in all types of settings, including homes, hospitals, clinics, nursing homes, and institutions. Whatever the age, the effects, and demands of the illness, or the setting, the nurse must make every effort to promote wellness in the client with a chronic illness, with a focus of care that emphasizes what is possible rather than what can no longer be.

Effects of Illness on the Family

You will rarely give nursing care to a client who does not have some form of support system. The system usually comprises family members but also may include, or comprise, significant others, peers, and friends.

When an illness occurs, roles change for both the client and the family. The following are several examples of family reactions to, and influences on, illness of a member. This brief introduction to the family in health and illness serves to demonstrate that consideration of the family is an integral component in nursing care.

- A chronic illness creates stress for the client and family because it may require lifelong alterations in roles, life-style, frequent hospitalizations, economic problems, and decreased social interactions among members.

Health-Style: A Self-Test

All of us want good health. But many of us do not know how to be as healthy as possible. Health experts now describe *life-style* as one of the most important factors affecting health. In fact, it is estimated that as many as seven of the ten leading causes of death could be reduced through common-sense changes in life-style. That's what this brief test, developed by the Public Health Service, is all about. Its purpose is simply to tell you how well you are doing to stay healthy. The behaviors covered in the test are recommended for most Americans. Some of them may not apply to people with certain chronic diseases or disabilities, or to pregnant women. Such people may require special instructions from their physicians.

Cigarette Smoking

If you <u>never</u> smoke, enter a score of 10 for this section and go to the next section on *Alcohol and Drugs*.

	almost always	sometimes	almost never
1. I avoid smoking cigarettes.	2	1	0
2. I smoke only low tar and nicotine cigarettes *or* I smoke a pipe or cigars.	2	1	0

Smoking score: _____

Alcohol and Drugs

	almost always	sometimes	almost never
1. I avoid drinking alcoholic beverages *or* I drink no more than one or two drinks a day.	4	1	0
2. I avoid using alcohol or other drugs (especially illegal drugs) as a way of handling stressful situations or the problems in my life.	2	1	0
3. I am careful not to drink alcohol when taking certain medicines (for example, medicine for sleeping, pain, colds, and allergies), or when pregnant.	2	1	0
4. I read and follow the label directions when using prescribed and over-the-counter drugs.	2	1	0

Alcohol and drugs score: _____

Eating Habits

	almost always	sometimes	almost never
1. I eat a variety of foods each day, such as fruits and vegetables, whole grain breads and cereals, lean meats, dairy products, dry peas and beans, and nuts and seeds.	4	1	0
2. I limit the amount of fat, saturated fat, and cholesterol I eat (including fat on meats, eggs, butter, cream, shortenings, and organ meats such as liver).	2	1	0
3. I limit the amount of salt I eat by cooking with only small amounts, not adding salt at the table, and avoiding salty snacks.	2	1	0
4. I avoid eating too much sugar (especially frequent snacks of sticky candy or soft drinks).	2	1	0

Eating habits score: _____

Exercise and Fitness

	almost always	sometimes	almost never
1. I maintain a desired weight, avoiding overweight and underweight.	3	1	0
2. I do vigorous exercises for 15 to 30 minutes at least three times a week (examples include running, swimming, brisk walking).	3	1	0
3. I do exercises that enhance my muscle tone for 15 to 30 minutes at least three times a week (examples include yoga and calisthenics).	2	1	0
4. I use part of my leisure time participating in individual, family, or team activities that increase my level of fitness (such as gardening, bowling, golf, and baseball).	2	1	0

Exercise/fitness score: _____

Stress Control

	almost always	sometimes	almost never
1. I have a job or do other work that I enjoy.	2	1	0
2. I find it easy to relax and express my feelings freely.	2	1	0
3. I recognize early, and prepare for, events or situations likely to be stressful for me.	2	1	0
4. I have close friends, relatives, or others whom I can talk to about personal matters and call on for help when needed.	2	1	0
5. I participate in group activities (such as church and community organizations) or hobbies that I enjoy.	2	1	0

Stress control score: _____

Safety

	almost always	sometimes	almost never
1. I wear a seat belt while riding in a car.	2	1	0
2. I avoid driving while under the influence of alcohol and other drugs.	2	1	0
3. I obey traffic rules and the speed limit when driving.	2	1	0
4. I am careful when using potentially harmful products or substances (such as household cleaners, poisons, and electrical devices).	2	1	0
5. I avoid smoking in bed.	2	1	0

Safety score: _____

(continued)

Health-Style: A Self-Test (continued)

What Your Scores Mean to You

Scores of 9 and 10

Excellent! Your answers show that you are aware of the importance of this area to your health. More important, you are putting your knowledge to work for you by practicing good health habits. As long as you continue to do so, this area should not pose a serious health risk. It's likely that you are setting an example for your family and friends to follow. Because you got a very high test score on this part of the test, you may want to consider other areas where your scores indicate room for improvement.

Scores of 6 to 8

Your health practices in this area are good, but there is room for improvement. Look again at the items you answered with "Sometimes" or "Almost never." What changes can you make to improve your score? Even a small change can often help you achieve better health.

Scores of 3 to 5

Your health risks are showing! Would you like more information about the risks you are facing and about why it is important for you to change these behaviors? Perhaps you need help in deciding how to successfully make the changes you desire. In either case, help is available.

Scores of 0 to 2

Obviously, you were concerned enough about your health to take the test, but your answers show that you may be taking serious and unnecessary risks with your health. Perhaps you are unaware of the risks and what to do about them. You can easily get the information and help you need to improve, if you wish. The next step is up to you.

Where Do You Go from Here

Start by asking yourself a few frank questions: *Am I really doing all I can to be as healthy as possible? What steps can I take to feel better? Am I willing to begin now?* If you scored low in one or more sections of the test, decide what changes you want to make for improvement. You might pick that aspect of your life-style where you feel you have the best chance for success and tackle that one first. Once you have improved your score there, go on to other areas.

If you already have tried to change your health habits (to stop smoking or exercise regularly, for example), don't be discouraged if you haven't yet succeeded. The difficulty you have encountered may be due to influences you've never really thought about—such as advertising—or to a lack of support and encouragement. Understanding these influences is an important step toward changing the way they affect you.

There's help available. In addition to personal actions you can take on your own, there are community programs and groups (such as the YMCA or the local chapter of the American Heart Association) that can assist you and your family to make the changes you want to make. If you want to know more about these groups or about health risks, contact your local health department or the National Health Information Clearinghouse. There's a lot you can do to stay healthy or to improve your health—and there are organizations that can help you. Start a new "health-style" today!

For assistance in locating specific information on these and other health topics, write to the National Health Information Clearinghouse:

National Health Information Clearinghouse
P.O. Box 1133
Washington, DC 20013

(Reprinted with permission of the National Health Information Clearinghouse.)

- Parents of a sick child often react with blame, overprotection, and severe anxiety.
- Family members of clients requiring intensive care often feel alone and frightened. They may also feel guilty and imagine the worst possible outcome.
- The reactions of family members to the hospital experience will vary; some want to be there all the time, whereas others avoid visiting.
- Family members need information about the client's care and health status, both in the hospital and at home. They often rely on the nurse for answers, for emotional support, and for feeling a part of the care given.

Nursing Care as Preventive Care

Levels of Preventive Care

The current focus of health care is on preventive care. Leavell (1965) describes the three levels of preventive care as (1) primary, (2) secondary, and (3) tertiary.

Primary Level **Primary preventive care** is directed toward health promotion and specific protection against illness. Activities at this level may focus on individuals or groups. Examples of primary-level activities are immunizations, family planning services, dental care teaching, poison-control information, and accident prevention education.

Secondary Level Secondary preventive care focuses on health maintenance for clients experiencing health problems or on prevention of complications or disabilities. Examples of activities for this level are carrying out nursing actions for hospitalized clients (eg, skin care, giving medications, or exercising arms and legs); assessing children for normal growth and development; teaching breast self-examination; and encouraging regular medical and dental screenings and care.

Tertiary Level Tertiary preventive care is aimed at helping rehabilitate clients and restore them to a maximum level of functioning after an illness. Nursing activities on a tertiary level include teaching a diabetic client how to recognize and prevent complications or referring a woman to a support group after removal of a breast due to cancer.

Nurse as Role Model

Nurses who strive to be competent practitioners learn early that they must take care of their own health to be able to give effective nursing care to others. Not only does good personal health enable nurses to practice more efficiently, it also enables them to serve as health models for clients and their families. Nurses can help clients acquire new health behaviors by modeling the very behaviors that are important to the clients' well-being.

It is difficult for nurses to be sincerely attentive to the needs of clients when their own needs are not being met. Because no one is perfectly healthy or "whole" all of the time, it is important that as nurses prepare for professional practice they spend time getting to know themselves. From this self-knowledge should come a commitment to pursue holistic health actively. To help you begin your self-knowledge, take the self-test in the accompanying display. As you develop skills as a nurse and work directly with clients, you may want to use this self-test to help your clients learn a new health-style.

In summary, the most effective nurse serves as a role model of healthy self-care behaviors. In Units VII and VIII, a list of health care goals for the nurse under the heading Nurse as Role Model precedes text exploring how nurses can help clients. Taking the time to see how many of these goals you can meet right now will give you some idea of how effective you will be as a role model for your clients. The results may also spur you to develop new health behaviors.

The wellness promotion guides highlighted throughout the text may be useful to you as well as to your clients. These guides can be used to assess and identify both strengths and increased risk for alterations in health. The guides can also serve as the basis for teaching self-care to clients.

KEY POINTS

- Health and illness are relative processes, defined by each person. Wellness, or the achievement of maximum function and strength, is possible even when a person has been diagnosed as being ill.
- Health and illness relationships and interactions can be described by the use of models such as the health–illness continuum, high-level wellness model, agent–host–environment model, and health-belief model.
- Wellness levels are influenced by the dimensions that compose the whole person, by needs, and by self-concept. These factors are interrelated and affect actual and potential health–illness status and behaviors.
- People at risk for an illness can be identified through a health-risk appraisal. If a person is identified at risk for illness, nurses can support life-style practices that support health.

- Acute illnesses occur rapidly, have a relatively short time span, and may be either self-treated or require medical intervention. The person with an acute illness progresses from the onset of symptoms to recovery through certain definite stages.
- Chronic illnesses more often have a slow onset, cause permanent change, and require long-term medical care. The increasing number of older adults, accompanied by an increase in chronic illnesses, means that nursing care of the chronically ill will become even more important in the 21st century.
- Nursing care for clients in both health and illness must include their family members. Illness results in altered expectations and reactions from family members.
- Nurses carry out wellness promotion activities on primary, secondary, and tertiary levels.

BIBLIOGRAPHY

Ambrosio, E. (1991). Poor housing, poor health. *Canadian Nurse, 87*(5), 22–24.

American Public Health Association. (1990). *Healthy people 2000: National health promotion and disease prevention objectives.* Washington, DC: Author.

Bestard, S., & Courtenary, M. (1990). Focusing on wellness. *Canadian Nurse, 86*(11), 24–25.

Birchfield, M. (1985). *Stages of illness: Guidelines for nursing care.* Bowie, MD: Brady Communications.

DeYoung, L. (1985). *Dynamics of nursing* (5th ed.). St. Louis: Mosby.

Dimond, M., & Jones, S. (1983). *Chronic illness across the life span.* Norwalk, CT: Appleton-Century-Crofts.

Dunn, H. (1961). *High-level wellness.* Arlington: Beathy.

Edelman, C., & Mandle, C. (1990). *Health promotion throughout the life span* (2nd ed.). St. Louis: Mosby.

Gallagher, L. P., & Kreidler, M. C. (1987). *Nursing and health: Maximizing human potential throughout the life cycle.* Norwalk, CT: Appleton & Lange.

Hames, C., & Joseph, D. (1986). *Basic concepts of helping: A wholistic approach* (2nd ed.). New York: Appleton-Century-Crofts.

Harrison, M., O'Connor, A., & Weaver, L. (1991). Canadian nurses and smoking. *Canadian Nurse, 87*(7), 28–31.

Kaufman, J. S., Fox, R., & Swearengen, P. (1990). How a support group can help your chronically ill patient. *Nursing, 20*(10), 65–66.

Leavell, H., & Clark, E. G. (1965). *Preventive medicine for the doctor in the community* (3rd ed.) New York: McGraw-Hill.

Maslow, A. (1968). *Toward a psychology of being* (2nd ed.). New York: Van Nostrand Reinhold.

Mathus-Kraft, C., & York, L. (1989). The hospital as wellness educator. *Nursing Management, 20*(1), 72.

McCann-Flynn, J. B., & Heffron, P. B. (1988). *Nursing: From concept to practice* (2nd ed.). East Norwalk, CT: Appleton & Lange.

Miller, J. F. (1983). *Coping with chronic illness: Overcoming powerlessness.* Philadelphia: Davis.

Murray, R. B., & Zentner, J. P. (1989). *Nursing assessment and health promotion through the lifespan* (4th ed.). Norwalk, CT: Appleton & Lange.

Niknian, M., Lefebvre, C., & Carleton, R. A. (1991). Are people more health conscious? A longitudinal study of one community. *American Journal of Public Health, 81*(2), 205–207.

Pollock, S. E. (1986). Human responses to chronic illness: Physiologic and psychosocial adaptation. *Nursing Research, 35*(2), 90–95.

Rosenstock, I. (1974). Historical origin of the health belief model. *Health Education Monographs, 2,* 334.

Shugars, D. A., O'Neil, E. H., & Bader, J. D. (Eds.). *Healthy American: Practitioners for 2005—An agenda for action for U.S. health professional schools.* Durham: Pew Health Professions Commission.

Suchman, E. (1965). Stages of illness and medical care. *Journal of Health and Human Behavior, 6,* 114.

Woods, N. F., Yates, B. C., & Primomo, J. (1989). Supporting families during chronic illness. *Image: Journal of Nursing Scholarship, 21*(1), 46–50.

World Health Organization. (1947). *Constitution.* Geneva: Author.

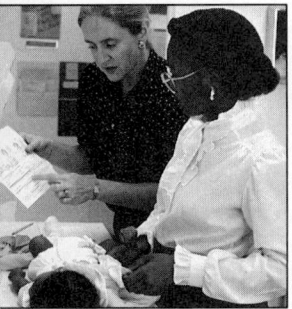

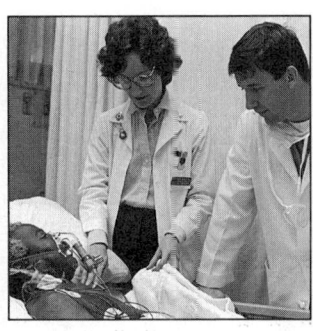
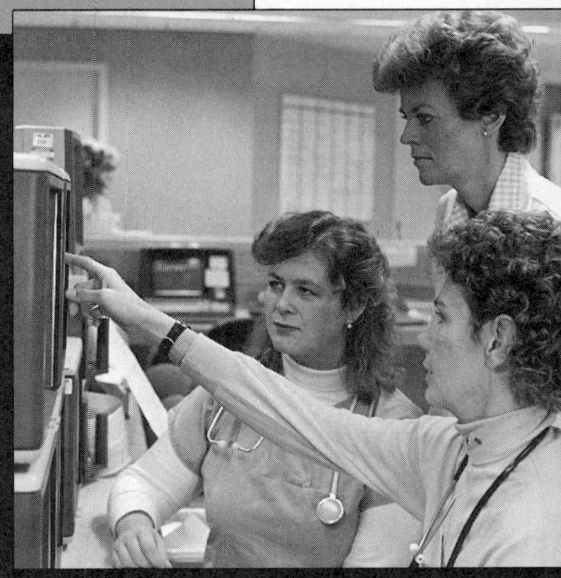

OBJECTIVES

After studying this chapter, the learner should be able to:

Define key terms used in the chapter.

Compare and contrast inpatient and outpatient health care settings.

Discuss the services provided by community health care agencies and in community settings.

Describe government health care agencies and services.

Describe the roles of health care team members.

Discuss various private insurance, group plans, and federal support in the United States and Canada.

Discuss trends and issues affecting the health care delivery system.

KEY TERMS

crisis intervention centers
day-care centers
diagnosis-related groups
health maintenance organization
hospice
inpatient
Medicaid
Medicare
outpatient
preferred provider arrangement
preferred provider organization
Public Health Service

The Health Care System

3

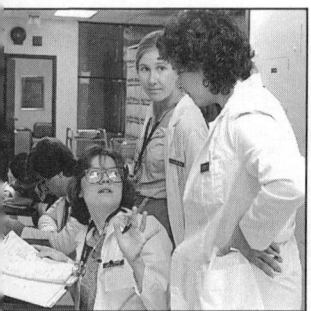

Nurses, clients, and health care settings are all part of a vast and complicated system—the health care system. This system comprises all the institutions, agencies, policies, payment plans, and people that provide health care services to others. This chapter provides a broad introduction to the settings, the members of the health care team, and the economics and selected issues and trends of the health care system in the mid-1990s.

Types of Health Care Settings

Nurses provide care to clients in a wide variety of health care settings. Figure 3-1 illustrates the variety of settings available; Table 3-1 lists the nursing functions performed in the types of settings described in this section.

Inpatient Settings

When people enter a health care setting and stay for a period ranging from more than 24 hours to many years, they are said to be **inpatients.** This section discusses two types of institutions in which people are given inpatient care: (1) hospitals and (2) extended-care facilities.

Hospitals   Hospitals have been the traditional setting for providing care for people who were too ill to care for themselves at home, required surgery or complicated treatments, or were having babies. These individuals were admitted to the hospital and were not discharged until they were fully recovered or had used all of the services available within the hospital. As a result of federal regulations and other health care reimbursement policies, this is no longer true. With the trend toward discharging clients earlier in their hospital stay, hospitals more often focus on the acute care needs of the client. Along with this acute care focus has come a proliferation of services offered by the hospital and aimed at the **outpatient**—the person who requires health care services but does not need to stay in the institution for those services.

Hospital size ranges from as few as 20 beds to large medical centers with hundreds of beds. Various services are provided, depending on the size and location of the

hospital. Most hospitals provide inpatient care, surgery, diagnostic tests, emergency care, a pharmacy, and client education. Other services provided within the hospital setting might include intensive care units, obstetrical care, social services, outpatient clinics and surgery, educational programs, and long-term skilled nursing facilities. Hospitals may provide care for all types of illnesses and trauma, or may specialize. Specialty hospitals, or special units in general hospitals, meet the varied needs of clients, including those clients needing rehabilitation, children, clients requiring psychiatric or drug dependency care, clients who have been burned, and clients with diabetes.

Hospitals are classified as public or private, and as for-profit or not-for-profit. Public hospitals, which are not-for-profit institutions, are financed and operated by local, state, or national agencies. Many clients admitted to a public hospital do not have health insurance, and services are provided at no cost or little cost. Private hospitals may be for-profit or not-for-profit and are operated by communities, churches, businesses or corporations, and charitable organizations. Most clients cared for in private hospitals have some type of personal health insurance or health care plan.

Canadian hospitals receive funding from federal and provincial sources. Clients have basic health insurance specific to the province in which they reside. In addition, some clients have private health insurance plans or health plans through employment that provide extended coverage and additional benefits.

Government hospitals such as the Veterans Administration (VA) hospitals and military hospitals also provide care. VA hospitals provide health care services to veterans and military hospitals provide care to members of the armed forces and their immediate families.

Nurses employed in the hospital setting may have many roles. Although most nurses are direct care providers, other roles include manager of other members of the health care team that provides client care, administrator, clinical nurse specialist, client educator, in-service educator, and researcher.

Extended-Care Facilities   Extended-care facilities provide care for periods ranging from days to years. Institutions that provide extended care are usually independent but may be associated with a hospital. Included in this category are intermediate and long-term care facilities, skilled care facilities, nursing homes, retirement centers, and residential institutions that provide care for mentally and developmentally or physically disabled clients.

Extended care facilities have proliferated, primarily because of two factors. First, clients are being discharged from the hospital earlier in their recovery period and often require care that is beyond the scope of home care. Second, the numbers of older adults is increasing; an estimated 21% of the total population will be older than age 65 years by 2040 (Riffer, 1985b). Many of these older adults will not have any caregivers, will no longer be able to carry out activities of daily living independently, or will not want to continue to maintain a home. Because clients entering extended care facilities require so many levels of care, it is difficult to generalize about services provided.

In some instances, the older adult may choose to move into a retirement center that provides health care services only when needed. Others, entering a nursing home, may require complete care for as long as they live. Those individuals entering convalescent centers only remain until they are considered recovered. The nurse's role in an extended care facility is much the same as in the hospital setting. Nurses provide direct care, supervise others, administrate, and teach. Because most clients in extended care facilities are elderly, increasing numbers of gerontology nurse specialists are contributing their knowledge and expertise to the care of these clients. Almost all extended care facilities require that skilled nursing care must be available at all times. Hence, the care given to clients can only be performed by or under the direct supervision of a licensed nurse.

Outpatient Settings

Individuals who do not require inpatient care can receive treatment, care, and education on an outpatient basis. The services provided include surgical procedures, diagnostic tests, medications, physical therapy, counseling, and health education. Outpatient services are also rapidly expanding and are provided by hospitals, physicians' offices, ambulatory care centers, and clinics.

Physicians' Offices Physicians provide primary health care services in their offices through diagnosis and treatment of minor illnesses, minor surgical procedures, obstetric care, well-child care, counseling, and referrals. Many offices contain laboratory and x-ray facilities. Although some doctors are general practitioners who treat all types of illness, many physicians specialize in one type of illness or surgery. A nurse in a physician's office makes health assessments, assists the physician, and provides health

F I G U R E   3 - 1

In recent years, the number and variety of health care settings have increased dramatically.

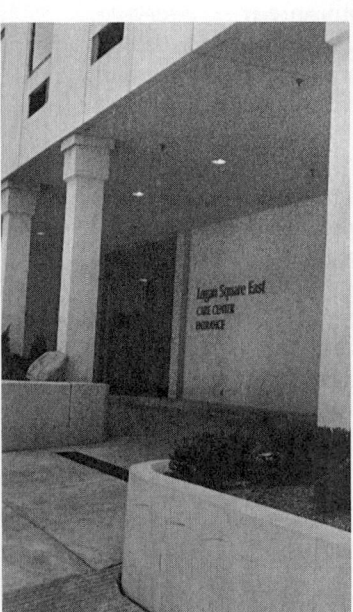

Women's health-care clinics

Long-term independent living care facilities

Multi-facility health-care systems

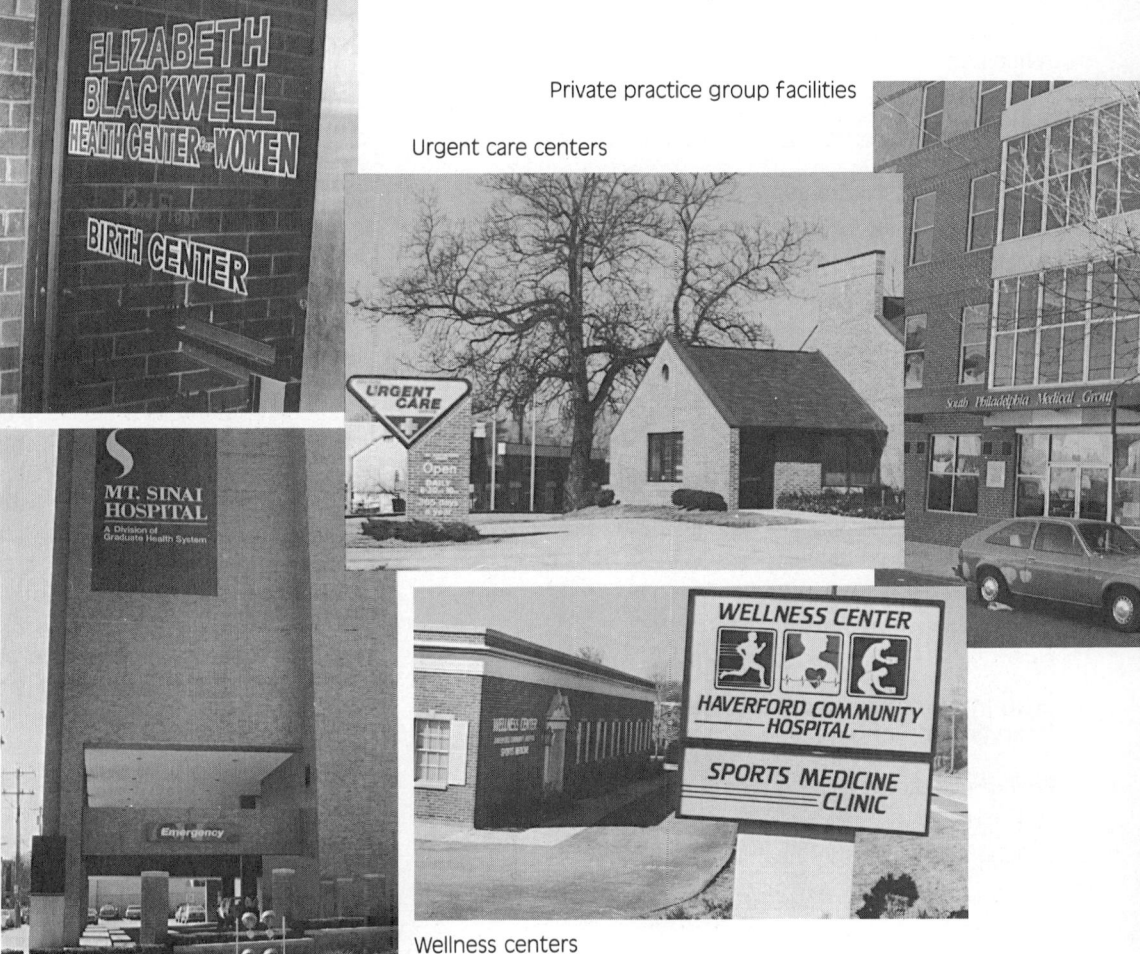

Private practice group facilities

Urgent care centers

Wellness centers

T A B L E 3 - 1

Nursing Functions in Various Health Care Settings

Hospital

Provides direct nursing care

Assesses and monitors client status

Teaches client and family

Develops nursing care plans

Evaluates care given

Coordinates care given by others

Serves in administrative capacity

Provides staff education

Conducts or participates in research activities

Provides expert knowledge and skill in specialty areas

Coordinates discharge planning

Extended-Care Facilities

Provides direct care

Coordinates care given by others

Serves in administrative capacity

Provides expert knowledge and skill in gerontology and rehabilitation

Physician's Office, Clinics, and Ambulatory Care Centers

Makes health assessments

Assists the physician

Teaches client and family

Provides health promotion and wellness education

Provides direct nursing care

Provides expert knowledge and skill for a variety of health-related client needs

Home Care Agencies and Day-Care Centers

Provides direct nursing care education and support

Teaches client and family

Provides support for family members

Coordinates care given by others

Crisis Intervention and Drug and Alcohol Intervention Centers

Provides counseling and teaching

Makes referrals

Collaborates with other health care team members

Hospice

Provides counseling and support for client and family

Serves as coordinator of services

education. Some offices include a nurse practitioner, who makes assessments and cares for clients who require health maintenance or health promotion activities.

Clinics and Ambulatory Care Centers   Clinics and ambulatory care centers may be found in hospitals, or may be provided as a freestanding service by a group of physicians who work together. Clinics and ambulatory care centers are also located in low-income areas and in shopping malls or other community settings. Many of these settings offer walk-in services so that appointments are unnecessary, and they are also open at times other than traditional office hours. A special type of ambulatory care center is an urgent-care center, which provides emergency care services. Nurses who work in clinics and ambulatory care centers have the same roles as those who work in physicians' offices. In some instances, nurse practitioners have established their own independent outpatient service.

Community Health Care Settings

Community health care settings provide health care services to clients within a defined area, such as a small town or a neighborhood in a large city. Community settings provide services within the agency itself, in the client's home, and through day-care centers for children and elderly people. Other types of community settings are crisis intervention centers, community agencies, and drug and alcohol rehabilitation programs and organizations. Community settings may also focus on special needs, such as the older adult or terminally ill clients.

Agencies Providing Home Care   Care for clients may be provided in their homes through community health departments, visiting nurses' associations, and home health agencies. These agencies provide many different health-related services, including skilled nursing assessment and direct care. Many agencies also conduct clinics to provide immunizations for infants and children; screenings for sexually transmitted diseases (STDs) or tuberculosis; and verification of need and voucher distribution for milk and food for women and children with low incomes. Nurses who work in this type of setting do assessments and provide physical care, administer medications, teach, and support family members. They also work closely with physicians and other health care providers such as speech therapists, occupational therapists (OTs), and respiratory therapists (RTs) to plan and provide client care.

Day-Care Centers   Day-care centers have a variety of purposes. Some centers care for infants and children who are healthy but need care while parents work. Elder-care centers provide a place for adults to socialize and to receive care while family members work. Some day-care centers also provide health-related services and care to people who do not need to be in a health care institution but cannot be at home alone. Such centers include centers for elderly people; clients requiring physical rehabilitation; clients with special needs (eg, cerebral palsy); and clients who are in drug and alcohol programs. Nurses who work in day-care centers administer medications and treatments, conduct health screenings, teach, and counsel.

Crisis Intervention Centers Crisis intervention centers may be freestanding or may be part of a hospital. They typically provide 24-hour services and hot lines for people who are suicidal, who are abusing drugs or alcohol, and who require psychologic or psychiatric counseling. These centers also provide information and services for victims of rape and physical abuse. Nurses who work in crisis intervention centers must have strong communication and counseling skills, and must be thoroughly familiar with community resources specific to the needs of clients being served.

Community Agencies Community agencies offer health and human services to a variety of clients. They are often operated by volunteers. Community agencies are primarily financed by private donations, grants, or fund-raisers (although some may charge minimal fees). Examples of this type of agency are Meals on Wheels, which supplies meals to elderly and homebound people; transportation services for elderly and physically disabled people, hearing contact people for hearing impaired clients, and shopping or housecleaning services.

Other types of not-for-profit voluntary community agencies found in the United States and Canada include such agencies as the Heart Association and the Lung Association. Physicians and nurses are often active members of these organizations and provide health screenings and educational programs.

Drug and Alcohol Treatment Centers and Organizations Centers that specialize in services for clients requiring physical or emotional rehabilitation and for treatment of any type of drug dependency may be freestanding or may be associated with a hospital. The goal is to return clients to optimal health and to the community as productive members of society. Centers that focus on rehabilitation use a health care team comprising physicians, nurses, physical therapists (PTs), OTs, and counselors.

Hospice Hospices are special services available to terminally ill individuals and their families. The hospice agency may be public or private and may provide both inpatient and home care. These agencies are committed to maintaining quality of life and dignity in the dying person by providing an environment that encourages open communication, symptom management, and comfort measures for the client, and that supports the family during and after death of the client. Many hospice agencies are developed and supervised by nurses but use trained volunteers to supply emotional and physical support, assist with transportation and household care, serve as liaison between client and health care providers, and provide short-term respite care for family members who are primary caregivers.

NURSING TODAY Challenges and Solutions

Nursing in the Community

Challenges

- Family violence and child abuse is a major problem facing people today and one that we will face in the future.
- Acquired immune deficiency syndrome is a major health problem in both urban and rural areas.
- In many rural counties, there is no physician and no ambulatory care. Physicians who are available are increasingly refusing to care for poor people.
- Years of drought and farm foreclosures have increased the number of homeless people in rural areas of the United States.
- Insufficient funding to provide the health care services that are needed is a major concern.

Nursing Solutions

- District of Columbia nurses, represented by the American Nurses' Association, launched a campaign to save public health in the district. Volunteers made speeches at neighborhood gatherings, community forums, and church groups; contacted the media; and lobbied elected and appointed officials.
- The Ohio Nurses' Association Community Health Assembly has published guidelines for nurses interested in developing programs to deal with adolescent sexuality and pregnancy.
- Nurses in Fargo, North Dakota, operate Health Care of the Homeless as part of the Community Health Center. Nurses volunteer to staff a free clinic for 2 hours three times weekly.
- A nurse practitioner is the care coordinator for HUG (Help Us Grow) in Nashville. HUG is part of the Tennessee Department of Health and Environmental program aimed at making health care and social services accessible to pregnant and postpartum women up to 6 months after delivery and to infants younger than age 2 years. Emphasis is on health life-styles, self-esteem, and parenting.

(Selbe, T. [September, 1990]. Nurses drive public health. *American Nurse*, 1.)

Government Agencies

VA hospitals, public hospitals, and military hospitals all come under the umbrella of government-supported and government-operated health care. Governmental agencies are financed by national, state, local, or provincial taxes. City taxes help support city hospitals and public health clinics; state and provincial taxes help support state mental health hospitals; and national taxes aid in financing national health and welfare programs such as the Canadian Department of Health and Welfare.

Public Health Service   The **Public Health Service** (PHS) is a federal health agency that falls under the direction of the U.S. Department of Health and Human Services. A similar health service is provided by the Department of Health and Welfare in Canada. PHS is a multifaceted program that covers a wide range of services. It is the medical branch of the U.S. Coast Guard and the principal source of native American health care through the Indian Health Services. The amount of direct client care provided by PHS is more limited than in the past.

PHS supplies funds to health centers that provide care to migrant workers and to community agencies that supply health care to the poor or uninsured. The principal budget of PHS goes to grant programs for poor and uninsured individuals.

The Centers for Disease Control (CDC) in Atlanta and the National Institutes of Health (NIH) are both part of PHS. CDC focuses on the epidemiology, prevention, control, and treatment of communicable diseases such as STDs. NIH is engaged in various health research activities and includes The Nursing Research Center.

PHS also supplies health care professionals (eg, nurses, physicians, dentists, and pharmacists) to the U.S. Department of Justice to provide care in federal prisons. The service is also involved to varying degrees in drug and alcohol abuse and mental health programs within the state. PHS activities vary from area to area. In most cases, they focus on community needs and attempt to meet those needs whenever possible.

Canadian Health Services   The types of governmental health care services and agencies available in Canada are similar to those in the United States. The major difference between the two systems is the way that health care is financed.

The Canadian health care system is financed by health care plans within each province. These plans cover all Canadian residents for most of their necessary hospital care and physicians' fees. These provincial health insurance plans are financed by federal and provincial taxes, employers, or by personal policies.

Voluntary Agencies

Voluntary health care agencies are strictly nonprofit. Their functioning depends on volunteers, although health care professionals such as nurses and physicians are part of the system as volunteers, coordinators, and resource people. Voluntary agencies include Lupus Alert, Inc., National Multiple Sclerosis Society, Red Cross, Canadian Lung Association, and the Canadian Heart Foundation. These agencies are actively involved in promoting health through the prevention and detection of specific illness such as cancer and lung diseases. They also support research related to the specific illness about which the agency is concerned. Some voluntary agencies help people pay for the cost of equipment, respite care, or home nursing care for short periods. Financially, these agencies are supported by private donation, fund-raising, and federal grants. They can be found at community and national levels.

Home Care

Home health care is that component of a continuum of comprehensive health care in which health services are provided to individuals and families in their places of residence for the purpose of promoting, maintaining or restoring health, or of maximizing the level of independence while minimizing the effects of disability and illness, including terminal illness. Caring for the sick at home is not a new phenomenon. Modern community health nursing practice developed from a history of providing health care to sick and indigent individuals in their homes. Home health care has become a highly specialized area of health care that requires professionals with great skill and creativity (Fig. 3-2).

Home health services are provided by a variety of agencies with an employed staff or on a contractual basis. Ser-

F I G U R E   3 - 2

Caring for the sick at home is not new but has become a highly specialized area of health care and a major component of a continuum of comprehensive health care. (Photo by Robert Coldwell, courtesy of Community Home Health Services of Philadelphia.)

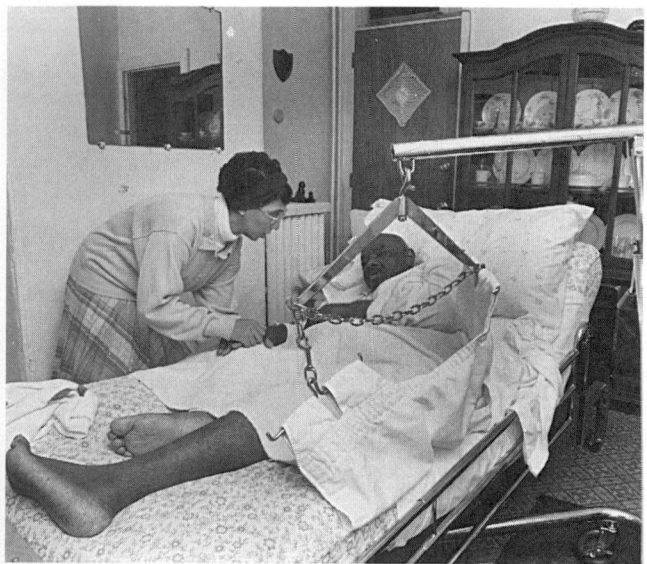

vices include skilled care (eg, nursing, physical therapy, speech therapy, or occupational therapy); social services (to coordinate financial and long-term placement issues); counseling for family and client; and personal services (eg, home health aide, housekeeper, or companion). An agency can be hospital based, freestanding, for-profit, voluntary, not-for-profit, or official. For an agency to receive government reimbursement from the Medicare program, it must be Medicare certified and must adhere to the guidelines set forth by the Health Care Financing Administration (HCFA).

The importance of home health care is evidenced by many factors, including the following:

- The prospective payment system of reimbursement (DRGs), which encourages early discharge from the hospital, has created a new acutely ill population who need skilled care at home.
- There is a greater percentage of elderly people living longer with multiple chronic illnesses who are not institutionalized.
- With more sophisticated technology, people can be kept alive and relatively comfortable in their own homes.
- Health care consumers demand that services be humane and that provisions be made for a dignified death at home.

Cost containment is an important factor in home health care. Services must be carefully coordinated and planned to ensure reimbursement. Reimbursement is affected by three levels of care in home health services: (1) intensive, (2) intermediate, and (3) maintenance.

Intensive-level care indicates that a client's condition warrants close observation, monitoring, or treatment, and requires skilled care (eg, a client who needs sterile dressing changes to a large abdominal wound that is draining copious amounts of purulent discharge). This client's family needs the services of a nurse to assess the wound for healing or infection, to monitor the amount and type of drainage, to perform the dressing changes, and to teach the caregiver the procedure. This family also needs to be educated about medications, high-protein diet, and vitamins to promote wound healing, fluid balance, and complications of immobility. The client may also be receiving intravenous antibiotics (Fig. 3-3).

Intermediate- or rehabilitative-level care indicates the client with an expected change or improvement in function, warranting skilled services (eg, a client with a stroke who no longer needs nursing services but may still need physical or speech therapy). This level is reimbursed by insurance.

Maintenance-level care indicates a client for whom there is no expected change in condition. This client's family needs assistance with personal care and homemaker services. Such care is not reimbursed by Medicare and most other insurance carriers. These services are usually paid out of pocket by the family or by state grants through Area Agencies on Aging.

To have skilled services reimbursed by Medicare, the client must meet the following major criteria:

- The client must be homebound.

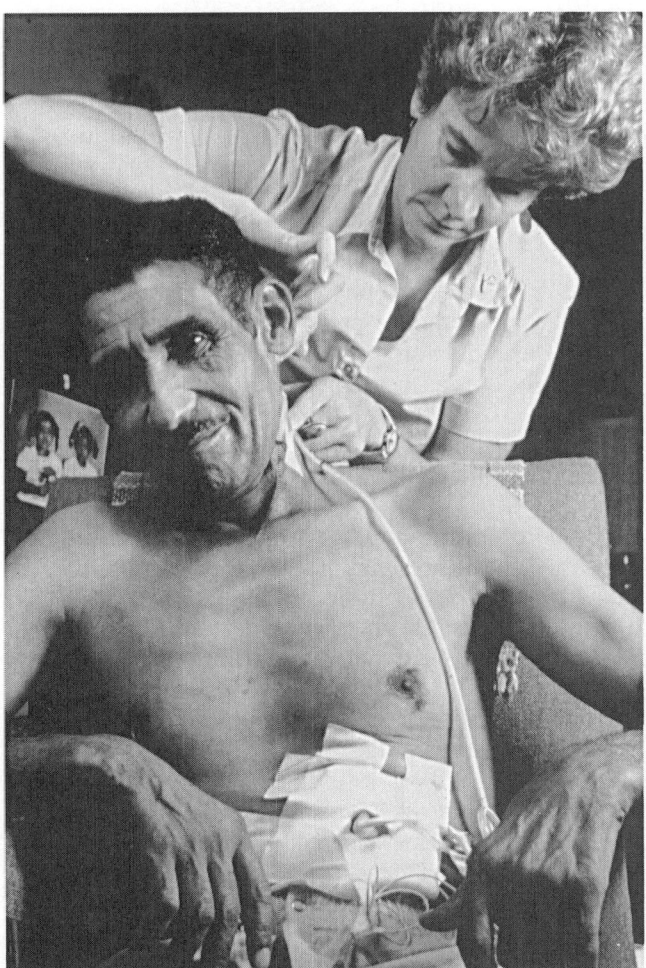

FIGURE 3-3

Intensive-level home health care requires the services of a highly skilled professional. The client requiring sterile dressing changes, monitoring of indwelling catheters or tubes, and special training for the caregiver needs intensive-level care. (Photo by Robert Coldwell, courtesy of Community Home Health Services of Philadelphia.)

- The care must be intermittent.
- There must be a responsible physician ordering the care.

Health Care Team

Many different health care providers care for the client who enters the health care system (Fig. 3-4). The primary goal of each member of the health care team is to promote wellness and restore health. All members collaborate to plan and deliver individualized and holistic care to meet client needs. Increased technology and knowledge of medical care also increases the specialized training, education, and services provided to clients. Included in this section is a discussion of each member of the health care team (other than nurses) with whom you will be working most often.

Physician   The physician is primarily responsible for the diagnosis of illness and the medical or surgical treatment of that illness. Physicians are granted the authority to admit clients to health care settings by the setting itself (eg, by the board of a hospital) and to practice care within that setting by writing orders.

Individuals become physicians after extensive education and clinical practice, and by passing a licensing examination. Depending on the curriculum completed, a physician may become a Doctor of Medicine (M.D.) or a Doctor of Osteopathy (D.O.). Physicians may specialize in the treatment of one type of illness or a specific type of surgery, or may be general practitioners.

Physician's Assistant   A physician's assistant (PA) has completed specific courses of study as preparation for providing support to the physician. The PA's responsibilities usually depend on the physician supervising the activities.

In most states, a nurse is not legally bound to follow a PA's orders unless they are cosigned by a physician. This is an important aspect to investigate if PAs are employed by hospitals in your area. PAs do not practice in Canada.

Physical Therapist   A PT seeks to restore function or prevent disability or further disability in the mobility of a client after an injury or an illness. The PT uses various techniques to treat clients, including massage, heat, ice packs, water, sonar waves, exercises, and electricity. Most PTs are also educated in the use of psychologic strategies to motivate clients.

To become a physical therapist, an individual must complete 4 years of college and obtain a baccalaureate degree in physical therapy. The person also must pass a state licensing examination. In some areas, a college graduate with a degree in another area may enroll in a 6- to 12-month certificate program to become a candidate for the state licensing examination for PTs.

Respiratory Therapist   An RT has been trained and educated to administer techniques that will improve pulmonary (lung) function and oxygenation. RTs may also be responsible for administering a variety of tests that measure lung functioning and for educating the client about the use of various devices and machines prescribed by the physician.

Occupational Therapist   An OT is licensed to assist the physically challenged client to adapt to limitations. The OT may use a variety of adaptive devices and strategies to aid a client in carrying out activities of daily living. The person must complete 4 years of college in the field of occupational therapy before taking the licensing examination for OTs.

Speech Therapist   A speech therapist is trained to help hearing-impaired clients speak more clearly, to assist a stroke victim to relearn how to speak, and to correct or modify a variety of speech disturbances in children and adults. Four years of college study in speech therapy is required to become a speech therapist.

Dietitian   Generally, a registered dietitian (RD) is responsible for managing and planning for the dietary needs of clients. The RD is knowledgeable about all aspects of nutrition and its effects on the body. An RD can adapt specialized diets for the individual needs of clients, counsel and educate individual clients, and supervise the dietary services of the entire facility. Dietitians are a valuable resource for nurses.

A dietitian's education includes 4 years of college in an approved, coordinated undergraduate program in dietetics. The person then must pass a registration examination to become an RD. Another educational option is 4 years of college with an approved dietetics major and 1 year in a dietetics internship, followed by the registration examination.

Pharmacist   A pharmacist is licensed to formulate and dispense medications. The pharmacist is also responsible for keeping a running file of all client medications and for informing the physician when a potential or actual medication error in prescribing has occurred or when prescribed drugs may interact adversely. The pharmacist is an excellent resource for both clients and nurses for any information related to medications. A pharmacist must complete at least 4 years of college with a major in pharmacology before taking the licensing examination.

Social Worker   A social worker counsels clients and family members and also informs them of and refers them to various community resources. A social worker usually has obtained a baccalaureate or master's degree in social work.

Chaplain   Most agencies employ a chaplain to give spiritual support and guidance to clients and their families. The chaplain can also refer a client to a priest, minister, or rabbi of the client's own religious denomination.

Economics of Health Care Delivery

Health care is expensive, with costs continuing to increase. Few U.S. citizens can afford to pay for health care from personal resources. To finance health care delivery, private organizations and federal agencies have developed health care insurance, prepaid health care programs, and federally funded services to pay costs.

Private Insurance

Personal health care can be financed by private insurance, through large, nonprofit, tax-exempt organizations (eg, Blue Cross and Blue Shield) or through smaller private for-

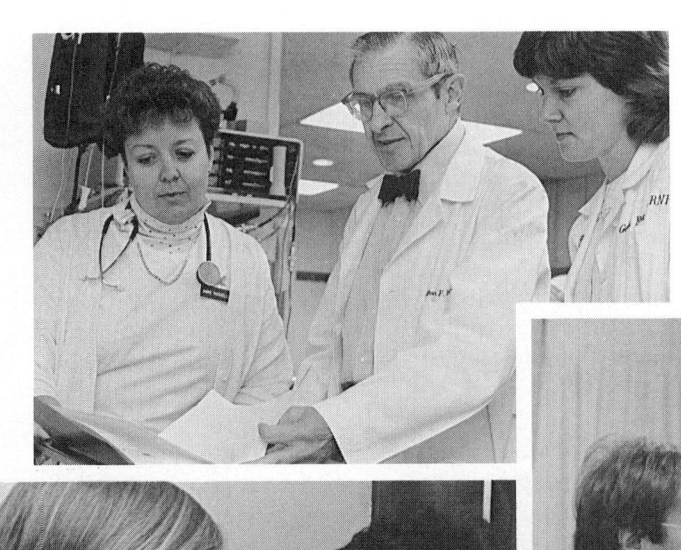

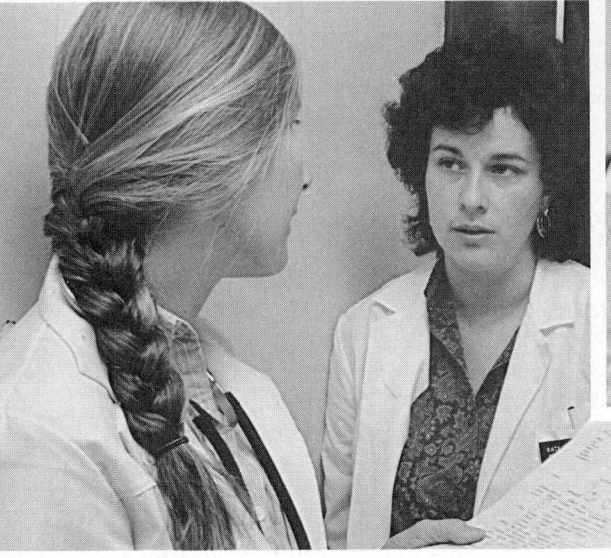

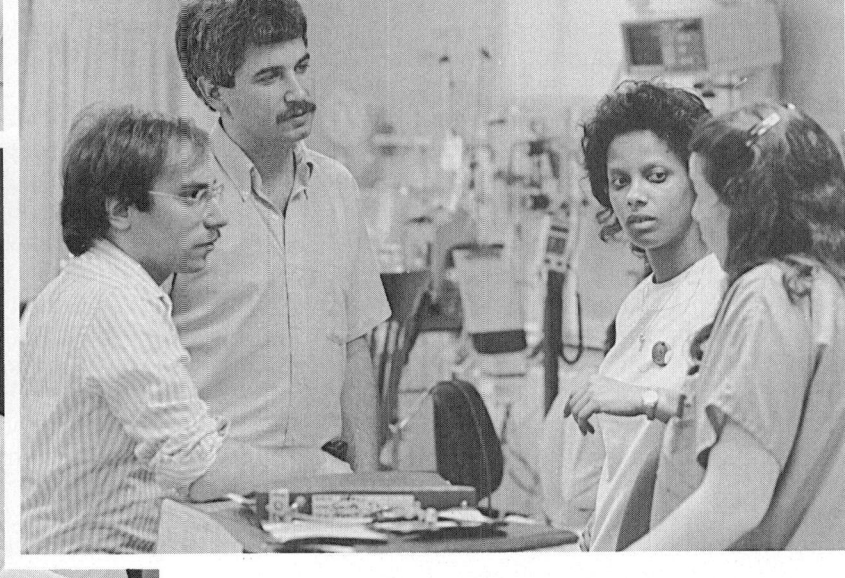

FIGURE 3-4

Quality health care results from the collaborative efforts of a team of professionals, many fulfilling specialized functions.

profit insurance companies. To be insured, members pay monthly premiums either by themselves or in combination with their employer. These plans usually pay about 80% of health care costs.

Group Plans

Group plans for financing health care in the United States include HMOs, PPOs, and PPAs. Enrollment in these plans is voluntary. An individual pays a fixed rate on either a monthly or annual plan and, in turn, receives financial coverage for all the health care necessary to maintain wellness and prevent illness. HMOs are especially interested and active in preventive health care and the maintenance of health.

Health Maintenance Organizations   HMOs were developed as alternative health care systems. In an effort to help control spiraling health costs, the U.S. Congress passed the Health Maintenance Organization Act in 1973. This act helped finance the development of HMOs such as the Kaiser-Permanente Medical Program, which began in California. Kaiser-Permanente is expanding into other states and more private agencies are developing HMOs.

Some HMOs offer almost unlimited resources to the client. They own and operate hospitals, clinics, physicians' offices, laboratories, and various other facilities. A person insured by an HMO plan is restricted to using HMO facilities and member physicians, except in some emergency situations. To maintain and increase cost effectiveness, HMOs may also place further limitations on a client's use of the system. Second opinions may be required for elective surgical procedures and a physician specialist may be consulted only if the client's primary HMO physician agrees and recommends the appointment. These limitations are effective methods for improving cost containment and keeping health care expenditures lower than average.

An HMO subscriber pays monthly or annual premiums and generally receives all health care free as long as it is obtained through the HMO. For some services, such as a physician's office visit, the subscriber may need to pay a minimal fee in addition to the premiums.

A more recent development in HMOs is the use of an independent practice association (IPA) model. The IPA model permits HMOs to contract individually with local, independently practicing physicians. This arrangement allows the HMO to expand its client base by adding physicians to an approved provider list.

Preferred Provider Organizations and Preferred Provider Arrangements PPOs and PPAs are almost synonymous, the primary difference being that PPOs involve organizations of health care providers and PPAs can be arranged with individual health care providers.

According to Fox (cited in Powills and Weinberg, 1985, p. 43), *PPA* may be used to describe "any arrangement whereby clients are channeled to specific providers." A PPA is a system in which the subscriber receives more extensive benefits if a designated preferred provider, either hospital or physician, is used. Unlike an HMO subscriber, a PPA subscriber is not necessarily limited to the use of preferred providers.

A PPA plan may be based on limited or unlimited participation. A limited PPA plan restricts subscribers to the use of only preferred providers of health care. An unlimited PPA plan allows all providers in the area who accept a contractual agreement to participate in the PPA. The payer, usually an insurance company, makes the decision whether to base the PPA plan on a limited or unlimited agreement.

In general, PPAs establish lower health care prices. They also use cost controls such as preadmission certification, second surgical opinion, and client length-of-stay reviews. An increasing number of commercial insurance companies and Blue Cross and Blue Shield are offering PPA plans to subscribers.

Because HMOs, PPAs, and PPOs assume the financial loss or gain of the health care services used by their clients, they encourage preventive health care to avoid the higher costs of illness and hospitalization. For the same reason, these plans carefully monitor the quality and quantity of the health care delivered to clients. They also place limitations on the use of high-cost procedures and require certain guidelines to be followed when a higher-cost procedure is recommended by a physician. Some people do not like these plans because they use a selective contracting approach, mandating subscriber use of specific institutions and health care providers. Some consumers dislike the lack of control they have in making decisions relating to personal or family health.

Long-Term Care Insurance A recent development in the health care insurance market is the growing interest in long-term care (LTC) insurance. In general, a minimal amount of LTC is paid for by private insurance. Most LTC (about 90%) is paid for by Medicaid and out-of-pocket spending. Medicare pays for a small percentage of LTC. The "graying of America," the steady increase in the population of people aged 65 years and older, has become a major concern within the health care financing area.

Some commercial insurance companies offer LTC benefits. Promoters of LTC insurance have developed models of plans that would cover a variety of services such as nursing home care and home care as well as other services that would help prevent the institutionalization of elderly, debilitated, and chronically ill people. Adult day-care centers and respite care would also fall under these types of services and would be covered by benefits.

Federal Government Health Care Support

United States As health insurance programs grew and prospered, it soon became apparent that a portion of the population (eg, poor, elderly, and physically or mentally challenged people) did not have access to health insurance and ultimately to health care. In 1965, the U.S. government became involved in health insurance when it enacted legislation creating Medicare for elderly and physically challenged people and Medicaid for poor people.

Medicare Medicare is a U.S. federal health insurance program for people aged 65 years or older, people of any age with permanent kidney failure, and certain physically challenged individuals. It is run by HCFA. Local Social Security Administration offices can supply all the necessary information about the program. It is financed partly through the Social Security (FICA) tax.

Medicare has been set up in two parts: (1) hospital insurance and (2) medical insurance. *Hospital insurance* helps pay for inpatient hospital and skilled nursing facility care, home health care, and hospice care. It is financed partly through the FICA tax. *Medical insurance* helps pay for necessary physicians' services, outpatient hospital and home health services, and a variety of other medical supplies and services. Applying for the medical insurance portion of the plan is voluntary. It is financed from the monthly premiums paid by the people who have enrolled in it and from general federal revenues.

The full cost of some services is not covered by Medicare; it is recommended that clients subscribe to supplemental insurance policies offered by private insurance companies. Also, because Medicare is federally funded, benefits may change annually according to decisions made concerning the federal budget.

Physicians and facilities are voluntary Medicare providers. Therefore, no physician or health institution is forced to care for Medicare clients. This voluntary agreement process may be jeopardized because some states are considering denying licensure renewal to physicians who do not care for Medicare clients (*Medicare Handbook,* 1990).

Medicaid Medicaid is the federally funded health insurance program for people with low incomes. Current budgetary considerations are forcing state and federal agencies to trim Medicaid expenditures. The rapid growth of an aging population and an increase in the number of poor people, many of whom are women and children, are draining the Medicaid budget. For survival, the Medicaid programs are implementing reforms such as reduced benefits, or are placing clients into use-control systems such as PPAs.

Diagnosis-Related Groups In 1983, Medicare converted to a prospective payment plan labeled **diagnosis-related groups** (DRGs). This plan pays the hospital a predetermined, fixed rate that is determined by the medical diagnosis or specific procedure involved rather than by the actual cost of hospitalization and care. DRG charges are based on an analysis of recent charges for care, with rates updated annually.

DRGs were implemented by the federal government in an effort to control rising health care costs. The plan pays only the amount of money preassigned to a diagnosis (eg, an appendectomy); if the cost for hospitalization is greater than that assigned, the hospital must absorb the additional cost. However, if costs are less than that assigned, the hospital makes a profit. Although there are a large number of DRG categories, they cannot cover all admissions accurately or comprehensively. Therefore, unusually costly or lengthy hospital care cases (called *outliers*) require additional documentation and support for the circumstances of each case.

Canada The Canada Health Act became law in 1984. It clarifies and defines the conditions of Canadian health insurance—universality, accessibility, comprehensiveness, and portability among provinces. The organization and services vary from province to province. However, "the health and physician insurance services exist to finance, administer, and regulate the provisions of federal and provincial legislation regarding hospital and medical care" (Storch, 1985). The general areas of involvement of provincial governments are approval of hospitals and budgets, approval of claims and payments, data collection, inspection and consultation, and licensing and financial assistance for hospital and nursing home construction. Other benefits supplemental to medical insurance may be administered by the particular provincial government.

Trends and Issues in the Health Care Delivery System

Many questions have arisen about the health care delivery system as it currently exists. These questions are debated at the local, state, and federal level as well as by health care providers and consumers of health care services. A few of the issues that influence trends in health care are discussed in this section. In your career as a nurse, you may find that some questions are answered, but you will also discover that more problems arise. As a nurse, it will be important for you both personally and professionally to be knowledgeable about all the aspects of the health care delivery system.

Focus on Self-Care and Wellness

Health awareness and the desire for personal involvement in one's own health care has strongly influenced the delivery of health care services in society. People are becoming convinced that it is more important to remain healthy than it is to neglect one's health and then treat a resulting illness or injury. This belief has far-reaching influences on the way we live. Stress management programs, nutritional awareness, exercise and fitness programs, and antismoking and antidrug campaigns are all examples of this trend. Equally as important in the health of all members of society are measures such as promoting the wearing of seat belts, promoting automobile and airplane safety, controlling smog, and eliminating hazardous wastes.

A public interest in self-care has evolved into a strong force in terms of the education and services provided by health care professionals. Consumers of health care are better educated about health, prefer to control and make decisions about their own personal health, and want to be active participants in planning and implementing health care.

Consumer Movement

A **consumer** is someone who uses a commodity or service. Consumers of health care services have become better educated about the services they require and the services that are available. They have also become concerned about the access to services and the cost of those services. As a result of a consumer movement in health care, consumers have questioned escalating costs and the proliferation and duplication of services and, in some instances, changes are being made. Consumers have become actively involved in the administration of health care agencies and have helped develop standards for care, client rights, and cost-containment measures as protection for clients when they enter a health care setting. A negative aspect of the consumer movement has been an increase in malpractice lawsuits, resulting in high malpractice insurance rates (especially for physicians) and the necessity to carefully document care given; the increased paperwork often serves to take the nurse away from actual client care.

Cost Containment

The health care system is experiencing a financial crisis. Health costs have increased dramatically, and some analysts believe that cost-containment measures have been implemented too late to effectively reverse the current upward swing in health costs. The actual short-term and long-term results of these cost-containment measures remain to be seen. The health care industry has functioned in a specific manner for many years and has become big business. The process of change can often be difficult.

Historically, the health care system and the financial arrangements for paying for health care encouraged the use of expensive and sometimes inappropriate or ineffective health services. Many insurance plans paid for inpatient hospital care but not for ambulatory outpatient care. Therefore, to receive payment, clients were often hospitalized unnecessarily. Health care has also focused on the treatment of illnesses instead of on their prevention because preventive strategies often were not covered by a client's health insurance policy.

Third-party reimbursement effectively insulated clients from knowing the actual cost of their health care. Because the insurance company was responsible for pay-

COMPUTER APPLICATIONS IN NURSING

Computer Use in Hospitals to Reduce Health Care Costs

Hospitals use a wide variety of computer applications to benefit consumers of health care, including the following examples:

- Automated patient classification systems, used to determine staffing needs
- Direct on-line nursing documentation
- Computerized nursing care plans
- Automated staff scheduling
- Computer generated medication documentation records

- Results of diagnostic tests available through unit computers
- Order processing directly by way of computer entry
- Complex analysis of budget and position control related to patient acuity

These functions save time for nurses and administrators, provide data for research, improve accuracy and documentation of care, and reduce costs of hospitalization for clients.

---

ing the incurred bills, the client was often bypassed in this process and seldom saw the bills for the cost of the care received.

The increased competition among hospitals further fueled the increase in health costs. Technologically, people have made amazing advances in health care, but as new machines and more advanced and expensive procedures are developed and used, clients' expectations of hospital resources will also increase. The media is constantly informing the public of new and innovative treatment modalities. As a result, consumers expect these services to be available in "their" hospital. To attract clients, hospitals invest huge sums of money in technologically advanced equipment. Supporters of cost-containment measures are encouraging hospitals to cooperate with each other and to share resources rather than compete with each other.

Fragmentation of Care

Increased health care research has resulted in an upward spiral of technology and knowledge. In effect, this means that health care providers can no longer keep up with all of the advances made, so that specialization has become almost the rule rather than the exception. What does this mean for the client?

A physician who is a general practitioner diagnoses and treats a variety of common health problems. However, a client who requires diagnosis and treatment for a more complex problem is usually referred to a physician who is a specialist. For example, a diabetic client with a heart condition may be cared for by his or her family physician, a cardiologist, and an endocrinologist. The hospitalized client not only comes in contact with many different health care providers (eg, registered nurses, licensed practical nurses, nursing assistants, nurse specialists, PTs, dietitians, and students) but also is frequently seen by other physician specialists called in on consultation or to do surgery. It is no wonder that the client becomes confused about care and treatments. This fragmentation of care can result in the loss of continuity of care, resulting in conflicting plans of care, too much or too little medication, and higher health care costs.

Increasing Numbers of Older and Chronically Ill Adults This topic is a major issue in health care delivery. The older adult, and particularly those over age 70, are the most rapidly growing segment of our population. As people age, there is an associated increase in chronic illnesses. This presents two problems. First, these clients require more health care in both inpatient and outpatient settings. As a result, hospitals are increasingly filled with older men and women who are in the acute or terminal stages of one or more chronic illnesses. Second, these clients need additional doctor's visits, more medications, and more health-related supplies, but they often have difficulty affording these needs, especially if they are on a fixed income. This problem may be further compounded by a lack of transportation, a scarcity of family members or support systems, and a desire for independence that interferes with compliance with health care regimens. Many of these needs are also found in the growing number of people with AIDS. Evidently, much needs to be done to meet the special health care needs of the older population.

Health Care: A Right or a Privilege? Two major factors that influence health care provision in the United States are (1) the ability to pay and (2) location of facilities. Poor or uninsured people, minorities, and elderly people often are faced with inadequate access to health care services, as are residents of rural areas. In the United States, 37 to 39 million people currently have no or inadequate insurance. Although many people assume that all people have a right to health care, consider these questions:

Do indigent people who do not take care of themselves deserve the same health care as the employed person with insurance?

Who provides funds for the health care needs of the homeless population?

Is the person who goes on national television asking for an organ donation for his or her child any more deserving than the person who has been waiting months for just such a transplant?

Are you willing to pay increased insurance premiums so that the drug addict who overdoses can have intensive care?

If 20 people need a heart transplant and only one heart is available, who decides who gets another chance at life?

These are only a few of the questions being raised, and there are no easy answers. The issue of who gets health care and, in turn, who pays the bills, will be of major importance to society as we move into the 21st century. The question of availability of care to all people is being addressed by nursing in an agenda for health care reform drawn up by the American Nurses' Association, the National League for Nursing, state nurses' associations, the American Association of Colleges of Nursing, and specialty nursing organizations. The major components of the agenda include the following:

- A restructured health care system
- A federally defined standard package of essential health care services available to all U.S. citizens and residents
- A phase-in of essential services
- Planned change to anticipate health service needs that correlate with changing national demographics
- Steps to reduce health care costs
- Insurance reforms

In addition, the health care reform proposed by nursing professionals, called "the core of care," calls for a shift from a focus on illness and cure to an orientation toward wellness and care.

KEY POINTS

- The health care system comprises institutions, agencies, members of the health care team, and both public and private health care financing systems.
- Hospitals provide a wide variety of inpatient services and are classified as either private or public, for-profit or not-for-profit.
- Extended-care facilities provide inpatient services through long-term care facilities, skilled care facilities, nursing homes, retirement centers, and residential institutions.
- Outpatient services are increasing rapidly and are provided by hospitals, physician's offices, ambulatory care centers, and clinics.
- Community care settings include home care, day-care centers, crisis intervention centers, agencies, rehabilitation centers, and hospices.
- Government agencies are also a part of the health care system, providing funding, research, and information to meet community and national needs.
- Members of the health care team collaborate to promote client wellness and to restore health to clients who require health care services.

- Health care costs are financed through health care insurance, prepaid health care programs, and federally funded programs and services.
- Medicare is a federal health insurance program in the United States for people aged 65 years or older, people with permanent kidney failure, and certain physically challenged individuals. Medicaid is a federally funded health insurance program for people with low incomes.
- A prospective payment plan, referred to as DRGs, pays a predetermined fixed rate regardless of actual hospitalization costs. With private insurance, an insurance company pays a portion of the medical bills.
- Current societal issues influencing health care delivery focus on wellness promotion, maintenance of health care for the older adult, cost containment, and consumer rights. Clients are better educated about health matters, prefer more control and more participation in decision making about personal health, and are becoming active participants in planning and implementing health care.

BIBLIOGRAPHY

ABCs of DRGs. (1985). *RN, 48*(6), 55–58.

Aday, L. A., Fleming, G. V., & Anderson, R. (1984). *Access to medical care in the U.S.: Who has it, who doesn't.* Chicago: Pluribus.

Aiken, L. H. (1990). Charting the future of hospital nursing. *Image: Journal of Nursing Scholarship, 22*(2), 72–77.

Allison, S., & Latham, G. (1991). Same-day admission surgery. *Canadian Nurse, 87*(11), 25.

Brickfield, C. F. (1985). Long-term care financing solutions are needed now. *American Health Care Association Journal, 11*(6), 11–15.

Brucker, M. C., & MacMullen, N. J. (1985). Understanding health insurance (making it work for the patient and you). *Nursing Success Today, 2*(12), 7–9.

Buzath, J., Lievaart, B., & Schow, E. (1992). Political action: Choice or obligation? *Canadian Nurse, 88*(2), 35–36.

Capuzzi, C., & Garland, M. (1990). The Oregon plan: Increasing access to health care. *Nursing Outlook, 38*(6), 260–263, 286.

Curtin, L. L. (1989). Hospitals 1990: Back to the future . . . or else. *Nursing Management, 20*(12), 7–8.

Deane, R. T. (1986). Looking at Medicare after the promise. *Provider, 12*(6), 25–27.

Drew, J. C. (1990). Health maintenance organizations: History, evolution, & survival. *Nursing and Health Care, 11*(3), 145–149.

Evans, R. (1984). *Strained mercy: The economics of Canadian health care.* Toronto: Butterworth.

Fiesta, J. (1990). The "nurses do everything" dilemma. *Nursing Management, 21*(4), 24–25.

Friedman, E. (1985). Increasing numbers of Americans lack health insurance. *Hospitals, 59*(4), 21.

Gage, L. (1985). Interview: Public hospitals in a private market. *Hospitals, 59*(4), 114–116.

Gale, B. J., & Steffl, B. J. (1992). The long-term care dilemma: What nurses need to know about Medicare. *Nursing and Health Care, 13*(1), 34–41.

Hamilton, C. L., & Neubauer, B. J. (1989). Hospice nursing: Serving ambivalent clients. *Nursing and Health Care, 10*(6), 320–322.

Hamilton, C. L., & Wilson, C. N. (1989). The new Medicare catastrophic coverage act: Will it affect nursing? *Nursing and Health Care, 10*(1), 31–34.

Hull, M. M. (1991). Hospice nurses: Caring support for caregiving families. *Cancer Nursing, 14*(2), 63–70.

Joel, L. A. (1987). Reshaping nursing practice. *American Journal of Nursing, 87*(6), 793–795.

Johnson, P. A. (1990). A national health insurance program: A nursing perspective. *Nursing and Health Care, 11*(8), 416–429.

Kickbusch, I. (1986). Health promotion: A global perspective. *Canadian Journal of Public Health, 77*(5), 321–326.

King, M. L. (1992). Care management. *Canadian Nurse, 88*(4), 15–17.

Lambert, C. E., Jr., & Lambert, V. A. (1989). *Perspectives in nursing: The impacts on the nurse, the consumer, and society.* Norwalk, CT: Appleton & Lange.

Last, J. M. (1986). Achieving health care for all. *Canadian Journal of Public Health, 77*(6), 384–385.

LeClair, M. (1975). The Canadian health care system. In S. Andreopoulous (Ed.). *National health insurance: Can we learn from Canada?* (pp. 11–92). New York: Wiley.

LTC insurance needs increased awareness. (1986). *Contemporary Long-Term Care,* June, 26–30, 63.

McCormick, B. (1986). What's the cost of nursing care? *Hospitals, 60*(2), 48–52.

Medicare handbook (Pub. No. HCFA 10050). (1990). Baltimore, MD: U.S. Department of Health and Human Services.

Phillips, E. K., Fisher, M. E., MacMillan-Scattergood, D., & Baglioni, A. J. (1989). DRG ripple and the shifting of care to home health. *Nursing and Health Care, 10*(6), 325–327.

Powills, S. E., & Weinberg, W. (1985). PPAs: A new payment system evolves. *Hospitals, 59*(9), 43–46.

Rantz, M. J. (1990). Inadequate reimbursement for long-term care: The impact since hospital DRGs. *Nursing and Health Care, 11*(9), 470–472.

Riffer, J. (1985a). Diversification push drives day care rise. *Hospitals, 59*(5), 68.

Riffer, J. (1985b). Elderly: 21 percent of the population by 2040. *Hospitals, 59*(5), 41–44.

Rooks, J. P. (1990). Let's admit we ration health care—then set priorities. *American Journal of Nursing, 90*(6), 39–43.

Rozovsky, L. (1979). *Canadian hospital law* (2nd ed.). Ottawa: Canadian Hospital Association.

Rozovsky, L. (1980). *The Canadian patient's book of rights.* Toronto: Doubleday Canada.

Ruderman, A. (1986). Marketing health promotion in Canada: An idea whose time has come. *Canadian Journal of Public Health, 77*(5), 315–317.

Sandhu, B. K., & Duquette, A., & Kerouac, S. (1992). Care delivery modes. *Canadian Nurse, 88*(4), 18–20.

Scott, K. (1991). Northern nurses and burnout. *Canadian Nurse, 87*(10), 18–21.

Slauenwhite, C., DeWitt, P., & Grivell, M. (1991). Independent nurse practitioners. *Canadian Nurse, 87*(10), 24.

Smith, S. L., & Elesha-Adams, M. (1989). Allocating nursing resources in ambulatory care. *Nursing Management, 20*(1), 61–64.

Storch, J. (1985). The Canadian health care delivery system: Policies, programs, services. In M. Stewart, et al. (Eds.), *Community health nursing in Canada* (pp. 33–48). Toronto: Gage.

Weingart, M. (1991). Commercially managed healthcare: An experience. *Nursing Management, 22*(1), 40–42.

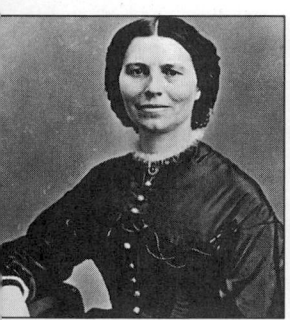
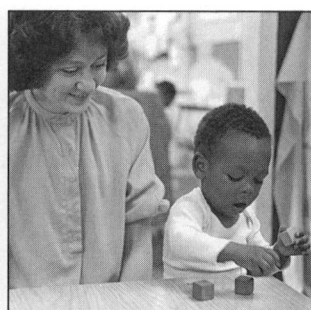

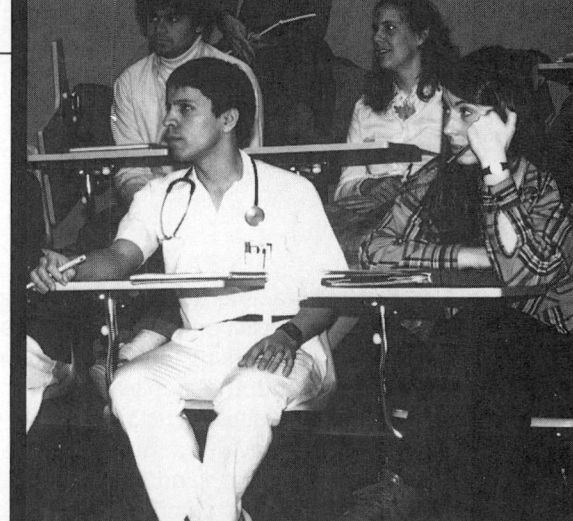

OBJECTIVES

After studying this chapter, the learner should be able to:

Define key terms used in the chapter.

Describe the underlying processes and characteristics of nursing theory.

Define the four common components of nursing theory.

Summarize the historical background, cultural influences, and value of nursing theory.

Discuss selected nursing theories, including definitions, assumptions, beliefs, and applications to nursing practice.

KEY TERMS

adaptation theory
concept
conceptual framework or model
developmental theory
general systems theory
nursing theory
philosophy
process
theory

Theoretical Base for Nursing Practice

4

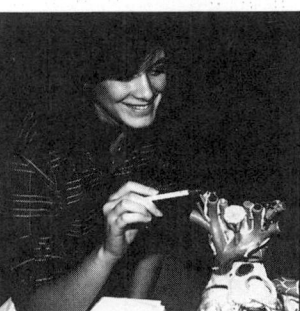

Nursing is a unique health care discipline in which a service, based on knowledge and skill, is provided to others. Nursing therefore has two parts—a body of knowledge and the application of that knowledge through nursing practice. The body of knowledge, called a *knowledge base*, provides a rationale for everything that a nurse does. As you learn and practice nursing, you will use rationales from many different areas, such as anatomy, physiology, chemistry, nutrition, psychology, and sociology. You will also use a knowledge base and rationale developed specifically for nurses, allowing you to know what nursing care is and why and how it is given. This chapter discusses how the nursing knowledge base—also known as **nursing theory**—has been developed and how it is used to give safe and knowledgeable nursing care.

Introduction to Theory

Each individual collects, organizes, and arranges facts to build a knowledge base that defines his or her personal reality. A similar organization and a structure of facts and events are present in large bodies of knowledge, through philosophies, concepts, theories, and processes.

Philosophy is the study of wisdom, fundamental knowledge, and the processes used to develop and construct our perceptions of life. Philosophy both provides a viewpoint and implies a system of values and beliefs. Each individual develops a personal philosophy to give meaning to experiences and to direct behavior and attitudes. An individual may develop a personal philosophy through learning from interpersonal relationships, through formal and informal educational experiences, through religion and culture, and from the environment.

The philosophy of each nurse and the philosophies of schools of nursing and of health care institutions form the basis of giving nursing care. As nurses give care, teach, and work with others, they reflect both a personal and a professional philosophy through values and beliefs about concepts such as goodness, wellness, health, illness, accountability, and ethics. In the same way, nursing education and nursing practice settings provide education or client care based on philosophical beliefs about humans, health, teaching and learning, and standards of client care.

Concepts can be compared with ideas: they are abstract impressions from the environment organized into symbols of reality. Concepts describe objects, properties, and events, and the relations among them. A group of concepts that follows an understandable pattern makes up a **conceptual framework or model.** Concepts can be thought of as the individual bricks and boards used to build a house, with the conceptual framework being the blueprint that specifies where each brick and board should go.

A **theory** is a group of concepts that form a pattern of reality. A theory is a statement that explains or characterizes a process, an occurrence, or an event, and is based on observed facts but lacks absolute or direct proof. Theories arrange a group of related statements or concepts so that they give meaning to a series of events. Theories can be tested, changed, or used to guide research or to provide a base for evaluation. They are derived through two principal methods: (1) *deductive reasoning*, in which one examines a general idea, after which one considers specific actions or ideas; and (2) *inductive reasoning*, where the reverse process is used—one identifies a specific idea or action and then makes conclusions about general ideas. Nursing theorists use both of these methods.

A **process,** which is the action phase of a conceptual framework or a theory, is a series of actions, changes, or functions that bring about a desired result. During a process, one takes systematic and continuous steps to meet a goal and uses both assessments and feedback to direct actions to meet the goal. A particular theory or conceptual framework with its own specific definitions directs the way in which these actions are carried out.

The nursing process consists of applied nursing theories and concepts. The delivery of nursing care within the nursing process is directed in an institution by specific conceptual frameworks and theories.

Nursing Theory

Nursing theory, as defined by Barnum (1990), "attempts to describe or explain the phenomenon (process, occurrence, or event) called nursing." Nursing theory differentiates nursing from other disciplines and activities in that it serves the purposes of describing, explaining, predicting, and controlling desired outcomes of nursing care practices.

Basic Processes in the Development of Nursing Theories

Nursing theories are often based on and influenced by other broadly applicable processes and theories. The ideas and principles of the theories that follow are basic to many nursing concepts and are a part of the nursing literature. It is important that nurses understand these theories and their terminologies so they can develop their own knowledge base in nursing. The following is a brief description of the major points of each theory.

General Systems Theory   General systems theory has been used by a wide range of disciplines since it emerged in the 1920s. Its primary theorist, Ludwig von Bertalanffy, developed the theory so that it could be universally applied. This theory explains the breaking of whole things into parts and then learning how the parts work together in "systems." It includes the relationship between the whole and the parts and defines concepts about how the parts will function and behave. These concepts may be applied to different kinds of systems, for example, to molecules in chemistry, cultures in sociology, organs in anatomy, and health in nursing.

Key points in general systems theory are as follows:
- A system is a set of interacting elements, all serving the common purpose of contributing to the overall goal of the system; the whole system is always greater than the sum of its parts.
- Systems are hierarchical in nature and comprise interrelated subsystems that work together in such a way that a change in one element could affect other subsystems as well as the whole.
- Boundaries separate systems both from each other and from their environments.
- A system communicates with and reacts to its environment through processes that enter the system (input) or are transferred to the environment (output).
- An open system allows energy, matter, and information to move freely between systems and boundaries, whereas a closed system does not allow input from or output to the environment (no known closed systems exist in reality).
- To survive, open systems maintain balance through feedback.

Stress/Adaptation Theory   Adaptation theory defines **adaptation** as the adjustment of living matter to other living things and to environmental conditions. Adaptation is a dynamic or continuously changing process that effects change and involves interaction and response. Human adaptation occurs on three levels—the internal (self), the social (others), and the physical (biochemical reactions). See Chapter 9 for more information on stress and adaptation.

Developmental Theory   Developmental theory states that the process of growth and development of humans is orderly and predictable, beginning with conception and ending with death. Although the pattern is one of definite stages, the progress and behaviors of an individual within each stage are unique. The growth and development of an individual are influenced by heredity, temperament, emotional and physical environment, life experiences, and health status.

Several theorists are important to developmental theory, but only two are mentioned briefly because their work is often used to develop nursing theory and to organize nursing practice. Eric Erikson based his theory of psycho-social development on the process of socialization, emphasizing how individuals learn to interact with the world. Erikson recognized the role of social, biologic, and environmental factors in development and defined specific tasks or conflicts to be accomplished or overcome during what he defined as the eight stages of life. See Chapter 10 for more information on developmental theory.

Abraham Maslow divided his theory of human needs by the physical and psychosocial needs considered essential to human life, rather than by chronologic age, as Erikson did. Maslow defined five levels of need (physiologic well-being; physical safety; affection, love, and relationships; self-esteem; and self-actualization) existing in a hierarchy, with several needs being able to exist simultaneously. See Chapter 7 for more information on the theory of human needs.

As you continue in your nursing education and practice, you will learn how systems, adaptation, and developmental theories are used in planning and giving holistic care to clients. The discussion of specific nursing theories will enable you to better understand the knowledge base used to develop the concepts unique to nursing.

Basic Characteristics of Nursing Theory

Nursing theories identify and define interrelated concepts specific to nursing and clearly state the relation between these concepts. Nursing theories must be logical in nature; they should use orderly reasoning and describe relations that are developed using a logical sequence. Theories must also be consistent with the basic assumptions used in their development. Nursing theories should be simple and general; simple terminology and broadly applicable concepts ensure their usefulness in a wide variety of nursing practice situations. Nursing theories should also increase the nursing profession's body of knowledge by generating research. Furthermore, nursing theory should guide and improve practice.

Nursing theory is valuable in research, education, and practice. In addition, nursing theory guides nurses by providing a knowledge base, organizing concepts, providing guidelines for practice, and identifying nursing care goals (Chinn & Jacobs, 1987; Torres, 1990).

Common Components in Theories of Nursing

Four concepts common to nursing theory that influence and determine nursing practice are (1) person, (2) environment, (3) health, and (4) nursing. Each of these concepts is defined and described by a nursing theorist, and although these concepts are common to all nursing theories, both the definitions and the relations among them may differ greatly from one theory to another. (These theories are discussed later in this chapter.) Of the four concepts, the most important is that of the person. The focus of nursing, regardless of definition or theory, is the person (Fig. 4-1).

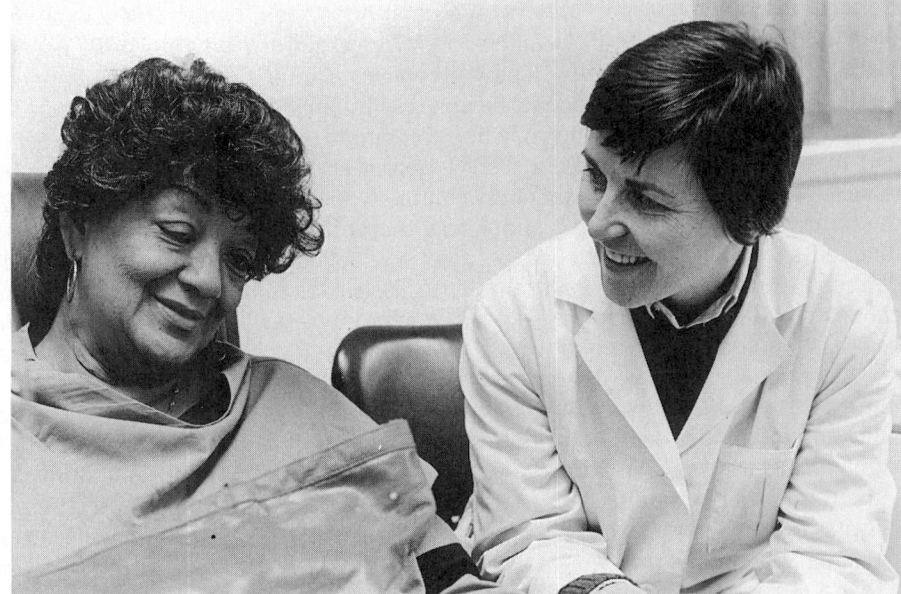

FIGURE 4-1

Four concepts common to all nursing theories are person, environment, health, and nursing. The most important concept and the focus of nursing is the person. (Photo by Gates Rhodes, courtesy of School of Nursing, University of Pennsylvania.)

Nursing Theory and Nursing Practice

Historical Perspectives and Influences

Nightingale's Definition and Belief Florence Nightingale, the nurse who established the theoretical base of nursing, developed and published a philosophy and a theory of health and nursing that has served as a solid foundation for the nursing profession. Her contributions to nursing theory included identifying the role of the nurse in meeting the client's personal needs; recognizing the importance of environmental influences on the care of sick people; elevating the standards and acceptance of nursing by developing sound principles of nursing education, as well as by demonstrating efficient and knowledgeable nursing care; defining nursing practice as separate and distinct from medical practice; and differentiating between health nursing and illness nursing (Dolan, Fitzpatrick, & Herrmann, 1983).

Cultural Influences on Nursing Certain cultural influences have affected nursing as we currently know it. Although since the beginning of time both men and women have given comfort and assistance to sick people, until the past two decades, nursing essentially had been considered "women's work." In the 18th and 19th centuries, women were viewed as subservient and inferior to men. However, after Nightingale established an occupation for educated women and facilitated improved attitudes toward nursing, the role of the woman as nurse became more favorably accepted.

Despite Nightingale's belief in the uniqueness of nursing, the training of nurses was carried out primarily under the direction and control of the medical profession (Kalish & Kalish, 1986). Because the conceptual and theoretical basis for nursing practice came from outside the profession, nursing has struggled for years to establish its own identity and to receive recognition for its significant contributions to health care.

Nursing in the United States

Influences of Educational Frameworks on Nursing Practice Most schools of nursing established in the United States were adapted from Nightingale's model. There was no planned educational curriculum; rather, learning came from lectures by physicians and by practical experience acquired through caring for sick people in the hospital (Dolan, Fitzpatrick, & Herrmann, 1983). This service orientation for nursing education remained the strongest influence on nursing practice until the 1950s. Rather than developing a body of knowledge specific to nursing, nursing care was carried out under the control and direction of the hospital administration and the physicians practicing in that hospital. Nursing care was based on traditional ideas about following orders, as well as on common wisdom about caring for others based on either "common sense" or widely accepted scientific principles (Chinn & Jacobs, 1991). It is no wonder that nursing knowledge remained undeveloped and fragmented for so long.

Developing a Scientific Base for Nursing During the first half of the 20th century, a change in the structure of society resulted in a change of roles for women and, in turn, in nursing. As a result of World War I and World War II, women increasingly entered the work force, became more independent, and sought higher education. At the same time, nursing education began to focus on education instead of on training, and nursing research was conducted and published. As women became more assertive, nursing's need for a clearly defined identity of unique contributions to the health care system emerged. In the 1950s, the idea of nursing as a science became more generally accepted, and philosophical beliefs and a knowledge base for nursing practice began to evolve. The nursing practice currently used by nurses is one that increasingly focuses on giving effective client care based on sound rationales from nursing knowledge.

Evolution of Nursing Theory

Research and Publishing in Nursing

Beginning in the 1950s, as great advances were made in technology and medical research, nursing leaders realized that research into the practice of nursing was necessary to meet the health needs of modern society. Increasing numbers of nurses began to conduct nursing research and write articles telling other nurses how to carry out nursing research. Two major developments in nursing theory were made during the 1950s: (1) the first research journal, *Nursing Research,* was published in 1950 (and continues today); and (2) as ideas were published, they served as a basis for theory development (Chinn & Jacobs, 1991; Kalish & Kalish, 1986).

Educational Advances in Nursing

Beginning in the 1960s, college- and university-based baccalaureate programs in nursing began to increase in both number and enrollment. At the same time, master's and doctoral programs in nursing were established. This upward trend in education for nurses was reflected in the nursing literature; more attention was given to the consideration and formulation of knowledge specific to nursing.

Value of Nursing Theory

Broad Goals of Nursing Theory Nursing theory provides a rational and knowledgeable reason for nursing actions, based on organized, written descriptions of the reality of nursing. Additionally, nursing theory gives nurses the knowledge base necessary for them to act and respond appropriately in nursing care situations; provides a base for discussion; and, ideally, provides resolution of current nursing issues. Furthermore, nursing theory allows the nurse who knows and practices theory to have better problem-solving skills, so that nursing actions are organized, considered, and purposeful. Nursing theory also prepares the nurse to question assumptions and values in nursing, thus further defining nursing and increasing the knowledge base.

Applying Theory to Practice Nurses have difficulty agreeing on what nursing really is; however, if theory-based nursing is practiced, direction is provided that allow nurses to work toward a common goal, with the ultimate outcome being improved client care.

Improving and Facilitating Communication Nursing is based on communication with others—clients, other health care team members, community members—as well as with nurses practicing in a variety of specialty settings. Because concepts are both abstract and highly individualized, verbal communication with others can be interpreted in many ways. As ideas are developed and words are defined, nurses build a knowledge base and a common terminology to use in communicating with other professionals.

Improving Autonomy of Nursing The term *autonomy* means independence and self-governance. As a discipline, nursing is in the process of defining its own independent functions and contributions to health care. The development and use of nursing theory provide autonomy in interdependent ways:
- Having a body of knowledge specific to the discipline allows members of that discipline to be viewed by others as experts; this, in turn, gives nurses authority to carry out actions.
- Actions carried out and based on sound rationale are trusted and respected.

FIGURE 4-2

Florence Nightingale developed and published a philosophy and theory of health and nursing that has served as a solid foundation for the nursing profession. (Photo courtesy of the Center for the Study of the History of Nursing, University of Pennsylvania.)

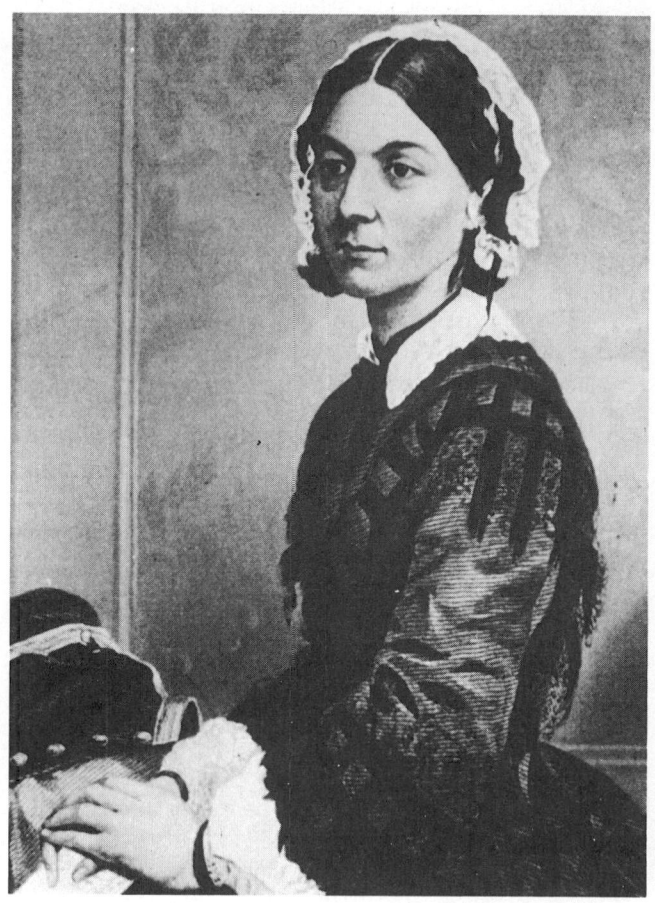

- Nursing theory makes nursing care visible, leading to increased internal control by nurses.
- As nurses demonstrate that nursing care does indeed make a difference and that nursing services are valuable, the discipline becomes more independent.

Conceptual and Theoretical Frameworks for Nursing

Theorists and Their Models

The theories and conceptual models included in this section have been selected because they represent different approaches to defining the reality of nursing and because they are used in a variety of educational, research, and practice settings. They are arranged in alphabetical order as a means of organization only. Accompanying each theory or model is a brief summary of the central theme, basic assumptions, definitions, and applications in nursing. The information is summarized in Table 4-1. Students who find a particular framework relevant and useful are encouraged to explore the literature to learn more about the theory or model and the theorist.

Dorothy E. Johnson: Behavioral Systems Model

Dorothy Johnson believes that nursing care is directed toward caring for the whole client to facilitate effective and efficient behaviors necessary to prevent illness. Her behavioral systems model integrates systems, developmental, and needs theories into a specific nursing focus. Johnson believes the four goals of nursing are to assist the person:
- Whose behavior is commensurate with social demands
- Who is able to modify his or her behavior in ways that support biologic imperatives
- Who is able to benefit, to the fullest extent during illness, from the physician's knowledge and skill
- Whose behavior does not give evidence of unnecessary trauma as a result of illness

Johnson views nursing as being separate from medicine in that medicine focuses on pathologic changes in the ill person, whereas nursing focuses on the behaviors of the person. She sees the nursing role as being complementary to the medical role. Nurses, giving care, supply functional requirements to the client through protection, nurturance, and stimulation. She views humans as individuals who act in ways that make up a behavioral system specific to each person. Within this behavioral system are seven interrelated subsystems. Changes in one subsystem affect all the others. The seven subsystems are as follows:

Attachment or "affiliative": This is the first behavioral subsystem to develop, initially allowing the infant to attach (bond) to a significant caregiver and continuing through life with other individuals. These attachments provide a sense of security.

Dependency: The behaviors in this subsystem precipitate nurturing by others and result in approval, attention, and physical assistance.

Ingestive: Behaviors surrounding the intake of food belong in this subsystem, including social and cultural factors.

Eliminative: The behaviors in this subsystem are involved with the excretion of waste products from the body and also relate to physical control and social situations.

Sexual: The behaviors in this subsystem are cultural and gender behaviors related to procreation and gratification.

Aggressive: In this subsystem, the behaviors are concerned with protection and self-preservation.

Achievement: Behaviors that attempt to control the environment, including intellectual, physical, creative, mechanical, and social skills, belong in this subsystem.

Johnson believes that both the internal and external environments of the system need to be orderly and predictable to maintain homeostasis. If the subsystems are out of balance, "tension" and disequilibrium result. Nursing, as part of the external environment, can help the client return to a state of balance.

Imogene M. King: Open Systems Framework

Imogene King developed both a conceptual framework (open systems) and a theory of goal attainment derived from the framework. She used many sources to develop these bodies of knowledge.

Some assumptions are basic to this framework:
- The focus of nursing is the care of humans.
- The nursing goal is the health of individuals and health care for groups.
- Humans are in constant interaction with their environment.

Within the framework are three interacting systems, each of which is defined and has relevant concepts:

Personal systems: Each individual is a personal system. The concepts defined in personal systems are perception, self, growth and development, body image, space, and time.

Interpersonal systems: Interpersonal systems are formed as humans interact. The concepts are interaction, communication, transaction, role, and stress.

Social systems: Social systems include families, religious groups, educational systems, work systems, and peer groups. The concepts are organization, authority, power, status, and decision making.

King developed the conceptual framework and defined the concepts based on the belief that individuals actively interact with others and objects in the environment and are changed as a result of the experiences. King describes her theory of goal attainment as the interpersonal system in which two people come together in a health care organization to help or be helped to maintain a state of health that

Theorists and Their Conceptual Models

Theorist	Central Theme	Definitions			
		Person	Environment	Health	Nursing
Johnson's behavioral systems model	The human as a behavioral system	Humans with two major systems: biologic and behavioral	Society as the environment in which an individual exists, influencing the individual's behavior	Purposeful, adaptive responses (physical, mental, emotional, social) to internal and external stimuli to maintain balance and comfort	Primary goal is to foster balance within an individual, specific to the behavioral system, when illness occurs
King's open systems framework and theory of goal attainment	Interrelationships of concepts and the process of human interactions	Humans are open systems who are social, rational, perceiving, controlling, purposeful, and action and time oriented	Not specifically defined	Dynamic life experience of a human, implying continuous adjustment to stressors in the internal and external environment through optimal use of one's resources to achieve maximum potential for daily living	A process of human interactions between nurse and client whereby each perceives the other and the situation, and, through communication, together set goals, explore means, and agree on means to achieve goals
Leininger's transcultural care model	A model that provides cultural specific care consistent with nursing science and knowledge	Caring beings capable of being concerned about, holding interest in, or having regard for other people's needs, well-being, and survival	The culture of each individual, group, or society	A state of well-being that is mainly known and expressed in cultural meanings and ways	A learned humanistic art and science that focuses on personalized care behaviors and processes that are directed toward promoting and maintaining health behaviors or recovery from illness. These behaviors and processes have physical, psychocultural, and social significance or meaning.
Levine's theory of nursing	Conservation, the holistic person	A living being who continually interacts with his or her environments and adapts to change	The health care system, including the nurse	Maintenance of the unity and integrity of the client	A discipline that focuses on the human and the complexity of his or her relationships with the environment; the essence of nursing is human interaction
Neuman's health care systems model	A health care systems model for a total person approach to client problems	Each human is a total person as a client system and is a composite of biologic, psychologic, sociocultural, and developmental variables	Those internal and external forces that surround humans and with which they constantly interact	Views health as levels of wellness or stable lines of defense	A unique profession, concerning itself with all the variables affecting human response to stressors, with a primary concern for the total person

(continued)

TABLE 4 - 1 *(continued)*

Theorists and Their Conceptual Models

Theorist	Central Theme	Definitions			
		Person	Environment	Health	Nursing
Orem's self-care model	Nursing and self-care activities	Humans with physical, psychologic, interpersonal, and social components, meeting self-care needs through learned behavior	Modern society's values and expectations	Wellness in the integrity of the individual; illness results in the person's inability to maintain self-care	The giving of direct assistance to a person who is unable to meet his or her own self-care needs, developed through nursing education and experiences
Rogers' science of unitary man [sic]	Unitary human and his or her life processes; nursing science	Humans who are unified beings with individuality, in continuous exchange of energy with the environment	All of the patterns that exist external to the individual	Not specifically defined	An art and a science directed toward the unitary human and concerned with the nature and direction of human development
Roy's adaptation model	The person in constant interaction with a changing environment	A biopsychosocial being that is basically good	All the conditions, circumstances, and influences surrounding and affecting the development of organisms	A state or process of being or becoming an integrated and whole person	A theoretical system in which knowledge prescribes a process of analysis and action related to the care of the ill or potentially ill person
Watson's theory of caring	Nursing as a human science and human care	A person who is in need of the caring process to attain or maintain health or die a peaceful death; the person has personal, internal, and mental-spiritual mechanisms to allow the self to be healed.	Human life—the spiritual–mental–physical being in the world, which is continuous in time and space	The unity and harmony within the mind, body, and soul; the degree of congruence between the self as perceived and the self as experienced	An art and science of a human-to-human care process with a spiritual dimension; nursing comprises knowledge, thought, values, philosophy, commitment, and action

permits functioning in roles. A nurse (having special knowledge and skills) and a client (with self-knowledge and personal problems) interact to identify problems and to establish and achieve goals. Based on this theory, King offers several propositions, including the following:

- If perceptual accuracy is present in nurse–client interactions, transactions will occur.
- If nurse and client make transactions, goals are attained.
- If goals are attained, effective nursing care will occur.
- If nurses with special knowledge and skills communicate appropriate information to clients, mutual goal setting and goal attainment will occur.

Madeline Leininger: Transcultural Care Diversity and Universality

Leininger's theoretical/conceptual model of nursing is based on the belief that nursing is a transcultural care profession, with care being the central area of concern for nursing. Nursing is believed to be an art and a science that provides culture-specific care to individuals and groups to promote or maintain health behaviors or recovery from illnesses.

Within the model are the following three types of culturally based nursing actions:

Cultural care preservation (maintenance): Those culturally based actions that help the individual preserve or maintain favorable health and caring lifeways.

Cultural care accommodation (negotiations): Those culturally based actions that reflect ways to adapt, negotiate, or adjust to the health and caring lifeways of others.

Cultural care repatterning (reconstruction): Those reconstructed or altered designed to help clients change meaningful health or life patterns.

The model is based on a substantial number of propositions and assumptions. A selected sample are as follows:

- Culture is the blueprint for thought and action and is the dominant force in determining health-illness caring patterns and behaviors.
- Cultural values vary among all humans and groups of humans.
- Human caring is a universal phenomenon that is expressed differently in all cultures.
- Caring unifies the intellectual and practical dimensions of nursing.

Myra E. Levine: Theory of Nursing

Myra Levine based her theory of nursing on the belief that the essence of nursing is human interaction. Assumptions that define the theory are as follows:

Condition: Clients entering the health care system are in a state of illness or altered health.

Responsibilities: The nurse is responsible for recognizing the client's organismic response (ie, changes in behavior or level of body function) as the client adapts or attempts to adapt to the environment (environment equals illness and nurse). The four levels of response are (1) fear, (2) stress, (3) inflammatory, and (4) sensory.

Functions: Nursing functions include interventions to promote adaptation to illness and evaluation of interventions as supportive or therapeutic. Supportive interventions help maintain the present health state and prevent further illness. Therapeutic interventions promote healing and restore health.

The foundation for all nursing intervention, as defined by Levine, consists of four conservation (meaning to maintain balance) principles that support the goal of nursing, which is to maintain or restore a person to a state of health:

Conservation of energy: Balancing energy intake and output to avoid excessive fatigue (rest, nutrition, exercise)

Conservation of structural integrity: Maintaining or restoring the structure of the body (promoting healing)

Conservation of personal integrity: Maintaining or restoring a sense of identity and self-worth (recognition of unique qualities)

Conservation of social integrity: Recognizing the client as a social being (especially with significant others)

Levine's theory is focused on one person—the client. This theory has major implications in acute-care settings, where nursing interventions are supportive or therapeutic.

Betty Neuman: Health Care Systems Model

Neuman's model, the *total person approach,* can be used to provide an organized approach to a variety of nursing problems and for understanding humans and their environment. The model focuses on the client system's reaction to stress and the factors of reconstitution or adaptation. The person is an open system interacting with the environment. Surrounding each person are internal and external factors that are stressors. Over a lifetime, the person becomes a "normal line of defense" who uses biologic, psychologic, sociocultural, and developmental skills to deal with stressors. Stressors cause the line of defense to react or respond as the total person. The stressors may be extrapersonal, interpersonal, or intrapersonal. The effect of the stressors on the system is individualized and depends on such variables as the number of stressors, how long they last, and the system's coping skills.

Nursing interventions can be carried out on three preventive levels. When the stressor is identified but no reaction has occurred, interventions can decrease the degree of reaction or increase the line of defense. This is called *primary prevention.* When the reaction has already happened, *secondary prevention* is carried out, with interventions aimed at treating symptoms and reducing reactions. After active treatment, *tertiary prevention* strengthens the lines of defense through education and uses the system's total resources to prevent further occurrences.

Dorothea E. Orem: Self-Care Model

The nursing model of Dorothea Orem is based on the belief that the individual has a need for self-care actions and that nursing can assist in meeting that need to maintain life, health, and well-being. The model is widely used in all areas of nursing. *Self-care*, as defined by Orem, consists of the activities that individuals carry out on their own behalf. These actions are deliberate, having pattern and sequence, developed from day-to-day living. The ability of the individual to perform self-care is called *self-care agency* and is usually carried out by adults. Infants, children, and aged, ill, and disabled people require complete care or help with self-care activities. Three categories of *self-care requisites* (the purposes of actions directed toward the provision of self-care) follow:

Universal self-care requisites: These are common to all humans and are associated with maintaining life, health, and well-being. They include air, water, food, elimination, activity and rest, solitude and social interaction, prevention of hazards, and promotion of human functioning.

Developmental self-care requisites: These include maintaining conditions to support life and human development.

Health deviation self-care: This is required in illness, injury, or as a result of medical tests or treatments to correct a condition.

Orem suggests that a person needs nursing when the person has a health-related self-care deficit. The areas of nursing practice are:

- Entering into and maintaining nurse–client relationships with individuals, families, or groups
- Determining if and how clients can be helped through nursing
- Responding to clients' requests and needs
- Giving direct help to clients and families
- Coordinating and integrating nursing with the client's daily living, other health care activities, and social or educational services required

Orem has defined three nursing systems on the premise that the nursing system depends on the self-care needs and abilities of the client. In the first system, the nurse gives total care to meet all needs. In the second, both the nurse and the client perform care measures. In the third, the client can carry out self-care activities but requires assistance.

Martha E. Rogers: Nursing— A Science of Unitary Man

Martha Rogers has written a complex theory of nursing. The goal of this theory is to develop a science of nursing that would provide a growing body of theoretical knowledge applicable in nursing practice to the achievement of meaningful service to humanity.

Rogers' theory is built on a knowledge base of the history of humanity and of the universe (anthropology, sociology, astronomy, religion, philosophy, history, and mythology). Based on the belief that humans are the center of nursing's purpose, Rogers' theory considers the total individual, describing the human life process and explaining and predicting the nature and direction of human development. Both systems and developmental theories are a part of Rogers' theory.

Rogers' basic assumptions about humans are as follows:

- Humans are unified wholes that are more than a sum of their parts.
- Humans are constantly interacting with their environment.
- Anything that occurs in life is unique because no two things in life can ever be repeated in an identical manner or under identical circumstances.
- Humans develop patterns of behaving, and their behavior becomes predictable.
- Humans are distinctive in their capacity for abstract thought, imagery, and emotion.

Nursing concepts are derived and nursing science principles are identified from these basic assumptions. Based on these assumptions, Rogers identifies four building blocks:

Energy fields: Both the human and the environment are viewed as energy fields; there is a constant exchange of energy between the two that is essential to life.

Openness: This is based on the belief that the universe consists of open systems.

Pattern and organization: These are identifying characteristics of the energy field that is undergoing continuous change.

Four-dimensionality: This is a characteristic of both human and environmental fields.

Sister Calista Roy: Roy's Adaptation Model

Sister Calista Roy (1984) developed the adaptation model of nursing. This model is widely used as a philosophical base and conceptual model in nursing education. The adaptation model is essentially a systems model. The assumptions basic to this model are as follows:

- Each person is a biophysical being and an integrated whole. All body systems are balanced to produce a functioning person with biologic, psychosocial, and social needs. Constant interaction with the changing environment of the modern world subjects the person to continual changes and stressors.
- Each person uses both innate and acquired mechanisms to cope with changes and adapt individually, with either positive or negative responses. The adaptation level reached is the result of three classes of stimuli—the primary cause of the change, other situational factors, and beliefs and past experiences shaping the response.
- Each person responds to needs (requirements within the individual stimulating a response to maintain integrity) in one or more of four modes—physiologic, self-concept, interdependent behaviors, and role-function.
- Each person's position on the health-illness continuum changes in relation to the effectiveness of coping to maintain an adaptive state.

As defined by Roy, response to a decrease in body integrity creates a need state, and the individual responds with an act or behavior. The physiologic mode involves oxygenation and circulation, fluid and electrolyte balance, nutrition, rest and activity, and regulation of temperature, hormones, and sensory function. The self-concept mode is concerned with the perception of one's physical self and personal self, including personality, moral and ethical beliefs, and values. The interdependence mode involves social relationships, including both the need to be interdependent and the need for support by others. The role-function mode involves the behaviors of a person in each role taken on in life (Rambo, 1984).

In Roy's model, all nursing activity is aimed at promoting the individual's adaptation to health and illness in all four adaptive modes. This model guides the nurse in using observation and interviewing skills to make an individualized assessment of each person, and serves as a guide in planning and carrying out nursing actions.

Jean Watson: Nursing—Human Science and Human Care

Jean Watson's theory and philosophy of caring is based on the values of kindness, concern, love of self and others, and respect for the spiritual dimension of the person. In nursing as a human science (Watson, 1988), *human caring in nursing* is defined as an art and a science in which caring is a human-to-human process demonstrated through a therapeutic interpersonal interaction.

The basic assumptions of Watson's theory of nursing are as follows:

- A person's mind and emotions are windows to the soul. Although nurses give physical care and carry out procedures, the nurse's presence in the relationship transcend the physical and material world, facilitating the client to develop a higher sense of self.
- Although a person's body is confined in time and space, the mind and soul transcends time and space and may be an indicator of the spiritual evolution of humans.
- A nurse may have access to a person's inner self, provided the physical body is not perceived and treated as separate from the mind, emotions, and sense of self.
- People need each other in a caring, loving way. Love and caring are needs that are often overlooked. We need to love, respect, and care for ourselves with dignity before we can respect, love, and care for others and treat them with dignity (Watson, 1988, pp. 50–51).

Within the theory, optimal health is the attainment of all needs, but even when the scientists in medicine believe that nothing can be done for a client, the nurse can provide care by providing comfort measures and instilling hope. Caring is the mechanism by which nurses help individuals and groups reach self-actualization, maintain or attain health, or die a peaceful death. Holistic, individualized care is given through transpersonal caring, which is a human art, a human science, and the moral ideal of nursing.

Application of Conceptual and Theoretical Frameworks

The aims of nursing, described in Chapter 1, are the same for all nursing theorists, but the values, assumptions, and beliefs individualize each framework when giving nursing care. The brief case study that follows illustrates how the conceptual and theoretical frameworks discussed in this chapter apply to an individual requiring nursing care.

 CASE STUDY

Julie Smith is an 18-year-old college freshman. She has an academic scholarship and is active in music and art activities. When Julie came home for winter vacation, her parents were alarmed to see her so thin. Her mother cooked all of Julie's favorite foods, but Julie refused to eat more than a few bites, saying that she was "too fat."

The mother finally convinced Julie to go to the doctor. The examination showed that Julie weighed only 85 pounds; she had lost more than 20 pounds in 4 months. After tests showed no disease process, the doctor diagnosed anorexia nervosa.

Based on Johnson's model, nursing care for Julie would initially focus on ineffective functioning within or between the behavioral subsystems. The nurse would carry out planning and implementation to give Julie the external support necessary to modify her behaviors, return to a state of equilibrium, and regain effective functioning of her whole system.

Based on King's theory, nursing care for Julie would use communications and mutual participation in the plan of care. The nurse and Julie would mutually interact to identify problems, set goals, and carry out planned activities. An effective plan of care would result in Julie's self-fulfillment and health maintenance.

A nursing care plan for Julie, when using Leininger's model as a framework, would be based on Julie's cultural values, beliefs, and health practices. Using that knowledge, the nurse would provide nursing interventions that have physical, psychocultural, and social significance for Julie. If Julie's cultural practices were different from those of the nurse, it would be important for the nurse to remember that nurses should not value the health care practices of their own culture to the exclusion of the client's culture.

Levine's theory would emphasize the nurse's interventions necessary to help Julie adapt to and reach a state of health. A holistic assessment of Julie would provide information about strengths and weaknesses and would allow a nursing diagnosis. The plan of care would include supportive or therapeutic interventions that are evaluated in terms of their effect on Julie's health status.

Using Neuman's model, the plan of care for Julie would be based on a total person approach. Assessments and interventions would focus on Julie's perceptions, responses, and resources relative to stressors in her environment and to the variables affecting her responses. Goals and interventions would be mutually designed for all three levels of preventive nursing care: (1) strengthening the flexible line of defense, (2) facilitating wellness, and (3) maintaining a maximum level of wellness. Nursing interventions should reduce the degree of Julie's reaction to stressors.

Using Orem's framework, the nurse would first assess and analyze Julie's ability to maintain therapeutic self-care and then would identify deficits to determine why nursing is needed. Based on this information, the nurse would design a system that would be most effective in overcoming the self-care deficits. The nurse then would implement the system to help Julie change conditions in herself or in her environment, and meet her self-care requirements.

When planning and giving nursing care to Julie using Roger's theory, the nurse would become an integral part of the environment that is focused on Julie as a whole person, working toward achieving optimal health. The plan of care would be based on an analysis of Julie's interactions with the environment, including past and present experiences as well as behavioral patterns and developmental level. Nursing activities would be directed toward modifying variations in the behavior patterns and life processes so that Julie could reach her total potential as a human.

Using Roy's model, the nurse would focus on promoting Julie's adaptive responses to improve health. A nursing process would be used first to assess behaviors affecting Julie's health and then to make a nursing diagnosis, stating the desired adaptive behaviors. The goals of the nursing care plan would be derived through mutual agreement with Julie. The nursing interventions planned and carried out would be aimed at altering the environmental stimuli so that an adaptive response could be made, or at increasing Julie's coping ability to make healthy adaptive responses.

The care of Julie, based on Watson's theory, would be based in participative, interpersonal experiences between Julie and her nurse. The nurse would pass on to Julie feelings that have been lived through, realized, or learned. As Julie experienced these same feelings, she would be able to facilitate self-healing and discover inner power and control.

The application of conceptual and theoretical frameworks of nursing provides a focus for nursing care activities. The person receiving care is the central theme, but the way each theorist defines that person, the environment, health, and nursing gives the methodology of nursing a unique focus specific to a particular theory or model. The ultimate goal of each framework, however, is holistic client care, individualized to meet needs, prevent illness, and promote wellness.

KEY POINTS

- Nursing is a combination of a body of knowledge and the application of that knowledge through nursing practice.
- Large bodies of knowledge organize and structure both facts and events into philosophies, concepts, and theories. These bodies of knowledge are then put into action by a process. In nursing, this is the nursing process.
- Nursing theories define concepts and relations specific to nursing, using orderly reasoning and logical sequence. They should be both understandable and widely applicable.
- Nursing theories provide for the improvement of nursing practice through nursing research.
- Florence Nightingale's philosophy and theory of nursing provided the base for modern nursing.

- Nursing theory describes or explains nursing and usually includes the concepts of person, environment, health, and nursing.
- Nursing theories are often based on other processes and theories, including general systems, adaptation, and human development.
- Changes in society during the 20th century led to improvement and advances in nursing education, nursing research, and nursing practice.
- Nursing theory provides rationale for nursing actions, gives direction to all aspects of nursing, improves communications, and provides autonomy for the profession of nursing.
- Individual theories and conceptual models provide an organizing framework that can be applied to nursing practice.

BIBLIOGRAPHY

Barnum, B. (1990). *Nursing theory: Analysis, application, evaluation* (3rd ed.). Boston: Little, Brown.

Chinn, P., & Jacobs, M. (1991). *Theory and nursing: A systematic approach* (3rd ed.). St. Louis, MO: Mosby.

Dolan, J. A., Fitzpatrick, M. L., & Herrmann, E. K. (1983). *Nursing in society: A historical perspective.* Philadelphia: Saunders.

Fawcett, J. (1989). *Analysis and evaluation of conceptual models of nursing* (2nd ed.) Philadelphia: Davis.

Fitzpatrick, J., & Whall, A. (1983). *Conceptual models of nursing: Analysis and application.* Bowie, MD: Brady Communications.

George, J. (Ed.). (1990). *Nursing theories: The base for professional practice* (3rd ed.). Englewood Cliffs, NJ: Prentice-Hall.

Hekton, L. M. (1989). Martha E. Rogers: A life history. *Nursing Science Quarterly, 2*(2), 63–73.

Huch, M. H. (1988). Theory-based practice: Structuring nursing care. *Nursing Science Quarterly, 1*(1), 6–7.

Johnson, D. (1959). The nature of a science in nursing. *Nursing Outlook, 7*(5), 291–294.

Kalish, P., & Kalish, B. (1986). *The advance of American nursing* (2nd ed.). Boston: Little, Brown.

Kim, H. (1983). *The nature of theoretical thinking in nursing.* Norwalk, CT: Appleton-Century-Crofts.

King, I. (1971). *Toward a theory for nursing: General concepts of human behavior.* New York: Wiley.

Leininger, M. M. (1978). *Transcultural nursing: Concepts, theories, and practices.* New York: Wiley.

Leininger, M. M. (1979). *Transcultural nursing.* New York: Masson.

Leininger, M. M. (1988). Leininger's theory of nursing: Cultural care diversity and universality. *Nursing Science Quarterly, 1*(4), 152–160.

Levine, M. (1973). *Introduction to clinical nursing* (2nd ed.). Philadelphia: Davis.

Malenski, V. M. (1986). *Explorations on Martha Roger's science of unitary human being.* Norwalk, CT: Appleton-Century-Crofts.

McCann/Flynn, J. B., & Heffron, P. B. (1988). *Nursing from concept to practice* (2nd ed.). East Norwalk, CT: Appleton & Lange.

Melies, A. I. (1989). *Theoretical nursing: Development and progress.* Philadelphia: Lippincott.

Neuman, B. (1989). *The Newman systems model.* Norwalk, CT: Appleton & Lange.

Nevin-Haas, M. (1992). Checking the fit. *Canadian Nurse L'Infirmiere, 88*(2), 33–34.

Orem, D. (Ed.). (1979). *Concept formalization in nursing: Process and product* (2nd ed.). Boston: Little, Brown.

Orem, D. (1991). *Nursing: Concepts of practice* (4th ed.). St. Louis: Mosby–Year Book.

Rambo, B. (1984). *Adaptation nursing: Assessment and intervention.* Philadelphia: Saunders.

Riehl, J., & Roy, C. (1980). *Conceptual models for nursing practice* (2nd ed.). Norwalk, CT: Appleton-Century-Crofts.

Rogers, M. (1970). *The theoretical basis of nursing.* Philadelphia: Davis.

Roy, C. (1984). *Introduction to nursing: An adaptation model* (2nd ed.). Englewood Cliffs, NJ: Prentice-Hall.

Stevens, B. (1978). *Theory development: Why, why, how?* New York: National League for Nursing.

Thibodeau, J. (1983). *Nursing models: Analysis and evaluation.* Monterey, CA: Wadsworth Health Sciences.

Torres, G. (1990). The place of concepts and theories within nursing. In J. B. George (Ed.). *Nursing theories: The base for professional practice* (pp. 1–12). Norwalk, CT: Appleton & Lange.

Waley, L., & Wong, D. (1991). *Nursing care of infants and children* (4th ed.). St. Louis: Mosby.

Watson, J. (1985). *Nursing: Human science and human care.* Norwalk, CT: Appleton-Century-Crofts.

Watson, J. (1987). Nursing on the caring edge: Metaphorical vignettes. *Advances in Nursing Science, 10*(1), 10–17.

Watson, J. (1988). *Nursing: Human science and human care: A theory of nursing* (Pub. No. 15–2236). New York: National League for Nursing.

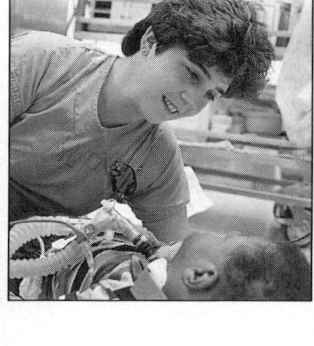
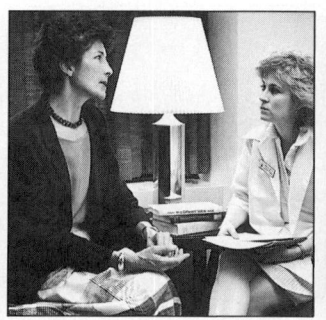
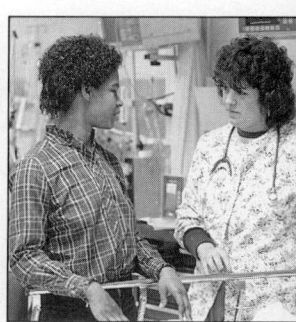

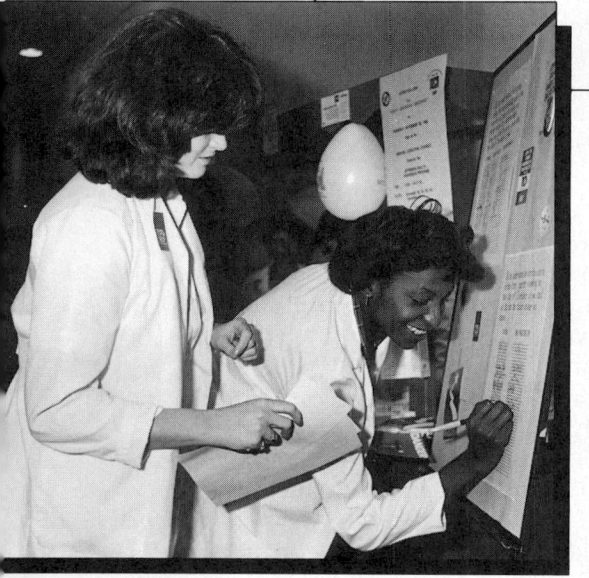

Values and Ethics in Nursing

OBJECTIVES

After studying this chapter, the learner should be able to:

Define key terms used in the chapter.

List five common modes of value transmission.

Identify the seven basic values essential in the practice of nursing.

Describe seven steps in the valuing process.

Use values clarification strategies in clinical practice.

Identify three sources of standards for professional ethical conduct.

Describe nursing practice that is consistent with the code of ethics for nursing.

Describe three typical concerns of the nurse advocate.

Recognize ethical issues as they arise in nursing practice.

Use an ethical framework and decision-making process to resolve ethical problems.

Identify four functions of institutional ethics committees.

KEY TERMS

advocacy
attitude
autonomy
beliefs
beneficence
biomedical ethics
confidentiality
deontologic
ethic of caring
ethics
ethics committee
fidelity
justice
morals
nonmaleficence
nursing ethics
paternalism
respect for persons
utilitarian
value
values clarification
value system
veracity

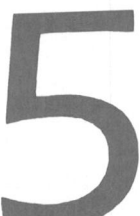

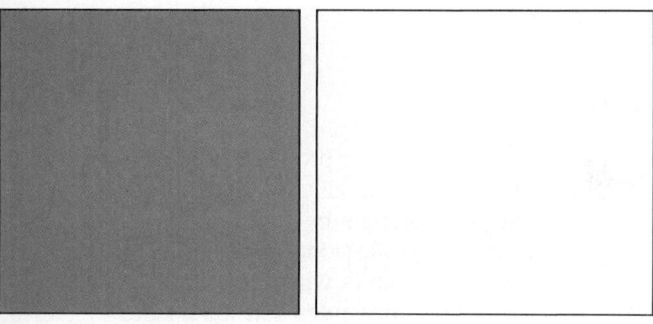

The unique nature of nursing places nurses at the bedside and in groups of professionals where sensitive decisions are made about the best way to treat illness and solve health care problems. Often the question confronting the nurse is not "how do I do this?" but rather "should I do this?" The more science and technology increase the options available to clients and health care professionals, the more frequently nurses will find themselves asking, "Just because we can do this, *should we,* here and now, for this client?" The answer to this and other ethical questions is too important for nurses to base their responses on some intuitive, opinionated, or self-imposed sense of right and wrong.

This chapter explores the influence of values on human behavior and the ethical dimensions of nursing practice. Nurses who understand how clients' values and their own values shape nurse–client interactions and who continually develop sensitivity to the ethical dimensions of nursing practice are best able to provide quality care.

Values

A **value** is a personal belief about worth that acts as a standard to guide one's behavior. A **value system** is an organization of values in which each value is ranked along a continuum of importance; a value system often operates as a personal code of conduct.

Because attitudes and beliefs also influence human behavior, it is important to distinguish them from values. An **attitude** is a feeling or an emotion, generally including positive or negative judgment, toward people, objects, or ideas. **Beliefs** refer to a special class of intellectual attitudes based primarily on faith as opposed to fact.

A person's values influence beliefs about human needs, health, and illness; the practice of health behaviors; and human responses to illness. Nurses who work effectively with clients are sensitive to how a client's values and their own values influence their interactions.

Types of Values

The following six basic types of values underlie a person's interests and motives (Feldman & Newcomb, 1969):

Theoretical: The theoretical person values truth and tends to be empirical, critical, and rational.

Economic: The economic person is interested in what is practical and useful.

Aesthetic: The aesthetic person values beauty, form, and harmony.

Social: The social person values humans in terms of love, and is kind, sympathetic, and unselfish.

Political: The political person values power.

Religious: The religious person values unity.

Although each person's value orientation is a unique blend of these six types of values, one of the types usually predominates. The accompanying display illustrates different nursing responses to the problem of understaffing based on these six value types. Identifying one's own orientation as well as that of others helps the nurse understand how and why people perceive situations differently and choose different courses of action.

Development of Values

An individual is not born with values. Rather, values are formed over a lifetime from information from the environment, family, and culture. As children observe actions, they quickly learn what has high and low value for family members. If the parents spend a good portion of each day cooking and the family spends a long time eating and talking at the table, the children learn to value food and the good times it represents. Similarly, children learn helpfulness is a good and respected quality if praised when helping parents, grandparents, and siblings.

Common modes of value transmission include the following:

Modeling: Children learn what is of high or low value by observing parents, peers, and significant others. Thus, modeling may lead to socially acceptable or unacceptable behavior.

Moralizing: Children are taught a complete value system by parents or an institution (eg, church or school) that allows little opportunity for children to weigh different values.

Laissez-faire: Children are left to explore values (no one set of values is presented as best for all) and to develop a personal value system. This approach is often accompanied by little or no guidance and can lead to confusion and conflict.

Rewarding and punishing: Children are rewarded when demonstrating values held by parents and punished when demonstrating unacceptable values.

Responsible choice: Children are encouraged to explore different values and to weigh their consequences. Support and guidance are offered as children develop a personal value system.

Values Essential to the Professional Nurse

In 1985, the American Association of Colleges of Nursing undertook a project that included the identification of values essential to the practice of professional nursing. The group identified seven values (aesthetics, altruism, equal-

Basic Value Orientations and Related Interests and Motives

Situation: Nurses on a 21-bed surgical unit are upset because nursing management has no plans to replace two full-time nurses who transferred out of the unit. Understaffing has resulted, and other nurses are frequently asked to work extra shifts. The nurses have varying views of the situation.

Theoretical Orientation

"Let's begin keeping some data about how many clients we have, what level of nursing care they need, how many nurses are on duty each shift, how often we work doubles. If we have the figures to prove we can't give quality care while understaffed this way—can show that clients are actually at risk—management will have to listen!"

Economic Orientation

"I do the best I can and then I go home *on time* and forget about this place. It's just a job. If it gets much worse I'll find a better job somewhere else."

Aesthetic Orientation

"I just live one day at a time and judge each day on its own merit. I try to keep our environment nice even in stressful times, like bringing flowers for the nurses' station and a radio for the lounge."

Social Orientation

"We've just got to find a way to give better care or die trying. The clients deserve more. I try to do my part by working overtime without pay and doing double shifts even when I'm tired. I'm afraid I may be headed for burnout."

Political Orientation

"The longer we put up with these working conditions, the longer we'll have them. I say we need action and we need it now. If we could just unite we'd make them listen to us fast!"

Religious Orientation

"I try to be a source of strength for both my clients and my colleagues. There seems to be an awful lot wrong with the system and no one is happy. Let's see what we can do, as individuals and together, to improve things."

Value Neutrality

In an effort to encourage health care professionals to respect and accept the individuality of clients, some educators have advised that professionals be "value-neutral" and "nonjudgmental" in their professional roles. Thus the nurse has a "commitment to clients whether or not the nurse and the clients hold the same values. The nurse does not assume that personal values are right and should not judge the client's values as right or wrong depending on their congruence with the nurse's personal value system" (Steele & Harmon, 1983, p. 27). This kind of thinking enables a nurse to care for a client with different values. For example, a nurse who strongly believes that any premarital or extramarital sex is wrong may offer competent and compassionate nursing care to a young female prostitute with active herpes lesions. On the other hand, if the same client, following education, indicates that she is unconcerned about whom she might infect in future sexual encounters, the nurse is in no way bound to be nonjudgmental about this response. In this case, it would not be morally permissible for the nurse to view this behavior with indifference. Because not all values are equal, nurses may have a moral obligation to respond to a client whose values may lead to harm for the client or others.

Values Clarification

Values clarification is a process by which people come to understand their own values and value system. "It is a process of discovery and allows the person to discover through feelings and analysis of behavior what choices to make when alternatives are presented, and to identify whether or not these choices are rationally made or are the result of previous conditioning" (Steele & Harmon, 1983, p. 13). Values clarification has a beneficial application to nursing.

Values theorists most often describe the process of valuing as having seven steps centered on three main activities: (1) choosing, (2) prizing, and (3) acting (Raths, Simon, & Harmin, 1978; Simon, 1972). When one values something, one:

Chooses
- Freely
- From alternatives
- After careful consideration of the consequences of each alternative

Prizes
- With pride and happiness
- With public affirmation

Acts
- With incorporation of the choice into one's behavior
- With consistency and regularity on the value

Values Clarification by the Nurse

For example, if respect for human dignity is a value that characterizes your nursing practice, you:

ity, freedom, human dignity, justice, and truth) and related attitudes and personal qualities. These values are defined, and examples given, in the accompanying display.

Essential Values of the Professional Nurse, With Examples of Attitudes and Personality Qualities*

Aesthetics

Qualities of objects, events, and people that provide satisfaction

Appreciation
Creativity
Imagination
Sensitivity

- Adapts the environment so it is pleasing to the client
- Creates a pleasant work environment for self and others
- Presents self in a manner that promotes a positive image of nursing

Altruism

Concern for the welfare of others

Caring
Commitment
Compassion
Generosity
Perseverance

- Gives full attention to the client when providing care
- Assists other personnel in providing care when they are unable to do so
- Expresses concern about social trends and issues that have implications for health care

Equality

Having the same rights, privileges, or status

Acceptance
Assertiveness
Fairness
Self-esteem
Tolerance

- Provides nursing care based on the client's needs irrespective of personal characteristics†
- Interacts with other providers in a nondiscriminatory manner
- Expresses ideas about the improvement of access to nursing and health care

Freedom

Capacity to exercise choice

Confidence
Hope
Independence
Openness
Self-direction
Self-discipline

- Honors individual's right to refuse treatment
- Supports the rights of other providers to suggest alternatives to the plan of care
- Encourages open discussion of controversial issues in the profession

Human Dignity

Inherent worth and uniqueness of an individual

Consideration
Empathy
Humaneness
Kindness
Respectfulness
Trust

- Safeguards the individual's right to privacy
- Addresses others as they prefer to be addressed
- Maintains confidentiality of clients and staff
- Treats others with respect regardless of ground

Justice

Upholding of moral and legal principles

Courage
Integrity
Morality
Objectivity

- Acts as a health care advocate
- Allocates resources fairly
- Reports incompetent, unethical, and illegal practice objectively and factually

Truth

Faithfulness to fact and reality

Accountability
Authenticity
Honesty
Inquisitiveness
Rationality
Reflectiveness

- Documents nursing care accurately and honestly
- Obtains sufficient data to make sound judgments before reporting infractions of organizational policies
- Participates in professional efforts to protect the public from misinformation about nursing

*Values are listed in alphabetic rather than priority order.

†From American Nurses' Association. (1976). *Code for nurses*. Washington, DC: Author.

(Essentials of college and university education for professional nursing. [1986]. Washington, DC: American Association of Colleges of Nursing.)

Choose
- Freely choose to believe in the worth and uniqueness of each individual
- Realize that you have other options (that you could treat with dignity only those people who are most like you)

- Believe that respecting each person's human dignity yields the best consequences for you and for all of society

Prize
- Feel proud and happy with your choice (you especially enjoy when clients let you know they appreciate your

Steps in the Valuing Process

Case: A male client with high blood pressure

Choosing

1. Freely
Rehospitalized for high blood pressure after abruptly stopping his antihypertensive medication, the client decides from now on to take his medication as prescribed.

2. From Alternatives
After a teaching–learning session with a nurse, the client understands he has basically three options:
- Comply with prescribed treatment regimen.
- Refuse to take the medication but try harder to control his blood pressure through diet, exercise, and stress management.
- Refuse to take his medication and assume a "we'll see" attitude.

3. After Consideration of the Consequences
The client understands the *probable* consequences of these options:
- Compliance with the treatment regimen will yield the best control of high blood pressure (but may cause some annoying side effects).
- Diet, exercise, and stress management may reduce his blood pressure somewhat but did not yield sufficient control in the past.
- High blood pressure may result in serious complications such as stroke, kidney disease, or impaired vision.

Prizing

4. With Pride and Happiness
The client states, "Now that I understand high blood pressure better and know what I can do to control it, I feel more in charge of my life—and I like that!"

5. With Public Affirmation
The client states to his wife, "I guess I was wrong to stop taking that medicine when I blamed it for how lousy I was feeling. You can bet that won't happen again. If you ever hear me complaining about my pills, remind me to see my doctor right away."

Acting

6. With Incorporation of the Choice into One's Behavior
After discharge from the hospital, the client takes the medication as prescribed.

7. With Consistency and Regularity on the Value
The client seeks to understand any new medication he is prescribed (ie, reason for the medication, possible side effects, consequences of noncompliance) and successfully manages the treatment regimen; he feels proud of his new knowledge and self-care abilities.

---

care and when nursing colleagues and supervisors compliment you on interpersonal skills)
- Are able to defend this value when someone's human dignity is being ignored

Act
- Incorporate this value into your practice
- Attempt consistently to respect human dignity in both your personal and professional life

As you become more conscious of this value, you will be sensitive to those of your actions that are inconsistent with it. You may feel uncomfortable after gossiping with other nurses during break about a client no one likes; you realize that this behavior contradicts your basic respect for human dignity. Thus, values clarification is a "process by which we increase the likelihood that our living in general, and a decision in particular [to respect human dignity], will, first, have a positive value for us, and, second, for the society we serve" (Kirschbaum, 1977).

The nurse interested in values clarification strategies is referred to the book by Steele and Harmon (1983), who offer numerous exercises for nurses seeking to clarify their personal and professional values. Another reference is an article by Uustal (1978), who offers 10 strategies designed to increase your awareness and appreciation of yourself, and to explore selected values conflicts and ethical dilemmas in nursing.

Clinical Applications

Unless the nurse is comfortable with change and believes that health is important enough to merit learning a new treatment regimen, client education is doomed to failure. The accompanying display illustrates how the steps in the valuing process can be used to assist a male client with high blood pressure take charge of his health and manage his medications. Other clinical examples follow.

Client Places Low Value on Health and Health Behaviors
You become frustrated when repeated attempts to teach or counsel a 26-year-old pharmaceutical salesperson meet with failure. Although hospitalized with a serious duodenal ulcer, all he can talk about is his job and meeting his sales quota.

Values Clarification First help this client identify his basic life values. Ask him, "What three things are most important to you in life?" or have him rank the following behaviors in terms of how he would most likely spend an unexpected free day:

_____ Enjoy some quiet time alone (eg, thinking, reading, listening to music)

_____ Spend time with family, friends

_____ Do something active (eg, hiking, playing ball, swimming)

_____ Watch television

_____ Volunteer time and energy to help someone else

_____ Use time for my job

_____ Other _____

Discuss what these rankings indicate about his values. Determine whether his rankings would be different if he were asked how he *wished* he would spend the free day versus how he would *most likely* spend it.

Choosing After exploring with this client how values might affect other aspects in his life (ie, long-term effects of stress related to his present preoccupation with job performance), counsel him to choose his key values freely. It would be a positive sign if health were among these values, but it might not be.

Prizing Use affirmation to reinforce the client's wellness-promoting values and, when possible, enlist the support of family members. For example: "Your wife seemed so happy yesterday when you told her you decided to quit smoking. You can see how much she loves you and values your health."

Acting Assist the client to plan new behaviors consistent with the values he has chosen and to think of ways those behaviors can be incorporated into his life. "Once you get home, how will your life be different?" "You said you wanted to begin to take time for yourself—how are you going to do this?"

Values of Client and Family Members Conflict You sense a growing tension while counseling the young parents of a child with asthma. Questioning ("You seem uncomfortable with what I'm saying now. Is there something wrong?") reveals that the wife is a confirmed smoker and cat lover who has told her husband that even if these behaviors are hurting their child, she is unwilling to give them up.

Values Clarification Suggest that both parents complete the following "values voting" exercise (the format of the exercise was adapted from Uustal, 1978). Then share with one another what factors influence their behavior.

Where do you stand on the following issues? (Indicate your responses in the following manner: SA, strongly agree; A, agree; D, disagree; SD, strongly disagree; U, undecided.)

_____ A parent's primary obligation is to meet the needs of his or her child.

_____ Each member of a family is entitled to pursue personal pleasures—even if these are not in the best interest of all.

_____ Pleasure is more important than health.

_____ The choices one family member makes can dramatically affect other family members (positively and negatively).

This exercise will help the parents to evaluate their basic values, explore areas of conflict, and, perhaps, move toward joint choosing, prizing, and acting on several health-promoting values.

Ethics

Ethics is systematic inquiry into the principles of right and wrong conduct, of virtue and vice, and of good and evil as they relate to conduct. Many people use the term *ethics* when describing the professional ethics incorporated into a code of professional conduct, such as nursing codes of ethics. **Morals,** although similar in meaning to ethics, usually refers to personal standards of right and wrong. It is important to distinguish ethics from law, custom, and institutional practices. Ethical considerations logically precede legal and social considerations. Just because an action is legal or customary does not make it "right."

As nurses assume increasing responsibility for managing care, it is critical that they be prepared to recognize the ethical dimensions of this care and to participate competently in ethical decision making. In a national study of baccalaureate nursing students before graduation and 1 year after graduation (Cassells, Redman, & Jackson, 1986), 72% of respondents reported having been involved in an ethical issue in clinical practice. In order of frequency, these issues were as follows:

- Clients refusing treatment (73%)
- Moral dilemmas in caring for clients with a poor prognosis (72%)
- Issues regarding resuscitation or discontinuation of lifesaving treatment (67%)
- Issues of informed consent (54%)
- Evaluation of client's competency to make own decisions (50%)
- Issues regarding withholding information from clients (46%)
- Allocation of scarce resources (12%)

Ethics offers the nurse a means to look at and evaluate alternative courses of right action using basic moral concepts and principles.

Professional Ethical Conduct

Nurses, in their quest for high-quality care, determine and clarify their values, develop professional ethical behavior, and learn ethical decision-making skills. The study of professional ethical behavior begins in nursing school, continues in formal and informal discussions with colleagues and peers, and culminates when nurses "try on" and make their own the behaviors of role models who practice professional nursing that is consistent with high ethical standards. Where do nurses learn the standards for profes-

sional ethical behavior? Nursing codes of ethics and patient's bills of rights specify many aspects of professional behavior. Theories of ethics also provide assistance in making ethical decisions. These topics are discussed in the following sections.

Nursing Codes of Ethics

A professional code of ethics provides a framework for making ethical decisions and sets forth professional expectations. Nursing codes of ethics inform both nurses and society of the primary goals and values of the profession. Reflected in the codes are universal moral principles such as **respect for persons; autonomy** (self-determination); **beneficence** (doing good); **nonmaleficence** (avoiding

---

Three Codes of Ethics for Nurses

International Council of Nurses Code for Nurses*

The fundamental responsibility of the nurse is fourfold—to promote health, to prevent illness, to restore health, and to alleviate suffering.

The need for nursing is universal. Inherent in nursing is respect for life, dignity, and rights of humans. It is unrestricted by considerations of nationality, race, creed, age, sex, politics or social status.

Nurses render health services to the individual, the family, and the community and coordinate their services with those of related groups.

Nurses and People

The nurse's primary responsibility is to those people who require nursing care.

The nurse, in providing care, promotes an environment in which the values, customs, and spiritual beliefs of the individual are respected.

The nurse holds in confidence personal information and uses judgment in sharing this information.

Nurses and Practice

The nurse carries personal responsibility for nursing practice and for maintaining competence by continual learning. The nurse maintains the highest standards of nursing care possible within the reality of a specific situation.

The nurse uses judgment in relation to individual competence when accepting and delegating responsibilities.

The nurse, when acting in a professional capacity, should at all times maintain standards of personal conduct that reflect credit on the profession.

Nurses and Society

The nurse shares with other citizens the responsibility for initiating and supporting action to meet the health and social needs of the public.

Nurses and Coworkers

The nurse sustains a cooperative relationship with coworkers in nursing and other fields. The nurse takes appropriate action to safeguard the individual when his or her care is endangered by a coworker or any other person.

Nurses and the Profession

The nurse plays the major role in determining and implementing desirable standards of nursing practice and nursing education.

The nurse is active in developing a core of professional knowledge.

The nurse, acting through the professional organization, participates in establishing and maintaining equitable social and economic working conditions in nursing.

American Nurses' Association Code for Nurses†

1. The nurse provides services with respect for human dignity and the uniqueness of the client unre-

* Adapted from International Council of Nurses. (1973). ICN *Code for nurses: Ethical concepts applied to nursing.* Geneva, Imprimeries Populaires.

† From American Nurses' Association. (1985). *Code for nurses.* Kansas City, MO: Author.

‡ This represents only one element of the code—values. Obligations, which provide more specific direction for conduct than do values by spelling out what a value requires under particular circumstances, and limitations, which describe exceptional circumstances in which a value or obligation cannot be applied, are provided with each value in the publication.

harm); **veracity** (truth-telling); **confidentiality** (respecting privileged information); **fidelity** (keeping promises); and **justice** (treating people fairly). These principles should be compatible with the nurse's personal value system and moral code. Other functions of professional nursing codes include the following:

- Indicating nursing's acceptance of the responsibility and trust with which it has been invested by society
- Providing guidance for conduct and relationships in carrying out nursing responsibilities consistent with the ethical obligations of the profession and with high quality in nursing care
- Providing a means for the exercise of professional self-regulation (American Nurses' Association [ANA], 1985, pp. i to iv)

Codes are effective in accomplishing their goals only to the extent that they are upheld by members of the profession. Code requirements may exceed legal requirements. Although violations of the law subject a nurse to civil or criminal liability (see Chapter 6), violations of the code of ethics may result in reprimands, censure, suspension, and expulsion.

Codes of ethics for nursing include the International Council of Nurses (ICN) *ICN Code for Nurses* (adopted in 1953 and revised in 1965 and 1973); the ANA *Code for Nurses With Interpretive Statements* (adopted in 1950 and revised in 1968, 1976, and 1985); and the Canadian Nurses Association (CNA) *Code of Ethics for Nursing* (adopted in 1980 and revised in 1991). Ethical statements in the codes are given in the display.

---

stricted by considerations of social or economic status, personal attributes, or the nature of health problems.

2. The nurse safeguards the client's right to privacy by judiciously protecting information of a confidential nature.
3. The nurse acts to safeguard the client and the public when health care and safety are affected by the incompetent, unethical, or illegal practice of any person.
4. The nurse assumes responsibility and accountability for individual nursing judgments and actions.
5. The nurse maintains competence in nursing.
6. The nurse exercises informed judgment and uses individual competence and qualifications as criteria in seeking consultation, accepting responsibilities, and delegating nursing activities to others.
7. The nurse participates in activities that contribute to the ongoing development of the profession's body of knowledge.
8. The nurse participates in the profession's efforts to implement and improve standards of nursing.
9. The nurse participates in the profession's efforts to establish and maintain conditions of employment conducive to high quality nursing care.
10. The nurse participates in the profession's effort to protect the public from misinformation and misrepresentation and to maintain the integrity of nursing.
11. The nurse collaborates with members of the health professions and other citizens in promoting community and national efforts to meet the health needs of the public.

Canadian Nurses Association Code of Ethics for Nursing Clients†§

I. A nurse treats clients with respect for their individual needs and values.
II. Based on respect for clients and regard for their right to control their own care, nursing care reflects respect for the right of choice held by clients.
III. The nurse holds confidential all information about a client learned in the health care setting.
IV. The nurse is guided by consideration for the dignity of clients.
V. The nurse provides competent care to clients.
VI. The nurse maintains trust in nurses and nursing.
VII. The nurse recognizes the contribution and expertise of colleagues from nursing and other disciplines as essential to excellent health care.
VIII. The nurse takes steps to ensure that the client receives competent and ethical care.
IX. Conditions of employment should contribute in a positive way to client care and the professional satisfaction of nurses.
X. Job action by nurses is directed toward securing conditions of employment that enable safe and appropriate care for clients and contribute to the professional satisfaction of nurses.
XI. The nurse advocates the interests of clients.
XII. The nurse represents the values and ethics of nursing before colleagues and others.
XIII. Professional nurses' organizations are responsible for clarifying, securing, and sustaining ethical nursing conduct. The fulfillment of these tasks requires that professional nurses' organizations remain responsive to the rights, needs, and legitimate interests of clients and nurses.

§From Canadian Nurses Association. (1991). *Code of ethics for nursing.* Ottawa, Ontario: Author.

Introduction

The American Hospital Association presents *A Patient's Bill of Rights* with the expectation that observance of these rights will contribute to more effective patient care and greater satisfaction for the patient, his physician, and the hospital organization. Further, the Association presents these rights in the expectation that they will be supported by the hospital on behalf of its patients, as an integral part of the healing process. It is recognized that a personal relationship between the physician and the patient is essential for the provision of proper medical care. The traditional physician–patient relationship takes on a new dimension when care is rendered within an organizational structure. Legal precedent has established that the institution itself also has a responsibility to the patient. It is in recognition of these factors that these rights are affirmed.

A Patient's Bill of Rights

1. The patient has the right to considerate and respectful care.

2. The patient has the right to obtain from his physician complete current information concerning his diagnosis, treatment, and prognosis in terms the patient can be reasonably expected to understand. When it is not medically advisable to give such information to the patient, the information should be made available to an appropriate person in his behalf. He has the right to know by name the physician responsible for coordinating his care.

3. The patient has the right to receive from his physician information necessary to give informed consent prior to the start of any procedure and/or treatment. Except in emergencies, such information for informed consent should include but not necessarily be limited to the specific procedure and/or treatment, the medically significant risks involved, and the probable duration of incapacitation. Where medically significant alternatives for care or treatment exist, or when the patient requests information concerning medical alternatives, the patient has the right to such information. The patient also has the right to know the name of the person responsible for the procedures and/or treatment.

4. The patient has the right to refuse treatment to the extent permitted by law, and to be informed of the medical consequences of his action.

5. The patient has the right to every consideration of his privacy concerning his own medical care program. Case discussion, consultation, examination, and treatment are confidential and should be conducted discreetly. Those not directly involved in his care must have the permission of the patient to be present.

6. The patient has the right to expect that all communications and records pertaining to his care should be treated as confidential.

7. The patient has the right to expect that within its capacity a hospital must make reasonable response to the request of a patient for services. The hospital must provide evaluation, service, and/or referral as indicated by the urgency of the case. When medically permissible, a patient may be transferred to another facility only after he has received complete information and explanation concerning the needs for and alternatives to such a transfer. The institution to which the patient is to be transferred must first have accepted the patient for transfer.

8. The patient has the right to obtain information as to any relationship of his hospital to other health care and educational institutions insofar as his care is concerned. The patient has the right to obtain information as to the existence of any professional relationships among individuals, by name, who are treating him.

9. The patient has the right to be advised if the hospital proposes to engage in or perform human experimentation affecting his care or treatment. The patient has the right to refuse to participate in such research projects.

10. The patient has the right to expect reasonable continuity of care. He has the right to know in advance what appointment times and physicians are available and where. The patient has the right to expect that the hospital will provide a mechanism whereby he is informed by his physician or a delegate of the physician of the patient's continuing health care requirements following discharge.

11. The patient has the right to examine and receive an explanation of his bill regardless of source of payment.

12. The patient has the right to know what hospital rules and regulations apply to his conduct as a patient.

No catalogue of rights can guarantee for the patient the kind of treatment he has a right to expect. A hospital has many functions to perform, including the prevention and treatment of disease, the education of both health professionals and patients, and the conduct of clinical research. All these activities must be conducted with an overriding concern for the patient and, above all, the recognition of his dignity as a human being. Success in achieving this recognition assures success in the defense of the rights of the patient.

(American Hospital Association. [1972]. *A patient's bill of rights*. Chicago: Author. Copyright © 1972, AHA.)

A Client's Bill of Rights

The American Hospital Association developed *A Patient's Bill of Rights* in 1972 (see the accompanying display). The bill of rights includes the rights and responsibilities of the client while receiving care in the hospital. A number of other bills of rights have emerged recently, such as the Pregnant Patient's Bill of Rights, the Indian Patient's Bill of Rights, a Nursing Home Bill of Rights, and the Veterans Administration Code of Patient Concern. Each of these bills of rights emphasizes a specific aspect of client rights within a particular health agency. These bills of rights imply a code of ethics the nurse observes professionally.

Theories of Ethics

Ethical theories are systems of reflection that attempt to explain how we ought to live and why. These theories may be broadly categorized as action guides that answer the question, "What ought I to do?" or character guides that answer the question, "What kind of person ought I to be?" Action guides fall into two main categories:

   Utilitarian: The rightness or wrongness of an action depends on the consequences the action produces.

   Deontologic: An action is right or wrong independent of the consequences it produces.

Biomedical Ethics   When general ethical theories are applied to the field of biomedicine, the result is **biomedical ethics.** Examples of contemporary issues bioethicists are studying include the ethical implications of gene therapy, the new reproductive technologies, physician-assisted suicide, treatment withdrawal—including nutrition and hydration, and the rationing of health care.

Nursing Ethics: An Ethic of Caring   Nursing ethics was traditionally viewed as a subset of medical ethics. In the 1980s, however, ethicists began to acknowledge the unique domain of nursing ethics, that is, the ethical issues and analysis used by nurses to make ethical judgments. Nurse ethicists currently are arguing that the value foundations of nursing ethics are based on the exchange of human caring that occurs between client and nurse, in contrast to medical ethics, which focuses on models of "client-good" or rights-based autonomy (Fry, 1989a). Nursing ethics complements medical ethics and advocates attending and relating to people in a way that protects them from being reduced to the moral status of objects.

> In other words, the ideals of human caring that are rooted in receptivity, intersubjective relatedness, and human responsiveness help to counteract the medical ethic of rational principle, fairness, and equity that objectifies, detaches, and distances the professional from the subjective world of human experience. (Watson & Ray, 1988, p. 2)

Advocacy

Nursing has traditionally held that its primary commitment is to the client, and more recently has claimed client advo-

---

National Reference Center for Bioethics Literature

Kennedy Institute of Ethics
  Georgetown University
  Washington, DC 20057
  Toll-free telephone number: 800-MED-ETHX

   A specialized collection of library resources concerned with contemporary biomedical issues in the fields of ethics, philosophy, medicine, nursing, science, law, religion, and the social sciences.
   Call for bioethics information; BIOETHICSLINE searches (computerized data base); search strategies; reference help; publication orders.

---

cacy as a legitimate nursing role. **Advocacy** is the protection and support of another's rights (advocacy is discussed in Chapter 22). Nurses who wish to practice in this tradition:

- Ensure that their loyalty to an employing institution or to a physician does not compromise their primary commitment to the client.
- When making an ethical decision, place more weight on the good to be produced for the individual client than on the greatest good for the greatest number (utilitarianism).
- Evaluate carefully in each situation the competing claims of autonomy (self-determination) and client well-being.

   When respecting autonomy, the nurse respects and supports the client's right to make decisions. Informed consent is described in Chapter 6. When promoting client well-being, the nurse acts in the best interests of the client. Ideally, both autonomy and client well-being are promoted in each nurse–client interaction; however, conflicts sometimes arise. For instance, if an elderly male client with a serious chronic lung disease, who understands well the danger of smoking asks the nurse to get him a pack of cigarettes, the nurse must decide whether to respect his autonomy and follow his wishes or to promote his medical well-being. Nurses sensitive to the need to promote both client autonomy and well-being may often experience conflict, but they are more likely than other nurses to succeed in securing the client's genuine best interests.

Types of Moral and Ethical Problems

The nurse in clinical practice is actively involved in resolving ethical issues. Three types of moral and ethical problems faced by nurses are as follows:

   Moral uncertainty: The nurse is unsure of which moral principles or values apply.

   Moral dilemmas: Two (or more) clear moral principles apply but support mutually inconsistent courses of action.

   Moral distress: The nurse knows the right thing to do but institutional constraints make it nearly impossible to pursue the right actions. (Jameton, 1984, p. 6)

Moral and ethical problems may arise between nurses and clients, nurses and physicians, and nurses and other nurses. As you read through the mini-cases that follow, try to determine your response. A process of ethical decision making follows.

Nurses and Clients

Troublesome nurse–client situations that can result in ethical distress for nurses include **paternalism** (acting for clients without their consent to secure a good or prevent harm), deception, confidentiality, allocation of scarce nursing resources, informed consent, and conflicts between the client's and nurse's interests.

Paternalism An alert elderly client who is at high risk of falling refuses to call the nurse for assistance getting out of bed. The nurse must decide whether to obtain an order to restrain the client. Does preventing potential harm justify violating the client's right to autonomy and make it acceptable for the nurse to act as a "parent" and choose an action the client does not want because it is believed to be in the client's best interest?

Deception A postoperative client asks the student nurse who is about to administer an intramuscular injection for pain, "Is this your first shot?" It is the student's first injection and the student is anxious. Would the student's intent to decrease the client's anxiety justify telling the client, "No, I've given several before"?

Confidentiality A nurse asks a middle-aged woman who is crying quietly, "Would you like to share what's troubling you?" The woman tells the nurse she has no idea how she will pay for this hospitalization because she entered the country illegally 2 months ago and is trying to earn enough money to help her family back home. She begs the nurse not to tell anyone. If the nurse believes this anxiety is interfering with the client's recovery, would it be ethical to break the woman's confidence to obtain help for her?

Allocation of Scarce Nursing Resources A nurse has just been pulled from your unit, leaving it understaffed. Among your clients are a 33-year-old man recovering from a heart attack who is being discharged in the morning (he tells you he still has many questions); an elderly client who is close to death; and a woman with cancer who has been vomiting all day and who is in severe pain. You know you cannot meet everyone's needs well. How do you "distribute" your nursing care? (You really *like* the client who is going home in the morning.)

Informed Consent A resident is attempting to perform a spinal tap on an adolescent who you know dislikes the resident. After one failed attempt, the adolescent tells the resident to stop. The resident asks you to administer an antianxiety medication to the client so the resident can get the spinal tap done quickly. Should you administer the medication knowing the client no longer consents to the procedure?

Conflicts Between the Client's and Nurse's Interests Nurses are taking turns caring for a client who is positive for the human immunodeficiency virus. One nurse, who is nursing her 8-month-old infant, refuses to take her turn, fearing she will transmit the disease to her baby. The other nurses tell her she must take care of the client because none of them is willing to take her turn. Is a nurse ever justified in refusing to nurse a client assigned to his or her care?

Nurses and Physicians

Nurse–physician situations can also result in ethical distress for nurses. Common problems include disagreements about the proposed medical regimen, conflicts regarding the scope of the nurse's role, and physician incompetence.

Disagreements About the Proposed Medical Regimen In the nursing home where you work, any client who loses a significant amount of weight (more than 10% of usual body weight) is automatically subjected to an exhaustive battery of tests (including a complete gastrointestinal [GI] series) to determine whether there are any physical causes for the weight loss (eg, tumor). You strongly object to one client being put through these tests because she has made it clear that she wants to die and will starve herself to death if that is the only way she can do it. The medical director insists that the client undergo the diagnostic studies because there is a long history of client family dissatisfaction with the medical care. The director wants to avoid causing further dissatisfaction. Are you responsible for preparing the client for these diagnostic studies and scheduling them? Are there grounds for refusing to participate?

Conflicts Regarding the Scope of the Nurse's Role A young woman needing surgery that will result in a permanent colostomy tells the nurse how afraid she is and how much she dreads getting used to "the thing." The nurse is certain this client would benefit greatly from the help of the young staff enterostomal therapist (ET), who also has a colostomy. However, when this suggestion is mentioned to the surgeon, the surgeon tells the nurse that he does his own teaching and counseling for all his clients and does not "believe" in ETs. He points out that the nurse's duty here is to carry out his orders. Does it fall within the scope of nursing to recommend the ET to the woman? Is the nurse morally obligated to make this recommendation to the client?

Physician Incompetence A nurse who works in the operating room notices that a pediatric surgeon who has been on the staff for several years and done excellent work seems all of a sudden not to be concentrating during surgery and to be making more mistakes than usual. Rumors have been circulating about a problem with cocaine abuse following the surgeon's divorce. The parents of one pediatric client

CHAPTER 5 Values and Ethics in Nursing 71

The first ethical dilemma that I encountered as a nursing student occurred in my junior year. I was working in a geriatric unit of a hospital caring for an elderly woman with severe rheumatoid arthritis and acute gastrointestinal (GI) bleeding. As I spent time talking with her, I became aware of her unique personality and life style. Before her hospitalization she lived alone for 15 years; she had never married and had no children. She treasured her privacy and solitude and made this clear in the hospital. Her behavior as a patient reflected her previous life style.

When the issue of whether she should sit inside or outside her hospital room arose, there was great conflict. She clearly did not want to be in the view of others. It made her feel uncomfortable, nervous, and upset. If she had to sit in a chair, she wanted it to be placed in her room. Despite this, some nurses believed that she should be forced to sit in the hall with other clients. They perceived her behavior as "reclusive" and "abnormal" and wanted her to learn to associate with others. Her illness had progressed so greatly that it was clear she would not be returning to her home. Because she would soon become a permanent resident of a nursing home, she needed to learn how to interact with others—even if she didn't want to. Her desire to sit alone was not accepted as suitable to her needs. The nurses decided that disregarding her wishes was in her best interests.

I was overcome with a feeling of confusion. I asked myself, "Who is right?" Is it appropriate to force a grown woman who cries openly at the thought of being "stared at" to sit in the hall? Wouldn't this be ignoring her personality? Or, on the other hand, was this a necessary therapeutic intervention? She was going to be placed in a nursing home and would eventually have to learn how to be around others. She would not be able to live a life of isolation. Which was the "greater good"?

I searched textbooks, journals, and magazines for the solution. I needed to find an answer. Much to my dismay my research yielded no clear-cut answer. There were readings that supported the decision to place her in the hall as well as readings that supported her being allowed to remain in her room. I discovered that the hard thing about clinical ethics is that you ultimately have to make a decision—and that hopefully it is a decision with which you can live. After much reflection I found the answer—in myself.

—Deborah A. Schuster, Georgetown University,
Washington, DC

dissatisfied with the progress the client is making ask the nurse for an opinion about the surgeon. Should the nurse voice personal concerns? Is the nurse morally obligated to report the physician to the proper hospital authority for investigation?

Nurses and Other Nurses

Some of the most difficult ethical problems nurses encounter result from nurse–nurse interactions and may be complicated by obligations of friendship. Problems include claims of loyalty and nurse incompetence.

Claims of Loyalty A nurse working the 11 PM to 7 AM shift tells the other nurse on the unit, "I just made rounds and everyone is OK. Please cover for me while I catch an hour of sleep. I had an awful day." She neglects to tell the nurse who is covering that it was mentioned in report that one client needed special monitoring. This client dies unexpect-

edly while the nurse sleeps. When she wakes up and discovers the death, she begs the other nurse, her friend, not to ever tell anyone she was sleeping. "The client could have died anyway between my rounds."

Nurse Incompetence When you make your morning rounds, a client tells you that one of the nurses fondled her body and made suggestive remarks during the previous night shift. You suspect that the client may simply be trying to cause trouble and because you like the nurse in question, find it hard to believe the client. What should you do?

Nurses and Institutional and Public Policy

As nurses assume increased responsibility for decision making at all levels of care, the institutional and public policy arenas offer unique dilemmas. Two current examples are short-staffing and health care rationing.

Short-Staffing The nursing shortage has resulted in chronic understaffing on the unit where you work. You believe that clients are now at risk because there simply are not enough nurses to provide quality care. Some nurses are talking about forming a union and going on strike. Because yours is the only major hospital in a rural area, you are unsure if striking is a morally legitimate option. What do you do?

Health Care Rationing In the United States, 37 to 39 million people are uninsured or underinsured and have limited access to health care. Whether each person has a "right" (is entitled to) basic health care continues to be the subject of debate. There are plans for rationing health care that could limit the options available to the elderly, the poor, the terminally ill, and to those in society whom many view as having limited "social value." What moral obligation do you have to contribute to this debate? How might you ensure that your voice and the nursing viewpoint are heard?

Ethical Decision Making

This section on developing analytical skills may be helpful to you in working out your response to the ethical problems previously described.

Decision making cannot be based on emotional content; rather, it requires intellectual problem solving. Several models of ethical decision making are available in the literature, most of which have similar steps. The model described here is a six-step process proposed by Jameton (1984):

1. Identify the problem.
2. Gather data.
3. Identify options.
4. Think the ethical problem through: Consider basic conventional principles of professional ethics and determine whether they address the issue and resolve the problem; if this fails, see if any reflective ethical considerations clarify and resolve the problem.
5. Make a decision.
6. Act and assess.

These steps are illustrated in the accompanying case study. The following text will help you better understand the fourth step.

Conventional Principles and Values

Conventional principles are "rules for action, related principles, ideals, standards, and values . . . commonly used as standards . . . and followed in practice" (Jameton, 1984, p. 71). Examples of conventional principles of nursing practice include the following:

- Nurses have an obligation to be competent.
- The good of clients should be the nurse's primary concern.
- Nurses should not use their positions to exploit others.
- Nurses should be loyal to one another.

Unfortunately, many nurses find themselves in situations in which conventional principles conflict or are otherwise deficient in resolving ethical dilemmas. The staff nurse who suspects that his or her colleague and friend is both stealing and abusing narcotics will need to report this even if this is being disloyal.

Basic Moral Concepts

When conventional principles fail to provide nurses with a guide to action, the nurse needs to explore ethical values and principles in a deeper and broader way. Jameton (1984) has identified five basic moral concepts:

Respect for persons: This involves having empathy for others (listening and understanding) and not using people as a means to an end.

Justice: Distributive justice of the allocation of goods and services is the type of justice most relevant to health care, including how much of national resources should be devoted to health care, which aspects of health care should receive the most resources, and which clients should have access to these resources. Models for distributing the burdens and benefits of society include:

  To each equally
  To each according to merit
  To each according to past or future social contribution

 COMPUTER APPLICATIONS IN NURSING

Computer Software for Ethics Case Analysis

Dr. Ethics is a unique computer program that analyzes the ethical implications of case studies in clinical medicine and recommends resolutions that can be used as the starting point for ethical dialogue. The program has a large collection of codes of ethics (including the International Council of Nurses [1973] *Code for Nurses* and American Nurses' Association [1985] *Code for Nurses With Interpretive Statements*) that can be accessed as the user works on an ethical case, fills out a grant form, or takes a quiz. This interactive expert-system is available for both Macintosh and IBM platforms.

InterActive Software
P.O. Box 52012
Knoxville, TN 37950-2012
(615) 523-2436

A Case Study Using a Six-Step Process for Resolving the Ethical Problem

Case: Jean W. is a labor and delivery room nurse in a small community hospital that serves both private clients and clinic clients. Jean has always felt that certain members of the obstetrics–gynecology medical staff have treated these two groups of clients differently. On this particular morning, Jean is caring for a woman who is scheduled for an elective cesarean delivery. The woman (who is a clinic client) has made it very clear that she wants to be awake for the delivery and has requested epidural or spinal anesthesia. Jean is dismayed when the anesthesiologist enters the delivery room because the anesthesiologist's success rate with epidural anesthesia is poor. The anesthesiologist unsuccessfully attempts to perform an epidural block. After waiting 20 minutes for results, the obstetrician is growing impatient and instructs the anesthesiologist to put the client to sleep. Jean feels the rights of this client are being violated but is unsure of what her response should be.

Step 1: Identify the Problem

State the problem clearly: unsure of ethical issue; two or more moral principles are in conflict; object to proposed course of action.

Identify your relationship to the decision.

Identify time parameters.

Jean W. objects to the obstetrician's intent to disregard the client's wish to be awake for her delivery; she is aware of no good reasons justifying this course of action.

The nurse will be a participant in carrying out the decision.

The decision for this case must be made immediately; it would be helpful to plan to avoid situations like this in the future.

Step 2: Gather Data

Describe the situation that gives rise to the problem: main people involved (their views and interests); client's overall nursing, medical, and social situation; relevant legal, administrative, and staff considerations.

The client is in stable medical condition (elective cesarean delivery, not an emergency) and has made it very clear that she wishes to be awake for the delivery. The client is not a private-paying client of the obstetrician. The nurse believes her role is to promote/protect the client's interests; she knows of no reason in this case why the client's preferences should be disregarded.

The anesthesiologist has a poor success record with epidural anesthesia.

The obstetrician seems to want to complete delivery quickly. In the past, he has seemed to give more weight to following wishes of private clients as opposed to clinic clients. He is the head of the obstetrics–gynecology department; he believes nurses should obey physicians unquestioningly.

Nurses have in the past expressed dissatisfaction with the different levels of care being provided to private and clinic clients, but no one to date has formally addressed the concern.

Step 3: Identify Options

Identify all the possible courses of action open to you and weigh the outcomes of each; consider immediate consequences to the people involved as well as long-term consequences to the institution and society.

The nurse can say nothing to the obstetrician and help with the delivery. If asked by the client later why she needed to be put to sleep, the nurse can (1) tell the truth, (2) refer her to the obstetrician, (3) express sympathy that she could not be awake, or (4) say nothing. *Outcome:* The client's wishes are disregarded; delivery occurs in record time and the obstetrician is happy; the nurse fulfills obligation to physician and hospital but feels she has betrayed the client's trust. *Long-term outcome:* There is a good probability the same problem will happen again.

Or

(continued)

A Case Study Using a Six-Step Process for Resolving the Ethical Problem (continued)

The nurse can remind the obstetrician that the client was adamant about wanting to be awake and suggest that a different anesthesiologist be called in. If the obstetrician agrees, the client may get her wish and everyone is satisfied with the outcome (the nurse must still decide how to prevent recurrence of this dilemma). If the obstetrician refuses and insists that the client be put to sleep, the nurse can (1) refuse to participate (if another nurse is unavailable or unwilling to replace her, the nurse has abandoned the client and harm may ensue); or (2) participate and proceed as above or resolve to speak to the obstetrician in a "cool moment" after the delivery to see how to avoid this problem in the future. If the nurse does not get satisfaction with the obstetrician, then she must decide whether to move through the proper administrative channels. Depending on the institution and people involved, the nurse may be affirmed or censored for this move. *Long-term outcome:* Future clients may be helped by the nurse following through with her concerns.

Or

The nurse can say nothing and assist with this delivery, believing it to be the wisest course of action for the time being, but resolve to take the steps above to correct the perceived injustice. *Outcome:* There is no benefit for the present client but potential benefit to future clients.

Step 4: Think the Ethical Problem Through

See if conventional principles of professional ethics address and resolve the problem; if not, see if broader ethical principles and theories clarify and resolve the problem. Rely on those principles you judge most important and of which you feel most sure.

Basic conventional principle: The good of clients should be the nurse's primary concern strongly suggests that the nurse should act, but it does not address the nurse's obligation to do so if she feels it would jeopardize her own good (job security).

Basic moral principle: Respect for persons would suggest that the client's autonomy (right to self-determination) should be respected unless there is strong justification for not doing so. *Equality* would suggest that whether a client pays the obstetrician privately should have no bearing on the quality of care received.

Step 5: Make a Decision

Choose a course of action that best reflects your considered judgment; consultation with an institutional ethics committee or other staff may be helpful.

Jean W. feels from past interactions with this obstetrician that her speaking up will not influence his decision to have the client put to sleep. She decides to speak with the obstetrician after the delivery and follow up with whatever approach is necessary to avoid recurrence.

Step 6: Act and Assess

Act and compare the actual outcome with what you considered and hoped for in advance. How can you improve the decision process next time?

Jean W. will never know if speaking up would have resulted in the client's wishes being respected. Although she is dissatisfied with the outcome of this case, she hopes to prevent this from happening to other clinic clients in the future. In this instance, a hospital committee was formed to study the problem and make recommendations. If Jean W. had been told to "mind her own business" unless she wanted trouble, she would have to make a decision weighing client benefit on one hand with potential personal risk or harm on the other.

To each according to what can be acquired in a free market

To each according to need

To each according to need, from each according to ability

Values: These underlie the goods and purposes sought in life; relevant to health care is whether there are some values that take precedence over others and the role values play in shaping client decisions and professional behavior.

Rights: These are justified claims on others not to interfere with what we have or are doing (negative rights) or to provide something (positive rights). Associated with rights are responsibilities. In health care, this issue most often focuses on identifying what clients are entitled to but do not always receive.

Responsibility: Before making moral judgments, it is necessary to identify who is responsible for what; as the nurse's professional role is expanding, nurses are becoming both morally and legally responsible for more aspects of client care. (Jameton, 1984, pp. 124–145)

Nurses and Ethics Committees

An increasing number of health care institutions have developed ethics committees whose chief functions include education, policy making, case review, and consultation. These committees are uniquely equipped to deal with the complexities of modern medicine because they are multidisciplinary, provide a forum where radically divergent views can be aired without fear of repercussion, and provide links to the law, to technology and its problems, and to social mores (Cranford & Roberts, 1986). Nurses bring an important voice to the ethics committee. When cases are being reviewed, nurses can help to ensure that the technical facts are understood, that the appropriate decision makers have been identified, that the client's medical and overall best interests have been identified, and that the course of action selected from the alternatives is justified by sound ethical principles. The nurse's strong background in interpersonal communications has the potential to contribute unique knowledge of the client and family to the discussion and to facilitate the ethics committee's group dynamics.

KEY POINTS

- Knowing whether to perform a nursing action ("should I?") is often as important as knowing how to perform the action.
- A value is a belief about worth that acts as a standard to guide behavior. Values influence beliefs about human needs, health and illness, the practice of health behaviors, and human responses to health and illness.
- Values are formed over a lifetime from information a person receives from the environment and from the family and culture. Common modes of value transmission are modeling, moralizing, laissez-faire, rewarding and punishing, and responsible choice.
- The American Association of Colleges of Nursing identified altruism, aesthetics, equality, freedom, human dignity, justice, and truth as essential values for the practicing nurse.
- Although it is important for nurses to respect the value orientations of others, not all values are equal. Nurses may find themselves morally obligated to respond to client values likely to cause harm to the client or others.
- Values clarification is a process by which people come to understand their own values and value system. The process of valuing is centered on choosing, prizing, and acting.
- Ethics offers the nurse a means to look at and evaluate alternative courses of right action using basic moral concepts and principles. It reduces the likelihood that nursing actions to resolve ethical problems will be based solely on intuition, opinions, and self-interest.

- The nursing codes of ethics (ICN, ANA, CNA) provide a framework for making ethical decisions and set forth professional expectations. They inform both nurses and society of the profession's primary goals and values. Codes are effective only when upheld by members of the profession.
- Theories of ethics offer moral guides to action and to character. Nursing ethics currently is recognized as a distinct set of applied ethics. An ethic of caring takes as its unique moral position attending and relating to a person in such a way that the person is protected from being reduced to the status of moral objects.
- Nurses who are sensitive to the need to promote both client autonomy (self-determination) and client well-being may experience ethical conflict, but are more likely than other nurses to be successful in securing the client's genuine best interests.
- Ethical problems faced by nurses include moral uncertainty, moral dilemmas, and moral distress.
- One of several processes for resolving ethical problems in nursing is the following six-step process: (1) identify the problem; (2) gather data; (3) identify options; (4) think the ethical problem through (explore conventional principles and basic moral concepts); make a decision; and act and assess.
- Nurses often serve on institutional ethics committees whose chief functions include education, policy formation, case review, and consultation.

BIBLIOGRAPHY

American Association of Colleges of Nursing. (1986). *Essentials of college and university education for professional nursing*. Washington, DC: Author.

American Nurses' Association. (1985). *Code for nurses with interpretive statements*. Kansas City, MO: Author.

American Nurses' Association. (1988). *Ethics in nursing: Position statements and guidelines*. Kansas City, MO: Author.

Anonymous. (1989). Blowing the whistle on incompetence: One nurse's story. *Nursing, 19*(7), 47–50.

Beauchamp, T. L., & Childress, J. F. (1989). *Principles of biomedical ethics* (3rd ed.). New York: Oxford University Press.

Benjamin, M., & Curtis, J. (1992). *Ethics in nursing* (3rd ed.). New York: Oxford University Press.

Bishop, A. H., & Scudder, J. R. (1990). *The practical, moral, and personal sense of nursing*. Albany: State University of New York Press.

Botter, M. L., & Dickey, S. B. (1989). Allocation of resources: Nurses, the key decision makers. *Holistic Nursing Practice, 4*(1), 44–51.

Brown, C. (1990). Limiting care: Is CPR for everyone? *AACN Clinical Issues Critical Care Nursing, 1*(1), 161–168.

Canadian Nurses Association. (1991). *Code of ethics for nursing*. Ottawa, Ontario: Author.

Cassells, J. M., Redman, B. K., & Jackson, S. S. (1986). Generic baccalaureate student satisfaction regarding professional and personal development prior to graduation and one year post graduation. *Journal of Professional Nursing, 2*(2), 114–127.

Chally, P. S. (1990). Theory derivation in moral development. *Nursing and Health Care, 11*(6), 302–306.

Condon, E. H. (1991). Nursing and the caring metaphor: Gender and political influences on an ethics of care. *Nursing Outlook, 40*(1), 14–19.

Cranford, R. E., & Roberts, J. C. (1986). Biomedical ethics committees. *Primary Care, 13*(2), 327–341.

Donovan, N. M. (1991). Confidentiality vs. duty to warn: Whose life is it anyway? *Nursing and Health Care, 12*(8), 432–436.

Feldman, K. A., & Newcomb, T. M. (1969). *Impact of college on students*. San Francisco: Jossey-Bass.

Fry, S. T. (1989a). The role of caring in a theory of nursing ethics. *Hypatia, 4*(2), 88–103.

Hanvey, L. (1990). Values in maternal and newborn care. *Canadian Nurse, 86*(9), 22–23.

Husted, G. L., & Husted, J. H. (1991). *Ethical decision making in nursing*. St. Louis: Mosby.

International Council of Nurses. (1973). *ICN code for nurses: Ethical concepts applied to nursing*. Geneva: Imprimeries Populaires.

Jameton, A. (1984). *Nursing practice: The ethical issues*. Englewood Cliffs, NJ: Prentice-Hall.

Kirschbaum, H. (1977). *Advanced values clarification*. La Jolla, CA: University Associates.

Levine-Ariff, J. (1990). Preventive ethics: The development of policies to guide decision-making. *AACN Clinical Issues Critical Care Nursing, 1*(1), 169–177.

Lindsay, E. (1991). Life at all costs. *Canadian Nurse, 87*(3), 16–18.

MacIntosh, J. (1989). Ethics and an ethical dilemma: To resuscitate or not. *Canadian Critical Care Nursing Journal, 6*(1), 20–22.

Melroe, N. H. (1990). "Duty to warn" vs. "patient confidentiality": The ethical dilemma in caring for HIV-infected clients. *Nurse Practitioner, 15*(2), 58, 60, 65ff.

Neil, R., & Watts, R. (1990). *Explorations in the feminist perspectives: Caring and nursing*. New York: National League for Nursing.

Noddings, N. (1984). *Caring: A feminine approach to ethics and moral education*. Berkeley, CA: University of California Press.

Oddi, L. F., & Cassidy, V. R. (1990). Participation and perceptions of nurse members in the hospital ethics committee. *Western Journal of Nursing Research, 12*(3), 307–317.

Pence, T., & Cantrall, J. (Eds.). (1990). *Ethics in nursing: An anthology*. New York: National League for Nursing.

Raths, L. E., Simon, S. B., & Harmin, M. (1978). *Values and teaching* (2nd ed.). Columbus: Charles E. Merrill.

Royal College of Nursing of the United Kingdom. (1980). *Guidelines on confidentiality in nursing*. London: Author.

Rozovsky, L. E. (1980). *The Canadian patient's book of rights*. Toronto: Doubleday Canada.

Salladay, S. A., & McDonnell, M. M. (1992). Facing ethical conflicts. *Nursing, 22*(2), 44–47.

Scanlon, C., & Fleming, C. (1990). Confronting ethical issues: A nursing survey. *Nursing Management, 21*(5), 63–65.

Silva, M. C. (1984). The American Nurses' Association code for nurses: Purposes, content, and enforceability. *Health Matrix, 2*(2), 55–63.

Silva, M. C. (1990). *Ethical decision making in nursing administration*. New York: Appleton-Lange.

Simon, S. B. (1972). *Values clarification: A handbook of practical strategies for teachers and students*. New York: Hart.

Steele, S. M., & Harmon, V. M. (1983). *Values clarification in nursing* (2nd ed.). Norwalk, CT: Appleton-Century-Crofts.

Taylor, C. (1990). Ethics in health care and medical technologies. *Theoretical Medicine, 11*, 111–124.

Uustal. D. B. (1978). Values clarification in nursing: Application to practice. *American Journal of Nursing, 78*(12), 2058–2063.

Watson, J., & Ray, M. A. (Eds.). (1988). *The ethics of care and the ethics of cure: Synthesis in chronicity* (Pub. No. 15-2237). New York: National League for Nursing.

Yeo, M. (1991). *Concepts and cases in nursing ethics*. Lewiston, NY: Broadview Press.

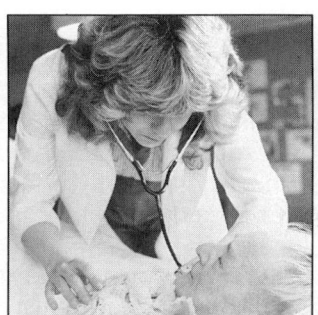
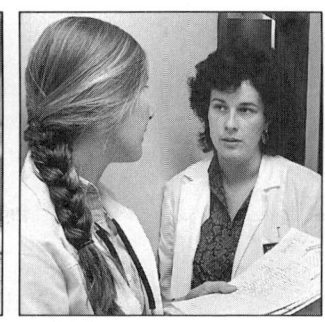
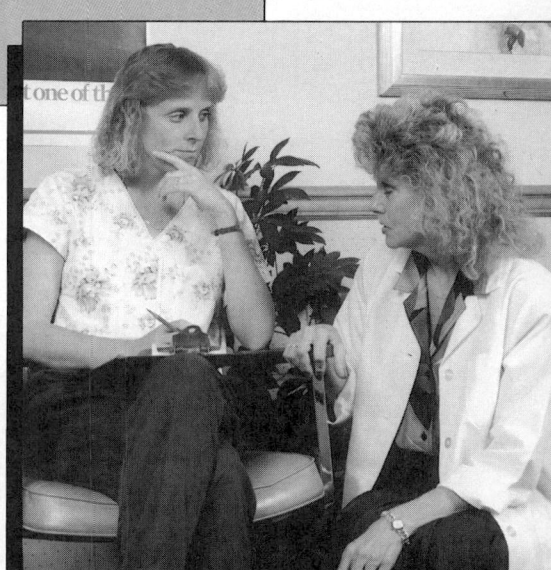

OBJECTIVES

After studying this chapter, the learner should be able to

Define key terms used in the chapter.

Define *law* and describe its four sources.

Describe the professional and legal regulation of nursing practice.

Identify the purpose of credentialing, using as examples accreditation, licensure or registration, and certification.

Identify grounds for suspending or revoking a license or registration.

Differentiate intentional torts (assault and battery, defamation, invasion of privacy, false imprisonment, fraud) and unintentional torts (negligence).

Evaluate personal areas of potential liability in nursing.

Describe the legal procedure once a plaintiff files a complaint against a nurse for negligence.

Describe the roles of the nurse as defendant, fact witness, and expert witness.

Use appropriate legal safeguards in nursing practice.

Explain the purpose of incident reports.

Describe laws affecting nursing practice.

Identify two types of advance directives.

KEY TERMS

accreditation
advance directive
assault
battery
certification
civil law
common law
contract
credentialing
crime
defamation of character
defendant
durable power of attorney
    for health care
expert witness
fact witness
false imprisonment
felony
fraud
incident report
informed consent
invasion of privacy
law
liability
licensure
litigation
living will
malpractice
misdemeanor
negligence
plaintiff
public law
risk management
standard of care
statutory law
tort

Legal Implications of Nursing

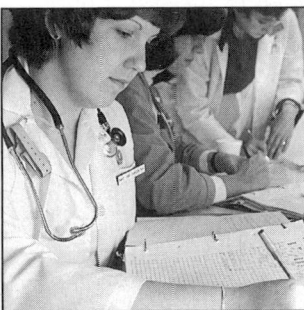

As the roles and duties of nurses have expanded in the current health care system, so too has their legal accountability. In the past, many nurses worked under the supervision of a physician, few carried liability insurance, and even if a nurse's actions were the direct cause of harm to a client, primary liability for the nursing action fell on the employing agency or physician. Currently, nurses independently assess and diagnose clients and plan, implement, and evaluate nursing care. Full legal responsibility and accountability for these nursing actions rest with the nurse. A steadily increasing number of nurses are being named as litigants in negligence cases and being brought to court to defend their practice.

It has never been more crucial for nurses to carefully document their actions and take part in other malpractice prevention practices. Nurses who wish to avoid legal conflicts must develop trusting nurse–client relationships (satisfied clients rarely sue); practice within the scope of their competence; and identify potential liabilities in their practice and develop prevention strategies.

Legal Concepts

Definition of Law

A **law** is a standard or rule of conduct established and enforced by the government of a society. Laws are intended chiefly to protect the rights of the public. **Public law** is a law in which the government is directly involved. It regulates the relationships between individuals and the government. Also, an important body of public law describes the powers of the government in authority. Private law, also called **civil law,** regulates the relationships among people. Civil law includes laws relating to contracts, ownership of property, and the practice of nursing, medicine, pharmacy, and dentistry.

Sources of Laws

Four sources of law exist at both the federal and state (provincial) level—constitutions, statutes, administrative law, and common law.

Constitutions Federal and state constitutions indicate how their governments are created and given authority and state the principles and provisions for establishing specific laws. Although they contain relatively few laws (called constitutional laws), they serve as guides to legislative bodies.

Statutes A **statutory law** is enacted by a legislative body. In the United States, statutory laws must be in keeping with the federal constitution and with the constitution of the state as well. Nurse practice acts are an example of statutory laws.

Administrative Law Executive officers (eg, the president of the United States or prime minister of Canada, state governors or provincial premiers, or city mayors) administer various agencies that, among other functions, are responsible for law enforcement. These agencies have power to make administrative rules and regulations, in conformity with enacted law, which act as laws and are enforceable. Boards of nursing are administrative agencies at the state level. Rules and regulations they adopt are administrative laws. One example of a municipal administrative agency is a city's board of health.

Common Law The government provides for a judiciary system, which is responsible for reconciling controversies. It interprets legislation at the local, state (province), and national level as it has been applied in specific instances and makes decisions concerning law enforcement. A body of law known as **common law** has evolved from these accumulated judiciary decisions. Common law is thus court-made law. Most law in the area of malpractice is court-made law. The exception is in the province of Quebec, where a civil law system is in effect.

Common law is based on the principle of *stare decisis,* or "let the decision stand." After a decision has been made in a court of law, that decision becomes the rule to follow when other cases involving similar circumstances and facts arise. The case that first sets down the rule by decision is called a *precedent.* Court decisions can be changed but only when strong justification exists. Common law helps prevent one set of rules from being used to judge one person and another set to judge another person in similar circumstances.

Litigation

A lawsuit is a legal action in a court. **Litigation** is the process of a lawsuit. The person or government bringing suit against another is called the **plaintiff.** The one being accused of a crime or tort (defined later) is called the **defendant.** The defendant is presumed innocent until proven guilty of a crime or tort.

The two levels of courts in the United States are (1) trial court and (2) appellate court. The trial court, the first-level court, hears all the evidence in a case and makes decisions on facts, usually through a jury. The appellate court only hears cases questioning a point of law decided by the trial court. No witnesses testify at the appellate court level. The opinions of appellate judges are published and become common law (Fiesta, 1988).

Professional and Legal Regulation of Nursing Practice

Nurses who engage in the safe practice of their profession respect both the voluntary and legal controls that map the boundaries of nursing practice. Both these controls are designed to provide quality health care and to protect society from unsafe nursing practice (Fig. 6-1).

Voluntary standards, developed and implemented by the nursing profession itself, are not mandatory but are used as guidelines for peer review. Professional nursing organizations continually reassess the functions, standards, and qualifications of their members. The organizations are guided by their own assessment of society's need for nursing and by the public's expectations of nursing. Examples of voluntary standards include the American Nurses' Association (ANA) and Canadian Nurses Association (CNA) standards of practice (see Chapter 1), profes-

sional standards for the accreditation of education programs and service organizations, and standards for the certification of individual nurses in general and specialty areas of practice.

Legal standards are developed by legislative action and are implemented by authority granted by the state (or province) to determine minimum standards for the education of nurses, to set requirements for licensure or registration, and to decide when a nurse's license may be suspended or revoked. Examples of legal standards include state and province nurse practice acts and rules and regulations of nursing.

Credentialing

Nursing has taken several steps to ensure the competence of its practitioners, including the credentialing process. **Credentialing** refers to ways in which professional competence is ensured and maintained.

Three processes are used for credentialing in nursing. The first is **accreditation,** which is the process by which an educational program is evaluated and then recognized as having met certain predetermined standards of education.

FIGURE 6-1

Diagram of proposed professional and legal regulation of nursing practice showing the separation of and parallels between professional and legal regulatory processes. (American Nurses' Association. [1987]. *The scope of nursing practice.* Kansas City, MO: Author, p. 5.)

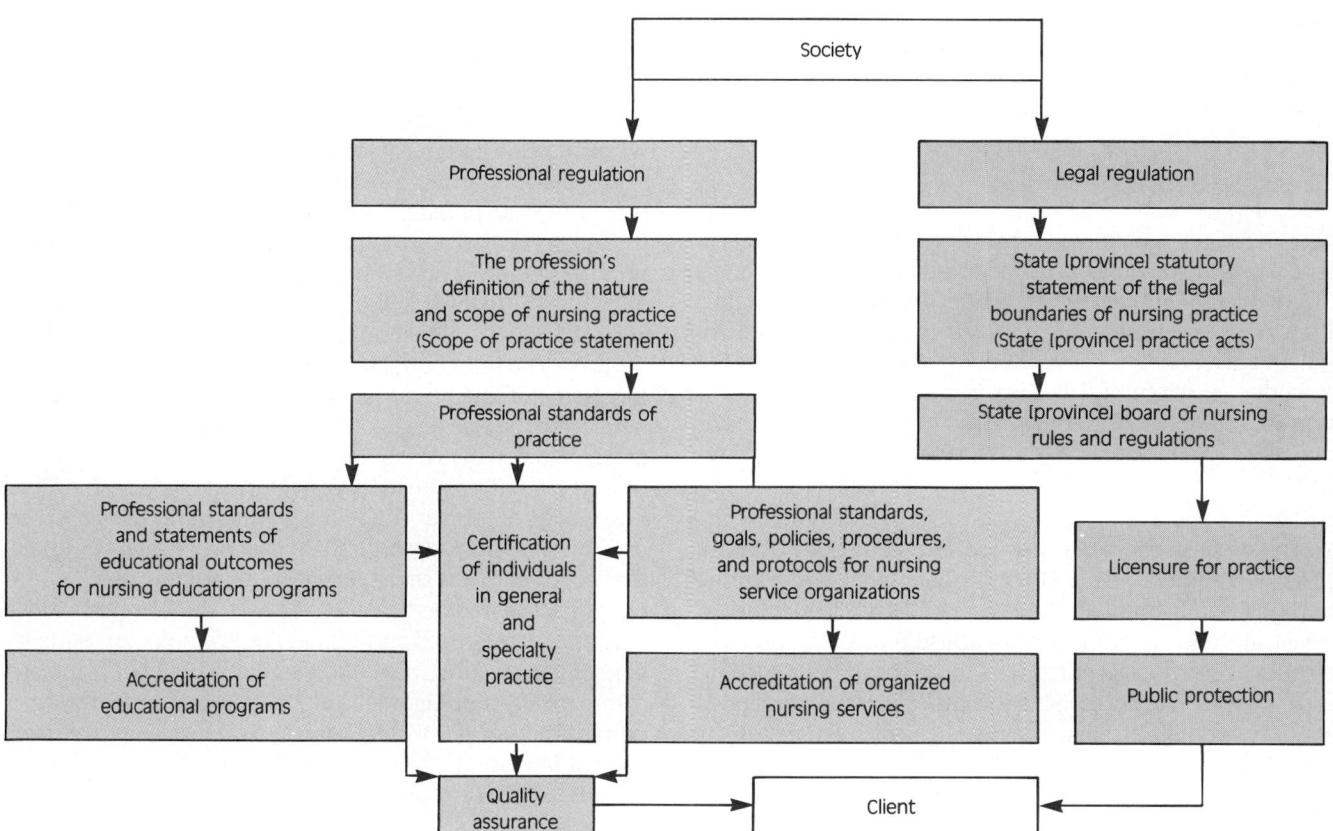

The second is **licensure,** which is the process by which a state determines that a candidate meets certain minimum requirements to practice in the profession of his or her choice and grants a license to do so. The third is **certification,** which is the process by which a person who has met certain criteria established by a nongovernmental association is granted recognition.

Accreditation

Constitutions provide governments with the responsibility of securing the public welfare. Legislative bodies have used this principle to enact laws that provide certain controls on occupational and professional groups. One function of these laws is to see that schools preparing practitioners maintain certain minimum standards of education. Nursing is one group operating under state (or province) laws that aim to promote the general welfare by determining minimum standards of education through accreditation of schools of nursing. In each Canadian province there is an approval mechanism for certifying schools of nursing. In the United States, state-approved, or accredited, educational programs in nursing include practical or vocational, associate degree, diploma, baccalaureate, and graduate programs in nursing.

Legal accreditation of a school preparing nursing personnel should not be confused with voluntary accreditation. The National League for Nursing (NLN) is a voluntary agency that accredits schools when they meet certain criteria established by NLN. Most schools choose to seek this voluntary accreditation, and many prospective students prefer selecting a school that has been accredited by NLN. Accreditation by NLN of educational programs to prepare nurses is not a legal requirement for a school to exist. State accreditation is a legal requirement.

Licensure and Registration

Licensure is a specialized form of credentialing that has a legal basis in laws passed by a legislative body. A *license* is a "legal document that permits a person to offer to the public his [or her] skills and knowledge in a particular jurisdiction, where such practice would otherwise be unlawful without a license" (Creighton, 1986a, p. 9). Licensure and registration are mandatory in Canada. Both must be renewed periodically. Licensure and registration are discussed in Chapter 1.

Licensure or Registration Revocation   The State Board of Nurse Examiners in the United States (or the registering body in Canada) may revoke or suspend a nurse's license or registration for drug or alcohol abuse (currently the most frequent reason). Other reasons for revocation or suspension of a license or registration include fraud, deceptive practices, criminal acts, previous disciplinary action by other state boards, gross or ordinary negligence, and physical or mental impairments, even those resulting from aging (Northrop, 1986).

Once earned, a license to practice is a property right and may not be revoked without due process. This includes notice of the investigation, a fair and impartial hearing, and a proper decision based on substantial evidence. Critical to a nurse's successful defense are early legal counsel, use of character and expert witnesses, and thorough preparation for all proceedings.

Certification

Many U.S. professional organizations offer nursing certification, including two primary organizations, (1) the American Association of Critical-Care Nurses, which represents the specialty with the largest number of certified nurses, and (2) ANA, which began certifying nurses in 1974. Although certification is voluntary, nurse specialists are increasingly becoming certified. Certification programs also exist in Canada.

Crimes and Torts

A **crime** is a wrong against a person or his or her property, but the act is considered to be against the public as well. In a criminal case, the government, called "the people," prosecutes the offender. When a crime is committed, the factor of intent to commit wrong is present in most cases. However, people who break certain laws are guilty of a crime, whether or not there was intent. For example, failure to observe the Federal Food, Drug, and Cosmetic Act may constitute a crime.

In most cases, criminal law is statutory law and only infrequently, common law. Crimes are classified as felonies or misdemeanors. A **misdemeanor** is a less serious crime than a felony. Misdemeanors are commonly punishable with fines or with imprisonment for less than 1 year, or with both, or with parole. A **felony** is punishable by imprisonment in a state or federal penitentiary for more than 1 year.

A **tort** is also a wrong committed by a person against another person or his or her property. Torts generally result in civil trials. In most instances, the court in a civil case will settle damages with money but rarely by imprisonment. Torts may be intentional or unintentional acts of wrongdoing. Some of the intentional torts for which nurses may be held liable include assault and battery, defamation of character, invasion of privacy, false imprisonment, and fraud. A person committing an intentional tort is considered to have knowledge of the permitted legal limits of his or her words or acts. Violating these limits is grounds for prosecution. Unintentional torts are referred to as **negligence.**

An act generally considered a tort, may, because of its severity, be classified as a crime. For example, gross negligence that demonstrates the offender is guilty of complete disregard for another's life may be tried as both civil and criminal action. It is then prosecuted under criminal as well as civil law. By its very nature, a wrong tried as a crime implies a more serious offense with more legal implications than a tort.

Intentional Torts

Assault and Battery

Assault is a threat or an attempt to make bodily contact with another person without that person's consent. **Battery** is an assault that is carried out and includes every willful, angry, and violent or negligent touching of another person's body or clothes or anything attached to or held by that other person. Forcibly removing a client's clothing, administering an injection after the client has refused it, and shoving a client into a chair are all examples of battery. When a nurse needs to defend himself or herself or others from an assaultive client, only those actions necessary for self-protection or the aid of another are permitted (Creighton, 1986c).

Every individual has the right to be free from invasion of his or her person, and the adult client who is alert and oriented has the right to refuse any aspect of treatment. The fact that treatment is desirable does not allow the nurse or physician to proceed without the consent of the client or to go beyond the limits to which the person has consented.

Informed Consent   Every person is granted freedom from bodily contact by another person unless consent has been granted. In hospitals and other health care settings, a signed informed consent form is needed on admission (for routine treatment); for each specialized diagnostic procedure or medical or surgical treatment; and for experimentation involving clients. The consent must be written, be signed by the client or person legally responsible for the client, and be for the procedure performed. A signed consent is not needed in an emergency if there is an immediate threat to life or health, experts agree that it is an emergency, and the client is unable to consent and the legally authorized person cannot be reached. Although some value informed consent as a protection against lawsuits, the central values underlying **informed consent** include the promotion of a client's well-being and respect for the client's self-determination (President's Commission for the Study of Ethical Problems in Medicine and Biomedical and Behavioral Research, 1982). Elements of informed consent include disclosure, comprehension, competence, and voluntariness (see the display entitled Checklist to Ensure Informed Consent).

Obtaining an informed consent is the responsibility of the person who will execute the diagnostic or treatment procedure or conduct the research study. The nurse's role is to confirm that a signed consent is in the client's chart and to respond to any questions the client has about the consent. In some instances, the nurse may be responsible for having the client sign the consent form after the physician has explained to the client the procedure, its risks and benefits, and alternative treatments. The documentation of the consent process through the use of a printed consent form should not be confused with the actual explanation given to the client and the informed consent itself. When documenting consent, the nurse should assess if the client understands what he or she is signing and report to the physician any problems. Nurses often find themselves in a position where they question the client's understanding of the proposed procedure and its risks, or the client's ability to voluntarily consent to the procedure. Impediments include effects of anxiety, pain, medication, depression, and

---

Checklist to Ensure Informed Consent

Disclosure

1. Patient has been informed of current medical status and course of treatment.
2. Patient has been informed of the risks and benefits of various treatment alternatives.
3. Patient has been told that no outcomes can be guaranteed.
4. Patient has been given a professional opinion as to the best alternative.

Comprehension

5. The nurse has been innovative in transmitting information to aid understanding.
6. Interior impediments to comprehension (eg, anxiety, pain, and medication) have been assessed.
7. Exterior impediments to comprehension (eg, transcultural barriers, terminology, and speed of presentation) have been assessed.

Competence

8. The nurse has assessed competence in terms of the abilities of the client, considering age, education, and emotional stability.
9. The nurse has assessed the requirements of the task.
10. The nurse has assessed the possible deleterious effects of the client's decision.
11. The client possesses a set of values and goals that make possible reasonably consistent choices.
12. The client is able to communicate and understand the information presented.
13. The client has the ability to reason and deliberate.

Voluntariness

14. The nurse had determined that the client has not been forced to consent.
15. The nurse has been careful to avoid coercive influences by herself/himself or others.
16. The nurse has been careful to avoid subtle manipulation of the client by herself/himself or others.

(Taylor, C., & Hobaugh, R. [1986]. *Dimensions in Critical Care Nursing, 5*[2], 98–105.)

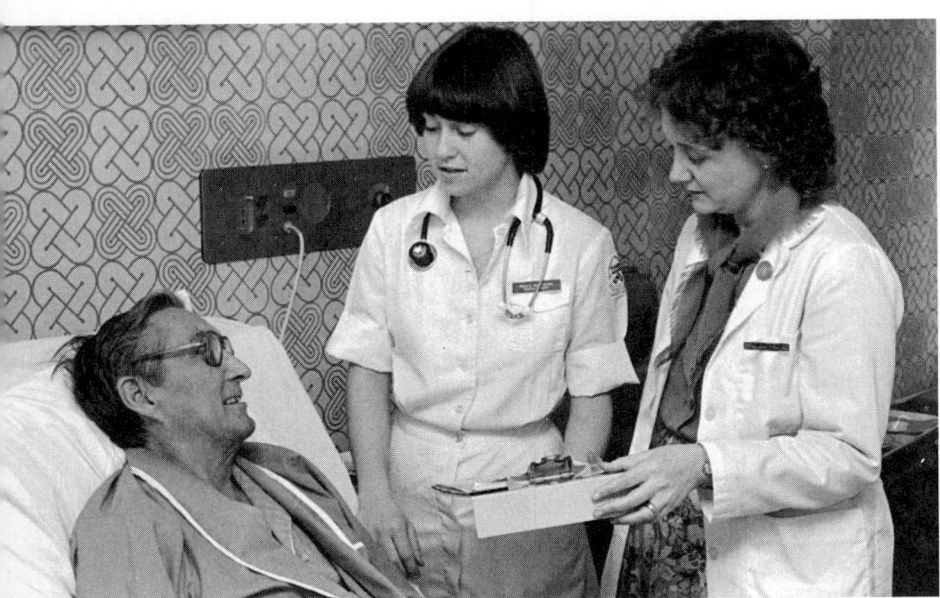

Elements of informed consent include disclosure, comprehension, competence, and voluntariness. The documentation of the consent process through the use of a printed consent form does not substitute for the actual explanation given to the client and the informed consent itself. (Photo by Gates Rhodes, courtesy of School of Nursing, University of Pennsylvania.)

temporary or permanent states of disorientation and confusion. The nurse signs the consent form as a witness to having seen the client sign the form, not to having obtained the consent (Fig. 6-2).

Consequences of not obtaining a valid consent include charges of battery against the nurse, doctor, and hospital (the hospital has a duty to protect clients and is responsible for its employees' actions). A client's refusal to sign a consent should be documented and the client should be informed of the possible consequences of the refusal. The client should sign a release form indicating his or her refusal to consent and releasing the nurse, physician, and hospital from responsibility for outcomes of this act. This statement should be witnessed.

Defamation

Defamation of character is an intentional tort in which one party makes derogatory remarks about another, diminishing the other party's reputation. *Slander* is an untruthful, oral statement about a person that subjects that person to ridicule or contempt. *Libel* is written defamation. Defamation of character is grounds for an award of civil damages. Damages are awarded on the basis of the degree of harm done to the plaintiff. Nurses who make false statements about their clients or co-workers run the risk of being sued for slander or libel. A person charged with slander or libel may not be liable if it can be proved that his statement was made not to injure another but for a nonmalicious, justifiable purpose (eg, proof of consent, truth, privilege, or fair comment).

Invasion of Privacy

The U.S. Supreme Court has interpreted the right against invasion of privacy as inherent in the federal constitution. It holds that the Fourth Amendment protects citizens by giving them the right of privacy and the right to be left alone. Disclosure of confidential information whenever a client's problem is inappropriately discussed with a third party may be construed as **invasion of privacy** and may subject the nurse to liability. The nurse's intimate knowledge of the client increases legal risk in this regard.

Currently, no uniformity exists in the Canadian laws dealing with the right to privacy, although two provinces have statutory laws that protect the right to privacy (Storch, 1982).

Certain acts by nurses could constitute invasion of privacy, as the following examples illustrate:

- Unnecessary exposure of clients while moving them through health-agency corridors or while caring for them in rooms they share with others
- Talking with clients in rooms that are not soundproof
- Discussing information concerning clients with people not entitled to the information (eg, with the client's employer or the press)
- Pressing the client for information not necessary for care planning
- Interacting with the client's family in ways not authorized by the client
- Using tape recorders, dictating machines, computer banks, and the like, without taking precautions to ensure the client's confidentiality
- Preparing written or oral class assignments about clients without concealing their identity
- Carrying out research without taking proper precautions to ensure the anonymity of clients

At times an individual's right to privacy may conflict with other rights such as the public's right to information. For example, although the client with acquired immunodeficiency syndrome (AIDS) has the right not to publicize the diagnosis, some contend that health care professionals caring for the client have the right to know that the client has AIDS so that they can protect themselves and other clients. When in doubt about disclosing confidential information, the nurse should consult the nursing supervisor, ethics committee, or public relations department of the institution.

False Imprisonment

Unjustified retention or prevention of the movement of another person without proper consent can constitute **false imprisonment**. For example, only a reasonable amount of restraint should be used in circumstances that warrant it. The indiscriminate and thoughtless use of restraints on a client can constitute the act of false imprisonment.

A person cannot be legally forced to remain in a health agency, such as a hospital, if he or she is of sound mind, even when health practitioners believe the person should remain for additional care. Health agencies have special forms to use when a client insists on being discharged against medical orders. The person's signature indicates that the agency cannot be held responsible for any harm that may result from the client's leaving. People who are mentally ill may be committed to a psychiatric institution for treatment without their consent (involuntary commitment) only when it can be proven that they are harmful to themselves or others.

Fraud

Fraud is willful and purposeful misrepresentation that could cause, or has caused, loss or harm to a person or property. Misrepresentation of a product is a common fraudulent act. In nursing, people fraudulently misrepresenting themselves to obtain a license to practice may be prosecuted under nurse practice acts. Also, misrepresenting the outcome of a procedure or treatment may constitute fraud.

Unintentional Torts

Negligence and Malpractice

Negligence is defined as performing an act that a reasonably prudent person under similar circumstances would not do, or conversely, failing to perform an act that a reasonably prudent person under similar circumstances would do. As the definition implies, an act of negligence may be an act of omission or commission. **Malpractice** is the term generally used to describe negligence of professional personnel.

Elements of Liability   Liability consists of four elements that must be established to prove that malpractice or negligence has occurred—duty, breach of duty, causation, and damages. Duty refers to an obligation to use due care (what a reasonably prudent nurse would do) and is defined by the standard of care appropriate for the nurse–client relationship. Breach of duty is the failure to meet the standard of care. Causation, the most difficult element of liability to prove, refers to the failure to meet the standard of care

TABLE   6 - 1

Examples of Elements of Liability	
Element	**Example**
Duty	Hospital staff nurses are responsible for
	• Accurate assessment of clients assigned to their care
	• Alerting responsible health care professionals to changes in a client's condition
	• Competent execution of safety measures for clients
Breach of duty	• Failure to note and report that an elderly client assessed as alert on admission is exhibiting periods of confusion
	• Failure to execute and document use of appropriate safety measures (eg, upper and lower bedside rails, use of restraints if necessary, assisted ambulation)
Causation	• Failure to use appropriate safety measures; this failure causes the client to fall while attempting to get out of bed, resulting in a fractured left hip
Damages	• Fractured left hip, pain and suffering, lengthened hospital stay, and need for rehabilitation

(breach)—this failure actually causes the injury. Damages are the actual harm or injury resulting to the client. Examples of these four elements are presented in Table 6-1.

Standards of Care   To determine negligence, a standard of care is devised by deciding what a reasonably prudent person would or would not have done under similar circumstances.

Each nurse is responsible for following the standards of care for his or her particular area of practice. For example, the labor and delivery nurse must understand how standards for nursing practice differ from those for medical obstetric practice (nurse practice act); be familiar with specific standards for obstetric nursing (eg, Standards of the Nurses' Association of the American College of Obstetricians and Gynecologists); and execute the nursing responsibilities detailed in the hospital's policies and procedures and in the job description. If hospital policy dictates an assessment of each woman in the early stages of labor every 30 minutes, the nurse must adhere to this standard unless the nurse documents a reason for doing otherwise.

Table 6-2 lists areas of potential liability associated with each of the ANA standards of clinical nursing practice. Although any nurse can make an error, nursing errors can result in serious outcomes for the client, as is illustrated in the examples.

Malpractice Litigation

When a client believes that he or she has been injured through the negligence of a nurse or other health care professional and pursues legal action, one of three outcomes usually ensues:

T A B L E 6 - 2

Areas of Potential Liability for Nurses		
Standards of Care*	**Areas of Potential Liability**	**Examples**
Standard I: Assessment		
The nurse collects client health data.	• Incomplete data base obtained (occurs frequently when client is too ill at admission to respond to questions) • Significant omissions or errors in recording data base • Failure to note in the client's plan of care (and to execute) need for more frequent nursing assessments • Failure to recognize and to report significant changes in the client's condition	• Child too weak to be weighed on admission; chart contains no record of client's weight; dosage of postoperative antibiotic therapy (which should be calculated on child's weight) too small to prevent infection; abscess develops • No record of client's allergies on chart; medication administered that led to anaphylactic shock • Previously alert client was exhibiting periods of confusion; found beating roommate with a hairbrush • Mother's labor is failing to progress, nurses unaware of signs of fetal distress; obstetrician not informed; irreversible cerebral damage to fetus • Healthy client making slower than usual post-anesthesia recovery; signs of developing cerebrovascular accident (slurred speech, difficulty moving extremities, falling to one side) present and unnoted
Standard II: Diagnosis		
The nurse analyzes the assessment data in determining diagnoses.	• Failure to identify priority nursing diagnosis critical to the client's care • Nursing diagnosis incorrectly developed and "labels" the client negatively	• Nowhere in the client's plan of care was it noted that the client had a history of choking on food ("impaired swallowing") and that close supervision was indicated during meals; client aspirated brussel sprout and died • Homosexual male client without AIDS admitted for gallbladder surgery questions the few interactions he has with staff, nursing diagnosis on cardex reads "High Risk for Violence: Directed at Others (AIDS), related to homosexuality."

*From American Nurses' Association. (1991). *Standards of nursing practice.* Kansas City, MO: Author.

• All parties concerned work toward a fair settlement.
• Case is presented to a malpractice arbitration panel (in the United States).
• Case is brought to trial court.

The steps involved in malpractice litigation where the case is brought to the trial court are shown in Figure 6-3. The nurse may be involved in legal proceedings as a defendant, a fact witness, or an expert witness.

Nurse as Defendant When a nurse is named a defendant, it is important to work closely with an attorney while preparing the defense. The attorney representing the nurse's interests will be secured either by the nurse (if carrying personal liability insurance) or by the employing hospital or institution. Recommendations for the nurse defendant include the following:

• Do not discuss the case with anyone at your hospital (in the United States, the nurse may discuss the case with the risk manager).
• Do not discuss the case with the plaintiff.
• Do not discuss the case with the plaintiff's lawyer.
• Do not discuss the case with anyone testifying for the plaintiff.
• Do not discuss the case with reporters.
• Do not alter the client's records. Tampering with a chart is the worst mistake you can make—you may well ruin your defense.
• Do not hide any information from your lawyer.
• Do not go to the witness stand unprepared.
• Do not be discourteous on the witness stand.
• Do not volunteer any information (Mandell, 1987a).

The National Nurses Claims Data Base (see accompanying

Standards of Care*	Areas of Potential Liability	Examples
Standard III: Outcome Identification		
The nurse identifies expected outcomes individualized to the client.	• No indication in nursing care plan that nurses were aware of and sensitive to the client's health care priorities	• Obese client with a history of impaired circulation continually refuses to ambulate after major abdominal surgery; client dies following a massive pulmonary embolism; plan of care showed no concern or attempt to compensate for client's lack of mobility
Standard IV: Planning		
The nurse develops a plan of care that prescribes interventions to attain expected outcomes.		
Standard V: Implementation		
The nurse implements the interventions identified in the plan of care.	• Client's record contains no documentation of attempts to teach appropriate self-care measures to client and family • Nursing interventions deviate from usual standard of care (understaffing, indifference on part of nurse, inexperience of nurse, faulty or scarce equipment or resources)	• Male client discharged from short-procedure unit on crutches; falls first day home, refracturing leg; alleges his not receiving instructions for crutch-walking caused fall; client record contains no documentation of client education • Skin breakdown on frail, elderly client worsens with eventual muscle deterioration; sepsis; nurses seem confused about treatment regimen for pressure ulcers; treatment is inconsistent
Standard VI: Evaluation		
The nurse evaluates the client's progress toward attainment of outcomes.	• No evidence in plan of care and nursing notes that nurses evaluated whether the client achieved target goals • Client discharged before key goals are met and without follow-up instructions	• Male client newly started on insulin therapy discharged without understanding the relationship among food, exercise, and insulin and after giving himself the insulin only once—no referral made to visiting nurse; client readmitted after 2 weeks with dangerously low blood sugar following overdose with insulin

display) may provide helpful information to nurse defendants.

Nurse as a Fact Witness A nurse who has knowledge of the actual incident prompting the legal case may be called on by either attorney to testify as a **fact witness.** It is critical that fact witnesses, who are placed under oath, base their testimony only on first-hand knowledge of the incident and not on assumptions. The nurse will be asked if the testimony is based on independent recollection of the incident or on documentation in the client record. The nurse may testify, "I do not remember Ms. Jones but I see from review of her record that I cared for her on the evenings of June 10, 13, 14, and 17." When in doubt about the facts of the incident, the nurse should simply testify, "I do not remember that." New research into memory is showing that people

National Nurses Claims Data Base

The National Nurses Claims Data Base (NNCDB) was set up by ANA in 1987 to provide information to the profession about professional liability claims and incidents involving nurses. Information from the NNCDB:
• Is available to nurses who need help in defending themselves against liability suits
• Assists the nursing profession in negotiating with insurance companies, assuring nurses adequate and available coverage
• Provides data for development of programs that teach nurses how to avoid malpractice

To obtain a form to report a claim to the NNCDB, call ANA at 1-800-274-4ANA.

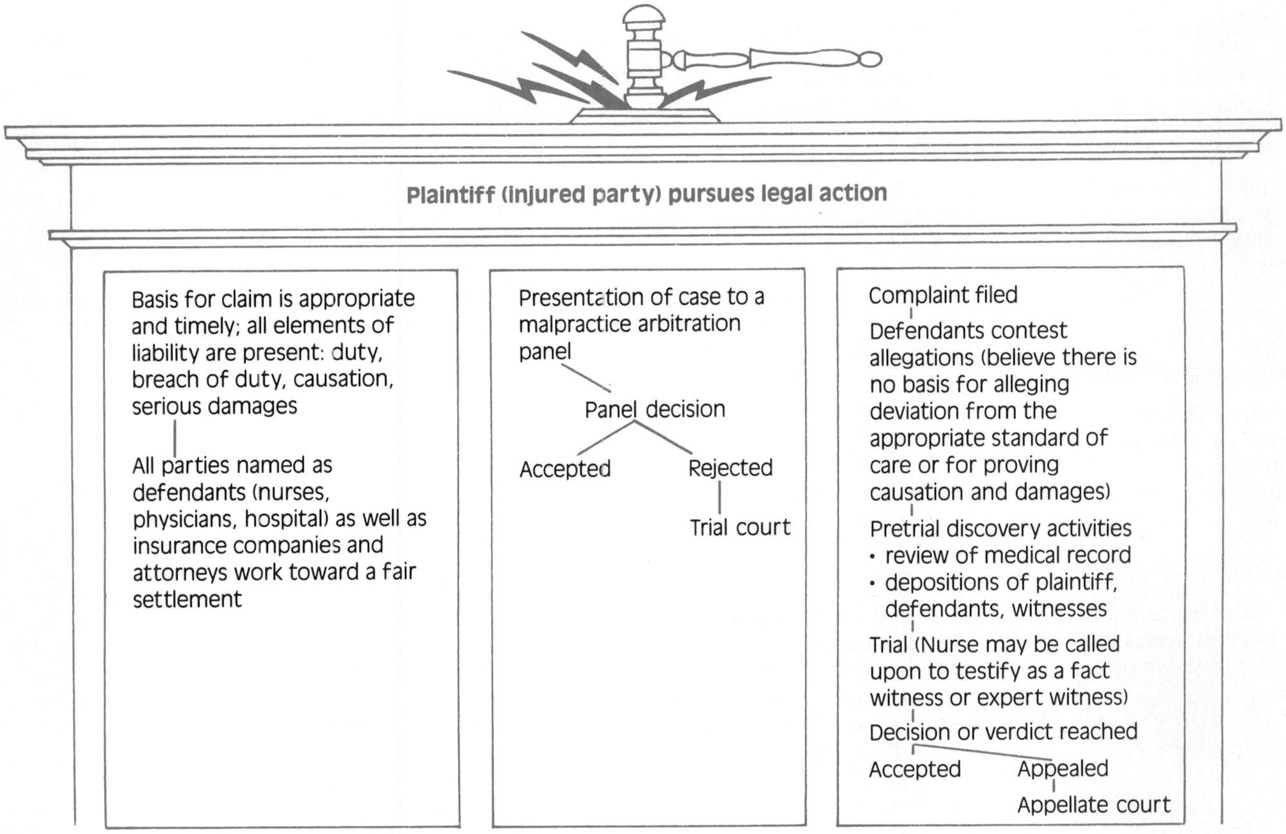

FIGURE 6-3

Civil legal procedure in malpractice litigation.

often remember things differently from the way they were and challenges the value of the eyewitness memory. Thus, accurate documentation remains the nurse's best defense.

Nurse as an Expert Witness The role of a nurse called on by either attorney to testify as an **expert witness** is to explain to the judge and jury what happened based on the client's record and to offer an opinion whether the nursing care met acceptable standards. Nurse expert witnesses need a solid educational background and strong clinical experience comparable with those of the nurse defendant. An understanding of the legal aspects of nursing and malpractice liability and knowledge of the state (or province) nurse practice act and the standard of nursing care where the incident occurred are also necessary.

Legal Safeguards for the Nurse

Contracts

A **contract** may be defined as the exchange of promises between two parties. The law of contracts provides a remedy for a breach of contract so that the person who suffers from a broken contract may be compensated for any resulting loss. For a contract to be legally enforceable, it must contain real consent of the parties, a valid consideration, a lawful purpose, competent parties, and the form required by law (Creighton, 1986a, p. 35).

Practicing nurses enter into legally valid and binding contracts with both their employers and their clients. It is thus important that they understand and are able to fulfill the terms of their agreement before giving consent.

Competent Practice

Competent practice remains the nurse's most important and best legal safeguard (Fig. 6-4). Each nurse is responsible for making sure that educational background and clinical experience are adequate to fulfill the nursing responsibilities described in the job description. Legal safeguards include the following:

- Respecting legal boundaries of practice
- Following institutional procedures and policies
- "Owning" personal strengths and weaknesses; seeking means of growth, education, supervised experience, and discussions with colleagues
- Evaluating proposed assignments; refusing to accept responsibilities for which the nurse is unprepared
- Keeping current

- Respecting client rights and developing rapport with clients
- Keeping careful documentation
- Working within the institution to develop and support management policies

Competent practice includes developing sensitivity to common sources of client injury, such as falls, use of restraints, and malfunctioning equipment, and then taking specific measures to prevent client injury. Table 6-3 lists the most frequent allegations against nurses and related prevention tips for nurses and hospitals.

Client Education

U.S. courts affirm the client's right to know and view client education as the legal duty of the nurse. Standards for client education are derived from national professional standards and from state nurse practice acts in the United States and provincial nurse practice acts in Canada, as well as the local standards described in hospital policies, procedure manuals, and job descriptions. Special forms for documenting the nurse's assessment of the client's learning needs and for subsequent teaching are available at some agencies. Failure to conduct or document the assessment of learning needs and teaching may later be construed as negligence.

General guidelines for the nurse wishing to execute client education responsibilities competently include the following:

- Determine in your practice setting what specific aspects of client education are the responsibility of nursing. Consult your job description and be familiar with agency policies regarding client education and its documentation.
- Remember that an important aim of nursing is to assist clients in managing their own care. Discuss the nursing care plan with the client and family and iden-

tify their learning needs and learning readiness. Document the teaching plan as part of the nursing care plan. Document all nursing efforts to educate the client and family about health care management and also document the client's response. If a client refuses health education or refers the nurse to a family member (eg, "Talk to my wife about my pills, she'll be giving them to me at home"), document this on the client's record. If client education greatly increases the client's anxiety and the client requests not to be given any more information, the nurse should document the client's initial response to teaching, the client's request that it be stopped, and, if the nurse complied, the reason for doing so.

- Because lack of time is a frequently offered reason for failing to document client education, nurses should assess what type of client documentation is routinely offered on their unit. If possible, they should develop forms or checklists that will facilitate rapid documentation. For example, preoperative checklists have greatly facilitated the recording of preoperative teaching and are often introduced as evidence in court that preoperative teaching was done. Other successful models include forms for documenting diabetic teaching, teaching after a myocardial infarction, and teaching postpartal and baby care to mothers. The teaching role of the nurse is discussed in Chapter 21.

Executing Physician's Orders

Nurses are legally responsible for carrying out the orders of the physician in charge of a client unless an order is one that would lead a reasonable person to anticipate injury if it were carried out. Guidelines when executing orders follow:

1. Be familiar with the parties, designated in your nurse practice act, who can legally write orders for

(Text continues on p. 90)

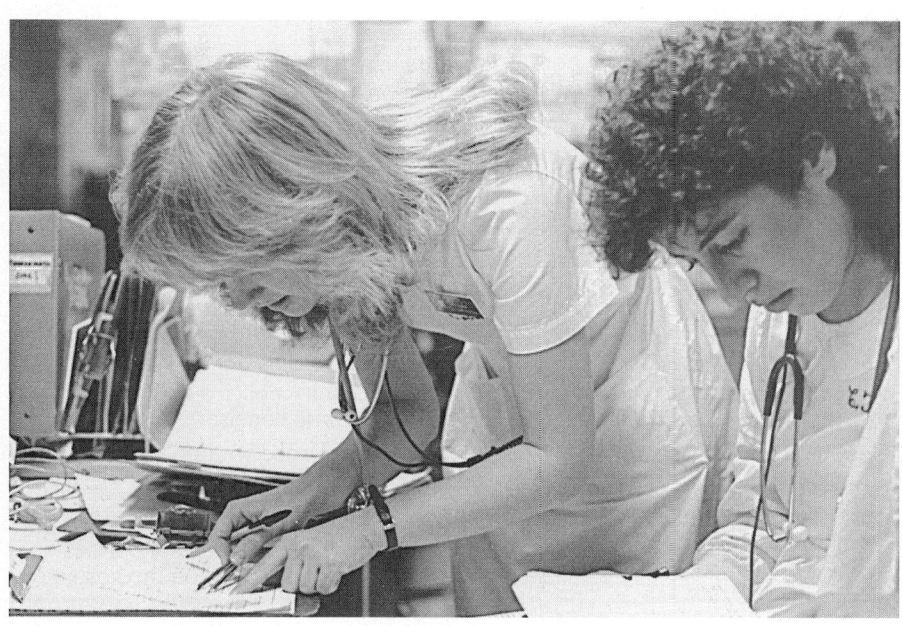

F I G U R E 6 - 4

Competent practice is the nurse's most important legal safeguard. Careful documentation is the key to competent practice. (Photo by Gates Rhodes, courtesy of School of Nursing, University of Pennsylvania.)

TABLE 6-3

Nursing Malpractice Prevention

Most Frequent Allegations Against Nurses	Prevention Tips for Nurses	Prevention Tips for Hospitals
1—Failure to Ensure Patient Safety	1—Monitor patient in a timely manner. 2—Provide assistance for those patients who require it when they need to use the lavatory or shower. 3—Keep bedrails raised for patients who are medicated or confused. 4—Use restraints appropriately.	1—Maintain an adequate level of staff. 2—Clearly define criteria for use of bedrails and restraints. 3—Provide education to nurses on patient safety.
2—Improper Treatment or Performance of Treatment	1—Question treatments you believe are improper. 2—Use proper techniques when performing procedures. 3—Follow hospital procedures when performing treatments. 4—Seek consultation for treatments beyond your abilities. 5—Update your clinical skills through continuing education classes.	1—Design a clear procedure for nurses to follow if they feel the medical treatment is inappropriate. 2—Provide resources for nurses to consult regarding treatments. 3—Provide appropriate procedures for nursing treatments.
3—Failure to Monitor and to Report	1—Follow physician's orders regarding monitoring of patient. 2—Report any requested information or significant changes in a patient's condition. 3—Perform appropriate and timely nursing assessments.	1—Verify nursing assessment skills. 2—Maintain an adequate nurse–patient ratio.
4—Medication Errors and Reactions	1—Verify any questionable medical orders. 2—Verify patient's name before administering medication. 3—Listen to patient's objections regarding medication. 4—Refer to *Physician's Desk Reference* for any questions on appropriate dosages, side effects, and reactions.	1—Provide a clear policy on verbal and written medication orders. 2—Provide current *Physician's Desk Reference* to each nursing unit. 3—Provide inservice education on medications and clear protocols regarding their administration.
5—Failure to Follow Hospital Procedure	1—Know your hospital's procedures. 2—If you must deviate from a procedure, discuss the incident with your supervisor and decide on the appropriate action. 3—Advise the appropriate person of any procedures that need to be revised.	1—Provide necessary policies and procedures that are clear and concise. 2—Measure compliance with policies and procedures. 3—Keep policies and procedures updated. 4—Recognize legal implications of policies and procedures for the nurse and the hospital.

Most Frequent Allegations Against Nurses	Prevention Tips for Nurses	Prevention Tips for Hospitals
Other Common Issues In Lawsuits		
6—Documentation	1—Document significant information about your patients objectively and factually. 2—Be time specific about the information, such as when you performed actions, made observations, or performed patient assessments. 3—Document legibly, spell correctly, and use only hospital-approved abbreviations.	1—Support the best possible method of charting, such as flow charts or computerized charting. 2—Develop standardized nursing care plans that can be customized for individual clients. 3—Routinely evaluate the quality of documentation.
7—Equipment Use	1—Learn how to operate equipment in a safe and appropriate manner. 2—In teaching patients to use equipment, follow a predetermined procedure. 3—Provide home care patients with the telephone number of a 24-hour backup hospital or home care service in case of emergency. 4—Have clients demonstrate their competence with equipment before allowing them to use it.	1—Provide orientation and ongoing in-service programs for nurses expected to use equipment, especially when it is updated or modified. 2—Have a system in place for the documentation of training sessions (ie, what was covered, who attended). 3—Verify that employee nurses and agency personnel know how to use any applicable equipment before assigning them to a particular patient.
8—Adverse Incidents	1—When adverse incidents occur, complete the appropriate documentation and report the incident to the designated individual. 2—Don't assume, voice, or record any blame for the incident.	1—Clearly delineate the institutional chain of command for reporting instances where patient care is at issue. 2—Provide a policy for how adverse incidents will be handled. 3—Provide a loss prevention program that identifies potential liabilities, guards against patient injuries, and maximizes the defense of the institution and its employee nurses.
9—Clients With HIV	1—Be conscious of actions that could result in a lawsuit: • Discrimination in treatment • Nosocomial (in hospital) transmission of the virus • Breach of confidentiality • Participation in testing a patient for HIV without first obtaining informed consent. 2—Follow hospital procedures for care of patients with infectious diseases.	1—Provide clear guidelines for nurses in caring for patients with infectious diseases. 2—Make sure the guidelines are consistent with national standards such as those established by the Centers for Disease Control. 3—Advise nurses about any state laws affecting care of patients with HIV.

(Reprinted with permission from *American Nurse,* June 1989, p. 28.)

the nurse to execute (in many states, a physician's assistant cannot legally write orders for the nurse).

2. Attempt to have all physician's orders in writing. Verbal and telephone orders should be countersigned within 24 hours. To eliminate errors caused by telephone orders:
   - Limit telephone orders to true emergency situations in which there is no alternative.
   - Designate the nurses who may take telephone orders (those who have more education and experience, such as a primary nurse).
   - Repeat a telephone order back to the physician.
   - Document the order, its time and date, the situation necessitating the order, the physician prescribing and reconfirming the order as it is read back, and your name; indicate if the order is a VO (verbal order) or TO (telephone order).
   - When telephone extensions make this possible, have two nurses listen to a questionable telephone order, with both nurses countersigning the order.

3. Question any physician order that is:
   - Ambiguous
   - Contraindicated by normal practice (eg, dose of medication that is abnormally high)
   - Contraindicated by the client's present condition (eg, as a client's present condition improves, he or she may no longer need aggressive forms of treatment)

It is good practice for the nurse to double check any order a client questions.

Documentation

Documentation is discussed in Chapter 18, and thus only the legality of documentation is discussed in this chapter. Although most nurses prefer to spend their time interacting with clients rather than writing in a client's record, careful documentation is a critical legal safeguard for the nurse. Documentation must be accurate, complete, and entered in a timely fashion. The presumption of the law is that if something was not documented, it was not done. This includes even routine acts such as taking vital signs, repositioning clients, and using side rails.

Nurses should be sure that the nursing care plan is a part of the client's permanent record. Institutions should have flow sheets or some type of documentation form that enables nurses to check off routine aspects of care rapidly and completely. The nurse should write a comprehensive nursing note for each client problem the nurse addressed during his or her time of duty. The note should include the current nature of the problem, how the nurse intervened, the client's response, and, when appropriate, future priorities for care. Once a problem is noted, nursing documentation should evidence continuity of care until the problem is resolved.

A common problem reported by nurses is not knowing how to document an incident, for example, when the nurse believes the client needs medical attention and intervention but the responsible physicians are not responding to calls for assistance. In this case, the best legal safeguard for the nurse is to document the facts of the incident, being careful not to make incriminatory statements such as, "Anyone could see we were losing this client rapidly" or "Once again, Dr. Jones was unavailable when her client needed her." The note should document the time the physician was called and the time of response or lack of response, and the subsequent nursing response (eg, nursing supervisor notified). Such a note documents that the nurse is carefully assessing the client, recognizing significant cues, and reporting them appropriately. The nursing supervisor should write the next note after reviewing the case and choosing a course of action. Client noncompliance with the therapeutic regimen should also be documented along with the nurse's attempts to increase compliance.

Adequate Staffing

Understaffing is a problem that results in reduced quality of nursing care and may jeopardize client safety. Temporary management solutions to understaffing, such as floating nurses from one unit to another or asking nurses to work overtime or double (back-to-back) shifts, are ineffective because they further jeopardize client safety. A nurse on an understaffed hospital unit will be held to a professional standard of judgment with respect to accepting responsibility for work and for delegating nursing responsibilities to others. If client injury results, the hospital employer and nurse employee will most likely be named as codefendants (Creighton, 1986b).

Professional Liability Insurance

Although a nurse's best legal safeguard is always competent practice, the increasing number of malpractice claims naming nurses as defendants make it wise for nurses to carry their own liability insurance. Nurses may obtain this insurance through ANA, through provincial nursing associations in Canada, and through other sources.

Reasons ANA lists for purchasing a personal professional liability insurance policy are as follows:

Protection of the nurse's best interests: If the nurse is named defendant in a malpractice action along with the hospital, a conflict of interest could arise between the nurse and the hospital. Nurses have no assurance of their best interest being represented unless they have their own coverage, which provides their own attorney.

Limitations of employer's coverage: Most health care facilities carry "claims made" insurance, which means if the nurse is no longer working there or the facility closes, the nurse is not covered when a claim is filed.

Care or advice given outside of work: An employer's policy only covers the nurse within the confines of the work setting.

Risk Management Programs

In the hope of reducing malpractice claims, many health care institutions have initiated risk management programs designed to identify, analyze, and treat risks. Elements of a comprehensive **risk management** program include:

Safety program: The aim is to provide a safe environment in which the basic safety needs of clients, employees, and visitors are met.

Products safety program: The aim is to ensure safe and adequate equipment; this involves ongoing equipment evaluation and maintenance.

Quality assurance program: The aim is to provide quality health care to clients; this involves ongoing evaluation of all systems used in the care of the client.

Nurses with legal questions often find hospital risk managers a helpful resource.

Incident Reports

An **incident report** is a tool used by health care institutions to document the occurrence of anything out of the ordinary that results in or has the potential to result in harm to a client, employee, or visitor. It is the chief means of identifying risks. More harm than good results from ignoring mistakes. Incident reports improve the management and treatment of clients by identifying high-risk patterns and initiating in-service programs to prevent future problems. These forms also make all the facts about an incident available to the institution in case of litigation.

The nurse responsible for a potentially or actually harmful incident or who witnesses an injury is the one who fills in the incident form. This form should contain the complete name of the person or people involved and the names of all witnesses; a complete factual account of the incident; the date, time, and place of the incident; pertinent characteristics of the person or people involved (eg, alert, ambulatory, asleep) and of any equipment or resources being used; and any other variables believed to be important to the incident. A physician completes the incident form with documentation of the medical examination when there has been actual or potential injury to a client, employee, or visitor.

In some states, the incident report may be used in court as evidence. The nurse documenting a client incident should include a complete account of what happened in the client's record; additionally, the nurse should prepare the incident report. However, documentation on the client record should not include the fact that an incident report was filed. In Canada, incident reports are on file in the institution.

Good Samaritan Laws

Good Samaritan laws are designed to protect health practitioners when they give aid to people in emergency situations. For example, a physician at the scene of an automobile accident may give emergency care without fear of legal suit if such care appears necessary, unless care is given in a grossly negligent manner.

Forty-eight states and the District of Columbia have Good Samaritan laws, although the laws vary considerably. Nurses are covered in some states but not in others. Good Samaritan legislation exists in four Canadian provinces and covers both physicians and nurses. So far, there appears to be no common law resulting from decisions based on these statutes.

No person has a legal obligation to help another, and a health practitioner, as any other person, may choose to help or to leave the scene of an emergency. However, in many situations, there would appear to be an ethical responsibility to assist. When health practitioners assist a person in an emergency situation and consent for the care is impossible, they are expected to use good judgment in determining whether an emergency exists and to give care that a reasonably prudent person with a similar background and in a similar circumstance would give.

Student Liability

Student nurses are responsible for their own acts of negligence if these result in client injury. Moreover, they are held to the same standard of care that would be used to evaluate the actions of a registered nurse (RN). Legal responsibilities of student nurses include careful preparation for each new clinical experience and a duty to notify their clinical instructor if they feel in any way unprepared to execute a nursing procedure. For no reason should a student attempt a clinical procedure if unsure of the correct steps involved in its application. The student nurse is responsible for being familiar with agency policies and procedures.

A hospital may also be held liable for the negligence of a student nurse enrolled in a hospital-controlled program because the student is considered an employee of the hospital. The status of students enrolled in college and university programs is less clear, as is the liability of the educational institution in which they are enrolled and the health care institution offering a site for clinical practice.

Nursing instructors may share a student's responsibility for damages in the event of client injury if the student's assignment called for clinical skills beyond the student's competency or the instructor failed to provide reasonable and prudent clinical supervision. Because the status of clients can change rapidly, especially in an acute-care setting, students should notify their instructor or a staff member of any significant changes in the client's condition, even if they are unsure of the meaning of these changes.

Most nursing programs require students to carry personal professional liability insurance. School policies provide coverage only for clinical nursing done for educational purposes. Moreover, student nurses who work as nursing assistants or in some other health care role are legally permitted to offer only the services contained in their job description. Even if they feel confident with medication administration, catheter insertion, and other professional nursing acts, they risk disciplinary action when they perform these procedures outside the supervised clinical practice setting.

Laws Affecting Nursing Practice

Occupational Safety and Health

The Occupational Safety and Health Act of 1970, commonly known as OSHA, set legal standards in the United States in an effort to ensure safe and healthful working conditions for men and women. The act is intended to reduce work-related injuries and illnesses. It has affected health care agencies and has increased certain responsibilities for many nurses. Occupational health and safety acts are provincial statutes in Canada. The following examples illustrate situations that could violate standards, if care is not taken, because of the potential threat to worker safety:

• Use of electrical equipment
• Use of isolation techniques for clients with infectious diseases and the management of contaminated equipment and supplies
• Use of radiation, such as infrared or ultraviolet radiation; sound or radio waves; and laser beams
• Use of chemicals, such as those that are toxic or flammable

The law, which continues to be updated, is specific concerning its applications, and fines can be severe when infractions are noted. Nurses can assist in implementing this law by promoting health and safety precautions wherever they work. Nurses employed in industrial settings have a particularly important role in conforming to the law's requirements.

Reporting Obligations

The unique nature of nurse–client interactions frequently results in the nurse's having knowledge (eg, of child abuse, rape, or a communicable disease) that a state (or province) requires to be reported. Legislation varies in this regard and the nurse is responsible for knowing what needs to be reported in the local area and to what authority.

Controlled Substances

Both the United States and Canada have special laws governing the distribution and use of **controlled substances** (drugs with abuse potential), such as narcotics, depressants, stimulants, and hallucinogens. Drug abuse laws are specific and violations are considered criminal acts. Nursing responsibilities for controlled substances include their storage in special locked compartments and documentation responsibilities.

Wills

State and provincial laws regulate requirements for a will. The person who makes a will is called the *testator*. A will describes intentions a testator wishes carried out upon his or her death. A person who receives money or property from a will is called a *beneficiary*. Nurses are occasionally asked to witness a testator's signing of his or her will.

The nurse should be familiar with the certain guidelines concerning a will and witnessing the testator's signature:

• The witness should feel sure that the testator is of sound mind, that is, the testator knows what he or she is doing and is free of the influence of drugs that could likely distort his or her thinking.
• The witness should feel sure that the testator is acting voluntarily and is not being coerced in any way concerning the terms of his or her will.
• Witnesses should watch the testator sign his or her will and they should sign in the presence of each other. State law indicates how many witnesses must acknowledge the testator's signature on a will. Two or three witnesses are most commonly required.
• Witnesses to the signature on a will do not need to read it, but they should be sure that the document being signed is a will and not some other type of document.
• In most states, a person who is a beneficiary in a will is disqualified to act as a witness to the testator's signature.

Legal Issues Related to Dying and Death

Legal responsibilities for the dying or deceased client are discussed in Chapter 13. Advance directives and do-not-resuscitate (DNR) orders are discussed in this chapter.

Advance Directives

Decisions about health care are becoming increasingly complex, and clients, family members, and health care professionals alike are all voicing frustration as they grapple with complex decisions about prolonging life. Some of the most difficult cases involve clients who are no longer able (competent) to indicate their treatment preferences. Two kinds of written **advance directives** can minimize difficulties by allowing individuals to state in advance what their choices would be for health care should certain circumstances develop. **Living wills** provide specific instructions about the kinds of health care that should be provided or forgone in particular situations (Fig. 6-5) A **durable power of attorney for health care** appoints an agent the person trusts to make decisions in the event of the appointing person's subsequent incapacity (Fig. 6-6). In Canada, a public trustee is appointed on behalf of people who do not have family support and who require financial and health decisions to be made.

Many means have been suggested to ensure that adult clients have an opportunity to learn about and use advance directives to indicate their wishes about life-prolonging treatment and to appoint surrogate decision makers should they lose decision-making capacity. Nurses have an important role to play in facilitating this dialogue. In the United States, the Patient Self-Determination Act of 1990 requires all hospitals to inform their clients of advance directives. Because the status of advance directives varies from state to state (or province to province) it is important for nurses to be familiar with federal and state (or province) law concerning these directives. Nurses can also be instrumental in developing institutional policies that ensure that clients on admission are encouraged to talk with family, significant others, and health care professionals about their treatment preferences.

Do-Not-Resuscitate or No-Code Orders

To prevent the improper use of cardiopulmonary resuscitation, which is designed to prevent unexpected death, some physicians will write DNR, or no-code, orders on the chart of a terminally ill client if the client or family has expressed

FIGURE 6-5

A living will. (President's Commission for the Study of Ethical Problems in Medicine and Biobehavioral Research. *Deciding to forego life-sustaining treatment* [pp. 314–315]. Washington, D.C.: U.S. Government Printing Office.)

"LIVING WILL"*

DECLARATION

Declaration made this _____ day of _____ 19_____.

I, _____, being of sound mind, willfully and voluntarily make known my desires that my dying shall not be artificially prolonged under the circumstances set forth below, and do declare:

If at any time I should have an incurable injury, disease, or illness certified to be a terminal condition by two (2) physicians who have personally examined me, one of whom shall be my attending physician, and the physicians have determined that my death will occur whether or not life-sustaining procedures are utilized and where the application of life-sustaining procedures would serve only to artificially prolong the dying process, I direct that such procedures be withheld or withdrawn, and that I be permitted to die naturally with only the administration of medication or the performance of any medical procedure deemed necessary to provide me with comfort or care or to alleviate pain.

In the absence of my ability to give directions regarding the use of such life-sustaining procedures, it is my intention that this declaration shall be honored by my family and physician(s) as the final expression of my legal right to refuse medical or surgical treatment and accept the consequences of such refusal.

I understand the full import of this declaration and I am emotionally and mentally competent to make this declaration.

Signed _____

Address _____

_____

I believe the declarant to be of sound mind. I did not sign the declarant's signature above for or at the direction of the declarant. I am at least 18 years of age and am not related to the declarant by blood or marriage, entitled to any portion of the estate of the declarant accord-

ing to the laws of intestate succession of the _____ _____ or under any will of the declarant or codicil thereto, or directly financially responsible for declarant's medical care. I am not the declarant's attending physician, an employee of the attending physician, or an employee of the health facility in which the declarant is a patient.

Witness _____
Address _____
_____

Witness _____
Address _____
_____

ss.:

Before me, the undersigned authority, on this _____ day of _____, 19_____, personally appeared _____, _____, and _____, known to me to be the Declarant and the witnesses, respectively, whose names are signed to the foregoing instrument, and who, in the presence of each other, did subscribe their names to the attached Declaration (Living Will) on this date, and that said Declarant at the time of execution of said Declaration was over the age of eighteen (18) years and of sound mind.

[SEAL]
My commission expires:

_____
Notary Public

*Check requirements of individual state statute.

DURABLE POWER OF ATTORNEY FOR HEALTH CARE*

I, _____
hereby appoint:

_____
name

_____
home address

_____

_____
home telephone number

_____
work telephone number

as my agent to make health care decisions for me if and when I am unable to make my own health care decisions. This gives my agent the power to consent to giving, withholding or stopping any health care, treatment, service, or diagnostic procedure. My agent also has the authority to talk with health care personnel, get information, and sign forms necessary to carry out those decisions.

If the person named as my agent is not available or is unable to act as my agent, then I appoint the following person(s) to serve in the order listed below.

1. _____
   name

   _____
   home address

   _____

   _____
   home telephone number

   _____
   work telephone number

2. _____
   name

   _____
   home address

   _____

   _____
   home telephone number

   _____
   work telephone number

By this document I intend to create a power of attorney for health care that shall take effect upon my incapacity to make my own health care decisions and shall continue during that incapacity.

*Check requirements of individual state statute.

My agent shall make health care decisions as I direct below or as I make known to him or her in some other way.

(a) STATEMENT OF DESIRES CONCERNING LIFE-PROLONGING CARE, TREATMENT, SERVICES, AND PROCEDURES:

_____

_____

_____

_____

_____

_____

_____

(b) SPECIAL PROVISIONS AND LIMITATIONS:

_____

_____

_____

_____

_____

_____

_____

_____

BY SIGNING HERE I INDICATE THAT I UNDERSTAND THE PURPOSE AND EFFECT OF THIS DOCUMENT.

I sign my name to this form on _____
                                              (date)

My current home address: _____

_____

_____
(You sign here)

their wish for a peaceful death without heroic measures. Many physicians are reluctant to write these orders, especially when this issue is a source of conflict between the client and family or between individual family members. In these cases, a physician who believes the client will not benefit from resuscitative measures may verbally indicate to the nurse that only a slow-code should be called, that is, in the case of cardiopulmonary or respiratory arrest, calling a code and resuscitating the client are to be delayed until these measures will be ineffectual. The legality of no-code and slow-code orders is not well established and is generally decided on a case-by-case basis. It is likely that a nurse could be charged negligent in the event of a slow-code and resultant client death.

WITNESS

I declare that the person who signed or acknowledged this document is personally known to me, that he/she signed or acknowledged this durable power of attorney in my presence, and that he/she appears to be of sound mind and under no duress, fraud, or undue influence. I am not the person appointed as agent by this document, nor am I the patient's health care provider or an employee of the patient's health care provider.

First Witness

Signature: _____

Home Address: _____

Print Name: _____

Date: _____

Second Witness

Signature: _____

Home Address: _____

Print Name: _____

Date: _____

(AT LEAST ONE OF THE ABOVE WITNESSES MUST ALSO SIGN THE FOLLOWING DECLARATION.)

I further declare that I am not related to the patient by blood, marriage, or adoption, and, to the best of my knowledge, I am not entitled to any part of his/her estate under a will now existing or by operation of law.

Signature: _____

Signature: _____

I further declare that I am not related to the patient by blood, marriage, or adoption, and, to the best of my knowledge, I am not entitled to any part of his/her estate under a will now existing or by operation of law.

Signature: _____

Signature: _____

FIGURE 6-6

Durable Power of Attorney for Health Care. (From Barbara Mishkin, Hogan and Hartson.)

KEY POINTS

- As the roles and duties of the nurse have expanded, so too has the legal accountability of the nurse.
- Laws are standards or rules of conduct established and enforced by the government of a society to protect the rights of the public. Laws may be constitutional, statutory, administrative, or common.

- Voluntary standards regulating nursing practice are developed and implemented by the nursing profession itself. These standards include the ANA and CNA standards of practice, professional standards for the accreditation of education and service programs, and certification standards.

- Legal standards are mandatory and are developed by legislative action controlling professional conduct. They include the nurse practice acts and rules and regulations of nursing.
- Credentialing is the process of ensuring and maintaining professional competence. Credentialing involves accreditation, licensure or registration, and certification.
- A nurse whose license is suspended or revoked because the nurse engaged in drug and alcohol abuse or other acts of unprofessional conduct is entitled to due process of law.
- Intentional torts for which the nurse may be liable include assault and battery, defamation of character, invasion of privacy, false imprisonment, and fraud.
- Every individual has the right to be free from invasion of person, and thus consent is needed for all diagnostic, treatment, or research procedures. The person performing the procedure is responsible for obtaining informed consent. Documenting the informed consent may be delegated to nursing.
- Negligence is defined as performing an act that a reasonably prudent person under similar circumstances would not do or as failing to perform an act.

- Legal safeguards for the nurse include understanding and fulfilling the terms of contracts with employers and employees, competent practice, thorough client education, safe execution of physician orders, careful documentation, professional liability insurance, and participation in risk management programs.
- The client's record should never be tampered with in an attempt to prepare a better defense.
- Competent practice includes respecting legal boundaries of nursing, following institutional procedures and policies, owning personal strengths and being aware of weaknesses, evaluating proposed assignments, keeping current, respecting client rights and developing rapport with clients, providing careful documentation, and working with nursing management to develop and implement programs to improve quality care and decrease risks of client injury.
- Student nurses are legally responsible for their own acts of negligence resulting in client injury. They are held to the same standard of care that would be used to evaluate the actions of an RN.
- Nurses need to be knowledgeable about specific laws affecting nursing practice. These include laws regulating occupational health and safety, reporting obligations, controlled substances, wills, and legislation related to dying and death.

BIBLIOGRAPHY

American Nurses' Association. (1990). *Liability prevention and you: What nurses and employers need to know.* Kansas City, MO: Author.

American Nurses' Association. (1991). *Position statement on nursing and the patient self-determination act.* Kansas City, MO: Author.

American Nurses' Association. (1992). *Position statement on foregoing artificial nutrition and hydration.* Washington, DC: Author.

American Nurses' Association. (1992). *Position statement on nursing care and do-not-resuscitate decisions.* Washington, DC: Author.

Anderson, M. et al. (1991). The living will issue: Who has the right to choose? *Canadian Nurse, 87*(10), 37–39.

Brown, C. (1990). Limiting care: Is CPR for everyone? *AACN Clinical Issues in Critical Care Nursing, 1*(1), 161–168.

Calfee, B. E. (1991). Protecting yourself from allegations of nursing negligence. *Nursing, 21*(12), 34–39.

Collins, H.L. (1987). Certification: Is the payoff worth the price? *RN, 50*(7), 36–44.

Cournoyer, C. P. (1985). Protecting yourself legally after a patient's injured. *Nursing Life, 5*(2), 18–22.

Creighton, H. (1986a). *Law every nurse should know* (5th ed.). Philadelphia: Saunders.

Creighton, H. (1986b). Understaffing. *Nursing Management, 17*(4), 24, 27–28; *17*(5), 14, 16.

Creighton, H. (1986c). When can a nurse refuse to give care? *Nursing Management, 17*(3), 16, 18–20.

Cushing, M. (1990). Law and orders. . . . How you carry out medical orders. *American Journal of Nursing, 90*(5), 29–30, 32.

DeMilliano, M. (1984). 8 Common charting mistakes to avoid. *Nursing Life, 4*(3), 30–32.

Fiesta, J. (1988). *Law and liability for nurses* (2nd ed.). Albany: Delmar Publishers.

Fine, E.R.J. (1982). What to do when the doctor's wrong. *Nursing Life, 2*(6), 22–24.

Hall, J. K. (1990). Understanding the fine line between law and ethics. *Nursing, 20*(10), 34–40.

Houston, C. S. (1988). Living wills: A solution to the prolonged act of dying? *Canadian Medical Association Journal, 139*, 241–243.

Johnson, L. G. (1990). Preparing for a deposition. *Nursing, 20*(7), 44–47.

Killian, W. H. (October 1990). Nursing students face liability risk too. *American Nurse, 13*.

Mandell, M. (1986). Ten legal commandments for nurses who get sued. *Nursing Life, 6*(3), 18–21.

McWilliams, R. M. (1990). Reflections on being an expert witness. *Today's OR Nurse, 12*(1), 17–19, 26–28.

Murphy, E. K. (1990). Incident reports may or may not be privileged information. *AORN Journal, 51*(3), 851–852, 854.

Murphy, E. K. (1991). Informed consent doctrine. *Nursing Outlook, 39*(1), 48.

Need for liability protection keeps growing: An interview

with Pat McLean, manager, Canadian Nurses Protective Society. (1992). *RN,* April/May, 8–10.

Norman, J. (1990). Dr. Grant liked to pull a disappearing act. *Nursing, 20*(3), 110, 112, 114.

Northrup, C. E. (1985). Student nurses and legal accountabilities. *Imprint, 32*(4), 16, 18–20.

Northrup, C. E. (1986). Unprofessional conduct and licensure revocation. *Nursing Outlook, 34*(1), 48.

Northrup, C. E. (1987). *Legal issues in nursing.* St. Louis: Mosby.

Pazola, K. J., & Gerberg, A. K. (1990). Privileged communication: Talking with a dying adolescent. *MCN: American Journal of Maternal–Child Nursing, 15*(1), 16–21.

President's Commission for the Study of Ethical Problems in Medicine and Biomedical and Behavioral Research. (1982). *Making healthcare decisions: A report* (vol. 1). Washington, DC: U.S. Government Printing Office.

Quinley, K. M. (1990). Legal side: Twelve tips for defending yourself in a malpractice suit. *American Journal of Nursing, 90*(1), 37–38, 40.

Rabinaw, J. (1989). Where you stand in the eyes of the law. *Nursing, 19*(2), 34–42.

Roach, M. S. (1990). The need for distinction. *Canadian Nurse, 86*(8), 28–29.

Rozovsky, L. E. (1989). The nurse as "Good Samaritan." *Canadian Operating Room Nursing Journal, 7*(3), 20–21.

Rozovsky, L. E., & Rozovsky, F. A. (1986). The legal dilemma: Getting caught between a rock and a hard place. *Canadian Critical Care Journal, 3*(1), 15–16, 19.

Storch, J. (1982). *Patient's rights: Ethical and legal issues in healthcare and nursing.* Toronto: McGraw-Hill Ryerson.

Streim, J. E., Siebers, M. J., Hill, S. L., Bauwens, S. F., Meyer, M., & Vincent, M. O. (1989). Planning in advance for critical care. *American Journal of Nursing, 89*(1), 37–41.

Taylor, C., & Hobaugh, R. (1986). The role of the critical care nurse in developing informed consent. *Dimensions of Critical Care Nursing, 5*(2), 98–105.

U. S. Special Committee on Aging. (1989). *A matter of choice: Planning ahead for health care decisions.* Washington, DC: American Association of Retired Persons.

Weiler, K. (1990). The law and nursing. *Imprint, 37*(1), 23–24.

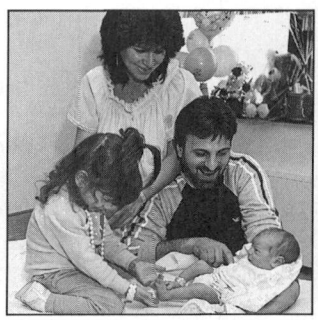 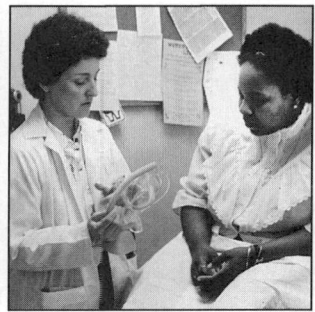  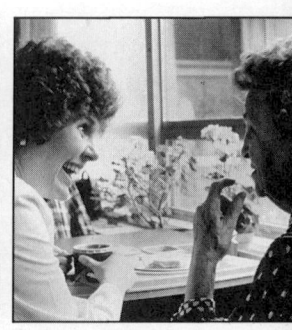

The Client: Concepts for Holistic Care

The chapters in Unit II focus on the client—the person receiving health care from the nurse. Concepts necessary in providing holistic care for the client as an individual and as a member of a family and community include basic needs, culture and ethnicity, and stress and adaptation. By considering all aspects of the individual, nurses can provide health care oriented toward wellness and can maximize the client's strengths to reach his or her potential.

In Unit II, Maslow's hierarchy of basic human needs provides a framework for prioritizing nursing actions and for understanding the relation between the ability to meet needs and the social environment. Family structures and functions are examined; the influence of the family and the community on health and illness is described. Consideration of cultural and ethnic factors in client care expands the nurse's holistic perspective of the client.

Stress and adaptation have great importance for nurses who are themselves subject to stress and who care for clients experiencing physiologic and psychological stressors. Stress affects basic need attainment, is influenced by sociocultural environments, and may either promote health or precipitate illness. Nursing actions to reduce stress, facilitate wellness, and promote coping must be individualized and holistic.

Unit II provides the knowledge necessary to understand the integration of basic human needs, sociocultural influences, and stress and adaptation—factors that make up the composite whole of each individual client—into nursing care, which will make that care holistic and individualized.

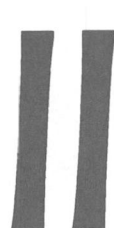

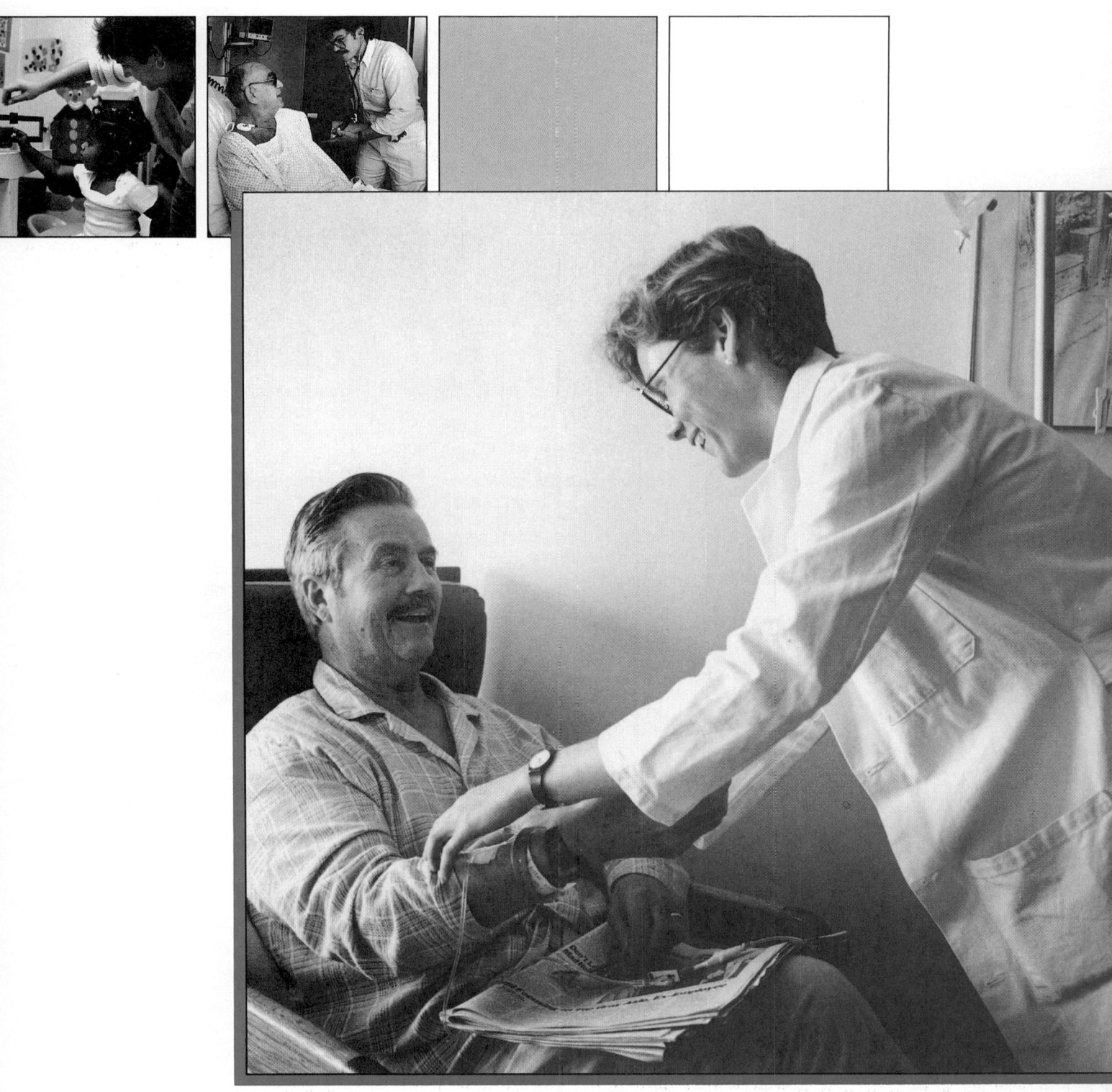

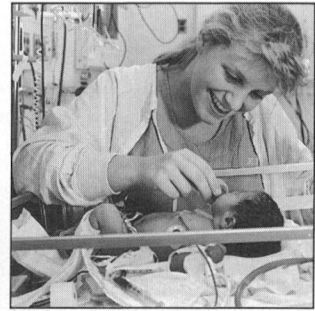
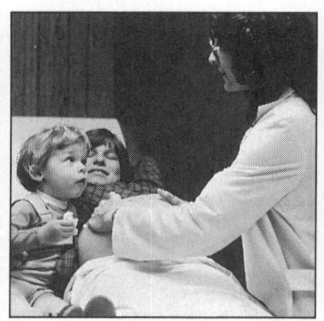

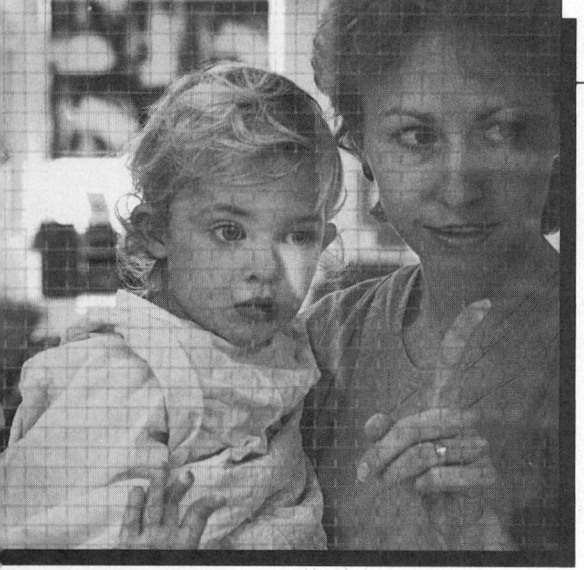

Basic Human Needs: Individual, Family, and Community

OBJECTIVES

After studying this chapter, the learner should be able to:

Define key terms used in the chapter.

Describe each level of Maslow's hierarchy of basic human needs.

Discuss nursing actions necessary to meet needs for each level of Maslow's hierarchy.

Discuss family concepts, including family roles, structures, functions, developmental stages, tasks, and health risk factors.

Identify aspects of the community that affect individual and family health.

Describe nursing interventions to promote and maintain wellness in the individual as a member of a family and as a member of the community.

KEY TERMS

basic human needs
blended family
cohabiting family
community
extended family
hierarchy of basic needs
love and belonging needs
nuclear family
physiologic needs
safety and security needs
self-actualization need
self-esteem need
single-parent family
step family
traditional family

7

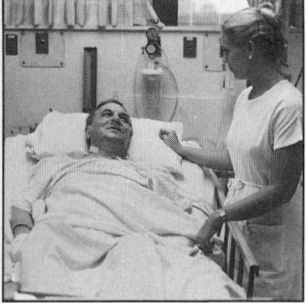

Humans are complex organisms, influenced by and responsive to both internal and external environments. Our behaviors, our feelings about self and others, our values, and the priorities we set for ourselves are all the result of physiologic and psychosocial needs. These needs are common to all people and are essential to the health and survival of all people, so they are labeled **basic human needs**. Basic human needs are met or unmet in a variety of ways. Some needs are met independently, but most require relationships and interactions with other people for partial or complete fulfillment. Need satisfaction largely depends on an individual's social environment, especially a person's family and community.

Holistic nursing care is based on the consideration of all of the dimensions affecting human needs in health and in illness. Chapter 2 provided an introduction to the dimensions of the whole person and the interaction of human needs with those dimensions. This chapter discusses how basic human needs affect the individual, the family, and the community.

Individual

In nursing, we are concerned with the physical and psychologic needs of each individual client. Abraham Maslow (1968) developed a hierarchy of basic human needs (Fig. 7-1) that is used to determine the needs of the client that are the most important at any given time. Certain needs are more basic than others and must at least be minimally met before other needs can be considered.

Levels of Needs

Maslow's hierarchy of basic needs is useful in understanding the relationships of basic human needs and in establishing priorities of care. The hierarchy is based on the theory that something is a basic need if:

- Its absence results in illness
- Its presence prevents illness or signals health
- Meeting an unmet need restores health
- If it is unmet, it is preferred over other satisfactions
- There is a feeling of something missing when the need is unmet
- There is a feeling of satisfaction when the need is met

Maslow arranged the hierarchy of basic human needs to illustrate that certain needs are more basic than other needs. Although all of the needs are present within each person all of the time, the person strives to meet certain of the needs (at least to a minimal level) before attending to other needs. The five levels of needs, with physiologic needs being the most basic, are as follows:

Level 1: Physiologic needs
Level 2: Safety and security needs
Level 3: Love and belonging needs
Level 4: Self-esteem needs
Level 5: Self-actualization needs

Nursing care is often directed toward meeting unmet needs. Maslow's hierarchy provides a framework for nursing assessment and for understanding the needs of clients at all levels so that interventions to meet needs become a part of the care plan. For example, in caring for a person coming into the emergency department with a heart attack, the nurse's immediate concern would be physiologic needs (ie, oxygen and pain relief). However, at the same time, safety needs (eg, following proper precautions with oxygen use and ensuring the person does not fall off the examining table) and love and belonging needs (eg, letting a family member stay with the person, if possible) are major considerations.

The nursing activities that you will learn as you progress through your education are aimed at meeting basic human needs of clients. The following discussion describes each level of need.

FIGURE 7-1

Maslow's hierarchy of basic human needs.

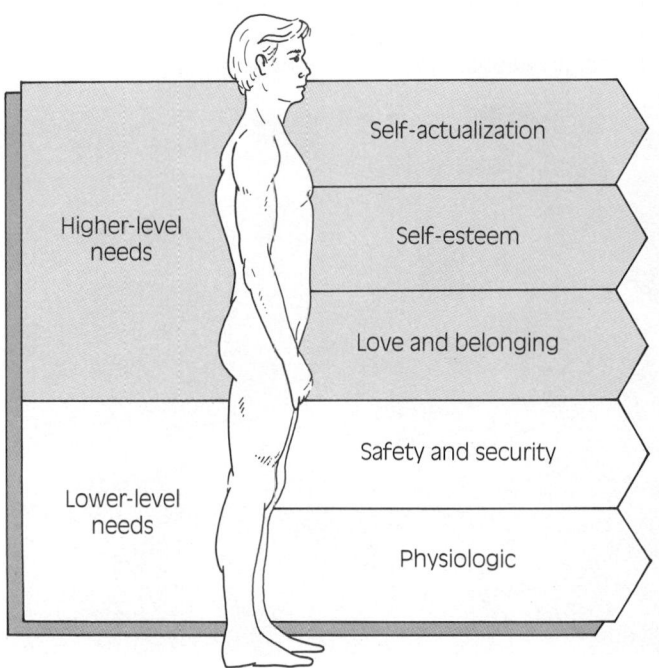

Physiologic Needs

Physiologic needs, located at the base of the hierarchy of needs, have the highest priority. **Physiologic needs**—oxygen, food, water, temperature, elimination, sexuality, physical activity, and rest—must be minimally met to maintain life. Most healthy children and adults meet their physiologic needs, but physiologic needs are often a major part of the nursing care plan for young, old, disabled, and ill people who require assistance in meeting these needs.

Oxygen is the most essential of all needs; all body cells require oxygen for survival. Oxygenation of body cells is carried out primarily by the respiratory and cardiovascular systems, and any alteration in their structure and function can result in increased need for oxygen. This need may be acute (necessitating cardiopulmonary resuscitation) or chronic (requiring special positioning, treatments, and teaching). Nurses evaluate oxygen needs by continual assessment of skin color, vital signs, and responsiveness.

Physical activity and rest are also basic physiologic needs. Physical activity is accomplished by intact and functioning neuromuscular and bony systems. Immobility, with disuse of muscles and bones, affects all other basic needs. Rest and sleep allow time for the body to rejuvenate and be free of stress. Individual requirements for rest and sleep vary widely, but the effects of deprivation have been well documented. Factors that influence sleep are age, environment, exercise, stress, and drug use. Clients entering the health care setting often need increased rest and sleep but are unable to meet these needs without or because of the nurse's interventions.

F I G U R E   7 - 2

By teaching the mother to feed her infant by gavage, the nurse is helping to fulfill the need for love and belonging of both mother and child. (Photo by Gates Rhodes, courtesy of School of Nursing, University of Pennsylvania.)

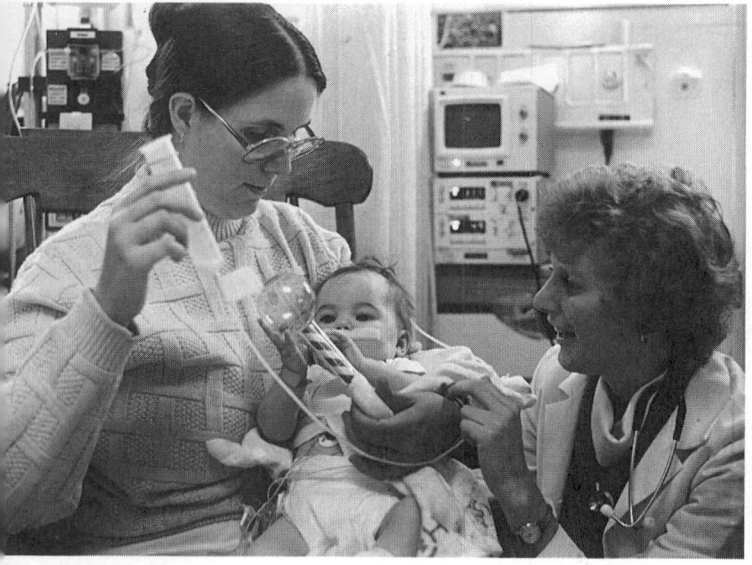

Safety and Security Needs

Safety and security needs come next in priority and involve both physical and emotional components. *Physical safety* means protecting a person from potential harm or actual harm. Nurses carry out a wide variety of activities to meet clients' physical safety needs, for example:

- Handwashing and using sterile techniques to prevent infection
- Using electrical equipment properly
- Giving medications knowledgeably
- Using skill and rationale to transfer and ambulate clients
- Teaching parents about household chemicals that are dangerous to children

Emotional safety and security involves trusting others and being free of fear, anxiety, and apprehension. Clients entering the hospital may have increased emotional security needs; often they fear the unknown and depend on others through no fault of their own. Nurses can meet such needs by encouraging religious practices that give peace, allowing as much independent decision making and control as possible, and carefully explaining new and unfamiliar procedures and treatments.

Love and Belonging Needs

All humans have a basic need for love and belonging. Following physiologic and safety and security needs, this is the next priority of need and is often called a higher level need. **Love and belonging needs** include the understanding and acceptance of others in both giving and receiving love, and the feeling of belonging to others—friends, peers, families, neighborhoods, and communities.

People who perceive that their love and belonging needs are unmet often have a sense of loneliness and isolation. They may withdraw physically and emotionally, or they may become overly demanding and critical. Often these behaviors are a signal (or cue) that unmet needs are present. Nurses should always consider love and belonging needs in their care plan. Some nursing interventions to meet this need are as follows:

- Including family and friends in the care of the client (Fig. 7-2)
- Establishing a nurse–client relationship based on mutual understanding and trust (through demonstration of caring, communication, and respect for privacy)
- Referring clients to groups that focus on problems (such as cancer support groups or AA)

Self-Esteem Needs

The next highest priority on the hierarchy is **self-esteem need**—the need for a person to feel good about himself or herself, to feel pride and a sense of accomplishment in what the person does, and to believe that others also hold that person in high regard. Self-esteem gives the individual confidence and independence.

Many factors affect self-esteem. When a person's role changes (eg, through job loss or through loss of a child who has just moved out of the home), self-esteem can be seriously altered because responsibilities and relationships have also changed. Other changes that may affect self-esteem are a change in body image, such as a gain in, or loss of, weight; an injury; or a growth spurt during puberty. Nurses must remember that the person's perception of the change—rather than the actual change itself—is what affects that individual's self-esteem.

Nurses can meet clients' self-esteem needs by accepting values and beliefs, encouraging clients to set attainable goals, and facilitating support by family or significant others. These actions will promote a sense of worth and self-acceptance.

Self-Actualization Needs

The highest level on the hierarchy of needs is **self-actualization need**—the need for an individual to reach his or her potential through full development of the individual's unique capabilities. In general, each lower level of need must be met to some degree before this need can be satisfied. The process of self-actualization is one that continues throughout life. Maslow lists the following qualities that indicate achievement of one's potential:

- Acceptance of self and others as they are
- Focus of interest on problems outside of self
- Ability to be objective
- Feelings of happiness and affection for others
- Respect for all people
- Ability to discriminate between good and evil
- Creativity as a guideline for solving problems and carrying out interests

To meet clients' self-actualization needs, the nurse must focus on strengths and possibilities, rather than on problems. Nursing interventions are aimed at caring for the total person (holistic care); providing a sense of direction and hope; and engaging in teaching that is aimed at maximizing potentials.

Applying Maslow's Theory

Maslow's hierarchy of basic needs can be applied to the assessment, planning, implementation, and evaluation of client care. Several nursing diagnoses, approved by the North American Nursing Diagnosis Association, are based on the levels of needs. (The five steps of the nursing process are discussed in Unit IV.) The hierarchy can be used with all ages, in all health care settings, and in both health and illness. It provides a vehicle for holistic nursing care—identifying unmet needs as they become health care needs and considering all dimensions. The hierarchy of basic needs allows the nurse to place the client on the health–illness continuum and to incorporate the health models into meeting needs.

As the nurse identifies and carries out interventions to meet needs, he or she must remember that this is only a framework or guideline, and that, in actuality, each individual sets priorities and meets needs on the level most important to that person. Additionally, basic human needs are related and may require nursing actions at more than one level at a given time.

Family

Almost every person is a member of a number of groups, such as a group of friends, a work group, a church group, or a school group. Each of these groups is concerned with a specific part of the person's life and is important to the person. However, only one group is concerned with all parts of a person's life and with meeting his or her physical, emotional, and social needs. That group is the family.

What Is a Family?

A **family** can be simply defined as any group of people who live together. Families exist in all sizes and configurations and are essential to the health and survival of the individual family members, and to society as a whole. The family serves as a buffer between the needs of the individual family member and the demands and expectations of the society in which it exists. The role of the family is to meet the needs of its members while also meeting the needs of society (Friedman, 1992).

Duvall (1977) defined family as two or more people who are related through blood, marriage, adoption, or birth. Friedman (1992) expanded that definition by describing a family as comprising two or more people who are emotionally involved with each other and live close together. This definition includes more of the different types of current family structures in which members may be unrelated either biologically or legally.

Family Structures

No one commonly accepted form of family structure currently exists. The following discussion briefly introduces the many different types of family structures.

Traditional Family The **traditional family** comprises a father, a mother, and their children (Fig. 7-3). The father and mother are married, and all members of the family live in the same house until the children leave home as young adults. The traditional family may comprise biologic parents and children, adoptive parents and children, surrogate parents and children, or stepparents and children.

Fitting within the broad traditional family definition are couples without children, and couples with grown children who no longer live at home. The **blended family** is also a traditional family, although it comprises family units who join together to form a new family structure. Children in a blended family live most often with one birth parent and one non–birth parent in a unit called a **step family**.

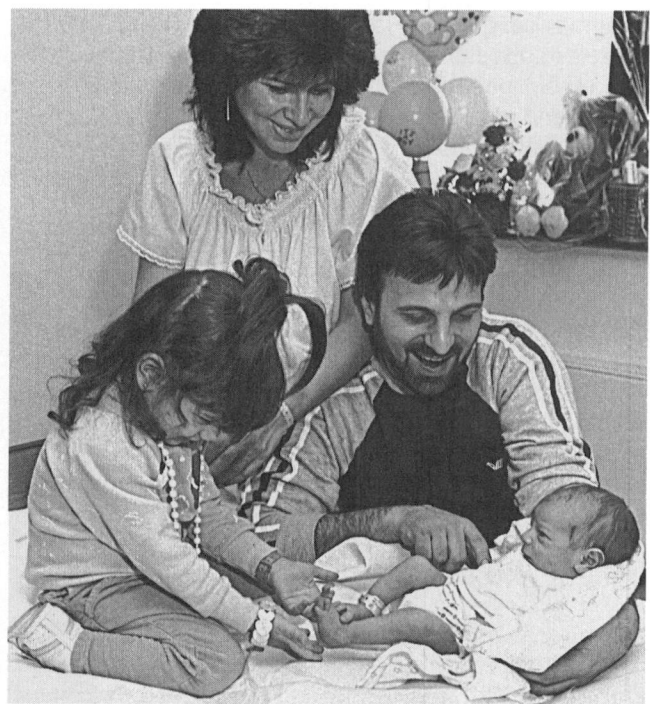

FIGURE 7-3

The members of this nuclear family—mother, father, and child—celebrate the new addition to their family. (Photo by Don Walker, courtesy of Thomas Jefferson University Hospital.)

In the traditional **nuclear family**, the father is the family member who goes to work, providing economic security, whereas the mother stays at home, providing physical and emotional safety and security. This family group usually lives in close geographic proximity to relatives, such as aunts, uncles, and grandparents, who are a part of the **extended family**. Although this was the accepted family structure for many years, that has changed.

The traditional family unit still has the same form (ie, mother, father, and children), but the roles of the members have changed considerably. Two major factors have caused this change: (1) increased education and career opportunities for women and (2) changes in the U.S. economy—changes requiring that families earn additional income to maintain a desired standard of living. As a result, two-career families, in which both parents work outside the home, have become the norm instead of the exception. When both parents work, there is usually a blending of tasks, with the father taking a more active role in housework and child care and the mother contributing to economic support.

With changes in the traditional family structure have come other influences on the needs of family members. Considerations for the family, and for nursing care, include support systems (in our mobile society, family members may live hundreds or thousands of miles away); availability of child care; time for leisure and recreation; and changing role models.

Single-Parent Families Single parents may be never married, separated, divorced, or widowed. Most often, the single parent is divorced or widowed, but increasing numbers of never-married men and women are choosing to become parents. The single-parent family, however, is most often headed by women. Nearly 95% of all single parents are women; single parents compose more than 16% of North American families (U.S. Bureau of the Census, 1984).

Single parents have many special problems and needs, including financial concerns; role shifts (ie, being both father and mother, remarriage or relationships with the opposite sex); and social stigma. These problems are important considerations when planning and implementing nursing care (Friedman, 1992).

Alternate Family Structures Some families do not meet the definition of traditional or single-parent families but do meet the criteria previously outlined. It is critical for nurses to remember that there are no absolute "rights" or "wrongs," and that one individual's values must not be imposed on another person. Acceptance of family members and relationships is essential to holistic, individualized client care. Alternate family structures include the following:

Cohabiting families: This form includes those individuals who choose to live together for a variety of reasons—relationships, financial need, or changing values. Cohabiting families include unmarried adults living together, communal or group marriages, and gay and lesbian families.

Single adults: Although the single person is not living with others, he or she is part of a family of origin, usually has a social network with significant others, or may even regard a pet as family. Most single adults living alone are found in two age groups: (1) the young adult who has achieved independence and enters the work force and (2) the elderly person, left alone through death of a spouse.

Family Functions

The family provides a set of functions important to the needs of the individual family members and to society as a whole. The family provides the individual with the necessary environment for development and social interactions; it also provides new and socialized members for society. Five major functions of the family are as follows:

Physical: The family provides a safe, comfortable environment necessary to growth, development, and rest or recuperation.

Economic: The family provides financial aid to family members, and also meets monetary needs of society.

Reproductive: The family gives birth to children.

Affective and coping: The family provides emotional comfort to members. It also helps members establish an identity and maintain that identity during times of stress.

Tasks for Family Survival and Continuity

- Providing shelter, food, clothing, and health care
- Allocating resources (money, time, space) according to each member's needs
- Determining individual roles and responsibilities in the support, management, and care of the home and family members
- Ensuring socialization of members through the internalization of increasingly mature roles in the family and in society
- Establishing socially acceptable ways of interacting, communicating, and expressing feelings (eg, affection, aggression, sexuality)
- Rearing children (natural, adopted) and then releasing them appropriately
- Relating to the community (school, church, work, neighborhood) and establishing rules for relatives, guests, friends
- Maintaining morale and motivation, rewarding achievement, meeting personal and family crises, setting attainable goals, and developing family loyalties and values

(Duvall, E. [1977]. *Marriage and family development* [5th ed.]. Philadelphia: Lippincott.)

Socialization: The family teaches; transmits beliefs, values, attitudes, and coping mechanisms; provides feedback, and guides problem solving (Friedman, 1992).

Developmental Tasks of Families

Duvall (1977) has identified stages of the family life cycle and critical family developmental tasks. Duvall's theory, based on Erikson's theory of psychosocial development (defined in Chapter 10), states that all families have certain basic tasks for survival and continuity, and also have specific tasks related to each stage of development throughout the life of the family. The basic tasks defined in the display entitled Tasks for Family Survival and Continuity are closely related to the functions of the family. They are included here because they expand those functions previously discussed.

The developmental tasks of the family are related to sequential stages in the life of a family. Seven stages and related developmental tasks are identified in Table 7-1. If developmental tasks are not met, societal disapproval and intervention may occur in areas such as child abuse, police actions, welfare agencies, or health departments (Edelman & Mandle, 1990). The successful mastery of each developmental stage is important to adaptation and family growth through successive stages.

Family in Health and Illness

Health care activities, health beliefs, and health values are learned as part of a family. In health and illness, as well as in other areas of life, the individual reflects behaviors learned as a family member. When a person enters the health care system, he or she brings his or her own personal behaviors and needs, but the person also brings (in a sense) his or her

TABLE 7-1

Family Stages and Tasks	
Stage	**Task**
Beginning family	Establishing a mutually satisfying marriage
	Planning to have or not have children
Childbearing family (see Fig. 7-3)	Having and adjusting to infant
	Supporting needs of all three members
	Renegotiating marital relationship
Family with preschool children	Adjusting to costs of family life
	Adapting to needs of preschool children to stimulate growth and development
	Coping with parental loss of energy and privacy
Family with school-age children	Adjusting to the activity of growing children
	Promoting joint decision making between children and parents
	Encouraging and supporting children's educational achievements
Family with teenagers and young adults	Maintaining open communication among members
	Supporting ethical and moral values within the family
	Balancing freedom with responsibility for teenagers
	Releasing young adults with appropriate ritual and assistance
	Strengthening marital relationship
	Maintaining supportive home base
Postparental family	Preparing for retirement
	Maintaining ties with older and younger generations
Aging family	Adjusting to retirement
	Adjusting to loss of spouse
	Closing family home

(Data from Duvall, E. [1977]. *Marriage and family development* [5th ed.]. Philadelphia: Lippincott; and Aldous, J. [1975]. *The developmental approach to family analysis.* Minneapolis: University of Minnesota Press.)

E X A M P L E S O F N U R S I N G D I A G N O S E S

The Family

The following nursing diagnoses are examples of those that might be appropriate for the family as client.

- Altered Family Processes related to hospitalization of ill family member
- Ineffective Family Coping, Disabling, related to domestic abuse of wife by alcoholic husband
- High Risk for Violence/Directed at Others related to birth of premature infant to parents who lack information about care and previous history of abuse of own children
- Anxiety related to lack of knowledge about extended-care facilities for placement of elderly mother with Alzheimer's disease

- Impaired Verbal Communication related to recent move to the US and inability to understand English
- Health-Seeking Behaviors: High-Level Wellness Concerns related to lack of knowledge about health promotion practices for all family members
- Impaired Home Maintenance Management related to difficulty in caring for children and self secondary to loss of job and substandard housing
- High Risk for Trauma related to lack of knowledge of household hazards
- High Risk for Altered Parenting related to unrealistic expectations of child by parent.

family, too. Friedman (1992) has clearly identified the importance of family-centered nursing care, based on the following rationale:

- The family comprises interdependent members who affect each other. If some form of illness occurs in one or more members, all other members become a part of the illness. Nursing assessment and interventions must consider the whole family to be holistic.
- A strong relationship exists between the family and the health status of its members; therefore, the role of the family is essential in every level of nursing care.
- The level of wellness of the family and, in turn, each member, can be significantly improved through health promotion activities.
- Illness or disease in one family member may indicate the same problem in other members; through assessment and intervention, the nurse can assist in improving the health status of all family members.

Risk Factors

Family patterns of behavior and the environment provided by the family, the environment in which the family lives, and genetic factors can place family members at a higher risk for health problems. It is important for nurses to assess these factors before developing nursing care plans or plans for health promotion. Typical questions that should be included in a family assessment are as follows:

- What is the family structure?
- What is the socioeconomic level?
- What is the ethnic background and religious affiliation of family members?
- Who cares for children if both parents work?
- What health practices are common (eg, type of foods eaten, times eaten, immunizations, bedtime, exercise)?
- What habits are common (eg, does one or more members smoke, drink to excess, or use drugs)?
- How does the family cope with stress?

- Do close friends or family members live nearby, and can they help if necessary?

When conducting a health assessment for a family, the nurse should consider the following risk factors:

Life-Style
- Lack of knowledge about sexual and marital roles, leading to teenage marriage and pregnancy; divorce; sexually transmitted diseases; child, spouse, or elder abuse; and lack of prenatal or child care.
- Alterations in nutrition, either more or less than body requirements at any age
- Chemical dependency, including the use of alcohol, drugs, and nicotine
- Inadequate dental care and hygiene
- Unsafe or unstimulating home environment

Psychosocial Factors
- Inadequate child care resources when both parents work, both for preschool and school-age children
- Inadequate income to provide safe housing, food, clothing, and health care
- Conflict between family members

Environmental Factors
- Lack of knowledge or finances to provide safe and clean living conditions
- Work or social pressures, which add to stress
- Air, water, or food pollution

Developmental Factors
- Families who have new babies, especially if support systems are unavailable
- Elderly people, especially those living alone or on a fixed income
- Unmarried, adolescent mothers who lack personal, economic, and educational resources

Biologic Factors
- Birth defects

- Mental retardation
- Genetic predisposition to certain diseases, including cardiovascular diseases and cancer

Nursing Interventions to Promote Wellness

The role of the nurse in reducing risk factors is primarily focused on activities that promote health for all family members at any level of development. Each person has a personal definition of health, based on family beliefs and values about health and illness. By providing interventions that emphasize wellness, the nurse can assist both the individual and the family meet basic human needs. Examples of nursing interventions to promote wellness in the family are shown in Table 7-2. Nurses may carry out the activities or may refer the individual or family to groups for additional education.

The family is the primary educational and support structure for the individual. The family, as a social unit, provides the environment and relationships necessary to meet physiologic and psychosocial, individual basic human needs. Health beliefs and practices are learned within the family context and are strongly influenced by the family's developmental level. Health promotion activities and nurs-

ing interventions can reduce the risk of illness and facilitate healthy behaviors at any age within the family life cycle.

Community

A person, as an individual and as a member of a family, belongs to the community. The community environment affects the ability of the individual to meet basic human needs. This section of the chapter discusses the community as it relates to basic human needs, including influences on health and illness.

A **community** can be defined in a variety of ways, but the most basic definition is that a community is a specific population (or group of people) living in a specified geographic area under similar regulations and having common values, interests, and needs. Within a community, people interact and share resources.

The community has a strong influence on the health promotion and illness prevention of its individuals and families (Fig. 7-4). Just as the family has risk factors for the health of individual members, so does the community have risk factors involving resources, economics, and services.

TABLE 7-2

Nursing Interventions to Promote Family Health and Wellness	
Family Developmental Level	**Nursing Interventions and Referrals**
Couple and child-bearing family	Family planning clinics
	Prenatal classes
	Immunization information
	Poison-prevention programs
Family with school-age children	Vision and hearing screenings
	Dental health information
	Parent support groups
	Communicable disease control
Family with adolescents	Alcohol and drug abuse information
	Accident prevention programs
	Sex education
	Nutrition support groups
	Mental health programs
Family with middle-aged adults	Blood pressure screenings
	Exercise classes
	Stress reduction programs
	Specific support groups (stop smoking, Alcoholics Anonymous, coping with grief)
Family with older adults	Screening for chronic diseases (hypertension, glaucoma, diabetes)
	Retirement information
	Home safety programs
	Pharmacology information

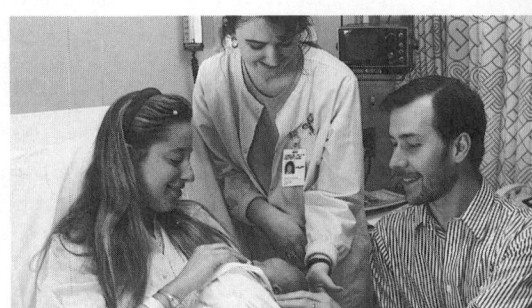
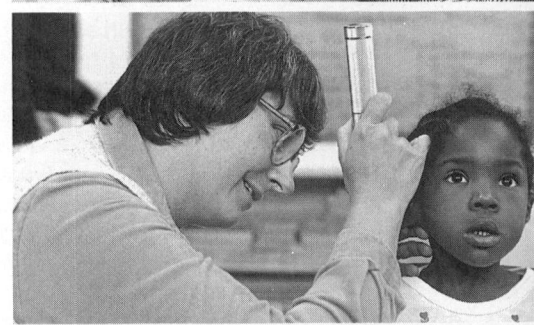
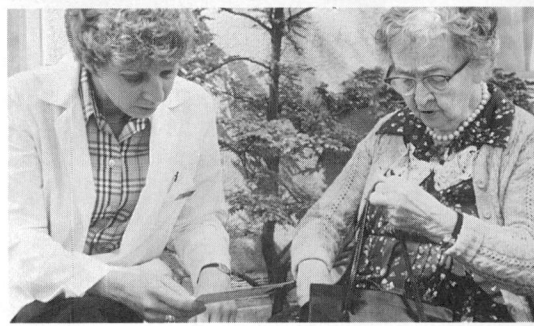

R E S E A R C H   I N   N U R S I N G   Making a Difference

Basic Human Needs: Individual, Family, Community

Basic human needs are met, largely through the relationships and interactions a person has with his or her family members. Nursing interventions are planned and implemented to include family members in meeting needs of not only the individual who requires health care but also the family who loves that individual and will most often provide care after dismissal from the acute-care setting. Research to identify the most effective way to meet individual and family needs continues to increase our knowledge base and the effectiveness of our care.

Related Research

Bull, M. J. (1990). Factors affecting family care-giver burden and health. *Western Journal of Nursing Research,* 12(6), 758–776.

The trend toward decreased length of in-hospital stay results in an increased need for assistance from family members to manage care during recovery at home. The purpose of the study was to identify factors that influence family caregiver burden and health outcomes during transition from hospital to home, and to identify variables that might be incorporated into a model of caregiver burden. Study findings could be useful in assessing family needs, functional abilities, and feelings about care before discharge; they could also assist the nurse in developing interventions that focus on caregiver well-being.

Gillis, A. J. (1990). Nurses' knowledge of growth and developmental principles in meeting psychosocial needs of hospitalized children. *Journal of Pediatric Nursing,* 5(2), 78–87.

The purpose of the study was to assess the knowledge of pediatric nurses about growth and development principles in meeting health care needs of hospitalized children and their families. The nurses who responded to the questionnaire reported a deficit in knowledge about principles of growth and development necessary to meet psychosocial needs of children and their families when planning care. It is suggested that both student nurses and practicing nurses be given increased experiences in integrating knowledge when providing care to children and their families during illness and hospitalization.

Price, M. D., Forrester, A. F., Murphy, P. A., & Monaghan, J. F. (1991). Critical care family needs in an urban teaching medical center. *Heart and Lung,* 20(2), 183–188.

When an individual is admitted to an intensive care unit, family members experience extreme stress and have a variety of needs. The study described needs of 213 family members to serve as a base for the development of appropriate nursing interventions. Two major needs were identified: (1) to have honest, intelligible, and timely information, and (2) to feel confident that their family member is being cared for by competent and caring people. These findings support the importance of providing accurate information and supportive caring to family members during the crisis.

Gaynor, S. E. (1990). The long haul: The effects of home care on caregivers. *Image: Journal of Nursing Scholarship,* 22(4), 208–212.

The purpose of this investigation was to examine the effects and implications in women who care for a spouse with a long-term illness or disability. Findings showed that feelings of perceived burden were highest in women who had provided care for extended periods, as was the number of reported illnesses. Younger women reported poorer emotional health. Based on the study, it is suggested that chronic illness should be regarded as a disease that involves all members of the family, and that education of family members about caregiving, respite care, and home care services should be included in nursing care plans.

Summary

It is evident from these studies that nurses cannot care for the client in isolation, but must also include members of the family in every aspect of care, no matter what the age of the client or the setting where care is provided. The needs of each individual are intertwined with the needs of the family and the community, and each aspect must be included when providing nursing care. Nursing research will continue to identify the most effective assessments and interventions to meet individual and family needs; as a result, nursing care to meet those needs will become even more holistic.

Nursing assessments and interventions would not be comprehensive and individualized if the community influence were not also considered.

Community Risk Factors

It is not within the scope of this book to discuss community health nursing as a whole. However, because the community provides the environment affecting health and illness, it is important to discuss environmental factors influencing the safety and security of the individuals within that community. The following are community factors affecting health:
- Number and availability of health care institutions and services
- Housing codes and police and fire departments

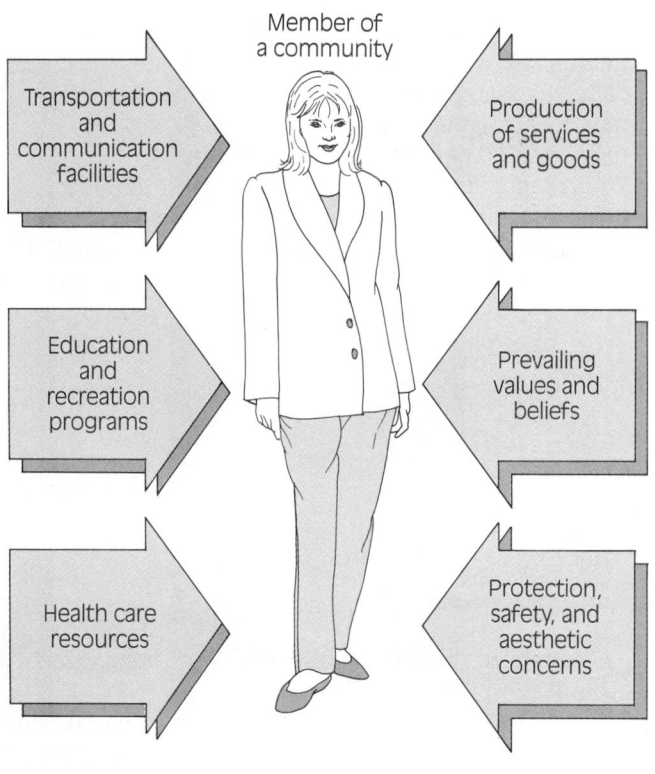

Member of a community

Transportation and communication facilities

Production of services and goods

Education and recreation programs

Prevailing values and beliefs

Health care resources

Protection, safety, and aesthetic concerns

F I G U R E 7 - 4

Many characteristics of a community influence the health of its members. This diagram shows six categories of characteristics that influence the health of a member of a community.

- Nutritional services for low-income infants, mothers, school lunch programs, and elderly people
- Zoning regulations separating residential and industrial areas
- Waste disposal services and locations
- Air and water pollution regulations
- Food sanitation guidelines
- Health education services and dissemination
- Recreational opportunities
- Prevalence of violent crimes or drug use

To illustrate how the community can affect individual and family needs, consider the following examples:

- Maria, aged 19 years, lives in an inner-city, two-room apartment with her 6-month-old baby girl. The apartment lacks adequate heat and sanitation. Maria's husband has left her, and she does not have family living in the United States. Maria rarely leaves her apartment because she fears the street gangs and drug addicts who live around her. She has never taken her baby to a local clinic for checkups, because she speaks only Spanish and does not want to ask her neighbors for directions.
- Jan, aged 22 years, lives in a small house in a rural area of the midwestern United States. She is married, and has a 2-year-old son. Her husband works at a local factory, and Jan works part-time at a clothing store. Both Jan and her husband have family members who live nearby, and they see them often. Jan, her husband, and her son all have regular health assessments.

These two different examples are given to demonstrate that the community plays a major role in the health of the people who live within it. Maria and her daughter are at much greater risk for illness than are Jan and her family. Even if the two women had identical health care needs, a plan of care would reflect different interventions because of their community environments.

Nursing in the Community

Nurses carry out a variety of activities that involve community health, designed to promote wellness and prevent illness. Nurses promote wellness as individuals, as caregivers within institutional settings, and as community-based health care providers.

As individuals, nurses provide community services as volunteers in health-related activities (eg, screenings, educational programs, or blood drives) and as role models for health practices and life-styles. Nurses working in health care institutions include community influences in developing individualized nursing care plans and in making referrals to community agencies and support groups. Community-based nurses are employed in many different kinds of health-related practice settings, including home health care, community health centers, school nursing, occupational nursing, and independent nursing practice.

K E Y P O I N T S

- Basic human needs are common to all people and are essential to health and survival. Many needs are met through a person's social environment, specifically the person's family and community.
- Maslow's hierarchy of basic human needs describes five levels of needs: (1) physiologic, (2) safety and security, (3) love and belonging, (4) self-esteem, and (5) self-actualization.

- Physiologic needs have the highest priority and are the base of the hierarchy. These needs include oxygen, food, water, temperature, elimination, sexuality, physical activity, and rest.
- Safety and security needs include a physical component, involving protection from potential or actual harm, and an emotional component, including trust and freedom from fear.

- Love and belonging needs include both giving and receiving love, and having a sense of belonging to others.
- Self-esteem needs focus on a person's feeling good about himself or herself and believing that others also hold that person in high regard.
- Self-actualization needs are the highest level of need and are met when a person achieves his or her potential.
- The family, the basic social unit of society, serves as a buffer between the needs of society and the needs of individual members. Many different family structures (or forms) exist, but all families carry out the same functions—physical, economic, reproductive, affective and coping, and socialization.

- The family life cycle has definite stages and developmental tasks.
- Family-centered nursing care incorporates basic human needs, family concepts, and risk factors into nursing interventions to promote wellness.
- The community provides an environment that is an integral component of individual needs and family functions. Holistic nursing care integrates community risk factors and influences in all types of health care settings.

BIBLIOGRAPHY

Aldous, J. (1975). *The developmental approach to family analysis.* Minneapolis: University of Minnesota Press.

Anderson, K. H., & Tomlinson, P. S. (1992). The family health system as an emerging paradigmatic view for nursing. *Image: Journal of Nursing Scholarship, 24*(1), 57–63.

Bull, M. J. (1990). Factors affecting family care-giver burden and health. *Western Journal of Nursing Research, 12*(6), 758–776.

Cetinski, G., & Milne, R. (1991). Family caregivers. *Canadian Nurse, 87*(1), 33–34.

Danielson, C. B., Hamel-Bissel, B. P., & Winstead-Fry, P. W. (1992). *Families, health, and illness: Perspectives on coping and interventions.* St. Louis: Mosby–Yearbook.

Duvall, E. (1977). *Marriage and family development* (5th ed.). Philadelphia: Lippincott.

Edelman, C., & Mandle, C. (1990). *Health promotion throughout the lifespan* (2nd ed.). St. Louis: Mosby–Year Book.

Friedman, M. (1992). *Family nursing: Theory and assessment* (3rd ed.). Norwalk, CT: Appleton & Lange.

Gaynor, S. E. (1990). The long haul: The effects of home care on caregivers. *Image: Journal of Nursing Scholarship, 22*(4), 208–212.

Gillis, A. J. (1990). Nurses' knowledge of growth and developmental principles in meeting psychosocial needs of hospitalized children. *Journal of Pediatric Nursing, 5*(2), 78–87.

Healthy people: *The Surgeon General's report on human promotion and disease prevention* [abridged]. (1990). Washington, DC: American Public Health Association.

Johnson, S. (1986). *Nursing assessment and strategies for the family at risk: High-risk parenting* (2nd ed.). Philadelphia: Lippincott.

Leahey, M., Stout, L., & Myrah, I. (1991). Family systems nursing. *Canadian Nurse, 87*(2), 31–33.

Maslow, A. (1968). *Toward a psychology of being* (2nd ed.). New York: Van Nostrand–Reinhold.

Meierhoffer, L. L. (1992). Nurses battle family violence. *American Nurse, 24*(4), 1, 7–8.

Pender. N. (1987). *Health promotion in nursing practice* (2nd ed.). Norwalk, CT: Appleton-Century-Crofts.

Price, M. D., Forrester, A. F., Murphy, P. A., & Monaghan, J. F. (1991). Critical care family needs in an urban medical center. *Heart and Lung, 20*(2), 183–188.

U.S. Bureau of the Census. (1984). *Household and family characteristics* (Popular Report's Series P-20, No. 398). Washington, DC: U.S. Government Printing Office.

Woods, N. F., Yates, B. C., & Primomo, J. (1989). Supporting families during chronic illness. *Image: Journal of Nursing Scholarship, 21*(1), 46–50.

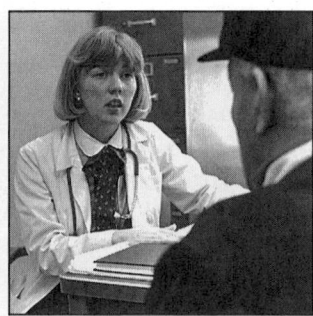
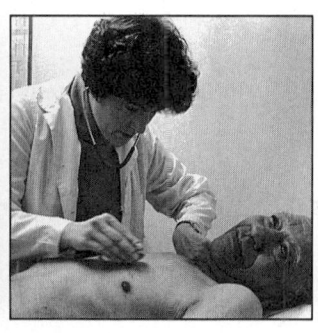

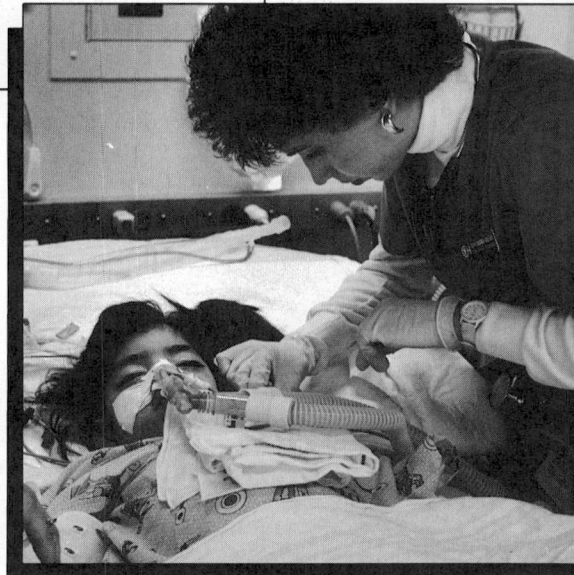

Culture and Ethnicity

OBJECTIVES

After studying this chapter, the learner should be able to:

Define key terms used in the chapter.

Discuss the concepts of culture, ethnicity, race, and stereotyping.

Describe cultural and ethnic characteristics that influence health care, including gender roles, language and communication, orientation to space and time, food and nutrition, socioeconomic factors, importance of family, physical and mental characteristics, spiritual characteristics, and perceptions of illness and health.

Compare and contrast the culture of the health care system with the broad concept of culture.

Identify the factors that affect the interaction of the nurse and the client in terms of health care values.

Discuss the guidelines that are useful in practicing transcultural nursing care.

Use knowledge of specific cultural and ethnic factors in providing holistic, individualized nursing care to clients.

KEY TERMS

cultural assimilation
cultural imposition
culture
culture shock
dominant group
ethnicity
ethnocentrism
minority group
personal space
race
stereotyping
subculture
transcultural nursing
yin and yang

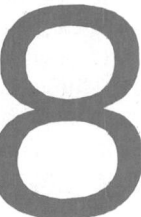

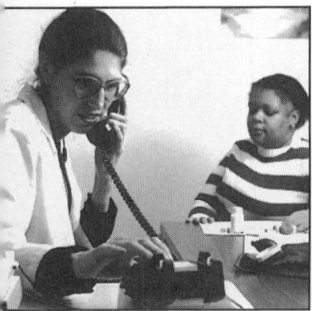
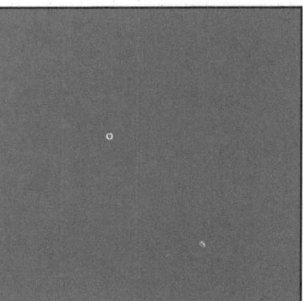

We live in a society that is made up of widely diverse groups of people. The groups include people of different racial and ethnic backgrounds, people with different sexual orientations, and people from different socioeconomic backgrounds. These groups and subgroups are called cultures.

One's culture influences one's behavior in both health and illness because of genetic characteristics and the values and beliefs we learn from our families and communities. Nurses must maintain an open and honest interest in the cultural characteristics, values, and lifeways of clients so that holistic, individualized care can be planned and implemented.

This chapter focuses on the concepts of culture and ethnicity, including definitions of terms and a discussion of various characteristics that are culturally based and influence nursing care. It also provides a broad introduction to the major cultural and ethnic groups in North America, and examines the importance of integrating transcultural nursing concepts into one's daily practice of nursing.

Concepts of Culture and Ethnicity

Culture

Culture, broadly defined, is the set of values, beliefs, and traditions that are held by a specific social group and handed down from generation to generation. Culture also is the beliefs, habits, likes and dislikes, and customs and rituals learned from one's family (Spector, 1991). As described by Leininger (1990), "culture includes all human activities taking material and nonmaterial forms and expressions . . . the political, economic, social, religious, educational, philosophical, technological, and environmental contexts in which human beings live and function" (p. 535). The concepts of culture include the following:

- Culture guides behavior into acceptable ways for the people in a specific group. As such, culture originates and develops within the social structure through interpersonal interactions.

- Culture is learned by each new generation through both formal and informal life experiences. Language is the primary means of transmitting culture.
- The practices of a particular culture often arise because of the group's social and physical environment.
- Cultural practices and beliefs are adapted over time, but they mainly remain constant as long as they satisfy needs.
- Culture influences the way people of a group view themselves, have expectations, and behave in response to certain situations. Because a culture is made up of individuals, differences within cultures as well as across cultures are found.

Within a culture are subgroups, or subcultures. The **subcultures** are made up of people with a distinct identity but who have certain ethnic, occupational, or physical characteristics that are found in the larger culture. For example, nursing is a subculture of the larger health care system culture, and teenagers and older adults are regarded as subcultures in North America.

Cultures have dominant groups and minority groups. A **dominant group** is the group within the culture that has the authority to control the value system and determine the rewards of the system. The dominant group usually is (but does not have to be) the largest group in a society (for example, white middle-class people are the dominant group in North America). A **minority group** usually has some physical or cultural characteristic (such as race, religious beliefs, or occupation) that identifies the people within it as different; those people believe that they are discriminated against because of that characteristic. Groups who have been vocal in expressing this belief in North America are members of non-Caucasian ethnic groups, homosexuals, and women.

Cultural Assimilation

Because minority groups live within the dominant group, many of their members lose the cultural characteristics that made them different. This process is called **cultural assimilation** or *cultural acculturation.* Mutual cultural assimilation can occur, with some characteristics of both groups being traded. For example, when the Vietnamese came to the United States they learned to speak English, and Americans learned to cook with the vegetables preferred by the Vietnamese. In this way, almost all of us have gained from the many cultures in which we have lived and grown up. Although we seldom think about it, the clothes we wear, the foods we eat, the music we enjoy, the slang we use, and the leisure activities we practice are all areas in which we have become acculturated.

Ethnicity

Ethnicity is the sense of identification that a cultural group collectively has, largely based on the group's common heritage. One belongs to a specific ethnic group either through birth or through adoption of characteristics of that group.

People within an ethnic group share common and unique cultural and social beliefs and behavior patterns, including language and dialect, religious practices, literature, folklore, music, political interests, food preferences, and employment patterns.

Race

Although *ethnicity* often is used interchangeably with **race**, these terms are not the same. Classifying people by race is a way of categorizing them into subgroups according to specific physical characteristics, such as skin pigmentation, body stature, facial features, and hair texture. Although there has been a blending of physical characteristics through the centuries, the three major classifications by race are Caucasian, Negroid, and Mongoloid.

Stereotyping

When one assumes that all members of a culture or ethnic group act alike, **stereotyping** is at work. Common stereotypic beliefs are that all Italians are emotional, that all Germans are stoic, and that men never cry. Stereotyping may be positive or negative. Negative stereotyping includes racism, ageism, and sexism. These are beliefs that certain races, ages, or genders are inherently superior to others, leading to discrimination against those considered inferior. Stereotyping often is done by members of the dominant group about the minority group in a culture (Fig. 8-1).

Cultural and Ethnic Influences on Health Care

North America is multicultural and multiethnic. As such, there is a wide diversity of people in almost every populated area. This means that it is important for us, as nurses, to be aware of and sensitive to the needs of a culturally diverse client population. This section deals with general considerations in transcultural care; specific values and behaviors of different groups are discussed later in the chapter.

Gender Roles

In many cultures, the male is the dominant figure. In cultures where this is true, males make decisions for other family members as well as for themselves. For example, if approval for medical care is needed, the man gives it, no matter which family member is involved. In cultures where the male is dominant, the female usually is passive. In African-American families, however, as well as in many Caucasian families, the female often is dominant.

Knowledge of the dominant member of the family is an important consideration in planning nursing care. If the dominant member is ill and can no longer make decisions, the whole family probably is anxious and confused. If a nondominant family member is ill, he or she may require help in verbalizing needs, particularly if they differ from those the dominant member perceives as being important.

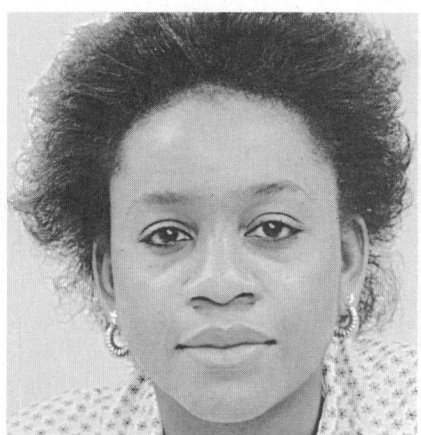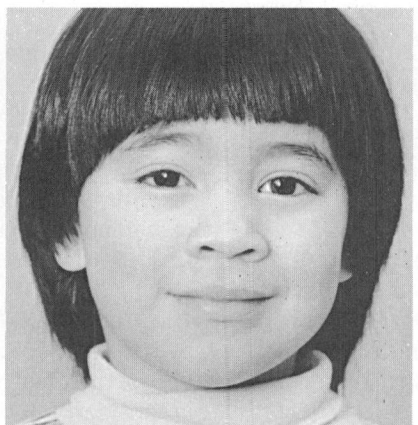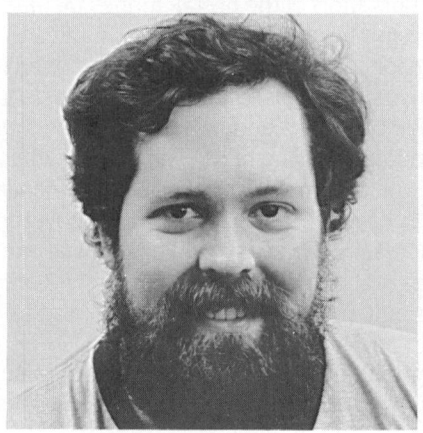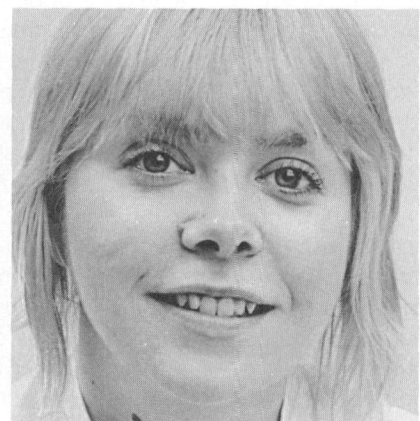

FIGURE 8-1

Identifying one's own prejudices is the first step toward eliminating them. Think about the assumptions you make about the people in these images.

Language and Communication

When people from another part of the world move to North America, they may speak their own language fluently, but have difficulty speaking the language of their new country. This is especially true of the women in the family, many of whom do not work outside the home, and of groups of people who live in proximity to others who speak the same language. The English language, with all its peculiarities, is especially difficult for many foreign-born people to learn.

Most Americans do not learn a second language; as a result, communication problems can arise during health care activities. This problem is not unique to non–English-speaking clients; even in different regions of the United States certain dialects or word meanings can cause differences in understanding. Consider how difficult it must be to describe symptoms or give a personal health history when you do not understand the questions being asked. Something as simple as showing the nurse where you hurt is an impossibility if you do not know what is being said.

Nurses who work in an area that has a high population of residents who speak a language other than English need to learn pertinent words and phrases in that language. Many agencies have an interpreter, or one can be found in the community. Sometimes a family member or friend can translate for the nurse. It is important to select an interpreter who has knowledge of the health care system to avoid misinterpretation of questions and answers. Many family members are protective and may not be the most reliable means of transferring information. Nurses may find themselves talking in a louder tone of voice to a client who does not understand what is being said; it is important to remember that this is a communication problem, not a hearing problem. Chapter 20 provides information on communicating with non–English-speaking clients.

Orientation to Space and Time

Personal space is the area surrounding a person that is regarded as part of the person. This area, individualized to each person and to different cultures and ethnic groups, is the distance maintained from others during communications. When one's personal space is not taken into consideration, one may become uncomfortable or even angry. With nursing care, which involves physical contact and close communications, it is important to know cultural personal space preferences. As examples, people of Arabic and African origin commonly sit and stand close to one another when talking, whereas people of Asian and North American descent are more comfortable talking with some distance between themselves and others.

Most people and almost all institutions in North America value promptness and punctuality. When arriving for an appointment, doing a job, or carrying out an activity, being on time and getting the job done are viewed as important. This is not true in some other cultures. For example, in some South Asian cultures, being late is considered a sign of respect. In addition, although most of middle-class North America is future-oriented (including activities that not only promote health in the present, but also in the future), other cultures are more concerned with the present or the past. This means that client teaching may have to be adapted; as an example, if a client is to take a medication twice a day at home, the teaching plan should focus on taking the pill twice a day (for example, one in the morning and one in the evening), rather than on taking it at 9 AM and 9 PM.

Food and Nutrition

The way foods are prepared and the foods that are eaten often are culturally related. Certain food groups serve as staples of the diet based on culture, and remain so even when members of that culture are living in a country that is not their own. For example, rice and vegetables are the staples of Asians and Chinese, and pasta is a staple of Italians. Mexican Americans favor beans and tortillas, whereas Puerto Ricans try to eat a balance of hot, cold, and cool foods (the classification is based on type of foods and not temperature of foods).

Clients in the hospital setting often do not have much of a choice of foods. This means that people with cultural food preferences may not be able to select appealing foods, and thus may be at risk for less than adequate nutrition. When assessing the cause of decreased appetite in clients, the nurse should determine if the problem is one of culture. It may be possible for family or friends to bring in foods that satisfy nutritional needs and still meet dietary restrictions.

Socioeconomic Factors

The amount of money a person or family has or does not have affects the way the person or family meets basic needs and maintains health. A major problem in North America is poverty, which leads to other problems concerning health care financing, care of infants and children, and the homeless. All these areas are of concern to nursing.

The Culture of Poverty There has been much debate over the true definition of poverty. In terms of economics, a person or family whose income falls below the poverty line is considered poor. The U.S. Census Bureau has stated that "a family is poor if it falls short of the pretax money income needed to purchase a minimum amount of goods and services" (Moccia & Mason, 1986). On the other hand, it has been stated that poverty is "a relative term that reflects a judgment made on the basis of standards prevailing in the community. The standards change in time and place; what is judged poverty in one community might be regarded as wealth in another" (Spector, 1991). No matter how poverty is defined, it is an increasingly devastating epidemic—one that has evolved into a culture of its own. At highest risk are families headed by single mothers, elderly people, and future generations of those now living in poverty.

The so-called feminization of poverty threatens to raise the number of people who are living at poverty level. The

I was doing my maternity rotation, and was assigned to labor and delivery. The patient I was given spoke no English—she and her husband were from Central America and had been in the United States for only 2 months. She was being given Pitocin I.V. to induce labor.

When I arrived at 7 AM, the night nurse was giving a report about my patient to the day nurse. The night nurse was frantic—no one understood the couple, all efforts to locate a translator had come up empty, and, quite frankly, she had no idea exactly what condition this woman was in. The day nurse did not speak Spanish either, so she was no better off.

I quickly began to think back on my 2 years of Spanish. Could I be of any help to this couple? I wondered. Would I remember enough to communicate with them about giving birth? Then I decided (quite nervously) that any little bit of communication at this point was better than none, so I spoke up. I told both nurses that I spoke some Spanish, and asked if I could be of any help. The night nurse literally hugged me (she had really been upset)!

I began by telling the expectant couple that I was a nursing student and that I spoke some Spanish. We exchanged introductions and then I asked the woman some assessment questions. Nothing I said was complicated—all of my sentences were short and simple, but who needed more than that? The key, as far as I was concerned, was not to impress anyone (including myself), but to help this couple.

Then the couple asked me some questions. They had heard about "cutting open the stomach" to delivery a baby. I naturally assumed that they meant a cesarean delivery. They looked so afraid, but I had to be honest. They wanted to know how it was done and why. The words I could not remember or did not know I acted out. They looked so relieved when I was finished.

The man said that they thought *all* babies were born this way in our country. He said that they had never heard of this procedure until coming to the United States. No wonder they were so frightened!

The doctor came in, examined the woman, and said that she was fully dilated. The doctor asked me if I could possibly teach a crash course in Lamaze breathing to the patient. She also asked me if I would stay throughout the delivery because she would need assistance in translating directions to the patient. Of course I said yes.

The woman was understandably terrified. I told her that t was normal to be afraid, and that I would be with her during the delivery. She took my hand and whispered, "Muchas gracias." I had never felt more useful than I did at that moment. Even though I had been afraid to try using my Spanish, I had anyway. I don't believe I will ever hesitate to try it again.

—A. Kelly Gaylor, Holy Family College,
Philadelphia

---

number of female-headed households is increasing as a result of divorce, abandonment, unmarried motherhood, and changes in abortion laws. Because many households depend on two incomes for economic survival, a single woman supporting a household is at a financial disadvantage. The number of single-parent families headed by women is closely associated with the increasing number of children living in poverty and the number of homeless families with children.

The expanding population of elderly people has contributed to problems with poverty. Most elderly people live on fixed incomes, which often do not keep up with inflation, and many (particularly widows) are on the borderline of poverty or have already slipped into the poverty culture.

In some cases the culture of poverty is passed from generation to generation. This seems to be especially true in such groups as migrant farm workers, families living on welfare, and people who live in isolated areas of

Appalachia. Poverty cultures have the following characteristics:

- Feelings of despair, resignation, and fatalism
- Day-to-day attitude toward life with no hope for the future
- Unemployment and need for financial or government aid
- Use of escape valves such as alcohol and drugs
- Unstable family structure with abusiveness and abandonment
- Decline in self-respect and retreat from community involvement

Effects of Poverty on Health Care   Poverty has long been a barrier to health care. It prevents many people from adequately meeting their basic human needs. Lack of affordable or adequate housing is a problem frequently experienced by poor people. When low-income housing is available, it often is associated with low-cost maintenance, sometimes resulting in the absence of such necessities as running water, heat, and electricity. To stretch their available money and to pool resources, many poor people live in crowded conditions, with several families living together in one household.

Research has demonstrated that crowded living conditions foster impersonalization, correlate with higher crime rates, and lead to psychological problems, such as schizophrenia, alienation, and feelings of worthlessness (Spector, 1991). They also contribute to an increased incidence of disease and illness because of the proximity of people, the sharing of utensils and belongings, poor sanitation, and other poor health habits. The health effects of such conditions are numerous:

- Poor people get sick more often than people in higher-income groups.
- When poor people are ill, they usually experience more complications and complications of greater severity.
- Recovery time is longer for poor people.
- Poor people are less likely to regain their preillness level of functioning (Kotelchuck, 1985).

Access to health care facilities frequently necessitates transportation, which many times is neither affordable nor available to poor people. Their access to health insurance also is frequently limited, and commonly a choice must be made between purchasing food and purchasing health care. In 1968, Canada introduced a national health insurance program aimed at ensuring Canadian citizens equal access to health care regardless of age, economic status, creed, or ethnic origin. Despite this program and a high-quality health care system, people's health remains directly related to their economic status. Those in the upper-income group live longer and are freer of disability than those in the lower-income group (Storch, 1982). Other barriers to health care include isolation, language or communication difficulties, seasonal occupations, migration patterns, depersonalization, and institutional prejudice (Spector, 1991).

Family Support

Many cultural and ethnic groups have large extended families and consider the needs of any family member to be equal to or greater than their own, and who are unwilling to share with those outside the family (including health care providers) private information about family members. Other cultural groups have great respect for the elders in the family, and would never consider institutional care for them. Including the family in planning care for any client is a major component in nursing care to meet individualized needs, especially if those needs can be met only through consideration of all members of the family.

Physical and Mental Health

Differences and similarities in physiologic and psychological characteristics are found among cultural and ethnic groups. These characteristics influence the health and illness status of group members.

Physiologic Characteristics   Researchers theorize that past generations slowly adapted to their surrounding environment. Dark-skinned people developed lighter skin as early populations moved to colder northern climates where there is less sunlight throughout the year compared with equatorial climates. Lighter skin is better able to use the vitamin D from sunlight than darker skin. It also is theorized that a person's nose shape and size evolved according to the climate in which the person lived (Henderson & Primeaux, 1981). From a scientific and anthropologic point of view, these adaptations were logical changes necessary for improving the lives and well-being of human beings. Some of these biologic variations were effective adaptations for a particular period or for living in a certain environment.

Once a person is removed from the environment that encouraged the biologic variation to occur, the variation could have a detrimental effect on health and well-being. The results of various studies have shown that certain ethnic groups have particular characteristics that make them more prone to developing specific diseases and conditions. These conditions may be acquired as a result of environmental factors, or they may be inherited. Some of the variations are discussed in the next section.

Keloid Formation   Keloids result from the overgrowth of connective tissue that occurs during the healing process after an injury, surgery, or other type of connective tissue damage. People of African heritage are much more likely to develop keloids. Rather than healing flush with the surrounding skin tissue, the wound of a person with a tendency toward keloid formation heals with a rough, lumpy, or elevated scar.

Lactase Deficiency   Milk and many milk products contain lactose, a sugar. The enzyme lactase must be present in the body to break down lactose during digestion. Without lactase, the lactose ferments in the intestines, resulting in gas (flatus), diarrhea, and abdominal bloating and cramping. About 70% of African Americans, 90% of Native Americans, and 3% to 10% of the white population have a lactase deficiency (Porth, 1990).

People with a lactase deficiency have to get their calcium and protein requirements from alternative sources because they are not able to tolerate regular milk products. Special milk and milk products are available for them. Also, they may tolerate sharp cheeses (aged more than 60 days) and fermented milk products, such as yogurt, buttermilk, and sour cream (Henderson & Primeaux, 1981).

Sickle Cell Anemia   The sickle cell trait originally served as a protective mechanism against malaria. Sickle cell anemia is most common in people with African or Mediterannean ethnic backgrounds. People with sickle cell anemia have sickle-shaped red blood cells (RBCs) that break down more rapidly than normal-shaped RBCs. The sickle shape also prevents the RBCs from moving easily through the smaller vessels in the body. This factor can lead to the smaller vessels being clogged by the RBCs, which can cause many potentially serious problems. Sickle cell carriers can be identified by a blood test.

Tay-Sachs Disease   People of Eastern European Jewish descent may carry a gene for a hereditary disorder called Tay-Sachs disease. A child born with this progressive disease has a short life span, usually less than 2 years. There is no cure or treatment for this devastating disease. Carriers of the disease can be identified by serum analysis.

G6PD Deficiency   Glucose-6-phosphate dehydrogenase is an enzyme normally found in RBCs. G6PD deficiency affects about 10% of the black population. The deficiency is sex-linked and carried on the X female chromosome. A person with this deficiency has RBCs that are unable to maintain a cell membrane. Without this protective membrane, RBCs are easily destroyed (hemolyzed) by various oxidant drugs, such as aspirin, ascorbic acid, probenecid, sulfa drugs, and vitamin K, and by fava beans (also called horse or broad beans). This destruction results in anemia, which may be severe and life-threatening, and in elevated bilirubin levels (a result of the hemolyzed RBCs), which causes jaundice (yellowing of the skin and sclerae).

Thalassemia   A genetic disorder, thalassemia affects the hemoglobin in the RBCs. The production of the alpha or beta globin chains is defective, and disrupts RBC function. This disorder is most commonly found in people of Mediterranean, Asian (especially Chinese), and African origin.

Sarcoidosis   Much more prevalent in the black population, sarcoidosis involves the formation of multiple tubercles or nodules on various parts of the body, most commonly the lymph nodes, liver, spleen, lungs, skin, eyes, and small bones of the feet and hands. These nodules eventually form into fibrous tissue. Skeletal muscle involvement can result in muscle atrophy (wasting). If the myocardium is involved, major cardiac problems can result.

Gout   Gout is most commonly found in men, especially those of Puerto Rican or Filipino descent. Excessive quantities of uric acid are found in the blood and may be deposited in joints and cartilage. The deposition of uric acid results in swelling, inflammation, and pain in the affected area. The uric acid crystals eventually may permanently damage the joints. These crystals also predispose the person to the formation of renal calculi (kidney stones).

Psychological Characteristics   In most situations, a person relates the behaviors of another person to her or his own familiar culture. This process usually is multidirectional; for example, in a health care setting, the client is evaluating the attitudes and actions of the health care provider at the same time the health care provider is gathering perceptions about the behavior of the client. It is important to remember that what may seem reasonable and important to a client may seem ridiculous and irrelevent to a nurse. The reverse perception also is apparent: Practices a nurse perceives as logical and effective may seem senseless, incompetent, or even dangerous to a client.

Most mental health norms have been based on research and observations made of white, middle-class people. Many ethnic groups have their own norms or acceptable patterns of behavior concerning psychological well-being and psychological reactions to certain situations. For example, members of the Puerto Rican culture may be close-mouthed about personal and family affairs, making effective psychotherapy difficult to achieve. Many traditional Chinese people consider mental illness a stigma; therefore, seeking psychiatric help is a disgrace to the family. Traditionally, Chinese people prefer to avoid or minimize any type of conflict, so the use of any direct confrontation during psychotherapy may not work as well as expected. Also, Chinese people traditionally have been taught that the expression of strong emotions results in disharmony and imbalance between the body's energy forces (**yin and yang**), and is considered a sign of weakness. As a result of this belief, therapy involving the venting of strong feelings and emotions may be unacceptable to the client. In situations of extreme stress or high anxiety, some Puerto Ricans may demonstrate hyperkinetic seizure activity known as *ataques*. This behavior is a culturally accepted reaction.

Culture Shock   **Culture shock,** or the feelings a person experiences when placed in a different and often strange culture, may result in psychological discomfort or disturbances. The patterns of behavior a person found acceptable and effective in his own culture often are not adequate in the new one. The person may then feel foolish, fearful, incompetent, inadequate, embarrassed, humiliated, and inferior. These feelings eventually can lead to frustration and anxiety.

As a reaction to these perceptions of inadequacy and inferiority, a person experiencing culture shock may become angry. If the anger is suppressed, it may build up and eventually result in hostility. Hostility may be overt (openly expressed) or covert (hidden). Covert hostility may be expressed in various ways. The hostile person may be categorized by health professionals as uncooperative.

Reaction to Pain Health care researchers maintain that the expressions and behaviors exhibited by people in pain are culturally prescribed. Some cultures allow and even encourage the open expression of emotions experienced by a person in pain, whereas other cultures frown on the open and free expression of emotions. The main concern of nurses in this area of cultural expression is the categorization of clients as the ideal client. A client who quietly and stoically deals with pain may have her pain reduction needs ignored by nurses. It often is assumed that a client who does not complain of pain is not experiencing any great degree of pain. Nurses should be sensitive to other signals of discomfort, such as holding or applying pressure to the painful area, self-restriction of activities that intensify the pain, and uncontrollable, spontaneous expressions of discomfort, such as facial grimacing and moaning. Clients who freely express their discomfort should not be classified as constant complainers whose requests for pain relief sometimes seem excessive. Pain is a warning from the body that something is wrong, and every complaint of pain should be carefully assessed.

Folk Medicine

Values and beliefs about illness, health, and illness care are developed as a direct result of cultural and ethnic influences. The folk medicine system classifies illnesses as natural or unnatural. Natural illnesses are caused by dangerous agents, such as cold air or impurities in the air, water, or food. Unnatural illnesses are punishments for failing to follow God's rules, resulting in evil forces or witchcraft causing physical or mental health problems (Giger & Davidhizar, 1991).

Folk Healers In some cultures the power to heal is thought to be a gift from God bestowed on certain people. It is believed that these special people, healers, know what is wrong with a client through divine intervention and experience. A client who is familiar with such healers may perceive modern health care providers as incompetent because they have to ask many questions before they can treat an illness. A folk healer may prescribe one dose of a boiled herbal tea as a treatment. Someone who is accustomed to this type of treatment may find it difficult to take a succession of pills that are not even steeped in hot water. Folk healers traditionally are less expensive, usually more accessible, and more understanding of the client's cultural and personal needs, and they speak the client's language.

Traditional Folk Medicine Having knowledge and understanding of traditional folk remedies used by culturally different clients greatly improves and enhances effective nursing care and facilitates a safe return of the client to a state of wellness or health.

A common mode of treatment in many cultures is the use of herbs. In fact, many medications used today have a basis in herbs or other plant sources that have been used for centuries to cure illnesses. A problem may arise when a client is being cared for by both an herbalist and a physician. The herbalist may be prescribing an herb and the physician a drug, both of which have the same action. The client may be overmedicated or undermedicated because of the double prescription.

In most instances, the nurse should not discourage the client's use of traditional folk medicine unless it is harmful to the client's health and well-being or decreases the effectiveness of the nursing and medical care planned. Incorporating the client's traditional health care beliefs into the care plan is an effective way to gain his trust and cooperation. For example, if a client would traditionally drink an herbal tea to alleviate symptoms of an illness, there is no reason why both the herbal tea and the medications prescribed by the physician cannot be used as long as the tea is

EXAMPLES OF NURSING DIAGNOSES

Culture and Ethnicity

The following nursing diagnoses are examples of those that might be appropriate for the client who is a minority within a dominant culture.

- Impaired Verbal Communication related to language barrier between client and family and caregivers
- Ineffective Family Coping related to recent move to this country and distance from extended family
- Social Isolation related to inability to verbally communicate with neighbors and lack of transportation

- Spiritual Distress related to inability to maintain usual contact with members of a spiritual group
- Anticipatory Grieving related to loss of usual environment and support systems
- Powerlessness related to social isolation and social displacement
- High Risk for Altered Self-Esteem related to recent change in role responsibility

safe to drink and the ingredients do not interfere with or exaggerate the action of the medication.

Transcultural Nursing

Madeleine Leininger (1990), whose theory of transcultural care is described in Chapter 4, defines **transcultural nursing** as follows:

> Transcultural nursing is a formal area of study and practice focused on a comparative study of human cultures with respect to discovering universalities (similarities) and diversities (differences) as related to nursing phenomena of care (caring), health (wellness), or illness patterns within a cultural context and with a focus on cultural values, beliefs, and lifeways of people and institutions, and using this knowledge to provide culture-specific or universal care practices.

When the nurse provides transcultural nursing care, it means that the care is planned and implemented in a way that is sensitive to the needs of individuals, families, and groups representing the diverse cultural populations within society. When cultural diversity is recognized and respected, cultural sensitivity is present and nursing care is provided that accepts the significance of cultural factors in health and illness. To provide transcultural care, the nurse must be aware that the health care system itself is a culture, and that cultural imposition and ethnocentrism must be avoided.

The Culture of Health Care

The health care system (described in Chapter 3) is a culture with customs, rules, values, and a language of its own. As you progress through your education, you will be acculturated into the culture of the health care system and will develop values of health and health care. Many of the customs and rules are typical of the society in which we live; for example, cleanliness and punctuality are valued behaviors. The display outlines some common cultural norms of the health care system.

Nursing is the largest subculture of the health care system. Most nurses are members of, and have the same value systems as, the dominant middle class in North America. According to Boyle and Andrews (1989), the typical American nurse is "white, middle-class, Anglo-Saxon, Protestant, female, and socialized into a subculture labeled 'health care professional, subdivision nurse' " (p. 50). When the nurse, with a particular set of cultural values about health, interacts with a client who has his or her own particular set of cultural values about health, the following factors affect the interaction:
- The cultural background of each participant
- The expectations and beliefs of each about health care
- The cultural context of the encounter (for example, hospital, clinic, home)
- The degree of agreement between the two persons' sets of beliefs and values (Boyle & Andrews, 1989)

Cultural Imposition and Ethnocentrism

Cultural imposition, described by Leininger (1991) as "one of the most serious problems in the health field" (p. 36), is the tendency for health personnel to impose their beliefs, practices, and values on people of other cultures because they believe that their ideas are superior to those of another person or group (Leininger, 1970). When health professionals assume that they have the right to make choices and decisions for clients, clients respond

---

**Cultural Norms
of the Health Care System**

Beliefs
- Standardized definitions of health and illness
- Omnipotence of technology

Practices
- Maintenance of health and prevention of illness
- Annual physical examinations and diagnostic procedures

Habits
- Charting
- Frequent use of jargon
- Use of a systematic approach and problem-solving methodology

Likes
- Promptness
- Neatness and organization
- Compliance

Dislikes
- Tardiness
- Disorderliness and disorganization

Customs
- Professional deference and adherence to the pecking order found in autocratic and bureaucratic systems
- Use of certain procedures attending birth and death

Rituals
- Physical examination
- Surgical procedure
- Limiting visitors and visiting hours

in the same way that minority cultures respond to dominant cultures: by becoming passive, resistive, angry, or noncompliant.

Closely related to cultural imposition is ethnocentrism. **Ethnocentrism** is the belief that one's own ideas, beliefs, and practices are the best, superior, or most preferred to other lifeways (Leininger, 1970). To overcome this practice, the nurse must carefully and critically examine his or her own values and beliefs, and be willing to understand health and illness from the cultural viewpoint of the client receiving care.

Providing Transcultural Care

A major theme of transcultural nursing care is to focus on the caring practices of various cultures. Caring is a universal phenomenon, even though the forms and manifestations may vary among cultures. Caring practices are the protecting and assisting activities related to health and performed as part of a culture.

Nursing care can become complicated when the client and the nurse have distinctly different cultural norms. The nurse's role is to understand the client's needs and to adapt care to meet those needs. Unless the nurse is willing to carefully examine and clarify his or her own attitudes and values and to be sensitive to others who are "different," the use of cultural concepts to provide holistic care will be unsuccessful.

Sometimes a nurse is placed in a cultural bind: The nurse's cultural upbringing influences values and beliefs, and the nurse is expected to adopt the customs of the nursing profession and at the same time accommodate the folkways and norms of individual clients. A careful merging of modern and traditional cultural beliefs is a necessary prerequisite for safe, considerate, and successful nursing care of all clients.

Once cultural awareness and sensitivity in planning client care have been attained, it is easier to recognize the client's use of traditional folk medicine and its importance. When caring for a client who subscribes to such a practice, the nurse takes this circumstance into account during assessment and planning.

Cultural Assessment The most effective way to identify specific factors that influence behavior is to do a cultural assessment of the client. The primary informant should be the client, if possible. If the client is not able to respond to the questions, a family member or a friend can be consulted.

Client differences in values, religion, dietary practices, family lines of authority, family life patterns, and beliefs and practices related to health and illness can be anticipated. Research has made it possible to obtain this anticipatory information before initiating contact with the client, with the reminder that information about specific cultures is general in content and must be individualized according to each client once interaction has begun.

Holistic Health Care Rationale for cultural nursing is the fact that the nursing profession values holistic and comprehensive approaches to providing care. Holistic health care takes into consideration the whole person interacting in his environment. With the philosophy of holistic health care, the knowledge and use of cultural factors cannot be ignored because a person's culture is an integral part of his life and, therefore, of holistic nursing care. A client can be placed in jeopardy if a health care professional lacks cultural awareness or sensitivity.

Considerations for Transcultural Care Table 8-1 lists cultural factors that affect nursing care for specific cultures. The following guidelines are useful in practicing transcultural nursing care:

- Become conscious of the role of cultural influences in your own life. Objectively examine your own beliefs, values, practices, and family experiences. As you become more sensitive to the importance of these factors, you also will become more sensitive to cultural influences in others' lives.
- Identify biases in your own life. How do they affect your feelings about others? How could they affect your nursing care of others?
- Learn about the varieties of cultures and some general observations about variables in their health care.
- Learn as much as possible about the belief system and practices of people in your community and, specifically, of clients in the area in which you work. Cultural practices and beliefs are deeply rooted and must be considered in planning health care for it to be successful.
- Display an accepting, nonjudgmental, objective attitude about clients' cultural beliefs.
- Practice techniques of observation and listening to acquire knowledge of beliefs and values of clients to whom care is being given. Some people, especially those of minority cultures, may have been belittled and subjected to ridicule and insults, and may be hesitant to discuss their beliefs and practices. The topic must be approached carefully. If the nurse is motivated by sincerity, respect, and concern, his or her attitude conveys this, and most clients respond positively. On the other hand, if the nurse is motivated by curiosity and has a condescending attitude, most clients respond negatively.
- Incorporate factors from the client's cultural background into health care whenever possible and when the practices are not considered harmful to health. To ignore or contradict the client's background may result in refusal of care or noncompliance with prescribed therapy.
- Keep in mind that health practices are part of the overall culture and that changing them may have widespread implications for the person. An accurate understanding of these implications is essential before such a change is implemented. The nurse also needs

RESEARCH IN NURSING Making a Difference

Cultural Differences Influence Nursing Care

In today's society, with people of many cultures freely moving about the world, it is essential that nurses be familiar with the values and beliefs of cultures that differ from their own. Individualized assessments and interventions can be made only if cultural influences and factors are integrated into planning for holistic care. The studies described here are examples of this critical element of nursing practice.

Related Research

Jezewski, M. A. (1990). Culture brokering in migrant farmworker health care. *Western Journal of Nursing Research, 12*(4), 497–513.

Many migrant farm workers do not possess the health-seeking means of entering the health care system, and require a broker, or go-between. This article describes the process by which brokering by nursing facilitated access to health care in this population. Barriers to seeking health care were found to be decreased financial resources, inability to effectively communicate health care needs, and lack of cultural sensitivity on the part of the health care provider. Use of the theory that emerged from the data that was collected provides nurses with guidelines for facilitating health care in subculture populations.

Munet-Vilaro, F., & Vessey, J. A. (1990). Children's explanation of leukemia: A Hispanic perspective. *Journal of Pediatric Nursing, 5*(4), 274–282.

Cultural background affects the experience of and response to illness in children as well as in adults. In this study, 23 Hispanic children between ages 8 and 12 with the medical diagnosis of acute lymphocytic leukemia were interviewed to ascertain their perception of this ill-

ness. Content analysis of the information led to the following findings: (1) children tended to explain their illness in terms of symptoms and adverse effects of treatment; (2) Hispanic parents did not give the children much information about the illness; (3) all advice from physicians was held in high esteem; and (4) family members were more comfortable in confiding to the nurse.

Davis, A. J., & Slater, P. V. (1989). U.S. and Australian nurses' attitudes and beliefs about the good death. *Image: Journal of Nursing Scholarship, 21*(1), 34–39.

This study was conducted to ascertain the values and beliefs of nurses about euthanasia in the United States and Australia. The ethical questions raised about the right to determine one's own death are major issues in the health care system today. From responses to vignettes during interviews, the investigators found that nurses from these two countries did not agree on what was done or what should be done. These differences are suggested as the result of such factors as differences in health care systems, the role of the law in health care decisions, the social position of nursing, and the relationships nurses have with family members.

Summary

Cultural diversity in clients and in nurses themselves is increasingly being recognized as an essential component of the practice of nursing. No matter the age-group or the population, nursing interventions to meet the needs of the client and family must be planned based on cultural or ethnic background. As nursing advances into the 21st century, this component of caring must become an integral part of nursing education and nursing practice.

to provide the necessary support and reinforcement for the client if a change in a health practice with a cultural basis is considered necessary.

- Do not force the client to participate in care that conflicts with their values. If the client is forced to accept it, the care may even be harmful because resulting feelings of guilt and alienation from a religious or cultural group are likely to threaten the client's well-being.
- Accommodate the cultural dietary practices of clients as much as possible. Dietary departments in many hospitals supply clients with meals that are consistent with special dietary practices. Families may be encouraged to bring food from home for clients with particular preferences when this practice does not violate hospital policy. Teaching clients and families about therapeutic diets also can be done within the

framework of particular cultural practices.
- Take into consideration the cultural role of the family member who makes most of the important decisions. In some cultures, it is the husband or father, whereas in others it is the grandmother or another respected elder. To disregard this fact or to proceed with nursing care that is not approved by this person can result in conflict or in disregard for what has been taught. The nurse should be careful to involve this person in the nursing care planning.
- Seek assistance of a respected family member, member of the clergy, or folk medicine practitioner as indicated so that the client is more likely to accept familiar health care services. Acknowledging the role of the person's folk medicine practitioner can be an

(Text continues on p. 124)

TABLE 8-1

Cultural Factors That Affect Nursing Care

White Middle Class

Family
- Nuclear family is highly valued.
- Elderly family members may live in a nursing home when they can no longer care for themselves.

Folk and Traditional Health Care
- Self-diagnosis of illnesses
- Use of over-the-counter drugs (especially vitamins and analgesics)
- Dieting (especially fad diets)
- Extensive use of exercise and exercise facilities

Values and Beliefs
- Youth is valued over age.
- Cleanliness
- Orderliness
- Attractiveness
- Individualism
- Achievement
- Punctuality

Common Health Problems
As a result of the high value placed on achievement:
- Cardiovascular diseases
- Gastrointestinal diseases
- Some forms of cancer
- Motor vehicle accidents
- Suicides
- Mental illness
- Chemical abuses

Nursing Considerations
- Careful assessment of client's use of over-the-counter medications (observe for signs and symptoms of toxic medication levels, especially fat-soluble vitamins)
- Nutritional assessments of dietary habits

African American

Family
- Close and supportive extended-family relationships
- Develop strong kinship ties with nonblood relatives from church or organizational and social groups
- Family unity, loyalty, and cooperation are important.
- Usually matriarchal

Folk and Traditional Health Care
- Varies extensively and may include spiritualists, herb doctors, root doctors, conjurers, skilled elder family members, voodoo, faith healing

Values and Beliefs
- Present oriented
- Members of the African-American clergy are highly respected in the black community.
- Frequently highly religious

Common Health Problems
- Hypertension (precise cause unknown, may be related to diet)
- Sickle cell anemia
- Skin disorders; inflammation of hair follicles, various types of dermatitis and excessive growth of scar tissue (keloids)
- Lactose enzyme deficiency resulting in poor toleration of milk products
- Higher rate of tuberculosis
- Diabetes mellitus
- Higher infant mortality rate than in the white population

Nursing Considerations
- Many African-American families may still use various folk healing practices and home remedies for treating particular illnesses.
- Special care may be necessary for the hair and skin.
- Special consideration should be given to the sometimes extensive and frequently informal support networks of clients (ie, religious and community group members who offer assistance in a time of need).

Asian

(Beliefs and practices vary, but most Asian cultures share some characteristics.)

Family
- Welfare of the family is valued above the person.
- Extended families are common.
- A person's lineage (ancestors) is respected.
- Sharing among family members is expected.

Folk and Traditional Health Care
- Theoretical basis is in Taoism, which seeks a balance in all things.

Values and Beliefs
- Strong sense of self-respect and self-control
- High respect for age
- Respect for authority
- Respect for hard work
- Praise of self or others is considered poor manners.
- Strong emphasis on harmony and the avoidance of conflict

- Good health is achieved through the proper balance of yin (feminine, negative, dark, cold) and yang (masculine, positive, light, warm).
- An imbalance in energy is caused by an improper diet or strong emotions.
- Diseases and foods are classified as hot or cold and a proper balance between them will promote wellness (eg, treat a cold disease with hot foods).
- Many Asian health care systems use herbs, diet, and the application of hot or cold therapy. Also, many Asians believe that there are points on the body that are located on the meridians or energy pathways. If the energy flow is out of balance, treatment of the pathways may be necessary to restore the energy equilibrium.

Acumassage—Technique of manipulating points along the energy pathways
Acupressure—Technique for compressing the energy pathway points
Acupuncture—Technique by which fine needles are inserted into the body at energy pathway points

Nursing Considerations
- Some members of Asian cultures may be upset by the drawing of blood for laboratory tests. They consider blood to be the body's life force, and some do not believe that it can be regenerated.
- Some members believe that it is best to die with the body intact, so they may refuse surgery except in dire circumstances.
- Members of many Asian cultures seldom complain about what is bothering them. Therefore, the nurse must carefully assess the client for pain or discomfort by observing for nonverbal signs of discomfort, such as facial grimacing or wincing and holding of the painful area.
- Some Asians consider it polite to give a person the responses the person is expecting. Therefore, misinformation may be transmitted to the questioner in an effort, on the client's part, to be respectful.
- Some members may move from physician to physician in an attempt to be cured of an illness, but to avoid insulting or embarassing a physician, they will not inform him or her that they are going to another physician. This can result in confusion, inaccuracies, and overmedication.
- Some Asians may refuse to have diagnostic studies done because they believe that a skilled and competent physician can diagnose an illness solely through a physical examination.
- Some members may have a difficult time understanding the importance of taking a regimen of medications because many of their folk treatments involve the ingestion of one dose of herbal mixtures.
- Dietary counseling may be necessary if the client is on a salt-restricted diet because many Asian foods have a high salt content related to the use of soy sauce.

Hispanic, Mexican American

Family
- Familial role is important.
- *Compadrazgo:* special bond between a child's parents and his or her grandparents
- Family is the primary unit of society.

Folk and Traditional Health Care
- *Curanderas(os):* frequently folk healers who base treatments on humoral pathology—basic functions of the body are controlled by four body fluids or "humors":
      Blood—hot and wet
      Yellow bile—hot and dry
      Black bile—cold and dry
      Phlegm—cold and wet
- The secret of good health is to balance hot and cold within the body; therefore, most foods, beverages, herbs,

Common Health Problems
- Tuberculosis
- Communicable diseases
- Malnutrition
- Suicide
- Various forms of mental illness
- Lactose enzyme deficiency

Values and Beliefs
- Respect is given according to age (older) and sex (male).
- Roman Catholic Church may be very influential.
- God gives health and allows illness for a reason; therefore, may perceive illness as a punishment from God. An illness of this type can be cured through atonement and forgiveness.

Common Health Problems
- Diabetes mellitus and its complications
- Poverty and resultant problems, such as poor nutrition, inadequate medical care, poor prenatal care
- Lactose enzyme deficiency

(continued)

T A B L E 8 - 1 (continued)

Cultural Factors That Affect Nursing Care

Folk and Traditional Health Care (continued)
and medications are classified as hot (*caliente*) or cold
(*fresco, frio*) (a cold disease will be cured with a hot
treatment).

Nursing Considerations
- It may be difficult to convince an asymptomatic client that he or she is ill.
- Special diet considerations are necessary if the client believes in the hot/cold theory of treating illnesses.
- Diet counseling may be necessary at times because many members have a normal diet that is high in starch.

Hispanic, Puerto Rican

(Since the Jones Act of 1917, all Puerto Ricans are American citizens.)

Family
- *Compadrazgo*—same as in Mexican-American culture

Folk and Traditional Health Care
- Similar to that of other Spanish-speaking cultures

Common Health Problems
- Parasitic diseases, such as dysentery, malaria, filariasis, and hookworms
- Lactose enzyme deficiency

Values and Beliefs
- Place a high value on safeguarding against group pressure to violate a person's integrity (may be difficult for Puerto Ricans to accept teamwork)
- Close-mouthed about personal and family affairs (psychotherapy may be difficult to achieve at times because of this belief)
- Proper consideration should be given to cultural rituals such as shaking hands and standing up to greet and say goodbye to people.
- Time is a relative phenomenon; little attention is given to the exact time of day.
- *Ataques*—culturally acceptable reaction to situations of extreme stress, characterized by hyperkinetic seizure activity

Nursing Considerations
- It may be difficult to teach Puerto Rican clients to follow time-oriented actions (eg, taking medications, keeping appointments).

important way of building trust. If invited, folk medicine practitioners can work closely with professional health practitioners in the interest of the client and family. Such efforts promote mutual understanding, respect, and cooperation.
- Use past transcultural experiences as a guide, but never as the solution to all transcultural solutions.
- Learn from your mistakes and do not repeat them. All nurses make mistakes at some time when caring for

culturally different clients. Inadvertent mistakes are just that, but repeated mistakes are careless and disrespectful; they adversely affect the nurse's interaction with clients and coworkers.
- Treat each person as an individual. What was true of one person will not be true of another, even if they are from the same cultural background. View each person as an individual with rights, and help the client retain dignity.

KEY POINTS

- Culture is the set of values, beliefs, and traditions held by a specific social group that is learned and handed down from generation to generation.
- One's culture guides behavior, is primarily transmitted through language, and can be adapted over time.

- Ethnic groups are made up of people who share common and unique cultural and social beliefs and social patterns.

Native Americans

(Each tribe's beliefs and practices vary to some degree.)

Family
- Families are large and extended.
- Grandparents are official and symbolic leaders and decision makers.
- A child's namesake may become the same as another parent to the child.

Folk and Traditional Health Care
- Medicine men (shaman) are heavily used.
- Heavy use of herbs and psychological treatments, ceremonies, fasting, meditation, heat, and massages

Common health problems
- Alcoholism
- Suicide
- Tuberculosis
- Malnutrition
- Communicable diseases
- Higher maternal and infant mortality rates than in most of the population
- Diabetes mellitus
- Hypertension
- Gallbladder disease

Nursing Considerations
- The family is expected to be part of the nursing care plan.
- Note taking often is taboo because it is considered an insult to the speaker because the listener is not paying full attention to the conversation. Good memory skills often are required by the nurse.
- Indirect eye contact is acceptable and sometimes preferred.
- It often is considered rude or impolite to indicate that a conversation has not been heard.
- A low tone of voice often is considered respectful.
- A Native American client may expect the caregiver to deduce the problem through instinct and not through asking many questions and history taking. If this is the case, it may help to use declarative sentences rather than direct questioning.

Values and Beliefs
- Present oriented. Taught to live in the present and not to be concerned about the future. This time consciousness emphasizes finishing current business before doing something else.
- High respect for age
- Great value is placed on working together and sharing resources.
- Failure to achieve a personal goal frequently is believed to be the result of competition.
- High respect is given to a person who gives to others. The accumulation of money and goods often is frowned on.
- Some Native Americans practice the Peyotist religion in which the consumption of peyote, an intoxicating drug derived from mescal cacti, is part of the service. Peyote is legal if used for this purpose. It is classified as a hallucinogenic drug.

- Stereotyping, which occurs when the assumption is made that all members of a culture or ethnic group act alike, often is practiced by the dominant group about a minority group in a culture.
- As members of a minority group live within a dominant group, cultural characteristics often are lost through assimilation.
- A wide variety of cultural and ethnic characteristics affect transcultural nursing care. These characteristics include family member roles, communications, nutrition, and income levels.
- Poverty has a major influence on health and illness, affecting health-related behaviors. This issue is made even more complex because of the increased number of families headed by single women, of elderly people, and of homeless families.

- Certain physiologic and psychological characteristics that are found in specific cultural and ethnic groups are risk factors for illness.
- The health care system is a culture, with nursing being the largest subculture.
- As part of the health care system, which has its own values and behaviors, nurses must be aware of the tendency of health care professionals toward cultural imposition and ethnocentrism.
- Guidelines for transcultural nursing care help the nurse accept the values, beliefs, and behaviors of others. Holistic nursing care requires that cultural influences and factors be integral components of an individualized plan of care.
- When nurses provide transcultural care, they demonstrate cultural sensitivity by recognizing and respecting cultural diversity.

BIBLIOGRAPHY

Adams, R., Briones, E. H., & Rentfro, A. (1992). Cultural considerations: Developing a nursing care delivery system for a Hispanic community. *Nursing Clinics of North America, 27*(1), 107–117.

Ailinger, R. L. (1985). Beliefs about treatment of hypertension among Hispanic older persons. *Topics in Clinical Nursing, 7*(3), 26–31.

American Nurses' Association. (1991). *Philosophical statement on ethics and human rights.* Kansas City, MO: Author.

American Nurses' Association. (1991). *Position statement on cultural diversity in nursing practice.* Kansas City, MO: Author.

An Asian patient: How does culture affect care. (1991). *Journal of Christian Nursing, 8*(3), 5–9.

Boyle, J. S., & Andrews, M. M. (1989). *Transcultural concepts in nursing care.* Glenview, IL: Scott, Foresman.

Brink, P. J. (1984). Value orientations as a cultural assessment tool in cultural diversity. *Nursing Research, 33*(4), 198–203.

Capers, C. F. (1985). Nursing and the Afro-American client. *Topics in Clinical Nursing, 7*(3), 11–17.

Davis, A. J., & Slater, P. V. (1989). U. S. and Australian nurse's attitudes and beliefs about the good death. *Image: Journal of Nursing Scholarship. 21*(1), 34–39.

Elliott, J. L. (Ed.). (1983). *Two nations: Many cultures—ethnic groups in Canada.* Ontario: Prentice-Hall.

Flaskerud, J. H., & Rush, C. E. (1989). AIDS and traditional health beliefs and practices of Black women. *Nursing Research, 38*(4), 210–214.

Fong, C. M. (1985). Ethnicity and nursing practice. *Topics in Clinical Nursing, 7*(3), 1–10.

Friedman, M. M. (1990). Transcultural family nursing: Application to Latino and black families. *Journal of Professional Nursing, 5*(3), 214–222.

Galanti, G. (1991). *Caring for patients from different cultures: Case studies from American hospitals.* Philadelphia: University of Pennsylvania Press.

Geissler, E. M. (1991). Transcultural nursing and nursing diagnoses. *Nursing and Health Care, 12*(4), 190–203.

Giger, J. N., & Davidhizar, R. E. (1991). *Transcultural nursing: Assessment and intervention.* St. Louis: Mosby.

Henderson, G., & Primeaux, M. (1981). *Transcultural health care.* Menlo Park, CA: Addison-Wesley.

Jezewski, M. A. (1990). Culture brokering in migrant farmworker health care. *Western Journal of Nursing Research, 12*(4), 497–513.

Kotelchuck, R. (1985). Poor diagnosis, poor treatment. *Health PAC Bulletin, 16*(1), 8.

Leininger, M. (1970). *Nursing and anthropology: Two worlds to blend.* New York: John Wiley & Sons.

Leininger, M. (1978). *Transcultural nursing: Concepts, theories, and practices.* New York: John Wiley & Sons.

Leininger, M. (1990). Transcultural nursing: A worldwide necessity to advance nursing knowledge and practice. In J. C. McCloskey & H. K. Grace (Eds.), *Current issues in nursing* (3rd ed., pp. 534–541). St. Louis: Mosby.

Leininger, M. (1991). Becoming aware of types of health practitioners and cultural imposition. *Journal of Transcultural Nursing, 2*(2), 32–39.

Lipson, J. G., & Meleis, A. I. (1985). Culturally appropriate care: The case of immigrants. *Topics in Clinical Nursing, 7*(3), 48–56.

Louie, K. B. (1985). Providing health care to Chinese clients. *Topics in Clinical Nursing, 7*(3), 18–25.

Malone, R. E. (1990). The challenge of Third World nursing. *American Journal of Nursing, 90*(7), 32–37.

Meleis, A. I., Lipson, J. G., & Paul, S. M. (1992). Ethnicity and health among five middle eastern immigrant groups. *Nursing Research, 41*(2), 98–103.

Moccia, P., & Mason, D. J. (1986). Poverty trends: Implications for nursing. *Nursing Outlook, 34*(1), 20–24.

Muecke, M. A. (1983). Caring for Southeast Asian refugee patients in the USA. *American Journal of Public Health, 73*(4), 431–438.

Munet-Vilaro, F., & Vessey, J. A. (1990). Children's explanation of leukemia: A Hispanic perspective. *Journal of Pediatric Nursing, 5*(4), 274–282.

Porth, C. M. (1990). *Pathophysiology: Concepts of altered health states.* (3rd ed.). Philadelphia: Lippincott.

Rairdan, B., & Higgs, B. (1992). Transcultural nursing: The Hmong. *American Journal of Nursing, 92*(3), 52–55.

Rosenbaum, J. N. (1991). A cultural assessment guide. *The Canadian Nurse, 87*(4), 32–33.

Secundy, M. G. (Ed.). (1992). *Trials, tribulations, and celebrations: African-American perspectives on health, illness, aging, and loss.* Yarmouth, ME: Intercultural Press.

Sobralske, M. C. (1985). Perceptions of health: Navajo Indians. *Topics in Clinical Nursing, 7*(3), 32–39.

Spector, R. E. (1991). *Cultural diversity in health and illness.* (3rd ed.). New York: Appleton & Lange.

Spector, R. E. (1986). Sociocultural influences on children's health. In G. Scipien, et al. (Eds.), *Comprehensive pediatric nursing* (3rd ed., pp. 35–46). New York: McGraw-Hill.

Storch, J. (1982). *Patients' rights: Ethical and legal issues in health care and nursing.* Toronto: McGraw-Hill Ryerson.

U.S. Bureau of the Census. (1984). *Current population reports: Money income and poverty status of families and persons in the United States.* Washington, DC: U.S. Government Printing Office.

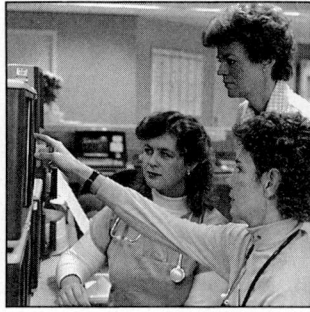
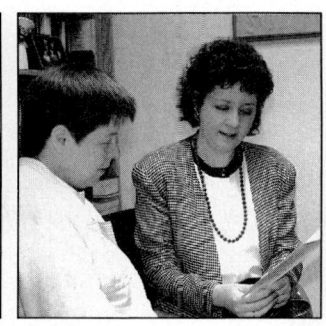
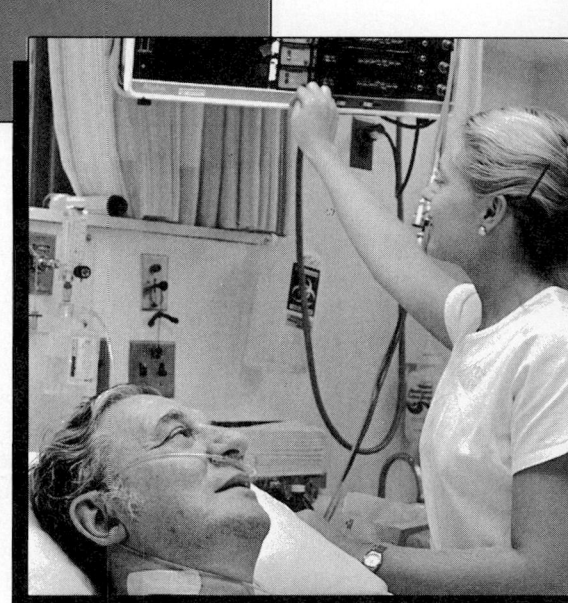

OBJECTIVES

After studying this chapter, the learner should be able to:

Define key terms used in the chapter.

Describe the mechanisms involved in maintaining physiologic homeostasis.

Explain the interdependent nature of stressors, stress, and adaptation.

Compare and contrast developmental and situational stress, incorporating the concepts of physiologic and psychosocial stressors.

Describe the physical and emotional responses to stress, including mind–body interaction, local adaptation syndrome, general adaptation syndrome, and coping and defense mechanisms.

Discuss the effects of short- and long-term stress on basic human needs, health and illness, and the family.

Integrate knowledge of healthy lifestyle, support systems, stress management techniques, and crisis intervention into nursing care plans.

Recognize and effectively cope with stress unique to the nursing profession.

KEY TERMS

adaptation
anxiety
burnout
caregiver burden
coping mechanisms
crisis
crisis intervention
defense mechanisms
developmental crisis
fight-or-flight response
general adaptation syndrome
homeostasis
inflammatory response
local adaptation syncrome
psychosomatic disorcers
reflex pain response
situational stress
stress
stressor

Stress and Adaptation

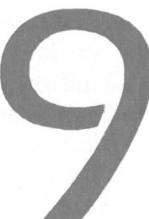

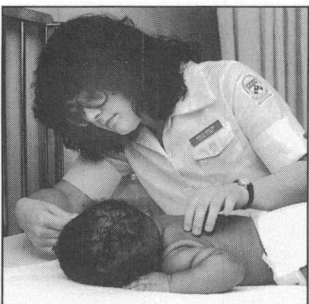

Stress has become part of life; the word is used by almost everyone. Books and magazines are filled with articles about stress; they discuss everything from the negative stressful effects that may be involved in performing one's job to the positive stressful effects of celebrating holidays. Television advertisements for over-the-counter remedies promise fast relief from stress headaches and upset stomachs. Stress is blamed for excessive weight gain, drinking, and smoking as well as for divorce and child abuse. Being "stressed out" is common, and taking "stress breaks" to do physical exercise is recommended in many work settings. With stress being so much a part of everyday life, it is easy to see that any additional problem—such as a health problem—increases the stress and its effects on the person experiencing the problem.

It is important for nurses to understand the concepts and dimensions of stress as they provide nursing care to clients in all types of settings. Nurses themselves are subject to increased stress from the demands of their career, and they need to know healthy ways of responding. This chapter discusses stress from a holistic perspective, including both physical and psychological stress. Major components to be discussed are homeostasis, stress and adaptation, and nursing actions to promote stress reduction.

Homeostasis

Our bodies are always interacting with a constantly changing environment. That environment can be divided into two parts: the external environment, which surrounds our bodies, and the internal environment, which includes the mechanisms that regulate body functions and the fluids that surround body cells. To maintain health, the body's internal environment must remain in balance within a fairly narrow range. Various physiologic mechanisms within the body respond to internal changes to maintain the essential balance in a process called **homeostasis**.

The concept of homeostasis was introduced by W. B. Cannon in 1939, but throughout history, the belief that health is the result of a balanced state has been present. This belief was written about and discussed by some of the most important people in medical history, including Hippocrates (the father of medicine) and Claude Bernard (the father of physiology). The knowledge that the human body responds to an ever-changing environment originally focused on the life processes that occur within the body, such as heart rate, blood pressure, and water balance. The definition of homeostasis has been expanded to include both the internal and the external environment, and physiologic *and* psychological balance.

Physiologic Homeostasis

Long before you entered nursing you knew that sweating when you were hot and shivering when you were cold were ways to maintain a stable body temperature. This part of the chapter summarizes the homeostatic mechanisms that regulate the body's internal environment.

Regulation of the homeostatic mechanisms is primarily controlled by the autonomic nervous system and the endocrine system (Fig. 9-1). Involved to a lesser degree are the respiratory, cardiovascular, gastrointestinal, and renal systems. These mechanisms are self-regulating, come into action without conscious thought, and usually function to correct abnormal conditions. They can be compared, on a simple level, to the relation of a thermostat to a furnace. When the temperature in a house falls below the preset temperature on the thermostat, the thermostat turns on the furnace, which heats the house to the desired temperature and then shuts off.

The regulatory mechanisms of the body are constantly reacting to change to maintain health. When a person is ill, injured, or subjected to long-term stress, the mechanisms continue to try to restore balance, but they may either become ineffective or lose their normal control. The result is increased illness or death.

The body systems, with homeostatic mechanisms, are summarized in Table 9-1. Their actions and effects are only briefly described, and are much more complex than shown. They are important in understanding the consequences of both short- and long-term stress and make material presented later in this chapter more meaningful.

Psychological Homeostasis

To remain healthy, humans also must maintain psychological homeostasis, or a state of mental well-being. As discussed in Chapter 7, each person needs to feel loved and that he or she belongs, to feel safe and secure, and to have self-esteem. When these needs are not met or a threat to need attainment occurs, the person uses homeostatic measures in the form of coping or defense mechanisms to return to emotional balance. Additional information about psychological homeostasis is included later in this chapter.

Basic Concepts of Stress and Adaptation

As with any concept or process, one must first understand the meaning of the terms used. Although the concepts are discussed in greater detail in the next section, it is impor-

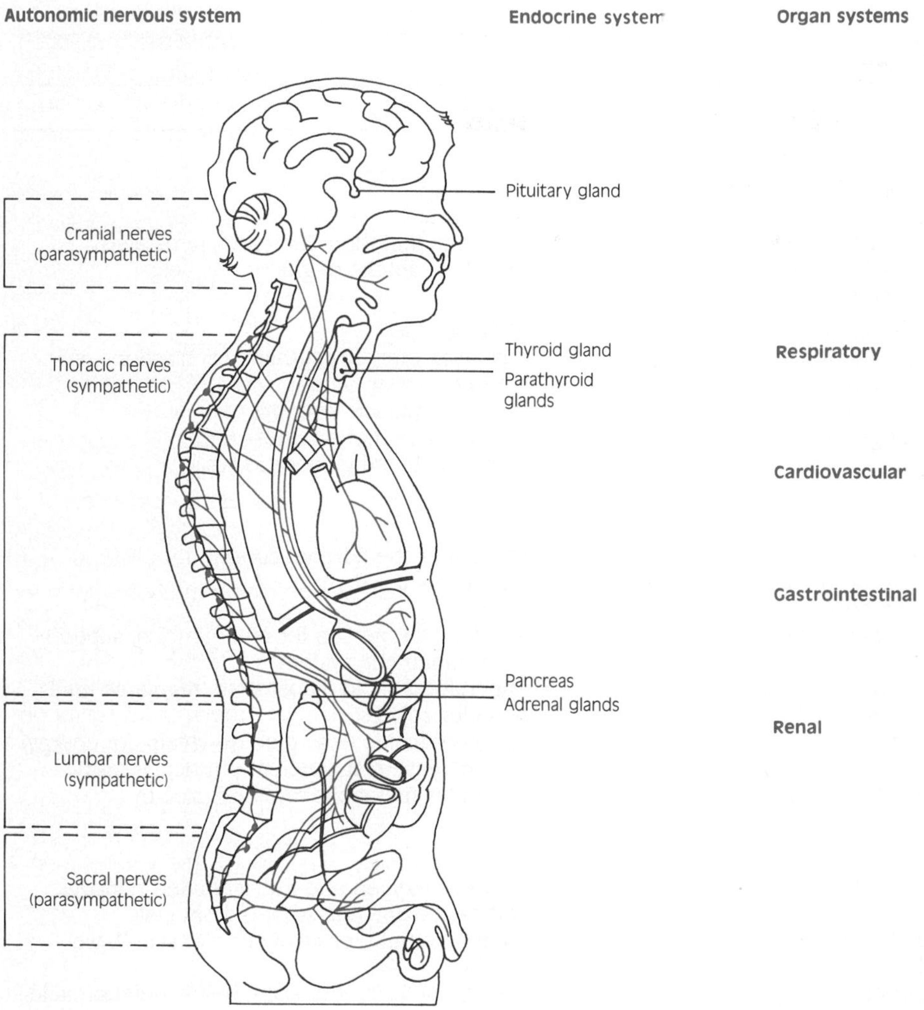

Autonomic nervous system   Endocrine system   Organ systems

Pituitary gland

Cranial nerves
(parasympathetic)

Thoracic nerves
(sympathetic)

Respiratory

Thyroid gland

Parathyroid
glands

Cardiovascular

Gastrointestinal

Pancreas
Adrenal glands

Lumbar nerves
(sympathetic)

Renal

Sacral nerves
(parasympathetic)

FIGURE 9-1

Homeostatic regulators of the body.

tant to first know the definitions of stress, stressors, and adaptation.

Definitions

Stress All of us experience varying levels of stress every day. In fact, a person's responses to stress are necessary to life (as seen in homeostasis). Stress has both positive and negative effects, and is produced by a change in the environment that is perceived as a challenge, a threat, or a danger (Smeltzer & Bare, 1992). Stress has a holistic effect—it affects the whole person in all the human dimensions (physical, emotional, intellectual, social, and spiritual). The perception of stress as well as the responses to it are highly individualized, not only from person to person but also from one time to another in the same person. Because stress is individualized and holistic, there is no commonly accepted definition or measurement. Most simply, **stress** is a condition in which the human system responds to changes in its normal balanced state.

Stressor A **stressor** is anything that causes a person to experience stress. It is a change in the person's balanced state. Stressors may be either internal (such as an illness, a

hormonal change, or fear) or external (such as loud noise or cold temperature). As with stress, the perception and effects of the stressor are holistic and highly individualized. Stressors are neither positive nor negative, but rather have positive or negative effects as the person responds to change (Fig. 9-2).

Coping and Adaptation When a person is in a threatening situation, immediate responses are made. Those responses, which often are involuntary, are called coping responses. The change that takes place as a result of the response to a stressor is **adaptation**. Adaptation is, to some degree, an ongoing process as a person strives to maintain balance in both the internal and the external environment (Fig. 9-3). Although it is easier to explain coping and adaptation in terms of the individual, adaptation also occurs in families and groups. Adaptation results in the following:
- Optimal functioning in all dimensions
- Normal growth and development
- Normal reactions to physical and emotional stress
- Ability to tolerate changing situations

To summarize, stress, stressors, and adaptation are individualized and holistic. The process is constant and dynamic, and essential to physical, emotional, and social

T A B L E   9 - 1

Homeostatic Regulators of the Body		
System	**Action**	**Effect**
Autonomic Nervous		
Parasympathetic—Functions under normal conditions and at rest		
(Cranial and sacral nerves)	• Regulates heart rate • Stimulates secretion of digestive juices and digestive tract smooth muscle • Stimulates insulin secretion	• Slows rate • Improves digestion, increases peristalsis • Increases uptake of glucose by cells
Sympathetic—Functions under stress conditions to bring about the fight-or-flight response		
	• Stimulates heart rate and force • Dilates skeletal muscle blood vessels • Dilates blood vessels to the brain • Stimulates release of glycogen stores	• Increases rate, strengthens contractions, increases cardiac output • Increases muscle strength • Increases mental alertness • Increases blood glucose levels
Endocrine		

Pituitary	• Secretes hormones:
	    Adrenocorticotropic hormone (ACTH)
	    Thyroid-stimulating hormone (TSH)
		• Stimulates the adrenal cortex
		• Stimulates the thyroid

Adrenals	• Medulla produces epinephrine and norepinephrine • Cortex secretes mineralocorticoids, glucocorticoids, and androgens	• Prepares the person for emergencies; supports the sympathetic system • Mineralocorticoid aldosterone regulates fluid and electrolytes • Glucocorticoids raise glucose levels (for energy) and increase resistance to physical stress
Thyroid	• Secretes thyroid hormone and calcitonin	• Regulates metabolic rate and growth
Other		
Cardiovascular	• Serves as transport system and pump	• Provides oxygen and nutrients and removes carbon dioxide and wastes from cells
Renal	• Filters, excretes, and reabsorbs metabolic products and water	• Maintains fluid, electrolyte, and acid–base balance
Respiratory	• Intake and output of oxygen and carbon dioxide	• Necessary for metabolism; helps maintain acid–base balance
Gastrointestinal	• Takes in food and fluids • Eliminates waste products	• Energy sources; maintains fluids and electrolytes

well-being. Stress and adaptation are major components in health and illness, and strongly influence nursing care.

Dimensions of Stress and Adaptation

Source of Stress Although there are an infinite number of sources of stress, they can be categorized into two broad areas that create major demands for adaptive responses. The areas are (1) developmental and (2) situational.

Developmental stress or a **developmental crisis** occurs as a person progresses through the normal stages of growth and development from birth to old age. Developmental crises are fully described in the next unit. Within each stage, certain tasks must be achieved to resolve that crisis and reduce the stress. Examples of developmental stress include the following:
• The infant learns to trust others.
• The toddler learns to control elimination.
• The school-age child socializes with peers.

• The adolescent strives for independence.
• The middle adult accepts physical signs of aging.

Situational stress is different from developmental stress. It does not occur in predictable patterns as one progresses through life. Rather, situational stress can occur at any time, although the ability to adapt may be strongly influenced by a person's developmental level. Examples of situational stress (or crises), which may be either positive or negative, include the following:
• Illness or accidents
• Marriage or divorce
• Loss (belongings, relationships, family member)
• New job
• Role change

To further illustrate the positive or negative aspects of situational stress, consider pregnancy as an example. A young married couple may be overjoyed at the prospect of becoming parents, whereas an unmarried teenager may be panic-stricken when she discovers she is pregnant. In this

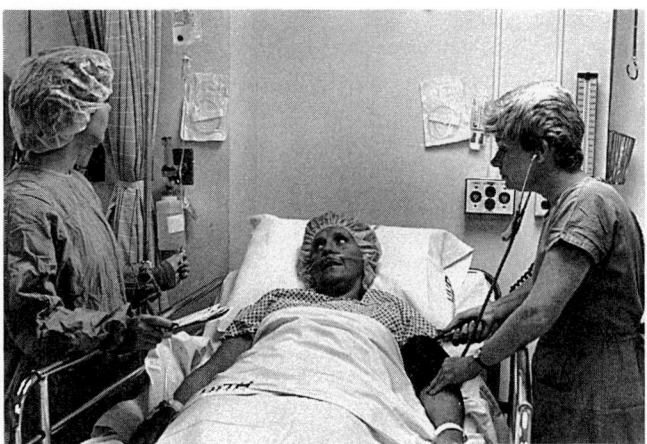

FIGURE 9 - 2

Preoperative preparation of the client can represent situational stress for the nurse as well as the client. What stressors can you imagine might affect the preoperative client and the nursing staff preparing the client for surgery? (Photo by Denise Angelini, courtesy of the School of Nursing, University of Pennsylvania.)

case, the situations and the developmental levels of the young couple and the teenager will have a major impact on the adaptations made. The physical and psychosocial capacities to cope with the situation depend not only on the stage of maturation but also on the support systems available.

Stressors We are constantly bombarded with stressors, and we adapt to the changes to maintain a normal or healthy state. However, if the stressors increase in number or intensity, a person's physical or psychological balance is impaired, and illness may result.

Physiologic stressors have both a specific effect and a general effect. The specific effect is seen in alteration of normal body structure and function. The general effect is the stress response, discussed in the next section. The accompanying display lists the agents considered to be primary physiologic stressors.

Primary Physiologic Stressors

Chemical agents	Infectious agents
• Drugs	• Viruses
• Poisons	• Bacteria
• Toxins	• Fungi
Physical agents	Faulty immune system
• Heat	Genetic disorders
• Cold	Nutritional imbalances
• Radiation	Hypoxia
• Electrical shock	
• Trauma	

Factors influencing stress management

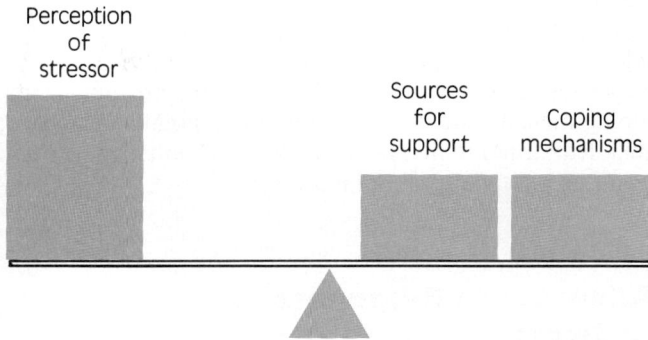

A balance is achieved when the perception of the stressful event is realistic and support and coping mechanisms are adequate

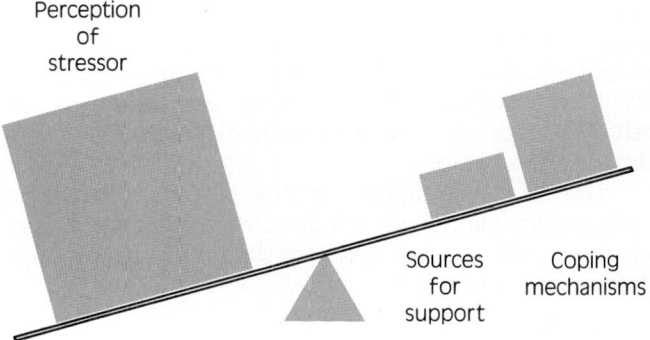

An imbalance can occur if the perception of the event is exaggerated or if sources for support or coping mechanisms are inadequate

FIGURE 9 - 3

A realistic perception of a stressful event, sources for emotional support, and appropriate coping mechanisms are components of a system of balances during stress.

There is an almost infinite variety of *psychosocial stressors,* and they become so much a part of our daily lives that we often overlook them. To illustrate the many types of psychosocial stressors, consider the following categories, summarized from work by Antonovsky (1979):
• Accidents and their survivors, which cause stress for the victim, the person who caused the accident, and the families of both
• Experiences of family members and friends
• Horrors of history, such as Nazi concentration camps, famine in Africa, and the effects of the atomic bomb on Hiroshima
• Fear of aggression or mutilation from others, such as muggings, rape, murder, and terrorist attacks
• Events of history that are brought into our homes through television, such as wars, earthquakes, and violent threats to the lives of world figures
• Developmental and life crises

- Rapid changes in our world and the way we live, including changes in economic and political structures and technology

Psychosocial stressors may be either actual or the result of a person's perception of a threat. The person's responses are continuous, and include the individualized coping mechanisms that are used to respond to anxiety, guilt, fear, frustration, and loss. The mechanisms serve to maintain psychological homeostasis.

Adaptation: Responses to Stress

Each person constantly encounters physical, psychological, or social changes in the internal and external environment. The perception of these changes may be conscious or unconscious. If the person has the necessary resources, adaptation takes place, and balance is maintained. If the resources cannot reestablish balance, a state of stress will result. The responses that are made and the degree of stress that is produced depend on the nature, intensity, and duration of the stressor.

This section examines adaptive responses to stress, including the mind–body interaction, the local adaptation syndrome, the general adaptation syndrome, and coping/defense mechanisms.

Mind–Body Interaction

Consider the following examples of mind–body interaction.

- Tomorrow you are scheduled to take a final examination, and you must make a passing score to pass the course and remain in the nursing program. After being awake most of the night, you are unable to swallow any food for breakfast, have a rapid heartbeat, are filled with feelings of apprehension, and have diarrhea.
- Since his wife was killed in a car accident, Tom Green has been the sole support of his 4-year-old son, who is mentally retarded. Tom has been coming to the neighborhood health clinic with increasing frequency the past 5 months, complaining of weight loss, headaches, and stomach pain.

These two examples illustrate the relation between psychological and physiologic stress and reinforce the holistic and individualized nature of stress. In the first example, as you begin the test and discover that you know most of the answers, your symptoms rapidly disappear. Tom's stress, however, is always present and long-term, causing increased risk for developing an illness.

Why does this happen? Although the exact cause is not well understood, it is thought that humans react to threats of danger as if the threats were actual stressors. A person perceives the threat on an emotional level, and the body prepares itself to either resist or run away and avoid the danger (the **fight-or-flight response**). Each person reacts in her or his own way. For example, some may have chronic diarrhea, and others may develop asthma. These illnesses are real but are called **psychosomatic disorders** because the physiologic alterations are thought to be at least partially caused by psychological influences.

Another component of mind–body interaction is the impact of life change on a person. Researchers have found that the number of changes a person has in his or her life (both positive and negative) has a positive correlation with the onset of illness. A life change can be defined as an event in a person's life that requires energy for adaptation. When energy is expended to adapt to the event, the person's resistance to illness is lowered. The Social Readjustment Rating Scale, shown in Table 9-2, is used to measure the stress of life changes. Some figures on the scale may vary, depending on geographic location. A high score does not mean that the person is ill, but it does indicate the risk of illness.

Physiologic Responses to Stress

As we have seen, there are both physical and emotional components in the response—or adaptation—to stress. The physiologic responses are the local adaptation syndrome and the general adaptation syndrome.

Local Adaptation Syndrome   The **local adaptation syndrome** (LAS) is a localized response of the body to stress. It does not involve the entire body but rather involves a body part (tissue, organ) only. The stress precipitating the LAS may be traumatic or pathologic. LAS is an adaptive response, primarily homeostatic, and short-term. Although the body is capable of exhibiting many localized stress responses, two of the most common that influence nursing care are the reflex pain response and the inflammatory response.

The **reflex pain response** is a response of the central nervous system when pain is the stimulus. It is rapid and automatic, serving as a protective mechanism to prevent injury. The reflex depends on an intact, functioning neurologic reflex arc and involves both sensory and motor neurons. For example, if you step into a bathtub of hot water, your skin senses the heat and immediately sends a message to the spinal cord. In turn, the message is sent to a motor nerve, which activates the muscles in your leg, and you quickly withdraw your foot. All of this happens before you consciously realize that the water is too hot to be safe.

The **inflammatory response** is a localized response to injury or infection. It serves to localize and prevent the spread of infection and so promote wound healing. When you cut your finger, you often develop the symptoms of the inflammatory response: pain, swelling, heat, redness, and changes in function. There are three phases in the inflammatory response.

1. In the first phase, bleeding initially is controlled by vasoconstriction (or narrowing) of the blood vessels at the injury site. After the bleeding has been controlled, histamines are released and capillary permeability increases, allowing increased blood flow and white blood cells to the area. The blood flow

TABLE 9-2

Social Readjustment Rating Scale*		
Rank	Life Event	LCU Value
1	Death of spouse	100
2	Divorce	73
3	Marital separation	65
4	Jail term	63
5	Death of close family member	63
6	Personal injury or illness	53
7	Marriage	50
8	Fired at work	47
9	Marital reconciliation	45
10	Retirement	45
11	Change in health of family member	44
12	Pregnancy	40
13	Sex difficulties	39
14	Gain of new family member	39
15	Business readjustment	39
16	Change in financial state	38
17	Death of close friend	37
18	Change to different line of work	36
19	Change in number of arguments with spouse	35
20	Mortgage over $10,000	31
21	Foreclosure of mortgage or loan	30
22	Change in responsibilities at work	29
23	Son or daughter leaving home	29
24	Trouble with in-laws	29
25	Outstanding personal achievement	28
26	Wife begins or stops work	26
27	Begin or end school	26
28	Change in living conditions	25
29	Revision of personal habits	24
30	Trouble with boss	23
31	Change in work hours or conditions	20
32	Change in residence	20
33	Change in schools	20
34	Change in recreation	19
35	Change in church activities	19
36	Change in social activities	18
37	Mortgage or loan less than $10,000	17
38	Change in sleeping habits	16
39	Change in number of family get-togethers	15
40	Change in eating habits	15
41	Vacation	13
42	Christmas	12
43	Minor violations of the law	11

*The Social Readjustment Rating Scale is an example of a tool used by health practitioners for identifying persons at risk for developing health problems. The scale is based on the premise that change requires adjustment, and excessive adjusting is a causative factor in illness. A value has been assigned to common changes in one's life, called life change units or LCUs. The LCU values are an indication of the amount of adjusting required by each change. The sum of the LCUs is an indication of the total amount of adjusting required of an individual at a particular time. The higher the cumulative score, the greater the amount of adjustment required, and the greater the likelihood of life crisis within 1 to 2 years, including health problems. An LCU score of 150 to 199 is thought to be an indicator of probable mild life crisis. A score of 200 to 299 is predictive of moderate life crisis, and a score of 300 or more is a predictor of major life crisis.

(Holmes, R. H., & Rahe, R. H. [1967]. The social readjustment rating scale. *Journal of Psychosomatic Research, 5*[11], 213–218.)

then returns to normal, but the white blood cells remain to help resist infection.
2. During the second stage, exudate (made up of fluid, cells, and inflammatory by-products) is released from the wound. The amount of exudate depends on the size, location, and severity of the wound.
3. During the third and final stage, damaged cells are repaired by either regeneration (replacement with identical cells) or formation of scar tissue. Some body tissues (skin, bone) are easily reproduced, and regain their former function; others (nervous system, intestines) do not regenerate but rather form nonfunctional scar tissue.

General Adaptation Syndrome The **general adaptation syndrome** (GAS) is a biochemical model of stress developed by Hans Selye. The concept of stressors as factors that cause stress also was made by Selye (1976). The GAS describes the body's general response to stress and serves as part of the knowledge base essential to all areas of nursing care.

There are three stages in the GAS. They are described in the following narrative and shown in Figure 9-4.
1. In the first stage, the *alarm reaction,* a person perceives a specific stressor, and various defense mechanisms are activated. The perception of threat may be conscious or unconscious. The autonomic nervous system initiates the fight-or-flight response, and hormone levels rise to fully prepare the body to react. This phase of the alarm reaction, called the *shock phase,* is characterized by an increase in energy levels, oxygen intake, cardiac output, blood pressure, and mental alertness. (If you think of the last time you narrowly missed wrecking your car, you will easily be able to identify these body reactions!) During the second phase of the alarm reaction, *countershock,* there is a reversal of body changes.
2. The second stage of the GAS is *resistance.* Having perceived the threat and mobilized its resources, the body now attempts to adapt to the stressor. Vital signs, hormone levels, and energy production return to normal. If the stress can be managed or confined to a small area (LAS), the body regains homeostasis. If the damage to the body is too great (for example, when there is severe injury and bleeding or a major illness such as cancer or a heart attack), the adaptive mechanisms fail, and the third phase of the GAS begins.
3. The third stage, *exhaustion,* is the result of exhaustion of the adaptive mechanisms. Without defense against the stressor, the body may either rest and mobilize its defenses to return to normal or reach total exhaustion and die.

Although the alarm stage is short-term (from minutes to hours), the length of the resistance and exhaustion stages varies greatly, depending on such variables as the severity and duration of the stressor, the previous health of the person, and the immediacy and effectiveness of health care interventions.

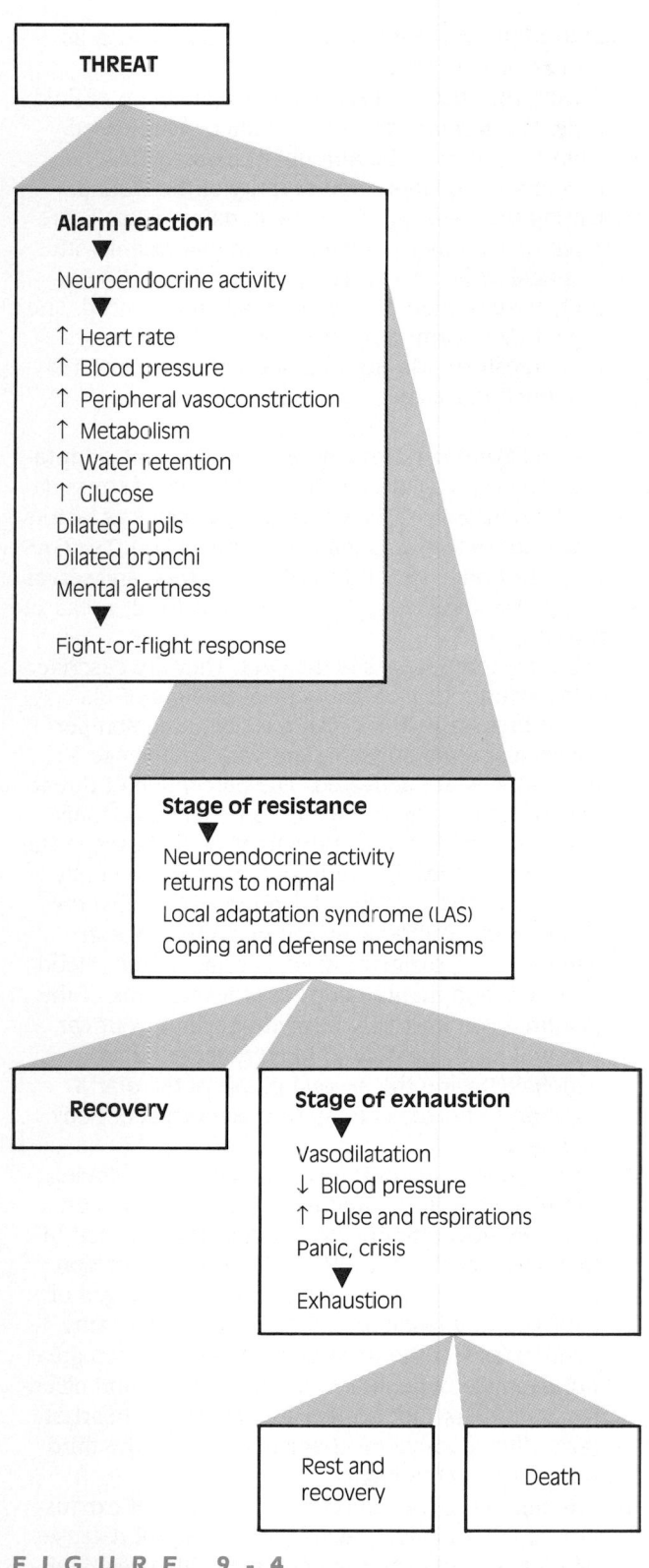

The general adaptation syndrome (general response to stress).

The GAS is a physiologic response to stress, but it is important to remember that the response is the result of both physical and emotional stressors. The stages occur in both physical and psychosocial damage to the body. Ob-

vious examples are seen in clients after severe injury or in those who have an illness, but GAS also is a factor in mental illness, social isolation, and loss (or lack) of human relations.

Psychosocial Responses to Stress

Humans respond to threat—and stress—psychologically as well as physically. Various emotional responses may be made, but the response most common in the human experience is anxiety. Anxiety is experienced from birth to death by all people, and involves one's body, self-perceptions, and social relationships (Stuart & Sundeen, 1991). **Anxiety** is a vague sense of impending doom or apprehension that appears to have no reason. (In contrast, fear is a response to a real stressor.) It is precipitated by the unknown and is present before all new experiences, serving as a threat to one's identity and self-esteem.

There are four levels of anxiety, each having different effects. The levels are as follows:

Mild anxiety: Present in day-to-day living; increases alertness and perceptual fields and motivates learning and growth

Moderate anxiety: Narrows the person's perceptual fields so that the focus is on immediate concerns, with inattention to other communications and details

Severe anxiety: Creates a very narrow focus on specific detail; causes all behavior to be geared toward getting relief

Panic: Causes the person to lose control and experience dread and terror. The resulting disorganized state is characterized by increased physical activity, distorted perceptions and relations, and loss of rational thought. This level of anxiety can lead to exhaustion and death.

At a mild level, anxiety can have a positive effect. For example, mild anxiety about an upcoming examination can motivate you to do the required reading and review. Anxiety beyond that level is regarded as negative, with unpleasant effects. In an attempt to neutralize, deny, or counteract the anxiety, a person develops individualized patterns of coping (Stuart & Sundeen, 1991).

Coping Mechanisms   Mild anxiety often is handled without conscious thought. **Coping mechanisms** include the following:

- Crying, laughing, sleeping, and cursing
- Physical activity and exercise
- Smoking and drinking
- Lack of eye contact and withdrawal
- Limiting relationships to those with similar values and interests

Moderate, severe, and panic levels of anxiety are greater threats and involve more complex coping mechanisms as the person strives to reduce the stress and anxiety. Coping mechanisms are categorized as task-oriented reactions or defense mechanisms.

Task-oriented reactions involve consciously thinking about the stress situation and then taking action to solve problems, resolve conflicts, or satisfy needs. These reactions, as defined by Stuart and Sundeen (1991), are as follows:

Attack behavior: Occurs when a person attempts to overcome obstacles to attack a problem; may be constructive, with assertive problem solving, or destructive, with feelings and actions of aggressive anger and hostility

Withdrawal behavior: Involves physical withdrawal from the threat, or emotional reactions such as admitting defeat, becoming apathetic, or feeling guilty and isolated

Compromise behavior: Usually constructive; involves the substitution of goals or negotiation to partially fulfill one's needs

Many of these behaviors are learned, and are based on past experiences and sociocultural influences and expectations.

Defense Mechanisms If the mechanisms used to cope with stress are not successful, other reactions called **defense mechanisms** often are used to protect the self. These mechanisms protect one's self-esteem and are useful in mild to moderate anxiety. They do, if used to extreme, distort reality and create problems with relationships. At that point, the mechanisms become maladaptive instead of adaptive.

Defense mechanisms are summarized here. You will learn more about them in the curriculum component that focuses on mental health and illness.

Compensation occurs when a person substitutes what is perceived as a good or a strength for a perceived weakness. A person may compensate for blindness by perfecting other senses.

Denial occurs when a person refuses to acknowledge the presence of a condition that is disturbing. An ill person uses denial when refusing to accept a diagnosis or prognosis.

Displacement occurs when a person can satisfy a need, blocked by one type of behavior, by using another type of behavior. For example, a person who is angry with a coworker displaces anger by kicking a chair.

Introjection occurs when a person internalizes some part of the external world and keeps it intact in the psyche. After the death of a loved one, for instance, a person may internalize the deceased person or some attribute of the deceased person.

Projection occurs when a person's undesirable impulses are attributed to another person or object. For example, a person carelessly trips over an article on the floor and blames the article for the accident.

Rationalization occurs when a person gives questionable behavior a logical or socially acceptable explanation. It amounts to behavior justification. A client may be rationalizing when an appointment with a health care practitioner is forgotten and the client explains that the practitioner is incompetent and the client does not want to continue seeing such a person.

Reaction formation occurs when a person gives a reason for behavior that is opposite from its true cause. An example is the parent of an unwanted child who overindulges the child.

Regression occurs when a person returns to an earlier method of behaving. Children often demonstrate regressive behavior, such as soiling diapers and demanding a bottle, when they are ill.

Repression occurs when a person excludes an anxiety-producing event from the conscious awareness. People tend to forget the unpleasantness of the past and remember only the good times.

Sublimation occurs when a person consciously expresses an unacceptable or impossible impulse or feeling in a more acceptable way. A woman who has chosen to be celibate and forgo motherhood may sublimate her maternal drives by working with children, by breeding pets, or by nurturing plants.

Suppression occurs when a person consciously turns attention away from a perceived threat. "If I let myself give in to this headache, I'll never accomplish what I must do today."

Effects of Stress

Stress affects all of the human dimensions. It has a strong influence on the attainment of basic human needs; it is a factor in health and illness; and it becomes a component in family reactions to illness. Long-term or prolonged stress, as well as crisis situations, seriously affects a person's physical and emotional health. Each of these areas are discussed in this section.

Interactions With Basic Human Needs

Basic human needs, described in Chapter 7, are common to all people. Stress, too, is common to all people. Both need attainment and the adaptation to stress require energy, respond to internal and external environments, and motivate behaviors. As a person strives to meet basic human needs at each level, stress can serve as either a stimulus or a barrier.

Basic human needs and responses to stress are individualized; both are modified by sociocultural backgrounds, priorities, and past experiences. In all people, the failure to meet needs results in imbalance in homeostatic mechanisms and, eventually, illness.

Stress affects a person and his or her attainment of basic human needs in the following ways:

Physiologic Needs
- Exhibits change in appetite
- Demonstrates change in activity pattern
- Experiences change in sleep pattern
- Undergoes change in elimination pattern

Safety and Security Needs
- Feels threatened and nervous
- Focuses on stressor, resulting in inattention, which may cause accidents

- Uses ineffective coping mechanisms (smoking, drinking) that are harmful to physical and emotional health

Love and Belonging Needs
- Is withdrawn and isolated
- Blames others for own faults
- Becomes overly dependent on others
- Demonstrates physical or emotional violence toward family members

Self-Esteem Needs
- Becomes a workaholic
- Exhibits behaviors that draw attention to oneself
- Has increasing complaints of physical illness

Self-Actualization Needs
- Refuses to accept reality
- Centers on own problems
- Demonstrates lack of control

Stress In Health and Illness

The health-illness continuum (described in Chapter 2) also integrates stress. Wellness and homeostatic balance are at one extreme of the continuum; exhaustion and death are at the other extreme.

Stress in a healthy person may promote health and prevent illness. For example, the fear of developing lung cancer may motivate a person to stop smoking, or anxiety about baby care may prompt prospective parents to attend prenatal classes and read child care books. Stressors in health also facilitate normal growth and development, provide the stimulus for learning constructive adaptive behaviors, stimulate problem-solving abilities, encourage social relationships, and help develop spiritual strength.

The effects of stress on a sick or injured person are, in contrast, usually negative. Stress can cause illness; illness causes stress. The presence of an illness or a disability demands new coping skills at a time when homeostasis is out of balance. Additionally, people who enter the health care setting are subjected to stressors unique to the situation.

Adaptation to acute and chronic illness involves two sets of adaptive tasks: (1) *general tasks* (as in the case of any situational stress) that involve maintaining self-esteem and personal relationships and preparing for an uncertain future, and (2) *illness-related tasks,* which include the following (Moos, 1985):
- Losing independence and control
- Handling pain and incapacitation
- Facilitating body function recovery
- Dealing with the hospital environment
- Developing relationships with caregivers
- Controlling symptoms
- Carrying out medical treatment
- Confronting economic and family problems

Nursing interventions designed to reduce stress and promote coping must be individualized and holistic. Considerations include the person's major concern, specific illness, sociocultural background, and available resources.

For example, one elderly woman may be anxious about the cost involved in repairing her hip fracture, whereas her roommate, with the same injury, is seriously concerned about the care of her cats while she is in the hospital. Or, as another example, two women (Mary and Jane) have entered the hospital with the medical diagnosis of breast cancer. Mary is worried about possible disfigurement and death, but she believes that with the help of surgery and chemotherapy, she can overcome the cancer. Jane, on the other hand, comes from a community that has strong fundamental religious beliefs. She believes that the cancer is a punishment from God and refuses any form of medical treatment.

As a nurse, it is important to remember that each situation is different, that each person perceives and reacts to stressors in an individual manner, and that there is no one best way to cope with a given situation.

Family Reactions to the Stress of Illness

The stress that affects a person who is ill also affects the person's family members or significant others. Viewing the family as a system, the behavior of the individual is influenced by the family, and any alterations in the individual's behavior in turn affects the family. The family thus is an integral part in the assessment, planning, and nursing interventions for stress.

The family of a person with an acute or chronic illness is subjected to various stressors, including the following:
- Changes in family structure and roles
- Isolation from the loved person
- Loss of control over normal routines
- Anger and feelings of helplessness and guilt
- Lack of information about care
- Concern for future economic stability

The family, both as individuals and as a unit, uses many of the same coping and defense mechanisms previously described. Family members may be overly protective, deny the seriousness of the illness, or blame the hospital staff for the client's condition or behaviors. On the other hand, the family can provide the social support necessary to help the client manage and adapt to stress. Emotional support from family members allows open expression of feelings and meets love and belonging needs. The inclusion of family members in problem solving, teaching-learning activities, and physical care helps both the client and the family to maintain their self-esteem and feeling of worth.

Prolonged Stress

Prolonged or long-term stress is a serious threat to physical and emotional health. As the duration, intensity, or number of stressors increases, a person's ability to adapt is lessened. The failure of adaptive mechanisms also is influenced by a person's level of wellness and past experiences with stress.

Long-term stress affects physical status, increasing the risk of disease or injury; recovery and return to normal function also are compromised by prolonged stress. High levels of stress are associated with cardiovascular disease, gastrointestinal disorders, and cancer. It is believed that these diseases are the result of various factors, including the effects of the fight-or-flight response, eating patterns, life-style, and coping mechanisms. A person who reacts to stress by overeating, smoking, becoming chemically dependent, or becoming hyperactive puts additional strain on a body prepared to react to threat. Homeostasis cannot be maintained, and illness results.

Reactions to home care of family members for long periods also cause prolonged stress. Called **caregiver burden**, this stress response includes chronic fatigue, sleep problems, and increased incidence of stress-related illnesses, such as high blood pressure and heart disease.

Prolonged stress also can seriously threaten mental health. As coping or defense mechanisms become ineffective, a person may try less effective coping patterns or maladaptive defense mechanisms. As anxiety increases despite these measures, the person may experience difficulties on the job, with personal relationships, and with self-esteem. These problems in turn act as stressors, and mental illness may result.

Crisis

A **crisis** occurs when coping and defense mechanisms that have been used to solve problems and adapt to change are no longer effective. This failure produces high levels of anxiety, disorganized behavior, and an inability to function adequately. A crisis situation is the result of a person's perception of and emotional response to a loss of self-esteem (or threat of a loss) from such events as illness, a change in status, a failure in school, or a verbal put-down.

The acute period of a crisis is self-limiting, lasting from 4 to 6 weeks. By that time, the threat is reduced, and the person has found some method of coping to reduce the emotional imbalance (Rambo, 1984). A person in crisis needs immediate help. Crisis intervention is discussed in the next section.

Nursing Actions to Promote Stress Reduction

Stress is a fact of life and must be integrated into plans of care in health promotion and maintenance for clients of all ages. Various stress reduction methods are included in this part of the chapter, but keep in mind the individualized nature of stressors and stress. The methods used should be carefully selected, based on each person's physical and emotional characteristics, family and social structure, and previously used coping mechanisms.

Activities of Daily Living

A person's normal life-style greatly influences perceptions and reactions to stressors. The person who is overweight, sedentary, and chronically tired is at increased risk to develop an illness as a result of stress. (These factors also are stressors, and further increase the risk.) Exercise, rest, and good nutrition are important components in stress reduction.

Regular *exercise* helps to maintain physical and emotional health. The benefits of exercise include an improved musculoskeletal system, more effective cardiovascular function, weight control, and relaxation. Exercise improves one's general sense of well-being, relieves tension, and enables one to better cope with day-to-day stressors. General health guidelines recommend that an exercise program consist of 30 to 45 minutes of activity three or four times a week. People who are overweight, chronically ill, or over age 35 should have a thorough physical examination before beginning such a program. The type of exercise can be individualized to what one enjoys most—for example, walking, jogging, bicycling, swimming, or participating in sports such as golf or tennis.

Rest and sleep allow the body to maintain homeostasis and restore energy levels. Adequate rest can provide "insulation" against stress, but stress may interfere with one's

---

EXAMPLES OF NURSING DIAGNOSES

Stress and Adaptation

The following nursing diagnoses are examples of those that might be appropriate for the client experiencing stress.

- Anxiety related to lack of knowledge about perioperative procedures
- Fear related to care of infant secondary to loss of previous child from sudden infant death syndrome
- Decisional Conflict related to use of contraceptive measures and religious beliefs
- Ineffective Individual Coping related to conflict between the need for medical treatment and culture
- Defensive Coping related to inappropriate evaluation of own behaviors

- Altered Health Maintenance related to use of alcohol, tobacco, and food in response to stress
- Health-Seeking Behaviors related to verbalized need for healthy stress reduction techniques
- Powerlessness related to inability to control environment while hospitalized
- Altered Sexuality Patterns related to ineffective coping with career requirements
- Sleep Pattern Disturbance related to anxiety response to change in income after loss of job

ability to sleep. Relaxation techniques can be helpful in health and illness in facilitating rest and sleep. Hospitalized clients may require additional nursing interventions to relieve pain and promote comfort to get needed rest.

Nutrition plays an active role in maintaining the body's homeostatic mechanisms and in increasing resistance to stress. Obesity and malnutrition are major stressors, and greatly increase the risk of illness. People of all ages are encouraged to maintain a normal body weight and to follow guidelines established by the U.S. Senate Committee on Nutrition and Human Needs. These guidelines include the following recommendations:

- Reduce intake of salt, refined sugar, animal fat, and cholesterol.
- Eat more fruit, vegetables, and whole grains.
- Eat less red meat and more fish and poultry.

Support Systems

As previously discussed, the client's family plays an important role in helping the client cope with stress. This support also can be provided by other social support systems.

Support systems provide emotional support that helps a person identify and verbalize feelings associated with stress. Other valuable contributions include providing information and services, maintaining positive self-concept, and establishing an avenue for new relationships and social roles. Additionally, families and support groups provide an accepting environment, allowing the person to explore problem-solving methods and try out new coping skills.

There are support groups for almost every situation, for example:

Alcoholics Anonymous
Overeaters Anonymous
Weight Watchers
Parents Without Partners
Reach to Recovery (cancer)
Ostomy clubs
Child abuse support groups
Sudden infant death support groups
Stroke clubs
Assertiveness training groups

N U R S I N G   T O D A Y   Challenges and Solutions

The Homeless

Challenges

- Homeless youth include runaways—usually from chaotic, poor, or violent families—and "graduates" from foster care. Many of these adolescents have attempted suicide and been expelled from school, and use drugs. To live on the streets, they sleep in abandoned buildings, panhandle, sell drugs, and become prostitutes.
- Many homeless single adults have psychological problems (such as anxiety and depression) or use drugs. Although they are known to the criminal justice system, most of the crimes involve misdemeanors. The typical homeless single adult is a male in his mid-30s, has never been married or divorced, and is of average educational level, with blacks and Hispanics overrepresented.
- Families are the fastest-growing segment of the homeless population. Most are headed by single mothers with children under the age of 16. The average age of the mother is 27, there is an average of two to three children in the family, and most receive Aid to Families with Dependent Children. Drug abuse, especially of crack, is epidemic among homeless mothers. Many children do not go to school, and have developmental delay.
- Living on the street results in exposure to the elements, poor nutrition, and lack of sleep. Living in shelters increases the risk of tuberculosis. Trauma and rape are everyday occurrences. Death is more common in infants and children and in those with AIDS. Pregnancy is twice as common in homeless adolescent females, and babies born to addicted mothers are learning to walk in hospital cribs because they have been abandoned. Many babies are of lower birth weight, do not receive immunizations, and have higher levels of lead in their bodies.

Nursing Solutions

- A nurse in New York City established a drop-in center and soup kitchen for homeless mentally ill women.
- A nurse-managed shelter in Boston provides on-site primary health services for the homeless.
- Nurses in Washington, DC, have established a shelter to serve as an infirmary, clinic, and detoxification unit.
- A clinic that provides primary care, social services, and transportation has been established by nurses on Skid Row in Los Angeles.
- At each of the St. Francis Residences in New York City, nurses coordinate the health care and nurture community bonds for the homeless living there.
- A nurse in Georgia persuaded the Georgia General Assembly to fund a clinic for the homeless, run by the Georgia Nurses' Foundation.
- Volunteer nurses from the third district of the Minnesota Nurses' Association organized a nursing clinic for the homeless.

(Data from Rafferty, M. [1989]. Standing up for America's homeless. *American Journal of Nursing, 89*[12], 1614–1617; and Rafferty, M. [1989]. How nurses are helping the homeless. *American Journal of Nursing, 89*[12], 1618–1619.)

Stress Management Techniques

Stress creates emotional distress, often having outward symptoms. All of us have had experiences with stress and know how we feel and how we react. One person may have tension headaches; another becomes irritable; another clenches his fists. Many people take drugs (legal and illegal), drink or smoke to excess, or eat compulsively. These behaviors can be modified and adaptive mechanisms strengthened through specific techniques aimed at managing stress. Only a few techniques are included here, but the literature is filled with stress reduction methods. Students are encouraged to learn different methods they can use for themselves and for varied clinical situations.

Relaxation Relaxation techniques are useful in many situations: childbirth, pain, anxiety, sleeplessness, illness, anger (and other uses are being discovered). Relaxation promotes a body reaction opposite to that of the fight-or-flight response, decreasing respiratory, pulse, and metabolic rates; blood pressure; and energy use.

Relaxation can be taught to individuals or groups, and is especially helpful because it allows a person to control feelings and behaviors. Various techniques are used, but each involves rhythmic breathing, reduced muscle tension, and an altered state of consciousness (Stuart & Sundeen, 1991). Two relaxation activities are discussed in the display. Relaxation also is discussed as a pain relief measure in Chapter 32.

Meditation Meditation has four components: (1) quiet surroundings, (2) a passive attitude, (3) a comfortable position, and (4) a word or mental image to focus on. A person practicing meditation closes his or her eyes, relaxes each of the major muscle groups, and repeats the selected word silently with each exhalation. Alternatively, the person may focus on a pleasant scene and mentally place himself or herself in it while breathing slowly in and out. This exercise should be performed for 20 to 30 minutes twice a day.

Anticipatory Guidance Anticipatory guidance focuses on psychologically preparing a person for an unfamiliar or painful event. Nurses use this technique to teach clients about procedures and the surgical experience. When clients know what to expect, their anxiety is reduced and their coping mechanisms are more effective. For example, before changing a dressing, teaching would include all the information about the pain involved—onset, severity, cause, methods of relief. With this knowledge, the client feels less threat and tolerates the procedure more easily.

Guided Imagery In guided imagery, a person creates an image in his mind, concentrates on the image, and becomes less responsive to stimuli (including pain). The nurse sits by the client and uses a scene or an experience that the client has described as happy, pleasant, or peaceful. The client is then "guided" through the image. For example, using a soothing, soft voice, the nurse might start as follows: "You are floating in your swimming pool. The water is cool and comfortable. Birds are singing in the trees. The roses are perfuming the air." As the client becomes more and more focused on the scene, the nurse will only need to verbally "paint the picture" at intervals.

Biofeedback Biofeedback is a method of gaining mental control of the autonomic nervous system, and thus regulating body responses, such as blood pressure, heart rate, and headaches.

A measurement device (eg, skin temperature sensors) is used, and the client tries to voluntarily control the readings through relaxation and conscious thought. The feedback from the change in readings teaches the person to control physiologic functions that normally are considered involuntary responses. The process is long-term and still being researched.

Crisis Intervention

As defined earlier, a crisis is a situation that cannot be resolved by usual coping mechanisms. As a result, a person is unable to function normally and requires interventions to regain equilibrium. **Crisis intervention** is a five-step problem-solving technique designed to promote a more adaptive outcome, including improved abilities to cope with future crisis (Fig. 9-5). The steps are as follows:

1. *Identify the problem.* This may be more difficult than it appears; the cause of the crisis often is difficult for the person to accurately identify. Until it is clear, a solution is impossible.
2. *List alternatives.* All possible solutions to the problem need to be listed. An appropriate solution to a problem is much more likely if a substantial number of options are considered.

Relaxation Activities

Deep Breathing

- Sit comfortably and place your hands on your stomach. Inhale slowly and deeply, letting your stomach expand as much as possible. Hold your breath for a few seconds.
- Exhale slowly through your mouth, blowing the air out through pursed lips. When your stomach feels empty, repeat the cycle.
- Repeat three or four times each session.

Progressive Muscle Relaxation

- Tighten your hand into a fist and notice how it feels; hold the tension for a few seconds.
- Loosen the grip on your muscles, relax your muscles, and let the tension slip away.
- Continue through each muscle group—hands, arms, shoulders, face, chest, back, stomach, legs, feet.

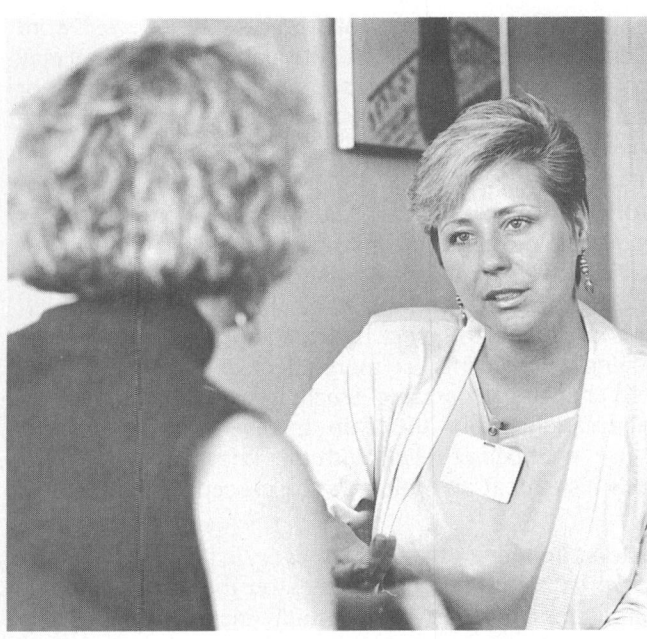

3. *Choose from among alternatives.* Each option needs to be carefully considered, using a ''what would happen if I—'' approach. The alternative chosen will be highly individualized, based on priorities and values.
4. *Implement a plan.* The alternative chosen is put into action. It may be necessary to provide support and encouragement so that action is taken.
5. *Evaluate the outcome.* In this final step, the effectiveness of the plan needs to be carefully considered. If it did not work as well as expected, another alternative needs to be chosen. If it did work, it has the positive benefit of improving self-confidence and future problem solving.

FIGURE 9-5

In crisis intervention, it is important for the nurse to help clients recognize their own stress levels and to encourage accepting what cannot be changed and changing what cannot be accepted. (Photo by Robert Neroni, courtesy of Thomas Jefferson University.)

RESEARCH IN NURSING Making a Difference

Stress and Adaptation

The concepts of stress and adaptation are important to nurses as they plan and implement client care to promote wellness, maintain or regain health, and facilitate coping. A wide variety of studies have been done to determine how people respond to stressors and adapt to changes in both health and illness. Information from research can be applied in clinical practice to more holistically meet client needs.

Related Research

Hamucharurnkui, S., & Vinya-Nguag, P. (1991). Effects of promoting patients' participation in self-care on postoperative recovery and satisfaction with care. *Nursing Science Quarterly, 4*(1), 14–20.

 The purpose of this experimental study was to test the effectiveness of clients' participation in self-care in facilitating recovery from surgery and in increasing satisfaction with care. Using a framework of nursing theories derived by Orem and King, clients in the experimental group carried out self-care activities through nurse–client interactions. This group had significantly less pain and distress, used fewer pain medications, ambulated more, had fewer complications, and had greater satisfaction with care than did the clients in the control group.

Davis, L. L. (1990). Illness uncertainty, social support, and stress in recovering individuals and family caregivers. *Applied Nursing Research, 3*(2), 69–71.

 The recovery from a major illness or injury is a stressful period for clients and families. In this study, Davis found higher stress levels in recovering clients who had higher levels of uncertainty about their illness, less social support, and a lower use of personal resources. Family caregivers had increased stress when they perceived less social support and available resources. It was suggested that stress during the recovery period, especially for caregivers, may be related to concerns about managing uncertainties of the future.

Pollock, S. E., Christian, B. J., & Sands, D. (1990). Responses to chronic illness: Analysis of psychological and physiological adaptation. *Nursing Research, 39*(5), 300–304.

 This study was conducted to determine whether adaptive responses of adults with three chronic illnesses (arthritis, multiple sclerosis, and hypertension) were significantly different. It was found that although physiologic adaptation was significantly different among the groups, psychological adaptation did not differ. Conclusions were that psychological adaptation to a chronic illness is not dependent on a specific medical diagnosis.

Summary

These studies are indicative of the trends in nursing care toward client self-care, involvement of families in client care, and chronic illness. They illustrate the effectiveness of nursing interventions in reducing postoperative stress, the importance of social support and resource use by recovering clients, and the commonality of adaptation to the stress of a chronic illness.

The major factor in helping clients adapt to high levels of stress is to identify and plan for the individuality of each situation. The following suggestions are useful:

- Help the person recognize his or her own stress level and specific responses to stress.
- Encourage a philosophy of accepting what cannot be changed and changing what cannot be accepted.
- Encourage the person to accept help from others—and to give support to others when needed.
- Encourage active but deliberate involvement in problem solving and decision making.
- Be an active listener, increasing therapeutic relationships and communications.
- Provide health teaching about developmental crises and threatening events.

Stress Management for Nurses

Nursing involves activities and interpersonal relationships that often are stressful (Fig. 9-6). The activities identified by Kinzel (1982) as being most stressful include the following:

- Having to assume responsibilities for which one is not prepared
- Working with unqualified personnel
- Working in an environment in which supervisors and administrators are not supportive
- Caring for a client during a cardiac arrest, or for a client who is dying
- Experiencing conflict with peers

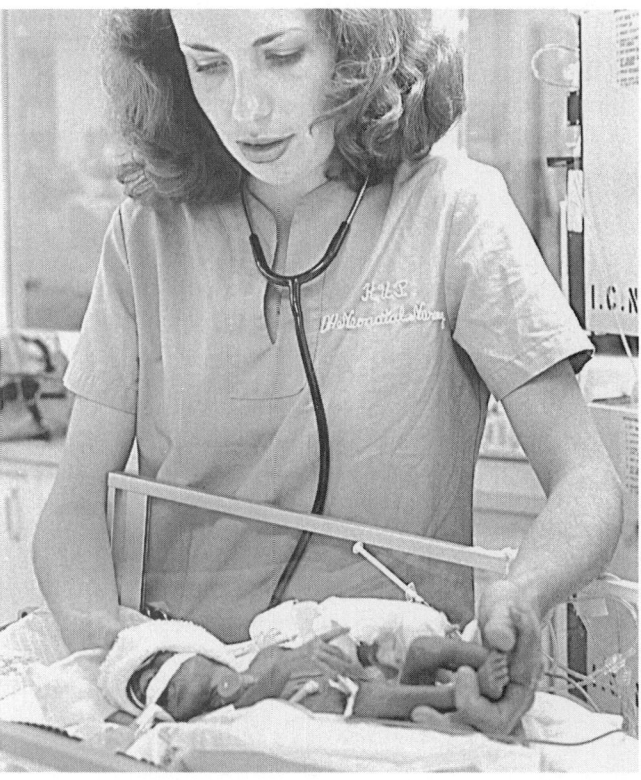

FIGURE 9-6

Some nursing specialties can be more stressful than others. To prevent burnout and alleviate stress, a nurse may need to work in another area of nursing, temporarily or permanently. (Photo by Gates Rhodes, courtesy of School of Nursing, University of Pennsylvania.)

▼ PROMOTING WELLNESS

Stress and Adaptation

Use the assessment checklist to determine how well you are adapting to stress. Then develop a prescription for self-care by choosing appropriate behaviors from the list of suggestions.

Assessment Checklist

almost always	sometimes	almost never	
☐	☐	☐	1. I have realistic perceptions of new situations, self, and others.
☐	☐	☐	2. I understand my own personal physical and emotional responses to stress.
☐	☐	☐	3. I anticipate and prepare for change.
☐	☐	☐	4. I have the ability to satisfactorily solve problems and make decisions.

Self-Care Behaviors

1. Accept as positive indicators of growth the changes that come with different parts and stages of life.
2. Maintain an open mind about change—change what you can, and accept what you cannot change.
3. Avoid self-defeating behaviors to cope with stress, such as smoking, alcohol, and drugs.
4. Practice methods of stress management that work best for you: relaxation techniques, exercise, hobbies.
5. Set realistic goals.
6. Develop problem-solving strategies for use in stressful situations.
7. Accept help from others.
8. Take life one day at a time.

The stress is even greater for two groups: new graduates, who must adjust to an environment different from what they experienced as students, and nurses who work in settings such as intensive care and emergency care.

The anxiety is further complicated by the expected behavior of nurses: Even though they may have strong negative feelings and reactions, their role does not include behaviors and verbal expressions that are less than positive and supportive.

Most nurses thoroughly enjoy their work and cope with the physical and emotional demands effectively. Some, however, are overwhelmed, and develop symptoms of anxiety and stress. The complex of behaviors exhibited is called professional burnout. **Burnout** can be compared with the exhaustion stage of anxiety, and is characterized by a wide range of behaviors. Some nurses try to become supernurses, expecting perfection in themselves and others. Some withdraw and do only minimal work; still others resort to drugs or alcohol. A large number of nurses who are unable to handle the stress leave the profession.

What can nurses do to help reduce stress and prevent burnout? The first step in preventing a stress level high enough to cause burnout is to identify and accept the stress. The same stress reduction techniques that are used for clients have positive benefits for nurses. Other suggested activities to reduce stress are as follows:

- Get involved in constructive change, particularly if organizational activities cause you stress.
- Take time for relaxation—use break time to practice a relaxation technique that works, and go off the unit for lunch.
- Carry out a regular exercise program—walk, jog, play tennis, play golf, join an aerobic dance class.
- Give yourself some time each day to unwind, relax, and do what you want—soak in a bubble bath, listen to music, read a novel.
- Learn something new—learn to knit, cane chairs, speak a foreign language, cook gourmet food.
- Develop assertive skills—learn to say no to additional tasks and accept the fact that no one person is perfect or indispensable.

Nurses need to accept that they have the same needs and are as individual as their clients. By recognizing the early signs of stress and taking steps to reduce the stress, nurses will continue to be effective, productive, and self-satisfied in the profession.

KEY POINTS

- Homeostasis, or a healthy balanced state, is maintained by various physiologic and psychological mechanisms. Physiologic mechanisms are largely involuntary responses of the autonomic and endocrine systems, necessary to health maintenance. Psychological balance is maintained through the use of coping or defense mechanisms.
- Stress, stressors, and adaptation are all interrelated parts of a process. *Stressors* (a challenge, a danger, or a threat) cause *stress* (a change in the balanced state). A person *adapts* through a series of responses. Each component is highly individualized and holistic in effect.
- Stress may be developmental or situational; stressors may be physiologic or psychosocial. Physiologic stressors have both a general and a specific effect. Psychosocial stressors affect us constantly in day-to-day living.
- The relation between physical and emotional stress is illustrated by the mind–body interaction, in which the perception of a threat on an emotional level results in the fight-or-flight response by the body. Resulting illnesses are called psychosomatic disorders.
- Life-changing events have an impact on health. The Social Readjustment Rating Scale can be used to predict risk of illness.
- The LAS is a localized body response to traumatic or pathologic stress that helps to maintain homeostasis and adaptation. Two examples of the LAS are the reflex pain response and the inflammatory response.
- The inflammatory response occurs in response to injury or infection, serving to prevent the spread of infection and promote wound healing through regeneration of tissue or formation of scar.
- The GAS is a biochemical model that describes the body's general response to stress. There are three stages to the GAS: alarm reaction, stage of resistance, and stage of exhaustion. The stages occur in response to both physical and emotional stress.
- The most common psychological response to stress is anxiety. Anxiety, precipitated by new experiences and the unknown, is a threat to self-esteem and identity. Anxiety has four levels: mild, moderate, severe, and panic.
- Coping mechanisms are largely unconscious methods of attempting to adapt to stress.
- Higher levels of stress may require psychological adaptation by coping with task-oriented reactions (attack, withdrawal, or compromise behavior) or defense mechanisms. Many of these behaviors are learned, based on past experiences and sociocultural environment.
- Stress can interfere with basic need attainment, disrupting homeostasis and causing illness.
- Stress can promote health and learning, but the stress of illness imposes additional burdens on a person who is out of balance. Adaptation to illness involves general tasks and illness-related tasks. Nursing interventions to reduce the stress of illness must be individualized and holistic.

- Stress affects the family as well as the individual. Families use varied coping methods and provide an important support system for the ill person.
- Prolonged stress affects both physical and mental health.
- Crisis results from ineffective coping, leading to severe anxiety, disorganized behavior, and malfunction.
- Nurses can promote health through the use of stress reduction teaching and methods, including healthy life-style, support groups, stress management techniques, and crisis intervention.

- Nursing is a stressful occupation. Nurses may become overwhelmed by the demands made on them and may develop symptoms of burnout. They can practice stress management techniques both on and off the job to help prevent stress and to improve career satisfaction.

BIBLIOGRAPHY

Antonovsky, A. (1979). *Health, stress and coping.* San Francisco: Jossey-Bass.

Breakwell, G. M. (1990). Are you stressed out? *American Journal of Nursing, 90*(8), 31–33.

Davis, L. L. (1990). Illness uncertainty, social support, and stress in recovering individuals and family caregivers. *Applied Nursing Research, 3*(2), 69–71.

DiMotto, J. (1984). Relaxation. *American Journal of Nursing, 84*(6), 754.

Donovan, M. (1980). Relaxation with guided imagery: A useful technique. *Cancer Nursing, 3*(1), 27–32.

Eakes, G. G. (1990). Grief resolution in hospice nurses: An exploration of effective methods. *Nursing and Health Care, 11*(5), 242–248.

Grainger, R. D. (1990). Managing fatigue. *American Journal of Nursing, 90*(3), 13.

Grey, M., Cameron, M. E., & Thurber, F. W. (1991). Coping and adaptation in children with diabetes. *Nursing Research, 40*(3), 144–149.

Haak, M. (1988). Stress and impairment among nursing students. *Research in Nursing and Health, 11*(2), 125–134.

Hames, C., & Joseph, D. (1986). *Basic concepts of helping: A wholistic approach* (2nd ed.). New York: Appleton & Lange.

Humucharurnkui, S., & Vinya-nguag, P. (1991). Effects of promoting patients' participation in self-care on postoperative recovery and satisfaction with care. *Nursing Science Quarterly, 4*(1), 14–20.

Johnson, B. (1989). *Psychiatric–mental health nursing: Adaptation and growth* (2nd ed.). Philadelphia: Lippincott.

Kinzel, S. L. (1982). What's your stress level? *Nursing Life, 2*(2), 54–55.

McCranie, E., Lambert, V. A., & Lambert, C. E., Jr. (1987) Work stress, hardiness, and burnout among hospital staff nurses. *Nursing Research, 36*(6), 374–378.

Miller, J. (1985). Inspiring hope. *American Journal of Nursing, 85*(1), 22–25.

Moos, R. (1985). *Coping with physical illness* (2nd ed.). New York: Plenum.

Pasquali, E., et al. (1989). *Mental health nursing: A holistic approach* (3rd ed.). St. Louis: Mosby.

Pollock, S. E. (1989). The hardiness characteristic: A motivating factor in adaptation. *Advances in Nursing Science, 11*(2), 53–62.

Pollock, S. E., Christian, B. J., & Sands, D. (1990). Responses to chronic illness: Analysis of psychosocial and physiological adaptation. *Nursing Research, 39*(5), 300–304.

Rambo, B. (1984). *Adaptation nursing: Assessment and interventions.* Philadelphia: Saunders.

Robinson, L. (1990). Stress and anxiety. *Nursing Clinics of North America, 25*(4), 935–943.

Ryan, J. (1984). The neglected crisis. *American Journal of Nursing, 84*(10), 1257–1258.

Selye, H. (1976). *The stress of life.* New York: McGraw-Hill.

Smeltzer, S., & Bare, B. (1992). *Brunner and Suddarth's Textbook of medical–surgical nursing* (7th ed.). Philadelphia: Lippincott.

Sorenson, E. S. (1990). Children's coping responses. *Journal of Pediatric Nursing, 5*(4), 259–267.

Sparacino, J. (1982). Blood pressure, stress and mental health. *Nursing Research, 1*(2), 89–94.

Stokes, S., & Gordon, S. (1988). Development of an instrument to measure stress in the older adult. *Nursing Research, 37*(1), 16–19.

Stuart, G., & Sundeen, S. (1991). *Principles and practices of psychiatric nursing* (4th ed.). St. Louis: Mosby.

Wakefield, M. (1992). Stress control for nurses. *Canadian Nurse, 88*(4), 24–25.

Wyka, G., & Caraulia, S. (1986). Crisis intervention: Stopping push before it comes to shove. *Nursing, 11*(16), 44–45.

Yu, L. C., Mansfield, P. K., Packard, J. S., Vicary, J., & McCool, W. (1989). Occupational stress among nurses in hospital settings. *American Association of Occupational Health Nursing, 37*(4), 121–129.

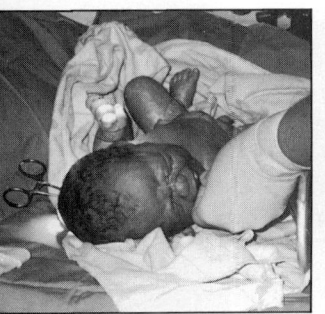 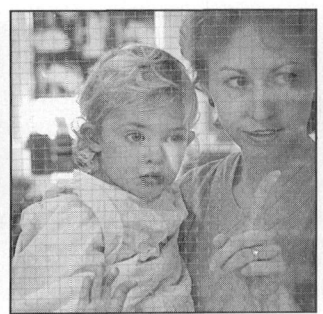  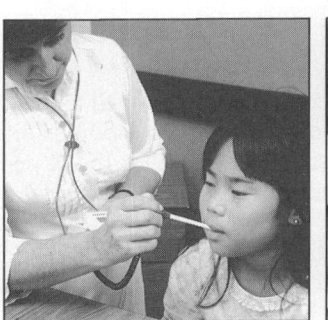 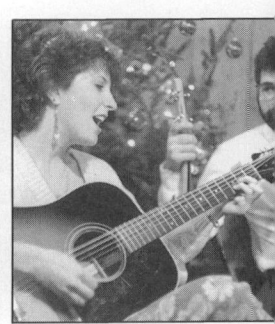

Promoting Wellness Across the Life Span

Nurses give care to clients of all ages and at all stages of growth and development. Unit III explores the impact of developmental stages and tasks on nursing care for clients and families throughout the entire life span from conception to death.

Developmental theories provide guidelines for giving individualized client care, with consideration for physiologic, cognitive, psychosocial, moral, spiritual, and family components of each individual. Each person progresses through life in well-defined stages, with critical tasks and common health needs and problems. The chapters in this unit follow the sequential stages of growth and development, describing factors that influence normal development, common age-related health problems, and the role of the nurse in preventing illness and promoting health.

With increasing numbers of the population over age 65, the health needs of older adults are a major nursing concern and will continue to be so. Chapter 12 discusses formal age-related changes, common myths and realities of the older age group, and the nurse's role in promoting wellness and coping with change.

Death, as the final stage of life, requires nursing interventions to meet individual and family needs, and to facilitate coping with loss and grief.

Unit III provides a comprehensive picture of growth and development throughout life, enabling the nurse to individualize care and meet needs for clients in all stages of life.

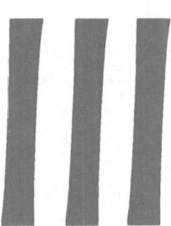

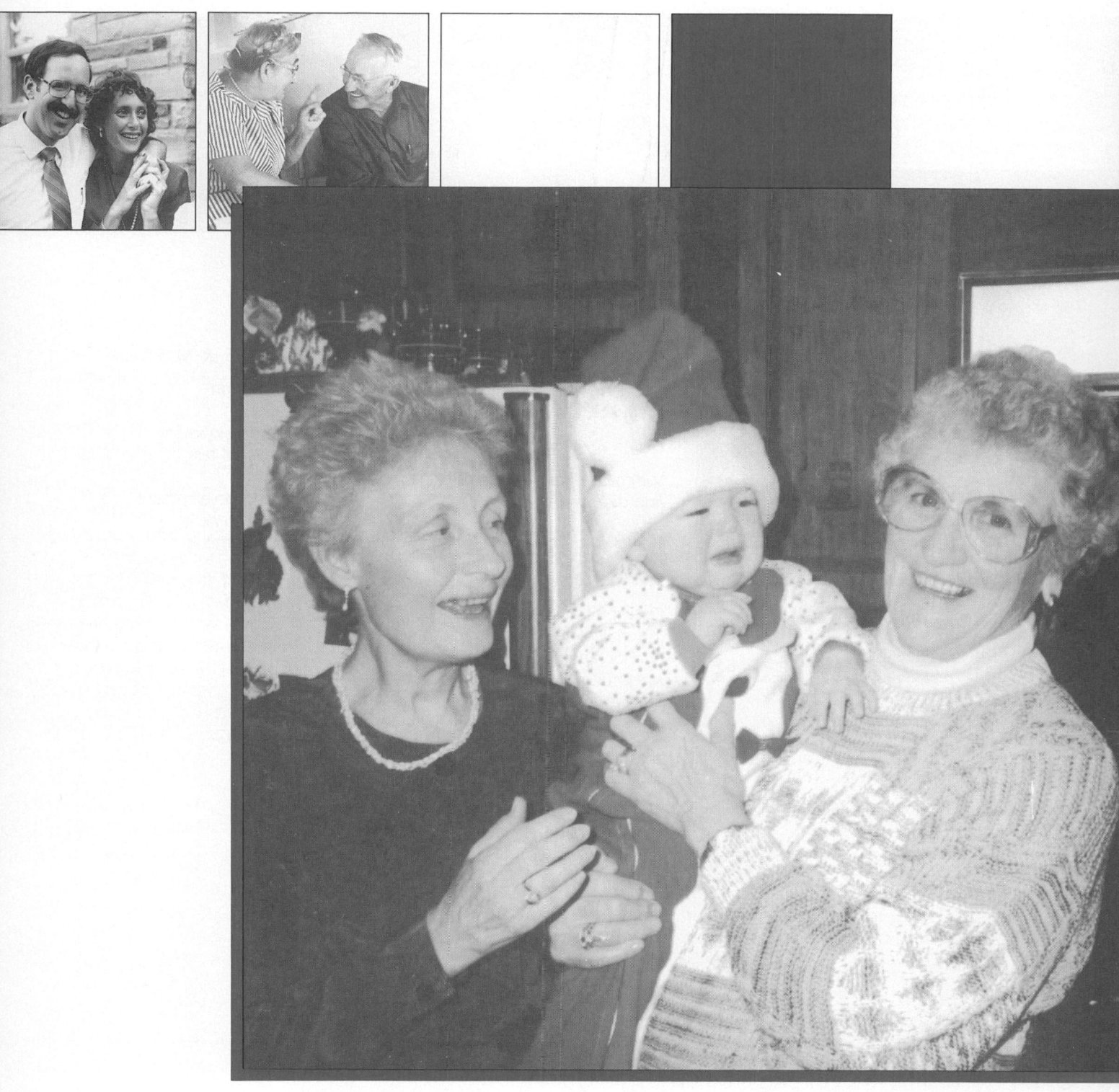

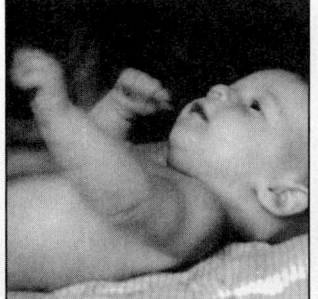
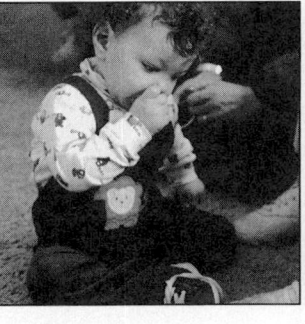

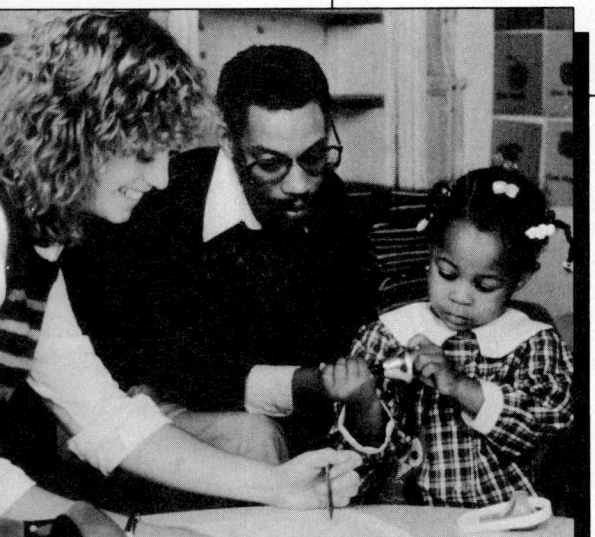

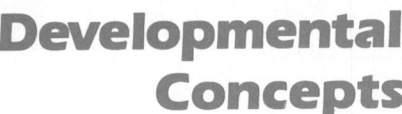

Developmental Concepts

OBJECTIVES

After studying this chapter, the learner should be able to:

Define key terms used in the chapter.

Summarize basic principles of growth and development.

Discuss the theories of Freud, Erikson, Havighurst, Piaget, Kohlberg, Gilligan, and Fowler.

Describe the importance of incorporating multiple theories of growth and development in assessing and planning nursing care for individuals and families.

Describe the dynamics of family in providing nursing care.

List implications for nursing practice that uses a knowledge base of growth and development.

KEY TERMS

accommodation
assimilation
cognitive development
developmental task
faith
growth and development
moral development
psychosocial theory

10

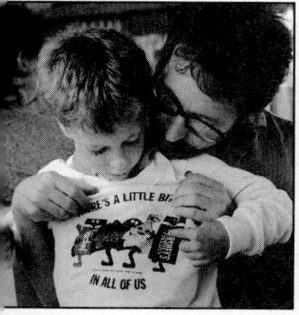

As caregivers, nurses promote health and wellness for people from birth to death. All people, regardless of age, have unique health care needs that result from the physical, emotional, intellectual, social, spiritual, and cultural aspects of their developmental level. To plan and give holistic and individualized care, the nurse must understand typical behavior for each developmental level.

Physical development has a predetermined genetic base because of inheritance patterns carried on chromosomes. Thus, the unborn child begins life with specific physical attributes, either properly formed or malformed. Environmental factors from birth through the early years of growth provide initial psychological and social contact through positive or negative parenting experiences. As environmental influences expand beyond the immediate caregivers or family, psychosocial experiences increase and affect development. Cognitive, moral, and spiritual growth are fostered through contact within families, schools, and communities. Information derived from multiple theories of human and family development assist the nurse in perceiving these interrelated variables at designated stages throughout life.

This chapter presents basic principles of growth and development to serve as a foundation for understanding the human being at various life stages. Major theories examining cognitive, psychosocial, spiritual, and moral development are discussed. In addition to reviewing theories specific to the individual's development, the family and its influence on personal development are briefly discussed.

The Nature of Human Growth and Development

The human processes of **growth and development** are the result of two interrelated factors—heredity and environment. Humans simultaneously grow and develop in physical, cognitive, psychosocial, moral, and spiritual dimensions, with each dimension being an essential part that makes up the whole person. Development is a dynamic and continuous process, characterized by a series of ascents, plateaus, and declines as one proceeds through life. Each phase of development also has a period of disequilibrium, when adjustment to internal and external demands are more difficult, and a period of equilibrium, when adjust-

ment to demands is more easily made (Erikson, 1963; Mussen, Conger, & Kagan, 1974). If adjustments are not made in the appropriate level of development, one may have difficulties during a later stage of life.

Principles of Growth and Development

Although growth and development in each of the dimensions are individualized, certain generalizations can be made about the nature of human development. These generalizations form the principles that serve as guidelines for understanding growth and development. The broad generalizations are as follows:

Growth and development are orderly and sequential as well as continuous and complex. All humans experience the same growth patterns and developmental levels. As these patterns and levels are individualized, a wide variation in biologic and behavioral changes is considered normal. Within each developmental level, certain milestones are identified, for example, the time the infant rolls over, crawls, walks, and begins to say his or her first words.

Growth and development follow regular and predictable trends. Cephalocaudal (proceeding from head to tail) development is the first trend, with the head and brain developing first, followed by the trunk, legs, and feet. Photographs of an infant in utero show the large size of the head compared with the rest of the body (Fig. 10-1). The second trend is proximodistal development, which means that growth progresses from gross motor movements (such as learning to lift one's head) to fine motor movements (such as learning to pick up a toy with the fingers). The last trend is that development of the body is symmetrical, with both sides of the body developing equally.

Growth and development are both differentiated and integrated. As nerve pathways develop, they become more specialized, allowing the growing child to respond to different stimuli. Throughout the life span, each new learned activity builds on previous learning and abilities, so that increasingly complex tasks can be accomplished. For example, the toddler learning to use a spoon combines motor skills, hand–eye coordination, cognitive patterning, and social imitation from watching others to repeat an act when appropriate (Fig. 10-2). As children grow and develop, the task of learning to use a spoon becomes basic, forming the foundation for learning more advanced skills that require manual dexterity.

Different aspects of growth and development occur at different stages and at different rates, and can be modified. For example, muscles and bones both grow most rapidly during the first year of life; during the toddler and preschool years, bone growth slows but muscle fibers increase in size and strength. The most intense period of speech development is between ages 3 and 5 (Fig. 10-3). Sexual maturity begins during the preadolescent years and progresses into the adult years, but is based on gen-

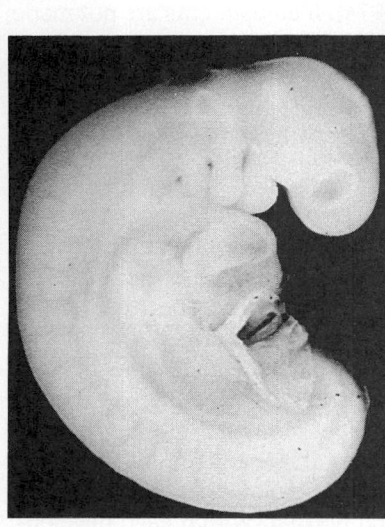
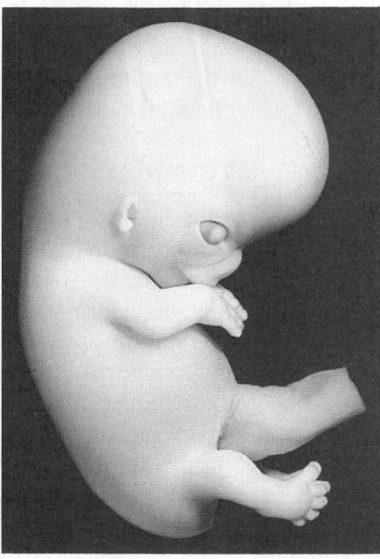
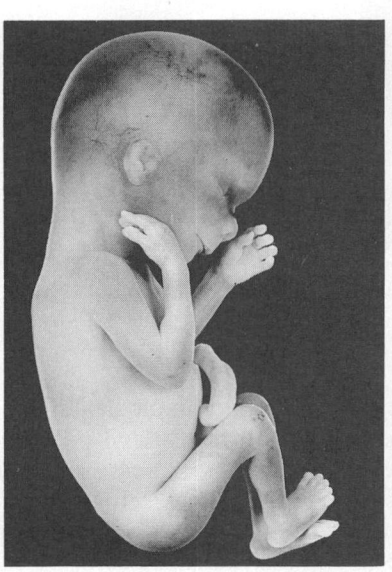

F I G U R E   1 0 - 1

Three stages of human development in utero—at about 4, 8, and 16 weeks—showing the development first of the head and then the trunk and limbs. (Courtesy of the Carnegie Institute, Washington, DC.)

der and sex role identity established from birth. Many factors can modify growth and development, including nutrition, love and affection from caretakers, and illnesses.

The pace of growth and development is specific for each person. Both physical and psychological skills and maturation vary between and among people. For example, while learning to walk, a child may concentrate energies on the task and temporarily slow down in language development. Cultural variations also may be seen; Oriental and Asian children tend to be smaller than Caucasian children of the same age. In addition, one's genetic heredity places re-

strictions on the upper limits that can be achieved in growth and development.

Overview of Developmental Theories

Researchers have studied human development and behavior since the beginning of the 20th century, and have developed classic theories to explain human responses that are expected at certain ages during life. Although a psychological approach is common to all developmental theories,

F I G U R E   1 0 - 2

The toddler learning to use a spoon is integrating hand–eye coordination, cognitive patterning, and social imitation in mastering the task.

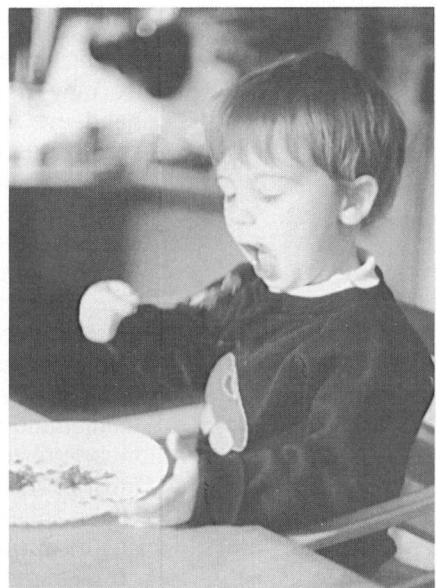
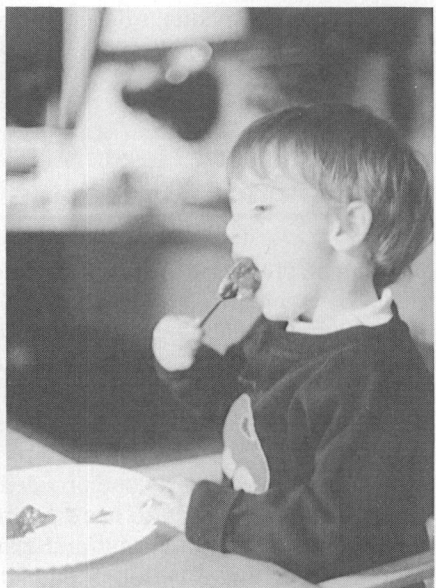

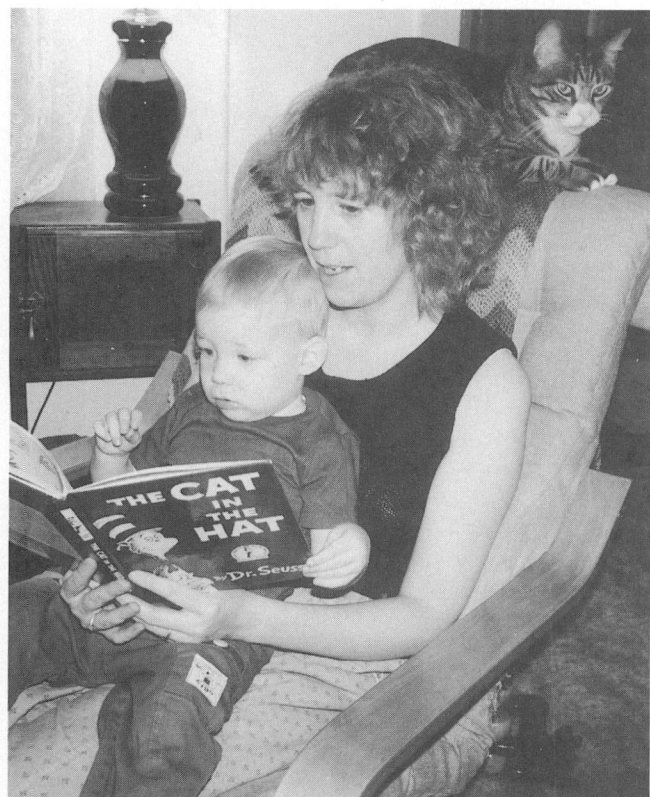

F I G U R E   1 0 - 3

Speech development is greatest between the ages of 3 and 5 years; it is fostered by interaction and communication with caregivers. (Photo by William Boehm.)

each theory focuses on a different influence. The theories discussed in this section examine cognitive, social, and instinctual influences on human growth and development.

Psychoanalytic Theory: Sigmund Freud

Freud's theory (Freud, 1923) stressed the impact of instinctual human drives on determining behavior. The primary concepts of the theory are the unconscious mind, the id, the ego, the superego, and stages of development based on sexual motivation. Freud identified the underlying stimulus for human behavior as sexuality, which he called libido. Libido was defined as general pleasure-seeking instincts rather than purely genital gratification.

Major Components of Freud's Theory

Unconscious mind: Contains memories, motives, fantasies, and fears that are not accessible to recall but directly affect behavior.

Id: Part of the psyche concerned with self-gratification by the easiest and quickest available means.

Ego: Conscious part of the psyche that serves as a mediator between the desires of the id and the constraints of reality so that one may live effectively within one's social, physical, and psychological environment. The ego includes one's intelligence, memory, problem solving, separation of reality from fantasy, and incorporation of experiences and learning into future behavior. Development of the ego in the first year of life allows the infant, by 6 months of age, to view self as separate from others and to begin to alter behaviors in response to cues. Ego development continues throughout life.

Superego: Part of the mind that represents one's conscience and develops from the ego during the first year of life as the child learns praise versus punishment for actions. The ego represents the internalization of rules and values so that socially acceptable behavior is practiced.

A further contribution of Freud's theory was the description of defense mechanisms, which are means of unconscious coping when the id's impulses cannot be satisfied so as to reduce stress in the conscious mind. Defense mechanisms are discussed in Chapter 9. In addition, Freud described a series of developmental stages through which all people must pass (Table 10-1).

Freud's Stages of Development

Oral stage (ages 0 to 18 months): The infant's pleasures center around gratification by using the mouth for sucking and satisfying hunger.

Anal stage (ages 8 months to 4 years): This stage begins when neuromuscular control is developed to allow control of the anal sphincter. Toilet training is a crucial issue that requires delayed gratification as the child compromises between enjoyment of bowel function and limits set by social expectations.

Phallic stage (ages 3 to 7 years): The child has increased interest in gender differences, one's own gender, and conflict and resolution of that conflict with the parent of the same sex (named the Oedipus complex in boys and the Electra complex in girls when intimate sexual possessiveness of the oppo-

T A B L E   1 0 - 1

Freud's Stages of Psychosexual Development		
Stage	**Age**	**Sexual Activity**
Oral	0–18 months	Sucking, swallowing, chewing, biting
Anal	8 months–4 years	Expulsion and retention of waste products
Phallic	3–7 years	Masturbation
Latent	5–12 years	—
Genital (adult sexuality)	12–20 years	Masturbation, sexual intercourse, feelings for others

(Data from Fong, C., & Resnick, R. [1980]. *The child: Development through adolescence.* Menlo Park, CA: Benjamin/Cummings)

site-sex parent is shown). Curiosity about the genitals and masturbation increases.

Latency stage (ages 5 to 12 years): This stage marks the transition to the adult sexuality or genital stage during adolescence. Increasing sex role identification with the parent of the same sex prepares for adult roles and relationships.

Genital stage (ages 12 to 20 years): At this stage, sexual interest can be expressed in overt heterosexual relationships. Sexual pressures and conflicts cause turmoil as the adolescent makes adjustments in relationships.

Psychosocial Theory: Erik Erikson

Erikson's (1963) developmental theory was based on work by Freud, but was expanded to include cultural and social influences in addition to biologic processes. **Psychosocial theory** is based on four major organizing concepts: (1) stages of development, (2) developmental goals or tasks, (3) psychosocial crises, and (4) the process of coping (Newman & Newman, 1975). Erikson believed that development is a continuous process made up of distinct phases characterized by the achievement of developmental goals that are affected by the social environment and significant others.

Erikson identified eight stages that progress from birth to old age and death (Table 10-2). Each stage is characterized by a developmental crisis that has to be mastered, with polarities that indicate the possibility of successful or unsuccessful resolution of the crisis. Unsuccessful resolution at any one stage may delay progress through the next stage, but mastery can occur later.

Erikson's Stages of Development

Trust versus mistrust—infancy: The infant learns to rely on caregivers to meet basic needs of warmth, food, and comfort so that trust in others is formed. Mistrust is the result of inconsistent, inadequate, or unsafe care (Fig. 10-4).

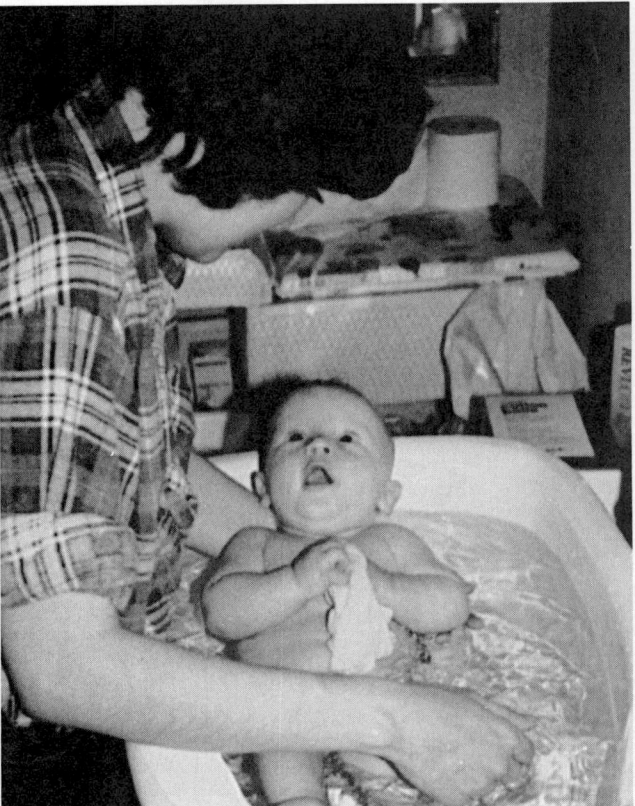

F I G U R E   1 0 - 4

Infants develop a sense of trust and security as they learn that they can rely on their caregivers to fulfill their needs. (Photo by Patrick O'Kane.)

T A B L E   1 0 - 2

Erikson's Stages of Psychosocial Development		
	Developmental Crisis	**Stage**
Stage I	Trust vs mistrust	Infancy
Stage II	Autonomy vs shame and doubt	Toddler years
Stage III	Initiative vs guilt	Preschool years
Stage IV	Industry vs inferiority	School-age years
Stage V	Identity vs role confusion	Adolescence
Stage VI	Intimacy vs isolation	Young adulthood
Stage VII	Generativity vs stagnation	Middle adulthood
Stage VIII	Ego integrity vs despair	Later adulthood

Autonomy versus shame and doubt—toddler (ages 1 to 3): As motor and language skills develop, the toddler learns from the environment and gains independence through encouragement from parents to feed, dress, and toilet self. If the parents are overprotective or have expectations that are too high, shame and doubt, as well as feelings of inadequacy, may develop in the child.

Initiative versus guilt—preschool (ages 4 to 6): Confidence gained as a toddler allows the preschooler to have initiative in learning, so that new experiences are actively sought out and the how and why of activities are explored. If restrictions or reprimands for seeking new experiences and learning are experienced, guilt results, and the child becomes hesitant to attempt more challenging skills in motor or language development.

Industry versus inferiority—school-age: Focusing on the end result of achievements, the school-age child gains pleasure from finishing projects and receiving recognition for accomplishments (Fig. 10-5). If the child is not accepted by peers or cannot meet parental expectations, a feeling of inferiority and lack of self-worth may develop.

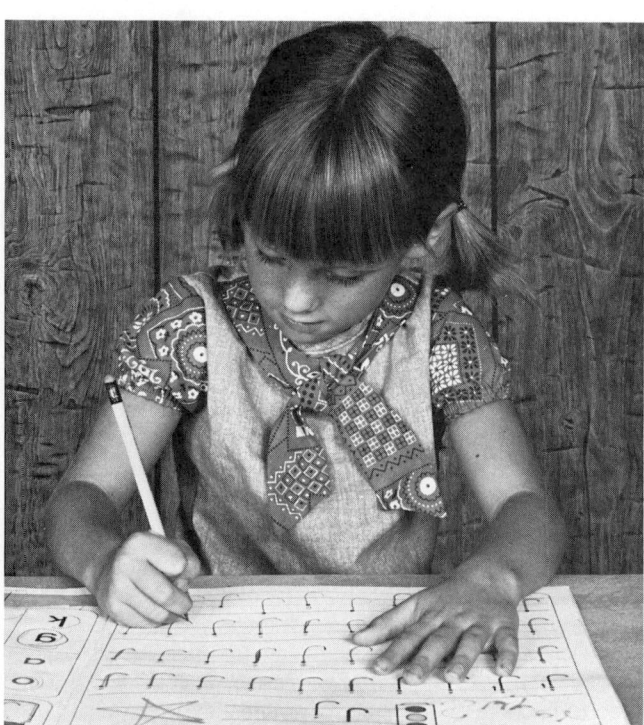

FIGURE 10-5

School-age children focus on the end results of accomplishments—recognition and praise from family, teachers, and peers—developing a sense of competition and industry.

Identity versus role confusion—adolescence: As many changes occurs in his or her body, the adolescent is in transition from childhood to adulthood. Hormonal changes produce physiologic growth of secondary sex characteristics and mood swings. Trying on roles and even rebellion are considered normal behaviors in acquiring a sense of who one is and what direction one will take in life. Role confusion occurs when the adolescent is unable to establish identity and a sense of direction.

Intimacy versus isolation—young adulthood: The tasks for the young adult are to unite self-identity with identities of friends, and to make commitments to others (Fig. 10-6). Fear of such commitments results in isolation and loneliness.

Generativity versus stagnation—middle adulthood: The middle adult years are a time of concern for the next generation as well as involvement with friends and community. There is a desire to make a contribution to the world. If this task is not met, stagnation results, and the person becomes self-absorbed and obsessed with her or his own health needs, or regresses to an earlier level of coping.

Ego integrity versus despair—later adulthood: As one enters one's older years, reminiscence of life events provides a sense of fulfillment and purpose. If one believes that one's life has been a series of failures or missed directions, a sense of despair may prevail.

Developmental Tasks: Robert J. Havighurst

Havighurst (1972) believed that living and growing are based on learning, and that a person must continuously learn to adjust to changing societal conditions. He described learned behaviors as **developmental tasks** that occur at certain periods in life. Successful achievement leads to happiness and success in later tasks, whereas unsuccessful achievement leads to unhappiness, societal disapproval, and difficulty in later tasks. The developmental tasks arise from maturation, personal motives and values that determine occupational and family choices, and civic responsibility. Table 10-3 summarizes the developmental tasks described by Havighurst.

Cognitive Development: Jean Piaget

Piaget, a Swiss psychologist, developed a theory of **cognitive development** from infancy through adolescence. Piaget believed that learning occurred as a result of the internal organization of an event, which formed a mental schemata, and served as a base for further schemata as one grew and developed. Intellectual growth, as described by Piaget, was a continual restructuring of knowledge to progress to higher levels of problem solving and critical thinking. Two continual processes of assimilation and accommodation stimulate intellectual growth in the child. **Assimilation** is the process of integrating new experiences into existing schemata; **accommodation** is an alteration of thought processes to correlate more complex information

FIGURE 10-6

Establishing intimacy in young adulthood involves integrating self-identity and identities of others, and establishing relationships based on commitment, which necessitates self-sacrifice and compromise. (Photo by Tracy Baldwin.)

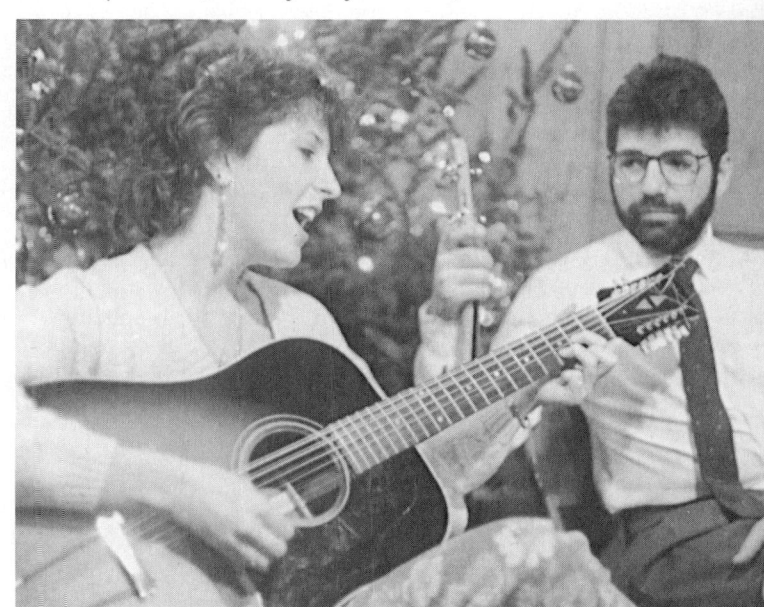

TABLE 10-3

Developmental Tasks Described by Robert J. Havighurst

Infancy and Early Childhood	Middle Childhood	Adolescence
Learning to walk	Learning physical skills necessary for ordinary games	Achieving new and maturer relations with age-mates of both sexes
Learning to take solid foods	Building wholesome attitudes toward oneself as a growing organism	Achieving a masculine or feminine social role
Learning to talk	Learning to get along with age-mates	Accepting one's physique and using the body effectively
Learning to control the elimination of body wastes	Learning an appropriate masculine or feminine social role	Achieving emotional independence from parents and other adults
Learning sex differences and sexual modesty	Developing fundamental skills in reading, writing, and calculating	Preparing for marriage and family life
Forming concepts and learning to describe social and physical reality	Developing concepts necessary for everyday living	Preparing for an economic career
Getting ready to read	Developing conscience, morality, and a scale of values	Acquiring a set of values and an ethical system as guide to behavior—developing an ideology
	Achieving personal independence	Desiring and achieving socially responsible behavior
	Developing attitudes toward social groups and institutions	

Early Adulthood	Middle Age	Later Maturity
Selecting a mate	Assisting teenage children to become responsible and happy adults	Adjusting to decreasing physical strength and health
Learning to live with a marriage partner	Achieving adult social and civic responsibility	Adjusting to retirement and reduced income
Starting a family	Reaching and maintaining satisfactory performance in one's occupational career	Adjusting to death of a spouse
Rearing children		Establishing an explicit affiliation with one's age-group
Managing a home	Developing adult leisure-time activities	Adopting and adapting social roles in a flexible way
Getting started in an occupation	Relating oneself to one's spouse as a person	Establishing satisfactory physical living arrangements
Taking on civic responsibility	Accepting and adjusting to the physiologic changes of middle age	
Finding a congenial social group	Adjusting to aging parents	

(Havighurst, R. J. [1972]. *Developmental tasks and education* [3rd ed.]. New York: Longman.)

TABLE 10-4

Jean Piaget's Theory of Cognitive Development

Stage	Age
Sensorimotor	0–24 months
Reflective	0–1 month
Primary circular reactions	1–4 months
Secondary circular reactions	4–8 months
Coordination of secondary schemata	8–12 months
Tertiary circular reactions	12–18 months
Invention of new means through mental combinations	18–24 months
Preoperational	2–7 years
Preconceptual	2–4 years
Intuitive	4–7 years
Concrete operational	7–11 years
Formal operational	11+ years

(Piaget & Inhelder, 1969). Four stages of cognitive development were described by Piaget (Table 10-4).

Piaget's Stages of Cognitive Development

Sensorimotor stage (birth to 24 months): During this period, the child progresses through a series of developmental stages, for example:

0 to 1 month—demonstrates basic reflexes, such as sucking (Fig. 10-7)

1 to 4 months—discovers enjoyment of random behaviors (such as smiling or sucking thumb) and repeats them

4 to 8 months—relates own behavior to change in environment, such as shaking a rattle to hear the sound (Fig. 10-8)

8 to 12 months—coordinates more than one thought pattern at a time to reach a goal, such

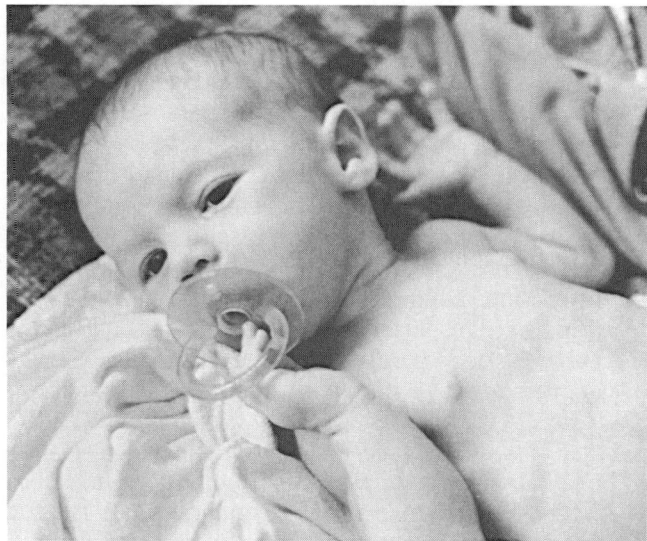

FIGURE 10-7

During the first month of life, the infant has no understanding of the environment and can respond only by exercising basic reflexes such as sucking. (Photo by Tracy Baldwin.)

FIGURE 10-8

From about age 4 months, the infant can begin to relate his own behavior as causing a change in the environment, and from about age 8 months, can integrate more than one thought pattern to obtain a purposeful goal. (Reeder, S. J., & Martin, L. L., [1991]. *Maternity nursing* [17th ed.]. Philadelphia: Lippincott.)

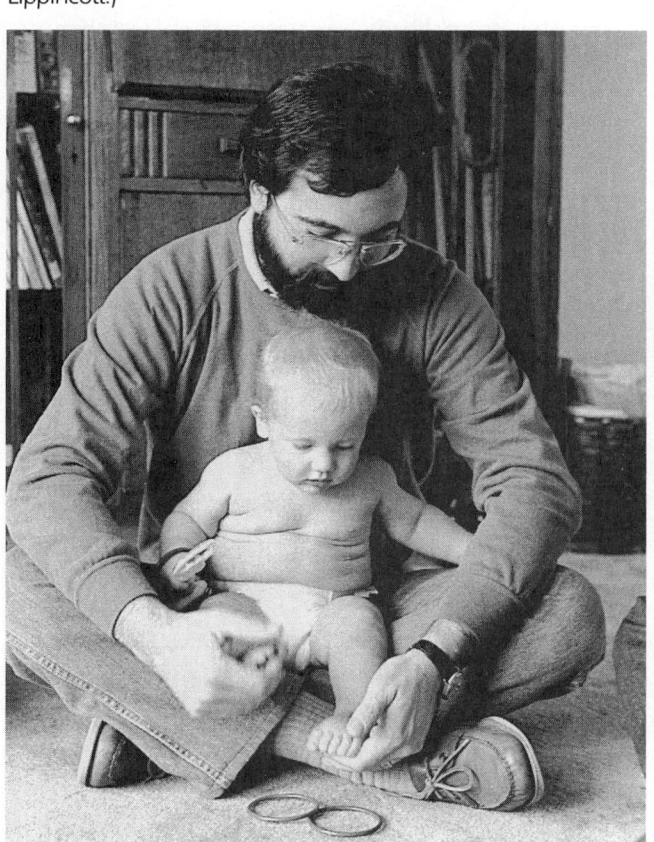

as repeatedly throwing an object on the floor; only objects in sight are considered permanent

12 to 18 months—recognizes the permanence of objects, even if out of sight; can understand simple commands

18 to 24 months—begins to develop reasoning and can anticipate events

Preoperational stage (ages 2 to 7): This stage is characterized by the beginning use of symbols, through increased language skills and pictures, to represent the preschooler's world (Fig. 10-9). This stage is divided into two parts: the preconceptual stage (ages 2 to 4) and the intuitive stage (ages 4 to 7). Play activities during this time allow the child to better understand life events and relationships.

Concrete operational stage (ages 7 to 11): During this time, children learn by manipulating concrete or tangible objects, and can classify articles according to two or more characteristics. Logical thinking is developing with an understanding of reversibility, relations between numbers, and loss of egocentricity. Another characteristic of this stage is the ability to incorporate another's perspective.

Formal operational stage (age 11 or older): This stage is represented by the use of abstract thinking and deductive reasoning. General concepts are related to specific situations and alternatives are considered. The world is evaluated by testing beliefs in an attempt to establish values and meaning to life (Fig. 10-10).

FIGURE 10-9

The preschool child's development is characterized by the beginning use of symbols through language and pictures, an ability to learn simple sequences, and a basic ability to categorize objects. (Photo by Gates Rhodes, courtesy of School of Nursing, University of Pennsylvania.)

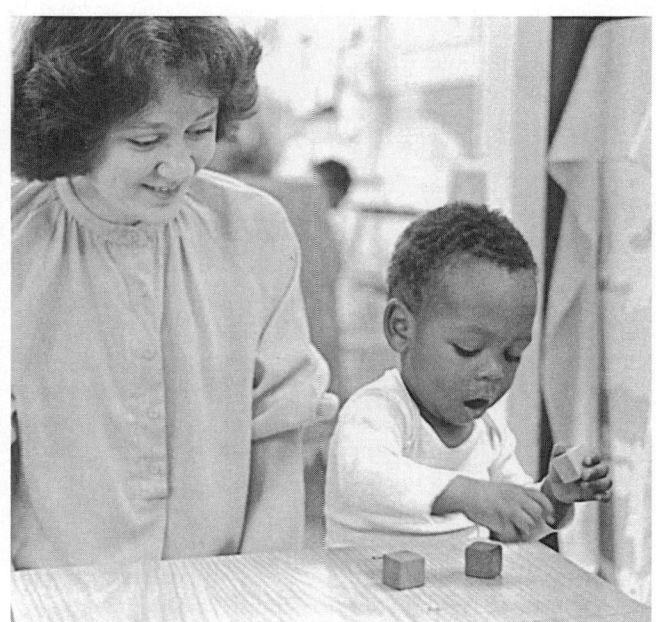

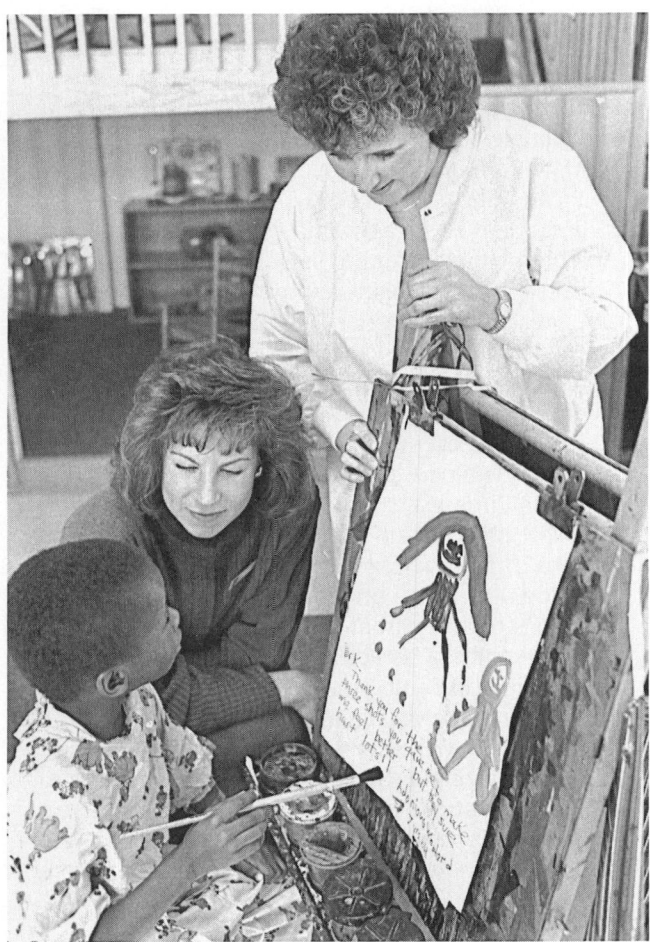

F I G U R E   1 0 - 1 0

Abstract reasoning is required for a child to understand that painful medical treatments given now will make him feel better later. A child who is not old enough to have reached the formal operational stage, in which abstract reasoning develops, may require special attention from the health care staff to understand the uncomfortable experiences of his hospital stay. (Photo by Don Walker, courtesy of Thomas Jefferson University Hospital.)

Moral Development: Lawrence Kohlberg and Carol Gilligan

Lawrence Kohlberg Kohlberg (1969) developed a theory of **moral development** with levels that closely follow Piaget's theory of cognitive development. Each level is further divided into two separate stages.

Kohlberg's Levels of Moral Development

Preconventional level: This level follows intuitive thought, and is based on external control as the child learns to conform to rules imposed by authority figures. At stage 1, *punishment and obedience orientation,* the motivation for choices of action is fear of physical consequences of authority's disapproval. As a result of the consequences, a perception of goodness or badness develops. At stage 2, *instrumental relativist orientation,* the thought of receiving a reward overcomes fear of punishment, so actions that satisfy this desire are selected.

Conventional level: This level is obtained when the person becomes concerned with identifying with significant others and shows conformity to their expectations. Values and ideals supported by family and friends are respected, regardless of consequences. Stage 3, *"good boy–good girl" orientation,* is when the person strives for approval in an attempt to be viewed as "good." Stage 4, *"law and order" orientation,* is when behavior focuses on following social or religious rules as a respect for authority. In his later work, Kohlberg maintained that many adults are at this stage because they think abstractly and view themselves as members of society (Duska & Whelan, 1975).

Postconventional level: This level is associated with moral judgment that is rational and internalized into one's standards or values. Stage 5, *social contract, utilitarian orientation,* supports that correct behavior is defined by the legal rights of society. Laws can be changed, however, to meet society's needs, while maintaining respect for self and others. Stage 6, *universal ethical principle orientation,* represents the person's concern for equality for all human beings, which is guided by personal opinions and standards, regardless of those set by society or laws. Justice may be internalized at an even higher level than society. Few adults ever reach this stage of development.

Kohlberg recognized that moral development is influenced by cultural effects on perceptions of justice in interpersonal relationships. The beginnings of moral development are witnessed in parent and child communications during the early childhood years, as the young child tries to please her parents. The concept of morality emerges as a subset of a person's beliefs or values and governs choices made throughout life. Rules and regulations established by society eventually are challenged and evaluated as a person either accepts societal rules into her own internal set of values or rejects them.

Carol Gilligan Gilligan (1977, 1982) originally did work with Kohlberg. As she listened to women discuss their own real-life moral conflicts, she recognized that there was a conception of morality from the female viewpoint that was not represented in Kohlberg's work.

In Gilligan's theory, males and females have different ways of looking at the world. Males are more likely to associate morality with obligations, rights, and justice. Females are more likely to see moral requirements emerging from the needs of others within the context of a relationship. This moral orientation of females is called the *ethic of care,* which develops through three levels. Each level ends with a transitional period—a time when the female considers new approaches to moral considerations and moves to a new level.

Gilligan's Levels of Moral Development

Level 1—Selfishness: In the first level, the focus is on needs of the self. "Should" and "would" are the same. Morality is seen as sanctions by society. Relationships often are disappointing, and as a result, a woman may choose to isolate herself to avoid getting hurt. The transition that follows this level is characterized by the move from selfishness to responsibility—a move that integrates the responsibility to care for self with the desire to care for others.

Level 2—Goodness: Moral judgment is based on shared norms and expectations, and societal values are adopted. Acceptance by others becomes critical, and the ability to protect and care for others is seen as the defining characteristic of female goodness. This characteristic is upheld through beliefs that one is responsible for the actions of others, but that others are responsible for the choices that are made. As self-sacrifice is examined, the second transition occurs, with the woman asking if her own needs are not also important. A shift from goodness to truth (as well as a new conception of goodness) takes place.

Level 3—Nonviolence: A changed understanding of self and a redefinition of morality allow the woman to reconcile selfishness and responsibility. Nonviolence (the injunction against hurting) governs all moral judgments and actions. Care becomes a universal obligation toward self and toward others. Moral problems usually are considered within the context of maintaining relationships and response, and of promoting the welfare or preventing the harm of others.

Gilligan developed a theory of moral development that views females as developing a morality of response and care, and males as developing a morality of justice. Research will facilitate further development of this theory and increase knowledge about human development.

Faith Development: James Fowler

Fowler (1981) has developed a developmental theory of the spiritual identity of humans, based on work by Piaget, Kohlberg, and Erikson. He describes **faith** as follows (1981, p. 4):

> Faith is not always religious in its content or context. . . . Faith is a person's or group's way of moving into the force field of life. It is our way of finding coherence in and giving meaning to the multiple forces and relations that make up our lives. Faith is a person's way of seeing him or herself in relation to others against a background of shared meaning and purpose.

TABLE 10-5

Comparison of Psychosocial and Faith Stages

Erikson's Psychosocial Stages	Fowler's Faith Stages
Trust vs mistrust	Undifferentiated (infancy)
Autonomy vs shame and doubt	Intuitive-projective (early childhood)
Initiative vs guilt	
Industry vs inferiority	Mythical-literal (school years)
Identity vs role confusion	Synthetic-conventional (adolescence)
Intimacy vs isolation	Individuative-reflective (young adulthood)
Generativity vs stagnation	Conjunctive (midlife)
Ego integrity vs despair	Universalizing

(Data from Fowler, J. W. [1981]. *Stages of faith: The psychology of human development and the quest for meaning.* New York: Harper & Row, 1981)

Faith, therefore, is not necessarily religious, but it comprises the reasons one finds life worth living.

Fowler's theory is composed of prestage and six stages of faith development. The age when a certain stage exists varies, but the sequence does not. Equilibrium, or the plateau of faith development, can occur at any stage, beginning with stage 2.

In the organization of the stages of faith development, Fowler explained a triadic relationship between self, shared causes or values, and others, which is the unifying factor in all stages and is based on trust. During the prestage, called *undifferentiated faith,* trust, courage, hope, and love compete with threats of abandonment and inconsistencies in the infant's environment. The strength of faith in this stage is based on the relationship with the primary caregiver. Table 10-5 compares Erikson's psychosocial stages with Fowler's faith stages.

Fowler's Stages of Faith Development

Stage 1—Intuitive–projective faith: This stage is most typical of the 3- to 7-year-old child. Children imitate religious gestures and behaviors of others, primarily their parents. They follow parental attitudes toward religious or moral beliefs without a thorough understanding of them. Imagination in this stage leads to long-lived images and feelings that must be questioned and reintegrated in later stages (Fig. 10-11).

Stage 2—Mythical–literal faith: This stage predominates in the school-age child with increased social interaction. Stories represent religious and moral beliefs, and existence of a deity is accepted. Perspectives of others can be appreciated, as well as the concept of reciprocal fairness.

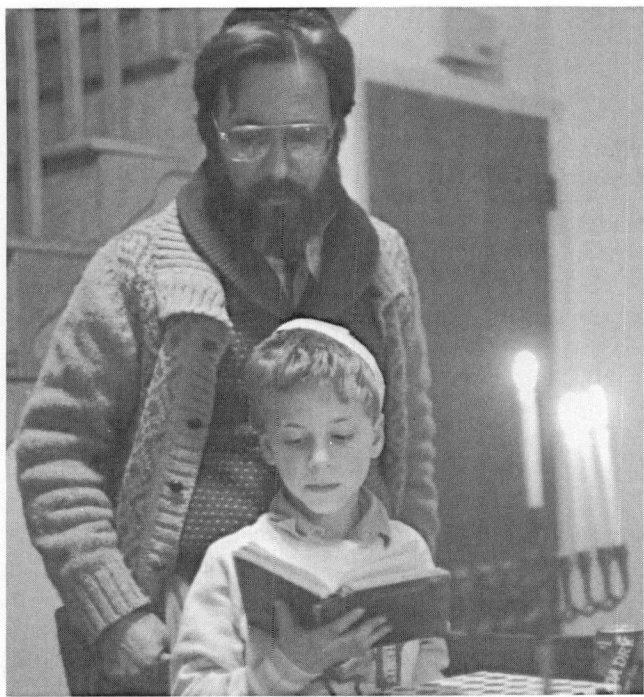

FIGURE 10-11

In the earliest stage of faith development, the child imitates religious gestures and behaviors of his parents and others. Images and feelings experienced in early years will be reevaluated and reintegrated in later stages.

Stage 3—Synthetic–conventional faith: This is the characteristic stage for many adolescents. As the person experiences increasing demands from work, school, family, and peers, the basis for identity is complex. An ideology has emerged but has not been closely examined until now. The person begins to question some of the life-guiding values or religious practices in an attempt to stabilize his own identity.

Stage 4—Individuative–reflective faith: This stage is critical for older adolescents and young adults because the responsibility for their commitments, beliefs, and attitudes becomes their own. Many adults do not construct this stage, and for some people, it does not emerge until they are in their 30s or 40s. Searching for self-identity no longer defined by the boundaries of faith compositions of significant others is a primary concern.

Stage 5—Conjunctive faith: This stage integrates other viewpoints about faith into one's understanding of truth. One is able to see the paradoxical nature of the reality of one's own beliefs. Along with this realization, the divisions of faith development among people become apparent.

Stage 6—Universalizing faith: This stage involves overcoming paradoxes noted in stage 5, and makes tangible the values of absolute love and justice for

humankind. The faith relationship noted in stage 6 is characterized by total trust in the principle of being and the existence of the future, whether derived from the Judeo-Christian image of faith or otherwise.

Applying Growth and Development Principles and Theories to Nursing

In review, the complex and interrelated elements that contribute to the phenomenon of human development constitute not only biophysical factors, but also factors of personality development. The theories presented from Freud, Erikson, Havighurst, Piaget, Kohlberg, Gilligan, and Fowler give knowledge of the evolution of cognitive, psychosocial, moral, and spiritual development. In relating to the whole person, all the components of development need to be evaluated to understand certain life events or concerns.

Although these theorists have brought a great deal of insight into the process of human development, some limitations exist in each theory. Therefore, in planning holistic nursing care for clients with diverse needs, backgrounds, and ages, nurses should assess the client and support decisions for interventions on rationale from multiple theories of development so as to provide comprehensive health promotion. A few examples are discussed here.

While interviewing a young mother with her first child the nurse senses a frustrated single parent as the mother reviews the task of rearing her 14-month-old child alone. Based on Freud, the nurse can relate the behaviors typical of the oral stage of development for the infant. Havighurst and Erikson support the stage of gaining independence in learning to walk for the toddler. Recognizing that the mother may be limited in her support system, the nurse may need to assess further to identify problems with intimacy and a feeling of generativity. In planning care for this young mother, the nurse anticipates needed emotional support and health teaching about the normal toddler years. The mother's anxiety level and the child's attempts to investigate the environment through locomotion and oral exploration place them at risk for injury from falls or aspiration. The nurse has a primary role in prevention through client education based on astute observation and knowledge of child development.

A 16-year-old girl is admitted to the nursing unit after having sustained multiple injuries in a motor vehicle accident. The injuries include several deep facial lacerations and a fractured femur. The young woman is stabilized, medicated for pain, and placed in traction. The nurse notices the girl crying quietly in her room. Realizing the importance of self-identity for the adolescent (Erikson, 1963), the nurse approaches the girl and asks if she would like to talk. Initially seeming hesitant, the girl is able to discuss her fears of scar formation on her face and comments from her friends. The nurse can assist by allowing the girl to share her feelings and by encouraging her to talk with her physician to find out the possible outcome after healing occurs.

A 70-year-old man fell and fractured his hip while repairing the exterior of his home. Having been the traditional head of his household, he now is troubled by needing others, including his wife, to care for him. He appears withdrawn, refusing to talk and eating poorly. Reflecting on Havighurst's and Erikson's theories, the nurse knows that the man may be fluctuating between feelings of nonadjustment and acceptance of declining health and a sense of ego integrity.

These few situations demonstrate the application of growth and development theories to the practice of nurs-

ing. Health care needs change quickly as a person grows and passes through life. These needs are unique for each person but include certain similarities at specific periods. The nurse is faced with the dynamic tasks of planning care based on both general and unique health needs of a client and continually revising aspects of care in the evolution of the growth process or alteration in health status.

Family Dynamics

The functions, structures, and developmental tasks of the family are discussed with human needs in Chapter 7; the establishment of a family is discussed in Chapter 11 in

---

RESEARCH IN NURSING   Making a Difference

Growth and Development

Knowledge of normal growth and development is part of the knowledge base of nursing and is used to recognize normal patterns as well as to identify variations from normal. Although this is important for any age-group, it is especially critical in the nursing care of both healthy and ill children and adolescents.

Related Research

White, M. A., Williams, P. D., Alexander, D. J., Powell-Cope, G. M., & Conlon M. (1990). Sleep onset latency and distress in hospitalized children. *Nursing Research, 39*(3), 134–139.

This research investigated the effects of different strategies to promote sleep in 94 hospitalized 3- to 8-year-old children. Children in this study had increased distress and took longer to go to sleep with parent presence or association of a voice with a parent or other family member. Based on this study, it is recommended that nursing strategies be developed to facilitate sleep, such as using a stranger-recorded story at bedtime and modifying the environment by dimming lights and reducing noise.

DeMaio-Esteves, M. (1990). Mediators of daily stress and perceived health status in adolescent girls. *Nursing Research, 39*(6), 360–363.

The purpose of this study was to test the effects of daily stress, introspectiveness, and coping efforts on perceived health status in adolescent girls. A sample of 159 teenagers completed the study, with results that supported the strong influence of daily stress on negative perceptions of health. As stress increased, so did thoughts and feelings about self, which served to facilitate coping with stressors and positively influencing health perception.

Sorenson, E. S. (1990). Children's coping responses. *Journal of Pediatric Nursing, 5*(4), 259–267.

Although a major goal of nurses is to facilitate positive coping, little is known about individual coping strategies, especially from the child's perspective. This study of well children ranging in age from 8 to 11 years was done to identify and describe coping responses. Among findings were that the most common response to daily stressors was submission or endurance and that mothers were viewed as the most common coping support source. In addition, girls tended to respond emotionally, whereas boys responded by physical aggression. It is suggested that nurses consider the value of each child's unique perception of stress as care is given.

Janes, B., & Morse, J. (1990). Adolescent girls' perceptions of and preparation for menarche. *Canadian Journal of Nursing Research, 22*(2), 47–58.

Although menarche marks the transition of girl to woman, little is known about the menarche experience. This study was conducted to determine how adolescent girls view the preparation they receive for menarche and how they cope with menstruation in daily life (especially at school). Data supported that these girls were not as well prepared as they could be. Suggestions include increasing education by community health nurses and school health nurses to both adolescent girls and their mothers.

Summary

Nurses are in a unique position in the health care field to facilitate optimal growth and development in children and adolescents. Recognition of the importance of principles of growth and development and use of those principles as a base for individualized nursing interventions is essential. Nursing research, conducted to describe and explore experiences from a developmental framework, can provide increased knowledge and more effective nursing care.

the section dealing with the young adult. The family is mentioned in this chapter because the study of growth and development would not be complete without noting the interrelationship between an individual and the family. Family dynamics, a major environmental influence, begins with conception and continues throughout life.

Along with structural variety, families are the product of cross-cultural principles. Because of the diversity of ethnic groups that have immigrated to the United States, the nurse is exposed to different perspectives on the management of health and illness. Religious practices, dietary restrictions, child rearing, and care of elderly people are affected by certain cultural beliefs. Friedman (1992) stated that culture circumscribes and guides the ways in which societies and ethnic groups solve their problems and derive meaning from their lives. (Culture and ethnicity are discussed in Chapter 8, and spirituality is discussed in Chapter 41.)

The family plays a vital role in wellness promotion and illness prevention. The family inflicts values and cultural influences on decisions regarding interpretation of illness. A health problem or developmental crisis of any family member can affect the remainder of the unit. Health practices, whether positive or negative, often are shared in the family, being learned by younger members. Sometimes the family may even be the cause of illness of individual members. It is well known that heart disease, arthritis, alcoholism, and emotional disorders, to list only a few examples, run in families. Alterations in coping and communication patterns may predispose families to dysfunctional means of relating to one another.

Applying Family Dynamics to Nursing

The nurse has a responsibility to assess not only the health needs of individual members of the family, but also the demands placed on the total family in meeting every member's needs. The nurse can then function as a catalyst in planning appropriate interventions and teaching, and as a collaborator with other health care professionals (social workers, psychologists, physicians, clergy) in achieving optimal family wellness.

Marilyn M. Friedman (1992) describes the family using a structural-functional approach. The functions of the family include (1) affective (meeting psychosocial needs of the family, (2) socialization, (3) reproduction, (4) family coping, (5) economics, and (6) provision of physical necessities. The family uses four structural components to fulfill these functions: (1) role structure, (2) value systems, (3) communication patterns, and (4) decision making. Through four basic structural components, the family strives to obtain these goals. Friedman has devised a family assessment tool that comprises these four components to information to plan family nursing care. These components include role structure, value systems, communication patterns, and power or decision-making structure.

With a thorough family assessment, the nurse can identify or assist families in identifying the priorities of their health care needs. Analysis of data collected can lead to the development of nursing diagnoses to systematically organize a plan of care with selected interventions. Through mutual goal setting with family members, the nurse guides the evaluation process in helping the family meet developmental needs and quality levels of health for its members.

Implications for Nurses

General guidelines for incorporating principles and theories of growth and development and family dynamics into daily practice of nursing care are listed below. They are given as suggestions for working with all ages.

- Be knowledgeable concerning the various stages of cognitive, psychosocial, moral, and spiritual development. Be prepared to support developmental stages typical of certain ages.
- Maintain flexibility in assessing people, and respect the uniqueness of each person. Although the literature describes development typical of a particular age, not everyone fits into an exact mold.
- Although development follows an order of succession, the rate of progress differs among people in certain life stages. Anticipate possible regression during difficult periods or times of crisis, accepting and supporting a person's return to a forward progression in development.
- Become cognizant of environmental and cultural influences because of their strong effect on development, especially psychosocial development. A deprived environment can be detrimental, whereas an enriched environment enhances development.
- Assess each person with an awareness that within each stage of development, a person may retain some behaviors of a previous stage, attain goals of the current stage, and begin to exhibit behaviors of the next stage. There is a time of transition to the next stage with no definite beginning or ending to the particular stage of development.
- Remember that clients are members of families and that the family unit can have both positive and negative influences on the development of individual members. Attempt to support good family relationships and healthy environments that assist members to reach their greatest potential for growth.
- Provide client teaching to individuals and their families to aid in their understanding of periods of development.
- Aid clients in setting priorities for family health. Conflicts can occur when they try to meet their own needs, their children's needs, and those of aging parents.
- Be ready to provide health care to clients who suffer from illnesses or failure to meet developmental goals. Collaborate with other members of the health care team in providing care to prevent or minimize disruption of development and to promote optimal wellness throughout life.
- Prepare environments and experiences that are developmentally challenging.

KEY POINTS

- Nurses provide care to all ages in the life continuum; this care involves both individuals and their families.
- Growth and development theories, taken together, involve all aspects of life: physiologic, cognitive, psychosocial, moral, spiritual, and family dimensions.
- Principles of growth and development state that the processes are (1) orderly and sequential, (2) continuous and complex, (3) specific for each person, (4) influenced by environmental factors, (5) directed by regular trends, and (6) quantitative and qualitative, and that they (7) become integrated, (8) have vulnerable periods, (9) have rates and patterns that can be modified, and (10) occur at different stages and at different rates.
- Freud's psychosexual theory explains ego development through predictable id–superego conflicts.
- Erikson identifies personality development in a series of stages from birth to later adult years, when critical tasks must be mastered.
- Havighurst focuses on the concept of learning in order to understand growth and development.
- Piaget's theory describes cognitive development from infancy through adolescence based on assimilation, accommodation, and formation of schemata.
- Kohlberg presents a theory of moral judgment of reasoning that begins in early childhood years. Gilligan developed a theory of moral development in females that is based on caring and responsibility.
- Fowler defines faith or spirituality as comprising meaning for life, which includes values, beliefs, and, possibly, religious affiliation.
- Each developmental theory explains a portion of the process of development and provides part of the nurse's understanding of the total being and coping abilities. Such theories are limited by their specific focus and the theorist's beliefs about growth and development.
- The family plays a vital role in promoting wellness and preventing illness. Both positive and negative health practices are shared in the family and learned by younger members. Health problems affect the family unit.

BIBLIOGRAPHY

Billingham, K. A. (1982). *Developmental psychology for the health care professions.* Boulder: Westview.

Coles, R. (1990). *The spiritual life of children.* Boston: Houghton & Mifflin.

DeMaio-Esteves, M. (1990). Mediators of daily stress and perceived health status in adolescent girls. *Nursing Research, 39*(6), 360–363.

Duska, R., & Whelan, M. (1975). *Moral development: A guide to Piaget and Kohlberg.* New York: Paulist.

Erikson, E. H. (1963). *Childhood and society* (2nd ed.). New York: Norton.

Flanagan, O., & Jackson, K. (1987). Justice, care, and gender: The Kohlberg–Gilligan debate revisited. *Ethics 97,* 622–637.

Fong, B. C., & Resnick, M. R. (1980). *The child: Development through adolescence.* Menlo Park, CA: Benjamin/Cummings.

Fowler, J. W. (1981). *Stages of faith: The psychology of human development and the quest for meaning.* New York: Harper & Row.

Fowler, J. W. (1991). *Weaving the new creation: Stages of faith and the public church.* San Francisco: HarperCollins.

Freud, S. (1923/1974). *The ego and the id.* London: Hogarth.

Friedman, M. M. (1992). *Family nursing: Theory and assessment* (3rd ed.). Norwalk, CT: Appleton & Lange.

Gilligan, C. (1977). In a different voice: Women's conceptions of the self and of morality. *Harvard Educational Review, 47,* 481–517.

Gilligan, C. (1982). *In a different voice.* Cambridge, MA: Harvard University Press.

Havighurst, R. J. (1972). *Developmental tasks and education.* New York: David McKay.

Janes, B., & Morse, J. (1990). Adolescent girls' perceptions of and preparation for menarche. *Canadian Journal of Nursing Research, 22*(2), 47–58.

Kempe, H., & Helfer, R. E. (1968). *The battered child.* Chicago: University of Chicago Press.

Klaus, M. H., & Kennell, J. H. (1982). *Parent–infant bonding.* St. Louis: Mosby.

Kohlberg, L. (1969). Stage and sequence: The cognitive–developmental approach to socialization. In D. Gaslin (Ed.). *Handbook of socialization: Theory and research* (pp. 347–380). Chicago: Rand McNally.

Mott, S. R., Fazekas, N. F., & James, S. R. (1990). *Nursing care of children and families: A holistic approach* (2nd ed.). Menlo Park, CA: Addison-Wesley.

Mussen, P. H., Conger, J. J., & Kagan, J. (1974). *Child development and personality* (4th ed.). New York: Harper & Row.

Newman, B. M., & Newman, P. R. (1975). *Development through life: A psychosocial approach.* Homewood, IL: Dorsey.

Parker, R. S. (1990). Measuring nurse's moral judgments. *Image: Journal of Nursing Scholarship. 22*(4), 213–218.

Piaget, J., & Inhelder, B. (1969). *The psychology of the child.* New York: Basic Books.

Sorenson, E. S. (1990). Children's coping responses. *Journal of Pediatric Nursing, 5*(4), 259–267.

White, M. A., Williams, P. D., Alexander, D. J., Powell-Cope, G. M., & Conlon, M. (1990). Sleep onset latency and distress in hospitalized children. *Nursing Research, 39*(3), 134–139.

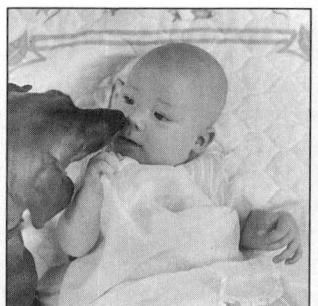
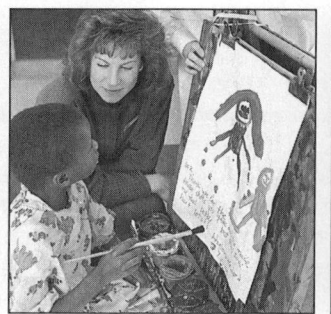
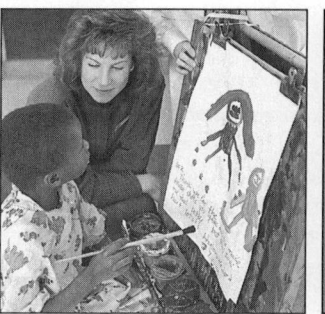

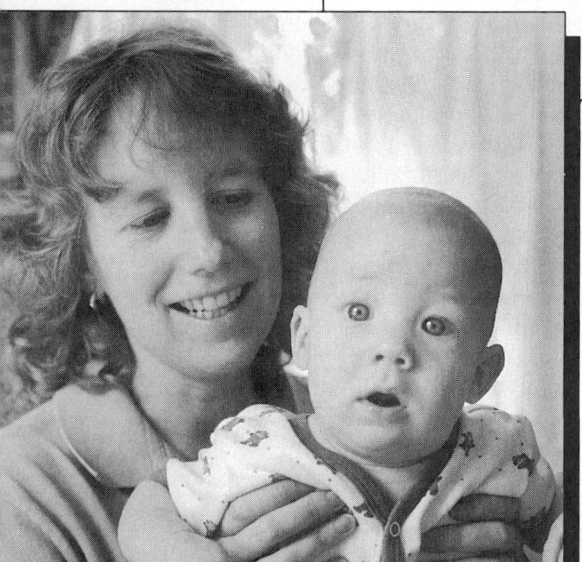

Conception Through Midlife

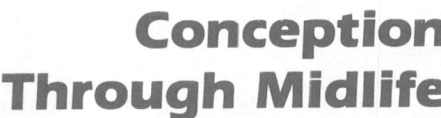

OBJECTIVES

After studying this chapter, the learner should be able to:

Define key terms used in the chapter.

Summarize major physiologic, cognitive, psychosocial, moral, and spiritual development for each age period conception through the middle adult years.

List common health problems of each age period from conception through middle adulthood.

Describe nursing actions to promote wellness at each developmental level.

Discuss the adult developmental theories of Gould, Levinson, and Erikson.

KEY TERMS

andropause
anorexia nervosa
attachment
bulimia
child abuse
Denver Developmental
   Screening Test
failure to thrive
infant
menopause
negativism
neonate
play
prelinguistic phase
preschooler
regression
school-age child
separation anxiety
sudden infant death syndrome
temperament
toddler
trimester
widowhood

11

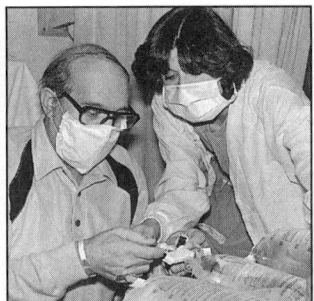

Growth and development occur throughout each person's life span. Knowledge of sequential growth and developmental milestones provides the base for planning and implementing holistic, individualized nursing care to maximize strengths and promote wellness for clients and their families.

This chapter continues the discussion of theories of development introduced in Chapter 10, with specific information relating to various stages of growth and development. Included are the sequential developmental stages that occur from conception to adolescence as well as the developmental stages of the young to middle adult years. (Development of the older adult is discussed in Chapter 12.) Although developmental milestones are briefly presented, the chapter focuses primarily on providing information that is necessary as the nurse promotes optimal functioning, growth, and wellness for clients of any age.

Environmental and Nutritional Influences

Environmental and nutritional factors influence all stages of development. The effect of each can occur independently, but they are more likely to be interrelated. The following examples illustrate the interrelations:

- Infants who are malnourished in utero develop fewer brain cells than do infants who have had adequate prenatal nutrition (May & Mahlmeister, 1990).
- Substance abuse by the mother during pregnancy increases the risk of congenital anomalies, low birth weight, and prematurity in neonates (Martin & Reeder, 1991).
- Federally sponsored school meal programs support the belief that learning is enhanced when nutrition is adequate.
- Failure to thrive, a condition of early infancy, has been linked to both nutritional and emotional deprivation.
- Child abuse is an extreme example of physical and emotional harm or deprivation, leading to deficits in physical or psychosocial development, or both.
- Substance abuse among adolescents is associated with an increased incidence of teenage pregnancy, violence, accidents, and suicide. Abuse of alcohol (as well as abuse of other drugs) is more prevalent in teens who have poor family relationships, low self-esteem, and poor social skills.
- The workplace can be an area of exposure to toxins, increasing the risk of illness in adults.

Childhood

The period from conception to adolescence is divided into different stages but can be considered childhood. Included within this time span are prenatal development, the neonate, the infant, the toddler, the preschooler, and the school-age child. Each of these stages is discussed in this section, including physiologic, psychosocial, and cognitive development; common health problems; and the nurse's role in meeting health care needs. Nursing's focus on wellness for the child is described in the display.

Conception and Prenatal Development

Human growth and development begin at the moment the ovum is fertilized by the sperm. The fertilized ovum, or *zygote,* contains the full complement of genetic information provided by each parent that determines gender and influences personality, intellect, and physical and psychological traits. The growth and development of the fetus are orderly and continuous, and proceed in three stages:

1. The *preembryonic stage* lasts for about 3 weeks. The zygote implants in the uterine wall, and has three distinct cell layers:

    The *ectoderm,* the outer cell layer, which becomes the brain, spinal cord, nervous system, and outer body parts (skin, hair, nails)

    The *endoderm,* the inner cell layer, which becomes the respiratory system, the digestive system, the liver, and the pancreas

    The *mesoderm,* which becomes the skeleton, connective tissue, cartilage, and muscles and the circulatory, lymphoid, reproductive, and urinary systems

2. The *embryonic stage* occurs from the 4th through the 8th week. Rapid growth and differentiation of the germ cell layers take place, and by the end of this period, all basic organs have been established, the bones have begun to ossify, and some human features are recognizable. Because this is a period of such rapid growth and change, the fetus is especially vulnerable to any factor that might cause congenital anomalies.

3. The *fetal stage* is from 9 weeks to birth. Continued growth and development of all body organs and systems take place. By the time birth occurs, the average neonate weighs 7½ lb (3.4 kg) and is 20 inches (50.8 cm) long.

Neonate (Birth to 28 Days)

At birth, the neonate must adapt to extrauterine life, and must make several significant physiologic adjustments to do so. Although these adjustments occur in all body systems, the most important occur in the respiratory and circulatory systems. Assessment of the neonate is done immediately after birth. There are several measurement scales, but the Apgar is the one most commonly used.

NURSING TODAY Challenges and Solutions

The Child

Challenges

- The United States has one of the highest infant mortality rates in the world, with 40,000 babies dying each year.
- One in four children are born into poverty.
- More than 2 million children are abused and neglected each year.
- More than 1 million children run away from home each year and are then exposed to malnutrition, crime, prostitution, drugs, and AIDS.
- The youth of the nation face problems of homelessness, pregnancy, drug abuse, illness, and violent death.

Nursing Solutions

- In Washington, DC, nurses in the pediatric unit of one hospital serve as surrogate parents for "boarder babies"—babies who have been abandoned by their parents. The nurses provide love and clothing and celebrate birthdays and holidays.
- A clinic in Topeka serves the health care needs of children of families who are uninsured.
- School nurses in Denver serve as primary health care providers for a population of children who face poverty, violence, gang activities, suicide, pregnancy, homelessness, and parenting issues. The nurses provide professional services, care, support, security, and resources.
- In Boston, nurses are dealing with the growing child abuse problem by serving as advocates for the children and their families and by conducting research into abuse at day-care centers and on maternal use of drugs and child abuse.

(Children's needs challenge RNs. [1991]. *American Nurse*, June, 1.)

The Apgar rating scale, developed in 1953, is applied to neonates at 1 minute and 5 minutes after birth. Each category (Table 11-1) is rated as 0, 1, or 2. The rating for each category is then totaled to a maximum score of 10. Normal neonates score between 7 and 10. Neonates who score between 4 and 6 require special assistance; those who score below 4 are in need of immediate life-saving support.

Physiologic Development The physical characteristics of the neonate include those shown in Figure 11-1 and the following:
- Has reflexes that allow sucking, swallowing, blinking, sneezing, and yawning
- Has labile temperature control that responds quickly to environmental temperatures
- Is alert to the environment, sees color and form, hears and turns toward sound, can smell and taste, and is sensitive to touch and pain

- Can eliminate both stool and urine
- Will drink breast milk, glucose water, and plain water

The neonate also inherits a transient immunity from infections as a result of immunoglobulins that cross the placenta. Breast-feeding provides further protection against bacterial and viral infections through immunoglobulins and leukocytes in breast milk. The high lactose content in breast milk, combined with limited protein, promotes an acid environment that is unsuitable for bacterial growth (Scipien et al., 1990). Antibodies secreted in breast milk help to control some viral infections.

Common Health Problems Particular difficulties related to the birth process, the transition to extrauterine life, or *congenital anomalies* may necessitate intervention by health care personnel. Breathing difficulties are common, especially if the neonate has been sedated by drugs given to the mother during labor and delivery. The premature neo-

TABLE 11-1

Apgar Scoring Chart			
Sign	**0**	**1**	**2**
Heart rate	Absent	Slow (less than 100 beats/min)	Over 100 beats/min
Respiratory effort	Absent	Slow, irregular	Good, crying
Muscle tone	Flaccid	Some flexion of extremities	Active motion
Reflex irritability	No response	Weak cry or grimace	Vigorous cry
Color	Blue, pale	Body pink, extremities blue	Completely pink

nate is vulnerable to *respiratory distress syndrome* because of the relative immaturity of lung function. The neonate delivered by cesarean birth is at risk for respiratory difficulties because of excess mucus in the lungs. Therefore, frequent suctioning is common in the cesarean-delivered neonate.

Incompatibility between the blood group of the mother and that of the infant requires prompt care at the time of birth. Congenital malformations, such as cleft palate and cleft lip, spina bifida, and Down syndrome, present profound and long-term health problems. Neonates who are born with *congenital syphilis* and drug addiction require special care. Birth traumas, which may result in temporary symptoms, are of concern because the parents need to be reassured that the symptoms will disappear. Examples include *caput succedaneum*, *molding*, bruises from the use of forceps during delivery, and *subconjunctival hemorrhage*.

Parents also need help to understand the nonthreatening nature of *physiologic jaundice*, which commonly is present during the neonate's first days.

The neonate born to a mother who smokes cigarettes, drinks alcohol, or uses drugs is of special concern. These substances may cause developmental deficits as well as complications during birth. Nicotine doubles the risk of low birth weight. Fetal alcohol syndrome in the infant of the mother who drinks is believed to be a leading cause of birth defects, including growth retardation, developmental delay, and impaired intellectual ability. The maternal use of cocaine, crack-cocaine, and heroin increases the probability of congenital anomalies, prematurity low birth weight, and withdrawal syndromes (Bennett & Woolf, 1991).

Cocaine or crack-cocaine use brings about abrupt changes in the mother's blood pressure, resulting in nu-

FIGURE 11-1

Reflexes and behaviors of the neonate. (Reeder, S. J., & Martin, L. L. [1991]. *Maternity nursing* [17th ed.]. Philadelphia: Lippincott.)

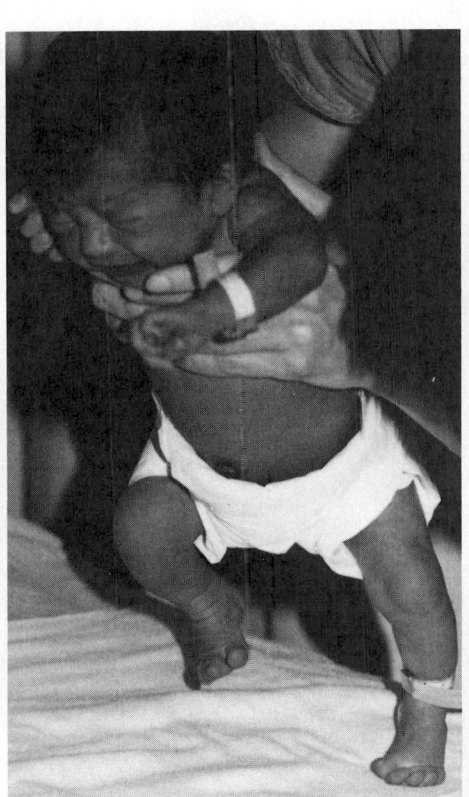

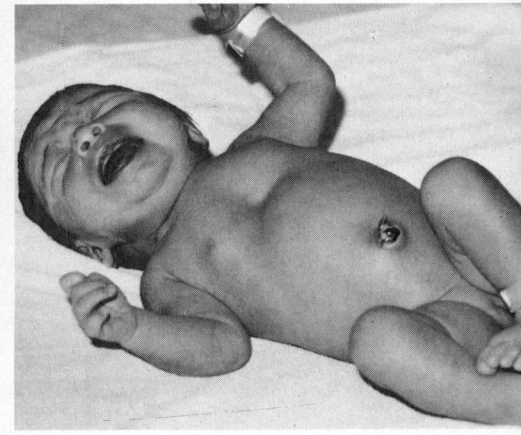

Stepping reflex

Active crying state

Moro reflex

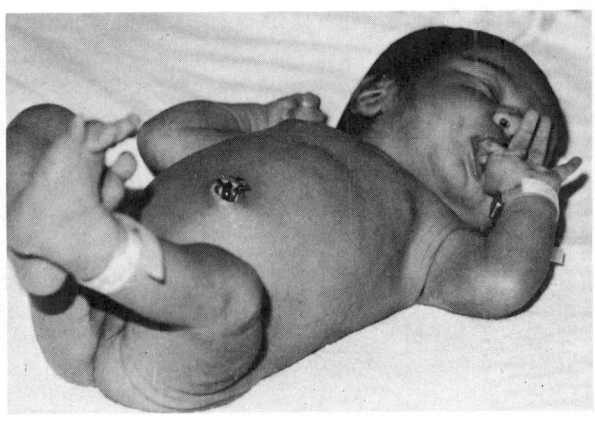

Quiet alert state

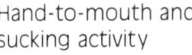

Hand-to-mouth and sucking activity

Initial play behavior by infants is centered on self: repetitive hand play, babbling, and cooing

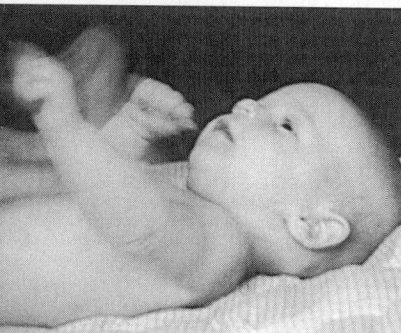

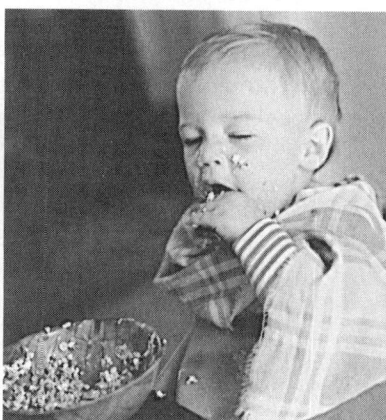

Developmental tasks of the first year include: taking solid food, learning to walk and talk

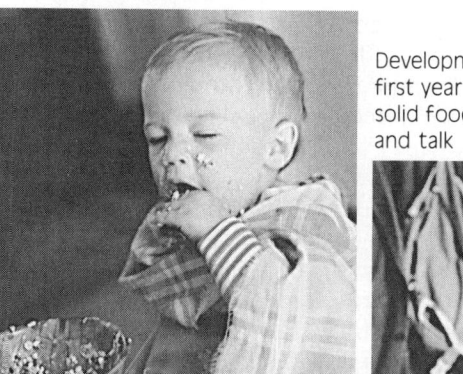

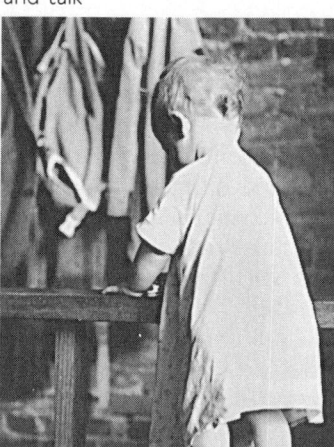

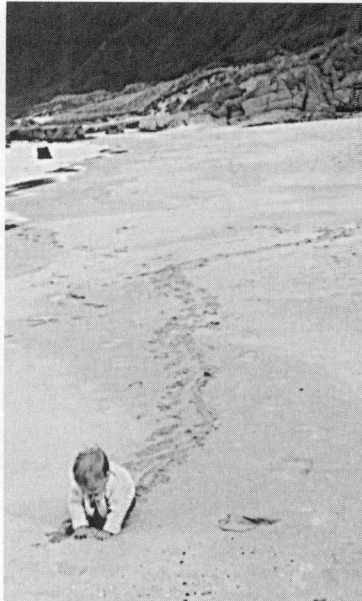

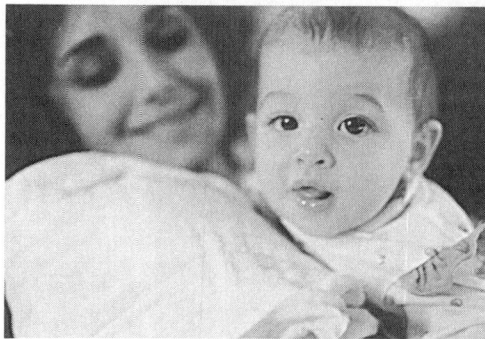

Erikson describes the psychosocial development prominent in infancy as "Trust vs Mistrust"

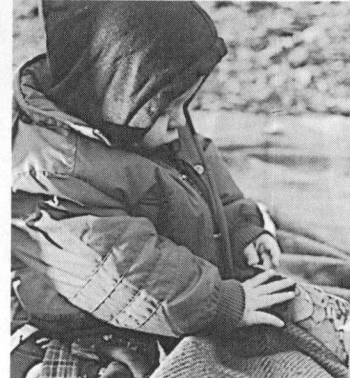

As the infant enters the second half of his first year, play will begin to involve manipulation of objects and the environment

F I G U R E   1 1 - 2

Development during the first year of life.

merous small strokes in the developing fetus. When they are born, "crack babies" are lethargic, hypersensitive to noise or stimuli, and unable to focus visually, and they have diarrhea. The number of neonates born with this syndrome, which may last for 2 to 3 weeks after birth, is increasing. The long-term effects are not fully known (Bobak, Jensen, & Zalar, 1989).

Infant: 1 Month to 1 Year

At the end of the first month, the neonate becomes an **infant** and is so until the first birthday (Fig. 11-2).

Physiologic Development   The physical characteristics of the infant include the following:
- Brain grows to about half the adult size.
- Body temperature stabilizes.
- Motor abilities develop to allow using building blocks, trying to feed self, crawling, and walking.
- Eyes begin to focus and fixate.

- Heart doubles in weight; the heart rate slows and blood pressure rises.
- Deciduous teeth begin to erupt at 4 to 6 months.
- Birth weight usually triples by 1 year; at 1 year, the average male baby weighs 22 lb (10 kg) and the average female baby weighs 21 lb (9.5 kg). Length increases by 50%.

Growth Patterns   The adequacy of rate and totality of growth in the infant and toddler is assessed by comparison with standardized growth charts. Several such charts are available; each is gender specific because the growth rates of boys and girls differ. Care should be taken in making comparisons for the following reasons:
- Each child has individual variations and short-term spurts and lags in growth.
- Atypical infants, such as those who are premature or have low birth weight, are not addressed.
- Growth charts may be ethically and socioeconomically weighted in favor of white, middle-class children.

The **Denver Developmental Screening Test** (DDST) is commonly used as a screening test for quickly and inexpensively determining atypical developmental patterns in infants and children. The following critical areas of development are assessed in the DDST:

- Gross motor behavior and skills
- Fine motor behavior and skills
- Language acquisition
- Personal and social interaction

The test isolates problem areas that require more precise assessments. The student is referred to pediatric textbooks for further information about this test.

Cognitive Development The infant from birth to 1 year is in the sensorimotor stage of development described by Piaget (see Chapter 10). Language development is in what is referred to as the **prelinguistic phase**. Babies begin to coo and make pleasurable sounds soon after birth, and by age 12 months, they can convey wishes through a few key words. Language development has several consistent characteristics, regardless of the specific language being learned. They are as follows:

- Use of syllable repetition (such as ma-ma, da-da, bye-bye)
- Identical early phonetic expressions (babbling sounds)
- Imitation of sounds and intonations spoken by caregivers

Psychosocial Development Based on the developmental theories discussed in Chapter 10, the infant has the following characteristics:

- Is in the oral stage (Freud), striving for immediate gratification of needs and having a strong sucking need
- Develops trust (Erikson, 1963) when the caregiver can be counted on to provide food when the infant is hungry. Trust also is facilitated by diaper-changing, warmth, and comforting.
- Meets developmental tasks (Havighurst) by learning to take solid food, walk, and talk

Other components of psychosocial development in the neonate and infant include attachment, play, and temperament.

Attachment is "an active, affectionate, reciprocal relationship between two people" (Papilia & Olds, 1986, p. 154). It can be differentiated from *bonding*. Bonding, described by Klaus and Kennell (1982), occurs during a sensitive period in the first few hours after birth (although bonding also may occur later in the first few months) and is necessary for later attachment. Bonding may be considered the initial fusing of two persons, and attachment, the long-term maintenance and strengthening of the fused state.

Play allows the infant and child to discover the environment and begin to learn how to control it. Beginning as soon as the baby is aware of sensations and the pleasure they produce, play progresses from self-pleasure to interaction with others. The two dimensions of play are social play and cognitive play. Social play is motivated by a desire for fun, pleasure, and relationships with others. Cognitive play is motivated by the desire to learn.

Temperament is primarily inborn, although it is influenced by environment. Characteristics of temperament allow description of a baby and child as "easy," "slow to warm," and "difficult" (Thomas, Chess, & Birch, 1968). The "easy" infant sleeps, eats, and eliminates easily; smiles spontaneously; and cries in response to significant needs. The "slow to warm" infant is more passive and distant. The "difficult" infant has volatile and labile responses, often is a restless sleeper, is highly sensitive to noises, and eats poorly. These traits remain fairly consistent throughout one's life. The behavior of caregivers as they care for the baby can influence both positively and negatively the degree to which temperament will dictate behavioral style.

Common Health Problems Various health problems in infancy may require the intervention of health care personnel. Gastroenteritis and food allergies are common. Skin disorders, such as diaper dermatitis (diaper rash), seborrheic dermatitis (infant dandruff), prickly heat rash, and thrush (infection of the oral mucous membrane by the fungus *Candida albicans*), also are common.

Safety concerns must be addressed during infancy. The relative immobility of the infant makes susceptibility to suffocation a possibility. The swallowing reflex matures progressively from birth, but until it is fully developed, aspiration is a risk. As the infant becomes more mobile, the risk of falls increases. Preventive measures against such safety hazards must be taught to new parents. In addition, the use of special car safety seats and restraints for infants is mandated by law in most states.

Several health problems in infancy are significant enough for further discussion. These are infant colic, failure to thrive, and sudden infant death syndrome.

Infant Colic *Colic* is "acute, paroxysmal abdominal pain caused by spasmodic contractions of the intestine during the first 3 months of life" (Miller & Keane, 1987, p. 275). The exact cause of colic is not known, but the following factors have been associated with this problem: swallowing excess air, feeding too rapidly, overfeeding, ingestion of excess carbohydrates, overexcitement, allergies, emotional distress in the infant, and anxiety in the primary caregiver.

Failure to Thrive **Failure to thrive** results in severely inadequate physiologic development (particularly height and weight) in an infant. This condition is thought to be related to disturbed infant–primary caregiver interaction. Although this relation appears to be present in most instances, underlying physical causes must first be ruled out. If the cause is deemed to be psychosocial, then the dynamics commonly involve inadequate nutritional intake related to caregiver ignorance and lack of concern for emotional nurturing. Specialized health intervention usually is warranted.

Child Abuse

Child abuse is the "intentional nonaccidental physical or sexual abuse of a child by a parent or other caregiver entrusted with his or her care" (Freiberg, 1987, p. 255). Most child abuse begins in infancy. More than 1 million cases of child neglect or abuse are reported each year. When serious physical abuse that results in permanent injury or death occurs, the term battered child syndrome is used; fatal battering most often occurs in children under age 5. Sexual abuse accounts for about 20% of all reported child abuse, with 25% of sexual abuse being done to preschoolers.

Although abuse occurs in all ethnic groups and in all levels of society, certain factors increase the potential for abusive behavior:

- Parents under stress from unemployment, depression, poor social and marital relationships, substance abuse, or health problems
- Parents who were themselves abused
- Children who cry frequently, have sleep difficulties, wet the bed, are hyperactive or aggressive, who have difficult temperaments, or who have physical, emotional, or cognitive disabilities

- Lack of knowledge about parenting and normal behaviors of children
- Lack of family and social support for the caregivers

Health care professionals must recognize and report abuse of children and provide interventions for high-risk families. In some states, education about child abuse is mandated for nurses and other health care providers. In Canada, there is mandatory reporting of child abuse and maltreatment. The long-term treatment of abused children and their families is complex and multidisciplinary. A team approach may be used, most often using community health nurses, social workers, early childhood educators, and mental health professionals. Specific resources by state may be found in the publication (for purchase) *The National Directory of Children and Youth Services* from:

American Association for Protecting Children of the American Humane Society
9725 East Hampden Avenue
Denver, CO 80231

TABLE 11-2

Promoting Wellness in Infancy

Areas of Concern	Preventive Teaching
Accident prevention	• Associate common accidents to developmental abilities of the infant. • Encourage relaxed, slow feeding and regular "bubbling" (burping) to prevent aspiration. • Emphasize that bottles should not be propped and left with an unattended infant. • Emphasize the use of bumper pads and keeping crib sides up at all times to prevent injury related to bumping or falling. • Teach the correct usage of infant car seats. • Emphasize never leaving an infant unattended on a table, chair, or regular bed. • Teach proper positioning of infant for sleeping, and discourage the use of pillows to prevent suffocation.
Nutrition and feeding methods	• Assist the mother with the initiation and maintenance of breastfeeding. • If bottle feeding, provide information on the preparation of formula at feeding, expulsion of air from the bottle, nipple type and hole size, and positioning for an effective feeding experience. • Emphasize the significance of emotional nurturing during feeding. • Discuss the age at which solid foods are needed (ie, 5 to 6 months). • Discuss the sequence of solid foods (ie, cereals, vegetables, fruits, meats, and protein products).
Infections	• Encourage prompt attention for infections. • Encourage completion of required immunizations of infancy.
Hygiene and skin care	• Teach proper infant bathing techniques (ie, washing eye from inner to outer canthus, washing genitals last, umbilical cord care). • Discuss the proper use of creams, oils, and powders. • Describe the nature of infant skin and its susceptibility to disturbance. • Teach diapering and hygienic practices related to the disposal of products of elimination. • Teach care related to hair, nails, and genitals (particularly circumcised males).
Developmental performance	• Provide accurate information about development norms. This can prevent unrealistic expectations in caregivers and assist in isolating and treating developmental delays earlier.
Emotional attachment	• Encourage intimate child–caregiver contact in the crucial period immediately after birth. • Provide information about the sequence of normal attachment behaviors in infants. • Reassure concerned caregivers that attachment feelings occur at different rates for different caregivers and infants.

Sudden Infant Death Syndrome **Sudden infant death syndrome** (SIDS) is the sudden death of an infant or a young child, unexpected by history, in which a post mortem examination fails to reveal a cause of death. The general risk is 2 out of every 1000 live births, with SIDS causing about one-third of all deaths between ages 1 week and 1 year. The highest incidence occurs in the 3rd and 4th months of life. Increased risk is found in families who are poor or live in crowded housing, during cold months of the year, and during infant sleep periods. Maternal health, smoking, and nutrition are all being investigated as contributing factors. Other research is examining infectious diseases, genetic factors, apnea (periods of no breathing), sleeping position, and types of bedding.

Child Abuse The incidence of reported cases of **child abuse** has increased dramatically and is a cause of national concern. Health care workers are in an excellent position to recognize families at risk and offer interventions (see accompanying display).

Role of the Nurse in Health Care The most essential role of the nurse in meeting health care needs of the infant is the prevention of illness and the promotion of wellness through teaching family members. Teaching may range from providing basic information about prevention of diaper rash to facilitating grieving in parents who have lost a baby to SIDS. Examples of specific areas of preventive teaching for parents of infants are given in Table 11-2.

Immunization against contagious diseases begins during the first year of life and should follow a regular schedule, as outlined in Table 11-3.

Toddler: 1 to 3 Years

Physiologic Development Physiologic development continues steadily during the **toddler** years, but the pace is considerably slower than that during infancy (Fig. 11-3). Growth and development include the following:

- Rapid brain growth; increase in length of long bones of the arms and legs; growth of muscles
- Can use fingers to pick up small objects
- Can walk forward and backward, run, kick, climb stairs, and ride a tricycle
- Drinks from a cup and uses a spoon
- At age 2, is typically four times the birth weight, averaging 30 to 35 lb (13.6 to 15.9 kg) and 23 to 37 inches (58.4 to 94 cm) in height
- Is able to have bladder control during the day and sometimes during the night (2½ to 3 years)
- Can turn pages in a book and, by age 3, can draw stick people

Cognitive Development As discussed in Chapter 10, the toddler is in Piaget's last two stages of sensorimotor development, thereby beginning to understand object permanence, following simple commands, and anticipating events. The toddler is able to understand self as separate

TABLE 11-3

Schedule of Immunizations	
Name	**Schedule**
Diphtheria, tetanus, pertussis (DPT)	Three doses 2 months apart the first year, followed by a booster 1 year later (15 to 18 months) and another booster (of DT only) when entering school
Polio (OPV, IPV)	Doses at 2, 4, and 6 months with another booster when beginning school (oral polio vaccine [OPV] used in the United States; inactivated polio vaccine [IPV] used in Canada)
Measles, mumps, rubella	One dose at 15 months in the United States and at 12 to 15 months in Canada

(Data from Foster, R., Hunsberger, M., & Anderson, J. [1989]. *Family-centered nursing care of children.* Philadelphia: Saunders.)

from others, and the perception of body image begins. As part of body image development, several body parts can be identified and named, and gender identity is present.

Language begins at about age 1, with the use of single or bisyllable sounds. Around age 2, children begin to use short sentences.

Psychosocial Development Based on psychosocial theories, the toddler has the following characteristics:

- Is in Freud's anal stage, as increased muscle development and sphincter control encourage the child to focus on the pleasure of sphincter contraction and relaxation. Freud believed that caregiver fixation on toilet training could result in adults who were either excessively messy or excessively clean.
- Enters Erikson's stage of autonomy versus shame and doubt. Independence in feeding, walking, dressing, and toileting as well as the ability to verbally express wishes facilitate autonomy. Children who do not feel autonomous may be reluctant to explore and fearful of activities and people.
- Has the developmental task (Havighurst) of learning to control the elimination of urine and feces; begins to learn sex differences, form concepts, and learn language, and learns to distinguish right from wrong

Toddlers may exhibit **separation anxiety**, **negativism**, and **regression**. Separation anxiety occurs when a child is afraid of being sent away from those people who are loved and serve as security. Negativism (characteristically expressed by saying no) is the result of the toddler's effort to have some measure of control over the environment. Regression, or behavior that is more characteristic of a younger age, can occur at any time in response to stressful circumstances. The most common regressive behaviors are excessive clinging to caregivers, loss of control over elimination, and the use of more infantile speech patterns.

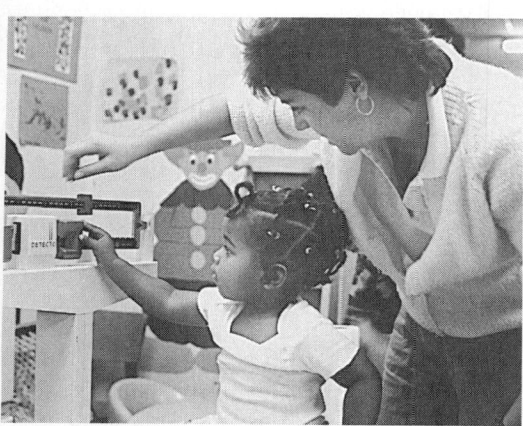

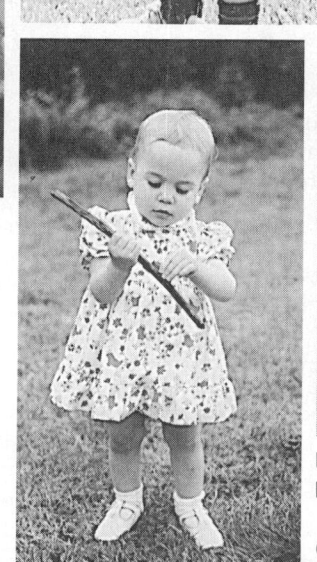

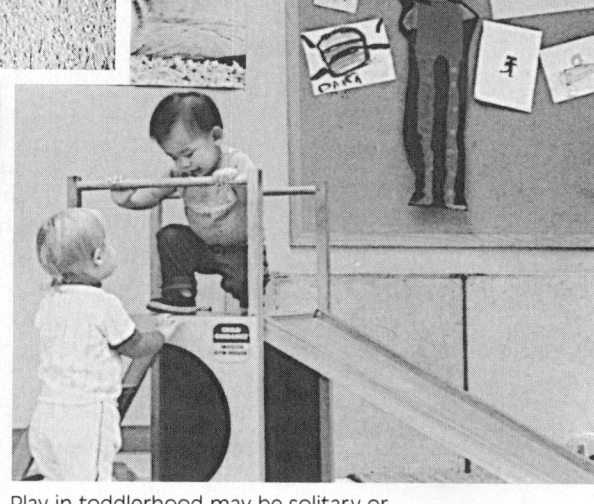

A broad stance and protruding abdomen are characteristic of the physical development of the toddler

Cognitive abilities in toddlerhood include mastery of seeing oneself as separate from others and perception of body image

Play in toddlerhood may be solitary or parallel

Gross motor skills are prominent in toddlerhood

F I G U R E   1 1 - 3

Characteristics of development in the toddler.

Common Health Problems   Accidents, such as motor vehicle accidents, poisonings, burns, drownings, aspiration, and falls, remain the major cause of death in toddlerhood. Dental problems can occur, especially if the toddler is allowed to go to sleep with a bottle of milk or sweetened liquid in his mouth (Foster, Hunsberger, & Anderson, 1989). Respiratory tract and middle ear infections are common. Some surgeries, such as repair of a cleft lip and palate, may be done in the toddler years. Surgery to repair most congenital anomalies is not done until later childhood.

Role of the Nurse in Health Care   The role of the nurse in wellness promotion continues, as shown by the examples in Table 11-4. A significant part of teaching is in helping caregivers find the means of helping their toddler through encouraging health independence while setting firm limits.

Preschooler: 3 to 6 years

At around age 3, the chubby toddler begins to give way to the leaner and better coordinated **preschooler**. Although growth and development are slower than in infancy and toddlerhood, they are still steady (Fig. 11-4).

Physiologic Development   The physical characteristics of the preschooler include the following:
- Head is close to adult size by age 6.
- Motor abilities include skipping, throwing and catching a ball, copying figures, and printing letters and numbers.
- Full set of 20 deciduous teeth is present, but baby teeth begin to fall out and are replaced by permanent teeth.

- Average weight at ages 5 to 6 is 45 lb (20.4 kg), with boys being slightly heavier than girls.

Cognitive Development   The preschooler is in Piaget's preoperational stage of development (see Chapter 10). Passing through the preconceptual and the intuitive phases, the child demonstrates the following transitional changes:

- Egocentrism decreases as socialization with other children increases and ability to express self verbally improves.
- Play is more related to real-life events (rather than fantasy).
- Basic curiosity results in constant questions and improved reasoning ability.

Language development is seen in more elaborate and grammatically correct sentences, with 6- to 18-word sentences becoming common by age 6 (Papilia & Olds, 1986). The incessant use of "why?" increases the child's knowledge, encourages further conversations, and develops language abilities.

Preschoolers clearly identify themselves as male or female, can understand basic body functions, and have a curiosity about sex differences. This curiosity often leads to "playing doctor," which is normal behavior for the age. Many children in this age-group want to look special or dressed up, and gain increased self-esteem through compliments about appearance.

Psychosocial Development   Based on psychosocial theories of growth and development (see Chapter 10), the preschooler has the following characteristics:

- Is in Freud's phallic stage, with the biologic focus being primarily genital. The child has a sexual desire for the opposite-sex parent but, as a means of defense, strongly identifies with the same-sex parent; as a result of this conflict resolution, the superego and conscience begin to develop.
- Is in Erikson's stage of initiative versus guilt. Inner turmoil is created when natural curiosity is pitted against a constant examination of the propriety of one's actions by a rigid conscience. Realistic self-limits are learned through social interactions.

TABLE 11-4

Promoting Wellness in Toddlerhood	
Areas of Concern	**Preventive Teaching**
Accident prevention	• Explain how the autonomy needs of the toddler need to be met with an eye to safety. • Suggest locking poisons out of child's reach. • Suggest safety plugs for electric outlets. • Advise to block stairs with a gate and then help the child learn how to maneuver stairs. • Advise not allowing toddler to have small, hard food items like popcorn, peanuts, raw carrots, hard candy, or balloons, which may cause aspiration. • Discourage the toddler from running with food in his mouth. • Encourage the proper use of car seats. • Advise never to leave the child unattended near water. • Suggest teaching toddler of dangers in clear, simple terms (eg, stove hot). • Advise against tossing child into the air or swinging child by the arms.
Toilet training	• Explain developmental tasks necessary for toilet training. • Correct misconceptions about mastery of this task. • Suggest some helpful literature for caregivers.
Negativism	• Help caregivers understand the normality of negativism in toddlerhood and its meaning from the child's point of view
Feeding and nutrition	• Suggest that food be provided in forms the toddler can manipulate independently. • Advise caregivers to not be concerned abut the messiness of toddler eating habits because the independence gained by the child is more important. • Provide soft finger foods that the child can eat while playing. • Reassure caregivers that short anorexic periods are common in toddlerhood.
Hygiene and dental care	• Emphasize the teaching of good hygiene habits (eg, handwashing after toileting or before eating). • Suggest teaching the toddler how to brush his teeth (with assistance). • Encourage caregivers to take the toddler with them for dental appointments as an observer. Many dentists encourage this.
Infections	• Encourage caregivers to attend to respiratory tract infections promptly because of the high correlation between such infections and otitis media. • Encourage the completion of initial immunization schedule and any necessary boosters.
Play habits	• Encourage the selection of toys that emphasize gross motor skill and creativity. • Advise parents that sharing is not likely to occur and that parallel play is an important precursor to interactive play.

Basic curiosity results in questioning and an
improved reasoning ability in the preschooler

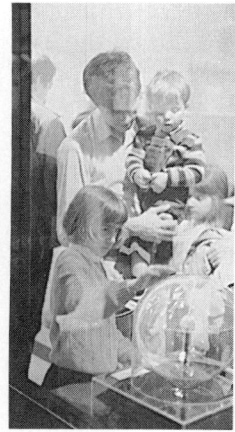 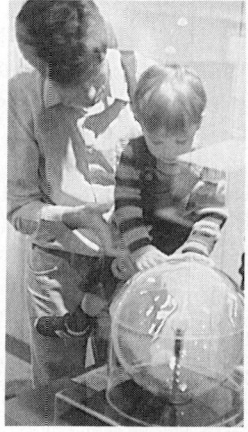 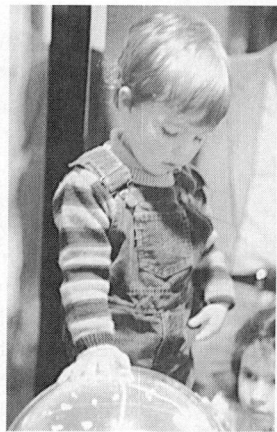 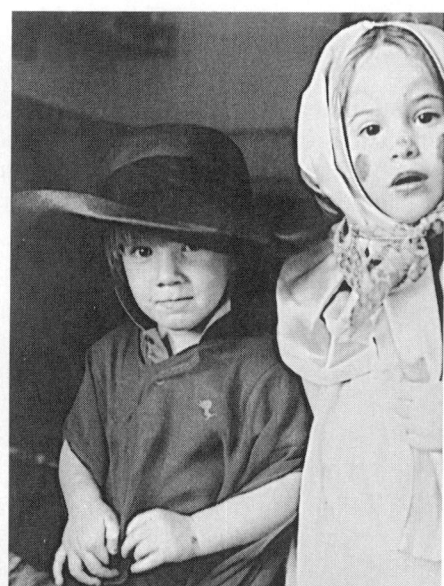

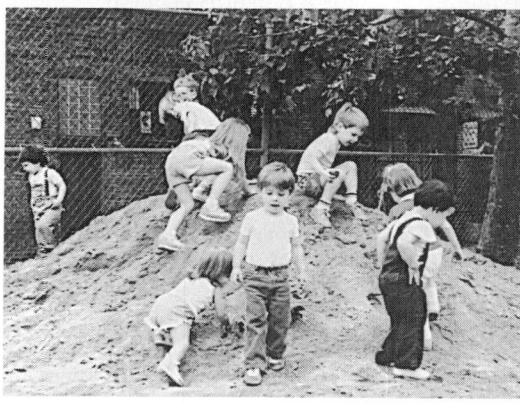

Preschooler play is associative and cooperative
in its social dimension and cognitive development is demonstrated in constructive and
pretend play

Symbolic play gradually becomes more related
to real life events

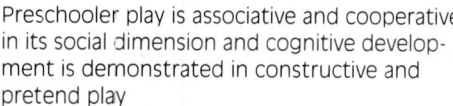

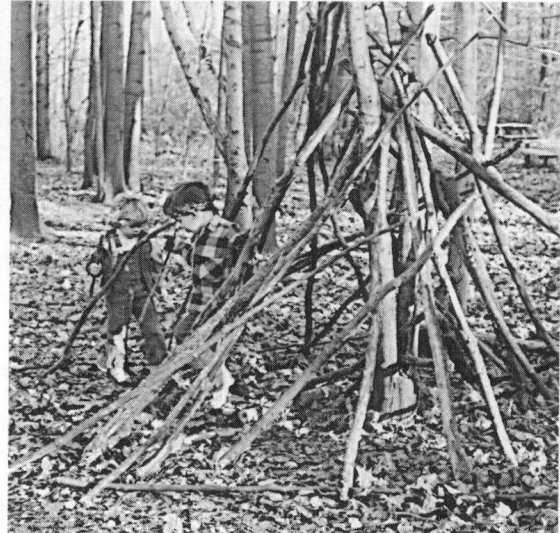

F I G U R E   1 1 - 4

Characteristics of development in the preschooler.

- Has four developmental tasks (Havighurst): to learn sex differences and modesty, to describe social and physical reality through concept formation and language development, to get ready to read, and to learn to distinguish right from wrong.

The preschooler often has fears. The primary task of becoming more socially oriented can cause many fears, with shyness and fear of new places common. Two other common fears during the preschool years are fear of the dark and fear of having nightmares, which often are made worse by the child's own fertile imagination and ability to fantasize. Support and validation of feelings by caregivers are essential.

Moral and Spiritual Development Kohlberg's preconventional phase of moral reasoning dominates this age. The focuses of this stage for the preschooler are as follows:
- Obeying rules to avoid punishment

- Obeying rules because it is in one's self-interest to do so; for example, a reward will be forthcoming.

The cognitive, psychosocial, and moral development of the preschooler provide the base for spiritual development, as described by Fowler. The preschooler attends activities at church or synagogue with the family but does not understand the religious concepts. The concept of a deity is literal, with God being viewed as a human male. Imagination of concepts such as heaven, hell, and holy spirits is incomprehensible but often frightening.

Common Health Problems Preschoolers continue to have some of the health problems that are common in toddlerhood. Communicable diseases and respiratory tract infections are frequent, especially with increased socialization at nursery schools and day care. Preschoolers are prone to accidents because of their increased curiosity about the world.

TABLE 11-5

Promoting Wellness in Preschoolers

Area of Concern	Preventive Teaching
Accident prevention and safety	• Advise that preschoolers, now out of car seats, need to learn how to use seat belts. • Advise that clear boundaries regarding where tricycles or bicycles can be ridden need to be given. • Teach simple road safety (eg, looking both ways before crossing the street). • Encourage education of children regarding strangers and block parent programs. • Encourage education about sexual abuse (ie, explaining to child what is and is not appropriate touching by an adult). • Swimming lessons can begin and basic water safety taught. • Teach the dangers of matches, and practice home fire safety drills.
Infections	• Advise that these are an inevitable result of increased socialization. • Advise teaching children sound hygiene practices such as hand washing after toileting, correct disposal of tissues after use, nonsharing of items like eating utensils. • Keep immunizations current.
Sleep disorders	• Explain to caregivers the commonality of this problem among preschoolers. • Suggest that relaxed bedtime rituals and a night light can help. • Advise that comforting and warm reassurance are needed when a child is awakened by nightmares.
Dental hygiene	• Teach that preschoolers should be brushing their teeth and flossing with caregiver assistance. • Advise that a dental visit at this time is useful for teaching dental hygiene and overcoming fear of the unknown.
Play habits	• Advise caregivers that make-believe play and imaginary friends are common and normal in the preschool years. • Encourage caregivers to promote socialization through neighborhood play groups and nursery school.
Self-esteem	• Encourage caregivers to provide opportunities to make new discoveries and gain a sense of autonomy by experiencing neighborhood and preschool activities. • Advise to avoid frequent criticism and overprotectiveness. • Teach caregivers the importance of providing opportunities for the child to plan and carry out activities, and giving appropriate praise for accomplishments.

Some congenital disorders, such as *hypospadias, inguinal hernias*, and cardiac anomalies, will require surgery at this time. Dental caries become common if teeth are neglected. As language becomes more sophisticated, speech disorders may become apparent.

Role of the Nurse in Health Care Table 11-5 provides examples of areas of concern and preventive teaching in promoting wellness in preschoolers. When caring for the preschool child who is scheduled for surgery or requires hospitalization, the nurse must recognize that fear of pain and body mutilation as well as separation anxiety are important considerations.

The nurse can allay some fears by explaining procedures in language the child can understand and by being honest about how much pain a procedure will cause. Many health care institutions have preprocedure visits for the child having surgery so that he or she can become familiar with the setting and with the activities that will be done. Allowing the child to practice procedures on a doll and encouraging the child to openly express feelings also are beneficial. Encouraging caregivers to take an active role in the child's care helps to reduce fear and separation anxiety.

School-Age Child: 6 to 12 Years

The **school-age child** is sturdy, strong, and usually lean. Physical growth during this time is relatively slow but continues steadily, with both refinement and subtle changes taking place (Fig. 11-5).

Physiologic Development Physiologic development of the school-age child includes the following:
• Brain reaches 90% to 95% of adult size; by age 12, the nervous system is almost completely matured, resulting in coordinated body movements.
• Motor abilities progress from the ability to hold a pencil and print words at age 6 to the ability to write in script and in sentences at age 12.
• Sexual organs grow but are dormant until late in this period, when hormonal changes begin.
• All permanent teeth are present, except for the second and third molars by age 12.
• Height increases 2 to 3 inches (5.1 to 7.6 cm) and weight increases 3 to 6 lb (1.4 to 2.7 kg) a year.

Cognitive Development The school-age child is at Piaget's concrete operational stage of development, organizing

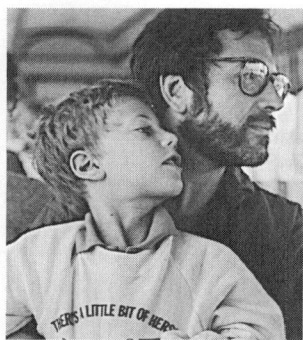

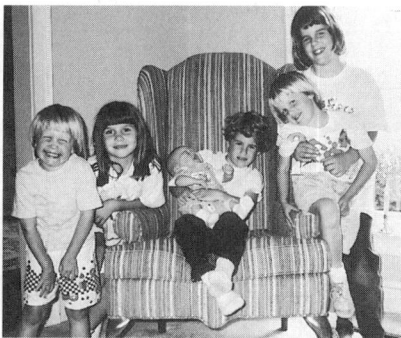

The school-age child has limited interest in members of the opposite sex and strong identification with one's own sex is dominant

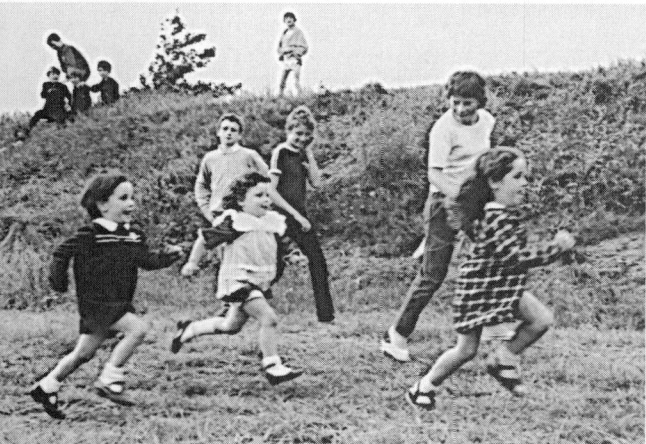

Play involves development of skills, games with rules, and competitive activities

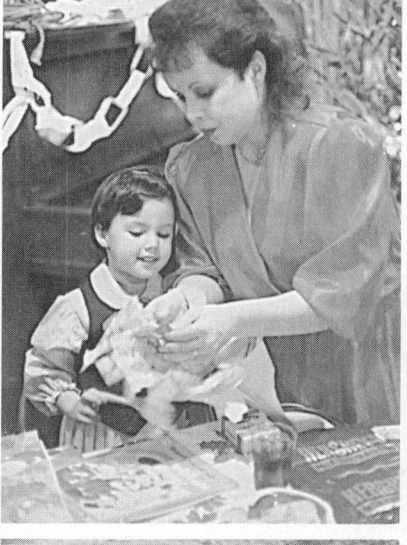

Total play gives way to productivity in the school-age child

Fine motor coordination develops

FIGURE
11 - 5

Characteristics of development in the school-age child.

facts about the environment to use for problem solving. During this period, the child has the following characteristics:

- Thinks logically and develops concepts of mass, volume, weight, and measurement
- Deals best with actual objects and people, but relates concepts and compares events
- Uses inductive reasoning to solve new problems
- Generalizes about people, places, and things
- Develops classification systems
- Develops an awareness and understanding of other people's feelings and points of view
- Understands reversal of events

The school-age child has well-developed language skills, using language in a more sophisticated manner. The ability to store information in long-term memory and retrieve it in the remembering (recall) process is more efficient.

Body image, self-concept, and sexuality are interrelated. Sexual development results in a strong need to clearly understand body function and to have accurate information about sexuality.

Psychosocial Development The psychosocial development of the school-age child, based on the theories discussed in Chapter 10, are as follows:

- In the latency stage of Freud's theory, with psychosocial energies being channeled toward strong identification with own sex
- In the industry versus inferiority stage of Erikson's theory, illustrated by the focus of the child on learn-

ing useful skills and thereby developing positive self-esteem. A sense of identity begins to emerge and values are integrated. The emphasis is doing, succeeding, and accomplishing.

- Has the following developmental tasks (Havighurst):
  - Learning physical game skills
  - Learning appropriate masculine or feminine social role
  - Developing fundamental skills in reading, writing, and calculating
  - Developing concepts necessary for everyday living
  - Achieving personal independence
  - Developing conscience, morality, and a scale of values

Peer relationships become the major gauge for determining status, skill, and personableness. Peer groups in middle childhood help prepare the child for getting along in the larger world and teach appropriate sex role behavior. They also act as transition modes for the child as he or she leaves the total caregiver influence and heads toward adult independence.

Moral and Spiritual Development Most of the middle childhood years are spent in the conventional phase of moral development. Behavior is based on familial and peer group beliefs, and conformity to the norm is common. Following school regulations, respecting teachers, and viewing justice as a means of fair play are all important.

In Fowler's theory, school-age children view religious faith as a relationship that involves reciprocal fairness. They take part in rituals of their faith with a basic understanding of the rituals' significance. The importance of spiritual beliefs and the possibility of life after death are believed, even if not totally understood.

Common Health Problems Accidents continue to be common in the school-age child. With increased interactions through school, communicable conditions such as scabies, impetigo, and head lice are more prevalent. Drug and alcohol abuse, although not as common as in adolescence, has been documented in children as young as age 8 (Salkind & Ambron, 1987).

Role of the Nurse in Health Care The nurse's role in promoting wellness for the school-age child involves individual and family teaching, which may be conducted by the school nurse. Table 11-6 provides examples of nursing activities specific to this age-group.

T A B L E   1 1 - 6

Promoting Wellness in School-Age Children	
Area of Concern	**Preventive Teaching**
Accident prevention	• Emphasize traffic safety. • Encourage the use of seat belts. • Emphasize bicycle, skateboard, and scooter safety. • Teach children to take water safety programs.
Communicable conditions	• Encourage proper hygiene habits, including not sharing personal items like combs. • Home visit may be required to discuss home health practices if a child has a communicable condition like pediculosis. • Advise of common treatment methods for conditions like scabies, impetigo, and pediculosis. • Teach about STDs, including AIDS.
Substance abuse	• Early preventive teaching about alcohol, nicotine, and street drugs that includes guidance for families is essential.
Sexuality	• Sex education needs to begin as early as age 7 or 8. • Families need encouragement to talk about sex at home. • Caregivers need encouragement to answer questions honestly and correctly. • Menstruation needs to be discussed by at least age 8 because some girls menstruate as young as age 9.
Mental health concerns: School phobia Depression and suicide	• Nurse needs to work with teachers and families so that they learn to recognize behavior that indicates mental health difficulties. • Nurse can provide referral for specialized assistance.
Physical fitness	• Teach good food choices that are lower in fat, salt, and sugar, but avoid strenuous dieting if child is overweight. An estimated 25% of all children are obese. • Emphasize the importance of physical activity: Children should exercise nonstop for at least 20 to 25 minutes three times a week.
Self-esteem	• Teach caregivers to encourage independent activities and social interactions, and to be sure that successes are greater in number than failures. • Provide the child with positive statements that demonstrate being valued, important, and loved.

E X A M P L E S   O F   N U R S I N G   D I A G N O S E S

Childhood

The following nursing diagnoses are examples of those that might be appropriate for the child from infancy through school age.

- Diarrhea related to incompatibility with formula used for bottle-feeding
- Altered Growth and Development related to lack of stimulation and fear of pain secondary to abusive episodes by caretakers
- High Risk for Injury related to maturational age of hospitalized child

- Health-Seeking Behaviors related to verbalized desire by parents to seek information about community resources for a family fitness program
- High Risk for Infection related to frequent exposure at school
- High Risk for Injury related to lack of knowledge about proper use of bicycles, skateboards, and roller blades.

F I G U R E   1 1 - 6

Characteristics of adolescent development.

Athletic activities and skills are important to both sexes in adolescence

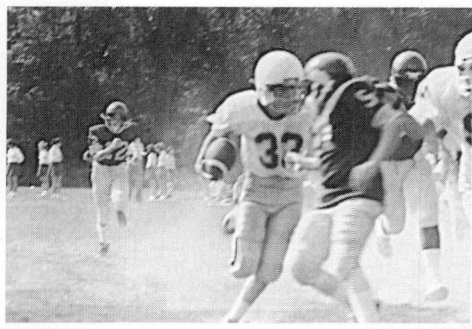

A primary developmental task of adolescence is to achieve new and more mature relationships with peers of both sexes

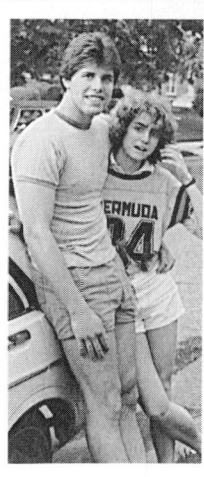

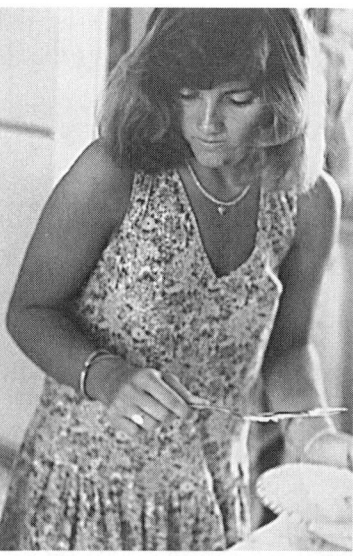

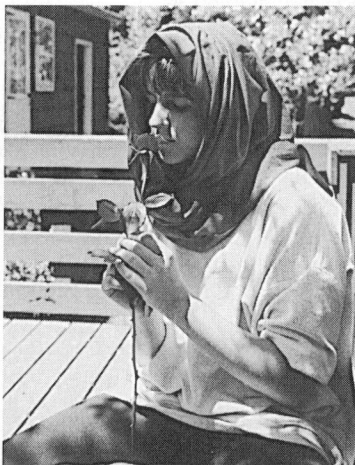

Physical appearance is extremely important to the adolescent

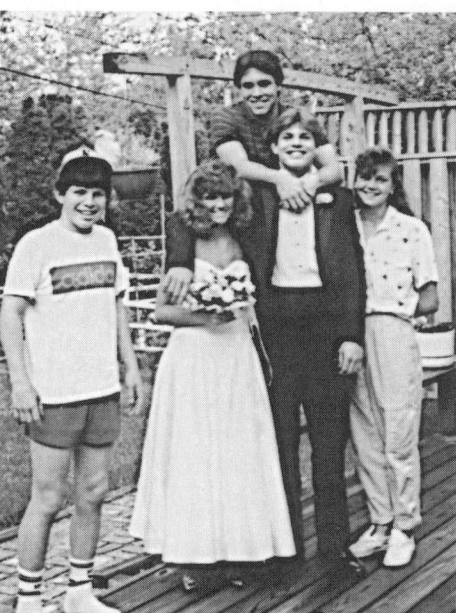

The prom is an opportunity to practice formal adult social skills among one's peers

The development of self-identity in adolescence involves "trying out" different roles and self-images, even if only in play

Adolescence: 12 to 18 Years

The **adolescent** years are, among other things, a time of rapid physical growth, reproductive maturity, and emotional development (Fig. 11-6). This is a time of change as the child becomes an adult. Although a time span is defined, each person is different. Some people enter adolescence at age 11 or 12 and go on into the middle or late 20s; others enter at age 14 and end within a year (Freiberg, 1987). Physical, cognitive, and social factors are critical in determining the length of the adolescent period.

Physiologic Development The changes that take place in the adolescent's body transform him or her from a child to an adult in appearance. The physiologic development includes the following:

- The feet, hands, and long bones grow rapidly, accompanied by an increase in muscle mass (especially in males).
- Primary and secondary development occurs, with maturation of the genitalia (Fig. 11-7); presence of body hair (Fig. 11-8); breast development (Fig. 11-9) and menstruation in females; facial hair growth, voice changes, and spermatogenesis in males.
- **Puberty** begins at age 10 or 11 for girls (with menstruation usually beginning between ages 11 and 14) and at age 12 or 13 for boys.
- Sebaceous and axillary sweat glands become active.
- Full adult size is reached, although some males may continue to grow into the 20s.

A true assessment of adolescent development would be incomplete without an expansion of the profound changes in reproductive functioning. **Puberty** can be divided into the following three stages:

Prepubescence: Secondary sex characteristics begin to develop but the reproductive organs do not yet function.

Pubescence: Secondary sex characteristics continue to develop and ova and sperm begin to be produced by the reproductive organs.

Postpubescence: Reproductive functioning and the development of secondary sex characteristics reach adult maturity.

The developmental occurrences at each stage are described in Table 11-7.

Cognitive Development According to Piaget, adolescence is the stage when the cognitive development of formal operations is developed. Deductive, reflective, and hypothetical reasoning are possible, and abstract concepts can be handled. Long-term goals can be set as the concept of time, its passage, and the future become real.

These abilities can make problem solving difficult for the adolescent, and challenging the decision making of adults is common. Egocentrism returns, and imaginary audiences and daydreaming are used.

Psychosocial Development Based on developmental theories (see Chapter 10), the adolescent has the following characteristics:

- Is in Freud's genital stage. The libido reemerges in a mature, adult form. Freud believed that this new state upsets the delicate balance of the id, ego, and superego, so that intellectualization becomes the common mechanism used to justify behavior.

FIGURE 11-7

Maturational stages of male genital development.

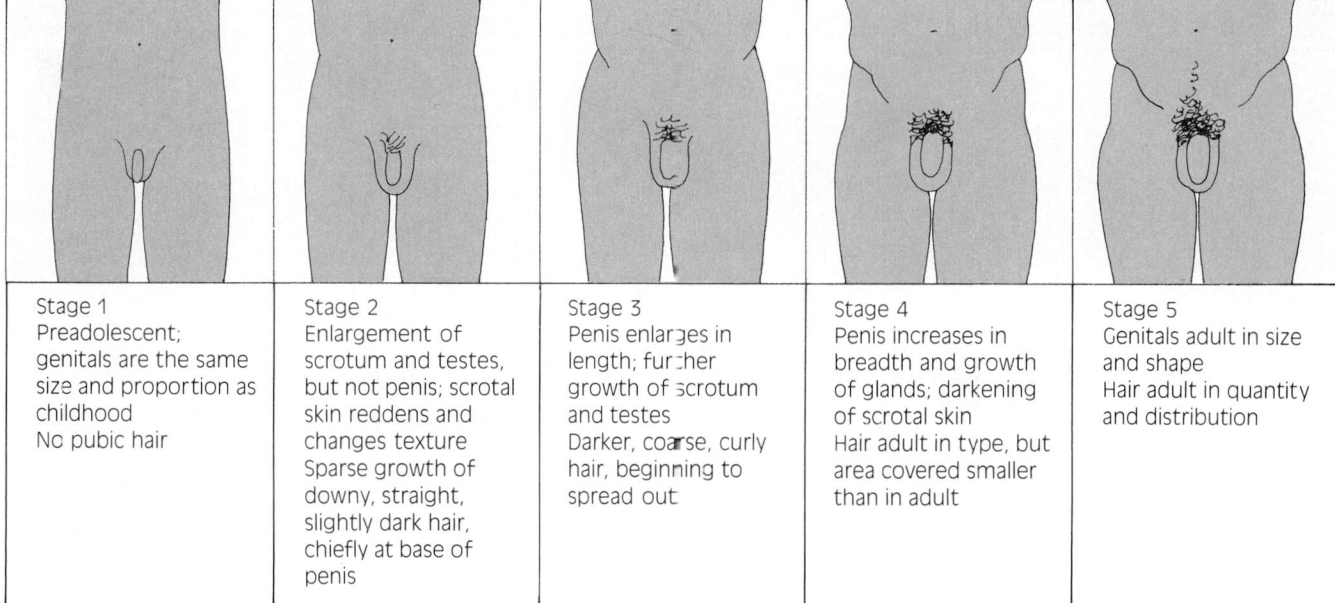

Stage 1	Stage 2	Stage 3	Stage 4	Stage 5
Preadolescent; genitals are the same size and proportion as childhood No pubic hair	Enlargement of scrotum and testes, but not penis; scrotal skin reddens and changes texture Sparse growth of downy, straight, slightly dark hair, chiefly at base of penis	Penis enlarges in length; further growth of scrotum and testes Darker, coarse, curly hair, beginning to spread out	Penis increases in breadth and growth of glands; darkening of scrotal skin Hair adult in type, but area covered smaller than in adult	Genitals adult in size and shape Hair adult in quantity and distribution

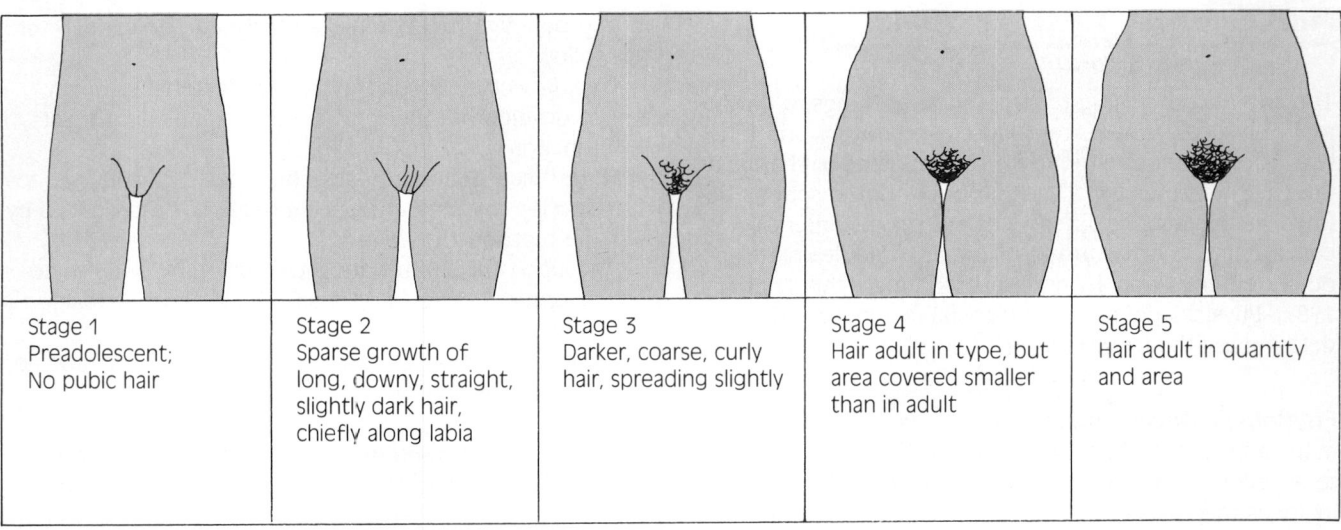

| Stage 1
Preadolescent;
No pubic hair | Stage 2
Sparse growth of
long, downy, straight,
slightly dark hair,
chiefly along labia | Stage 3
Darker, coarse, curly
hair, spreading slightly | Stage 4
Hair adult in type, but
area covered smaller
than in adult | Stage 5
Hair adult in quantity
and area |

F I G U R E   1 1 - 8

Maturational stages of female pubic hair development.

F I G U R E   1 1 - 9

Maturational stages of female breast development.

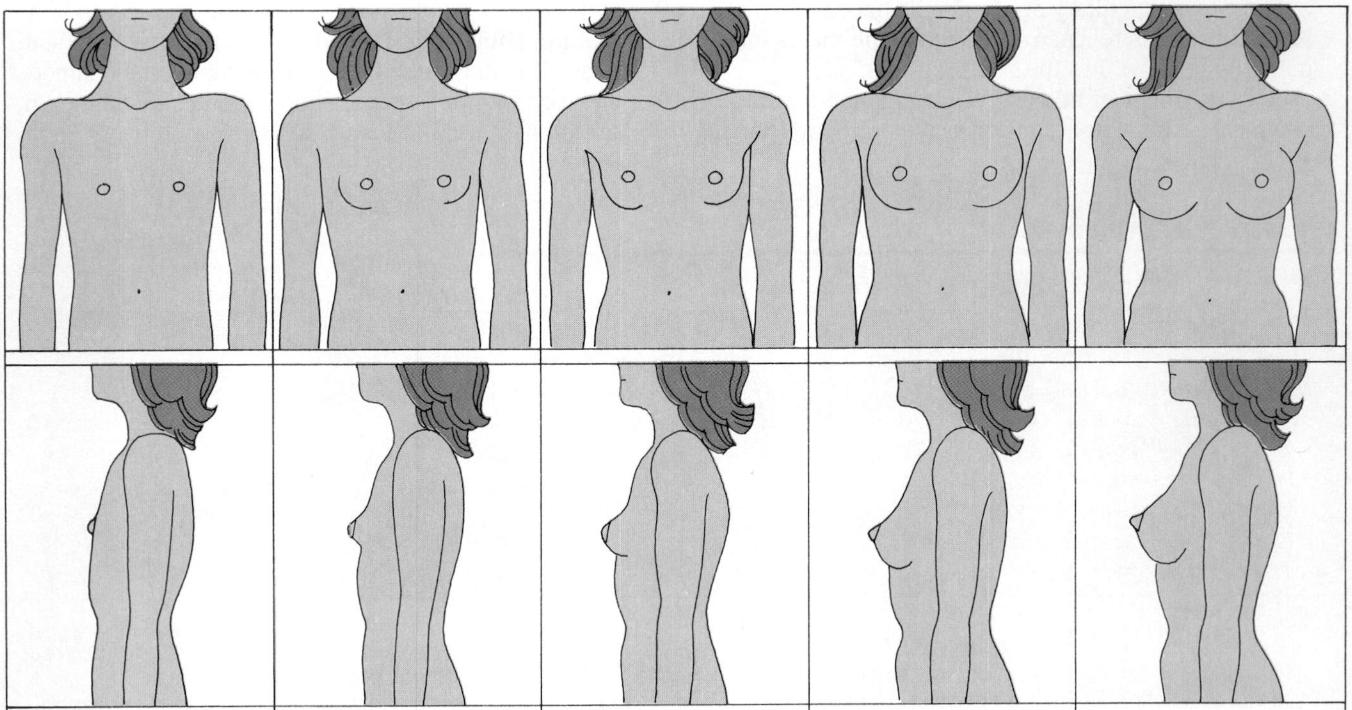

| Stage 1
Preadolescent;
elevation of papilla
only | Stage 2
Breast bud stage;
elevation of breast
and papilla as small
mound; enlargement
of areolar diameter | Stage 3
Further enlargement
of breast and areola
with no separation of
their contours | Stage 4
Projection of areola
and papilla to form
secondary mound
above level of breast | Stage 5
Mature; projection of
papillae only;
recession of areola
into contour of breast |

TABLE 11-7

Adolescent Sexual Development		
Stage	**Males**	**Females**
Prepubescence	• Progressive enlargement of testicles, seminal ducts, prostate gland • Enlargement and reddening of the scrotal sac • Increase in length and circumference of penis • Appearance of downy pubic hair	• Progressive enlargement of the ovaries • Ripening of graafian follicles • Rounding of the hips • Appearance of breast buds • Enlargement of the fallopian tubes, vagina, and uterus • Appearance of downy pubic hair
Pubescence	• Increase in amount, pigmentation, and curling of pubic hair • Growth spurt involving peak pace of height and weight increase • Deepening of the voice due to growth of larynx • Testicles enlarge • Scrotum grows and its pigmentation increases • Penis grows in length and circumference • Spermatogenesis begins	• Increase in amount, pigmentation, and curling of pubic hair • Growth spurt involving peak pace of height and weight increase • Menarche • Axillary hair appears • Vulva and clitoris enlarge • Breast tissue develops • Ovulation begins
Postpubescence	• Completion of sexual growth and development • Fertility	• Completion of sexual growth and development • Fertility

• Tries out different roles, personal choices, and beliefs, according to Erikson, in the stage called identity versus role confusion. Self-concept is being stabilized, with the peer group acting as the influential body.
• Has the following developmental tasks, defined by Havighurst:
  • Achieving new and maturer relationships with both males and females of the same age
  • Achieving a masculine or feminine social role
  • Accepting one's personal appearance
  • Acquiring a set of values and an ethical system as a guide to behavior
  • Achieving emotional independence from significant adults
  • Preparing for a career

Moral and Spiritual Development The child enters adolescence with a law-and-order orientation, and may never progress beyond that point. Some people may enter the postconventional stage, during which moral judgments are made on the basis of universal beliefs.

The adolescent can think in the abstract, and may question beliefs and practices that no longer serve to stabilize identity or purpose. It is not uncommon for the adolescent to temporarily abandon traditional religious practices.

Common Health Problems Although adolescence is the time of life when one reaches maximum physiologic development and health, a wide variety of health problems can occur. Wellness promotion in the adolescent focuses on nutrition, relationships with self and others, and safety.

Accidents Accidents are the leading cause of death in adolescents. Motor vehicle accidents are the most common

cause of mortality and often are related to the use of alcohol or other drugs.

Substance Abuse Although the use of illegal drugs (such as marijuana) is reported to be decreasing, the use of alcohol remains a significant part of adolescent risk-taking behavior. In addition, the use of crack-cocaine, a relatively inexpensive and highly addictive drug, has reached epidemic proportions in major cities.

Suicide The suicide rate in adolescents has increased drastically over the past 30 years, with suicide being more prevalent in teenagers than in any other age-group. Although girls attempt suicide more often than boys, boys are more likely to complete it. Depression is a possible contributing factor.

Pregnancy The United States leads the developed countries in the number of pregnancies among adolescents aged 15 to 19 (Martin & Reeder, 1991). These pregnancies are physically, psychologically, and economically costly for the teenage mother, the infant, the family, and society. Most teen mothers are poor, do not complete high school, and are at high risk for complications involving the pregnancy and the infant. In addition, infant and child care costs to the public are in excess of $1 billion per year (Edelman, 1987).

Nutritional Difficulties Fad dieting and socialization that involves fast foods are common among adolescents. In the short run, such nutritional imbalances are harmless. For those adolescents who are obsessed with body image (particularly females), severe eating disorders can result. The most common are **anorexia nervosa** (compulsive dieting to the point of self-starvation) and **bulimia** (a destructive cycle of binge eating followed by self-induced vomiting in an effort to prevent weight gain). The psychodynamics of these conditions are complex but almost always involve severe family dysfunction. Although these disorders were once considered uncommon, they now affect 10% to 15% of young women between ages 12 and 25 (Salkind & Ambron, 1987).

Sexually Transmitted Diseases   Adolescents who engage in sexual intercourse are at a higher risk for contracting **sexually transmitted diseases** (STDs) and their complications than are adults. Lack of knowledge, lack of psychosocial maturity, embarrassment, and the denial of the need to plan ahead and use condoms are the most common reasons for this increased risk. Gonorrhea is the most prevalent STD among adolescents of both sexes. Trichomonal and monilial infections, as well as human papillomavirus, are common in adolescent girls. Chlamydial infections occur in both sexes, as does syphilis and herpes simplex type II (genital herpes).

None of these STDs have such serious implications for individuals and society as a whole as acquired immune deficiency syndrome (AIDS) does. Although AIDS can be transmitted through means other than sexual contact (eg, blood transfusions and intravenous drug use), transmission is primarily through sexual intercourse. The incidence of AIDS is predicted to increase; it currently is a major cause of death in North America.

Role of the Nurse in Health Care   Areas of concern in adolescence and preventive teaching activities are found in Table 11-8. Teaching often is done by the school nurse. Perhaps one of the more significant activities of the nurse during this period is that of facilitating healthy family relationships. Mutual respect, open communications, and accurate information exchange among family members pave the road for a healthy transition from adolescence to adulthood.

Young and Middle Adulthood

Growth and development continue as a sequence of predictable patterns throughout life. As long as a person lives, he or she learns, adapts, and changes. The theorists discussed in Chapter 10 defined growth and developmental stages and tasks in all dimensions of the individual across

TABLE 11-8

Promoting Wellness in Adolescents	
Area of Concern	**Preventive Teaching**
Substance abuse	• Advise adolescents of statistics about substance abuse. • Discuss the risks of substance abuse. • Discuss the physical consequences of substance abuse. • Discuss the psychosocial consequences of substance abuse. • Assist in preparing strategies for saying no to substance use.
Motor vehicle accidents	• Encourage driver education classes for adolescents. • Discuss the relation of alcohol consumption and motor vehicle accidents.
Suicide	• Assist teachers and caregivers to identify risk factors and data indicative of suicide risk (eg, decreased school performance, social withdrawal). • Advise adolescents with depression where to seek help (eg, psychiatrist, community clinics, crisis centers).
Nutrition	• Discuss healthy eating habits. • Discuss dangers of excessive or nutritionally unsound dieting. • Help caregivers and teachers recognize "risk" students. • Advise adolescents who legitimately need to lose weight to consult a physician or respected weight loss organization (eg, Weight Watchers).
Sex education	• Provide factual information about physical and psychosexual development. • Discuss the nature and prevention of STDs. • Discuss safe sex practices in relation to STDs, particularly AIDS. • Assist with developing strategies for saying no to sexual activity for those who wish. • If adolescent is or intends to become sexually active, discuss responsible sexual behavior and birth control. • Provide assistance to pregnant adolescents by: Discussing options Encouraging medical care Encouraging psychosocial counseling
Self-esteem	• Teach caregivers that normal behavior includes belonging to a peer group, the desire to be like everyone else, and trying on different roles (which may include hairstyles, clothing, and jewelry). • Keep lines of communication open. • Encourage caregivers to facilitate independence while providing love and consistent rules.

EXAMPLES OF NURSING DIAGNOSES

Adolescence

The following nursing diagnoses are examples of those that might be appropriate for the adolescent client.

- High Risk for Injury related to lack of knowledge about automobile safety
- High Risk for Injury related to use of street drugs and poor impulse control
- Impaired Social Interaction related to divorce of parents and social isolation

- Self-Esteem Disturbance related to obesity and failure in school
- Altered Parenting related to adolescent single parent without financial or parental support
- High Risk for Infection related to frequent sexual contacts without use of condoms
- Altered Health Maintenance related to alcohol and tobacco use

---

the life span. Theories also have been developed to describe adult growth and development. Included here is a summary of the theories most commonly used for the young and the middle adult.

Adult Developmental Theories

Erikson's Developmental Crises Erikson (1963) describes two major crises, with related tasks, for the young and the middle adult. They are described in Table 11-9. If the developmental tasks are not accomplished and the crisis is not resolved, the young adult becomes isolated and self-absorbed; the middle adult experiences a sense of stagnation and loss. Adults who do not achieve the tasks satisfactorily tend to focus on themselves, becoming overly concerned with their physical and emotional health needs.

Levinson's Individual Life Structure Levinson and co-workers (1978) based their theory on what they call "individual life structure," centered around the belief that the pattern of life at any point in time is formed by the interaction of three components—the self (values, motives), the social and cultural aspects of one's life (family, religion,

career, ethnic background), and the particular set of roles in which one participates (eg, husband, daughter, friend, student). When anything changes in one component, the whole life structure must then reorganize. According to Levinson, the major periods in young and middle adult life are as follows:

Early adult transition (ages 18 to 22): The major concerns are to break away from one's family, make initial career choices, establish intimate relationships, and select personal values, goals, and life-style.

Entering the adult world (ages 22 to 28): The person now builds on previous choices; there may be a transient quality to occupational choices and friendships.

Settling down (ages 30 to 40): The person invests energies in those areas of life most personally important (family, work, community) and strives to gain status, respect from others, and a sense of authority.

Midlife transition (ages 40 to 45): At this time of life, there is a reappraisal of goals and values. The person may choose to either continue or reorganize and change the established life-style.

TABLE 11-9

Developmental Tasks of Young and Middle Adulthood	
Young Adult (20–30 years)	**Middle Adult (40–60 years)**
Stage/Crisis	
Intimacy versus isolation	Generativity versus stagnation
Tasks	
• Selecting a life partner • Choosing an occupation or a career • Establishing independence from parents • Establishing intimate relationships • Establishing a social network • Forming a personal philosophical and ethical structure	• Establishing and guiding the next generation • Accepting middle-age changes • Adjusting to the needs of aging parents • Being comfortable with spouse • Reevaluating goals and accomplishments

Pay-off years (ages 45 to 65): This is a time of maximum influence, self-direction, and self-approval.

Gould's Transformation Gould (1972) believes that a central theme for the adult years is "transformation," with specific beliefs and developmental phases. According to this theory, adults exhibit the following characteristics:

Ages 18 to 22: They believe that they have established control of themselves but could be pulled back into the family

Ages 22 to 28: They feel established as adults and separate from the family but believe that they must demonstrate their competence as independent adults to their parents. They want to enjoy the present but also build for the future.

Ages 29 to 34: They no longer perceive the need to prove themselves and become more accepting of self. Marriages and careers are well established, but questions about life in general are present.

Ages 35 to 43: They continually look inward and question self, values, and life. They see time as having an end, and believe that there is little time left to shape the behavior of adolescent children.

Ages 43 to 50: They believe their personalities are set. They accept life span as having definite boundaries. They have a special interest in spouse, friends, and community.

Ages 50 to 60: They have decreased negativism and increased feelings of self-satisfaction. Spouses become valued companions. There is a realization of mortality and a concern for health.

Although theorists divide adult life into various age-groups by developmental stages and tasks, it is fairly common to use two major adult age-groups. The remainder of the chapter deals with the young adult (ages 20 to 40) and the middle adult (ages 40 to 60). Chapter 12 focuses on the changes and special needs of older adults.

Young Adulthood: The 20s and 30s

The young adult is considered to have reached maturity—to have completed physical growth and to have developed internal and external controls and values acceptable to society. There are no specific measurements of maturity of the average adult person. Each person is an individual, and a wide range of normal values and behaviors are considered healthy.

Physiologic Development The young adult has well developed and coordinated organ systems, functioning at peak efficiency. Although some normal changes begin to take place during the latter part of the period, for the most part, physical changes are minimal. The major exception is in the pregnant woman. Table 11-10 compares the physical development of the young adult with that of the middle adult.

Psychosocial Development Although physical growth and development are minimal, there are major psychosocial developmental requirements for the young adult. Included in psychosocial development are the major tasks of vocational and relationship choices (Fig. 11-10).

Choosing a Vocation The decision to enter the world of work is strongly influenced initially by the need to become independent of one's family and to be self-sufficient. The

TABLE 11-10

Physiologic Development: Young and Middle Adult		
Assessment	**Young Adult**	**Middle Adult**
General body structure	• Weight evenly distributed (wide normal individual variations)	• Fatty tissue redistributed; men tend to develop abdominal fat, women thicken through the middle • Weight gain
Skin and hair	• Skin smooth with decreased acne • Hair resilient and evenly distributed	• Dry skin • Wrinkle lines appear on the face • Gray hair appears • Men may begin to lose hair on the head
Cardiovascular	• Well developed with peak efficiency	• Cardiac output starts to decrease • Increased fatigue
Musculoskeletal	• Maximum tone, strength, coordination	• Gradual decrease in muscle mass, strength, and agility • Loss of calcium from bones, especially in post-menopausal women
Sensory	• Normally full visual and hearing acuity	• Changes in visual acuity, especially for near vision (presbyopia) • Diminished hearing acuity, especially for high-pitched sounds
Reproductive	• Fully developed • Females have regular menstrual cycles • Males' sexual maturity remains at a peak	• Decreasing hormone production resulting in menopause or andropause

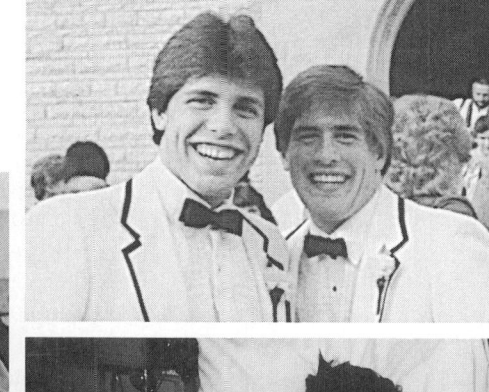

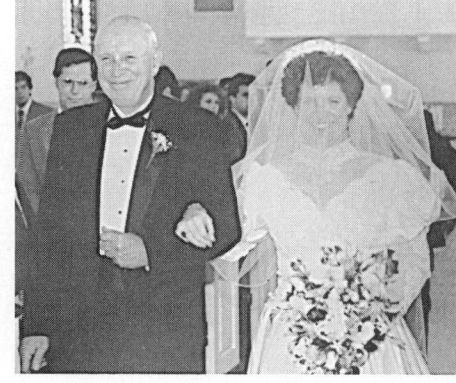

The primary tasks of young adulthood involve establishing intimate relationships and a social network, choosing an occupation or career, establishing a home, parenting, and forming a personal philosophical and ethical structure

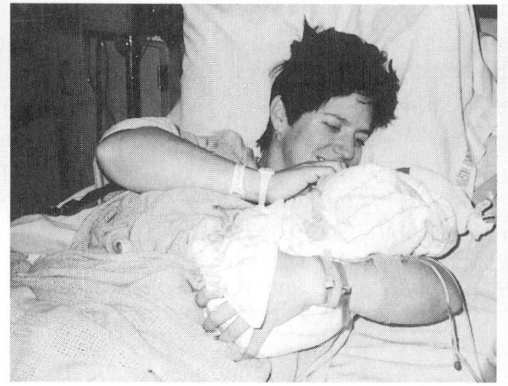

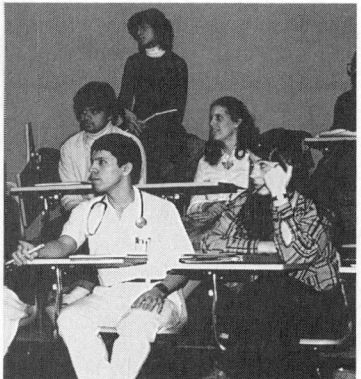

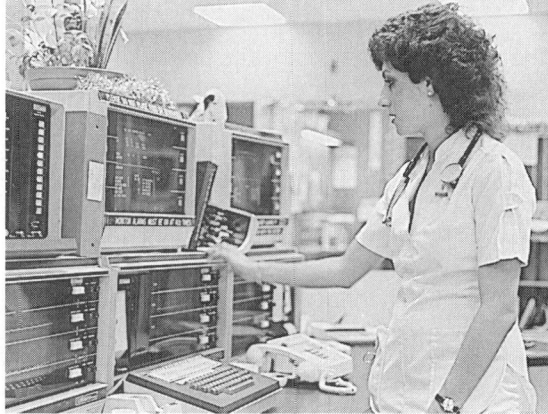

FIGURE 11-10

Developmental tasks of the young adult center around establishing intimate relationships and a home and getting started in an occupation.

choice of an occupation or a career also is guided by the desire to get married, to raise a family, and to become part of the community.

Occupational and career choices are largely tied to educational choices. Many careers necessitate education beyond high school level. Adults learn from both informal and formal experiences, and are largely goal-directed learners. If the identified goals are to increase career opportunities, maintain financial stability, and pursue upward mobility, the adult will be motivated to learn and change. The major factor in achieving satisfaction with one's vocational choice is the belief that one is functioning to capacity and making a contribution to society.

Choosing Relationships The developmental tasks of the young adult are centered around choosing a mate and establishing a family. In today's society, an increasing number of young adults choose to remain single or to live together in heterosexual or homosexual relationships. The accepted societal norm is still to fall in love with a member of the opposite sex, get married, and establish a family.

Establishing a Family The childbearing family is a whole entity even though the physiologic changes take place in the woman. The physiologic and psychological adaptations and needs of pregnancy are described here because they are a major area in the young adult's life.

Physiologic and Psychosocial Adaptations of Pregnancy The physiologic adaptations of pregnancy are summarized in Table 11-11; psychosocial adaptations and tasks are included in the following discussion.

Pregnancy may be considered a period of developmental crisis during which certain tasks must be completed for

TABLE 11-11

Physiologic Adaptations of Pregnancy

System	Normal Changes
Reproductive system	• Uterus enlarges to result in a 500 to 1000-fold increase in capacity. • Cervix has increased vascularity and mucous production. • Ovaries stop producing ovum, but produce hormones to maintain pregnancy. • Vagina increases in size, vascularity, and secretions. • Breasts increase in size and nodularity and begin to secrete colostrum.
Respiratory system	• Oxygen consumption and tidal volume increase. Breathing changes from abdominal to thoracic as pregnancy advances.
Cardiovascular system	• Blood volume increases to 30% to 50% above pregestational level. Blood flow to kidneys and uterus increases.
Gastrointestinal system	• Nausea and vomiting may occur during first trimester. Intestines and stomach are displaced by the growing baby; gastric emptying time and intestinal motility are decreased.
Urinary tract	• Enlarging uterus puts pressure on the kidneys, ureters, and bladder.
Skin	• Changes in skin pigmentation are common, especially on the face and abdomen.
Skeletal system	• Accentuated lumbosacral spinal curve and postural changes accommodate the increased size and weight of the uterus.
Metabolic changes	• Average weight gain is 25 to 30 lb. • Water retention increases. • Protein, carbohydrate, and iron needs increase.

acceptance and coping by the expanding family. The completion of the tasks is influenced by the psychosocial, cultural, and educational dimensions of the prospective parents. The gestational period can be considered 9 months long, with each 3-month period called a **trimester**. The psychosocial needs of the pregnant woman, by trimester, are as follows:

First trimester: The verification of pregnancy may raise conflicting emotions in the woman. Her reactions are influenced by such factors as whether the pregnancy was planned or unplanned, how the baby will affect her career goals, and how significant others accept her pregnancy. The tasks to be achieved are acknowledgment and acceptance of the pregnancy by self and others. If these tasks are met satisfactorily, the woman will have increased self-esteem and accept her new role as a mother.

Second trimester: During the second trimester, body changes and fetal movement actualize the baby's presence. The woman can visualize herself as a mother, and the tasks to be achieved are to focus attention on her pregnancy and to assume responsibility for fetal well-being.

During this period, visible body changes can result in altered body image, with either positive or negative effects. The woman commonly has mood swings. Concerns during the second trimester include normal development and health of both the baby and self, mothering capabilities, family acceptance, adjustments to the addition of a new baby, and labor and delivery of the baby. These concerns often lead to participation in prenatal classes by both parents.

Third trimester: During the third trimester, physical and emotional changes, combined with altered body image and fatigue, can cause lowered self-esteem and irritability. The woman now centers on maternal tasks and the maternal role. She makes plans for the baby (room, clothes) and prepares herself for the labor and delivery process. During the latter months of pregnancy, the woman's need for love and attention increases.

Psychosocial Needs of the Prospective Father The needs of the prospective father must be assessed too. Considerations for the father include the following:
• Learning the physical and psychological changes of pregnancy
• Accepting his supportive role in meeting maternal dependency needs
• Understanding alterations in sexual need and activity during pregnancy
• Exploring feelings about the developing fetus
• Learning about the birthing process
• Accepting his own feelings about the actual birth

In today's world, both parents are active participants in child care. They may share a leave of absence from work so that both can take turns caring for the baby and continuing in their respective careers. No longer are love and caring for children considered "women's work"; the result is stronger family unity and a greater acceptance of individual needs and goals.

Cognitive, Moral, and Spiritual Development The young adult has the ability to solve problems and carry out logical reasoning. The ability to learn is enhanced throughout adult life by educational and life experiences. The young adult, as compared with the adolescent, is creative in thought, objective, realistic, and less self-centered. Although learning takes place in various settings, the young adult often actively seeks formal educational opportunities, both as a post–high school choice and as a means of changing directions in careers.

Young adults who have satisfactorily mastered previous levels of moral development (as defined by Kohlberg in Chapter 10) enter the conventional level. At the conventional level, the person is concerned with maintaining expectations, and values conformity, loyalty, and social order. An estimated 80% of adults do not move beyond this stage, or do so only as middle adults (Murray & Zentner, 1989).

Spiritually, the young adult focuses on reality and may ask questions about spirituality. This individuating-reflective period (as defined by Fowler) brings discovery of the meaning of values as they relate to the achievement of social purposes and to the acceptance of the value systems of others.

Common Health Problems   The 20s and 30s normally are a time of good health, but physical and emotional problems can result from life-style, developmental, or situational crises; family history; and the environment. Even if an illness does not appear at this age, the person is at increased risk later in life.

Life-Style   Various risk factors are present in the way a young adult chooses to live. Some actual and potential health hazards of life-style are as follows:

Violent death: Accidents are the leading cause of death in young adults; suicide ranks third. Alcohol is associated with most motor vehicle accidents.

Relationships: Sexual experimentation and changing social values may result in unwanted pregnancy or STDs. STDs include genital herpes, gonorrhea, syphilis, and AIDS.

Drug abuse: Drug abuse is a major threat to the health of young adults. Prolonged use of various substances can cause death, physical and emotional problems, and disease. Commonly abused substances are nicotine, alcohol, marijuana, amphetamines, and cocaine.

Diet and exercise: Young adults require fewer calories than adolescents because growth is completed. Fast foods and busy life-styles often are a way of life, resulting in increased caloric intake and minimal exercise. As a result, obesity can become a health problem.

Developmental or Situational Stressors   The young adult has to deal with many stressors as a result of choices about life-style, occupation, and relationships. Family-centered stressors may be related to both positive and negative factors: marriage, divorce, parenthood, death of a parent. The increased stress may precipitate mental or physical health problems, aggravated by ineffective coping mechanisms

such as substance abuse, child abuse, spouse abuse, decreased nutrition and rest, and risk-taking behavior. Problem areas for the young adult include the following:

- An increasing number of men and women are choosing to remain single. This singlehood status has advantages and disadvantages. Being single gives one the freedom to come and go as one chooses, to have more autonomy, and to spend money and time as one wishes. On the other hand, external pressures to marry and the desire for love, to belong, and to raise a family may make the young adult question the decision to remain single.

- The decision by young married couples to have children may be delayed until careers are established, or there may be no children by choice. If children are desired, infertility (the inability to conceive after 1 year of coitus without contraception) may add even more stress.

- Divorce is common in our society, with rates being highest for those marrying young, having low income, and having low educational levels. It separates children from their families, has long-term emotional costs, and increases the number of single-parent families headed by women.

- Women who are married, have a job or career, and have a family must contend with multiple roles. The desire to be superwoman and do all things well is physically and emotionally exhausting.

- Women who have postponed having children may realize in their middle to late 30s that their so-called biologic clock is winding down; an increasing number of women in this age-group are having a first child.

Family History   A family history of chronic diseases such as hypertension, heart disease, and diabetes increases a person's risk of developing the disease.

Environment   The young adult may be exposed to environmental pollutants at work. He or she may be at increased risk of becoming ill or injured because of economic difficulties, poor housing and hygiene, and increased probability of accidents. Additionally, the young adult, actively spending leisure and work time in contact with others, increases his or her exposure to acute infectious disease.

Nurse's Role in Health Care   Many activities that promote health are discussed in Chapter 2. As with any client, the nurse must consider each young adult as an individual, taking a holistic view of special needs and influences on health maintenance. Nursing considerations specific to the young adult are as follows:

- Teaching the need for regular physical examinations and dental care, including screenings for diseases most common to this age
- Teaching preventive health practices related to nutrition, rest, substance use, and stress-related illnesses
- Providing information about sexuality, pregnancy, and health of the reproductive system through self-breast

and self-testicular examination, birth control, and prevention of STDs
- Providing and supporting safety education in the workplace and in activities of daily living

Acute illness in the young adult is more of an annoyance than of serious consequence. If the young adult is hospitalized, he or she usually is strongly motivated to recover and to resume normal activities. The nurse must remember that independence and self-sufficiency are important to the young adult; the dependent sick role is not easily accepted. Health care will be facilitated if the young adult is informed and involved in decisions about care.

Although chronic illnesses are less common, their occurrence in the young adult can lead to delayed development, loss of independence, and permanent changes in personal and career goals.

Middle Adulthood: The 40s and 50s

The middle adult years are a time of change in both physical and psychosocial dimensions. The changes are gradual and individualized. As the normal life span increases, most people in this age-group still consider themselves young in relation to the older population. Visible signs of aging and an awareness of time left to live, however, make the middle adult evaluate achievement of goals and influence adaptation to older age.

Physiologic Development The early years of this period of life are marked by maximum physical development and functioning. As time passes, gradual physiologic changes—both internal and external—occur. These are not pathologic changes, but rather normal changes that result from aging. Self-image and self-concept must be altered to successfully adapt to and accept these normal changes. The physical development of the middle adult is outlined in Table 11-10.

The hormonal changes that take place in midlife affect men and women differently. Women undergo a change called **menopause**, a gradual decrease in ovarian function, with subsequent depletion of estrogen and progesterone. This change usually occurs between ages 40 and 55. With the cessation of ovulation, menstrual periods stop (either gradually or abruptly); most women also experience hot flashes, mood swings, and fatigue. The whole process lasts for several years, and on completion, the woman is no longer able to become pregnant. Men do not have physical symptoms from the decreased levels of hormones, called **andropause**. Androgen levels diminish slowly; the man may have some loss of sexual potency but is still capable of reproduction.

Psychosocial Development The middle adult years usually are a time of increased personal freedom, economic stability, and social relationships. They also are a time of increased responsibility and an awareness of one's own mortality (Fig. 11-11). One is faced with the realization that half of one's life is over and many things are still undone. This realization can lead to developmental crises and situational stressors.

Role Transition Various changes can take place during the middle years. These changes include changes in relationships within a marriage, with children who are becoming adults, and with aging parents.

Relationships with one's spouse may go through contrasting changes. Although this usually is a time of security and stability, with stronger emotional commitment and sharing, it also may be a time of disenchantment. The husband or wife may develop negative, critical feelings and attitudes as a result of changes in physical appearance, energy levels, and sexual needs and abilities. Dissatisfaction with achievement of career and family goals contributes to the stresses placed on the marriage. Extramarital affairs and divorce may be the result.

Widowhood (the status change resulting from the death of a husband or wife) may take place in the middle years. The loss of a spouse is a major crisis and a threat to self-concept, as well as a major role change. A multitude of changes may occur, including reduced income, changes in life-style and social relationships, and the need for help to work through the loss and grief.

The middle-aged adult is caught in the middle of a "generation sandwich." Children often are independent

EXAMPLES OF NURSING DIAGNOSES

Young to Middle Adult

The following nursing diagnoses are examples of those that might be appropriate for the young to middle adult client.
- Altered Health Maintenance related to lack of knowledge of language and health care system
- Altered Family Processes related to seriously ill father
- Decisional Conflict related to career choice
- Anxiety related to lack of knowledge about surgical procedure

- Diversional Activity Deficit related to change in life-style after early retirement
- Fatigue related to long-term care of chronically ill parent
- Altered Sexuality Patterns related to prenatal and postpartum changes
- Sleep Pattern Disturbance related to hospitalization
- Health-Seeking Behaviors related to request for stress management techniques

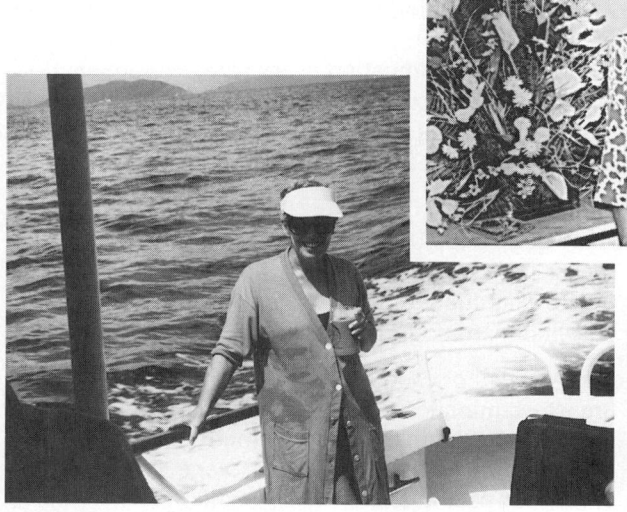

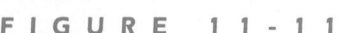

FIGURE 11-11

The middle adult years are characterized by greater expendable wealth, renewed relationship with one's spouse, and expanded social relationships.

and married, and have children of their own. Although much has been written about the *empty-nest syndrome* (resulting from the last child leaving home), most middle-aged parents welcome the space, time, and independence when freedom from parenting occurs. As involvement and responsibility for children are decreasing, there may be an increasing need to become involved in caring for aging parents and other family members. The physical aging or death of a parent makes one's own aging and inevitable death a reality.

Midlife Transition This phenomenon does seem to occur in both men and women in their late 30s to early 40s. The transition involves changes in physiology, work, and family relationships. The following areas of one's life may be questioned:

- Women may choose to go to school, get a job, or change their career. Conversely, women who have been immersed in a career may decide in their early 40s to have children and stay at home.
- Men may become workaholics, spending little time with family or in leisure activities. Many men may choose to make a career change, often with increased emphasis on job satisfaction.
- As the 50s approach, questions about retirement and economic security become more prevalent, with increased interest in examining benefits of financial and retirement plans.
- Although one may not feel that one is aging, the realization that others consider the middle adult years as being older can be stressful.

Cognitive, Moral, and Spiritual Development Cognitive and intellectual abilities of the middle adult change little from those of the young adult. There often is increased motivation to learn, especially if the knowledge gained can be immediately applied and has personal relevance. Problem-solving abilities remain throughout adulthood, although response time may be slightly longer. This is due not to a decrease in ability but rather to a longer memory search of increased amounts of material and to a desire to think a problem through before responding.

Morally, the middle adult may either remain at the conventional level or move to the postconventional level, especially if the person has had sustained responsibility for the welfare of others and has consistently applied ethical principles developed in adolescence. At this level, the adult believes that the rights of others take precedence, and takes steps to support those rights.

As with moral development, not all adults progress to Fowler's paradoxical-consolidative state of spiritual development. Fowler believes that only some people reach this stage, and only after age 30. Most middle adults are less rigid in beliefs and have increased faith and trust in spiritual strength.

Common Health Problems The middle adult, like the young adult, is subject to physical and emotional health problems from life-style, developmental or situational crisis, family history, and the environment. Both acute and chronic illnesses may occur, but with increased age, recovery time is longer. This is a result of slower and more prolonged responses to stressors, more pronounced reactions to an illness, and the possibility of more than one illness being present at a time (Schuster & Ashburn, 1986).

The leading causes of death in the middle adult years are motor vehicle accidents, occupational accidents, suicide, and chronic disease (cancer in women and heart attacks in men). Major health problems are cardiovascular and pulmonary diseases, cancer, rheumatoid arthritis, diabetes mellitus, obesity, alcoholism, and depression.

The risk of developing these common health problems often is a result of the combination of life-style and aging. As one gets older, energy requirements decrease. The middle adult tends to maintain eating patterns and caloric intake while, at the same time, having less physical activity. This trend can result in obesity and atherosclerosis, with increased risk for high blood pressure, coronary artery disease, renal failure, and diabetes. Additionally, smoking and alcohol consumption put the person at greater risk for developing lung cancer, chronic respiratory problems, liver disease, and peptic ulcer disease.

Chronic illness in the middle adult has a major impact on self-concept and may precipitate changes in life structure. For example, after a serious heart attack, a man may face changes in his family role, his earning capacity, and his social relationships. All of these changes are a source of great stress.

Middle age does not automatically result in physical and emotional health problems. Most men and women remain healthy throughout their lives, but knowledge of proper preventive health care and the special needs of this age-group can lead to improved quality and quantity of life.

Nurse's Role in Health Care The nurse plays a major role in promoting health in the middle adult by teaching, serving as a role model, and encouraging self-care responsibilities.

The following health promotion activities are recommended:

All Middle Adults
- Complete physical examination every 2 years
- Annual dental examination
- Eye examination every 1 to 2 years, including a test for glaucoma
- Maintenance of current immunizations
- Annual examination of fecal material for the presence of blood
- Digital rectal examination every year
- Regular self-testicular examination and regular prostate examinations
- Cancer screening for women, as recommended by the American Cancer Society

Adults Aged 20 to 40
- Breast self-examination every month
- Breast examination by a physician every 3 years
- Baseline mammogram between ages 35 and 39

Adults Aged 40 or Older
- Breast examination by a physician yearly
- Self-breast examination every month
- Mammogram every 1 to 2 years to age 49 and then every year past age 50

All Women
- If age 18 or older and for sexually active people, pelvic examination and Papanicolaou test yearly
- After three or more consecutive normal annual tests, Pap tests may be done less frequently at the physician's discretion

The middle adult should be taught the importance of proper nutrition, rest, and exercise, as well as the dangers of substance abuse. Referrals to support groups and individual counseling may be necessary to strengthen the coping mechanisms and allow acceptance of personal and family changes.

Although the young and middle adult years are a time of change, they also are the period of life when a person is at optimal physical and psychosocial functioning. Having successfully met developmental tasks, the adult is ready to enjoy the rest of life. A sense of continuity and adaptability, achieved from the beginning of the 20s to the end of the 50s, is essential to satisfactorily meeting developmental tasks of aging and to the enjoyment of one's remaining years.

KEY POINTS

- Heredity dictates an individual child's growth potential, whereas environment and nutrition influence the degree to which that potential will be reached.
- Growth and development in childhood begin rapidly, increase at a slower, steady pace in the middle, and end rapidly.
- The development of higher levels of moral and spiritual reasoning is directly related to higher levels of cognitive ability.
- The family is an integral part of a child's growth and development.
- Healthy development occurs if the tasks of each stage are completed before entering the next stage.

- The nurse's role in child health care is focused on preventive teaching.
- An understanding of childhood development is essential to understanding adulthood.
- Growth and development continue as a sequence of predictable patterns throughout the adult life span.
- Erikson, Levinson, and Gould have described major developmental stages and tasks for the young and the middle adult.
- The young adult has reached optimal physical development, but major psychosocial adaptation centers around choosing a vocation and defining relationship choices.

- Establishing a family (and the expanding family group) creates special tasks and needs for the young adult.
- During the middle adult years, visible signs of aging and an awareness of mortality appear. Various role changes may occur, and midlife crisis may precipitate changes in life-style.

- Both young and middle adults are generally healthy, but increased risk for illness results from life-style, developmental or situational crises, family history, and the environment.
- Nursing considerations to promote health and prevent illness in adulthood focus on teaching self-care activities and the importance of regular physical examinations.

BIBLIOGRAPHY

Bee, H., & Mitchell, S. (1984). *The developing person: A lifespan approach.* New York: Harper & Row.

Bennett, E. G., & Woolf, D. (Eds.). (1991). *Substance abuse* (2nd ed.). Albany: Delmar.

Bobak, I. M., Jensen, M. D., & Zalar, M. K. (1989). *Maternity and gynecologic care: The nurse and the family* (4th ed.). St. Louis: Mosby.

Boynton, P. R. (1989). Health maintenance alteration: A nursing diagnosis of the elderly. *Clinical Nurse Specialist, 3*(1), 5–10.

Burke, P. J. (1987). Adolescent's motivation for sexual activity and pregnancy prevention. *Issues in Comprehensive Pediatric Nursing, 10,* 161–171.

Catanzaro, M. (1990). Transitions in midlife adults with long-term illness. *Holistic Nursing Practice, 4*(3), 65–73.

Children's needs challenge RNs. (1991). *American Nurse,* June, 1.

Edelman, M. W. (1987). Teenage pregnancy: An epidemic takes its toll. In A. R. Cohn & L. A. Leach (Eds.). *Generations.* New York: Pantheon.

Engle, W. (1973). The development from sound to phoneme in child language. In C. A. Ferguson & D. I. Slobin (Eds.). *Studies of child language development.* New York: Holt, Rinehart, & Winston.

Erikson, E. (1963). *Childhood and society.* New York: Norton.

Foster, R., Hunsberger, M., & Anderson, J. (1989). *Family-centered nursing care of children.* Philadelphia: Saunders.

Freiberg, K. L. (1987). *Human development: A lifespan approach* (3rd ed.). Boston: Jones & Bartlett.

Gould, R. (1972). The phases of adult life: A study in developmental psychology. *American Psychiatry, 129,* 33–43.

Hogan, R. (1985). *Human sexuality: A nursing perspective.* Norwalk, CT: Appleton-Century-Crofts.

Hughes, F. P., & Noppe, L. D. (1990). *Human development across the lifespan.* New York: Merrill.

Klaus, M. H., & Kennell, J. H. (1982). *Parent–infant bonding.* St. Louis: Mosby.

Levinson, D., J., Darrow, C. N., Klein, E. B., Levinson, M. H., McKee, B. (1978). *The seasons of a man's life.* New York: Knopf.

Marchoen, A., & Brumagne, M. (1985). Loneliness among children and young adolescents. *Developmental Psychology, 21*(11), 1025–1031.

Martin, L., & Reeder, S. (1991). *Essentials of maternity nursing: Family, newborn and women's health.* Philadelphia: Lippincott.

May, K. A., & Mahlmeister, L. R. (1990). *Comprehensive maternity nursing: Nursing process and the childbearing family* (2nd ed.). Philadelphia: Lippincott.

Miller, B., & Keane, C. (1987). *Encyclopedia and dictionary of medicine, nursing and allied health* (4th ed.). Philadelphia: Saunders.

Mott, S., Fazekas, N., & James, S. (1990). *Nursing care of children and families* (2nd ed.). Menlo Park, CA: Addison-Wesley.

Murray, R., & Zentner, J. (1989). *Nursing assessment and health promotion through the life-span.* Englewood Cliffs, NJ: Prentice-Hall.

Myers, N., & Perlmutter, M. (1978). Memory in the years from 2 to 5. In P. Ornstein (Ed.). *Memory development in children.* Hillsdale, NJ: Erlbaum.

Nelson, K. (1973). *Structure and strategy in learning to talk.* Monographs of the Society for Research in Child Development, 38.

Papilia, D., & Olds, S. (1989). *Human development* (4th ed.) New York, McGraw-Hill.

Salkind, N., & Ambron, S. (1990). *Child development* (6th ed.). New York: Holt, Rinehart & Winston.

Santrok, J., & Yussen, S. (1989). *Child development: An introduction* (4th ed.). Dubuque: Brown.

Schuster, C., & Ashburn, S. (1986). *The process of human development: A holistic life-span approach* (2nd ed.). Boston: Little, Brown.

Scipien, G., & Barnard, M. (1990). *Comprehensive pediatric nursing.* St. Louis: Mosby–Year Book.

Sheehy, G. (1976). *Passages: Predictable crisis of adult life.* New York: Dutton.

Stern, M., Northman, J. E., & VanSlyck, M. R. (1984). Father absence and adolescent "problem behaviors": Alcohol consumption, drug use and sexual activity. *Adolescence, 19*(74), 301–312.

Stuart, G., & Sundeen, S. (1991). *Principles of psychiatric nursing* (4th ed.). St. Louis: Mosby.

Thomas, A., Chess, S., and Birch, H. G. (1968). *Temperament and behavior discussed in children.* New York: New York University Press.

Waechter, E., Phillips, J., & Holaday, B. (1985). *Nursing care of children.* Philadelphia: Lippincott.

Whaley, L., & Wong, D. (1991). *Nursing care of infants and children* (4th ed.). St. Louis: Mosby.

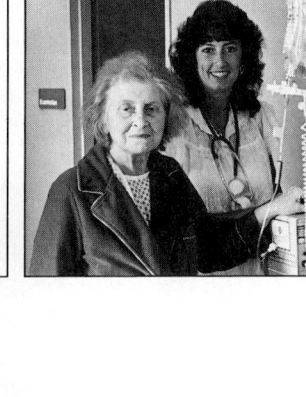

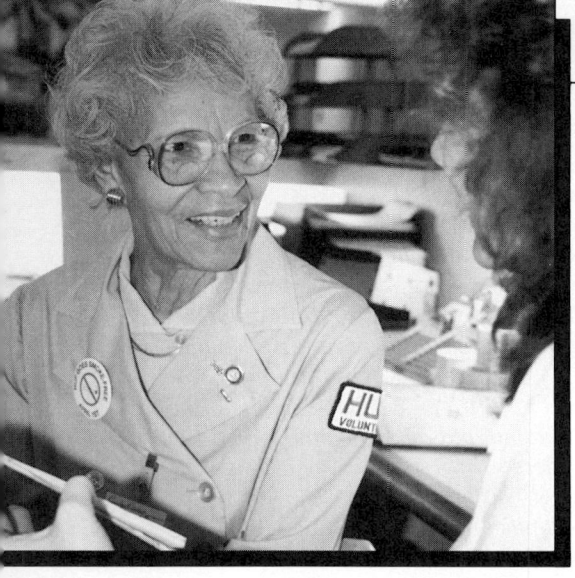

The Older Adult

12

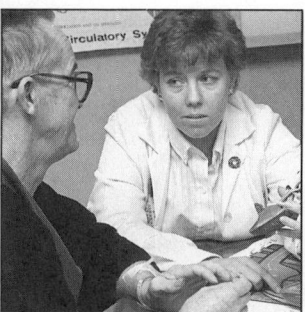
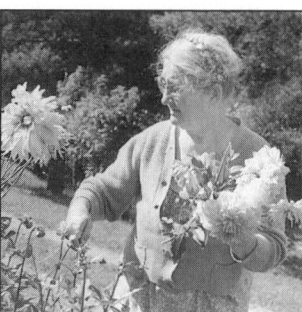

Growth and development continue as one ages, with no specific age or experience that causes a person to feel old versus young. Aging is gradual, characterized by continued development, maturation, and adaptation in all areas of life. Our society has arbitrarily labeled the **older adult** as one over age 65. Although all people over age 65 often are grouped together, this group is diverse, representing various economic, sociocultural, and experiential backgrounds.

The population of the United States and Canada is growing older. With this shift in age comes increased health care needs in both acute and long-term settings. As the health care system changes to meet these needs, the nurse will care for more older adults—both well and ill—in various settings. It is essential, therefore, that nurses understand the concepts of growth and development as they relate to older adults. Illness, functional disabilities, and hospitalization cause major disruptions in the growth and development of any person, but they can be particularly devastating to an elderly person.

The nurse recognizes that these disruptions are small in relation to the whole of life experiences. It is within the nurse's role to promote wellness, prevent illness, restore health, and facilitate coping with life experiences and to assist the client to challenge and complete developmental tasks successfully to reach individual potentials as a unique human being.

Aging: A Paradox in Society

The older adult population is the most unique and diversified group in today's society because its members have lived the longest and have participated in and adapted to complex societal changes. Within the life span of the older adult, society has developed largely from a rural agricultural base, through industrialization, into a service-oriented, high-technology base. Consider that in 1900, a 20-mile trip meant an all-day undertaking—probably in a horse-drawn wagon. Today a person can fly across the continent in less time and with considerably less effort. Most older adults have lived through the trauma of one or two world wars. Most had parents with strong ethnic ties to another country, and many were immigrants themselves. The older adult has lived through the Great Depression of the 1930s and developed self-sufficiency. Major societal changes, such as the enactment of Social Security and Medicare, necessitated adaptations and helped to shape the values and life-styles of older adults (Fig. 12-1).

With advancing age, further adaptations become necessary because of physical or mental limitations, retirement, loss of a spouse or family members, or changing income. The older adult is faced with numerous role changes that may be directly related to chronologic age or health status. Lost roles must be replaced with new roles and activities that are acceptable and satisfying to the person.

Elderly people are thus facing a world that has necessitated both slow and abrupt adaptations. It is a time to reach one's potential and to satisfy long-range goals that may have been delayed because of other responsibilities. Willingly or unwillingly, it also can be a time to turn over to others "productive" tasks such as career or community leadership. Research has shown that most older adults do adjust and adapt to new roles (Costa et al., 1991), and most are satisfied with their lives and with what they have. Depending on the older adult's adaptability and supportive resources, older adulthood may promote feelings of happiness, peace, and understanding, or of sorrow, conflict, and confusion.

Ageism: Common Stereotypes

The older adult has been the victim of ageism. **Ageism** is a form of prejudice, like racism, in which older adults are stereotyped by characteristics found in only a few members of their group. Fundamental to ageism is the view that elderly people are different from "me" now and will remain different from "me" in the future; therefore, they do not experience the same desires, needs, and concerns (Hendricks & Hendricks, 1986). Perhaps this viewpoint developed with the post–World War II baby boom and the emphasis on a youth-oriented society, along with a tendency to deny our own aging and mortality. Industrialism and technologic advancements have placed a high priority on productivity, so that retired people may be said to have "outlived their usefulness." Along with this, the younger generations often have lost ties to the older generation because of increased mobility of the nuclear family, and thus lack experiences with older relatives and their friends.

Elderly people may be *incorrectly* depicted as being rigid or narrow-minded, unable to learn, unreliable because of memory loss, too old for sex, or childlike and dependent. Many people fear advancing age because of the pervasive views that elderly people are poor, lonely, in frail health, and able to look forward only to institutionalization in a nursing home. These descriptors, which are discussed in this chapter, are not true for most older adults (Fig. 12-2).

Changing Values With a Graying Population

Based on information compiled by the U.S. Senate Special Committee on Aging (1987–1988), about 29.2 million people are age 65 or older. It is projected that by the year 2000, half of the aging population will be age 75 or older, and that

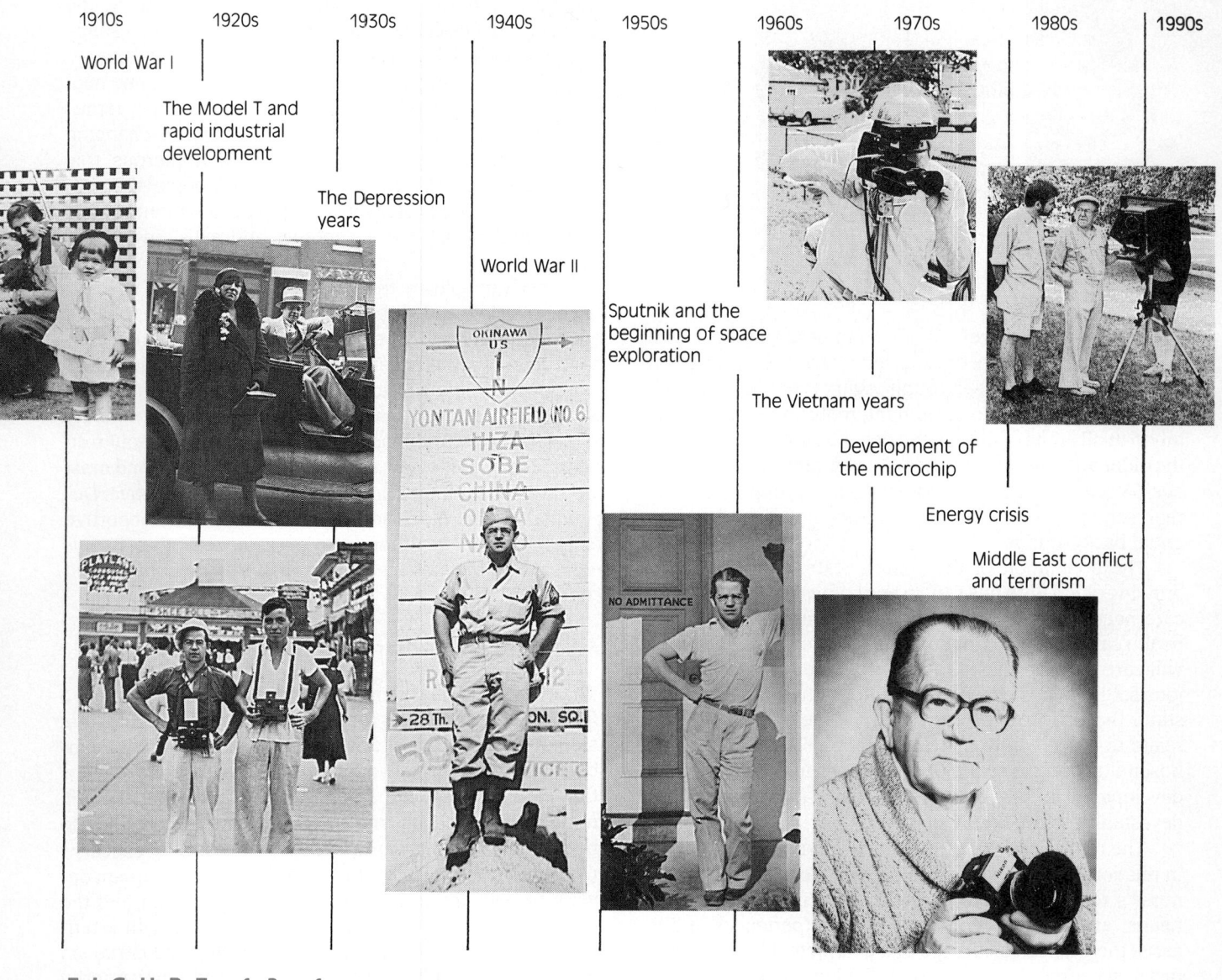

1910s   1920s   1930s   1940s   1950s   1960s   1970s   1980s   **1990s**

World War I

The Model T and
rapid industrial
development

The Depression
years

World War II

Sputnik and the
beginning of space
exploration

The Vietnam years

Development of
the microchip

Energy crisis

Middle East conflict
and terrorism

F I G U R E   1 2 - 1

The older adult population is a unique group with vast and diverse experience. Images from one man's life highlight some of the social events and change that this population group has experienced.

by 2040, about 20% of the total population will be age 65 or older. These shifts in population are the result of an increased life expectancy and a decrease in birth rates. On the average, North American women can now expect to live to age 78 and men, to age 71.

This age shift in the population is influencing all of society and helping to shape social, political, and health care issues. Older adults are emerging as a strong social and political force. Consider such organizations as the American Association of Retired Persons, which provides educational and community service programs for those over age 50 and lobbies for legislative change in issues regarding the older adult at state and federal levels. Other examples include the proliferation of retirement planning magazines, media advertisements for health and life insurance, and retirement centers.

Who Is the Older Adult?

Contrary to myth, most older adults adjust well, and continue to live active, independent, and productive lives. Most are satisfied with their lives, finding retirement and old age more enjoyable than they had anticipated. Three fourths live in their own homes, and one third of these live alone. Because of their longer life span, there are 1.5 times as many older women as older men. Most older adults maintain close ties with their families, and have incomes above the poverty level (AARP, 1990; Kovar, 1986).

Functional Health Versus Disease   Most older adults regard themselves as healthy, and deny severe limitations in activities. Most are never institutionalized, nor do they suffer the effects of senility. *Healthy*, however, does not necessarily mean without disease. More than 80% of older adults suffer from at least one chronic illness. Like younger adults, they define their health in relation to how well they function—that is, whether or not they can engage in their usual and desired daily activities. This functional health definition includes a person's ability to remain self-reliant, to "make do," and to maintain a sense of control and independence over self and environment.

Older adulthood is a general term that encompasses everyone over age 65. **Old-old** and **frail-old** are terms used to identify people over age 75; this group is the fastest-growing segment in the population. In 1984, there were 2 million people over age 85 still living in the community (Kovar, 1986). In fact, only 5% of all older adults live in nursing homes, but 40% of those who do are over age 85 (Ebersole & Hess, 1990). The old-old have special significance for nursing care because they are more likely to need help with mobility and basic activities of daily living. They may need increasing assistance to maintain a safe and comfortable living environment. The older the person, the more likely that he or she needs family and community support to maintain functional health.

Family and Reverse Roles   Spouse and other family members are natural support systems who help the older adult maintain functional health and independence and meet developmental tasks of old age. Supportive assistance may include the provision of transportation, food, shelter, social interactions, and even complex medical and nursing treatments. Significant others, such as close friends and neighbors, also may take on tasks formerly assumed to be the responsibilities of the traditional family. Contrary to common stereotypes, families do feel a responsibility toward their elders; most live within an hour of each other and have visited within the past week (Hendricks & Hendricks, 1986).

Not all families can assist an aged member satisfactorily because of such factors as geographic distance, low income, poor health, strained marital relationships, and infringement on career or life-style. Adult children may feel "sandwiched" between responsibilities for their own children and careers and the needs of elderly parents. It can be a guilt-ridden and emotionally draining time for all involved when physical or emotional illness reverses roles and strains family resources.

The nurse must recognize that the whole family is the client, and assess the family for capabilities and limitations in assisting the aged member. The nurse can help ease the strain by listening to client and family concerns and by validating the importance of family needs. The nurse assists the client and family to find workable solutions, and may refer the family to community support services.

Growth and Development Throughout the Life Span

The principles of growth and development apply to people of all ages. As discussed in Chapter 10, the process of growth and development involves a series of changes that usually occur in an orderly and predictable sequence, but at variable rates. The onset and the effect of those changes are influenced by numerous biologic, psychosocial, and environmental factors. Each person is, therefore, unique. In old age, growth hastens the physiologic decline first encountered in middle adulthood. Development and maturation continue, however, throughout older adulthood, depending

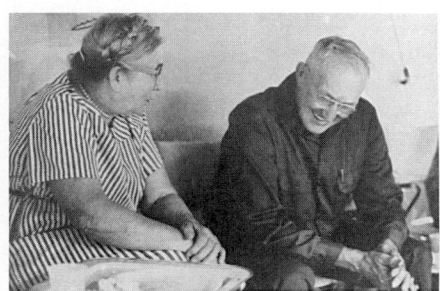
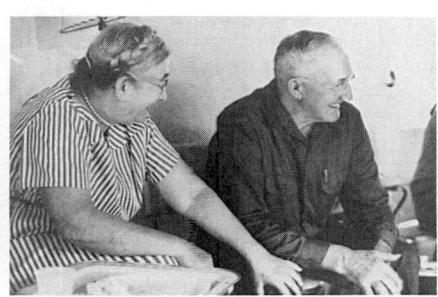
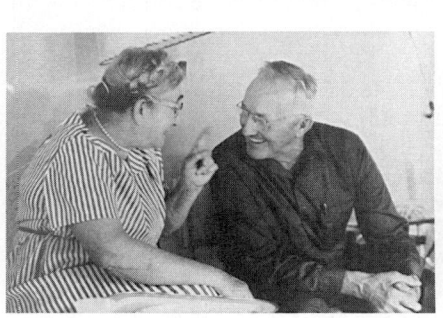
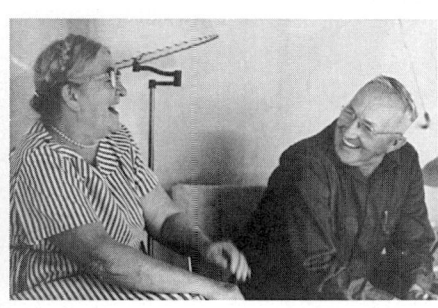

F I G U R E   1 2 - 2

Stereotypical images of the older adult as narrow-minded, forgetful, sexless, and dependent are untrue for most of the older adult population. This couple exhibits the vitality, sensuality, joy, and playfulness of a young couple. (Photos by Karen Baldwin.)

FOCUS ON THE OLDER ADULT

Normal Physiologic Changes of Older Adulthood

General Status

- Progressively decreasing efficiency of physiologic processes results in a fragile balance and hinders the body's ability to maintain homeostasis.
- Physical or emotional stressors cause the older adult to be more vulnerable because of decreased physiologic reserves.
- The older adult may continue to engage in all activities of middle age but intuitively adjusts to a modified pace and more frequent rest periods.

Integumentary

- Wrinkling and sagging of skin occur with decreased skin elasticity; dryness and scaling are common.
- Balding becomes common in men, and women experience thinning of hair also; hair loses pigmentation.
- Skin pigmentation and moles are common, although the skin may become pale because of loss of melanocytes.
- Nails typically thicken and become brittle and yellowed.

Musculoskeletal

- Decreases in subcutaneous tissue and weight commonly are found in the old-old.
- Muscle mass and strength decrease.
- Bone demineralization occurs, and bones become porous and brittle.
- Joints tend to stiffen and lose flexibility, and range of motion may decrease.
- Overall mobility commonly slows and posture tends to stoop. Height decreases slightly.

Neurologic

- The central nervous system responds more slowly to multiple stimuli. Hence, the cognitive and behavioral response of the older adult may be delayed.
- Rate of reflex response decreases.
- Temperature regulation and pain perception become less efficient.
- The sense of balance declines, and fine movements may become more difficult.
- Sleep at night typically shortens and the older adult may awaken more easily. Cat naps become common.

Special Senses

- Diminished visual acuity (*presbyopia*) occurs, with increased sensitivity to glare and decreased ability to adjust to darkness. Cataracts may further obscure vision.
- Diminished hearing acuity (*presbycusis*) occurs, particularly diminished pitch discrimination in the presence of environmental noises.
- The senses of taste and smell are decreased.

Cardiopulmonary

- Blood vessels become less elastic and often rigid and tortuous. Venous return becomes less efficient. Fatty plaque deposits continue to occur in the linings of the blood vessels. Lower-extremity edema and cooling may occur, particularly with decreased mobility.
- The body is less able to increase heart rate and cardiac output with activity.
- Pulmonary elasticity and ciliary action decrease so clearing of the lungs becomes less efficient. Respiratory rate may increase, accompanied by diminished depth.

Gastrointestinal

- Digestive juices continue to diminish and nutrient absorption decreases.
- Malnutrition and anemia become more common.
- With reduced muscle tone and decreased peristalsis, constipation and indigestion are common complaints.

Dentition

- Tooth decay and loss continue for most older adults.
- Eating habits may change, particularly if the older adult lacks teeth or has ill-fitting dentures.

Genitourinary

- Blood flow to the kidneys decreases with diminished cardiac output.
- The number of functioning nephron units decreases by 50%; waste products may be filtered and excreted more slowly.
- Fluids and electrolytes remain within normal ranges, but the balance is fragile.
- Bladder capacity decreases by 50%. Voiding becomes more frequent; two or three times a night is usual. A decrease in bladder and sphincter muscle control may result in stress incontinence or incomplete bladder emptying.
- About 75% of men over age 65 experience hypertrophy of the prostate gland; surgery may be required if urinary retention occurs.
- There is atrophy, decrease of secretions, and thinning of the older woman's genital tract.

to a great extent on a person's sense of self-concept and prior ability to adapt.

Physiologic Theories

Growth refers to biologic processes that result in physical change. In older adulthood, the process of aging becomes progressively more rapid. There are numerous theories that describe how and why aging occurs, but none is universally accepted. The genetic theory of aging explains that life span depends to a great extent on genetic factors. Genes within the organism control "genetic clocks" that determine the occurrence and rate of metabolic processes, including cell division. The wear-and-tear theory explains that organisms wear out from increased metabolic functioning, and that cells become exhausted from continual energy depletion in adapting to stressors (Schuster & Ashburn, 1986). There is no agreement as to why some people, even within families or similar environments, age much more rapidly than others. Although internal processes may in part predetermine aging, other factors, such as drugs, nutrition, and smoking, also may play a role.

Physiologic Status In the older adult, all organ systems undergo some degree of decline in overall functioning, and the body becomes less efficient (see the display titled Normal Physiologic Changes of Older Adulthood). Body functions that require integrated activity of several organ systems are affected the most. For example, renal function, which depends on cardiac output and the condition of the vascular system, declines by about 50% from age 30 to age 80 (Schuster & Ashburn, 1986). The most commonly encountered chronic disorders are cardiovascular disorders such as hypertension and coronary artery disease, cancers, and skeletal disorders such as arthritis and osteoporosis.

Functional Status There is growing evidence that aging is not synonymous with disease and disability. Although 80% of older adults have one or more chronic disorders, their ability to adapt determines whether they are ill or healthy. Most continue their activities from middle age and adapt intuitively to gradual limitations of aging. It may take longer to complete any given activity, or the activity may need to be modified. An older adult with arthritis may need to use an electric can opener rather than a manual one; a person with coronary artery disease may need 3 hours to mow the lawn, with intermittent rest periods, rather than 1 hour (Fig. 12-3).

The greatest threat to the health of older adults is that the physiologic reserve of the various organ systems is gone. When illness occurs, increased physical and emotional stress places an older adult at risk for complex reactions. An older adult is more likely to develop complications and to require longer to recover. For instance, an elderly client with a hip fracture is at high risk for pneumonia and skin breakdown because of immobility, decreased ability to expel pulmonary secretions, and thinner, more fragile skin. The nurse knows that the older client has less reserve, and works to maintain normal functioning. Complications are

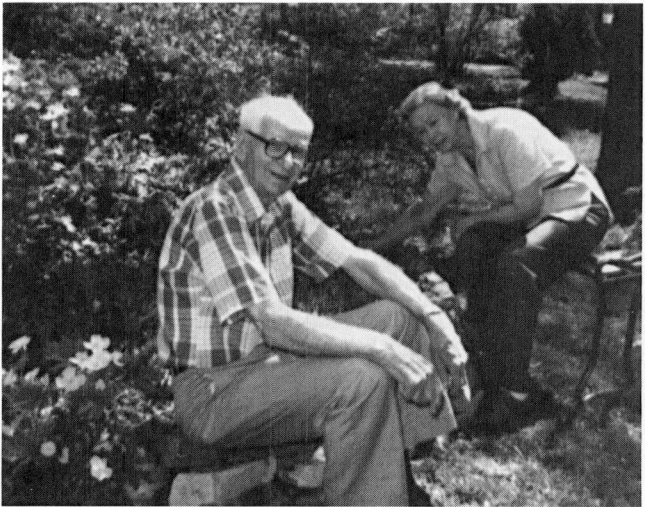

FIGURE 12-3

This couple, married 61 years, enjoy gardening together. They've found that they can continue most activities of middle age with only minor adjustments.

prevented by careful assessment of the symptoms and by assisting the client to cough and deep breathe, turn, and carry out personal hygiene.

Cognitive Development

The term *cognition* is used to indicate cerebral functioning, including the ability to perceive and understand one's world. Cognition does not change appreciably with aging. An older adult continues to learn and problem solve, and intelligence and personality remain consistent (see the display titled Cognitive Status of the Older Adult). It is normal for an older adult to take longer to respond and react, particularly in new or unfamiliar surroundings. Knowing this, the nurse should slow the pace of care and allow the older

---

Cognitive Status of the Older Adult

- Intelligence increases into the 60s, and learning continues throughout life.
- Cognitive functioning is related to use. Reasoning ability and abstract thought remain astute, particularly for usual situations and familiar experiences.
- Processing and reaction times increase and may be evident in slower and seemingly more deliberate responses.
- There is a decreased capacity for adaptation, especially in stressful or unfamiliar environments and with impaired senses.
- Recent memory loss may occur, but long-term memory remains intact.

client extra time to ask questions or complete activities. In the United States, of the 25 million people over age 65, only 5% suffer from a serious mental impairment, and only 10% experience a moderate loss of memory (Dychtwald, 1986). Mild short-term memory loss is common, but can be remedied by an older adult with the use of notes, schedules, and calendars.

When serious mental impairment occurs, the effect on the client and family can be devastating. **Dementia** describes various organically caused disorders that progressively affect cognitive functioning. Of the dementias that affect older adults, **Alzheimer's disease** is the most common. It affects brain cells, and is characterized by patchy areas of the brain that degenerate, or break down. A person with Alzheimer's disease faces a progressively serious and ultimately fatal disorder. At first, forgetfulness and impaired judgment may be evident. Over a period of several years, the person becomes progressively more confused, forgetting family and becoming disoriented in familiar surroundings. When the ability to perform simple activities of daily living is lost, the person requires constant supervision and care, often in a nursing home. There is no effective medical treatment for Alzheimer's disease. Comprehensive and empathetic nursing care are important. The nurse directs nursing care to ensure the client's safety and to meet basic needs of nutrition and fluids, elimination, and hygiene. Both the client and family need emotional support and teaching, and may benefit from community resources that can ease the family's burden.

In the health care field, sometimes confusion and depression in an older adult are mistaken for permanent dementias. Drug interactions, circulatory or metabolic problems, or even nutritional deficiencies are likely to be the real cause. An older adult also may become confused when too many changes or losses occur at one time or when she or he is moved to a radically different environment. Sometimes a type of confusion called **sundowning syndrome** occurs, in which an older adult habitually becomes confused with darkness. The nurse can assist other members of the health team in determining the cause of the client's confusion and in helping to reorient the client. For example, the nurse uses **reality orientation** to redirect the client's attention to what is real in the environment. Nursing interventions include the use of calendars and clocks, calling the client by name, and talking about the client's family and the season. The client also is encouraged to make decisions, to promote a sense of control over the environment. The nurse must remember that many older adults have hearing and visual impairments. These impairments can be counteracted by speaking clearly and slowly, looking directly at the client, and repeating instructions. The environment should be well lighted but without glare.

Developmental Theories

Development continues throughout the life span; new tasks associated with older adulthood are identified, and new behavioral patterns emerge. An early controversial psychosocial theory, called the *disengagement theory*, maintained that an older adult withdraws from societal interactions because it is mutually desired and satisfying for both the individual and society (Schuster & Ashburn, 1986). Later studies have shown that isolation is not desired or acceptable, and that as societal interactions decrease, a healthy older adult increases close relationships with family and friends (Berkman, 1983). According to the *activity theory*, successful aging involves the ability to maintain high levels of activity and functioning. An older adult may substitute activities but does not slow down or disengage from society. The *identity–continuity theory* assumes that healthy aging is related to the ability of the older adult to continue similar patterns of behavior that existed in young to middle adulthood (Schuster & Ashburn, 1986).

Most theorists agree that a person's self-concept is relatively stable throughout adult life. An older adult who has developed a strong sense of self-identity and has successfully met challenges earlier in life will probably continue to do so. This person substitutes new roles for old roles and perhaps continues former roles in a new context. For example, the business manager, on retirement, may continue to use leadership talents in community organizations. Older adults with a strong self-concept typically describe themselves as being healthier than others or "young for my years." On the other hand, events that accompany aging can threaten a person's self-concept. Depending on the person's outlook on life and past ability to cope, events such as retirement, loss of health or income, and isolation can be devastating. For example, the retired teacher whose sense of identity was closely tied to career may suddenly find that friends, income, and sense of accomplishment are lost and, consequently, may feel a great loss of control and self-identity.

Erikson: Psychosocial Development   Erikson identifies ego-integrity versus despair and disgust (Erikson, 1980) as the last stage of human development, which begins around age 60. The older adult continues to look forward, but now also looks backward, and begins to reflect on his or her life. It is a time for realization of a "wholeness" perspective, with an inner search for meaning and order of the life cycle. The older adult searches for emotional integration and acceptance of the past and present, as well as acceptance of physiologic decline without fear of death. The nurse is familiar with older adults who like to retell stories or past events. This phenomenon is called **life review** or **reminiscence** and has been identified worldwide. In a sense, it is a way for an older adult to relive and restructure life experiences, and is part of achieving ego-integrity (Fig. 12-4).

As with other developmental stages identified by Erikson, ego-integrity is facilitated when the older adult has successfully accomplished tasks earlier in life. It can be a time to look backward with pride and without regrets and forward with optimism and enthusiasm. A person who regrets the past and sees current problems as insurmountable may despair. This person may view life as a series of unresolved problems and missed opportunities, and feel

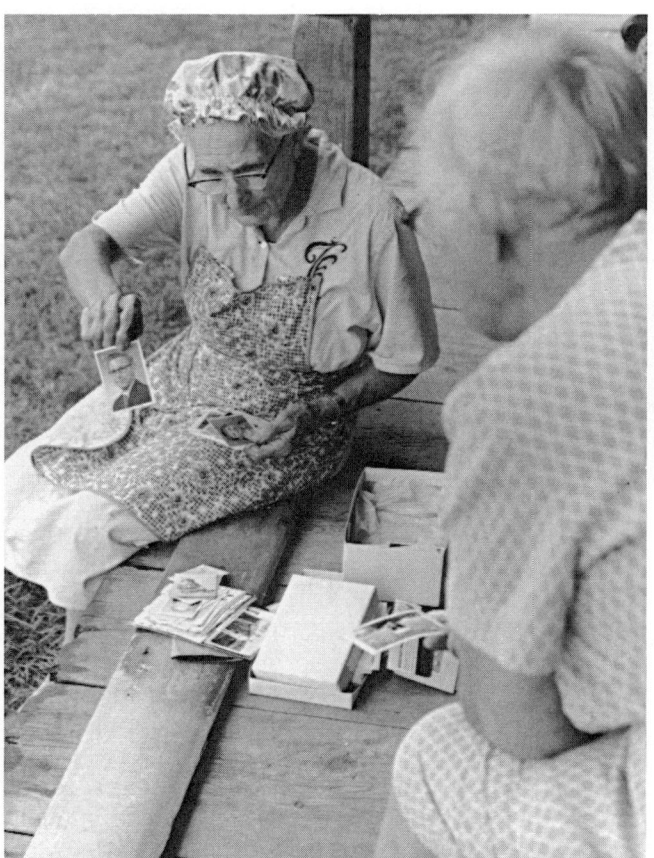

FIGURE 12-4

Reminiscing is a culturally universal phenomenon of aging. It is a way for the older adult to reassess life experiences and further develop a sense of accomplishment, fulfillment, and reward in life. (Photo by Karen Baldwin.)

worthless or hopeless. The despairing person may want to do things over but fears the lack of time before death.

Tasks of midlife continue or resurface. The older adult still strives to guide the coming generations and to leave something behind (generativity versus stagnation). The need for love and closeness continues (intimacy versus isolation), as does a strong sense of who one is in relation to family and community (identity versus role diffusion). Because of physical and social changes associated with aging, the older adult is repeatedly faced with the need to adapt and to again face already completed tasks.

Havighurst: Developmental Tasks   According to Havighurst, the major tasks of old age are primarily concerned with the maintenance of social contacts and relationships. Successful aging depends on a person's ability to be flexible and adapt to new age-related roles. The person must find new and meaningful roles in old age while maintaining reasonable comfort within the social customs of our times (Ebersole & Hess, 1991). The developmental tasks that, according to Havighurst, are associated with "later matu-

rity" (Havighurst, 1972) are listed in the accompanying display. Also, a discussion of each task follows.

Adjusting to Declining Physical Strength and Health   As stated earlier, most older adults gradually modify their lifestyles to accommodate for declining vigor and strength. Rest periods become more frequent; at the same time, continued activity is important for maintaining all physiologic functions. An older adult is at high risk for accidents and falls, and may need to curtail driving or use a cane or other aid to remain mobile. Modification in diet and prescribed medications may be necessary, and because of chronic illness, an older adult may need to adjust to living with pain. With severe illness, loss of independence over oneself and one's environment can occur. The loss of health is difficult to adjust to because it affects every aspect of life.

Adjusting to Retirement and Reduced Income   Retirement brings a change in a person's concept of time. An older adult must learn to occupy leisure time in a way that maintains self-esteem and is personally satisfying. Retirement is considered the hallmark of old age, and satisfaction with retirement is closely tied to income and the relationships one has outside of work. Most older adults manage on smaller incomes after retirement, but about 21% live at or near the poverty level (AARP, 1990). Lack of finances can affect an older adult's ability to meet all needs, from adequate medical care and housing to social and creative interests.

Adjusting to Changes in the Health of One's Spouse   When one's spouse becomes ill or dies, numerous and difficult adjustments must be made. An older adult may face new roles for the first time. A husband may begin to cook meals; a wife may learn to handle family finances. These role changes come at a time when stress is already high. Physical care can be overwhelming if the other spouse also is in poor health. Adaptations may occur in living conditions and life-style, and the spouse may need to plan social and recreational events alone.

Havighurst's Developmental Tasks of Later Maturity

- Adjusting to declining physical strength and health
- Adjusting to retirement and reduced income
- Adjusting to changes in health of one's spouse
- Establishing an explicit affiliation with one's age-group.
- Adopting and adapting social roles in a flexible way
- Establishing satisfactory physical living arrangements

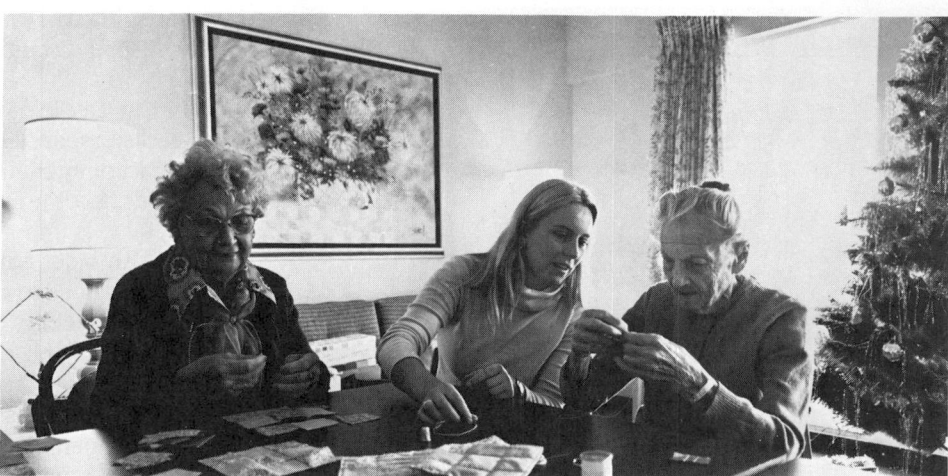

F I G U R E 1 2 - 5

Social relationships and satisfying leisure activities remain important throughout life. These women are making holiday gifts to help support their community nutrition center.

The need for love and belonging does not diminish with age, and may become acute with the loss of one's spouse. We are sexual beings, and our sexual behavior does not necessarily stop in old age. Sexuality encompasses who we are, and older adults are no exception. Like younger adults, older adults need to express intimacy physically by touching and emotionally by sharing joys, sorrows, ideas, and values.

Establishing an Explicit Affiliation With One's Age-Group With an aging population, social organizations for older adults are becoming more numerous. For example, most communities have senior citizens' centers that offer meals, social and informational programs, and other activities for a nominal fee. Other organizations offer the opportunity for travel, cultural events, and political involvement. Affiliation with other people of the same age allows older adults to share common interests and concerns and find status among their peers. It should not be assumed, however, that older adults want to associate only with others of the same age (Fig. 12-5).

Adopting and Adapting Social Roles in a Flexible Way Social roles change with the developmental tasks and adjustments of older adulthood, but the need to feel valued, useful, and productive continues. An older adult may develop new hobbies or increase involvement in community, church, or family affairs. He or she may do volunteer work or even launch into a new career. If an older adult cannot adjust and form new relationships, social isolation can become a problem. **Social isolation** is a sense of being alone and lonely because of fewer meaningful relationships. It may occur because of declining health or income, transportation problems, or ageism. Whatever the cause, prolonged social isolation has been correlated to declining health and higher mortality (Berkman, 1983).

Establishing Satisfactory Physical Living Arrangements The ability to function safely and independently at home depends a great deal on functional health, transportation, income, and family. An older adult, for example, may need assistance with home repairs, housecleaning, or grocery shopping. Architectural barriers, such as steps, may need to be modified. Easy access to medical and recreational facilities and churches may become more important. In urban areas, fear of crime may necessitate changes in living arrangements. Many older adults in poor health may be able to continue living at home with some assistance from visiting community nurses or with the aid of other services, such as home-delivered meals and senior transportation.

Most older adults prefer to live in their own homes. It is difficult to move from one's home. Moving in with adult children creates changes in roles and authority. When moving to an extended-care facility, such as a nursing home, the loss of one's home and, sometimes, possessions and the need to conform to the routines of institutional living can be traumatic for the client and family. Some people, however, choose to move for convenience, social relationships, or needed health care.

Retirement centers and senior citizens' housing have recently flourished. For those who need health care, alternative methods of care have become available. Examples of **alternative care** are respite care facilities, which allow the family a needed rest by temporarily housing and caring for an ailing older family member, and day-care centers, which provide a safe, stimulating environment during the day, when family members must work. The nurse must be knowledgeable about which health care and social services are available in the client's community so that the client and family can be informed. Thus, the nurse can effectively work with other members of the health care team to ensure that the client gets needed services.

Gerontology and the Health Care System

Knowledge of aging has increased dramatically in the past 40 years. **Gerontology** is the scientific and behavioral study of all aspects of aging and its consequences. Normal changes that occur with aging are the result of complex

RESEARCH IN NURSING Making a Difference

The Older Adult

As the population of North America continues to age, the health care needs of the older adult are increasingly a focus of nursing research. The studies described here are a representative sample that illustrate the recognition by nursing that the older adult requires interventions tailored to meet needs in both health and illness.

Related Research

Hardy, M. A. (1990). A pilot study of the diagnosis and treatment of impaired skin integrity: Dry skin in older persons. *Nursing Diagnosis, 1*(2), 57–63.

This pilot study of 15 elderly long-term care residents was conducted to identify indicators of dry skin as well as nursing interventions to treat dry skin in the older adult. Based on findings, Hardy suggested that flaking and scaling are valid indicators of dry skin, whereas a bathing intervention to promote moisture retention may be effective in treating dry skin.

Mitchell, G. J. (1990). The lived experience of taking life day-by-day in later life: Research guided by Parse's emergent method. *Nursing Science Quarterly, 3*(1), 29–36.

Taking life day by day as one ages is a common experience. Ten persons over age 75, living in Canada, were interviewed and discussed the meaning of this experience. Findings of the study support that taking life one day at a time is a way of living health that enhances one's quality of life as one grows older.

Naylor, M. D. (1990). Comprehensive discharge planning for hospitalized elderly: A pilot study. *Nursing Research, 39*(3), 156–161.

This study compared the effects of comprehensive discharge planning by a gerontologic nurse specialist with the hospital's general discharge planning procedure. Findings from the study reinforce the need for continued studies on the effect of comprehensive discharge planning for the older adult in terms of client length of stay, rehospitalization for care, and cost of care outcomes.

Lenihan, A. A. (1988). Identification of self-care behaviors in the elderly: A nursing assessment tool. *Journal of Professional Nursing, 4*(4), 285–288.

The purpose of this study was to develop and test a nursing assessment interview tool that would enable nurses to identify self-care practices of the elderly living at home. The author suggested that use of this tool in a national survey of noninstitutionalized elderly people would provide data about the prevalence of self-care practices and capacities among them. In turn, this would allow nurses to more effectively do discharge planning, provide community-based programs and services, and organize nursing practice and education around functional assessment and care planning for the older adult.

Summary

Research aimed at promoting wellness and optimal functioning at all levels of health and illness in the aging population is critical to nursing. A focus on self-care activities that promote physical and psychological health, as well as the development of specific nursing assessments and interventions to meet health care needs of the older adult, provides direction for future health promotion and illness prevention strategies.

interactions among genetics, biologic systems, and physical and social environments. Disease complicates a person's ability to adapt and maintain **functional health** (the ability to carry out usual and desired daily activities). Mental or physical decline in the older adult often may not be directly related to the aging process, but rather result from the absence of supportive care and services that could prevent disease and maintain the older adult's ability to function.

The aging population has greatly strained a health care system that has traditionally focused on cures and acute disease processes. For the older client with chronic disorders, the focus of care should include the client's and family's goals and promote functional health and independent

living to the greatest extent possible. Gerontologic, or gerontic, nursing does just that. **Gerontologic nursing** combines basic knowledge and skills of nursing with a specialized knowledge of aging in both illness and health (Fig. 12-6).

Meeting Health Care Needs of the Older Adult

As the population of older adults increases, nurses will be increasing the amount of time they spend providing care for this population. The older adult who requires care to prevent illness and promote wellness is found in all types of health care settings, including hospitals, long-term care facilities, emergency departments, outpatient surgeries,

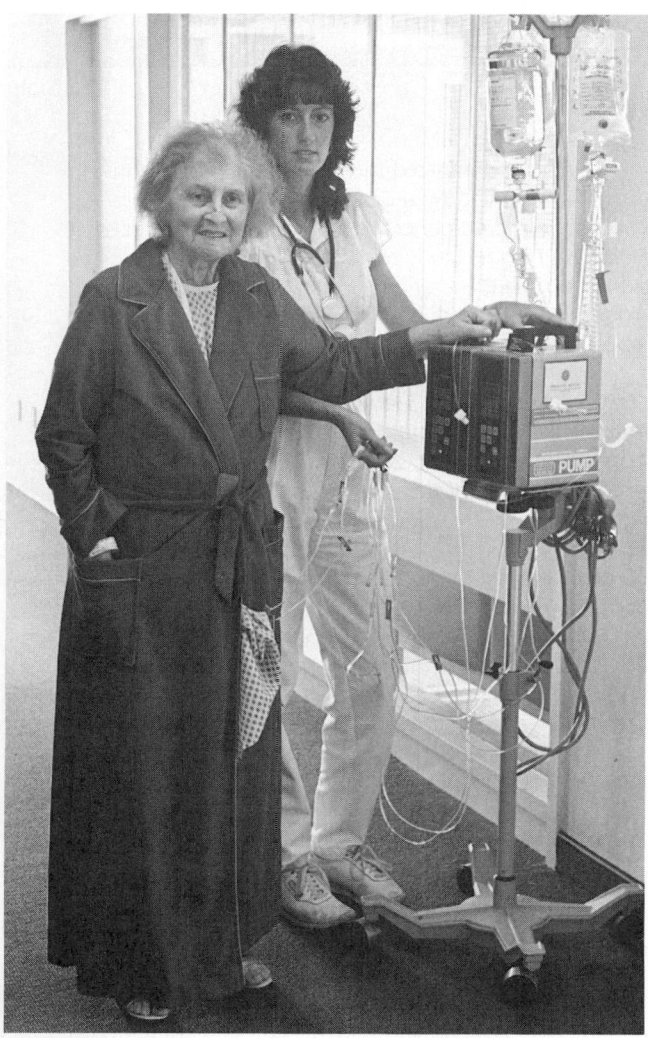

F I G U R E 1 2 - 6

The hospitalized older adult requires nursing interventions to prevent complications and to promote a return to wellness. (Photo by Denise Angelini, courtesy School of Nursing, University of Pennsylvania.)

and home health care agencies. The nursing care that is planned and implemented for the older adult should be based on the following factors (Eliopoulos, 1990, p. 11):
- Most elderly people are not impaired, but are functional in the community, thereby benefiting from wellness-oriented interventions.
- Elderly people are more vulnerable to physical, emotional, and socioeconomic problems than people in other age-groups, and may require special attention to health promotion and maintenance.

    This section provides a broad introduction to the health care needs of the older adult in terms of chronic illness, accidental injuries, and acute illness.

Chronic Illness and the Older Adult As a person ages, the probability and incidence of his or her becoming ill increase. One or more chronic illnesses occur in almost 90% of all older people (Eliopoulos, 1987). The most common illnesses are heart disease, cancer, hypertension, arthritis, and diabetes mellitus. Other causes of illness or disability include acute illnesses, such as fractures and pneumonia; motor vehicle accidents; and falls. These acute illnesses or accidents may cause chronic health problems.

    Although illness affects all dimensions of a person, no matter what age, older adults have to contend with a variety of problems as they live with chronic illness. Although aging is a normal process and chronic illness is a pathologic process, both often occur at the same time. The problems of aging and the problems of chronic illness interrelate to increase problems in all areas of one's life, including—but not limited to—self-care, life-style, economics, social factors, and living arrangements. Consider the following:
- Chronic illness limits activities in about 15% of the population, but almost 50% of adults over age 65 have limitations as a result of one or more chronic illnesses.
- Meeting the expense of health care often is difficult for older adults and their families. Medication costs with chronic illness continue for the rest of a person's life, with multiple medications being the rule rather than the exception. Hospitalization costs continue to rise, and the price of high-quality long-term care may well be beyond the client's or family members' ability to pay. In addition, special diets, special equipment, or medical supplies increase economic difficulties.
- Family members must learn how to cope with the needs of the ill person: Included are personal hygiene, medication administration, special diets, elimination, activities of daily living, and recognition of symptoms that necessitate medical attention. Family members also must adapt to psychological stressors in the form of changes in communications, changes in roles (for example, the elderly mother in effect becomes the child), and changes in their own life-style as they become the caregivers.

Injuries in the Older Adult As described by Myers and Sharpe (1990), injuries that occur in the older adult "are a serious problem in terms of mortality, morbidity, changes in level of self-care, suffering, length of hospitalization, costs, and quality of life" (p. 109). An older adult is at increased risk for accidental injury because of changes in vision and hearing, loss of mass and strength of muscles, slower reflexes and reaction time, and decreased sensory ability. In addition, the effects of chronic illness and medication may make an older adult more prone to accidental injuries.

    The older population of North America, with reduced income, often live in inadequate housing situated in neighborhoods with heavy traffic and high crime rates. They may be isolated from family members, and many live alone. Combined with normal changes of aging and the effects of any illness, elderly people not only are at increased risk, but

The first and most difficult client I ever encountered as a student was an elderly man who had chronic obstructive pulmonary disease. I entered his room to introduce myself and to explain that I would be his student nurse for the day. The client told me that the last thing he needed or wanted was a student nurse to "bother him all day." He went on to explain that he had already told his "real nurse" this and that I should go and "find another patient."

After leaving the room, the last thing I wanted to do was to enter it ever again. I went to the instructor and related to her what the client had said. She decided that it would be an educational experience for me to deal with this client and to remain his nurse. I took a few minutes to think about how I would explain this to the client, remain calm, and avoid bursting into tears.

I went back to the client's room. I told him that I was still his student nurse for the day, but I would come into his room only when I had to perform a task essential to his care. I then reassured him that his regular nurse also would be in to take care of him. The client appeared reassured and stopped mumbling under his breath.

I kept my promise and entered the room only when there was a purpose. The client remained terse and unfriendly the entire day, but when I told him I would be leaving for the day, he did say, "Thank you for every-thing. It wasn't as bad as I thought it was going to be." As I left for the day, I thought the same thing.

—Stacy A. Maillie, Delaware County Community College, Media, Pennsylvania

also have a more difficult time regaining health after an injury.

The most serious threats are injuries that result from falls. Falls may occur in the home, community, or health care institution. Hip fracture is the most common consequence of a fall, with surgery to repair the hip the most common surgery for people over age 75. Hip fracture and the resultant surgery mean that the person must be hospitalized, has increased risk for disability and death, and often has permanent limitations, even after recovery.

Acute Care Needs of the Older Adult An older adult who enters the hospital for surgery or acute care has special, age-related needs. These areas of concern, with related nursing actions, are outlined in Table 12-1, using functional health patterns as a framework.

Nursing Implications

Although specific nursing care adapted to the needs of the elderly client is described throughout this text, general implications for care are included here. The nurse must recognize physiologic and psychosocial interrelationships and view the older client holistically.

Illness can severely disrupt an older adult's ability to function independently. The ill client is under increased physical and emotional stress, which increases the risk for complications because of the lack of physiologic reserves. When a client is hospitalized or institutionalized, family and community interactions are severely inhibited. The acute-care environment itself adds new stressors, such as diagnostic tests, treatments, and surgery. In the face of new and unfamiliar routines and sensory stimulation, prior coping skills may not work, and an older client probably feels less able to understand and control the new environment. An elderly client is more likely than a younger client to suffer multisystem dysfunctions, *iatrogenic* complications caused by medications or treatments, accidents such as falls, and increasing dependence and confusion.

Major nursing care goals are to assist the elderly client to function as independently as possible and to continue to develop individual potentials. The nurse works with the family and other disciplines to prevent complications of illness, to secure a safe and comfortable environment, and to promote the client's return to wellness. General guidelines for nursing care are as follows:
- Maintain the client's physiologic reserves. Carefully assess the client so that complications caused by the stress on other body systems are discovered early.
- Prevent multisystem complications. Include nursing care that maintains physical integrity and function, such as skin care and planned rest and activity times.

TABLE 12-1

Meeting Needs of the Hospitalized Older Adult

Area of Concern	Nursing Actions
Health Perception and Health Management	
Health concerns	• Review with client perceptions of current health status, health problems, and medications taken.
Safety practices	• Age-related sensory deficits (eg, sight, hearing) and slower response times may require special safety practices to prevent injury. These may include leaving a light on at night and ensuring that call lights are answered immediately.
Nutrition and Metabolism	
Chewing ability	• Check to see if client has lost or damaged teeth; if he has dentures, check if they fit well and are available. Be sure that food is appropriate to client's ability to chew.
Dietary intake	• Assess height, weight, eating patterns, and food choices. The older adult is at risk for alterations in nutrition (either as excess weight or as malnutrition).
Elimination	
Bladder elimination	• Ask about frequency of urine elimination; reduced bladder capacity with aging can result in more frequent need to empty bladder. • Provide assistance as necessary, and ensure that floor is uncluttered, that toilet is easily accessible, that lighting is sufficient, and that call light is within reach. • The inability to control urine is not a normal age-related change. If client is incontinent of urine, perform further assessments.
Bowel elimination	• Changes in diet and activity, the effects of medications and surgery, and loss of privacy can all contribute to changes in bowel elimination. • Know client's normal time for bowel elimination, and assist with toileting. Provide privacy. • Ensure that diet (staying within ordered dietary guidelines) has necessary fluid and fiber content to promote normal elimination. If client does not eat well or complains of lack of appetite, assess for constipation.
Activity and Exercise	
Impaired activity	• Assess ability to walk; consider normal activity levels and any impairment from illness or surgery. If client uses a walker or cane at home, be sure assistive device is available. • Consider effects of illness, surgery, and medications on strength and motor function. Changes in nutrition, fluids, and electrolytes may increase fatigue and loss of strength (already decreased by age-related changes in cardiac output, lung changes, and degenerative changes in the musculoskeletal system).

• Provide a safe and uncluttered environment with comfortable temperatures and good lighting. If the environment is unfamiliar, orient the client to routines and equipment. Closely observe the client for his or her ability to protect against falls and other accidents.

• Slow your pace of care. Allow the client extra time to carry out activities, particularly those that require physical coordination, such as grooming and eating.

• Encourage independence. Do not help the client if your assistance benefits a time factor only. Keep your client and family informed and involved as much as possible.

• Beware of the stereotype of ageism. Treat each client as a unique person. Although many older clients have similar needs, factors such as background, interests, capabilities, values, and life-style may differ greatly.

• Promote continued development. Assist the client and family to accept physical limitations. Work with them to adapt the environment so that functional health is maintained. Ask yourself the following questions:
  • Does the client have obvious developmental lags that need to be further identified?
  • Is the client or family deprived of normal needs or activities because of institutionalization?
  • Is the client deprived of normal learning experiences because of physical or sensory limitations?
  • How can we help the client or family to find creative alternatives to accomplish developmental tasks?

• Be familiar with the resources available in your facility and community. Work with the health care team to provide assistance needed and desired by the client and family.

Area of Concern	Nursing Actions
Cognition and Perception	
Cognitive abilities	• Slow down pace of activity and wait for responses; although intellectual ability is not affected with age, reaction and response times often are. • Repeat teaching as many times as necessary, especially if short-term memory is impaired. • Assess levels of vision and hearing. If client wears glasses or hearing aid, be sure it is used. Ensure that glass lenses are clean and that hearing aid batteries are strong.
Sleep and Rest	
Sleep pattern changes	• Assess normal time of going to bed and getting up, bedtime rituals, number of hours slept, and nap schedule. Sleep may be impaired with hospitalization as a result of unfamiliar environment, pain, anxiety, and the effect of medications. • Encourage activity and exercise within ordered limits during the daytime. Discourage excessive naps.
Sexuality	
Perceptions of self as male or female	• One's sexual self-concept includes feelings about self as an attractive man or woman. Assist as necessary with hygiene, hair care, oral care, makeup, and clean bedclothes. Be sure environment is clean and odor-free.
Love and belonging	• Provide interventions that demonstrate genuine caring; ask preferred name, listen carefully, show respect for belongings, provide touch in various ways.
Coping and Stress	
Response to stress	• Be aware that illness and hospitalization are major stressors and may further impair the ability to recover from illness or injury. • Assess client's sources of strength and ensure that (as much as possible) those are available; include cultural and spiritual values and needs. • Encourage use of support systems, including family, friends, pets.
Self-Concept	
Altered self-concept	• Carry out interventions to maintain or improve physical function, and to maintain appearance. Illness, pain, and changes in grooming and dress can all lower self-esteem. • Encourage display of small photographs or personally relevant items that provide familiar components of one's life or life-style. • Set mutual goals with client as progress toward wellness is made. • Facilitate client's role as an active decision maker.

EXAMPLES OF NURSING DIAGNOSES

Older Adult

The following nursing diagnoses are examples of those that might be appropriate for the older adult client.
• Social Isolation related to lack of transportation and death of husband
• Self-Care Deficit: Toileting related to weakness and visual deficits
• Constipation related to lack of exercise and diet low in fiber

• Pain in Knee Joints related to degenerative arthritis
• High Risk for Injury related to cluttered environment, weakness, and sensory impairment
• Noncompliance in Taking Medication for High Blood Pressure related to adverse effects of medications
• Spiritual Distress related to inability to practice spiritual rituals while in the hospital

KEY POINTS

- Aging is a gradual process. Older adulthood is characterized by continued development and adaptation. The older adult population is the most unique and diversified group in our society.
- Ageism is a form of prejudice in which the older adult is incorrectly stereotyped as being different from other members of society. Also, aging is not synonymous with disease.
- Most older adults adjust well to aging and continue to live active, independent, and productive lives. Most older adults regard themselves as healthy, although almost 90% have one or more chronic disorders.
- The spouse and family are natural support systems who typically help the older adult maintain health and independence.
- Gerontologic nursing is a specialty field within the nursing profession, with specialized knowledge of aging in both health and illness that can benefit all nurses.
- In older adulthood, physiologic aging becomes more rapid, with all organ systems showing decline in efficiency. The lack of physiologic reserves places the elderly client at risk for multisystem complications.
- The older adult continues to learn and problem solve; intelligence and personality remain consistent after middle age.
- According to Erikson, ego-integrity versus despair is the last stage of human development. The older adult continues to look forward but also reflects back on life experiences to find meaning and acceptance.
- Havighurst views the major tasks of older adulthood to be primarily concerned with social relationships and roles.
- A major goal of nursing care is to help the client promote functional health; the nurse does this by working with the client, family, and health care team.

BIBLIOGRAPHY

American Association of Retired Persons. (1990). *A Profile of Older Americans, 1990.* Washington, DC: Program Resources Dept., AARP, Pub. No. PF3049 (1290), D996.

American Nurse's Association. (1976). *Standards for gerontological nursing practice.* Kansas City, MO: Author.

Beam, I. M. (1984). Alzheimer's disease: Helping families survive. *American Journal of Nursing, 84*(12), 228–232.

Berkman, L. F. (1983). The assessment of social networks and social support in the elderly. *Journal of the American Geriatric Society, 31*(12), 228–232.

Berry, A. L., & Davignon, D. R. (1991). Changes with age. In M. Patrick, S. Woods, R. Craven, R. Rokosky, & P. Bruno (Eds.). *Medical–surgical nursing: Pathophysiological concepts* (2nd ed.). Philadelphia: Lippincott.

Boynton, P. R. (1989). Health maintenance alteration: A nursing diagnosis of the elderly. *Clinical Nurse Specialist, 3*(1), 5–10.

Burggraf, V., & Dolan, B. (1985). Assessing the elderly: System by system. *American Journal of Nursing, 85,* 974–984.

Burke, M. M., & Walsh, M. B. (1992). *Gerontologic nursing: Care of the frail elderly.* St. Louis: Mosby–Year Book.

Costa, P. T., McCrae, R. R., & Norris, A. H. (1981). Personal adjustment to aging: Longitudinal prediction from neuroticism to extraversion. *Journal of Gerontological Nursing, 36,* 78–85.

Dychtwald, K. (1986). *Wellness and health promotion for the elderly.* Rockville, MD: Aspen.

Ebersole, P., & Hess, P. (1991). *Toward healthy aging: Human needs and nursing responses* (3rd ed.). St. Louis: Mosby.

Eliopoulos, C. (1987a). *Gerontological nursing* (2nd ed.). Philadelphia: Lippincott.

Eliopoulos, C. (1987b). *A guide to the nursing of the aging.* Baltimore: Williams & Wilkins.

Eliopoulos, C. (1990). *Caring for the elderly in diverse care settings.* Philadelphia: Lippincott.

Erikson, E. (1980). *Identity and the life cycle.* New York: Norton.

Fuller, J., & Schaller-Ayers, J. (1990). *Health assessment: A nursing approach.* Philadelphia: Lippincott.

Gallagher, L. P., & Kreidler, M. C. (1987). *Nursing and health: Maximizing human potential throughout the life cycle.* Norwalk, CT: Appleton & Lange.

Golightly, C. D., Bossenmaier, M. M., McChesney, J. A., Williams, B. S., & Wyble, S. J. (1984). Planning to meet the needs of the hospitalized elderly. *Journal of Nursing Administration, 14*(5), 29–39.

Hardy, M. A. (1990). A pilot study of the diagnosis and treatment of impaired skin integrity: Dry skin in older persons. *Nursing Research, 1*(2), 57–63.

Havighurst, R. J. (1972). *Developmental tasks and education* (3rd ed.). New York: Longman.

Hawranik, P., & Kondratuk, B. (1986). Depression in the elderly. *Canadian Nurse, 82*(9), 30–34.

Hendricks, J., & Hendricks, C. D. (1986). *Aging in mass society: Myths and realities* (3rd ed.). Boston: Little, Brown.

Kovar, M. G. (1986). Aging in the eighties: Preliminary data from the supplement on aging to the national health interview survey. *Vital and Health Statistics of the National Center for Health Statistics,* No. 115, January/June, 1984.

Lenihan, A. A. (1988). Identification of self-care behaviors in the elderly: A nursing assessment tool. *Journal of Professional Nursing, 4*(4), 285–288.

Matteson, M. A., & McConnell, E. S. (1988). *Gerontological nursing: Concepts and practice*. Philadelphia: Saunders.

Mattice, M., & Mitchell, G. J. (1990). Caring for confused elders. *Canadian Nurse, 86*(11), 16–18.

Mitchell, G. J. (1990). The lived experience of taking life day-by-day in later life: Research guided by Parse's emergent method. *Nursing Science Quarterly, 3*(1), 29–36.

Myers, A. H., & Sharpe, A. (1990). Risks and prevention. In C. Eliopoulos (Ed.). *Caring for the elderly in diverse care settings* (pp. 110–145). Philadelphia: Lippincott.

Nagley, S. J. (1986). Predicting and preventing confusion in your patients. *Journal of Gerontological Nursing, 12*(3), 27–31.

Naylor, M. D. (1990). Comprehensive discharge planning for hospitalized elderly: A pilot study. *Nursing Research, 39*(3), 156–161.

Rice, E. M. (1989). Contributing factors to confusion in the hospitalized elderly. *Advancing Clinical Care*, May/June, 8–14.

Schuster, C. S., & Ashburn, S. S. (1986). *The process of human development: A holistic life-span approach* (2nd ed.). Boston: Little, Brown.

Seymour, M. (1991). Too old for care. *Canadian Nurse, 87*(11), 26–27.

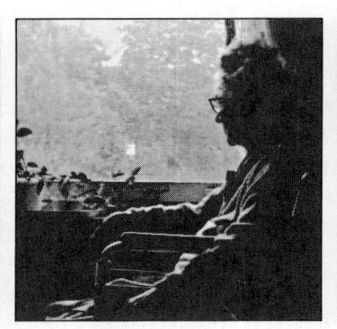
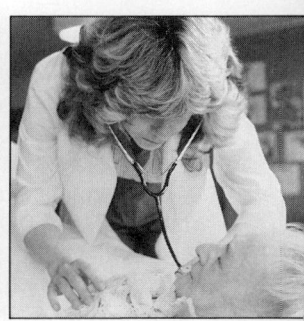
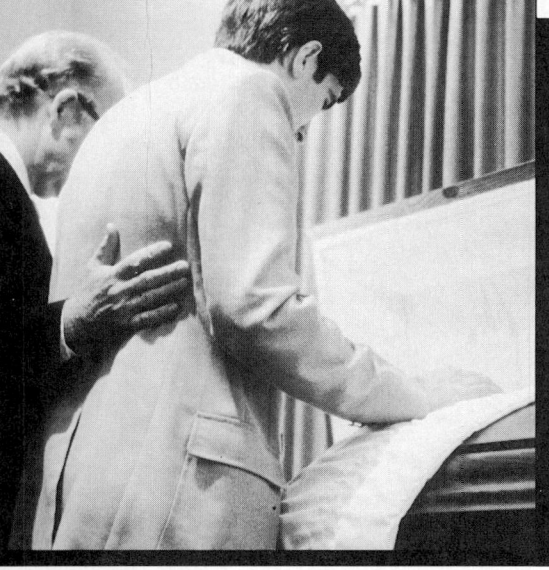

Loss, Grief, and Death

13

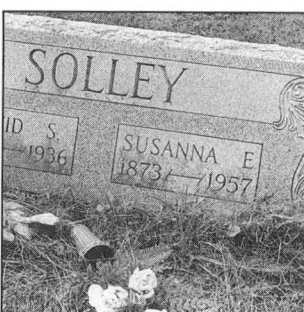

There is the potential for loss, grief, and death at any stage of one's life. This is especially true for a person who experiences alterations of health and for his family. A wide variety of losses may occur, including loss of a body part or function, loss of one's ability to care for oneself, loss of one's role as head of a family, and death, which may be the most difficult loss of all. This chapter is included as part of the section on human development because at some point in each person's life, loss will be experienced and can affect the developmental stages of life.

Death often is as difficult for health care providers as it is for the surviving family members. The goals of health care focus on health maintenance and health restoration, with an emphasis on facilitating maximum potential in wellness. One of the functions of the nurse is, however, to facilitate coping with disability and death. The nurse often is the key person in providing support and care when loss or death occurs. To provide effective care, the nurse must have accepted his or her own feelings about death, and understand the stages of grieving and dying.

Loss and Grieving

Loss

Loss occurs when a valued person, object, or situation is changed or made inaccessible so that its value is diminished or removed. There are several types of loss, all of which may be experienced at some time by everyone. **Actual loss** can be recognized by others as well as by the person sustaining the loss; loss of a limb, of a spouse, of a valued object such as money, and of a job are all examples of actual loss. **Perceived loss** is felt by the person but is intangible to others; loss of youth, of financial independence, and of a valued environment are examples of perceived loss. Directly related to actual and perceived loss are **physical loss** and **psychological loss**. A person who loses an arm in an automobile accident suffers from both the physical loss of the arm and the psychological loss that may be caused by an altered self-image and the inability to return to his or her occupation. These losses are simultaneously physical, psychological, and actual. A person who is scarred but does not lose a limb may suffer a perceived and psychological loss of self-image.

Another type of loss is **anticipatory loss**, in which a person displays loss and grief behaviors for a loss that has yet to take place. Anticipatory loss often is seen in families of terminally ill clients, and serves to lessen the impact of the actual loss of a family member.

Loss can have a tremendous impact on a person's development, and age affects a person's reaction to loss (see Factors Affecting Grief, later in this chapter). Although most adults can accept death on an intellectual level, they may have trouble dealing with it on an emotional level. The loss of a friend, a pet, or a job may help a person anticipate and cope with the loss of a spouse or other loved one.

Grieving

Grieving is the emotional reaction to loss. It occurs with loss caused by separation as well as with loss caused by death. Many people who divorce experience grief, and loss of a body part, a job, a house, or a pet may cause grief. **Bereavement** is the state of grieving during which a person goes through grief reaction. **Mourning** is the period of acceptance of loss and grief during which the person learns to deal with the loss.

Bereavement, which is experienced by both the client and the family, may have profound health consequences that require additional care. Bereaved people often neglect their health to an extreme, whereas mourning is characterized by a return to more normal living habits.

Grief Reactions   **Grief** is the emotional pain caused by a loss. Reactions to both grief and dying are similar. The stages of these reactions overlap and vary among individuals. One person may skip a reaction stage, whereas another may repeat an earlier stage. Each person is different, and clients and family members may be at different reaction stages.

Engel (1964) was among the first to define stages of grief. Engel's six stages are (1) shock and disbelief, (2) developing awareness, (3) restitution, (4) resolving the loss, (5) idealization, and (6) outcome. *Shock and disbelief* usually are defined as refusal to accept the fact of loss, followed by a stunned or numb response: "No, not me." *Developing awareness* is characterized by physical and emotional responses such as anger, feeling empty, and crying: "Why me?" *Restitution* involves the rituals surrounding loss, and with death includes religious, cultural, or social expressions of mourning, such as funeral services. *Resolving the loss* is dealing with the void left by the loss, and *idealization* is the exaggeration of the good qualities of the person or object lost, followed by acceptance of the loss and a lessened need to focus on it. *Outcome* is the final resolution of the grief process, including dealing with loss as a common life occurrence.

Kübler-Ross (1969), considered a pioneer in the study of grief and death reactions, defined five stages of reaction similar to those of Engel: (1) denial and isolation, (2) anger, (3) bargaining, (4) depression, and (5) acceptance. Kübler-Ross's work is discussed in greater depth under "Stages

205

Grief and Death Reactions

Engel's Six Stages of Grief Reactions

1. Shock and disbelief
2. Developing awareness
3. Restitution
4. Resolving the loss
5. Idealization
6. Outcome

Five Stages of Kübler-Ross' Grief and Death Reactions

1. Denial and isolation
2. Anger
3. Bargaining
4. Depression
5. Acceptance

---

of Dying," later in this chapter. Other works in the grief process literature include that of Clark (1984), who describes three stages of grief, and Martocchio (1985), who describes five grief groupings. More important than the actual stages of any given grief reaction is the idea that grief *is* a process and that it varies from person to person.

Normal Versus Dysfunctional Grief Both normal and dysfunctional grief may be delayed, and normal grief may be either abbreviated or anticipatory. *Abbreviated grief* is of short duration but is genuine; *anticipatory grief* occurs before the actual loss, as in the extended terminal illness of a family member. **Dysfunctional grief** is abnormal or distorted; it may be either unresolved or inhibited. In *unresolved grief*, a person may have trouble expressing feelings of loss or may deny them; unresolved grief also describes a state of bereavement that extends over a lengthy period. In *inhibited grief*, a person suppresses feelings of grief and may instead manifest somatic symptoms.

Factors That Affect Grief and Death

Many factors, including age, family relationships, socioeconomic position, and cultural and religious influences, affect a person's reaction to and expression of grief, and like the stages of grief reaction, they vary from person to person.

Developmental Considerations Children do not understand death on the same level as adults do, but their sense of loss is just as great. Both terminally ill children and their siblings are more likely to talk and ask questions about

death in an attempt to understand it (Foster, Hunsberger, & Anderson, 1989). Terminally ill children of all ages require parental love and support, as well as social interaction with other children. Death of a parent or another significant person can retard a child's development or may cause the child to regress developmentally; children need to go through the same grief reactions as adults do to accept such a loss and maintain emotional well-being.

The loss of a parent by a middle-aged adult helps to prepare the adult for the loss of a spouse or significant other and to accept his or her own eventual death. Elderly people may lose a spouse, or friends and relatives their own age. As this happens, they reminisce about life, put their lives and the purpose of living in perspective, and prepare themselves for their own inevitable death.

Family Roles within families are important factors that affect reactions to and expressions of grief. For example, the eldest sibling may feel a need to "be strong," and therefore may not grieve openly; a person who loses a spouse may display the same type of behavior to "protect the children."

The death of a child usually is a devastating experience for her or his family. The family needs time to accept the reality of the situation, opportunities to talk and to be listened to, and the experience of expressing themselves behaviorally in a nonjudgmental environment. The family of a terminally ill child may express feelings of guilt for wondering if they were responsible for the impending death. A sibling may suppress a guilt feeling for having wished the ill child (or a parent) dead.

Socioeconomic Factors A bereaved family may suffer more acutely if there is no health or life insurance or pension after the death of the family provider. Such families face not only the loss of a loved one, but also an economic loss that may further disrupt family life. Elderly people especially may be placed in a difficult position, since the death of a spouse may result in a source of retirement income for the surviving spouse being either diminished or cut off. This reduction in income may lead to loss of home, community, and support systems.

Cultural Influences Both the physical and the emotional manifestations of grief may be culturally influenced. Schulz (1978) defined the clinical symptoms of grief as repeated somatic distress, tightness in the chest, choking or shortness of breath, sighing, empty feeling in the abdomen, loss of muscle power, and intense subjective distress. Other symptoms include vomiting, dizziness, fainting, fatigue, weight loss, headaches, and chest pains (Gonda & Ruark, 1984).

Culture also influences a person's expression of grief. In many families in the Western culture, grief is a private matter that is shared only with the family. As such, many people internalize their feelings of grief and may not express their grief or feelings of loss to others. On the other hand, cultural background may necessitate that the client's and family's public display be emotional and distressed, with loud weeping and moaning.

Although sex roles have become more unified in the past few decades, male and female reaction to death may differ. The widow who has a job may not be as emotionally distraught as the woman who has needed her husband for support. Likewise, the widower who has not taken care of the children or the house may view the future more bleakly than the man who has cooked meals and changed diapers. Some ethnic traditions may be ingrained in certain people, and the woman may be expected to be weak and need support, whereas the man may be expected to be emotionally supportive. This varies from culture to culture and from person to person.

Religious Influences Faith and religious practices play an important role in the expression of grief, and provide comfort and solace to the person experiencing loss. Many people who have put spiritual matters in the background of their lives have found death to be an impetus for a return to earlier practices of religion. At the same time, others may blame God for the death of their loved one and turn away from God.

Cause of Death Death may result from various causes, and the grief response often depends on the cause. Many deaths are sudden and involve shock as well as normal grieving in the survivors. *Death from disease* generates several types of response, including belief that the death is a punishment (for example, when acquired immunodefi-

ciency syndrome was first diagnosed in homosexuals and drug users), terror and panic (when people are reminded of the devastation caused by plagues of earlier centuries), and guilt (when family and friends believe that they could have prevented the death). *Accidental death* often is associated with feelings of bad luck. The guilt response can be enormous, especially when children die as the result of an accident. *Death while defending a country* usually is viewed by most of society as honorable and necessary. *Violent deaths* occur daily, especially in the larger cities of North America. Suicide accounts for a great number of violent deaths; in fact, among teenagers, it has become a major concern. It also is believed that many accidental deaths are actually suicides.

Dying

Needs of the Dying

A client who is dying has various options available about care before and after death. See the Dying Person's Bill of Rights in the display. A client's wishes should, if possible, be followed. She or he may choose to die at home, in a hospital or nursing home, or in a hospice (discussed in Chap. 3). The client and the family should take an active role in planning for care. Such planning takes the client's preferences into consideration, facilitates the acceptance of death by the client and the family, and provides interventions to meet holistic needs.

The Dying Person's Bill of Rights

I have the right to be treated as a living human being until I die.

I have the right to maintain a sense of hopefulness however changing its focus may be.

I have the right to be cared for by those who can maintain a sense of hopefulness, however changing this might be.

I have the right to express my feelings and emotions about my approaching death in my own way.

I have the right to participate in decisions concerning my care.

I have the right to expect continuing medical and nursing attention even though "cure" goals must be changed to "comfort" goals.

I have the right not to die alone.

I have the right to be free from pain.

I have the right to have my questions answered honestly.

I have the right not to be deceived.

I have the right to have help from and for my family in accepting my death.

I have the right to die in peace and dignity.

I have a right to retain my individuality and not be judged for my decisions which may be contrary to beliefs of others.

I have the right to discuss and enlarge my religious and/or spiritual experiences, whatever these may mean to others.

I have the right to expect that the sanctity of the human body will be respected after death.

I have the right to be cared for by caring, sensitive, knowledgeable people who will attempt to understand my needs and will be able to gain some satisfaction in helping me face my death.

(Created at the workshop *The Terminally Ill Patient and the Helping Person*, in Lansing, Michigan, sponsored by the Southwestern Michigan Inservice Education Council and conducted by Amelia J. Barbus, Associate Professor of Nursing, Wayne State University, Detroit.)

Impact of Terminal Illness

Diagnosis In the case of a **terminal illness**, the physician usually is responsible for deciding what and how much the client should be told. The nurse, social worker, clergyman, or others in the service professions may be involved with this decision and in discussing the client's condition with him or her. Most clients want to know their prognosis as soon as possible, so that they can both come to grips with it and take care of business and personal affairs. All who are involved with the client's care should know exactly what the client and the family have been told; members of the client's health care team need to communicate among themselves.

Impact on Client Many clients realize without being told that they are suffering from a terminal illness; this realization often is picked up from nonverbal communication by their families and by health care professionals. Clients must be allowed to go through the stages of the grieving process and to make decisions about their care, and be supported in all decisions. An adult client has the right to refuse treatment and should be offered this option.

Impact on Family The family of a terminally ill client should be encouraged to participate in planning the client's care. Health care personnel should be available to discuss the client's condition with family members and should offer support and care as the family begins the grieving process. The family may want to make arrangements with the client for funeral or memorial services; this is contingent on which stage of grief both client and family members have progressed to.

Stages of Dying

Although each person reacts to the knowledge of impending death or to loss in his or her own way, there are similarities in the psychosocial responses to the situation. World-renowned authority Dr. Elisabeth Kübler-Ross has studied the emotional responses to death and dying in depth, and her findings have been used extensively by the nursing and other helping professions.

The stages of dying, much like the stages of grief, may overlap, and the duration of any stage may range from as little as a few hours to as long as a period of months. The process varies from person to person. Some people may be in one stage for such a short time that it seems as if they skipped that stage. Sometimes a person returns to a previous stage.

According to Kübler-Ross, the stages of dying are (1) denial and isolation, (2) anger, (3) bargaining, (4) depression, and (5) acceptance.

Denial and isolation: In the denial and isolation stage, the client denies that he or she will die, may repress what is discussed, and may isolate self from reality. The client may think, "They made a mistake in the diagnosis. Maybe they mixed my records with someone else's."

Anger: The client expresses rage and hostility in the anger stage and adopts a "why me?" attitude. "Why me? I quit smoking and I watched what I ate. Why did this happen to me?"

Bargaining: The client tries to barter for more time. "If I can just make it to my son's graduation I will be satisfied. Just let me live until then." Many clients put their personal affairs in order, make wills, and fulfill last wishes, such as trips, visiting relatives, and so forth. It is important to meet these wishes, if possible, because bargaining helps clients move into later stages of dying.

Depression: In the depression stage, the client goes through a period of grief before death. The grief is characterized by crying and not speaking much. "I waited all these years to see my daughter get married. And now I may not be here to see her walk down the aisle. I can't bear the thought of not being there for the wedding—and to see my grandchildren."

Acceptance: When the stage of acceptance is reached, the client feels tranquil. She or he has accepted death and is prepared to die. The client may think, "I've tied up all the loose ends—made the will, made arrangements for my daughter to live with her grandparents. Now I can go in peace knowing everyone will be fine."

Meeting the Needs of Grieving and Dying People

The nurse's aims in caring for the dying client and the grieving family include facilitating coping of the dying person and family and promoting wellness and preventing illness of the family. Nursing care to facilitate coping and promote wellness is outlined and summarized in the display titled Nursing Care to Facilitate Coping in Grief and Death.

Clarifying One's Own Feelings

Holistic care of the terminally ill client and family almost always involves some personal emotional investment. It is unrealistic and unfair to expect nurses to handle circumstances surrounding death without feelings. The best policy seems to be taking the time to explore one's own feelings and express them. The nurse who neglects to deal with personal feelings about life, dying, and death is in a questionable position to analyze and consider the needs of clients facing death. Therefore, a nurse's own feelings play a major role in determining how he or she cares for a client with a terminal illness. The following are some personal questions the nurse should use to help clarify feelings about finiteness of self:

• If I could control the events that result in my own death, where would I want to be? What cause of death

Nursing Care to Facilitate Coping in Grief and Death

- Assess the knowledge base of the client and family pertaining to the client's illness and previous care. Determine their perception of the present situation, strengths, and weaknesses.
- Assess the client and family for strengths and weaknesses and use these in planning care.
- Assess coping behaviors and priorities of needs.
- Use information gathered during family assessment to plan client care and anticipate potential family concerns.
- Encourage the client and family to take an active role in planning and providing care.
- Let your genuine concern and caring show. Do not be afraid to cry with the client and family.
- Encourage questions and respond positively.
- Meet with the family before the client arrives in the unit. Describe the environment and equipment being used for other clients as well. Reinforce that equipment is present for prevention and early detection of problems.
- Remain with the family during the first visit to provide additional information and support.
- Plan with the health care team to be consistent in discussions with client and family as to terminology and what and how much is being said.
- Use simple terminology in explaining care, treatment, and progress. Do not use generalizations.
- Maintain good communications at all times. Use both verbal and nonverbal communication in assessing and giving care and be an understanding listener.
- Develop a trusting relationship between the client and family and self.
- Be patient in explaining the condition, treatment, and progress of the client. Sometimes information must be repeated or information sessions must be divided.
- Be as realistic as possible, being aware of coping mechanisms and needs for hope.
- Encourage independence as long as possible. Be creative in finding self-care activities for the client.
- Encourage the family to bring pictures and other familiar and favorite items from home.
- Support the client psychologically by being present, by listening, and by touching.
- Arrange for visits by the client and family's spiritual advisor, if desired. Pray with the client, if asked, and discuss faith and beliefs if appropriate.
- Consider the client as a unique individual and special to the family when discussing issues.
- Ensure the family that the best possible care is being given to the client. Emphasize that the health care personnel are experienced and have special training to provide expert care.

- Give regular progress reports to family and notify them of changes in the client's condition.
- Review the agency's policy for visiting hours to determine if it is adequate for the family.
- Suggest simple things the family can do to provide care for the client.
- Remind family members to take care of themselves: eat, rest, and exercise. Tell them where the chapel is, if appropriate.
- Indicate a place where family members may relax if they must leave the client's room during nursing care or so the client can sleep.
- Help the family to understand the needs and emotions of the dying person.
- Prepare the family for the client's death by discussing the normalcy of the grieving process.
- Allow the client to go through the stages of dying and the family to go through the stages of grief. Accept these stages and do not be judgmental. Offer support where needed.
- Support the family as adjustments in roles are made. Be prepared to make referrals and suggest support groups when needed.
- If the prognosis is poor, allow adequate time to be with the family. Establish time to meet again.
- Meet with family and physician to discuss extraordinary measures and advanced life-support systems.
- Speak to the client (including the comatose client) when performing care.
- Encourage the family to discuss among themselves or with the client ethical and legal concerns, organ donations, support systems, the will, and the funeral arrangements.
- Discuss follow-up visits with the family before the death. Set a date for such visits after the death.
- On the client's death, encourage the family to express their feelings, but do not tell them what they should feel and do.
- Perform nursing responsibilities: care of the body, ensuring the attending physician's signature is on the death certificate, placing identification tags on the body and shroud. Tags are also placed on dentures and eyeglasses.
- Provide sympathetic support to the family. Do not rush them out of the hospital. Provide a private place for them to begin their grieving, especially in sudden deaths.
- Allow the family to talk about the person as much as they want to. Encourage them to discuss special qualities and memories.
- Reassure them they did everything they could and that the medical care was the best. State other true and positive things about care.

(Assembled and adapted from a variety of sources, including Bouman, C. [1984]. Identifying priority concerns of families of ICU patients. *Dimensions in Critical Care Nursing, 3*[5] 316–317; and Schmidt, I. [1979]. *Parent Bereavement Outreach*. Santa Monica, California.)

would I choose? Whom would I want to have present during my terminal illness?

- What fears do I have about death?
- How would I answer these same questions for a client for whom I have been caring?
- How could I improve the quality of care for a terminally ill client for whom I am caring?
- If I were a member of the client's family, what things would I want a nurse to do for me?

Assessing Needs

The nursing process, discussed in Unit IV, is a helpful tool in the nursing care of a dying client and the grieving family. Before client and family needs (Table 13-1) are met, the nurse must assess for strengths and weaknesses in coping and in relationships.

The nurse assesses the knowledge base of the client and family. If this is a chronic illness, how have they dealt with its problems in the past? What do they know about the disease process, the treatment, and the prognosis? Each family member is assessed for reactions to the illness or death, recognizing the individual differences mentioned earlier. Which stage of grieving is each in?

Each person can be cared for according to the individual stage, remembering that all stages are normal and acceptable for a period of time. The reaction process is a highly personal one, and the nurse should not try to force movement from one stage to another.

The nurse determines whether the client and family have developed good coping behaviors. Is the coping functional or dysfunctional? Coping mechanisms are discussed in Chapter 9.

Explaining the Client's Condition and Treatment

All involved health care personnel should know exactly what the client and family have been told. Telling them different things puts the nurse and other team members at cross purposes and sets up distrust in the family. Because clients and families often direct questions about the client's prognosis to the nurse, it is up to the nurse to take the initiative in determining a means to be consistent in terminology, prognosis, and description of progress.

The client's condition and treatment should be explained to both the client and the family. Patience is required during explanations. They may be so grieved by the diagnosis that they do not hear all the information that is shared with them. The nurse can question them to learn how much they have retained. Then the information they missed can be repeated. Care options, as well as the expected outcomes of each option, should be fully explained.

Providing Open Communication

Communication is a lifelong need up to the moment of death and should be maintained at all times with the client and family.

T A B L E   1 3 - 1

Needs of Grieving Families	
Hope	• That the best care possible will be provided for their loved one • That there is a place after death where suffering and pain cease
Participating	• In some way in what is happening • By giving some form of care • By feeling free to either stay at or leave the bedside • By sharing in mutual decision making with the health care staff and the loved one
Being informed	• By the medical and nursing staff on a regular basis • So that choices and decisions can be made • And having the right to ask questions
Support	• By having fears and concerns acknowledged, accepted, and understood • So that anger, tears, denial, and decisions are accepted • In coping with change • To allow feelings of closeness and openness with the one who is dying
Spiritual needs	• To be comforted by those who share a common faith • To have prayer as a support • To gain strength and comfort from God and from others

(Data from Carson, V. B. [1989]. *Spiritual dimensions of nursing practice*. Philadelphia: Saunders.)

To develop meaningful communications, the nurse must develop a trusting relationship with the client. This relationship is explored throughout this text. The nurse needs to develop listening skills and the ability to recognize both verbal and nonverbal cues given by the client and family. These skills are discussed in Chapter 20.

The nurse should be willing to openly discuss the client's fears and doubts and to serve as a nonjudgmental listener. A caring nurse feels at ease in crying with the grieving person and sharing experiences with fears, loneliness, and death. This allows the griever the freedom to express his or her deepest concerns. Nonverbal communication is equally important. A smile, a touching hand or stroke, and eye-to-eye contact are all meaningful. The warmth behind the gesture and the honest concern of the nurse are what count.

The sense of hearing is believed to be the last sense to leave the body; many clients retain a sense of hearing almost to the moment of death. It is kind and thoughtful of the nurse to speak to the comatose client and to encourage family members to do likewise. The nurse should explain to the client the nursing care being given and the noises in the unit.

Promoting Self-Care and Self-Esteem

The client should be encouraged to retain independence and decision making as long as possible. If strong enough, the client should be allowed to help with light housekeeping and kitchen duties early in the course of care. Personal hygiene practices and self-feeding also should be managed by the client as long as possible. Once the client is confined to bed, the creative nurse and family should attempt to find self-care activities the client can perform. When physical abilities fail, determining when to take medication, for example, may be all the control the client can retain.

Having familiar objects in view can help make the client feel more comfortable and secure. Whether the client is at home or in a health care agency, it is desirable to have the environment reflect personal preferences. This gives the client some degree of control when health and other activities of daily living have slipped out of the client's reach, and supports self-esteem.

Allowing Family Members to Assist in Care

Allowing family members to assist in nursing care can be beneficial to both the client and the family members: The client is comforted by having loved ones near, and family members are comforted by knowing that they helped comfort the client. Family members providing nursing care to the client must be supervised by the nurse.

Family members may not want to provide care themselves but want to know what to expect and how they can psychologically aid the client. The nurse can help by explaining the client's condition, what treatment the client is undergoing, and what result the family can expect from the treatment. Knowing the facts may help family members to better cope with impending loss.

Meeting Client Needs

Physiologic Needs *Physiologic care* of the client involves meeting physical needs such as personal hygiene, pain control, nutritional and fluid needs, movement, elimination, and respiratory care. *Personal hygiene* includes cleanliness of the skin, hair, mouth, nose, and eyes. Frequent baths and linen changes may be necessary. The mouth and nose should be kept free of mucus, and secretions should be wiped from the eyes. The physician will determine the medication and dosage needed for *pain control*, but the client's wishes should be considered. (See Chap. 32 for a further discussion of pain control.) Some clients prefer and are able to control their own medication. Many dying clients suffer from malnutrition and dehydration, so *nutritional and fluid needs* must be addressed. The client may require intravenous feeding but should be encouraged to take sips of water if still able to swallow. Periodic *movement* also should be allowed; regular changes of position help prevent decubitus ulcers. Problems with *elimination* include the development of incontinence, constipation, and urinary retention. Absorbent pads or a nearby bedpan may be used for incontinent clients; laxatives or enemas may be used for relieving constipation; and catheterization may be required for urinary retention. Bed linens should be changed often. *Respiratory care* can be provided by repositioning the conscious client in semi-Fowler's position; the unconscious client should be positioned in a semiprone position that allows drainage of saliva and mucus. Oxygen therapy may be necessary for some clients.

Psychological Needs When people speak of their fears of death, responses typically include fear of the unknown, pain, separation, leaving loved ones, loss of dignity, loss of control, and unfinished business. Kübler-Ross believes that there is still another, more overwhelming and more significant fear that often is repressed and unconscious: that of the catastrophic destructive force that has befallen a person and that the person cannot change. Kübler-Ross points out that terminally ill people communicate this fear of a destructive force but do so largely through symbolic language. A person may use nonverbal language, such as a facial expression, a particular kind of hand clasp, or, in the case of children, through drawings and manner of play with toys. Verbal communication also may be used symbolically.

A fear of isolation, of having to face death alone, is a primary concern of the dying client. The nurse supports the client by indicating his or her presence, giving full attention, and showing that he or she cares. The presence of family members in the room should be encouraged. Reminiscences should be shared.

Spiritual Needs Many terminally ill clients find great comfort in the support they receive from their religious faiths. The nurse should aid in obtaining the services of clergy as each situation indicates.

Although not all clients follow specific spiritual or religious beliefs, most require some form of *spiritual care*. Most clients need to feel that their lives have meaning; many feel a need for hope in the face of death. The nurse should not impose his or her beliefs on the client, but should let the client know that the client's beliefs are important. The nurse should arrange for visits from a spiritual adviser if this is desired. Spiritual needs are discussed more fully in Chapter 41.

Meeting Family Needs

The nurse can provide care for the *family facing loss* by listening to the family's concerns. Family members need to verbalize their worries and fears, and nurses and other health care personnel can provide support by being non-judgmental listeners. Likewise, nursing care of the *grieving family* involves communication and listening. Application of communication skills discussed in Chapter 20 and earlier in this section aids the nurse in being a nonjudgmental listener; feedback to the family can be provided by summarizing or paraphrasing, without questioning the validity of the family's emotions. All family members, including children, should be part of the grieving process.

In some instances, the nurse spends more time with the relatives than with the client, such as when the client becomes comatose. Family members may need to be reminded to get rest and to eat. Too many visitors may tire the client, and when explanations are offered, most relatives readily understand this. When they want to remain at the hospital, they should be directed to a quiet place where they may relax.

THROUGH THE EYES OF A STUDENT

Before witnessing the death of a client for the first time, I thought I had it all figured out. I had thought about it carefully and decided that I would be able to view death in a rational and clinical manner. I was still worried about it, though, because I knew that my emotions might override even my best rational thinking.

Mrs. Gram was a client on the urology floor where I was doing my medical–surgical clinical rotation. She was being treated for extensive complications of long-term, untreated diabetes mellitus. She was unable to communicate, but I sensed by her eye contact that she was aware of what was going on around her. It was nearly the end of our clinical day when I heard shouting coming from Mrs. Gram's room. As nurses and students poured into the room, I took my place, out of the way, to watch and listen. I wasn't ready for the barrage of thoughts and feelings that hit me in the next five minutes. Mrs. Gram had died—that was clear. The shouting was that of her daughter, who, in essence, was giving her mother permission to die without worrying about the ones she was leaving behind. Mr. Gram was calling for someone to do something when his daughter turned to him and said, "No, Daddy, we have to let her go—she just can't do this anymore!"

I was numb, desperately trying to hold on to my clinical viewpoint. Other students were at the bedside trying to get a blood pressure or a pulse, but I couldn't bring myself to do something I believed was disrespectful and an intrusion on her peaceful passage. When the others left, I went to the bedside to hold Mrs. Gram's hand and say a short prayer. I left the room in silence. Late that night, I cried.

As much as I had tried to condition myself for this experience, I still had not been ready for it. My instructor assured me that every person's reaction to death is different and that each is highly personal. She pointed out that as I develop my nursing career, there will be many first reactions, personal dilemmas, and ethical decisions with which I will have to come to terms. This particular experience gave me a good look inside myself to see the nurse I am to become. I liked what I saw.

—Janelle Selby, Southeast Missouri State University,
Cape Girardeau, Missouri

The reality of death can be made less painful by preparing the family ahead of time. When the process has been explained to the family, they are better prepared to understand the needs of and to support the dying person.

The steps of the grieving process should be explained to all family members ahead of time, so that they will recognize the specific stages as they experience them and understand that the process is normal. They will be able to recognize that other members of the family are going through the same stages, perhaps at different times. This preparation allows for better understanding and communication within the family.

Death creates a change in family roles. As one person (the dying person) leaves a role, adjustments must be made within the family to compensate. Each member plays a part in that compensation. The nurse can help with these adjustments.

Meeting Self Needs

The nurse who cares for a client for an extended period will undergo a grief reaction when the client dies. Grief after the death of a client is natural, and the nurse should allow himself or herself to go through the grieving process, rather than shut off the grief. The nurse also should address personal health needs.

Death

Before death occurs, the client and family should have an opportunity to discuss what will happen after death, review the client's will, and discuss ethical and legal issues of concern.

Ethical and Legal Dimensions

Ethical and legal implications of nursing are discussed in Chapters 5 and 6. Religious beliefs and practices concerning spiritual beliefs and medical procedures are summarized in Chapter 41. The following issues and their implications should be discussed with the family and their wishes made known to the physician.

End-of-Life Treatment Decisions Multiple treatment options and sophisticated life-support technologies, which at times make it difficult to draw the line between promoting life and needlessly prolonging the dying process, complicate health care decision making for clients and health care professionals alike. The increasing popularity of the "managed death" concept and calls to legalize physician-assisted suicide and physician administered lethal injections ("aid in dying") pose new ethical challenges. As clients and families struggle with end-of-life treatment decisions, they are increasingly looking to nurses for informa-

Signed by the donor and the following two witnesses in the presence of each other:

_____ _____
Signature of Donor   Date of Birth of Donor

_____ _____
Date Signed   City and State

_____ _____
Witness   Witness

This is a legal document under the Uniform Anatomical Gift Act or similar laws in all 50 states.

For further information call

Delaware Valley TRANSPLANT PROGRAM

800 **KIDNEY-1**
2401 Walnut St., Suite 404
Philadelphia, PA 19103

UNIFORM DONOR CARD

Print or type name of donor

In the hope that I may help others, I hereby make this anatomical gift, if medically acceptable, to take effect upon my death. The words and marks below indicate my desires.
I give: a)_____any needed organs or parts
        b)_____only the following organs or parts

Specify the organ(s) or part(s)

for the purpose of transplantation, therapy, medical research or education;
        c)_____my body for anatomical study if needed

Limitations or special wishes, if any

F I G U R E   1 3 - 1

Organ donor card.

tion, advice, and support. Advance directives are discussed in Chapter 22.

Organ Donations Clients who express a wish to donate functional organs, such as hearts, corneas, livers, lungs, and kidneys, can fill out an organ donor consent card (Fig. 13-1). The family of a deceased client also may decide to donate the client's functional organs. The nurse should be able to review options and provide consent forms to interested clients and their families.

Autopsy An **autopsy** is an examination of the organs and tissues of a human body after death. Consent for autopsy is a legal requirement. The closest surviving family member or members usually have the authority to determine whether or not an autopsy is performed. Some religious groups prohibit autopsies except for legal purposes.

It commonly is the physician's responsibility to obtain permission for an autopsy. Sometimes the client may grant this permission before death. The nurse can assist by explaining the reasons for an autopsy. Many relatives find comfort when they are told that the knowledge gained from an autopsy may contribute to advancements in medical science as well as establish the exact cause of death.

If death is caused by accident, suicide, homicide, or illegal therapeutic practice, the coroner must be notified, according to law. The coroner may decide that an autopsy is advisable, and can order that one be performed, even though the client's family has refused consent. In many cases, a death that occurs within 24 hours of admission to the hospital must be reported to the coroner.

Clinical Signs of Death

The clinical signs of *impending* or *approaching* death include inability to swallow; pitting edema; decreased gastrointestinal and urinary tract activity; bowel and bladder incontinence; loss of motion, sensation, and reflexes; elevated temperature but cold or clammy skin; cyanosis; lowered blood pressure; noisy or irregular respiration; and Cheyne-Stokes respirations. The client may or may not lose consciousness.

Death was defined in 1981 by the President's Commission for the Study of Ethical Problems in Medicine and Biomedical and Behavioral Research as follows:

Death is present when an individual has sustained either (1) irreversible cessation of circulatory and respiratory functions, or (2) irreversible cessation of all functions of the entire brain, including the brain stem.

Another definition of *death* proposed by a Harvard University committee states that the following characteristics must be present for at least 24 hours before death can be declared:

- Lack of receptivity and responsiveness
- Lack of movement or breathing
- Lack of reflexes
- Flat encephalogram

Nursing Responsibilities

When a client dies, the nurse's responsibilities include caring for the client's body, caring for the family, and discharging specific legal responsibilities. The latter involve ensuring that a death certificate is issued and signed, labeling the body, and reviewing organ donation arrangements, if any.

Care of the Body After the client has been pronounced dead, the nurse is responsible for preparing the body for discharge. The body is placed in normal anatomic position to avoid pooling of blood, soiled dressings are replaced, and tubes are removed. In most cases, it is unnecessary to wash the body; the mortician normally attends to this. Some religions strictly forbid washing of the body, whereas in others, it must be performed by a special person. In cultures in which the family's washing of the deceased's body is considered the last service a family can give a loved

one, the family should be given the necessary supplies and left alone in the room with the body. If an autopsy is to be performed, any tubes that were in place should not be removed. In such cases, the nurse should follow the hospital's policy.

The nurse is legally responsible for placing identification tags on both the shroud or garment the body is clothed in and the ankle to ensure that the body can be identified even if it is separated from its shroud. The nurse also should place an identification tag on the client's dentures or other prostheses to ensure that these are received by the mortician. The client's body may have to be placed in the hospital's morgue refrigerator if mortuary arrangements were not made before the client's death. *The importance of proper and complete identification cannot be overemphasized*.

If the client died of a communicable disease, the body may require special handling to prevent the spread of that disease. Requirements for such handling usually are specified by local law and are contingent on the disease-causing organism, mode of transmission, and other characteristics.

Care of the Family After a client has died, the nurse provides support and care to the client's family. In most cases, this involves listening to the family's expressions of grief, loss, and helplessness. Because comforting words often are difficult to find, the nurse should offer solace and support by being an attentive listener. Family members may need to see the client's body to fully accept the death; in such cases, the nurse should arrange for family members to view the body before it is discharged to the mortician.

Sudden death creates unique problems for the family. In the case of sudden injury or illness, the physical needs of the client are paramount to the health care team. This means that family members are not provided as much emotional support or information as they would be if the client's illness were prolonged; nor are they permitted to exercise as many options regarding the client's care. The family that loses a member unexpectedly has not had an opportunity to begin the grieving process or to share in grieving with the deceased person. Family members should be allowed to express grief and given emotional support. Most often the family is in the emergency department waiting room when death is confirmed. They are stunned, bewildered, and numb. They should not be rushed from the waiting room, but rather provided a private place to begin their grieving. The nurse should acknowledge their shock and listen to their grief. The family needs guidance in making plans and help in making decisions.

It is proper for the nurse who was caregiver or who took care of the client for a prolonged period to attend the funeral. It also is appropriate for the nurse to make a follow-up call to the client's family after the funeral or memorial service to offer both concern and care for the family's well-being. Follow-up visits are important to give support to the family. If the nurse assesses that the family is not coping well (dysfunctional grief), appropriate referral should be made.

RESEARCH IN NURSING   Making a Difference

Loss and Grieving

Nurses offer support to individuals and families who have an actual or a potential loss as an important aspect of facilitating coping. Assessments of reactions to grief and interventions to meet physical and emotional needs of clients and families can be made even more meaningful and individualized based on research findings. The following examples investigated reactions to loss in various situations.

Related Research

Hall, B. A. (1990). The struggle of the diagnosed terminally ill person to maintain hope. *Nursing Science Quarterly, 3*(4), 177–184.

This study explored the concept of hope in 11 men who had been diagnosed with AIDS. Hall concluded that hope is as important immediately before death as it is at any other time in one's life. She also found evidence suggesting that professional caretakers often perceive hope in the terminally ill as a form of denial. Based on these findings, nursing interventions are recommended that promote life in those facing death by discussions about the meaning and quality of their lives.

Murphy, S. A. (1990). Preventive intervention following accidental death of a child. *Image: Journal of Nursing Scholarship, 22*(3), 174–179.

This study was done to test a preventive intervention program for bereaved parents after accidental death of their adolescent or young adult children. Information and emotional support was given to one group at 2 to 6 months after loss and to another group at 7 to 13 months after loss. Both groups reported therapeutic benefits of the intervention; however, different emotional needs were identified within each period. The authors recommended use of the intervention in community support groups.

Carter, S. L. (1989). Themes of grief. *Nursing Research, 38*(6), 354–358.

The author of this investigation interviewed 30 adults who had experienced the death of a loved one, and used the results to identify themes of grief. The core themes were being stopped, hurting, missing, holding, and seeking. Nurses can use these findings to anticipate a broad range of responses from the bereaved and to accept individualized needs during the bereavement process.

VanDongen, C. J. (1990). Agonizing questioning: Experiences of survivors of suicide victims. *Nursing Research, 39*(4), 224–229.

Interviews of 35 adult survivors of family suicide victims provided information about their experiences after the loss. All the participants reported that they were struggling with questions relating to the suicide, centering around "Why did this happen?" Findings of the study support that survivors of sudden, violent death have difficulty achieving the tasks of grieving. As a result, nursing interventions are necessary to facilitate coping.

Summary

The implications of nursing research in these areas focus on the need for nursing interventions to facilitate coping with impending death and with loss after the death of a loved one. Although nurses may more traditionally provide immediate support in the hospital setting, these studies illustrate the need for nursing care in all health care settings and on a long-term basis.

Care of Other Clients   Because it is not unusual for a nurse to provide care to more than one client at a time, after the death of one client, the nurse must continue to provide care to the other clients. Other clients often are aware of a death and may need to be consoled; this is particularly true of a client who has shared a room with the deceased client. Other clients may have grief reactions and should be supported through the grief process by the nurse. Death of a client may cause depression in other clients and may make them more aware of their own future deaths.

Death Certificate   Both U.S. and Canadian laws require that a death certificate be prepared for each person who dies. The laws specify what information needs to be supplied. Death certificates are sent to local health departments, which compile many statistics from the information. The mortician assumes responsibility for handling and filing the death certificate with proper authorities. A physician's signature is required on the certificate, as well as that of the pathologist, the coroner, and others in special cases. The nurse's responsibility is to ensure that a death certificate has been signed by the physician.

KEY POINTS

- Everyone experiences losses at various points in the life continuum. Such losses can be actual, perceived, physical, psychological, or anticipatory. Loss can have an effect on the developmental stages of the human life span, especially in children.
- Grief is the emotional response to loss, and grief reactions can be divided into identifiable stages. Grief can be manifested both emotionally and physically, and grief reactions are influenced by development, family and socioeconomic factors, and religious and cultural influences.
- Dying clients have various needs, ranging from the need for open communication to physiologic, psychological, and spiritual needs. They should maintain self-care as long as possible.
- Families of dying clients also need open communication, and may want to assist the nurse in providing care. This is considered a healthy experience for both client and family members.
- Like grief, dying can be broken down into identifiable and overlapping stages.

- Clients and families increasingly look to nurses for information, advice, and support when making end-of-life treatment decisions. Nurses need to recognize the ethical, spiritual, and legal ramifications of these decisions.
- Although there is no exact definition for death, the clinical signs of approaching or impending death can be recognized.
- The nurse should provide emotional support for the grieving family by being an attentive, nonjudgmental listener and a good communicator.
- The nurse has specific responsibilities at the time of a client's death, including ensuring that a death certificate is issued, caring for the body, placing identification tags on the shroud and body, ensuring that the body is discharged to the proper party, and caring for the family.
- The nurse should provide care to other clients who are affected by the loss.

BIBLIOGRAPHY

Archer, D. N., & Smith, A. C. (1988). Sorrow has many faces: Helping families cope with grief. *Nursing, 18*(5), 43–45.

Beaudoin, S. J. (1990). Caring and surviving: Coping with patient death. *Canadian Nurse, 86*(7), 19–20.

Carpenito, L. J. (1992). *Nursing diagnosis: Application to clinical practice* (4th ed.). Philadelphia: Lippincott.

Carson, V. B. (1989). *Spiritual dimensions of nursing practice.* Philadelphia: Saunders.

Carter, S. L. (1989). Themes of grief. *Nursing Research, 38*(6), 354–358.

Clark, M. D. (1984). Healthy and unhealthy grief behaviors. *Occupational Health Nursing, 32*(12), 633–635.

Corr, C. A., & Corr, D. M. (1983). *Hospice care: Principles and practice.* New York: Springer-Verlag.

Dugan, D. O. (1987). Death and dying: Emotional, spiritual, and ethical support for patients and families. *Journal of Psychosocial Nursing, 25*(7), 21–29.

Dying well? A colloquy on euthanasia and assisted suicide. (1992). *Hastings Center Report, 22*(2).

Eakes, G. G. (1990). Grief resolution in hospice nurses: An exploration of effective methods. *Nursing and Health Care, 11*(5), 242–248.

Engel, G. L. (1964). Grief and grieving. *American Journal of Nursing, 64*(9), 93–98.

Foster, R. L., Hunsberger, M. M., & Anderson, J. (1989). *Family-centered nursing care of children.* Philadelphia: Saunders.

Gifford, B. J., & Cleary, B. B. (1990). Supporting the bereaved. *American Journal of Nursing, 90*(2), 48–53.

Gonda, T. A., & Ruark, J. E. (1984). *Dying dignified: The*

health professional's guide to care. Menlo Park, CA: Addison-Wesley.

Grassman, D. (1992). Turning personal grief into personal growth. *Nursing, 22*(4), 43–47.

Hall, B. A. (1990). The struggle of the diagnosed terminally ill person to maintain hope. *Nursing Science Quarterly, 3*(4), 177–184.

Hutchings, D. (1991). Spirituality in the face of death. *Canadian Nurse, 87*(5), 30–31.

Johnson, S. H. (1986). *Nursing assessment and strategies for the family at risk: High-risk parenting* (2nd ed.). Philadelphia: Lippincott.

Kübler-Ross, E. (1969). *On death and dying.* New York: Macmillan.

MacDonald, B. (1990). Death with dignity. *Canadian Nurse, 86*(11), 24–25.

Martocchio, B. C. (1985). Grief and bereavement: Healing through hurt. *Nursing Clinics of North America, 20*(2), 327–341.

Murphy, P. (1990). Helping Joanne die with dignity: A nursing profile in courage. *Nursing, 20*(9), 44–49.

Murphy, S. A. (1990). Preventive intervention following accidental death of a child. (1990). *Image: Journal of Nursing Scholarship, 22*(3), 174–179.

Oerlemans-Bunn, M. (1988). On being gay, single, and bereaved. *American Journal of Nursing, 88*(4), 472–476.

Portenoy, R. K. (1991). Special issue on medical ethics: Physician-assisted suicide and euthanasia. *Journal of Pain and Symptom Management, 6*(5).

President's Commission for the Study of Ethical Problems in

Medicine and Biomedical and Behavioral Research. (1981). *Defining death*. Washington, DC: U.S. Government Printing Office, Pub. No. 81-600150.

Rosenbaum, J. N. (1991). Widowhood grief: A cultural perspective. *Canadian Journal of Nursing Research, 23*(2), 61–76.

Ryan, P. F., Cote-Arsenault, D., & Sugarman, L. (1991). Facilitating care after perinatal loss: A comprehensive checklist. *Journal of Obstetric, Gynecologic, and Neonatal Nursing, 20*(5), 385–389.

Schulz, R. (1978). *The psychology of death, dying and bereavement*. Reading, MA: Addison-Wesley.

Stephany, T. M. (1990). A death in the family. *American Journal of Nursing, 90*(4), 54–56.

Ufema, J. (1990). Meeting the challenge of a dying patient. *Nursing, 21*(2), 42–46.

VanDongen, C. J. (1990). Agonizing questioning: Experiences of survivors of suicide victims. *Nursing Research, 39*(4), 224–229.

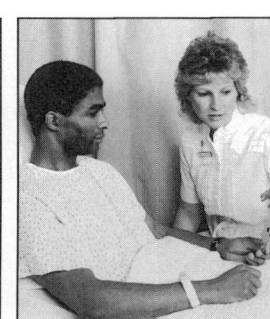
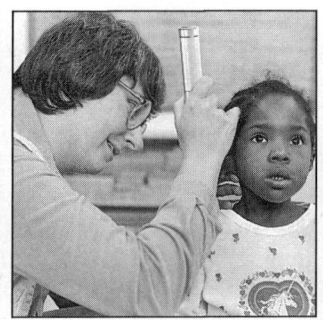
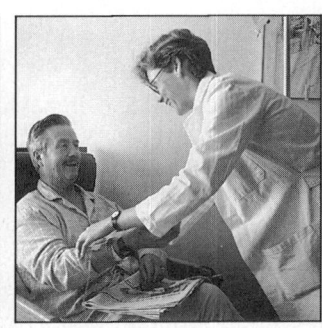

The Nursing Process

The nursing process is a systematic, client-centered, goal-oriented method of caring that provides a framework for nursing practice. Unit IV discusses each of the five steps of the nursing process—assessing, diagnosing, planning, implementing, and evaluating. The use of nursing process skills allows the nurse to apply knowledge and skills in meeting client needs while giving holistic, individualized care.

The steps are not actually separate items but rather are parts of a whole, used to identify needs, establish priorities of care, maximize strengths, and resolve actual or potential alterations in human responses to health and illness, thereby promoting wellness to the highest level possible for each client.

Assessment, the systematic and continuous collection and communication of data, allows analysis of data to identify problems and strengths of clients. During planning, the nurse and client mutually set goals and agree on nursing interventions necessary to meet the established goals. The nurse implements the plan of care, adapting to each individual, and documents nursing actions and client responses. After implementation, the nurse and client evaluate the effectiveness of the plan, based on achievement of goals, and determine if the plan should be continued, modified, or terminated.

The nursing process is nursing practice in action. Unit IV provides the information necessary for the beginning application of the nursing process; as knowledge and skills are learned and practiced (both as students and as nurses), the process becomes an integral component of each nurse–client interaction. The outcome is comprehensive and individualized nursing care.

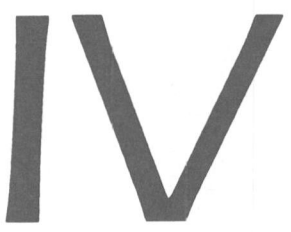

IV

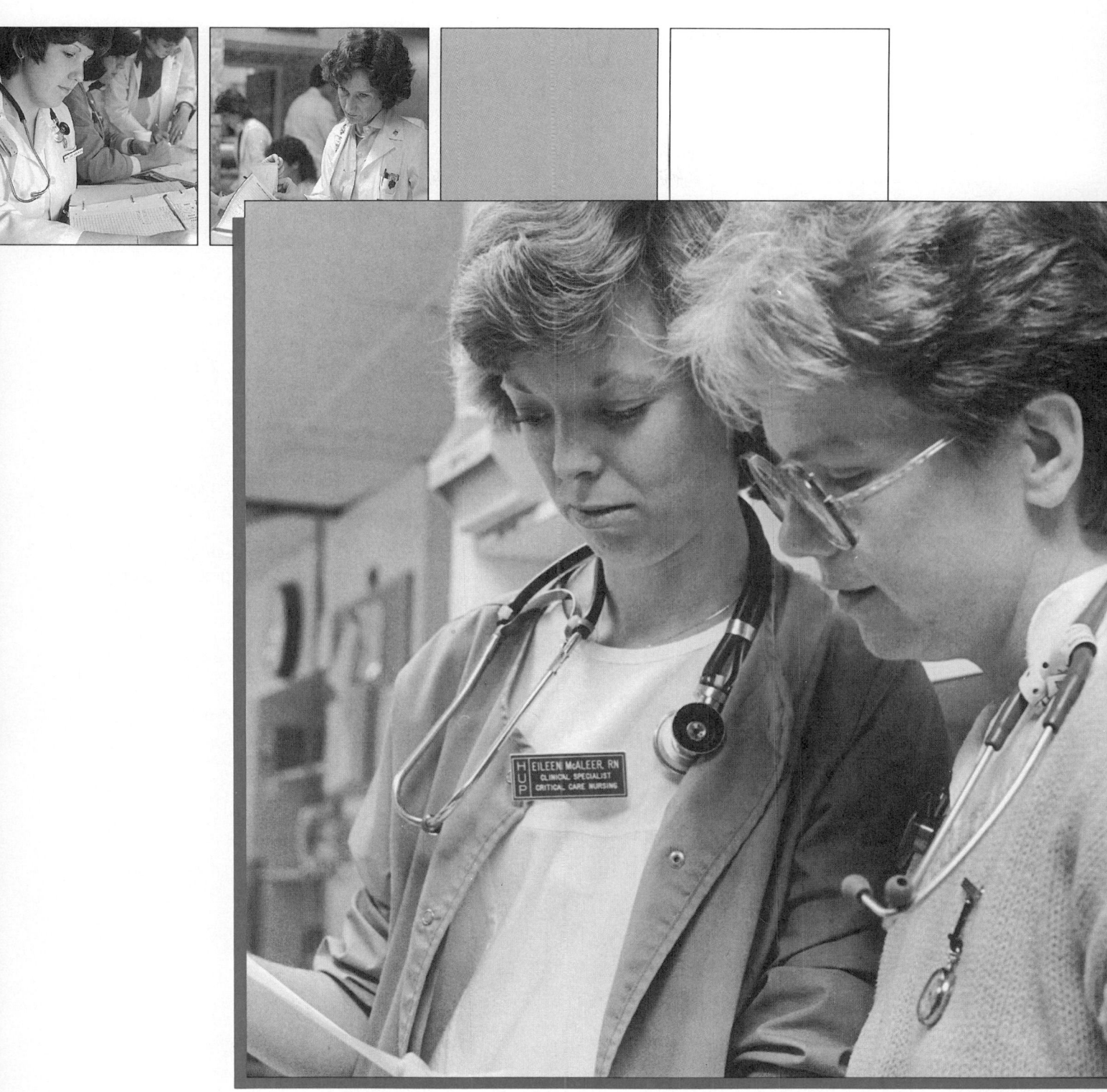

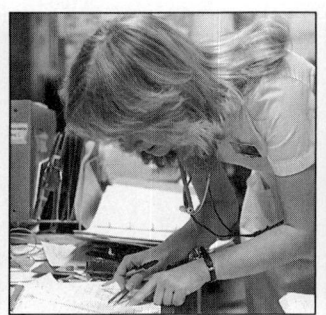
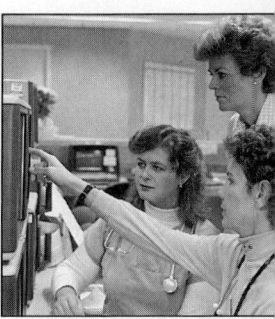

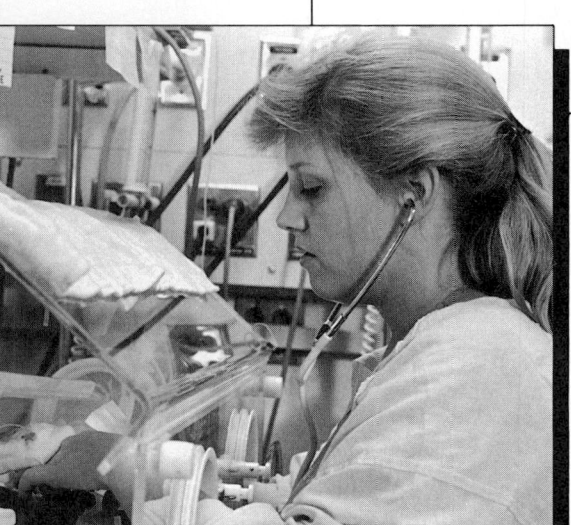

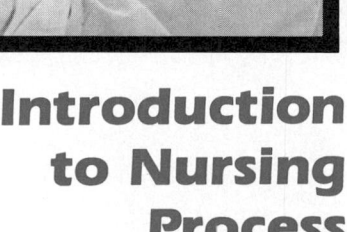

Introduction to Nursing Process

14

O B J E C T I V E S

After studying this chapter, the learner should be able to:

Define key terms used in the chapter.

Describe the historic evolution of the nursing process.

Describe the nursing process and each of its five steps.

List five characteristics of the nursing process.

List three client and three nursing benefits of using the nursing process correctly.

K E Y   T E R M S

assessing
diagnosing
evaluating
implementing
intuitive problem solving
nursing process
planning
scientific problem solving
trial-and-error problem solving

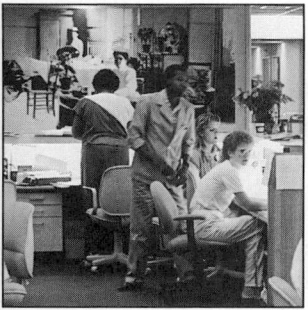
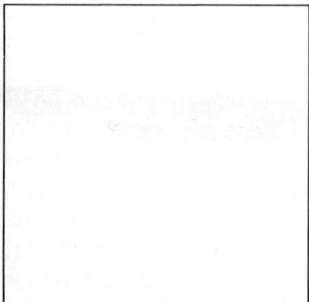

Traditionally, nurses have prided themselves on comforting those who are ill and on executing with precision such tasks as dressing wounds, administering medications, and bathing, feeding, and ambulating clients. Many of these tasks were ordered by physicians, and few nurses would have characterized their "work" as being independent, scientifically based, or creative.

The health care delivery system has changed, and nursing has changed with it. Nurses now work with well and ill clients in both private and institutional settings. In addition to their role as caregiver, nurses fill specialized roles as care managers—coordinators, teachers, counselors, advocates, and researchers. Nurses are responsible for a unique dimension of health care, "the diagnosis and treatment of human response to actual or potential health problems" (American Nurses' Association, 1980), and as such are knowledgeable, competent, and independent professionals who work collaboratively with other health care professionals to design and deliver holistic care.

As the practice of nursing became more complex, nurses began to study the *process* of nursing to both understand and improve the means nurses use to accomplish their aims.

Historic Perspective

Since the term *nursing process* was first used by Hall in 1955, many nurses have struggled to define exactly what constitutes the "work of nursing" and what makes nurses successful. In the 1960s, nursing theorists began to describe nursing as a distinct entity among the health care professions, and also delineated specific steps in a process approach to nursing practice. In 1967, Yura and Walsh published the first comprehensive book on nursing process, in which they described four steps in the nursing process—assessment, planning, intervention, and evaluation. They viewed the element of nursing diagnosis as the logical conclusion of the assessment phase, whereas Gebbie and Lavin (1974) made nursing diagnosis a separate step in the process. These and other studies led to the development of the five-step nursing process commonly used today—assessment, diagnosis, planning, implementation, and evaluation.

The steps of the nursing process were legitimated in 1973, when the American Nurses' Association Congress for Nursing Practice developed *Standards of Practice* to guide nursing performance. These standards were revised in 1991 and appear in Chapter 1. The standards for nursing practice were quickly reflected in revised nurse practice acts in many states.

The Joint Commission on Accreditation of Healthcare Organizations requires that care be documented according to the nursing process, and the National League for Nursing mandates that educational programs incorporate the nursing process as their cognitive process. In 1982, the state board examinations for professional nursing practice underwent major revisions. One of the organizing concepts used in the revisions was nursing process. The revised examinations are structured to test the practitioner's ability to assess clients; to diagnose health problems amenable to nursing therapy; and to plan, implement, and evaluate nursing care. The examinations had previously organized content on a medical model, structured according to medical specialities—medicine, surgery, maternity, pediatrics, and psychiatry.

Evolution of Nursing Diagnosis

The term *nursing diagnosis* first appeared in the literature in the 1950s. In 1976, Aspinall described nursing diagnosis as "the weak link" in nursing process. As early as 1966, Hammond wrote that nurses need both to be competent in information-seeking strategies and to have a good background of theoretical knowledge with which to conduct the search for cues and evaluate evidence—all resulting in accurate diagnosing. Key elements in the evolution of nursing diagnosis as an integral component of nursing process include the following:

- In 1972, the New York State Nurse Practice Act identified diagnosing as part of the legal domain of professional nursing; practice acts in many other states have been revised similarly since then.
- In 1973, the American Nurses' Association's *Standards of Practice* included diagnosing as a function of professional nursing.
- Also in 1973, Gebbie and Lavin of St. Louis University called the First National Conference on Classification of Nursing Diagnoses, beginning a national effort to identify, standardize, and classify health problems treated by nurses. Conferences are held every 2 years, and much progress has been made in defining, classifying, and describing nursing diagnoses.

At its first meeting in 1973, the National Group, since renamed the North American Nursing Diagnosis Association (NANDA), appointed a task force to accomplish the following goals:

- Gather information and disseminate it through the Clearinghouse for Nursing Diagnosis.
- Encourage educational activities at regional and state levels to promote the implementation of nursing diagnoses. These activities include conferences to orga-

nize nurses to identify additional diagnostic labels and workshops to teach nurses about nursing diagnoses.

- Promote and organize activities to continue the development, classification, and scientific testing of nursing diagnosis. These activities include planning national conferences, identifying criteria for accepting diagnoses, surveying current research activities, and exploring varied methods for classification.

Description of Nursing Process

The **nursing process** is a systematic method that directs the nurse and client as they together (1) determine the need for nursing care, (2) plan and implement the care, and (3) evaluate the results. The steps in this client-centered, goal-oriented process are interrelated; each of the five steps depends on the accuracy of the step preceding it. The process provides a framework that enables the nurse and client to do the following:

- Systematically collect client data (assessing)
- Clearly identify client strengths and problems (diagnosing)
- Develop a holistic plan of individualized care that specifies both the desired client goals and the nursing actions most likely to assist the client to meet those goals (planning)
- Execute the plan of care (implementing)
- Evaluate the effectiveness of the plan of care in terms of client goal achievement (evaluating)

In each step of the process, the nurse and client work together as partners; the client's health state and resources influence the client's level of participation. When the client is an infant, unconscious, or uncooperative, the steps of the process are worked through with the help of a family member or support person.

The primary purpose of the nursing process is to help the nurse manage each client's care scientifically, holistically, and creatively (Fig. 14-1). To do this successfully, the nurse needs many intellectual, interpersonal, and psychomotor skills, as well as the willingness to use these skills creatively when working with clients to promote wellness, to prevent disease or illness, to restore health, and to facilitate coping with altered functioning. Many of these skills are described in the units that follow.

Steps of the Nursing Process

The five steps of the nursing process are shown in Figure 14-2. Each step is briefly described here and discussed in greater detail in the chapters that follow. Those who want to study nursing process or any of its steps in greater detail should consult one of the nursing texts that deals exclusively with nursing process (eg, Alfaro, 1990; Atkinson & Murray, 1990; Griffith-Kenney & Christensen, 1990; Iyer, Taptich, & Bernocchi-Losey, 1991; LaMonica, 1985; Marriner, 1983; Pinnell & de Meneses, 1986; and Yura & Walsh, 1988).

Assessing

The first step in the nursing process, **assessing**, is the systematic and continuous collection, validation, and communication of client data. Data collection guidelines reflect the nursing theory of the particular institution. (Nursing theory is discussed in Chap. 4.) In general, nurses are concerned with how human functioning is enhanced by health promotion and compromised by illness and suffering. The remaining steps of the nursing process depend on complete, accurate, and relevant data.

During the assessment step of the nursing process, the nurse does the following:

- Establishes the data base, which includes nursing history, physical assessment, review of the client record and nursing literature, and consultation with the client's support people and health care professionals

F I G U R E   1 4 - 1

The nursing process achieves for the client scientifically based, holistic, individualized care; the chance to work collaboratively with nurses; and continuity of care.

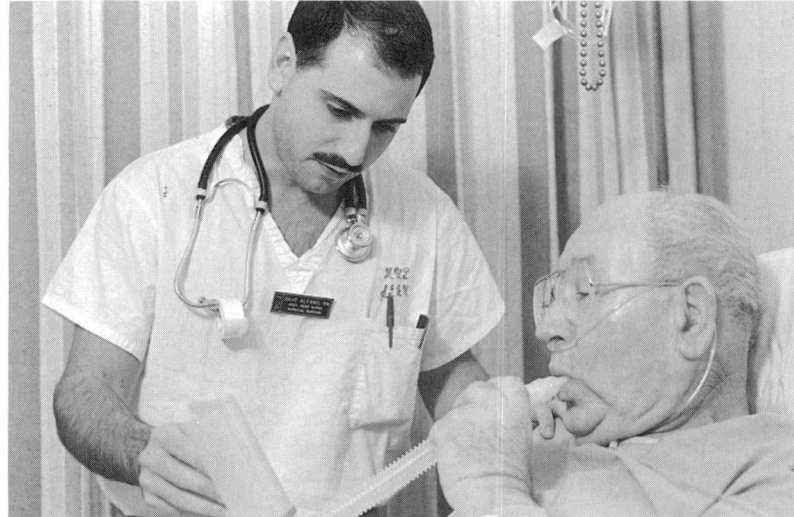

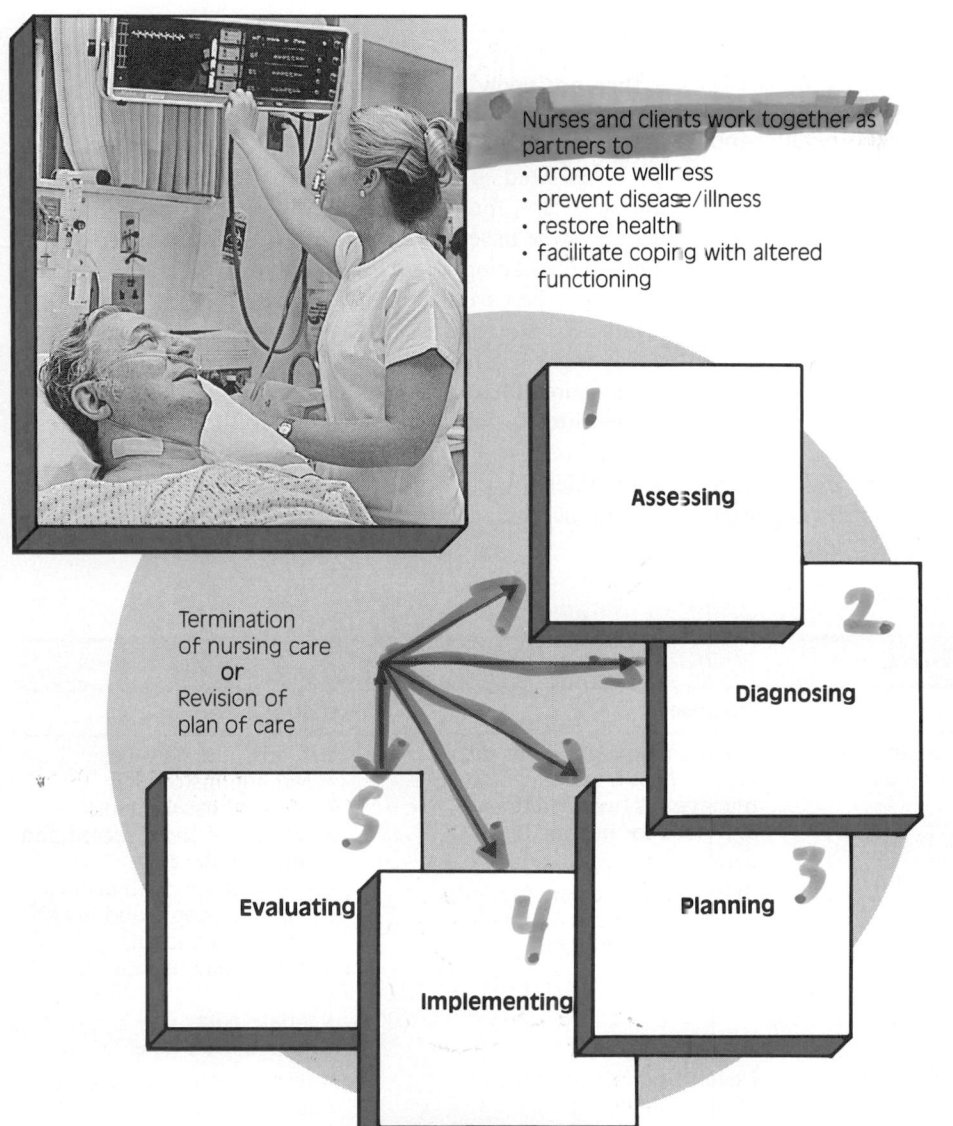

Nurses and clients work together as partners to
• promote wellness
• prevent disease/illness
• restore health
• facilitate coping with altered functioning

Termination
of nursing care
or
Revision of
plan of care

1 Assessing

2. Diagnosing

3 Planning

4 Implementing

5 Evaluating

FIGURE 14-2

The nursing process. The nursing process is a systematic method that directs the nurse and client as, together, they determine the need for nursing care (assessing and diagnosing), and then plan, implement, and evaluate care. The steps in this client-centered, goal-oriented process are interrelated, and each of the five steps depends on the accuracy of the step preceding it. Evaluation, the fifth step in the process, leads either to the termination of nursing care or to revision of the plan of care after each preceding step in the process has been evaluated. (Photo by Gates Rhodes, courtesy of School of Nursing, University of Pennsylvania.)

• Continuously updates the data base
• Validates data
• Communicates data

• Formulates and validates nursing diagnoses
• Develops a prioritized list of nursing diagnoses

Diagnosing

Diagnosing is analysis of client data to identify data clusters that indicate actual or potential health problems, factors that contribute to or cause these problems, and coping patterns or strengths of the client.

The nurse next determines if each health problem is best treated by nursing or by another health discipline. When data analysis reveals an actual or potential health problem that nursing intervention can prevent or resolve, the problem is termed a *nursing diagnosis*. During the diagnosis step of the nursing process, the nurse does the following:

• Interprets and analyzes client data
• Identifies client strengths and client health problems

Planning

Planning is the establishment of client goals by the nurse working with the client that prevent, reduce, or resolve problems identified in the nursing diagnoses, and the determination of related nursing interventions most likely to assist the client in achieving these goals. In addition, a comprehensive plan of care also specifies (1) the nursing assistance needed by the client to meet human needs, and (2) the nursing interventions dictated by the plan of medical care. During the planning step of the nursing process, the nurse does the following:

• Establishes priorities
• Writes client goals and develops an evaluative strategy
• Selects nursing measures
• Communicates the plan of nursing care

Implementing

Implementing is simply the carrying out of the plan of care. It includes all actions performed by nurses to promote wellness, prevent disease or illness, restore health, and facilitate coping with altered functioning. During the implementing step of the nursing process, the nurse does the following:

- Carries out the plan of nursing care
- Continues data collection and modifies the plan of care as needed
- Documents care

Evaluating

Evaluating is the measuring of the extent to which client goals have been met. The nurse and the client together measure how well the client has achieved goals specified in the plan of care, and nurse and client identify factors that either positively or negatively influenced goal achievement. Client response to the plan of care determines whether nursing care should be continued as is, modified, or terminated. If evaluation points to a need to modify nursing care, then the accuracy, completeness, and relevance of the assessment data, as well as the appropriateness of client diagnoses, goals, and nursing interventions, should all be carefully reviewed and modified. During the evaluation step of the nursing process, the nurse does the following:

- Measures the client's achievement of desired goals
- Identifies factors that contribute to the client's success or failure
- Modifies the plan of care, if indicated

An overview of the steps of the nursing process is pre-

T A B L E   1 4 - 1

Overview of the Nursing Process

Component	Description	Purpose	Activities
Assessing	Collection, validation, and communication of client data	Make a judgment about the client's health status, ability to manage his own health care, and need for nursing Plan individualized holistic care that draws on client strengths and is responsive to changes in the client's conditions	1. Establish the data base • Nursing history • Physical assessment • Review of client record and nursing literature • Consultation with client's support people and health care professionals 2. Continuously update the data base 3. Validate data 4. Communicate date
Diagnosing	Analysis of client data to identify client strengths and health problems that independent nursing intervention can prevent or resolve	Develop a prioritized list of nursing diagnoses	1. Interpret and analyze client data 2. Identify client strengths and health problems 3. Formulate and validate nursing diagnoses 4. Develop prioritized list of nursing diagnoses
Planning	Specification of (1) client goals to prevent, reduce, or resolve the problems identified in the nursing diagnoses; and (2) related nursing interventions	Develop an individualized plan of nursing care	1. Establish priorities 2. Write goals and develop an evaluative strategy 3. Select nursing measures 4. Communicate plan of nursing care
Implementing	Carrying out the plan of care	Assist clients to achieve desired goals—promote wellness, prevent disease and illness, restore health, facilitate coping with altered functioning	1. Carry out the plan of care 2. Continue data collection and modify the plan of care as needed 3. Document care
Evaluating	Measure the extent to which the client has achieved the goals specified in the plan of care, identifying factors that positively or negatively influenced goal achievement; revise the plan of care if necessary	Continue, modify, or terminate nursing care	1. Measure how well the client has achieved desired goals 2. Identify factors that contribute to the client's success or failure 3. Modify the plan of care (if indicated)

Illustration of the Steps of the Nursing Process

Assessing

You are checking on a client who had abdominal surgery yesterday and hear that the client has considerable pain. "It kept me up all night." The client has been reluctant to ask for any pain medication, fearing effect of the drug. "I don't want to become a junkie." The client's blood pressure and pulse rate are slightly elevated.

Diagnosing

You analyze the data above and write the nursing diagnosis: *Pain related to a fear of taking pain-relieving medications.* The client agrees that this is becoming a problem.

Planning

You decide to work with the client to achieve the goal: *By 3:00 PM client reports sufficient relief of pain to enable him to rest and to get out of bed to go to the bathroom.* The client wants to accomplish the goal. You identify teaching as the primary nursing intervention.

Implementing

After asking the client about his experiences with pain-relieving medications, you explain that although many of these drugs are addictive when abused, there is no harm if they are taken as prescribed postoperatively. You also explain that it is important for him to experience enough pain relief to be able to cough and deep breathe, ambulate, and do other things important to his recovery. You suggest that the medication will be most effective if taken before his pain peaks and becomes intense. You administer the prescribed medication for pain when the client indicates that he is willing to give it a try.

Evaluating

After enough time has elapsed for the medication to take effect, you check back with the client to evaluate whether or not he has obtained relief and met his goal. If the client is satisfied and you both feel comfort is no longer a problem, you terminate the plan of care for this diagnosis. If the client still feels pain or is dissatisfied with the medication, each of the preceding steps of the nursing process is reevaluated, and necessary changes are made in the plan of care.

sented in Table 14-1; the accompanying display gives examples of each of the steps.

Documenting the Nursing Process

More than ever before, nurses are aware of the need to document nursing care. Legally speaking, a nursing action not documented is a nursing action not performed. Each chapter in this unit offers specific documentation guidelines for nursing process activities. It is helpful to practice documentation while learning any given nursing activity; like any other nursing skill, documentation improves with practice. Examples of nursing documentation, nursing assessments, care plans, and notes are provided throughout this text.

Problem Solving and the Nursing Process

One of the strengths of the nursing process is that it is based on a methodology that is familiar to most nursing students—problem solving. Problem solving is a basic life skill; identifying a problem and then taking steps to resolve it is a matter of common sense. Different approaches to problem solving yield different results, some of which are more successful than others.

The **trial-and-error method** of problem solving involves testing any number of solutions until one is found that works for that particular problem. This method is not efficient for the nurse and can be dangerous to the client; it is, therefore, not recommended as a guide for nursing practice.

The **scientific method** of problem solving is a systematic seven-step problem-solving process that involves (1) problem identification, (2) data collection, (3) hypothesis formulation, (4) plan of action, (5) hypothesis testing, (6) interpretation of results, and (7) evaluation, resulting in conclusion or revision of the study. This method is used most correctly in a controlled laboratory setting, but is closely related to the more general six-step problem-solving process commonly used by health care professionals as they work with clients. The relation between both of these methods and the nursing process is shown in Table 14-2.

Intuitive Problem Solving

For years, nurse theorists and educators have argued that clinical judgments should be based on data alone (the scientific method), in an attempt to establish nursing as a science, worthy of the respect of other professions. Controversy has recently been sparked by nurses both studying

TABLE 14-2

Comparison of Steps in the Problem-Solving Process, the Scientific Method, and the Nursing Process

Problem-Solving Process	Scientific Method	Nursing Process
1. Problem encountered	1. Problem identification	1. Assessing
2. Data collection	2. Data collection	
3. Exact nature of problem specified	3. Hypothesis formulation	2. Diagnosing
4. Plan of action determined	4. Plan of action developed to test hypothesis	3. Planning
5. Plan of action carried out	5. Hypothesis testing	4. Implementing
6. Outcomes of the plan evaluated and the plan continued, modified, or terminated	6. Interpretation of results	5. Evaluating
	7. Evaluation resulting in conclusion or revision of the study	

and writing about the role of **intuitive problem solving** in clinical decision making. Many veteran nurses can describe situations in which an "inner prompting" led to a quick nursing intervention that saved a client's life. Benner (1984, p. 295) describes intuition as "direct apprehension of a situation based upon a background of similar and dissimilar situations and embodied intelligence or skill." Schraeder and Fischer (1986, p. 161) credit to intuitive perception "a wide range of experience, from the sudden, inexplicable feeling that 'something is wrong,' to recognizing the teaching moment, when to offer encouragement, and when it is most helpful simply to listen."

Advocates of intuition recommend the following:

- Welcoming flashes of intuition as additions to logical reasoning, rather than disruptions
- Validating intuitions: when an intuition cannot be validated (eg, when the nurse senses that something is wrong with the client, although there are no clinical signs), careful monitoring of the client should be initiated
- Furthering nursing research to help find ways (1) to cultivate intuition and its typical results (accurate, early diagnosis; vigilant monitoring; better client care) and (2) to document the information intuition supplies (Rew, 1987)

Beginning nurses must use nursing knowledge and scientific problem solving as the basis of care they give; intuitive problem solving comes with years of practice and observation. If the beginning nurse has an intuition about a client, the information should be discussed with the supervisor.

Characteristics of Nursing Process

Various words and phrases have been used to describe the nursing process; key descriptors include *systematic*, *dynamic*, *interpersonal*, *goal-oriented*, and *universally applicable*.

Systematic

A quick look at the many and varied activities of any nurse on a busy day might lead one to conclude that nursing is little more than the execution of countless haphazard tasks. A closer look will reveal that each nursing task is part of an ordered sequence of activities. Moreover, each activity depends on the accuracy of the activity that precedes it, and influences the actions that follow it. Without a complete and accurate data base, the nurse cannot identify client strengths and problems; lacking knowledge of these, it is impossible for the nurse and client to develop a plan of care based on realistic and valued client goals. Unless the goals are well written, nursing actions and evaluation will be meaningless. The nursing process directs each step of nursing care in a sequential, ordered manner.

Dynamic

Although the nursing process is presented as an orderly progression of steps, in reality there is great interaction and overlapping among the five steps. No one step in the nursing process is a one-time phenomenon; each step is fluid and flows into the next step. In some nursing situations, all five stages occur almost simultaneously. When a nurse discovers that a client is choking on food and cannot speak or breathe, the nurse quickly identifies the problem and takes steps to dislodge the food particle blocking the airway—all the while evaluating the effectiveness of the intervention. In other instances—for example, child abuse—the nursing team may labor over each step of the nursing process as nurses work with the family to resolve complex problems. As well as being dynamic, the nursing process is continually open to change; at any point, new client data may cause the plan of care to proceed in an entirely different direction.

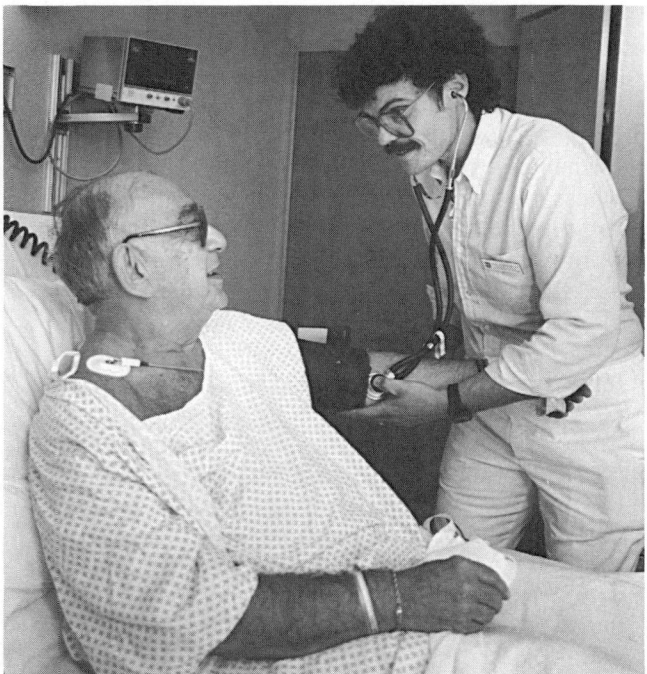

FIGURE 14-3

One characteristic of the nursing process is that it ensures that nursing is client centered rather than task oriented. (Photo by Robert Neroni, courtesy of Thomas Jefferson University.)

Interpersonal

Always at the heart of nursing is the human being. Nursing exists as a profession because some people require assistance as they respond to health and illness. The nursing process ensures that nurses are client-centered rather than task-centered. Rather than simply walking into a client's room to take vital signs, the nurse thinks: "How is Mr. Warner today? Any new data that indicate a need to modify his plan of care? Are our nursing actions helping him to achieve his goals? How can we better help him?"

The nursing process encourages nurses to work together to help clients use their strengths to meet all their human needs. This is different from viewing the client as a "problem to be solved" and interacting mechanically to provide the solution. Working intimately with clients helps nurses to explore their own strengths and limitations and to develop themselves personally and professionally.

Goal Oriented

Countless good things can be accomplished for most clients, ranging from improving their oral hygiene to helping them cope with the demands of being a new parent, recover from an acute medical illness, live with chronic pain,

or prepare for death. Likewise, it would take hundreds of pages to list and describe all the nursing actions a nurse might perform for a client. Moreover, nurses and clients often differ in the importance they attach to selected goals. The nursing process offers a means for nurses and clients to work together to identify specific goals related to wellness promotion, disease and illness prevention, health restoration, and coping with altered functioning, which are most important to the client, and to match them with the appropriate nursing actions. Once these are recorded in the plan of care, each nurse can quickly determine the client's priorities and begin nursing with a clear sense of how to proceed. The client benefits from continuity of care, and each nurse's care moves the client closer to goal achievement.

Universally Applicable

Once nurses have a working knowledge of the nursing process, they find that they can practice nursing with well or ill people, young or old, in any type of practice setting. Efforts made by the student nurse to master nursing process will result in the student's possession of a valuable tool that can be used with ease in any nursing situation.

What should be clear from the preceding discussion on nursing process is that it provides a framework for all the nurse's activities. With each nurse–client interaction, it is important to assess the client, note any significant alterations in health status, determine if the nursing action is helping the client achieve his or her goals, and modify the plan of care as necessary. Thus, the nurse who feeds a pediatric client through a special tube as ordered by a physician continually assesses how the child is responding to the feeding and if the child or family will be able to manage the feedings independently when the child is discharged. Depending on the results of the nursing assessment, new nursing diagnoses may be needed, as may additions to the plan of care. The nursing process offers direction for *all* the activities carried out by the nurse when caring for clients.

Benefits of the Nursing Process

When used properly, the nursing process achieves for the client scientifically based, holistic, individualized care; the opportunity to work collaboratively with nurses; and continuity of care. Nurses who use the nursing process in a thoughtful and systematic way achieve a clear and efficient plan of action by which the entire nursing team can achieve results for clients; the satisfaction that they are making an important "difference" in the lives of their clients; and the opportunity to grow professionally as nurses evaluate the effectiveness of interventions and variables that contribute positively or negatively to the client's goal achievement.

KEY POINTS

- The nursing process is a systematic method that directs the nurse and client as they together determine the need for nursing care (assessing and diagnosing) and then plan, implement, and evaluate care.
- The primary purpose of the nursing process is to help the nurses manage each client's nursing care scientifically, holistically, and creatively.
- In each step of the nursing process, the nurse and client work together as partners. The client's health state and resources influence the client's level of participation.
- Assessment is the systematic and continuous collection, validation, and communication of client data.
- Diagnosing is the analysis of client data to identify (1) data clusters that indicate actual or potential problems in the way the client is responding to health or illness, (2) factors that contribute to or cause these problems, and (3) coping patterns or other strengths the client can draw on to prevent or resolve the problem.
- During the planning step of the nursing process, the nurse, working with the client, (1) develops client goals that, if achieved, prevent, reduce, or eliminate the problems specified in the nursing diagnoses; and (2) identifies the nursing interventions most likely to achieve these goals.

- Implementation is simply the carrying out of the plan of nursing care. It includes all the actions performed by the nurse to promote wellness, prevent disease and illness, restore health, and facilitate coping with altered functioning.
- During evaluation, the nurse and client measure how well the client has achieved the goals specified in the plan of care and identify factors that positively or negatively influenced goal achievement. Client responses to the plan of care determine if nursing care is to be continued without change, modified, or terminated.
- Underlying the science and art of nursing is a successful blend of the scientific problem-solving method and the intuitive method.
- The nursing process is systematic, each step depending on the accuracy of the previous step and influencing the steps that follow. The steps of the nursing process are interrelated; each step is fluid and moves into the next.
- The nursing process is an interpersonal process that is always client-centered rather than task-centered. As nurses help clients to use their strengths to meet all their human needs, nurses themselves grow personally and professionally.
- A goal-oriented process, the nursing process offers a means for nurses and clients to work together to identify the specific health goals that are most important to the client—and to match these with the appropriate nursing interventions.

BIBLIOGRAPHY

Alfaro, R. (1990). *Application of nursing process: A step-by-step guide* (2nd ed.). Philadelphia: Lippincott.

American Association of Colleges of Nursing (1986). *Essentials of college and university education for nursing.* Washington, DC: Author.

American Nurses' Association (1980). *Nursing: A social policy statement.* Kansas City, MO: Author.

American Nurses' Association Congress for Practice (1973; revised 1991). *Standards of practice.* Kansas City, MO: Author.

Aspinall, M. J. (1976). Nursing diagnosis: The weak link. *Nursing Outlook, 24*(7), 433–436.

Atkinson, J., & Murray, M. E. (1990). *Understanding the nursing process* (4th ed.). New York: Macmillan.

Benner, P. (1984). *From novice to expert.* Menlo Park, CA: Addison-Wesley.

Gebbie, K., & Lavin, M. A. (1974). Classification of nursing diagnosis. *American Journal of Nursing, 74,* 250–253.

Griffith-Kenney, J. W., & Christensen, P. J. (1990). *Nursing process: Application of theories, frameworks, and models* (3rd ed.). St. Louis: Mosby.

Hall, L. E. (June 1955). Quality of nursing care. Address given at the Department of Baccalaureate and Higher Degree Programs of the New Jersey League for Nursing. *Public Health News.* New Jersey: New Jersey State Department of Health.

Hammond, K. R. (1966). Clinical inference in nursing: A psychologist's point of view. *Nursing Research, 15,* 27–38.

Hill, L., & Smith, N. (1990). *Self-care nursing: Promotion of health* (2nd ed.). East Norwalk, CT: Appleton & Lange.

Iyer, P., Taptich, B., & Bernocchi-Losey, D. (1991). *Nursing process and nursing diagnosis* (2nd ed.). Philadelphia: Saunders.

Kobert, L., & Folan, M. (June 1990). Coming of age in nursing: Rethinking the philosophies behind holism and nursing process. *Nursing and Health Care, 11*(6), 308–312.

LaMonica, E. (1985). *The humanistic nursing process.* Monterey, CA: Wadsworth.

Marriner, A. (1983). *The nursing process: A scientific approach to nursing* (3rd ed.). St. Louis: Mosby.

Mauksch, I. G., & David, M. (1972). Prescription for survival. *American Journal of Nursing, 72*(12), 2189–2193.

McHugh, M. K. (1987). Has nursing outgrown the nursing process? *Nursing, 17*(8), 50–51.

McHugh, M. K. (Ed.) (1987). Nursing process. *Holistic Nursing Practice, 1*(3).

Pinnell, N., & de Meneses, M. (1986). *The nursing process.* Norwalk, CT: Appleton-Century-Crofts.

Rew, L. (1987). Nursing intuition: Too powerful—and too valuable—to ignore. *Nursing, 17*(7), 43–45.

Ryan-Wenger, N. M. (1990). A nursing process methodology. *Nursing Outlook, 38*(40), 190–193.

Schraeder, B. D., & Fischer, D. K. (1986). Using knowledge to make clinical decisions. *MCN, 11*, 161–163.

Valega, T. M. (1984). It's time for nurses to begin nursing nurses. *Nursing and Health Care, 5*(6), 331–335.

Yura, H., & Walsh, M. B. (1967;1988). *The nursing process: Assessing, planning, implementing, evaluating* (5th ed.). Norwalk, CT: Appleton-Century-Crofts.

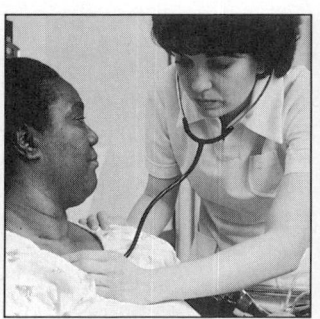
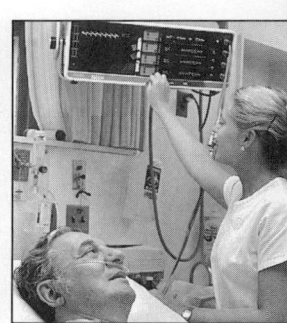

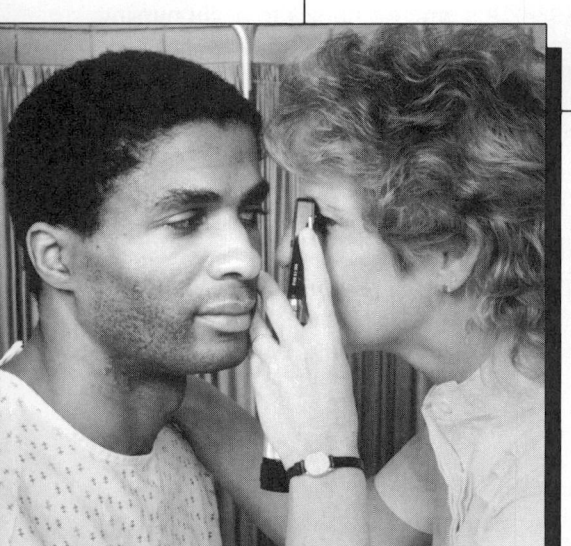

Assessing

OBJECTIVES

After studying this chapter, the learner should be able to:

Define key terms used in the chapter.

Describe the purpose of the initial nursing assessment and of ongoing nursing assessments.

Differentiate a nursing assessment from a medical assessment.

Differentiate objective and subjective data.

Describe the purpose of nursing observation, interview, and physical assessment.

Obtain a nursing history using effective interviewing techniques.

Identify five sources of client data useful to the nurse.

Differentiate comprehensive admission assessments from focused assessments.

Plan client assessments by identifying assessment priorities and structuring the data to be collected systematically.

Identify common problems encountered in data collection, noting their possible cause.

Explain when data need to be validated and several ways to accomplish this.

Describe the importance of knowing when to report significant client data and of proper documentation.

Obtain complete, accurate, factual, and relevant client data.

KEY TERMS

assessing
data
data base
interview
nursing history
objective data
observation
physical assessment
subjective data
validation

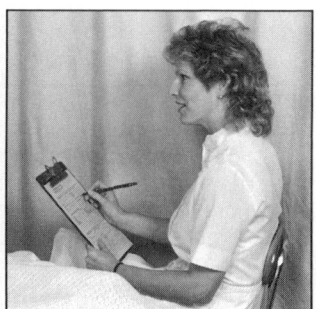

which targets data pointing to pathology, nursing assessments focus on client responses to health problems. Is there, for example, interference with meeting basic human needs? Can the client perform activities of daily living? Although sometimes the findings of a nursing assessment contribute to the identification of a medical diagnosis, the unique focus of nursing assessments is on the client's responses to actual or potential health problems.

Assessing is the systematic and continuous collection, validation, and communication of client data; these **data** reflect how health functioning is enhanced by health promotion or compromised by illness. A **data base** (or baseline data) includes all the pertinent client information collected by the nurse and other health care professionals; as such, it enables a comprehensive and effective plan of care to be designed and implemented for the client. The collection of client data is a vital step in the nursing process because the remaining steps depend on complete, accurate, factual, and relevant data.

The initial comprehensive nursing assessment results in a data base that enables the nurse to make a judgment about a client's health status, ability to manage his or her own health care, and need for nursing; refer the client to a physician or other health care professional, if indicated; and plan and deliver individualized, holistic nursing care that draws on the client's strengths. In addition to an initial assessment of the client, ongoing assessments are made by the nurse. Ongoing nursing assessment alerts the nurse to changes in the client's responses to health and illness, and suggests necessary changes in the plan of nursing care or care offered by other health care professionals.

During the assessment step of the nursing process, the nurse establishes the data base by interviewing the client to obtain a nursing history; the nurse may also perform a nursing examination to collect data. Other sources of client information used by the nurse include the client's support people, the client record, the client's health care professionals, and nursing and other health care literature. After the nurse has established the data base, data about the client are collected continuously because the client's health status can change quickly. Questionable data are verified (validated) as part of the assessment step of the nursing process. All pertinent data are recorded and, when appropriate, verbally communicated to the responsible person, so that it can best benefit the client (Fig. 15-1).

Unique Focus of Nursing Assessment

When nurses make nursing assessments, they do not duplicate medical assessments. Unlike the medical assessment,

Data Collection

Types of Data

There are two types of data—objective and subjective. **Objective data** are information perceived by the senses; data observed by one person can be verified by another person observing the same client. Examples of objective data are an elevated temperature reading (101°F), skin that is moist, and refusal to look at or eat food. Objective data also are called signs or overt data.

Subjective data are information perceived only by the affected person; these data cannot be perceived or verified by another person. Examples of subjective data are feeling nervous, nauseated, or chilly and experiencing pain. Subjective data also are called symptoms or covert data (Table 15-1).

Characteristics of Data

When collecting and recording client data, it is important to be complete, accurate, factual, and relevant.

Complete   To the extent that it is possible, all the client data needed to understand a client health problem and develop a plan of care to maximize wellness should be identified. For example, knowing that a client has lost weight is meaningless until the nurse discovers (1) if the weight loss was intentional or unintentional, (2) if it was related to a change in eating or exercise patterns or to some underlying pathology, and (3) how the client views and is responding to the weight loss.

Accurate and Factual   Both the client and the nurse may intentionally or unintentionally misrepresent or distort client information. For example, a client who values being thin may describe a weight gain of several pounds as the onset of obesity. Nurses concerned with accuracy and fact continually verify what they hear with what they observe using other senses and validate all questionable data. When nurses suspect that personal bias or stereotyping is influencing their data collection, it is appropriate for them to consult with another nurse. It also is best to describe observed behaviors rather than the interpretation of the behavior. Such a description may read: "Client frequently is observed lying with his face to the wall. Attempts to engage him in conversation fail. He refused lunch today and ate

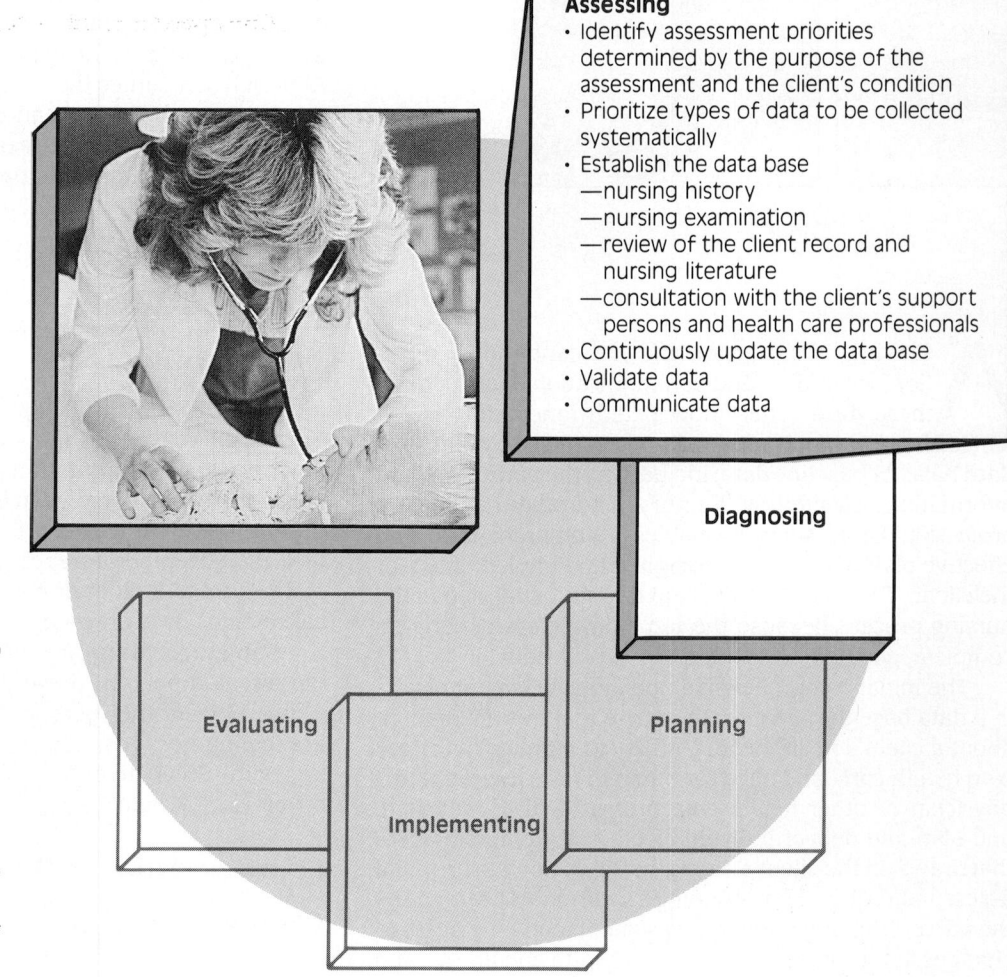

Assessing
- Identify assessment priorities determined by the purpose of the assessment and the client's condition
- Prioritize types of data to be collected systematically
- Establish the data base
  —nursing history
  —nursing examination
  —review of the client record and nursing literature
  —consultation with the client's support persons and health care professionals
- Continuously update the data base
- Validate data
- Communicate data

Diagnosing

Planning

Implementing

Evaluating

F I G U R E 1 5 - 1

Assessing. The primary source of client information is the client. Resources include the client's support people, the client record, information from other health care professionals, and information from nursing and health care literature. (Photo by Gates Rhodes, courtesy of School of Nursing, University of Pennsylvania.)

only soup for dinner." "Client is depressed," conversely, is the nurse's interpretation of the client's behavior; it is not a factual statement. Recording the client's behaviors factually allows other health care professionals to explore causes of the behavior with the client.

T A B L E 1 5 - 1

Comparison of Objective and Subjective Data

Objective Data	Subjective Data
32-year-old man Height: 5′8″. Weight: 9/18/88—224 lb 2/4/89—202 lb	"I'm beginning to feel better about myself now that I'm losing weight and I seem to have more energy."
Posterior, left midcalf is warm and red.	"My leg hurts when I walk."
Client observed fidgeting with bed covers; facial features are tightly drawn.	"I'm so afraid of what they might find when they cut me open tomorrow."

Relevant Because recording comprehensive data can become an endless task, one challenge facing nurses is to determine *what type* of data and *how much* data to collect for each client. This chapter describes ways to do this. The aim is to record concisely all pertinent data. Often only experience teaches nurses what data are needed in specific cases.

Learning how to collect, validate, and communicate data that are complete, accurate, factual, and relevant is the focus of the remainder of this chapter.

Data Collection Methods

Common methods used in the collection of data in nursing include observation, interview, and physical assessment.

Observation

Observation is the conscious and deliberate use of the five physical senses to gather data. The skilled nurse uses each nurse–client interaction to observe and interpret meaningful stimuli (data). Student nurses can develop such observation skills by training themselves to carefully observe the following each time they encounter a client:

- What are the client's current responses (physical and emotional) to his or her situation? Be alert to signs of distress—difficulty breathing, bleeding, pain, heightened anxiety—as well as to anything out of the ordinary—sudden eruption of rash, changes in levels of consciousness, and so forth.
- What is the client's current ability to manage his or her care (need for additional information or nursing assistance)?
- What is the immediate environment? Consider the safety of the environment—side rails, spills on floor—as well as the functioning of equipment (intravenous therapy, oxygen, drains). Who are the people in the room? What are the temperature and odor of the room?
- What is the larger environment (hospital or community)?

Interview

Nursing History An **interview** is a planned communication. During the assessment step of the nursing process, the nurse interviews the client to obtain a nursing history. Ideally, the nursing history captures the uniqueness of the client and records this, so that care planning may be patterned to meet the client's individual needs. The nursing history should, therefore, be obtained as soon as possible after a client presents for care, and should be followed by the nursing physical assessment. The **nursing history** should clearly identify client strengths and weaknesses, health risks such as hereditary and environmental factors, and potential and existing health problems. The focus of the nursing history is on getting to know the *person.* Data included in the nursing history are listed in the accompanying display.

Strong interviewing skills are needed to obtain the necessary client data and to communicate concern for the client. A brief discussion of the work of each phase of the interview follows.

Phases of the Interview The four phases in the nurse–client interview are preparatory phase, introduction, working phase, and termination. More detailed information on interviewing techniques can be found in Chapter 20.

Preparatory Phase Before initiating the interview, the nurse prepares to meet the client by reading current and past records and reports, when available. During this phase, it is important not to let stereotypes and prejudices predetermine the nurse–client relationship. If the nurse is aware of personal prejudices, those prejudices can be dealt with constructively. Professional nurses learn to approach clients with open minds and to be sensitive to the human needs that underlie diverse behaviors.

During the preparatory phase, the nurse should ensure that the environment in which the interview is to be con-

---

Components of a Nursing History

- Client's profile: name, age, sex, marital status, religion, occupation, education
- Client's reason for seeking health care
- Client's normal health habits and patterns and any need for nursing assistance
- Client's current state of health, functioning of body systems, and past medical and surgical history
- Meaning client attributes to health and illness and characteristic response or coping patterns
- Client's developmental history, family history, environmental history, and psychosocial history
- Client and family's expectations of nursing and of the health care team
- Client and family's ability and willingness to participate in the plan of care
- Client's personal resources and deficits

---

ducted is private and relaxed. Unless the client wants to have family members or friends present during the interview, the nurse should interview the client alone, either in the client's room or in a quiet office.

Both the seating arrangement and the distance between nurse and client are important (Fig. 15-2). Chairs placed at right angles to each other and about 3 to 4 ft (0.9 to 1.2 m) apart facilitate an easy exchange of information. If the client is in bed, placing a chair at a 45-degree angle to the bed is helpful. If the nurse stands at the foot or side of the client's bed and physically talks or looks down at the client,

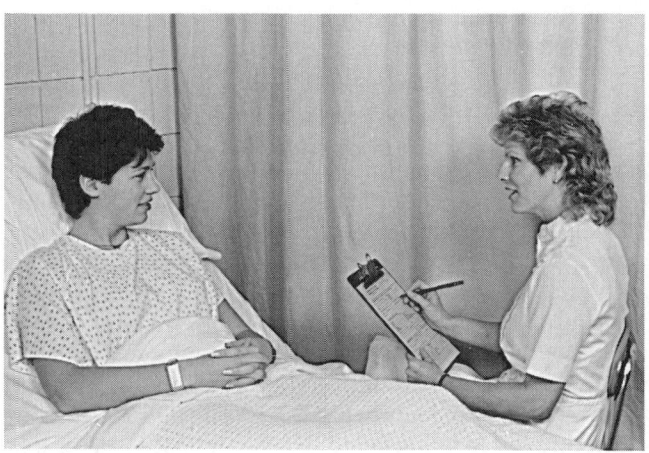

F I G U R E   1 5 - 2

In the interview, both the seating arrangement and the distance from the client are important in establishing a relaxed and comfortable environment for data collection. (Photo © Ken Kasper.)

a superior–inferior relationship is communicated, and can defeat the interview. Whenever possible, it is best to communicate with clients at eye level.

The interview should be scheduled when both the nurse and the client are free of concerns and distractions, so they can concentrate on the task. Ten to 15 minutes may be all that is necessary in some circumstances, whereas an hour or more may be required in others. Information can be gathered in several meetings, especially if the nurse notices that the client is tiring or is in pain.

Introduction The interview's introduction is critical because it sets the tone not only for the remainder of the interview, but also for every nurse–client interaction that follows. At the end of this phase of the interview, the client should know the name of her primary nurse and what she can expect of nursing; should sense that the nurse is competent and cares about him or her; and should know what is expected of him or her in terms of developing the plan of care and participating in its execution.

The nurse initiates the interview by stating his or her name and status, identifying the purpose of the interview, and clarifying the roles of nurse and client. A typical introduction might run like this: "Good afternoon, Miss Komer. My name is Lisa Gray, and I'll be your primary nurse while you are in the hospital. Right now I'd like to ask you a few questions about yourself so that we can plan your nursing care together. Feel free to respond only to those questions you feel comfortable answering, and know that your responses will be treated confidentially by the staff. This will take about 20 minutes. Is this time convenient for you? Do you need anything before we start?"

The initial impression the nurse creates is critical, especially with clients who are new to the health care environment. All nurses that the client encounters in the future may be judged in light of this first impression. When the nurse communicates respect and genuine concern for the client, the client is then encouraged to discuss health concerns and problems freely. The interpersonal qualities of a respectful presence, professionalism, and caring invite the client's confidence and inspire hope that help is available.

During the introduction, it is important for the nurse to assess the client's comfort and ability to participate in the interview. It also is appropriate to discuss confidentiality. The client should know where the data being recorded are stored, how they will be used, and who has access to them. Some nurses record data on the appropriate form while with the client, whereas other nurses take notes and complete the form later. Writing should not interfere with the sharing of information during the interview. If a contractual agreement clearly identifying the responsibilities of both client and nurse is indicated, terms are discussed at this time (see also Chapter 6).

Working Phase During the working phase of the interview, the nurse gathers all the information needed to form the subjective data base. The accuracy, completeness, and relevancy of the data base depend on the nurse's use of the interviewing and basic communication techniques discussed in Chapter 20. The communication techniques highlighted below are important ingredients of a successful interview.

- Focus on the client during the interview, demonstrating interest and concern: use the client's name, use eye contact appropriately, avoid rushing the client.
- Listen to the client attentively, using reflection and paraphrase to communicate to the client that he or she is being understood.
- Ask about the client's main problem first, using terminology the client understands; save personal or delicate questions for when a rapport is established. Defer less important questions until a later interview if the client is too ill or upset to communicate easily.
- Pose questions and comments to the client in the manner best suited to produce the desired communication (see Chapter 20):
  - Closed questions elicit specific information.
  - Open-ended questions allow the client to verbalize freely.
  - Reflective questions encourage the client to elaborate on thoughts and feelings.
  - Direct questioning may be used to validate information, to clarify information, or to place events into a meaningful sequence.
- Avoid comments and questions that impede communication (see Chapter 20)—cliches, questions that require a yes or no answer only, intimidating why or how questions, probing questions, giving advice, using judgmental comments, changing the subject, giving false assurance.
- Use silence and touch appropriately.

Many client variables can positively or negatively affect the outcome of an interview. Table 15-2 identifies client variables that can negatively influence an interview unless the nurse responds appropriately.

Termination The successful interview is concluded carefully. A client should be advised that the interview is coming to an end. It is helpful to recapitulate the interview, highlighting key points. Both the client and the nurse should be satisfied that the important data are recorded. A helpful strategy is to ask the client after the summary: "Is there anything else you would like us to know that will help us plan your care?" This gives the client an opportunity to add data the nurse did not think to include.

Before leaving the client, it is helpful to alert the client as to what she can expect within the next 24 hours. The client also should know when the nurse will reestablish contact: "Thank you for answering these questions, Miss Komer. Please feel free to keep us informed of anything you think we should know. I'll be leaving soon, but when I return tomorrow morning, I'll discuss your plan of care. This afternoon will be busy for you: Some blood tests and a chest x-ray have been ordered. Your evening will probably

During my chronic medical–surgical rotation, my clinical group was placed on an oncology floor. My first thought was, "Oh no, not the cancer floor!" The word *fear* didn't even begin to describe how I felt. These clients had enough problems without some "green" nursing student aggravating them all day. I kept thinking these people are extremely ill and won't want to be bothered by my intruding questions.

Nonetheless, I knew I had to do it. Not only did I have to take care of this client all day, I had to develop a data base and care plan. I knew I would have to do a lot more than give him his morning care and leave him alone. I would have to carry on an extended conversation with this patient to get all the information I needed.

As if all of this wasn't enough to make me throw in the white flag, when my client assignment was given, I discovered my client was a male and only 1 year older than me. A 28-year-old man with terminal cancer—this was too scary!

Clinical day came, as I knew it would, and I was shaking. I walked in that room and together the client and I planned his care. I explained to him the things I needed to talk about with him and I couldn't believe it—he didn't tell me to go away! We talked at length about his disease process and how it had affected his plans and goals. He opened up to me about his spirituality, his relationships with friends and family, and other personal subjects. Periodically he would cringe, and I could tell, it was time for a break. He was hurting too badly to go on at that time.

At the end of that day, my view point was totally different than it had been that morning. I walked away from that room and off that floor feeling like I had made a difference for this person. We had shared a lot and he seemed so appreciative for the time I took to talk with him. The amazing part was that all I had to do was just be myself and allow him to do the same and our day flowed smoothly. The lesson I learned here was important for me: Keep calm and hold onto compassion and nursing offers many rewards!

—Nancy E. Driskill, Southeast Missouri State University,
Cape Girardeau, Missouri

---

be quiet. Do you have any questions? Is there anything else I can do for you before I leave?

Physical Assessment

Physical assessment is the examination of the client for *objective data* that may better define the client's condition and help the nurse in planning care. The physical assessment normally follows the nursing history and interview, and may verify data gathered during the history or yield new data. There has been a great deal of controversy about nursing's role in the physical assessment of the client caused by concern that this is a duplication of medicine's role. Physicians traditionally have performed the intake physical assessment, which commonly is the mechanism of entry into the health care delivery system as well as the basis for medical treatment. Some nurses in expanded roles are performing comprehensive intake physical assessments, which identify health and illness states, and are then recommending or prescribing appropriate follow-up

care. In any case, all nurses conduct select aspects of physical assessment for nursing purposes.

Unlike the physical assessment performed by the physician to identify pathology and its cause, the nursing physical assessment focuses primarily on the client's functional abilities. If a neurologic deficit is present, the nurse is concerned with identifying how this deficit affects the client's reasoning and sensorimotor abilities. For example, the client who has had a cerebrovascular accident (stroke) is examined to determine his ability to comprehend and communicate information; his ability to execute the tasks of everyday life also should be assessed.

Purposes of the nursing physical assessment include the appraisal of health status, the identification of health problems, and the establishment of a data base for nursing intervention (Fig. 15-3).

Nurses practicing in different settings may use different physical assessment techniques for different purposes. Nurses in the coronary care unit use sophisticated high-technology assessment techniques, whereas nurses in a

T A B L E   1 5 - 2

Client Variables That Can Negatively Influence an Interview and Suggested Nursing Responses		
Client Variables	**Effect on Interview**	**Nursing Response**
High anxiety	Client may speak rapidly or incoherently and may jump from one topic to another; client may deny or misrepresent what he is experiencing.	Normalize anxiety: "Many people find it difficult to talk about their health and become anxious"; approach client gently, speak slowly and softly; underscore importance of the client sharing what he is experiencing so nurses can help.
Pain	Client offers clipped responses and yes or no answers whenever possible; overriding concern is pain relief.	Do everything possible to make client comfortable before the interview, including obtaining an order for and administering pain medication; if pain persists, obtain only vital data and defer remainder of interview until client is more comfortable.
Language difficulty (client not fluent in nurse's language because speaks a different language, has a limited education, or fears saying the "wrong thing")	Vital client data will not be communicated; client may mistakenly be labeled "indifferent" or "noncommunicative."	Speak clearly (do not raise voice) using simple language; whenever possible obtain the assistance of an interpreter (family member may help but if client data are confidential a stranger may be preferable).
Previous negative experience with nurses or health care delivery system	Client is aloof, unwilling to participate in interview; general attitude: "Why should I waste my time telling you anything . . . it won't do me any good."	"I know other people who have had a tough time with nurses or the system . . . life isn't perfect . . . but how about giving us a chance this time to show you what nurses can do? Communicate respect for the client and competence.
Unrealistic expectations of health care professionals	Client expects nurses and other health care professionals to magically know everything about him or her and to "take care" of him or her; "surrenders" himself or herself to the system—"you know best" attitude.	Communicate clearly that no one knows or understands the client like the client does, and invite him or her to become involved in his or her care; "No two persons are alike and unless you tell me a little more about yourself and how you are feeling, there is no way we'll be able to plan good care."

rehabilitation center use a wide range of physical assessment skills that focus on identifying functional and nonfunctional response patterns to disabilities.

The nursing physical assessment involves the examination of all body systems in a systematic manner; a head-to-toe format commonly is used. These data may be documented on a separate nursing physical assessment tool, or incorporated into a combined data base assessment form, as shown on pages 238 to 242. Nurses also may use physical assessment skills to evaluate selected systems.

Techniques   Four methods are used to collect data during a physical assessment—inspection, palpation, percussion, and auscultation. These techniques and the basic skills the student must learn to perform physical assessment are described in Chapter 24.

Sources of Data

Client   The client is the primary and usually the best source of information. Unless specified otherwise, it is as-

sumed that the data recorded in the nursing history have been collected from the client. Most clients are willing to share information when they know it will be helpful in planning their care. Although data collected from the client usually are accurate, the nurse should be alert to certain difficulties. For example, a client who is acutely ill may not be able to communicate adequately if her pain is severe or if her consciousness is altered in any way. An emotionally upset client may distort information: A client who is fearful because he thinks that the illness may threaten his work or life may deny certain symptoms or deliberately give misleading facts. If the nurse becomes aware that the client's report of symptoms differs from physical findings or data obtained from other sources, it is important to note this and to explore the cause of the discrepancy. The client with limited mental capacity or a very young client cannot be relied on to report accurately. Children, elderly people, and people with decreased mental capacity or impaired verbal ability should be encouraged to respond to interview questions as best they can. Bypassing these clients and automatically turning to a family member, friend, or caregiver

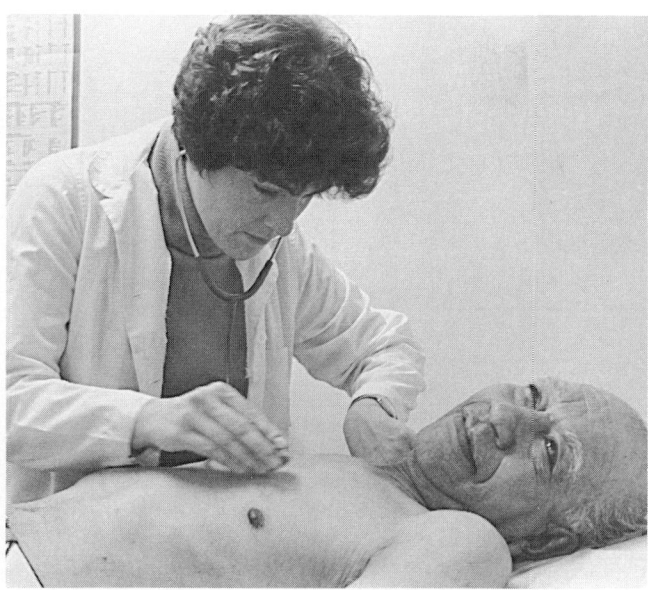

FIGURE 15-3

The physical examination should include appraisal of health status, identification of health problems, and the establishment of a data base for nursing intervention. (Photo by Gates Rhodes, courtesy of School of Nursing, University of Pennsylvania.)

for information communicates powerfully that the nurse either has no time for the client to express his or her needs or doubts the client's ability to communicate these needs.

Support People Family members, friends, and caregivers are especially helpful sources of data when the client has limited capacity to share information with the nurse or when the client is a child. Husbands and wives can supply information concerning their spouses. Friends may accompany a client to a health agency, and often can supply useful information. Care must be taken to determine that the client does not object to data being gathered from friends, and that the friends want to participate. Also, the nurse is cautioned that there should be a clear understanding by the client, family, and friends of the confidentiality of the data collected. Whenever data are gathered from support people, this should be indicated in the nursing history.

Client Record Records prepared by different members of the health care team provide information essential to comprehensive nursing care. The nurse should review records early when gathering data—in some instances, before the first contact with the client. Such a review helps to focus the nursing assessment and to confirm and amplify information obtained from other sources.

The client's hospital record or chart, which lists such information as age, sex, occupation, religious preference, next of kin, and financial status, is one type of record. The hospital record includes information entered by various

health care professionals, such as the physician, social worker, dietitian, physiotherapist, and laboratory technicians. Nurses who want their care to be supportive of the client as he or she responds to changes in health status must be familiar with the many sections of the client record other than the documentation of the nursing care plan and nursing notes. The following are important sources of data for the nurse.

Medical History, Physical Examination, and Progress Notes These sources record the findings of physicians as they assess and treat the client; they focus on identifying pathology and its cause and on determining the medical regimen that will best treat the problem.

Consultations The client's physicians may invite specialists to assess and work with the client; the focus is on documenting findings that help establish a medical diagnosis or on planning and executing the medical regimen.

Reports of Diagnostic Studies Reports of laboratory studies and other diagnostic tests, such as x-rays, offer the nurse objective data that can either confirm or conflict with data collected during the nursing history or examination. Results of diagnostic studies are helpful to physicians in establishing a diagnosis and in monitoring the client's response to treatment. The results of these same studies also may be helpful to nurses in evaluating the success of nursing interventions.

Reports of Therapies by Other Health Care Professionals Other health care professionals who interact with the client also record their findings and note any progress the client is making in their specific areas—for example, nutrition, physical therapy, or speech therapy. These reports help the nurse to better assess the client's progress in general and are useful when determining the client's ability to return home and manage care independently.

Records of previous admissions for health care and records from other health agencies, such as a social service agency or a home health care agency, also are valuable sources of data. They contain information about the client's previous medical or surgical problems and response patterns, which may be important determinants of the current plan of care.

Health Care Professionals Nurses can learn a great deal about a client's normal health habits and patterns and her or his response to illness by talking with other nurses, physicians, social workers, and other members of the health care team (Fig. 15-4). Although such communication is always important, it can be critical when clients are transferred from home to institution, from institution to institution, or from one hospital to another. The only way to ensure continuity of care is to make special efforts to share pertinent information.

(Text continues on p. 243)

BRONSON METHODIST HOSPITAL
Kalamazoo, Michigan

Medical/Surgical-Critical Care Admission Assessment

A. DEMOGRAPHIC DATA

Name: *Margaret Tembra*

Prefers to be called: *Mrs. Tembra* Age: *72*

Date: *9/2/92* Time of arrival to unit: *2:00 pm*

Mode of admission: *wheelchair*

I.D. bracelet on and coincides with addressograph: ☑ Yes ☐ No Information given by: *patient and her daughter Lisa*

If unable to reach next of kin/legal guardian, contact: *Barbara Tembra* Phone: *634-5221*

Valuables (list and state disposition): *eye glasses (at bedside); purse taken home by daughter Lisa; no other valuables*

Admitted from: ☑ Home ☐ Nursing Home ☐ Assisted Living ☐ Foster Care ☐ Senior Citizens' Apartments ☐ Other

Facility Name: ______ Adm. Medical Diagnosis: *T.I.A.*

B. VITAL SIGNS

Ht: *5' 2"* Wt: *63.6* Kg

Temp: *98.2 °F* ☑ Oral ☐ Ax. ☐ Rectal

Pulse: *88* ☐ Reg. ☑ Irreg.

Resp.: *18* ☑ Reg. ☐ Irreg.

BP: Left: *184/120*
☑ Lying ☐ Sitting ☐ Standing

Right: *180/120*
☑ Lying ☐ Sitting ☐ Standing

C. ORIENTATION TO UNIT

(The following have been explained):

Call system/bed-bathroom	☑ Yes ☐ N/A	Floor restrictions	☑ Yes ☐ N/A
Bed operation/siderails	☑ Yes ☐ N/A	Visitation Policy	☑ Yes ☐ N/A
Bathroom/bedpan-urinal	☑ Yes ☐ N/A	Lounge	☑ Yes ☐ N/A
TV/CH2/telephone	☑ Yes ☐ N/A	Newspaper/mail	☑ Yes ☐ N/A
Meal/cafeteria hours	☑ Yes ☐ N/A	Siderails policy	☑ Yes ☐ N/A
Smoking policy	☑ Yes ☐ N/A	Chaplain services	☑ Yes ☐ N/A

Signature: *Margaret Tembra*

D. Health Patterns Assessment: Complete information, **including patient's words.** Indicate N/A if non-applicable. Circle, code, or check all other findings as appropriate.

1. HEALTH PERCEPTION/HEALTH MANAGEMENT

Reason for hospitalization/chief complaint: *"I fell in the kitchen this morning and couldn't move my left leg for awhile; I've also been having 'headaches'."*

Recent illness/exposure to communicable disease: *—*

Previous hospitalizations/surgeries: *about 1965 gall bladder surgery; hospitalized for high blood pressure 1985*

What other health problems have you had? *—*

Things done to manage health: *"I drink lots of water, eat fruit and avoid fried foods. I try not to worry so much."*

Statement of patient's general appearance (include condition of hair, skin, nails): *Alert, medium-built, well-nourished female; appears anxious about hospitalization: voice low, grabs daughter's hand; neat appearance; skin pale, cool and dry; gray hair-thin; scalp clean; thick nails; adequate cappillairy refill.*

Tobacco use: ☐ Yes ☑ No ☐ Used to smoke:

EtOH use: *none*

Allergies: ☐ Yes (list with reaction experienced) ☑ No

Food: *—*

Medications/anesthetics: *—*

Other (e.g., wool, tape, pollens): *regular soaps cause skin to be excessively dry*

FORM 102 (Revised 10/84) — Page 1

Patient's Name: _Tembra, Margaret_   Hospital No.: _4629 F_   Date: _9/2/92_

Medications: (e.g., prescript., non-prescript.) ☑Yes ☐No Did you bring? ☐Yes ☑No Taken home? ☐Yes ☐No ☐N/A

NAME	DOSE	SCHEDULE	REASON	PRESCRIBING PHYSICIAN
hydralazine	?	OD	high blood pressure	Dr. Skomar
aspirin	ꝉꝉ	PRN	headaches	—
metamucil	1 Tbsp	PRN	constipation	—

Have you been taking your medication(s) as prescribed? _yes_

OTHER PERTINENT DATA: _—_

	SCT	initials

NUTRITION / METABOLIC

2. Special diet? _—_   Supplements: _—_

Pattern of daily food/fluid intake: _Drinks at least 5-6 glasses H₂O daily + juices + tea;_ _↓ fried, fatty foods; likes baked or broiled meat, vegetables + fruit, "sweet_ _tooth."_

Appetite: _"very good"_   Wt. loss/gain: _—_

Nausea/Vomiting: _—_

GI pain: _—_

Condition of oral mucous membranes: _pink, moist_

Dental condition: _dentures clean_   Dentures: ☑Upper ☑Lower ☐Partial ☐N/A

Skin: ☐Warm ☑Dry ☑Cool ☐Moist ☐Other: _pale_

Turgor: ☑Supple ☐Firm ☐Fragile ☐Dehydrated ☐Other: _____

Color: ☐Pink ☑Pale ☐Dusky ☐Cyanotic ☐Jaundiced ☐Mottled ☐Other: _____

Edema: _+ 1 ankles_

Wounds/drains/dressings: _____

Skin problems (description and location): _Skin on legs and upper arms dry + scaley;_ _scratch marks; reddened area under left breast – skin intact._

I.V.'s: _____ ☐N/A

OTHER PERTINENT DATA: _—_

	SCT	initials

ELIMINATION

3. Abd. tenderness/guarding/distention: _—_

Bowel sounds: _present all 4 quadrants_   Stoma (type): _—_

Any problems with hemorrhoids/involuntary stool? _hx hemorrhoid 2° straining / constipation_

Usual bowel pattern (frequency, character, consistency, etc.): _stools tend to be hard and dry --_ _q 2-3 days_   Date of last BM: _9/1/89_

If problem, describe: _occasional (1x/wk) constipation_

Use of anything to manage bowels (e.g., laxatives, enemas, suppositories, "home remedies", anti-diarrheals): _↑ fluids, ↑ fruit, metamucil; dislikes bran_

Usual urinary pattern (frequency, character, amount, incontinence, nocturia, etc.): _5-6 x per day;_ _up once at night to void_   Last void (time): _"this AM"_

If problem, describe: _—_

Perspiration/nocturnal sweats: _—_

OTHER PERTINENT DATA: _—_

	SCT	initials

4.

CARDIO-VASCULAR STATUS

Peripheral pulses: *palpable, strong* ☐ N/A

Neurovascular check (e.g., capillary refill): *↓ sensation (hot/cold sharp/dull) L leg; rapid capillary refill*

Chest pain/radiation: *—*

Jugular vein distention: ☐ Yes ☑ No
Hx of murmur: ☐ Yes ☑ No
Pacemaker: ☐ Yes ☑ No
Presence of A-V Shunt: *—* ☑ No
Arterio-venous bruit: _____ ☑ N/A
Monitor/rhythm: _____ ☑ N/A
Hemodynamic monitoring: *—* ☑ N/A

Tembra, M., 4269 F

RESPIRATORY STATUS

Respiratory pattern: ☑ No problem ☐ Dyspnea ☐ Nocturnal Dyspnea ☐ S.O.B. at rest
☐ S.O.B. on exertion: *—* ☐ Other: *—*
Lung sounds: *clear* Use of accessory muscles? ☐ Yes ☑ No
Cough/production: *—* O₂ supplement: _____ ☑ N/A
Resp. tubes (e.g., ET, trach, chest/describe secretions/drainage): *—* ☑ N/A
Ventilatory assistance: _____ ☑ N/A

ACTIVITIES OF DAILY LIVING/MOBILITY STATUS

Use the **Activity Level Code** below to assess admission statuses:

	ADL Status	**Mobility Status**

0—total independence
1—assist with device
2—assist with person
3—assist with device & person
4—total dependence

Feeding *set up tray* Meal Preparation *—*
Bathing *2* Cleaning *—*
Dressing *0* Shopping *—*
Grooming *0* Laundry *—*
Toileting *1* Other *—*

Bed mobility *2*
Cart transfer *bedrest*
Chair/toilet transfer *bedrest*
Ambulation *bedrest*
R.O.M. *2*

Handedness: ☑ Right ☐ Left
Able to use? ☑ Yes ☐ No
Reasons for ADL/Mobility limitations: *Bedrest ordered during diagnostic work-up; At present able to move all 4 extremities* ☐ N/A
Devices used for assist: *Bed pan* ☐ N/A
Do you need assistance with transportation? ☐ Yes ☐ No If "Yes", specify: *—*
Where do you plan to be discharged? *home* Will you need assistance? ☐ Yes ☑ No
If "Yes", describe: _____
OTHER PERTINENT DATA: *—*

| SCT | initials |

5.

Level of consciousness: *Alert* Oriented to: ☑ Person ☑ Place ☑ Time
Behaviors (describe): *Face reflects concern about 's morning's paralysis & hospitalization*
Hx of epilepsy/seizures/Parkinson's, etc.: *—*

REFLEXES

Reflexes: ☑ No problem ☐ Problem (If "No problem", do not complete this section.)
Eyes: Pupil size: r *O* l *O* Equal? ☑ Yes ☐ No Reaction to light: r ✓ l ✓
Accommodation: r ✓ l ✓ Deviation: _____
Handgrasp: r ✓ l ✓ Gag: ✓ Swallow: ✓
Movement of extremities: *↓ strength and ↓ movement left lower extremity*

SENSORIUM

Eyes/sight: ☐ No problem ☑ Deficit: *"blurry vision" at times* Aid: *eyeglasses*
Ears/hearing: ☐ No problem ☑ Deficit: *"hard" of hearing" Ⓛ ear* Aid: *none*
Nose/smell: ☑ No problem ☐ Deficit: _____
Tongue/taste: ☑ No problem ☐ Deficit: _____
Skin/touch: ☑ No problem ☐ Deficit: _____
Numbness/tingling: ☐ No problem ☑ Deficit: *left leg "feels queer - pins and needles"*
Dizziness: ☐ No problem ☑ Deficit: *feels "slightly dizzy - unsteady"*

FORM 102 (Revised 10/84) — Page 3

Patient's Name: _Tembra, M._   Hospital No.: _4269 F_   Date: _9/2/9̶2̶_

COGNITIVE/PERCEPTUAL

PAIN

Pain: ☐ No problem ☑ Problem (If "No problem", do not complete this section.)

If "Problem", describe location, type, intensity, onset, duration: _headaches – began about 6 months ago – of increasing frequency and severity; at present occur 1-2x/wk, last 1-2 days_

Methods of pain management: _Asprin, other OTC extra strength pain relievers only helps "a little"_

COGNITION

Primary language: _English_   Speech deficit: _—_   Aid: _—_

Any learning difficulties? _—_

OTHER PERTINENT DATA: _—_

_____

| | SCT | initials |

6.

SLEEP/REST

Usual sleep/rest pattern: _11 pm – 7 am_

Adequate? ☑ Yes ☐ No   Factors affecting sleep/rest: _gets up to void once during night_

Methods to promote sleep: _—_

Hx of sleep disturbances: _—_

OTHER PERTINENT DATA: _—_

| | SCT | initials |

7.

SELF-PERCEPTION SELF-CONCEPT

Are there any ways you feel differently about yourself since you've been ill/hospitalized? _"never questioned my health" expresses fear_

Description of non-verbal behaviors: _quiet speech, wrinkled brow, wants daughter near_

OTHER PERTINENT DATA: _daughter reports mother has been very independent, strong woman – rarely ill_

| | SCT | initials |

8.

ROLE/RELATIONSHIP

Marital status: _Widowed_   Children: _3_

Do you live? ☐ Alone ☑ With family ☐ Other: _lives with daughter Lisa & her family_

Family feelings regarding hospitalization: _Concern_

Who are the people that will help you most at this time? _2 daughters: Lisa, Barbara_

Are you presently employed? ☐ Yes ☑ No Occupation: _____ ☐ N/A

Are you presently in school? ☐ Yes ☑ No Will illness/hospitalization interfere? _____ ☐ N/A

Upon discharge, if necessary, will you be able to afford?

   Medications: ☑ Yes ☐ No   Supplies: ☑ Yes ☐ No   Medical Care: ☑ Yes ☐ No

OTHER PERTINENT DATA: _Husband died 8 months ago – moved in with daughter 6 months ago after selling family home – High Stress_

| | SCT | initials |

9.

SEXUALITY/REPRODUCTIVE

Female: ☐ N/A   Menopausal: ☑ Yes ☐ No   Menstrual pattern: _____ ☐ N/A

Problems/changes: _____

Date of L.N.M.P. _____ ☑ N/A   Possibly pregnant? ☐ Yes ☐ No ☐ N/A

Pregnancy history: _G 3 P 3_

Use of birth control measure ☐ Yes ☐ No ☑ N/A   Type: _____

Any problems with use? _____

Monthly self-breast exam? ☐ Yes ☑ No ☐ N/A

Vaginal discharge/bleeding/lesions: _—_

Receiving medical attention? ☐ Yes ☑ No ☐ N/A

OTHER PERTINENT DATA: _—_

| | SCT | initials |

Male: ☑ N/A   Prostate problems? _____

Monthly self-testicular exam? ☐ Yes ☐ No ☐ N/A

Penile discharge/bleeding/lesions: _____

Receiving medical attention? ☐ Yes ☐ No ☐ N/A

OTHER PERTINENT DATA: _____

| | | initials |

FORM 102 (Revised 10/84) — Page 4

COPING/STRESS

10. Have you experienced any recent stressful situations in addition to your illness/hospitalization? ☑Yes ☐No

If "Yes", please describe briefly: _In past year:_
death of husband
sale of family home
relocation with daughter

Are there any ways we can be of assistance? _"can't think of any"_

How do you usually manage stresses? _talk with friends, pray_
"I used to share everything with my husband"

What do you do for relaxation? _used to crochet, watch TV_

Support groups/counselling resources used: _____

Were they helpful? _____ ☐N/A

OTHER PERTINENT DATA: _misses husband very much_

SCT	initials

Tembra, M. 4269F

VALUE/BELIEF

11. Will illness/hospitalization interfere with any of the following?

Spiritual or religious practices? ☐Yes ☑No

Cultural beliefs or practices? ☐Yes ☑No

Familial traditions? ☐Yes ☑No

If "Yes", to any of the above, please describe briefly: _____

Would you like your clergy or hospital chaplain to be contacted? ☑Yes ☐No ☐N/A _daughter will contact minister_

OTHER PERTINENT DATA: _____

SCT	initials

IMPRESSIONS

E. Include: a. Possible nursing diagnostic concept labels to consider for care planning.

   b. Possible referral resources to consider for discharge planning needs.

   c. Other pertinent information

a. _Diagnostic labels: Colonic Constipation, High Risk for Impaired Physical Mobility, High Risk for Altered Health Maintenance Related to Knowledge Deficit: TIA → stroke management, disturbance in self-concept, skin integrity impairment_

b. _Social Service Referral_
referral to home minister

	initials

DATE	TIME	INITIALS	SIGNATURES	
9/2/92	2:00 pm	SCT	S. Carol Taylor, RN	(1st Adm. R.N.)
				(2nd Adm. R.N.)
				(3rd Adm. R.N.)
				(4th Adm. R.N.)

FORM 102 (Revised 10/84) — Page 5

©1984 Bronson Methodist Hospital. All rights reserved.

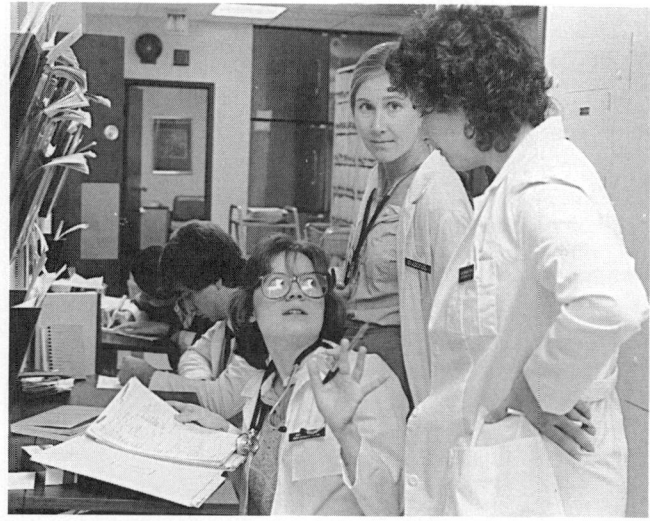

FIGURE 15-4

Nurses can learn a great deal about a client's normal health habits and patterns and responses to illness by talking with other nurses, physicians, social workers, and other members of the health care team. This exchange of information is particularly important when clients transfer from one health care setting to another or to home.

Nursing and Other Health Care Literature To obtain a comprehensive client data base, it may be necessary to consult the nursing and related literature on specific health problems. For example, if a nurse has not cared for a client with Paget's disease before, it is important for him or her to read about the clinical manifestations of the disease and its usual progression in order to know what to look for when assessing the client. In addition to information concerning the medical diagnoses, treatment, and prognosis, a literature review offers the nurse important information about nursing diagnoses, developmental norms, and psychosocial and spiritual practices that is helpful when assessing clients.

Planning Data Collection

Comprehensive Versus Focused Data Collection

Nursing assessments include both the comprehensive admission assessment (data base assessment) and the focused assessment. *Data base assessment* usually is performed during the nurse's initial contact with the client. The nurse collects data concerning *all aspects* of the client's health, establishing priorities for ongoing focused assessments. A data base nursing assessment structured according to Gordon's 11 functional health patterns appears in the accompanying display. *Focused assessment* may be done during the initial assessment if client health problems surface, but it is routinely part of ongoing data collection. The focus is on gathering data about a *specific problem* that has already been identified (Alfaro, 1990, p. 20).

Assessment Priorities

Before beginning to collect data on any client, the nurse should have a good sense of the type of data needed to best develop a satisfactory plan of care. Client data of interest to the nurse include the following:
• Client profile (name, address, age, sex, race, culture, religion, education, occupation)
• Client's developmental stage and ability to meet developmental tasks
• Family, psychosocial, and environmental histories
• Health beliefs, habits, patterns (how client meets basic human needs)
• Client's responses (physical and emotional) to health and illness (functioning of each major body system)
• Meaning client attaches to health and illness
• Presence of risk factors
• Client resources—internal (eg, coping strengths) and external (eg, support people, adequate finances, availability of health care)
• Client's expected and preferred modes of treatment (past experiences with health care professionals)
The purpose for which the assessment is being performed offers the best guidelines as to what type and how much data to collect.

Assessment priorities are influenced by the client's health orientation, developmental stage, and need for nursing.

Health Orientation Wellness assessments, such as Health-Style: A Self-Test in Chapter 2, may be used by nurses to assist clients to identify potential and actual health risks and to explore habits, behaviors, beliefs, attitudes, and values that influence levels of wellness (Pinnell & deMeneses, 1986). Hill and Smith (1990) offer nurses who are interested in wellness a variety of specialized assessment tools that focus on relationships; psychological, environmental, and physical self-care; relaxation; spirituality; humor and play; movement and exercise; sleep and dreams; nutrition; and sexuality. These assessments are very different from the comprehensive admission assessments of clients being hospitalized for treatment in terms of the type of client data gathered.

Developmental Stage Nursing assessments are modified according to the developmental needs of clients. For example, when assessing an infant, special attention is given to weight gain and physical growth, feeding and elimination problems, sleep–activity cycles, and the parenting skills of caregivers. When children are hospitalized, it is similarly important to note how independent the child is with basic care measures (toileting, hygiene, dressing, eating), what words the child uses to indicate the need to void and defecate, play preferences, and so forth.

Need for Nursing   Whether nurses will be interacting with the client for a short or a long period (same-day surgery versus surgery that necessitates a long recovery in an intensive care unit) and the nature of nursing care needed by the client (assistance with the birth of a baby versus support and care throughout a terminal illness) powerfully influence the type of data the nurse collects. A general guideline when assessing clients is to gather only data that are helpful when planning and delivering care. Thus it would be inappropriate to collect a detailed sexual history on a client admitted to the hospital overnight after a slight concussion. Conversely, the nurse who fails to ask a pregnant woman admitted to the hospital for observation because of bleeding during her first trimester if she has any questions about resuming sexual activity once she gets home is doing the client a great disservice.

Practical Considerations   Data already collected from the client and communicated in the client record should not be repeatedly sought from the client unless there is a need to validate this data. Repetitious questioning can be annoying to the client and may cause the client to wonder about the lack of communication among health care professionals. A careful review of the client record before interviewing the client avoids this problem.

Before meeting a new client, it is helpful to take a minute to carefully think about the type of data needed to plan quality care. After the comprehensive nursing assessment has been completed, client health problems dictate assessment priorities for future nurse–client interactions.

Structuring the Assessment

Having now studied the different types of data about clients that nurses collect, it is easy to see the need to structure data collection systematically. Using systematic guidelines specifically developed for a nursing assessment ensures that comprehensive, holistic data are collected for each client and lead easily to the formulation of nursing diagnoses. Once the nurse internalizes the assessment guidelines, it is easier for her or him to focus on the client during the assessment rather than worry about what to assess next.

Most schools of nursing and health care institutions have developed their own structured assessment guidelines, many of which are based on a selected nursing theory. Gordon (1987) proposes a standardized structure for delineating the basic areas of assessment that is applicable to all clients and compatible with all nursing theories. This framework (see display) identifies 11 functional health patterns and organizes client data into these patterns.

Problems Related to Data Collection

Common problems encountered during data collection include inappropriate organization of data base, omission of

---

Functional Health Patterns

Health-perception–health-management pattern: Describes client's perceived pattern of health and well-being and how health is managed

Nutritional-metabolic pattern: Describes pattern of food and fluid consumption relative to metabolic need and pattern indicators of local nutrient supply

Elimination pattern: Describes patterns of excretory function (bowel, bladder, and skin)

Activity-exercise pattern: Describes pattern of exercise, activity, leisure, and recreation

Cognitive-perceptual pattern: Describes sensory-perceptual and cognitive pattern

Sleep–rest pattern: Describes patterns of sleep, rest, and relaxation

Self-perception–self-concept pattern: Describes self-concept pattern and perceptions of self (eg, body comfort, body image, feeling state)

Role-relationship pattern: Describes pattern of role-engagements and relationships

Sexuality-reproductive pattern: Describes client's patterns of satisfaction and dissatisfaction with sexuality pattern; describe reproductive patterns

Coping–stress-tolerance pattern: Describes general coping pattern and effectiveness of the pattern in terms of stress tolerance

Value-belief pattern: Describes patterns of values, beliefs (including spiritual), or goals that guide choices of decisions

(Gordon, M. [1987]. *Nursing diagnosis: Process and application* [2nd ed., p. 93]. New York: McGraw-Hill.)

---

pertinent data, irrelevant or duplicate data, erroneous or misinterpreted data, too few data acquired from client, interpretation of data recorded rather than observed behavior, and failure to update data base. Table 15-3 lists these problems and describes possible causes and remedies.

Data Validation

Validation is the act of confirming or verifying. The purpose of validating is to keep data as free from error, bias, and misinterpretation as possible. Validation is an important part of assessment because invalid information can lead to inappropriate nursing care.

Validation of all data is neither possible nor necessary; the nurse needs to decide which items need verification.

TABLE 15-3

Common Problems of Data Collection, Possible Causes, and Suggested Remedies

Problem	Possible Causes	Suggested Remedies
Data base inappropriately organized	Failure to plan for the assessment by identifying needed data; use of inappropriate tools for data collection	Review the guidelines for specifying pertinent data. Consider modifying tool for data collection or select an alternative tool.
Pertinent data omitted	Not following up on clues during data collection; inappropriate guidelines	Identify potentially relevant factors in advance of collection. Practice interview strategies.
Irrelevant or duplicate data collected	Failure to identify specific purpose of data collection; failure to review available client records; use of inappropriate tools for data collection	Determine specific purpose of data collection for each client. Consider existing data before initiating collection. Consider modifying data collection tool or selecting alternative.
Erroneous or misinterpreted data collection	Failure to observe carefully or validate during data collection; interviewer prejudices or stereotypes	Sharpen observation skills by independently observing the same situation with a peer and compare notes afterward. Role play several validation techniques.
Too little data acquired from client	Failure to establish sufficient rapport or use appropriate communication techniques with client; failure to know what information is wanted	Review and practice communication techniques discussed in Chapter 20. Role play several explanations of purpose of data collection. Identify general data desired before collection.
Interpretation of data is recorded rather than the observed behavior	Nurse jumps to hasty conclusion about client's behavior and deprives others of exploring with the client possible causes of the behavior; deficient validation.	Review the distinction between data and interpretation of data. Practice documenting observed client behavior concisely.
Failure to update the data base	Erroneous belief that assessment is concluded once the initial data base is recorded; low priority attached to ongoing data collection	Recollect that it is impossible to give quality individualized care without knowledge of changes in the client's status. Ongoing data collection is critical to the deletion or modification of old problems and the identification of new problems.

For example, data needs to be verified when there are discrepancies: A client tells the nurse he is fine and has no concerns, but the nurse notes that he demonstrates tense body musculature and seems curt in his responses. There is a discrepancy between what the person is saying and what the nurse is observing, and so validation is necessary to determine accuracy. Validation in this instance may take the form of the nurse saying, "You tell me you feel fine, but right now your body and behaviors are telling me something else. I wonder why this is?"

Data also need verification when they lack objectivity. For example, a nurse suspects that the client hears from one ear but does not seem to hear well from the other. The nurse should validate the data before proceeding, and should determine whether the client does indeed have a hearing problem. Suspicions are not objective. In this instance, the nurse needs to test the client's hearing in both ears. Speaking toward the ear that is suspected to hear well, the nurse explains, "It seems to me that you hear better out of one ear than the other. I would like to test this. I'll bring a watch slowly toward your right ear first and then toward your left. Please look straight ahead and tell me when you first hear the watch ticking." The nurse then records how far the watch was from each ear when the client first heard it ticking.

The nurse may validate data as they are collected or at the end of the data-gathering process. When it is clear that the data are correct, the nurse is ready to analyze the data and formulate nursing diagnoses—the next step of the nursing process.

Data Communication

The client data collected by the nurse, both initially and as client contact continues, are of no benefit to the client and the health care team unless they are appropriately communicated. Appropriate communication involves correct timing and proper documentation.

Timing

Immediate verbal communication of data is indicated whenever assessment findings reveal a critical change in

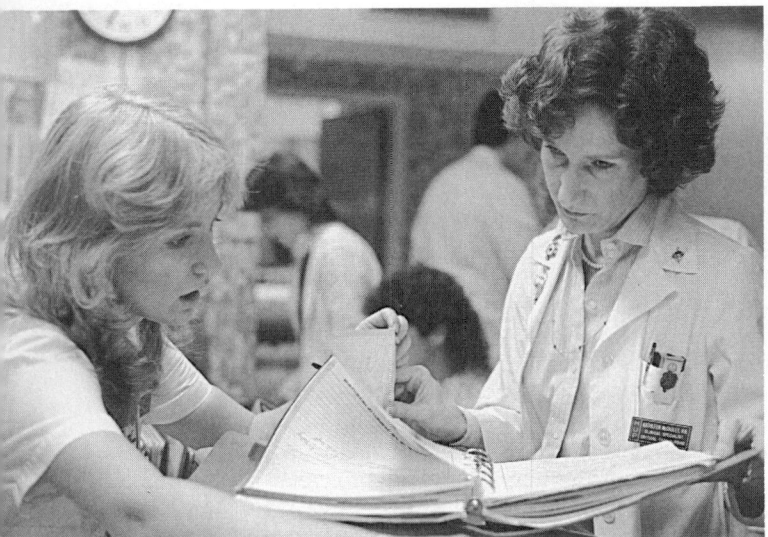

FIGURE 1 5 - 5

Immediate verbal communication of data is indicated whenever assessment findings reveal a critical change in the client's health status. (Photo by Gates Rhodes, courtesy of School of Nursing, University of Pennsylvania.)

Legal Alert

Nurses are responsible for alerting the appropriate health care professional whenever assessment data differ significantly from the client's baseline, indicating a potentially serious problem. Interventions for which the nurse may be legally responsible include increasing the frequency of assessments and initiating necessary changes in the treatment regimen.

Documentation

The initial data base should be recorded in ink, using the designated agency forms, the same day the client is admitted to the agency. If, for any reason, important data cannot be obtained during the initial assessment, this needs to be documented so that it is obtained as soon as possible. Objective and subjective client data should be summarized and written, so that data communicate a unique sense of the client and are comprehensive, concise, and easily retrievable. The data should be written legibly, and good grammar and only standard medical abbreviations should be used. To facilitate quick data retrieval, data should be presented under clearly marked headings.

Whenever possible, subjective data should be recorded using the client's own words. Quotation marks should be used: "I feel tired from the moment I first get up in the morning. Any more it seems I have no energy at all." Client reports also may be paraphrased: Client reports feeling dyspneic, "hard to catch my breath" when walking one flight of stairs.

The tendency to record data using nonspecific terms that are subject to individual definition or interpretation—adequate, good, average, normal, poor, small, large—should be avoided. One nurse's sense of what constitutes an average fluid intake may be very different from that of another nurse. It is important to be specific.

An increasing number of health care settings now use computerized documentation systems—many of which facilitate documentation by allowing for the entry of client data at the client's bedside.

the client's health status that necessitates the involvement of other nurses or health care professionals (Fig. 15-5). The nurse who observes an elevated temperature of 103.2°F (39.5°C) in a client scheduled for surgery that morning must report this to the charge nurse and to the surgeon, who will probably cancel surgery. Failure to communicate this finding could result in the client's receiving preoperative sedation, being taken to the operating room, and even having the surgery performed. Similarly, a nurse who hears a client making suicidal remarks must communicate this information to the health care team, so that all are alerted to the client's danger and suicide precautions may be taken immediately.

The nurse who is unsure of the significance of a particular finding is well advised to consult with another nurse. In some situations, years of experience are needed to accurately distinguish significant from nonsignificant findings. Neither ignorance nor the fear of appearing less than competent justifies failure to report critical data.

KEY POINTS

- Assessing is the systematic and continuous collection, validation, and communication of client data. A data base is all the pertinent client information collected by the nurse and other health care professionals that enables a comprehensive and effective plan of care to be designed and implemented for the client.

- Ongoing nursing assessment alerts the nurse to changes in the client's responses to health and illness and suggests necessary changes in the plan of care.

- Unlike medical assessments, whose primary purpose is to define the existence of medical problems and identify the underlying pathology, nursing assessments are focused primarily on client responses to health problems.
- Objective data are perceptible to the senses and verifiable by another person observing the same data. Subjective data can only be perceived by the affected person and cannot be perceived or verified experientially by another.
- Common methods used for collecting data in nursing are observation, interview, and physical assessment. Observation is the conscious and deliberate use of the five senses to gather data. Skilled nurses observe clients for significant data during each nurse–client interaction.
- Strong interviewing skills are needed by the nurse to obtain a comprehensive nursing history that captures the unique qualities and characteristics of the client in a way that makes individualized care planning possible.
- During the nursing physical assessment, the nurse assesses the client for objective data to better define the client's condition and help the nurse in planning care. The nursing examination focuses primarily on the client's functional abilities.
- The primary source of client data is the client. Unless otherwise specified, it is assumed that the data recorded in the nursing history are from the client. Other important sources of client data are the client's support people, the client record, other health care professionals, and the nursing and related health care literature.

- A data base nursing assessment is done during the nurse's initial contact with the client, and involves collecting data about all aspects of the client's health. A focused assessment may be done during any nurse–client interaction. Its purpose is to gather data about a specific problem.
- Before beginning to collect data, the nurse should have a good sense of the type of data needed to best develop a satisfactory plan of care. Assessment priorities are influenced by the client's health orientation, developmental stage, and need for nursing.
- Using systematic assessment guidelines specifically developed for a nursing assessment ensures that comprehensive, holistic data are collected for each client and that those data easily lead to the formulation of nursing diagnoses.
- Problems related to data collection include inappropriate organization of data base, omission of pertinent data, irrelevant or duplicate data, erroneous or misinterpreted data, too little data acquired from the client, interpretation of data recorded rather than observed behavior, and failure to update data base.
- Validation is the act of confirming or verifying. The purpose of validation is to keep data as free from error, bias, and misinterpretation as possible. Data need to be verified when they contain discrepancies and lack objectivity.
- Client data collected by the nurse, both initially and as client contact continues, are of no benefit to the client and the nursing and health care teams unless they are appropriately communicated. It is important to learn when significant data need to be communicated verbally immediately and how to document data.
- Client data should be summarized and written so that they communicate a unique sense of the client and are comprehensive, concise, and easily retrievable.

BIBLIOGRAPHY

Alfaro, R. (1990). *Application of nursing process: A step-by-step guide.* Philadelphia: Lippincott.

American Nurses' Association (1980). *Nursing: A social policy statement.* Kansas City, MO: Author.

Bates, B. (1992). *A guide to physical examination* (5th ed.). Philadelphia: Lippincott.

Braverman, B. G. (1990). Eliciting data from the patient who is difficult to interview. *Nursing Clinics of North America, 25*(4), 743–750.

Catherman, A. (1990). Biopsychosocial nursing assessment: A way to enhance care plans. *Journal of Psychosocial Nursing, 28*(6), 31–33.

Cormier, L. S., Cormier, W. H., & Weisse, R. J. (1984). *Interviewing and helping skills for health professionals.* Monterey, CA: Wadsworth.

Davis, A. J. (1984). *Listening and responding.* St. Louis: Mosby.

Doe, J. (1991). Tunnel vision. *Nursing, 21*(10), 55–56.

Farrell, J. (1980). The human side of assessment. *Nursing, 10*(4), 74–75.

Fields, W. L., & McGinn-Campbell, K. M. (1983). *Introduction to health assessment.* Englewood Cliffs, NJ: Reston.

Gordon, M. (1987). *Nursing diagnosis: Process and application* (2nd ed.). New York: McGraw-Hill.

Hill, L., & Smith, N. (1990). *Self-care nursing: Promotion of health* (2nd ed.). East Norwalk, CT: Appleton & Lange.

Laschinger, H. S. (1990). Helping students apply a nursing conceptual framework in the clinical setting. *Nurse Educator, 15*(3), 20–24.

Malasanos, L., Barkauskas, V., Moss, M., & Stoltenberg-

Allen, K. (1989). *Health assessment* (4th ed.). St. Louis: Mosby.

McPhetridge, L. M. (1968). Nursing history: One means to personalize care. *American Journal of Nursing, 68*(1), 68–75.

Parish, L. (1986). Communicating with hospitalized children. *Canadian Nurse, 82*(1), 21–24.

Parker, K. (1986). Health works: An adolescent assessment tool. *Canadian Nurse, 82*(1), 28–31.

Pinnell, N., & deMeneses, M. (1986). *The nursing process.* Norwalk, CT: Appleton-Century-Crofts.

Smith, C. E. (1984). With good assessment skills you can conduct a solid framework for patient care. *Nursing, 14*(12), 26–31.

Stewart, C. J., & Cash, W. B. (1991). *Interviewing principles and practice* (6th ed.). Dubuque: Brown.

Wolff, H., & Erickson, R. (1977). The assessment man. *Nursing Outlook, 25*, 103–107.

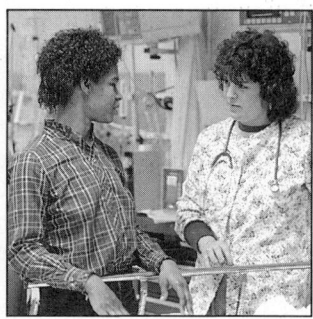
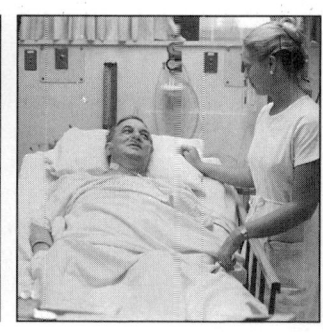
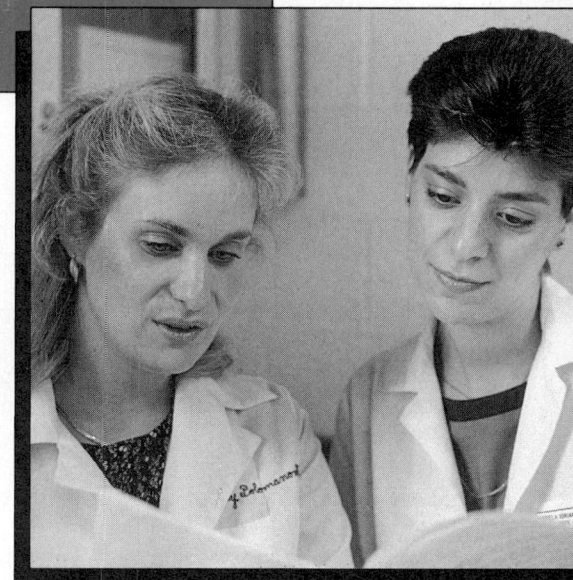

OBJECTIVES

After studying this chapter, the learner should be able to:

Define key terms used in the chapter.

Describe the term nursing diagnosis, distinguishing it from a collaborative problem and a medical diagnosis.

Describe the four steps involved in data interpretation and analysis.

Use the guidelines for writing nursing diagnoses when developing diagnostic statements.

List four advantages of using the NANDA-approved list of nursing diagnoses.

Describe means to validate nursing diagnoses.

Develop a prioritized list of nursing diagnoses using identifiable criteria.

Describe the benefits and limitations of nursing diagnoses.

KEY TERMS

actual problems
collaborative problem
cue
data cluster
diagnosing
health problem
medical diagnosis
nursing diagnosis
possible problems
potential problems
wellness diagnosis

Diagnosing

16

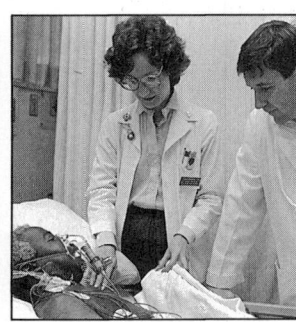

Once the nurse has collected and recorded the client data, the work of diagnosing begins—the second step in the nursing process. The purpose of diagnosing is to identify (1) actual and potential problems in the way the client responds to health or illness, (2) factors that contribute to or cause the problems (etiologies), and (3) strengths the client can draw on to prevent or resolve the problems.

During the diagnosing step of the nursing process, the nurse interprets and analyzes data gathered from the nursing assessment. These data help the nurse identify client strengths and health problems. A **health problem** is a condition related to health that necessitates intervention if disease or illness is to be prevented or resolved, and if coping and wellness are to be promoted.

When health problems are identified, the nurse must decide which health care professional can best treat the problem. Actual or potential health problems that can be prevented or resolved by independent nursing intervention are termed **nursing diagnoses**. The nurse formulates and validates nursing diagnoses, and lists these nursing diagnoses by priority (Fig. 16-1).

A brief history of the evolution of nursing diagnosis can be found in Chapter 14. Now an accepted and essential step in the nursing process, nursing diagnosis was initially confused with medical diagnosis, and this sparked great controversy. Although the confusion has been resolved, many nurses have been slow to understand and describe the "work" of diagnosing. Several books have been written to describe the relation of diagnosing to the other steps in the nursing process (see Bibliography).

Unique Focus of Nursing Diagnosis

During the diagnosing step of the nursing process, the nurse identifies what it is about the client that is nursing's unique concern (ie, what it is about the client that gives rise to the need for nursing, as opposed to the need for medicine or for physical therapy). Nursing diagnoses are, therefore, written to describe client problems that nurses can treat independently. As nurses interpret and analyze client data,

they may identify health problems that are better treated by physicians (medical diagnoses) or by nurses working with other health care professionals (collaborative problems). In such a case, the nurse reports the findings to the physician or other appropriate health care professional and works collaboratively with him or her on resolving the problem (Fig. 16-2).

Nursing Diagnosis Versus Medical Diagnosis

Medical diagnoses identify diseases, whereas nursing diagnoses focus on identifying unhealthy responses to health and illness. Medical diagnoses describe problems for which the physician directs the primary treatment, as opposed to nursing diagnoses, which describe problems treated by nurses within the scope of independent nursing practice. A medical diagnosis remains the same for as long as the disease is present; a nursing diagnosis may change from day to day as the client's responses change. These distinctions are in keeping with the differing foci of medical and nursing practices.

Nursing Diagnosis Versus Collaborative Problems

Nursing diagnoses also must be distinguished from collaborative problems. Together, nursing diagnoses and collaborative problems constitute the range of responses that nurses treat, and as such define the unique nature of nursing (see Fig. 16-2). Carpenito defines **collaborative problems** as "certain physiologic complications that nurses monitor to detect onset or changes in status. Nurses manage collaborative problems utilizing physician-prescribed and nursing-prescribed interventions to minimize the complications of the event" (1992, p. 38).

Unlike medical diagnoses, collaborative problems represent situations that are the primary responsibility of nurses. Unlike nursing diagnoses, collaborative problems represent situations in which the prescription for definitive treatment comes from both nursing and medicine. "When the nurse writes client outcomes that require delegated medical orders for goal achievement, the situation is not a nursing diagnosis but a collaborative problem" (Carpenito, 1992, p. 41). Because collaborative problems deal with potential complications, it is important that they be identified early so that the related nursing care, which is preventive, can be instituted early. Figure 16-3 shows collaborative problems identified by a nurse caring for a client with ovarian cancer. These problems are related to a medical disease, a medical treatment, and a diagnostic study. Alfaro recommends that whenever possible, collaborative problems should be described using the term *potential complication*. The problem and its cause should be linked by using *secondary to* or *related to. Example:* Potential Complication: Anorexia → Cachetic Syndrome secondary to ovarian cancer (Alfaro, 1990, p. 81).

Table 16-1 shows how nurses successfully interpreted different clusters of data that lead to the identification of a nursing diagnosis, collaborative problem, and medical di-

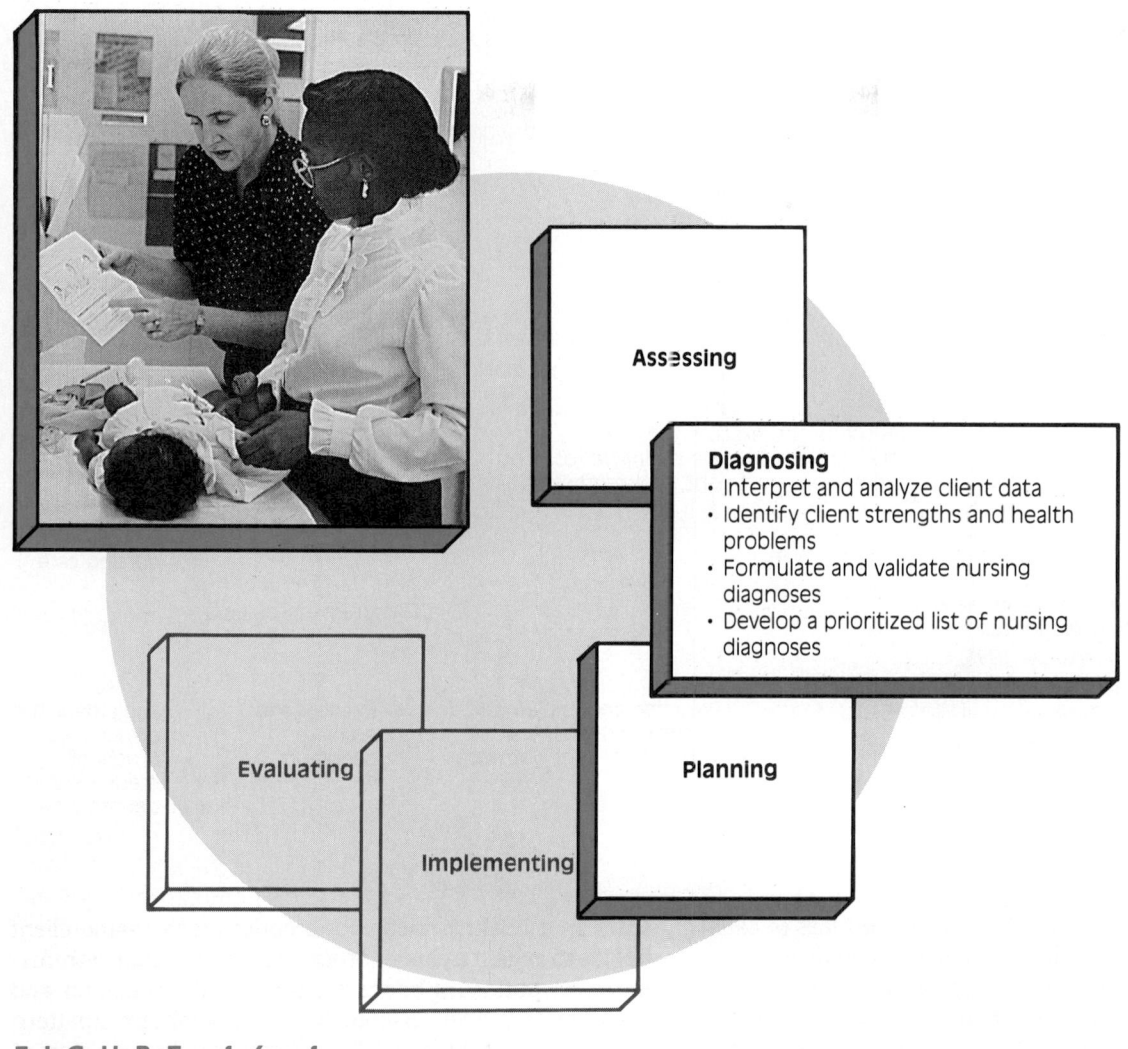

Assessing

Diagnosing
- Interpret and analyze client data
- Identify client strengths and health problems
- Formulate and validate nursing diagnoses
- Develop a prioritized list of nursing diagnoses

Evaluating

Planning

Implementing

F I G U R E   1 6 - 1

Diagnosing. *Diagnosing is the interpretation and analysis of client data to identify client strengths and health problems that independent nursing intervention can prevent or resolve. Nursing diagnoses may change from day to day as the client's responses to health and illness change.* (Photo by Gates Rhodes, courtesy of School of Nursing, University of Pennsylvania.)

agnosis. In the first example, a nursing diagnosis was identified and successfully treated. In the next example, the nurse identified a collaborative problem and initiated intervention within the scope of her practice. When this failed to resolve the problem, a physician was contacted to order medication or a catheterization. In the last example, the nurse's early detection and reporting of the problem to the physician led to the physician's prompt medical diagnosis of cystitis and successful antibiotic therapy.

Data Interpretation and Analysis

Most experienced nurses begin the work of interpreting and analyzing data while they are still collecting (assess-

ing) it. The term **cue** often is used to denote significant data or data that influence decisions. Such significant data should raise a red flag for the nurse, who then looks for patterns or clusters of data that signal an actual, potential, or possible nursing diagnosis.

Recognizing Significant Data

Sorting out *healthy* client responses from those that are *not healthy* is not as clear-cut as it may seem. To avoid erroneously labeling selected client health patterns as unhealthy while failing to detect actual unhealthy behavior, nurses must be familiar with comparative standards to be used in data interpretation and analysis.

Comparing Data to Standards A standard or a norm is a generally accepted rule, measure, pattern, or model that

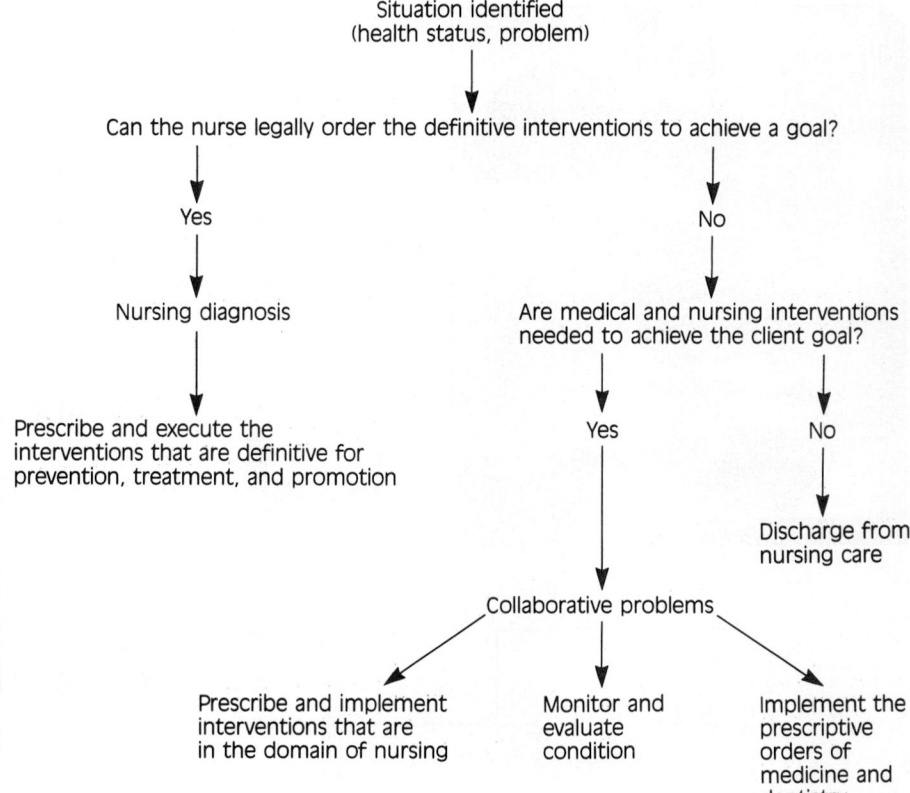

FIGURE 16-2

Differentiation of nursing diagnoses from collaborative problems. (© 1990, 1988, 1985. Lynda Juall Carpenito. Used with permission. Carpenito, L. J. [1992]. *Nursing diagnosis: Application to clinical practice* [4th ed., p. 40]. Philadelphia: Lippincott.)

can be used for comparing data in the same class or category. For example, when determining the significance of a client's blood pressure reading, appropriate standards include normative values for the client's age-group, race, and illness category. The client's own normal range, if known, is an important standard. A pressure of 150/90 may be high for someone whose pressure normally is 120/70, but it may be normal for a person with hypertension. Examples of how standards may be used to identify significant cues follow below (Gordon, 1987, p. 191):

- Changes in a client's usual health patterns that are unexplained by expected norms for growth and development
- Deviation from an appropriate population norm
- Behavior that is nonproductive in the whole-person context
- Behavior that indicates a developmental lag or evolving dysfunctional pattern

Recognizing Patterns or Clusters

A **data cluster** is a grouping of client data or cues that points to the existence of a client health problem. Nursing diagnoses should always be derived from clusters of significant data, rather than from a single cue. The danger of deriving a nursing diagnosis from a single cue is illustrated in the following example. The nurse who diagnoses a woman recovering from gallbladder surgery with ineffective coping may have misinterpreted the client's use of

tears as a healthy release of emotion. If the same client begins to exhibit a cluster of significant cues, such as refusing to eat, preferring bed rest to scheduled ambulation, and reporting increasing discomfort, then an unhealthy pattern is emerging. Table 16-2 offers examples of how clusters of significant data lead to formulation of accurate nursing diagnoses.

Identifying Strengths and Problems

The next step in analyzing data is to determine client strengths and problems.

Determining the Client's Strengths If a client appears to meet a standard, the nurse then concludes that the client has a strength in that particular area, and that this strength contributes to the client's level of wellness. For example, a person who has a history of maintaining a well-balanced diet usually is better able to cope with illness than a person who has a history of eating poorly.

Client strengths may include healthy physiologic functioning, emotional health, cognitive abilities, coping skills, interpersonal strengths, and spiritual strengths. Resources such as the presence of support people, adequate finances, and a healthy environment may all contribute to client strengths. Many people take their strengths for granted, and may not know how to use them effectively when responding to illness. Discussing observed strengths with

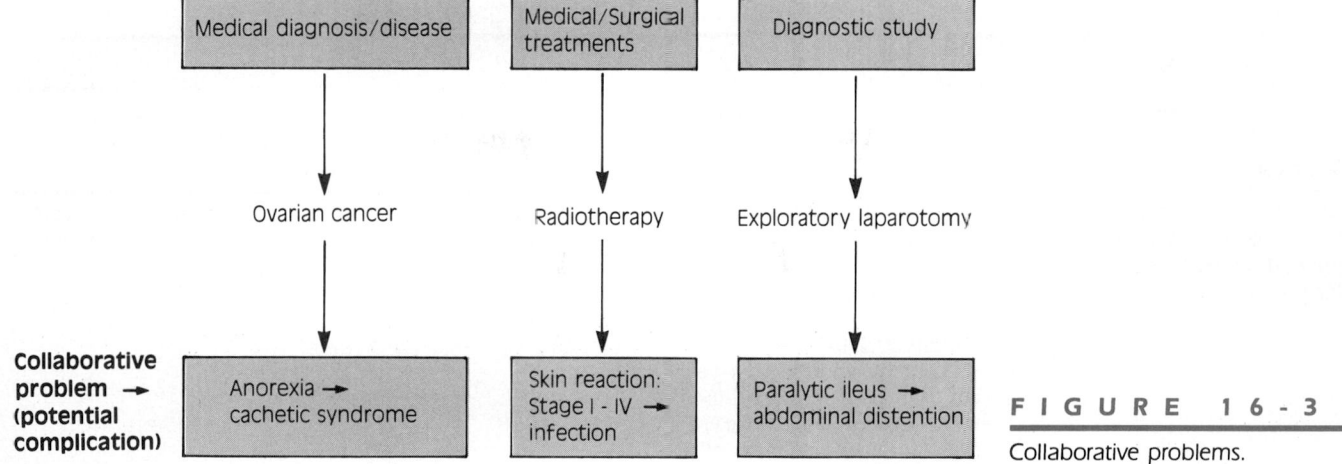

FIGURE 16-3

Collaborative problems.

TABLE 16-1

A Comparison: Nursing Diagnosis, Collaborative Problem, Medical Diagnosis			
	Nursing Diagnosis	**Collaborative Problem**	**Medical Diagnosis**
Definition	A nursing diagnosis is a clinical judgment about individual, family, or community responses to actual or potential health problems or life processes. Nursing diagnosis provides the basis for selection of nursing interventions to achieve outcomes for which the nurse is accountable (NANDA)	Certain physiologic complications that nurses monitor to detect onset of changes in status (Carpenito)	Traumatic or disease condition or syndrome validated by medical diagnostic studies
Focus	Monitoring human responses to actual and potential health problems	Monitoring pathophysiologic responses of body organs or systems	Correcting or preventing pathology of specific organs or body systems
Sample data cluster	56-year-old mother of seven; 5'4", 167 lb; "Whenever I sneeze lately, I dribble urine. This is embarrassing"	42-year-old woman; 1 hour after delivery; spinal anesthesia; 1500 mL fluid infused in past 4 hours without client voiding; unable to void	"Whenever I have to urinate it burns terribly. I also feel like I have to go all the time—real bad." Small, frequent voidings, cloudy urine; T—100.8°F
Diagnostic statement	Stress Incontinence related to degenerative changes in pelvic muscles and structural supports associated with advanced age, obesity, gravid uterus	Potential complication: urinary retention secondary to fluid overload and effects of anesthesia	Cystitis
Select nursing responses	Teach Kegel exercises to increase muscle tone; explore client's willingness and motivation to pursue weight reduction and exercise program; evaluate need for bladder-training program	Monitor for signs of increasing urine retention; offer bedpan and encourage voiding with running water, warm water dripped over perineum, etc; if no result, administer physician-prescribed medication; if no result, perform physician-prescribed catheterization	Report signs and symptoms to physician; obtain urine culture; report results to physician; administer appropriate physician-prescribed antibiotic

T A B L E 1 6 - 2

Diagnosing

Data Interpretation and Analysis		Formulation of Tentative Nursing Diagnosis	Validation of Nursing Diagnosis
Significant Cues	Sample Data Clusters		
Change in a client's usual health patterns that is unexplained by expected norms for growth and development	• "I guess I lost about 20 to 30 pounds over the last 6 months—I think I've just been too busy to eat." • Height: 5'8" • Weight: 102 lb • 35-year-old mother of 4-year-old twin boys; returned to work (executive secretary) for first time since delivery of twins 7 months ago	Altered Nutrition: Less Than Body Requirements, related to stress of new job; role conflict and demands	Accurate diagnosis: Client validates this diagnosis, agreeing with contributing factors
Deviation from an appropriate population norm	• Teacher notices and reports frequency of bruises on third-grade boy who is repeatedly observed alone during recess periods and who is withdrawn in classroom • In conversation with the school nurse, one parent remarks: "That boy brings out the worst in me! I don't know why but I often have to smack him hard to make him listen."	High Risk for Violence (Child Abuse) related to ? etiology (deficient parenting skills?)	Incomplete diagnosis: Additional data collection yields new information: • Father out of work for past 18 months • Father was abused as a child Diagnosis restated: High Risk for Violence (Child Abuse) related to increased family stress and father's history of being abused
Behavior that is nonproductive in the whole-person context	• Fiancé abruptly terminated relationship 3 months before established wedding date • Noticeable change in physical appearance; frequently wears same clothes; makeup, jewelry, hair-styling are absent; strong body odors present • No desire to be with others; goes home (lives alone) immediately after work • Stopped attending aerobics classes	Self-Esteem Disturbance related to feeling rejected by fiancé	Premature diagnosis resulting from incomplete data collection. Client has a long history of major depressive states one of which may have resulted in the breakup of this relationship. Medical diagnosis and treatment indicated. Changes in appearance are indicative of depressive state. Need to explore related nursing diagnoses.
Behavior indicating developmental lags or evolving dysfunctional patterns	• Admitted to nursing home 2 months ago • "I have nothing to live for anymore . . . why don't I die?" • Wishes to remain in room seated in chair—will only ambulate with great urging • Anything requiring movement has become "too much bother." • Decreased muscle mass, tone, and strength; reduced joint mobility	Impaired Physical Mobility related to difficult transition to nursing home	Accurate but routinized diagnosis that may result in staff's acceptance of status quo unless a more specific cause is identified

clients and counseling clients about ways to develop and use their strengths are important nursing measures.

Determining the Client's Problem Areas A person who does not meet a certain health standard probably has a limitation in this aspect of health status, and may profit from professional services. For example, a person who has a long history of constipation is probably in need of care to help overcome this problem. As stated previously, the nurse makes a decision about whether the data represent a nursing diagnosis or a collaborative problem, or whether it should be reported to the physician because it might contribute to the identification of a medical diagnosis.

Determining Problems the Client Is Likely to Experience It is important for the nurse to identify potential health problems. For example, the nurse notes that a client has signs of a wound infection, but laboratory test results show that the client's white blood cell count has not increased, as is usual when such an infection is present. The nurse concludes that the body apparently is not building up normal defenses to combat the infection. The nurse then predicts the problems this client is likely to encounter, such as a longer than normal healing period. This prediction has implications for nursing care, such as measures related to the client's diet, fluid intake, urine output, and mobility.

When determining strengths and problems, it is helpful to determine if the client agrees with the nurse's identification of a problem and is motivated to work toward its resolution.

Reaching Conclusions

The nurse reaches one of four basic conclusions after interpreting and analyzing the client data. Different nursing responses are possible for each conclusion:

No problem
- No nursing response indicated
- Reinforce client's health habits and patterns
- Initiate health promotion activities to prevent disease or illness or to promote a higher level of wellness
- Wellness diagnosis may be indicated.

Possible problem
- Collect more data to confirm or disconfirm suspected problem

Actual or potential nursing diagnosis
- Unable to treat because client denies problem and refuses treatment (make sure client understands possible outcomes of this stance)
- Begin planning, implementing, and evaluating care designed to prevent, reduce, or resolve the problem

Clinical problem other than nursing diagnosis
- Consult with appropriate health care professional and work collaboratively on problem
- Refer to medicine

Formulating and Validating Nursing Diagnoses

Writing Nursing Diagnoses

Once the nurse recognizes a cluster of significant client data indicating a health problem that can be treated by independent nursing intervention, it is time to write the nursing diagnosis. Most nursing diagnoses are written either as two-part statements listing the client's problem and its cause or as three-part statements that also include the problem's defining characteristics (Table 16-3).

Those just beginning to write nursing diagnoses may find it helpful to consult the list of health problems accepted by the North American Nursing Diagnosis Association (NANDA) for testing and study. The NANDA list is a beginning list of suggested terms for suggested health problems that may be identified and treated by nurses. Each of the diagnostic category labels accepted by NANDA consists of three components: (1) the title or label that provides a name for the diagnosis that is a concise description of the health problem, (2) causative and contributing factors, and (3) defining characteristics. There are distinct advantages to nurses' use of common terminology when formulating nursing diagnoses.

First, using a nationally accepted list of diagnoses helps nurses communicate with one another. Nursing knowledge is easier to teach and learn if authors, faculty, and clinicians all use the same terminology. Second, using common terminology facilitates the use of computers in nursing because nurses are able to retrieve records according to nursing diagnoses rather than according to medical diagnoses and therefore are able to collect data to further nursing research. Third, using a nationally accepted list of diagnostic categories provides a method for reimbursement according to nursing activities related to nursing diagnoses rather than to those related only to medical diagnoses. Fourth, all nurses can work together toward testing and refining the diagnostic categories to identify assessment criteria and nursing interventions to improve nursing care (Alfaro, 1990, p. 70).

Pocket-sized handbooks of NANDA-approved nursing diagnoses are available, and may be of great help to the student who is unfamiliar with this grouping of problem statements. Nurses who encounter different health problems within the scope of their practices that they believe to be nursing diagnoses may submit these to the NANDA Diagnosis Review Committee.

Problem The purpose of the problem statement is to describe the health state or health problem of the client as clearly and concisely as possible. Because this section of the nursing diagnosis identifies what is unhealthy about the client and what the client would like to change in his or her health status, it suggests client goals. NANDA recommends use of the following quantifiers when writing the

T A B L E 1 6 - 3

Formulation of Nursing Diagnosis Statements			
	Definition	**Purpose**	**Example**
Problem	Identifies what is unhealthy about the client, indicating the need for change (clear, concise statement of the client health problem)	Suggests the client goals (expectations for change)	Bathing/Hygiene Self-Care Deficit ↓ related to ↓
Etiology	Identifies the factors that are maintaining the unhealthy state or response (contributing or causative factors)	Suggests the appropriate nursing measures	Fear of falling in the tub and obesity ↓ as manifested by ↓
Defining characteristics	Identify the subjective and objective data that signal the existence of the problem (cues that reflect the existence of a problem)	Suggest evaluative criteria	Strong body and urine odor, unclean hair: "I'm afraid I'll fall in the tub and break something." (5'4", 170 lb)

Examples:

Two-part diagnostic statement: Bathing/Hygiene Self-Care Deficit related to fear of falling in tub and obesity

Three-part diagnostic statement: Bathing/Hygiene Self-Care Deficit related to fear of falling in tub and obesity, as manifested by strong body and urine odor, unclean hair, statement of fearing fall in tub, and height and weight: 5'4", 170 lb

problem statement: altered, impaired, depleted, deficient, excessive, dysfunctional, disturbed, ineffective, decreased, increased, acute, chronic, and intermittent.

Etiology The etiology identifies the physiologic, psychological, sociologic, spiritual, and environmental factors believed to be related to the problem as either a cause or a contributing factor. Because the etiology identifies the factors that are maintaining the unhealthy client state and preventing the desired change, the etiology directs nursing intervention. Unless the etiology is correctly identified, nursing actions may be inefficient and ineffective. For example, a diabetic client who is frequently admitted to the hospital with hyperglycemia and who has a poor history of dietary and pharmacologic management is diagnosed to be noncompliant. Assuming that the noncompliance is related to a knowledge deficit and then channeling all nursing activities and energies into teaching the client how to manage the diabetes is useless if the noncompliance is actually a result of the client's decreased will to live.

Defining Characteristics The subjective and objective data that signal the existence of the actual or potential health problem are the third component of the nursing diagnosis. NANDA has identified defining characteristics for each accepted nursing diagnosis, and familiarity with these characteristics assists nurses in recognizing clusters of significant data. Table 16-3 defines the three components of a nursing diagnosis statement and shows how they affect client goals, nursing measures, and evaluation. Other examples of nursing diagnosis statements are found throughout the book.

Guidelines for Writing Nursing Diagnoses

1. Phrase the nursing diagnosis as a client problem or alteration in health state rather than as a client need.
2. Check to make sure that the client problem precedes the etiology and that the two are linked by the phrase *related to*.
3. Defining characteristics, when included in the nursing diagnosis, should follow the etiology and be linked by the phrase *as manifested by*.
4. Write in legally advisable terms.
5. Use nonjudgmental language.
6. Be sure the problem statement indicates what is unhealthy about the client or what the client wants to change (enhance).
7. Avoid using defining characteristics, medical diagnoses, or something that cannot be changed in the problem statement.
8. Reread the diagnosis to make sure the problem statement suggests client goals and that the etiology will direct the selection of nursing measures.

Common errors in writing nursing diagnoses are shown in Table 16-4, along with suggestions for correcting them.

What Is Not a Nursing Diagnosis

The nursing diagnosis statement is written in terms of a client problem, alteration in health state, or client strength *for which nursing provides the primary therapy*. The following are not nursing diagnoses: medical diagnoses, medical pathology, diagnostic tests, treatments, or equipment. Similarly, although all the following need to be considered

Nursing Diagnoses, North American Nursing Diagnosis Association, April 1992

Activity Intolerance
Activity Intolerance, High Risk for
Adjustment, Impaired
Airway Clearance, Ineffective
Anxiety
Aspiration, High Risk for
Body Image Disturbance
Body Temperature, High Risk for Altered
Breastfeeding, Effective
Breastfeeding, Ineffective
Breastfeeding, Interrupted*
Breathing Pattern, Ineffective
Cardiac Output, Decreased
Caregiver Role Strain*
Caregiver Role Strain, High Risk for*
Communication, Impaired Verbal
Constipation
Constipation, Colonic
Constipation, Perceived
Coping, Defensive
Coping, Ineffective Individual
Decisional Conflict (Specify)
Denial, Ineffective
Diarrhea
Disuse Syndrome, High Risk for
Diversional Activity Deficit
Dysreflexia
Family Coping: Compromised, Ineffective
Family Coping: Disabling, Ineffective
Family Coping: Potential for Growth
Family Processes, Altered
Fatigue
Fear
Fluid Volume Deficit
Fluid Volume Deficit, High Risk for
Fluid Volume Excess
Gas Exchange, Impaired
Grieving, Anticipatory
Grieving, Dysfunctional
Growth and Development, Altered
Health Maintenance, Altered
Health-Seeking Behaviors (Specify)
Home Maintenance Management, Impaired
Hopelessness
Hyperthermia
Hypothermia
Incontinence, Bowel
Incontinence, Functional
Incontinence, Reflex
Incontinence, Stress
Incontinence, Total
Incontinence, Urge
Infant Feeding Pattern, Ineffective*
Infection, High Risk for
Injury, High Risk for
Knowledge Deficit (Specify)
Noncompliance (Specify)
Nutrition, Altered: Less than Body Requirements

Nutrition, Altered: More than Body Requirements
Nutrition, Altered: Potential for More than Body
  Requirements
Oral Mucous Membrane, Altered
Pain
Pain, Chronic
Parental Role Conflict
Parenting, Altered
Parenting, High Risk for Altered
Peripheral Neurovascular Dysfunction, High Risk
  for*
Personal Identity Disturbance
Physical Mobility, Impaired
Poisoning, High Risk for
Post-Trauma Response
Powerlessness
Protection, Altered
Rape Trauma Syndrome
Rape Trauma Syndrome: Compound Reaction
Rape Trauma Syndrome: Silent Reaction
Relocation Stress Syndrome*
Role Performance, Altered
Self-Care Deficit
  Bathing/Hygiene
  Feeding
  Dressing/Grooming
  Toileting
Self-Esteem, Chronic Low
Self-Esteem, Situational Low
Self-Esteem Disturbance
Self-Mutilation, High Risk for*
Sensory-Perceptual Alterations (Specify) (visual,
  auditory, kinesthetic, gustatory, tactile, olfactory)
Sexual Dysfunction
Sexuality Patterns, Altered
Skin Integrity, High Risk for Impaired
Skin Integrity, Impaired
Sleep Pattern Disturbance
Social Interaction, Impaired
Social Isolation
Spiritual Distress
Suffocation, High Risk for
Swallowing, Impaired
Therapeutic Regimen, Ineffective Management of*
Thermoregulation, Ineffective
Thought Processes, Altered
Tissue Integrity, Impaired
Tissue Perfusion, Altered (Specify Type) (renal,
  cerebral, cardiopulmonary, gastrointestinal,
  peripheral)
Trauma, High Risk for
Unilateral Neglect
Urinary Elimination, Altered
Urinary Retention
Ventilation, Inability to Sustain Spontaneous*
Ventilatory Weaning Response, Dysfunctional*
Violence, High Risk for: Self-Directed or Directed at
  Others

*New diagnoses from 1992 conference.

T A B L E   1 6 - 4

Common Errors in Writing Nursing Diagnoses and Recommended Corrections

Error	Example	Correction	Example
Writing the diagnosis in terms of needs and not response	Needs assistance with bathing related to bed rest	Write the diagnosis in terms of response rather than need	Self-Care Deficit: Bathing related to immobility
Making legally inadvisable statements	Noncompliance due to hostility toward nursing staff (the words *due to* imply a direct cause-and-effect relationship)	Use "related to" rather than "due to" or "caused by" to link the etiology to the problem statement	Noncompliance related to hostility toward nursing staff (denotes a relation between the problem and etiology but not necessarily a causal relation)
	Spouse Abuse related to husband's immaturity and violent temper	Write diagnosis in legally advisable terms: statements that may be interpreted as libel or that imply nursing negligence are legally hazardous to all the nurses caring for the client	High Risk for Violence: Spouse Abuse related to husband's reported inability to control behavior.
	Impaired Skin Integrity related to client's lying on back all night		Impaired Skin Integrity related to mobility deficit
Identifying as a problem a client response that is not necessarily unhealthy	Mild Anxiety related to impending surgery	Include in the problem statement of the nursing diagnosis only client responses that are unhealthy or that the client wants to change	No need for nursing diagnosis: Mild anxiety before surgery is a healthy response that motivates preoperative self-care behavior
Identifying as a problem signs and symptoms of illness	Cough related to long history of smoking	Avoid including signs and symptoms of illness in the problem statement of the nursing diagnosis	Ineffective Airway Clearance related to 20-year history of smoking

(Common errors adapted from Mundinger, M. O., & Jauron, G. D. [1975]. Developing a nursing diagnosis. *Nursing Outlook, 23*[2], 94–98. Guidelines for writing nursing diagnoses adapted from Iyer, P., Taptich, B., & Bernocchi-Losey, D. [1991]. *Nursing process and nursing diagnoses* [2nd ed.]. Philadelphia: Saunders)

when identifying nursing diagnoses, they do not belong as such in the diagnosis statement: therapeutic client needs, therapeutic client goals, a single sign or symptom, or an *unvalidated* nursing inference. Examples of these items, frequently and erroneously placed in nursing diagnoses, appear in Table 16-5. Illustrations are derived from clients with diabetes mellitus.

Actual, Potential (High Risk), and Possible Nursing Diagnoses

Client health problems may be **actual** (problem is present), **potential** (problem may occur), and **possible** (problem may be present). A potential nursing diagnosis is written when the health problem is likely to occur unless the nurse intervenes in a particular way. NANDA-approved diagnoses once designated as "potential" were labeled "high risk" in 1992:

A high risk nursing diagnosis is a clinical judgment that an individual, family or community is more vulnerable to develop the problem than others in the same or similar situation. High risk nursing diagnoses are supported by risk factors that guide nursing interventions to reduce or prevent the occurrence of the problem.

A possible nursing diagnosis is written when the nurse suspects that a health problem exists but needs to gather more data to confirm the diagnosis (Carpenito, 1992, p. 22).

An actual nursing diagnosis for a client who has experienced vomiting, diarrhea, and excessive diaphoresis for 3 days is *Fluid Volume Deficit related to abnormal fluid loss*. If the diarrhea persists and weakness interferes with the client's normal perineal hygiene, he may be at risk for skin breakdown. This is written as the potential diagnosis *High Risk for Impaired Skin Integrity*. If the nurse suspects that a

Error	Example	Correction	Example
Identifying as a client problem or etiology what cannot be changed	Alterations in Bowel Elimination: Permanent Colostomy related to cancer of bowel	Express the problem statement and etiologic factors in terms that can be changed; otherwise, nursing energies are being directed to a hopeless task	Self-Care Deficit: Care of Colostomy, related to severe anxiety about cancer and feelings of powerlessness
	Grieving related to death of spouse		Dysfunctional Grieving related to inability to accept death of spouse
Identifying environmental factors rather than client factors as a problem	Cluttered Home related to inability to discard anything	Express the problem statement in terms of unhealthy client responses rather than environmental conditions	High Risk for Injury related to cluttered home (inability to discard anything)
Reversing clauses	Knowledge Deficit related to alteration in parenting	Avoid reversing the problem statement and etiologic statement	Altered Parenting related to knowledge deficit: Child growth and development, discipline
Having both clauses say the same thing	Alteration in Comfort related to pain (pain *is* the comfort alteration—what is contributing to the pain?)	Be sure that the *two* parts of the diagnosis do not mean the same thing	Unrelieved Incisional Pain related to fear of addiction
Including value judgments in the nursing diagnosis	Poor Home Maintenance Management related to laziness	Write the diagnosis without value judgments; avoid words such as poor, inadequate, abnormal, unhealthy	Impaired Home Maintenance Management related to low value ascribed to home safety and cleanliness
Including the medical diagnosis in the diagnostic statement	Impaired Home Maintenance Management related to arthritis	Do not include the medical diagnosis in the nursing diagnosis statement	Impaired Home Maintenance Management related to mobility, endurance, and comfort alterations

disturbance of self-concept also is present but lacks the necessary data (defining characteristics) to confirm this, it can be written as a possible diagnosis: *Possible Disturbance in Self-Concept*. This alerts other nurses to the need to collect more data about the client's self-concept.

Wellness Diagnoses

A persistent critique of nursing diagnoses that focus exclusively on client health problems is their limited applicability in nursing settings that primarily deal with healthy clients. To remedy this concern, **wellness diagnoses** were proposed and are now readily accepted. According to NANDA (1990), a "wellness diagnosis is a clinical judgment about an individual, family, or community in transition from a specific level of wellness to a higher level of wellness" (p. 117). The diagnostic statement for wellness diagnoses is a one-part statement that contains the label *Potential for En-*

hanced followed by the desired higher-level wellness. Examples include Potential for Enhanced Family Coping, Potential for Enhanced Health Maintenance, Potential for Enhanced Parenting, Potential for Enhanced Self-Esteem.

Validating Nursing Diagnoses

Once a tentative nursing diagnosis is formulated, it should be validated. Price (1980, p. 670) indicates that an affirmative response to each of the following questions validates a tentative diagnosis:
- Is my data base sufficient, accurate, and derived from some concept of nursing?
- Does my synthesis of data (significant cues) demonstrate the existence of a pattern?
- Are the subjective and objective data I used to determine the existence of a pattern characteristic of the health problem I defined?

T A B L E   1 6 - 5

What a Nursing Diagnosis Is Not, and Why		
What a Nursing Diagnosis Is Not	**Example**	**Rationale**
Medical diagnosis	Diabetes mellitus	Although there is nursing care associated with medical illnesses, the illness is not primarily amenable to nursing intervention. Nursing's concern is the *person* who has the illness and the effect of the illness on human functioning.
Medical pathology	Hypoglycemia	Nurses need to understand the pathology underlying disease states to plan appropriate nursing care, but once again, nursing's focus is the person, not the pathology. The person's response to hypoglycemia, how hypoglycemia affects human functioning— these are the domain of *nursing* diagnoses.
Diagnostic tests, treatments, equipment	Fasting blood glucose Insulin therapy Insulin syringe Infusion pump	Nursing's concern is the person's response to the diagnostic study, treatment, or equipment. If the need for insulin therapy reveals a knowledge deficit or self-care deficit, this becomes the nursing diagnosis, not insulin therapy in and of itself.
Therapeutic client needs	Needs to learn the relation among diet, exercise, and insulin	The diagnosis should be written as a client health problem rather than a client need. *Example:* Altered Health Maintenance (Diabetic Care) related to lack of knowledge of relation among diet, exercise, and insulin.
Therapeutic nursing goals	To develop therapeutic diabetic self-care behaviors	The diagnosis should be written from the client perspective rather than the nursing perspective and phrased as a client health problem. *Example:* Self-Care Deficit: Diabetic Self-Care Behaviors, related to decreased value on life and decreased motivation to learn.
A single sign or symptom	After successfully administering own insulin for 3 days client tells nurse, "You give me my shot today."	A nursing diagnosis is not developed until a pattern or cluster of significant cues is detected. The signs and symptoms lead to the identification of the problem statement but are not the problem statement. In this situation, no nursing diagnosis is indicated until further data collection, interpretation, and analysis take place.
An *unvalidated* nursing inference	Above incident leads to the nursing inference: Noncompliance related to depression	This is a premature nursing diagnosis that may not accurately reflect a client problem. More data and the validation of the tentative nursing diagnosis (nursing inference) are needed before the diagnoses can be recorded.

- Is my tentative nursing diagnosis based on scientific nursing knowledge and clinical expertise?
- Is my tentative nursing diagnosis able to be prevented, reduced, or resolved by independent nursing action?
- Is my degree of confidence above 50% that other qualified practitioners would formulate the same nursing diagnosis based on my data?

In addition, clients who are able to participate in decision making should be encouraged to validate the diagnosis. "It seems to me that bathing has become a problem now that you are afraid of falling in the tub. What's your sense of this?" Table 16-2 lists possible outcomes of validating tentative nursing diagnoses.

Prioritizing Nursing Diagnoses and Documentation

To develop a prioritized list of nursing diagnoses, the nurse needs guidelines for ranking diagnoses as high, medium, or low priority. High-priority diagnoses pose the greatest threat to the client's well-being. Non–life-threatening diagnoses are ranked as medium priorities, and diagnoses that are not specifically related to the current illness and prognosis are of low priority. In all levels, psychosocial needs must be considered as well as physiologic needs. Three helpful guides suggested by Atkinson and Murray (1990) for prioritizing client problems are Maslow's hierarchy of human needs, client preference, and anticipation of future problems.

Maslow's Hierarchy of Human Needs

Because lower needs must be met before a person can focus on higher ones, client needs may be prioritized according to the following hierarchy: physiologic needs—safety needs—love and belonging needs—self-esteem needs—self-actualization needs. *Example:* A geriatric client who is incontinent of urine and sitting in a wet disposable brief (physiologic need) will be unable to participate fully in a music therapy diversional activity (self-esteem need).

Client Preference

It is best to first meet the needs the client thinks are most important, if this order does not interfere with other vital therapies. *Example:* A woman is admitted to an orthopedic unit with a fractured pelvis and multiple lacerations after an automobile accident. The morning after the accident she complains of pain and needs assistance with bathing and attention to her lacerations, but she refuses to do anything until she calls home to find out who is caring for her 15-month-old twins.

Anticipation of Future Problems

The knowledge base of the nurse must be tapped to consider the potential effects of different courses of nursing action. Assigning low priority to a diagnosis the client wants to ignore when this can result in harmful future consequences for the client may be nursing negligence. *Example:* An obese client with multiple sclerosis and greatly decreased limb strength who spends most of her day in bed may see no value in diet modification and position changes. The nurse who is alert to the potential serious problem of pressure ulcers would assign high priority to this diagnosis, and incorporate weight management and position changes into the plan of care, despite the client's reluctance to do so.

Once the prioritized list of nursing diagnoses is developed, the nurse documents this on the nursing care plan. Depending on the documentation system in use, nursing diagnoses also may be recorded on the multidisciplinary problem list at the front of the client record.

Nursing Diagnosis: A Critique

The current nursing diagnosis literature contains many examples of nurses writing about how using nursing diagnosis has improved their clinical practice; one also finds articles that detail the many benefits nursing diagnosis brings to the profession. Conversely, there are articles that point out the limitations of nursing diagnosis and that urge nurses to be cautious; so an uncritical use of nursing diagnosis does not restrict their practices.

The primary benefit that nursing diagnosis offers the client is the individualization of client care. For example, nurses may be caring simultaneously for three women who have had a modified radical mastectomy because of breast cancer. Although the postoperative nursing management of these women will be similar, priorities of care may differ. A prioritized list of nursing diagnoses enables nurses to direct their energies toward these differing client priorities:

Client A: Body Image Disturbance
Ineffective Individual Coping
Client B: Pain
Self-Care Deficit
Client C: High Risk for Sexual Dysfunction
Powerlessness

The use of nursing diagnosis also allows clients to be informed and willing participants in their care as they validate their diagnoses and assist in prioritizing them.

Improved communication among nurses and other health care professionals is probably the most important benefit that accurate, up-to-date diagnoses—expressed in well-defined and standardized terminology—offer nurses. This communication aids in planning, charting, client data retrieval, health team conferences, change-of-shift reports, and health care follow-up. It also promotes nursing accountability for the problems that nurses diagnose.

Among the other benefits that nursing diagnoses offer the profession is help in defining the domain of nursing to health care administrators, legislators, and other health care providers; this is important when seeking funding for nursing and reimbursement for nursing services. Nursing diagnoses also are used to define curriculum content and to direct specialization and advancement in nursing and nursing research.

When the diagnostic process is used incorrectly, a client may be "misdiagnosed." Premature diagnoses based on an incomplete data base, erroneous diagnoses resulting from an inaccurate data base or a faulty data analysis, and routinized diagnoses resulting from the nurse's failure to tailor data collection and analysis to the unique needs of the client are common sources of error. Failure to modify diagnoses and to identify new diagnoses as the client's status changes also may be problems. Failures in diagnosis lead to failures in nursing care. All of the above are not so much limitations of nursing diagnosis as they are limitations of the nurses who are diagnosing incorrectly.

Nurses who are inexperienced in working with diagnoses may become frustrated because attempts to standardize nursing diagnoses are still in the early stages, and confusion exists about the need to standardize and the best way to do it. Individual nurses working together at any one time may have different exposures to nursing diagnoses and may differ widely in their commitment to the use of nursing diagnoses in practice. Once nurses master skills in developing nursing diagnoses and begin to use them to direct care, it is believed that these difficulties will be minimized.

More serious criticisms of nursing diagnosis are raised by nurses who claim that a classification of standardized nursing diagnoses limits nursing, curbing nurses' originality and ability to think things through.

Although some nurses believe that diagnosis offers a valued shortcut to practice, critics find this offensive, and respond that rather than invest nursing's energies in perfecting a shortcut, nurses need to change the working conditions that interfere with in-depth problem solving and thoughtful nursing care.

Critics of diagnostic labeling point out that instead of identifying what is unique and positive about nursing, nursing diagnoses make a clear statement that nurses are concerned about what is deviant, wrong, or pathologic (Hagey & McDonough, 1984). The ever-changing and dynamic human person with a need for nursing care becomes objectified (Gebbie, 1984).

Nurses who are sensitive to transcultural issues raise important concerns about the cultural limitations of the NANDA diagnoses. Foremost among these concerns is that NANDA diagnoses and behaviors assume that the client is "wrong" and the provider is "right," and deny the validity of cultural and health care beliefs and practices that are different from those of the nurse (Geissler, 1991). Examples of nursing diagnoses that often are misused in labeling such cultural deviations as abnormal include Impaired Verbal Communication, Impaired Social Interaction, and Noncompliance.

In conclusion, nursing diagnosis has become a valued and essential step in the nursing process. Used correctly, it is a powerful tool for individualizing client care, and ensures that nursing's energies are being used in the most efficient way to meet client needs. Nurses who are as concerned about the art and spirit of nursing as they are about its science are careful to avoid labeling clients in a way that objectifies them or limits the potential range of nurse–client interactions.

KEY POINTS

- The purpose of diagnosing is the identification of (1) problems in the way the client is responding to health or illness, (2) factors that contribute to or cause these problems (etiologies), and (3) strengths the client can draw on to prevent or resolve the problems.
- Actual or potential health problems that independent nursing intervention can prevent or resolve are termed nursing diagnoses.
- Once significant client data are detected, the nurse looks for data clusters that signal a client strength or problem, and checks out these findings with the client.
- The interpretation and analysis of client data may lead to the identification of nursing diagnoses or collaborative problems (best treated by nurses working together with other health care professionals) or, when shared with a physician, may contribute to medical diagnoses.
- Most nursing diagnoses are written as either two-part statements that contain the client problem and its etiology connected by the words *related to*, or as three-part statements that include the problem's defining characteristics.
- A wellness diagnosis is a one-part statement that contains the label *Potential for Enhanced* followed by the desired higher-level wellness.
- The problem identifies what is unhealthy about the client, indicating the need for change. It suggests the client goals. The etiology identifies the factors that are maintaining the unhealthy state or response and suggests the appropriate nursing intervention. The defining characteristics are the subjective and objective data that initially signaled the existence of the problem. They suggest evaluative criteria.
- Although nursing care may be related to the following, they are not nursing diagnoses and should not appear in the diagnostic statement: medical diagnosis, medical pathology, diagnostic tests, treatments, equipment, therapeutic client needs, therapeutic client goals, a single sign or symptom, and *unvalidated* nursing inferences.
- Other sources of error when writing nursing diagnoses include making legally inadvisable statements, reversing the clauses, identifying environmental factors rather than client factors as the problem, identifying as a client response what is not necessarily unhealthful, having both clauses say the same thing, and identifying as a client problem what cannot be changed.
- Three helpful guides for prioritizing client problems are Maslow's hierarchy of human needs, client preference, and anticipation of future problems.

BIBLIOGRAPHY

Alfaro, R. (1990). *Application of nursing process: A step-by-step guide*. Philadelphia: Lippincott.

American Nurses' Association (1980). *Nursing: A social policy statement*. Kansas City, MO: Author.

Aspinall, M. J. (1976). Nursing diagnosis: the weak link. *Nursing Outlook, 24*(7), 433–436.

Atkinson, J., & Murray, M. E. (1990). *Understanding the nursing process* (4th ed.). New York: Macmillan.

Carlson, J., Craft, C., & McGuire, A. (1990). *Nursing diagnosis*. Philadelphia: Saunders.

Carnevali, D. L., Mitchell, P. H., Woods, N. F., & Tanner, C. A. (1984). *Diagnostic reasoning in nursing*. Philadelphia: Lippincott.

Carpenito, L. J. (1985). Diagnostics: Actual, potential, or possible? *American Journal of Nursing, 85*(4), 485.

Carpenito, L. J. (1992). *Nursing diagnosis: Application to clinical practice* (4th ed.). Philadelphia: Lippincott.

Carroll-Johnson, R. M. (Ed.). (1991). *Classification in nursing diagnosis: Proceedings of the ninth conference*. Philadelphia: Lippincott.

Doenges, M. E., Jeffries, M. F., & Moorehouse, M. F. (1989). *Nursing care plans: Guidelines for planning patient care* (2nd ed.). Philadelphia: Davis.

Dossey, B., & Guzzetta, C. E. (1981). Nursing diagnosis. *Nursing, 11*(6), 34–38.

Dougherty, C. M. (Ed.). (1985). Symposium on nursing diagnosis. *Nursing Clinics of North America, 20*(4).

Fitzpatrick, J. J., Kerr, M. E., Saba. V. K., Hoskins, L. M., Hurley, M. E., Milles, W. C., Rottkamp, B. C., Warren, J. J., & Carpenito, L. J. (1989). Translating nursing diagnosis into ICD code. *American Journal of Nursing, 89*(4), 493–495.

Gebbie, K. M. (Ed.). (1975). *Summary of the second national conference.* St. Louis: Clearinghouse for Nursing Diagnoses.

Gebbie, K. M. (1984). Nursing diagnosis: What is it and why does it exist? *Topics in Clinical Nursing, 5*(4), 1–9.

Gebbie, K. M., & Lavin, M. A. (1973). *Summary of the first national conference.* St. Louis: Mosby.

Geissler, E. M. (1991). Transcultural nursing and nursing and nursing diagnosis. *Nursing and Health Care, 12*(4), 190–192, 203.

Gordon, M. (1976). Nursing diagnosis and the diagnostic process. *American Journal of Nursing, 76*(8), 1298–1300.

Gordon, M. (1987). *Nursing diagnosis: Process and application* (2nd ed.). New York: McGraw-Hill.

Gordon, M. (1992). *Manual of nursing diagnosis: 1993–1994.* St. Louis: Mosby–Yearbook.

Hagey, R. S., & McDonough, P. (1984). The problem of professional labeling. *Nursing Outlook, 32*(3), 151–157.

Hammond, K. R. (1966). Clinical inference in nursing: A psychologist's view point. *Nursing Research, 15*(1), 27–38.

Hardy, E. (1983). The diagnostic wheel: Identifying care that is unique to nursing. *Canadian Nurse, 79*(3), 38–40.

Hurley, M. (Ed.). (1986). *Classification of nursing diagnoses: Proceedings of the sixth conference.* St. Louis: Mosby.

Iyer, P., Taptich, B., & Bernocchi-Losey, D. (1991). *Nursing process and nursing diagnosis* (2nd ed.). Philadelphia: Saunders.

Kelly, M. A. (1985). *Nursing diagnosis source book.* Norwalk, CT: Appleton-Century-Crofts.

Kim, M. J., McFarland, G. K., & McLane, A. M. (Eds.). (1984). *Classification of nursing diagnosis: Proceedings of the fifth national conference.* St. Louis: Mosby.

Kritek, P. B. (1985). Nursing diagnosis in perspective: Response to a critique. *Image: Journal of Nursing Scholarship, 17*(1), 3–8.

Lindsey, A. M. (1990). Identification and labeling of human responses. *Journal of Professional Nursing, 6*(3), 143–150.

Lunney, M. (1982). Nursing diagnosis: Refining the system. *American Journal of Nursing, 82*(3), 456–459.

Martens, K. (1986). Let's diagnose strengths, not just problems. *American Journal of Nursing, 86*(2), 192–193.

McLane, A.M. (Ed.). (1987). *Classification of nursing diagnoses: Proceedings of the seventh conference.* St. Louis: Mosby.

Mehmert, P. A., Dickel, C. A., & McKeighen, R. J. (1989). Computerizing nursing diagnosis. *Nursing Management, 20*(7), 24–30.

Mitchell, G. J. (1991). Nursing diagnosis: An ethical analysis. *Image, 23*(2), 99–103.

Mundinger, M. O., & Jauron, G. D. (1975). Developing a nursing diagnosis. *Nursing Outlook, 23,* 94–98.

North American Nursing Diagnosis Association. (1990). *Taxonomy I revised with official diagnostic categories.* St. Louis: Author.

Nursing Diagnosis Newsletter. [Now a journal: *Nursing Diagnosis*]. North American Nursing Diagnosis Association.

Orem, D. (1991). *Nursing: Concepts of practice.* (4th ed.). St. Louis: Mosby–Year Book.

Popkess, S. (1981). Diagnosing your patient's strengths. *Nursing, 11*(7), 34–37.

Porter, E. J. (1986). Critical analysis of NANDA nursing diagnosis taxonomy I. *Image: Journal of Nursing Scholarship, 18*(4), 136–139.

Price, M. R. (1980). Nursing diagnosis: Making a concept come alive. *American Journal of Nursing, 80*(4), 668–674.

Rasch, R.F.R. (1987). The nature of taxonomy. *Image: Journal of Nursing Scholarship, 19*(3), 147–149.

Roberts, S. L. (1990). Achieving professional autonomy through nursing diagnosis and nursing DRGs. *Nursing Administration Quarterly, 14*(4), 54–60.

Rogers, M. (1970). *An introduction to the theoretical basis of nursing.* Philadelphia: Davis.

Roy, C. (1976). *Introduction to nursing: An adaptation model.* Englewood Cliffs, NJ: Prentice-Hall.

Shamansky, S. L., & Yanni, C. R. (1983). In opposition to nursing diagnosis: A minority opinion. *Image: Journal of Nursing Scholarship, 15*(2), 47–50.

Stolte, K. M. (1986). Nursing diagnosis and the childbearing woman. *MCN, 11,* 13–15.

Tartaglia, M. J. (1985). Nursing diagnosis: Keystone of your care plan. *Nursing, 15*(3), 34–37.

Vincent, K. G., & Coler, M. S. (1990). A unified nursing diagnostic model. *Image: Journal of Nursing Scholarship, 22*(2), 93–95.

Weber, G. (1991). Making nursing diagnosis work for you and your client: A step-by-step approach. *Nursing & Health Care, 12*(8), 424–430.

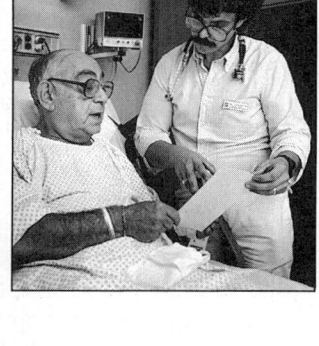
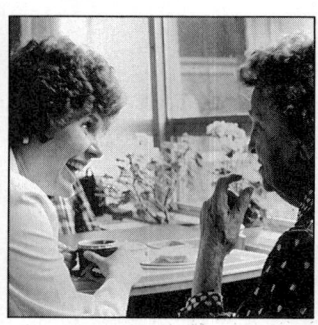

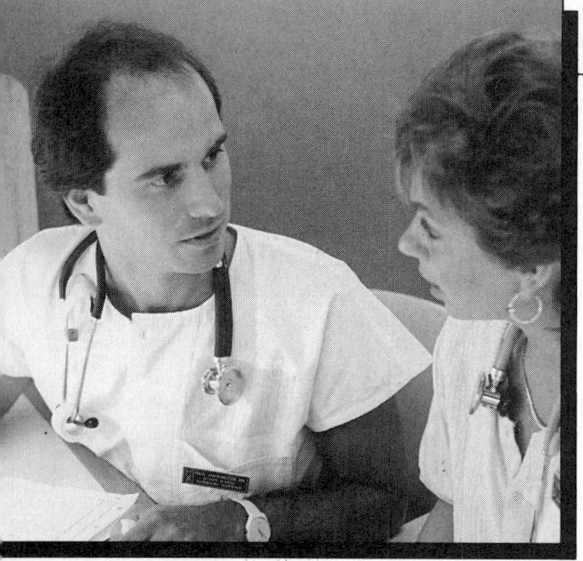

Planning

OBJECTIVES

After studying this chapter, the learner should be able to:

Define key terms used in the chapter.

Describe the purpose and benefits of planning.

Identify three elements of comprehensive planning.

Prioritize client health problems and nursing responses.

Describe how client goals and nursing orders are derived from nursing diagnoses.

Develop a plan of nursing care with properly constructed goals and related nursing orders.

Use criteria to evaluate planning skills.

Describe five common problems related to planning, their possible causes, and remedies.

KEY TERMS

client goal (objective, outcome)
computerized nursing care plan
criteria
discharge planning
goal
Kardex care plan
nursing care plan
nursing order
planning
standardized care plan

17

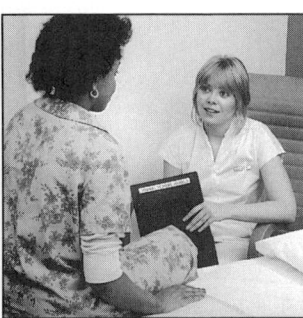

After the nurse collects and interprets client data, identifies client strengths and health problems, and prioritizes nursing diagnoses, it is time to plan for nursing action. During the **planning** step of the nursing process, the nurse works with the client and family to (1) develop client goals that, if achieved, prevent, reduce, or eliminate the problems specified in the nursing diagnoses, and (2) identify the nursing interventions that are most likely to assist the client in achieving these goals.

Elements of planning (outlined in Fig. 17-1) include the following:

- Establishing priorities
- Writing goals and developing an evaluative strategy
- Selecting related nursing measures
- Communicating the plan of nursing care

It is important that the nurse, client, and family work together as much as possible during planning. If the goals specified in the plan of care are not valued by the client or do not contribute to the prevention, resolution, or reduction of the client's problems, then the plan of care may be meaningless. Goal writing can, therefore, be a critical skill for the nurse who hopes to successfully intervene with clients.

In this chapter, planning is explored as a conscious, deliberate step in the nursing process. Informal planning, however, is such an integral component of nursing practice that it often happens without nurses being aware that they are planning. It is the link between the identification of a client strength or problem and the appropriate nursing response. When a nurse on a busy surgical unit learns that a postoperative client is complaining of incisional pain and quickly reshuffles priorities to allow time to assess the course and qualities of the pain and what nursing measures can be implemented to reduce discomfort, planning has occurred. When the postpartum nurse on the 3-to-11 shift realizes on the evening before discharge that he or she has not seen a particular father hold his new daughter and makes a mental note to observe the father–daughter interactions that evening and facilitate their bonding, planning has occurred. When a nurse in a geriatric day-care center hears a client choking and rushes to his side to perform the Heimlich maneuver if it becomes necessary, planning has occurred. Informal planning on a more conscious level is illustrated by a hospice nurse who ponders how to best support a client with terminal cancer who is gradually relinquishing her hold on life. When nurses find formal plan-

ning burdensome and are satisfied with this type of informal planning, they are depriving themselves and their clients of the benefits related to formal planning.

Some of the reasons for developing a formal plan of care are to individualize care, to set priorities, to facilitate communication among nursing personnel, to promote continuity of care, to coordinate care, to evaluate the client's responses to nursing care, and to promote the nurse's professional development. Prerequisite skills for the nurse who designs effective plans of care are a sound knowledge of nursing (including standards for professional nursing practice); the ability to collect, interpret, and analyze client data, develop nursing diagnoses, construct client goals, and select appropriate nursing interventions; creativity; sensitivity to the unique needs of the client; and the ability to communicate clearly and concisely. Computer skills also are becoming a necessity for the nurse.

Unique Focus of Nursing Planning

The primary purpose of the planning step of the nursing process is to design a plan of care for the client that, once implemented, results in the prevention or resolution of client health problems. A comprehensive plan of care also specifies any routine nursing assistance the client requires to meet basic human needs (eg, assistance with hygiene or nutrition) and describes appropriate nursing responsibilities for fulfilling the medical plan of care. For example, physicians may delegate to nurses caring for a surgical client the redressing of the surgical incision, the administration of prescribed medications and intravenous therapy, and responsibility for scheduling laboratory studies. The creative and innovative nurse learns to design a plan of care that incorporates his or her independent and collaborative responsibilities. Because nursing is concerned with the client's responses to health and illness, the plan of care is supportive of nursing's broad aims—to promote wellness, prevent disease and illness, promote recovery, and facilitate coping with altered functioning.

Comprehensive Planning

There are three basic types of planning critical to comprehensive nursing care—initial, ongoing problem oriented, and discharge. The nurse who develops a comprehensive plan of care on the client's day of admission and then fails to update the plan and to anticipate discharge needs has done the client a great disservice. This is probably the most common problem related to planning.

Initial Planning   The *initial plan* is developed by the nurse who performs the admission nursing history and the physical assessment. Comprehensive in nature, this plan

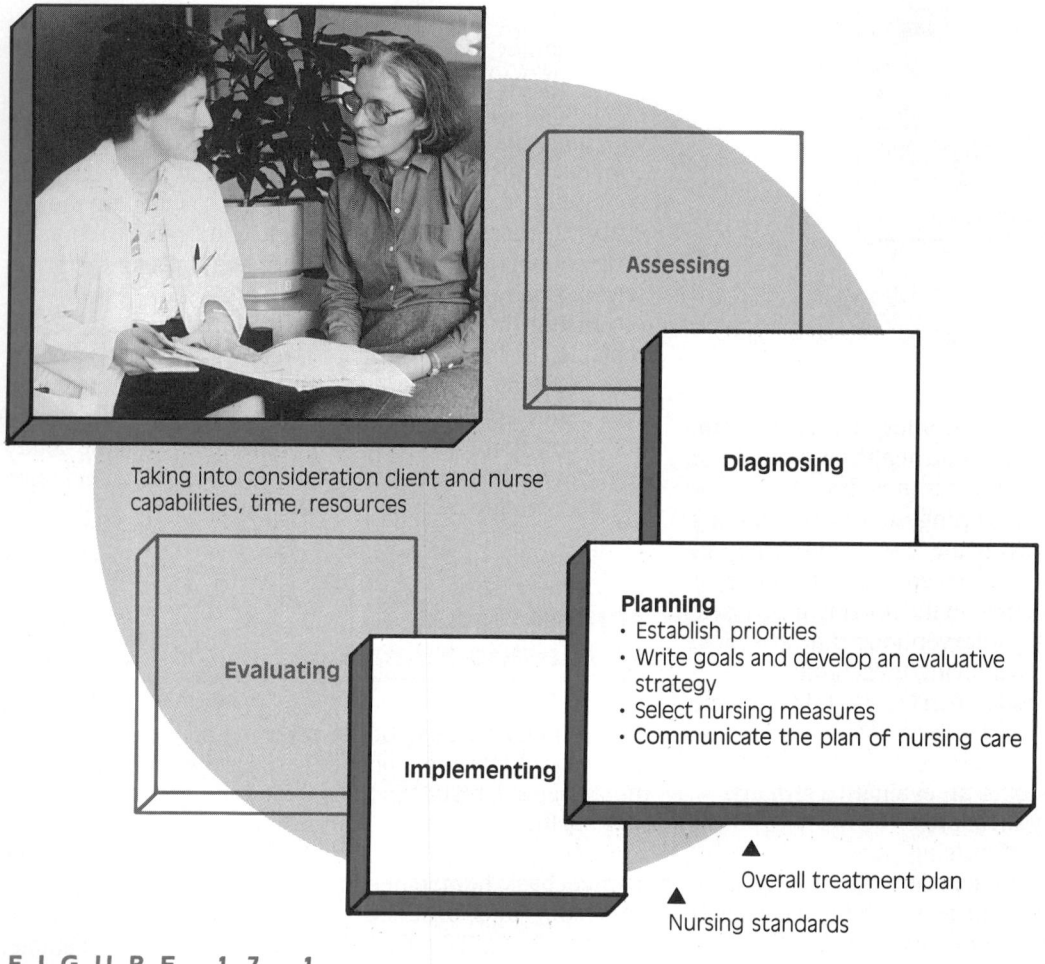

Taking into consideration client and nurse capabilities, time, resources

Assessing

Diagnosing

Planning
- Establish priorities
- Write goals and develop an evaluative strategy
- Select nursing measures
- Communicate the plan of nursing care

Evaluating

Implementing

▲ Overall treatment plan
▲ Nursing standards

F I G U R E   1 7 - 1

Planning. The nurse and client work together to develop client goals and identify the nursing interventions most likely to assist the client to meet the goals. It is important for the plan of care to be consistent with nursing standards, congruent with other planned therapies, and realistic in terms of the client and nurses' abilities or resources. (Photo by Gates Rhodes, courtesy of School of Nursing, University of Pennsylvania.)

addresses each problem listed in the prioritized nursing diagnoses and identifies appropriate client goals and the related nursing care. Standardized plans can provide an excellent basis for the initial plan *if the nurse tailors them to meet individual client needs.* Resources for standardized plans include computerized plans, textbooks with prepared care plans, and agency-developed plans. By using such standardized plans, the nurse is free to direct time and expertise to individualizing the plan.

Ongoing Planning   *Ongoing, problem-oriented planning* is carried out by any nurse who interacts with the client. Its chief purpose is to keep the plan up-to-date. The work of ongoing planning includes stating nursing diagnoses more clearly (both the problem statement and the cause) and developing new diagnoses as indicated by newly collected

and analyzed data; making previously developed client goals more realistic and developing new goals as needed; identifying those nursing actions that will best accomplish the client goals, given a better knowledge of the client; and using and documenting client responses to nursing actions to direct further planning.

At this stage of planning, standardized plans may be useful in working up new diagnoses, but the emphasis clearly is on individualizing the plan to meet unique client needs. For example, the standard nursing order "force fluids" would be rewritten as "offer 60 mL cranberry or orange juice between meals, and keep fresh water at bedside." A preliminary order such as "explore with the client existing supports" may be replaced with "keep daughter Barbara informed of mother's progress and coach her in effective support strategies (Barbara Clems, 448–3211)."

Discharge Planning Discharge planning is best carried out by the nurse who has worked most closely with the client and family, possibly in conjunction with a nurse or social worker who has a broad knowledge of existing community resources. Comprehensive discharge planning begins when the client is admitted for treatment. Careful planning ensures that the teaching and counseling skills of the nurse are used to help the client and family develop sufficient knowledge of the health problem and the therapeutic regimen to competently execute the necessary self-care behaviors at home. Discharge planning is further discussed in Chapter 28.

Establishing Priorities

Before developing or modifying the plan of care, it is helpful to review the prioritized list of nursing diagnoses to determine if they are correctly ranked as high priority (greatest threat to client's well-being), medium priority (non–life-threatening), and low priority (not specifically related to current illness and prognosis). Guidelines for establishing these priorities, such as Maslow's hierarchy of human needs, client preferences, and anticipation of future problems, are presented in Chapter 16.

When planning nursing care for each day, it is helpful to consider the following:

- Have changes in the client's health status influenced what are considered the most important threats to the client's well-being? For example, a client who was admitted to the hospital with the tentative medical diagnosis of unexplained weight loss has now been found to have ovarian cancer; this requires a new set of priorities for care.
- Have changes in the way the client is responding to health and illness or the plan of care affected those nursing diagnoses that can be realistically addressed? For example, the nurse may have identified ineffective individual coping as a high-priority diagnosis for the client after he learned of the medical diagnosis, and planned to initiate counseling. But if the client adamantly requests to be left alone for a day to think

things through, the nurse has to modify priorities of care for that day.

- Are there relations between problems, such that one must be worked on before another one can be resolved?
- Can several client problems be dealt with together?

After answering these questions, the nurse ranks problems in the order in which they will be addressed. Setting priorities enables the nurse to make sure that time and energy are being directed to the client's most important problems.

Writing Goals and Developing Evaluative Strategies

A **goal** is an aim or an end. A **client goal** describes an expected client outcome. The words goal, objective, and outcome often are used interchangeably. In some practice settings, the term *goal* or *objective* is used to describe what is wanted and the term *outcome* is used to describe the results achieved.

Deriving Goals from Nursing Diagnoses

Goals are derived from the problem statement of the nursing diagnosis. For each nursing diagnosis in the plan of care, at least one goal must be written that, if achieved, demonstrates a *direct resolution* of the problem statement (Table 17-1).

Other goals that contribute to the resolution of the problem may be written. For example, for the nursing diagnosis Nutritional Alteration: More Than Body Requirements, related to excessive snacking and inactivity, in addition to the goal "by 12/6/93, the client will reach target weight: 122 lb," the following goals are appropriate: "By 6/6/93, the client will identify 10 low-calorie snack foods he is willing to try; the client will have 3-day diet recall consistent with nutritionally balanced 1500-calorie diet; the client will report incorporating three periods of vigorous exercise into each week." The difference between these goals and the goal that the client reach his target weight is that whereas the achievement of these goals may contribute to the resolution of the problem, they also may be achieved without the problem being resolved and the client's plan of care may mistakenly be terminated. Remember, *at least one goal per nursing diagnosis must directly resolve the problem statement in the nursing diagnosis.*

Long-Term Versus Short-Term Goals

Goals may be either long-term or short-term. Simply defined, long-term goals require a longer period (usually more than a week) to be achieved than do short-term goals. Long-term goals also may be used as discharge goals, in which case they are more broadly written and communicate to the entire nursing team the desired end results of

---

T A B L E   1 7 - 1

Examples of Goals to Relieve Problems	
Problem Statement of the Nursing Diagnosis	**Related Client Goal**
Pain	By end of shift client reports pain is absent or diminished
Altered Nutrition: More Than Body Requirements	By 12/6/93, client reaches target weight of 122 lb
Impaired Physical Mobility	Before discharge, client ambulates length of hallway independently

Examples of Long- and Short-Term Goals

Client on Bed Rest From Nursing Home

Long-Term Goal
Mrs. Goldstein returns to the nursing home pain-free with her incision healed and her left leg in good alignment.

Short-Term Goals
- Whenever observed, client will be lying in bed with legs in correct alignment (abductor pillow in place if ordered).
- Before discharge, Mrs. Goldstein's hip incision will show signs of healing (skin surfaces approximate, free from signs of infection—redness, swelling, heat, purulent drainage).
- Whenever observed, client will report that comfort measures and medication are satisfactorily managing pain.

Active Client from Private Home

Long-Term Goal
Mrs. Siverstein returns home to her husband pain-free with incision healed, fully mobile (full weight-bearing on left leg), and capable of independent activities of daily living.

Short-Term Goals
- By 1/28/93, the client will verbalize willingness to participate in physical therapy program.
- By 2/4/93, the client will ambulate (with nursing assistance and walker) to bathroom (full weight-bearing).
- By 2/11/93, the client will ambulate with nursing assistance only (no walker) in her room.
- Goals for incision and pain relief same as for Mrs. Goldstein.

nursing care for a particular client. For example, two elderly women, both aged 77, are on a nursing unit after undergoing similar operative procedures for fractured left hips. Whereas one woman has spent the past 2 years in bed in a nursing home, the other woman fractured her hip at the YMCA where she swims daily. Their nursing care should not be the same because it is directed to different long-term goals, although their short-term goals may be similar (see sample goals).

Cognitive, Psychomotor, and Affective Goals

Goals may be categorized according to the type of change they describe for the client. *Cognitive goals* describe increases in client knowledge or intellectual behaviors. *Example:* By 6/12/93, the client will list three benefits of continuing to apply moist compresses to leg ulcer after discharge. *Psychomotor goals* describe the client's achievement of new skills. *Example:* By 6/12/93, the client will correctly demonstrate application of wet-to-dry dressing on leg ulcer. *Affective goals* describe changes in client values, beliefs, and attitudes. Difficult both to write and to evaluate, affective goals may be critical to the resolution of a complex client problem. *Example:* By 6/12/93, the client will verbalize valuing health sufficiently to practice new health behaviors to prevent recurrence of leg ulcer. In this example, even if the client intellectually grasps the reasons for taking care of her leg and can competently redress her ulcer, unless she is motivated to take care of herself, her knowledge and skills will not result in healthy outcomes (Fig. 17-2).

Guidelines for Goal Writing

When developing client goals, the nurse and client look at the problem statement of the nursing diagnosis and ask "What client changes or outcomes will result in the prevention or resolution of this problem?" The answer, when carefully worded, becomes the client goal. (See Guidelines for Writing Goals.) One of the most important considerations in goal writing is encouraging the client and family to be as active in goal development as their abilities and interest permit. The more involved they are, the greater the probability that the goals will be achieved.

Each client goal must have a *subject*, which is the client or some part of the client; a *verb*, which indicates the action the client will perform; and **criteria**, which describe in *observable, measurable terms* the expected client behavior (must include a time criterion—such as 4/6/93, before discharge, after viewing film, whenever observed—specifying the targeted time or date by which the goal should be achieved).

The following are examples of properly constructed client goals:
- By end of shift, client's 24-hour fluid intake will total at least 1800 mL.
- At next visit, 12/23/93, the client will correctly demonstrate relaxation exercises.

It may be helpful to include special conditions when writing a goal if this information is important for other nurses (eg, "Before discharge, client ambulates independently in hallway, using Philadelphia collar to support cervical vertebrae.").

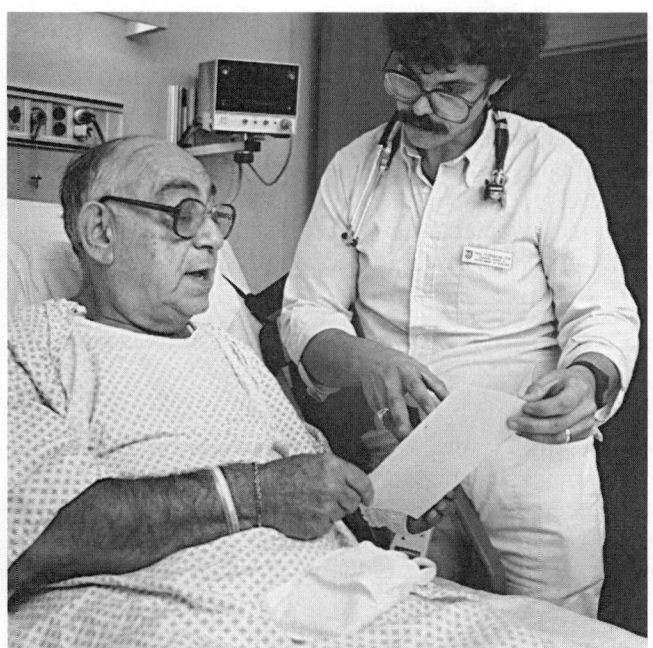

FIGURE 17-2

What cognitive, psychomotor, and affective goals might be set for a client who must learn new eating patterns after a heart attack? (Photo by Robert Neroni, courtesy of Thomas Jefferson University.)

Common Errors

Common errors when writing client goals include the following:

- Expressing the *client* goal as a *nursing* goal. *Incorrect:* Offer Mr. Myer 60 mL fluid every 2 hours while awake. *Correct:* Mr. Myer will drink 60 mL fluid every 2 hours while awake, beginning 2/24/93.
- Using verbs that are not *observable* and *measurable*. *Incorrect:* Mrs. Gaston will know how to bathe her newborn. *Correct:* After attending the infant care class, Mrs. Gaston will correctly demonstrate the procedure for bathing her newborn. Verbs to be avoided when writing goals include *know, understand, learn, become aware.* Verbs that are helpful when writing goals that are observable and measurable are shown in the accompanying display.
- Including more than one client behavior in short-term goals. *Incorrect:* Client will list dangers of smoking and stops smoking. *Correct:* By next meeting, 3/11/93, the client will (1) identify three dangers of smoking and (2) describe a plan he is willing to try to stop smoking. By 6/20/93, the client will report that he no longer smokes.
- Writing goals so vaguely that other nurses are unsure of the goal of nursing care. *Incorrect:* Client will cope better. *Correct:* After initial interview, 10/20/93, the client will (1) describe two new coping strategies he is willing to try and (2) demonstrate decreased incidence

of previously observed noneffective coping behaviors (chain smoking, withdrawal behavior, heavy alcohol consumption).

Developing Evaluative Strategy

Chapter 19 deals specifically with the evaluative component of the nursing process. During the planning step, an evaluative strategy must be identified and incorporated into the formal plan of care. Having client goals written on the plan is meaningless unless nurses evaluate whether these goals have been achieved. The nurse should record the date the goal was written and the date the goal is achieved. Students learning how to evaluate the effects of nursing care may find it helpful to write an evaluative statement (see display), which includes a statement about the achievement of the desired goal (goal met, goal partially met, goal not met) and lists an actual client behavior as evidence supporting the statement. If indicated, recommendations for revising the plan of care can be included in the evaluative statement (Atkinson & Murray, 1990).

> ### Guidelines for Writing Goals
>
> - Derive each set of goals from only one nursing diagnosis.
> - Make sure that at least one of the goals clearly shows a direct resolution of the problem statement in the nursing diagnosis and that other goals contribute to the prevention or resolution of the problem.
> - Write goals that are valued by the client and family.
> - Check to make sure the goals are supportive of the total treatment plan.
> - Write goals that are brief, specific (clearly describe an observable, measurable behavior), and phrased positively.
> - Remember that each short-term goal can contain only one client behavior.

> ### Verbs Helpful in Writing Goals
>
> | | |
> |---|---|
> | define | prepare |
> | identify | design |
> | list | verbalize |
> | describe | choose |
> | explain | select |
> | apply | inject |
> | use | perform |
> | demonstrate | |

Evaluative Statement

Documents that client has met, partially met, or not met the goal.

Goal Statement

Beginning 6/8/93, the client will ambulate half the length of hallway with assistance three times daily.

Evaluative Statement

6/8/93 Goal partially met; client refused to ambulate in the morning but did walk to the bathroom once in the afternoon with the assistance of one nurse.

Recommendation: Review reason for progressive ambulation with client; assess motivation to increase independence.

M. Stenulis, RN

Identifying Options

After the client goals are written, the nurse identifies various nursing measures to help the client achieve the goals. The effectiveness of the nurse is directly proportional to his or her command of varied nursing strategies. Consider the nursing options identified by three nurses when they are told that a woman 2 days after cesarean delivery is complaining of pain in her incisional area.

Nurse A
• Check to see what type of pain medication is ordered, and give it if the time interval is sufficient.

Nurse B
• Assess the quality of the pain, and use this time to communicate support by means of expression and squeeze of hand.
• Administer analgesic if indicated.
• Assess effectiveness of the analgesic ordered.

Selecting Nursing Measures

Deriving Nursing Measures from Nursing Diagnoses

Nursing measures, like client goals, are derived from the nursing diagnosis. But whereas the problem statement of the diagnosis suggests the client goals, it is the cause of the problem that suggests the nursing measures (Fig. 17-3). The effective nurse selects nursing measures that specifically address factors that cause or contribute to the client's problems.

For example, many factors may contribute to obesity such as deficient nutritional knowledge, convenience of high-calorie fast foods, lifetime snacking habits, limited food budget, little exercise, and low self-esteem. The nurse working with a client who wants to lose weight could attempt to deal with all these factors, but this approach would be inefficient. When a carefully developed nursing diagnosis identifies the specific factors that contributed to a particular client's weight problem, nursing measures can be selected to deal directly with these factors.

For example, nursing measures for the client with the diagnosis *Altered Nutrition: More Than Body Requirements, related to lifetime snacking habits and heavy reliance on high-calorie fast foods* might include education about the fat content and calories in fast foods and an exploration of ways the client could change eating habits to eat more nutritionally balanced meals with fewer calories. Thus not every client with a weight problem is nursed the same way. The art of nursing involves the careful tailoring of select nursing measures to the individual needs of the client.

F I G U R E   1 7 - 3

Deriving client goals and nursing orders from nursing diagnoses.

1st part of the nursing diagnosis
(problem statement)

• identifies the unhealthy response
• indicates what should change

↓

• suggests client goals (expectations for change)

2nd part of the nursing diagnosis
(etiology)

• identifies factors causing or contributing to the undesirable response and preventing desired change

↓

• suggests *nursing measures*

Nurse C
- Assess quality of the pain and explore the possibility of contributing factors such as the effects of increased gas in the abdominal area or concern about the newborn, herself, or other family members.
- Use empathic listening (possibly touch) to communicate support and to encourage the mother to share her concerns.
- Change her position in bed.
- Offer a back rub.
- Loosen the dressing over the incisional area.
- If appropriate, suggest activity that will distract attention from the pain (eg, watching a film of newborn care or listening to music).
- Give the prescribed medication for pain and observe its effect.
- When administering the medication, use the power of positive suggestion to enhance its effectiveness: "This will start taking the pain away in about 10 minutes and will help you relax."

It is possible that the client simply needs her prescribed analgesic to achieve the goal: "Client reports minimal to no pain whenever assessed." In this case, all three nurses would have been effective in meeting the client's need for nursing care. It also is possible that the prescribed medication was not working, or that the pain was compounded by the mother's fears about caring for her new baby or by her worries that the baby will ruin her relationship with her husband.

The more varied the options available to the nurse, the more effective the nursing response will be. In different situations, a skilled nursing procedure, an appropriate use of silence, respectful listening, humor, teaching, counseling, and touch can all be effective nursing strategies. The nurse who is task oriented and satisfied to meet every client problem with a mechanical procedure is limiting her effectiveness.

Students who want to develop a varied repertoire of nursing skills can actively seek assistance from nursing instructors and nurse practitioners. Nurses can learn valuable strategies by watching their successful colleagues and observing and talking with them about what it is they do that is different; by talking with clients and families about the nursing care they find most helpful; and by researching the nursing literature for suggestions to improve care.

Selecting From Options

From the list of options, nurses select those nursing measures they believe will best assist the client to meet goals. There are broad guidelines the nurse can use when selecting nursing measures. The nursing measures selected must be:
- Tailored to the client
- Consistent with standards of care, such as American Nurses' Association/Canadian Nurses Association standards of practice, nurse practice acts, institutional standards, standards of accrediting agencies (eg, Joint Commission of Accreditation of Healthcare Organizations [JCAHO])
- Realistic in terms of the abilities, time, and resources available to the nurse and client
- Compatible with the client's values, beliefs, and psychosocial background
- Valued, whenever possible, by the client and family
- Compatible with other planned therapies

Even if a nursing measure meets these criteria, there is no guarantee it will result in the client's successfully achieving a goal. What may be successful for one client may not work for someone else. Nurse researchers are now attempting to establish a statistical pattern for predicting the probability of success of select nursing measures. The competent nurse uses research findings (science of nursing) and knowledge of the client (art of nursing) to select effective nursing measures. Ongoing consultation with nurse colleagues and continuing education are among the best means to explore new and creative nursing approaches to client problems.

Writing Nursing Orders

Nursing orders communicate to the entire nursing staff the specific nursing measures that are to be implemented for the client (Fig. 17-4). Well-written nursing orders:
- Clearly and concisely describe the nursing action to be performed (answer the questions who? what? where? when? and how?)

F I G U R E   1 7 - 4

What comprehensive nursing orders might be written for teaching a client to use a TENS unit on discharge from the hospital? (Photo by Denise Angeloni, courtesy of School of Nursing, University of Pennsylvania.)

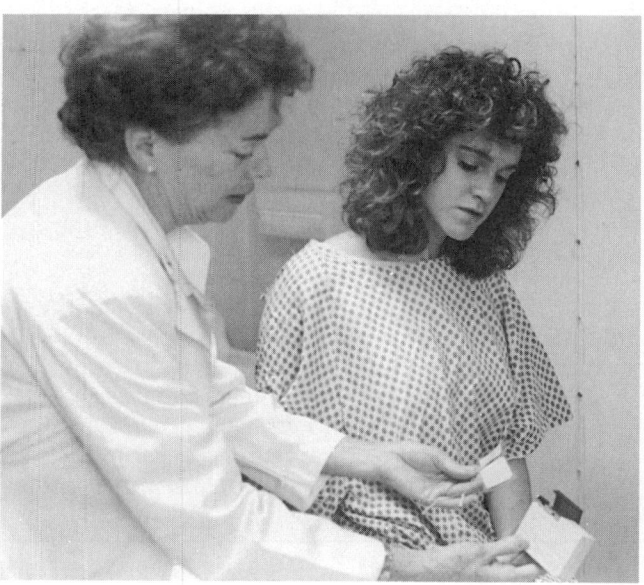

- Are dated when the order is written and when the plan of care is reviewed
- Are signed by the nurse prescribing the order
- Use only those abbreviations accepted in the institution (these usually are found in the policy manual; a list of commonly accepted abbreviations appears in Chapter 18)
- Refer the nurse to the agency's procedure manual or other literature for the steps of routine, lengthy procedures

The following are examples of nursing orders:

- Offer client 60 mL water or juice (prefers orange or cranberry juice) every 2 hours while awake.
- Instruct client on necessity of carefully monitoring fluid intake and output; needs to be reminded every shift to report fluid intake.
- Offer assistance with toileting (walk with client to bathroom) every 2 hours while client is awake; client has diminished sensation of full bladder.

The set of nursing orders written to assist a client to meet a goal must be comprehensive. Comprehensive nursing orders specify what *observations* need to be made and how often; what *nursing measures* need to be done and when they must be done; and what *teaching, counseling, and advocacy needs* clients and families have.

Many sets of nursing orders are deficient, in that they fail to indicate what the ongoing assessment priority needs to be in relation to a specific problem or goal. Clearly noting assessment priorities helps all nurses to be more sensitive to important client data. For example, when assisting a client who wants to lose weight to reach the target weight,

appropriate nursing orders would include the following: 6/17/93—Continue to assess (1) client's motivation to participate in weight loss program, and (2) factors that positively or negatively influence weight loss.

Similarly, it often is assumed that all clients have the same teaching needs. Nothing is farther from the truth. In fact, many clients come to the hospital with an excellent knowledge base (which may be greater than that of the nurse for a particular disease). Their need for nursing may be a need for counseling as they learn to live with a chronic illness. Comprehensive nursing orders relate to individual client needs.

Writing the Nursing Care Plan

The **nursing care plan** (plan of nursing care, client care plan) is the written guide that directs the efforts of the nursing team as they work with clients to meet health goals. Care plans offer many benefits to the client, nurse, nursing unit, nursing administration, and nursing profession. These are highlighted in the display. Primarily, nursing care plans ensure that the nursing team works efficiently to deliver holistic, goal-oriented, individualized care to clients. A well-written nursing care plan:

- Represents an adequate philosophy of nursing; advances nursing's four aims: promotes wellness, prevents disease and illness, promotes recovery, facilitates coping with altered functioning
- Is tailored to the individual characteristics and needs of the client
- Clearly identifies (1) any nursing assistance the client needs to meet basic human needs, (2) nursing diagnoses and related client goals and nursing orders, and (3) nursing responsibilities for fulfilling the medical plan of care
- Directs the nurse's assessment priorities, caregiving behaviors, and teaching, counseling, and advocacy behaviors
- Is based on scientific principles and incorporates findings of nursing research
- Meets developmental, psychosocial, and spiritual needs of the client, as well as physiologic needs
- Addresses discharge needs of the client and family
- When appropriate, is compatible with the medical plan of care and that of the interdisciplinary team

Formats for Care Plans

Many suggestions for care plans appear in the nursing literature. Each school of nursing and each health care institution has its own format, which may reflect a particular nursing theory. Common to all formats is a minimum of three columns for documenting nursing diagnoses, client goals, and nursing orders. Formats differ in the way they handle assessment data and nursing evaluation.

Guidelines for Developing the Nursing Care Plan

The nursing care plan:
- Is initiated on the day of admission
- Is developed by the nurse who best knows the client (primary nurse) and added to by other members of the nursing team
- Provides for client and family participation as much as possible
- Is signed and dated by the nurse developing the plan
- Is written in ink (if not computerized) and kept as part of the client's permanent record
- Clearly specifies nursing diagnoses, client goals, nursing orders, and evaluation strategies
- Uses standardized symbols, abbreviations, and key phrases specified in the agency's policy manual, as opposed to lengthy descriptions
- Refers nurses to agency procedure manuals for specific steps in routine nursing procedures
- Is updated consistently to reflect changes in client status and related needs for nursing care

Benefits of Nursing Care Plans

For the Client

- Provide quality care
- Monitor progress
- Ensure consistency and continuity

For the Nurse

- Communicate information
- Organize care
- Evaluate care

For the Clinical Unit

- Make assignments
- Organize time-related activities
- Direct shift report
- Evaluate nurse performance

For Administration

- Secure resources
- Distribute resources
- Evaluate nursing practice

For Nursing

- Educate practitioners
- Develop professionalism
- Define nursing parameters
- Test and develop theory
- Research

(Shea, H. [1984]. The nursing care plan dilemma: Suggestions for resolution. *Canadian Nurse, 80*[9], 44–46.)

Institutional Care Plans

Many health care institutions use a **Kardex care plan** in which the plan of care for each client is recorded on a 6 × 11–inch card and placed in a central Kardex file. In addition to abbreviated background information on the client, the Kardex file usually contains three types of information—nursing care related to basic human needs, nursing care related to nursing diagnoses, and nursing care related to the medical plan of care.

Nursing Care Related to Basic Human Needs The plan should be abbreviated and make readily available to caregivers client data concerning health habits and patterns obtained from the nursing history and modified appropriately by current treatment orders. This information is useful to caregivers only if it is kept current as the client's condition changes. Any nurse should be able to find on the nursing Kardex the instructions she or he needs to confidently and competently provide care.

Nursing Care Related to Nursing Diagnoses The plan contains goals and nursing actions for every nursing diagnosis, as well as a place to note client responses to the plan of care. This section is the heart of the care plan because it represents the independent component of nursing practice. If well developed, it demonstrates the clinical competence of the nurse (knowledge of the science of nursing), sensitivity to the individual needs of the client, and creativity. Development of this portion of the plan is nursing's challenge.

Nursing Care Related to the Medical Plan of Care The plan also records medical orders for treatment and diagnostic studies that involve nursing care. At one time, Kardexes were a bookkeeping system for medical orders.

Computerized Nursing Care Plans In an increasing number of institutional settings, nurses are using computer software programs to generate **computerized nursing care plans** (CNCPs). Once the nurse identifies an appropriate nursing diagnosis, a series of screens follows for selecting from lists of goals, causes, and interventions. Benefits of using CNCPs are highlighted in the accompanying display. At least one nurse researcher is studying the negative impact the development and use of CNCPs have on the professionalization of staff nurses. Harris (1990) cautions that the computerized system for client care planning and the larger system in which it is embedded contribute to the loss of autonomy, loss of individualization of care, and loss of nursing expertise. Individual nurses as well as researchers have to respond to Harris' challenge, "does a lot of nursing time spent in procedural, rule-governed, step-by-step thinking processes destroy part of the nurse's ability to care, to empathize, to intuit, to gain insight, to function in the expert mode?" (p. 73).

Student Care Plans

The care plans that students are required to develop often are more detailed than those found in practice settings. The aim is to assist students to assimilate each of the five steps of the nursing process. Although care plan formats vary from one nursing program to another, most are designed so that the student can systematically proceed through each interrelated step in the nursing process, and many use a five-column format.

The sample student care plan given here demonstrates a plan developed for the client whose admission assessment form is in Chapter 15. This 72-year-old woman was admitted to the hospital after experiencing a ministroke (transient ischemic attack) at home. Her condition is stable, and the three prioritized diagnoses developed on the plan address her inability to deal with this new medical diagnosis and to prevent a major stroke (high priority), ineffective coping (medium priority), and constipation (low priority). In the past year, her husband died and she sold her home and moved in with her daughter.

(Text continues on p. 276)

Student Care Plan

Assessment	Nursing Diagnosis	Goal
Subjective data: "Will I get a stroke now? I don't think I could handle that."	High Risk for Alteration in Health Maintenance Response to TIA and Stroke Prevention related to knowledge deficit	Before discharge, the client will: • Describe the terms *TIA* and *stroke*, identifying the underlying disease process, causes, symptoms, and treatment
Objective data: Admitting diagnosis: TIA BP: 184/120		

Strengths: Past pattern of adhering to prescribed health behaviors.		After discussion with the physician and nurse, the client will:
		• Correctly describe the treatment plan:
		  • Medications (drugs, intended effect, dose, time, route)
		  • Dietary modifications
		  • Exercise prescription
		  • Signs and symptoms to report
		  • Follow-up appointment date

Subjective data: Husband died 8 months ago; moved in with daughter 6 months ago after selling family home Daughter reports mother has been a very independent strong woman in the past—seemed to "crumple" after husband's death. History of headaches	Ineffective Individual Coping related to illness, recent death of husband and relocation with daughter	Beginning 9/7/93, the client will: • Verbalize her feelings related to the loss of her husband, loss of family home, loss of health
Objective data: Clutches daughter's hand		• Identify coping patterns that have helped her in the past • Identify three personal strengths and three outside supports that will help her now
Strengths: History of handling life stressors well		
Limitations: In the past, her husband was her primary support.		Before discharge, the client will: • Verbalize that she feels "okay" (sufficiently in charge of her life) about returning home

Nursing Orders

Assess what the client knows about TIA and stroke (correct any misinformation). Assess learning needs, readiness to learn, and factors that will influence learning.

Plan teaching and learning sessions to involve family members designated by client.

Include in the teaching plan a description of TIA and stroke, the underlying disease process, causes, symptoms, and treatment plan.

Once the treatment plan has been developed, make sure the client and family understand it (teaching) and *value* the prescribed lifestyle modification (counseling).

Once a shift, primary nurse to sit at client's bedside for at least several minutes to communicate caring and to explore with the client her current stressors and the adequacy of her coping response.
- Assess factors compounding her losses.
- Reinforce her personal strengths and support systems; counsel her to tap into these now.
- Suggest local support groups if indicated.

Primary nurse to explore with daughter, Lisa, how her mother's moving in with her has affected the family. Recommend support systems.

Scientific Rationale

Each person's learning needs are different; each person learns in own unique way; learning is dependent on readiness.

The more support people knowledgeably committed to the plan of care, the greater the probability the client will achieve goals.

New self-care behaviors are dependent on knowledge.

New self-care behaviors are dependent on motivation. Unless the client is committed to stroke prevention and values this outcome, she will not follow the treatment plan.

The nurse's unhurried, attentive, and caring presence communicates to the client that she is important to the nurse and that the nurse values her well-being. It is an invitation to the client to become actively involved in recovery. Also, it is logical to explore adequacy of past and current coping mechanisms before suggesting new approaches.

Adult children of aging parents are frequently experiencing overwhelming stress as they try to deal with own and their parents' problems. Supporting this family *is* supporting the client indirectly.

Evaluation

9/10/93 Goal not met. Client says her head is "too old" to learn all this stuff. Equates stroke with death.

Revision: Reteach content in simpler terms. Reassess learning readiness.

C. Taylor, RN

9/10/93 Too early to evaluate.

C. Taylor, RN

9/10/93 Goal partially met. Client speaks freely about how much she misses her husband and how fearful this hospitalization makes her. When asked about living with her daughter, she becomes uncharacteristically quiet.

C. Taylor, RN

9/10/93 Goal met. Client talks about how everything seemed better in the past after she talked it over with her husband and God.

C. Taylor, RN

9/10/93 Goal not met. Client couldn't think of anything about herself that is healthy or strong. Says "maybe" her family can help her now.

Revision: Counsel regarding personal strengths. Help her to experience them.

C. Taylor, RN

9/11/93 Too early to evaluate.

C. Taylor, RN

(continued)

Student Care Plan (*Continued*)

Assessment	Nursing Diagnosis	Goal

Subjective data: "I move my bowels every 2 or 3 days; get constipated at least once a week. Often Metamucil helps."
"I drink plenty of fluids and even fruits and vegetables."
History of hemorrhoids secondary to straining
 	
Objective data: No bowel movement in past 4 days
On bed rest since hospitalized
	Colonic Constipation related to decreased physical activity and long-term laxative use (Metamucil)	Beginning 9/7/93, the client will:
		• Pass soft, formed stool every 1 to 3 days without use of laxatives
		
		By 9/10/93, the client will:
		• Verbalize the importance of the following natural aids to bowel elimination:
		  • Daily intake of foods high in bulk
		  • Daily fluid intake of 8 to 10 glasses
		  • Regular time for elimination
		  • Daily physical exercise: walking

Assessing   In the assessment column, the student records the assessment data that led to the establishment of each diagnosis. Recording these data helps to link specific defining characteristics with diagnostic problem statements. On some care plans, pertinent assessment data are recorded in the nursing diagnosis column.

Diagnosing   Priorities are assigned to each diagnosis, and these are recorded in the nursing diagnosis column. For each diagnosis, a clear and concise problem statement is followed by an etiology statement that identifies contributing factors.

Planning   The planning column contains the expected changes in client health status or in client behaviors (ie, the client goals). If achieved, these resolve the problem statement in the nursing diagnosis.

Implementing   Sets of nursing orders are written for each client goal. These specify *what* nursing interventions are to be performed, *how* they are to be performed, *when* they are to be performed, and by *whom* they are to be performed. In many nursing programs, students are asked to document the source of the nursing orders they propose. Although a student may be able to "pull from her head" some nursing strategies, developing the practice of consulting the nursing literature on select client problems is a sure means to increase nursing knowledge. Some programs also require

students to provide a scientific rationale for the orders they propose. A succinct rationale statement demonstrates that the student is consciously choosing a nursing intervention because of its high probability to effect the desired change.

Evaluating   Incorporating evaluative statements on the plan of care clearly communicates the message that nursing care is never complete until client goal achievement is evaluated. Just as some say that teaching has not occurred if learning does not take place, so nursing care is incomplete if the desired client goals are not achieved.

Care Plan Controversies

The 1991 JCAHO Standards for Nursing Care created some controversy within the profession by eliminating the need for every client to have in his or her medical record a handwritten care plan representing all or most of the care to be provided. Although a handwritten plan of care is no longer a prerequisite for accreditation, it is equally clear that there is to be documentation of client assessments, diagnoses, nursing interventions, and client response. Alternate documentation modalities include CNCPs, preprinted care plans, standards of care, and care plans in progress notes (Carpenito, 1991).

What is important is that a client's nursing care is

Nursing Orders	Scientific Rationale	Evaluation
Monitor bowel elimination patterns; identify causative factors of constipation and successful corrective measures.	This client's elimination problems will not be resolved until all the specific causes of her constipation and successful corrective measures are identified. Needs to be an ongoing assessment priority.	9/10/93 Goal met. Soft, formed stool passed every 2 to 3 days. *C. Taylor, RN*
Explain the importance of adhering to a regular time for defecation (client suggests after breakfast)—adhere to this in the hospital.	This encourages positive use of circadian rhythms.	
When given medical clearance, assist client with progressive ambulation. Recommend that she include brisk walking into daily health habits (build strength to 20- to 30-minute brisk walk daily).	Peristalsis is stimulated by physical exercise.	9/10/93 Goal met. Client correctly related value of four natural aids to elimination. Questions whether or not she will be strong enough to walk. *Revision:* Encourage assisted ambulation.
Explain the long-term effects of laxative abuse on the bowel and discourage their use.	Laxative abuse leads to decreased peristaltic response to food and loss of intestinal tone	*C. Taylor, RN*
Reinforce the client's adequate fluid intake and ingestion of high-bulk foods such as fresh fruits and salad.	Commenting on these positive self-care behaviors reinforces them.	

directed and provided by a registered nurse who has the knowledge, skills and compassion to prescribe, delegate and coordinate that care; that the client and persons most significant to the client are involved in the care decisions; and that the hospital systems and structures support the registered nurse and the other members of the nursing staff in their efforts to provide nursing care of the highest possible quality. (Parsek, 1991, p. 6)

Problems Related to Planning

Some of the problems student nurses encounter while developing nursing care plans include goals stated too generally, goals not developed from specific nursing diagnoses, nursing orders not written clearly, failure to involve the client in the planning process, and failure to update the plan of care.

COMPUTER APPLICATIONS IN NURSING

Computer-Generated Nursing Care Plans

Computerized care plans allow nurses to address client care problems at the nurse's station. These programs are set up so that reference texts are edited and individualized before the care plan is saved on the disk and printed. One such program describes the client's medical symptoms, nursing diagnosis, client goals, measurable outcomes, and nursing interventions. There is also space for documenting the care given.

Benefits of the computerized care plans include:
- Expanded knowledge base

- Documentation of direct care and independent nursing interventions (eg, teaching, emotional support)
- Improved recordkeeping with resultant improvement in audits and quality assurance
- Documentation by all members of the health care team with printouts for the client's record and for change-of-shift report
- Reduction of time spent on paperwork; in some studies, as much as 2 hours of professional care hours for each new admission

KEY POINTS

- During planning, the nurse works with the client and family to (1) develop client goals that, if achieved, prevent, reduce, or eliminate the problems specified in the nursing diagnoses; and (2) identify the nursing interventions most likely to help the client achieve these goals.
- Conscious, deliberate planning individualizes care, helps communication among nurses, identifies priorities of care, promotes continuity of care, coordinates care, facilitates evaluation of the client's responses to care, and promotes the nurse's professional development.
- The three types of planning essential to comprehensive nursing care are initial, ongoing problem oriented, and discharge.
- When planning care, the nurse reviews the prioritized list of nursing diagnoses to see that diagnoses are ranked according to the level of threat they present to client well-being. Any changes in the client's health status or in the way the client is responding to health and illness or the treatment plan may signal the need to reestablish client priorities.
- A client goal describes an expected client behavior. Client goals are derived from the problem statement of the nursing diagnosis, and once achieved, they contribute to the prevention or resolution of this problem.
- Each client goal must have a subject (the client or some part of the client), a verb (which clearly indicates the action the client is expected to perform), and criteria that describe in observable, measurable terms the expected client behavior.
- Client goals should be valued by the client, be supportive of the total treatment plan, be brief, be specific, and be stated positively.
- Nursing measures are derived from the etiology of the nursing diagnosis. The effective nurse chooses from various possible nursing interventions and nursing measures that specifically address factors that cause or contribute to the client's problems.
- Effective nursing measures are tailored to the client; consistent with standards of care; realistic in terms of the abilities, time, and resources available to the nurse and client; compatible with the client's values, beliefs, and psychosocial background; valued by the client; and compatible with other planned therapies.
- Nursing orders clearly and concisely describe the nursing action to be performed; are signed by the nurse prescribing the order, and dated; use acceptable abbreviations, symbols, and key phrases; and refer nurses to procedure manuals for the steps of lengthy, routine procedures.
- Comprehensive nursing orders specify what observations need to be made and how often, what nursing measures need to be done (how they are to be done and when), and the teaching, counseling, and advocacy needs of clients and families.
- The nursing care plan is the written guide that directs the efforts of the nursing team as they work with clients to meet health goals. Primarily, nursing care plans ensure that nursing care is goal-oriented and individualized.
- The nurse who best knows the client develops the plan of care within 24 hours of the client's admission. The plan is written in ink (part of the client's permanent record) and signed and dated by the nurse who developed the plan.
- Many institutions use a Kardex system of care planning, which specifies nursing care related to basic human needs, prioritized nursing diagnoses, and the medical plan of care. Each client's 6 × 11-inch Kardex care plan is placed in a central Kardex file.
- Most student care plans are designed to help students systematically proceed through each of the five steps of the nursing process. The assessment data establishing and validating nursing diagnoses often are recorded on the plan, scientific rationales and references may be requested for the nursing order chosen, and evaluative statements are documented.
- Common problems related to planning include stating goals vaguely, failing to develop goals from the problem statement of the nursing diagnosis, writing vague nursing orders, failing to involve the client and family in care planning, and failing to update the plan of care as the client's status and needs change.

BIBLIOGRAPHY

Atkinson, L. D., & Murray, M. E. (1990). *Understanding the nursing process* (4th ed.). New York: Pergamon.

Boatwright, D., & Crummette, B. D. (1987). How to plan and conduct a patient care conference. *Nursing, 17*(12), 64.

Bower, F. L. (1982). *The process of planning nursing care: A theoretical model* (3rd ed.). St. Louis: Mosby.

Brider, P. (1991). Who killed the nursing care plan? *American Journal of Nursing, 91*(5), 35–38.

Carnevali, D. L. (1983). *Nursing care planning: Diagnosis and management* (3rd ed.). Philadelphia: Lippincott.

Carpentino, L. J. (June 1991). Has JCAHO eliminated care plans? *American Nurse,* 6.

Carpentino, L. J. (1991). *Nursing care plans and documentation.* Philadelphia: Lippincott.

Carpentino, L. J. (1992). *Nursing diagnosis: Application to clinical practice* (4th ed.). Philadelphia: Lippincott.

Gulanick, M., Klopp, A., Galanes, S., Gradishar, D., & Puzas, M. K. (Eds.) (1990). *Nursing care plans: Nursing diagnosis and intervention* (2nd ed.). St. Louis: Mosby–Year Book.

Harris, B. L. (1990). Becoming deprofessionalized: One aspect of the staff nurse's perspective on computer-mediated nursing care plans. *Advances in Nursing Science, 13*(2), 63–74.

Lederer, J. (1990). *Care planning pocket guide: A nursing diagnosis approach* (3rd ed.). Menlo Park, CA: Addison-Wesley.

Matthewman, J. (1987). Combining care worker and Kardex. *American Journal of Nursing, 87*(6), 852–854.

Mayers, M. G. (1983). *A systematic approach to the nursing care plan.* E. Norwalk, CT: Appleton-Century-Crofts.

McFarland, G. K., & McFarlane, E. A. (1989). *Nursing diagnosis and intervention: Planning for patient care.* St. Louis: Mosby.

Parsek, J. D. (September 1991). Did JCAHO abolish care plans? Yes! *American Nurse,* 6.

Rogers, B. R. (1981). Care planning: A comment on the Canadian experience. *Canadian Nurse, 77*(7), 34–35.

Shea, H. (1984). The nursing care plan dilemma: Suggestions for resolution. *Canadian Nurse, 80*(9), 44–46.

Ulrich, S. P., Canale, S. W., & Wendell, S. A. (1990). *Nursing care planning guides: A nursing diagnosis approach* (2nd ed.). Philadelphia: Saunders.

Vasey, E. K. (1979). Writing your patient's care plan . . . efficiently. *Nursing, 9*(4), 67–71.

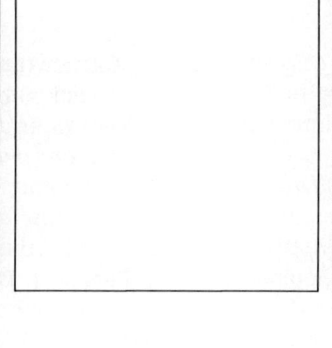
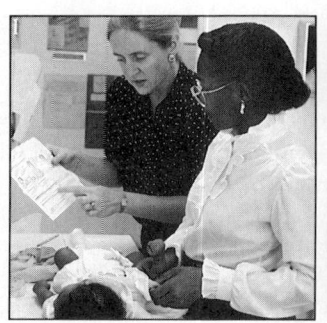
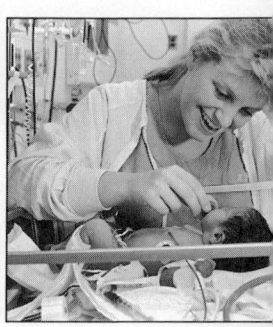

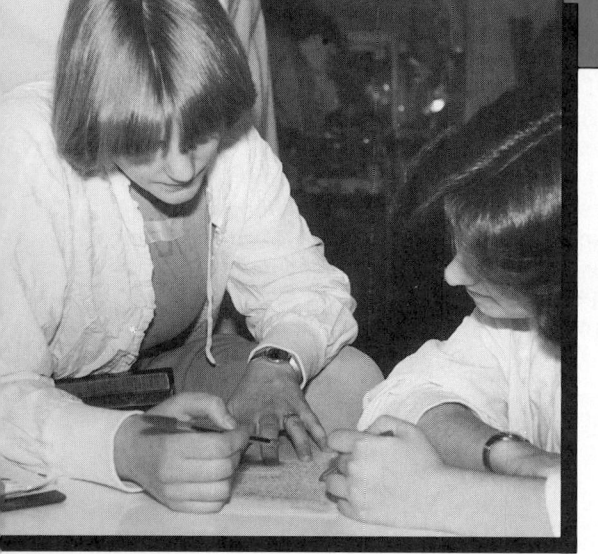

Implementing and Documenting

18

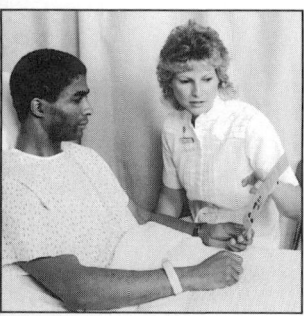

During the **implementing** step of the nursing process, all the nursing actions developed during the planning step are carried out. The purpose of implementation is to assist the client in achieving desired health goals—promote wellness, prevent disease and illness, restore health, and facilitate coping with altered functioning. The plan of care is best implemented when clients who are able and willing to participate have maximum opportunities to provide self-care. Family members and other support people, as well as other health care professionals, also can become involved in the successful implementation of the plan of care. During the implementation step, the nurse continues to collect data and to modify the plan of care as needed (Fig. 18-1). All activities are documented according to the form used in the nurse's institution.

Unique Focus of Nursing Implementation

In all nurse–client interactions, the nurse is concerned with both the client's response to health and illness and the client's ability to meet basic human needs. Whereas other health care professionals focus on selected aspects of the client's treatment regimen, the nurse is concerned with how the client is responding to the plan of care in general.

Types of Nursing Interventions

When implementing the plan of care, the nurse functions independently, dependently, and collaboratively.

Independent interventions or nursing actions involve carrying out nurse-prescribed orders written on the nursing plan of care, as well as any other actions that nurses initiate without the direction or supervision of another health care professional and that are the result of their assessment of client needs. Nurses are legally accountable for the assessments they make and for their nursing responses.

Dependent interventions or nursing actions involve carrying out physician-prescribed orders. Nurse practice acts make it clear from whom nurses can receive orders. Nurses are accountable for the dependent orders they implement and are thus responsible for the clarification of any questionable order.

Collaborative or **interdependent interventions** or nursing actions are those performed jointly by nurses and other members of the health care team. Because nurses are being increasingly respected as competent colleagues with a unique knowledge of the client, they are becoming more and more involved in collaborative ventures with the health care team.

To underscore the fact that nurses are always responsible for their actions, some nurses have moved away from the terminology independent and dependent nursing interventions, and replaced these terms with "nurse-initiated" or "nurse-prescribed" and "physician-initiated," or "physician-prescribed" interventions, respectively.

All these actions may be illustrated with reference to the care received by a depressed client with data indicative of a gastrointestinal blockage. If the physician orders a series of gastrointestinal studies, it is nursing's responsibility to prepare the client by executing the physician's orders for cleansing the bowel. These nursing actions are dependent interventions. If the nurse senses that the client seems unusually fearful of what the outcome of the studies will be, and plans to explore the client's fears and follow-up with appropriate teaching and counseling, then the nurse is involved in independent nursing actions. When a multidisciplinary team conference is held to discuss the client's failure to progress, the nurse works collaboratively with the psychiatrist, gastroenterologist, social worker, and pastoral counselor to develop a comprehensive plan of care; these are collaborative or interdependent nursing actions.

Practicing nurses as well as students beginning clinical experience may be surprised when they evaluate how much of their day is devoted to independent nursing practice (care organized by nursing diagnosis) and how much is spent carrying out dependent functions (medically delegated care—disease management, medical orders, and so forth). Using a circle, divide your day into segments that represent independent nursing practice, dependent nursing practice, collaborative nursing practice, continuing education, and other activities. How your circle is divided illustrates your priorities, as well as the range of nursing interventions possible in your particular practice setting (Fig. 18-2).

Protocols and Standing Orders

Protocols and standing orders may expand the scope of nursing practice in certain clearly defined situations. **Protocols** are written plans that detail the nursing activities to be executed in specific situations. Although some protocols specify routine aspects of nursing care (eg, protocols that describe nursing responsibilities when a client is admitted to or discharged from the institution), other protocols include **standing orders** that empower the nurse to initiate actions that ordinarily require the order or supervision of a physician. Examples include admission protocols for obstetrics and gynecology clients, protocols for bowel pro-

281

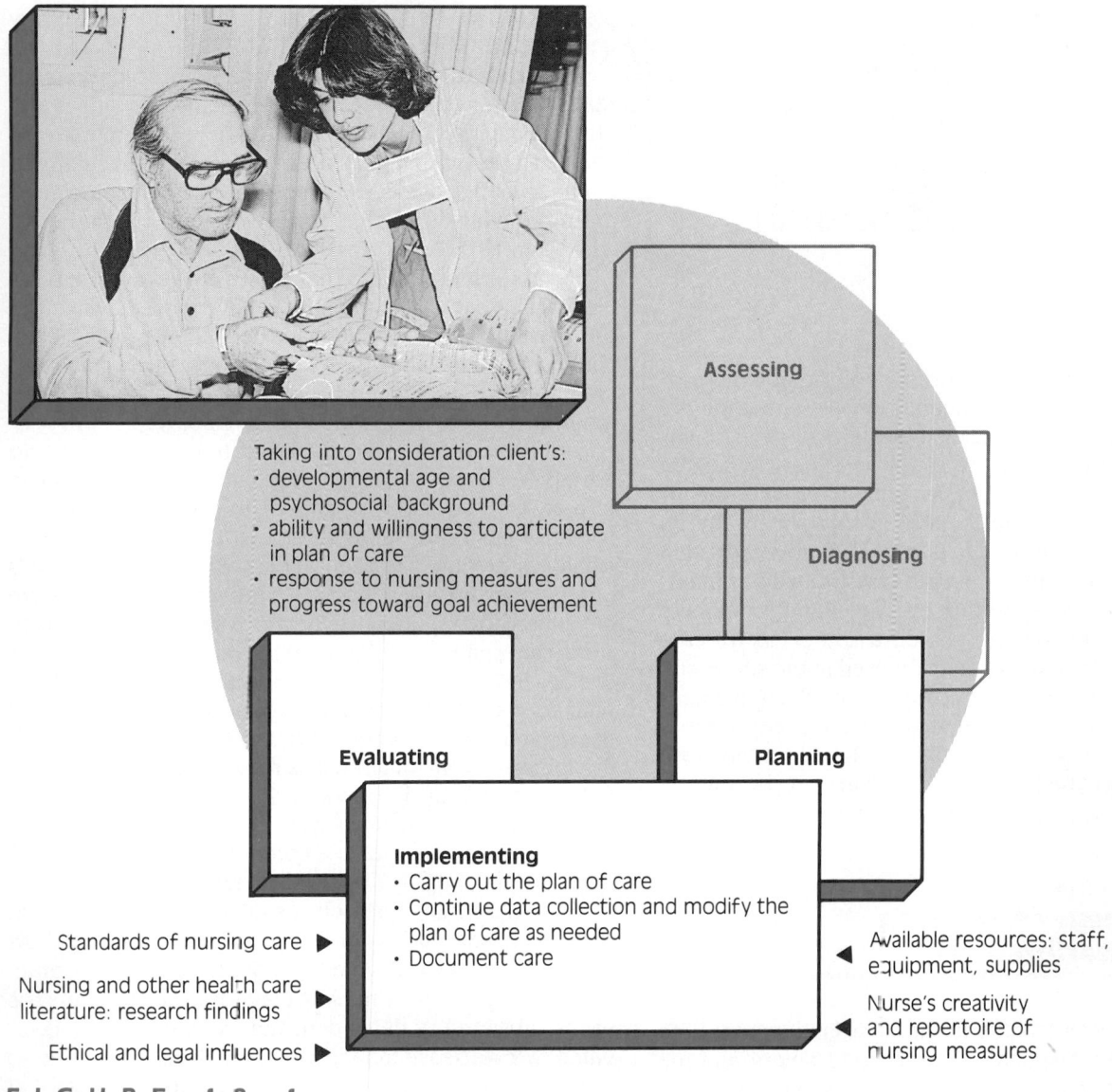

Taking into consideration client's:
- developmental age and psychosocial background
- ability and willingness to participate in plan of care
- response to nursing measures and progress toward goal achievement

Assessing

Diagnosing

Evaluating

Planning

Implementing
- Carry out the plan of care
- Continue data collection and modify the plan of care as needed
- Document care

Standards of nursing care ▶

Nursing and other health care literature: research findings ▶

Ethical and legal influences ▶

◀ Available resources: staff, equipment, supplies

◀ Nurse's creativity and repertoire of nursing measures

F I G U R E 1 8 - 1

Implementing. Implementing is simply the carrying out of the plan of care, which is modified in response to client changes. Numerous variables influence the way the plan of care is implemented (see arrows). (Photo by Gates Rhodes, courtesy of School of Nursing, University of Pennsylvania.)

grams that allow the nurse to select and administer necessary bowel interventions, standard orders for narcotic overdoses that specify the agents the nurse is to administer to reverse respiratory depression in an emergency, and standard orders for pain management that enable the nurse to select the strength of the medication to be given within preset ranges.

The Nurse as Coordinator

One of nursing's major contributions to the health care team is that of the role of coordinator. It is easy for care to become fragmented when clients are seen by numerous specialists—each interested in a different aspect of the client. At best, clients complain that no one person really knows them and can talk with them about what is going on and how it will affect them in the future. At worst, the orders of the different specialists may conflict with one another and be counterproductive. Therefore, it is important for nurses to make rounds with other health care professionals and to read the results of consultations that clients have had with various specialists. The nurse can then interpret the specialists' findings for clients and family members, prepare clients to participate maximally in the plan of care both before and after discharge, and serve as a liaison among the members of the health care team.

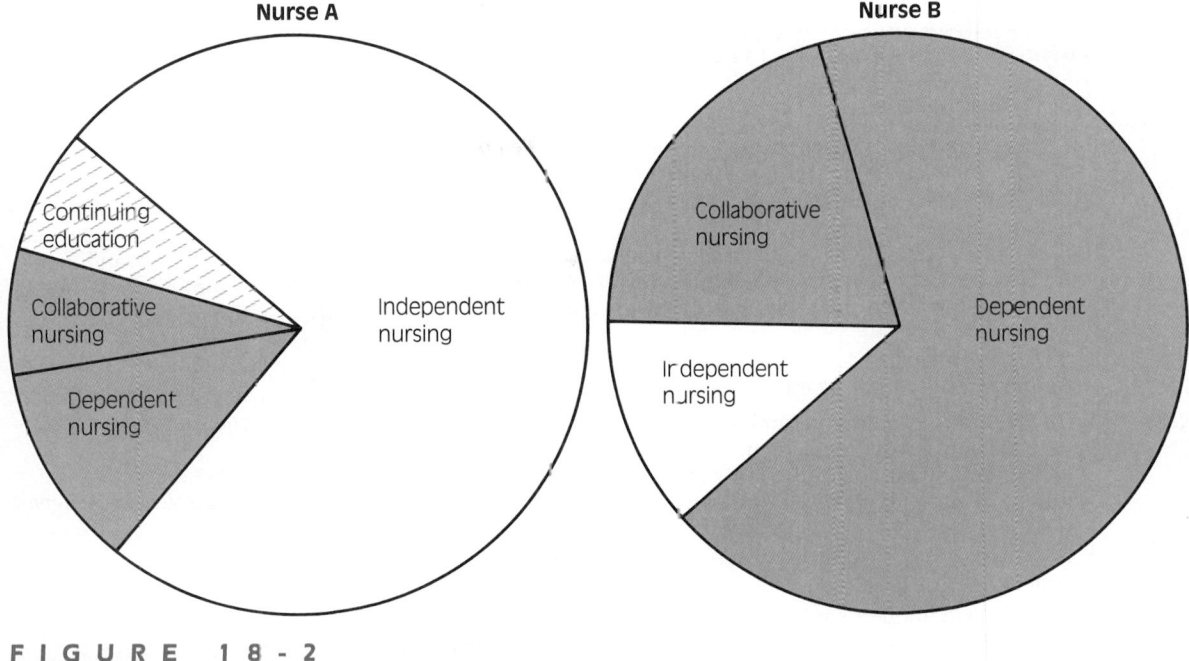

Nurse A

Continuing education

Collaborative nursing

Independent nursing

Dependent nursing

Nurse B

Collaborative nursing

Dependent nursing

Independent nursing

FIGURE 18-2

Division of nursing time. These circles illustrate the way two nurses in different practice settings spend their work day. This time division quickly indicates the emphasis on independent, dependent, and collaborative nursing.

Carrying Out the Plan of Care

When carrying out the plan of care, nurses use specialized abilities to (1) determine the client's need for nursing assistance, (2) promote self-care, and (3) assist the client to achieve health goals.

Prerequisite Nursing Skills

When implementing the plan of nursing care, nurses use intellectual, interpersonal, and technical skills. Each nurse possesses a unique blend of these skills and is effective to the extent that his or her abilities are able to match the client's need for nursing care.

Intellectual Skills Nurses use cognitive abilities to (1) think critically about nursing situations, bringing to bear pertinent nursing theory; (2) design plans of care that enhance client strengths and resolve problems (problem-solving and decision-making skills and creativity); and (3) develop a work environment that promotes nursing excellence.

Interpersonal Skills Because nursing involves interaction with other people, interpersonal skills are essential. These include communicating competence and caring, eliciting the trust that allows the professional nurse–client relationship to develop, teaching, and counseling (Table 18-1). Communication skills are presented in Chapter 20.

Technical Skills Technical skills include the ability to execute both simple and complex nursing procedures, which often require the skillful use of equipment and supplies. Giving a client a bath, assessing vital signs, administering an injection, irrigating and packing a wound, and suctioning a tracheostomy are all examples of technical skills.

Examples of the nursing skills necessary to implement select plans of nursing care are presented at the end of each clinical chapter in this text.

Determining the Need for Assistance

Although most people are capable of independently meeting basic human needs, illness and the stress of diagnostic and therapeutic measures may interfere with a person's usual practice of self-care abilities. A careful nursing assessment of the client's abilities to independently meet human needs is indicated. Nursing often has failed clients by doing too much for them and by encouraging negative, sick role behaviors, such as inappropriate dependence. Conversely, there is a time and a place for the "tender loving care" that says to a client, "I know you may be able to do this for yourself, but just this once, how about if I do it and we'll talk!" Challenging a client's best self-care effort while meeting the universal human need to feel important and loved is an important component of the art of nursing.

The nursing care plan should include specific instructions for any nursing assistance the client needs to meet basic human needs, including the need for forceful nursing encouragement to promote greater independence in functioning. When routines of self-care are indicated (eg, colos-

T A B L E   1 8 - 1

Professional Nursing Relationships: Key Tasks and Skills

Relationship	Key Tasks	Necessary Skills
Nurse–client	• Communicate to the client that someone is concerned about him or her (as well as the disease) and is interested in how this change in health state will affect his or her overall well-being. • Create an environment in which the client can commit his or her energies to health promotion or restoration or peaceful dying, confident that basic human needs are being addressed. • Challenge the client to maximally develop self-care abilities that promote holistic health.	• Repertoire of therapeutic interpersonal behaviors—attending, listening, interviewing, nonverbal communication, therapeutic communication, touching, facilitating, coaching • Ability to establish trusting nurse–client–family relationships • Demonstrated competence in the nursing roles of caregiver, teacher, counselor, advocate
Nurse–client–family	• Develop in the client and family the knowledge, attitude, and skills that will enable them to respond to the self-care challenge of their health or illness state. • Intervene as appropriate to promote healthy family functioning. • Educate the family to be wise and assertive health care consumers.	
Nurse–nurse	• Support one another's efforts to deliver quality nursing care; work collaboratively with nursing administration to improve quality care. • Provide creative leadership—formally or informally—to make the nursing unit a satisfying and challenging place to work. • Supervise the nursing care given by other nursing personnel; affirm the nursing strengths of others and constructively address the nursing deficiencies encountered. • Enhance the professional development of self and other nurses through active participation in professional organizations.	Communication Teaching/counseling/advocacy Assertiveness Collaboration Coordination Group process Organization Leadership Delegation Change strategies Problem solving Decision making Conflict resolution
Nurse–health care team	• Communicate clearly nursing's perspective regarding the client and family to the health care team. • Coordinate the inputs of the multidisciplinary team into a comprehensive plan of care. • Serve as a liaison between the client and family and the health care team, as necessary.	

tomy management), instructions should include the time of the procedure, the equipment used, the process, and the level of client involvement. Continuity of nursing care is essential to the client's development of a comfortable routine.

Promoting Self-Care: Teaching, Counseling, and Advocacy

If clients and their families want to participate actively in seeking wellness, preventing disease and illness, recovering health, and learning to cope with altered functioning, it is important that they possess effective self-care behaviors. Nurses sensitive to the importance of clients learning to direct and manage their own care use nurse–client interactions for both planned and spontaneous teaching, counseling, and advocacy. These nursing roles are described in Chapters 21 and 22. For example, while caring for a child recently diagnosed as having cystic fibrosis, the nurses work continuously with the parents and sib-

lings, helping them to develop the knowledge and skills that will enable them to care for the child on discharge. Referring families such as this to a community support group or other resources further enhances the self-care behaviors being developed.

Assisting Clients to Meet Health Goals

In this phase of the implementation process, the nursing team carries out the nursing orders detailed in the nursing plan of care. If the plan of care is well constructed, carrying out its orders is the nurse's most important task and should receive top priority. The nursing actions planned to promote client goal achievement and the resolution of health problems should be carefully executed. See implementation guidelines in the accompanying display.

Because understaffing continues to be a problem in many practice settings, it is important that nurses learn to use time wisely and to maximize each client encounter. A client bath can be simply that, or it can be an opportunity to

As I walked toward the hospital for my first day of clinical as a student nurse, I suppressed a desire to turn around and run away. My heart was pounding, my mouth was dry, and my stomach was in knots. This was it! Nursing was what I had been working toward for years. I was so excited and so scared at the same time. Apprehension welled up inside me. At that moment I felt everything would go wrong; my biggest fear was of failure; I was afraid of making a huge mistake.

As much as I wanted to be a nurse, I was equally afraid of what was ahead; what if I wasn't cut out to do this? What if I failed? All these feelings surfaced as the hospital loomed ahead.

The way I felt, I didn't know if I could go through with this first day—or any day for that matter. There was so much work, stress, and learning ahead of me I felt overwhelmed. How would I handle clients? Would I ever graduate? What if I make a life-threatening mistake?

I was about to enter a world that was new and different, and deep down inside I knew I wanted to be part of it. I knew that after the first-day jitters were over, my desire to be a registered nurse would remain. This was just the beginning, and even though my road was going to be bumpy, the end reward was going to be extremely good. As I entered the front door of the hospital, I entered, still nervous, into my new world.

One of my first clients was a woman from a nursing home. She had a history of Alzheimer's disease. When I was assigned this client, I knew that I was not going to have a good day. I had been introduced to this client the week before, when I had orientation. She was sitting in a gerry chair in the hallway where she sang at the top of her lungs and threw tissues on the floor. Occasionally, she would curse at a person passing by. This was definitely going to be a challenging day.

I took a deep breath and entered her room. At her bedside I introduced myself to her. With a few choice words she told me to get out of her room. I tried to ignore her response and prepared her breakfast tray. She proceeded to throw her scrambled eggs around the room. I was really having a bad day. After I took the tray away from her and finished cleaning up the mess, it was time for preconference. At preconference, my instructor told me we were going to "tub," or bathe, my client. I had visions of a grand fiasco in the tub room, and I dreaded giving her the bath.

My instructor and I took her to the tub room by wheelchair. Once we convinced her to get in the tub, she did nothing but yell that it was cold. We started the water and she yelled even louder. I knew everyone could hear her in the hallway as she cursed and yelled, but as the bath proceeded she quieted down and stopped fighting me. We completed the bath and wheeled her back down the hall to her room. I bundled her up in blankets and put her in the gerry chair in the hallway. She was so relaxed from the bath that she let me brush her hair and put it in a ponytail. While I was brushing her hair, she fell asleep. I did my chart until her lunch arrived. When I set her up for her lunch and told her I would be leaving, she thanked me, and it made my day. All the struggling I went through all day with her and she thanked me. When I went home I felt really good about helping her. During all my worrying about the day being a fiasco and the embarrassment of having a client yell at me, I had lost sight of the client herself and what she needed me to do for her. By her thanking me at the end of the day, I realized that when my clinical instructor forced me to do something for my client that the regular staff of the hospital wouldn't do, I was meeting her basic needs, and my client recognized that.

—Jeanene C. Smith, Delaware County Community College,
Media, Pennsylvania

GUIDELINES FOR NURSING CARE

Implementation

- Before implementing any nursing action, reassess the client to determine if the action is still needed.
- Approach the client competently. Know how to perform the nursing action, why the action is being performed, and potential adverse responses. Have all equipment and supplies ready.
- Approach the client caringly. Explain the nursing action using language the client understands. Communicate genuine concern for what the client is experiencing.
- Modify nursing interventions according to the client's (1) developmental and psychosocial background, (2) ability and willingness to participate in the plan of care, and (3) responses to previous nursing measures and progress toward goal achievement.

- Check to make sure that the nursing actions selected are consistent with standards of care and within legal and ethical guides to practice.
- Always question that the nursing action selected is the best of all possible alternatives. Consult colleagues and the nursing and related literature to see if other approaches might be more successful. Evaluate the effectiveness of the action selected noting any factors that positively or negatively influenced the outcome.
- Develop a repertoire of skilled nursing interventions. The more options one can choose from, the greater the likelihood of success.

---

gather additional focused data, to communicate concern for what the client is experiencing and to offer support, and to teach and counsel as appropriate. How the nurse uses the 30 minutes that he or she is in the client's room for the bath determines how effective the nurse is in helping the client to achieve his or her goals.

Variables That Influence Implementation   When working with clients to achieve the goals specified in the nursing plan of care, remember that nothing about the plan of care is fixed. Some of the most important variables that influence the way the plan of care is implemented follow.

Client Variables   Ideally, the client is the primary determinant of how nursing measures are implemented. Successful nurses modify their nursing actions according to the client's (1) changing ability and willingness to participate in the plan of care and (2) previous responses to nursing measures and progress toward goal achievement. Other important client variables are developmental stage and psychosocial background.

Many nurses who have studied development believe that they have addressed the developmental needs of a client simply by identifying the client's developmental stage on the plan of care. What the developmental tasks related to this stage are and how this is related to nursing care seldom are considered. Stereotypes about developmental stages and tasks also influence the care that clients receive. For example, the same student nurse who recommends that the parents of a premature infant make a tape of their voices to stimulate the infant in the neonatal intensive care unit also works weekends in a nursing home where the developmental needs of elderly people are routinely violated. This student has never thought to question the staff's selection of a radio station that plays rock music, or other

staff actions—humorous comments about "romances" among some of the residents, infantilizing some residents by calling them cute names or putting bright, big bows in their hair, or planning childish group activities that many of the clients find demeaning. Perhaps the greatest violation is the belief that all elderly people have to do is wait to die, that there are no developmental challenges for this age-group.

In implementing a comprehensive and holistic plan of care, nurses must find creative ways to meet developmental needs. This is of greatest importance when clients are separated from their families and home environments for long periods.

The same is true of the psychosocial needs of clients. Although few nurses would claim that people from all socioeconomic groups and cultures are the same, some practice nursing as if this were so. When choosing nursing measures, it is important to consider and respect the client's background. Therefore, although it is good to teach a malnourished client to include more protein in his diet, if the client has a marginal income, lives alone in one room, and has little interest in and facilities for cooking, teaching that ends with the recommendation above is terribly inadequate.

Nurse Variables   Nurse variables that influence the implementation of the plan of care include the nurses' levels of expertise, creativity (ability to match client needs with specific nursing strategies), willingness to provide care, and available time.

Resources   The most elaborately designed plan of care is doomed to failure on a chronically understaffed or undersupplied nursing unit. Adequate staff, equipment, and supplies are all important determinants of client care.

Current Standards of Care   All nursing actions that are selected when implementing the plan of care must be consistent with standards for practice. Each nurse is responsible for learning the standards that dictate practice in his or her specialty. Failure to practice according to these standards may result in a charge of negligence.

Research Findings   Nurses concerned about improving the quality of nursing care use research findings to enhance their nursing practice. Reading professional nursing journals and attending continuing education workshops and conferences are excellent ways to learn about new nursing strategies that have proven effectiveness.

Ethical and Legal Guides to Practice   It is impossible to practice good nursing today and be ignorant of the laws and regulations that affect health care and the ethical dimensions of clinical practice. As the nurse implements the plan of care, sincere motivation to benefit the client and a conscientious attempt to implement nursing orders well are no longer sufficient. Each nurse is responsible for developing sensitivity to the ethical and legal dimensions of practice, and moral and legal accountability are inherent in the practice of professional nursing. Chapters 5 and 6 deal specifically with the ethical and legal dimensions of practice. Hospital risk managers and ethics committees are increasingly available institutional resources for nurses.

Guide for Students

Student nurses trying in advance to organize their nursing care for a particular clinical day can use the guidelines for student clinical responsibilities in the display to help identify the nursing measures for which they will be responsible. Once these have been identified, working out a time schedule may provide clear direction for the clinical day and ensure that the client's needs are met.

Continuing Data Collection

An important nursing intervention is ongoing data collection. In every client encounter, the nurse needs to be sensitive to both subtle and dramatic changes in the client's condition or response to this condition. These assessment findings are used to update and revise the plan of care. Sensitivity to how the client is responding to nursing measures and to the client's progress toward goal achievement allows the nurse to modify nursing measures appropriately.

Communicating Care

The communication process and specific communication techniques are discussed in Chapter 20. This section explores how nurses communicate with other nurses and

---

Guidelines for Student Clinical Responsibilities

To organize clinical responsibilities, check:
1. Client profile
2. Name by which client wishes to be addressed
3. Client's current health status
   - Any physical or emotional changes indicating the need to modify the plan or care?
4. Routine assistance client needs to meet basic human needs
   - Note any special safety precautions needed
5. Priorities for nursing care
   - Prioritized nursing diagnoses, client goals, and related nursing interventions
   - Medical orders that need to be implemented
   - Interdependent or collaborative nursing responsibilities
6. Special "events" of the day that may require special observation of the client, teaching, preparation, or aftercare
   - Diagnostic tests
   - Consultations with specialists
   - New therapies (physical therapy, medications, surgery, radiotherapy, and so forth)
7. Special teaching, counseling, or advocacy needs
8. Special needs of the family

---

members of the health care team about the client. Effective communication among health care professionals is essential to the coordination and continuity of care. Communicating effectively enables personnel to supplement and complement one another's services and to avoid duplications and omissions in care.

Discussing, reporting, and documenting are the primary means of communication used in health care. **Discussion** is a verbal exchange between two or more persons often used to pool information for the purpose of clearly identifying a problem or developing a strategy for its resolution. For example, one nurse may ask another if he or she has noticed that a client seems to be getting little relief from the prescribed pain medication. If the other nurse concurs, the discussion proceeds to how this can best be remedied.

Reporting is the oral, written, or computer-based communication of client data with the purpose of informing others. A laboratory report, for example, may communicate to the health care team that a client's cardiac enzymes are normal or that a biopsy of breast tissue revealed no malignant or atypical cells. A nurse's shift report or nursing note may communicate the progress a client is making toward goal achievement.

Documentation is the written, legal record of all pertinent interventions with the client—assessing, diagnosing, planning, implementing, and evaluating. Purposes of documentation include the following: (1) to record and communicate pertinent information about the client, (2) to obtain reimbursement from the government and insurance companies, and (3) to provide a legal document that can be used in various legal proceedings.

The Joint Commission for the Accreditation of Healthcare Organizations specifies that nursing care data related to client assessments, the nursing diagnoses or client needs, nursing interventions, and client outcomes are permanently integrated into the clinical information system (1992). Each health care institution has policies that specify the nurse's recording and reporting responsibilities. Each nurse is accountable to practice according to these standards.

Client Record

The client record or chart is a compilation of a client's health care information. It is the only legal document that provides a comprehensive picture of the nursing care given to the client. This record is composed of various forms on which information pertaining to the client has been recorded by different groups of health care professionals. The forms usually are placed in a binder or folder and kept where they are easily accessible to health care practitioners.

Purposes of Client Records   Client records serve many purposes.

Communication   The client record helps health care professionals from different disciplines who interact with the client at different times to communicate with one another.

Care Planning   Each professional working with the client has access to the client's baseline and ongoing data, and can see how the client is responding to the treatment plan from day to day. Modifications of the plan of care are based on this data.

Audit   Charts may be reviewed to evaluate retrospectively (after the client's discharge) the quality of care received and the competence of the nurses providing that care. For example, in a nursing audit, a committee decides in advance certain standards of care they want to evaluate (eg, pertaining to nursing assessment, nursing documentation, or safety measures). A number of charts are then randomly selected and reviewed to see if they give evidence of the nurse's meeting the selected standards of care. If deficiencies are found, inservice can be used to remedy them and improve the quality of care.

Research   The record may be studied by researchers who are hoping to learn from the study of similar cases how best to recognize or treat other clients' health problems.

Education   Health care professionals reading a client's chart can learn a great deal about the clinical manifestations of particular health problems, effective treatment modalities, and factors that affect client goal achievement.

Legal Document   Client records are legal documents that may be entered into court proceedings as evidence; as such, they play an important role in implicating or absolving health practitioners charged with improper care. The record also can be used in accident or injury claims made by the client.

Historic Document   Because the dates of entries on records are specified, the record has value as a historic document. Years later, information may become pertinent concerning a client's past health care.

Nursing Entries on the Client Record   When the nursing process is fully implemented, nursing documentation on the client's permanent record includes the following:

Concise, comprehensive nursing assessment—Initial data base obtained from the nursing history and physical assessment and ongoing focused assessments

Up-to-date care plan individualized to the client—Identifies prioritized nursing diagnoses, related client goals and nursing orders, and the status of goal achievement—formats vary

Narrative notes—Deal with client problems identified in the plan of care; include a description of the status of the problem, related nursing interventions, client responses, and revisions in the plan of care

Flow sheets—Record routine nursing interventions

Graphic sheets—Record, as indicated, the client's vital signs, weight, intake and output, serum glucose level, neurologic status, and so forth

Medication records—Record all medications administered to the client (drug, dose, route, time), nurse administering the drug, and, for some medications (eg, analgesics), the reason the drug was administered and its effectiveness

Discharge summary—Records status of each client problem and the teaching and counseling done to prepare the client for discharge

Although the client record is the only permanent legal document that details the nurse's interactions with the client, it is not unusual to find critical omissions of nursing documentation, meaningless repetitious entries, and inaccurate entries. Although these errors may go undetected and have no effect on the client, they also may seriously affect the care the client receives and cause legal problems for the nurse responsible. Adherence to the accompanying guidelines for documentation helps to prevent errors.

One out of four malpractice suits is decided from the client's record. Iyer (1991b) offers the following defensive charting suggestions to keep you legally safe:

* Don't tamper with medical records.
* Don't criticize other health care professionals in the chart.

GUIDELINES FOR NURSING CARE

Documentation

Content

- Enter information in a complete, accurate, relevant (concise), and factual manner.
- Record client findings (observations of behavior) rather than your interpretation of these findings.
- Avoid words such as *good, average, normal, sufficient*, which may mean different things to different readers.
- Avoid generalizations such as "seems uncomfortable today." A better entry would be "on a scale of 1 to 10, client rates back pain 7 to 9 today as compared with 4 to 5 yesterday; no change in vital signs."
- Note problems as they occur; record the nursing intervention and the client's response; update problems or delete as appropriate.
- Document all medical visits and consultations of which other nurses should be aware, either because of their impact on the client or because of the nursing care the client now requires.
- Carefully document the nursing response to questionable medical orders or treatment (or failure to treat). Factually record the date and time the physician was notified of the concern and the exact physician response. If this occurs by phone, have a second nurse listen to the conversation and cosign the note. If a nurse administrator was contacted, document this.
- Avoid the use of stereotypes or derogatory terms when charting.

Timing

- Follow agency policy regarding the frequency of documentation and modify this if changes in the client's status warrant more frequent documentation.
- Indicate in each entry both the time the entry was written and the time of pertinent observations or interventions. This is crucial when a case is being reconstructed for legal purposes.
- Document nursing interventions as close as possible to the time of their execution. The more seriously ill the client, the greater the need to keep documentation current. Never leave the unit for an extended break when caring for a seriously ill client until all significant information is recorded.
- Never document interventions before carrying them out.

Format

- Chart on the proper form as designated by agency policy.
- Print or write legibly. Use correct grammar and spelling.
- Use only approved abbreviations and symbols (see Table 18-2).
- Date and time each entry.
- Chart nursing entries chronologically on consecutive lines. Never skip lines. Draw a single line through blank spaces.
- Sign your first initial, last name, and title to each entry.
- Do not use dittos, erasures, or correcting fluids. A single line should be drawn through an incorrect entry and the words *mistaken entry* or *error in charting* should be printed above or beside the entry and signed. The entry should then be rewritten correctly.
- Each page of the record should be identified with the client's name and identification number.
- Follow agency policy pertaining to the color of ink and the type of pen or ink to be used.

- Document any comments that a client or family member makes about a potential lawsuit against a health care professional or the hospital.
- Eliminate bias from written descriptions of the client.
- Precisely document any information you report to the physician.
- Document any "potentially contributing client acts" (anything the client does or does not do that may contribute to his injury or explain why he is not responding to nursing or medical care).

Types of Records

Source-Oriented Client Records A source-oriented record is one in which each health care group keeps data on its own separate form. Sections of the record are designated for nurses, physicians, laboratory and x-ray personnel, and so on. Notations are entered chronologically, with the most recent entry being nearest the front of the record. An advantage of the source-oriented record is that each discipline can easily find and chart pertinent data. The main disadvantage is that data are fragmented, and it is difficult to track problems chronologically with input from different groups of professionals.

Although the specifics vary among health agencies, general characteristics of the source-oriented record essentially have remained the same. Types of forms typically used in a source-oriented client record are presented in Table 18-3. Figures 18-3 and 18-4 show various forms used in source-oriented records.

Problem-Oriented Client Records Another type of record used in many health agencies is the problem-oriented record or problem-oriented medical record, which was origi-

(*Text continues on p. 294*)

TABLE 18-2

Abbreviations and Symbols Commonly Used by Health Practitioners

Activities

AMB	ambulatory
BRP	bathroom privileges
CBR	complete bed rest
OOB	out of bed
up ad lib	up as desired

Assessment Data

abd	abdomen
BP	blood pressure
bx	biopsy
C	Celsius (centigrade)
cc	chief complaint
c/o	complains of
dx	diagnosis
F	Fahrenheit
GI	gastrointestinal
GU	genitourinary
h/o	history of
HPI	history of present illness
Imp	impressions
lt or Ⓛ	left
NAD	no apparent distress
neg	negative
P	pulse
PE	physical examination
PMH	past medical history
R	respirations
R/O	rule out
ROS	review of systems
rt or Ⓡ	right
RX	treatment
Sx	symptoms
T	temperature
WNL	within normal limits
⊕	positive
⊖	negative

Diseases

ASHD	arteriosclerotic heart disease
ASCVD	arteriosclerotic cardiovascular disease
BPH	benign prostatic hypertrophy
CA	cancer
CAD	coronary artery disease
CHF	congestive heart failure
COPD	chronic obstructive pulmonary disease
CVA	cerebrovascular accident
DM	diabetes mellitus
HTN (↑ BP)	hypertension
MI	myocardial infarction
PVD	peripheral vascular disease
STD	sexually transmitted disease

Diagnostic Studies

ABG	arterial blood gases
BE	barium enema
CBC	complete blood count
CO_2	carbon dioxide
C&S	culture and sensitivity
CXR	chest x-ray
ECG (EKG)	cardiogram
lytes	electrolytes
RBC	red blood cells
UA	urinalysis
UGI	upper GI
WBC	white blood cells

Symbols

>	greater than
<	less than
↑	increase
↗	increasing
↓	decrease
↙	decreasing
2°	secondary to
=	equal to
≠	unequal
♀	female
♂	male
°	degree

Orders

ā	before
ad lib	as desired
AMA	against medical orders
BM	bowel movement
BP	blood pressure
c̄ (C)	with
CPR	cardiopulmonary resuscitation
dc (disc)	discontinue
dx	diagnosis
DNR (no code)	do not resuscitate
hs	hour of sleep
I&O	intake and output
IV	intravenous
noc	night
NPO (npo)	nothing by mouth
NS (NlS)	normal saline
O_2	oxygen
od	daily
p̄	after
OT	occupational therapy
postop	postoperative
preop	preoperative
prep	preparation
PRN (prn)	as needed
PT	physical therapy
pt	patient
q	every
qs	quantity sufficient
ROM	range of motion
s̄ (S)	without
STAT	immediately
TPR	temperature, pulse, respirations
VS	vital signs
x	times

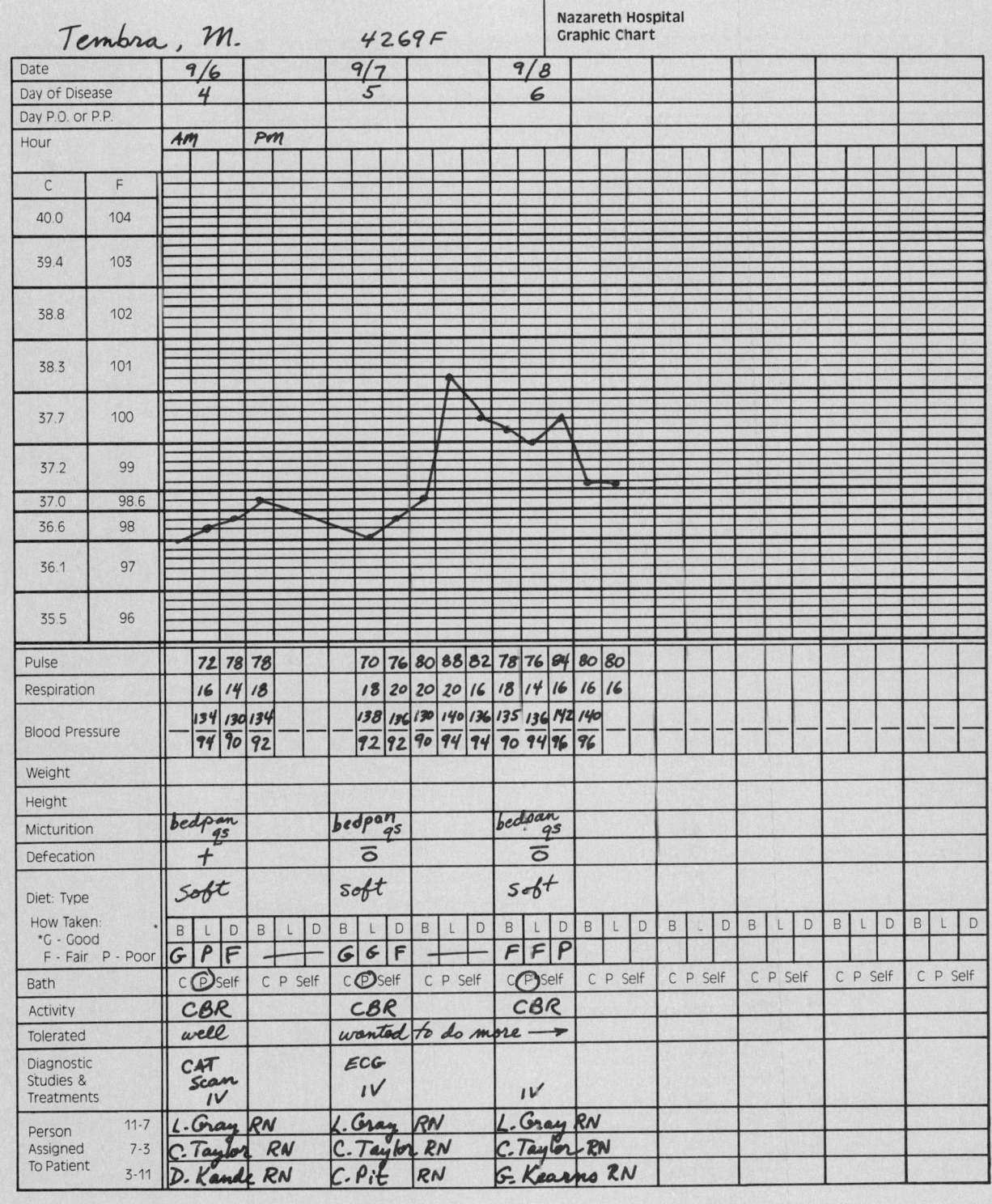

Tembra, M.   4269F

Nazareth Hospital
Graphic Chart

Date			9/6				9/7						9/8																
Day of Disease			4				5						6																	
Day P.O. or P.P.																														
Hour			AM	PM																										

C	F
40.0	104
39.4	103
38.8	102
38.3	101
37.7	100
37.2	99
37.0	98.6
36.6	98
36.1	97
35.5	96

Pulse			72	78	78		70	76	80	88	82	78	76	84	80	80														
Respiration			16	14	18		18	20	20	20	16	18	14	16	16	16														
Blood Pressure			134	130	134		138	136	130	140	136	135	136	142	140															
			94	90	92		92	92	90	94	94	90	94	96	96															
Weight																														
Height																														
Micturition			bedpan qs				bedpan qs						bedpan qs																	
Defecation			+				ō						ō																	
Diet: Type			Soft				soft						soft																	

How Taken: *G - Good F - Fair P - Poor	B	L	D	B	L	D	B	L	D	B	L	D	B	L	D	B	L	D	B	L	D	B	L	D	B	L	D	B	L	D
	G	P	F				G	G	F				F	F	P															

Bath	C Ⓟ Self	C P Self	C Ⓟ Self	C P Self	C Ⓟ Self	C P Self	C P Self	C P Self	C P Self
Activity	CBR		CBR		CBR				
Tolerated	well		wanted to do more →						
Diagnostic Studies & Treatments	CAT Scan IV		ECG IV		IV				

Person Assigned To Patient	11-7	L. Gray RN	L. Gray RN	L. Gray RN					
	7-3	C. Taylor RN	C. Taylor RN	C. Taylor RN					
	3-11	D. Kandt RN	C. Pit RN	G. Kearns RN					

FIGURE 18-3

Sample of graphic client record. (Courtesy of Nazareth Hospital, Philadelphia.)

T A B L E   1 8 - 3

Examples of Forms and Information in Source-Oriented Client Records

Form	Typical Client Information Entered on the Form
Admission sheet	Legal name, identification number Age, birthdate, sex Marital status Occupation and employer Religious preference Next of kin and person to notify in case of emergency Date, time, reason for admission Name of the attending physician Insurance information Discharge data
Admission nursing assessment	Results of nursing history and physical assessment
Graphic sheet (see Fig. 18-3)	Daily temperatures, pulse and respiratory rates, blood pressure (vital signs) Daily weight Special measurements, such as the patient's fluid intake and output
Activity flowsheet (see Fig. 18-4)	Diet and how client has eaten Bathing and skin care Activity level, safety measures Respiratory interventions Elimination Diagnostic measures, treatments Isolation
Nurse's notes (see Fig. 18-4)	Descriptions of pertinent observations of the client Statements that specify the nursing care, including teaching, received by the client and his or her responses to nursing care Statements that describe the client's condition and progress, or lack of progress, toward recovery and goal achievement Descriptions of the client's complaints and how the client is coping, or failing to cope, with them and nursing's response
Medication sheet	Name of prescribed medications administered on a regular basis Dosage of the medication administered Route by which the medication was administered, unless given orally Time medication was administered Name or initials of the person administering the medication
Medical history and examination sheet	Results of the physical examination performed by the physician Current medical condition Health history, including previous illnesses Family medical history Confirmed or tentative diagnosis Plan of medical therapy
Physician's order sheet	Orders for medications Orders for treatments Other directives pertinent to a particular client's care
Physician's progress notes	Interpretations of the client's pathology Responses of the client to medical therapy
Miscellaneous forms	Laboratory reports X-ray film reports Consultation reports Dietary requirements Results of social service consultations Types and results of physical, respiratory, and x-ray therapy

Shift	11-7:30 AM	7-3:30 PM	3-11:30 PM		Date	9/4/86 7 AM Pt. awake and
Diet or NPO	House = Soft	————————	⟶		Time	alert. Awoke at 2 AM to void —
Nutrition		BR ☑ G □ F □ P LU □ G □ F □ P □ Feed ☑ Self	Di □ G □ F □ P HS Snack ☑ □ Feed ☑ Self			unable to fall back asleep. Refused sedative. Rested quietly. Speech clear, moving all extremities. —
Bathing Skin Care	☑ Mouth Care □ Skin Care Keri lotion	□ S ☑ P □ C ☑ Mouth Care ☑ AM Care	☑ PM Care ☑ Mouth Care			—————— L. Gray. RN
Activity	☑ CBR ☑ Pos. q2° □ BRP □ BRP c̄ Asst. □ OOB Chair c̄ Asst. □ OOB Chair s̄ Asst. □ AMB c̄ Asst. □ AMB s̄ Asst.	☑ CBR ☑ Pos. q2° □ BRP □ BRP c̄ Asst. □ OOB Chair c̄ Asst. □ OOB Chair s̄ Asst. □ AMB c̄ Asst. □ AMB s̄ Asst.	☑ CBR ☑ Pos. q2° □ BRP □ BRP c̄ Asst. □ OOB Chair c̄ Asst. □ OOB Chair s̄ Asst. □ AMB s̄ Asst. □ AMB s̄ Asst.		9/4/86 10 AM	Prune juice + cup of hot water with breakfast. resulted in soft formed BM - about 1 hour p̄ breakfast (1st stool in 3 days). Keri lotion to dry skin on legs and arms. Strength seems to be increasing in left arm + leg. Performs lt. leg exercises independently. During
Resp. Assessment	☑ Cough/D. Breathe q2° □ Trach Care □ Suction Freq ___	☑ Cough/D. Breathe q2° □ Trach Care □ Suction Freq ___	☑ Cough/D. Breathe q2° □ Trach Care □ Suction Freq ___			bath talked about how much she misses her husband and her house. Explored feelings about participating
Treatments	Assisted Rom	P.T.	⟶			in support group for widows - recommended by her friends. Feels
Protective Precautions	□ Full ☑ Half	□ Full □ Half	□ Full □ Half			good about babysitting her 2 grandchildren.
Restraints	□ Posey □ Wrist □ Ankle □ None ☑ q2° Check □ Other	□ Posey □ Wrist □ Ankle ☑ None □ q2° Check □ Other	□ Posey □ Wrist □ Ankle ☑ None □ q2° Check □ Other			—————— C. Taylor, RN
Elimination Bowel Bladder □ Foley	bedpan voiding q5 □ Commode	↑BM Voiding q5 bedpan □ Commode □ Foley Care	□ Commode □ Foley Care		2 pm	Spent 30 min. teaching client + daughter Lisa about T.I.A. and stroke. Strong family history of PVD, CVA and MI. Reviewed importance
Diagnostic Studies +/or Specimens Obtained	—	CAT Scan	—			of dietary modifications, regular exercise and taking prescribed medication. Excellent motivation for self-care — S Taylor RN
Isolation Type	—	—	—		9/4/86	VS 98.8 - 78 - 18 136/92 Quiet this
Nursing Care Plan	☑ Reviewed □ Revised	☑ Reviewed □ Revised	☑ Reviewed □ Revised			evening. - Napping - Not hungry at dinner: states "Busy day"
Comments	awake @ 2am did not fall back to sleep	"when can I go home?" napped in pm	—			Moving all extremities; alert. Daughter Barbara says her mother wants to do "too much." Still afraid
Signature	L. Gray RN	C Taylor RN	D. Kands RN			T.I.A. automatically means stroke & death! — D. Kands RN.

Nazareth Hospital
Activity Flowsheet/Patient Care Notes

FIGURE 18-4

Sample of an activity flowsheet with client care notes. (Courtesy of Nazareth Hospital, Philadelphia.)

nated by Dr. Lawrence Weed in the 1960s. The **problem-oriented record** is organized around a client's problems, rather than around sources of information (see the example in Fig. 18-5). All health care professionals record on the same forms. The advantages of this type of record are that the entire health care team works together in identifying a master list of client problems and contributes collaboratively to the plan of care. Progress notes are clearly focused on client problems. Some nurses find that the SOAP method (**SOAP** = subjective data, objective data, assessment, plan) of charting focuses too narrowly on selecting problems, and are advocating a return to the traditional narrative format. Table 18-4 presents a summary of the four major parts of the problem-oriented record—the defined data base, problem list, care plans, and progress notes.

Charting by Exception **Charting by exception** is a shorthand documentation method that makes use of well-defined standards of practice; only significant findings or "exceptions" to these standards are documented in narrative notes. Benefits of this approach include decreased charting time (frees time for direct client care), greater emphasis on significant data, easy retrieval of significant data, bedside charting, standardized assessment, greater interdisciplinary communication, better tracking of important client responses, and lower costs. Widely billed as "a more efficient way to document," charting by exception is rapidly gaining advocates (Murphy & Burke, 1988, 1990; Comstock & Moff, 1991). Figure 18-6 shows one example of this type of charting.

Computer Records In an increasing number of health care institutions, comprehensive computer systems have revolutionized nursing documentation in the client record. Computer capacities are already in operation in which the nurse (1) calls up the admission assessment tool on the computer screen and keys in client data, which are automatically recorded; (2) develops the care plan using computerized care plans available for each North American Nursing Diagnosis Association–approved diagnosis; (3) adds to the client data base as new data are identified and modifies the plan of care accordingly; (4) receives a work list indicating the treatment, procedures, and medications necessary for the client throughout the shift; and (5) documents care immediately using the computer terminal at the client's bedside. Other ways in which computers are being

(*Text continues on p. 298*)

T A B L E 1 8 - 4

Organization of the Problem-Oriented Client Record

Part	Information

Data base (see Fig. 18-5A)	The data base is a compilation of all initial information about the client and includes the following:
	    Health state profile prepared by the nurse
	    Medical history and the physical examination, prepared by the physician
	    Social history
	    Initial diagnostic test results

Problem list (see Fig. 18-5B)	The multidisciplinary problem list itemizes major aspects of the client's life that require health attention and includes the following:
	    Socioeconomic, demographic, psychological, and physiologic problems
	    Each problem is labeled, numbered, and categorized as active or inactive

Plan of care (see Fig. 18-5C)	An initial plan is formulated for each specifically numbered problem on the problem list. The nursing plan, whether *therapeutic, diagnostic,* or *educational,* is expressed through nursing orders.

Progress notes (see Fig. 18-5D)
    Narrative progress notes
	Progress notes consist of narrative progress notes, flowsheets, and discharge notes, as follows: The narrative progress notes on the client follow the SOAP format, as follows:
	    S—Subjective information reported by the client
	    O—Objective observations made by health practitioners
	    A—Assessments drawn from new data
	    P—Plans or goals for action related to the client's problems

Flowsheets	Flowsheets are used for recording information that is monitored over time. This information provides data for making comparisons of a client's status at one time with his status later.

Discharge notes	Discharge notes are the entries made at the time an episode of the client's care is terminated and include the following information:
	    The date of the resolution of each problem, as had been described while using the
	        SOAP format
	    Referrals made for the client
	    Recommendations for unresolved or partially resolved problems

Summary of data base for client (18-5A)

72 year old, white, recently widowed female

brought to hospital after sudden fall caused by temporary paralysis of left leg; admitting diagnosis: transient ischemic attack (TIA), R/O cerebrovascular accident

treated for hypertension since 1985, otherwise in good health; history of headaches—once or twice a week (increasing in severity)—for last six months

ht 5'2"   wt 63.6 kg   98.2 F-88-18   BP L—184/120, R—180/120
↓ strength ↓ movement left lower extremity (LLE)

Problem List (18-5B)

XXXX Medical Center   4629F

Date	No.	Problem	Identified	Resolved
9/2/93	#1	transient ischemic attack (TIA) R/O cerebro-vascular accident	J. Gleer MD	
	#1A	impaired physical mobility related to weakness in left lower extremity	D. Kande RN	
9/4/89	#2	impaired adjustment related to major life stressors and decreased supports	D. Kande RN	

Plan of Care (18-5C)

Date	Problem
9/4/93	#2 Impaired adjustment related to major life stressors (including illness) and decreased supports Goal: Prior to discharge client reports feeling able to go home and take one day at a time Plan: *Diagnostic*: explore adequacy of client's usual patterns of coping and motivation to learn new strategies *Therapeutic*: 1) explain all tests/procedures to client who wants to know and understand what is happening to her 2) create a restful environment 3) talk with client's home minister (daughter will contact) *Educative*: Teach client new coping skills, e.g., relaxation exercises. Refer to community support group for widows. —D. Kande RN

Progress Notes (18-5D)

Date	Problem-Oriented Progress Notes
9/6/93	Impaired mobility related to weakness left lower extremity (LLE) **S** "My left leg still feels queer, pins and needles—but I can move it alright." **O** Able to lift left leg off bed, positive flexion, positive extension; muscle strength in LLE 3/5 (normal movement against gravity) **A** recovering mobility as strength returns **P** *therapeutic*: consult with physician about complete bed rest order; *diagnostic*: continue to monitor muscle strength and movement at least once/shift; be alert for any signs of recurrent TIA; *educative*: instruct not to try to get out of bed without assistance until diagnostic work-up is complete; reinforce need for safety precautions. —D. Kande RN

F I G U R E   1 8 - 5

Sample of a problem-oriented client record.

THE WILLIAMSPORT HOSPITAL & MEDICAL CENTER

Williamsport, Pennsylvania 17701-3198

FLOW SHEET

Nursing Intervention

Abbreviation Key		
AM = Morning	I = Independent	S = Sleeping
PM = Evening	A = Assist	W = Awake
	C = Complete	O = Patient off unit

* = Signature of assigned caregiver for shift

✓ = Within normal limits or performed
X = not within normal limits

	Dx #	Nursing Interventions	Date: 7/10 2400-0700	0800-1500	1600-2300	Date: 7/11 2400-0700	0800-1500	1600-2300
		Personal Care	PM - / * C. Taylor, RN	/ *	/ *	/ *	/ *	/ *
		Preps, preps & One-time Interventions	AM - A					
		Activity	Shave ⓐ groin					
			OOB + BRP					
		Safety Precautions	2400 ✓ 0100 ✓ 0200 ✓ 0300 ✓ 0400 ✓ 0500 ✓ 0600 ✓ 0700 ✓					
		IV hourly check	✓✓✓✓✓✓✓✓					
		Patient Check	S S S W S S W W					
	#3	skin care	✓					
	#4	K-pad	✓✓✓✓✓✓✓✓					
		Frequent Interventions						

✓ Addressograph

PAGE 2

MR - 6075 1/89

F I G U R E   1 8 - 6

Sample documentation of nursing care using charting by exception. (Courtesy of the Department of Nursing, Williamsport Hospital and Medical Center, Williamsport, PA.)

Nursing Diagnosis #	System	Date 7/10/93 Time 1200	7/10/93 1600	7/10/93 1800	7/10/93 2000	7/11/93 0200	
#1	Resp	X SOB c̄ exertion; lungs clear	→	Δ↑SOB; see progress notes	/	Δ less SOB	
#2	Fluid Status	X IV @ KVO; ↑PO fluids	/	Δ IV to heplock; ↑PO intake	/	D/C →	
#3	Skin	X reddened area on coccyx	/	/	↑	↑	
#4	musculoskeletal	X ©calf edematous, red, warm	→	→	Δ↑©calf pain - see progress notes	Δ K pad D/C'd per MD orders	
	Knowledge						
	Discharge Planning						
	Signature	c.T.	c.T.	c.T.	c.T.	c.T. c.T.	c.T.

/ = Assessment not currently required.
D/C = System no longer requires assessment

Δ = Change in condition.
X = New problem.

√ = Assessment within normal limits.
↑ = No change in condition since last assessment.

THE WILLIAMSPORT HOSPITAL & MEDICAL CENTER
Williamsport, Pennsylvania 17701-3198
FLOW SHEET
Nursing Assessment

COMPUTER   APPLICATIONS   IN   NURSING

Computerized Client Care

This story illustrates how often nurses use computer technology on a daily basis in given client care.

Tom Low, RN, arrives for work at 6:45 AM, following the schedule printed by the computer in the staffing office, and is assigned to a general surgery floor based on a computer-generated patient acuity needs assessment. After reading the computer printout on his assigned clients, he takes vital signs (using computerized equipment), monitors the flow of IV fluids (making sure the computerized flow and amount settings are correct), and gives medications (using a computer-based medication record to check and document administration). Unfamiliar with two medications, he reviews material from the computer medication data base before giving them. Tom then changes dressings, entering charges and ordering supplies on the computer.

One of Tom's clients has been having abnormal laboratory test results, so Tom calls up the result of today's tests to monitor changes. At the same time, he looks up the time for a scheduled surgical procedure for another client, so he will be sure to have time for preoperative teaching, using computer-assisted instruction.

After the morning care is completed, Tom sits down in front of the computer to document care given and to update care plans.

Not all of these computed applications are available in all health care settings, but the trend in today's high-tech society is toward automated resources to facilitate communications and improve clinical practice.

---

used in health care are highlighted throughout the text. The American Nurses' Association has been instrumental in developing the Computer-Based Patient Record Institute (CPRI) in response to a recommendation by the Institute of Medicine that a computer-based patient record be adopted by all health care providers and systems nationwide (Mulholland, 1992).

The increasing use of computerized client information systems to store client data has necessitated the development of policies and procedures to ensure the privacy and confidentiality of client information. Policies should specify what types of client information can be retrieved, by whom, and for what purpose. Client consent is necessary for the use and release of stored information.

Agency Policies   Most agencies have specific policies concerning client records. All who have access to the record (direct caregivers) are expected to maintain its confidentiality. At no time may a nurse give a client's chart to a family member or to any person other than an authorized caregiver. State laws differ as to whether the client has the legal right to review the chart. Most agencies grant student nurses access to client records for purposes of education. In this instance, the student assumes responsibility to hold the client information in confidence.

Agency policies also indicate which personnel are responsible for recording on each form in the record, and such policies also may describe the order in which the forms are to appear in the record. Additional policies may concern the frequency with which entries are to be made, whether routine care is recorded, the manner in which health personnel identify themselves after making an entry, which types of abbreviations are acceptable, and the manner in which an error in recording is handled.

The storage of client records is a function of the health agency's record department. Many client records are microfilmed for compact storage or are entered into a computer to expedite accessibility of information.

Other Communication Methods

Common methods for communicating among health practitioners other than by the client record include using face-to-face meetings, the telephone, a messenger, the written message, and the audiotaped message. Each of these methods has certain benefits and limitations, as detailed in Table 18-5. A brief discussion of three specific communication strategies frequently used by nurses—reporting, conferring, and referring—follows.

Reporting   To report is to give an account of something that has been seen, heard, done, or considered. For instance, hospital nurses report a summary of a client's condition and care when transferring clients from one unit to another (eg, from the recovery room to a surgical floor) and at the conclusion of each shift. Nurses also report to physicians and other health care professionals. Because the nurse is the one who is "with the client 24 hours a day," the nurse is responsible for determining significant changes in the client's condition and for reporting these findings to the appropriate team member. And finally, nurses often are asked by family members to report on the client's progress. (See Chap. 28 for transfer and discharge reporting guidelines.)

TABLE 18-5

Common Methods of Communication		
Method	**Advantages**	**Disadvantages**
Face-to-face meeting	• Message can be delivered immediately. • Nonverbal messages are readily conveyed. • Message can be clarified; receiver's questions can be raised and answered.	• Both the communicating and the receiving people must be available at the same time, in the same place. • Ordinarily there is no permanent record for later use.
Telephone conversation	• Message can be delivered immediately. • Message can be clarified; receiver's questions can be raised and answered. • Two parties need not be present in same place.	• Only the tone of voice and voice inflections can be communicated—no nonverbal messages. • Ordinarily there is no permanent record.
Written message	• Can be exchanged at times convenient for the people involved. • Record is available. • Time-efficient if message is understood.	• Message usually cannot be validated with the sender.
Audiotaped message	• Can be exchanged at times convenient for the people involved. • Record is available. • Time-efficient if information communicated is complete.	• Message usually cannot be validated with the sender.

Change-of-Shift Reports   A **change-of-shift report** ordinarily is given by a primary nurse to the nurse replacing him or her, or by the charge nurse to the nurse who assumes responsibility for continuing care of the client. The change-of-shift report may be given in written form or orally (Fig. 18-7) in a meeting or it may be audiotaped. Many charge nurses find that using a tape decreases the amount of time spent reporting and allows more time for last-minute details.

Typical information shared among nurses during a change-of-shift report includes the following:

- Basic identifying information about each client— name, room number, bed designation, and current diagnosis
- Current appraisal of each client's health status:
  - Changes in medical condition (results of pertinent diagnostic studies) and client's response to medical therapy
  - Where the client stands in relation to identified nursing diagnoses and goal achievement
- Current orders (especially any newly changed orders):
  - Nurse-prescribed orders
  - Physician-prescribed orders (changes in medications, intravenous fluids, diet, activity level)
- Summary of each newly admitted client, including his or her diagnosis, age, plan of therapy, and general condition
- Report of clients who have been transferred or discharged

It is important to avoid unprofessional comments about clients that could predispose oncoming nurses to view and respond to clients negatively.

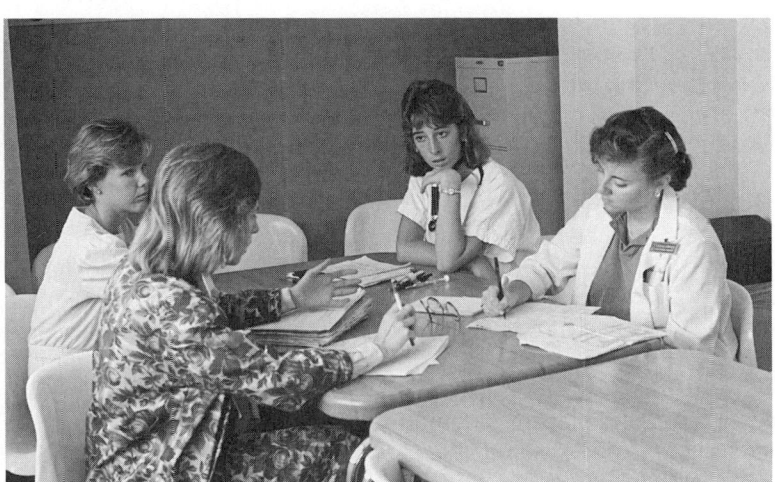

FIGURE 1 8 - 7

Oral change-of-shift report on a nursing unit. (Photo by Denise Angeloni, courtesy of University of Pennsylvania.)

COMPUTER APPLICATIONS IN NURSING

Bedside Terminals

Computerized patient care systems became available to nurses, physicians, and other care providers before the mid-1980s, usually from a centralized location on each nursing unit. Bedside terminals were introduced into the market to capture more immediately observed patient data and to improve nursing productivity by facilitating more timely monitoring procedures and more fully informed decision making. Few hospitals, however, have invested in bedside terminals. Herring and Rochman (1990) compared nursing on a test unit with bedside terminals with nursing on a control unit without terminals in three hospitals. They cite as benefits of computerized documentation the saving of considerable expense (fewer pre-printed documentation forms needed), better nursing and greater work efficiency, and improved system utilization. Reasons they gave for the improved quality of care included:

- Fewer errors of omission
- Greater accuracy and completeness of documentation
- Improved standardization of charting quality
- Increased accountability for charting and scheduling IVs
- More timely response to patient needs
- More accurate and up-to-date care plans
- Greater timeliness of tests and procedures
- More time available to provide patient education

(Herring, D., & Rochman, R. [1990]. A close look at bedside terminals. *Management, 21*[7].)

Conferring To confer is to consult with someone to exchange ideas or to seek information, advice, or instructions from another. A nurse may consult with another nurse, as when a team leader consults with a clinical specialist about a particular client's care. A school nurse may confer with a child's teacher or a psychologist about a behavior problem. A community health nurse and a physician may confer about a client's activity regimen. Health practitioners also confer to validate information. Both nurses and other health team members confer in groups to plan and coordinate client care. Such conferences also are commonly used for instructing students and practitioners.

Nursing Care Conference   A **nursing care conference** is a meeting of nurses to discuss some aspect of a client's care. For example, several nurses who have taken care of a generally uncooperative client may initiate a conference. This would allow each nurse an opportunity to offer his or her opinion about the client's problem and its cause, and then together they could discuss possible solutions to the problem.

Nurses may invite other health care practitioners to a nursing care conference to gain input concerning a particular client's care. For example, a dietitian may be invited to attend a conference when nurses meet to discuss problems relating to a client's diet. Nurses also participate in interdisciplinary team conferences.

Nursing Care Round   A **nursing care round** is a procedure in which a group of nurses visit selected clients individually at each client's bedside. The primary purposes of nursing care rounds are to gather information that helps to plan nursing care, to evaluate the nursing care the client has received, and to provide the client with an opportunity to discuss his or her care with those administering it. As each client is visited, the nurse assigned provides a short summary of the client's nursing diagnoses and goals and the care being given. There are two principal advantages of nursing care rounds over a discussion in a meeting room: Nursing personnel can actually see the client as a report of care is given, and clients can participate in discussions of their care.

It is important that nursing personnel use language the client can understand when holding discussions at the bedside. Otherwise, the client is likely to feel excluded and cannot intelligently participate in the discussion. Nurses also may make rounds with physicians to inform them of nursing's input.

Referring To refer is to send or direct someone for action or help. The process of sending or guiding someone to another source for assistance is called a referral. A client may be referred by a hospital to a community health nursing service for assistance with home care. A school nurse may refer a student to a hospital emergency department. A community health nurse may refer a problem to the Department of Health. A referral also may be used within a particular agency. For example, a hospital outpatient clinic may refer a client to the hospital's inpatient facilities.

Most health agencies have policies related to referrals.

An agency may have a special form that personnel are to use when making referrals. The policies usually indicate who may initiate a referral, how it is to be done, and so on.

Referrals are especially important in providing continuity of care for people who need a variety of services. It is essential that health practitioners to whom a client is referred are given information that is most useful to the continuity of care. The key question is, What would I want to know about this client if I were the person who had to continue his or her care? The client must know and approve of a referral to another agency or to other health personnel.

Nursing Oneself

It is difficult for nurses to be sincerely attentive to client needs when their own human needs are not being met. Because no one is perfectly healthy or "whole" all the time, it is important as nurses prepare for professional practice that they spend time getting to know themselves. In an excellent chapter on psychological self-care written for nurses, Hill and Smith (1990) describe psychological self-care as a constellation of activities practiced on a regular basis to promote psychological health. These include self-awareness, communication, time management, preparation for crisis and loss, developing and maintaining support systems, and concurrent practice of self-care in all areas. The characteristics of emotional health include self-esteem, self-knowledge, satisfying interpersonal relationships, environmental mastery, stress management, a positive body image, a sense of humor, and the ability to provide oneself with pleasure.

Nurses who want to be competent practitioners learn early to nurse themselves and other nurses before attempting to nurse clients. Not only does improved personal health enable the nurse to practice more efficiently, but it enables the nurse to be a health model for clients and their families. Nurses can help clients to imitate health behavior and eventually integrate it into daily life through the process of identification. Each clinical chapter contains a section titled "The nurse as role model," which you may find helpful.

KEY POINTS

- Implementing, the fourth step of the nursing process, is the carrying out of the plan of care. Its purpose is to assist clients to achieve desired health goals—to promote wellness, prevent disease and illness, restore health, facilitate coping with altered functioning.
- The plan of care is best implemented when clients who are able and willing to participate have maximal opportunity to do so.
- Whereas other health care professionals focus on select aspects of the client's treatment regimen, nursing is concerned with how the *person* is responding in general to the plan of care.
- Nurses implement independent (nurse-prescribed), interdependent (collaborative), and dependent (physician-prescribed) nursing actions.
- While carrying out the plan of care, nurses use intellectual, interpersonal, and technical skills. Nursing's first challenge is the determination of how much nursing assistance the client needs to reach desired goals.
- The nurse's teaching, counseling, and advocacy skills are used to assist clients to develop the self-care behaviors that enable them to direct and manage their own care.
- Nothing about the care plan or the way it is implemented is fixed. Client and nurse variables, as well as available resources, current standards of care, research findings, and ethical and legal guides to practice, may influence the plan's implementation.

- Ongoing data collection directs the revision of the plan of care.
- Nurses are responsible for documenting each step of the nursing process in the client record. Most health care institutions have standards for documentation that detail the nurse's responsibilities.
- The client record is the only legal document that provides a comprehensive picture of the nursing care given to the client.
- Each health care group keeps data on its own separate form in the source-oriented client record. In the problem-oriented record, recording is organized around the client's problems rather than around sources of information. Computer records have simplified nursing documentation in many ways. Use of computer terminals at the client's bedside enables nurses to document care immediately.
- Common methods of communication used by nurses other than the client record include reporting, conferring, and referring.
- Improved personal health enables nurses to practice more effectively and to be a health model for clients and their families.

BIBLIOGRAPHY

Afflerbach, D. (January 1986). A flow sheet that saves time and trouble. *RN, 49*(1), 42–44.

Albarado, R., McCall, V., & Thrane, J. M. (1990). Computerized nursing documentation. *Nursing Management, 21*(7), 64–65.

Allison, S., & Kinloch, K. (1981). Problem-oriented recording. *Canadian Nurse, 77*(11), 39–40.

Andreoli, K., & Musser, L. A. (1985). Computers in nursing care: The state of the art. *Nursing Outlook, 33*(1), 16–21.

Benner, P. (1984). *From novice to expert: Excellence and power in clinical nursing practice.* Menlo Park, CA: Addison-Wesley.

Benner P., & Wrubel, J. (1989). *The primary of caring: Stress and coping in health and illness.* Menlo Park, CA: Addison-Wesley.

Black, K., Sr. (1983). *Short-term counselling: A humanistic approach for the helping professions.* Menlo Park, CA: Addison-Wesley.

Blegen, M. A., Gardner, D. I., & McCloskey, J. C. (1992). Who helps you with your work? *American Journal of Nursing, 92*(1), 26–31.

Buckley-Womack, C., & Gidney, B. (1987). A new dimension in documentation: The PIE method. *Journal of Neuroscience Nursing, 19*(5), 256–260.

Bulechek, G. M., & McCloskey, J. C. (1987). Nursing interventions: What they are and how to choose them. *Holistic Nursing Practice, 1*(3), 36–44.

Burke, L., & Murphy, J. (1988). *Charting by exception: A cost effective quality approach.* Albany, NY: Delmar.

Cohen, M. R. (1987). Play it safe: Don't use these abbreviations. *Nursing, 17*(7), 46–47.

Comstock, L. G., & Moff, T. E. (1991). Cost-effective, time-efficient charting. *Nursing Management, 22*(7), 44–48.

Cournoyer, C. P. (1985). Protecting yourself legally after a patient's injured. *Nursing Life, 5*(2), 18–22.

DeMilliano, M. (1984). 8 common charting mistakes to avoid . . . quick review. *Nursing Life, 4*(3), 30–32.

Edelstein, J. (1990). A study of nursing documentation. *Nursing Management, 21*(11), 40–46.

Eggland, E. T. (1980). Charting: Document your care daily and fully. *Nursing, 10*(2), 38–43.

Ellis, J. R., & Hartley, C. L. (1991). *Managing and coordinating nursing care.* Philadelphia: Lippincott.

Fairless, P. R. (1986). Nine ways a computer can make your work easier. *Nursing, 16*(9), 55–56.

Gift, A. G., & Jacox, A. (Eds). (1990). Symptom management. *Nursing Clinics of North America, 25*(4), 849–986.

Glanze, W. D., Anderson, K. N., & Anderson, L. (Eds.) (1990). *Mosby's medical, nursing, and allied health dictionary* (3rd ed.). St. Louis: Mosby–Year Book.

Hansten, R., & Washburn, M. (1992). Delegation: How to deliver care through others. *American Journal of Nursing, 92*(3), 87–90.

Hansten, R., & Washburn, M. (1992). How to plan what to delegate. *American Journal of Nursing, 92*(4), 71–72.

Hill, L., & Smith, N. (1990). *Self-care nursing: Promotion of health* (2nd ed.). East Norwalk, CT: Appleton & Lange.

Iyer, P. W. (1991a). Thirteen charting rules to keep you legally safe. *Nursing, 21*(6), 40–45.

Iyer, P. W. (1991b). Six more charting rules to keep you legally safe. *Nursing, 21*(7), 34–39.

Iyer, P. W., & Camp, N. (1991). *Nursing documentation: A nursing process approach.* St. Louis: Mosby–Year Book.

Joint Commission on Accreditation of Healthcare Organizations. (1992). *Accreditation manual for hospitals.* Chicago: Joint Commission on Accreditation of Healthcare Organizations.

Jones, P., & Oertel, W. (1977). Developing patient teaching objectives and techniques: A self-instructional program. *Nurse Educator, 2*(5), 3–18.

Kilpack, V., & Dobson-Brassard, S. (1987). Intershift report: Oral communication using the nursing process. *Journal of Neuroscience Nursing, 19*(5), 266–270.

Knapp-Spooner, C., & Brett, J. (March 1992). Less is more: A med/surg flow sheet. *RN, 55*(3), 36–39.

Kohnke, M. F. (1982). *Advocacy: risk and reality.* St. Louis: Mosby.

Laing, M. (1981). Flow sheets: Meeting the charting challenge. *Canadian Nurse, 77*(11), 40–42.

Marrelli, T. M. (1992). *Nursing documentation handbook.* St. Louis: Mosby–Year Book.

McCloskey, J. C., & Bulechek, G. (Eds.). (1992). *Nursing intervention classification (NIC).* St. Louis: Mosby–Year Book.

McCloskey, J. C., & Bulechek, G. (1990). Classification of nursing interventions. *Journal of Professional Nursing, 6*(3), 151–157.

McConnell, E., O'Shea, S. S., & Kirchoff, K. T. (1989). RN attitudes towards computers. *Nursing Management, 20*(7), 36–40.

McGonigle, D. (1991). Establishing a nursing informatics program. *Computers in Nursing, 9*(5), 184–189.

Meintz, S. L., & Shaha, S. H. (1992). Our hand-held computer beats them all. *RN, 55*(1), 52–57.

Meyer, C. (April 1992). Bedside computer charting: Inching toward tomorrow. *American Journal of Nursing, 92*(4), 38–44.

Miller, P., & Pastorino, C. (1990). Daily nursing documentation can be quick and thorough. *Nursing Management, 21*(11), 47–49.

Mulholland, D. K. (April 1992). Electronic record will change practice. *American Nurse,* 13.

Murphy, J., & Burke, L. J. (1990). Charting by exception: A more efficient way to document. *Nursing, 20*(5), 65–69.

Neighbors, M., Eldred, E., & Sullivan, M. (1991). Nursing skills necessary for competing in the high-tech health care system. *Nursing and Health Care, 12*(2), 92–97.

Prescott, P. A., Phillips, C. Y., Ryan, J. W., & Thompson, K. O. (1991). Changing how nurses spend their time. *Image: Journal of Nursing Scholarship, 23*(1), 23–28.

Redman, B. K. (1984). *The process of patient education* (6th ed.). St. Louis: Mosby–Year Book.

Rich, P. L. (1985). With this flow sheet less is more. *Nursing, 15*(7), 25–29.

Rocerto, L. R., & Maleski, C. M. (1984). All about rights to medical records. *Nursing Life, 4*(4), 50–51.

Rutkowski, B. (1985). How DRG's are changing your charting. *Nursing, 15*(10), 49–51.

Schmitt, D., et al. (1990). Charting for accountability. *Nursing Management, 21*(11), 47–49.

Siegrist, L., Stocks, B., & Dettor, R. (1985). The PIE system: Complete planning and documentation of nursing care. *QRB, 11*(6), 186–189.

Simpson, R. L. (1991). Electronic patient charts: Beware the hype. *Nursing Management, 22*(4), 13–14.

Smith, C. E. (1986). Upgrade your shift reports with the three R's. *Nursing, 16*(2), 63–64.

Sundeen, S. J., Stuart, G. W., Rankin, E. D., & Cohen, S. A. (1989). *Nurse–client interaction: Implementing the nursing process* (4th ed.). St. Louis: Mosby–Year Book.

Valega, T. M. (1984). It's time for nurses to begin nursing. *Nursing and Health Care, 5*(6), 331–335.

Vaughan-Wrobel, B. D., & Henderson, B. S. (1982). *The problem-oriented system in nursing* (2nd ed.). St. Louis: Mosby.

Warne, M. A., & McWeen, M. C. (1991). Managing the cost of documentation: The FACT charting system. *Nursing Economist, 9*(3), 181–187.

Zangari, M. E., & Duffy, P. (1980). Contracting with patients in day-to-day practice. *American Journal of Nursing, 80*, 451–455.

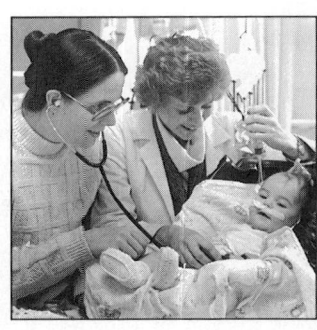

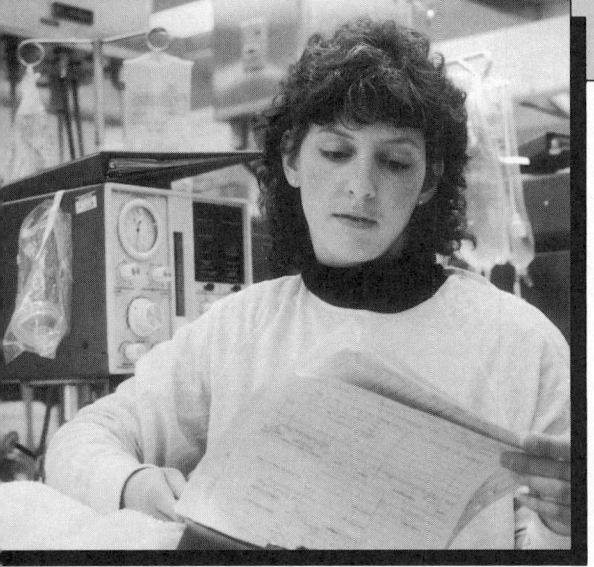

Evaluating

19

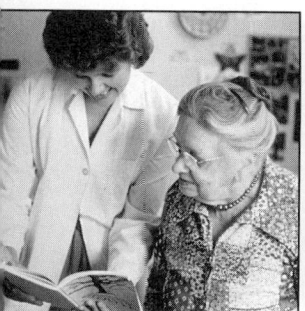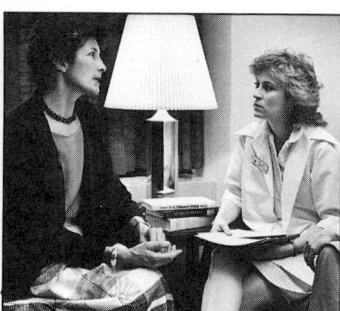

D uring the fifth step of the nursing process, **evaluating**, the nurse and client together measure how well the client has achieved the goals specified in the plan of care. While evaluating client goal achievement, the nurse identifies factors that contribute to the client's success or failure and, when necessary, modifies the plan of care. The purpose of evaluation is to allow client goal achievement to direct future nurse–client interactions. Based on the client's responses to the plan of care, the nurse decides to either (1) terminate the plan of care (each client goal is achieved), (2) modify the plan (client is having difficulty achieving goals), or (3) continue the plan of care (client simply needs more time to achieve goals). When evaluation points to the need to modify nursing care, each preceding step of the nursing process (assessing, diagnosing, planning, and implementing) is reviewed.

In summary, during the evaluation step of the nursing process, the nurse measures how well the client has achieved desired goals, identifies factors that contribute to the client's success or failure, and terminates, continues, or modifies the plan of care as needed (Fig. 19-1).

Unique Focus
of Nursing Evaluation

As members of the health care team, nurses are involved in many types of evaluation. Nurses measure how well individual clients have achieved desired goals, how effectively nurses help targeted groups of clients to achieve their specific goals, the competence of individual nurses, and the degree to which external factors, such as different types of health care services, specialized equipment or procedures, or socioeconomic factors, influence health and wellness. The client, however, is always the nurse's primary concern. A nurse may perform a nursing procedure competently, caringly, creatively, but if this nursing action does not help the client to reach desired goals, it is meaningless. Either directly or indirectly, the aim of all nursing evaluation is quality nursing care that aids client goal achievement. Therefore, the most important act of evaluation performed by the nurse is evaluating the client's goal achievement with the client.

Evaluation Criteria
and Standards

The classic elements of evaluation are identifying evaluative criteria and standards (what you are looking for when you evaluate), collecting data to determine if these criteria and standards are met, interpreting and summarizing findings, and taking appropriate action. In the nursing process, evaluative criteria are the client goals developed during the planning step. Because these goals reflect desired changes or outcomes in client behavior, and because nursing actions are directed toward these goals, it is logical that they be at the core of evaluation. Determining whether these goals have been met and then identifying the appropriate nursing response are the functions of evaluation.

Although the terms criteria and standard often are used interchangeably in the evaluation step, they have distinct definitions. **Criteria** are measurable qualities, attributes, or characteristics that specify skills, knowledge, or health states. They describe acceptable levels of performance by stating the expected behaviors of the nurse or the client.

Standards are acceptable, expected levels of performance by the nursing staff or other health team members. They are established by authority, custom, or consent (Griffith-Kenney & Christensen, 1990).

Measuring Client
Goal Achievement

Collecting Evaluative Data

The nurse collects evaluative data to determine whether the client has met the desired goals. Whereas the nurse collects data in the nursing assessment to identify client health problems, the nurse collects data in the evaluation step to determine whether the identified health problems were resolved through goal achievement.

Types of Goals The type of client data collected to support the goal achievement evaluation is determined by the nature of the goal. *Cognitive goals* involve increases in client knowledge; these goals may be evaluated simply by having clients repeat information or, at a higher level of performance, by having clients apply the new knowledge to their everyday situations. For example, having clients describe new dietary restrictions is very different from having them plan a weekly menu compatible with these restrictions. *Psychomotor goals* describe the client's achievement of new skills; they are evaluated by having the client demonstrate the new skill. *Affective goals* pertain to changes in client values, beliefs, and attitudes; affective goals are more complex to evaluate. Observation of client behavior and conversation are used to determine whether these affective goals have been achieved.

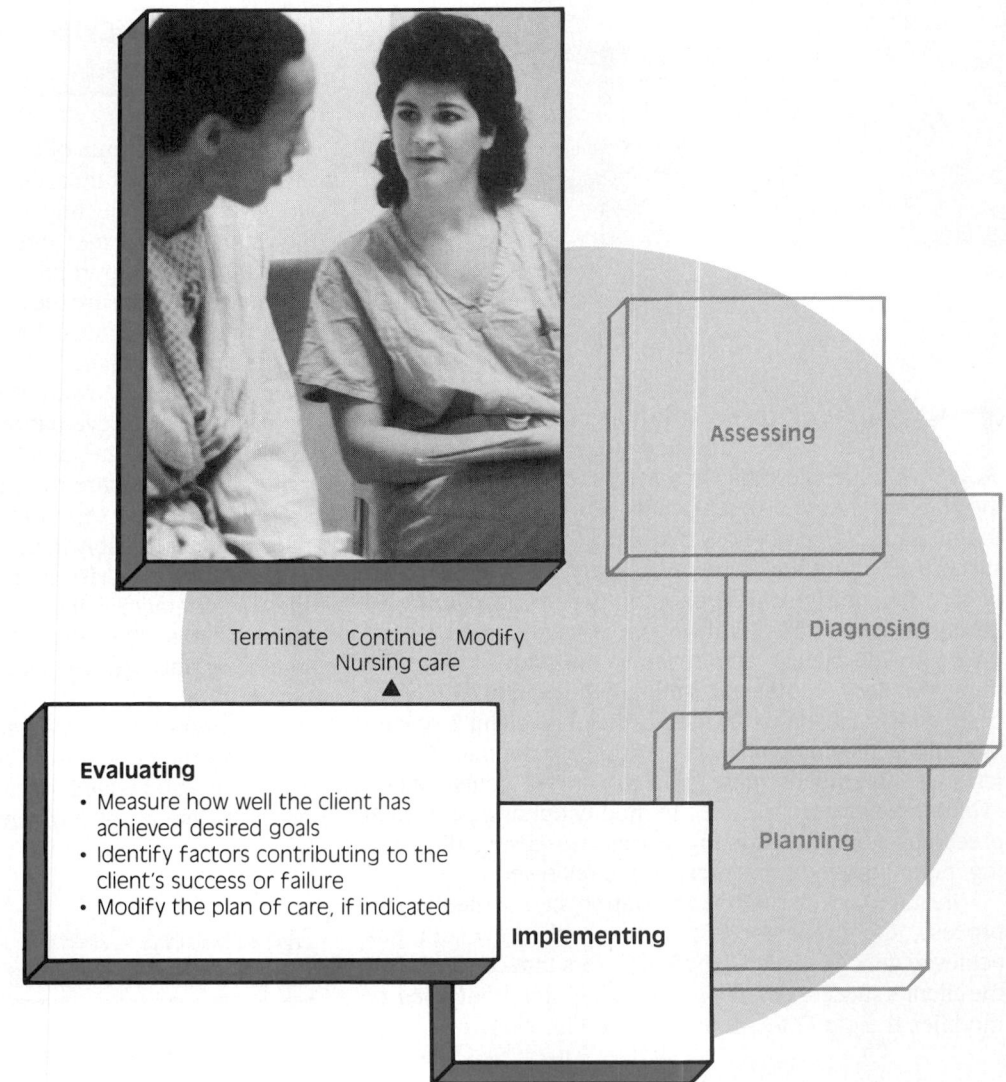

Evaluating. The nurse and client together measure how well the client has achieved the goals specified in the plan of care. Factors that contribute to the client's success or failure are identified, and the plan of care is modified if necessary. Client responses to the plan of care determine if nursing care is to be continued as is, modified, or terminated. (Photo by Gates Rhodes, courtesy of School of Nursing, University of Pennsylvania.)

Terminate Continue Modify
Nursing care

Evaluating
- Measure how well the client has achieved desired goals
- Identify factors contributing to the client's success or failure
- Modify the plan of care, if indicated

Implementing

Assessing

Diagnosing

Planning

In the final type of goal statement, *physical changes* in the client are the targeted outcome. To evaluate achievement of this type of goal, the nurse uses physical assessment skills to collect relevant data and compare these with previously acquired client data.

Samples of these goals are contained in Using Four Types of Goals in the Nursing Care Plan. The data collected to determine the degree of goal achievement are recorded in the related evaluative statement.

Time Criteria   In addition to knowing what type of data to collect to determine goal achievement, it is important to know when to collect the data. In properly constructed client goals, a time frame is established for determining whether the specified change in client behavior has been achieved. At the designated time, the nurse, in collaboration with the client, the family, and other members of the nursing team, evaluates the client's ability to demonstrate the desired behavior. If goals are developed in observable and measurable terms, the task of collecting data for eval-

uation becomes clear-cut. Examples of three types of time criteria follow:
- By 7/8/93, the client will walk the length of hallway with support of walker.
- Beginning 7/8/93, the client will demonstrate a weight loss of 3 lb per month until target weight (135 lb) is achieved (6/8/93, weight: 151 lb).
- Before discharge, parents will correctly demonstrate chest physiotherapy procedures for client.

It is important for nurses to evaluate client goal achievement as early as possible. Goal attainment, when celebrated with the client, usually results in the client's encouragement and leads to further goal achievement. When the client's failure to meet designated goals is detected early, the plan of care can be modified to redress the failure. The most common mistake nurses make in evaluation is waiting until the day the client is to be discharged before evaluating goal achievement. It is too late to do anything about the goals the client has not met at discharge.

This past summer, I was employed at a rehabilitation hospital as a nurse extern. I worked on the amputee unit, but this unit housed clients with chronic obstructive pulmonary disease and stroke clients as well as amputees.

One of my most memorable experiences was working with a woman who had had a left hemispheric stroke several years ago. She was admitted to the hospital because of her poor nutritional status. Her family couldn't get her to eat properly.

The client needed complete care. One had to bathe, dress, transfer, and feed her. She was on aspiration precautions and had to be encouraged to swallow. No matter who cared for her, she never spoke a word; she just stared at everyone.

As the weeks passed, she got some of her strength back. She tried to help herself as much as she could with the bathing, dressing, and eating. She would nod when one asked her a question, but still, not a word was spoken.

Finally, the day came for the client to be discharged. I was assigned to her that morning. I helped her wash, dress, and eat. I had her things packed to go home when her family came for her. They thanked me for all my help.

Just before they left, her husband told her to thank me. He said to her, "Go ahead and thank her. You can do it." In a raspy voice that hadn't spoke in weeks came "Thank you."

It was the best thank-you I have ever received.

—Maureen E. Scollon, Holy Family College, Philadelphia

Documenting Evaluation

Once data have been collected to determine client goal achievement, the nurse writes an evaluative statement to summarize the findings. Atkinson and Murray (1990) have suggested using a two-part evaluative statement on the nursing care plan to underscore the importance of evaluation. The evaluative statement includes a decision on how well the goal was achieved and all client data or behavior that support this decision. The nurse has three decision options—goal met, goal partially met, or goal not met. The nurse signs and dates the evaluative statement (see Using Four Types of Goals in the Nursing Care Plan).

$$\text{Evaluative statement} = \begin{matrix}\text{Goal met}\\\text{Goal partially met}\\\text{Goal not met}\end{matrix} + \begin{matrix}\text{Actual client}\\\text{behavior as}\\\text{evidence}\end{matrix}$$

Factors That Influence Goal Achievement

Numerous client, nurse, and health care system variables contribute both positively and negatively to client goal achievement. Identifying these variables allows the nurse to reinforce positive factors by drawing on them in the future and to deal with those factors that are creating problems. The more sensitive and responsive nurses are to these variables, the more rewarding their practices will be.

Examples of positive factors include a client's strong motivation to learn new health behaviors, a nurse who comes to work well rested and with a new care idea read in a nursing journal, and a health care institution that offers incentives for quality nursing and that staffs its nursing units well.

Once the nurse understands what is helpful to the client who is trying to reach desired goals, these factors often can be manipulated. For example, if a client is learning to ambulate independently after hip surgery and you notice that he seems to make his best effort when his wife is present, mention this observation to the wife and plan to ambulate the client at least once a day when the wife is present. Conversely, if the client seems more fearful when his wife is present note in the plan of care that ambulation is best attempted when the client's wife is not on the unit.

Table 19-1 presents common variables nurses encounter that can negatively influence client goal achievement. Tentative nursing approaches are suggested. What is important is that nurses become aware of the effects of these variables and respond creatively to them.

Modifying the Plan of Care

When evaluation reveals that the client has made little or no progress toward goal achievement, and attempts to identify the contributing factors point to problems with the plan of care, the nurse needs to reevaluate each preceding step

USING FOUR TYPES OF GOALS

In The Nursing Care Plan

Nursing Diagnosis:	High Risk for Altered Parenting related to no previous experience in childrearing (fear)
Assessment Data:	*Subjective:* "My husband and I are both afraid we won't know what to do when we get the baby home."
	Objective: Both parents are single children, report no childrearing experience; healthy newborn son delivered 2/4/93; first born
Strengths:	VIB (very important baby): parents are both 38; history of infertility with one miscarriage; strong motivation to learn and use good parenting skills; strong support network

Goals (Expected Outcomes)	Nursing Actions	Evaluative Statement (Actual Outcomes)
Before discharge, parents will demonstrate confidence in: • Holding baby • Diapering, dressing baby • Bathing baby • Feeding baby (Psychomotor objectives)	Assess both parents' knowledge of childrearing practices; identify and reinforce motivation to learn; correct any misinformation. Develop and implement at a time convenient for both parents a teaching plan to include: • The primary nurse role-modeling techniques for comfortably and safely holding, talking to, and dressing baby • Parents independently viewing videocassettes on: 　Baby care 　Baby bath 　Breast-feeding Followed by one-on-one discussion • Class for new parents: nurse to demonstrate baby bath and discuss general principles of care • Primary nurse observing mother and infant during initial feeding sessions and offering teaching and support as necessary Answer parents' questions and address related concerns.	2/6/93 Goal partially met. Both parents have correctly demonstrated safe techniques for holding, dressing, and bathing the baby. Mother is still concerned baby is not getting enough milk. *Revision:* Continue to spend time with mother and infant during feeding—provide positive reinforcement. *F. Morales, RN*
By 2/6/93, parents will report appropriate action to be taken if questions or problems arise after discharge: • Name and number of primary nurse • Name and number of pediatrician • LaLeche League contact and number (Cognitive objectives)	Assess parents' knowledge of infant problems frequently encountered by new parents. Inform parents of available community resources and describe appropriate action to take if questions or problems arise.	2/6/93 Goal met. Parents discussed some infant problems related to feeding, elimination, illness and reported appropriate community resource to contact. *F. Morales, RN*

(continued)

USING FOUR TYPES OF GOALS (continued)

In The Nursing Care Plan

Before discharge, parents will verbalize decreased anxiety in regard to caring for son. (Affective objective)	Assess parents' level of anxiety and potential negative effects on childrearing. Discuss this with parents.	2/6/93 Goal partially met. Except for concern about breastfeeding, *both* parents expressed feeling comfortable and eager to care for their son at home.
	Explore adequacy of parents' coping strategies—increased knowledge, practice in supportive environment, community resources. Counsel as necessary.	
		F. Morales, RN
	Compliment parents on new parenting skills. Allow for ventilation of anxiety or specific fears. Respond with teaching or emotional support as necessary.	
At 1 month postpartal telephone interview, 3/4/93 (by parents' report), the baby will demonstrate adequate: • Weight gain (birth weight, 7 lb 6 oz) • Sleep–wakefulness patterns • Comfort level indicating adequate parenting. (Physical objectives)	Use a 1-month postdelivery telephone interview to assess the adequacy of parenting skills. With positive report of growth and development, compliment (reinforce) the parents. With negative report, teach or counsel and refer as appropriate.	3/4/93 Goal met. Parents' report of baby's weight gain and behavior indicates good parenting skills. *F. Morales, RN*

of the nursing process for accuracy. After this study, new assessment data may need to be collected, diagnoses may be added or altered, goals may need to be modified or rewritten, nursing orders may be changed, and evaluation may be targeted more frequently. See the checklist in this chapter for help in evaluating your use of the nursing process. Table 19-2 suggests appropriate nursing responses to common problems encountered during evaluation.

Once the nurse has identified the factors that contribute to the client's failure to achieve goals, the evaluative statement can be used to suggest the necessary revision in the plan of care.

The following evaluative statement might be noted if the client fails to meet the behavior specified in the goal: "Client will participate in a minimum of two planned social activities per week beginning 9/20/93." "9/27/93 Goal not met. Resident refused to participate in any group activities this week." Many courses of action are then available to the nurse. Possible revision statements to follow the evaluative statement include the following:

Revision: This may not be a problem or concern for the resident. Evaluate and validate data pointing to the nursing diagnosis (delete or modify the nursing diagnosis).

Revision: Carefully determine the resident's need for activities and ability or desire to participate in activities (make the goal statement more realistic).

Revision: Reevaluate after 3 weeks; resident may need more time to adjust to being institutionalized and more encouragement (adjust time criteria in goal statement).

Revision: Make a special effort to familiarize yourself with the resident's interests, and match these with available programs and activities (change nursing interventions).

Evaluation Programs

In addition to each nurse's evaluation of client goal achievement and the subsequent modifications to the plan of care, many formal mechanisms exist to ensure quality nursing care. In the United States, regulatory agencies such as state boards of nursing, the Joint Commission on Accreditation of Healthcare Organizations (JCAHO), Professional Standards Review Organization, and the National

(Text continues on p. 315)

TABLE 19-1

Client, Nurse, and Health Care System Variables That May Detract From Quality Nursing Care	
Variables	**Possible Solution**
Client Variables	
Client who is physically and cognitively capable of self-care gives up—refuses to cooperate with therapeutic regimen or thwarts the regimen	Identify one nurse who is able to develop a trusting relationship with the client and determine the *reason* underlying the observed behavior: • No longer finds meaning and purpose in life • Overwhelming sense of powerlessness • Previous history of being "hurt," "exploited," "cheated" by the health care system • Inability to accept illness and related life-style changes Counsel appropriately. Use a team conference to develop a consistent plan of nursing care.
Client who quietly accepts whatever is done or not done for him or her; seldom communicates needs or dissatisfaction	Note on the plan of care the need to assess this client thoroughly because the client will probably not advocate for himself or herself. Educate the client to become a more assertive health care consumer.
Nurse Variables	
Nurse who sincerely desires to give 150% all the time and who becomes quickly frustrated when observing substandard care; may feel alienated from other staff; excellent candidate for burnout	Learn to give quality care during designated work period; leave on time; avoid the temptation to do the work of others; leave work concerns at work. After establishing a reputation for delivering quality nursing care, seek creative solutions for nursing problems (strategies to increase nursing resources, motivation, morale) and try them—hopefully with a support network. View concerns as challenges rather than overwhelming obstacles. Develop a realistic sense of how much nursing care and of what quality can be delivered with existing resources. If resources do not permit quality care, explore change strategies within the institution. If administration is not supportive, explore other practice settings.
Nurse with overwhelming outside concerns: • Preparation for marriage, childbirth, divorce • Illness (self or family members) • Role conflict (familial roles, school, work, and so forth) • New apartment, house	During periods of peak demand, may need to accept less than optimal performance at work. If this becomes the norm rather than the exception, carefully evaluate priorities. May need to cut work hours rather than "cheat" clients.
Nurse who is bored	After reflection, write down *personal* objectives related to work. Explore avenues within work setting for professional growth and development: Initiate changes in nursing unit to improve patient care and to stimulate peer development; join institutional committees; participate actively in staff development programs; develop patient and family support groups. Look for new position that offers new challenges within or outside the institution. Join professional organizations and participate actively. Evaluate educational goals and explore possibilities—continuing education programs and degree work.
Health Care System Variables	
Inadequate staffing	Develop and use a client classification system that incorporates an identification of the kind and amount of nursing services required. Record staffing patterns and relate to needs for nursing care and client outcomes. Clearly demonstrate and *document* that adequate staffing makes a difference. Present these data to nursing administration with the request for additional staff. If necessary, use professional bargaining unit.
Nursing administration has sold out nursing; insensitivity to nursing demands within the institution	It may be impossible to practice quality, progressive nursing in this environment. If there seems to be no hope for change after appropriate channels have been explored, look for a new practice setting. Evaluate the new setting on the basis of what experience has taught you.

TABLE 19-2

Common Problems Noted During Evaluation of the Nursing Process		
Problem	**Effect on Nursing Process**	**Nursing Response**
Assessing		
1. Data base is inaccurate.	1–3. Inaccurate nursing diagnoses. (Because the nursing diagnoses establish the client's *need* for *nursing*, inaccuracies here distort and may invalidate the entire plan of care.)	1. a. Identify the client or nurse variables responsible for inaccuracy. b. Revise the recorded data base.
2. Data base does not reflect changes in client condition.		2. Inservice the *entire* nursing staff on the importance of making assessment a priority in every client interaction as well as the *recording* of the new data obtained.
3. Data base is superficial: • Fails to communicate uniqueness of client. • Lacks sufficient detail on major problems or developments.		3. a. Rethink the critical relation between an adequate data base and quality care. b. Develop interviewing and physical assessment skills. c. Begin to identify the key data that need to be collected for specific nursing diagnosis and medical diagnosis and to assess client response to the therapeutic regimen (use of a nursing diagnosis handbook may be helpful).
Diagnosing		
1. General sense that nursing diagnoses are "common sense" and therefore do not need to be put in writing.	1. "Common sense" nursing, which fails to address client's real problems, may ensue. Lack of continuity of care.	1. Carefully develop and record priority nursing diagnoses for several clients and fairly evaluate whether or not this makes a difference in terms of the continuity of quality care.
2. General sense that nurses are too busy doing treatments, "passing meds," and doing paperwork to carefully develop nursing diagnoses.	2. Independent dimension of nursing practice remains underdeveloped; clients experience nurses as busy "doers" who are insensitive to their concerns.	2. Examine practice and see if *independent* nursing has a place; what percentage of every day is devoted to independent nursing functions? If this percentage is nonexistent or small, there understandably may be *no felt need* for nursing diagnoses—but a desperate need to revise practice priorities.
3. Nursing diagnoses are too vague to be helpful.	3. Routinized client care results; individualized client problems are overlooked.	3. a. Revise the problem statement to more accurately describe what is *unhealthy* about the client (the behavior that needs to be changed). b. Revise the etiology to more accurately identify what is making the problem a problem—this should be a guide to nursing intervention. c. Check NANDA lists.
4. Nursing diagnoses are not up to date.	4. Nurses will not value or use the plan of care, assuming that it does not address the client's ongoing priorities.	4. Have a process for periodically reviewing the plan of care to delete nursing diagnoses when problems have been resolved and to add a new diagnosis as needed.

(continued)

T A B L E   1 9 - 2 *(continued)*

Common Problems Noted During Evaluation of the Nursing Process

Problem	Effect on Nursing Process	Nursing Response
Planning		
1. The plan of care contains only the standard knowledge most nurses would know without a written plan.	1–2. Lack of personalized care; failure to address client's real problems; nursing staff works haphazardly on different priorities	1. Make use of standardized (computerized) plans as a basis for care planning. Devote nursing energies to *individualizing* this plan.
2. The long-term goal is vague, standard; fails to make clear the discharge goal for this client.		2. Practice writing specific long-term goals that clarify for all nurses the aim toward which all nursing care is directed (eg, client returns home ambulatory with walker, right hip incision healing, able to manage activities of daily living with minimal assistance from spouse).
3. The nursing goals, even if met, do not necessarily guarantee a resolution of the client problem.	3. Client problems are unresolved.	3. When writing goals, it often is helpful to develop short-term goals related to etiologic factors. Because the stated etiology may be incomplete or inaccurate, it is essential that at least *one goal* be written so that if it is achieved, the problem in the nursing diagnosis is resolved.
4. The goals are incorrectly developed.	4. Both the client and nurses may be unsure of the aims of care; progress toward goal achievement is difficult to evaluate.	4. After writing goals, check them against the following criteria: • Subject is the client or some part of the client. • The client behavior is stated in observable, measurable terms. • Criteria of acceptable performance are specified. • Time criteria are included in notes.
5. Nursing orders are superficial.	5. Client receives routinized care; lack of continuity of care; client goals may never be achieved. Each nurse must figure out a plan of nursing strategies.	5. Review nursing orders to ensure that they indicate the *specific* nursing strategies most likely to result in successful goal achievement *for this client* (eg, what comfort measures in particular are successful adjuncts to analgesic administration for a particular client?). In specifying the "who, what, when, where, how, and how much" of nursing actions, be sure to list the type of equipment and supplies needed in various treatments. As new client data are obtained, update nursing orders. Delete inappropriate or unnecessary orders.
6. The plan of care initiated on the day of admission fails to be updated.	6. Plan of care will not be consulted by nurses—if used, it will be to client's detriment.	6. If personal accountability for updating plan fails, develop a process on the nursing unit to ensure care plan review and revision.

(continued)

TABLE 19-2 *(continued)*

Common Problems Noted During Evaluation of the Nursing Process

Problem	Effect on Nursing Process	Nursing Response
Planning *(continued)*		
7. The plan of care addresses the immediate needs of the client but fails to anticipate discharge needs.	7. Client returns home unable to manage self-care activities.	7. Work hard at developing the ability to project yourself into the client's home after discharge. Learn to anticipate problems and concerns and prepare the client and family for these. Use all discharge resources in the institution. Learn from clients what their needs were after previous discharge.
Implementing		
1. Nurses are not aware of client priorities and the plan of care; lack of continuity; inefficient use of nursing resources.	1. Client fails to achieve goals.	1. a. Use shift report to update staff on status of priority nursing diagnosis and concomitant nursing care. b. Review plan of care and nursing notes before beginning care.
2. Nursing care becomes routinized and mechanized.	2. Client never has the sense that he or she is personally known by nurses.	2. Explore creative strategies to make quality nursing care on this particular unit a *challenge* rather than a *burden;* use ongoing education, problem-solving strategies by the nursing team, gaming, and other incentives.
3. Documentation is inadequate.	3. Because there is no complete written record of nursing care, *legally,* this care was never provided.	3. a. Develop the philosophy that quality nursing care *deserves* to be documented. Review legal reasons for careful documentation. b. Become familiar with the flow sheets and note format used within the work setting so that charting can be done quickly and comprehensively.
Evaluating		
1. It is not done.	1. Mastery of nursing process is stunted; severely limits accomplishment of nursing aims.	1. Develop the belief that quality nursing care does not happen automatically and that only ongoing evaluation will identify needed areas of revision. Devise an evaluative strategy and carry it out. Study its effect on quality of care after 6 months' implementation.

COMPUTER APPLICATIONS IN NURSING

Computerized Help in Quality Assurance

To perform its job, the hospital quality assurance department has to review large numbers of charts to identify strengths and weaknesses in client care and care documentation. As automated records become more common, the chart review process will change.

Currently, record review may take weeks while mountains of paper are shifted in the medical records department. The data frequently are scattered and incomplete, and trends are hard to detect and develop. In the future, nurses in quality assurance departments will be able to look at trends over a period of time and use those trends for forecasting and problem solving.

(Adapted from Walker, M.B., & Schwartz, C. [1984]. *What every nurse should know about computers.* Philadelphia: Lippincott. References: McHugh, M., & Schultz, S. [1982]. *Computer technology in hospital nursing departments: Future applications and implications. Proceedings of the Sixth Annual Symposium on Computer Applications in Medical Care.* Silver Spring, MD: IEEE Computer Society Press; Simpson, R.L. [1983]. *Nursing administrative applications: Proceedings of the Seventh Annual Symposium on Computer Applications in Medical Care.* Silver Spring, MD: IEEE Computer Society Press.)

Approaches to Quality Health Care: Inspection or Opportunity?

There are two distinct approaches to ensuring quality. *Quality by inspection* focuses on "finding the bad apples [deficient workers] and removing them." Although client satisfaction is important, the focus of quality by inspection is on the technical delivery of care and the competence of clinicians. Clinicians subject to this type of quality assurance tend to be angry or afraid, and expend their energies proving that they are not deficient or competent—in negative ways.

In contrast, *quality as opportunity* focuses on finding opportunities for improvement and fosters an environment that thrives on teamwork, with people sharing the skills and lessons they have learned. Mistakes are not viewed as being caused by lack of motivation or lack of effort on the part of workers, but rather as a result of problems in the system. Workers are viewed as doing the best they can, and are respected as trying hard, acting in good faith, and not willfully failing to do what they know is correct. In this work environment, clinicians respond with openness and a desire to learn because their integrity and self-worth are not threatened.

Donna Ambler Peters suggests a different way of looking at the quality of health care and its measurement. She reminds us that how well quality is measured is based on the beliefs we hold about health, the nurse–client relationship, our coworkers, and the health care system.

Without a personal commitment to quality and respect for oneself and others there is no means to achieve quality. There never will be sufficient financial resources, organizations artifice, or measurable standards to safeguard quality any other way. Each of us must care enough to make this happen—for ourselves, for our patients, and for our profession. (Peters, 1991, pp. 6–7)

Our goal should be to work in an environment in which quality measurements encourage our best efforts.

(Peters, D. [1991]. Measuring quality: Inspection or opportunity? *Holistic Nursing Practice, 5*[3], 1–7.)

Health Planning and Resources Development Act of 1975 require nurses to document that nursing standards are being implemented and maintained. Each of these agencies is concerned with quality care and quality control. The availability of fewer resources to treat clients in hospitals and the unavailability of sufficient alternative treatment settings pose a strong challenge to the nursing profession to find ways to avoid a compromise in quality of care. Numerous professional nursing organizations are meeting this challenge.

Quality Assurance

Specially designed programs that have as their aim the promotion of excellence in nursing are called **quality-assurance programs**. These programs may be as small as one conducted by the nurses on a small nursing unit or may have a scope as broad as that of an entire institution, state, province, or country.

Quality-assurance programs enable nursing to be accountable to society for the quality of care it provides. Such programs also are a response to the public mandate for professional accountability and the mandate of professional nursing law. They ensure professional survival, encourage nursing's fidelity to its moral and ethical responsibilities, and assist nursing to comply with other external pressures.

American Nurses' Association Quality-Assurance Program

The American Nurses' Association (ANA) in 1975 developed a model quality-assurance program consisting of seven steps: (1) identify values; (2) identify structure, process, and outcome standards and criteria; (3) measure the degree of attainment of criteria and standards; (4) make interpretations about strengths and weaknesses based on such measurements; (5) identify possible courses of action; (6) choose a course of action; and (7) take action. The ANA hoped that the model could be used at the local level to develop and implement quality-assurance programs.

The ANA model directs attention to three essential components of quality care—structure, process, and outcome. Different types of quality-assurance programs may focus exclusively on one component or on a mixture of components.

Structure This type of **structure evaluation** or audit is focused on the environment in which care is provided. Standards describe physical facilities and equipment; organizational characteristics, policies, and procedures; fiscal resources; and personnel resources.

Process The focus of the **process evaluation** is the nature and sequence of activities carried out by the nurse implementing the nursing process. Criteria make explicit acceptable levels of performance of nursing actions related to

client assessment, diagnosis, planning, implementation, and evaluation.

Outcome **Outcome evaluations** focus on measurable changes in the health status of the client or the end results of nursing care. Whereas the proper environment for care and the right nursing actions are important aspects of quality care, the critical element in evaluating care is demonstrable changes in client health status.

Nursing Audit

A **nursing audit** is a method of evaluating nursing care that involves a review of client records to assess the outcomes of nursing care or the process by which these outcomes were achieved. Successful nursing audits depend on careful nursing documentation.

Concurrent Versus Retrospective The evaluation of nursing care and client outcomes may be conducted while the client is receiving care (ie, a **concurrent evaluation**) or after the client has been discharged (ie, a retrospective evaluation). Concurrent evaluations are conducted by using direct observation of nursing care, client interviews, and chart review to determine whether the specified evaluative criteria are met.

Retrospective evaluations may use postdischarge questionnaires, client interviews (telephone or face to face), or chart review (nursing audit) to collect data. The type of retrospective audit most familiar to nurses working in hospitals is the JCAHO retrospective chart review. This accrediting body initially required hospitals to conduct a certain number of audits per year.

Self-Evaluation

Nurses who are sincerely committed to quality care learn early to make self-evaluation an integral part of their nursing practice. Self-evaluation skills promote professional development, enhance self-esteem, and develop self-awareness. The nurse who is just beginning to develop the caregiver role may find it helpful to conclude each caregiving experience with a brief moment of reflection that identifies and celebrates the nursing competencies that were skillfully used and targets competencies that need to be developed. This practice can keep one from becoming overwhelmed in the face of all that remains to be mastered and yet strongly motivated to learn new skills.

Identified in the case study that concludes each clinical chapter in this text are the specialized abilities the nurse needs to implement the plan of care. These abilities include intellectual, interpersonal, psychomotor, and organizational skills. It is helpful when planning care to try to identify the nursing resources that are needed to ensure that you will be able to meet each encounter's challenge. Nurses sensitive to mastering both the art and the science of nursing care evaluate their possession of the prerequisite knowledge and skills for each nurse–client encounter as well as their ability to perceive, respond to, and appreciate the uniqueness of each client. Quality care is each nurse's responsibility.

Summary

The cultivation of evaluation as a critical component of the nursing process ensures nursing's continued success in achieving desired changes in client health status. Only a firm commitment to evaluation enables nurses to answer the following questions:
- What are nursing's values?
- How can these be formalized in standards and evaluative criteria?

- What data exist to determine whether the specified evaluative criteria are being met?
- How can these data best be collected, analyzed, and interpreted?
- To what courses of action do the findings lead?

Nursing actions are far too valuable and costly resources today to be haphazardly implemented. Evaluation, carefully planned and executed, can direct and redirect these actions to maximize client benefit. This is the goal and challenge of nursing evaluation. Criteria that may be helpful in determining the adequacy of the evaluative component of the nursing process include the following:
- Evaluation of the client's achievement of desired goals
- Review of how the process is used and revision of the plan of care if necessary
- Participation in quality-assurance programs

Figure 19-2 provides a summary and overview of the evaluation step of the nursing process.

F I G U R E   1 9 - 2

Overview and summary of the evaluative component of the nursing process.

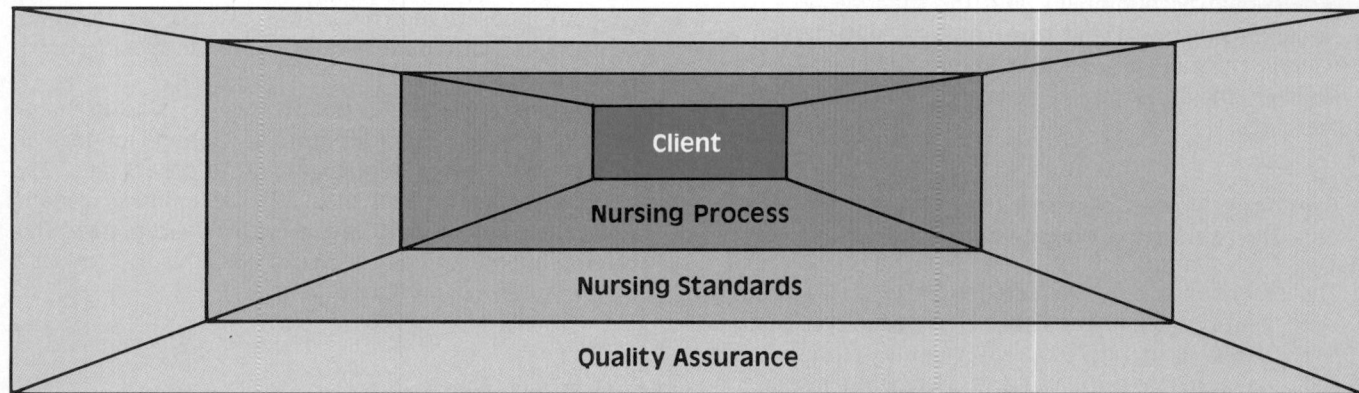

Why evaluate?

- Measure attainment of client goals
- Redirect plan of nursing care
- Enhance nursing's public image
- Ensure nursing's survival: *i.e.*, the selection and funding of nursing services in the competitive health care market

How to evaluate:

- Develop evaluative criteria
- Collect data and compare it to standards
- Summarize findings and make interpretations
- Identify courses of actions
- Take corrective action based on findings

Who is concerned about evaluation of nursing care?

- Nurses
- Clients
- Fiscal intermediaries
- Other health care professionals
- Community that determines allocation of resources to health care delivery

What do they want to know?

- What kinds of health and wellness problems nurses help clients to solve
- What nursing interventions are most successful in achieving desired client outcomes
- What it costs to achieve these results
- Are these the best nursing interventions and client outcomes considering the current status of the science and art of nursing and other health or health-related sciences

Types of evaluation:

- Determination of the client's degree of goal achievement
- Review of the use of nursing process
- Identification of and response to client, nurse, and health care system variables detracting from quality care
- Participation in quality assurance programs
  - structure/process/outcomes
  - concurrent/retrospective
  - institution/nurse/client

Checklist for Evaluating Your Use of the Nursing Process

Assessing

☐ The initial data base is obtained by means of a nursing history and nursing examination.

☐ Assessment data are documented:

  ☐ Accurately—Questionable data are validated.

  ☐ Completely—Use of a systematic guide ensures that recorded data describe (1) the client's functional ability to meet each basic human need and (2) responses to health and illness.

  ☐ Concisely—Irrelevant data and meaningless generalizations are avoided.

  ☐ Factually—Client behaviors are recorded rather than the nurse's interpretation of these behaviors.

☐ The initial data base communicates a "real sense" of the client that makes possible individualized care.

☐ Focused assessment data are recorded for each client problem.

☐ Data collection and documentation are ongoing and responsive to changes in the client's condition.

Diagnosing

☐ A prioritized list of nursing diagnoses is on the plan of care.

☐ Each nursing diagnosis describes an actual or potential client health problem that independent nursing intervention can prevent or resolve. Each nursing diagnosis:

  ☐ Is derived from an accurate and validated interpretation of a cluster of significant client data or "cues"

  ☐ Contains a precise problem statement describing what is unhealthy about the client and what needs to change—suggests client goals

  ☐ Identifies factors that contribute to the problem (etiology)—these suggest nursing interventions

  ☐ Uses nonjudgmental language and is written using legally advisable terms

☐ Old nursing diagnoses are deleted from the plan of care once resolved, and new diagnoses are added as soon as identified

Planning

☐ A comprehensive, individualized, and up-to-date plan of care that specifies client goals and nursing orders for each nursing diagnosis is developed with the assistance of the client and family.

☐ Planning is comprehensive:

  ☐ Initial

  ☐ Ongoing

  ☐ Discharge

☐ Long-term goals alert the entire nursing team to realistic client expectations after discharge.

☐ Short-term goals:

  ☐ When achieved, demonstrate a resolution of the problem specified in the nursing diagnosis

  ☐ Describe a single, observable, and measurable client behavior

  ☐ Are valued by the client and family

  ☐ Are realistic in terms of the resources of the client and the nurse

☐ Nursing orders:

  ☐ Clearly and concisely describe the nursing action to be performed (ongoing assessment; nursing treatments and procedures; teaching, counseling, advocacy)

  ☐ Are tailored to the client

  ☐ Are consistent with standards of care and supportive of other therapies

  ☐ Are effective in accomplishing the desired client goals

☐ The plan of care encourages client and family participation.

Implementing

☐ The client record contains daily documentation of the nursing measures used to (1) assist the client to meet basic human needs, (2) resolve health problems, and (3) implement select aspects of the medical plan of care.

☐ The plan of care is implemented:

  ☐ Competently

  ☐ Caringly

  ☐ Creatively

Evaluating

☐ Evaluative statements are recorded on the plan of care to document the client's level of goal achievement at targeted times.

☐ Ongoing evaluation of the client's responses to the plan of care are used to make decisions about terminating, continuing, or modifying nursing care.

KEY POINTS

- During evaluation, the nurse and client measure how well the client has achieved the goals specified in the plan of care. Factors that have positively or negatively influenced goal achievement are identified, and a decision is made to terminate, continue, or modify care.
- When evaluation points to the need to modify nursing care, each preceding step in the nursing process is reviewed for accuracy.
- The type of evaluative data collected to support the decision regarding goal achievement (goal met, partially met, or not met) is determined by the nature of the goal. Goals may be cognitive, psycho-motor, or affective, or they may describe physical changes in the client.
- It is important for nurses to evaluate client goal achievement as early as possible. Achievement, when celebrated with the client, encourages further goal achievement. Failure directs necessary revisions in the plan of care. Waiting until a client is about to be discharged to evaluate goals is the most common mistake nurses make in evaluation.
- Evaluative statements recorded on the plan of care alert the entire nursing staff to the client's level of goal achievement. Each evaluative statement includes a decision about how well the goal was achieved and the client data or behavior that supports the decision. The statement is dated and signed.
- Sensitivity to the client, nurse, and health care system variables that influence goal achievement enables the nurse to manipulate factors that will help the client reach desired goals.

- Common problems encountered during evaluation that may require a revision of the plan of care include inaccurate or incomplete data base, vague or missing nursing diagnoses, standardized plan of care, improperly developed nursing goals, superficial nursing orders, plan that is not kept up-to-date, failure to use evaluation to improve quality of nursing care, and insufficient communication among nurses.
- Historically, nursing has been a strong advocate for quality health care. The current availability of fewer resources to treat clients in hospitals and the unavailability of sufficient alternative treatment settings pose a serious challenge to nursing.
- Quality-assurance programs are evaluative programs designed to secure and implement excellence in nursing and health care. These programs may include process, structure, or outcome standards and have as their focus the client, the nurse, the institution, or the health care system.
- Quality-assurance programs enable nursing to be accountable to society for the quality of its service. They also are a response to the public mandate for professional accountability and the mandate of professional nursing law. They ensure professional survival, encourage nursing's fidelity to its moral and ethical responsibilities, and assist nursing to comply with other external pressures.
- Self-evaluation skills promote professional development, enhance self-esteem, and develop self-awareness.

BIBLIOGRAPHY

Allison, S., & Kinlock, K. (1984). Four steps to quality assurance. *Canadian Nurse, 77*(11), 36–38.

American Nurses' Association. (1975). *A plan for implementation of the standards of nursing practice*. Kansas City, MO: Author.

American Nurses' Association. (1976). *ANA quality assurance workbook*. Kansas City, MO: Author.

American Nurses' Association. (1991). *ANA's eight standards of nursing practice* (rev. ed.). Kansas City, MO: Author.

Atkinson, L. D., & Murray, M. E. (1990). *Understanding the nursing process* (4th ed.). New York: Pergamon.

Barba, M., Bennet, B., & Shaw, W. J. (1978). The evaluation of patient care through use of ANA's standards of nursing practice. *Supervisor Nurse, 9*(11), 42–53.

Best, M., Carswell, R. J. B., & Abbot, S. D. (1990). Self-evaluation for students. *Nursing Outlook, 38*(4), 172–177.

Bloch, D. (1975). Evaluation of nursing care in terms of process and outcome: Issues in research and quality assurance. *Nursing Research, 24*, 256–263.

Donabedian, A. (1980). *The definition of quality and its approaches*. Ann Arbor: Health Administration Press.

Donabedian, A. (1982). *The criteria and standards of quality: Explorations in quality assessment and monitoring*. Ann Arbor: Health Administration Press.

Griffith-Kenney, J. W., & Christensen, P. J. (1990). *Nursing process: Application of theories, frameworks and models* (3rd ed.). St. Louis: Mosby.

Joint Commission on Accreditation of Healthcare Organizations. (1993). *Accreditation manual for hospitals*. Chicago: Joint Commission on Accreditation of Healthcare Organizations.

Katz, J. M., & Green, E. (1992). *Managing quality: A guide to monitoring and evaluating nursing services*. St. Louis: Mosby–Year Book.

Koch, M. W., & Fairly, T. M. (1992). *Integrated quality management: The key to improving nursing care quality.* St. Louis: Mosby–Yearbook.

Laing, M., & Nish, M. (1981). Eight steps to quality assurance. *Canadian Nurse, 77*(11), 22–25.

Lang, N. M., & Krejci, J. W. (1991). Standards and holism: A reframing. *Holistic Nursing Practice, 5*(3), 14–21.

Peters, D. (1991). Measuring quality: Inspection or opportunity? *Holistic Nursing Practice, 5*(3), 1–7.

Phaneuf, M. (1976). *The nursing audit: Self regulation in nursing practice.* New York: Appleton-Century-Crofts.

Phaneuf, M. (1976). Quality assurance: A nursing view. *New Zealand Nursing Journal, 69*(2), 9–11.

Shiber, S., & Larsen, E. (1991). Evaluating the quality of caring: Structure, process, and outcome. *Holistic Nursing Practice, 5*(3), 57–66.

Tucker, S. M., Canobbio, M. M., Paquette, E. V., & Wells, M. E. (1992). *Patient care standards: Nursing process, diagnosis and outcome* (5th ed.). St. Louis: Mosby.

Wandelt, M. A., & Ager, J. W. (1974). *Quality patient care scale.* New York: Appleton-Century-Crofts.

Wandelt, M. A., & Slater, S. D. (1975). *Slater nursing competencies rating scale.* New York: Appleton-Century-Crofts.

Wright, D. (1984). An introduction to the evaluation of nursing care: A review of the literature. *Journal of Advanced Nursing, 9*(5), 457–467.

Yura, H., & Walsh, M. (1988). *The nursing process: Assessing, planning, implementing, and evaluation* (5th ed.). New York: Appleton & Lange.

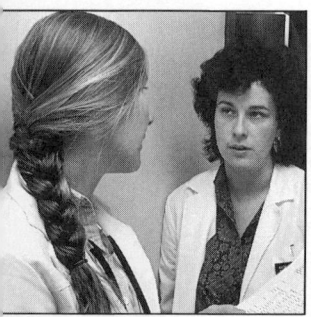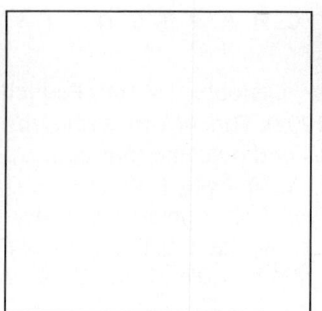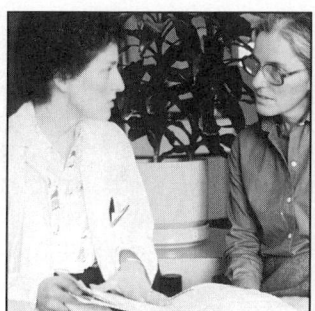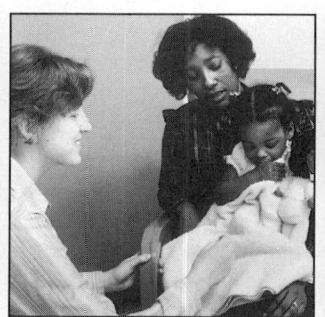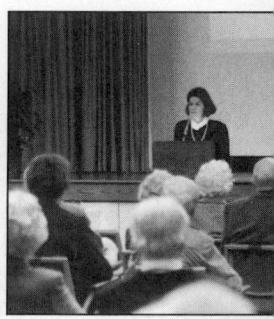

Roles Basic to Nursing Care

Communications

As health care providers, nurses function in a variety of roles to give holistic client care and to develop as members of the nursing profession. Unit V discusses the nurse's roles of communicator, teacher, counselor, leader, researcher, and advocate. These roles are interdependent, and each is an integral part of the broad nursing role of caregiver. The nurse uses these roles to help clients of all ages to meet needs along the health continuum.

To be effective as a caregiver, the nurse must be proficient in both the art and science of nursing roles. The role of the nurse as communicator is essential to each professional nursing role and is the heart of caring. Nursing is a person-centered service, based on relationships with clients, peers, and other members of the health care team. By developing effective interpersonal skills and using therapeutic communication skills, nurses are able to establish and maintain helping relationships with peers.

As teacher, the nurse uses communication skills to teach individuals and families. Teaching, implemented through the nursing process, is used to meet learning needs. As counselor, the nurse provides information, makes appropriate referrals, and assists the client in developing a systematic approach to problem solving and decision making. The nurse as leader practices assertive, self-directed nursing. Abilities for leadership and bringing about change begin with the student nurse and progress as the nurse develops self-confidence and skill in interpersonal relationships and experience in health care settings. As researcher, the nurse may conduct re-

search, use research findings to improve client care, or participate in research done by others. As advocate, the nurse combines all these roles to promote the right of clients to make their own decisions about health and life and to protect human and legal rights.

The content of Unit V enables beginning nurse caregivers to enrich their professional practice by integrating the professional nursing roles of communicator, teacher, counselor, leader, researcher, and advocate. Nursing practice, as a specialized and unique service to others, is based on the application of knowledge and skill presented in this unit.

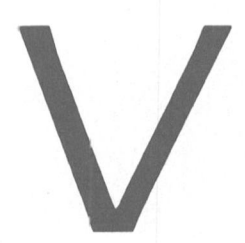

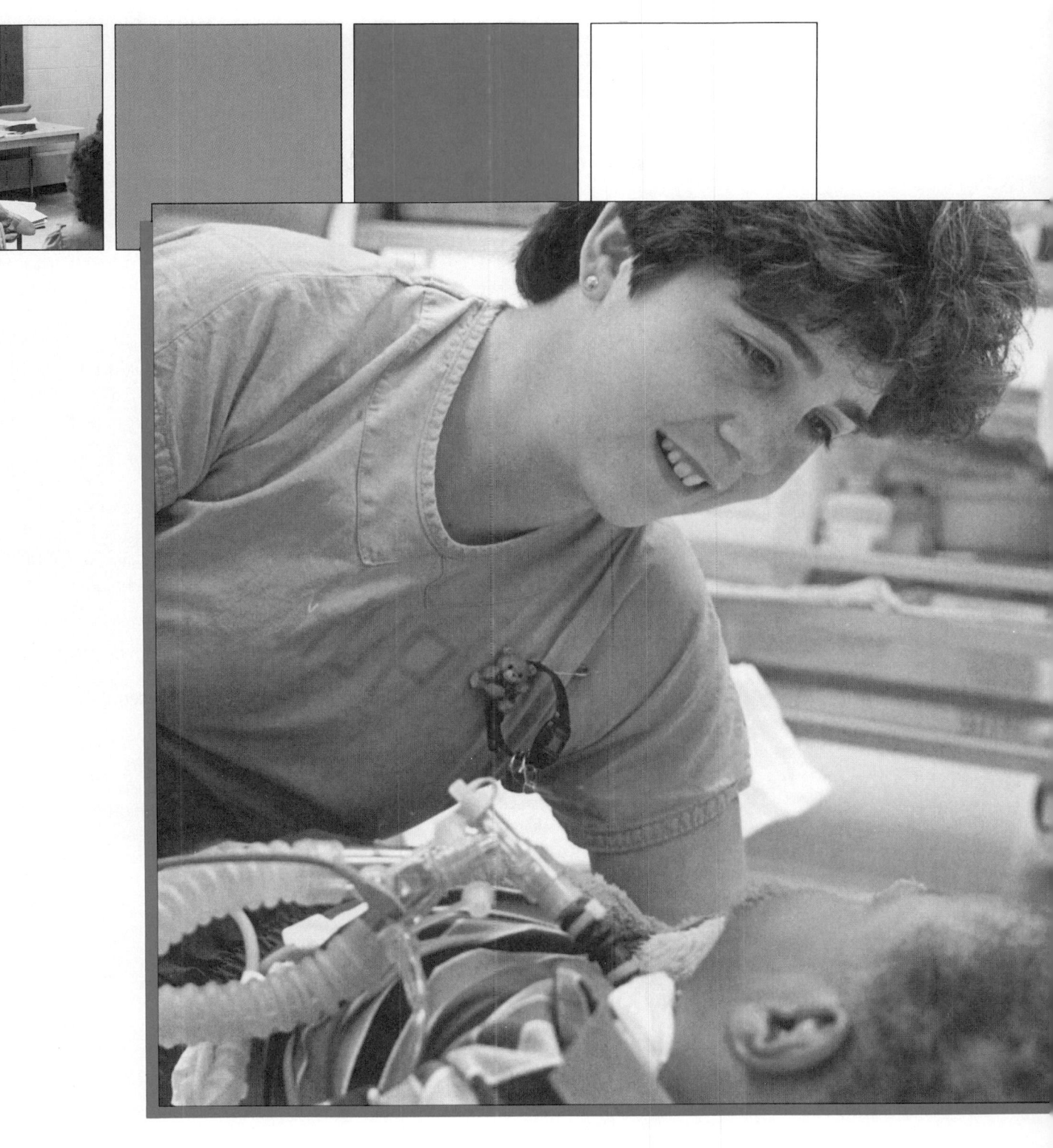

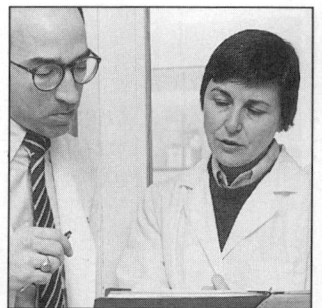
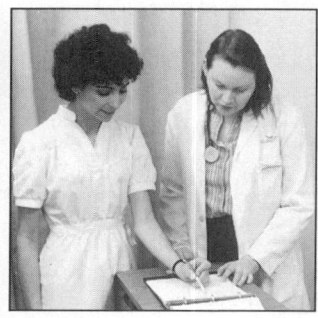

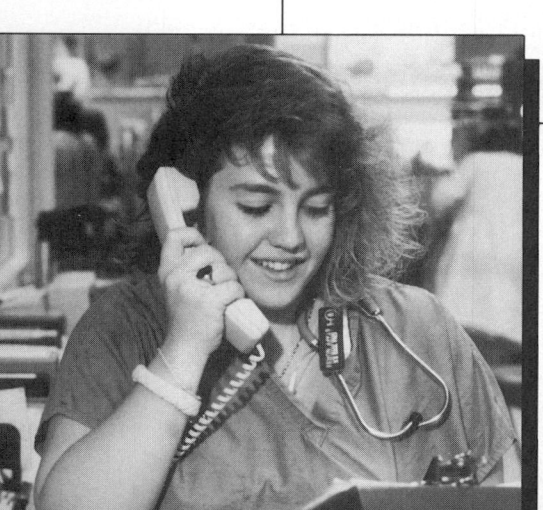

Communicator

OBJECTIVES

After studying this chapter, the learner should be able to:

Define key terms used in the chapter.

Describe the communication process.

List at least eight ways in which people communicate nonverbally.

Describe the interrelation between communication and the nursing process.

Identify client goals for each phase of the helping relationship.

Use each of the effective communication techniques when interacting with clients.

Evaluate self in terms of the interpersonal skills needed in nursing.

Describe how each of the ineffective communication techniques hinders communication.

Explain how to facilitate nurse–client interactions in special circumstances.

Establish therapeutic relationships with clients assigned to your care.

KEY TERMS

assertiveness
body language
channel
communication
empathy
feedback
helping relationship
interpersonal skills
interviewing techniques
language
message
nonverbal communication
rapport
receiver (decoder)
relationship
semantics
source (encoder)
therapeutic touch
verbal communication

20

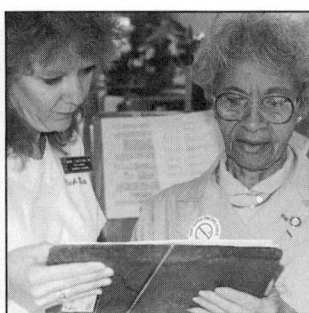

Any nurse who wishes to be an effective caregiver must first learn to communicate. Good communication skills enable nurses to get to know their clients and ultimately to diagnose and meet their needs for nursing care. The student nurse who sits face to face with a client for the first time and is charged with the responsibility of obtaining a comprehensive nursing history intuitively grasps the importance of the communicator role of the nurse. Communication skills are the building blocks of professional relationships: nurse–client, nurse–nurse, and nurse–physician (and other health team member). Many experienced nurses identify the quality of their interpersonal relationships as the single most significant element in determining their helper effectiveness. Studies have shown that on nursing units where nurses freely exchange ideas and information, problem solve together when something goes wrong rather than assigning blame, compliment one another, and use humor creatively, staff morale is high and clients demonstrate enhanced well-being and increased compliance with treatments and procedures.

Communication Process

Communication is a foundation for our way of life. Without some form of communication, it would be impossible to share family experiences, master an education, establish and maintain a government, and enjoy many current forms of entertainment. Humans by nature are social and meet needs in collaboration with others. Human relationships enable us to meet not only our physical and safety needs but also our psychosocial needs for love and belonging and self-esteem. The ability to communicate is basic to human functioning and well-being.

Communication is the process of sharing information or the process of generating and transmitting meanings. The two definitions are not in conflict because information is produced and has meaning before it can be shared. David K. Berlo (1960) is credited with the classic description of the communication process, which involves a source (encoder); message; channel; and receiver (decoder; Fig. 20-1). The function of the **source** or **encoder** is to prepare and send to the receiver a message that can be decoded with complete accuracy. The **message** is the actual physi-

cal product of the source or encoder. It might be a speech, interview, telephone conversation, chart, conversation, gesture, memorandum, or nursing note. The **channel** is the medium selected to convey the message and may target any of the receiver's senses. In a teaching session, a nurse may use auditory, visual, and tactile channels to communicate with a client. The **receiver (decoder)**, upon receiving the message, must translate it and make a decision about it. The nurse who is an effective communicator needs to consider the receiver at all times, seeking to select a message that appeals to the client's interests, is phrased in words the client understands, and requires minimal effort and time to decode. It is critical to look for verbal and nonverbal evidence—**feedback**—that the client received and understood the message. Noise, factors that distort the quality of a message, may interfere with communication at any point in the process. Some examples of noise include a distracted source or receiver, a room that is uncomfortably warm, a noisy television program, and pain.

Basic Characteristics of Communication

Communication is a reciprocal process in which both the sender and the receiver of messages participate simultaneously. The basic characteristics of communication are highlighted in the accompanying display.

To begin the process, more than one person must be involved and participants must establish a relationship. A person in isolation does not communicate; isolation not only may be physical but also may be self-imposed isolation from people and surroundings, as occurs in some mental and emotional illnesses. Also, two or more people next to each other, for instance in a checkout line in a market, do not necessarily communicate with one another. Some kind of relationship must exist between people for the communication process to occur.

Communication is continuous and reciprocal. Communicating people mutually and continuously send and receive messages, rather than having one person who only sends or one who only receives messages. These messages may be sent through verbal and nonverbal means. Nonverbal communication often helps a person understand subtle and hidden meanings in what is being said verbally. For instance, a person may respond to the question, "How are you?" by simply answering, "Fine." However, if this answer is accompanied by a rigid, tense facial expression, the true meaning of the response would need further investigation (Fig. 20-2).

Verbal and nonverbal communication occur simultaneously. Nonverbal communication is more likely to be involuntary. That is, it tends to be less under the control of the person sending the message than is verbal communication, hence the proverb, "What you do speaks so loudly I cannot hear what you say." Hence, nonverbal communication is generally considered a more accurate expression of true feelings. For instance, people may say they are well and that everything is fine when obvious appearances and

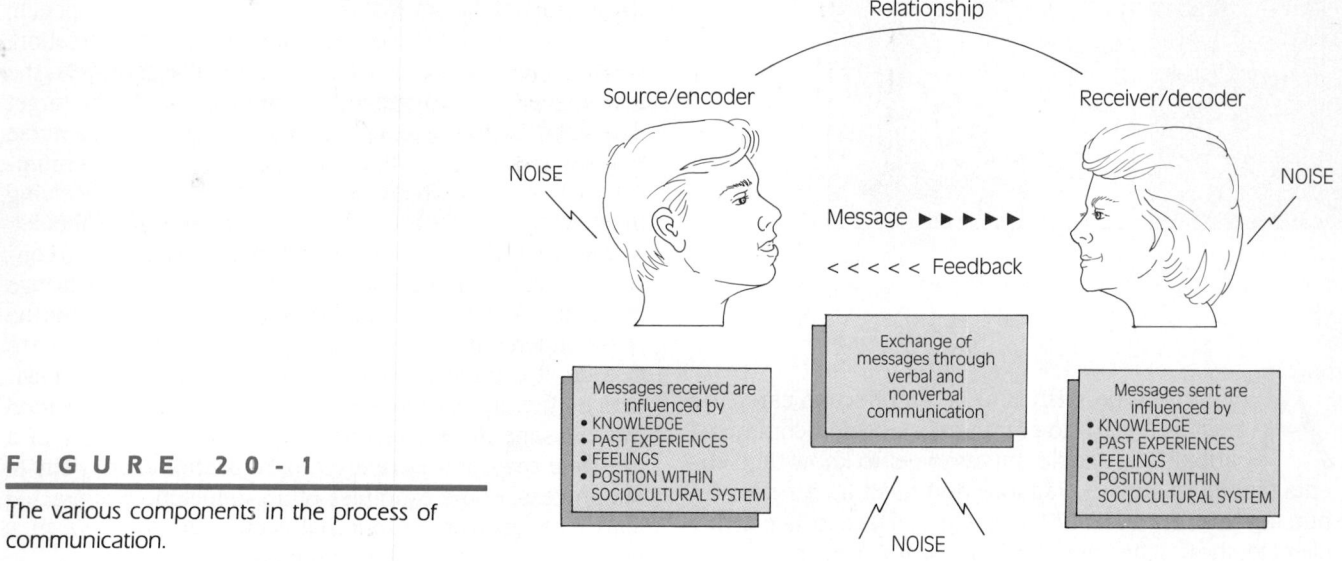

F I G U R E 2 0 - 1

The various components in the process of communication.

behavior show that all is not well. The nonverbal expression more accurately expresses the situation.

Communicating people respond to messages they receive. It is important to validate these responses—feedback—to learn whether a message was received accurately. Even the lack of a verbal response is feedback that requires validation. Perhaps the receiver was unable to

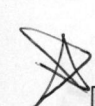

Basic Characteristics of Communication

- Communication requires at least two people who, as a result of communicating, establish a relationship with each other.
- Communication is continuous and reciprocal.
- Communicating people receive and send messages through verbal and nonverbal means.
- Verbal and nonverbal communications occur simultaneously.
- Communicating people respond to messages they receive.
- The message cannot always be assumed to mean what the receiver believes it to mean or what the sender intended it to mean.
- Exchanging messages requires knowledge.
- Past experiences influence messages sent, and interpretation by the receiver is based on past experiences.
- Communication is influenced by the way people feel about themselves, the subject matter being communicated, and others.
- A person's position within a sociocultural system may influence the process of communication.

---

comprehend the message or, more significantly, the message was met by inattention, disinterest, hostility, or anger. Thus, validation is also necessary to determine the accuracy of not only the message but also the meaning of the message. The message cannot always be assumed to mean what the receiver believes it to mean or what the sender intended it to mean.

The person sending a message must have knowledge to send, and the person receiving the message must have knowledge to understand what is sent. The levels of knowledge may not always be equal. For example, the nurse who teaches a client about diabetes must have knowledge about the disease and attempts to share that knowledge with the client. However, if the client does not understand the disease process or the terminology the nurse uses, the client will not receive the messages the nurse sends.

A person's past experiences influence what is sent, and interpretation by the receiver is based on past experiences as well. For example, what is a big meal, a small child, or a high temperature? Unless the sender and receiver's past experiences are similar in relation to the manner in which these adjectives are used, effective communication is difficult. Pain may mean one thing to a person who has suffered a great deal but something different to a person who has experienced little pain. The grief of death may have a different meaning to a person who has not experienced the loss of a loved one from that of the person who has.

Communication is influenced by the way people feel about themselves, the subject matter, and one another. The nurse who feels teaching is an important aspect of nursing care will communicate this feeling to clients. In contrast, the nurse who handles teaching as an unimportant chore is unlikely to share much information with the client. The client's motivation (or lack of motivation) to learn cannot help but influence the nurse. Also, a client who is anxious or angry may not hear what the nurse is saying no matter

MESSAGE

FIGURE 20-2

Research in communication has shown that words contribute only a small percentage to the communication of a message (*the colored area*). Nonverbal expression, tone, timing, context, the other characteristics of an exchange complete the message communicated.

how skillfully the nurse teaches the subject matter. Similarly, a nurse who is uncomfortable with a subject (eg, sexuality) will surely communicate his or her discomfort to the client.

A person's position within a sociocultural system may influence the communication process. Many people may feel intimidated in a health care environment especially if their socioeconomic status has made them feel powerless in the past. Conversely, some "power brokers" may act as if the entire health care system exists solely to cater to their needs. It is important for nurses to recognize these dynamics and to treat each client with respectful attention and care.

All of these characteristics compose the communication process. Other factors in communication of particular importance to nursing are forms of communications, the use of communication in therapy, and the development of communication skills.

Forms of Communication

People communicate in various environments involving a varying number of people. *One-to-one communication* occurs when only two people are involved in the communication process. A great deal of nursing situations involve the nurse and client in one-to-one communication.

Communication also occurs in *small groups* of 3 to 10 individuals. Nurses must learn to communicate effectively in small groups because they are often required to be members or leaders of such groups. *Large groups* comprise more than 10 people. Nursing instructors and students frequently experience the communication process in large groups. The nurse's role in teaching large groups is presented in Chapter 21. Attendance at social, religious, or political functions also involves large groups where communication may occur.

Communicating people receive and send messages through verbal and nonverbal means, which occur simultaneously. Learning about forms of communicating and developing skills in them are important parts of the nurse's education.

Verbal Communication

Verbal communication is an exchange of information using words, and includes both the spoken and the written word. Verbal communication depends on language. **Language** is a prescribed way of using words so that people can share information effectively. Language includes a common definition of words as well as a method of arranging the words in a certain order. The development of language is discussed in Chapter 11.

Both written and spoken forms of communication reveal a great deal about a person. The way a person pronounces certain words or uses particular phrases gives clues to such things as geographic or ethnic origins. Vocabulary, sentence structure, and spelling give indications of a person's intellectual development or educational level and may also indicate that English is a second language. Language helps nurses assess what clients know and feel. In turn, nurses must develop their own language skills to aid in reciprocal responses in the communication process.

The verbal form of communication is used extensively by nurses when speaking with clients, giving oral reports to other nurses, writing care plans, and recording in nursing progress notes. Other examples of verbal communication include public speaking, writing for publication, and composing signs and posters. In each of these examples, words and language are communicated to others.

Nonverbal Communication

Nonverbal communication is the exchange of information without the use of words. It is what is not said. Nonverbal communication is sometimes referred to as **body language**. There are various ways in which information is exchanged through nonverbal communication. It is generally accepted that nonverbal communication expresses more of the true meaning of a message than does verbal communication (Fig. 20-3). Therefore, nurses must be aware of both the nonverbal messages they send and the nonverbal messages they receive from clients. A great deal of variation exists in nonverbal communication, depending on one's individual or cultural patterns. Nurses working with clients from diverse cultural backgrounds should attempt to understand cultural variations to avoid misunderstanding nonverbal communication. The various forms of nonverbal communication follow.

Touch Tactile sense has been studied seriously as a form of nonverbal communication only within the past 3 or 4 decades. Touch expresses personal behavior and means different things to different people. Investigations have shown that tactile experiences are largely shaped by familial, regional, class, and cultural influences. Such factors as age and sex also play a role in individualizing meanings associated with touch. Despite its individuality, touch is viewed as one of the most effective nonverbal ways to express feelings such as comfort, love, affection, secur-

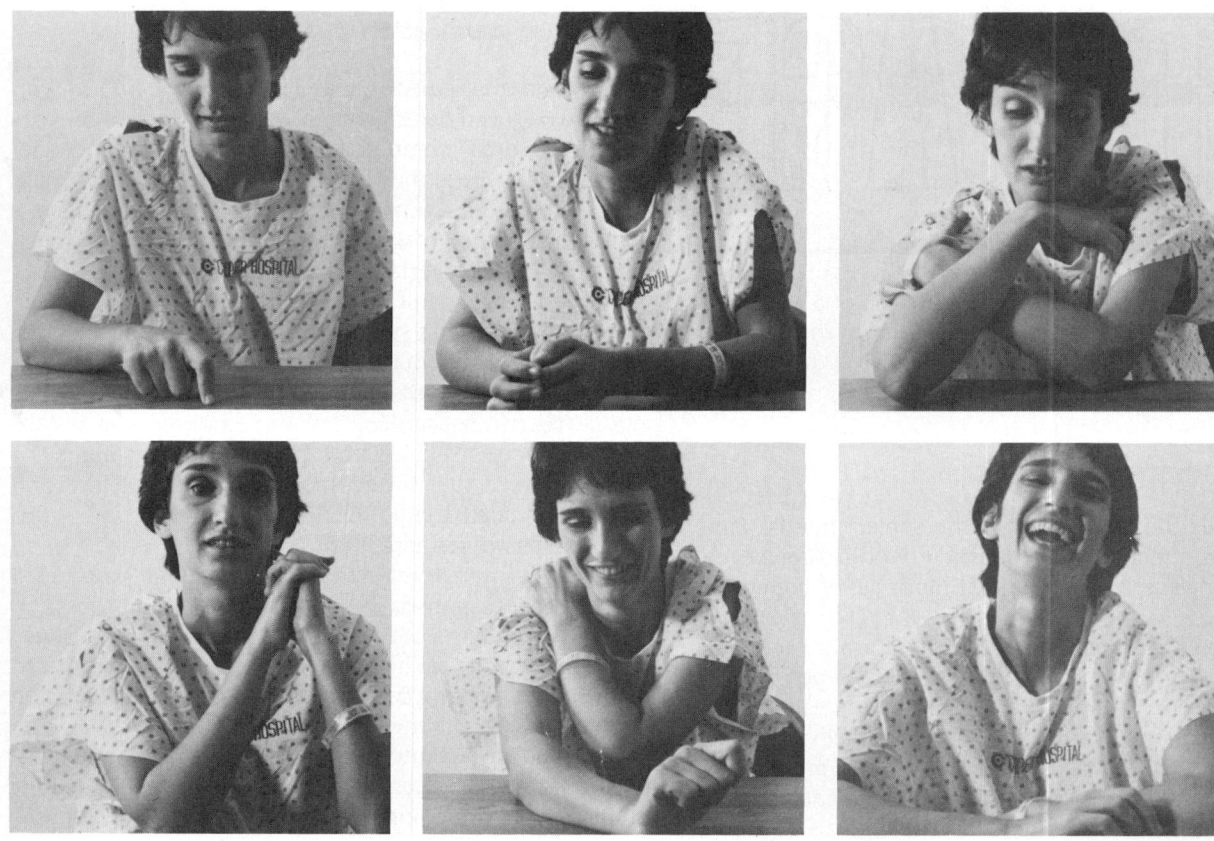

F I G U R E   2 0 - 3

Eye contact, the lack of it, facial expression, posture, gesture, and silence send nonverbal messages to the receiver. What messages do you receive from each of these photographs? (Photos by Charles Field. Barry, P. [1984]. *Psychosocial nursing: Assessment and intervention.* Philadelphia: Lippincott.)

ity, anger, frustration, aggression, excitement, and many others.

Eye Contact   Communication often begins with eye contact. A glance, for example, is often an attention-getting method to open conversation. Eye contact also suggests respect and a willingness to listen and to keep communication open. Lack of it often indicates anxiety or defenselessness or that a person is avoiding communication. However, young children and adolescents in some cultures are taught that it is disrespectful to look an adult in the eye. In other cultures, women are taught to avoid eye contact, or that out of respect, eye contact should not be made with a superior. In addition, the eyes themselves carry nonverbal messages. For example, the eyes fix in a stare during anger; they tend to narrow in disgust; and they ordinarily open wide in fear. A blank stare can indicate daydreaming or inattentiveness.

Facial Expressions   The face is the most expressive part of the body. Examples of the various messages facial expressions convey are anger, joy, suspicion, sadness, fear, and contempt. Some people have extremely expressive faces, whereas others mask their feelings, making it more difficult to determine what the person is really thinking. Nurses need to learn some control over their own facial expressions. For instance, a client with extensive burns may watch the nurse's reaction when burn dressings are changed for the first time. Any sign of repulsiveness or disgust would have grave implications for the client's self-image and recovery.

Posture   The way a person holds the body carries nonverbal messages. People in good health and with a positive attitude usually hold their bodies in good alignment. Depressed or tired people are more likely to slouch. Posture also often provides nonverbal clues concerning pain and physical limitations. For instance, a rigid, stiff appearance is a good indication of tension and pain.

Gait   A bouncy, purposeful walk usually carries a message of well-being. A less purposeful, shuffling gait often means the person is sad or discouraged. Certain gaits are associated with illness. For example, clients recovering from recent abdominal surgery usually walk slightly bent over and slowly and may need the assistance of handrails or a helping person.

Gestures Gestures using various parts of the body are capable of carrying numerous messages; for example, thumbs up means victory whereas thumbs down carries a negative connotation; kicking an object often expresses anger, as does a clenched fist; wringing the hands or tapping a foot usually indicates anxiety or anger; a waving hand serves to beckon someone to come, or, if waved in another way, signifies that someone should leave. Gestures are used extensively when two people speaking different languages attempt to communicate with each other.

General Physical Appearance Most illnesses cause at least some alterations in general physical appearance. Observing for changes in appearance is an important nursing responsibility in detecting a particular illness or in evaluating effectiveness of care and therapy. For example, the person with an insufficient intake of fluids has dry skin that wrinkles easily, eyes that may be sunken and dull in appearance, and poor muscle tone. On the other hand, the person in good health tends to radiate health status through general physical appearance.

Mode of Dress and Grooming A person's clothing and grooming practices carry significant nonverbal messages. For example, healthy people with good self-esteem tend to pay attention to details of dress and grooming, whereas those with low self-esteem show much less interest in them. People feeling ill often demonstrate little interest in personal appearance, and it is often a sign of returning health when interest in mode of dress and appearance begins.

Sounds Crying, moaning, gasping, and sighing are oral but nonverbal forms of communication. Such sounds can be interpreted in numerous ways. For example, a person may cry because of sadness or for joy. Gasping often indicates fear or pain. A sigh may be a sign of reluctant agreement to do something or a sign of relief.

Silence Periods of silence during communication often carry important nonverbal messages. The silence between two people may indicate complete understanding of each other or it may mean they are angry with each other. Silence and its possible uses and meanings are discussed later in this chapter.

Communication as a Component of Therapy

Communication and the Nursing Process

The nurse's ability to communicate with clients and with other nurses is essential to effective use of the nursing process. Knowledge of the communication process and of effective communication techniques is fundamental to all steps of the nursing process. At the same time, the nursing process provides the nurse with the guidance and direction needed to communicate with the client effectively.

Assessing Because the major focus of the assessment step is information gathering, verbal and nonverbal communication are essential nursing tools. Nurses use the written word to obtain data concerning their clients. Nurses often read their clients' records or charts before meeting them. The spoken word is used to give and receive reports

---

RESEARCH IN NURSING Making a Difference

Importance of Effective Communication for Families of Critically Ill Clients

Hickey, M. (1990). What are the needs of families of critically ill patients? A review of the literature since 1976. *Heart and Lung, 19*(4), 401–415.

Hickey found and analyzed eight research studies conducted since 1976 that explored the needs of the families of critically ill clients. Families consistently rated information needs as most important followed by needs for reassurance and convenience. The 10 most important needs that occurred with a frequency of 70% to 100% in all of the studies follow:

• To have questions answered honestly (100%)
• To know specific facts regarding what is wrong with client and his or her progress (100%)

• To know prognosis, outcome, and chance for recovery (90%)
• To be called at home about changes (90%)
• To receive information once a day (80%)
• To receive information in understandable explanations (80%)
• To believe that hospital personnel care about client (80%)
• To have hope (70%)
• To know exactly what/why things are being done for client (70%)
• To have reassurance that the best possible care is being given to client (70%)

to and from other health personnel. This is a common practice when admitting a client to a hospital unit. Nurses use one-to-one communication to obtain thorough nursing histories and physical examinations. Effective communication techniques, as well as observational skills, are used extensively during this phase. The data collected verbally and nonverbally are analyzed and then passed on to the appropriate people through oral and written communications.

Diagnosing Once a nurse formulates a nursing diagnosis, it must be communicated through the spoken and written word to other nurses as well as to the client. The written diagnosis becomes a permanent part of the client's record.

Planning The planning step requires the use of communication to share client objectives or goals and nursing orders with the client and other health care personnel. Because a nurse is rarely able to implement all parts of a plan alone, oral and written communication is relied on to inform others of what needs to be done to meet the set objectives or goals. Without communication, the nurse's plan would never proceed to the implementation phase.

Implementing Nurses assume many roles when they implement the care plan. Verbal and nonverbal communication allows nurses to enhance basic caregiving measures and to teach, counsel, and support clients and their families during the implementation phase. Even a simple nursing order such as "encourage to drink 100 mL of fluid every hour while awake" requires countless messages to be sent and received between the nurse and client. The nurse explains why fluids are important, what fluids are beneficial, and how often they are needed. The client, in turn, informs the nurse of his or her ability or inability to comply with the order. The client's verbal and nonverbal messages are assessed during each nurse–client interaction. Then, the implementation of the order is documented in the client's record.

Evaluating Nurses often rely on the verbal and nonverbal cues they receive from their clients to verify whether client objectives or goals have been achieved. Communication also facilitates the revision of parts of the care plan through the exchange of positive and negative messages between the nurse and the client.

Documenting Communication Any information required for the continual assessment of the client's needs and condition should be documented in the appropriate place, unless the information is confidential. This documentation serves to promote the continuity of care given by nurses and other health care providers. Because one nurse cannot provide 24-hour coverage for clients, significant information must be passed on to others through nursing progress notes and care plans. Documentation is discussed in Chapter 18.

Helping Relationship

One of the basic characteristics of communication is that people, as a result of communicating, establish a relationship with each other. Another characteristic is that communication is continuous and reciprocal. These characteristics work together to establish a helping relationship.

Most people entering the health care field do so because they want to help people. This is not accomplished through a random method but rather takes preconceived, purposeful paths, as evident in the steps of the nursing process. Another intentional system is the helping relationship, sometimes called the therapeutic relationship, which uses the nursing process (Fig. 20-4).

A **helping relationship** exists among many people who provide and receive assistance in meeting human needs in many walks of life. However, in this book, it refers to the helping relationships between nurses and clients. A helping relationship sets the climate for the participants to move toward common goals, which arise from human

F I G U R E   2 0 - 4

The helping relationship is dynamic, purposeful, and focused on achieving client-centered goals.

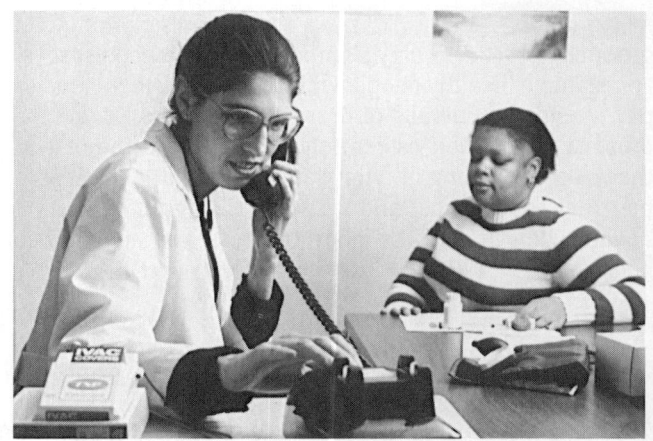

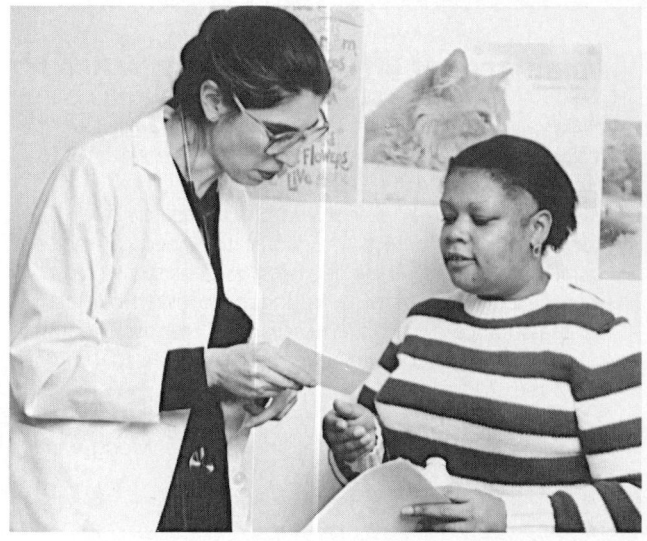

needs. Therefore, need gratification occurs as the result of a successful helping relationship.

When a nurse and client are involved in a helping relationship, the nurse assists the client to achieve goals that allow the client's human needs to be satisfied. The nurse is the helper and the client is the person being helped. The helping relationship between the nurse and client is sometimes called the nurse–client relationship.

Carative Factors   The quality of one's relationship with another person is the most significant element in determining helping effectiveness. "Of all the problems that can arise in nursing care, perhaps the most common is failure to establish rapport and a helping-trust relationship with the other person" (Watson, 1985, p. 24). Watson identified three "carative factors," which determine the quality of any helping relationship: (1) the formation of a humanistic-altruistic value system (ie, kindness, concern, love of self and others); (2) instillation of faith-hope; and (3) the cultivation of sensitivity to one's self and others. Other attitudinal processes the nurse brings to the successful relationship are congruence (genuineness); empathy (the ability to experience the other person's private world and feelings and to communicate this to the other); and nonpossessive warmth (unconditional positive regard).

Goals of the Helping Relationship   The goals of a helping relationship between a nurse and a client are determined cooperatively and are defined in terms of the client's needs. Broadly speaking, common goals might include increased independence for the person, greater feelings of worth, and improved physical well-being. Depending on the goal, the nurse selects nursing care activities that will move the person toward the goal. As the client's needs and goals change, so do the nursing care activities. The nurse also has many needs to be met, but in the helping relationship between the nurse and the client, the nurse's needs are temporarily set aside and the focus is on the client's needs.

Characteristics of the Helping Relationship   The helping relationship is intangible and therefore difficult to describe. However, most authorities agree that it has at least the following three basic characteristics:
- It is dynamic. Both the person providing the assistance and the person being helped are active participants to the extent each is able.
- It is purposeful and time limited. This means there are specific goals that are intended to be met within a certain period.
- The person providing the assistance in a helping relationship assumes the dominant role. The helping person must also assume responsibility for presenting self and his or her helping abilities as honestly as possible and should not convey the idea that he or she can provide more assistance than he or she is capable of offering.

Helping Relationship Versus Social Relationship

The difference between a helping relationship and a friendship must be emphasized. Helping relationships contain many of the qualities of a social relationship. They have in common the components of care, concern, trust, and growth, but they also possess major differences.
- The helping relationship does not occur spontaneously, as do most social relationships. It occurs for a specific purpose with a specific person.
- The helping relationship is characterized by an unequal sharing of information. The client shares information related to personal health problems, whereas the nurse shares information in terms of professional role. In a friendship, information sharing is more likely to be similar in quantity and type.
- The helping relationship is built on the client's needs, not on those of the helping person. In a friendship, needs of both participants are generally considered. A friendship may grow out of a helping relationship, but this is separate from the purposeful, time-limited interaction described as a helping relationship.

The helping relationship is ordinarily described as having three phases: (1) the orientation phase, (2) the working phase, and (3) the termination phase. In the helping relationship, the communication process follows the sequence of the nursing process. Both processes are continuous and reciprocal.

Orientation Phase

Ideally, the helping relationship between a nurse and a client is initiated when the nurse starts the data-gathering part of the nursing process. However, it can also be initiated at other times. In the orientation phase, the tone and guidelines for the relationship are established. The nurse and client meet and learn to identify each other by name. It is especially important that the nurse introduce himself or herself to the client. It may even be helpful for the nurse to write his or her name for the client. Failure to do so may result in the client becoming confused and mistrustful because of the number of health-agency personnel with whom most clients come in contact.

The following activities generally occur during the orientation phase of the helping relationship:
- The roles of both people in the relationship are clarified. It has been observed that a successful relationship is more likely to occur when the responsibilities assigned to each participant are known and accepted and when there is leadership present. In the nurse–client relationship, the nurse, by virtue of role, generally assumes leadership. Leadership does not mean control in the restrictive or manipulative sense but here implies taking the initiative to enlist the client's point of view. When cooperative planning occurs with consideration for the client's needs, the relationship between a nurse and a client is more likely to be mutually satisfactory.

- An agreement or contract about the relationship is established. The agreement is usually a simple verbal exchange or, occasionally, a written document, especially if the relationship extends over a long period. Elements in the agreement include the goals of the relationship; location, frequency, and length of the contacts; and the duration of the relationship. Depending on the purpose of the relationship, the agreement may also include the way in which personal information that the client may divulge will be handled.
- An orientation to the health care agency is provided. The nurse is responsible for seeing that the client is oriented to the health agency, its facilities, admission routines, and so on. The nurse identifies this orientation as one of the goals in the nurse–client helping relationship.

It is critical that trust begin to be established from the outset of the relationship. Some clients may engage in testing behavior, especially if they have had negative experiences in the past in their family or with other health care providers. The nurse's openness to and interest in the concerns of the client pave the way for trust to develop and communicate respect and care.

Working Phase

The working phase is usually the longest phase of the helping relationship. The nurse and the client work together to meet the client's needs. Interaction is the essence of the working phase. The nurse–client interactions that occur at this time are purposeful in that they have been designed to ensure achievement of mutually agreed upon health goals or objectives.

In the working phase, the nurse provides whatever assistance may be needed to achieve each goal. For example, an elderly client has a poor appetite and the goal is to increase food intake. The nurse discusses the idea of small, more frequent meals with the client. With the client's approval, the nurse makes the necessary arrangements. In another instance, a mother explains to a school nurse that she cannot afford dental care recommended for her child, although she would like to have the work done. The nurse asks if a referral to a social agency for financial assistance would be acceptable. With the mother's permission, the nurse contacts the agency.

When sentiments and feelings between people are unsatisfactory, the people often cannot work cooperatively toward achieving a common goal. When sentiments and feelings are satisfactory, the people can usually work together. In the preceding examples, satisfactory sentiments and feelings between the nurse and clients might have been the key aspects. The elderly person's relationship with the nurse may have allowed a positive response to the small, more frequent meals. The mother's feelings about the nurse may have allowed her to accept financial assistance for the dental care without feeling embarrassed.

In addition, the nurse as caregiver provides the client with whatever assistance may be needed to perform activities of daily living. For example, if a client with impaired mobility is unable to get out of bed except to use a bedside commode, the nurse needs to help with daily hygiene.

The nursing roles of teacher and counselor (see Chapter 21) are performed primarily during this phase. These roles involve motivating the client to learn and implement health-promotion activities, to comply with medical treatments such as medication regimens, and to express feelings about health problems, nursing care, any progress or setbacks, and any other areas of concern. This is where the nurse's interpersonal skills are used to their fullest (see the discussions of interpersonal skills and effective communication techniques later in this chapter). A breakdown of the helping relationship on one of these levels could result in serious consequences. For instance, a client began to break clinic appointments, although he had not appeared to lack interest in his health when he began visiting the clinic. When a community health nurse called on the client at home, he said, "The nurse at the clinic seems too busy; she just doesn't seem to care if I come or go. I don't like to go to that clinic." The lack of satisfactory interaction between the nurse and the client discouraged him from continuing the relationship, even at the expense of his health. Had the nurse–client interaction been satisfactory, breaking appointments probably would not have been a problem.

Satisfactory interaction preserves the integrity of people while promoting an atmosphere characterized by minimal fear, anxiety, distrust, and tension. People feel harmonious and contented with each other as they work cooperatively to reach common goals.

Termination Phase

The termination phase occurs when the conclusion of the initial agreement is acknowledged. This may happen at change-of-shift time, when the client is discharged, or when a nurse leaves on vacation or for employment elsewhere. The client and nurse examine the goals of the helping relationship for indications of their attainment or for evidence of progress toward the goals. If the goals have been reached, this fact should be acknowledged. Such acknowledgement generally results in a feeling of satisfaction for both the client and nurse. If the goals have not been reached, the progress can be acknowledged and either the client or the nurse may make suggestions for future efforts.

There ordinarily are feelings associated with the termination of a helping relationship. If the goals have been met, there is often regret about ending a satisfying relationship, even though a sense of accomplishment persists. If the goals have not been completely achieved, the client may experience anxiety and fear about the future. Whatever the feelings, the client should be encouraged to express emotions about the termination.

The nurse can prepare for the termination of the helping relationship in various ways. The thoughtful nurse can set the stage for the client to establish a helping relationship with another nurse, if appropriate. The nurse can assist the client transferring from one agency to another or from one unit in an agency to another by offering explanations concerning the transfer. In some instances, the nurse may introduce the client to personnel who will be giving care.

Occasionally, termination of the helping relationship produces emotional reactions. The client may feel angry, rejected by the nurse, or depressed and helpless, or may deny that a relationship ever really existed. Should such reactions occur, the nurse should help and support the client rather than impose feelings of guilt or wrong for having these views. However, emotional reactions of this sort are less likely to occur if the client has been involved in establishing goals and has been helped to anticipate termination of the helping relationship.

Table 20-1 summarizes goals for clients during the three phases of an effective helping relationship. Those wishing to explore the topic of interpersonal relations in nursing more fully are referred to the classic works of nursing theorists Orlando (1961), Paterson and Zderad (1976), Peplau (1952), Travelbee (1971), and Watson (1985).

Development of Communication Skills

Another basic characteristic of communication is that exchanging messages requires knowledge. Part of the knowledge provided by nursing education is developing communication skills. Although humans use communication all of their waking moments, the therapeutic use of communication requires training and practice. As students realize the importance of communication in helping relationships, they may feel awkward at first and feel the relationships are contrived. But as the merits of effective communication become evident through practice, nurses will feel more at ease with the process.

Effective Communication Techniques

Communication takes on many forms depending on the situation in which the communication occurs. If effective techniques are used appropriately, nurses can enhance the quality and purpose of any communication. At no time, however, should nurses put techniques of communication above the nurse–client relationship.

Conversational Skills

A good place to start is with conversation. *Conversation*, or the exchange of verbal communication, is a social interaction. As social beings, humans learn as children how to converse with others. Therefore, a person coming into nursing has had years of experience in communicating verbally. Even though this is the case, nurses can improve their communications with clients and achieve a more effective helping relationship by considering the following points:

- Control the tone of your voice so you are conveying exactly what you mean to say and not a hidden message. The nurse's tone should indicate an interest in the client and not boredom, patience and not anger, acceptance and not hostility, and so forth.
- Be knowledgeable about the topic of conversation and have accurate information. When possible, the nurse should be familiar with the subject of conversation before discussing it with the client. If the topic is an unfamiliar one, it is best to tell the client so. Convey confidence and honesty.
- Be flexible. The nurse may have selected to discuss a subject but learns the client wishes to discuss something else. It is better to follow the client's lead whenever possible. In due time, the nurse can return to the subject. For example, the nurse arrives at the client's bedside to administer a medication, but the client begins to talk about his or her diet. It is better to take a little time to allow the client to speak rather than to insist on carrying out a procedure when the time taken for the conversation is not contraindicated.
- Be clear and concise, and make statements as simple as possible. Clients are often anxious and will fail to receive the nurse's message unless the conversation is geared to a level the client understands. Stay on one subject at a time and say words concisely.
- Avoid words that may be interpreted differently. The study of the meaning of words is called **semantics**.

T A B L E 2 0 - 1

Summary of Client Goals for the Three Phases of the Helping Relationship		
Orientation Phase	**Working Phase**	**Termination**
The client will call the nurse by name.	The client will actively participate in the relationship.	The client will participate in identifying the goals accomplished or the progress made toward goals.
The client will accurately describe the roles of the participants in the relationship.	The client will cooperate in activities that work toward achieving mutually acceptable goals.	The client will verbalize feelings about the termination of the relationship.
The client and nurse will establish an agreement about: • Goals of the relationship • Location, frequency, and length of the contacts • Duration of the relationship	The client will express feelings and concerns to the nurse.	

Even when two people speak the same language, some words such as *love, hate, freedom*, and *liberty*—may have different meanings.

- Be truthful. The client will soon distrust the nurse if given false information. Admit not knowing and seek an answer rather than make a comment that is likely to be an error.
- Keep an open mind. An attitude of "I know better than the client" is quickly discerned by the client. Clients can make valuable contributions to their own health care.
- Take advantage of available opportunities. During most caregiving situations, the nurse can facilitate conversation that will make even the most routine task meaningful. For instance, when giving a bed bath to a client, a nurse can introduce the topic of the client's employment. This would allow the client to verbalize any positive or negative feelings about the job and the temporary absence from it. This could reduce the anxiety that often occurs with the loss of work. It is often comforting to know that someone understands and cares.

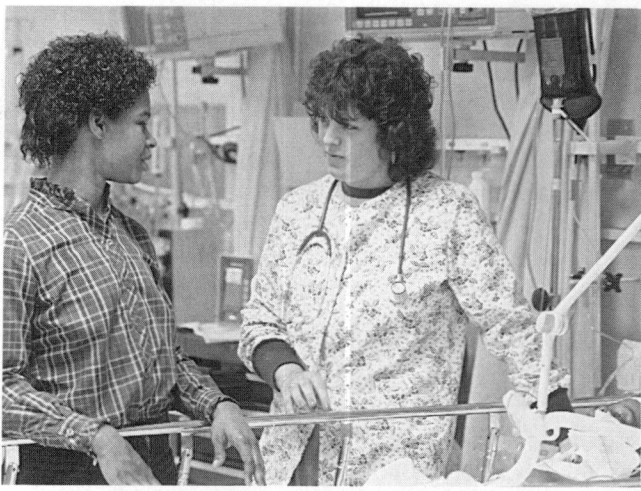

F I G U R E   2 0 - 5

Listening attentively, with concentration and genuine concern is key to productive communication. (Photo by Gates Rhodes, courtesy of School of Nursing, University of Pennsylvania.)

Listening Skills

Listening is a skill that involves both hearing and interpreting what is said. It requires attention and concentration to sort out, evaluate, and validate clues so that a person better understands the true meanings in what is being said. Listening requires concentrating on the client and what is being said (Fig. 20-5). The following recommended techniques may help improve listening skills:

- Whenever possible, sit when communicating with a client. Do not cross arms or legs; to do so is a type of body language that conveys a message of being closed to the client's comments.
- Be alert but relaxed, and take sufficient time so that the client feels at ease during the conversation. Keep the conversation as natural as possible, and avoid sounding overly eager.
- If culturally appropriate, maintain eye contact with the client, without staring, in a face-to-face pose. This technique conveys interest in the conversation and willingness to listen.
- Indicate that you are paying attention to what the client is saying by using appropriate facial expressions and body gestures. Be attentive to both verbal and nonverbal communication.
- Think before responding to the client. Responding impulsively tends to disrupt communication and listening.
- Do not pretend to listen. It is the rare client who is insensitive to an attitude of feigned attention, or to boredom and apathy.
- Listen for themes in the client's comments. Consider the following questions to help detect themes: What are the repeated themes in the person's speech and behavior? What topics does the client tend to avoid?

What subjects tend to make the client shift the conversation to other subjects? What inconsistencies and gaps appear in the client's conversation?

Use of Silence

The nurse can use silence appropriately by taking the time to wait for the client to initiate or continue speaking. During periods of silence, the nurse has the opportunity to observe the client without having to concentrate simultaneously on the spoken word.

Periods of silence during communication can carry a variety of meanings, including the following:

- The client may be demonstrating comfort and contentment in the nurse–client relationship. Continuous talking is unnecessary.
- The client may be trying to demonstrate stoicism and the ability to cope without help.
- The client may be exploring inner feelings, and conversation would disrupt these thoughts. In this situation, the client is really saying, "I need some time to think."
- The client may be fearful and use silence as an escape from a threat.

In due time, silence may be discussed with the client, especially if the nurse wishes to validate any speculation about its meaning. Fear of silence sometimes leads to too much talking by the nurse. Also, excessive talking tends to place the focus on the nurse rather than on the client.

Interviewing Techniques

The purpose of any interview is to obtain accurate and thorough information. In nursing, the interview is a major tool for collecting data during the assessment step of the

It was my first day of clinical rotation and I was assigned to Mr. Anderson, who was in his early nineties. He was in the hospital because he had had a second heart attack. Mr. Anderson had lived alone for 5 years after the death of his wife. He wanted to remain independent, but his daughter, who was herself in her late sixties, and his doctor believed that he would not be able to function well on his own any longer. Mr. Anderson was distressed about this belief.

Because it was my first day and, unlike some of my classmates, I had never worked in a hospital before, I felt insecure and nervous. There really wasn't a lot of work for us to do. We weren't allowed to give medication yet and my client was pretty self-sufficient. Because my skills were shaky, I took my time taking vital signs, assisted Mr. Anderson with his bath and toileting, and made his bed. After checking his chart, I began my nursing interview with him. I was overjoyed to discover that he was a real talker! His memory was tremendous—either that or he was a great improvisor! He recalled stories about his childhood and his wife with great detail and emotion. He smiled and laughed when he spoke of his daughter and grandchildren. He told me about his daughter's childhood illnesses as well as his own. We talked about the Depression and world wars and about music and art and education. He asked me about my family and I felt like I had made a friend.

The next day Mr. Anderson told me about his fears. He talked about losing his wife, about his health and body deteriorating, and about losing his independence and home. He despised having to be sent to a nursing home and having to depend on others. It hurt him a lot and made me sad. Mr. Anderson left on my second day, and as I said goodbye I wished I could do something for him.

I thought about him a lot since then and I've come to realize that in those 2 days that I knew Mr. Anderson, I did do something for him besides washing him and changing his sheets. I listened to him. Although his family had little time for him and the doctors quickly flew in and out of the room, I let him talk and heard all he said, both in words and in his eyes. He will always be a good memory for me.

—Kristina Hofmeister, Holy Family College, Philadelphia

nursing process (see Chapter 15). Consequently, every nurse needs to become proficient in the use of the communication techniques described previously, as well as in interviewing techniques, which are specifically designed to gather and validate information.

All interviews should be started with an explanation of the purpose of the interview. During the interview, the various interviewing techniques are used to obtain the information needed while remaining flexible in approach. The interview itself is a therapeutic interaction and may be an essential part of the orientation phase of the helping relationship. At the end of the interview, plans for further interactions can be made. The following interviewing techniques are useful in nearly all nurse–client interactions, especially the interview.

Open-Ended Question or Comment When obtaining a nursing history, the nurse uses this technique to allow the client a wide range of possible responses. It encourages free verbalization. The greatest advantage of this tech-

nique is that it prevents the client from answering with a simple yes or no. Consider the following example of an open-ended question and the response:

> *Nurse:* What did your doctor tell you about your need for this hospitalization?
>
> *Client:* He told me that my blood pressure is dangerously high and that I need some special tests done while I am here.

This open-ended question by the nurse allows the client to express what he or she understands to be true and yet is specific enough to prevent side-tracking from the issue at hand—the client's hospital admission. The nurse could continue with an open-ended comment such as

> *Nurse:* Yes . . . and . . .
>
> *Client:* Well, he thinks I could need a change in my blood pressure medicine too.

Now, the nurse has even more information from the client and can continue to seek more information. This should be done in a way that does not make the client feel as though the nurse is prying or probing.

Closed Question or Comment This technique allows limited choices in possible responses. It is used to gather specific information from a client and allows the nurse and client to focus on a particular area. The following is an example:

Nurse: What medicines have you been taking at home?
Client: Let me see, my doctor gave me a water pill and a blood pressure pill to take every day.

This technique gives the nurse the exact response that is being sought. Care should be taken to avoid the overuse of closed questions and comments because of the limiting effects they have on the client's responses.

Validating Question or Comment This type of question or comment serves to validate what the nurse believes is heard or observed. To continue the example used in the previous technique, the nurse could validate what was said as follows:

Nurse: At home you have been taking both a water pill and a blood pressure pill every day. Did you take them today?
Client: Yes. I took one of each with my breakfast.

The nurse is able to ascertain that the client has been taking the medication regularly, as well as the correct dosage that day. However, the overuse of questions and comments to validate information may lead the client to suspect that the nurse is not listening.

Clarifying Question or Comment By using this technique, a nurse can try to gain an understanding of a client's comment. An example follows:

Client: I have never needed to take medicine before in my life.
Nurse: Is this the first health problem you have had?
Client: Yes, I've always been healthy.

The overuse of this technique can lead the client to believe that the nurse is not listening or is unknowledgeable. However, when used appropriately, it can prevent possible misconceptions that could lead to inappropriate nursing diagnosis. For instance, by clarifying what the client's (in the example) health has been previously, the nurse can plan for what teaching will be necessary after a thorough assessment of what the client knows about his or her blood pressure problem (see Chapter 21).

Reflective Question or Comment This technique involves repeating what the person has said or describing feelings. It serves to encourage the client to elaborate on thoughts and feelings. An example of this technique follows:

Client: I've been really upset about my blood pressure and having to take these pills.
Nurse: You've been upset . . .
Client: I guess I'm worried about what could happen if my blood pressure gets too bad.

By saying this, the nurse has encouraged the client to expand this topic by expressing a more specific concern. Again, like previous techniques, the overuse of the reflec-

tive technique and using it mechanically may lead the client to believe the nurse is not listening or is uninterested.

Sequencing Question or Comment Sequencing is used to place events in chronologic order or to investigate a possible cause-and-effect relationship between events. This technique is evident in the following example:

Client: I don't feel like myself anymore since I've been taking my blood pressure medicine. I'm tired and don't have any energy.
Nurse: Your tiredness began after you started taking your medicine?

This type of question could lead to a possible contributing factor to the client's problem. Nursing assessment is facilitated when events leading to a problem are placed in sequence.

Directing Question or Comment It may become necessary at times to obtain more information about a certain subject brought up earlier in the interview or to introduce a new aspect of the current subject. In such an instance, the nurse can attempt to direct the client to the subject by using a technique similar to the following:

Client: Before I knew that I had high blood pressure, I was very active. I felt good at work and at home. I think the medicine is making me tired.
Nurse: When did your doctor start you on your current medication?
Client: I've been on them for 6 weeks.
Nurse: Have you been told about eating foods high in potassium when on this medication?
Client: My doctor gave me some special diet to follow, but I haven't looked at it. I hate diets.

In this way, the nurse has gained valuable information to consider in assessing the client's health status and educational needs.

Use of Touch

Because of the personal nature of touching, a nurse needs to weigh the beneficial versus the detrimental use of touch for each client. Touch can be a powerful therapeutic tool when used at the right time. However, anxiety or discomfort may result when a client does not understand the meaning of a tactile gesture or when the client simply dislikes being touched.

Touch is the most highly developed sense at birth. Tactile experiences of infants and young children appear essential for the normal development of self and awareness of others. It has also been found that many elderly people long for touch, especially when isolated from loved ones because of hospitalization or nursing home care. Many older people have no living family to provide them with the caring touch so necessary for the sense of well-being. In such an instance, a nurse can provide some special care by holding the client's hand (Fig. 20-6).

Many situations require the nurse to touch the client while implementing nursing care. Physical closeness be-

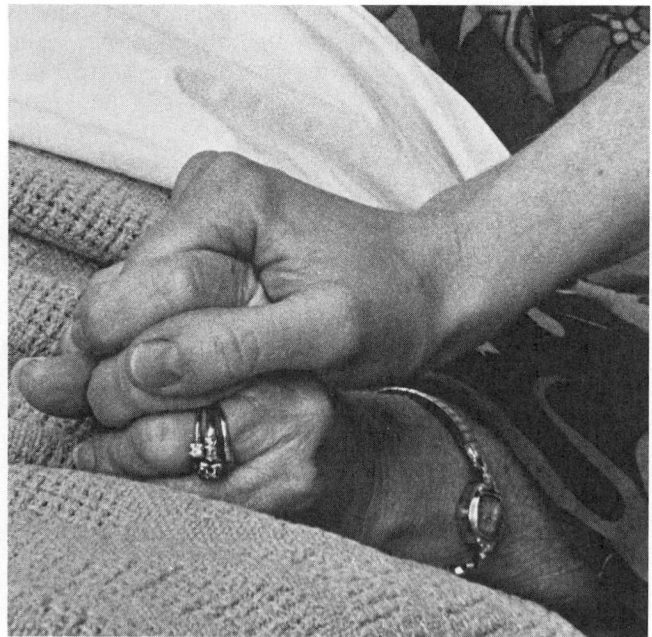

FIGURE 20-6

A reassuring handclasp uses touch to convey a message. Sometimes touch can be a more effective way of expressing concern and interest than verbal communication.

tween the client and the nurse is essential and inevitable. Therefore, every nurse needs to become comfortable with the judicious use of this nonverbal communication technique, so that security, rather than anxiety, will be promoted. Dexterity and sureness in the use of the hands help to assure the client of the nurse's expertise when measuring a blood pressure or giving an injection.

Interest has been growing in the phenomenon known as therapeutic touch. **Therapeutic touch** involves "unruffling," or unblocking, congested areas of energy in the body and redirecting this energy. After assessing a person's "energy field," the nurse uses therapeutic touch to promote comfort, relaxation, healing, and a sense of well-being in the client. Many nurses are studying therapeutic touch in nursing educational programs and through special courses or workshops. It is becoming a widely accepted form of therapy as well as a subject for nursing research.

Use of Humor

Humor has come to be increasingly valued in recent years as both an interpersonal skill for the nurse and as a healing strategy for clients. Nurses who are able to use humor effectively to maintain a balanced perspective in their work and to encourage clients to do the same have a valuable tool. Nurses with a sense of humor are able to laugh at themselves and to accept their failures, to confront the absurdities in everyday practice without falling apart, and to challenge clients to situate their current dilemma within the context of their bigger life experiences. Laughter releases excess physical and psychologic energy and it reduces stress, anxiety, worry, and frustration. Humor, like other interpersonal competencies, is a learned skill. When used inappropriately it can be destructive. Inexperienced nurses may find it helpful to identify nurses who use humor well and to "try on" behaviors they observe.

Interpersonal Skills

The skills required for positive relationships between people are referred to as **interpersonal skills**. In nursing, these

RESEARCH IN NURSING Making a Difference

Nonprocedural and Therapeutic Touch

Fisher, L., & Joseph, D. H. (1989). A scale to measure attitude about nonprocedural touch. *Canadian Journal of Nursing Research, 21*(2), 5–14.

Although nonprocedural touch is of major importance in nurse–client relationships, little has been done to investigate the client's attitude toward this form of touch. The authors designed a descriptive pilot study (convenience sample of 52) to develop and test an instrument to measure hospitalized clients' attitudes toward nursing use of nonprocedural touch. A 15-item Likert-type scale was used to determine if clients feel comforted emotionally by touch, feel comforted physically by touch, and value touch that is separate from required nursing care that involves touch. Data clearly demonstrated that clients

hold a positive attitude toward nonprocedural touch.

Heidt, P. R. (1990). Openness: A qualitative analysis of nurses' and patients' experiences of therapeutic touch. *Image: Journal of Nursing Scholarship 22*(3), 180–186.

Grounded theory was generated to explain the process of therapeutic touch for seven nurses and seven clients in the study. Opening to the flow of universal life energy was identified as the primary experience of therapeutic touch. The investigator invited further research on therapeutic touch using qualitative methodology to deepen an understanding of the inner experiences of both clients and nurses to experiences that facilitate the healing process.

skills are essential to the promotion of a nurse–client relationship that will be therapeutic for the client.

Warmth and Friendliness The helping relationship depends on the nurse's ability to begin the orientation phase successfully. A pleasant greeting accompanied by a smile can facilitate the initiation of this phase and allow the client to relax in the nurse's presence. By maintaining the qualities of warmth and friendliness throughout the helping relationship, the nurse conveys continuous acceptance of the client and interest in discussing the client's feelings and concerns.

Openness A person who is open conveys an attitude of acceptance, frankness, and lack of prejudice. This is an important quality for a nurse, because a client who feels the nurse is judging could hold back significant information. The nurse must also be open to supporting the client's strengths and promoting the client's growth.

Empathy Empathy is intellectually identifying with the way that another person feels. An empathic nurse is sensitive to the client's feelings and problems but remains objective enough to help the client work toward positive outcomes. A nurse who retains this quality can establish successful helping relationships without becoming the cold and stern nurse frequently portrayed in films and television.

Olson and Iwasiw (1989) investigated whether differences exist in staff nurses' verbal empathy in response to clients who experience pain, depression, anxiety, and anger. Analysis of 528 situations revealed that nurses most frequently identified the feelings of pain and anger and most frequently attempted to suppress the feelings of anxiety and anger. Further research is needed to identify strategies to help nurses develop empathic responses to depression, anxiety, and anger.

Competence Competent nurses are skilled in all aspects of nursing and are capable of meeting their client's health care needs through the use of technical, intellectual, and interpersonal skills. Nurses are responsible for evaluating their own strengths and for strengthening any weaknesses so that all clients will receive optimal care. Consequently, the clients develop trust in and respect for their nurses, facilitating helping relationships.

Consideration of Client Variables Nurses need to develop sensitivity to the variables presented by each client and the effects these factors have on communication. Attention to the following client variables can make the difference between effective and ineffective interactions.

Non–English-Speaking Clients Caring for non–English-speaking clients is common in many health care settings. If a particular non–English-speaking group is prominent in the community, nurses should learn some basic phrases in the language of that group (ie, phrases regarding eating, hygiene, elimination, or comfort). Language dictionaries are available that deal with commonly used phrases in health care settings. Such books should be made available on all nursing units. Many hospitals also keep lists of any personnel who speak second languages so that they may be used as translators when needed. This topic is discussed again at the end of this chapter.

Developmental Considerations It is imperative for nurses to understand the development of language as well as the intellectual and psychosocial developmental stages so they can communicate appropriately with clients of all ages. (These stages are presented in Chapters 10 and 11.) Knowing how each age group commonly perceives health, illness, and body functions guides nurses in their interactions with their clients. For instance, a 10-year-old child has a limited understanding of what an infection is and the nurse must explain this in simple terms so that the child cooperates with the treatment without being frightened. A teenager should be developing abstract thinking, so more detailed and accurate explanations can be given. Being familiar with commonly used slang usually helps nurses when communicating with teenagers. Communicating with adults can be complicated by many years of negative health-related experiences and inaccurate information. Nurses communicating with elderly clients must assess for any problems with hearing; sight (discussed later in this chapter); confusion; or depression, all of which could affect nurse–client interactions.

Sociocultural Differences Nurses need to develop skills in recognizing where a person is coming from in terms of cultural practices and economic influences, as well as personal habits or addictions. As an example, nurses working with expectant mothers must be familiar with street language so that they can determine whether the mothers have taken drugs during pregnancy, which affect the developing fetus. Also, because women in some cultures may speak of personal things only to their significant others, maternity nurses may have to talk with the client's partner about the postdelivery care that the mother is to receive.

It is best to use lay terminology when speaking with clients unless a client is known to be a health care professional. Use of medical terminology (ie, myocardial infarction for heart attack, cerebrovascular accident for stroke, or cholecystectomy for gallbladder operation) usually alienates clients and can inhibit further communication.

Occupation What a person does for a living gives a nurse a general idea of the person's skills, talents, interests, and economic status. However, stereotyping a person according to occupation can be misleading and should be avoided.

Assertive Skills

When interacting with clients, family members, other nurses, physicians, and other members of the health care team, it is important for nurses to communicate in a way that demonstrates respect for all parties in the communication. Assertive behaviors, which are one hallmark of professional nursing relationships, need to be distinguished from aggressive (ie, harsh, injurious, or destructive) and avoidance or acquiescent behaviors—both of which are the opposite of true assertive behavior. Chenevert (1983) equated learning to be assertive with learning to stand up for yourself and your clients, learning to trust your feelings and respect your opinions, and learning to like yourself. The key to assertiveness is open, honest, and direct communication. "I" statements, "I feel . . ." and "I think . . ." play an important role in assertive statements. See the accompanying display for examples of assertive and nonassertive speech.

Four basic components of the assertive response or approach are as follows: (1) empathic component, (2) description of feelings or situation, (3) expectation, and (4) consequences (Angel & Petronko, 1983). For example, the student who is feeling overwhelmed by her weekly clinical assignments may communicate the following to her instructor:

Empathy: "I guess it must be hard for you to make our clinical assignments each week and to know what each one of us needs."

Description: "I have to share with you that right now I feel so overwhelmed that I go home from clinical in tears each week."

Expectation: "I am wondering if we could talk about this. I am willing to work hard but I seem to need some help pulling everything together."

Consequences: "I expect to do well in clinical but I am afraid that if things continue the way they are right now, I may not last the semester. I would appreciate any help you can give me."

Characteristics of the assertive nurse's self-presentation include a confident, open body posture; eye contact; use of clear, concise "I" statements; and the ability to honestly share thoughts, feelings, and emotions. The assertive nurse's attitude toward work is characterized by working to capacity with or without supervision, the ability to remain calm under supervision, freedom to ask for help when necessary, the ability to give and accept compliments, and honesty in admitting mistakes and taking responsibility for them. Table 20-2 highlights some of the advantages and disadvantages of nonassertive and assertive behavior. Readers interested in developing assertive skills will find specific instructions, test situations, and assertive evaluation criteria in handbooks by Angel and Petronko (1983), Chenevert (1983), and Clark (1978).

Factors Promoting Effective Communication

In addition to the interpersonal and effective communication skills discussed, it is helpful for the nurse to consider several other factors that can affect the helping relationship. Controlling these factors helps promote what is referred to as a good **rapport**, which is a feeling of mutual trust experienced by people in a satisfactory relationship (Fig. 20-7).

Illustrations of Assertive and Nonassertive Speech

	Assertive	Nonassertive
Nurse to nurse	"I know we all lose track of time occasionally but I'm finding it harder and harder to cover for you when you take extra time for lunch. I don't think it's fair for your clients and I to have to wait an extra 30 minutes every day for you to come back from lunch. Can we talk about this?"	"Huh? No, I didn't really mind. Luckily I wasn't too busy today." Thought: "What a sucker I am. Now I'll have to grab a quick bite so that I can get back to the unit in time to do 2 PM treatments."
Nurse to physician	"I know we talked about Mr. Esposito's pain medication before but I've collected some new data. Even with the change in dosage he is only getting 1 to 1½ hours of relief. I believe a different analgesic agent might work better for him."	"Um . . . yes I know you already changed the dosage. It's just that I thought it still wasn't working. Maybe I didn't give it enough time. Thanks for listening to me anyway. I'm sorry to bother you with this."
Student nurse to preceptor	"Miss Cheng has a new order to be straight cathed. I reviewed the procedure but I'd sure appreciate your talking me through this because I've never done it before and I'm terrified."	"Uh . . . I'm sorry to be such a pain again. I have to do this cath and don't know where to begin. I know you must be busy, but, uh, is there any way you might have time for me?"

T A B L E   2 0 - 2

Advantages and Disadvantages of Assertive and Nonassertive Behavior		
Assertive Behavior	**Nonassertive (Passive) Behavior**	
Advantages	Advantages	Disadvantages
Increased sense of personal integrity and self-worth	"Comfortable" maintenance of status quo	Decreased sense of personal integrity and self-worth
Resolution of conflict	Avoidance of conflict (and thereby hostility and rejection)	No resolution of problem causing inner turmoil
Personal growth: independence, honesty, decision making	Avoidance of responsibility	Increased anxiety and stress and decreased health
Increased leadership ability	Commendation for being a team player (not rocking the boat)	Decreased sense of control (increased dependence)
		Increased feelings of inadequacy and insecurity → aggressive behavior

Specific Objectives Having a purpose for an interaction guides the nurse toward achieving a meaningful encounter with the client. One objective might be to do a quick head-to-toe physical assessment while greeting the client at the beginning of a shift. Another objective might be to discuss a client's feelings about newly diagnosed diabetes. The shortest encounter with a client can have an objective, even if it is as simple as conveying a feeling of friendliness to the client. Flexibility is essential at all times. Cues from the client should be followed to work toward meeting all needs.

F I G U R E   2 0 - 7

This nurse and young client are sharing an enjoyable moment. The nurse has established a rapport with the child, and they share a mutual trust. (Photo by Gates Rhodes, courtesy of School of Nursing, University of Pennsylvania.)

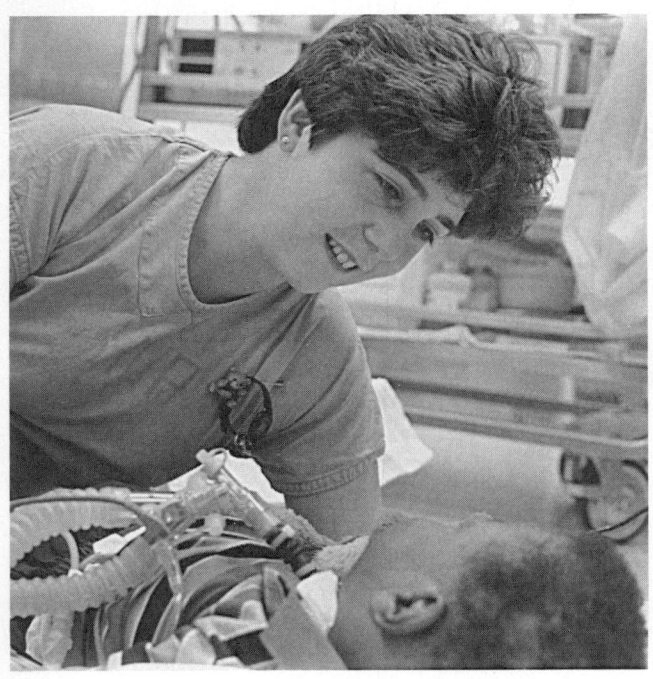

Comfortable Environment A comfortable environment, in which both the client and the nurse are at ease, helps to promote interactions. Such items as suitable furniture, proper lighting, and a moderate temperature are important. Also, effective relationships are enhanced when the atmosphere is relaxed and unhurried. If the nurse seems preoccupied and on the run, or if the client is ill at ease for fear of missing visitors or because of another commitment, communications are impaired.

Privacy It may not always be possible to carry out conversations with just the client and the nurse in a room. However, every effort should be made to provide sufficient privacy so that conversations cannot be overheard by others. Sometimes merely drawing the curtains around the bed or sitting in a corner of a waiting room or lounge can provide the sense of privacy so necessary for most interactions.

Confidentiality The confidentiality with which the information is to be treated should be established with the client. The nurse should indicate with whom the information the client gives will be shared. The client should know about the right to specify the people who may have access to the information. Failure to take this factor into account can be considered a breach of the client's right to privacy.

Client Focus Communication in the nurse–client relationship should focus on the client and the client's needs, not on the nurse or an activity in which the nurse is engaged. Consider the following example, in which the nurse's comment focuses on the client and the client's needs:

   Client: I don't know why these injections scare me, but they do.
   Nurse: You are afraid of these injections?

Now consider this example, in which the nurse's comment focuses on a nursing activity:

   Client: I don't know why these injections scare me, but they do.
   Nurse: Let's hurry and get this shot done. Then you won't have time to worry.

Use of Nursing Observations *Observation*, which involves both seeing and interpreting, is especially useful for validating information. For example, a nurse suspected that a client was afraid to hear the results of certain blood tests, but the client kept saying that the tests were unimportant. However, the nurse observed the client pacing in the corridor while appearing to be in deep thought. Observing the client's behavior helped validate the nurse's clue that the client was possibly fearful, and the client's assertion that he or she was unconcerned appeared to be a cover-up for true feelings.

Observation serves several important purposes:

- It helps the nurse become aware of nonverbal messages the client is sending.
- It serves as the primary source of information when a client is unable or unwilling to communicate verbally.
- It demonstrates caring and an interest in the client. (Clients often recognize when a nurse is unobservant and, rightly or wrongly, usually conclude that the nurse does not care.)

Optimal Pacing A nurse must consider the pace of any conversation or encounter with a client. For instance, it would be ineffective if the nurse rushed through a list of questions when obtaining a nursing history. It is more effective to let the client set the pace. The nurse can let the client know at the beginning of the interaction if time is limited. This way, the client will not feel that the nurse is rushing because of a lack of concern or personal interest.

Providing Personal Space Perceptions of personal space vary. Nurses must try to determine each client's perception of personal space because invasion of one's personal space can evoke uncomfortable feelings. Nurses can assess a client's personal space through careful observations of nonverbal communication. For example, some people like to be close to the person with whom they are speaking. They may also use touch during their conversations and seem comfortable with others in close proximity. Others back away from close encounters or become nervous when their personal space is invaded. It is important for nurses to be sensitive to personal space so that their clients feel comfortable during interactions.

Blocks to Communication

Failure to Perceive the Client as a Human Clients report that nothing is more discomforting than to be treated as an object of care rather than as Ms. Jan Bennett who happens to be undergoing surgery on her colon. What distinguishes nursing from other health professions is focus on the whole person, not just the illness or dysfunction.

Failure to Listen Clients may or may not feel able to speak freely to the nurse. Often the signs that they give indicating their readiness to talk are subtle. Nurses who walk into a client room with their own agenda and mind closed to the client's needs may miss valuable opportunities for important communication.

Inappropriate Comments and Questions Certain types of comments and questions should be avoided in most situations because they tend to impede effective communications. A description of each type follows.

Using Clichés A *cliché* is a stereotyped, trite, or pat answer. Most clichés tend to indicate that there is no cause for anxiety or concern, or they offer false assurance. Their use tends to be interpreted as a lack of real interest in what has been said. The only purpose a cliché serves is to break the ice when conversation begins. For example, even though the common question, ''How are you?'' could start a conversation, it can cause a problem if the person has reason to suspect that the nurse is not sincerely interested in how the client feels. The following are some commonly used clichés that are usually best left unsaid, because they tend to impede effective communications:

''Everything will be all right.''
''Don't worry. You will be just fine in another day or two.''
''Your doctor knows best.''
''Cheer up. Tomorrow is another day.''

Another type of cliché makes a sweeping generalization that does not necessarily apply to a specific client. It also tends to cut off communications and makes the person feel as though he or she is just another insignificant being. Consider the following examples:

''Men tolerate pain poorly. That must be why you are complaining of such severe pain.''
''Everybody is afraid of surgery. Why should you be any different?''
''You teenagers are all alike. You aren't being cooperative because you want to defy authority.''

Such comments rarely promote communication with clients to whom they are addressed.

Using Questions Requiring Only a Yes or No Answer Questions that can be answered by simply saying yes or no tend to cut off discussion, even when the person might wish to continue. Consider the following question:

Nurse: Did you have a good day?

The question almost begs for a noncommittal answer, which tells the nurse little. A better way to comment is as follows:

Nurse: Tell me about the kind of day you have had.

Another pitfall is to pose a question to which the client can say no when his or her answer could present a problem. Consider the following question that a nurse asks a postoperative client:

Nurse: Are you ready to get out of bed?

By offering the client the chance to say no, the nurse may have created difficulties if the client is to be out of bed.

There are times when questions that can be answered with yes or no are legitimate. The following are examples:

Nurse: Did you take your insulin before breakfast this morning?
Nurse: Do you have pain when I move your arm this way?

The problem arises when the nurse is seeking more detailed information or when the question may create difficulty.

Using Questions Containing the Words *Why* and *How*
Questions using *why* and *how* tend to be intimidating. Consider the following questions:

Nurse: Why were you not tired enough to sleep?

Nurse: How did you ever decide to go on a crash diet?

These two questions would be better stated as follows:

Nurse: What were you doing while you were unable to sleep?

Nurse: What things prompted you to decide to go on a crash diet?

Using Questions That Probe for Information Questions that appear to probe for information tend to cut off communication. Clients who are made to feel as though they are receiving the third degree become resentful and will usually stop talking and try to avoid further conversation. Although the nurse may feel more information is needed, it is better to follow the client's lead. Letting the client take the initiative allows the nurse to delve more deeply at a time when the client is ready. The person who says, "Let's get to the bottom of this" is likely to destroy conversation unless the client is ready to face the real cause of the problem.

Using Leading Questions A leading question suggests a response that the speaker wishes to hear. Leading questions tend to produce answers that may please the nurse but are unlikely to encourage the client to respond without feeling intimidated. Consider the following examples:

Nurse: You aren't going to smoke that cigarette, are you?

Nurse: You have been well cared for by your nurses, haven't you?

These questions beg the client to give an answer that pleases the nurse rather than to express thoughts.

Using Comments That Give Advice Giving the client advice often implies that the nurse knows what is best for the client and denies the client the right to make decisions and have feelings. Giving advice also tends to increase the client's dependence on health caregivers. However, advice does have a rightful place when it is requested, and the person giving the advice may have expert knowledge that the client does not.

Using Judgmental Comments Using judgmental comments tends to impose the nurse's standards on the client.

G U I D E L I N E S   F O R   N U R S I N G   C A R E

Communicating in Special Circumstances

Clients Who Are Visually Impaired

- Acknowledge your presence in the client's room.
- Identify yourself by name.
- Remember that the visually impaired client will be unable to pick up most nonverbal cues during communication. Speak in a normal tone of voice.
- Explain the reason for touching the client before doing so.
- Indicate to the client when the conversation has ended and when you are leaving the room.
- Keep a call light or bell within easy reach of the client.
- Orient the client to the sounds in the environment and to the arrangement of the room and its furnishings.

Clients Who Are Hearing Impaired

- Orient the client to your presence before initiating conversation. This may be done by gently touching the client or moving so you can be seen.
- Talk directly to the client while facing him or her. If the client is able to lip read, use simple sentences and speak in a quiet, natural manner and pace. Be aware of nonverbal communication.
- Do not chew gum or cover your mouth when talking with the client.
- Demonstrate or pantomime ideas you wish to express, as appropriate.
- Use sign language or finger spelling, as appropriate.

- Write any ideas that you cannot convey to the client in another manner.

An Unconscious Client

- Be careful of what is said in the client's presence. Hearing is believed to be the last sense lost, and therefore the unconscious client is often likely to hear even though there is no apparent response.
- Assume the client can hear you. Talk in a normal tone of voice about things you would ordinarily discuss.
- Speak with the client before touching. Remember that touch can be an effective means of communication with the unconscious client.
- Keep environment noises at as low a level as possible. This helps the client focus on the communication.

Clients Who Speak a Foreign Language

- Use an interpreter whenever possible.
- Use a dictionary that translates words from one language to another so that you can speak at least some words in the client's language.
- Speak in simple sentences and in a normal tone of voice.
- Demonstrate or pantomime ideas you wish to convey, as appropriate.
- Be aware of nonverbal communication. Remember that many nonverbal communication cues are universal.

Consider the comment of a nurse who noted that a young woman was crying:

Nurse: You aren't acting very grown-up. How do you think your husband would feel if he saw you crying like this?

The nurse judged the client as being immature, and the apparent hostility could end effective communication. A better comment in this situation might be as follows:

Nurse: I would like to help. Tell me what causes you to cry.

Consider the following exchange between a nurse and a client about to have surgery:

Client: I think I have a right to be afraid of this operation.

Nurse: Tell me what has made you afraid.

This client is likely to feel safe when allowed to express feelings without being judged.

Changing the Subject A quick way to stop conversation is by changing the subject. The client may be at a point of readiness to discuss something and can be expected to feel frustrated if put off by a change in the topic of conversation. The following example illustrates:

Client: When can I expect to be told about taking my own insulin?

Nurse: Let's discuss your diet now so that you will know what to eat when you get home. We can discuss your insulin some other time.

A nurse may also change the subject when feeling uncomfortable about the topic of conversation. For example, the client's needs are being met when the nurse allows the client to speak of impending death, thoughts of suicide, or a contemplated abortion. The nurse is ignoring the client when the subject is changed to meet the nurse's own needs.

Giving False Assurance It is easier and more pleasant to deal with positive outcomes than with negative ones. Through comments, the nurse may sometimes try to convince the client that things are going to turn out well even when knowing the chances are not good. False assurance leaves many clients with the impression that the nurse is not interested in their problems. Clichés are frequently used when a nurse gives a client false assurance. Unintentionally impeding communication may sometimes occur. Being aware of it and explaining with an apology to the client will help promote a return to effective communication.

Communication in Special Circumstances

There are certain situations in which special communication techniques are required for nurse–client interactions. Several special circumstances are discussed in the display entitled Recommended Guidelines for Nurses Communicating in Special Circumstances.

KEY POINTS

- Nurses communicate thoughts, ideas, experiences, and facts to other nurses, clients, physicians, other health care workers, and families as part of their promotion of wellness and prevention of illness.
- The communication process can be defined two ways: (1) the process of sharing information or (2) the process of generating and transmitting meanings. Communication, as a foundation of life, is a reciprocal process with simultaneous participation.
- People communicate one to one or in small or large groups by verbal and nonverbal communication.
- Nonverbal communication includes touch, eye contact, facial expressions, posture, gait, gestures, physical appearance, sounds, and silence.
- The ability of the nurse to communicate with others is essential to effective use of the nursing process.
- The three phases in the helping relationship are (1) orientation phase, (2) working phase, and (3) termination phase. A helping relationship is dynamic, purposeful and time limited, and involving one person in a dominant role.
- Effective communication techniques are conversational skills, listening skills, use of silence and touch, and interviewing techniques. The interview is a major tool for data collection in the assessment step of the nursing process.

- Interpersonal skills such as warmth and friendliness, openness, empathy, competence, and consideration of client variables are essential to a therapeutic nurse–client relationship.
- Assertive skills enable nurses to communicate with clients, nurses, and other members of the health care team in a direct, honest fashion that is respectful of the rights of all parties in the communication.
- In addition to effective communication skills and interpersonal skills, it is helpful for the nurse to consider other factors that benefit the helping relationship. These include having specific objectives, comfortable environment, privacy, confidentiality, client focus, as well as using nursing observations, allowing optimal pacing, and providing personal space.
- The nurse also needs to learn the ineffective techniques that need to be avoided.
- The nurse must develop communication skills for special circumstances, especially when the client is visually impaired, hearing impaired, unconscious, or speaks a foreign language.

BIBLIOGRAPHY

Angel, G., & Petronko, D. K. (1983). *Developing the new assertive nurse: Essentials for advancement.* New York: Springer-Verlag.

Arnold, E., & Boggs, K. (1989). *Interpersonal relationships: Professional communication skills for nurses.* Philadelphia: Saunders.

Bara, M. (1989). Assertive communication for effective leadership. *Canadian Nurse, 85*(9), 19–20.

Berlo, D. (1960). *The process of communication: An introduction to theory and practice.* New York: Holt, Rinehart, & Winston.

Brady, B. A. (1991). Using the right touch. *Nursing, 21*(5), 46–47.

Buxman, K. (1991). Making room for laughter. *American Journal of Nursing, 91*(12), 46–51.

Chenevert, M. (1988). *STAT: Special techniques in assertiveness training for women in the health professions* (2nd ed.). St. Louis: Mosby–Year Book.

Clark, C. C. (1978). *Assertive skills for nurses.* Wakefield, MA: Contemporary Publishing.

Estabrooks, C. A. (1989). Touch: A nursing strategy in the intensive care unit. *Heart and Lung, 18*(4), 392–401.

Fisher, L., & Joseph, D. H. (1989). A scale to measure attitude about nonprocedural touch. *Canadian Journal of Nursing Research, 21*(2), 5–14.

Harrison, L. L. (1990). Minimizing barriers when teaching hearing-impaired clients. *MCN: American Journal of Maternal–Child Nursing, 15*(2), 113.

Harrison, T. M. (1989). Assessing nurses' communication: A cross-sectional study. *Western Journal of Nursing Research, 11*(1), 75–91.

Heidt, P. R. (1990). Openness: A qualitative analysis of nurses' and patients' experience of touch. *Image: Journal of Nursing Research, 22*(3), 180–186.

Hickey, M. (1990). What are the needs of families of critically ill patients? A review of the literature since 1976. *Heart and Lung, 19*(4), 401–415.

Ingham, A. (1989). A review of the literature relating to touch and its use in intensive care. *Intensive Care Nursing, 5*(2), 65–75.

Kilkus, S. P. (1990). Self-assertion and nurses: A different voice. *Nursing Outlook, 38*(3), 143–145.

Liehr, P. R. (1989). The core of true presence: A loving center. *Nursing Science Quarterly, 2*(1), 7–8.

MacKay. (1990). *Empathy in helping relationship.* New York: Springer-Verlag.

May, C. (1990). Research on nurse–patient relationships: Problems of theory, problems of practice. *Journal of Advanced Nursing, 15*(3), 307–315.

Montagu, A. (1986). *Touching: The human significance of the skin* (3rd ed.). New York: Harper & Row.

Morse, J. M. (1989). Reciprocity for care: Gift-giving in the patient–nurse relationship. *Canadian Journal of Nursing Research, 21*(1), 61–73.

Norris, R. M. (1989). Commonsense tips for working with blind patients. *American Journal of Nursing, 89*(3), 360–361.

Olson, J. K., & Iwasiw, C. L. (1989). Nurses' verbal empathy in four types of client situations. *Canadian Journal of Nursing Research, 21*(2), 39–51.

Orlando, I. J. (1990). *The dynamic nurse–patient relationship: Function, process and principles.* New York: National League for Nursing.

Paterson, J., & Zderad, L. (1976). *Humanistic nursing.* New York: Wiley.

Peplau, H. (1952). *Interpersonal relations in nursing.* New York: Putnam.

Quinn, J. F. (1988). Building a body of knowledge: Research on therapeutic touch. *Journal of Holistic Nursing, 6*(1), 37–45.

Schoenhofer, S. O. (1989). Affectional touch in critical care nursing: A descriptive study. *Heart and Lung, 18*(2), 146–154.

Sundeen, S. J., Stuart, G. W., Rankin, E. D., & Cohen, S. A. (1989). *Nurse–client interaction* (4th ed.). St. Louis: Mosby.

Tennant, K. F. (1990). Laugh it off: The effect of humor on the well-being of the older adult. *Journal of Gerontological Nursing, 16*(12), 11–17.

Tovkar, M. K. (1989). Touch: The beneficial effects for the surgical patient. *AORN Journal, 49*(5), 1356–1361.

Travelbee, J. (1971). *Interpersonal aspects of nursing* (2nd ed.). Philadelphia: Davis.

Vanore-Black, N. (1990). Maintaining healthy relationships. *Holistic Nursing Practice, 4*(4), 39–45.

Watson, J. (1985). *Nursing: The philosophy and science of caring.* Boulder: Colorado Associated University Press.

Watson, J. B. (1988). Communication attitudes and aging. *International Journal of Aging and Human Development, 27*(1), 45–55.

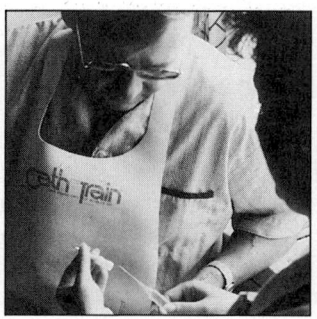
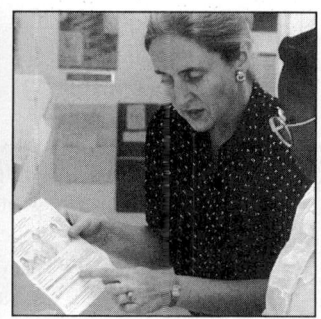
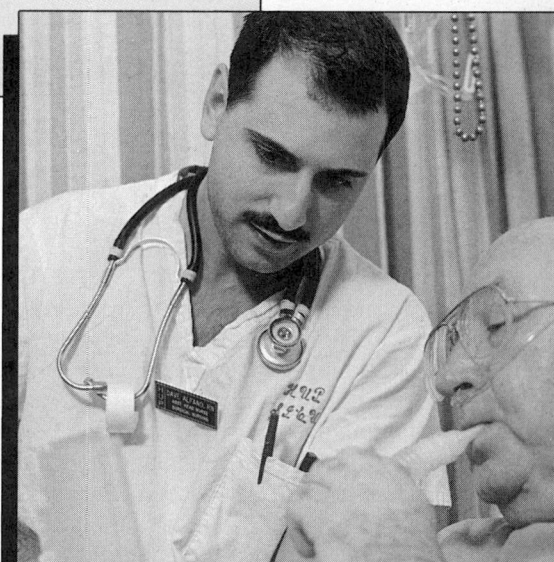

OBJECTIVES

After studying this chapter, the learner should be able to:

Define key terms used in the chapter.

Describe the teaching–learning process, including domains, developmental concerns, and specific principles.

Describe what factors should be assessed for the learning process.

Formulate diagnoses for identified learning needs.

Explain how to create a teaching plan for a client.

Describe what is involved in implementing a teaching plan.

Name three methods for evaluating learning.

Explain what should be included in the documentation of the teaching–learning process.

Discuss the nurse's role as a counselor.

Summarize how the nursing process is used to assist clients in problem solving.

Describe how to use the counseling role to motivate a client toward health promotion.

KEY TERMS

affective learning
cognitive learning
contractual agreement
counseling
developmental crisis
formal teaching
informal teaching
learning
learning readiness
literacy
negative reinforcement
noncompliance
positive reinforcement
psychomotor learning
situational crisis
teaching

Teacher and Counselor

21

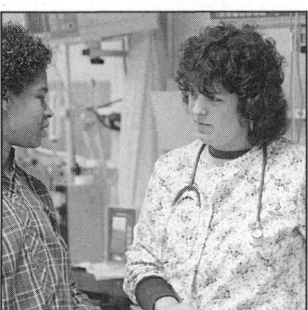

One of the means by which nurses apply communication skills is through the roles of teacher and counselor. They develop nursing skills by learning about the teaching–learning and counseling processes and by adapting the roles of teacher and counselor to nursing care. The roles of teacher and counselor overlap many other nursing roles. Because nurses have opportunities to teach and counsel clients and their families during many nursing care activities, teaching and counseling techniques are a necessary part of each nurse's repertoire of skills.

Nurses alternate between the roles of teacher and learner. Sometimes they themselves are pursuing new knowledge, skills, and values. For example, nurses are encouraged and sometimes required to attend staff development or in-service classes pertaining to current and new practices. More nurses are also choosing to pursue formal education for advanced degrees. At other times, nurses are facilitating learning in other people.

Trends in health care have made the roles of teacher and counselor even more important than previously. With the current trend for shorter hospital stays, clients and their families need more extensive instruction for home care. Both hospital nurses and home health care nurses must work together to ensure that clients receive the care they need. With effective methods of client teaching, both hospital and home recovery are expedited.

Conversely, as the importance of teaching in the hospital increases, the time for teaching decreases. Consequently, the quality of the teaching must be improved. Nurses must learn how to teach effectively and efficiently. As with all skills, teaching skills develop as the nurse matures in professional roles.

Aims of Teaching and Counseling

The basic purpose of teaching and counseling is to help clients and families develop the self-care abilities (ie, knowledge, attitude, and skills) that will enable them to maximize their functioning and quality of life (or dignified death). When skillfully used by nurses, teaching and counseling are powerful tools for achieving nursing aims.

Promoting Wellness

A higher level of wellness is possible for all. Nurses can help clients to value health and to develop specific health practices that promote wellness. Wellness teaching is varied and can range from teaching passive exercises to a client with left-sided paralysis to promoting joint flexibility or designing a safe exercise program for a young athlete.

Preventing Illness

Prevention, a major theme in health teaching and counseling, takes many forms. Nurses can counsel women of childbearing age about health practices that promote optimal fetal development, teach parents how to make their home safe for a toddler, or counsel individuals at high risk for heart disease, cancer, or communicable diseases.

Restoring Health

Once a client is ill, teaching and counseling are focused on developing self-care practices that will facilitate recovery. Preoperative and postoperative teaching, sexual counseling for a client recovering from a myocardial infarction, and life-style counseling for the client with an ostomy are all examples of teaching and counseling directed to restore health.

Facilitating Coping

Developmental life-style changes and acute, chronic, and terminal illness all place demands on clients and families that may become overwhelming. Nurses work not only with clients but also with their families and friends, to help them to come to terms with the illness and any life-style modifications it entails.

The nurse caregiver who is a skilled teacher and counselor can expect to effect the following outcomes:
- High-level wellness and related self-care practices
- Disease prevention or early detection
- Quick recovery from trauma or illness with minimal to no complications
- Enhanced ability to adjust to developmental life changes and acute, chronic, and terminal illness
- Family acceptance of the life-style changes necessitated by the illness or disability of a family member

General topics for health teaching are highlighted in the accompanying display.

Nurse as Teacher

Nurses assume the role of teacher when clients have identifiable learning needs. This teacher–learner relationship is enhanced by the continuance of the helping relationship (see Chapter 20), in which mutual respect and trust have been established. The nurse builds on this trust by sharing

Topics for Health Teaching and Counseling

Promoting Wellness

- Developmental and maturational issues
- Normal childbearing
- Hygiene
- Nutrition
- Exercise
- Mental health
- Spiritual health

Preventing Illness

- First aid
- Safety
- Immunizations
- Screening
- Identification and management of risk factors

Restoring Health

- Orientation to treatment center and staff
- Client's and nurses' expectations of one another

- The illness and physical condition: anatomy and physiology, etiology of problem, significance of symptoms, prognosis
- The medical and nursing regimens and how the client can participate in care
- Self-care practices the client and family needs to manage the client's condition independently

Facilitating Coping

- How the client's physical and mental condition affects other areas of functioning; life-style counseling
- Measures that maximize independence and enhance self-concept
- Stress management
- Environmental alterations
- Community resources
- Appropriate referrals (eg, physical therapy, occupational therapy, self-help groups, psychiatric–mental health counselor)
- Grief and bereavement counseling

---

information the nurse and client have mutually identified as important. The client may ask for this information or the nurse may initiate teaching as the result of assessment and diagnostic factors.

Teaching–Learning Process

How the human brain stores and retrieves information has not yet been fully determined. A person plays the role of learner throughout life, although what is learned and the ways learning occurs change according to developmental stages. Basic understanding of the teaching–learning process aids nurses in developing their own teaching and learning skills. The process is summarized in the display entitled Steps in the Teaching–Learning Process.

Teaching is a planned method or series of methods used to help someone learn. The person using these methods is the teacher. **Learning** is the process by which a person acquires or increases knowledge or changes behavior in a measurable way as a result of an experience. It is an internal experience that denotes an integration of thoughts, ideas, theory, and experience—past and present (LaMonica, 1985).

Learning Domains

Learning can be divided into three domains—cognitive, affective, and psychomotor (Bloom, 1956). **Cognitive learning** involves the storing and recalling of new knowledge and information in the brain (eg, the client states how salt affects blood pressure). When a physical skill has been acquired, the change that has occurred is called **psychomotor learning** (eg, the client demonstrates how to change dressings using clean technique). **Affective learning** includes changes in attitudes, values, and feelings (eg, the client expresses renewed self-confidence following physical therapy). These three areas of learning give the nurse-teacher a way of categorizing the learning that is planned for the client (see Planning: Client Goals).

Developmental Considerations

One of the major learning theories is Piaget's theory of intellectual development (see Chapter 10). By understanding the way children and adolescents develop learning abilities, a nurse can use this knowledge appropriately when teaching clients of all ages. For instance, if a 6-year-old girl must begin to take insulin every day, the nurses who are caring for her must recognize her limitations in understanding diabetes. Information should be simplified to provide only the most basic facts with accompanying concrete examples or demonstrations. At no time would a detailed discussion of the pathophysiology of diabetes be appropriate. The girl could be told that she needs a shot every day to keep her from getting sick or feeling funny. She could be allowed to play with the syringes and to give shots to a doll (Fig. 21-1).

A nurse who is teaching a sexually active 16-year-old girl about contraceptive methods needs to assess whether the young client has reached the stage Piaget refers to as *formal operations* (the ability to use logical reasoning to solve hypothetical problems). If the client's intellectual de-

Steps in the Teaching–Learning Process

Assess the Client's Learning Needs

1. Use all appropriate sources of information.
2. Identify the knowledge, attitude, or skills needed by the client and family.
3. Assess emotional and experiential readiness to learn.
4. Assess the client's ability to learn.
5. Identify client strengths.
6. Use Anticipatory Guidance

Diagnose the Learning Needs.

1. Be realistic.
2. Validate with client or family, or both.

Develop a Teaching Plan

1. Formulate measurable learner objectives.
   - Identify short- and long-term objectives.
   - Prioritize.
   - Determine who should be included (ie, family members, significant others).
   - Include the client in planning.
2. Create a teaching plan.
   - Match content with appropriate teaching strategies and learner activities.
   - Directly relate teaching content to the client's interests, resources, and patterns of everyday living.
   - Schedule within limits of time constraints.

- Decide on group versus individual teaching and formal versus informal.
- Formulate a verbal or written contract with the client.

Implement the Teaching Plan

1. Prepare the physical environment.
2. Gather all audiovisual materials and equipment.
3. Deliver content in organized manner using teaching strategies.
4. Be flexible.

Evaluate the Teaching–Learning

1. Evaluate completion of learner objectives.
   - Client's comments
   - Direct questioning
   - Observational skills
   - Return demonstration
   - Postdischarge follow-ups
2. Reinforce and celebrate learning.
3. Evaluate teaching.
   - Self-evaluation
   - Client questionnaires
4. Revise plan of learner objectives not met.
   - Alter content and teaching strategies.
   - Use motivational counseling if needed.
   - Reschedule teaching sessions.
5. Document the teaching–learning process.

F I G U R E   2 1 - 1

The teaching approach must be appropriate to the developmental age of the learner. Small children respond well to teaching strategies that permit them to participate actively. (Photo by Gates Rhodes, courtesy of School of Nursing, University of Pennsylvania.)

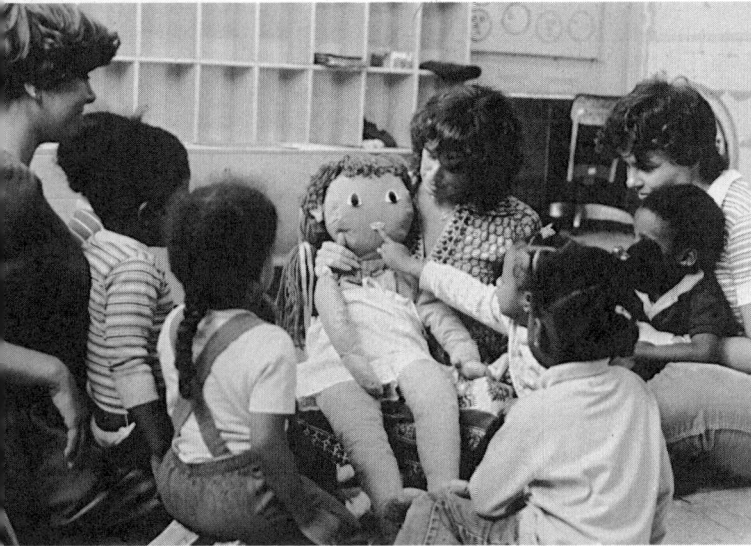

velopment is delayed and is still in the period of *concrete operations* (use of logical reasoning to solve concrete problems), she may be unable to think abstractly. That is, the adolescent may not perceive pregnancy as a real possibility and therefore may be unable to understand the need for contraception. If so, the nurse can alter the teaching plan to include audiovisual (AV) teaching aids that explain the topic in concrete terms.

Some adults have not attained the formal operations stage. The nurse must be alert to this possibility and teach or re-teach material as needed. For example, an adult taking an antibiotic may be unable to grasp the importance of taking the capsules at the prescribed times to maintain the proper blood level for the best effect. If the nurse sees that the client is not complying with the schedule, the effectiveness of the teaching and learning should be evaluated. Showing a simple diagram of how erratic scheduling affects the body could give the concrete information the client needs to be motivated toward taking the antibiotic as ordered. In this way, the teaching is altered to meet the client's intellectual development.

Motor development is also a concern in the teaching–learning process. The 6-year-old girl diagnosed with diabetes may not be expected to learn to give her own insulin shots if she lacks the fine motor skills needed to manipulate the equipment for insulin injections. On the other hand, a 13-year-old client could probably master the technique quickly.

Other developmental concerns related to the teaching–learning process are emotional maturity and psychosocial development. Chronologic age does not guarantee maturity. It is possible that a 13-year-old client could respond more maturely to health teaching than a 30-year-old client. A great deal depends on how the client has learned to respond to changes and stressful events in the past.

Adult Learners Many of the developmental concerns related to teaching and learning are exaggerated by age. As people age, their personalities as well as their learning abilities change. Most psychologists who have studied the teaching–learning process have based their work on children and adolescents, because a large amount of learning occurs early in life. The science of teaching—*pedagogy*—generally refers to the teaching of children and adolescents. In recent years, the study of teaching adults—*androgogy*—has become popular. This term emphasizes that adults need to be taught differently.

Knowles (1984) lists the following four assumptions concerning adult learners:

1. As a person matures, his or her self-concept is likely to move from dependence to independence.
2. The previous experience of the adult is a rich resource for learning.
3. The readiness to learn in an adult often is related to a developmental task or a social role.
4. The adult's orientation to learning is that material should be useful immediately, rather than at some time in the future.

Given these assumptions it is easy to see that androgogy has a problem or need-centered focus with immediate application of new material.

It is generally accepted that adults must believe they need to learn before they are willing to learn. Nurses often use their counseling skills (discussed later in this chapter) to motivate clients to participate in the teaching–learning process. Adults may need to be shown the necessity of learning new information, health practices, or skills.

Many adults are afraid of the teaching–learning process. This may be the result of a fear of failure, because many adults have not participated in formal educational programs since their school days. As aging occurs, adults often express a concern over memory loss, and being required to learn new material can threaten their feelings of self-worth. Consequently, the sensitivity and concern of the nurse in the helping relationship are the foundation for a nonthreatening learning environment for the adult client.

Adults may also resist learning because of preconceived ideas about the teaching–learning process and of others' expectations. Honest and open communication provides the adult learner with a preview of what will be involved. Many adults willingly participate in the process once they have received the reassurance that they are partners in the teaching–learning process. Retaining some control over what is taught and how it is taught gives adult learners the sense of control they are accustomed to in their daily living.

Some elderly clients are especially fearful and threatened by the idea of having to learn new information. They may often refer to the old adage, "You can't teach an old dog new tricks," as a defensive attempt to avoid failure or change. Nurses find that a slower approach is needed when introducing new material so that older clients do not become discouraged or overwhelmed.

Principles of Teaching–Learning

Several basic principles of teaching–learning serve as guidelines for a nurse assuming the role of teacher. They can be applied in situations in which the teaching–learning process is used to meet the needs of clients.

- The teaching–learning process is facilitated by the existence of a helping relationship (Fig. 21-2).
- Nurse-teachers need to be able to communicate effectively with individuals, small groups, and, in some instances, large groups.
- Knowledge of the communication process is necessary for the assessment of verbal and nonverbal feedback.
- A thorough assessment of clients and the factors affecting learning helps to diagnose their learning needs accurately.
- The teaching–learning process is more effective when the client is included in the planning of learner objectives.
- Unless the client values these objectives, little learning is likely to occur.
- The implementation of a teaching plan should include varied strategies for sensory stimulation, which apparently promote learning.
- Relating new learning material to clients' past life experiences is effective in helping to assimilate new knowledge.
- Proposed behavioral changes must always be realistic and explored in the context of the client's resources and everyday life-style.
- Careful attention should be paid to time constraints, scheduling, and the physical environment.
- Learner objectives provide the basis for evaluating whether learning has occurred.
- When learning objectives have not been met, careful reassessment provides ideas for changing the teaching plan for subsequent implementation.

Client teaching is approached most effectively by following the steps of the nursing process. The teaching–learning process and the nursing process are interdependent.

Assessing the Client's Learning Needs

Sources of Information

Clients are the best source of assessment information in most instances. By using effective interviewing techniques (see Chapter 20), a nurse can obtain the data needed to

RESEARCH IN NURSING Making a Difference

Client Adherence to Treatment Regimens

Many variables can influence the outcome of teaching–learning sessions. The challenge for nurses is to identify and use those factors that facilitate client adherence.

Related Research

Spees, C. M. (1991). Knowledge of medical terminology among clients and families. *Image: Journal of Nursing Scholarship, 23*(4), 225–229.

This descriptive correlational study investigated 25 hospitalized clients' and 25 family members' knowledge of 50 common medical terms. The results showed that clients and family members may not understand medical terms as well as nurses think they do and may need consistent assessment of knowledge in the context of patient teaching. In general, nurses need to make a conscious effort to use common terms and to explain all medical terms used in conversations with clients and families.

Two studies were conducted to examine the relation between medication regimen complexity and adherence among 178 older adults recently discharged from hospitals and 98 adults not recently hospitalized. Although the results did not show statistically significant correlations between these two groups, the results of both studies did indicate that more complex medication regimens result in reduced compliance among subjects. This prompted the investigators to question other factors that might affect compliance in older populations, such as less education or low motivation.

Summary

Further research is needed to investigate client, family member, and nursing factors that contribute to effective teaching–learning sessions that facilitate client adherence to treatment regimens.

Conn, V. S., Taylor, S. G., & Kelley, S. (1991). Medication complexity and adherence among older adults. *Image: Journal of Nursing Scholarship, 23*(4), 231–235.

FIGURE 21-2

The teaching–learning process is facilitated by the existence of a helping relationship and a teaching plan tailored to the client's learning needs. (Photo by Barbara Proud.)

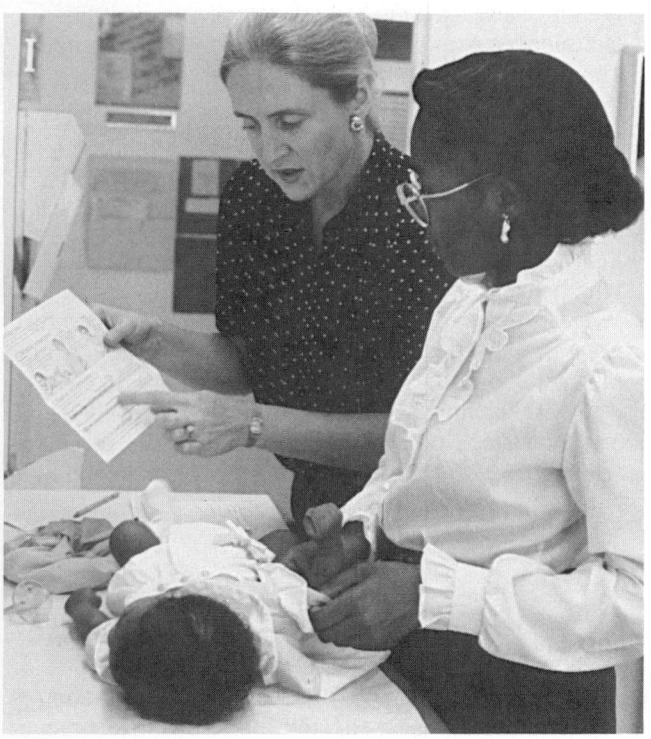

identify the client's learning needs. Relevant information can be obtained before actually meeting the client by reviewing the client's past and current medical records. These records provide a history of medical problems as well as documentation of the nursing assessments, nursing diagnoses, nursing physical examinations, and nursing interventions that have been performed.

The client's family and significant others are also valuable sources for assessment data. Sometimes the family or significant others are used for assessment data when the client is unable to communicate with the nurse because of health problems, language barriers, or impaired sensory functions. At other times, the family members or significant others may be the most appropriate source for certain information. For example, if seeking information pertaining to the use of salt in cooking, the nurse could speak with the person who prepares the meals in the client's home and then include that person in any teaching pertaining to food preparation. The client's permission should be secured before the nurse involves family members in the teaching–learning process.

Assessment Parameters

Four elements need to be considered in each assessment of client learning needs. The nurse first identifies what new knowledge, attitudes, or skills are necessary for clients and

Illiteracy

About 20% of adults are functionally illiterate (unable to read and write). Many have learned to compensate for this disability and may fool even experienced nurses. Never presume literacy in a client you are attempting to teach.

families to independently manage their health care. The second focus of assessment is on **learning readiness**, a concept signifying the client's willingness to engage in the teaching–learning process (emotional readiness; Fig. 21-3). The third focus is on experiential readiness to begin the challenge of learning. Readiness is distinguished from the client's physical ability to learn. The fourth focus of assessment is on client strengths, personal resources the nurse can assist clients to tap (Fig. 21-4). Many factors influence each of these elements and all should play a role in the assessment. These factors are highlighted in the accompanying display.

Diagnosing the Client's Learning Needs

When a lack of knowledge, attitude, or skill hinders a client's self-promotion of health, the nurse diagnoses the deficit. The nurse can use diagnoses or problem statements

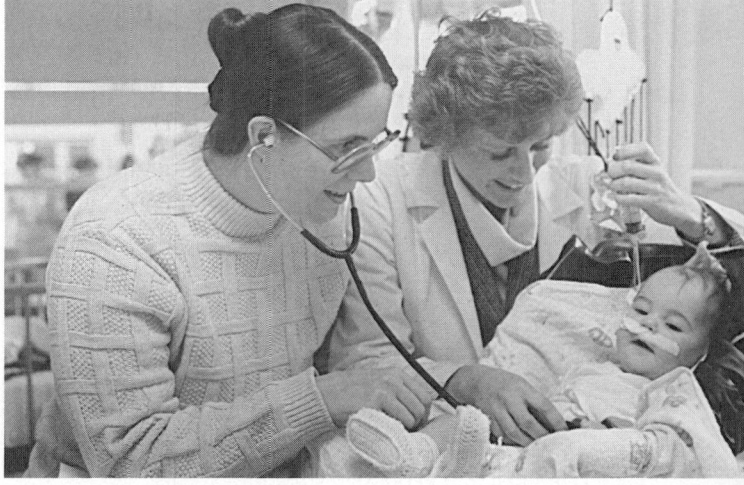

FIGURE 21-4

A client or family member will have more motivation to learn if the nurse focuses on the learner's interests and concerns. (Photo by Gates Rhodes, courtesy of School of Nursing, University of Pennsylvania.)

approved by the North American Nursing Diagnoses Association (NANDA) as a guide when diagnosing learning needs (see Chapter 16). If the nurse believes that the client's knowledge deficit is the primary problem, the nurse can write a diagnosis identifying a specific knowledge deficit as the problem followed by its etiology and the related signs and symptoms. For example:

Knowledge Deficit: Breastfeeding, related to inexperience as manifested by anxiety and multiple questions.

More often it is a knowledge deficit that results in an actual or potential problem; hence, the knowledge deficit is written as the etiology (second part of the diagnostic statement):

Infant at High Risk for Altered Nutrition: Less Than Body Requirements, related to mother's lack of knowledge about infant feeding and deficient learning readiness (as manifested by mother's quick frustration when breastfeeding, refusal to engage in learning process, and infant's weight loss).

Wellness diagnoses such as Potential for Enhanced Parenting or Potential for Enhanced Self-Esteem are written as one-part statements. Teaching and counseling are the primary nurse-prescribed interventions used to achieve related outcome criteria.

In addition to identifying the client's learning needs, nurses need to assess their own knowledge base and teaching skills. Nurses cannot teach information and skills to clients if the nurses lack the information and skills to be taught. Often, knowing where to find information or an appropriate resource person is the first step in correcting one's own knowledge deficits.

FIGURE 21-3

Anxiety is sometimes a positive motivating factor for learning. An anxious mother of a sick child may be receptive to the teaching of special techniques for the care of her child. (Photo by Gates Rhodes, courtesy of School of Nursing, University of Pennsylvania.)

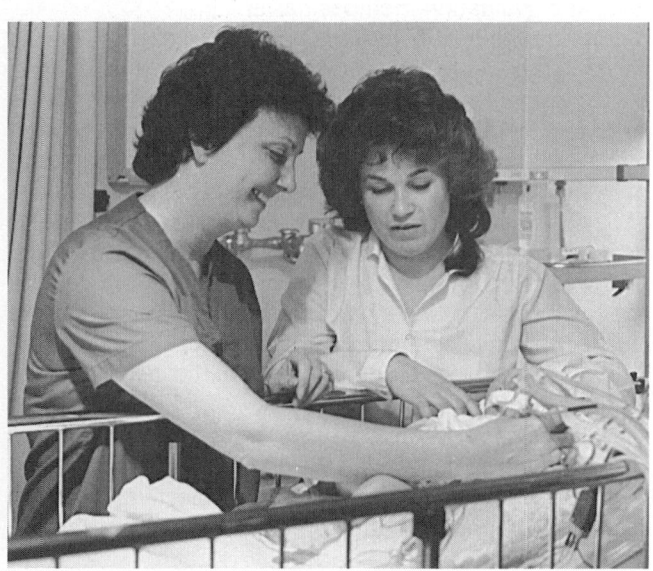

Assessment Parameters:
Factors That Affect Learning

Knowledge, Attitudes, and Skills the Client and Family Needs to Independently Manage Health Care

Readiness to Learn

- Emotional readiness
  Emotional health
  Motivation for learning
  Self-concept and body image
  Sense of responsibility for self
- Experiential readiness
  Social and economic stability
  Past experiences with learning
  Attitude toward learning
  Culture

Ability to Learn

- Physical condition
- Acuity of senses
- Developmental considerations
- Level of education
- Literacy
- Communication skills
- Primary language

Learning Strengths

- Successful learning in the past
- Above-average comprehension, reasoning, memory, or psychomotor skills
- High motivation
- Strong network
- Adequate financing

Planning

Planning for learning involves the development of a teaching plan. Teaching plans are similar to nursing care plans—both follow the steps of the nursing process. One type of teaching plan is given in Table 21-1 as an example to follow during the remaining steps of the teaching–learning process. Standardized teaching plans (some computerized) are available for major topics of health teaching. When using these plans, it is imperative to individualize the plan to the client's unique learning needs and abilities.

Thoughtful planning for a client's learning experiences maximizes the client's chances for learning while ensuring the most efficient use of the nurse's time and talents. Learner objectives are developed for each diagnosis of a learning need. The nursing orders become the content,

teaching strategy, and learner activity columns of the written plan. This phase requires thought and creativity. The nurse's efforts are rewarded when the client successfully completes objectives at the end of the implementation phase.

When planning for learning, the nurse and client together must decide who should be included in the learning sessions. When the client is a young child, one or both parents may be the primary learners. When the client is an adult, a spouse or close friend who will be giving the care that is to be learned may be included. For instance, the person who does the household cooking is usually asked to be present for any nutritional teaching. If the client is ill and unable to participate in the teaching–learning process, people who will provide care at home must be taught procedures. Teaching plans are developed according to the needs of the person being taught.

One nurse or several nurses can prepare and use a teaching plan. When two or more nurses plan and coordinate the implementation of the plan, it is referred to as *team teaching*. An advantage of team teaching is that the talents of more than one nurse are used to promote learning for the client. Several factors should be considered during the formulation of any teaching plan.

Learner Objectives

Learner objectives are written in the same manner as the client goals of the nursing process (see Chapter 17). When planning for the client's learning, it is best to determine first which of the three learning domains (cognitive, psychomotor, or affective) will be used when teaching. The nurse can then write learner objectives that reflect what learning is to occur. A well-constructed learner objective serves as a guide for planning evaluation methods.

Choosing the verb for a learner objective is probably the most difficult part when writing objectives (see the accompanying display). Yet, if chosen carefully, it makes the planning of content, teaching strategies, learner activities, and evaluation methods easier.

The number of objectives needed for each diagnosis varies. It is better to have several specific objectives than to try to use only one or two broad objectives. Many nurses state one long-term objective for each diagnosis followed by several specific objectives. For example, a long-term objective for the sample teaching plan could be as follows: "The client will be able to breastfeed her infant as long as desired without sore nipples." This objective could be met in 2 weeks or 2 years. Long-term objectives are general statements. On the other hand, the objectives written in the learner objective column of the sample teaching plan (see Table 21-1) are specific behaviors to be accomplished within a short time.

Clients and appropriate family members or significant others should be included in the planning of learner objectives. Once clients value the learning objectives, learning readiness is enhanced and compliance is maximized.

TABLE 21-1

Sample Teaching Plan

Diagnosis: High Risk for Impaired Skin Integrity: Nipples, related to knowledge and skill deficit (nipple care)

Signs and symptoms: Complains of sore nipples; first baby; 1 day after delivery; fair skin with freckles; no redness or cracking yet; no prenatal preparation

Learner Objective	Met	Content	Teaching Strategy	Learner Activity
The Client		Prevention and care of sore nipples		
Morning Session				
Begins protective measures immediately (psychomotor)	√ 8/10/93 L.S.	Protective measures: • Avoid soap • Avoid exposure to air and sunlight • Apply lanolin or vegetable oil • Avoid plastic liners in bra or bra pads	Lecture with discussion Audiovisual: Flip chart on breastfeeding	Read handout: Nipple Care
Explains why feedings should be shorter and more frequent (cognitive)	√ 8/10/93 L.S.	Preparation for breastfeeding: • Feed baby more frequently —Every 2 hours during day —Arrange for rooming in • Nipple roll before the feeding	Discussion Audiovisual: Flip chart on breastfeeding	Read handout: Sore Nipples
Demonstrates nipple rolling (psychomotor)	√ 8/10/93 L.S.		Return demonstration	
10 AM Session				
Demonstrates correct feeding technique and after care (psychomotor)	√ 8/10/93 L.S.	Breastfeeding the baby: • Start baby on less sore side • Hold the breast properly • Get baby onto areolar area • Position properly • Change position for each feeding • Remove baby from breast	Discovery: Guide through each step; assist as necessary	Read handout: Positioning Baby for Breastfeeding
Describes a feeling of improved comfort with each feeding (affective)	√ 8/10/93 L.S.	After the feeding: • Air dry nipples • Inspect for open or cracked areas • Apply lanolin or vegetable oil	Discovery	Borrow books on breastfeeding from client's reference shelf
Afternoon Session				
Explains the importance of good nutrition and rest at home (affective) List the signs of thrush (cognitive)	√ 8/10/93 L.S.	Considerations for home: • Maintain "demand" feedings • Ensure good nutrition • Get adequate rest • Know the signs and symptoms of thrush	Lecture with discussion Audiovisual: Poster	Refer to handouts at home as needed; call the maternity department's information number for any questions

---

Verbs That Can Be Used When Writing Learner Objectives

Cognitive Domain	Affective Domain	Psychomotor Domain
categorizes	answers	adapts
compares	chooses	arranges
composes	defends	assembles
defines	discusses	begins
describes	displays	changes
designs	forms	constructs
differentiates	gives	creates
explains	helps	manipulates
gives examples	initiates	moves
identifies	joins	organizes
labels	justifies	rearranges
lists	relates	shows
names	revises	starts
prepares	selects	works
plans	shares	
solves	uses	
states		
summarizes		
writes		

Content

Once the learner objectives are completed, the nurse needs to decide what information the client will need to complete those objectives successfully. This information is the content of the teaching plan. It is usually necessary to research the area to be taught to determine what information exists concerning the topic. Books, articles, and manuals are available in many nursing units for the nurse's research needs. It is becoming more common to have content that is already organized available for a variety of common health-teaching topics, thus shortening the required research time.

Nurses are concerned about what clients need to know about topics such as illness, procedures, medications, and surgeries. "How much should they know?" is a common topic for debate. It has been found that clients benefit from explanations of the physical sensations they will experience during a procedure. They appreciate advanced knowledge of what they will feel, taste, hear, see, and smell. See Table 21-1 for a sample teaching plan containing an example of content included for one client's learning needs.

Content explaining why certain treatments and medications are needed is included in a teaching plan. Information on the prevention of illness or its complications should also be covered. Compliance with the nursing and medical plans is a major objective for much of the health teaching done. People who have a basic understanding of their illness and its treatment will usually comply with the treatment more readily than those who do not understand their illness.

Teaching Strategies

The techniques used by a teacher to promote learning are *teaching strategies*. Teaching strategies are planned before the actual teaching sessions so that every content area can be matched with an effective teaching technique. The strategies chosen depend on the teacher's familiarity with the method, the availability of teaching aids such as AV and printed materials, the facilities for using AV materials, and factors in the client's learning, such as educational level and cultural background. The nurse must also consider age-appropriate methods for her client. For example, a 10-year-old will be receptive to a comic book on personal safety, whereas an adult could learn similar material by discussing the safety measures with the nurse.

Experts in the field of education generally agree that the use of a variety of teaching strategies aids learning. In addition, some methods are better suited to certain learning objectives. Table 21-2 gives suggested teaching strategies for the three learning domains. See Table 21-1 for the sample teaching plan, which shows how teaching strategies are varied for the learner objectives and content of that

---

T A B L E   2 1 - 2

Suggested Teaching Strategies for the Three Learning Domains

Cognitive Domain	Affective Domain	Psychomotor Domain
Lecture or discussion	Role modeling	Demonstration
Panel discussion	Discussion	Discovery
Discovery	Panel discussion	AV materials
AV materials	AV materials	Printed materials
Printed materials	Role playing	
Programmed instruction	Printed materials	
Computer-assisted instruction programs		

particular plan. Again, the nurse is free to use creativity in choosing the methods. However, the nurse should take care to stimulate as many of the client's senses as possible when teaching. Seeing, hearing, and touching are superior to hearing alone. Descriptions of common teaching strategies follow.

Role Modeling   The old saying, "Actions speak louder than words" explains why role modeling is effective. Clients watch their nurses closely; the nurse can use this opportunity to affect a client's behavior positively. For example, nurses who were formerly smokers can be role models for clients who are trying to quit smoking for health reasons.

Lecture   In the purest sense, a *lecture* is a presentation of information by the teacher to the learners. However, to be more effective, lectures usually include question-and-answer periods to allow for clarification of material. This strategy is often used to deliver information to a large group of clients. It is rarely used for individual instruction, without the addition of other strategies.

Discussion   Discussion involves the two-way exchange of information, ideas, and feelings between the teacher and the learners. It is an effective method when used by a nurse who is comfortable with leading a group and knowledgeable in group process (see Chapter 22). Also, it can be an effective method for one-on-one instruction.

Panel Discussion   This strategy involves the presentation of information by two or more people. Panel discussions

can be used to impart factual material but are also effective for sharing experiences and emotions. Debates are a form of panel discussion and allow for exposure of all aspects of a topic.

Demonstration   Demonstration of techniques, procedures, exercises, and the use of special equipment, combined with a lecture and discussion, is an effective strategy (Fig. 21-5). Evaluation of the client's learning can be done by a return demonstration. Practice sessions are often included for the learner. Models of body parts or practice models such as a resuscitation model are frequently used. When teaching breast self-examinations, the use of a breast model allows the learner actually to feel different types of lumps commonly found in breast tissue. Childbirth educators usually demonstrate the birth of a baby by using a pelvic model, knitted uterus, and a baby doll.

Discovery   In discovery learning, the nurse presents a problem or situation to the client or group of clients and then guides the clients to discovering the solution or approach. Discussion of other possible approaches and solutions can follow the client's own solutions. This is a good method for teaching problem-solving techniques and independent thinking. For instance, a nurse could give a group of diabetic clients a short description of a situation that includes signs and symptoms. The group would decide if the signs and symptoms indicate *hypoglycemia* (low blood sugar) or *hyperglycemia* (high blood sugar) and would choose what measures to take. Next, the nurse could discuss the group decision as a further learning experience. Even if the clients chose a poor resolution, the nurse could turn it into an effective learning experience.

Role Playing   This strategy gives the learner a chance to experience, relive, or anticipate an event. The nurse explains the scenario and then allows the client to play out the scene with the teacher or with one or more clients (Fig. 21-6). Role playing can be used to work through emotional traumas or to plan for possible traumas. For example, a nurse could help a teenage girl prepare herself to tell her mother about her pregnancy by letting the girl play her mother while the nurse plays the girl. This would help the client rehearse what she wanted to say and anticipate the emotional atmosphere that she will experience. Role playing is a good strategy for adults as well as for children. Puppets and dolls can help young children express negative feelings that have resulted from hospitalization and traumatic procedures.

AV Materials   The use of AV materials can be an effective teaching and learning tool. AV materials include films, filmstrips with or without audiotapes, slides, television programs, videotapes, overhead transparencies, flip charts, posters, and diagrams. Their use is a popular and effective teaching strategy when combined with a lecture or discussion. **Literacy**, the ability to read and write, should never be assumed in the client when using printed

FIGURE   2 1 - 5

Demonstration of techniques using practice models is an effective teaching strategy. Here, a nurse is increasing her own self-care knowledge and learning use of the model for teaching others self-care. (Photo by Don Walker, courtesy of Thomas Jefferson University.)

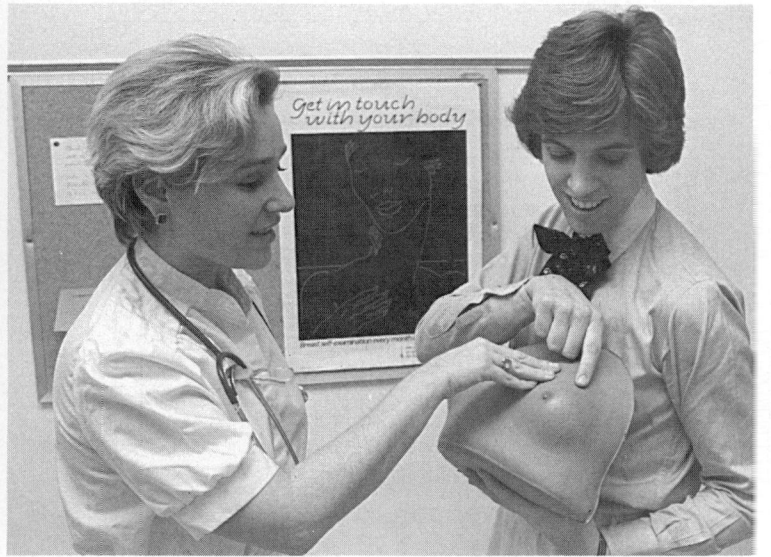

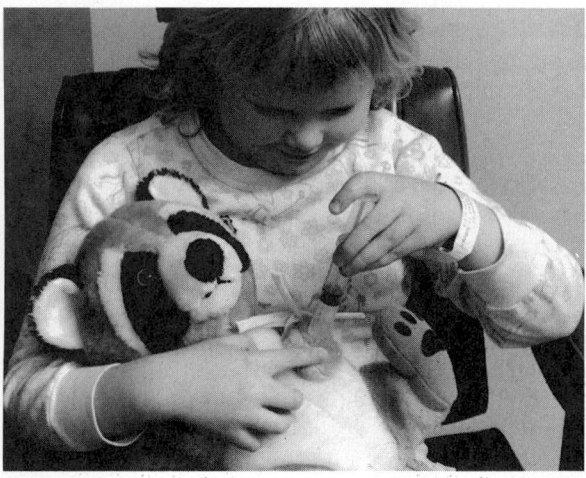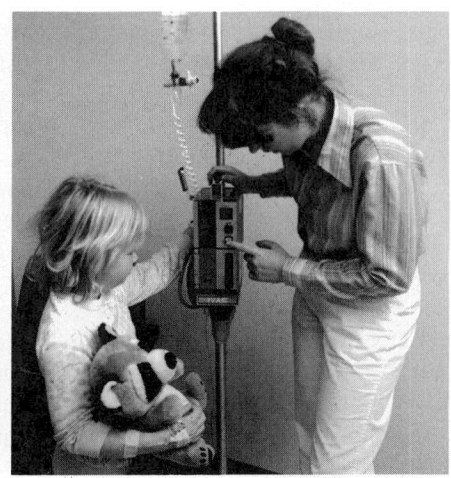

F I G U R E   2 1 - 6

The nurse preparing a child for an IV allows the child to role-play with her stuffed toy and a syringe, and demonstrates how the infusion control monitor works.

words. AV materials should never be the sole source of learning for the client. It is an accepted practice to allow the client to view an AV material alone but to precede and follow it with a discussion of the material.

Printed Material   The use of printed material depends on its availability to the nurse. Many nurses have contributed to written materials for distribution to clients. Writing pamphlets, instruction sheets, books, and comic books for health teaching can be rewarding as well as useful. As with AV materials, the nurse usually uses printed materials in conjunction with other strategies. Use of specially prepared games is a popular and fun way for clients to learn. Games

can be relatively easy to make. For instance, cards with pictures of foods can be used to develop a nutritional instruction game.

Programmed Instruction   Most programmed instruction books or booklets are prepared so that learners can use them independently of a teacher. However, educators generally agree that the teacher needs to spend time with the learner before and after the completion of the program to clarify information, answer questions, and provide the personal touch so needed for a learner's motivation. Because this is a self-paced strategy, it can be beneficial for many learners.

◆ C O M P U T E R   A P P L I C A T I O N S   I N   N U R S I N G

Computer-Assisted Instruction

Computer-assisted instruction (CAI) has proved to be a valuable tool in the teaching–learning process. Because learners actively interact with the computer, are self-directed, and receive immediate feedback, learning is facilitated and even fun. CAI can be used for all ages and in all types of teaching–learning situations. A brief list of topics, with content, is included as an example.

- The American Heart Association CPR course: Complete CPR course for training and certification
- Measuring blood pressure: Demonstrates the step-by-step procedure for students and the general public; uses animation to illustrate and reinforce material
- Healthy living: Determines risk factors, ways to stay healthy; includes individualized testing

- Wellness–illness continuum: Wellness–illness continuum and concepts; identifies risk factors
- Postoperative care simulation: Experiences in decision making and documenting care of postoperative clients
- Introduction to nursing diagnosis: Covers all areas necessary for understanding what a nursing diagnosis is, how to differentiate it from a medical diagnosis, and how to write a correctly formatted nursing diagnosis

The journal *Computers in Nursing* has regular features that review new computer software: "software reviews," "software exchanges," and "nibbles."

Computer-Assisted Instruction Programs The use of computer programs for teaching is still in its infancy but the possibilities are unlimited. Perhaps individual terminals will be made available in each client's room so that instruction will be available at any time. This method can even be personalized by programming the computer to address the learner by name and to give positive feedback when appropriate. Currently, this method is not widely used because of limited access. This technique is only acceptable when personal, human attention is also available.

Contractual Agreements

The use of contracts between nurses and clients is becoming a common practice in many health care settings. Usually the contracts are rather informal and not legally binding. A **contractual agreement** is a pact between two people made for the achievement of mutually set goals. When teaching a client, such an agreement can serve to motivate both the client and the nurse to do what is necessary to attain the client's learning objectives. The agreement serves to point out the responsibilities of both the teacher and the learner, thus emphasizing the importance of the mutual commitment. An example of a contractual agreement is given in the accompanying display. It is unnecessary for the contract to be typewritten; a handwritten agreement is acceptable. Informal oral contracts are also possible. Many teaching–learning contracts are verbal agreements between nurses and their clients regarding how and when learner objectives will be met. Contracts should be viewed as aids to learning and should never be intimidating. Nurses can redirect "failures" to meet contracted objectives into new learning and decision-making situations and boost self-esteem by rewarding objectives that were achieved.

Example of a Contractual Agreement Between a Nurse and a Client

I will participate in the learning activities needed to help me learn about my low-salt diet. During my hospital stay, I will attend the class on low-salt diets, read the materials given to me, and ask questions as I need to. I will work with S. Moore, RN, to plan my meals and food preparation at home. If I need help when I get home, I will contact S. Moore.

Jim Mall

I will provide Jim Mall with the experiences needed for him to follow his low salt-diet accurately.

S. Moore R.N.

Learning Activities

While planning teaching strategies, the nurse also decides what learning activities the client is to do independently. There are many ways that the client can preview new material or reinforce what has already been taught. Use of printed material, AV materials, and programmed instruction materials is often assigned in the learning activity column of the teaching plan. This column is used to guide the client in learning activities that can be done before, between, and after planned learning sessions.

Practical Considerations

Time Constraints Time constraints must be considered when planning for the client's learning. A problem for nurses is finding time to meet the client's learning needs. Priorities must be set so that essential content is taught thoroughly. Less important content is taught last so that the more important learner objectives are met within the time available. If time permits, the remaining content can be addressed. Note that in the sample teaching plan in Table 21-1, the client will be taught measures to use immediately.

To meet time constraints, nurses often plan together. Teamwork and cooperation allow the nurses to meet deadlines. If teaching must continue beyond the hospitalization, home visit, or clinic visit, the nurse can schedule additional learning opportunities through outpatient programs or referrals to community-based programs. Home health care nurses often receive referrals from hospital nurses to continue teaching begun during a client's hospitalization. Discharge planning needs to be started early to ensure continuity of teaching.

Scheduling It is better to plan for shorter, more frequent teaching sessions than for one or two longer sessions. Short sessions allow the client to digest the new material and prevent the client from becoming too tired or uncomfortable because of the current health problem. Sessions of 15 to 30 minutes are generally well tolerated. Usually, the more formal classroom programs last for more than 1 hour. In such cases, the nurse should provide breaks after every 50 minutes of class time. As with all nursing care, the client should be included in planning for the time and frequency of lessons.

Group Versus Individual Teaching The nurse must consider several factors when choosing the type of setting for the client. Some learner objectives are met more readily in a one-to-one encounter, whereas others are achieved more easily in a group. For example, the objective "The client will change the dressing using sterile technique" would be evaluated during a private session with the nurse. The objective, "The client will discuss feelings about returning home after a heart attack" might be met more easily in a group discussion with other clients with similar feelings to express.

Certain topics are learned well in group settings, particularly where a sense of comradeship is beneficial. For instance, people who are trying to lose weight for health reasons generally find that learning dietary and nutritional information with other overweight clients is less threatening and can actually be enjoyable. Other material, especially information of a personal nature, may be discussed more effectively with the nurse only.

The nurse should consult the client concerning preferences for group or individual instruction when such a choice is possible. Some people become extremely anxious in group settings, whereas others prefer to learn with others. In addition, the health status of the client can prevent attendance in a classroom setting, thus requiring bedside instruction. On the other hand, a client who is hospitalized may find the change of scenery beneficial to learning.

Formal Versus Informal Teaching   Most nurse—client interactions result in **informal teaching** being done by the nurse (Fig. 21-7). These unplanned teaching sessions are often effective because they deal with the client's immediate learning needs and concerns. Informal teaching often leads to additional planned, formal sessions. **Formal teaching** is the planned teaching done to fulfill learner objectives. Both forms are effective when the nurse uses them appropriately.

Implementing the Teaching Plan

Implementing the teaching plan requires use of interpersonal skills as well as effective communication techniques. Teaching the client can be a major part of the working phase of the helping relationship (see Chapter 20). The nurse must continually observe the client for additional assessment data that could alter the original teaching plan. This requires skill in adapting and reorganizing the teaching plan.

The nurse can facilitate learning in the client by continuing a warm and accepting approach. The nurse's attitude has more effect on the client than any other factor. The nurse must avoid a condescending attitude. Moreover, it is always best to avoid technical and medical terms unless the client has a background in this area. A nonthreatening teaching–learning atmosphere allows learning to occur.

The physical environment is another important consideration when implementing the teaching plan. Some preplanning may be needed to ensure adequate space, comfortable chairs, adequate lighting, and good ventilation. Privacy is also important, as is an environment free of distractions and interruptions.

During the implementation phase, the client as a learner must fulfill certain role functions. To avoid any misunderstandings, it is helpful to review the contractual agreement before implementing the teaching plan. The client is expected to listen, observe, and attempt to understand what is being taught.

Some people are uncomfortable in the role of learner; the nurse must assess this problem so that the client can be

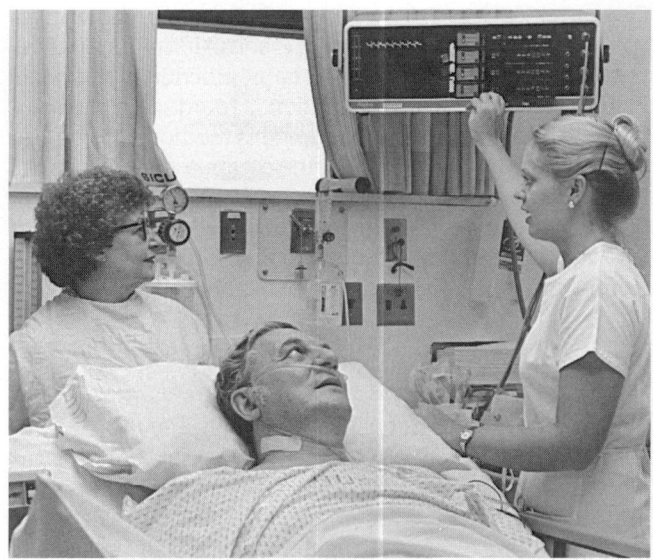

F I G U R E   2 1 - 7

Informal teaching occurs in most nursing interactions with the client and family. (Photo by Gates Rhodes, courtesy of School of Nursing, University of Pennsylvania.)

assisted to assume the role more easily. If special techniques or procedures must be learned (eg, colostomy care, self-injections, or eye medication instillation), the nurse can assure the client that it takes time and practice before anyone can perform new skills confidently.

The implementation phase may be as short as a few minutes, or the sessions may extend over days, weeks, or months, depending on what is being taught and to whom. This phase can be as simple as learning to check a pulse rate or as complex as CPR. As with all nursing care activities, teaching involves total concentration on the client.

The nurse needs to be prepared and organized before implementing the teaching plan. All teaching aids (eg, posters, films, or printed materials) should be gathered and organized before the actual teaching session. A disorganized teacher distracts the learner and has negative effect on the learning. If a procedure or skill is being taught, it is important to proceed in the correct sequence so that the client does not become confused.

An important nursing responsibility is to make each learning session interesting and enjoyable for the client. This is facilitated by an enthusiastic and positive attitude. In addition, the nurse can make learning fun through the creative use of planned teaching strategies. If the nurse approaches teaching positively, the client is more likely to approach learning in a similar way.

Evaluating Teaching–Learning

Evaluating Learning

It cannot be assumed that learning has occurred without some type of proof or feedback. The key to evaluation is the learner objectives written in the teaching plan (see Table 21-1), which describe what behaviors to measure. Methods for obtaining feedback of learning are discussed in the following section.

Methods of Evaluation Methods of evaluation vary. For instance, cognitive domain learning may be evaluated through oral questioning; affective domain, through the client's response; and psychomotor domain, by return demonstration. Consider the following learner objective from the cognitive domain: "The client will be able to describe what a blood pressure reading represents." To evaluate this, the nurse could say to the client, "Tell me what this blood pressure reading means to you." The client then has a chance to talk about the current reading while the nurse evaluates the client's understanding of it.

Sometimes the nurse can use observational skills to determine if the client is using the material learned. For example, observing what the client has ordered for lunch tells the nurse if dietary lessons are being put into practice. The nurse depends on observation when evaluating the client's psychomotor skills. The nurse observes any new technique or skill that the client demonstrates to determine if it is performed satisfactorily.

The client's comments can be used to decide whether learner objectives have been met. Sometimes a client verbalizes understanding of information taught, yet avoids further discussion of the topic. In such instances, the use of effective communication techniques when reintroducing the topic at a later time might provide the evaluation data needed.

F I G U R E   2 1 - 8

A return demonstration is an excellent method of evaluating learning. This client is demonstrating to himself and to the nurse that he is prepared to manage his peritoneal dialysis at home. (Photo by Gates Rhodes, courtesy of School of Nursing, University of Pennsylvania.)

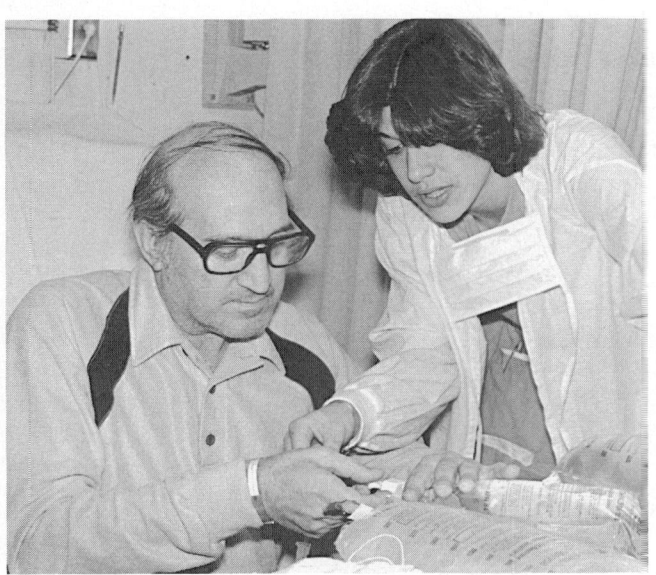

Using direct questions often provides an efficient method of evaluating learner objectives. The nurse simply asks the client a question to elicit a response that reflects the client's level of knowledge concerning a topic. This can also be used to evaluate the client's affective learning.

A return demonstration is an excellent evaluative method for the psychomotor domain (Fig. 21-8). Letting the client change his or her own dressing provides the nurse with concrete evidence of satisfactory or unsatisfactory performance of the procedure. Care must be taken to promote a nonstressful environment for the client's return demonstration.

Evaluation of learning may continue once the client has returned home. Home health care nurses may evaluate what was taught to the client in the hospital as well as what is being taught during home visits. Hospital nurses often check with family members or significant others after discharge to evaluate whether learner objectives have been met. Short-term objectives are usually evaluated while the client is still hospitalized.

Reinforcing and Celebrating Learning

Most people feel encouraged and supported when their efforts are acknowledged by another person, especially when the other person is trusted and valued. This is especially true in health care, where clients often feel overwhelmed by their illness. Nurses who recognize this dynamic can use **positive reinforcement** to affirm the efforts of clients who have mastered new knowledge, attitudes, or skills. Reinforcement may be as simple as a few words of acknowledgment—"You've mastered this diet quickly"; as spontaneous as a warm hug; or as planned as the entire staff joining to celebrate a client's independent ambulation. **Negative reinforcement**—criticism or punishment—generally is ineffective and, for the most part, undesirable behavior is best ignored. Behavior modification programs that reward desired behaviors and ignore undesired behaviors may be designed for some clients.

Evaluating Teaching

Nurses need to evaluate their teaching to capitalize on strengths and work on improving weaknesses. As all nursing roles, teaching requires a great deal of practice and experience. Even nurse educators agree that they are always learning better ways to promote learning in students. It is important to avoid becoming discouraged when evaluations of teaching are less than perfect.

It is best to evaluate one's own teaching effectiveness immediately after each session. This involves a quick review of how the nurse-teacher feels the implementation of the plan went. Mentally noting both the strengths and weaknesses of the teaching session helps the nurse when planning for subsequent sessions.

Nurses can also seek feedback from clients. A simple questionnaire can be used at the end of each teaching session or after discharge to evoke the client's perception of the nurse's teaching effectiveness. The questionnaire may be a standardized form used throughout the hospital or agency or a questionnaire prepared by the nurse-teacher. If it is an objective format, requiring only circles or check marks as answers, space should be provided for comments. The most honest and helpful evaluations are often those that are anonymous. Anonymity, however, is unnecessary and can sometimes bring forth harsh and nonproductive evaluations.

Revisions

During evaluation, nurses and clients may establish that revisions are needed in the teaching plan. A reassessment may indicate that some client factors were not considered in the original plan. Adjustments may be made accordingly to meet the client's needs. Often, the selection of a different teaching strategy is all that is needed for a client to successfully achieve learner objectives. Revision is a natural part of the teaching–learning process and should not be viewed negatively.

Neither the nurse nor the client has failed when an objective is not met. Most objectives can be met with a change in approach; however, learner objectives are sometimes unrealistic. Further assessment by the nurse may reveal that the content may be too complex or the time too short for successful achievement.

Documenting

Because teaching is such an important nursing responsibility, it must be documented in the client's record. Documentation of the teaching–learning process includes a summary of the learning need, the plan, the implementation of the plan, and the evaluation results. The evaluative statement is crucial and must show whether the client has displayed concrete evidence that learning has occurred. If the desired learning has not occurred, the nurse's notes should indicate how the problem was resolved. It is insufficient to document only what was taught. The charting has to show evidence that the client or significant other has learned the material taught. See Table 21-3 for an example of documentation.

Nurse as Counselor

Counseling is the interpersonal process of assisting clients to make decisions that promote their overall well-being. Often family members or significant others are included in the counseling sessions. Everyone participating must feel comfortable in the situation and surroundings.

The interpersonal skills of warmth, friendliness, openness, and empathy are necessary ingredients for successful counseling. The effective counselor needs to be a caring individual. Caring is based on humanistic philosophy (Watson, 1985), which is the core of nursing practice. A humanistic approach to counseling uses the caring process in helping the client strive toward the greatest health potential. Caring is important to all nursing roles but is fundamental in the counseling role.

Some nurses are full-time psychiatric or mental health counselors. The focus in this chapter is on the everyday counseling that is a basic component of each nurse's practice. This counseling involves listening carefully to the

---

TABLE 21-3

Example of Documentation to Meet a Learning Need

Date	Problem-Oriented Progress Note
8/10/93	#2 New Problem—High Risk for Impaired Skin Integrity: Nipples

S —Client stated that her nipples were sore during and after her new-born's first feeding

O —First day postpartum; client is fair skinned with freckles; no reddened areas, no cracking yet; no nipple preparation before delivery

A —At high risk to develop cracked, open areas; client lacks experience and knowledge of preventive measures

P —Develop teaching plan for nipple care

I —Teaching plan implemented

E —Client able to meet all of the objectives satisfactorily as recorded on the teaching plan; she currently is doing protective and preparatory care for her nipples; when breastfeeding, she uses the correct feeding technique with good aftercare; she states that her nipples are no longer sore, and she is able to explain what she should do when she goes home

R —None needed, but reinforcement of content will be continued

L. Sweeney, RN

questions, concerns, demands, and complaints of the client or family and then responding in an effective and facilitative manner. Appropriate responses may be difficult for the nurse to give at first but practice will help to develop these skills. Keep in mind that each nurse–client (or nurse–family) interaction is unique. A nursing response that works well with one client may intimidate or anger another. Sensitivity to the unique needs of each client and a willingness to get involved and make a difference is essential to effective counseling. Table 21-4 presents typical counseling situations that you might experience in your first year of nursing. Both effective and ineffective nursing responses are briefly analyzed. You may want to role-play these situations with a friend. It will quickly become apparent that the nurse who wishes to succeed as a caregiver and counselor needs to master the communication techniques described in Chapter 20.

The three types of counseling are short-term, long-term, and motivational. Following the descriptions of these three types is a discussion of strategies for dealing with uncooperative or noncompliant clients as well as a list of nursing diagnoses for which counseling is the primary intervention. Sometimes a client needs specialized counseling by nurses with advanced training or other health care professionals. In these cases, the best thing you can offer your client is a referral to the appropriate professional (eg, psychologist or psychiatrist, social worker, clergy, financial counselor, sex therapist, or occupational therapist).

Short-Term Counseling

Short-term counseling focuses on the immediate problem or concern of the client or family. It can be a relatively minor concern or a major crisis, but whatever the situation, it needs immediate attention (Fig. 21-9).

In counseling situations, the nurse does not tell the client what to do to solve the problem but instead assists and guides problem solving or decision making. Many people lack the knowledge and skills to approach a problem systematically. This is where the teaching and counseling roles can be combined to help the client solve the dilemma successfully.

The nursing process becomes an essential tool for the nurse in guiding and teaching the client. Nurses are educated to approach all nursing situations in a logical, systematic way. In a crisis situation, whether minor or major, the nurse can share problem-solving abilities with the client. The nursing process was used to organize the nurse–client counseling situation described in the accompanying display.

An example of when short-term counseling could be used is during a **situational crisis**, which occurs when a client faces an event or situation that causes a disruption in life. For example, a male client in the hospital finds out that his spouse has been involved in a car accident. His spouse only received a few scratches but their only car was demolished. The nurse is in an excellent position to help the client decide what can be done to solve this situational crisis. The nurse can guide the client in solving the travel, financial, and emotional difficulties that arise as a result of the accident. This holistic approach is especially necessary because the crisis could affect the client's recovery adversely.

Long-Term Counseling

Counseling is considered *long-term* when it extends over a prolonged period. A client may need the counsel of the nurse for daily, weekly, or monthly intervals. A client experiencing a developmental crisis may need long-term counseling. A **developmental crisis** can occur when a person is going through a developmental stage or passage. For example, many women going through menopause need the assistance of a nurse when adjusting to the changes they experience. Nurses can lead support groups for the purpose of group counseling.

Another example of long-term counseling occurs when a nurse counsels a client who is breastfeeding. The nurse may give assistance and guidance until the baby is weaned, which could be over 2 to 3 years. This type of counseling is often done over the telephone, which saves the client the inconvenience of traveling to meet with the nurse.

Many hospital specialty units provide clients with a telephone number to call for counseling after discharge. Clients are often relieved to know they can call to talk to a nurse at any time of the day or night. After experiencing the close observation and supervision of hospitalization, this telephone connection has helped many clients make the transition from acute care to home care.

Motivational Counseling

Motivational counseling involves discussing feelings and incentives with the client. Nurses often become frustrated because their clients do not seem to want to get better or to learn how to care for themselves. Perhaps individual clients may not have the inner drive or motivation to cooperate in their own health care. Clients often express the words, "I have nothing to live for." If the nurse has established a helping relationship with the client, he or she can help the client work through these feelings of despair. The nurse may be able to get the client to talk about what is generating disinterest in recovery. If a problem is identified, the nurse and client can use the problem-solving technique to work toward an acceptable solution (Fig. 21-10).

If a client shows an unwillingness to participate in learning activities, the nurse can assess any factors from the past or present that might be negatively influencing motivation for learning. Sometimes, if the nurse explains why certain knowledge is needed and the consequences of not learning the material, the client will become more receptive to the teaching–learning process. A trial learning session can be suggested to allow the client to see what the sessions will be like. If the nurse uses the nursing process

(Text continues on p. 362)

TABLE 21-4

An Analysis of Nursing Responses in Common Counseling Situations

Ineffective Response	Analysis	Effective Response	Analysis
Situation A: *You walk into the room of Ms. Goldstein, who learned earlier in the day that her tumor is malignant. She is crying.*			
"Oh cheer up! Tomorrow's got to be a brighter day."	Provides false reassurance; communicates insensitivity to client's feelings.	Touch forearm and sit next to her quietly. After several minutes, say, "I can't even begin to imagine how difficult this must be for you. Please let me know if there is anything I can do to help."	Uses touch, silence, and caring appropriately
Situation B: *You have been teaching 60-year-old Mr. Hyong diabetic self-care for 4 days and he is still asking the same questions and refusing to administer his own insulin or check his blood sugar.*			
"Well, I guess we are getting nowhere here. Is there anyone else who might be able to do this for you?"	Rejects client without first evaluating the teaching plan and exploring client variables that might be hindering learning.	"We may have a bit of a problem here. . . . I hear you asking the same questions every day. Let's see if together we can't figure out why this isn't making sense to you."	Enlists client in problem solving
Situation C: *The daughter of an elderly client with emphysema stops you at the nursing desk and starts screaming that none of the nurses is helping her mother.*			
"That's just not true! I was in your mother's room myself for a good part of the morning."	Gives a defensive response; may invite combat.	"I'm hearing a lot of concern from you about your mom and the care she is receiving. Tell me more about why you feel that the nurses aren't doing enough."	Affirms the daughter's concern and opens the door to communication that may reveal the daughter's true needs
Situation D: *One morning you walk into the room of an older resident who had withdrawn and become totally dependent on the nurses for basic care on her transfer into the nursing home. You are surprised to discover that she has washed and dressed herself—for the first time.*			
"Well, I'm happy to see that you have rejoined the ranks of the living. Did you wash off your glasses?"	Misses opportunity to celebrate the resident's achievement of an important goal.	Hugs resident warmly, looks her in the eye, and exclaims, "Don't you look wonderful today? What are you celebrating?" Defers an assessment of how thorough the morning care has been until later.	Rejoices spontaneously in the resident's achievement and reinforces this behavior. Gives the resident a reason to continue to make progress. Uses touch appropriately.
Situation E: *A 42-year-old male client who is in the step-down unit following a massive heart attack repeatedly tells you how pretty you are while you are assisting with his care. When you attempt to help him out of bed, he squeezes your breast.*			
Turn beet red, try to stammer a response, and flee the room.	Loses control of the situation. Is unable to meet the client's needs because own needs take precedence.	"Please stop. I am not comfortable with your remarks and I most certainly will not allow you to touch me like this. Often men feel like they need to test their virility and attractiveness after a serious illness. I am wondering if that might not be behind some of your behavior this morning?"	Retains control of the situation and keeps the focus on the client's needs. The nurse's second statement normalizes the client's behavior and gives him an opening to share his feelings. The nurse makes no judgment until all the data are in.

(continued)

Ineffective Response	Analysis	Effective Response	Analysis
Situation F:	*You are helping Mr. Stein, who has been on bed rest for 2 weeks because of a painful and debilitating illness, out of bed. A fiercely independent man, he is embarrassed to need your support and looks disgusted with himself when he steps on your foot.*		
"What's the problem, Honey? Haven't been eating your Wheaties?"	Uses terms of endearment, which often denote disrespect and condescension to clients, no matter in what spirit they are uttered.	"No problem Mr. Stein, my husband steps on my toes all the time when we go dancing!" After a few minutes . . . "It must be hard when you are used to doing everything for yourself to all of a sudden find yourself needing others for simple things . . . ?"	Uses humor and empathy appropriately; invites the client to share his feelings.
Situation G:	*Ms. Berretta recently underwent surgery resulting in a urinary diversion. She should be able to change her own ostomy bag by this time but she is still unwilling to look at the stoma, and participate alone in her care. The nurses are getting impatient with her "childish" refusals to learn.*		
"Really Helen, I'll do it myself but you'll be the loser once you get home with this thing and there's no one around to help."	Uses a threat in an attempt to coerce learning (negative reinforcement). Displays unwillingness to explore what is blocking Ms. Berretta's readiness to learn.	Before beginning Ms. Beretta's care: "I think we need to talk before your treatment today. You will be discharged soon and I want you to feel confident about caring for your stoma. I understand that until you can accept it, you don't want to learn anything about it. Would you like to talk about this with me or would you prefer me to make a referral to someone else?"	Communicates respect for client and sensitivity to her needs, without ignoring what is a real problem. Offers the possibility of a referral to another health care professional if the client so wishes.
Situation H:	*Ms. Congar is an alert 70-year-old woman who was admitted for a simple hypertension workup but has developed numerous complications and currently is in her fourth week of hospitalization. She has grown progressively more demanding and crotchety and now uses her call light several times each hour. She is a single woman without family or close friends.*		
Floor nurse to an agency nurse who does not know Ms. Congar: "Watch out for the witch in Room 52. Don't let her get to you . . . nothing pleases her."	Fails to see the client as a human with unique needs—the most effective block to communication.	Floor nurse to agency nurse: "We have really been having problems with Ms. Congar. She is so sick of being hospitalized right now that nothing pleases her. I try to make it a point to drop into her room frequently to see if she needs anything and then she doesn't use the light so often. Good luck."	Acknowledges a real problem but also offers a constructive solution; may be just enough information to help the agency nurse establish a meaningful relationship with the client, and thus be sympathetic to her needs.

Counseling for Human Immunodeficiency Virus Testing

More and more nurses are counseling persons who have been tested for human immunodeficiency virus (HIV). Legal pitfalls, however, can expose both the nurse and the health care institution to liability in such counseling situations. Killian (1990) recommends that nurses consider three basic principles: completeness, consistency, and confidentiality. Nurses new to counseling for HIV testing should become familiar with the Centers for Disease Control guidelines and any statutory and regulatory requirements in the nurse's state or province. Seek further assistance from hospital administration or risk management.

(Killian, W. H. [September 1990]. HIV counseling: Know the risks. *American Nurse*, 28.)

---

approach for counseling, a satisfactory change in the client's motivation may be achieved.

When a nurse assesses a motivational problem, assessing the client's cultural values is important. Often the way a person feels about something is strongly influenced by cultural background. For instance, if a person has grown up in a family where illness is perceived as an inevitable result of aging, it will be difficult to motivate that person to practice preventive measures for health. These problems seem insurmountable, yet a caring nurse can work toward helping the client become oriented toward promoting self-health. When discouraged, the nurse can seek counsel with a colleague to help solve client-centered problems.

Noncompliant Client When the nurse's best counseling efforts fail to produce motivation in the client to adhere to a treatment regimen, the client may be described as **noncompliant**. NANDA lists Noncompliance as one of its accepted diagnoses and defines it as a person's informed decision not to adhere to a therapeutic recommendation. It is critical that a client not be labeled noncompliant until exhaustive nursing energies have been invested in exploring possible factors that may be interfering with the client's learning readiness. Once it can be determined that a client understands his or her options and the probable consequences of noncompliance, than the nurse is ethically bound to respect the treatment decisions a competent person makes. An ethical consult may be helpful to the nurse who is unsure of the correct response in these cases.

Related Nursing Diagnoses

Numerous NANDA-approved nursing diagnoses exist for which counseling is the appropriate nursing intervention. Some of these diagnoses are as follows:

Altered Parenting
Altered Role Performance
Anxiety
Body Image Disturbance
Decisional Conflict (specify)
Defensive Coping
Dysfunctional Grieving
Fear
Health-Seeking Behaviors (specify)
Hopelessness
Impaired Adjustment
Impaired Social Interaction
Ineffective Denial
Ineffective Family Coping
Ineffective Individual Coping
Personal Identity Disturbance
Powerlessness
Self-Esteem Disturbance
Social Isolation
Spiritual Distress (Distress of the Human Spirit)

The nurse who is an effective teacher and counselor has two powerful tools to use in assisting clients to maximize their health potential and enhance their quality of living.

F I G U R E   2 1 - 9

Short-term counseling focuses on an immediate concern of the client. (Photo by Gates Rhodes, courtesy of School of Nursing, University of Pennsylvania.)

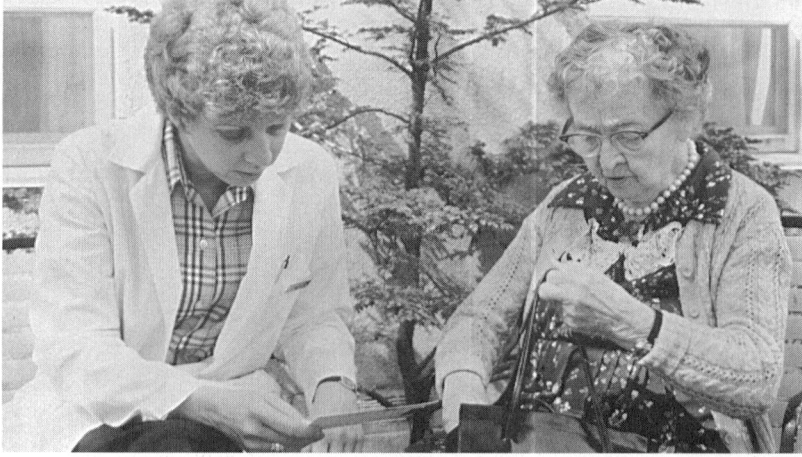

An Example of Problem Solving That Follows the Nursing Process

Situation

Monday, 7:30 PM, Amy Purcell has been admitted to the children's unit with dehydration resulting from diarrhea. Amy is responding well to IV fluids. Her mother is visibly distraught.

Assessing

Amy is doing well but will need 24 hours of IV therapy.
Amy and her twin sister Susan have never been separated from their parents or each other. They are 2 years old.
Ms. Purcell has no idea of who will care for Susan when Mr. Purcell goes to work in the morning.
The Purcells have no regular child-care arrangements and have no family members in the area.
Ms. Purcell wants to stay with Amy during her hospitalization.
The Purcells' neighbor is home during the day. Sometimes Amy and Susan play at her house.
There is a day-care center near their home, but Susan might be upset about going there. It's also expensive.
Mr. Purcell cannot afford to take Tuesday off but will take Wednesday morning off.
Insurance does not cover a private room, which would allow Susan to come to stay in the hospital too.

Diagnosing

Anxiety related to stress of daughter's hospitalization, need for child care for Susan, and uncertain resources

Planning Goal

Ms. Purcell will demonstrate decreased anxiety over the care of Susan during Amy's hospitalization.

Together, Ms. Purcell and the nurse have planned the following:
• The neighbor will come to the Purcell home to care for Susan when Mr. Purcell leaves for work on Tuesday morning.
• The neighbor will bring Susan to the hospital for the afternoon visiting hours to be with Ms. Purcell and Amy.
• Mr. Purcell will come to the hospital after work to have dinner with the family.
• Mr. Purcell will take Susan home for bedtime.
• On Wednesday morning, Mr. Purcell will take off work in the morning. He and Susan will go to the hospital to pick up Ms. Purcell and Amy.

Implementing

Plan implemented by the Purcells with support of the nursing staff.

Evaluating

Ms. Purcell told the nurse that she feels that both Amy and Susan did well with the care they received from their parents. The family's stress was minimized and she is relieved that everything went so well. The nurse decides that the goals were met.

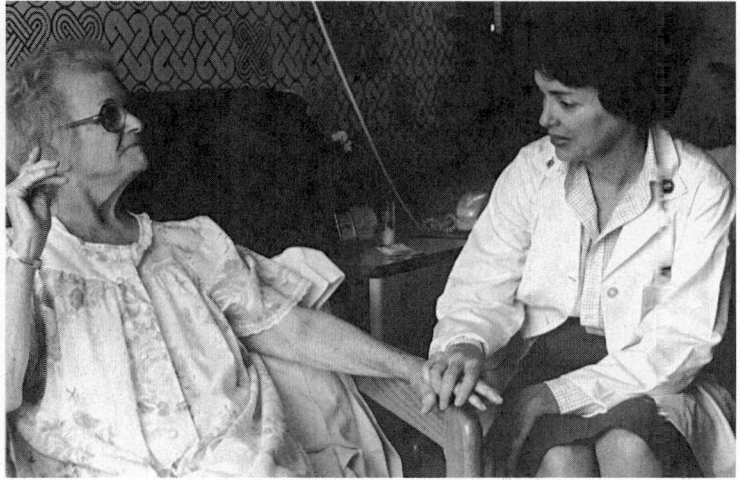

FIGURE 21-10

Motivational counseling involves discussing feelings and incentives with the client. Having established a helping relationship, the nurse can encourage the client to work through feelings that undermine the client's motivation. (Photo by Gates Rhodes, courtesy of School of Nursing, University of Pennsylvania.)

KEY POINTS

- Nurses use communication skills in their roles as teachers and counselors.
- The nursing roles of teacher and counselor require the use of the nursing process; the teaching–learning process follows the steps of the nursing process.
- With the trend of shorter hospital stays, clients and families need more extensive instruction for home care. However, as the importance of teaching increases, the hospital time for teaching decreases. Consequently, the quality of teaching must improve.
- The outcomes of effective teaching and counseling include high-level wellness and related self-care practices; disease prevention or early detection; quick recovery from illness with minimal to no sequelae; enhanced ability to adjust to developmental life changes and acute, chronic, and terminal illness; and family acceptance of the life-style changes necessitated by the illness or disability of a family member.
- Learning can be divided into the following three domains: (1) cognitive learning involves the storing and recalling of new knowledge and information in the brain; (2) psychomotor learning indicates a physical skill has been learned; and (3) affective learning involves changes in attitudes, values, and feelings.
- Assessment of learning needs focuses on the knowledge, attitude, and skills the client needs to independently manage health care; learning readiness; the physical ability to learn; and client strengths. Factors affecting each are explored, often in consultation with the family and significant others.

- Nursing diagnoses are developed that identify health problems related to client deficits in knowledge, attitudes, or skills.
- Teaching plans specify measurable learning objectives, related content, and specific teaching strategies and learning activities. A contractual agreement may facilitate learning.
- Implementing the teaching plan requires use of interpersonal skills as well as effective communication techniques. Teaching is part of the working phase of the helping relationship.
- The evaluation of learning provides the information needed for revisions and for documenting that learning has occurred. Positive reinforcement affirms and encourages learning.
- Counseling involves the nurse in teaching and assisting the client to learn problem-solving techniques.
- The three types of counseling are (1) short-term counseling, which focuses on an immediate problem; (2) long-term counseling, which extends over a prolonged period; and (3) motivational counseling, which involves discussing feelings and incentives with the client.
- Counseling may be needed for assisting the client through crises or for motivating the client to work toward health promotion.

BIBLIOGRAPHY

American Nurses Association. (1991). *Standards of clinical nursing practice.* Kansas City, MO: Author.

American Nurses' Association. (1991). *Position statement on nursing and the patient self-determination act.* Kansas City, MO: Author.

Aquilera, D. C. (1990). *Crisis intervention* (6th ed.). St. Louis: Mosby–Year Book.

Armstrong, M. L. (1989). Orchestrating the process of patient education: Methods and approaches. *Nursing Clinics of North America, 24*(3), 597–604.

Barnes, L. P. (1991). Teaching self-care to children. *MCN: American Journal of Maternal–Child Nursing, 16*(2), 101.

Bartlett, E. E. (Ed.). (1990). Current perspectives: Advances in nursing patient education research. *Patient Education and Counseling, 16*, 5–52.

Bartlett, E. E., & Jonkers, R. (Eds.). (1990). Current perspectives: Patient education—An international comparison. *Patient Education and Counseling, 15*, 101–170.

Bille, D. (1981). *Practical approaches to patient teaching.* Boston: Little, Brown.

Black, K. (1983). *Short-term counseling: A humanistic approach for the helping professions.* Menlo Park, CA: Addison-Wesley.

Bloom, B. S. (1956). *Taxonomy of educational objectives: The classification of educational goals.* New York: David McKay.

Canadian Nurses' Association. (1980). *A definition of nursing practice: Standards for nursing practice.* Ottawa: Author.

Cormier. L. S. (1986). *Interviewing and helping skills.* Boston: Jones & Bartlett.

Dennis, K. E. (1990). Patients' control and the information imperative: Clarification and confirmation. *Nursing Research, 39*(3), 162–166.

Gessner, B. A., & Armstrong, M. L. (Eds.). (1989). Patient teaching. *Nursing Clinics of North America, 24*(3), 583–693.

Hames, C., & Doyle, J. (1986). *Basic concepts of helping: A holistic approach* (2nd ed). New York: Appleton-Lange.

Hussey, L. C. (1991). Overcoming the clinical barriers of low literacy and medical noncompliance among the elderly. *Gerontological Nursing, 17*(3), 27–29.

Kelly, P. (1992). Counseling patients with HIV. *RN, 55*(2), 54–58.

Knowles, M. S. (1980). *The modern practice of adult education: From pedagogy to androgogy* (2nd ed.). Chicago: Follett.

Knowles, M. S. (1984). *The adult-learner: A neglected species* (3rd ed.). Houston: Gulf Publishing.

LaMonica, E. L. (1985). *The humanistic nursing process.* Monterey, CA: Wadsworth.

Lange, J. W. (1989). Developing printed materials for patient education. *Dimensions of Critical Care Nursing, 8*(4), 250–258.

Lipetz, M. J., Bussigel, M. N., Bannerman, J., & Risley, B. (1990). What is wrong with patient education programs? *Nursing Outlook, 38*(4), 184–189.

Lorig, K. (1992). *Patient education: A practical approach.* St. Louis: Mosby–Year Book.

Luker, K. (1989). Rethinking patient education. *Journal of Advanced Nursing, 14*(9), 711–718.

Luker, K. Focus on Patient Teaching [column]. *MCN: American Journal of Maternal–Child Nursing.*

Mann, K. V. (1989). Promoting adherence in hypertension: A framework for patient education. *Canadian Journal of Cardiovascular Nursing, 1*(1), 8–14.

Masten, Y., & Conover, K. P. (1990). Automated continuing education and patient education. *Computers in Nursing, 8*(4), 144–150.

McKerracher, B. (1990). How to lend support in a crisis. *Nursing, 20*(1), 62–64.

Merriam, S. B. (1988). Finding your way through the maze: A guide to the literature on adult learning. *Lifelong Learning: An Omnibus of Practice and Research, 11*(6), 4–7.

Merritt, S. L. (1989). Patient self-efficacy: A framework for designing patient education. *Focus on Critical Care, 16*(1), 68–73.

Murray, R. B., & Zentner, J. P. (1989). *Nursing assessment and health promotion strategies through the life span.* (4th ed.) Norwalk, CT: Appleton & Lange.

North American Nursing Diagnoses Association. (1990). *Taxonomy I revised—1990—with official diagnostic categories.* St. Louis: Author.

Rankin, S. H., & Stallings, K. D. (1990). *Patient education* (2nd ed.). Philadelphia: Lippincott.

Redman, B. K. (1992). *The process of patient education* (7th ed.). St. Louis: Mosby.

Resnick, B. M. (1991). Geriatric motivation: Clinically helping the elderly to comply. *Journal of Gerontological Nursing, 17*(5), 17–20.

Runions, J. (1988). Impediments to the practice of patient teaching. *Canadian Journal of Nursing Administration, 1*(2), 12–15.

Shofer, K. K. K., & Ward, C. J. (1990). The computerization of the patient education process. *Computers in Nursing, 8*(3), 116–122.

Theis, S. L. (1991). Using previous knowledge to teach elderly clients. *Gerontological Nursing, 17*(8), 34–37.

Watson, J. (1985). *Nursing: The philosophy and science of caring.* Denver: Colorado University Press.

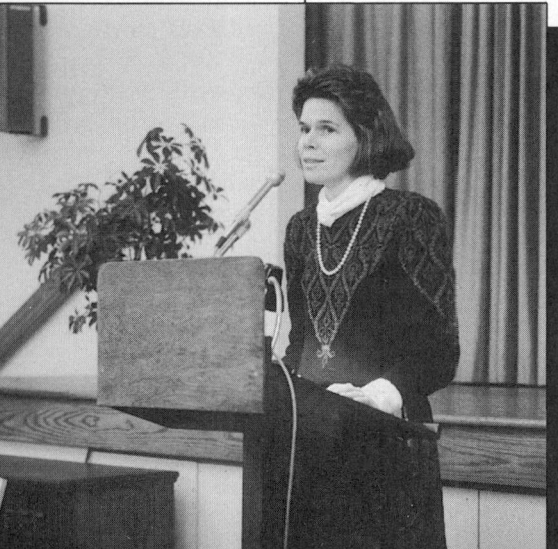
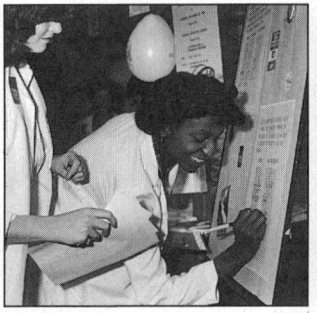

Leader, Researcher, and Advocate

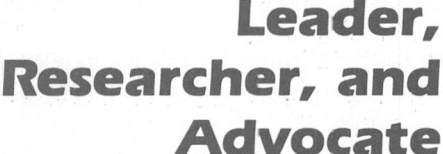

OBJECTIVES

After studying this chapter, the learner should be able to:

Define key terms used in the chapter.

Identify the qualities, four skills, and three styles of leaders.

List the four managerial functions.

Summarize the steps in the process of change.

Describe areas in which the beginning nurse can develop leadership skills that enhance the caregiver role.

Give an example of mentorship in nursing.

Compare the strengths and limitations of three sources of nursing knowledge.

Describe three ways the beginning nurse can use research to enhance the caregiver role.

Explain different ways nurse caregivers can be advocates for clients.

Describe the nurse advocate's role in situations requiring ethical decision making.

Explain how two types of advance directives promote client dignity and well-being.

KEY TERMS

advance directive
advocacy
assertiveness
autonomy
change
change agent
durable power of attorney for health
    care
group process
informed consent
knowledge
    authoritative knowledge
    scientific knowledge
    traditional knowledge
leadership
    autocratic leadership
    democratic leadership
    laissez-faire leadership
living will
management
mentorship
objectivity
planned change
power
preceptorship
professionalism
readiness
variables
    dependent variables
    extraneous variables
    independent variables

22

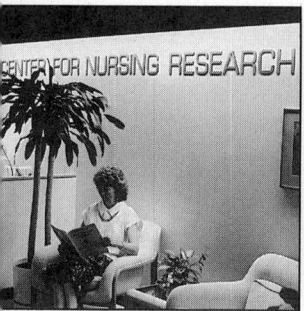
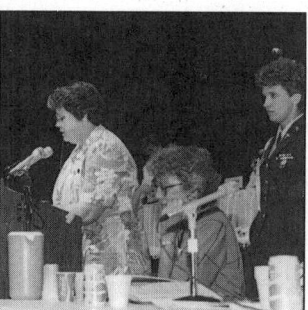

ood leaders must be advocates of client's rights to attain the ultimate goal of improved client care. Furthermore, good advocates need leadership skills to achieve positive changes for clients. Leadership and advocacy complement each other. Research gives a knowledge base to the leader and advocate. It adds the dignity of professionalism to teaching, counseling, and communication, all nursing skills applied to the leadership role.

Although many great nursing leaders have emerged throughout history, most nurses were kept in subordinate positions. However, this subordination has diminished gradually over the past several decades. Currently, most nurses feel more self-directed. This trend is expected to continue and accelerate as more nurses learn to apply their leadership skills in research and advocacy.

Although many nurses function as full-time leaders in institutional and professional groups or as full-time researchers or advocates, this chapter explores how the roles of leader, researcher and advocate enhance the basic caregiver role of the nurse.

Although it takes time and experience to develop these skills, the beginning nurse can monitor his or her progress by periodically reviewing the checklist provided to improve these skills.

Nurse as Leader

Leadership Dynamics

Leadership is the ability to direct or motivate others toward the achievement of predetermined goals; the leader may work toward influencing an individual or a group. Leaders have power, whether it is explicit or implied. Much of this power depends on the leadership style and how leadership responsibilities are fulfilled. The dynamics of leadership involve applying that power to growth or change. Nurses who use leadership skills can become proficient in effecting desired changes in many areas, including their clients' health patterns, the health care agency, the community, the nursing profession, and the health care system in general.

Leadership Qualities

Most people would agree that leaders should be dynamic, enthusiastic, and self-directed. They need to be comfortable with themselves (ie, have a positive self-image) and present themselves as role models to followers. Ideally they possess a vision that energizes the group and calls forth the best efforts of members. Critical thinkers and responsible decision makers, they commit high energy to goal achievement and are skilled in enlisting support and cooperation.

Leaders value learning and must be knowledgeable. Because it is impossible for nurse leaders to be knowledgeable about all aspects of the profession, they develop and use resources. They use each other and other health care workers as resources, respecting one another's expertise. Political awareness is also required of the nurse leader. Knowing how legislation at the local, state or province, and national levels affects health care allows the nurse to make informed decisions when voting for and supporting candidates.

Flexibility is a must for leaders. All nursing functions and roles require flexibility. The needs of clients, families, and the nursing team can change from minute to minute. A flexible, knowledgeable nurse is a welcomed team member.

Although aggression is rarely suited to the leadership role, leaders need assertiveness in nearly all leadership situations. It is used extensively when effecting change. Assertiveness is a learned quality all nurses can develop. (Assertiveness is discussed in Chapter 20.)

Leadership qualities exist in every nurse. With education and practice, these qualities can be developed to the point where a nurse is skilled in the many behaviors necessary for leadership. A discussion of each of these qualities and skills is beyond the scope of this text; the checklist earlier in the chapter provides an overview of how one might approach the role of leader.

Leadership Skills

The four basic types of skills needed for nursing leadership are as follows:

Communication skills—the ability to establish trusting interpersonal relationships with clients, peers, subordinates, and superiors that maximize goal achievement and enhance the personal growth of all participants

Problem-solving skills—the ability to analyze all sides of a problem, to explore multiple options, and to work to a creative solution; the ability to plan, implement, and stabilize change

Management skills—the ability to direct others toward goal achievement; this ability involves the recognition and fostering of unique talents and skills of others and ability to match these with necessary tasks, organizational skills, financial skills, and the ability to generate and use resources wisely (see accompanying display)

Checklist for the Beginning Nurse Who Wishes to Develop Leadership, Research, and Advocacy Skills

Basic Attitudes and Skills

Read the statements on the right and circle the appropriate response: (1) rarely characterizes me, (2) sometimes characterizes me, and (3) often characterizes me.

1 2 3   1. I am self-directed. I know what I want and take the necessary steps to get it.

1 2 3   2. I know my strengths and limitations and feel confident with who I am and who I am becoming.

1 2 3   3. I get an idea and energize others to help me "make it happen."

1 2 3   4. I coordinate or direct the activities of others, matching their abilities to the necessary task.

1 2 3   5. I reason objectively about a situation without letting my feelings or those of others bias my analysis.

1 2 3   6. Once I have identified a problem I work at it until I resolve it—to the extent that this is within my power.

1 2 3   7. When I need help, I know where to find it and ask for it.

1 2 3   8. I recognize the talents of others and offer sincere compliments.

1 2 3   9. I accept compliments and enjoy my success.

1 2 3   10. I confront individuals who are abusing my rights or those of others in my group.

1 2 3   11. I use assertiveness techniques when defending rights.

1 2 3   12. I am flexible and can change direction once I see the value of another course of action.

1 2 3   13. I follow an appropriate chain of command when problem solving.

1 2 3   14. I question how nursing interventions might be improved.

The higher your score the better. Reread the statements where you checked "1" and see how you might plan to improve in these areas.

Beginning Execution of Role Responsibilities: Leader, Researcher, Advocate

Read the list of behaviors on the right and check the appropriate box—met or not met.

MET   NOT MET

____   ____   1. Recognize some personal need you have been ignoring and take steps to ensure that it is met.

____   ____   2. Think of some group you belong to (eg, school, work, church, or social) whose members' needs are not being met and plan with other members to tackle the problem.

____   ____   3. Recognize the special advocacy needs of a client you believe is being underserved by the health care system. Become an advocate for this client.

____   ____   4. Find a nursing research study that recommends a specific type of care for one of your clients. Implement the recommendation and compare your findings with those of the researchers.

____   ____   5. Identify a researchable problem in your area of nursing practice. Describe what might make a good study.

____   ____   6. Join a professional nursing organization and become an active member.

____   ____   7. Analyze the media's portrayal of nurses in a specific television program, film, or book. Talk with a friend about how this portrayal of nursing influences your profession. Share your comments with the producer or author.

____   ____   8. Contact your legislator to share your views about pending legislation.

____   ____   9. Think about leaders you admire and respect; interview current nursing leaders; develop a plan for personal professional growth and development.

____   ____   10. Develop a mentoring relationship with a nursing leader.

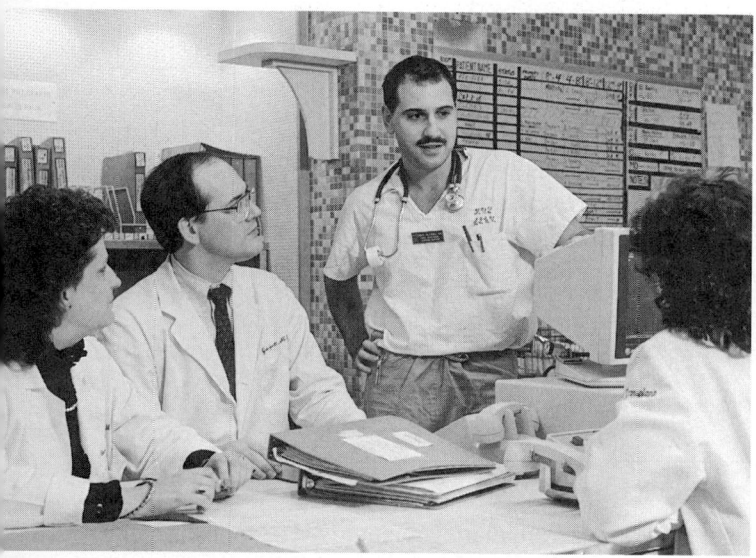

FIGURE 22-1

Leadership styles vary. The nurse should choose one that is comfortable and will be effective for the situation.

Self-evaluation skills—the ability to honestly assess one's effectiveness and to accept both praise and blame; the ability to direct personal professional growth and development

Leadership Styles

Three styles of leadership are commonly identified in the nurse's work settings—autocratic, democratic, and laissez-faire. Generally speaking, it is best for nurses to use the leadership style with which they are most comfortable if that style is effective for the task at hand and for the groups they are leading. The variables of the nurse's own personality, the group personality, and the tasks or objectives to be accomplished must be considered in each leadership situation.

Autocratic Leadership Autocratic leadership occurs when the leader assumes complete control over the decisions and activities of the group. The nurse with an autocratic personality can be described as "firm, insistent, self-assured, and dominating with or without intent, and keeps at the center of attention" (Douglass, 1992). There can be extremes in autocratic leadership, such as a leader who makes all the decisions for the workers or followers without consideration of the followers' ideas or feelings.

Many nurses are used to working under an autocratic leader. This approach has been used in most hospital settings until recently. It seems to have evolved from the military and religious images that nursing has developed historically. These images and this type of leadership are gradually being replaced by the democratic style of leadership, as nurses demand more participation in decision making.

Situation Nurse A has discovered that one of her clients is bleeding excessively from his surgical incision. She knows that he needs immediate attention, so she begins to give specific orders to another team member to attend to the needs of the other clients. She tells the registered nurse on her team to call the surgical resident to come as soon as possible. She implements a nursing plan of care to prevent further blood loss or complications.

Nurse A chose the autocratic style of leadership in this situation so that all of the necessary tasks would be accomplished immediately. Although she rarely uses this style, she implemented it effectively in this emergency situation.

Democratic Leadership Democratic leadership is characterized by a sense of equality among the leader and the followers. Decisions and activities are shared. The followers are encouraged to develop their skills and strengths within the group. The group and leader strive to work to accomplish mutually set goals. The leader needs to develop skills in group dynamics to apply this type of leadership effectively.

More nurses currently are working toward the democratic style of leadership. Nurses, as professionals, tend to respond well to this type when they are the followers and feel more comfortable when they are the leaders of democratic groups. Group satisfaction and motivation can be excellent benefits of this style.

Situation Nurse B, a head nurse, observes that staff members have not been documenting client teaching and learning in the nurse's progress notes. Nurse B is not sure why this has occurred but feels that this problem must be solved. He calls a staff meeting, and leads a discussion to seek information on possible causes and planning strategies.

Nurse B has decided that staff members need to be included in the problem-solving approach. He thinks the staff will be more motivated to document their teaching and the clients' learning if they have a say in how the changes will be implemented. Nurse B has used the democratic style of leadership.

Laissez-Faire Leadership In laissez-faire leadership, the leader has relinquished all power to the group. This encourages independent activity by the group members (Douglass, 1992). An outsider would be unable to identify the leader in such a group. This style depends on the strengths of the followers to direct the group activities.

This style is rarely seen in the hospital setting because task achievement is difficult when each nurse is working independently. However, it could be used effectively when the leader wants a problem to be solved completely by the group members. It has been successful in cases in which there is resistance to a certain policy or change and the leader allows the group to work to achieve an acceptable solution.

Situation Nurse C, a clinical coordinator, has read an interesting research study that supports a change in the cur-

COMPUTER APPLICATIONS IN NURSING

Computers as Office Assistance

Many nursing unit managers carry heavy responsibilities for planning, budgeting, and evaluating delivery of increasingly sophisticated levels of care. Computers are superbly adapted to assist with these chores. Two recent developments have brought the power and flexibility of the personal computer (PC) within the reach of middle managers: there has been a sharp decline in the price of computer hardware (a PC system can now be assembled for less than $2000), and sophisticated, user-friendly software has been developed. Three commonly used business software tools with multiple uses for nurse managers are (1) word processors, (2) spreadsheets for financial analysis, and (3) data base management systems used to store and analyze files of information.

(Tamarisk, N. K. [1990]. Personal computer databases for middle managers. *Management, 21*[7], 49–51.)

rent instructions being given to new mothers who are breastfeeding. The article, with a summary of findings, is posted in all of the nurses' stations in the maternity unit.

Nurse C is using a laissez-faire leadership style and is confident That the individual staff members are capable professionals who are concerned with keeping up with current research findings that they can use to improve their nursing care.

Leadership and Management

All nurses are leaders. Some nurses, because of their positions in the health care system, are also managers. The role of the nurse manager is to plan, organize, direct, and control available human, material, and financial resources to deliver quality care to clients and families.

Planning—identifying problems, developing goals, objectives, and related strategies

Organizing—pulling resources together to meet objectives

Directing—leading others in goal achievement

Controlling—implementing mechanisms for ongoing evaluation

Hersey and Blanchard (1977) substituted motivating for directing as one of the four management functions. This substitution is compatible with the recent shift in emphasis

"Four Rights" of Delegation

Delegating can be facilitated when you remember the "four rights" of delegation:

- The *right task* (the one that can be delegated)
- The *right person* (the one qualified to do the job)
- The *right communication* (clear, concise description of the objective and your expectations)
- The *right feedback* (evaluation in a timely manner, during and after the task is completed)

(Hansten & Washburn, 1992).

in organizations from management (used to control enterprises) to leadership (used to bring out the best in people and to respond quickly to changes; Naisbitt & Aburdene, 1990). Chief nurse executives have come to realize that nurse managers must be effective leaders to be successful. In all likelihood, nursing units with low morale, high turnover, and frequent physician and client complaints have unskilled leaders. Nursing managers who cannot create healthy group environments, who fail to define interpersonal issues that lower morale, and who are unable to develop a plan to resolve detrimental interpersonal issues lack leadership skills (Manthey, 1990).

Group Dynamics

A *group* exists when two or more people are gathered together. To be functional, the members must communicate with each other for the purpose of achieving a goal or purpose. When functional groups are observed or studied for their effectiveness or ineffectiveness, it is commonly referred to as *group dynamics*. Group dynamics involves the evaluation of whether a group was effective in making the changes that were planned. If the group was ineffective, the reason is investigated. Group dynamics also includes studying how the individual group members relate to each other during the process of working toward group goals. This observation can be done by the members themselves, the leader, or an outside observer. Much can be gained by the careful assessment of the dynamics or internal life of the group.

Types of Groups

Groups can be categorized by size—one-to-one, small, and large. Nurses, both professionally and personally, commonly belong to each of these types of groups. Many nursing situations involve the nurse and client in a one-to-one group—a collaborative situation in which the nurse maintains a leadership advantage.

Nurses participate in small groups as members and as leaders (Fig. 22-2). For example a nurse may lead a group of family members in discussing how they can meet their

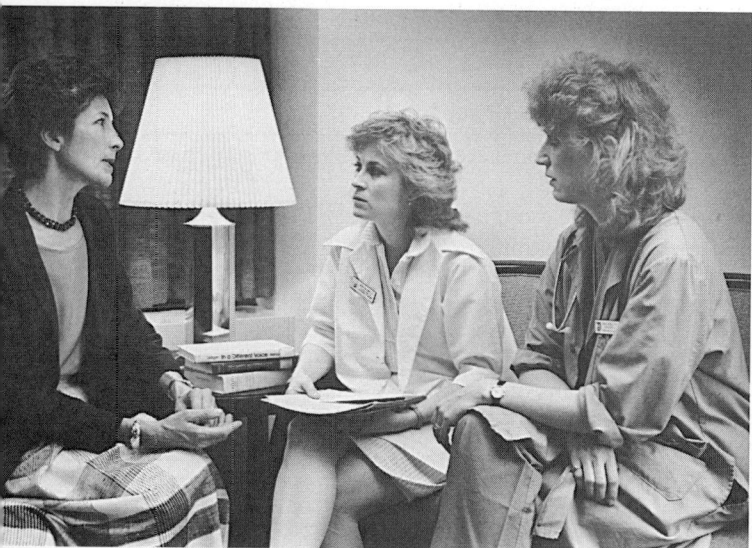

FIGURE 22-2

Nurses participate in small groups as members and as leaders. (Photo by Robert Neroni, courtesy of Thomas Jefferson University.)

mother's needs for supervision at home. The same nurse may also belong to the hospital safety committee and work toward achieving committee goals. In addition, many nurses choose to serve large groups of people through their involvement in community-based programs, such as community health-planning boards; health-promoting organizations (eg, American Red Cross, American Cancer Society, or American Heart Association); or even school board committees.

Groups can also be categorized as formal or informal. *Formal groups* usually stipulate membership requirements as well as group goals. The local chapter of the American Nurses' Association (ANA) is an example of a formal group. *Informal groups* have fewer rules and regulations, and sometimes none at all. A group of nurses gathered together during their lunch break is considered an informal group. A nurse who is discussing the hospital discharge policy with a group of clients in the lounge has formed an informal group.

Purpose of Groups

A group must have a purpose to bind its members together. The purpose may change and grow as the group develops or its membership changes. Most groups are formed for the purpose of effecting change, reflected in the group goals that are set. Some groups dissolve once the goals have been met; other groups may set new goals, thus continuing the group's existence.

The group's purpose may be clearly indicated by the group's name. Many formal groups have names that explain their purpose. Other groups may have more subtle or covert purposes, yet, on inspection, their mission becomes clear.

Roles of Group Members

Although effective leadership facilitates a group's achievement of its goals, the group's success or failure is largely a function of member behaviors. Ideally each group member uses his or her talents and interpersonal strengths to help the group accomplish its goals while maintaining sensitivity to the needs of individual group members. Group members who attempt to dominate or thwart the group process are confronted. Effective and ineffective groups are contrasted in Table 22-1. Member roles have been categorized as task-oriented roles whose focus is the work to be done; group-building or maintenance roles whose focus is the well-being of people doing the work; and self-serving roles, which advance the needs of individual members at the group's expense. Examples of these roles follow:

Task roles—information giver, information seeker, clarifier, coordinator, delegator, energizer, evaluator

Maintenance roles—active listener, harmonizer, trust builder, tension reliever, supporter

Self-serving roles—attention seeker, dominator, blocker, special pleader, withdrawer, aggressor (Benne & Sheats, 1948)

Effecting Change Through Leadership

Change is the process of transforming, altering, or modifying something. It may be planned, unplanned, or developmental. Nursing and the health care system are continually changing and evolving. Such factors as the increase in the number of chronically ill and elderly people, the increase in government intervention in health care, the rising cost of health care, and the changing patterns of health care delivery have helped provoke the need for innovation and change in health care.

Many theories of change exist but most are modifications of the classic theory of change proposed by Kurt Lewin in 1951. Lewin posited the following three stages of change:

Unfreezing: The need for change is recognized.

Moving: Change is initiated after careful process of planning.

Refreezing: Change becomes operational.

Planned change is a purposeful, systematic effort to alter or bring about change through the intervention of a change agent. Basic questions to consider before planning to make changes are highlighted in the accompanying display.

The eight steps in the process of change loosely follow the steps of the nursing process:

1. Recognize symptoms that indicate a change is needed and collect data.
2. Identify a problem to be solved through change. Analyze the symptoms and reach a conclusion. Note resistance or barriers to change and factors that promote the desired change.
3. Determine and analyze alternate solutions to the problem. Consider the advantages, disadvantages,

A Comparison of Effective and Ineffective Groups

Variable	Effective Group	Ineffective Group
Group identity	Members value and "own" the aims of the group; aims are clearly articulated	Group's aims are not of major importance to members
Cohesiveness	Members generally trust and like one another and are loyal to the group; high commitment; high degree of cooperation	Members often feel alienated from the group and from one another; low commitment; members tend to work better alone than with the group
Patterns of interaction	Honest, direct communication flows freely; members support, praise, and critique one another	Communication is sparing; little self-disclosure; self-serving roles (ie, dominator, blocker, or aggressor) may be unchecked
Decision making	Problems are identified, appropriate method of decision making is used (ie, individual, minority, majority, consensus, or unanimous); decision is implemented and followed through; group commitment to decision is high	Problems are allowed to build without resolution; little responsibility is shown for problem solving; group commitment to decision is low
Responsibility	Members feel strong sense of responsibility for group outcomes	Little responsibility for group felt by group members
Leadership	Effective style of leadership to meet desired aims	Ineffective leadership styles
Power	Sources of power are recognized and used appropriately; needs or interests of those with little power are considered	Power is used and abused to "fix" immediate problems; little attention to needs of powerless

and consequences of each alternative. An analysis of various proposed solutions to a problem may result in using a combination of alternatives.

4. Select a course of action from possible alternatives. It is best to avoid initiating too many courses of action and thereby dissipating resources and energy.

5. Plan for making a change. This step is critical to effect change successfully. Start by stating specific objectives, designing a plan for change, developing timetables, selecting people to assist with making the change, and anticipating how to stabilize change and how to deal with resistance to change. Unless a plan is clearly designed, effecting change is likely to be a chaotic experience.

6. Implement the selected course of action to effect change. The plan for change is then put into effect. During this period, flexibility is important to adapt to unforeseen problems.

7. Evaluate the effects of change by comparing them with objectives stated in the plan for change. Adjustments can be made in the plan as necessary after evaluation. If the results of evaluation indicate that the course of action selected to solve a problem has been unsuccessful, an adjustment or another course of action should be selected.

8. Stabilize the change. When a solution to a problem has been found, take measures to make the change permanent. Continue follow-up until the change is firmly established.

The same steps apply whether dealing with individuals or groups. Figure 22-3 illustrates the process of change.

Resistance to Change

Sometimes people resist change for various reasons. The leader must decide why there is resistance and what techniques will overcome the resistance.

Threat to Self People tend to view change in terms of how they are affected personally. Personal threats may include a loss of self-esteem, a belief that more work will be required, and a belief that social relationships will be disrupted. For example, when unit management was instituted in health agencies, many nurses resisted because they felt the unit clerks would take away their responsibilities, for example, transcribing physicians' orders.

Lack of Understanding The person who does not understand the nature of change is likely to resist. The involvement of people affected by change is important to overcome resistance. For example, nurses who do not realize the effectiveness of nursing care plans tend to resist preparing them because they believe they are not beneficial in providing client care.

Limited Tolerance for Change Some people simply do not like to function in a state of flux or disequilibrium. A person may understand the need for change but may be unable to cope emotionally with the change itself. For example, a nurse may resist change because of the confusion a change is likely to cause.

Basic Questions to Consider Before Effecting Change

- *What is amenable to change?* The answer to this question may reveal behavior not amenable to change.
- *How does the group function as a unit?* A change agent can make certain deductions concerning forces within a group favoring change and forces likely to resist change.
- *What resources are available to help make a change?* If specific resources are unavailable, adjustments must be made in keeping with available resources.
- *Is the person or group ready for change and, if so, at what rate can it be reasonably expected that change will be accepted?* The pace of change must be consistent with the person's or group's readiness to assimilate change. *Readiness* is possessing the ability to change.
- *Are the changes major or minor in nature?* A series of small changes may be more easily accomplished than one large change. Also, stability in one area in which change has just occurred is necessary before change begins in another area.

Disagreements About the Benefits of Change Resistance may occur when the information available to the change agent and those resisting change is different. If the information provided by people resisting change is more accurate and relevant than information held by the change agent, the resistance may be beneficial. As an example, consider a plan that had been effective in implementing home health care in a middle-class section of a city. The supervisor of community-health services proposed that the plan be implemented in a low-income neighborhood. The nurse in charge of the health program in the low-income area resisted, believing that a plan suitable for a middle-class section of the community could not be used in a financially and educationally disadvantaged neighborhood.

Fear of Increased Responsibility Many people are worried about having more complex responsibilities placed on them. This is especially true if they feel unprepared for the planned changes. The changes may seem overwhelming, so they respond by resisting.

Overcoming Resistance to Change

Nurses, in their leadership roles, find that they often must work to overcome resistance to change. Resistance can be subtle or distinct, gentle or aggressive. Responding to resistance is a leadership challenge in which a person's leadership qualities, leadership style, and knowledge of group

dynamics are combined to influence individuals toward a desired outcome. The nurse acting as an agent of change will find the following guidelines helpful for overcoming resistance to change:

- Explain the proposed change to all affected people in simple, concise language.
- List the advantages of the proposed change, both for an individual and for members of a group.
- Relate the proposed change to the existing beliefs and values of the person or group.
- Help overcome resistance by providing opportunities for open communication and feedback.
- Indicate clearly how the change will be evaluated.
- Introduce change gradually. Involve everyone affected by the change in the design and implementation of the process.
- Provide incentives for commitment to change. Incentives may be money, status, time off, or a better working environment.

Power

Nurses who wish to be effective change agents are sensitive to both the uses and abuses of power. **Power**, the ability

FIGURE 22-3

A planned change model demonstrating the logical process through which change is planned and implemented. (Spradley, B.W. [1980]. Managing change creatively. *Journal of Nursing Administration, 10*[5], 33.)

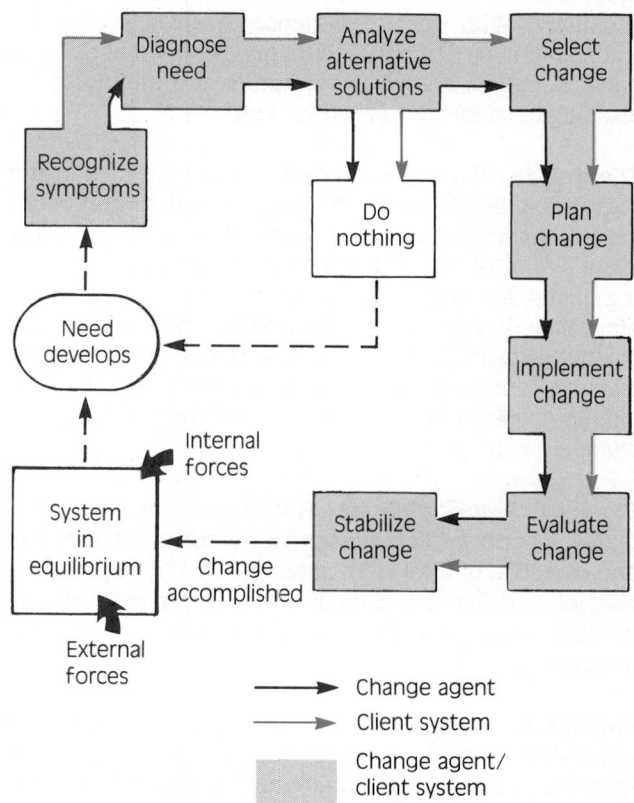

to influence others to achieve a desired effect, has many sources. Certain management positions within an institution, for example, director of nursing or charge nurse, have ascribed power associated with the role. Simultaneously, a group may attribute power to different individuals because of their expertise, leadership, or charisma. When introducing change, it is helpful to recognize and enlist the support of key power players who can then encourage others to become involved. Nursing leaders recognize the strengths and limitations of their own power and encourage the development and constructive use of power in others.

Leadership Skills and the Nurse's Caregiver Role

No one is born a leader. People develop leadership qualities through observations, knowledge, and experiences. Nurses develop their leadership qualities in the same way, although they may enter nursing with some background in leadership experiences.

Nursing students and beginning practicing nurses have some leadership responsibilities, but they are still working at developing skills and learning where and how to apply them. Fortunately, they have support systems for guidance.

Areas of Leadership

Leadership should be approached as any new role and skill is approached—slowly and carefully. The nursing student and beginning nurse should be prepared with all of the necessary tools or skills before attempting the new role. Initially, a nurse develops leadership skills in well-defined situations. With each experience, growth occurs and leadership is strengthened. It helps to remember that all nurse managers, nurse administrators, and nursing leaders also began as inexperienced nurses.

Client Care Even new graduate nurses have leadership responsibilities on the nursing unit where they work. Nursing leadership begins with nursing care of the individual client (Fig. 22-4). Nurses have to take the initiative in helping clients. Although clients are partners in their care planning, they do not have the knowledge base and skills to direct the plan. Through use of interpersonal skills and effective communication techniques, nurses lead their clients in acquiring new knowledge, solving problems, and changing behaviors.

Employee Responsibilities Nurses have specific tasks or duties to perform. These tasks are determined by the plan and objective of the health care agency. It is important to read job descriptions carefully and to continue to evaluate how institutional factors influence an individual's practice of nursing.

Managerial Responsibilities New graduate nurses use leadership techniques when they cover for the team leader's break. Gradually, new nurses assume increased leadership responsibilities as they become team leaders or

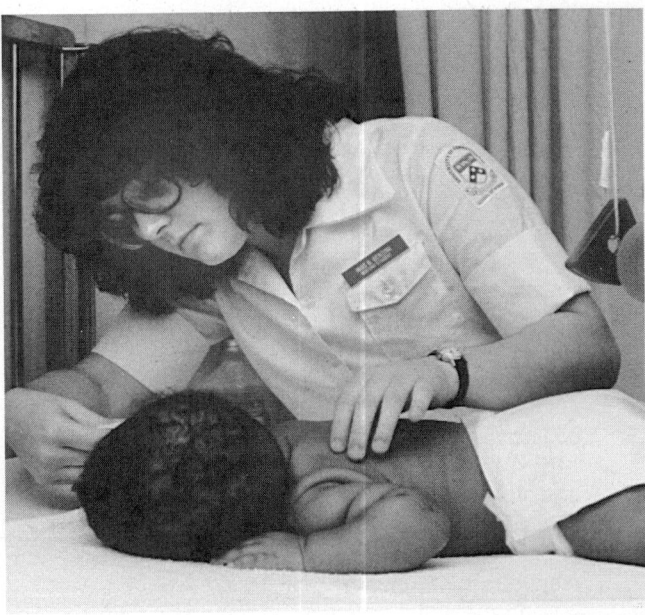

F I G U R E   2 2 - 4

Nursing leadership begins with nursing care of the individual client. (Photo by Gates Rhodes, courtesy of School of Nursing, University of Pennsylvania.)

primary nurses. The graduate nurse is responsible for one or two auxiliary personnel, and eventually the nurse may be in charge of an entire unit, which can include 3 to 10 nursing staff members and up to 60 clients.

Nursing Department The nursing team can also be viewed in the broader sense of the entire nursing department of a health care institution or agency. Nurses should have an interest in the functioning of the department. Using this knowledge, nurses can seek information or change through appropriate channels. The more nurses understand how the nursing department runs, the better able they are to constructively work toward the objectives of the department.

Employing Institution Nurses at all levels need to be knowledgeable about the administrative structure and functions of the employing institution. When problems arise concerning professional, unit, departmental, or institutional objectives, nurses must be able to use the proper channels of communication. These channels are structured according to the organization chart of the institution. The organization chart shows the relationships among the various administrative positions, the hospital departments, and the various job titles. Sometimes the nurse is referred to committees that deal with specific problems or to other hospital departments, such as public relations.

Research Nurses need to be concerned with the advancement of nursing as a profession. Of the many ways to promote nursing's evolution toward greater autonomy and strength, an important facet is nursing research (Fig. 22-5). The nurse as researcher is more fully discussed in the next section. Nurses have given, and will continue to give, comprehensive and cost-efficient care by using the research findings of their colleagues. Nurse researchers can provide staff nurses with invaluable information to use in client care, but staff nurses also contribute to nursing research by doing the following:

- Observing all nursing care activities to look for any area that needs improvement
- Questioning one's own practice to see if the rationale behind caregiving activities is sound
- Participating in the client-care research done by colleagues or nurse researchers
- Making suggestions for specific topics to be researched

Legislation Keeping informed concerning local, state or provincial, and national legislation allows nurses to write or call legislators before new laws are passed. Many nursing publications, newsletters, and papers have sections giving nurses specific information and guidelines on writing to elected officials concerning health-related legislation. ANA has lobbyists in Washington, DC, as well as in the state capitals. The potential influence of nurses in the continued improvement of health care is phenomenal (Fig. 22-6).

Public Image Nurses create the public's image of nursing whenever they interact with others and are recognized as a nurse. It is critical for beginning practitioners of nursing to understand the power they have to positively or negatively affect nursing's image. Because nurses are often portrayed negatively by the media (eg, as sex objects or as uncaring females), it is important that the public experience nurses who are intelligent, competent, and caring to reverse the media's image.

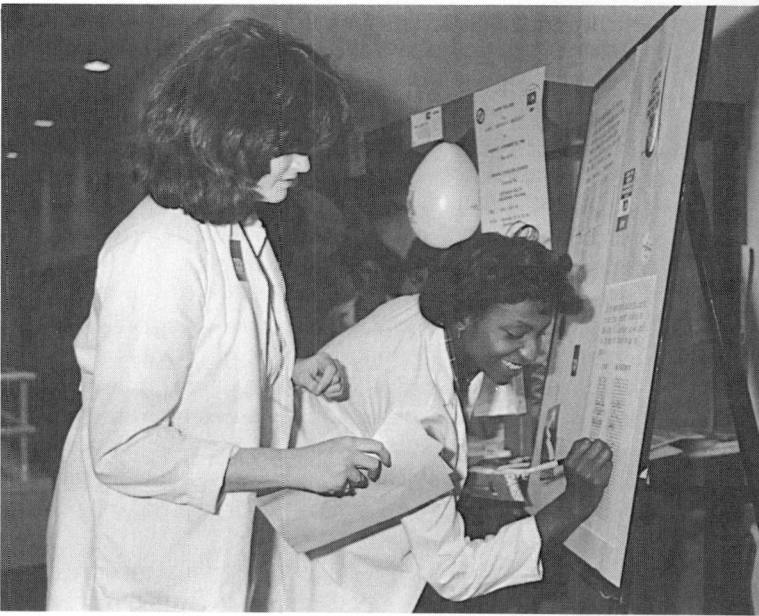

FIGURE 22-6

If all registered nurses (1.7 million in the United States alone) were active in movements for change and improvement in health care, they would command tremendous power and influence. (Photo by Robert Neroni, courtesy of Thomas Jefferson University.)

Kalisch and Kalisch (1983) recommend that nurses change negative portrayals of nursing in the media by organizing, monitoring the media, reacting to the media, and fostering an improved image. Certainly not all nurses are interested in joining a media watch group, but all nurses can practice nursing care in a manner that promotes a positive image of nursing.

Support for Leadership Training

Mentorship Mentorship is a relationship in which an experienced individual (the *mentor*) advises and assists a less experienced individual (*protégé* or *protégée*). This is an effective way of easing a new nurse into the leadership responsibilities that will be expected in the future. Mentors link with protégés or protégées by common interest and provide support, information, and network links. The relationship does not include financial reward.

Mentorship is used in all types of nursing positions. As a nurse climbs the ladder of leadership responsibility, a mentor who is experienced in management and administrative functions may be chosen. A mentor can be a critical factor in helping the less experienced nurse to successfully assume added responsibilities and position changes.

The role of mentor can be rewarding. Besides receiving the satisfaction of helping a newer nurse, the mentor is stimulated to further develop his or her own teaching, counseling, and leadership skills. Sometimes the mentor

FIGURE 22-5

Research is an important way to promote nursing's evolution toward greater autonomy and strength by contributing to improvement of the quality of health care.

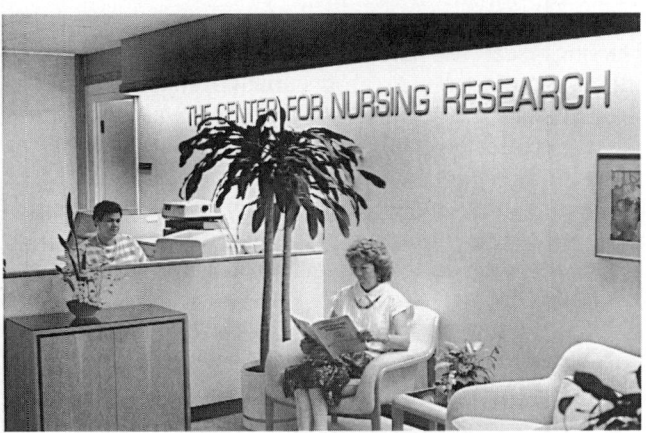

learns new knowledge and techniques when the newer nurse shares current information learned in school. Many mentorship relationships also become lasting friendships.

Preceptorship An alternate model is **preceptorship**. The *preceptor* (experienced nurse) is selected (and generally paid) to facilitate the orientee's transition to new responsibilities by way of teaching and guidance. The relationship is limited by the orientee's needs.

Nursing Organizations The many nursing organizations at the international, national, state or provincial, district, and local levels were discussed in Chapter 1. They are major forces for nursing leadership. These organizations have active groups in the United States and Canada. Membership and participation in professional organizations are important aspects of the nurse's leadership role (Fig. 22-7).

Continuing Education Many programs in developing leadership, managerial, and administrative skills are available to nurses. Courses can even be taken by mail correspondence. Periodicals and current books also provide continuing education for the emerging leader. Many of the continuing education programs and methods serve to prepare nurses before they assume higher levels of leadership; some are geared to nurses already in such positions. Consequently, it is wise to choose a program carefully so that your learning needs are correctly met.

Nurse as Researcher

While caring for victims of the Crimean War, Florence Nightingale kept careful and objective records. These records provided baseline data that she later used to determine which nursing interventions were most effective in treating her clients. Since that time, nursing research has taken many different pathways.

Nursing research was finally recognized by the public sector when the 1985 session of the U.S. Congress enacted legislation to establish a National Center for Nursing Research (NCNR) at the National Institutes of Health (NIH; see the accompanying display). Currently, increasing numbers of health care institutions are employing postgraduate nurses as researchers.

Studies on nursing education, administration, and practice all affect client care either directly or indirectly. Too often, practicing nurses mistakenly associate research with professions far removed from caring for clients at the bedside. This false impression has slowed the progress of practice-based nursing research. Yet much of what bedside nurses routinely do constitutes research. The nursing process (ie, assessing, diagnosing, planning, implementing, and evaluating) represents the basic framework of the research process.

Regardless of the specific direction nursing research takes, there will be an increased emphasis on its level of importance. Already schools of nursing have included research principles and methods in the basic curriculum for beginning nurses.

Professionalism of Nursing

Nursing research is fundamental to the recognition of nursing as a profession. As an occupation, nursing has been around since the beginning of time. Many argue however that the profession of nursing is still in its infancy. One of the essential elements that differentiates an occupation from a profession is the existence of a unique and distinct knowledge base. The ultimate goal of expanding nursing's body of knowledge is to learn improved ways to promote and maintain health. As health care and illness patterns change, nursing interventions must change. Ongoing practice-based research reflects the nursing profession's commitment to meet the ever-changing demands of health care consumers.

FIGURE 22-7

Membership and participation in professional nursing organizations help keep the individual nurse current on issues and recent developments, increase the strength of the group, and are important aspects of the nurse's leadership role. (Courtesy of the American Nurses' Association.)

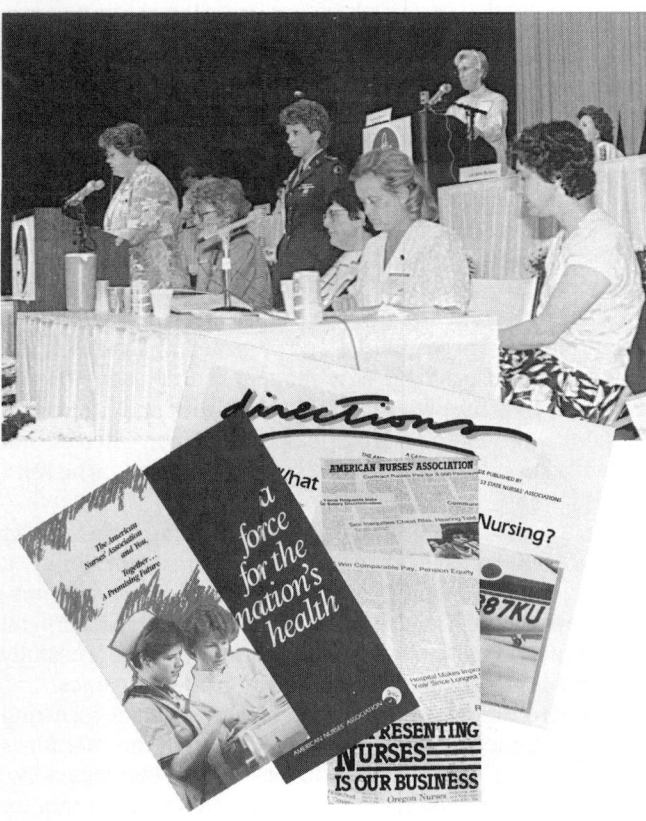

National Center for Nursing Research

The National Center for Nursing Research (NCNR), founded in 1986 within NIH to build a strong scientific base for nursing practice, created many new opportunities for nurse scientists to obtain funding for nursing research, research training, and career development. NCNR research priorities include

- Low birth-weight: Mothers and infants
- Human immunodeficiency virus infection: Prevention and care
- Long-term care for older adults
- Symptom management
- Information systems
- Health promotion for children and adolescents
- Technology dependency across the lifespan

(National Center for Nursing Research. (1990). *Facts about funding* [NIH Publication No. 90-3112]. Bethesda, MD: U.S. Department of Health and Human Services.)

Roots of Knowledge

How can nursing expand its knowledge base to meet the health care needs of clients? To answer this question, one must look to the roots of knowledge. Knowledge comes from a variety of sources. **Traditional knowledge** is that part of nursing practice passed down generation after generation. When questioned about this aspect of nursing practice nurses might reply, "We've always done it this way." Changing of bedclothes provides a practical illustration of how traditional knowledge has affected nursing practice. It is customary in acute-care settings to change a client's bedclothes daily whether soiled or not. There are no data to support this, yet virtually millions of hospital beds get changed daily because this practice is accepted as a necessary component of quality client care. Right or wrong, until this practice is challenged scientifically, it will remain a traditional part of client care.

Authoritative knowledge comes from an expert and is accepted as truth based on a perceived level of expertise, for example, when a senior staff nurse teaches a new graduate nurse an easier way of doing a technical procedure such as inserting an intravenous catheter. The senior nurse has gained knowledge through experience, and the new graduate nurse accepts it as truth based on a perceived authority within the experienced nurse. Authoritative knowledge remains unchallenged as long as the presumed authority maintains his or her perceived expertise.

Scientific knowledge is that knowledge arrived at through the scientific method. The term *research* implies the scientific approach to acquiring new knowledge. New ideas are tested and measured systematically using objective criteria. Scientific study implies the presence of control over **variables**—factors that might interfere with results (outcomes). Different types of variables compose a research study. **Independent variables** are the factors the researcher introduces into the study and can control. **Dependent variables** are those factors already in the situation that may respond to the interdependent variables. An example of scientific research that might be carried out at the bedside would be to measure the effects of two different skin emollients on opposite limbs of a client over the course of 2 days. The dependent variable in this example would be the client's limbs. The independent variable would be the skin emollients. With careful and objective data collection, the researcher might be able to determine which lotion elicited a better client result or outcome. By testing the results of the two emollients on the same client, the researcher would have maintained control within the study. Research as simple as this example could have vast implications on practice when results are shared among health care professionals. Scientific research relies on careful planning. If the emollients were tested on two clients, the results of the research might be affected by an unknown factor such as differing skin conditions in the two clients. These factors are called extraneous variables. **Extraneous variables** (ie, those that are not being studied) can sometimes result in inaccurate research findings.

Is one source of knowledge better than another? All sources of knowledge are useful to the collective body of knowledge that composes the nursing profession. Although these three methods provide nursing with important contributions, each has inherent strengths and limitations. Traditional and authoritative knowledge are practical to implement but are often based on subjective data. This limits their usefulness over a wide variety of practice settings. Scientific research is designed to achieve high levels of objectivity but is often costly, time-consuming, and can be impractical given the complexities surrounding client care. Scientific knowledge, because of its control and objectivity, however, can be generalized, making it highly useful in a variety of care settings. Acquiring new knowledge then is one reason why nurses must become more aware and involved in the research process.

Consumerism

The social climate of consumerism surrounding health care has increased the importance of nursing research as well. The health care marketplace is characterized by a rising concern over quality of care while assuring cost-containment. Consumers have become dissatisfied with unproven, costly treatments. Health care consumers demand effective methods of treatment at a reasonable cost. Nursing care, therefore, must focus on measurable results to assure the consumer of nursing's commitment to improve client care. Unless practice-based research is used to validate the effects of nursing interventions, consumers will not credit nursing for its important contribution.

Nursing Research Resources

Major nursing journals with a science or research focus
  Advances in Nursing Science
  Journal of Advanced Nursing
  Canadian Journal of Nursing Research
  Journal of Research in Nursing and Health
  Nursing Research
  International Journal of Nursing Studies
  Western Journal of Nursing Studies
Indexes of journal articles
  Cumulative Index to Nursing and Allied Health Literature (CINAHL)
  International Nursing Index
  Index Medicus
Secondary resources
  Annual Review of Nursing Research
  Review of Nursing Research in Nursing Education

Computerized literature searches of research*
  BIOETHICSLINE
  Cumulative Index to Nursing and Allied Health Literature (CINAHL)
  Educational Resources Information (ERIC)
  Medical Literature Analysis and Retreival System (MEDLARS)
  Psychological Abstracts (PsycINFO)
Individually subscribed computer bibliographic services†
  Knowledge Index (available through *DIAGLOG Information Services*)
  GRATEFUL MED (available through the National Library of Medicine)
  BRS Colleague (available through W.B. Saunders)

*To access these arsenals of information, you need the following four items: (1) a telephone line, (2) a computer, (3) a modem, and (4) communications software. To access the desired data base, the user needs to obtain a password and an account number.

Research Skills Basic to the Nurse's Caregiver Role

Relating Research to Practice   Unless the research findings of nurse researchers are used by practicing nurses to improve the quality of client care, clinical nursing research is for naught. As students develop clinical skills, it is critical they understand the scientific rationale that makes one course of action preferable to another. Throughout this text, Research in Nursing displays highlight current studies that have the potential to make a positive difference in nursing practice and client outcomes. Highlighted in the accompanying display are sources nurses can explore to find research studies pertinent to their concerns. Most librarians are willing to provide helpful introductions to these resources. As nurses develop their clinical and re-

N U R S I N G   T O D A Y   Challenges and Solutions

Gender Gap in Research

Challenges

- Although women comprise 51% of the population (and a larger majority of the elderly population), much of the current treatment methods are based on scientific research on males.
- Research is needed on the physiologic gender differences and gender-specific behaviors, and how these factors serve to prevent, stimulate, or reduce the risk of and or progression of diseases.
- More research is needed in the areas of mental health and reproductive health in women.

Nursing Solutions

The National Center for Nursing Research (NCNR) is currently funding the following women's health research projects:

- Development of a Center for Women's Health Research at the University of Washington.
- Research and training on developing better nursing techniques to help maintain or improve health during pregnancy including the promotion of infant health.
- A study of midlife women to identify the factors that affect a woman's decision to use hormone replacement therapy during menopause.
- A study of women's response to battering.

ANA Executive Director Barbara Redman, PhD, RN, FAAN, has called on the Bush administration to fund research on women's health issues and to include more women in clinical trials.

(Gender gap in research hit by ANA. [August 1991] *Pennsylvania Nurse*, 24.)

search skills, they will be better able to critique nursing research for validity, reliability, and applicability.

Identifying Researchable Problems Because it is the nurse as caregiver who works most immediately with clients and families, it is critical for caregivers to continually approach their practice with the question, "Is this the best way to achieve the desired client outcomes?" The questions, insights, and recommendations of caring, practicing nurses have assisted many nurse researchers to refine their studies in significant ways.

Protecting the Rights of Subjects Many nurses work in health care institutions in which clients are invited to participate in clinical research. Nurses with their focus on the overall well-being of the client play an important role in ensuring that client interests are not sacrificed to research interests. Nursing priorities on research units include determining that research studies have met appropriate scientific and ethical criteria before their implementation and protecting client rights. Specific rights of concern are **informed consent**, the client's right to knowledgeably consent to participate in the study without coercion (knowing that this consent may be withdrawn at any time) or to refuse to participate without jeopardizing the care that he or she will receive; the right to confidentiality; and the right to be protected from harm. Nurses caring for clients who are research subjects should be familiar with the ethical directives of the ANA (1985b) or Canadian Nurses' Association (1983) and *The Belmont Report* (National Commission for the Protection of Human Subjects of Biomedical and Behavioral Research, 1978).

Nurse as Advocate

Advocacy involves combining the three roles of teacher, counselor, and leader to form a new role through which the nurse protects and supports the client's rights. Nurses have always been advocates for clients' rights. This role is increasingly emphasized, perhaps because of clients' changing expectations and demands, as well as to the importance placed on an individual's rights by the nursing profession.

Advocacy requires that nurses inform the clients and then support them in their decisions (Kohnke, 1982). Nurses must recognize that clients have the right to make their own decisions. Through teaching and counseling, the nurse is able to give the client the information needed to make educated decisions about health care needs.

Many view advocacy as necessary only for those who cannot defend themselves. This is not true when considering the needs and rights of clients. Nearly all clients need a nurse advocate to provide the data needed for making informed decisions. Clients also need nurses to interpret what their rights are in given situations.

Client's Bill of Rights

As holism and holistic care became popular, clients began to demand their rights as health care consumers. In 1972, the American Hospital Association described *A Patient's Bill of Rights,* which includes the rights and responsibilities of the client to which the client is entitled while receiving care in the hospital. The bill has been widely disseminated, and in some hospitals, clients receive a copy on admission. (*A Patient's Bill of Rights* is discussed and reprinted in Chapter 5.)

In the United States, the Freedom of Information Act of 1967 and the Privacy Act of 1974 were enacted primarily to open personal government records to the people described in them. Medical records were included in this enactment. Clients in health agencies operated by the U.S. government (eg, the Department of Veterans' Affairs) and clients receiving Medicare are currently entitled to see their records. Although some specifics and interpretations of the laws have not been clarified, the trend is apparent: consumers are demanding their right to know about their health care and are seeking legislation to support this right. Nurses are responsible advocates of these client rights.

Advocacy Skills and the Nurse's Caregiver Role

People Requiring Advocacy

Most nurses would agree that a great deal of nursing time is spent representing clients' interests or guiding clients in protecting their own rights. The nurse is often involved as an intermediary between the client and the family, especially when the client and family have conflicting ideas about the management of health care situations (Fig. 22-8).

For instance, a male client with terminal cancer may want to go home to die. He has told this to his nurse. The client's family, however, has told the nurse that they cannot care for him at home. As an advocate, the nurse recognizes the rights of both the client and his family. The nurse then works to assist them in finding a solution that will benefit all concerned. By informing the family of the availability of home care and hospice care, the nurse has given them knowledge that may help satisfy the client's right to a dignified death. Most people on their own would have no way of getting the financial help needed for such care. The nurse has the resources available to help them and can arrange referrals from other health care workers, such as social workers, to achieve the desired outcomes.

Nurses may also serve as intermediaries between the client and the medical profession. Patricia Murphy (1990) documented a moving account of how nurses interceded for a 43-year-old woman with amyotrophic lateral sclerosis who was on a ventilator but wished to die. The client's primary physicians refused to help remove her from the ventilator and more than 20 other physicians declined to accept her as a client on learning what she wanted to do. After unsuccessful appeals for help to the county medical

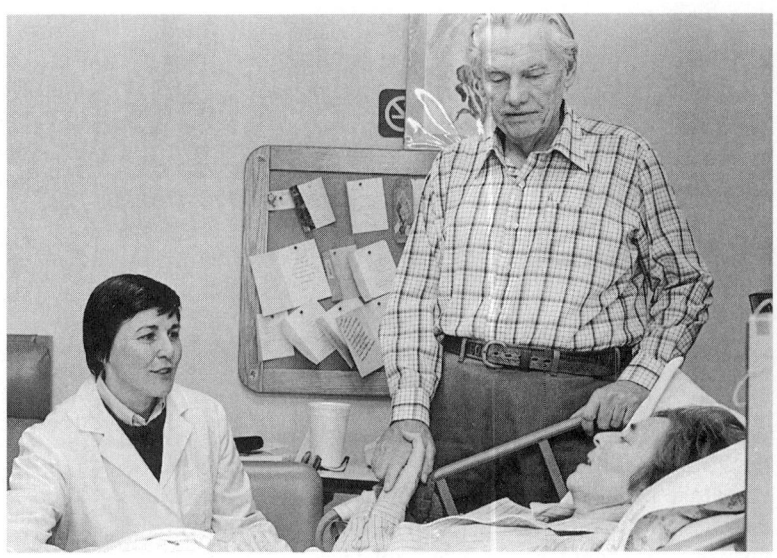

F I G U R E   2 2 - 8

The nurse acts as a client advocate to assist family members and the client with discussing all aspects of health care management.

society and her own attorney, the client's public health nurse, working with a supportive social worker, contacted her state nurses' association and finally secured the assistance she needed to help the client achieve her goal of a dignified death.

People with special advocacy needs include those who are uninformed concerning their rights and opportunities, people with sensory impairment, people who do not speak English, very young people, elderly people, seriously ill people, people who are mentally or emotionally impaired, and people with physical disabilities.

Advocacy Requires Assertiveness

To help clients attain their rights, nurses need to be assertive. Occasionally, they need to teach assertive techniques to their clients. Some individuals are intimidated in the health care environment, and even when they disagree with a physician's treatment plan, may feel unable to question or challenge the physician. Nurses can empower clients to claim and defend their right to knowledge, to respectful treatment, and to informed consent, by legitimizing these rights and by coaching clients in the assertiveness techniques that can help them secure these rights. Basic assertiveness techniques are described in Chapter 20.

Advocacy and Ethics

Advocacy is linked to the basic belief that making choices about health is a fundamental human right that promotes dignity and well-being. Ethical dilemmas may arise when people are unable or unwilling to make choices, or when they are not given the opportunity to do so. Faulty communication between clients, family members, and caregivers frequently contributes to these dilemmas. Nurses play an important advocacy role in educating the public about the value of written **advance directives**, which enable people to state how choices about health care should be made if certain circumstances (eg, terminal illness) develop. **Living wills** allow individuals to specify which kinds of health care they want provided or denied in particular situations. A **durable power of attorney for health care** designates someone else to make health care decisions in the event of the appointing individual's subsequent incapacity. Nurses should be familiar with laws pertaining to the status of advance directives. These vary from state to state or province to province. Sample advance directives are provided in Chapter 6.

Nurses as advocates must realize that they do not make the ethical decisions for their clients. Instead, they facilitate the clients' decision making. Nurses interpret findings for their clients; inform them of the various aspects to be considered; let them verbalize and organize their feelings; call in those people who should be involved in the decision making (eg, family, primary nurse, physician, or clergy); and help clients assess all of their options in relation to their beliefs. In this way, nurses advocate the right of clients to make their own decisions concerning health. It is important to recall that not all individuals want to make their own treatment decisions. The spirit of autonomy (self-determination) should not be violated by forcing it on anyone. Nurses sometimes advocate for clients by helping them to delegate a preferred decision maker whom they trust. In addition, in claiming to be a client advocate, nurses must be careful to clarify exactly what it is they mean by advocacy, because in most instances this is not simply supporting the client in all of his or her preferences. For example, if a client in the early stages of Alzheimer's disease with the support of her husband asked a nurse for help in terminating her life, the nurse would have excellent ethical grounds for refusing to advocate for this particular request. Advocacy is discussed in Chapter 5.

Advocacy and Political Action

A discussion of political action is beyond the scope of this text but no treatment of nursing advocacy would be complete without noting nursing's continuing voice in the political arena on behalf of those least well-served by the existing health care system. As the government becomes more involved in the delivery and funding of health care services and rationing plans speak seriously of age and other variables as criteria for limiting care, nurses must continue to advocate for the health care needs of those least empowered to do so for themselves, for example, homeless people, minorities, women, and children. Nurses represent a powerful block of voters whose potential for influencing health care legislation is just beginning to be tapped.

KEY POINTS

- Nurses have the basic qualities and skills for leadership; they need to work toward developing these qualities and skills.
- Nurses choose leadership styles according to their own personality traits, the objectives to be achieved, and the characteristics of the followers.
- Nurse leaders are responsible for effecting positive changes, managing client and staff activities, and using administrative knowledge appropriately.
- Nursing leadership is involved in working for the benefit of the client, the nursing team, the nursing profession, and society.
- Research provides an important step toward expanding the professional role of nursing, acquiring new knowledge to improve client care, and remaining competitive in the health care marketplace.

- Beginning nurses can use research findings to improve their care; identify researchable problems; and protect the rights of research subjects to informed consent, confidentiality, and freedom from harm.
- Making choices about health is a fundamental human right that promotes client dignity and well-being.
- As an advocate, the nurse informs the client of rights and supports client decisions concerning rights and health care choices.
- Assertiveness is a necessary tool for the nurse to use in both the advocacy and leadership role. Nurses may also need to teach assertiveness techniques to clients and families.
- Educating the public about the benefits of advance directives is an important nursing advocacy role.

BIBLIOGRAPHY

Leader

Adams, C. E. (1990). Leadership behavior of nurse executives. *Nursing Management, 21*(8), 36.

Barker, A. M. (1991). An emerging leadership paradigm. *Nursing and Health Care, 12*(4), 204–207.

Benne, K. D., & Sheats, P. (1948). Functional roles of group members. *Journal of Social Issues, 4*(2), 41.

Bennis, W. G., Benne, K. D., Chin, R., & Corey, K. E. (1976). *The planning of change* (3rd ed.). New York: Holt, Rinehart & Winston.

Brice-Stephens, N. (1989). 7 ways to sharpen your leadership skills. *Nursing, 19*(10), 130–136.

Brooten, D. A., Hayman, L. L., & Naylor, M. D. (1988). *Leadership for change: An action guide for nurses* (2nd ed.). Philadelphia: Lippincott.

Carnevale, F. A. (1991). Practice-based research on a unit level. *Canadian Nurse, 87*(10), 29–31.

Chenevert, M. (1985). *Pro-nurse handbook: Designed for the nurse who wants to thrive professionally.* St. Louis: Mosby.

Douglas, L. M. (1992). *The effective nurse: Leader and manager* (4th ed.). St. Louis: Mosby–Year Book.

Grohar-Murray, M. E., & DiCroce, H. R. (1992). *Leadership and management in nursing.* Norwalk, CT: Appleton & Lange.

Hamilton, E. M., Murray, M. K., & Lindholm, L. M. (1989). Effects of mentoring on job satisfaction, leadership behavior, and job retention of new graduate nurses. *Journal of Nursing Staff Development, 5*(4), 159–165.

Hansten, R., & Washburn, M. (1992). Working with people: How to plan what to delegate. *American Journal of Nursing, 92,*(4), 71–72.

Hardy, L. K. (1990). Education for nurse administrators. *Canadian Nurse, 86*(8), 32–34.

Hersey, P. (1989). *Situational leadership in nursing.* Norwalk, CT: Appleton & Lange.

Hersey, P., & Blanchard, K. (1977). *Management of organizational behavior: Utilizing human resources* (3rd ed.). Englewood Cliffs, NJ: Prentice-Hall.

Johnson, D. W., & Johnson, F. P. (1975). *Joining together: Group therapy and group skills.* Englewood Cliffs, NJ: Prentice-Hall.

Kalisch, B. J., & Kalisch, P. A. (1983). Improving the image of nursing. *American Journal of Nursing, 83*(1), 48–52.

Kilkus, S. P. (1990). Self-assertion and nurses: A different voice. *Nursing Outlook, 38*(3), 143–145.

Kinsey, D. C. (1990). Mentorship and influence in nursing. *Nursing Management, 21*(5), 45–46.

La Monica, E. L. (1983). *Nursing leadership and management: An experiential approach.* Monterey, CA: Wadsworth.

Lewin, K. (1951). *Field theory in social science.* New York: Harper & Row.

Manthey, M. (1990). Leadership: Accenting the positive. *Nursing Management, 21*(7), 40–42.

Mantle, J. (1992). Research and serendipitous secondary findings. *Canadian Nurse, 88*(1), 15–18.

Marriner-Tomey, A. (1992a). *Guide to nursing management* (4th ed.). St. Louis: Mosby–Year Book.

Marriner-Tomey, A. (1992b). *Transformational leadership in nursing.* St. Louis: Mosby–Year Book.

Naisbitt, J., & Aburdene, P. (1990). *Megatrends 2000: Ten new directions for the 1990's.* New York: Morrow.

Ouellet, D., & Elsner, C. (1992). Asking questions, researching answers. *Canadian Nurse, 88*(1), 33–35.

Perlman, D., & Takacs, G. J. (1990). The 10 stages of change. *Nursing Management, 21*(4), 33–38.

Risco, K. G., & Hakos, L. (April 1992). Caring for the caregiver: The art of mentoring. *Pennsylvania Nurse, 16.*

Rowland, H. S., & Rowland, B. L. (1991). *Nursing administration manual* (2 vols.). Gaithersburg, MD: Aspen.

Simpson, P. (1988). Motivational theories: Reflection on their application by nurse managers. *Canadian Journal of Nursing Administration, 1*(1), 16–19.

Sredl, D. (1988). What's your LQ . . . leadership quotient? *Nursing Management, 19*(10), 96Q, 96T, 96V.

Sullivan, E. J., & Decker, P. J. (1992). *Effective management in nursing* (3rd ed.). Redwood City, CA: Addison-Wesley Nursing.

Tamarisk, N. K. (1990). Personal computer databases for middle managers. *Management, 21*(7), 49–51.

Ward, M. J., & Price, S. A. (1991). *Issues in nursing administration: Selected readings.* St. Louis: Mosby.

Researcher

American Nurses' Association, Commission on Nursing Research. (1981a). *Guidelines for the investigative function of nurses.* Kansas City, MO: Author.

American Nurses' Association, Commission on Nursing Research. (1981b). *Research priorities for the 1980's: Generating a scientific basis for nursing practice.* Kansas City, MO: Author.

American Nurses' Association. (1985a). *Directions for nursing research: Toward the twenty-first century.* Kansas City, MO: Author.

American Nurses' Association. (1985b). *Human rights guidelines for nurses in clinical and other research.* Kansas City, MO: Author.

American Nurses' Association. (1987). *Research in nursing: Toward a science of nursing.* Kansas City, MO: Author.

American Nurses Association. (1991). *Position statement on nursing and the patient self-determination act.* Kansas City, MO: Author.

Anema, M. G. (1989). Ethical considerations in conducting clinical research. *Dimensions of Critical Care Nursing, 8*(5), 288–296.

Annas, G. J. (1992). *The rights of patients.* Totowa, NJ: Humana Press.

Bock, L. R. (1990). From research to utilization: Bridging the gap. *Nursing Management, 21*(3), 50–51.

Canadian Nurses Association. (1983). *Ethical guidelines for nursing research involving human subjects.* Ottawa: Author.

Davies, B. (1990). Clearing the vision through research. *Canadian Nurse, 86*(6), 20–22.

Fonteyn, M. E. (1990). The need for nurse involvement in critical care research. *Critical Care Nursing Quarterly, 12*(4), 1–4.

Larson, E., & McGuire, D. B. (1990a). Keys to research [column]. *MCN.*

Larson, E., & McGuire, D. B. (1990b). Patient experiences with research in a tertiary care setting. *Nursing Research, 39*(3), 168–171.

MacGuire, J. M. (1990). Putting nursing research findings into practice: Research utilization is an aspect of the management of change. *Journal of Advanced Nursing, 15*(5), 614–620.

National Commission for the Protection of Human Subjects of Biomedical and Behavioral Research. (1978). *The Belmont report: Ethical principles and guidelines for the protection of human subjects of research* (DHEW Publication No. [OS]78-0012). Washington, DC: U.S. Government Printing Office.

Newman, M. A., & Batey, M. (1991). The research–practice relationship. *Nursing Science Quarterly, 4*(3), 100–103.

O'Connor, A. (1989). Nursing research in Canada: Progress, problems, and prospects [editorial]. *Canadian Journal of Nursing Research, 21*(1), 1–2.

Pinch, W. J. (1989). Integrating research into practice. *Nurse Educator, 14*(3), 30–33.

Pringle, D. M. (1989). Another twist on the double helix: Research and practice. *Canadian Journal of Nursing Research, 21*(1), 47–60.

Sinclair, V. G. (1987). Literature searches by computer. *Image: Journal of Nursing Scholarship, 19*(1), 35–37.

Styles, M. (1990). A common sense approach to nursing research. *International Nursing Review, 37*(1), 203–206.

Tanner, C., & Lindeman, C. A. (1989). *Using nursing research* (Publication No. 15-2232:35-60). New York: National League for Nursing.

Thurston, N. E., Tenove, S. C., & Church, J. M. (1990). Hospital nursing research is alive and flourishing. *Nursing Management, 21*(5), 50–54.

Youngkins, J. M. (1991). The impact of one staff nurse's research. *MCN.*

Advocate

American Hospital Association. (1972). *A patient's bill of rights*. Chicago: Author.

Archer, S., & Gohner, P. (1982). *Nurses: A political force*. Monterey, CA: Wadsworth.

Beaman, J. (1989). Patient advocacy: Should I or shouldn't I? *Imprint, 36*(2), 155–157.

Bushy, A., & Smith, T. O. (1990). Lobbying: The hows and wherefores. *Nursing Management, 21*(4), 39–45.

Gadow, S. (1989). Clinical subjectivity: Advocacy with silent patients. *Nursing Clinics of North America, 24*(2), 535–541.

Gale, B. J. (1989). Advocacy for elderly autonomy: A challenge for community health nurses. *Journal of Community Health Nursing, 6*(4), 191–197.

Kohnke, M. F. (1982). *Advocacy: Risk and reality*. St. Louis: Mosby.

Murphy, P. (1990). Helping Joanne die with dignity. *Nursing, 20*(9), 45–49.

Sharf, B. F. (1988). Teaching patients to speak up: Past and future trends. *Patient Education and Counseling, 11*(2), 95–108.

U. S. Senate, Special Committee on Aging. (1989). *A matter of choice: Planning ahead for health care decisions*. Washington, DC: American Association of Retired Persons.

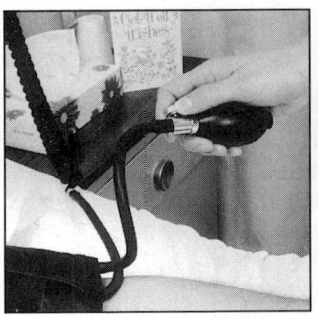 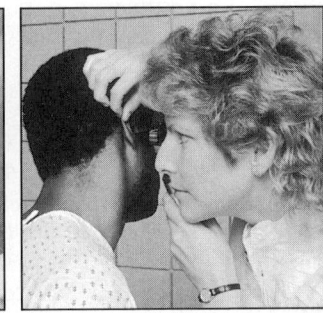 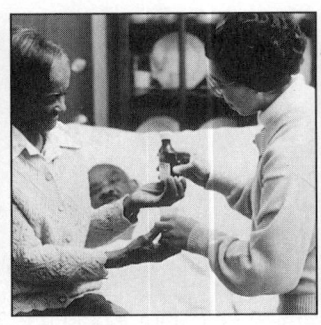 

Actions Basic to Nursing Care

Unit VI focuses on the actions basic to nursing practice—those commonly used to meet needs of clients of all ages, at any point on the health–illness continuum, and in both structured and nonstructured settings. Nursing assessment, including a health history and physical examination, provides a data base necessary to maintain or restore health as well as to promote wellness. Assessment is both an art and a science. The art of performing a skill is integrated into the science of nursing knowledge so that variations are identified and evaluated and necessary independent and interdependent nursing actions are implemented. Chapter 23 describes nursing responsibilities related to the assessment of vital signs and Chapter 27 outlines nursing responsibilities related to major diagnostic procedures.

Nurses are responsible for meeting basic human needs for physical safety and security. Chapter 25 discusses environmental safety and the nursing actions necessary to identify risk factors for all age groups and to implement teaching and other nursing measures to prevent accidents. Chapter 26 explains medical and surgical aseptic techniques to prevent and control the spread of microorganisms.

The realities of the health care system today have led to clients' spending fewer days in hospitals and have resulted in increasing numbers of community-based care options, including home care. Chapter 28 describes the challenging responsibilities of nurses who promote continuity of care by preparing clients, family members, and other members of the health care team for client admissions, transfers, and discharges. The importance of individualized discharge planning initiated at the time of admission and ongoing communication with care providers is emphasized.

Unit VI introduces the learner to the knowledge and skills basic to nursing practice in any setting. Using the nursing process, nurses make accurate assessments, ensure safety, prevent and control the spread of microorganisms, facilitate diagnostic testing, and responsibly promote continuity of care in the hospital, home, and community.

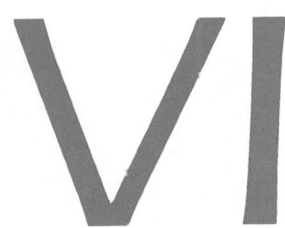

VI

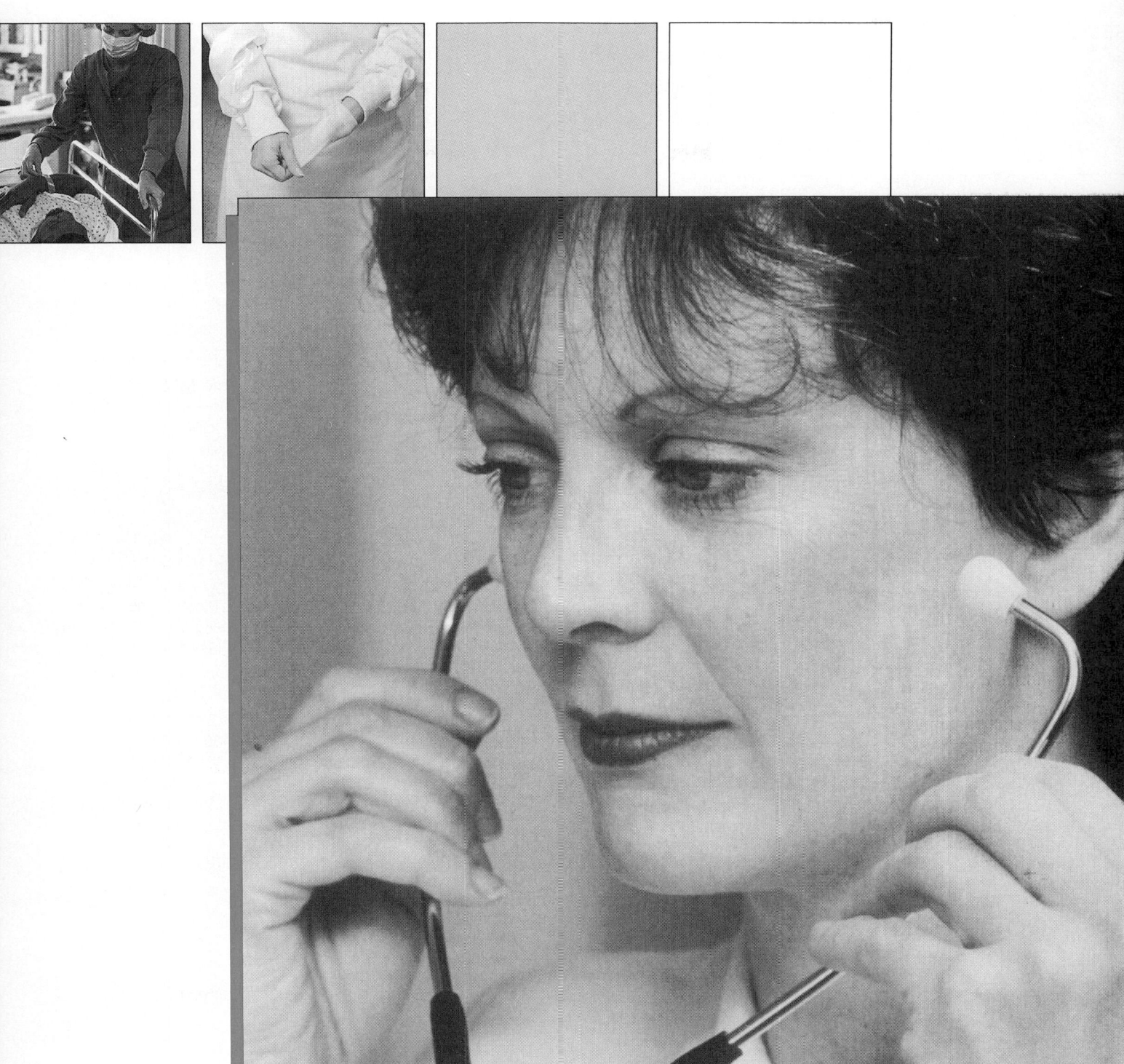

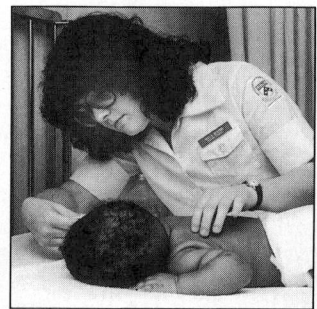

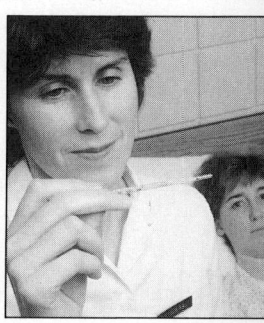

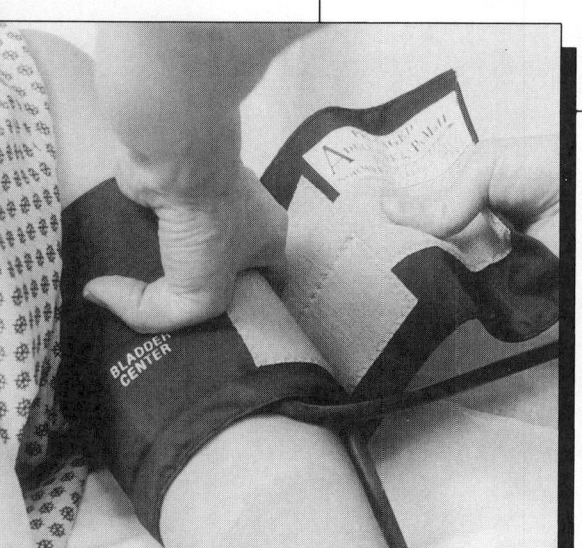
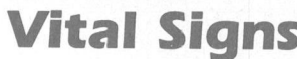

Vital Signs

OBJECTIVES

After studying this chapter, the learner should be able to:

Define key terms used in the chapter.

Discuss nursing responsibilities in assessing temperature, pulse, aspirations, and blood pressure.

Compare normal and abnormal vital sign assessments, including causes, effects, and implications of abnormal findings.

Describe the equipment necessary to assess vital signs.

Identify sites for assessing temperature, pulse, and blood pressure.

KEY TERMS

antipyretic
apnea
arrhythmia
bigeminal pulse
blood pressure
bradycardia
bradypnea
circadian rhythm
diastolic pressure
dyspnea
eupnea
expiration
hyperpyrexia
hypertension
hypotension
hypothermia
inspiration
Korotkoff sounds
lysis
orthopnea
orthostatic hypotension
pulse
pulse deficit
pulse pressure
pyrexia
respiration
sphygmomanometer
stertorous
stethoscope
stridor
systolic pressure
tachycardia
tachypnea
temperature
vital signs

23

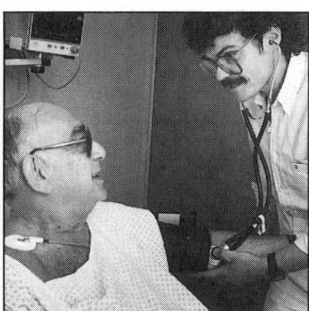

A basic nursing function in assessing the health status of an individual is taking the vital signs. **Vital signs** are a person's temperature, pulse, respiration, and blood pressure. The physiologic status of the body is reflected by these indicators of body function, which are normally regulated by the body through homeostatic mechanisms and fall within certain normal ranges. Any change from a person's normal pattern is considered indicative of a change in health.

Vital signs are taken and compared with accepted normal values and to the client's usual patterns in a wide variety of instances, including admission to a health care institution or agency, when giving medications that affect readings, before and after diagnostic and surgical procedures, before and after certain nursing interventions, and in emergency situations. It is an independent nursing action to take and record vital signs as often as the condition of a client requires such intervention.

Although vital signs are taken frequently, careful attention to details of the procedures and accuracy of the interpretation of the findings is extremely important. Each of the vital signs, with techniques and a discussion of normal and abnormal findings, is discussed in this chapter.

Frequency of Assessing Vital Signs

Assessing a person's vital signs is part of most agency admission procedures. These data provide part of the baseline information from which a plan of care is developed. It is recommended that on the person's admission, the nurse assess these signs whenever possible, rather than assigning the task to auxiliary nursing personnel who may have less knowledge about measuring these important health-status indicators.

After a client is admitted to a health agency, local policies govern when and how frequently vital signs are to be assessed. It is common policy for clients with elevated temperatures and for those who are in the postoperative period to have vital signs taken every 4 hours. Severely ill clients may have these observations made more frequently. In some self-care and psychiatric units, observations are made on the basis of the nurse's judgment. When a client does not have an elevated temperature or other vital-sign disturbances, there seems to be little justification for taking these signs several times a day. When the nurse visits in the home, the client's condition determines the frequency of obtaining data about vital signs.

The introduction of technologically advanced monitoring devices has made it possible to keep clients' vital signs under constant surveillance in critical care settings. The lives of many clients have been saved because continuous assessment of vital signs provides an accurate means of observing the effects of pathology and therapy.

Auxiliary personnel may obtain vital signs in some situations, but the nurse responsible for the client is ultimately accountable for these observations. If a client has untoward symptoms or demonstrates unexpected changes in vital signs, the nurse should double-check the measurements and further assess the client. The nurse should also be familiar with normal variations in vital signs that occur with age. These variations are described in the accompanying display.

Body Temperature

Physiologic Factors

Temperature refers to the hotness or coldness of a substance. Some living species are able to self-regulate the temperature of their body, whereas others are warmed and cooled by conditions in the environment. Humans are *homeothermic*, that is, they are warm-blooded and maintain body temperature independently of their environment. Cold-blooded animals are *poikilothermic*, meaning their body temperature is the same as their environment. Fish, frogs, and reptiles are poikilothermic animals.

Circadian Rhythm

It has been observed that environmental and physiologic processes occur in repeated cycles of time. Some events in humans appear to recur at 24-hour intervals. This cycling pattern is referred to as **circadian** (meaning nearly every 24 hours) **rhythm**. Predictable fluctuations in measurements of body temperature and blood pressure are examples of functions that exhibit a circadian rhythm. For instance, body temperature is usually approximately 0.6°C (1° to 2°F) lower in the early morning than in the late afternoon and early evening. This variation tends to be somewhat greater in infants and children. Current research indicates that the peak elevation of a person's temperature occurs in late afternoon, between 4 and 7 PM.

Temperature Regulation

The body temperature of a healthy person is maintained within a fairly constant range by the hypothalamus in the central nervous system. This structure is located at the base of the brain and plays an important role as the body's thermostat. It normally allows the body temperature to vary only about 1°F throughout the day. This constancy is referred to as the *set point*. The set point can be altered by

FOCUS ON THE OLDER ADULT

Normal Variations in Vital Signs With Aging

Temperature

- Changes in temperature regulation may necessitate a longer time for body temperature to register, and the actual body temperature may be normally lower.

Pulse

- Although pulse rate may not differ from that of the middle-aged adult, there may be an increased rate, and arrhythmias are more common.

Respirations

- As lung elasticity and gas exchange decrease with age, respirations are commonly more rapid and shallow.

Blood Pressure

- As age increases, the elasticity of arterial walls decreases, resulting in a higher systolic and diastolic blood pressure reading.
- Readings of 100 to 160 systolic and 60 to 95 diastolic are considered to be in the normal range.

---

the body's response to infectious agents, allergens, and inflamed tissue.

The hypothalamus has two parts: the *anterior hypothalamus* controls heat dissipation, and the *posterior hypothalamus* governs heat conservation. Thus, the set point is maintained through a balance of mechanisms involving heat production and heat loss. The following are examples of ways in which the body's thermal balance is maintained:

- Heat is produced through the metabolism of food. More heat is produced when metabolism is increased, and less when metabolism is decreased. For example, metabolism is increased when body temperature is elevated.

- Heat production is increased by the body's secretions of epinephrine, norepinephrine, and thyroxine.
- Exercise produces heat through muscle contraction.
- The body's surface, but not its internal structures, gains and loses heat physically from the sun, wind, and humidity in the environment.
- Heat is transferred primarily through physical processes of radiation, convection, evaporation, and conduction. These processes are defined and illustrated in Table 23-1.
- Heat is lost in small amounts through the urine, feces, and the process of warming and exhaling inspired air.
- Changes in vascularity of the skin modify body temperature. When blood is directed to the skin through

---

TABLE 23-1

	Radiation	Convection	Evaporation	Conduction
Mechanisms of Heat Transfer				
Definition	The diffusion or dissemination of heat by electromagnetic waves	The dissemination of heat by motion between areas of unequal density	The conversion of a liquid to a vapor	The transfer of heat to another object during direct contact
Example	The body gives off waves of heat from uncovered surfaces	An oscillating fan blows currents of cool air across the surface of a warm body	Body fluid in the form of perspiration and insensible loss is vaporized from the skin	The body transfers heat to an ice pack, causing the ice to melt
Illustration	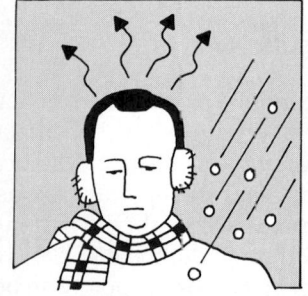	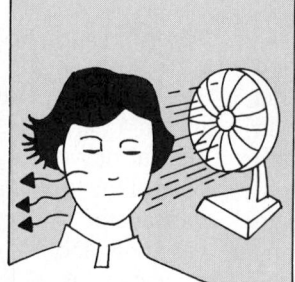	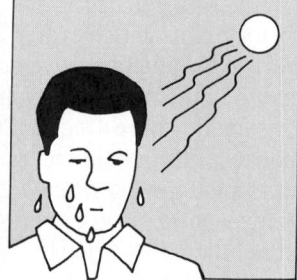	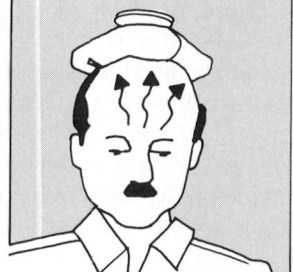

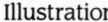

dilated vessels, heat loss is increased; when the skin vessels contract, heat is conserved.

- The contraction of smooth muscles when gooseflesh occurs and the involuntary movement of skeletal muscles when shivering is present produce heat and promote the circulation of blood that has been warmed through this process.

Normal and Abnormal Body Temperature

Normal Body Temperature

A thermometer is placed in a person's mouth to obtain an oral temperature, in the anal canal to obtain a rectal temperature, in an *axilla* (armpit) to obtain an axillary temperature, and in the esophagus to obtain a core temperature. Table 23-2 shows the average normal temperature standards for well adults at various body sites. The body's internal organs require a fairly constant inner or *core temperature* for optimal functioning, whereas the surface and periphery of the body can fluctuate widely while gaining or losing heat.

Variations normally occur in each person, and a range of 0.3° to 0.6°C (0.5° to 1.0°F) from the average normal temperature is considered to be within normal limits. However, wider variations from the average temperature have been found to be normal for certain people. Newborns and young children normally have a higher body temperature than adults.

Elevated Body Temperature

Pyrexia is an elevation of normal body temperature. The lay term is *fever*. **Hyperpyrexia** is a high fever, usually above 41°C (105.8°F), and survival is rare when the temperature reaches 44°C (110°F). Death is probably due to damaging effects to the respiratory center but may be due also to inactivation of body enzymes and destruction of tissue proteins.

Pyrexia is a common symptom of illness, and there is sufficient evidence to indicate that an elevation in temperature helps the body fight disease. In children, this response is often seen quickly. In the elderly person, pyrexia may be one of the later signs of illness, and the temperature may be elevated only 1° or 2°F above normal, even when pathologic processes are extensive.

It is generally theorized that when a fever occurs, the set point regulated by the hypothalamus is readjusted to a higher level. As a result, heat loss is decreased or heat production is increased, or both occur through the following mechanisms—shivering, constriction of surface blood vessels, and absence of sweating. After the body temperature rises to the new set point, heat loss mechanisms are again used to control the body temperature from rising to dangerous levels. Most fevers are self-limiting; the body temperature returns to normal range after the disease process is in check. Relieving a moderately elevated body temperature may reduce the body's defenses against disease as well as alter the ability to assess the person's progress.

The client with a fever usually experiences loss of appetite; headache; hot, dry skin; flushed face; thirst; and general malaise. Young children or people with high fevers may experience periods of delirium or seizures. Observing for other potentially dangerous signs that accompany a fever, such as dehydration, decreased urinary output, and rapid heart rate, are also important nursing assessments. The onset of an elevated body temperature may be sudden or gradual. Common terms used to describe the course of an elevated body temperature and its resolution are described in Table 23-3.

Antipyretic, or fever-reducing, drugs, such as aspirin or acetaminophen, may be necessary in certain circumstances. These drugs are believed to lower the elevated set point regulated by the hypothalamus. They do not affect body temperature when it is is within normal range. Body temperature may also be lowered through nonpharmacologic interventions. These interventions include alcohol or cold sponge baths, cool packs, and cooling blankets. The section on applications of heat and cold in Chapter 43 discusses measures used to reduce body temperature.

Subnormal Body Temperature

A body temperature below the lower limit of normal is called **hypothermia**. Death may occur when the temperature falls below about 34°C (93.2°F), but survival has been reported in isolated cases when body temperatures have

TABLE 23-2

Average Normal Temperatures for Well Adults in Various Body Sites				
Oral	Rectal	Axillary	Esophageal	Forehead*
37.0°c	37 5°C	36.5°C	37.3°C	34.4°C
98.6°F	99 5°F	97.6°F	99.2°F	94.0°F

*The manufacturer of Digitemp forehead thermometer (Hallcrest Products, 1820 Pickwick Lane, Glenview, IL 60025) says, "Most older children and adults have normal forehead temperatures between 93° and 95°F."

Common Courses of Pyrexia and its Resolution

Term	Definition	Illustration
Intermittent fever	The body temperature alternates regularly between a period of fever and a period of normal or subnormal temperature	
Remittent fever	The body temperature fluctuates several degrees, more than 2°C (3.6°F), above normal but does not reach normal between fluctuations	
Constant fever	The body temperature remains consistently elevated and fluctuates little, less than 2°C (3.6°F)	
Relapsing fever	The body temperature returns to normal for at least a day, but then fever recurs	
Resolution of pyrexia by crisis	An elevated body temperature returns to normal suddenly	
Resolution of pyrexia by lysis	An elevated body temperature returns to normal gradually	

fallen in the range of severe hypothermia (28°C or 82.4°F). This may happen to a person drowning in cold water or buried by snow. Because body functions are almost imperceptible at this range, health care personnel should attempt to warm hypothermic clients and continue resuscitation efforts.

Just as an elevated body temperature is a protective device for the body, a lowered body temperature may be beneficial also. Rates of chemical reactions in the body are slowed, thereby decreasing the metabolic demands for oxygen. Hypothermia as a form of therapy is discussed in clinical texts. Figure 23-1 illustrates the usual ranges of human body temperature.

Assessment Methods

Body temperature may be assessed by using a variety of devices. These are glass thermometers, electronic thermometers, disposable thermometers, temperature-sensitive patch or tape, and automated monitoring devices.

Glass Thermometer A glass thermometer with a mercury tip has traditionally been used to measure body temperature. This type of thermometer has two parts, as illustrated in Figure 23-2. The bulb contains liquid mercury, which expands when exposed to heat and rises within the stem. Most commonly, a long thin bulb is found on glass

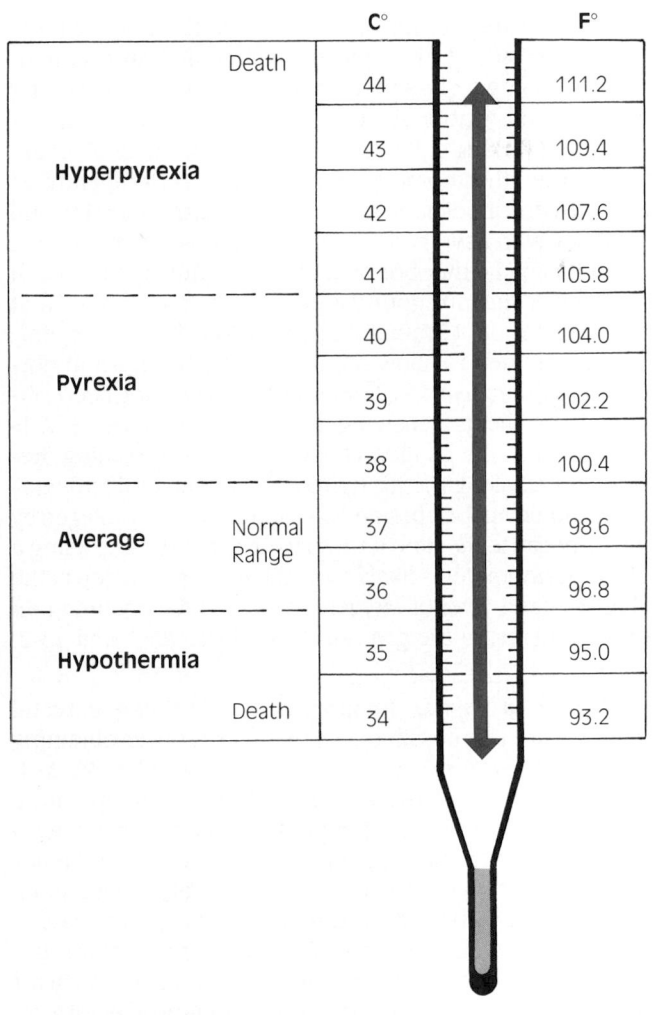

		C°		F°
	Death	44		111.2
Hyperpyrexia		43		109.4
		42		107.6
		41		105.8
Pyrexia		40		104.0
		39		102.2
		38		100.4
Average	Normal Range	37		98.6
		36		96.8
Hypothermia		35		95.0
	Death	34		93.2

F I G U R E   2 3 - 1

The range of human body temperature, as measured orally.

F I G U R E   2 3 - 2

The two glass thermometers on the top use the centigrade scale to measure temperature; the two on the bottom use the Fahrenheit scale. Note the blunt bulb on the rectal thermometers and the long, thin bulb on the oral thermometers. Either an oral or rectal thermometer may be used to obtain an axillary temperature, although the oral thermometer is generally preferred because of its larger bulb surface.

thermometers used to take oral temperatures and a blunt bulb is found on glass thermometers used to take rectal temperatures.

Glass thermometers are generally calibrated in either degrees of centigrade (Celsius [C]) or Fahrenheit (F). The range is about 34°C (94°F) to about 42.2°C (108°F). The degrees on a thermometer using the Celsius scale are subdivided into gradients of 0.1°; the subdivisions on a thermometer using the Fahrenheit scale are the equivalent of 0.2°. It is common practice to report the temperature to the nearest tenth of a degree when the mercury is a bit more or less from a line of calibration. Table 23-4 illustrates comparable centigrade and Fahrenheit temperatures and explains how temperatures are converted from one scale to the other.

Electronic Thermometer   Electronic thermometers measure body temperature in 25 to 50 seconds. Most have two nonbreakable temperature probes, one for oral use and one for rectal use. They are equipped with disposable probe covers, a feature that minimizes chances for cross infection and decreases cleaning chores. A sound indicates when the peak temperature has been recorded. This helps the nurse avoid wasting time. Various models are available. The technique for using an electronic thermometer is discussed later in this chapter.

Disposable Single-Use Thermometer   Disposable single-use thermometers register within seconds and are nonbreakable. Because they are used only once, they eliminate the danger of cross infection.

Temperature-Sensitive Patch or Tape   The temperature-sensitive patch or tape, commonly applied to the abdomen or forehead, changes color at different temperature ranges. This type of equipment is often used with well infants born at term. Newborns usually are incapable of achieving a fever; assessment of temperature at this age is primarily to

T A B L E   2 3 - 4

Equivalent Centigrade and Fahrenheit Temperatures*			
Centigrade	Fahrenheit	Centigrade	Fahrenheit
34.0	93.2	38.5	101.3
35.0	95.0	39.0	102.2
36.0	96.8	40.0	104.0
36.5	97.7	41.0	105.8
37.0	98.6	42.0	107.6
37.5	99.5	43.0	109.4
38.0	100.4	44.0	111.2

*To convert Centigrade to Fahrenheit, multiply by 9/5 and add 32. To change Fahrenheit to Centigrade, subtract 32 and multiply by 5/9.

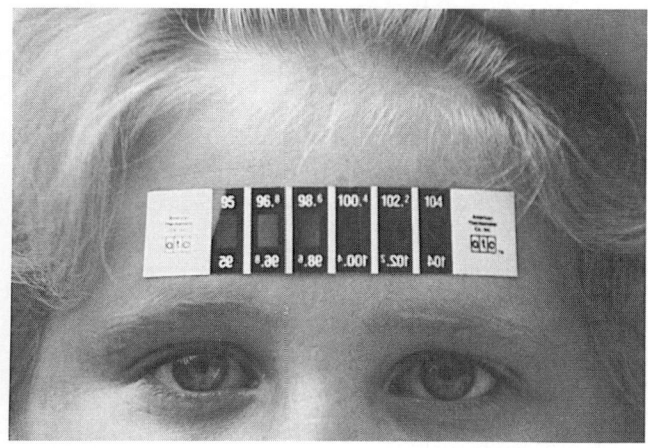

F I G U R E   2 3 - 3

This child has a thermometer patch on the forehead. The strip contains liquid crystals, which change colors as the temperature changes. The scale has been adjusted for converting skin-surface temperature to inner-body temperature. Although the calibration is not as detailed as that of a glass thermometer, this type of device is simple to use for a quick assessment. (Photo by Ken Timby.)

determine the infant's ability to regulate body heat. These devices may also be used when it is necessary to check the temperature of a toddler or young child who does not appear feverish (Fig. 23-3). A thermometer should be used to check the temperature if the color on the tape or patch indicates that the temperature is either above or below normal average range.

Automated Monitoring Device   Automated monitoring devices used in hospitals, usually in critical care areas, make it possible to simultaneously measure a client's body temperature, pulse, and blood pressure. Their use requires less task-oriented nursing time, especially when these assessments are obtained frequently.

Assessment Sites

Health agencies specify the site to be used for obtaining clients' temperatures. Most agencies measure temperature by the oral route. However, the nurse is expected to select and use alternative sites in certain situations. Factors affecting the site selection include such things as age of client, state of consciousness, amount of pain, and other care being provided at the time. It is customary to indicate the site that was used to obtain the temperature when recording the measurement within the client's record.

Obtaining an Oral Temperature   Obtaining oral temperatures is most common. One criterion for selecting an oral route is that the client must be able to close his or her mouth around the thermometer. Obtaining an oral temperature using a glass thermometer is contraindicated for unconscious, irrational, and seizure-prone clients, and for infants and young children because of the danger of breaking the glass thermometer in the mouth. Oral temperatures are also contraindicated for people with diseases of the oral cavity or who have had surgery of the nose or mouth. If a client has had either hot or cold food or fluids or has been smoking or chewing gum, it is generally recommended that a period of about 15 minutes elapse before an oral temperature is obtained to allow the oral tissues to return to normal. Traditionally, oral temperatures have not been obtained on clients receiving nasal oxygen because it is believed that the oxygen causes a false low reading. Research is challenging this opinion. However, oral temperatures should not be obtained on clients receiving oxygen by mask, because the time it takes to obtain a reading using a glass thermometer is likely to result in a serious drop in the client's blood level of oxygen. Measures for obtaining an oral temperature are given in Procedures 23-1 and 23-2.

Obtaining a Rectal Temperature   Obtaining a rectal temperature is a possible alternative whenever obtaining an oral temperature is contraindicated (Procedure 23-3). It is also recommended practice to check the temperature rectally if the client's oral temperature changes considerably and unexpectedly. Some hospitals require rectal readings on all clients with an elevated temperature. Obtaining a rectal temperature is contraindicated for clients having rectal surgery, diarrhea, and diseases of the rectum. Because the insertion of the thermometer can slow the heart rate by stimulating the vagus nerve, obtaining a rectal temperature is also often not recommended for people with certain heart diseases.

Using the rectum has been considered by some to be a more accurate way of measuring core temperature than the oral or axillary route. However, this opinion is being challenged by some authorities because studies have shown that the rectal temperature can be influenced by the presence of fecal matter, resulting in a false reading.

Obtaining an Axillary Temperature   An axillary temperature is generally obtained when both oral and rectal temperatures are contraindicated or when the sites are inaccessible. Some hospitals obtain temperatures by the axillary method on healthy newborns to avoid the potential for perforating the wall of the rectum with the thermometer. If the axilla has just been washed, obtaining the temperature should be delayed because the temperature of the water and the friction created by drying the skin can influence the temperature. Most authorities believe that when proper procedure is used, axillary temperatures are as accurate as oral or rectal temperatures.

For most clinical purposes, it would appear equally satisfactory to obtain an oral, a rectal, or an axillary tem-

(Text continues on p. 398)

PROCEDURE 23-1

Assessing Body Temperature by Oral Method: Glass Clinical Thermometer

Equipment

Oral thermometer   Pencil or pen
Soft tissues   Paper or flow sheet

Action	**Rationale**
1 Explain the procedure to the client.	An explanation encourages client cooperation and reduces client apprehension.
2 Gather equipment.	Gathering equipment provides for organized approach to task.
3 Wash your hands.	Handwashing deters the spread of microorganisms.
4 If the thermometer has been stored in a chemical solution, wipe it dry with a firm, twisting motion, using clean, soft tissue.	Chemical solutions may irritate the mucous membrane and may have an objectionable odor or taste. Soft tissue will approximate the surface, and twisting helps to contact the entire surface.
5 Wipe once from the bulb toward the fingers with each tissue.	Wiping from an area where there are few or no organisms to an area where organisms may be present minimizes the spread of organisms to cleaner areas.
6 Grasp the thermometer firmly with the thumb and forefinger, and with strong wrist movements shake the thermometer until the mercury line reaches at least 36°C (95°F).	Shaking the thermometer moves the mercury back into the bulb below the previously recorded measurement.
7 Read the thermometer by holding it horizontally at eye level, and rotate it between the fingers until the mercury line can be seen clearly.	Holding the thermometer at eye level facilitates reading. Rotating the thermometer aids in placing the mercury line in a position where it can be read best.
8 Place the mercury bulb of the thermometer well within the back of the right or left pocket under the client's tongue, and instruct the client to close his or her lips around the thermometer.	When the bulb rests deeply in the posterior sublingual pocket, it is in contact with blood vessels lying close to surface and can accurately measure body temperature.

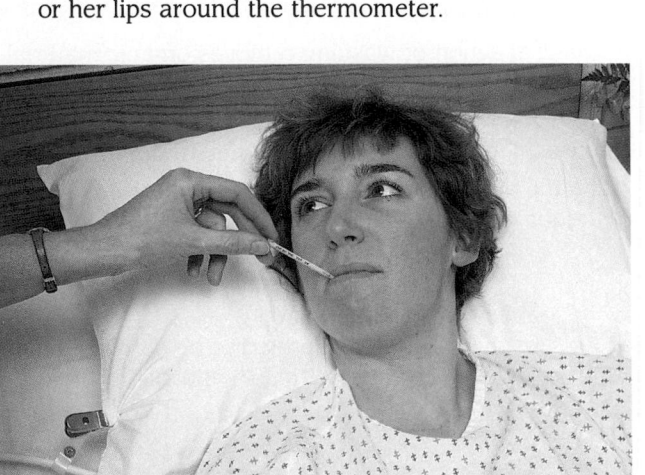

Action 8: Placing the thermometer.

(continued)

PROCEDURE 23-1 (continued)

Assessing Body Temperature by Oral Method: Glass Clinical Thermometer

Action	Rationale
9 Leave the thermometer in place at least 2 minutes. Check agency policy for recommended time interval.	Allowing sufficient time for the mercury to expand ensures an accurate measurement.
10 Remove the thermometer, and wipe it once from the fingers down to the mercury bulb, using a firm, twisting motion.	Cleaning from an area where there are few organisms to an area where there are numerous organisms minimizes their spread to cleaner areas. Friction helps to loosen matter from the surface.
11 Read the thermometer to the nearest tenth.	Mercury may rise a bit above or below a calibration on a thermometer.

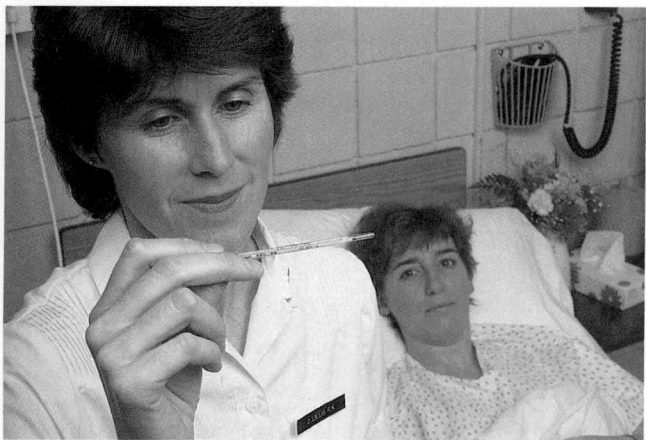

Action 11: Reading the thermometer. (Photos © Ken Kasper.)

Action	Rationale
12 Dispose of the tissue in a receptacle used for contaminated items.	Confining contaminated articles helps to reduce the spread of pathogens.
13 Wash thermometer in lukewarm soapy water. Rinse it in cool water. Dry and replace the thermometer in a container at the bedside.	Mechanical action of washing removes organic material and microorganisms.
14 Wash your hands.	Handwashing deters the spread of microorganisms.
15 Record temperature on flow sheet or paper. Report any abnormal findings to the appropriate person.	Recording the temperature provides accurate documentation.

Age Considerations

The axillary route or a temperature-sensitivity strip is the preferred method of evaluating the body temperature of a child younger than 6 years. This should also be the method of choice for a confused or disoriented adult.

Home Care Considerations

Reinforce differences in temperature reading depending on route used. Axillary temperature is generally a degree less than an oral measurement; a rectal temperature is usually a degree higher.

PROCEDURE 23-2

Assessing Body Temperature by Oral Method: Electronic Thermometer

Equipment

Thermometer with probe
Disposable probe cover

Soft tissues
Pencil or pen

Paper or flow sheet

Action

1 Explain the procedure to the client. Gather equipment.

2 Wash your hands.

3 Release the electronic unit from the charging area.

4 Remove the temperature probe from within the recording unit.

5 Attach a disposable cover over the temperature probe. Make sure it is secure.

6 Place the covered probe in the client's right or left sublingual pocket.

7 Hold the probe in place while it is in the client's mouth.

Rationale

An explanation encourages client cooperation and reduces client apprehension.

Handwashing deters the spread of microorganisms.

Charging sustains the power of the batteries when using the unit as a portable device.

Removal of the probe automatically prepares the machine to measure and record temperature.

A disposable cover prevents the transmission of organisms.

Thermometers placed in the middle area under the tongue have not registered as accurately as those placed in the areas to the sides.

If unsupported, the weight of the probe tends to fall away from the deepest areas under the tongue causing the measurement to be less reliable.

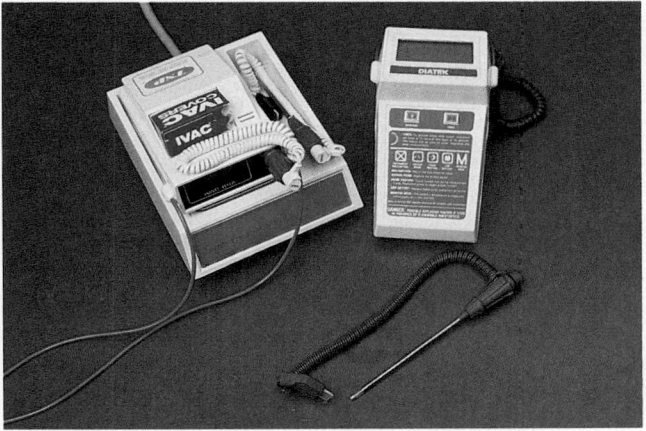

Two types of electronic thermometers and probes.

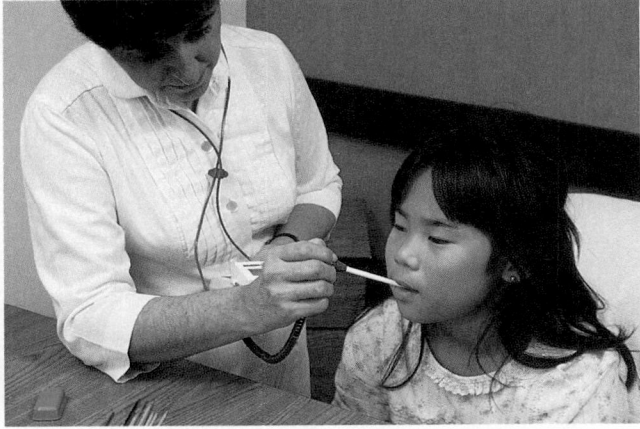

Actions 6 and 7: Placing and supporting the probe in place in the client's mouth.

8 Listen for a sound indicating that a maximum recording has been reached.

9 Remove the probe from the client's mouth, and note the numbers displayed on the electronic unit.

10 Press the probe release button while holding it over a receptacle, such as a wastebasket.

11 Return the probe to its storage location within the electronic unit.

A sound indicates that the unit is no longer sensing any further change in the measurement.

An electronic thermometer is not calibrated with multiple numbers. It displays only the measured temperature.

The release button frees the disposable cover from the probe without being touched by the nurse's hands.

The probe is protected from becoming broken if transported or stored within the recording unit.

(continued)

P R O C E D U R E   2 3 - 2   (continued)

Assessing Body Temperature by Oral Method: Electronic Thermometer

Action	Rationale
12 Wash your hands.	Handwashing deters the spread of microorganisms.
13 Record temperature on flow sheet or paper. Report any abnormal findings to the appropriate person.	Recording the temperature provides accurate documentation.
14 Return the electronic unit, and reconnect it to the source for charging the batteries.	Equipment needed by personnel for multiple patient use should be readily available.

Age Considerations

The axillary route or a temperature-sensitivity strip is the preferred method of evaluating the body temperature of a child younger than 6 years. This should also be the method of choice for a confused or disoriented adult.

Home Care Considerations

Reinforce differences in temperature reading depending on route used. Axillary temperature is generally a degree less than an oral measurement; a rectal temperature is usually a degree higher.

P R O C E D U R E   2 3 - 3

Assessing Body Temperature by Rectal Method: Glass Thermometer

Equipment

Rectal thermometer	Pencil or pen	Storage container	Disposable gloves
Soft tissues	Paper or flow sheet	Lubricant	(optional)

Action	Rationale
1 Explain the procedure to the client.	An explanation encourages client cooperation and reduces client apprehension.
2 Gather equipment.	Gathering equipment provides for organized approach to task.

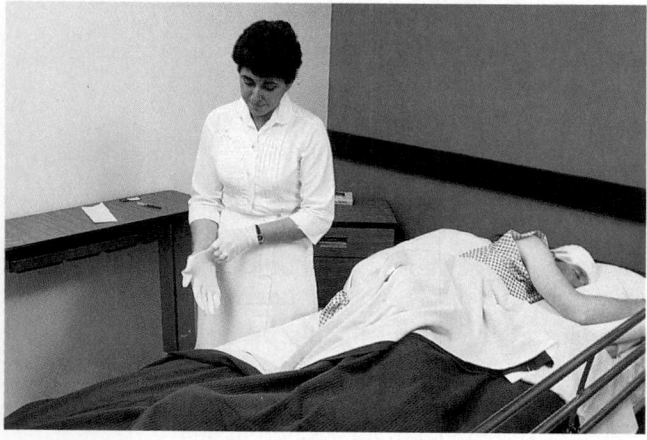

Action 3: Donning clean gloves.

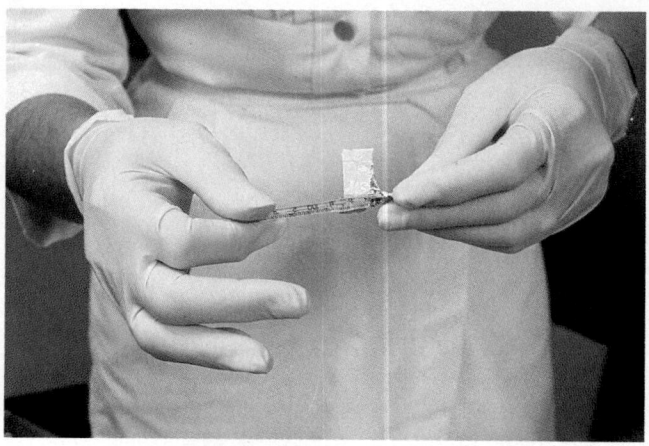

Action 5: Lubricating the mercury bulb.

(continued)

Assessing Body Temperature by Rectal Method: Glass Thermometer

Action	Rationale
3 Wash your hands. Don a disposable glove on your dominant hand or on both hands.	Handwashing deters the spread of microorganisms. Disposable glove protects the nurse from microorganisms in the feces.
4 Wipe, shake, and read the rectal thermometer.	A rectal thermometer requires the same preparation as an oral thermometer.
5 Lubricate the mercury bulb and an area approximately 2.5 cm (1 inch) above the bulb.	Lubrication reduces friction and thereby facilitates insertion, minimizing irritation or injury to the mucous membrane of the anal canal.
6 Provide for privacy. With the client on his or her side, fold back the bed linen and separate the buttocks so that the anal sphincter is seen clearly.	If not placed directly through the anal opening, the bulb of the thermometer may injure the adjacent tissue or cause discomfort for the client.
7 Insert the thermometer for approximately 3.8 cm (1½ inches) in an adult, 2.5 cm (1 inch) in a child, and 1.25 cm (½ inch) in an infant.	Insertion length must be adjusted according to the anatomical size of the client's rectum.
8 Permit the client's buttocks to fall in place while holding the thermometer in place for 2 to 3 minutes.	The thermometer may become displaced internally or externally if it is not held in place.
9 Remove the thermometer, and wipe it once with soft tissue from the fingers to the mercury bulb, using a firm, twisting motion.	Cleaning from an area where there are few organisms to an area where there are numerous organisms minimizes the spread of organisms. Friction helps to loosen the lubricant and fecal matter from the surface.
10 Wipe any residue of lubricant or stool remaining about the anus.	Removing lubricant and stool promotes the cleanliness and comfort of the client.
11 Read the thermometer and dispose of the tissue in a receptacle used for contaminated items.	Items containing organisms should be placed in containers for disposal to avoid transmitting them to other people.
12 Wash thermometer in lukewarm soapy water. Rinse in cool water. Dry and replace the thermometer in container marked ''rectal thermometer'' at the bedside. Remove the disposable glove from the inside out and discard the glove.	Mechanical action of washing aids in removal or organic material and microorganisms.

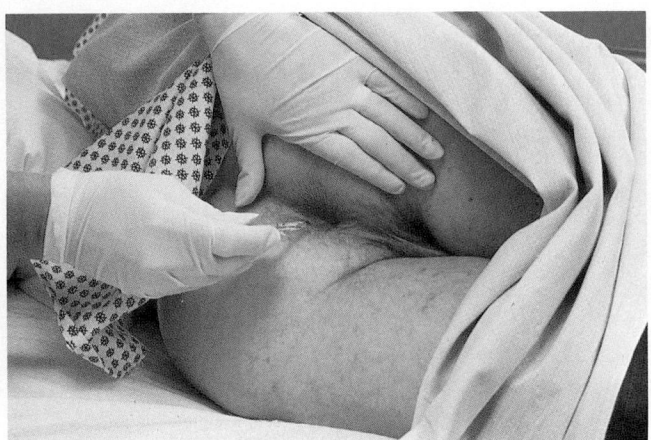

Actions 6 and 7: Separating the buttocks and inserting the thermometer.

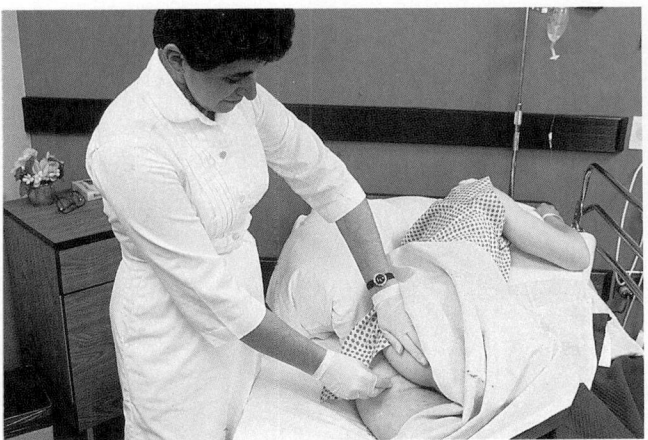

Action 8: Holding the thermometer in place.

(continued)

PROCEDURE 23-3 *(continued)*

Assessing Body Temperature by Rectal Method: Glass Thermometer

Action	Rationale
13 Wash your hands.	Handwashing deters the spread of microorganisms.
14 Record temperature on flow sheet or paper. Indicate that rectal route was used. Report any abnormal findings to the appropriate person.	Recording the temperature provides accurate documentation.

Age Considerations

The axillary route or a temperature-sensitivity strip is the preferred method of evaluating the body temperature of a child younger than 6 years. This should also be the method of choice for a confused or disoriented adult.

Home Care Considerations

Reinforce differences in temperature reading depending on route used. Axillary temperature is generally a degree less than an oral measurement; a rectal temperature is usually a degree higher.

perature provided proper technique is used and normal variations among the three methods are considered. Figure 23-4 shows the differences in normal body temperature depending on the site selected. Comparing the recordings using two different sites may also be a method for double-checking the validity of an unusual measurement. The procedure for obtaining an axillary temperature is described in Procedure 23-4.

Care of Equipment

If glass thermometers are used within a health care institution, each client has his or her own thermometer for the length of in-client care. The thermometer is kept in the client's room, usually in a container of liquid disinfectant. It is recommended that glass thermometers used for clients

with hepatitis (an infectious disease of the liver) and acquired immune deficiency syndrome be discarded when the client is discharged.

It is common practice in some agencies to have thermometers issued from a central supply unit. After being used one time for an individual client, they are returned for cleaning and disinfecting.

In the home, clean thermometers in lukewarm soapy water, rinse in cool water, and then store for reuse. If the thermometer is to be used by more than one person or if the person has a known or suspected infection transmitted by oral secretions, disinfect the thermometer with an appropriate solution after cleaning. The nurse should follow manufacturers' recommendations concerning the care and disposal of electronic and other types of thermometers and their sheaths.

F I G U R E   2 3 - 4

Comparison of normal adult axillary, oral, and rectal temperature ranges in Fahrenheit.

Axillary

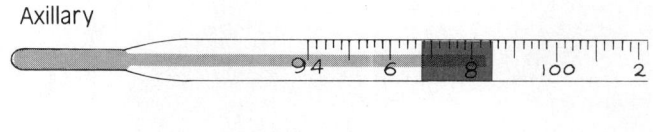

Oral

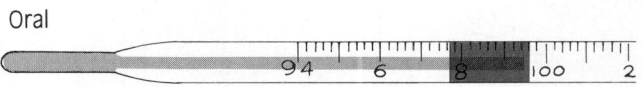

Rectal

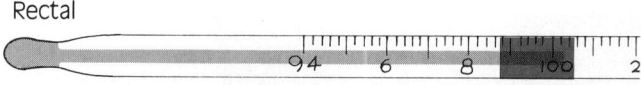

P R O C E D U R E   2 3 - 4

Assessing Body Temperature by Axillary Method: Glass Thermometer

Equipment

Thermometer   Pencil or pen
Soft tissues   Paper or flow sheet

Action	Rationale
1 Explain the procedure to the client.	An explanation encourages client cooperation and reduces client apprehension.
2 Gather equipment.	Gathering equipment provides for organized approach to task.
3 Wash your hands.	Handwashing deters the spread of microorganisms.
4 Provide privacy and move gown to expose axilla.	Moving the gown to expose axilla ensures accurate placement of thermometer.
5 Wipe the thermometer with a clean tissue if it has been stored in a chemical solution. Use a firm, twisting motion to remove the moisture.	Chemical solutions may irritate the skin. The presence of solution may alter skin temperature. Soft tissue and friction help remove the solution.
6 Shake and read the thermometer as suggested in Procedure 23-1.	The mercury must be below the calibrations of the previous recording to assess the current temperature accurately.
7 Place the bulb of the thermometer into the center of the axilla.	The deepest area of the axilla provides the most accurate temperature measurement.
8 Bring the client's arm down close to his or her body, and place the client's forearm over his or her chest.	Surrounding the bulb with the skin surfaces of the axilla reduces the amount of surrounding air and ensures a reliable measurement.

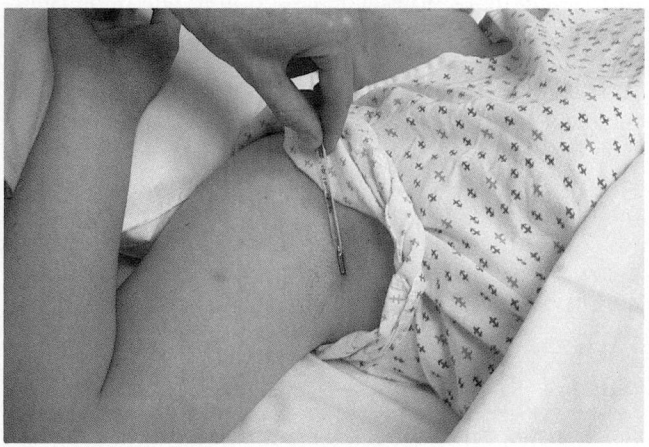

Action 7: Placing the bulb in the center of the axilla.

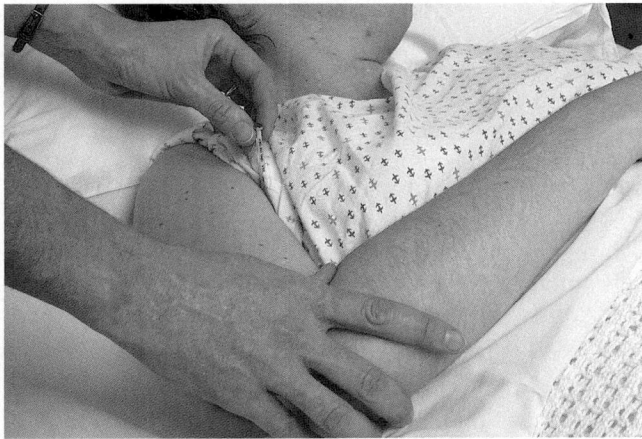

Action 8: Placing the client's arm close to the body. (Photos © Ken Kasper.)

9 Remain with the client and leave the thermometer in place for 10 minutes.	Additional time is required to ensure that the mercury expands to the maximum level of the client's temperature.
10 Remove and read the thermometer. Clean the thermometer and replace it in its location for reuse.	A thermometer that has been used for an axillary temperature should be cleaned before using it for another route and vice versa.

(continued)

Assessing Body Temperature by Axillary Method: Glass Thermometer

Action	Rationale
11 Wash your hands.	Handwashing deters the spread of microorganisms.
12 Record temperature on flow sheet or paper. Indicate axillary route. Report any abnormal findings to the appropriate person.	Recording the temperature provides accurate documentation.

Age Considerations The axillary route or a temperature-sensitivity strip is the preferred method of evaluating the body temperature of a child younger than 6 years. This should also be the method of choice for a confused or disoriented adult.

Home Care Considerations Reinforce differences in temperature reading depending on route used. Axillary temperature is generally a degree less than an oral measurement; a rectal temperature is usually a degree higher.

Pulse

Physiologic Factors

The stimulus for contraction of the heart starts in the **sinoatrial node** (SA node), which is in the upper part of the right atrium. Because this node sets the pace of the beat, it is often called the pacemaker.

Each time the left ventricle of the heart contracts to eject blood into an already full aorta, the arterial walls in the blood system expand, or distend, to compensate for the increase in pressure. This expansion of the aorta sends a wave through the walls of the arterial system that, on palpation, can be felt as a light tap. This sensation is called the **pulse**.

The quantity of blood forced out of the left ventricle with each contraction is called the *stroke volume*. The average amount of blood per contraction is 70 mL for an adult. The *cardiac output* is the amount of blood pumped per minute. This volume is determined by using the following formula:

cardiac output = stroke volume × pulse rate

Thus, the cardiac output of an adult with a stroke volume of 70 mL and a pulse rate of 72 beats per minute would be about 5000 mL. Many factors can affect both the heart rate, such as exercise, and the volume, such as a person's state of fluid balance. However, the body attempts to maintain a sufficient supply of blood to the cells at all times. For example, when the stroke volume decreases, such as when the blood volume is lowered because of hemorrhage, the contraction rate increases to maintain the same cardiac output. Conversely, in a physically fit athlete whose heart pumps a maximum volume of blood per stroke, the heart rate may be well at the low range or below the range of normal, yet the body cells remain adequately supplied.

Pulse Rate

The *pulse rate* is the number of pulsations felt in a minute. This rate ordinarily corresponds to the same rate at which the heart is beating. There are wide ranges for normal pulse rates. Rates differ as individuals age, gradually diminishing from birth to adulthood as shown in Table 23-5.

A rapid heart rate is called **tachycardia**. An adult has tachycardia when the pulse rate is 100 to 180 beats per minute. *Palpitation* means that the person is aware of his or her own heartbeat without having to feel for it over an artery. The pulse rate is ordinarily unduly rapid when palpitations are noted.

The term used to describe the heart rate when it falls below 60 beats per minute in an adult is called **bradycardia**. A slow pulse rate during illness is less common

T A B L E   2 3 - 5

Normal Pulse Rates per Minute at Various Ages		
Age	**Approximate Range**	**Approximate Average**
Newborn to 1 mo	120–160	140
1 to 12 mo	80–140	120
12 mo to 2 yr	80–130	110
2 to 6 yr	75–120	100
6 to 12 yr	75–110	95
Adolescence to adult	60–100	80

My first frightening clinical experience when I began nursing was the second week of my basic rotation. I went into my assigned client's room to take noon vital signs. I only got a pulse for a few seconds, and I kept losing it. I started getting nervous because I had no problem getting arm vital signs. Everyone in my group was getting ready to go to lunch. I went out of my client's room to tell my instructor that I couldn't get a good pulse—it kept fading in and out. My instructor and I entered my client's room. I went on the client's left side, and my instructor went on the right side. At this point, I was really nervous, because I kept thinking my instructor will get a pulse right away and I'll really feel stupid. She had a hard time getting a radial pulse, too. She told me to take an apical pulse. I was really nervous; I wasn't understanding what she was saying. In my mind, I was thinking axillary, so I put my hand near the client's axilla, feeling around for a pulse, and my instructor said, "Oh, you are trying for an axillary pulse. I think an apical would be easier to get." So then I am thinking, "She is going to fail me." She said, "Apical is near the heart." Then I thought, Oh... I can't believe this is happening to me." So I go and put my hand near the heart for an apical pulse. My instructor said to use the stethoscope. "You can get an apical pulse that way." I was so embarrassed. After I walked out of there, I couldn't believe that happened to me. I knew where the apical pulse was! I was so nervous, I thought axilla. This was my most frightening clinical experience, and I will never forget it.

—Elizabeth Ann McGrenra, Holy Family College, Philadelphia

than a rapid pulse rate, but, when present, bradycardia should be reported promptly.

The pulse rate is generally slower at rest and on awakening. Females generally have a slightly faster rate, about 7 to 8 beats per minute, than males. It has been noted that the body size and build of a person may affect the pulse rate. Tall, slender people often have a slower rate than short, stout ones.

The rate of the heartbeat, and thus the pulse as well, readily responds to impulses conducted along the autonomic nervous system. This system is subdivided into parasympathetic and sympathetic networks of nerves. Stimulation of the parasympathetic system decreases the heart rate. The drug digitalis, commonly used by clients with certain heart ailments, decreases the heart's contractions by stimulating the vagus nerve. Stimulation of the sympathetic system increases the heart rate. The following factors also contribute to an increase in the pulse rate:

- Pain
- Strong emotions, such as fear, anger, anxiety, and surprise
- Exercise, when the heart's compensatory ability attempts to meet the need for increased blood circulation
- Prolonged application of heat
- A decrease in blood pressure, such as occurs with blood loss, when the heart's compensatory ability attempts to meet the need for increased output of blood from the heart

- An elevated temperature, which usually causes an increase of about 7 to 10 beats per minute for each 0.6°C (1°F) of elevation above normal
- Any condition resulting in poor oxygenation of blood, for example, chronic pulmonary disease

Pulse Rhythm

The **pulse rhythm** is the pattern of the pulsations and the pauses between them. This rhythm is normally regular; that is, the beat and the pauses occur similarly throughout the time the pulse is being obtained. An irregular pattern of heartbeats is called an **arrhythmia**. Any irregularity in the heartbeat should be reported immediately. Common pulse rhythms are described and illustrated in Table 23-6.

Pulse Amplitude

The *pulse amplitude* describes the quality of the pulse in terms of its fullness and reflects the strength of the left ventricular contraction. It is noted by the feel of the blood flow through the vessel. Under normal conditions, the amplitude of each pulse beat is strong and feels similarly so at all areas where an artery can be palpated. A strong pulse can be obliterated with relative ease by exerting pressure over the artery, but it remains perceptible with moderate pressure. Table 23-7 presents a scale commonly used to describe pulse amplitude.

T A B L E   2 3 - 6

Various Pulse Rhythms

Term	Description	Illustration*

Regular   The pulsations and the pauses occur similarly throughout the entire minute

Normal

Tachycardia

Bradycardia

Arrhythmia   The pulsations or length of pauses occur with no pattern or predictability

Intermittent   A normal pulse rhythm is broken by periods of irregularity.

Bigeminal   A normal pulse rhythm of two beats is followed by a pause.

Premature beat   A heartbeat occurs before the normal one.

*Each vertical line represents one heartbeat.

TABLE 23-7

Pulse Amplitude

Number	Definition	Description
0	Absent pulse	No pulsation is felt despite extreme pressure
1+	Thready pulse	Pulsation is not easily felt and slight pressure causes it to disappear
2+	Weak pulse	Stronger than a thready pulse; light pressure causes it to disappear
3+	Normal pulse	Pulsation is easily felt, takes moderate pressure to cause it to disappear
4+	Bounding pulse	The pulsation is strong and does not disappear with moderate pressure

(Timby, B. K., & Lewis, L. W. [1992]. *Fundamental skills and concepts in patient care* [5th ed.]. Philadelphia: Lippincott, p. 255.)

Assessment Methods

Obtaining a Radial Pulse   Most commonly, the radial artery at the wrist is used for palpating the pulse because it is easily accessible. It is located on the inner, thumb-side of the wrist. Figure 23-5 shows its location and the position of the fingertips during assessment. If this site is inaccessible, select an alternative artery that does not require exertion or cause discomfort for the person, which could alter the pulse rate. Procedure 23-5 describes how to obtain the pulse rate using the site of the radial artery.

Obtaining an Apical Pulse   If a peripheral pulse is irregular, feeble, or extremely rapid, causing it to be difficult to assess accurately, the apical rate may be assessed. In the adult, the apical rate is counted by listening with a stethoscope over the apex of the heart. The contraction of the heart can be heard in the space between the fifth and the sixth ribs, about 8 cm (3 inches) to the left of the median line and slightly below the nipple, as illustrated in Figure 23-6. Nursing actions are given in Procedure 23-6. The apical rate of an infant is easily palpated with the fingertips.

Obtaining an Apical–Radial Pulse   When the radial pulse is irregular, the *apical–radial pulse rate* may be obtained by counting at the apex of the heart and at the radial artery simultaneously. The following techniques are recommended to obtain an apical–radial pulse rate:

- Two nurses are needed; one listens with a stethoscope over the apex of the heart for the heartbeat, and the other counts the rate at the radial artery.
- The client's chest wall is exposed so that the stethoscope can be placed directly on the skin of the chest wall.
- One watch with a sweep second hand is placed so that both nurses can read it conveniently and simultaneously.
- The nurses determine where they can best hear and feel the pulse and decide on a time to start counting, such as when the second hand on the watch is at a specified place.
- Both nurses count for 1 full minute and record their counts.

The difference between the apical and radial pulse rates is the **pulse deficit**.

Assessment Sites

The rate, rhythm, and amplitude of the pulse may be assessed by compressing an artery against an underlying bone with the tips of the fingers. The thumb is not used to
(Text continues on p. 406)

FIGURE 23-5

(*Left*) The location of the radial artery. (*Right*) The nurse is shown palpating the artery on a client.

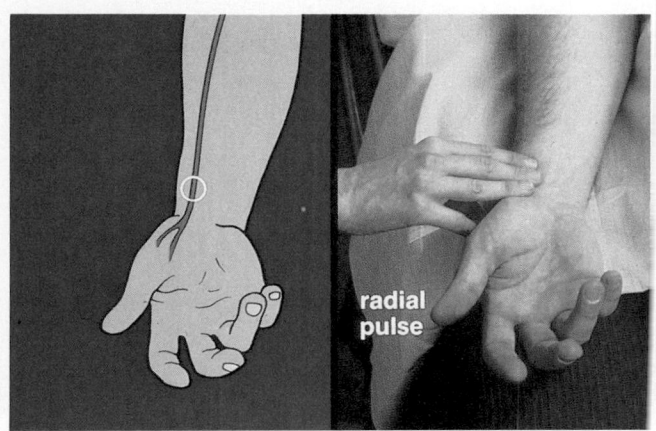

FIGURE 23-6

(*Left*) The site of the apical pulse at the apex of the heart. (*Right*) The nurse listens to the heartbeat using a stethoscope.

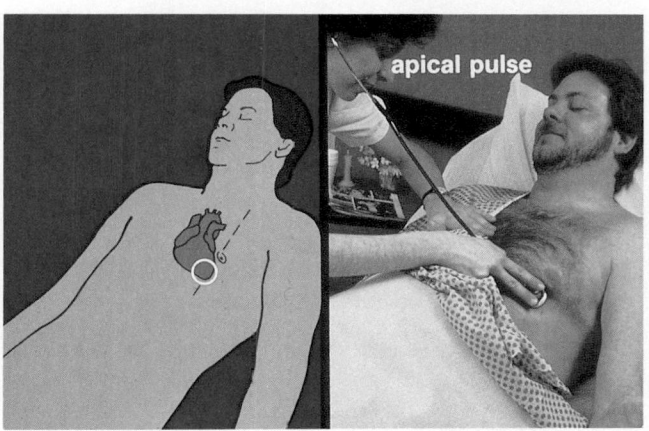

P R O C E D U R E   2 3 - 5

Assessing the Radial Pulse Rate

Equipment

Watch with second hand
  or digital readout

Pencil or pen
Paper or flow sheet

Action	Rationale
1 Explain the procedure to client.	An explanation encourages client cooperation and reduces client apprehension.
2 Gather equipment.	Gathering equipment provides for organized approach to task.
3 Wash your hands.	Handwashing deters the spread of microorganisms.
4 Have the client lie down and rest his or her arm alongside the body with the wrist extended and the palm of the hand downward. Or the client can sit with his or her forearm at a 90-degree angle to the body resting on a support and with the wrist extended and the palm of the hand downward.	These positions are ordinarily comfortable for the client and convenient for the nurse.
5 Place your first, second, and third fingers along the client's radial artery, and press gently against the radius; rest your thumb in apposition to fingers on the back of the client's wrist.	The fingertips, sensitive to touch, feel pulsation of the client's radial artery. If the thumb is used for palpating the client's pulse, the nurse's own pulse may be felt.
6 Apply only enough pressure so that the client's pulsating artery can be felt distinctly.	Moderate pressure allows the nurse to feel the superficial radial artery expand with each heartbeat. Too much pressure obliterates the pulse. If too little pressure is applied, the pulse is imperceptible.
7 Using a watch with a second hand, count the number of pulsations felt for 30 seconds. Multiply this number by two to obtain the rate for 1 minute.	Sufficient time is necessary to assess the rate, rhythm, and amplitude of the pulse.
8 If the pulse rate is abnormal in any way, palpate the pulse for a full minute or longer.	When the pulse is abnormal, longer counting and palpation are necessary to identify most accurately the unusual characteristics of the pulse.

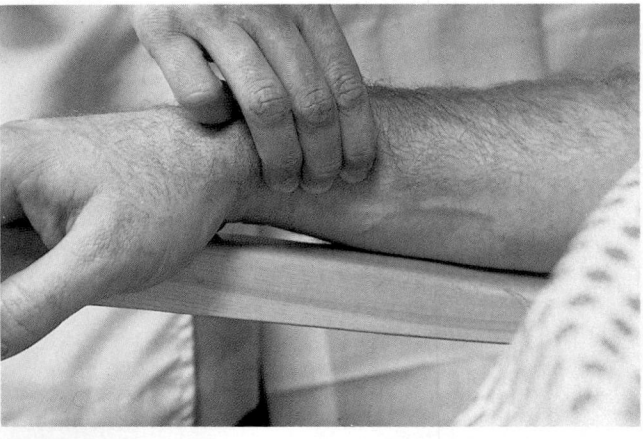

Action 5: Proper placement of the fingers along the radial artery.

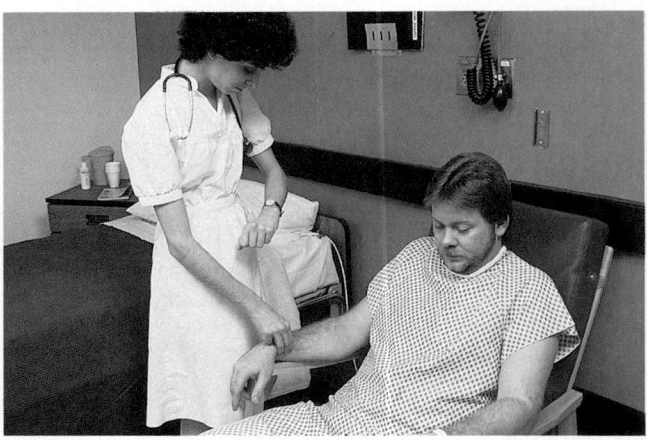

Action 7: Counting the pulsations felt for 30 seconds.

(continued)

PROCEDURE 2 3 - 5 *(continued)*

Assessing the Radial Pulse Rate

Action	Rationale
9 Assess rhythm, amplitude, and elasticity of the vessel wall while counting rate.	Irregularity in heart rate may disrupt the cardiac output. Amplitude of pulse indicates the quality of the heart's contraction. Elasticity of blood vessel does not affect the pulse rate but does reflect status of the vascular system.
10 Record pulse rate on flow sheet or paper. Report any abnormal findings to the appropriate person.	Recording the pulse rate provides accurate documentation.
11 Wash your hands.	Handwashing deters the spread of microorganisms.

Special Considerations

Inform the client of availability of digital pulse monitoring devices.

Instruct family members about techniques used to locate and monitor other peripheral pulse sites.

PROCEDURE 2 3 - 6

Assessing the Apical Pulse Rate

Equipment

Watch with second hand   Pencil or pen
   or digital readout   Paper or flow sheet
Stethoscope   Alcohol swab

Action	Rationale
1 Explain the procedure to the client.	An explanation encourages client cooperation and reduces client apprehension.
2 Gather equipment.	Gathering equipment provides for organized approach to task.
3 Wash your hands.	Handwashing deters the spread of microorganisms.
4 Use alcohol swab to cleanse ear pieces and diaphragm of stethoscope, if necessary.	Cleansing with alcohol deters transmission of microorganisms.
5 Assist client to sitting position in bed or on a chair if possible.	This position eases identification of site for nurse.
6 Provide privacy and move gown to expose upper chest area.	Moving the gown facilitates identification of site for placement of stethoscope.
7 Hold diaphragm of stethoscope against palm of hand for a few seconds.	Hand warms metal area of stethoscope which may be cold and may startle client.
8 Palpate fifth intercostal space and move to left midclavicular line. Place diaphragm over apex of heart.	This is point of maximal impulse, where heartbeat is easier to hear.
9 Listen for normal heart sounds, identified as "lub dub" beat.	These sounds occur as blood flows through heart valves.

(continued)

P R O C E D U R E 2 3 - 6 *(continued)*

Assessing the Apical Pulse Rate

Action	Rationale
10 Using a watch with a second hand, count the heartbeat for 30 seconds and multiply by two if rhythm is regular. Count for 60 seconds if regular rhythm is present.	Longer time interval allows for more accurate assessment of heart rate.

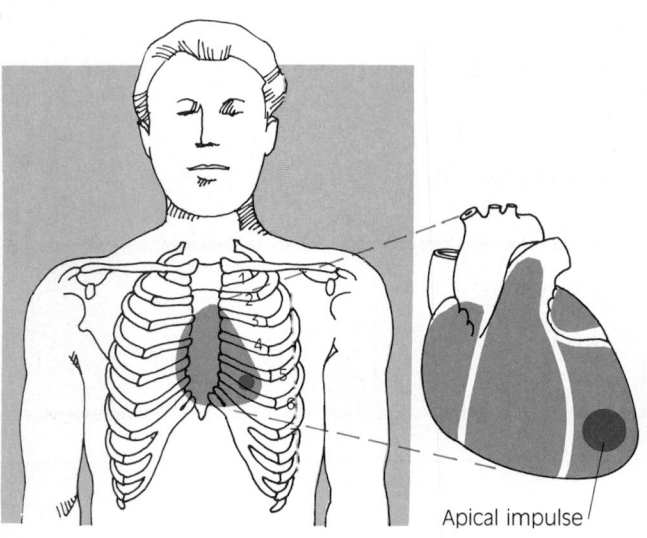

Schematic depiction of the thorax showing location of apical impulse.

Apical impulse

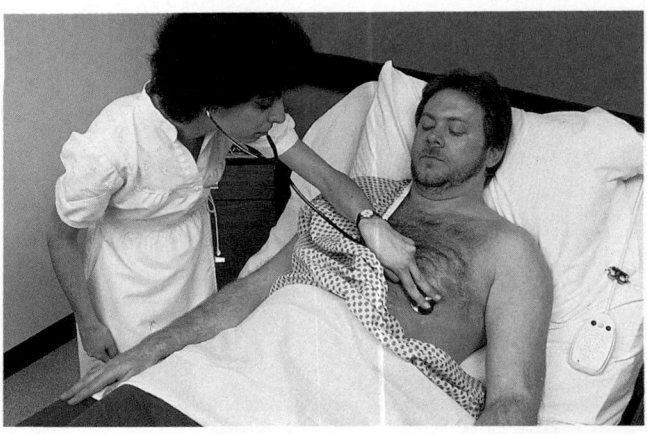

Action 10: Counting the heartbeat for 30 seconds.

Action	Rationale
11 Assess presence of any irregularity in heart rate and rhythm.	This assessment indicates adequacy of cardiac function.
12 Replace the client's gown and assist client to comfortable position.	Such action provides for privacy and comfort.
13 Record pulse rate on flow sheet or paper. Identify as apical rate. Report any abnormal findings to the appropriate person.	Recording the pulse rate provides accurate documentation.
14 Wash your hands.	Handwashing deters the spread of microorganisms.

Special Considerations

Inform client of availability of digital pulse monitoring devices.

Instruct family members about techniques used to locate and monitor other peripheral pulse sites.

---

compress an artery because the nurse would tend to feel his or her own pulse rather than that of the client.

The arteries located close to the skin surface are used most often. Most, but not all, are named for the bone to which each is adjacent. Common arteries used for assessment include the temporal, carotid, brachial, radial, femoral, popliteal, posterior tibial, and dorsalis pedis. Collectively, they are called *peripheral pulses* because they are distant from the heart. The location of these sites is illustrated in Figure 23-7.

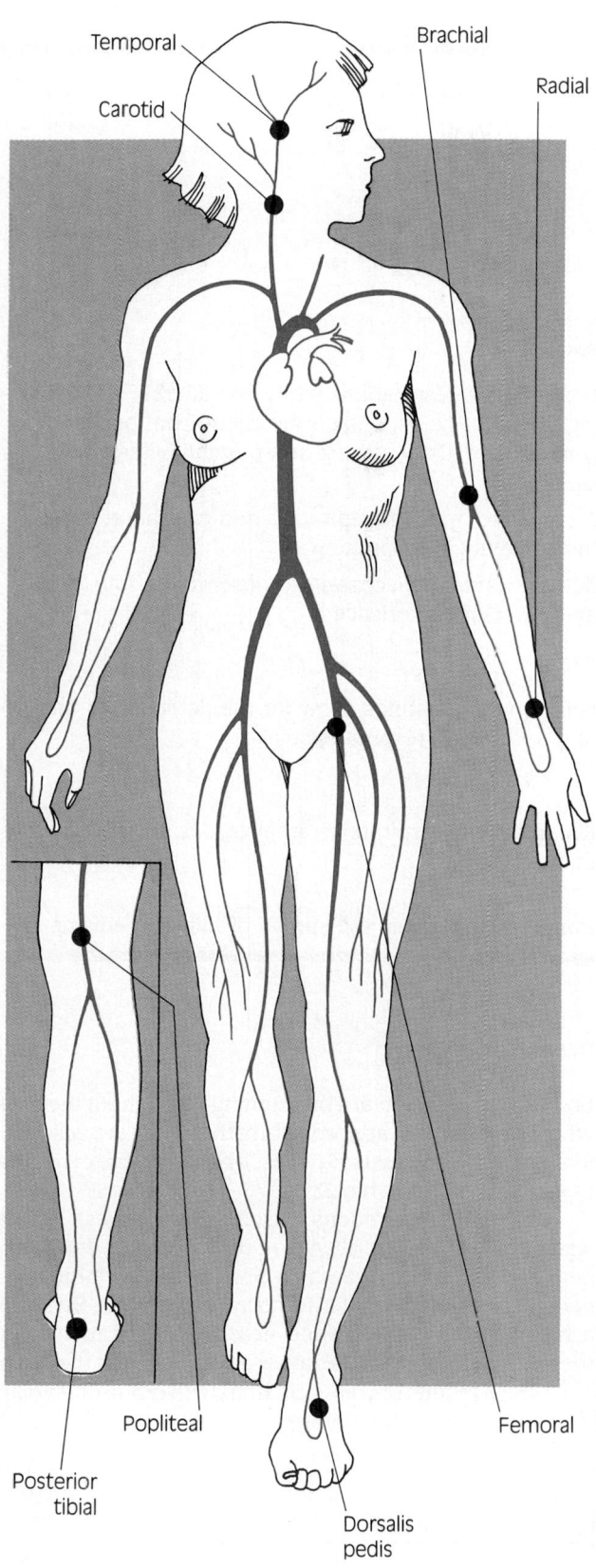

Temporal

Carotid

Brachial

Radial

Popliteal

Posterior
tibial

Dorsalis
pedis

Femoral

FIGURE 23-7

These arteries are located near the surface of the body. The pulse can be detected in any of these sites by light palpation.

Respiration

Respiration, in its broadest sense, begins with the act of breathing and includes the body's use of oxygen and the elimination of carbon dioxide. **Inspiration** or inhalation is the act of breathing in, and **expiration** or exhalation is the act of breathing out. *External respiration* includes lung ventilation, the absorption of oxygen, and the elimination of carbon dioxide. *Internal respiration*, sometimes called *tissue respiration*, includes the use of oxygen by body cells for the production of heat through oxidation and the liberation of energy from the food we eat.

Physiologic Factors

Respirations can be somewhat voluntarily controlled by activating or restricting muscles of the chest and diaphragm. This explains the ability of a person to control breathing when talking and singing. However, chemical receptors act as the primary involuntary regulator for respiration. As carbon dioxide accumulates in the blood, chemoreceptors in the aortic and carotid bodies dispatch impulses to the respiratory center in the medulla oblongata, and the rate and depth of respirations are increased. Despite a parent's panic when a child has a temper tantrum and holds his or her breath, chemical stimulation of respiration eventually overcomes the child's voluntary efforts to control it.

Assessment

Respiratory Rate

Under normal conditions, healthy adults breathe about 16 to 20 times each minute. Wider variations have also been observed in healthy people. The respiratory rate is more rapid in infants and young children. It has been noted that the relationship between the pulse rate and the respiratory rate is fairly consistent in well people, the ratio being one respiration to about four heartbeats.

During illness, the respiratory rate may vary from normal. When body temperature is elevated, the respiratory rate increases in response to the increased metabolic rate. Cells require more oxygen at this time and have a greater amount of carbon dioxide that must be removed. The rate increases as much as four breaths per minute with every 0.6°C (1°F) that the temperature rises above normal. Any condition involving an accumulation of carbon dioxide and a decrease in oxygen in the blood also tends to increase the rate and the depth of respirations.

Some conditions characteristically predispose to slow breathing. An increase in intracranial pressure depresses the respiratory center, resulting in irregular or shallow breathing, slow breathing, or both. Certain drugs also depress the respiratory rate (eg, morphine sulfate).

Procedure 23-7 describes how to obtain the respiratory rate.

P R O C E D U R E 2 3 - 7

Assessing the Respiratory Rate

Equipment

Watch with second hand
  or digital readout

Pencil or pen
Paper or flow sheet

Action	Rationale
1 While your fingertips are still in place after counting the pulse rate, observe the client's respirations.	Counting the respirations while presumably still counting the pulse helps to keep the client from becoming conscious of his breathing and possibly altering his usual rate.
2 Note the rise and fall of the client's chest with each inspiration and expiration.	A complete cycle of inspiration and expiration constitutes one act of respiration.
3 Using a watch with a second hand, count the number of respirations for a minimum of 30 seconds. Multiply this number by two to obtain the client's respiratory rate per minute.	Sufficient time is necessary to observe the rate, depth, and other characteristics.
4 If respirations are abnormal in any way, count the respiratory rate for a full minute. Repeat if necessary to determine the rate and characteristics of breathing.	Full-minute countings allow for the detection of unequal timing between respirations.
5 Record respiratory rate on flow sheet or paper. Report any abnormal findings to the appropriate person.	Recording the respiratory rate provides accurate documentation.
6 Wash your hands.	Handwashing deters the spread of microorganisms.

Respiratory Depth

In a state of rest, the depth of each respiration is about the same. The depth of respirations is generally described as ranging from shallow to deep. Periodically, each person automatically inhales deeply, filling the lungs with more air than inhaled with the usual depth of respiration.

Certain terms are used to describe the nature and depth of respirations. **Apnea** refers to periods during which there is no breathing. This is a serious situation in which brain damage and death can occur if breathing is suppressed for more than 4 to 6 minutes. **Dyspnea** is difficult or labored breathing. A dyspneic client is likely to demonstrate rapid, shallow breathing. Dyspneic clients usually appear to be anxious and worried as they experience the inefficient work of breathing. The nostrils flare as the client struggles to fill the lungs with air. Dyspneic people frequently find some relief if they assume an upright position. The condition of being able to breathe easier in this manner is known as **orthopnea**. A sitting or standing position uses gravity to lower organs in the abdominal cavity to fall away from the diaphragm. This gives more room for the lungs to expand within the chest, thus taking in more air with each breath.

Breath Sounds

Breath sounds are heard by listening throughout the chest with a stethoscope; abnormal breath sounds are described in Chapter 24. Terms used to describe the nature of respirations are given in Table 23-8.

Ordinarily, respirations are relatively noiseless. Several terms are used to describe the nature of sounds that can be heard as the client breathes. **Stertorous** breathing is a general term used to refer to noisy respirations. **Stridor** is a harsh, high-pitched sound heard on inspiration when there is a narrowing of the upper airway, such as the larynx or trachea. Infants or young children with croup often manifest stridor when breathing.

Blood Pressure

Physiologic Factors

Blood pressure refers to the force of the blood against arterial walls. Maximum blood pressure is exerted on the walls of arteries when the left ventricle of the heart pushes

TABLE 23-8

The Nature of Respirations

Term	Description	Illustration*
Eupnea	Normal respirations; the rate and depth are equal	
Tachypnea or polypnea	Fast respiratory rate	
Bradypnea	Slow respiratory rate	
Cheyne-Stokes	Gradual increase followed by gradual decrease in the depth of respirations, and then a period of apnea	
Biot's	Respirations of the same depth followed by a period of apnea	

*Each vertical line represents one respiration and its depth.

blood through the aortic valve into the aorta during systole. The highest pressure thus is called **systolic pressure**. When the heart rests (*diastole*) between beats, the pressure drops. The lowest pressure present on arterial walls at this time is called **diastolic pressure**. The difference between the two is called the **pulse pressure**.

Blood pressure is measured in millimeters of mercury (mm Hg) and is recorded as a fraction. The numerator is the systolic pressure; the denominator is the diastolic pressure. For example, if the blood pressure is 120/80, 120 is the systolic pressure and 80 is the diastolic pressure. The pulse pressure, in this case, is 40. The following factors are responsible for maintaining blood pressure. Deviations from normal blood pressure likely result from alterations in any one or more of these functions.

Peripheral Resistance Once blood leaves the heart, it is circulated through a continuous loop of blood vessels consisting of arteries, arterioles, capillaries, and veins. *Arterioles* are fine, elastic tubes with the capacity to contract or dilate to regulate the distribution of blood to various organs, tissues, or cells, depending on their moment-by-moment requirements.

Normally, arterioles are in a state of partial contraction; they are neither totally constricted nor fully relaxed. This semicontracted state is *peripheral resistance*. It creates a relatively constant level of restraint to blood flow. Peripheral resistance is one of the main factors affecting blood pressure.

Pumping Action of the Heart When increased amounts of blood are pumped into the arteries (ie, when cardiac output is increased), the arteries distend more, resulting in an increase in blood pressure. When less blood is pumped into the arteries (ie, when cardiac output is decreased), blood pressure falls. Hence, a weak pumping action results in a lower blood pressure than a strong pumping action.

Blood Volume When blood volume is low, as may occur with hemorrhage or dehydration, blood pressure is low because there is decreased fluid within the arteries. Increasing the quantity of blood increases the pressure because there is more fluid volume creating pressure within the arteries.

Viscosity of Blood Viscosity is the state of being sticky or gummy. The viscosity of the blood depends on the proportion of blood cells to plasma. The more viscid the blood, the higher the blood pressure. This occurs because the heart requires more force to move the concentrated fluid throughout the circulatory system.

Elasticity of Vessel Walls Arteries have a considerable quantity of elastic tissue that allows them to stretch. When the heart rests between each beat, the walls of the arteries recoil, although pressure in them does not drop to zero. The state of pressure keeps the blood entering the capillaries and veins in a continuous flow, not in spurts. Simultaneously, the arterioles, normally in a moderate state of contraction, offer certain resistance. Therefore, the elasticity of the walls, in addition to the resistance of the arterioles, helps to maintain normal blood pressure.

With age, the walls of arterioles become less elastic, which interferes with their ability to stretch and dilate. This can subsequently limit adequate blood flow and contribute to rising pressure within the vascular system.

Normal and Abnormal Blood Pressure

Normal Blood Pressure

Studies of healthy people indicate that blood pressure can be within a wide range and still be normal. Because individual differences are considerable, it is important to know what is the normal blood pressure for a particular person. A rise or fall of 20 to 30 mm Hg in a person's blood pressure is significant, even if it is within the generally accepted normal range. Table 23-9 offers a guide for average normal and hypertensive levels of blood pressure measurements for people of various ages.

The following factors influence blood pressure in the average healthy adult:

- A person's age influences his or her blood pressure.
- Normal fluctuations occur during the day. The blood pressure is usually lowest on arising in the morning, before breakfast, and before activity commences. The blood pressure has been noted to rise as much as 5 to 10 mm Hg by late afternoon, and it gradually falls again during sleep.
- A person's gender also influences blood pressure. Women usually have a lower blood pressure than men of the same age.
- Blood pressure has been observed to rise after the ingestion of food.
- Systolic blood pressure rises during periods of exercise and strenuous activity.

TABLE 23-9

Average and Hypertensive Blood Pressures According to Age		
Age	**Average Blood Pressure**	**Hypertensive Level***
Newborn	40 mm Hg systolic	Undetermined
1 mo	85/54 mm Hg	Undetermined
1 yr	95/65 mm Hg	≥110/75 mm Hg
6 yr	105/65 mm Hg	≥120/80 mm Hg
10–13 yr	110/65 mm Hg	≥125/85 mm Hg
14–17 yr	120/80 mm Hg	≥135/90 mm Hg
18+ yr	120/80 mm Hg	≥140/90 mm Hg

* Levels determined by the 1984 Joint National Committee on Detection, Evaluation, and Treatment of High Blood Pressure.

- Emotions, such as anger, fear, excitement, and pain, generally cause the blood pressure to rise, but the pressure falls to normal when the situation passes.
- A person's blood pressure tends to be lower when he or she is in a prone or supine position than when he or she is sitting or standing.

Because of the many factors that influence blood pressure, the measurements of a single blood pressure are not necessarily significant. People with a reading near or above the upper limits of normal should be reexamined to determine if the measurement persists. The U.S. Department of Health and Human Services, Public Health Service, has prepared recommended initial action and follow-up guidelines for subsequent blood pressure measurement (Fig. 23-8). The Canadian Heart Fund (Ontario Division) advises that, in adults older than age 18 years who are not being treated for hypertension, a diastolic pressure below 95 mm Hg is considered normal, diastolic pressure between 95 and 104 mm Hg is considered borderline elevation, and diastolic pressure above 104 mm Hg is definitely elevated. People found to have a diastolic pressure above 104 mm Hg are referred for evaluation and care (Ontario Heart Fund Foundation, 1983).

Hypertension

A person whose blood pressure is above normal for a sustained period is in a state of **hypertension**. When the cause of hypertension is due to known pathology, it is called *secondary hypertension*. *Primary* or *essential* hypertension is hypertension without a known cause.

Hypertension is a prevalent health problem. The public as well as health practitioners are becoming increasingly aware of the importance of having regular blood pressure measurements because of the many dangers associated with hypertension. Persistent diastolic hypertension is the most serious and most common blood pressure disturbance. It is a major cause of early death and serious disability in millions of people. Although the exact reason has not been determined, hypertension occurs almost twice as frequently in blacks as in whites.

Hypotension

A blood pressure below normal is called **hypotension**. A consistently low blood pressure, for example, a systolic reading of 90 to 115 mm Hg in an adult, appears to cause no ill effects. Rather, this is usually associated with longevity.

Orthostatic (postural) **hypotension** is a low blood pressure associated with weakness or fainting when rising to an erect position. It is the result of peripheral vasodilation without a compensatory rise in cardiac output. This type of hypotension can usually be prevented by arising and moving about slowly, especially after a period of bed rest. Ordinarily it can be corrected by lowering the head, which restores blood flow to the brain. Clients with postural hypotension (most of whom are elderly) require special monitoring.

Blood Pressure Classification* and Follow-Up Criteria

Diastolic Blood Pressure (mm Hg)	Systolic Blood Pressure (mm Hg)			
	Less than 140	140 to 159	160 to 199	200 or greater
Less than 85	Normal Blood Pressure	Borderline Isolated Systolic Hypertension	Isolated Systolic Hypertension	
	Recheck within 2 years†	1st occasion: Confirm within 2 months 2nd occasion: Evaluate or refer promptly to a source of care	Evaluate or refer to a source of care within 2 weeks	
85 to 89	High Normal Blood Pressure	Borderline Isolated Systolic Hypertension	Isolated Systolic Hypertension	
	Recheck within 1 year	1st occasion: Confirm within 2 months 2nd occasion: Evaluate or refer promptly to a source of care	Evaluate or refer to a source of care within 2 weeks	
90 to 104	Mild Hypertension	1st occasion: Confirm within 2 months 2nd occasion: Evaluate or refer promptly to a source of care		
105 to 114	Moderate Hypertension	Evaluate or refer to a source of care within 2 weeks		
115 or greater	Severe Hypertension	Evaluate or refer immediately to a source of care		

*Based on the average of two or more measurements on two or more occasions.

†Rechecking within one year is recommended on 2nd occasion and for individuals at increased risk (i.e., family history, obesity, blacks, oral contraceptive use, and high alcohol intake).

Source: 1984 Report of the Joint National Committee on Detection, Evaluation and Treatment of High Blood Pressure.

FIGURE 23-8

The recommended actions for various blood pressure readings given are those of the 1984 Joint National Committee on Detection, Evaluation, and Treatment of High Blood Pressure. (U.S. Department of Health and Human Services, Public Health Service, National Institutes of Health. [1984]. [NIH Publication No. NIH 80-1088]. Washington, D.C.: Author.)

Some drugs, such as meperidine hydrochloride (Demerol) cause hypotension. There are several illnesses associated with hypotension. For example, the blood pressure drops when a client is experiencing severe blood loss, burns, severe vomiting and diarrhea, or when cardiac output is impaired after a heart attack.

Assessment Methods

Sphygmomanometer

A **sphygmomanometer**, consisting of a cuff and a manometer, and a stethoscope are necessary for obtaining an indirect measurement of blood pressure.

Cuff The sphygmomanometer has a cuff that contains an airtight, flat, rubber bladder covered with cloth. It is important to select a bladder of the proper width to obtain an accurate blood pressure reading (Fig. 23-9). If it is too narrow, the reading could be erroneously high because the pressure is not evenly transmitted to the artery. This occurs,

FIGURE 23-9

It is important to select a cuff of an appropriate size to obtain an accurate blood pressure reading. Shown hear are three cuff sizes: a small cuff for a child or a small or frail adult, a normal adult size cuff, and a large cuff, called a leg cuff, for measuring blood pressure on a leg or for use on an obese adult.

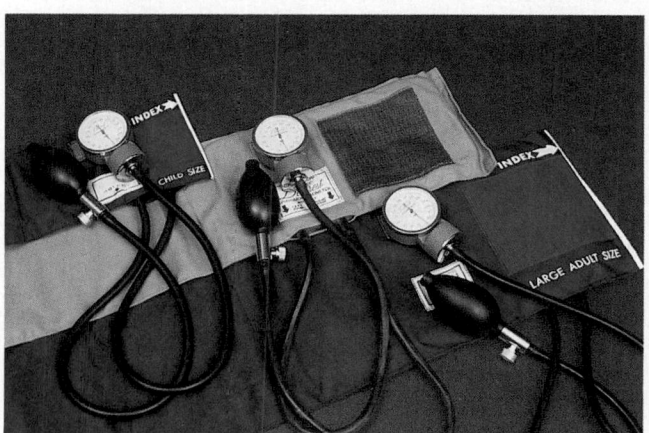

Recommended Bladder Sizes for a Blood Pressure Cuff

Arm Circumference at Midpoint* (cm)	Cuff Name	Bladder Width (cm)	Bladder Length (cm)
5–7.5	Newborn	3	5
7.5–13	Infant	5	8
13–20	Child	8	13
24–32	Adult	13	24
32–42	Large adult	17	32
42–50†	Thigh	20	42

* Midpoint of arm is defined as half the distance from the acromion to the olecranon. Use nonstretchable metal tape.

† In persons with very large limbs, the indirect blood pressure should be measured in the leg or forearm.

(Reproduced with permission. © "Recommendations for Human Blood Pressure Determination by Sphygmomanometers," 1967, 1980, 1987. Copyright American Heart Association.)

for example, when an average size bladder is used on an obese person. If a bladder is too wide, the reading may be erroneously low because pressure is being directed toward a proportionately large surface area. For example, using an adult cuff on the thin arm of a child may cause this to occur. Recommendations for the selection of an appropriate size cuff are given in Table 23-10.

Cuffs are closed around the limb with contact closures, such as nylon fabric that can be fastened to itself (Velcro) or hooks. Some long cuffs are applied by encircling the arm several times.

Two tubes are attached to the bladder within the cuff. One is connected to a manometer; the other is attached to a bulb used to inflate the bladder. The bladder is inflated to the extent necessary to obstruct the flow of blood through the artery. A needle valve on the bulb allows the operator to deflate the cuff while the pressure is being read.

Manometer A mercury *manometer* has a mercury-filled cylinder or tube calibrated in millimeters. When mercury rises in the tube, the upper or top surface of the mercury is a convex curve. The topmost point on the curved surface is called the *meniscus*. When determining blood pressure on the mercury manometer, the crest of the meniscus within the calibrated cylinder correlates with the pressure. If the meniscus is observed above eye level, the pressure reading appears higher than it really is. If the meniscus is lower than eye level, it appears lower than it really is. The apparent change of position of an object when observed from two different angles is called *parallax*. Figure 23-10 illustrates the meniscus and how pressure readings may be incorrect when the meniscus is above or below eye level.

Another type of manometer is called the *aneroid manometer*. It too has a cuff, but it is attached to a round, calibrated dial with a needle that indicates pressure. Figure 23-11 shows a mercury manometer and an aneroid anometer.

F I G U R E   2 3 - 1 0

A blood pressure reading should be made with the eye at the level of the meniscus as shown in the top drawing. The two drawings at the bottom illustrate how parallax can affect the accuracy of a reading when the line of sight is not level with the meniscus.

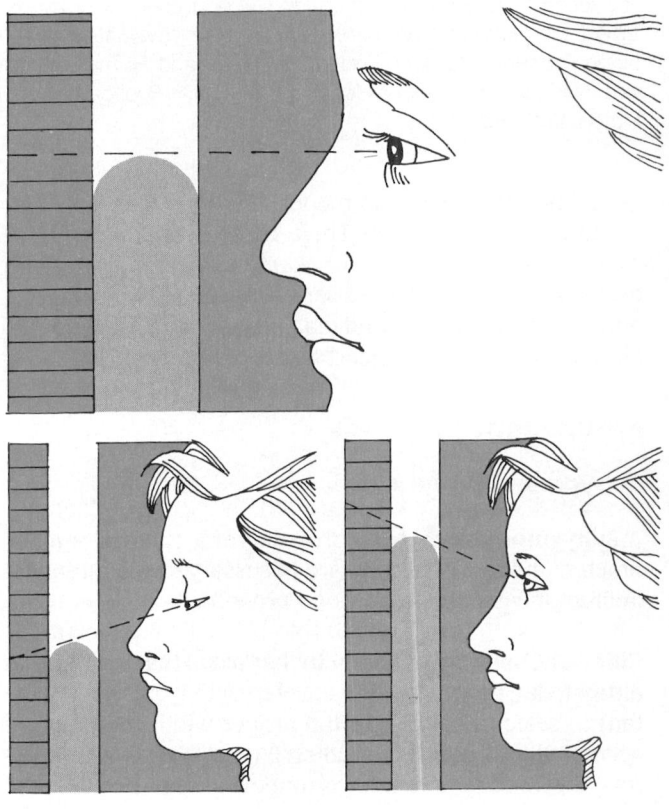

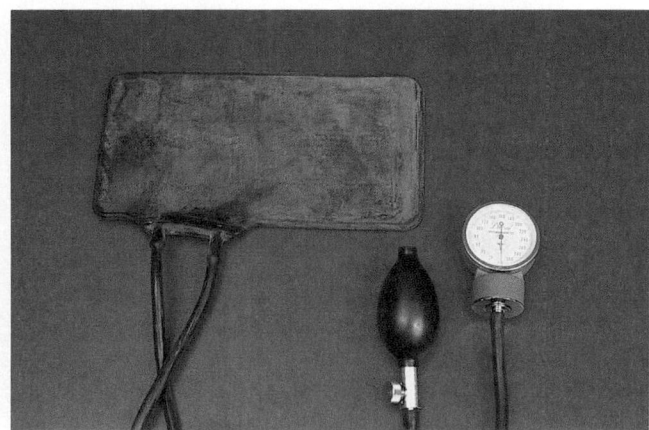

a hollowed, upright, curved appearance. Some acoustical stethoscopes have both.

The diaphragm is more useful for hearing high-frequency sounds because it is constructed to screen out low-frequency sounds. For example, the diaphragm is generally used for listening to respiratory sounds. The bell screens out high-frequency sounds and is more useful for hearing low-frequency sounds, such as those commonly made by the heart and the blood within the vessels. Figure 23-12 illustrates the bell and diaphragm of the acoustical stethoscope.

FIGURE   23-12

(A) Stethoscope. *(B)* Two sides of stethoscope amplifiers. (Photo © Ken Kasper.)

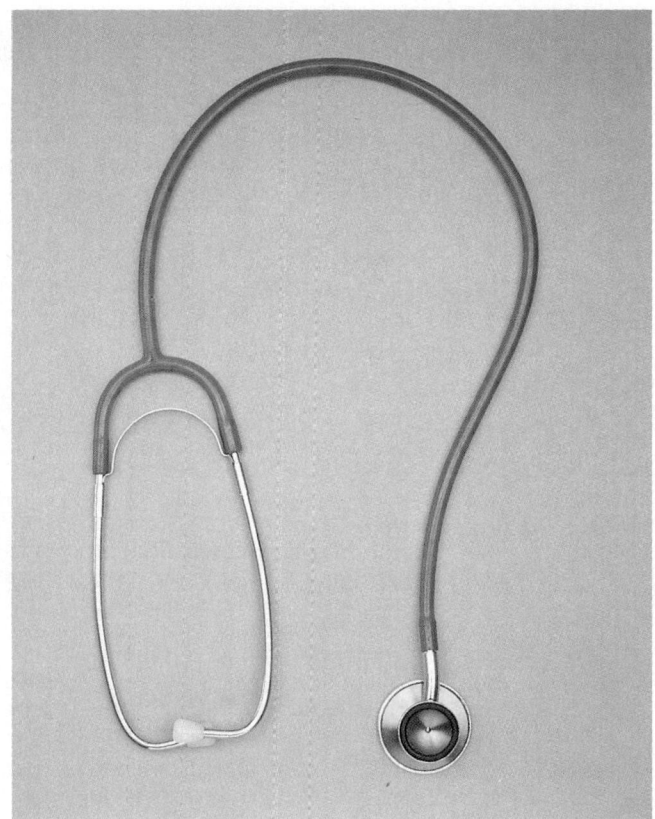

A

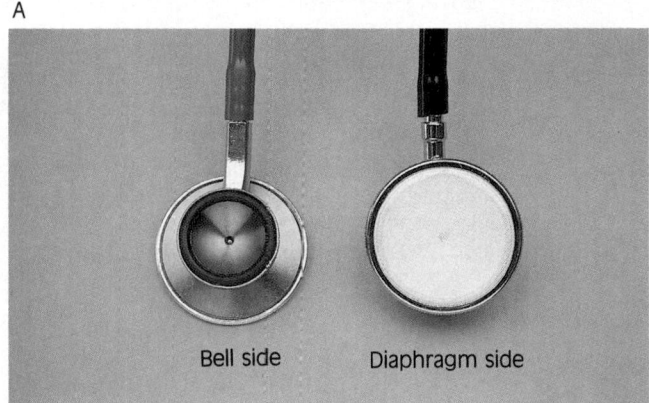

| Bell side | Diaphragm side |

B

FIGURE   23-11

An aneroid manometer (*top*) and a mercury manometer (*bottom*).

Stethoscope

Auscultation means listening for sounds within the body. The stethoscope is used to auscultate the sound heard directly over the artery as the pressure in the cuff is released and the blood is permitted to flow through the artery. The construction of the stethoscope magnifies the sounds in the artery as they are transmitted to the listener. The blood pressure reading is obtained by listening to the sounds and watching the manometer.

The acoustical stethoscope, the most common type used, has an amplifying mechanism connected to ear pieces by tubing. Examples of amplifying devices include a *diaphragm*, which is a large, flat disc, or a *bell*, which has

The ear tips of the stethoscope should be selected to fit the ear canals comfortably and snugly for the most effective auscultation. The tips should be sufficiently large to block out extraneous noises in the environment when the stethoscope is being used. The tips should be adjusted to be directed into the ear canal, not against the ear itself. The selection of an appropriate stethoscope for maximum efficiency during auscultation is an individual matter but should be considered carefully.

Korotkoff Sounds The series of sounds for which the nurse listens when measuring the blood pressure are called **Korotkoff sounds** and are described in Table 23-11. In some adults, each of these sounds is distinct, whereas in others, only the beginning and ending sounds are heard. It is important to determine institutional policy when recording blood pressure sounds, and to be consistent in taking and documenting the readings.

The first sound that is heard, which is the onset of phase I, represents the systolic pressure. It is recorded as the first number in the fraction; for example, if the blood pressure reading is 120/80, 120 is the systolic pressure. The second number (in this case 80) represents the diastolic pressure, which occurs when either a change in or cessation of the loud distinct sounds occurs. This occurs in either phase IV or phase V.

T A B L E 2 3 - 1 1

Korotkoff Sounds		
Phase	**Description**	**Illustration**
Phase I	Characterized by the first appearance of faint but clear tapping sounds that gradually increase in intensity; the first tapping sound is the systolic pressure	
Phase II	Characterized by muffled or swishing sounds; these sounds may temporarily disappear, especially in hypertensive people; the disappearance of the sound during the latter part of phase I and during phase II is called the auscultatory gap and may cover a range of as much as 40 mm Hg; failing to recognize this gap may cause serious errors of underestimating systolic pressure or overestimating diastolic pressure	
Phase III	Characterized by distinct, loud sounds as the blood flows relatively freely through an increasingly open artery	
Phase IV	Characterized by a distinct, abrupt, muffling sound with a soft, blowing quality; in adults, the onset of this phase is considered to be the first diastolic figure	
Phase V	The last sound heard before a period of continuous silence; the pressure at which the last sound is heard is the second diastolic measurement	

The blood pressure is most commonly recorded with two numbers written as a fraction, with the bottom number indicating either the change of the sound or the last sound heard. However, the American Heart Association (1987) recommends that in instances when both a change in the sounds and a cessation of the sounds are heard, all numbers be recorded. In this case, the blood pressure would be recorded as 120/80/64. If the sounds are heard all the way down to zero, the blood pressure recording would be 120/80/0. It is important to determine the procedure for recording blood pressure at each agency or institution so that readings are consistent.

Assessment Sites

Obtaining a Brachial Artery Blood Pressure Procedure 23-8 describes how to obtain the blood pressure with a mercury manometer while using the brachial artery. It is important to be conscientious in continuing to follow the recommended techniques to avoid the common errors identified in Table 23-12.

Obtaining a Popliteal Artery Blood Pressure When the client's brachial artery is inaccessible, the nurse can obtain the blood pressure using the popliteal artery in the leg. It can be expected that the systolic pressure is likely to be 10 to 40 mm Hg higher using this site. A cuff of proportionately larger size should be used. The client should be positioned on the abdomen or with the knee flexed if the client is in a supine position. The technique for assessment is essentially the same as when using the arm.

Alternate Techniques

Palpating the Blood Pressure Assessing the blood pressure through palpation is sometimes referred to as the *sensory detection method*. It requires only the use of the sphygmomanometer. The cuff is inflated 30 mm Hg above the point at which the pulsation in the artery disappears. As the air in the cuff is released, the nurse feels for the return of the pulse. Usually no diastolic pressure is recorded because the artery continues to pulsate as long as blood flows through it. Some home clients assess their blood pressure this way. Instead of palpating the artery, however, the person notes the pressure on the manometer when experiencing the onset and disappearance of the throbbing sensation. The measurements using this method have been fairly similar to other more sophisticated techniques for assessing blood pressure.

Use of the Doppler Ultrasound The blood pressure may also be taken with an ultrasound or Doppler apparatus, which amplifies sounds. This is especially useful if the sounds are indistinct or are inaudible with a regular stethoscope. Usually, the only measurement that can be obtained is the systolic reading. To use the Doppler, the nurse applies transmission gel to the probe, places the probe over the pulse point, and takes the reading.

Electronic Indirect Blood Pressure Meters Electronic blood pressure meters sense vibrations within the artery wall, record the pressure readings, and display them in digital numbers. These devices are helpful for people who wish to obtain their own blood pressure measurements. They are also advantageous for those people who have a hearing impairment because listening for Korotkoff sounds is unnecessary. No stethoscope is required. However, because of their delicate instrumentation, electronic machines should be recalibrated when readings are more than a few points different from the person's normal pattern. Clients using these devices at home should also have their blood pressure checked periodically by health personnel.

Direct Electronic Measurement It is possible to measure blood pressure directly through the insertion of a thin catheter into an artery (an **arterial line**). The tip of the catheter has the ability to sense pressures and transmit the informa-

(Text continues on p. 420)

TABLE 2 3 - 1 2

Blood Pressure Assessment Errors and Contributing Causes			
Error	**Contributing Causes**	**Error**	**Contributing Causes**
Falsely low assessments	• Hearing deficit • Noise in the environment • Viewing the meniscus from above eye level • Applying too wide a cuff • Inserting eartips of stethoscope incorrectly • Using cracked or kinked tubing • Releasing the valve rapidly • Misplacing the bell beyond the direct area of the artery • Failing to pump the cuff 20 to 30 mm Hg above the disappearance of the pulse	Falsely high assessments	• Using a manometer not calibrated at the zero mark • Assessing the blood pressure immediately after exercise • Viewing the meniscus from below eye level • Applying a cuff that is too narrow • Releasing the valve too slowly • Reinflating the bladder during auscultation

PROCEDURE 23-8

Assessing Blood Pressure

Equipment

Stethoscope   Pencil or pen
Sphygmomanometer   Paper or flow sheet
Blood pressure cuff   Alcohol swab
   of appropriate size

Action	Rationale
1 Explain the procedure to the client.	An explanation encourages client cooperation and reduces client apprehension.
2 Gather equipment.	Gathering equipment provides for organized approach to task.
3 Use alcohol swab to cleanse ear pieces and diaphragm of stethoscope, if necessary.	Cleansing stethoscope deters the transmission of microorganisms.
4 Wash your hands.	Handwashing deters the spread of microorganisms.
5 Select a blood pressure cuff of an appropriate size for the client.	A cuff that is too large or too small produces a false reading.
6 Delay obtaining the blood pressure if the client is emotionally upset, is in pain, or has just exercised, unless it is urgent to obtain the blood pressure.	Factors such as emotional upset, exercise, and pain alter usual blood pressure measurements.
7 Select appropriate arm for application of cuff (no intravenous infusion, breast or axilla surgery on that side, cast, arteriovenous shunt, or injured or diseased limb).	Measurement of blood pressure may temporarily impede circulation to a diseased or compromised extremity.
8 Have the client assume a comfortable lying or sitting position with the forearm supported at the level of the heart and the palm of the hand upward.	This position places the brachial artery on the inner aspect of the elbow so that the bell of the stethoscope can rest on it easily.
9 Expose the area of the brachial artery by removing garments, or move a sleeve, if it is not too tight, above the area where the cuff will be placed.	Clothing over the artery interferes with the ability to hear sounds and may cause inaccurate blood pressure readings. Tight clothing on the arm causes congestion of blood and possibly inaccurate readings.
10 Center the bladder of the cuff over the brachial artery, approximately midway on the arm, so that the lower edge of the cuff is about 2.5 to 5 cm (1 to 2 inches) above the inner aspect of the elbow. The tubing should extend from the edge of the cuff nearer the client's elbow.	Pressure in the cuff applied directly to the artery provides the most accurate readings. If the cuff gets in the way of the stethoscope, readings are likely to be inaccurate. A cuff placed upside down with the tubing toward the client's head, may give a false reading.
11 Wrap the cuff around the arm smoothly and snugly, and fasten it securely or tuck the end of the cuff well under the preceding wrapping. Do not allow any clothing to interfere with the proper placement of the cuff.	A smooth cuff and snug wrapping produce equal pressure and help promote an accurate measurement. A cuff too loosely wrapped results in an inaccurate reading.
12 Check that a mercury manometer is in a vertical position. The mercury must be within the zero area with the gauge at eye level. If an aneroid gauge is used, the needle should be within the zero mark.	Tilting a mercury manometer, inaccurate calibration, or improper height for reading the gauge can lead to errors in determining the pressure measurements.
13 Palpate the brachial or radial pulse by pressing gently with the fingertips.	Palpation allows for measurement of the approximate systolic reading.

(continued)

PROCEDURE 2 3 - 8 *(continued)*

Assessing Blood Pressure

Action	Rationale

Action

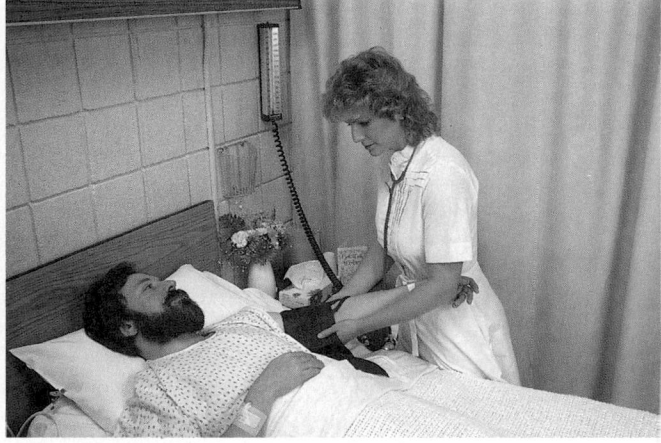

Actions 10 and 11: Centering the cuff over the brachial artery and wrapping smoothly and snugly.

14 Tighten the screw valve on the air pump.

15 Inflate the cuff while continuing to palpate the artery. Note the point on the gauge where the pulse disappears.

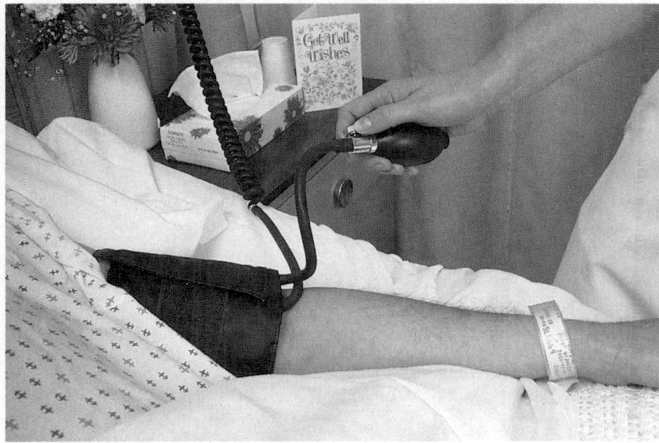

Action 14: Tightening the screw valve on air-pump.

16 Deflate the cuff and wait 15 seconds.

17 Assume a position that is no more than 3 feet away from the gauge.

18 Place the stethoscope earpieces in the ears properly.

Rationale

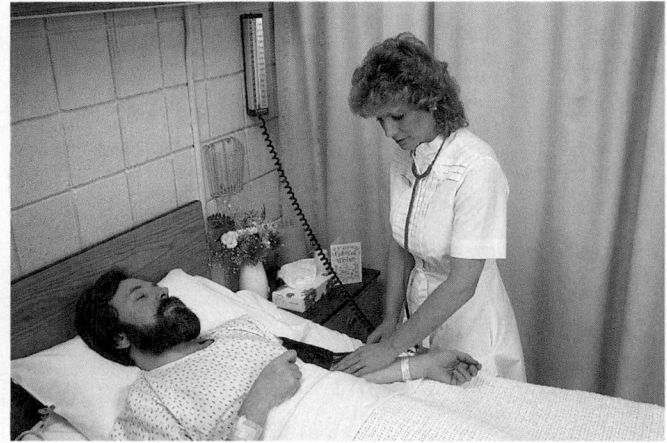

Action 13: Palpating the brachial artery.

The bladder within the cuff will not inflate with the valve open.

To identify the first Korotkoff sound accurately, the cuff must be inflated to a pressure above the point at which the pulse can no longer be felt.

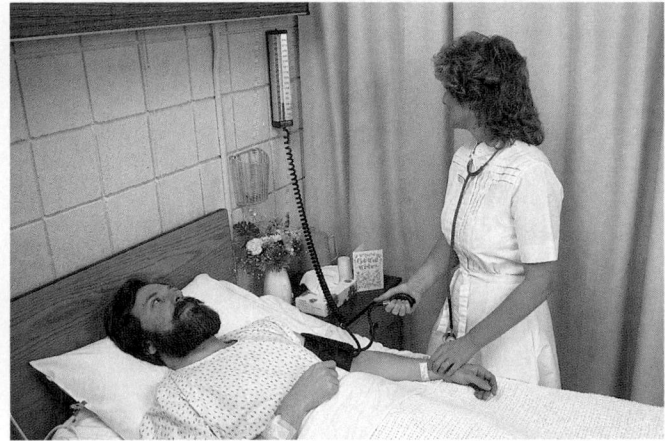

Action 15: Inflating cuff while palpating radial artery.

Allowing a brief pause before continuing permits the blood to refill and circulate through the arm.

A distance of more than about 3 feet can interfere with accurate readings of the numbers on the gauge.

The eartips should be directed downward and forward to fit the shape of the ear canal.

(continued)

P R O C E D U R E   2 3 - 8 *(continued)*

Assessing Blood Pressure

Action	Rationale
19 Place the bell or diaphragm of the stethoscope firmly but with as little pressure as possible over the artery where the pulse is felt. Do not allow the stethoscope to touch clothing or the cuff.	Having the bell or diaphragm directly over the artery makes more accurate readings possible. Heavy pressure on the brachial artery distorts the shape of the artery and the sound. Placing the bell or diaphragm away from clothing and the cuff prevents noise, which will distract from the sounds made by blood flowing through the artery.

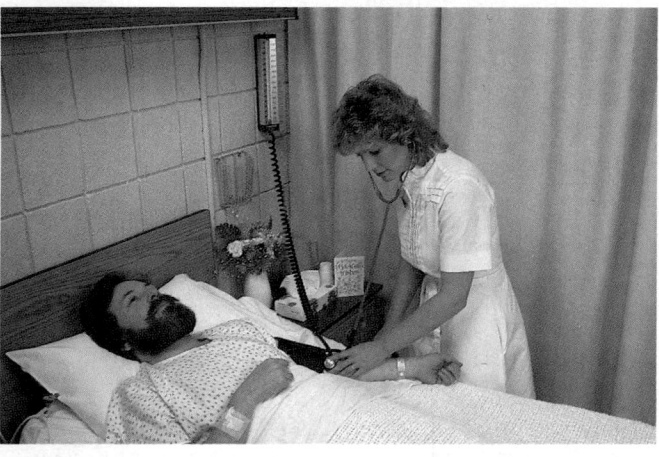

Actions 18 and 19: Placing amplifier of stethoscope over artery, reinflating cuff, and listening for disappearance of sound.

Action	Rationale
20 Pump the pressure 30 mm Hg above the point at which the pulse disappeared. Open the valve on the manometer and allow air to escape slowly (allowing the gauge to drop 2 to 3 mm per heartbeat).	Increasing the pressure above where the pulse disappeared ensures a period before hearing the first sound that corresponds with the systolic pressure. It prevents misinterpreting phase II sounds as phase I.
21 Note the point on the gauge at which there is an appearance of the first faint, but clear, sound that slowly increases in intensity. Note this number as the systolic pressure.	Systolic pressure is the point at which the blood in the artery is first able to force its way through the vessel at a similar pressure exerted by the air bladder in the cuff. The first sound is phase I of Korotkoff sounds.
22 Read the pressure to the closest even number.	It is common practice to read blood pressure to the closest even number.
23 Do not reinflate the cuff once the air is being released to recheck the systolic pressure reading.	Reinflating the cuff while obtaining the blood pressure is uncomfortable for the client and may cause an inaccurate reading. Reinflating the cuff causes congestion of blood in the lower arm, which lessens the loudness of Korotkoff sounds.
24 Note the pressure at which the sound first becomes muffled. Also observe the point at which the sound completely disappears. These may occur separately or at the same point.	The point at which the sound changes corresponds to phase IV of Korotkoff sounds and is considered the first diastolic pressure reading. According to the American Heart Association, this is used as the diastolic pressure recording in children. The last sound heard is the beginning of phase V and is the second diastolic measurement.

(continued)

Assessing Blood Pressure

Action

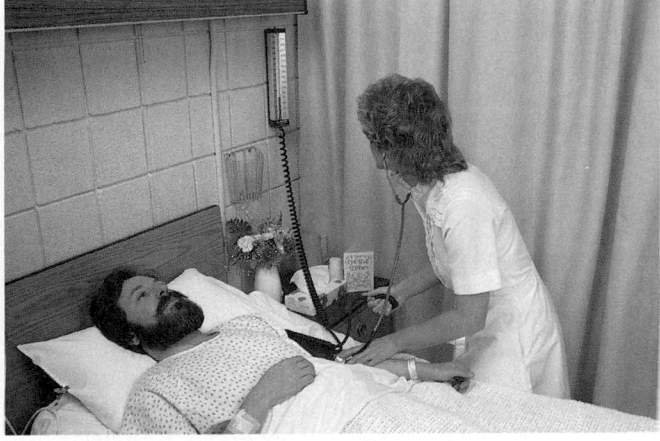

Rationale

Actions 20, 21, and 23: Listening for Korotkoff sounds and noting systolic and diastolic pressure readings. (Photos © Ken Kasper.)

25 Allow the remaining air to escape quickly. Repeat any suspicious readings, but wait 30 to 60 seconds between readings to allow normal circulation to return in the limb. Be sure to deflate the cuff completely between attempts to check the blood pressure.

False readings are likely to occur if there is congestion of blood in the limb while obtaining repeated readings.

26 If it is difficult to hear sounds when checking the blood pressure, raise the client's arm over his or her head for 15 seconds just before rechecking the blood pressure.

Raising the arm over the head helps relieve congestion of blood in the limb, increases pressure differences, and makes the sounds louder and more distinct when blood enters the lower arm.

27 Inflate the cuff while the arm is elevated and then gently lower the arm while continuing to support it.

Supporting the arm while it is lowered prevents altering the pressure in the manometer by as much as 20 to 30 mm Hg.

28 Position the stethoscope and deflate the cuff at the usual rate while listening for Korotkoff sounds.

The techniques used throughout the remaining assessment of blood pressure do not require any further modification.

29 Remove the cuff, clean and store the equipment.

Equipment that must be shared among personnel should be left in a manner ready for use.

30 Wash your hands.

Handwashing deters the spread of microorganisms.

31 Record the client's position, the arm that was used to obtain the blood pressure, and the readings that correspond to the systolic and diastolic readings. Compare to previous readings and report any abnormalities to the appropriate person.

Circumstances for assessing the blood pressure should be consistent for future comparisons.

Special Considerations

Use cuff size appropriate for limb circumference. Inform client that cuff sizes range from a pediatric cuff to a large thigh cuff and that a poorly fitting cuff may result in an inaccurate measurement.

Inform client about availability of digital blood pressure monitoring equipment. Though costly, most provide an easy-to-read recording of systolic and diastolic measurements.

tion to a machine that displays the systolic and diastolic pressure in a waveform. This technique is used exclusively in critical care areas.

Care of Equipment

It is important that equipment used for measuring blood pressure be in good repair and function accurately. Improperly functioning equipment is a major cause of inaccurate measurements. The nurse should check routinely to see that there are no air leaks in the rubber bladder, sphygmomanometer connectors, tubing, or valve. The mercury meniscus and the needle on the aneroid manometer should be checked to see that they are exactly on zero when the cuff is deflated for pressure to be measured accurately. The mercury manometer should be cleaned and checked at least annually to see that the mercury is free of foreign matter and air. The aneroid manometer must be checked for accurate calibration frequently against an accurate mercury manometer. Some authorities recommend weekly calibration for the aneroid manometer, whereas others suggest checking it every 6 months. Any time the accuracy of the equipment is questioned, it should be checked and repaired or replaced, as indicated.

K E Y   P O I N T S

- Assessing vital signs, a traditional nursing responsibility, involves obtaining temperature, pulse, respiration, and blood pressure as part of the baseline data from which a plan of care is developed.
- The frequency of assessing vital signs is governed by the health care agency's policies and the client's health status.
- Humans are warm blooded and maintain body temperature independently of their environment. The hypothalamus in the central nervous system maintains body temperature of the well human within a fairly constant range, called a set point.
- Pyrexia, or fever, an elevation of normal body temperature, is a common symptom of disease. Most fevers are self-limiting. On the other hand, hypothermia is a temperature below the lower limit of normal. Both may be means by which the body fights disease.
- Temperature may be assessed by glass clinical thermometer, electronic thermometer, disposable single-use thermometer, temperature-sensitive patch or tape, or automated monitoring device. Although most agencies measure temperature by the oral route, rectal and axillary routes are alternative sites.
- When the left ventricle of the heart contracts to eject blood into the filled aorta, arterial walls expand or distend; this expansion can be felt as a wave and is called the pulse. Pulse rate is the number of pulsations felt in a minute; pulse rhythm is the pattern of the pulsations and the pauses between them; and pulse amplitude describes the quality of the pulse.
- Arteries most commonly used for assessment are peripheral pulse or those close to the skin surface (ie, temporal, carotid, brachial, radial, femoral, popliteal, posterior tibial, and dorsalis pedis). The radial pulse at the wrist is most commonly used.
- Respiration is the act of breathing and includes the body's use of oxygen and elimination of carbon dioxide. Inspiration or inhalation is the act of breathing in. Expiration or exhalation is the act of breathing out.
- Healthy adults breathe about 16 to 20 times per minute with a fairly consistent relationship of pulse rate to respiratory rate of one respiration to about four heartbeats.
- Apnea refers to periods in which there is no breathing; dyspnea is difficult or labored breathing, demonstrated by rapid and shallow breathing. Dyspneic clients frequently are able to breathe easier in an upright position. Being able to breathe easier in this manner is known as orthopnea.
- Blood pressure refers to the force of blood against arterial walls. The highest pressure, exerted when the left ventricle of the heart pushes blood through the aortic valve into the aorta during systole, is called systolic pressure. When the heart rests (diastole) between beats, the pressure drops and the lowest pressure is called diastolic pressure. Blood pressure, measured in millimeters of mercury (mm Hg), is recorded as a fraction. The numerator is the systolic pressure; the denominator is the diastolic pressure (eg, 120/80).
- Deviations from normal blood pressure are likely due to alterations in any one or more of these functions: peripheral resistance, heart's pumping action, blood volume, blood viscosity, and elasticity of vessel walls.
- Blood pressure can be within a wide range and still be normal. Many factors influence a normal healthy adult's blood pressure.
- Hypertension is a state in which a person's blood pressure is above normal. Primary or essential hypertension has an unknown cause, whereas secondary hypertension is due to known pathologic factors. Blood pressure below normal is called hypotension. Orthostatic or postural hypotension is associated with weakness or fainting when rising to an erect position.
- A sphygmomanometer, consisting of a cuff and manometer, and a stethoscope are necessary for obtaining an indirect measurement of blood pressure. The series of sounds heard in this measurement are called Korotkoff sounds. They are written as fractions (eg, 120/80).
- Another site for assessing blood pressure is the popliteal artery. Blood pressure also can be assessed using palpitation, electronic indirect blood pressure meters, or direct electronic measurements.

STUDY QUESTIONS

1. An elevation of the body temperature above normal is labeled
   a. pyrexia
   b. hypothermia
   c. hypertension
   d. afebrile

2. For which of the following clients would you use an oral thermometer?
   a. a 6-month old infant
   b. a client receiving oxygen therapy
   c. a 42-year-old healthy female
   d. an unconscious client

3. Insertion of a rectal thermometer may cause a potentially harmful condition. This condition is
   a. an increase in heart rate
   b. a decrease in heart rate
   c. an involuntary loss of stool
   d. an increase in respirations

4. While taking an adult client's pulse, the nurse finds the rate to be 140. The nurse would report and document this finding as
   a. hyperthermia
   b. bradycardia
   c. palpitations
   d. tachycardia

5. A client complains of severe abdominal pain. When assessing the vital signs, the nurse would not be surprised to find
   a. an increase in the pulse rate
   b. a decrease in body temperature
   c. a decrease in blood pressure
   d. an increase in body temperature

6. The apical pulse is obtained by using
   a. a sphygmomanometer
   b. an electronic thermometer
   c. a stethoscope
   d. a Doppler apparatus

7. The difference between the apical and radial pulse rates is called the
   a. pulse deficit
   b. pulse amplitude
   c. ventricular rhythm
   d. heart arrhythmia

8. The normal respiratory rate in adults is considered to be
   a. 1 to 6 breaths per minute
   b. 16 to 20 breaths per minute
   c. 60 to 80 breaths per minute
   d. 100 to 120 breaths per minute

9. A client is having dyspnea. To facilitate respirations, the nurse would
   a. remove pillows from under the head
   b. elevate the head of the bed
   c. elevate the foot of the bed
   d. take the blood pressure

10. Blood pressure is the measurement of
    a. the flow of blood through the circulation
    b. the force of blood against arterial walls
    c. the force of blood against venous walls
    d. the flow of blood through the heart

11. With aging, blood pressure is often higher due to
    a. loss of muscle mass
    b. changes in exercise and diet
    c. decreased peripheral resistance
    d. decreased elasticity in arterial walls

12. A client has a blood pressure reading of 130/90 when visiting a clinic. The nurse would recommend
    a. follow-up measurements of blood pressure
    b. immediate treatment by a physician
    c. nothing, because the nurse considers this reading is due to anxiety
    d. a change in diet and exercise

13. In recording a blood pressure of 120/80, the 120 represents
    a. the pulse rate
    b. the diastolic pressure
    c. the systolic pressure
    d. the pulse deficit

14. It is important to have the appropriate cuff size when taking the blood pressure. A cuff that is too large or too small may result in
    a. an incorrect reading
    b. injury to the client
    c. prolonged pressure on the arm
    d. loss of Korotkoff sounds

15. A client has intravenous fluids infusing in the right arm. When taking a blood pressure on this client, the nurse would
    a. take the blood pressure in the right arm
    b. take the blood pressure in the left arm
    c. use the smallest possible cuff
    d. report inability to take the blood pressure

Answers With Rationale

1. The correct response is *a*. Pyrexia is an elevation of body temperature. Hypothermia is low body temperature. Hypertension is elevated blood pressure. Afebrile means that there is not an elevation of body temperature.

2. The correct response is *c*. Use of oral thermometers is contraindicated in infants, client's receiving oxygen therapy, and unconscious clients.

3. The correct response is *b*. Insertion of a rectal thermometer may stimulate the vagus nerve, which, in

turn, would decrease heart rate. This may potentially be harmful for clients with cardiac problems.

4. The correct response is *d*. A pulse rate of 100 to 180 beats per minute in an adult is tachycardia. Hyperthermia is high body temperature. Bradycardia is an adult pulse rate of below 60 beats per minute. The sensation one feels in being aware of the heartbeat is called palpitations.

5. The correct response is *a*. The pulse often increases when an individual is experiencing pain. Pain does not affect body temperature, and may increase (not decrease) blood pressure.

6. The correct response is *c*. The apical pulse can only be obtained by listening with a stethoscope.

7. The correct response is *a*. The difference between the apical and radial pulse rate is called the pulse deficit. The other responses are names given to volume and rhythm of the pulse.

8. The correct response is *b*. The normal respiratory rate for adults is 16 to 20 breaths per minute.

9. The correct response is *b*. Dyspnea is difficult respirations. Elevating the head of the bed allows the abdominal organs to descend, the diaphragm to have greater room for expansion, and facilities lung expansion. Any other intervention would not facilitate respirations.

10. The correct response is *b*. Blood pressure is the measurement of the force of blood against arterial walls. Other responses are incorrect in describing blood pressure.

11. The correct response is *d*. With aging, elasticity in arterial walls is decreased, contributing to an elevated blood pressure reading. The other responses may contribute to changes in readings, but they are not the physiologic base for blood pressure findings in the older adult.

12. The correct response is *a*. A single blood pressure reading that is mildly elevated is not significant, but the measurement should be taken again over time to determine if hypertension is a problem. The nurse would recommend a return visit to the clinic for a recheck.

13. The correct response is *c*—120 is the systolic pressure. The diastolic pressure is 80. The other responses relate to pulse rather than blood pressure.

14. The correct response is *a*. A blood pressure cuff that is not the right size may cause an incorrect reading. It will not cause injury or loss of sounds.

15. The correct response is *b*. The blood pressure should be taken in the arm opposite the one with the infusion. Blood pressure should not be taken in the arm with an intravenous infusion because the pressure of inflating the cuff may allow the artery to clot.

BIBLIOGRAPHY

American Heart Association. (1987). *Recommendations for human blood pressure determination by sphygmomanometers.* (Publication No. 701005). Kansas City, MO: Author.

Barker, E. (1990). Low blood pressure. *Nursing, 20*(11), 34–39.

Birdsall, C. (1985). How do you interpret pulses? *American Journal of Nursing, 85,* 785–786.

Boylan, A., & Brown, P. (1985a). Student observations: More than "doing the obs": The significance of pulse and blood pressure measurement. *Nursing Times, 81*(7), 24–25.

Boylan, A., & Brown, P. (1985b). Student observations: The pulse and blood pressure. *Nursing Times, 81*(7), 26–29.

Boylan, A., & Brown, P. (1985c). Student observations: Respiration. *Nursing Times, 81*(11), 35–38.

Boylan, A., & Brown, P. (1985d). Student observations: Temperature. *Nursing Times, 81*(16), 36–40.

Byra-Cook, C., Dracup, K. A., & Lazik, A. J. (1990). Direct and indirect blood pressure in critical care patients. *Nursing Research, 39*(5), 285–289.

Cashion, A. K., & Cason, C. L. (1984). Accuracy of oral temperatures in intubated patients: Effectiveness of the electronic thermometer. *Dimensions of Critical Care Nursing, 3*(6), 343–350.

Davis, C., & Lentz, M. J. (1989). Circadian rhythms: Charting oral temperatures to spot abnormalities. *Journal of Gerontological Nursing, 15*(4), 34–39.

Heidenreich, T., & Gieffre, M. (1990). Postoperative temperature measurement. *Nursing Research, 39*(3), 153–155.

Hohn, W. K., Brooks, J. A., & Hite, R. (1989). Blood pressure norms for healthy young adults: Relation to sex, age, and reported parental hypertension. *Research in Nursing and Health, 12,* 53–56.

Kennedy, W. C., Jr. (1990). Vital signs: Reading the essentials. *Journal of Emergency Medical Services. 15,* 26–30, 34, 36–39.

King, K. K., & Davis, B. K. (1986). Measuring blood pressure via sensory detection. *Journal of Gerontological Nursing, 12*(11), 8–11.

McCaffrey, M., & Ferrell, B. R. (1992). How vital are vital signs? *Nursing, 22*(1), 42–46.

Nations, L. E. (1986). Relationship of routine assessment of temperature and febrile illness. *Rehabilitation Nursing, 11,* 18–20.

Ontario Heart Fund Foundation. *Proposed guidelines for hypertension screening.* (1983). Ontario: Author.

Rudy, S. F. (1986). Take a reading on your blood pressure techniques. *Nursing, 16*(8), 46–49.

Samples, J. F., VanCott, M. L., & Long, C. (1985). Circadian rhythms: Basis for screening for fever: Routine temperature assessments in hospitals. *Nursing Research, 34*, 377–379.

Stone, S. (1986). A new concept in routine vital signs measurement. *Nursing Management, 17*(2), 28–29.

U.S. Department of Health and Human Services, Public Health Service, National Institutes of Health. (1988). *The 1988 report of the joint national committee on detection, evaluation, and treatment of high blood pressure* (NIH Publication No. 88–1088). Washington, D.C.: Author.

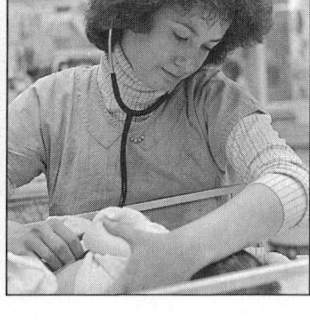
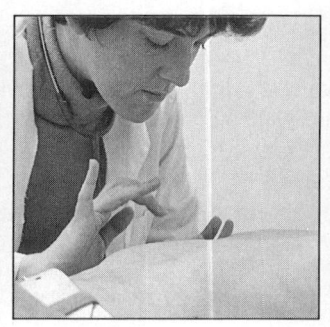

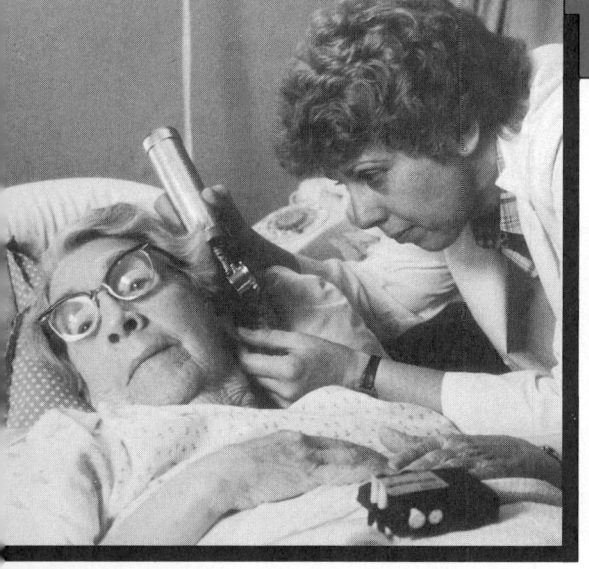

Nursing Assessment

OBJECTIVES

After studying this chapter, the learner should be able to:

Define key terms used in the chapter.

Identify the purposes of the nursing assessment.

Describe the techniques used during a nursing examination.

Discuss the importance of client preparation for a nursing assessment.

Identify equipment used in performing a nursing assessment.

Describe positioning used for each body system examination.

Conduct a nursing assessment of each body system in a systematic manner, identifying normal and abnormal findings.

Document significant findings in a concise, descriptive manner.

KEY TERMS

adventitious breath sounds
auscultation
bruits
bronchial sounds
bronchovesicular sounds
crackles
cyanosis
ecchymosis
edema
flushing
inspection
jaundice
nasal speculum
ophthalmoscope
otoscope
pallor
palpation
petechial
pleural friction rub
precordium
rales
rhonchi
thrills
tremor
tuning fork
turgor
vaginal speculum
vesicular breathing sounds
wheeze

24

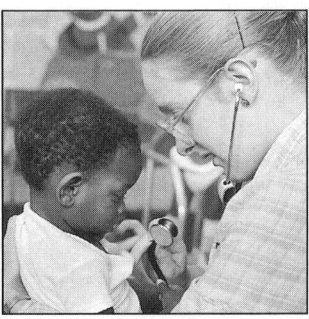

Nursing assessment is an integral component of holistic nursing care and is the basis of the nursing process. Client assessments are used to initiate and maintain care plans to promote an optimal level of wellness through interventions focused on prevention of illness, restoration of health, and facilitation of coping with disabilities or death.

The two components of nursing assessment are (1) a health history and (2) a physical assessment. The nurse uses communication skills and interviewing techniques during the health history to gather data to determine the client's health status. The physical assessment is a head-to-toe, system-by-system physical examination of the client by the nurse. Both subjective and objective data are collected during the health history and the physical assessment. The purposes of the nursing assessment are as follows:

- Establish a nurse–client relationship
- Gather data about the client's general health status, integrating physiologic, psychological, cognitive, sociocultural, developmental, and spiritual dimensions
- Identify client strengths
- Identify actual and potential health problems
- Establish a base for the nursing process

Health History

A **health history** is a collection of subjective and objective data that provides a detailed profile of the client's health status. A nurse collects the information through an interview with the client. The components of the health history and specific interviewing skills are found in Chapters 15 and 20. A sample health history is included at the end of this chapter to illustrate documentation of data.

Physical Assessment

The physical examination is done by using a head-to-toe sequence, but this can be adapted to meet the needs of the client being examined. This section discusses commonly used positions and techniques for the healthy adult. In the clinical setting, it is often necessary to modify the se-

quence, positions, and specific assessments to the client's energy level and physical state and to time constraints. Even when modified, the physical assessment should be conducted in an organized and knowledgeable manner.

General Guidelines

This section discusses the general guidelines for the physical assessment, including instrumentation, positioning, draping, preparation of the environment, client preparation, and techniques of physical examination.

Instrumentation

The instruments (or equipment) used during a physical assessment should be readily accessible, clean or sterile, in proper working order, and organized in the sequence of use (Fig. 24-1). Any equipment that will touch the client should be warmed (either with the examiner's hands or with warm water) before use. Although all of the instruments described may not be needed in an assessment, they are commonly used in the examination of clients. Additional equipment and supplies are listed in the accompanying display.

Ophthalmoscope An **ophthalmoscope** is a lighted instrument used for visualization of the interior structures of the eye. It consists of two parts—a body, containing the light source, and a detachable head, containing the magnifying lens used to bring the internal eye structures into focus. The magnification of the lens can be adjusted using a rotating dial. The head is placed into the body and secured. The round black dial located on the head, when depressed and

---

Instruments, Equipment, and Supplies Needed for a Physical Examination

Instrumentation	Equipment and Supplies
Blood pressure cuff	Alcohol swabs
Stethoscope	Cotton applicators
Ophthalmoscope	Disposable pad
Snellen's chart	Drape
Otoscope	Gauze dressing (4 × 4)
Nasal speculum	Gloves (sterile and non-
Scale	sterile)
Vaginal speculum	Lubricant
Tuning fork	Penlight
Percussion hammer	Safety pin
Neurologic hammer	Smells (1 or 2 vials for
	testing sense of smell)
	Tape measure
	Thermometer
	Tongue depressor

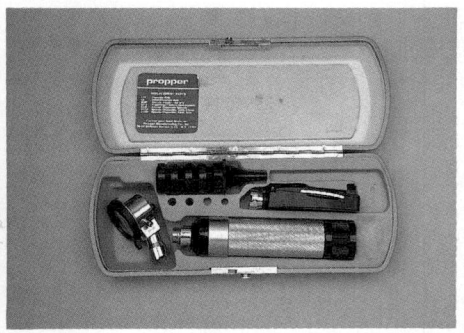

Ophthalmoscope
and otoscope set

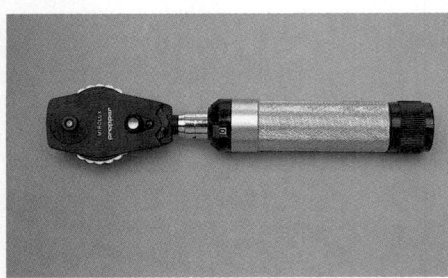

Ophthalmoscope

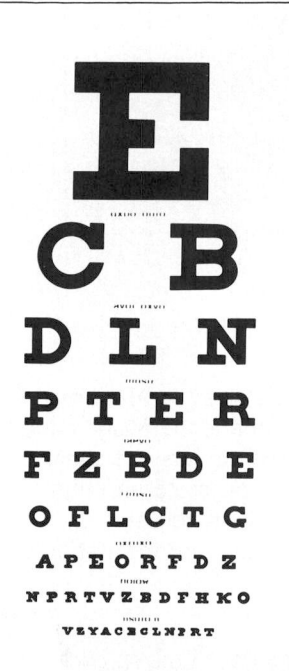

Snellen chart

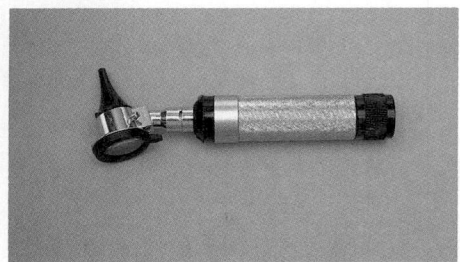

Otoscope

Nasal speculum

Neurologic hammer

Percussion hammer

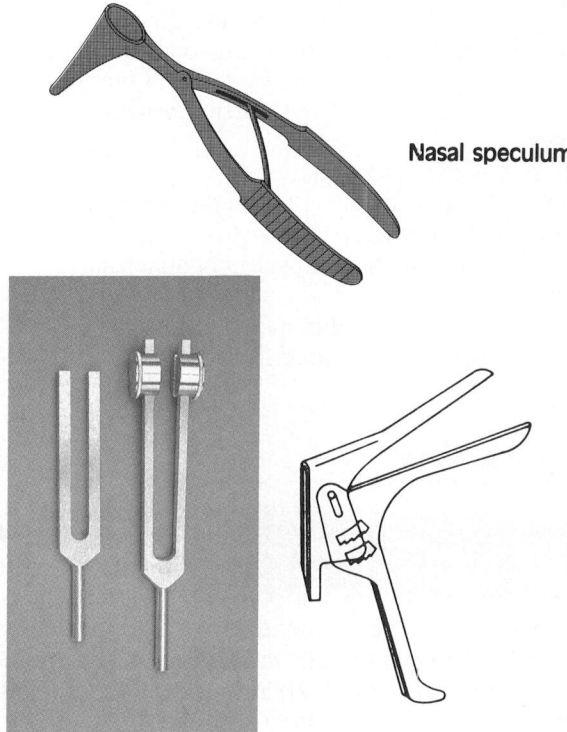

Tuning forks

Vaginal speculum

F I G U R E   2 4 - 1

Instruments used in the physical examination. (Photos © Ken Kasper.)

turned, provides illumination. At the beginning of the examination, the lens should be positioned at 0 diopters (the 0 magnification power of the lens). The numbers on the rotating dial range from −20 to +40, corresponding to the magnification power of the lens, with the negative numbers in red and the positive numbers in black. The system of negative and positive numbers compensates for near-sightedness and farsightedness and allows the examiner to visualize structures more distinctly.

Otoscope The **otoscope** is a lighted instrument used for examining the external ear canal and the tympanic membrane. The ophthalmoscope and otoscope heads are interchangeable on the same body. An attached speculum directs the light in a narrow beam to improve visualization of structures. The specula come in various sizes; the largest speculum that will extend into the client's ear canal is used.

Snellen's Chart Snellen's chart, which is used as a screening test for vision, consists of 11 lines of different size characters arranged with the line of largest characters at the top of the chart and the line of the smallest characters at the bottom. Scores ranging from 20/10 (the smallest line of characters) to 20/200 (the largest line of characters) are in the left-hand column and distances are in the right-hand column next to the numbers.

Nasal Speculum The **nasal speculum** is an instrument that allows visualization of the lower and middle turbinates of the nose. A penlight or flashlight is needed for illumination. The blades of the speculum are inserted about a ½ inch (1 cm) into the nares and opened so that they do not press on the septum. An alternative instrument that can be used to visualize the internal nares is the otoscope. The light is provided by the scope, and the shortest, widest speculum that will fit into the client's nares is used.

Vaginal Speculum A **vaginal speculum** is a two-bladed instrument used to examine the vaginal canal and cervix. The speculum is inserted into the vagina, and the speculum blades are opened, allowing visualization and examination of the vagina and cervix. Warming and lubrication of the speculum (either with warm water or with a water-soluble agent) are essential before insertion.

Tuning Fork A **tuning fork** is a two-pronged metal instrument used for testing auditory function and vibratory perception. The fork is activated by gently tapping the prongs of the tuning fork against the palm of the hand. Once activated, the fork is held at the base to avoid diminishing the sound or vibration produced by the prongs.

Percussion Hammer The *percussion hammer*, also called the *reflex hammer*, is an instrument with a rubber head used to test reflexes and determine tissue density. The hammer is held between the thumb and index finger to direct a brisk tap on the selected body area. A rapid downward and backward wrist action allows a quick and firm tap

to be made. The pointed end of the hammer is used for smaller areas.

Neurologic Hammer The *neurologic hammer* is similar to the percussion hammer. It is used to test reflexes during the neurologic assessment and features two additional pieces that unscrew from the base of the instrument—a soft brush and a sharp needle, both used for sensory discrimination.

Positioning

A variety of positions are used during a physical assessment (Fig. 24-2). It is important to consider the client's energy level and privacy; clients who are weak may require assistance with positioning, and uncomfortable or embarrassing positions should not be maintained for long periods. The examination should be organized so that several body systems can be assessed with the client in one position, thus minimizing unneeded and possibly tiring movements.

Sitting Position The client may sit upright in a chair, on the side of an examining table or bed, or, if physically unable to maintain an upright position, may lie supine in the bed with the head elevated. This position allows visualization of the upper body and facilitates full lung expansion. It is used to assess the head and neck, posterior and anterior thorax and lungs, breasts, heart, and upper extremities, and to take vital signs.

Supine Position In the *supine position*, the client lies flat on the back with legs together but extended and slightly flexed at the knees. The head may be supported with a small pillow. This position allows relaxation of abdominal muscles and can be used to assess the head and neck, anterior thorax and lungs, breasts, heart, abdomen, extremities, and peripheral pulses.

Dorsal Recumbent Position In the *dorsal recumbent position*, the client lies on the back with legs separated, knees bent, and soles of the feet flat on the bed. This position may be used for clients who have difficulty maintaining the supine position but should not be used for abdominal assessment because it causes abdominal muscles to contract. Areas that can be assessed in this position are the head and neck, anterior thorax and lungs, breasts, heart, extremities, and peripheral pulse.

Sims' Position In the *Sims' position*, the client lies on either the right or left side. The lower arm is behind the body and the upper arm is flexed at the shoulder and elbow. The knees are both flexed, with the uppermost leg more acutely flexed. The Sims' position is used to assess the rectum or vagina.

Prone Position In the *prone position*, the client lies on the abdomen, flat on the bed, with the head turned to one side. This position is difficult to assume for many clients. It is

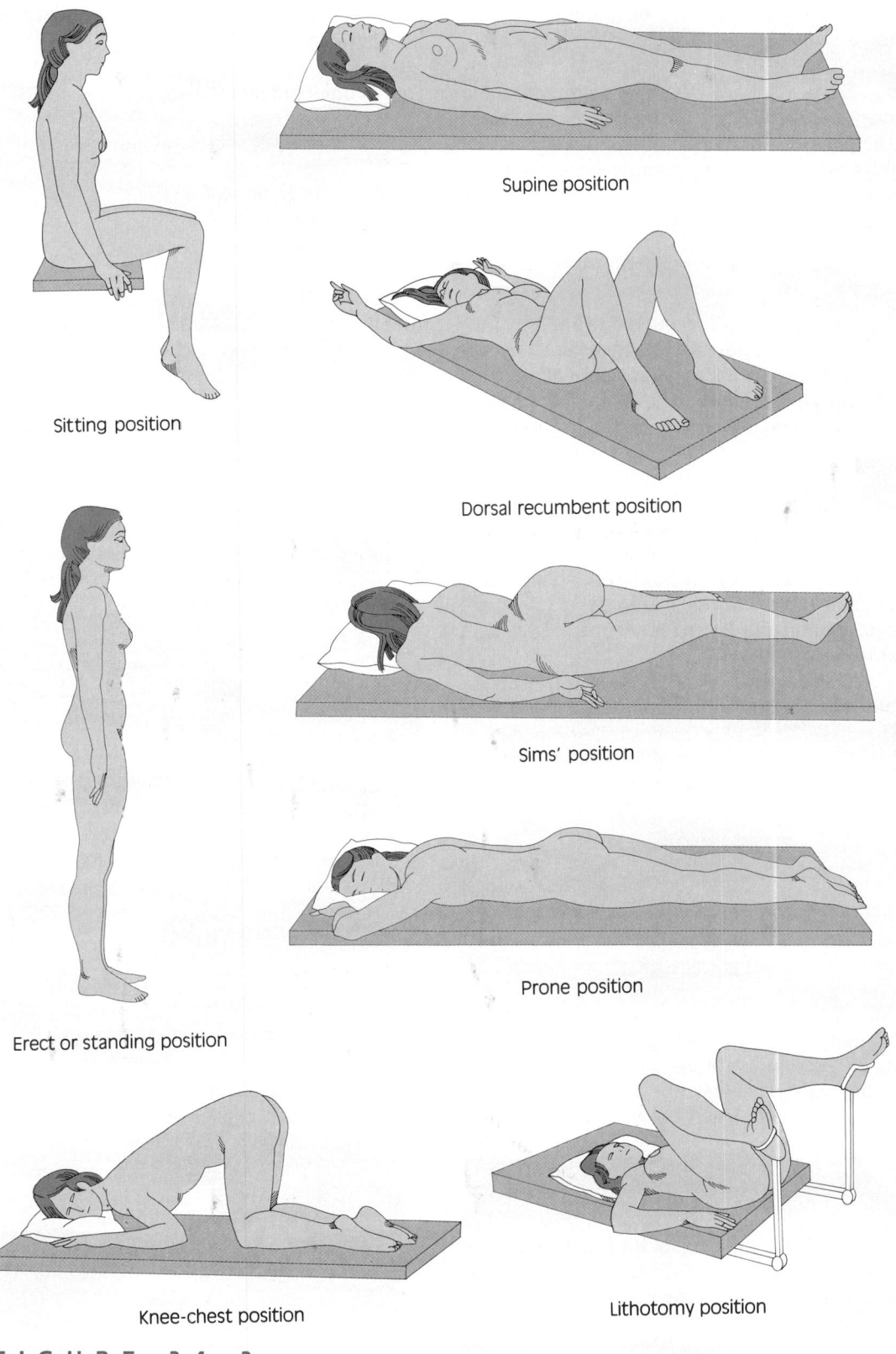

Sitting position

Supine position

Dorsal recumbent position

Sims' position

Prone position

Erect or standing position

Knee-chest position

Lithotomy position

FIGURE 24-2

Various client positions used during the nursing examination.

used to assess the hip joint and can be used to assess the posterior thorax.

Lithotomy Position In the *lithotomy position*, the client is in the dorsal recumbent position with the buttocks at the edge of the examining table and the feet supported in stirrups. This position is used for examination of the rectum and female genitalia. It is uncomfortable for older clients and is often embarrassing, so time spent in this position should be minimized.

Knee–Chest Position In the *knee–chest position*, the client kneels, using the knees and chest to bear the weight of the body. The body is at a 90-degree angle to the hips, with the back straight, the arms above the head, and the head turned to one side. The position is used for examination of the rectal area. The same precautions should be used as with the lithotomy position.

Erect Position The *standing*, or *erect, position* is also used in the nursing examination to assess posture, gait, and balance.

Draping

Draping during the physical assessment is primarily used to prevent unnecessary exposure, to provide privacy, and to keep the client warm. Drapes may be paper, cloth, or bed linens (eg, sheets and bath blankets). As the examination is conducted, only those body parts being assessed are exposed.

Preparing the Environment

An important consideration when conducting a physical assessment is preparation of the environment. The time for the assessment should be mutually agreed on by both the nurse and the client if at all possible and should not interfere with meals, treatments, or visiting hours. The client should be as pain free as possible.

Some agencies have a special examination room that provides a quiet, private space for assessment. If such a room is available, the nurse prepares the examination table, provides a gown and drape for the client, and gathers instruments and special supplies needed for the examination. If the area is accessible to others, an enclosure with a curtain or screen is essential.

Preparing the Client

Both physiologic and psychological needs of the client should be considered before and during the physical assessment (Fig. 24-3). The client is told that a physical assessment will be done by the nurse, that body structures will be examined, and that the assessments are painless. The client is asked to change into a gown and directed to a private dressing area. If necessary, the nurse assists the client with undressing. Once the client has donned the

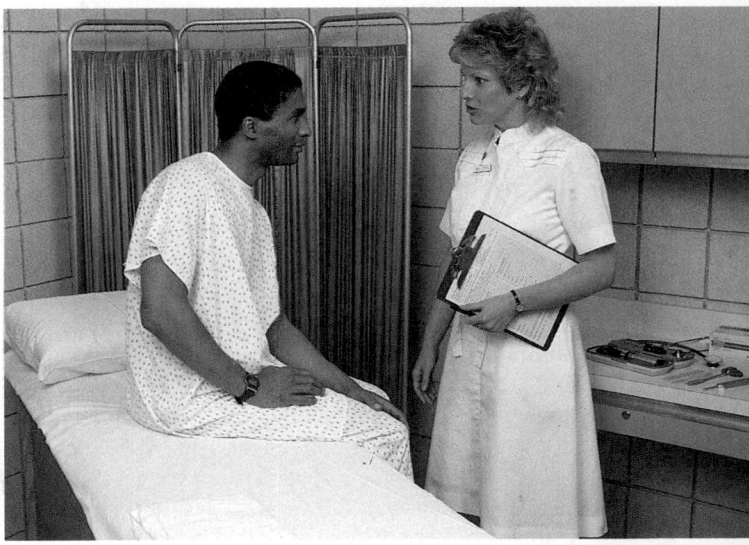

FIGURE 24-3

The physiologic and psychological needs of the client must be considered in preparation for the examination. Care is taken to provide for comfort, warmth, and privacy. A brief explanation of the examination before beginning and just before each stage alleviates client fear and anxiety and improves cooperation. (Photo © Ken Kasper.)

gown, he or she is asked to empty the bladder; this increases comfort during the examination and facilitates assessment of the abdomen. Even though the assessments are painless, the client may be anxious for various reasons. The nurse can help decrease the client's embarrassment, fear of possible abnormal physical findings, or fear of "failing" a test by explaining in general terms how and why the examination will be done and then explaining each assessment in greater detail as it is being done. The nurse should answer the client's questions directly and honestly.

Techniques

The four primary assessment techniques are (1) inspection, (2) palpation, (3) percussion, and (4) auscultation. These techniques are used to conduct a nursing examination of various body systems.

Inspection Inspection is the process of deliberate, purposeful observations performed in a systematic manner. Observations are made by using visual, auditory, and olfactory senses as tools for gathering data throughout the examination. Inspection begins at the time of initial contact with the client and continues throughout the entire examination. Adequate lighting, either natural or artificial, is essential for distinguishing color, texture, and moisture of body surfaces. A quiet environment eliminates extraneous noises and allows sounds to be heard without interference.

The nurse inspects each area of the body for size, color, shape, position, and symmetry, making observations of normal findings and any deviations from normal. A comparison of bilateral body parts during inspection is necessary for recognizing abnormal findings. Inspection may be combined with the palpation phase of the examination.

Palpation Palpation is a technique that uses the sense of touch. The hands and fingers are sensitive tools and are used to gather information about temperature, turgor, texture, moisture, vibrations, and shape. The dorsum, or back, of the hand and fingers is used for gross measure of temperature. When a discriminatory sense is needed for differentiating between texture, shape, fluid, size, consistency, and pulsation, the palmar surface of the fingers and finger pads is used. The sense of vibration is palpated best with the palm of the hand (Fig. 24-4).

General guidelines to follow during palpation include the following:

- The client should be provided with a warm, comfortable, and relaxed environment.
- The nurse's hands should be warm and fingernails short.
- Any area of tenderness is palpated last.

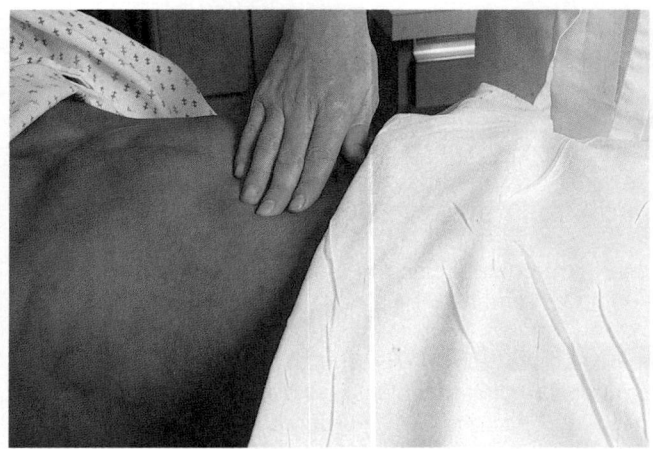

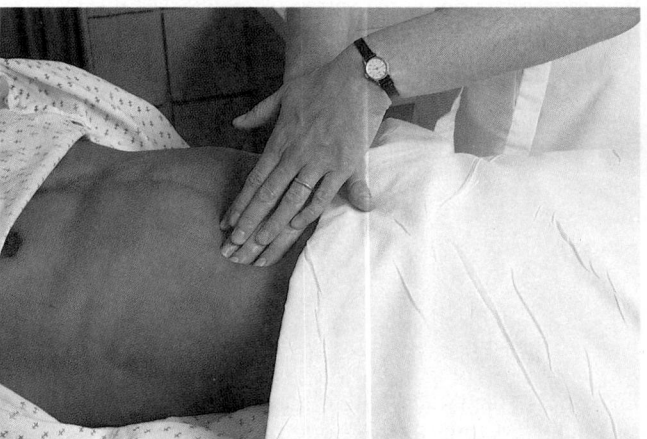

FIGURE 24-5

(*Top*) In light palpation, light pressure is applied by placing the fingers together and depressing the skin and underlying structures approximately ¹/₂ inch (1 cm). (*Bottom*) Deep palpation is used with caution. The skin and underlying structures are depressed approximately 1 inch (2 cm). (Photos © Ken Kasper.)

FIGURE 24-4

(*Top*) Palmar surfaces of the examiner's fingertips and finger pads are used for discriminatory sensation, such as texture, presence of fluid, or size and consistency of a mass. (*Bottom*) The dorsum, or back of hand, is used to assess surface temperature.

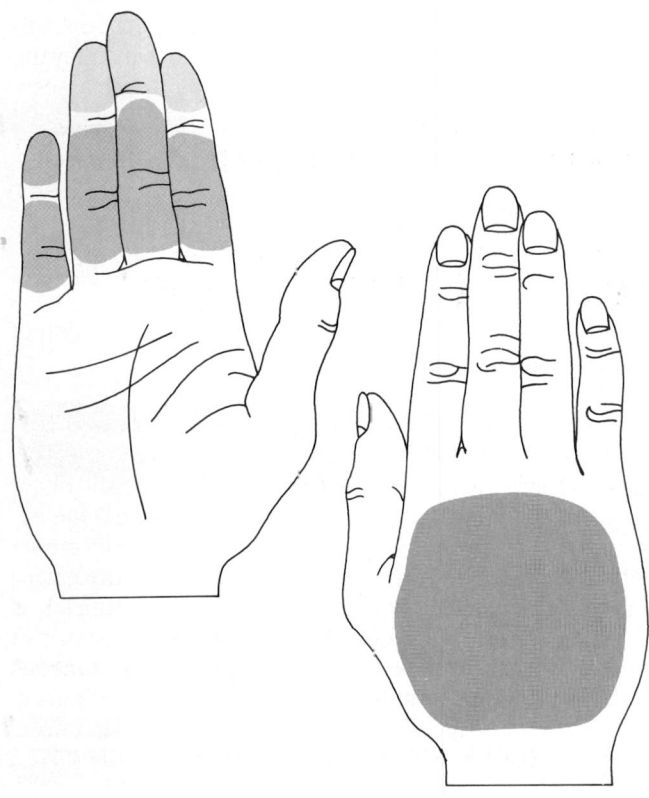

Light or deep palpation may be used and is controlled by the amount of pressure applied. For light palpation, apply light pressure by placing the fingers together and depressing the skin and underlying structures about ¹/₂ inch (1 cm; Fig. 24-5, *top*). For deep palpation, press inward about 1 inch (2 cm; see Fig. 24-5, *bottom*). Deep palpation, with the risk of possible internal injury, should be used with caution. Applying intermittent pressure to a specific area allows assessment of surface characteristics and underlying structures. Characteristics of masses, as determined by palpation, are described in Table 24-1.

Percussion Percussion is the act of striking one object against another for the purpose of producing sound. The sound waves produced by the striking action are known as **percussion tones** and are generated by body tissue. Per-

TABLE 24-1

Characteristics of Masses Determined by Palpation

Quality	Characteristics to Determine
Shape	Round Ovoid Tubular Irregular
Size	Measured in centimeters
Consistency	Firm Edematous Spongy Cystic
Surface	Smooth Nodular Granular
Mobility	Fixed or nonmobile Mobile
Tenderness	Amount of tenderness to touch
Pulsatile	Pulsation can or cannot be felt in the mass

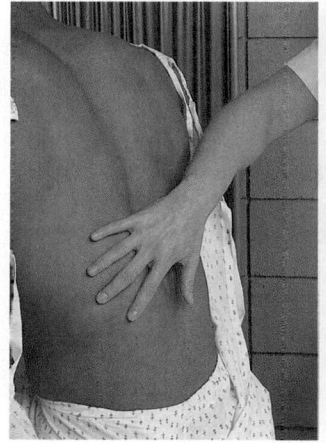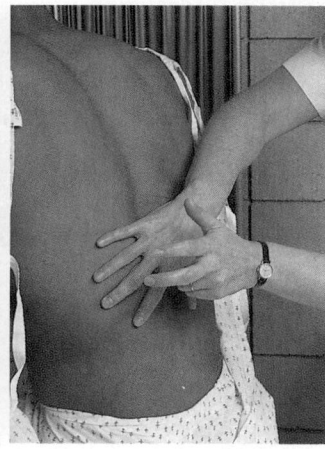

FIGURE 24-6

Percussion is used to assess the location, shape, size, and density of tissues. (Left) The nondominant hand is placed directly on the area to be percussed, and the middle finger placed firmly on the body surface. (Right) The tip of the middle finger of the dominant hand strikes the joint of the middle finger of the opposite hand. (Photos © Ken Kasper.)

cussion is used to assess the location, shape, size, and density of tissues.

The nurse uses both hands as the tools for producing sound waves. The nondominant hand is placed directly on the area to be percussed, with the fingers slightly separated and the middle finger placed firmly on the body surface (Fig. 24-6, *left*). The opposite hand (or dominant hand) is the striking force, which is initiated by sharp downward wrist movement with the forearm stationary and the wrist relaxed. The tip of the middle finger of the dominant hand strikes the joint of the middle finger of the opposing hand (see Fig. 24-6, *right*). This action produces a vibration that allows the nurse to discriminate among five different tones. The five percussion tones are as follows:

Tympany—loud drumlike sound that is illustrated by the sound produced by percussing a puffed-out cheek; heard when percussing the stomach, an air-filled organ

Resonance—moderate to loud, lower-pitched, hollow sound percussed over lung tissue

Hyperresonance—very loud, low-pitched sound with a booming quality; most often percussed over the emphysematous lung

Dullness—soft to moderate, high-pitched sound with a thud-like quality; percussed over the liver

Flatness—soft, high-pitched sound that is flat; usually percussed over muscle tissue

Table 24-2 summarizes percussion tones and their characteristics.

Auscultation   Auscultation is the act of listening to sound produced within the body using a stethoscope. Chapter 23 discusses types of stethoscopes, their uses, and specific characteristics.

Auscultation is performed by firmly placing the stethoscope against the body part being assessed. The diaphragm

TABLE 24-2

Percussion Tones and Their Characteristics

Tone	Relative Intensity	Relative Pitch	Relative Duration	Sample Location
Flatness	Soft	High	Short	Thigh
Dullness	Medium	Medium	Medium	Liver
Resonance	Loud	Low	Long	Normal lung
Hyperresonance	Very loud	Lower	Longer	Emphysematous lung
Tympany	Loud	*	*	Gastric air bubble or puffed-out cheek

*Distinguished mainly by its musical timbre.

(Bates, B. [1991]. A guide to physical examination and history taking (5th ed.). Philadelphia: Lippincott, p. 247.)

of the stethoscope is used to detect high-pitched sounds, such as normal lung and bowel sounds. The bell of the stethoscope is used to detect low-pitched sounds, such as those produced by the heart and vascular system.

Four characteristics of sound should be assessed by auscultation. They are (1) *pitch* (ranging from high to low); (2) *loudness* (ranging from soft to loud); (3) *quality* (eg, gurgling or swishing); and (4) *duration* (described as short, medium, or long).

General Survey

Components of the general survey, including self-image and self-concept, are assessed during the health history. Other data assessed in the general survey are the client's general appearance, vital signs, height, and weight.

General Appearance

Assessment of general appearance includes the following:
- Gender and race
- Body build, posture, and gait (note proportion of height to weight, erect or slumped posture, coordination of movements, pattern of gait)
- Hygiene, grooming (note cleanliness, body odors, appropriate dress for age and environment)
- Signs of illness (note posture, skin color, respirations, nonverbal communications of pain or distress)
- Affect, attitude, mood (note speech, facial expressions, ability to relax, eye contact, behavior)
- Cognitive processes (note speech content and patterns, orientation, appropriate verbal responses)

Vital Signs

Vital signs are measured to establish a data base and to detect actual or potential health problems. Vital signs are discussed in Chapter 23.

Height and Weight

In adult clients, the correlation (or ratio) of height and weight is an assessment of overall health and nutrition. An indication of body image can be assessed by asking the client his or her height and weight before actually doing the measurements. A large difference in perceived and actual measurements may indicate a potential problem in body image and self-concept. Both height and weight should be measured using accurate scales and measuring devices, and the client should remove shoes and heavy clothing if the measurements are taken before undressing. If the client is unable to stand erect, weight can be obtained by using a chair or bed scales. The client's actual height and weight can be compared to recommended average weights on a standardized chart as a general guideline for assessing nutritional status and health (see Chapter 33).

Assessment of Body Systems

This section discusses the assessment of each body system. Accompanying each system is a brief review of normal anatomy and physiology, factors for consideration during assessment, positions, assessment techniques, and common normal and abnormal findings. A completed assessment is included at the end of the chapter to illustrate documentation.

Integument

Skin

The skin is the external covering of the body and consists of three layers—the *epidermis*, or outer layer; the *dermis*, or middle layer; and *subcutaneous tissue*, or the innermost layer. The epidermis protects the body against environmental substances and helps regulate body temperature. The dermis, comprising vascular connective tissue and sensory nerve fibers, supports and separates the epidermis from adipose tissue and provides the sensations of pain, touch, and temperature. The subcutaneous layer of skin comprises sweat glands, fat, hair follicles, and blood vessels.

The skin is a general indicator of a client's health status and provides information that may be significant of an underlying pathology. When assessing the skin, it is helpful to know if the client has been exposed to harmful environmental materials or increased sun exposure, has had recent changes in skin condition, or is currently taking medications.

The skin is assessed by inspection and palpation. The examination begins with an overall assessment of the skin condition; specific areas of the skin can be assessed while performing other body system assessments. Adequate lighting is essential for accurate assessments.

Inspection   The skin is inspected through assessment of color, vascularity, and lesions. Body odors are also included in inspection (Fig. 24-7).

Color   The skin color varies among races and among individuals. Normally, skin color ranges from a pinkish white to various shades of brown, depending on the person's race. The skin areas that are normally exposed, such as the face and hands, may have a somewhat different color than areas that are usually covered by clothing, but generally the color is relatively constant. Special care must be taken to detect color changes in dark-skinned people, such as African Americans, Hispanics, native Americans, people of Mediterranean descent, and whites who are deeply suntanned. Some body areas of dark-skinned people, such as the palms of the hands and the soles of the feet, normally have less pigmentation than other areas of the body. Various terms used to describe abnormal appearance of the skin are summarized in Table 24-3.

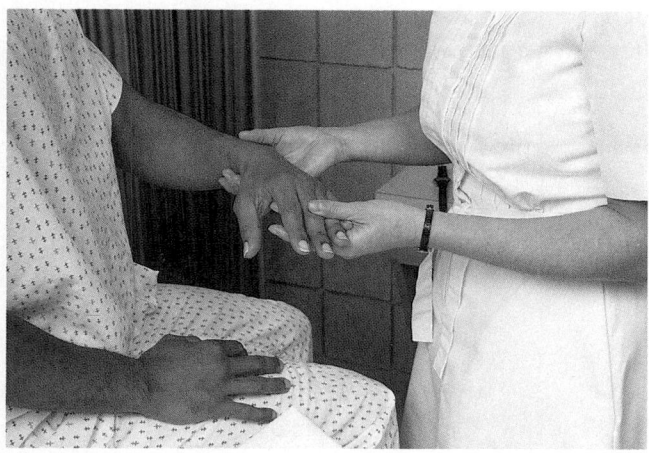

FIGURE 24-7

The skin is inspected for color, vascularity, and lesions.

Flushing is redness of the skin, as in sunburn. It is often associated with an elevated body temperature, and the face and the neck are more likely to be affected than other parts of the body. **Cyanosis** is a dusky bluish color of the skin, and, in dark-skinned people, can usually be detected more readily in the conjunctiva, lips, and inside the mouth. **Jaundice** is a yellow color of the skin. In adults, it is usually initially seen in the sclera of the eyes and then in the skin and mucous membranes. Jaundice in dark-skinned people is more difficult to observe because the sclera often has a normal yellowish color. **Pallor** is paleness of the skin, often resulting from an inadequate amount of circulating blood or hemoglobin, both of which cause inadequate oxygenation of the body tissues. Depending on severity, pallor may be visible over the entire skin surface; locally it is seen in the lips, nailbeds, mucous membranes, and conjunctiva. Pallor may be more difficult to assess in dark-skinned people.

Vascularity The skin is also inspected for vascularity, bleeding, or bruising, because these signs may be related to cardiovascular or liver dysfunctions. **Ecchymosis** is a collection of blood in the subcutaneous tissues, causing purplish discoloration. **Petechiae** are small hemorrhagic spots caused by capillary bleeding. Both of these abnormal findings should be assessed for location, color, and size.

Lesions The skin is assessed by inspection for the presence of lesions, which are areas of diseased or injured tissue (Table 24-4). Normally, the skin is smooth and without breaks in its continuity. Evidence of bruises, scratches, cuts, insect bites, and wounds should be noted. A *wound* is a break in the continuity of the skin and should be assessed and described as to size, shape, depth, location, and presence of drainage or odor. *Scars* are healed wounds (Wounds are discussed in Chapter 43). A *rash* is a skin eruption. The descriptive details of a rash include the type, size, elevation, coloring, and presence or absence of drainage or itching. The nurse should document the exact body surface areas involved.

Palpation The temperature, moisture, turgor, and texture of the skin are determined by palpation.

Temperature and Moisture The skin is normally warm and dry. An increase in skin temperature and moisture can indicate an elevation of body temperature. An excessive amount of perspiration, such as when the entire skin is moist, is called *diaphoresis*. When the body loses excess water—*dehydration*—the depletion of body fluids with dryness and loss of turgor occurs.

TABLE 24-3

Skin Color Assessment		
Color Variations	**Assessment Areas**	**Pathologic Causes**
Redness (erythema; flushing)	Facial area, localized area	Blushing, alcohol intake, fever, injury trauma, infection
Bluish (cyanosis)	Exposed areas, particularly the ears, lips, inside of the mouth, hands and feet, nailbeds	Cold environment, cardiac or respiratory disease (decreased oxygenation)
Yellowish (jaundice)	Overall skin areas, mucous membranes, and sclera	Liver disease (increase in bilirubin levels)
Paleness (pallor)	Exposed areas, particularly the face and lips, conjunctivae, and mucous membranes	Anemia (decreased hemoglobin)
	Overall skin areas, lips, nailbeds, conjunctivae	Shock (decreased blood volume)
Vitiligo	Whitish patchy areas on the skin	Depigmentation (congenital or autoimmune conditions)
Tanned or brown	Sun-exposed areas	Overexposure (increased melanin production), pregnancy (brown spots?)

T A B L E   2 4 - 4

Basic Types of Skin Lesions

Lesion Name	Description	Example
Primary Lesions*		
Circumscribed, Flat, Nonpalpable Change in Skin Color		
Macule	Lesion ≤1 cm	Petechiae, freckle
Patch	Lesion >1 cm	Vitiligo
Palpable Elevated Solid Masses		
Papule	Mass ≤0.5 cm	Mole
Plaque	Mass >0.5 cm	Coalesced papules
Nodule	Mass 0.5–2 cm; firmer than a papule	Nevus (wart)
Tumor	Mass >2 cm	Lipoma
Wheal	Irregular, superficial area of localized skin edema	Hives, mosquito bite
Circumscribed, Superficial Skin Elevations Formed by Free Fluid in a Cavity Within the Skin Layers		
Vesicle	Filled with serous fluid, ≤0.5 cm	Herpes simplex
Bulla	Filled with serous fluid, >0.5 cm	2nd-degree burn
Pustule	Filled with pus	Acne, impetigo
Secondary Lesions†		
Loss of Skin Surface		
Erosion	Loss of superficial epidermis, moist, nonbleeding surface	Moist area after rupture of a vesicle, as in chickenpox
Ulcer	Loss of epidermis and dermis, may bleed and scar	Stasis ulcer
Fissure	Deep linear crack, extends into dermis	Athlete's foot
Material on the Skin Surface		
Crust	Dried residue of serum, pus, or blood	Impetigo
Scale	Thin flake of exfoliated dermis	Dandruff, dry skin
Miscellaneous Lesions		
Lichenification	Thickened and roughened epidermis, with increased visibility of skin furrows	Atrophic dermatitis
Atrophy	Thinning of the skin, loss of skin furrows, shiny appearance	Arterial insufficiency
Excoriation	Scratch of the epidermis	
Scar	Fibrous tissue replaces tissue in the dermis or subcutaneous layer	
Keloid	Hypertrophied scar	
Other Common Skin Lesions, Not Technically Primary or Secondary		
Comedo	Plugged opening of a sebaceous gland, a hallmark of acne	Common blackhead
Telangiectasia	Small, dilated, red or bluish surface vessels; may be part of a basal cell carcinoma or skin injury from radiation	
Nevus	Flat to slightly elevated, round, evenly pigmented	Common mole

* May arise from previously normal skin.

† Result from changes in primary lesions.

Turgor Turgor (Fig. 24-8) is the fullness or elasticity of the skin. Normal turgor results in elasticity of the skin, allowing it to be picked up in a fold and to return to its shape when released. Difficulty in lifting a skin fold may indicate excess fluid in the tissues, or **edema**. Edema is characterized by swelling, with taut and shiny skin over the edematous area. If the area of edema is palpated with the fingers, an indentation may remain after the pressure is released. Edema may be described on a scale, as follows:

0 = none
+1 = trace
+2 = moderate
+3 = deep
+4 = very deep

When the client is dehydrated, normal skin elasticity and fullness are decreased and the skin fold returns to normal slowly. (This, however, is a normal finding in the elderly client.)

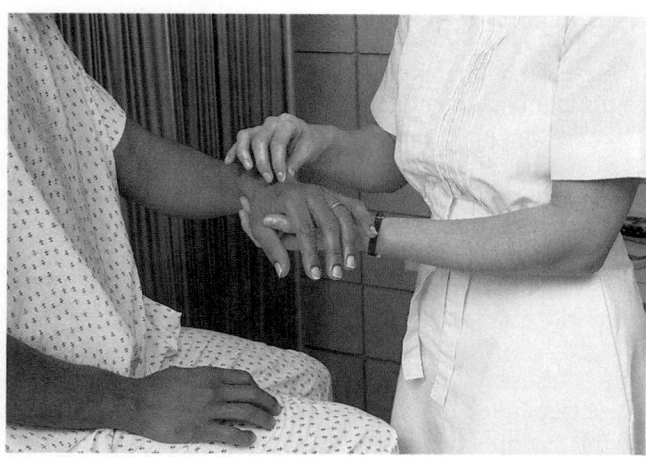

FIGURE 24-8

To assess skin turgor, a small fold of skin is picked up and then released to return to its normal shape. Difficulty in lifting a skinfold may indicate presence of edema. (Photo © Ken Kasper.)

Texture The texture of the skin may vary from smooth and soft to rough and dry. In the dehydrated client, the texture is loose and wrinkled and the mucous membranes are cracked and dry.

Nails

The nails are differentiated tissue but continuous extensions of the skin. The nails are inspected for shape, texture, and color. The shape of the nails should normally be somewhat convex and follow the natural curve of the finger. The angle between the nail and its base in the finger should be about 160 degrees. The texture of the nails should be smooth, and the nail base, when palpated, should be firm and not tender. Abnormal findings include indentations, called *Beau's lines*; infection (*paronychia*); increased brittleness and angulation; changes in the thickness or texture; and clubbing. Figure 24-9 illustrates nail abnormalities.

Hair and Scalp

The hair is normally resilient, evenly distributed, and neither excessively dry or oily. Hair is found on all body surfaces except the palms of the hands, the soles of the feet, and parts of the genitalia. Hair has various colors and textures. The hair is examined for color, texture, and distribution. Abnormal findings include unusual balding (*alopecia*) and excessive amounts of hair on the body (*hirsutism*). Decreased oxygenation of peripheral tissues, especially of the lower extremities, may cause the abnormal finding of loss of hair and thickened toenails.

The hair is separated to inspect the scalp for excessive dryness, scaliness, lumps, lesions, or lice. If any lumps or masses are palpated, note location, size, tenderness, and mobility.

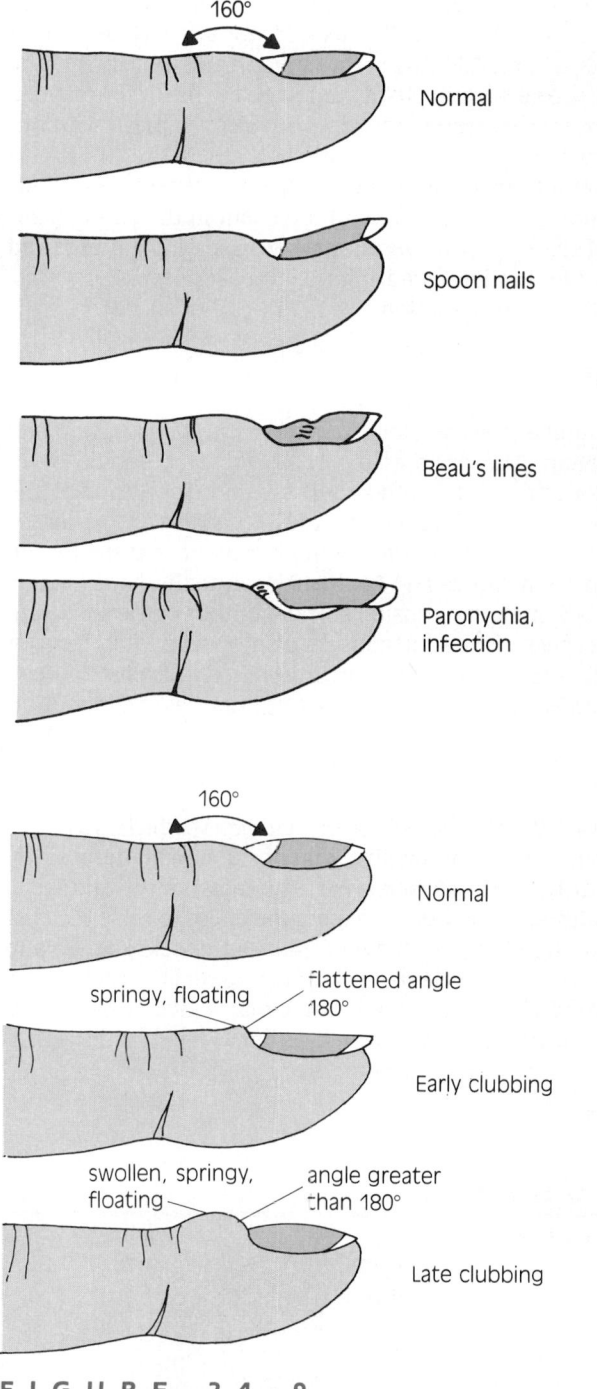

FIGURE 24-9

Examples of nail abnormalities.

Head and Neck

Assessment of the head and neck includes the skull, face, eyes, ears, nose and sinuses, mouth and pharynx, trachea, thyroid gland, and lymph nodes. The skull comprises bones that protect the brain and neurologic networks, which allow use of sensory and motor functions. The skull and facial cavities are covered by facial muscles, innervated by cranial nerves V and VII. The neck comprises vertebrae, ligaments, and muscles to provide support and movement. The trachea and thyroid gland are located in the anterior neck. An extensive arterial network provides the brain with nutrients and oxygen.

Structures of the head and neck are assessed by inspection and palpation, with the client in the sitting position. Factors for consideration while assessing the head and neck are possible head injury, increased levels of stress, and thyroid dysfunction.

Skull

The skull is assessed for size and shape by inspection and palpation. The parts of the head and face should be in proportion to each other and symmetric. Although the shape of the normal skull varies considerably, generally the shape is gently curved with prominences at the frontal and parietal bones (Fig 24-10). Abnormal findings include lack of symmetry, unusual size or contour of the skull, and tenderness. If the skull appears disproportionately large or small, it is measured for circumference. (Measuring head circumference is a normal part of infant assessment.)

Face

The face is examined for color; *symmetry*, which is a correspondence in contour, size, and position of bilateral sides; and distribution of facial hair. The facial nerve and facial muscles are assessed by asking the client to raise the eyebrows, tightly close the eyes, puff out cheeks, smile, and show the teeth. Edema of the face, especially around the eye (*periorbital edema*), and involuntary facial movements (tic or **tremor**) are abnormal findings.

FIGURE 24-10

Bones of the skull.

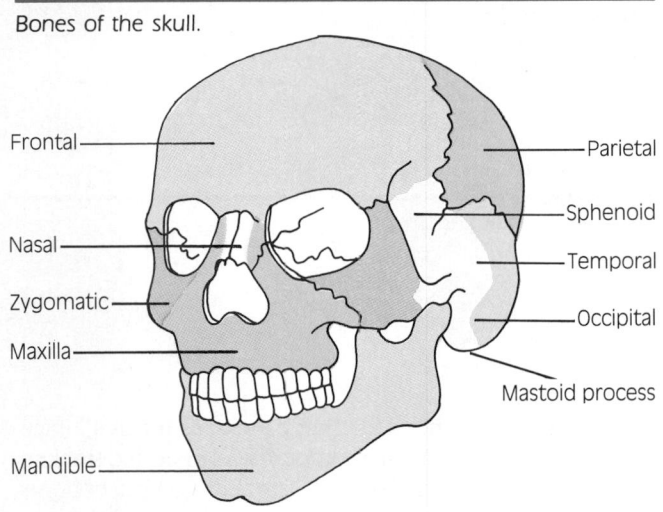

Frontal — Parietal
Sphenoid
Nasal — Temporal
Zygomatic — Occipital
Maxilla — Mastoid process
Mandible —

Eyes and Ears

The eyes and ears are sensory organs that transmit visual and auditory stimuli to the brain for interpretation. The eye muscles are attached to the eye and are innervated by cranial nerves III, IV, and VI. Cranial nerve testing is described later in this chapter with neurologic assessment. The equipment used in assessing the eyes and ears are a penlight, an ophthalmoscope or otoscope, an eye chart, a watch that ticks, and a tuning fork. The eyes and ears are primarily assessed by inspection.

Eye Assessments of the eye include external eye structures, pupils and iris, visual acuity, extraocular movements (EOMs), peripheral vision, and internal eye structures (Fig. 24-11). Factors for consideration while assessing the eye include age, use of corrective lens, artificial eye, allergies, pain, visual disturbances, and health-related factors such as high blood pressure or diabetes.

External Eye Structures External eye structures (Fig. 24-12) are assessed for position and alignment of the eyes, eyebrows, eyelids, eyelashes, lacrimal gland, and the pupils and iris. The position of the eyes is inspected for symmetry and parallel alignment. The eyebrows should have equal distribution, with the eyelashes curling outward. The eyelids are examined for color, edema, and equal coverage of the eyeball. The lacrimal glands are inspected and palpated for edema and pain.

Pupil and Iris The pupils are normally black, equal in size, round, and smooth, but may be pale and cloudy if the client has cataracts. Injury to the eye, glaucoma, and certain medications may cause the pupil to dilate (*mydriasis*); certain drugs can cause constriction (*miosis*); and unequal pupils may result from central nervous system injury or illness. The pupil is assessed for reaction to light and accommodation, and for convergence.

Assess *reaction to light* by following these five steps (Fig. 24-13):
- Ask the client to look straight ahead.
- Bring the penlight from the side of the client's face and shine the light on the pupil.
- Observe the pupil's reaction; normally it will constrict (*direct response*).
- Repeat the procedure and observe the other eye; normally it too will constrict (*consensual reflex*).
- Repeat the procedure with the other eye.

Accommodation is assessed by following these three steps (Fig. 24-14):
- Hold your forefinger, a pencil, or other straight object about 10 to 15 cm (4 to 6 inches) from the bridge of the client's nose.
- Ask the client to first look at the object, then at a distant object, then back to the object you are holding.
- Normally the pupil should constrict when looking at a near object and dilate when looking at a distant object.

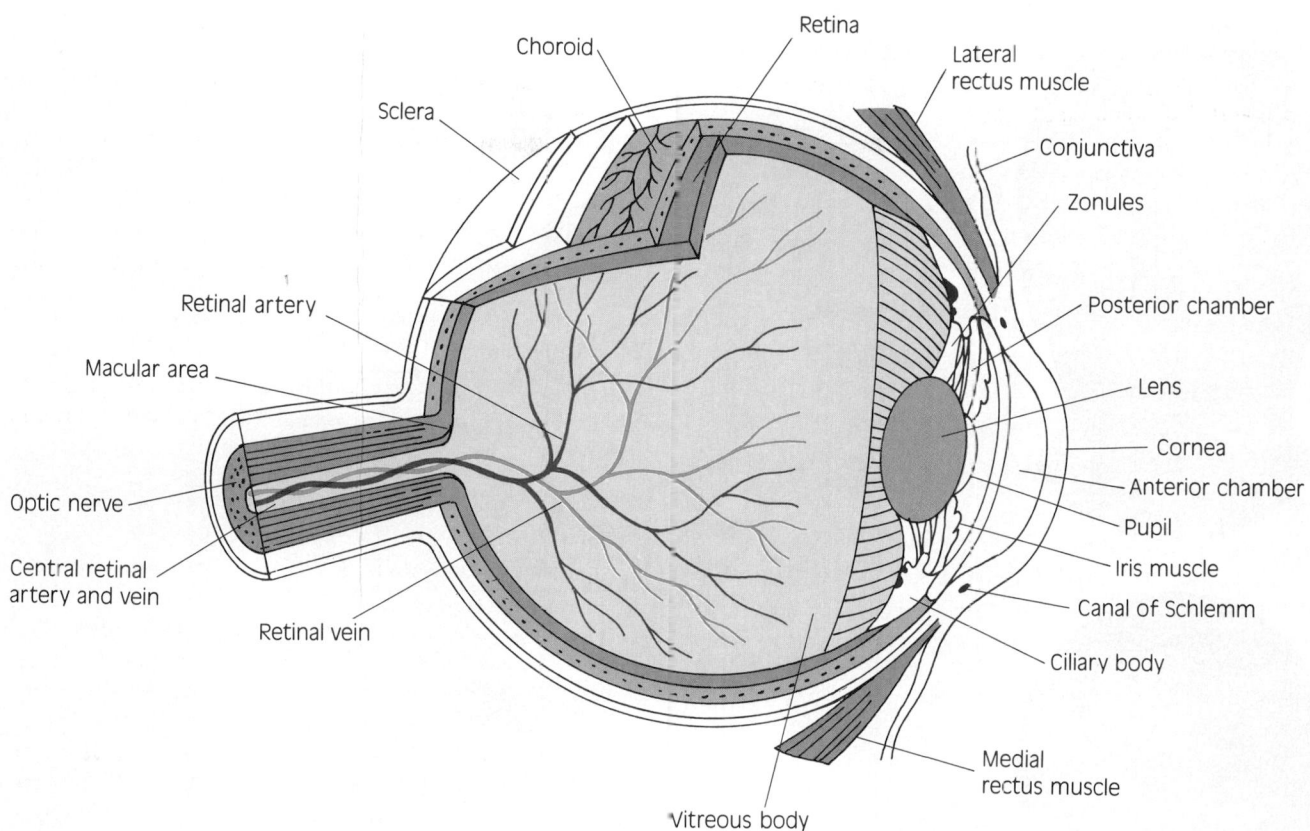

A cross section of the eye.

Convergence is assessed by moving your finger toward the client's nose; the client's eyes should normally converge (assume a cross-eyed appearance; Fig. 24-15).

Visual Acuity   Visual acuity is assessed by placing the client 20 feet from Snellen's chart and testing each eye. The client is asked to read the smallest possible line of letters, first with both eyes and then with one eye at a time. Visual acuity is measured by standardized numbers listed on the side of the chart. The numerator is 20, representing the distance from which a person with normal vision can read the lettering. The larger the denominator, the poorer the vision. Normal vision is 20/20. Visual acuity is recorded as the smallest line of letters that can be read accurately. If Snellen's chart is unavailable, the client may read from a newspaper or magazine for an estimate of visual acuity.

Extraocular Movements   EOMs are tested by assessing the eight cardinal fields of vision for coordination and alignment (Fig. 24-16). Normally both eyes move together, are coordinated, and are parallel. To assess EOMs, follow these three steps:
- Ask the client to sit or stand about 2 feet away, facing you, as you also sit or stand on eye level with the client.

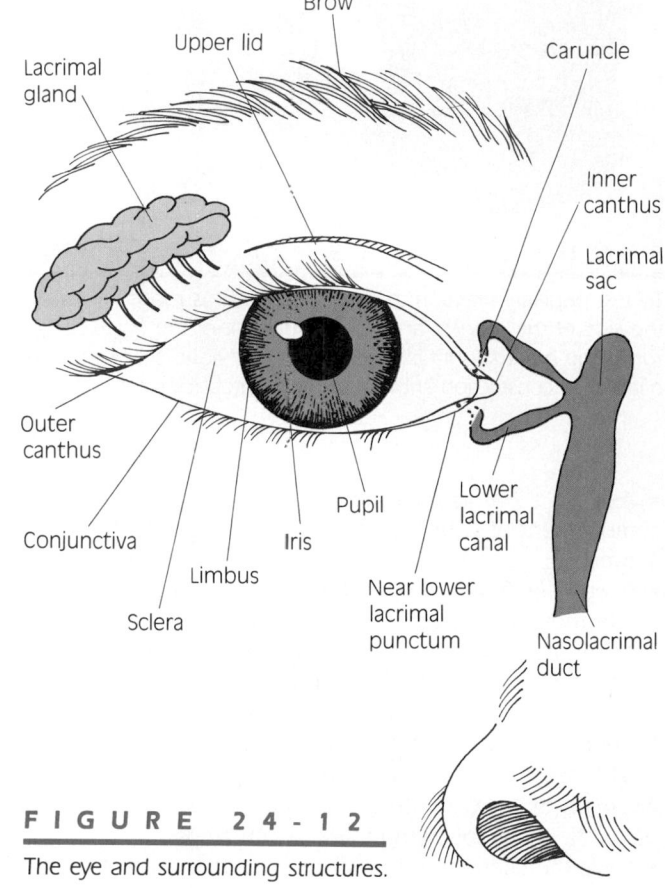

F I G U R E   2 4 - 1 2

The eye and surrounding structures.

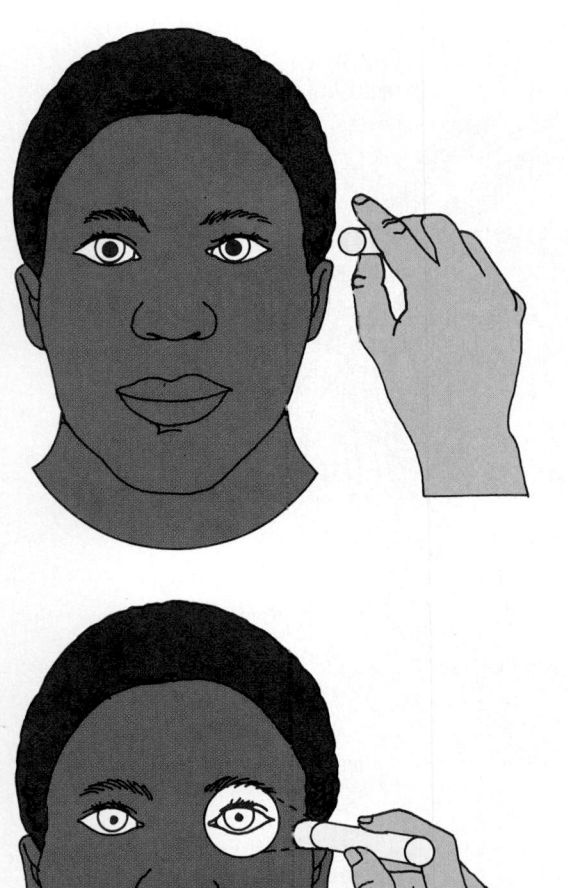

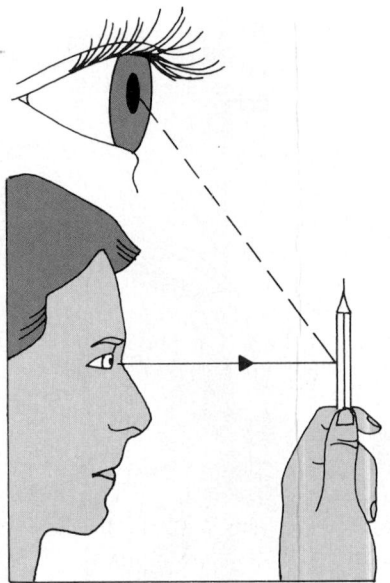

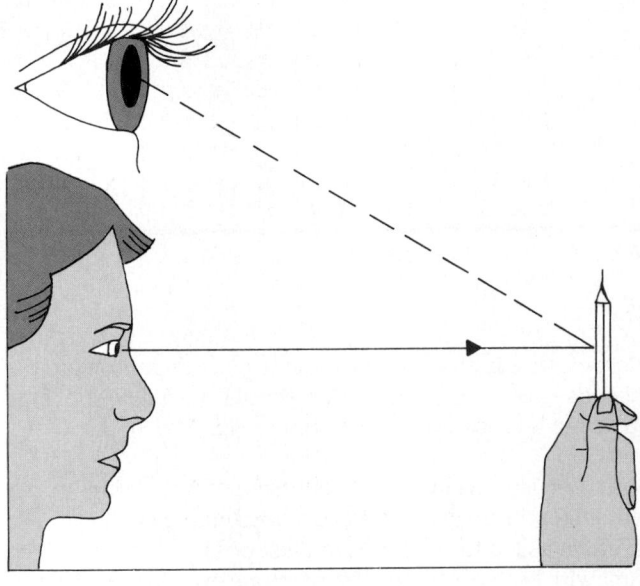

FIGURE 24-13

To test pupillary reaction to light, a penlight is moved from the side of the client's face (*top*) to in front of the eye (*bottom*). The pupil should constrict when the light is present. The dilation or constriction shown is exaggerated for clarity.

- Ask the client to hold the head still and follow the movement of your forefinger or a penlight with the eyes.
- Keep your finger about 1 foot from the client's face and move it through the cardinal positions—up and down, left and right, diagonally up and down to the left, diagonally up and down to the right.

Peripheral Vision   Tests for peripheral vision (or visual fields) assess retinal function and optic nerve function. Normally, the client will have full peripheral vision. Assess visual fields by following these seven steps:

- Have the client stand or sit about 2 feet away, facing you; ensure you are at eye level.

FIGURE 24-14

The normal pupil constricts when focused on a near object and dilates when focused on a far object. This is called accommodation.

- Ask the client to cover one eye with his or her hand or an index card.
- Ask the client to look directly at your nose, and fix his or her eyes on that spot.
- Cover your own eye opposite the client's closed eye.
- Hold your hand at arm's length to one side (right or left) and move your fingers into the visual fields from various peripheral points.
- Ask the client to tell you when he or she see your fingers (both you and the client should see your fingers at the same time).
- Repeat the procedure for the other eye.

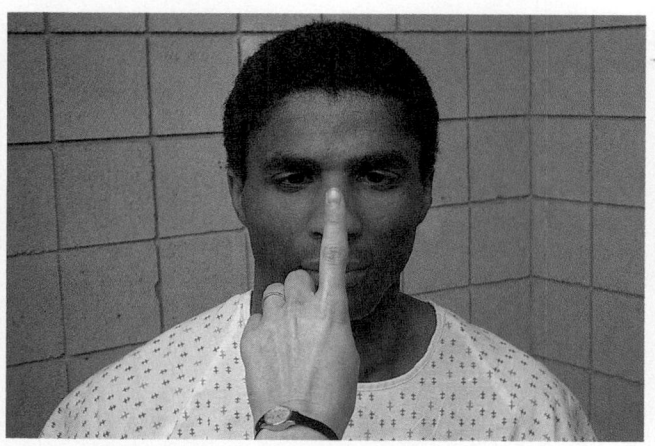

FIGURE 24-15

Convergence is assessed by moving your finger toward the client's nose. (Photo © Ken Kasper.)

Abnormalities of the external eye, pupil and iris, and visual assessment examination include asymmetry of position and alignment, inability to open and close the upper lids, scanty eyebrows and eyelashes, edema, redness or

FIGURE 24-16

Test extraocular movement of the eye by asking the client to hold his head still and follow the movement of your forefinger (top) through the cardinal positions of the eye (bottom). (Photo © Ken Kasper.)

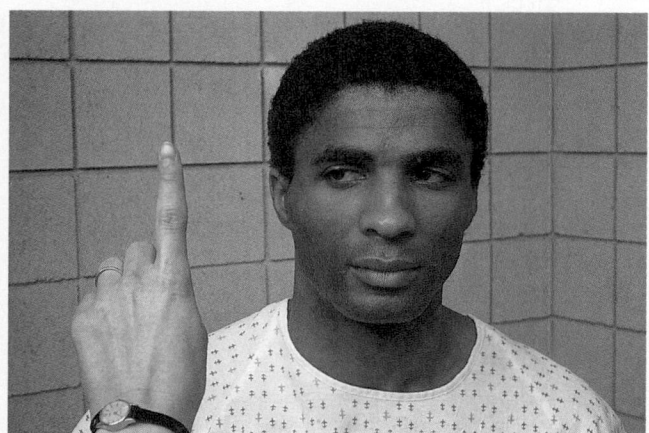

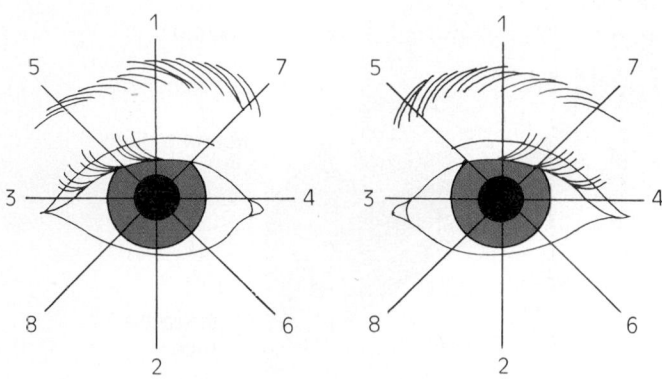

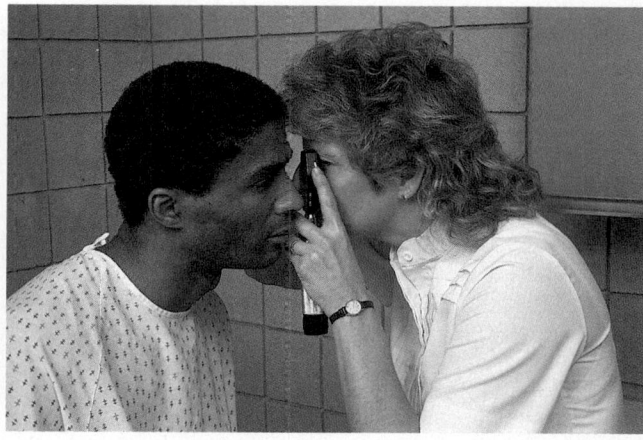

FIGURE 24-17

Examination of the internal structures of the eye using an ophthalmoscope. (Photo © Ken Kasper.)

drainage, decreased or absent pupillary response, inability of the eyes to accommodate or converge, and alterations in the visual fields.

Internal Eye Structures The internal eye (Fig. 24-17) is examined using the ophthalmoscope to assess the eye fundus, including the retina, optic nerve disc, macula, fovea centralis, and retinal vessels. Use of the ophthalmoscope takes practice and may not be a part of the nursing examination in some clinical settings. General guidelines of the examination are included in this chapter. Normal findings are a uniform red reflex; clear, yellow optic nerve disc; reddish retina; and light red arteries and dark red veins, the veins being about 1½ times as large as the arteries (Fig. 24-18). Guidelines for assessing the internal eye are listed in the accompanying Focused Assessment Guide.

FIGURE 24-18

The normal fundus as seen through an ophthalmoscope.

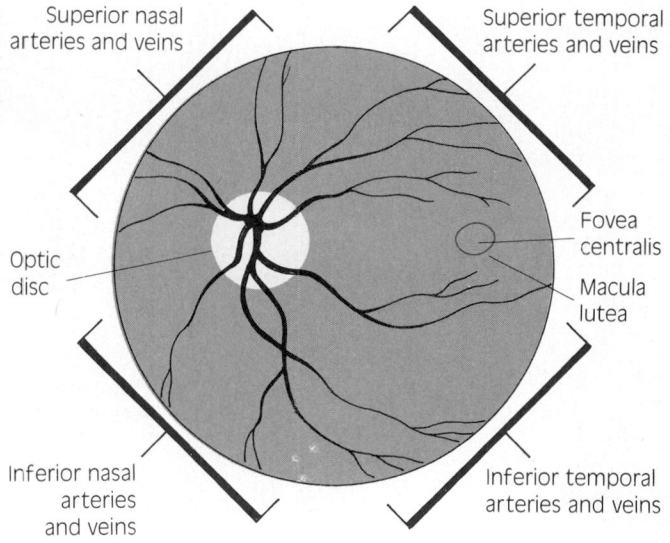

Superior nasal arteries and veins

Superior temporal arteries and veins

Optic disc

Fovea centralis

Macula lutea

Inferior nasal arteries and veins

Inferior temporal arteries and veins

F O C U S E D A S S E S S M E N T G U I D E

Internal Eye

General guidelines for assessment of the internal eye are as follows:

- Assemble the ophthalmoscope, beginning with the light setting at the large white light and the lens wheel at 0 setting.
- Darken the room and have the client remove glasses. Allow time for the client's pupils to dilate. The client should be sitting.
- Sit facing the client and ask him or her to look straight ahead during the examination.
- Keep both eyes open while looking through the ophthalmoscope viewer.
- Use your right hand and eye to examine the client's right eye, and your left hand and eye for the client's left eye.
- Shine the light on the pupil and observe the round red or orange glow (the red reflex).

- Focusing on the red reflex, slowly move the ophthalmoscope toward the client's eye.
- Rotate the lens wheel until internal eye structures are sharp and clear.
- Follow blood vessels toward the midline to locate the optic disc; note color, size, shape, margins, and central area (physiologic cup).
- Follow blood vessels outward to each of the four quadrants, assessing color, size, and pattern.
- Ask the client to look up, down, and from side to side, assessing the characteristics of the retina.
- Locate the macula by first locating the optic disc and then looking toward the client's temple for a small circular structure near the disc; note color, characteristics, and area of reflected light (fovea centralis).

Abnormal findings include cloudiness of the lens, narrowing of blood vessels, and changes in color and surface characterisitics.

Ear The ear comprises three major compartments. The external ear is made of cartilage covered with skin. The middle ear is an air-filled cavity that transmits sound from the tympanic membranes to the inner ear. The inner ear transmits sound impulses to cranial nerve VIII (Fig. 24-19).

Risk factors for consideration when assessing the ears are environmental hazards, such as exposure to chemicals, or uncontrolled loud noises. The use of corrective hearing devices should be included in the assessment documentation.

The client remains sitting while the nurse assesses the ears and hearing ability by inspection and palpation. An otoscope with a suitably sized ear speculum may be used to inspect the ear canal; a tuning fork is used in hearing acuity assessment.

F I G U R E 2 4 - 1 9

Internal structures of the ear.

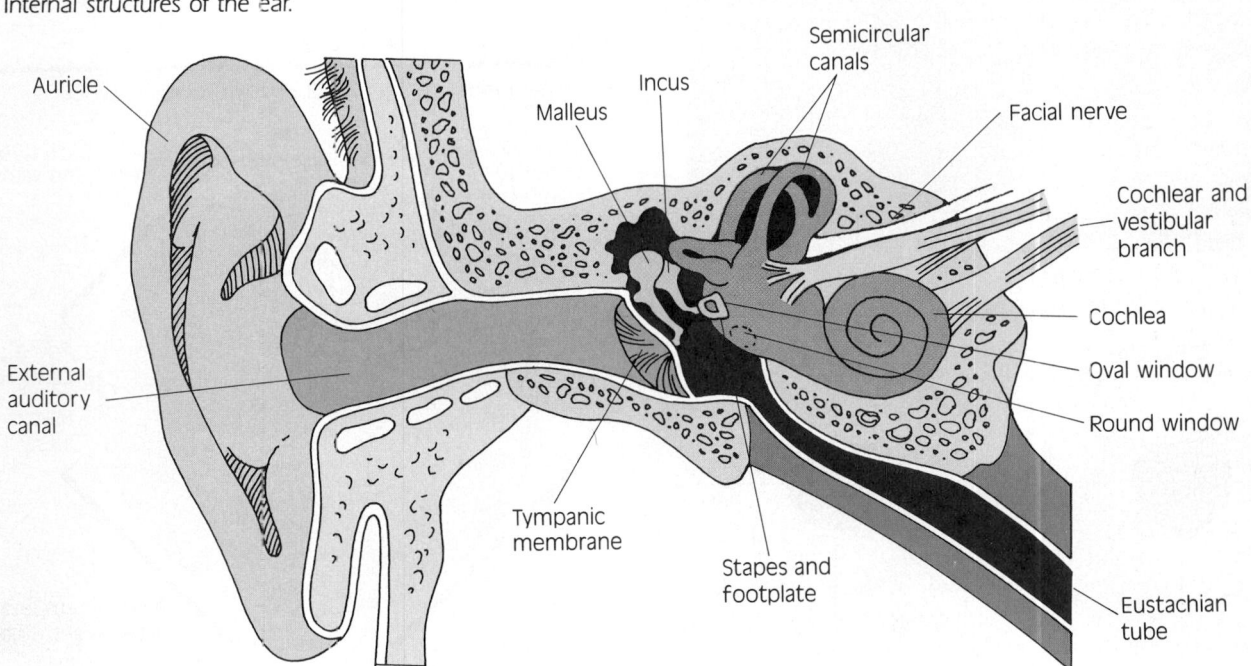

Auricle · Malleus · Incus · Semicircular canals · Facial nerve · Cochlear and vestibular branch · Cochlea · Oval window · Round window · External auditory canal · Tympanic membrane · Stapes and footplate · Eustachian tube

Hearing Hearing is assessed, one ear at a time, by determining if the client can hear the nurse's whispered voice or a ticking watch from a distance of 1 to 2 feet. The nurse must be certain the client is not lip-reading and assesses hearing acuity out of the line of vision. When hearing loss is found, a tuning fork or audiometer may be used for more precise assessments of hearing; audiometry is not generally used in routine physical assessment. Tuning fork tests are used to assess the type of hearing loss. Hearing loss may be *conductive*, that is, the result of a problem with the transmission of sound waves through the outer and middle ear; *sensorineural*, resulting from inner ear damage; or *mixed*, a combination of both. Weber's and Rinne's tests are used.

Weber's test is used to assess bone conduction. The three-step procedure is as follows:

- Hold the tuning fork at its base and strike it against the palm of the opposite hand so the fork vibrates.
- Place the base of the tuning fork on the center of the top of the client's head.
- Ask the client where the sound is heard best.

Clients with conductive hearing loss hear the sound better in the affected ear because bone transmits the sound directly to the ear. Normal findings would be sound heard in both ears or in the midline.

Rinne's test compares air conduction (AC) to bone conduction (BC). The four-step test is as follows:

- Activate the tuning fork.
- Hold the base of the tuning fork against the mastoid process of the client and ask the client to tell you when the sound can no longer be heard.
- Immediately place the still-vibrating tuning fork close to the external ear canal and ask if the client can hear the sound; the normal ear will do so.
- Repeat the test with the other ear.

Normally, air conduction is better than bone conduction (positive Rinne's test with AC exceeding BC). If the hearing loss is conductive, bone conduction will be the same or greater than air conduction.

External Ear The external ear is inspected for shape, size, and lesions. The external surfaces of the ear should be smooth, and the shape and size of the ears should be symmetric and proportionate to the head. The external ear is gently palpated for pain, edema, or presence of lesions (Fig. 24-20). Abnormal findings of the external ear include unequal height and size, uneven color, and lesions.

Ear Canal and Tympanic Membrane The otoscope is used to examine the ear canal and the tympanic membrane. The otoscope head is placed on the base, and the largest speculum that will fit into the client's ear comfortably is attached. The otoscope speculum is inserted as the client's head is slightly tilted away from the examiner. The client is in the sitting position. To achieve better visualization, the ear canal of the adult is straightened by gently pulling the pinna up and back (the ear canal is straightened in children younger than age 3 years by pulling the pinna

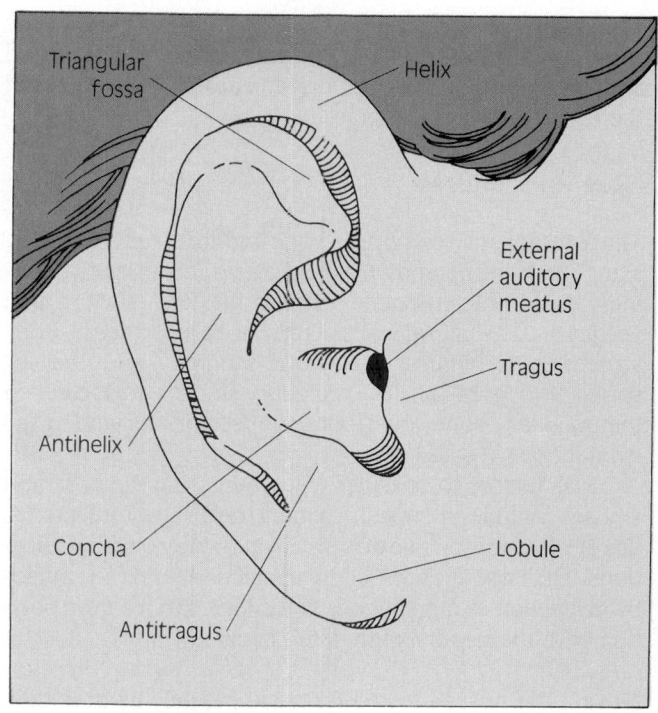

FIGURE 24-20

External structures of the ear.

down and back). The ear canal should be smooth and pinkish in color. It is examined for wax, discharge, and foreign bodies. The tympanic membrane should be intact and without redness or discharge. The membrane is translucent, shiny, and gray (Fig. 24-21). Typical abnormal findings in-

FIGURE 24-21

Normal tympanic membrane, as seen through an otoscope.

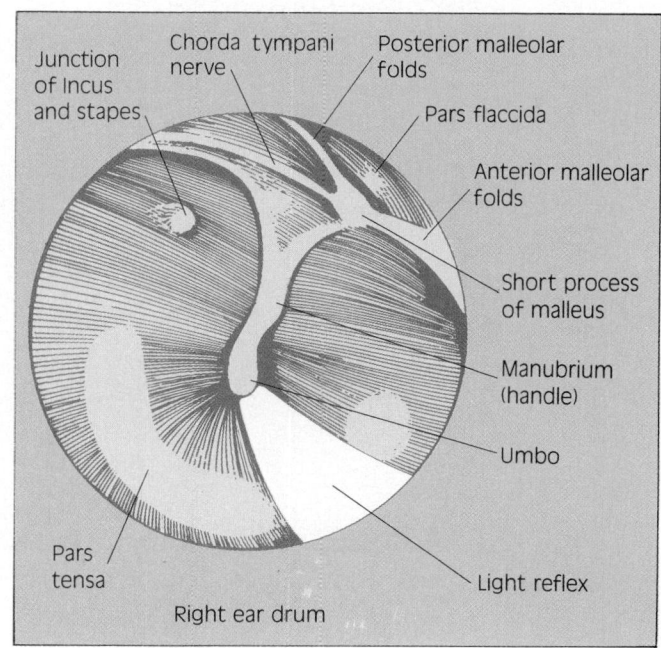

clude pain when manipulating the pinna, redness of the canal, nodules on the auricle, mastoid tenderness, a red and swollen eardrum, a perforated eardrum, wax plugs in the ear canal, and drainage.

Nose and Sinuses

The external nose comprises bone and cartilage covered by skin. The nose extends from the *nares* (or anterior openings) to the internal nose, divided into two cavities and vestibules. The lateral walls of the nose are formed by bony structures (*turbinates*) that warm, humidify, and filter inspired air (Fig. 24-22). The maxillary sinuses are located in the maxillary bone; the frontal sinuses are located in the frontal bone (Fig. 24-23).

Risk factors to consider when assessing the nose and sinuses include allergies, frequent respiratory infections, use of cocaine, and use of nasal drops, sprays, and medications. The nose is assessed by inspection, and the sinuses by inspection and palpation. The client is in a sitting position with the head slightly tilted back.

Nose The nose is tested for nasal patency by occluding one nostril at a time and asking the client to inhale through

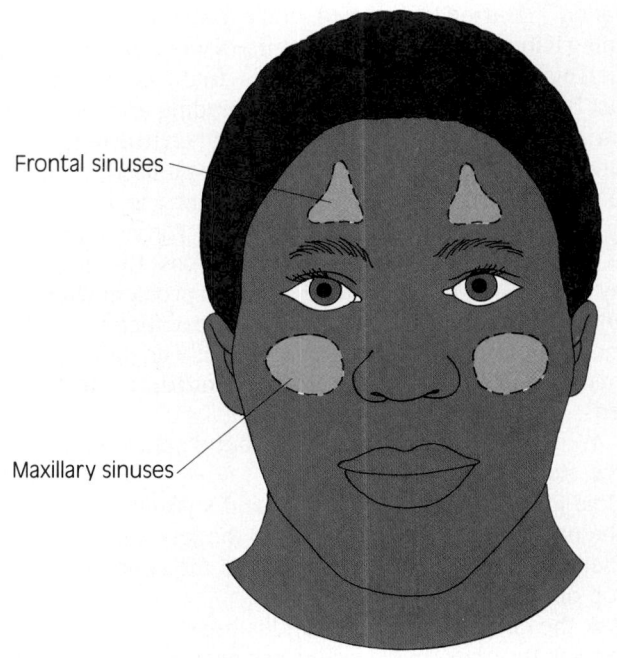

F I G U R E   2 4 - 2 3

Location of the frontal and maxillary sinuses.

the nose. Each nostril is inspected, using an otoscope with a short, wide tip or with a nasal speculum and penlight (Fig. 24-24). The mucous membranes are examined for color and the presence of exudate or growths. The nasal septum is inspected for intactness and deviation. Normally, the nasal mucosa is moist and redder than the oral mucosa. Abnormal findings that should be noted when assessing the nose are swelling of the mucosa, bleeding, discharge, perforation or deviation of the nasal septum, and polyps.

Sinuses The frontal and maxillary sinuses are examined for pain and edema. The frontal sinuses are palpated by

F I G U R E   2 4 - 2 2

Cross section of the nasal cavity.

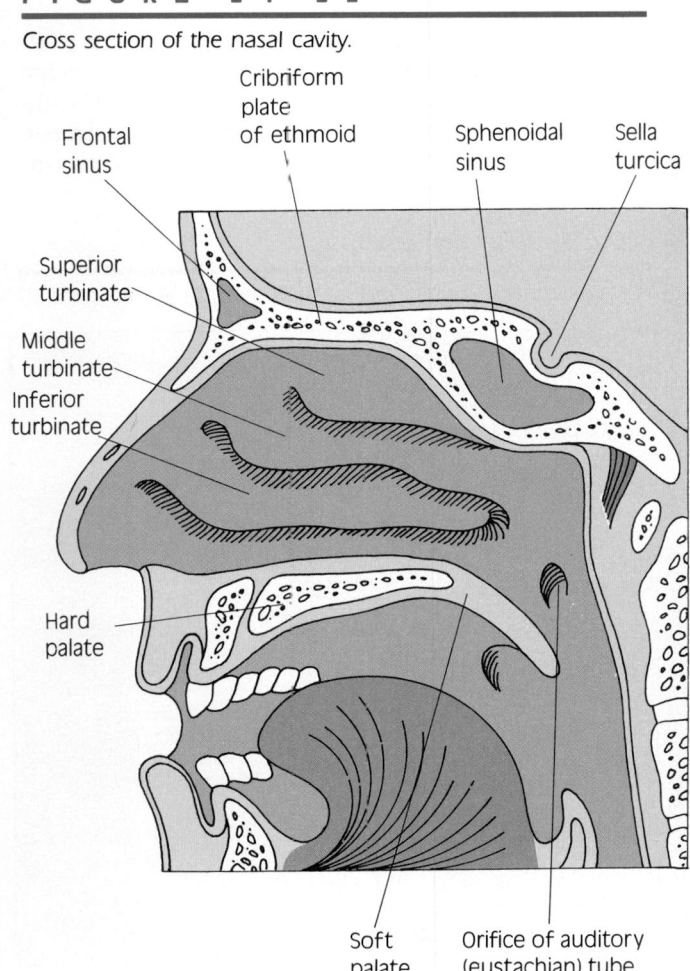

F I G U R E   2 4 - 2 4

Examination of the nasal passages using an otoscope with a wide speculum. (Photo © Ken Kasper.)

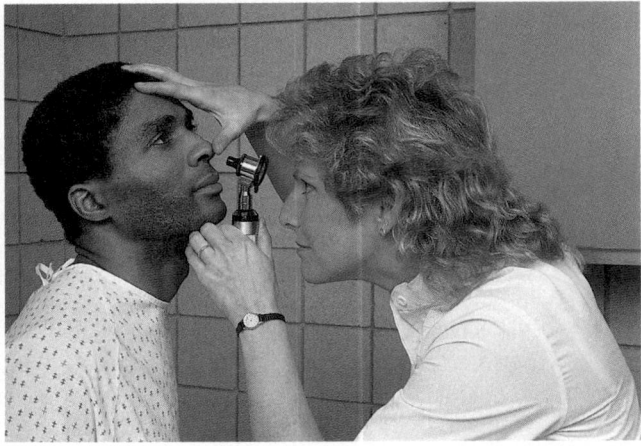

Equipment for assessment of the mouth and pharynx includes a penlight, a tongue blade, and gloves. The mouth and pharynx are assessed by inspection of the lips, gums and teeth, tongue, and hard and soft palates, using palpation if any abnormalities are noted during inspection. The client is in the sitting position with his or her head tilted backward and is instructed to open the mouth wide. The nurse should wear gloves when assessing a client's mouth.

The lips should be pink, moist, and smooth. The tongue and mucous membranes are normally pink in color, moist, and free of swelling or lesions. If the client wears dentures, they are removed for inspection of the gums and roof of the mouth. The gums should be pink and smooth. With the tongue relaxed on the floor of the mouth, the mucous membrane of the oropharynx is examined as the base of the tongue is depressed with a tongue depressor. The uvula normally is centered and freely movable. The tonsils, if present, are small, pink, and symmetric in size. The teeth should be regular and free of cavities or have dental restoration. Abnormal findings of the mouth and pharynx are pallor, cyanosis, redness and swelling of the mucous membranes; lesions of the mucosa and lips; swollen and red tonsils; swollen, red, and bleeding gums; poorly aligned, missing, or carious teeth; a hairy or fissured tongue; and paralysis of the tongue.

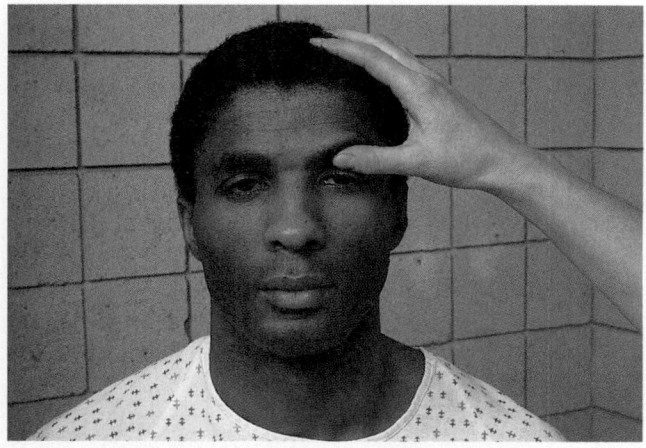

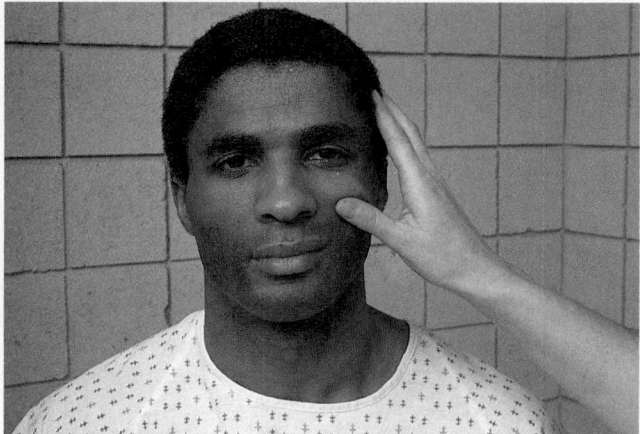

F I G U R E   2 4 - 2 5

(*Top*) The frontal sinuses are palpated by gently pressing upward on the bony prominences above each eye. (*Bottom*) The maxillary sinuses are palpated by applying gentle pressure on the bony prominences of the upper cheek. (Photos © Ken Kasper.)

gently pressing upward on the bony prominences located above each eye. The maxillary sinuses are palpated by gentle pressure on the bony prominences of the upper cheek (Fig. 24-25). Normally, the sinuses are not painful when palpated. Pain may be a finding if the sinuses are infected or obstructed.

Mouth and Pharynx

The mouth and pharynx comprise various structures—the lips, tongue, teeth, gums, hard and soft palate, salivary gland, the tonsillar pillars, and the tonsils (Fig. 24-26). The primary function of the mouth and pharynx is to allow passage of air, food, and liquids. Special properties of the mouth aid in digestion and vocalization. Risk factors for consideration during assessment include oral hygiene patterns, eating habits, use of dentures, use of smokeless tobacco, pipe smoking, and medications.

F I G U R E   2 4 - 2 6

Structures of the mouth.

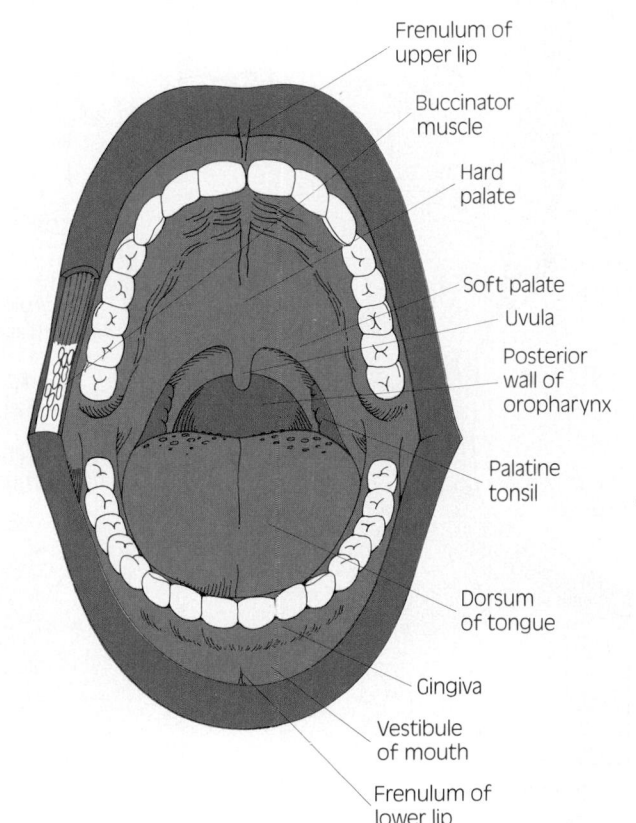

Frenulum of upper lip

Buccinator muscle

Hard palate

Soft palate

Uvula

Posterior wall of oropharynx

Palatine tonsil

Dorsum of tongue

Gingiva

Vestibule of mouth

Frenulum of lower lip

Neck

With the client in the sitting position, the neck (Fig. 24-27) is assessed by inspection and palpation. The neck should be slightly hyperextended. Risk factors to consider when assessing the neck include past injury, infections, and evidence or history of thyroid problems.

The neck is assessed for size and position of the trachea and thyroid (Fig. 24-28), range of motion, lymph nodes, and venous distention. Full range of motion is assessed by asking the client to tilt the head backward, forward, and side to side. The neck should be symmetric with full range of motion. No neck vein distention should be visible.

Trachea The trachea is palpated for alignment and position, which is normally midline at the suprasternal notch. Palpate by placing the thumb and forefinger on each side of the trachea at the suprasternal notch; an unequal space between the trachea and the sternocleidomastoid muscle on each side is an abnormal finding indicating tracheal displacement.

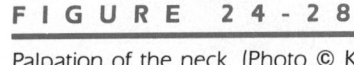

FIGURE 24-28

Palpation of the neck. (Photo © Ken Kasper.)

Thyroid The thyroid gland is assessed by palpation, but in many individuals is normally not palpable. The client is sitting, with the examiner using the posterior approach (Fig. 24-29). Palpate for size, shape, symmetry, tenderness, and presence of any nodules. Follow these five steps to palpate the thyroid gland:

- Standing behind the client, place your hands around the client's neck, with your fingertips over the lower half of the neck and trachea.
- Ask the client to swallow, and feel for enlargement of the gland as it rises.
- Palpate each lobe of the thyroid by having the client turn the head slightly toward the side to be examined; then gently displace the trachea with one hand.

FIGURE 24-27

Structures of the neck.

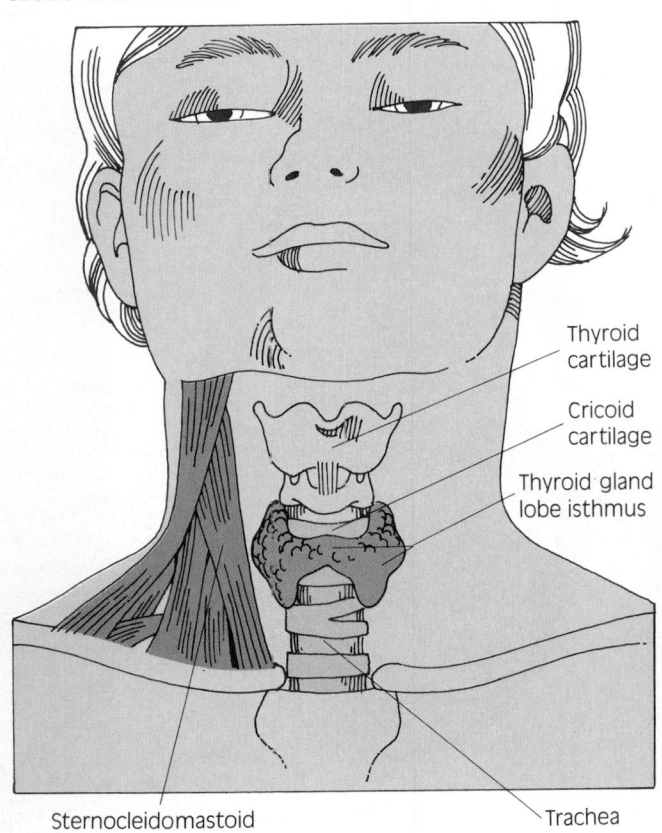

Thyroid cartilage

Cricoid cartilage

Thyroid gland lobe isthmus

Sternocleidomastoid muscle

Trachea

FIGURE 24-29

Examination of the thyroid. (Photo © Ken Kasper.)

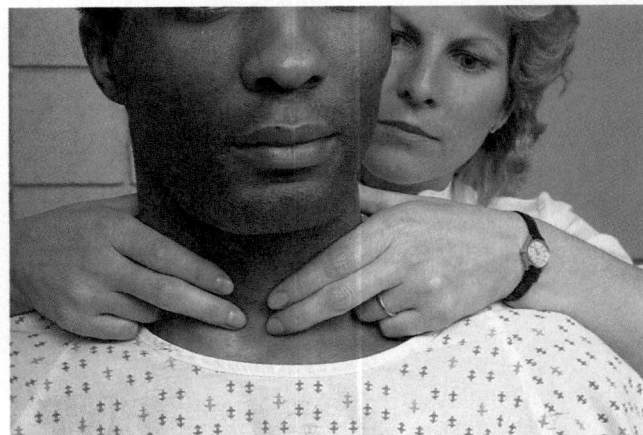

• Ask the client to swallow, and palpate the thyroid with your other hand.
• Repeat for the other side.

The thyroid gland should feel soft and should be without tenderness, enlargement, masses, or nodules.

Lymph Nodes The lymph nodes are palpated with the pads of the fingers for enlargement, tenderness, and mobility. The nodes form a chain with the preauricular and posterior auricular (located anteriorly and posteriorly to the ear); occipital (base of skull); tonsillar (upper lateral neck); submaxillary and submental (jaw line); superficial cervical and posterior cervical (lateral upper and lower portion of the neck); and supraclavicular (anterior upper to lower neck region; Fig. 24-30) nodes. The nodes are generally not palpable; if palpable, they should be small, mobile, and not tender. If palpable, assess location, size, consistency, mobility, and tenderness. Abnormal findings of the neck include limited neck movement, enlargement of veins, tracheal deviation, thyroid enlargement, and palpable lymph nodes. Consistent hoarseness should also be documented.

FIGURE 24-30

Location of the lymph nodes of the neck.

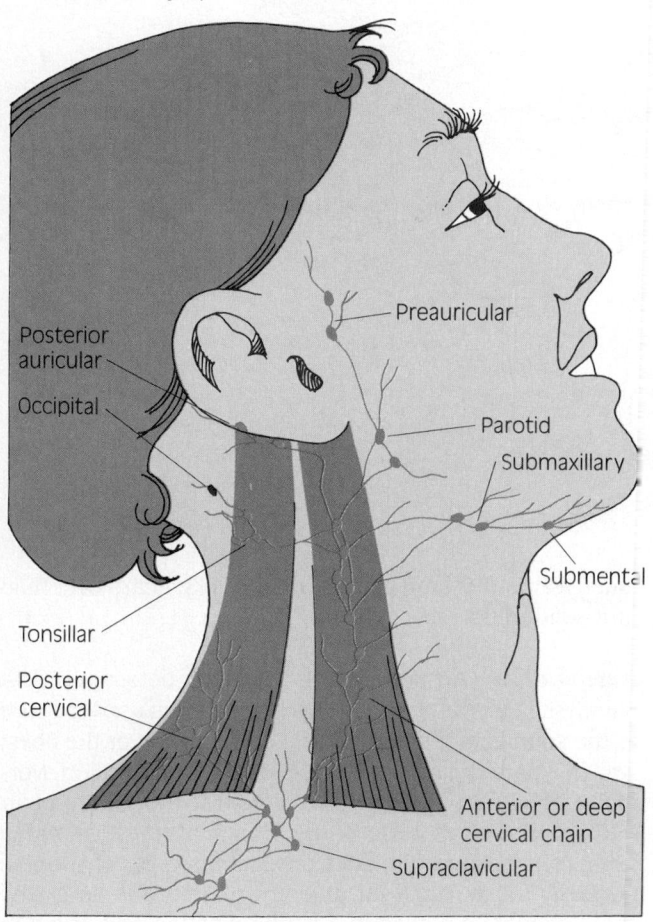

Thorax and Lungs

The thorax (Fig. 24-31) comprises the rib cage, cartilage, and muscles that enable the respiratory process to occur. The interior chest is divided into the right and left pleural cavities, with three lobes of lung tissue on the right and two lobes on the left. Air is inspired into the tracheobronchial system through the trachea, which branches into the right and left mainstem bronchi. Each bronchus branches into bronchioles, and then into the alveoli, where the exchange of oxygen and carbon dioxide occurs. Risk factors for consideration when assessing the thorax and lungs include environmental hazards, smoking, nutritional status, and frequent or chronic respiratory infections.

The equipment needed for this examination includes a stethoscope (warmed) and a tape measure. The environment should be warm and have adequate lighting. The techniques for this examination include inspection, palpation, percussion, and auscultation. The client is in a sitting position during the assessment.

Inspection Inspection begins with observation of the client's chest for color, shape or contour, breathing patterns, and muscle development. The color should be even and consistent with the color of the client's face. The shape or contour should have a downward equal slope at the rib cage. The chest should be symmetric, with the transverse diameter being greater than the anterior posterior diameter. If the contour of the chest changes, as in chronic lung disease conditions, the contour of the chest wall can be described as *barrel-chest* with noted increase in anterior posterior diameter (Fig. 24-32). The breathing patterns should be smooth and even, ranging from 12 to 20 breaths per minute. Abnormal findings during inspection include an increase in chest size and contour, abnormal breathing patterns with use of accessory muscles, and changes in skin color.

Palpation Palpation is used to detect areas of sensitivity, chest expansion during respirations, and vibrations (**fremitus**). The examiner uses the palmar surface of the hands to palpate the anterior and posterior thoracic landmarks (Fig. 24-33) in a sequential pattern for temperature, moisture, muscular development, and the presence of tenderness or masses. The same technique and sequence are used to test for tactile (vocal) fremitus, comparing bilateral sides. Normally, equal bilateral mild vibratory sensations will be palpated. The skin should be warm and dry, muscular development symmetric, and there should be no tenderness or masses. Chest expansion is determined by placing the hands over the anterior and posterior thorax and feeling the amount of movement during shallow and deep respirations. The thorax should expand symmetrically (Fig. 24-34). Abnormal findings during palpation may be cool, excessively dry or moist skin, muscle asymmetry, tenderness, masses, increased or decreased vibratory sensation, asymmetric thoracic expansion, and abnormal breathing patterns (Fig. 24-35).

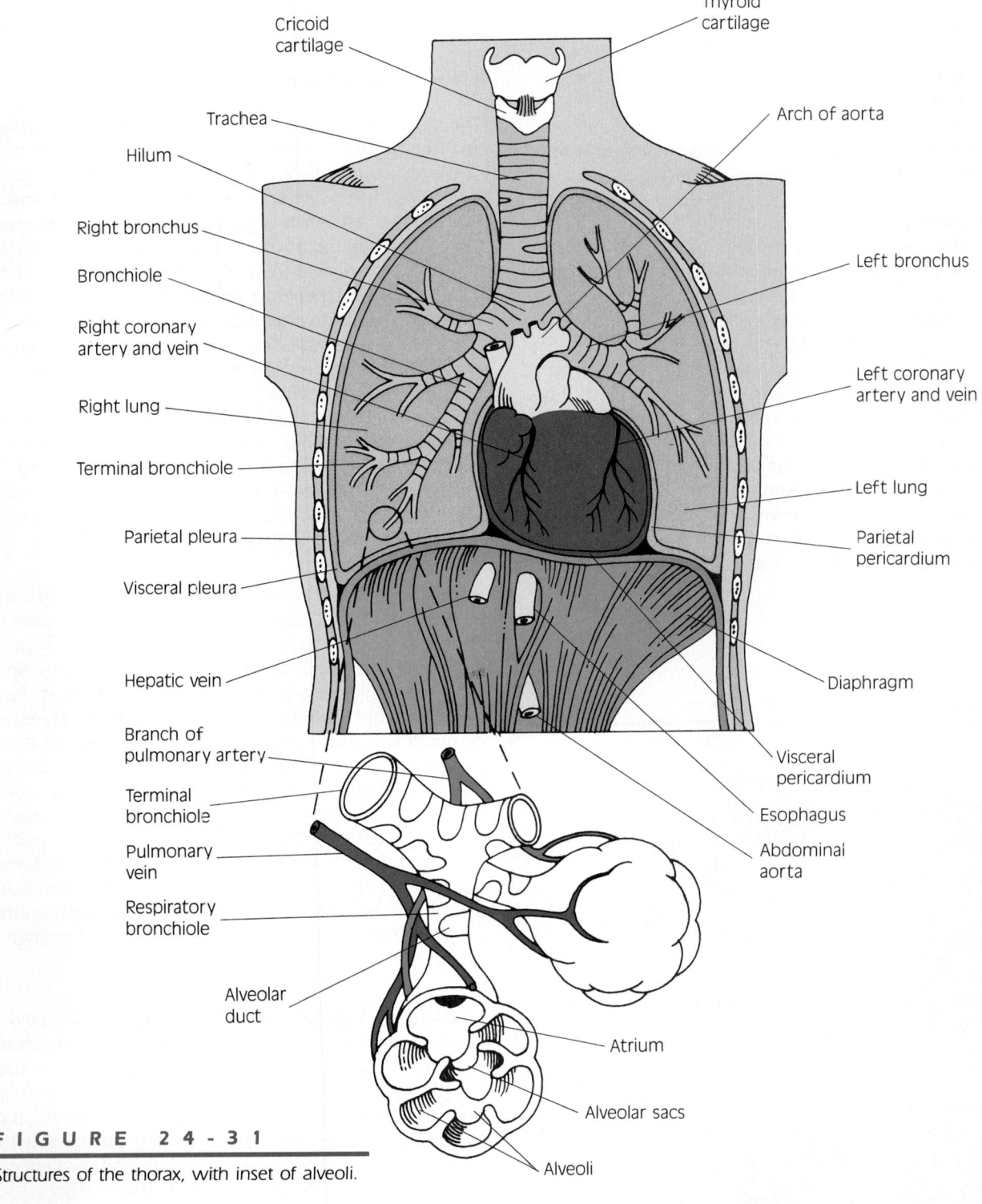

FIGURE 24-31

Structures of the thorax, with inset of alveoli.

Percussion   Percussion is used to determine lung position and size and to detect the presence of air, liquids, or solids within the lungs. The shoulder area and anterior and posterior thorax are palpated in a systematic pattern (see Fig. 24-33). The nurse listens for the intensity, pitch, duration, and quality of the sounds produced. When a normal air-filled lung is percussed, the sound is hollow, loud, low-pitched, and of long duration. This percussion tone is known as *resonance*. A *flat* tone will be heard over bony or well-developed muscle tissue. *Tympany*, a hollow sound, is percussed over the stomach. Percussion sounds that are abnormal over lung tissue are *hyperresonance*, heard over emphysematous lung tissue, and *dullness*, heard over fluid or a solid mass.

Auscultation   Auscultation is used to detect air flow within the respiratory tract. A stethoscope is used to listen to the sounds of inspiration and expiration over the chest wall in a pattern similar to that used with percussion. Normally, breath sounds result from the free movement of air into and out of all parts of the bronchial tree. The nurse listens for the duration, pitch, and intensity of the sounds; normally these vary over different parts of the lung. The client should be placed in a sitting position and asked to

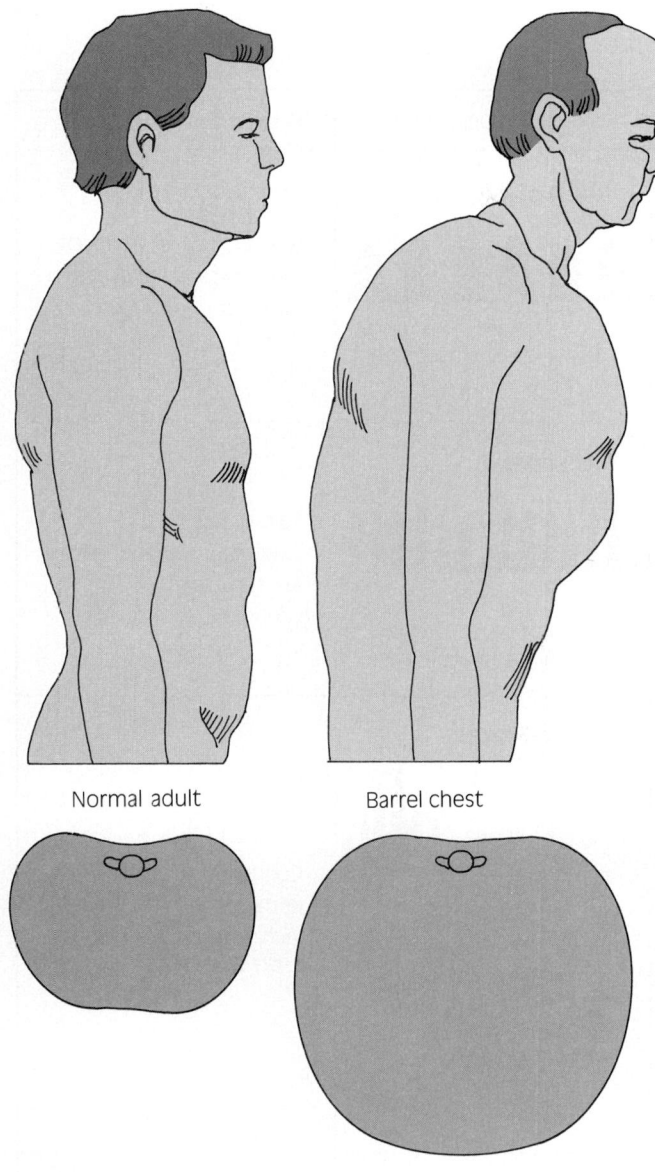

Normal adult   Barrel chest

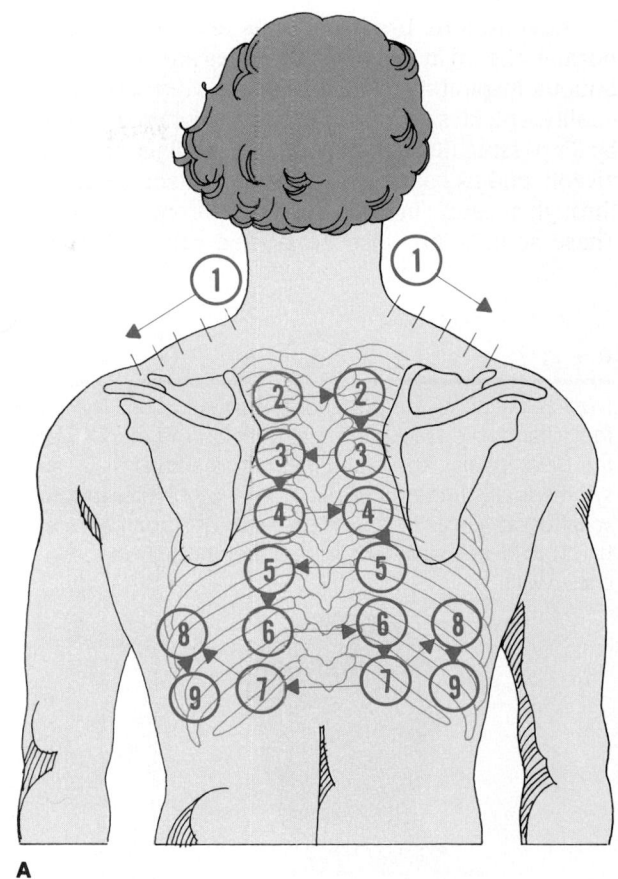

A

FIGURE 24-32

Profile and anteroposterior diameter of normal adult chest and barrel chest.

breathe slowly and deeply through the mouth. The warmed diaphragm of the stethoscope is placed over the thoracic landmarks, and breath sounds are auscultated in the same sequential pattern as used for palpation and percussion (see Fig. 24-33).

Normally, **bronchial sounds** are heard over the trachea and are high in pitch and intensity, with expiration being longer than inspiration. **Bronchovesicular sounds** are heard over the mainstem bronchus, and are moderate in pitch and intensity, with inspiration equal to expiration. **Vesicular breathing sounds** are soft, low-pitched sounds, heard over the normal lung tissue throughout the lung fields; inspiration is longer than expiration. (Fig. 24-36).

FIGURE 24-33

Anterior (A) and posterior (B) chest—landmarks and systematic sequence of examination. The pattern is used for palpation, percussion, and auscultation of the chest.

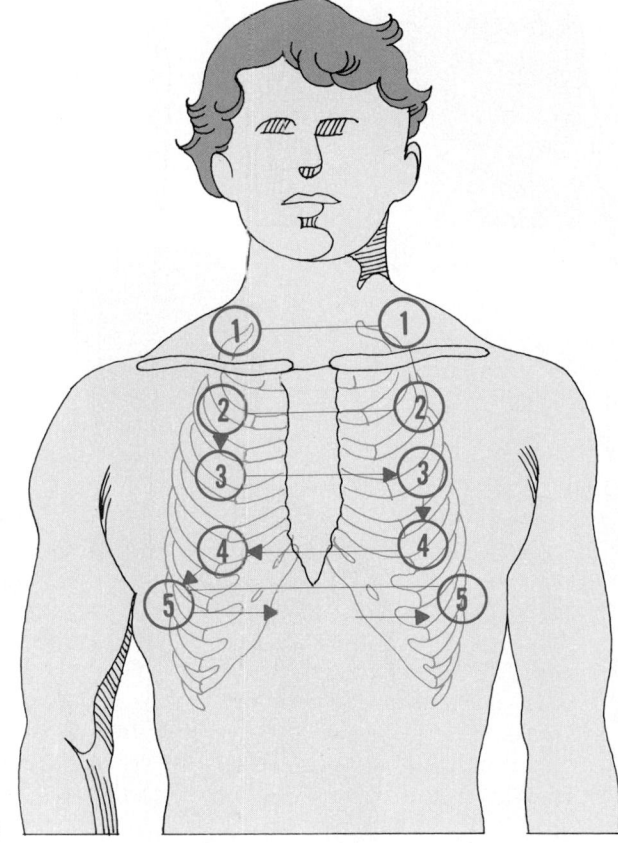

B

Adventitious breath sounds are breath sounds not normally heard in the lungs. **Crackles** are discrete, discontinuous, inspiratory sounds that have a dry or wet crackling quality. Crackles are described as fine when they are made by air passing through moisture in small air passages and alveoli, and as coarse when they are made by air passing through moisture in the bronchioles, bronchi, and trachea. These sounds may also be labeled **rales**. **Wheezes** are

FIGURE 24-34

(*Top*) Palpation of the posterior thorax excursion. The examiner's hands are placed symmetrically on the client's back. As the client inhales, the examiner's hands should move apart symmetrically. (*Bottom*) Palpation of the posterior thorax for vocal or tactile fremitus. The examiner uses the palms of the hands to detect vibrations transmitted through the lung to the chest wall.

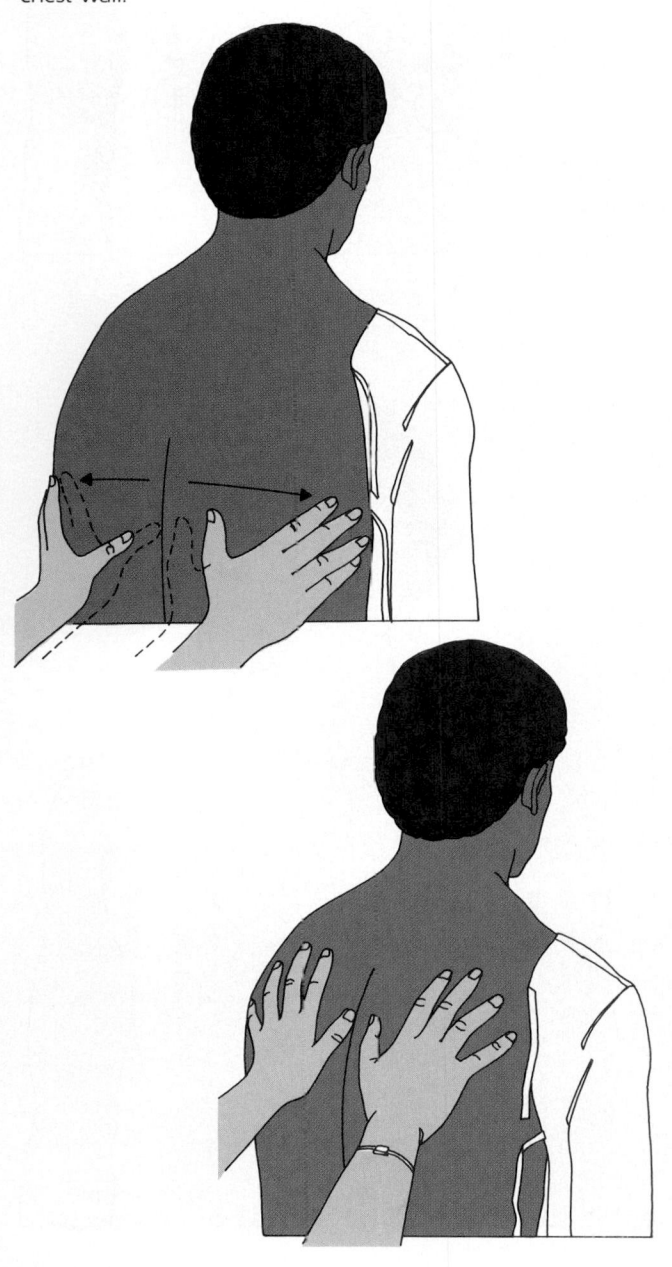

Pattern and Description	Pathological Conditions
Bradypnea Rate < 12 respirations per minute	Neurologic disturbance Electrolyte disturbance Infection
Tachypnea Persistent rate > 20 respirations per minute	Pain or injury Liver enlargement Ascites
Cheyne-Stokes Apnea Cyclic pattern of respirations which progress from slow and shallow to rapid and deep respirations with a gradual return to slow and shallow respirations followed by a period of apnea	Congestive heart failure Renal failure Increased intracranial pressure
Kussmal Faster and deeper respirations than normal without pauses	Diabetic ketoacidosis Metabolic acidosis Renal failure

FIGURE 24-35

Abnormal breathing patterns.

continuous sounds that originate in small air passages that are narrowed by secretions, swelling, or tumors. They may be inspiratory or expiratory and are high-pitched sounds. **Rhonchi**, or gurgles, are also continuous sounds, originating in large air passages that are narrowed (as with wheezes). Rhonchi are low-pitched and may be altered by coughing. A **pleural friction rub** is a grating sound, caused by an inflamed pleura rubbing against the chest wall (Fig. 24-37). If a productive cough occurs during auscultation, the sputum should be assessed for color, consistency, and amount.

Bronchial or Tubular

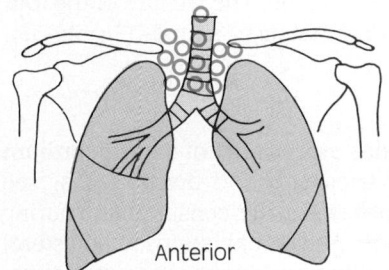

Anterior

Blowing, hollow sounds auscultated over the trachea

Ratio of inspiration to expiration

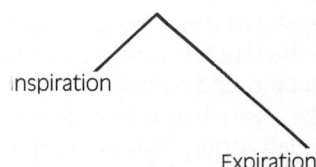

Inspiration

Expiration

Inspiration is shorter than expiration
Expiration is longer, lower, and
higher-pitched than inspiration

Bronchovesicular

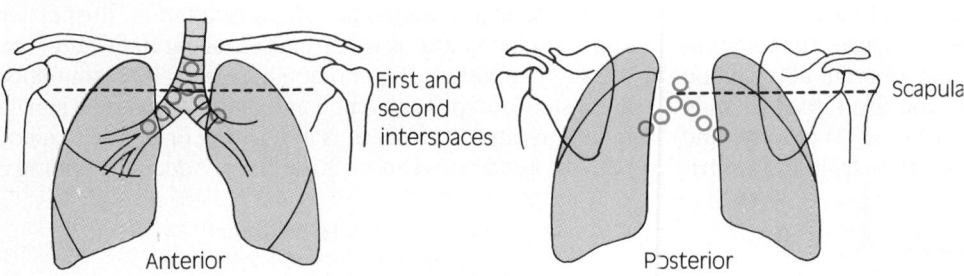

First and
second
interspaces

Anterior

Scapula

Posterior

Medium-pitched, medium intesity, blowing sounds auscultated over the
first and second interspaces anteriorly and the scapula posteriorly

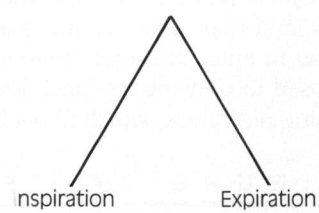

Inspiration   Expiration

Inspiration and expiration have
similar pitch

Vesicular

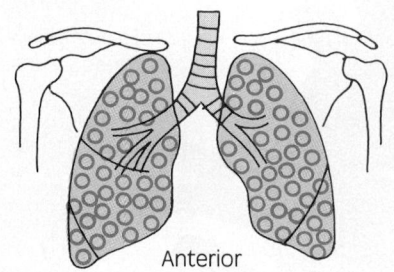

Anterior

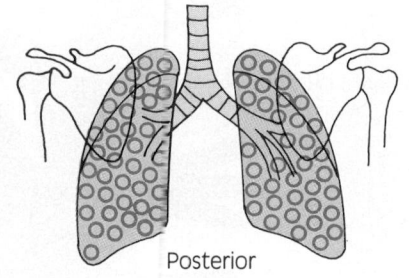

Posterior

Soft, low-pitched sounds auscultated over the lung periphery

Expiration

Inspiration

Inspiration is longer, louder, and
higher-pitched than expiration

FIGURE 24-36

Normal breath sounds.

FIGURE 24-37

Abnormal breath sounds.

Breath Sounds	Characteristics	Breath Sounds	Characteristics
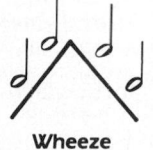 **Wheeze**	Musical or squeaking High-pitched and continuous sounds Auscultated during inspiration or expiration Occurs in small air passages	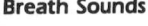 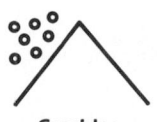 **Crackles**	Bubbling, crackling, popping Low- to high-pitched, discontinuous sounds Auscultated during inspiration Occurs in small air passages, alveoli, bronchioles, bronchi, and trachea
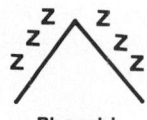 **Rhonchi**	Sonorous or coarse Low-pitched and continuous sounds Auscultated during inspiration or expiration Occurs in large air passages (Coughing may clear the sound)	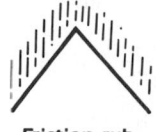 **Friction rub**	Rubbing or grating Loudest over lower lateral anterior surface Auscultated during inspiration and expiration

Cardiovascular and Peripheral Vascular Systems

The heart is a hollow, muscular, contractile organ that lies in the thoracic cavity behind the sternum to the left of the midline, and is enclosed in a sac known as the *pericardium*. The heart has four chambers: (1) the right atrium and (2) left atrium that both serve as receiving chambers, and (3) the right ventricle and (4) left ventricle that both serve as pumping chambers. The four chambers of the heart are connected by two sets of valves—the atrioventricular valve and the semilunar valve. The *atrioventricular valves*, located between the atria and the ventricles, are the tricuspid and mitral valves. The tricuspid valve leads from the right atrium to the right ventricle; the mitral valve is located between the left atrium and the left ventricle. These valves respond to pressure changes as they open to allow blood flow to enter into their chamber, and are forced to snap closed to prevent any backflow of blood. The aortic and pulmonic valves, which allow blood flow from the ventri-cles to the lungs and body, are known as *semilunar valves* because of their half-moon shape. The closure of the four valves is responsible for normal heart sounds (Fig. 24-38).

Heart

This examination includes assessment of the **precordium** (the aortic, pulmonic, tricuspid, and apical areas; see Fig. 24-38) and heart. Risk factors for consideration during this assessment include nutritional status, cholesterol levels, triglyceride levels, hypertension, congenital disorders, stress, use of tobacco, alcohol consumption, and use of medications.

The techniques used for assessment of the heart include inspection, palpation, and auscultation. (Inspection and palpation, although discussed separately here, are usually combined.) Equipment used in this examination are a stethoscope with a bell and diaphragm and a sphygmomanometer. The client is in a sitting or supine position with the head raised about 30 degrees. Adequate lighting is

FIGURE 24-38

View of the interior of the heart showing the atrioventricular and semilunar valves responsible for normal heart sounds.

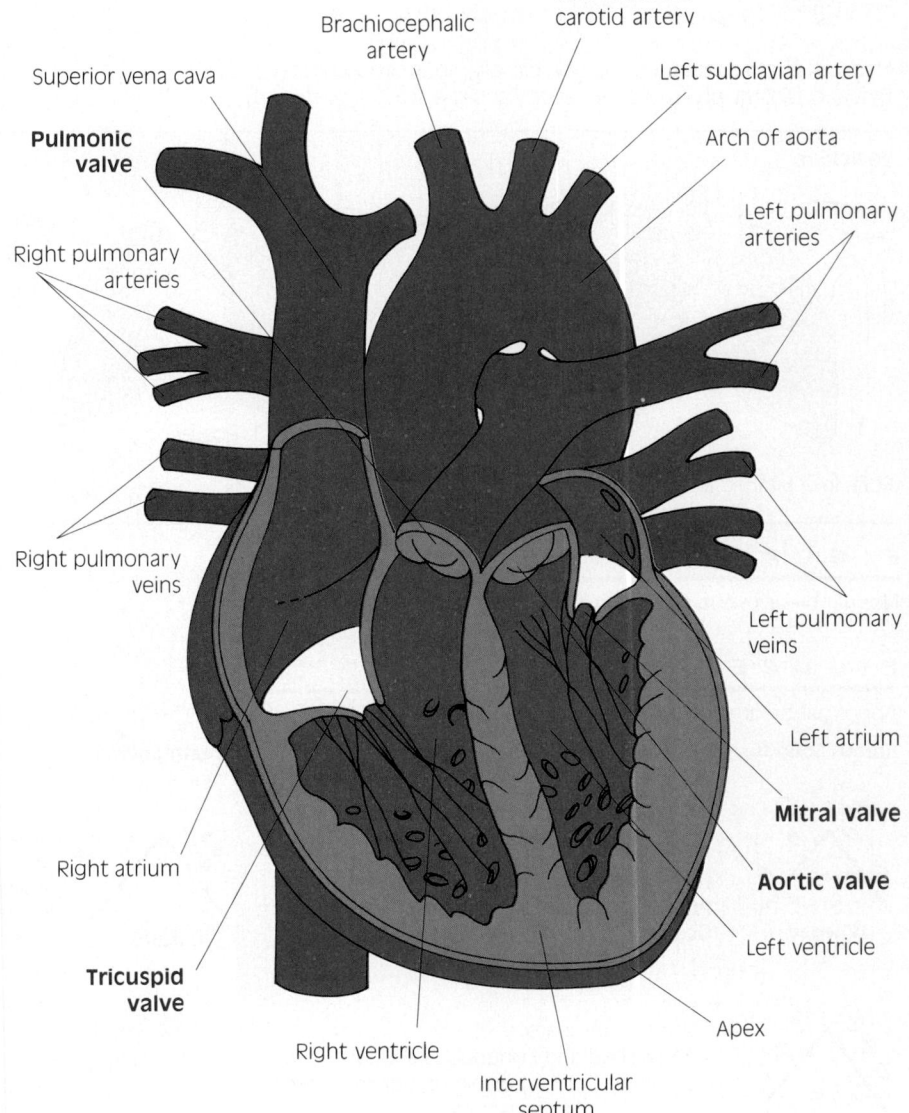

essential for inspection of color and pulsations. A quiet environment is necessary for accurate auscultation of heart sounds. The nurse is usually positioned at the right side of the client.

Inspection The neck and precordium are observed for visible pulsations. Generally, there are no visible pulsations, except the apical impulse (or the point of maximal impulse [PMI]), located approximately at the fourth or fifth intercostal space at the left midclavicular line. Inspect the epigastric area at the tip of the sternum for pulsation of the abdominal aorta. Findings of neck vein distention or visible pulsations in precordial areas other than the PMI are considered abnormal.

Palpation The precordium is palpated for the presence of pulsations. The nurse's hands, which should be warm, are used to gently palpate with the four fingers held together. Palpation proceeds in a systematic manner, with assessment of specific cardiac landmarks—the aortic, pulmonic, tricuspid, and mitral areas (Fig. 24-39).

Each area is palpated to determine if a pulsation is felt. Identify the PMI and record the apical impulse by interspace and relationship to the midsternal line or midclavicular line. Identify any precordial **thrills**, which are fine, palpable, rushing vibrations over the right or left second intercostal space; and *lifts* or *heaves*, which involve a rise along the border of the sternum with each heartbeat.

Normal findings include no pulsation palpable over the aortic and pulmonic areas, with a palpable pulsation at the PMI. Abnormal findings include visible pulsations, palpable thrill at the aortic, pulmonic, tricuspid, or mitral areas, and lifts or heaves.

Auscultation Auscultation is used to determine the heart sounds caused by closure of the heart valves. A systematic approach is used as the nurse attentively listens at all cardiac landmarks (Fig. 24-40). Auscultation is done systematically, beginning at the aortic area, then moving to the pulmonic, then to the tricuspid, and last to the apical areas. The client should breathe normally. The stethoscope diaphragm is first used to listen to high-pitched sounds, followed by use of the stethoscope bell to listen to low-pitched sounds. The nurse focuses on the overall rate and rhythm of the heart and the normal heart sounds (S_1 and S_2).

During auscultation, the first heart sound heard is the "lub" of "lub-dub." This sound occurs when the mitral and tricuspid valves close and corresponds with the onset of ventricular contraction (Fig. 24-41). The sound, low-pitched and dull, is called S_1, and is heard best at the apical area. The second heart sound, S_2, occurs at the termination of systole and corresponds with the onset of ventricular diastole. It is the "dub" of "lub-dub," and represents the closure of the aortic and pulmonic valves. The sound of S_2 is higher pitched and shorter than S_1. The two sounds occur within 1 second or less, depending on the heart rate.

Normal findings include S_1 to be louder at the tricuspid and apical areas, with S_2 louder at the aortic and pulmonic

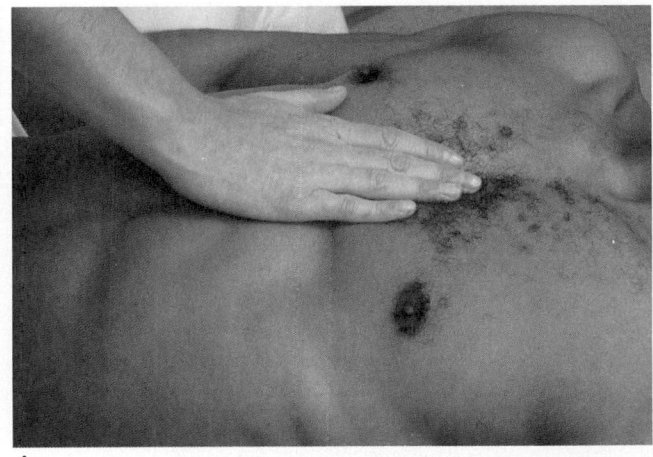

A

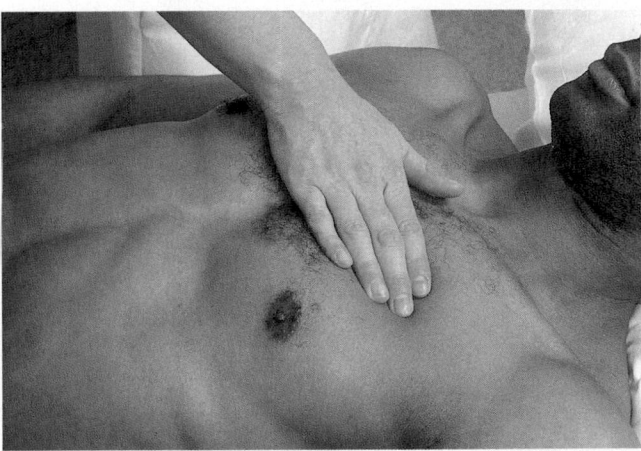

B

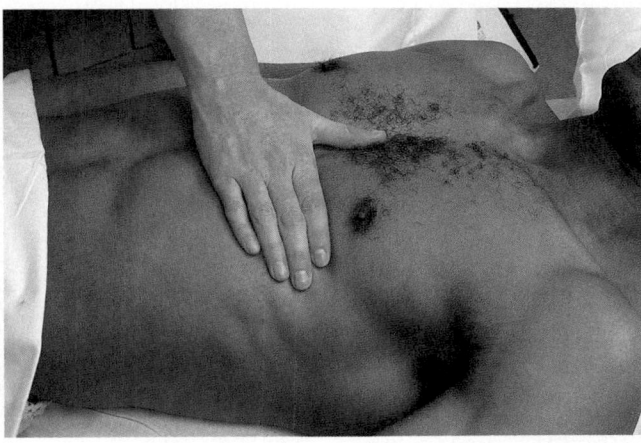

C

F I G U R E   2 4 - 3 9

Palpation of areas of the precordium: (A) aortic area, (B) pulmonic area, and (C) apical and tricuspic area. (Photo © Ken Kasper.)

areas. Abnormal findings include extra heart sounds at any of the cardiac landmarks, and abnormal rate or rhythm.

Extra heart sounds may be S_3, S_4, murmurs, or bruits. S_3, known as the *third heart sound*, often is represented by a "lub-dub-dee" pattern ("dee" being S_3); this sound is best

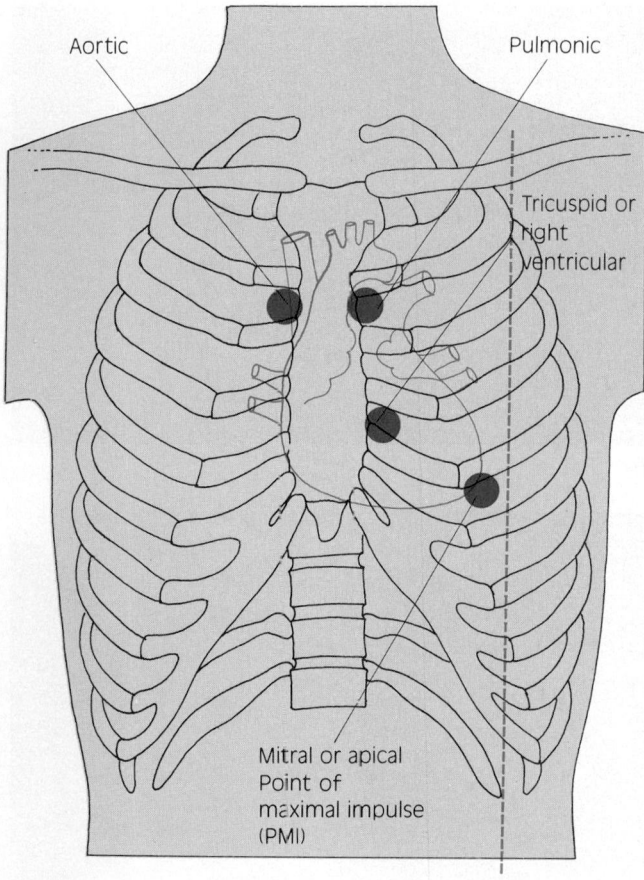

Pulmonic

Tricuspid or right ventricular

Mitral or apical
Point of
maximal impulse
(PMI)

FIGURE 24-40

Cardiac landmarks and sequence of examination using auscultation.

FIGURE 24-41

Heart sounds in relation to the cardiac cycle and an electrocardiogram.

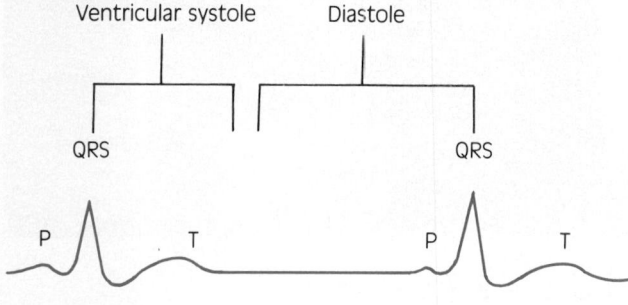

Ventricular systole   Diastole

QRS   QRS

P   T   P   T

Electrocardiogram

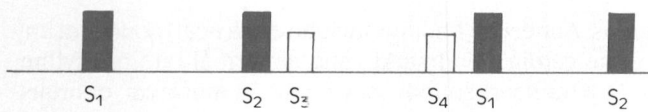

S_1 S_2 S_3 S_4 S_1 S_2

Heart sounds

heard with the stethoscope bell at the mitral area, with the client lying on the left side. S_3 is considered normal in children and young adults and abnormal in middle-aged and elderly adults. S_4 is the fourth heart sound, represented by "dee-lub-dub." S_4 is considered normal in elderly clients but abnormal in children and adults. Heart *murmurs* are extra heart sounds caused by some disruption of blood flow through the heart. The characteristics of a murmur depend on the adequacy of valve function, rate of blood flow, and the size of the valve opening. Table 24-5 illustrates the grading of heart murmurs. **Bruits** are sounds similar to murmurs and are heard over major blood vessels. The sound is indicative of a partially blocked or overextended artery, causing blood to swirl rather than flow straight. Bruits are most commonly heard over the carotid arteries, over the abdominal aorta, and over the femoral arteries.

Peripheral Vascular System

The *peripheral vascular assessment* includes measuring the blood pressure, assessing peripheral vascular pulses, and assessing peripheral vascular perfusion. Assessments are done by inspection and palpation, with the client in the sitting or supine position. Peripheral vascular assessments may be combined with assessment of other body areas.

Inspection   The skin of the extremities is inspected for color and temperature (as described previously for assessment of the integument); venous patterns; and edema. There should be no venous patterns evident (eg, varicosities, rashes, or ulcers) on the lower extremities. There should also be no edema present.

Palpation   To palpate peripheral pulses, use the pads of the index and middle fingers and palpate the pulse for rate, rhythm, amplitude, and symmetry. Palpate the carotid pulses (one at a time and with caution); the brachial pulses; the radial pulses; the femoral pulses; the popliteal pulses; the dorsalis pedis pulses; and the posterior tibial pulses. Figure 24-42 illustrates the palpation of each of these peripheral pulses.

TABLE 24-5

Common Grading System for Heart Murmurs	
Grade	**Description**
I	A murmur so faint that it can only be heard with great effort
II	A faint murmur but one that can be easily detected
III	A moderately loud murmur
IV	A very loud murmur that is usually associated with a thrill sound
V	An extremely loud murmur
VI	An exceptionally loud murmur that can be heard while the stethoscope is lifted off the skin

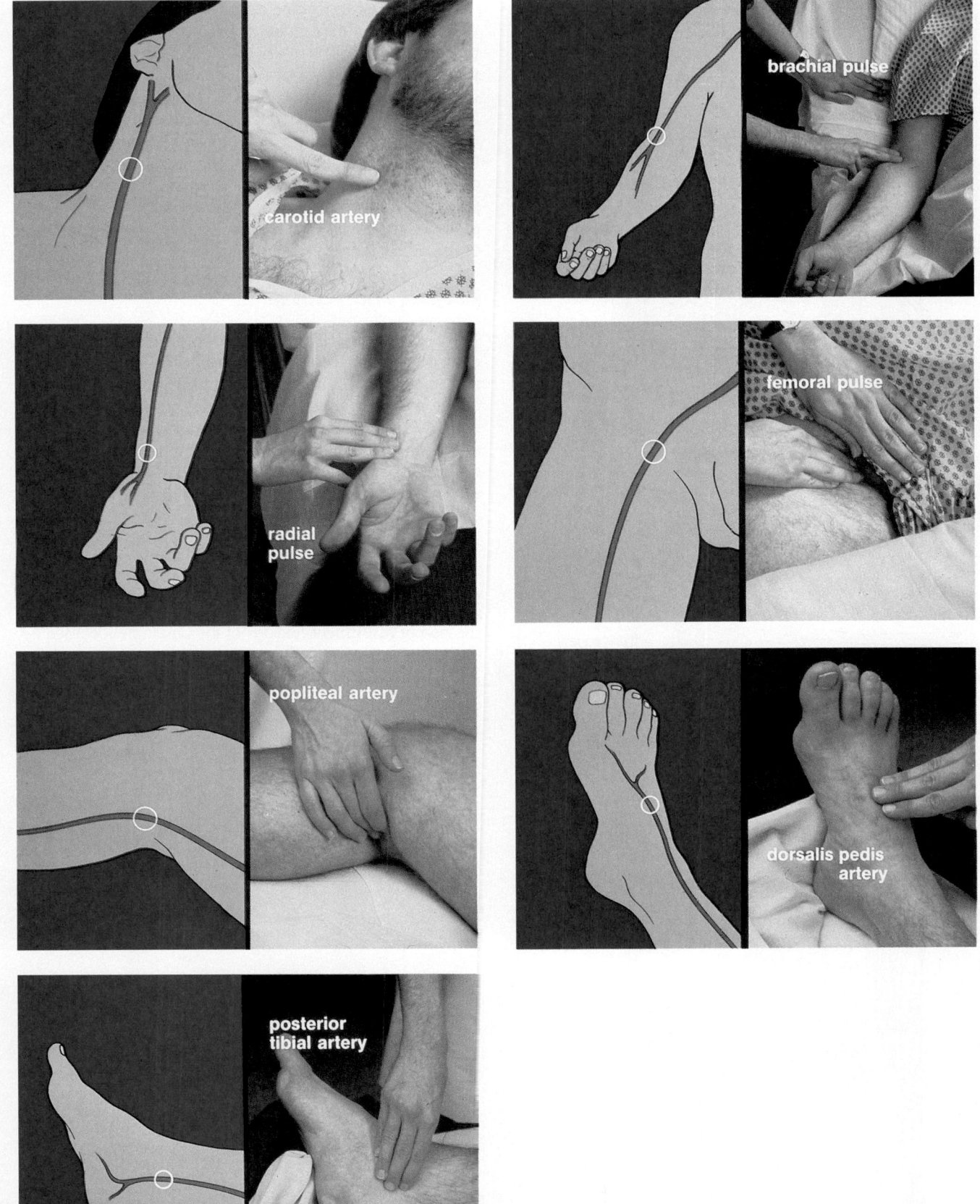

carotid artery

brachial pulse

radial pulse

femoral pulse

popliteal artery

dorsalis pedis artery

posterior tibial artery

FIGURE 24-42

Sites for palpation of peripheral pulses. (Lippincott Learning Systems.)

The pulse rate should range between 60 and 90 beats per minute, with a regular rhythm and strong and equal pulses bilaterally. It is unnecessary to determine rate on all peripheral pulses (eg, a strong palpable dorsalis pedis pulse is significant of good peripheral circulation). Abnormal findings include an increased or decreased rate, irregular rate, regularity with pauses or skipped beats, weak or thready pulse, forceful or bounding pulse, and asymmetry of pulses. Related abnormal assessments include cold, pale, cyanotic skin; edema; and varicosities. The blood pressure may be taken at this time or during the initial stage of the assessment.

Breasts and Axillae

The breasts are located on the anterior chest wall and extend from the second or third rib to the sixth or seventh rib. The breast comprises glandular, fibrous, and subcutaneous fatty tissue. The **areola**, a brown pigmented area, is located centrally on the breast and surrounds the nipple. Each breast comprises a lymphatic network that drains into the underlying axilla (Fig. 24-43). Although assessments and disorders focus on the female breast, both

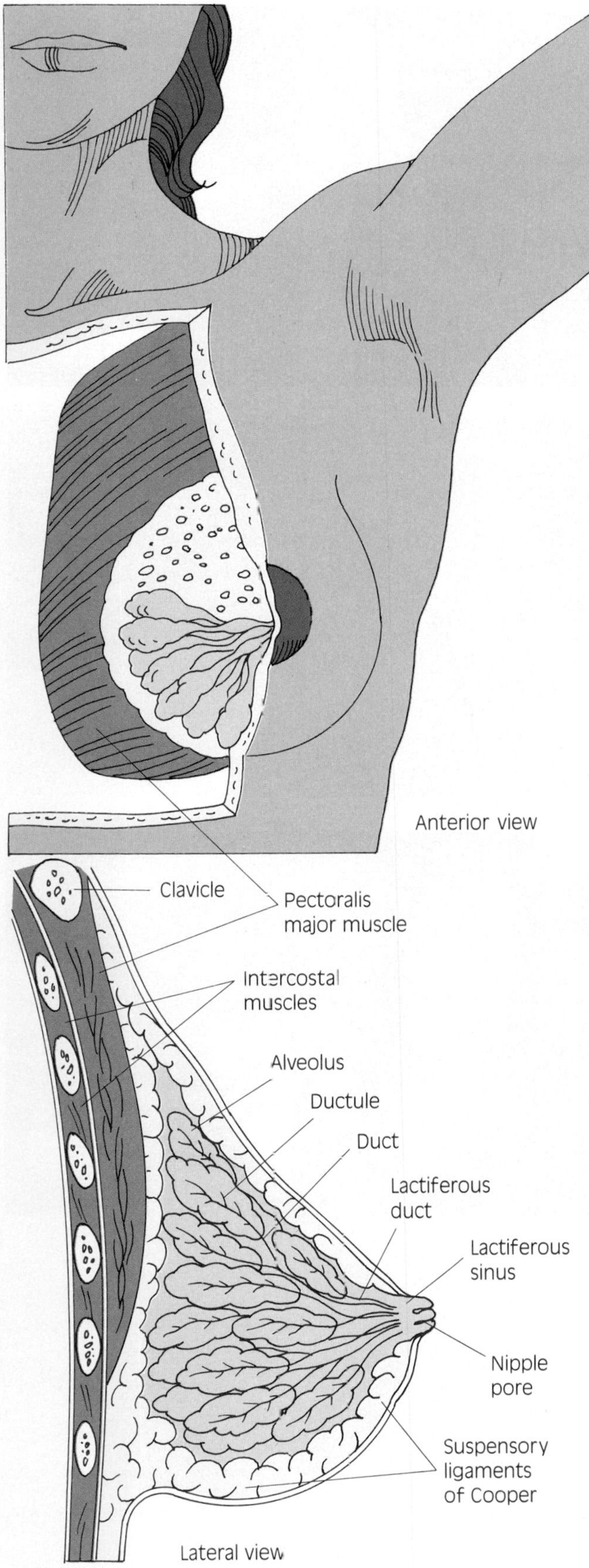

Anterior view

Clavicle

Pectoralis major muscle

Intercostal muscles

Alveolus

Ductule

Duct

Lactiferous duct

Lactiferous sinus

Nipple pore

Suspensory ligaments of Cooper

Lateral view

F I G U R E   2 4 - 4 3

Anterior and lateral views of the female breast.

F I G U R E   2 4 - 4 4

Location of assessment findings of the breast are identified by quadrant.

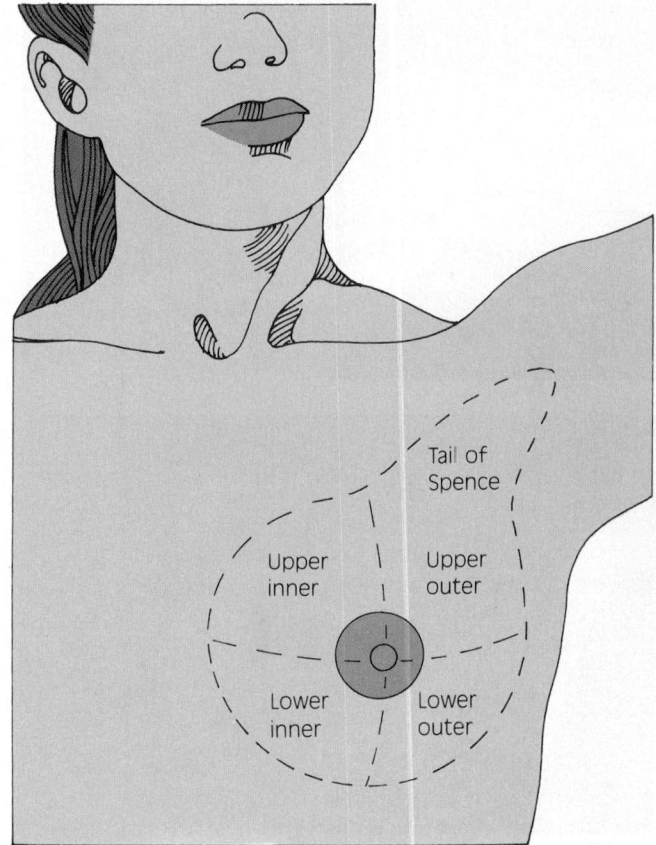

Tail of Spence

Upper inner

Upper outer

Lower inner

Lower outer

in size, round or oval, with a smooth surface. Montgomery's tubercles are a normal component of the areola. The nipples are normally everted. The skin is intact and without discharge.

Palpation The primary purpose of palpation is to detect any abnormal masses or lumps. The breast is divided into four quadrants: (1) the outer upper quadrant, (2) the outer lower quadrant, (3) the inner upper quadrant, and (4) the inner lower quadrant (Fig. 24-44). Using the pads of the first three fingers, each quadrant of each breast is palpated using a systematic method as the breast tissue is gently compressed against the chest wall (Fig. 24-45). The breast tissue should be smooth and firm with a granular consistency. If a mass is detected, the location, size, shape, consistency, and tenderness should be carefully assessed. The breasts are normally tender the week before the onset of menses. The nipple and areola are palpated, and the nipple is gently compressed between the thumb and forefinger to assess for discharge.

The axillary areas are palpated for lymph nodes, which normally are not palpable and are not tender. If any nodes are palpable, assess location, size, shape, consistency, tenderness, and mobility. The lymph nodes (Fig. 24-46) are the supraclavicular, subclavian, intermediate, brachial, scapular, mammary, and internal mammary. Abnormal findings when assessing the breast include presence of a lump, dimpling, nipple discharge, lesions, asymmetry, and palpable lymph nodes.

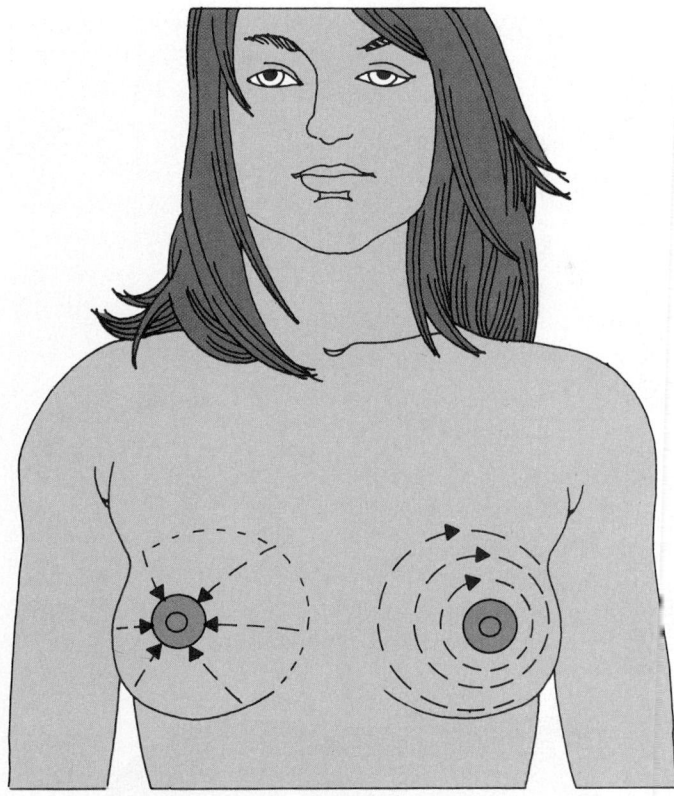

F I G U R E   2 4 - 4 5

Two techniques for palpation of the breast. (*Left*) Working in a clockwise direction, the examiner palpates the breast from the periphery toward the aureola at "hour" positions. (*Right*) The breast is palpated from the outer periphery in smaller and smaller circles moving toward the aureola.

male and female clients should have breast examinations. Men as well as women may have diseases of the breast.

Risk factors for consideration when assessing the breasts include age, changes in breast tissue, pain, discharge from the nipple, and knowledge and practice of breast self-examination (breast self-examination is discussed in Chapter 40). Inspection and palpation are the techniques used in the assessment. The client may be in a sitting or supine position. If sitting, the client should sit erect, arms at sides or abducted overhead. If supine, the client's hands are under the head.

Inspection The breasts and axilla are inspected for size, shape, symmetry, color, texture, and skin lesions. The breasts should be relatively symmetric, although variations are normal. The size varies among individuals. The shape of the breasts is round and smooth, and there should be no skin depressions (*retraction*) or puckering (*dimpling*). The color should be consistent with the rest of the skin, and the texture of the skin should be soft.

The areola and nipples are inspected for size and shape; the nipples are inspected for discharge, crusting, and inversion. The areolar and nipple areas should be equal

F I G U R E   2 4 - 4 6

Location of the cervical, axillary, and mammary lymph nodes.

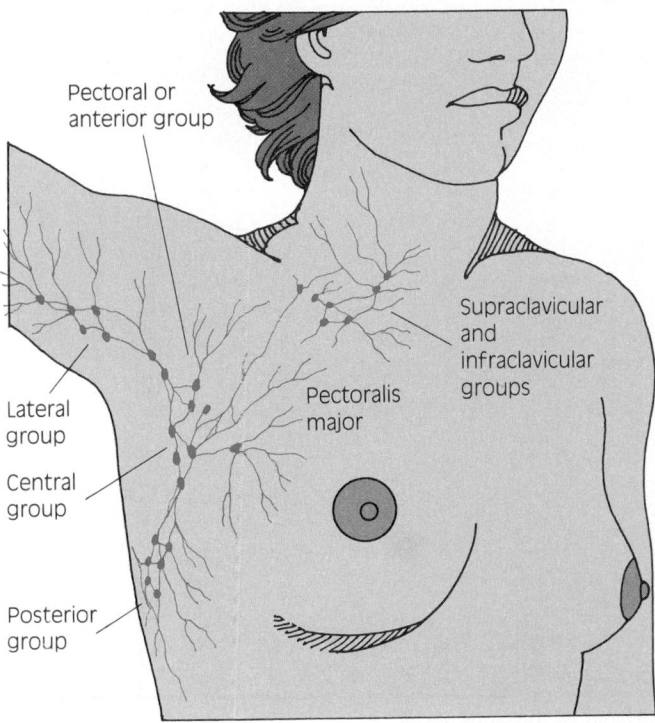

Pectoral or anterior group

Lateral group

Central group

Posterior group

Pectoralis major

Supraclavicular and infraclavicular groups

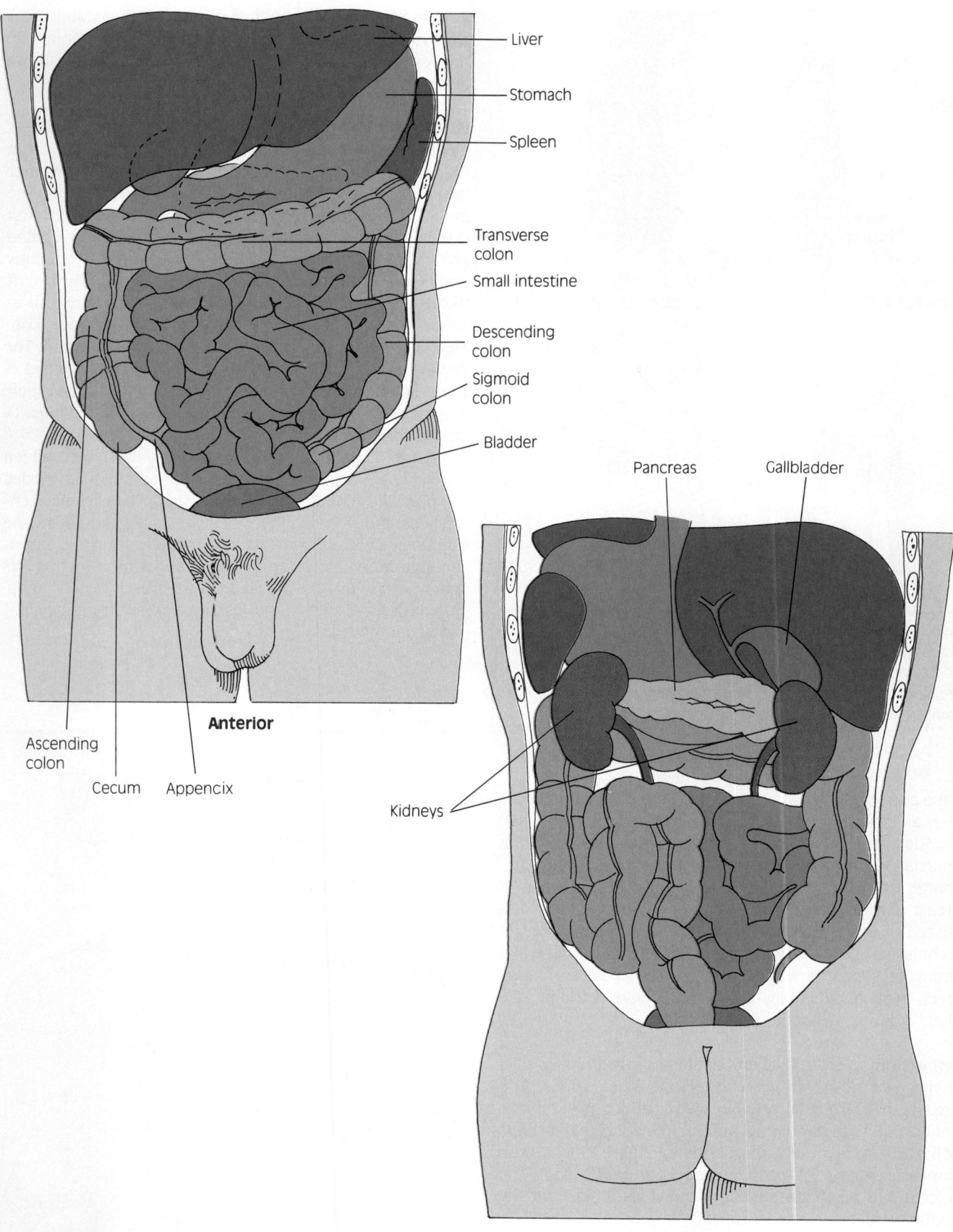

Liver

Stomach

Spleen

Transverse colon

Small intestine

Descending colon

Sigmoid colon

Bladder

Anterior

Ascending colon

Cecum

Appencix

Pancreas

Gallbladder

Kidneys

Posterior

F I G U R E   2 4 - 4 7

Organs of the abdominal cavity.

Abdomen

The abdominal cavity (Fig. 24-47) contains several vital organs. The stomach, the small intestine, and the large intestine ingest and digest food; absorb essential nutrients, electrolytes, and water; and excrete waste products. The liver, located in the right upper quadrant, is responsible for carbohydrate, fat, and protein metabolism. The gallbladder, located on the inferior surface of the liver, concentrates and stores bile. The pancreas lies behind the stomach and functions as an exocrine gland to produce hormones and digestive juices. The spleen is in the left upper quadrant above the kidney and functions as part of the reticuloendothelial system. The kidneys are responsible for filtration, reabsorption, and secretion of water and electrolytes and for eliminating wastes. The urinary bladder, located behind the symphysis pubis, collects and eliminates urine.

Factors to consider during assessment of the abdomen include nutrition, use of alcohol, stress, urine and stool characteristics, bowel habits, infectious diseases, trauma, and medications. A warm stethoscope, adequate lighting, and warm hands with short fingernails are needed for abdominal assessment. The client is placed in the supine position with the head slightly elevated and arms at sides. Small pillows may be placed under the head and knees. The client should have an empty bladder and be warm. These measures, as well as the position, help prevent contraction of the abdominal muscles.

To better locate organs and to make documentation more specific, the abdomen can be divided into four quadrants: (1) right upper, (2) right lower, (3) left upper, and (4) left lower (Fig. 24-48). Some examiners prefer to further divide the abdomen into nine sections: (1) right hypochondriac, (2) left hypochondriac, (3) right lumbar, (4) left lumbar, (5) right inguinal, (6) left inguinal, (7) epigastric, (8) umbilical, and (9) hypogastric.

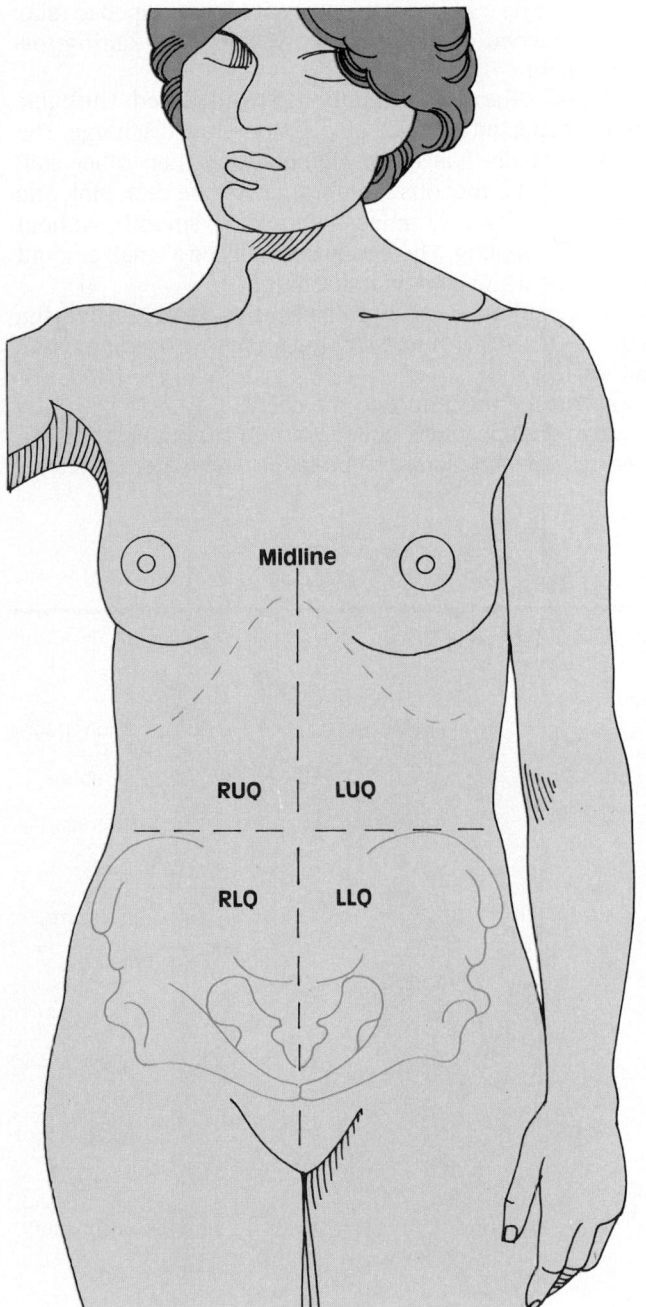

Midline

RUQ | LUQ

RLQ | LLQ

FIGURE 24-48

Diagram of abdominal quadrants and outline of underlying organs.

Right Upper Quadrant	Left Upper quadrant
Pylorus	Stomach
Duodenum	Spleen
Gallbladder	Left kidney and adrenal gland
Liver	Splenic flexure of the colon
Right kidney and adrenal gland	Body of pancreas
Hepatic flexure of the colon	
Head of the pancreas	

Right Lower Quadrant	Left Lower Quadrant
Cecum	Sigmoid colon
Appendix	Left ovary and fallopian tube (female)
Right ovary and fallopian tube (female)	Left ureter and lower kidney pole
Right ureter and lower kidney pole	Left spermatic cord (male)
Right Spermatic cord (male)	

Midline

Urinary bladder

Uretus (female)

The sequence of techniques used to assess the abdomen is inspection, auscultation, percussion, and palpation. Percussion and palpation stimulate bowel sounds and thus are done after auscultation of the abdomen.

Inspection The nurse inspects the abdomen while sitting at the right side of the client, allowing a tangential view that enhances shadows and contours. Inspection is made of skin color and surface characteristics, including the umbilicus, contour, symmetry, peristalsis, pulsations, and masses. The skin color may be slightly lighter than exposed areas. Fine white or silver lines (*striae*) may be visible and are caused by stretching from weight gain or pregnancy. The umbilicus should be centrally located and normally may be flat, rounded, or concave. The abdomen should be evenly rounded or symmetric, without visible peristalsis. In thin people, an upper midline pulsation may normally be visible.

Auscultation Auscultation is used to assess bowel sounds and vascular sounds. Auscultation is performed in a systematic manner, using the four quadrants as a guide. The stethoscope is warmed, and the flat diaphragm is placed lightly on the abdomen in one of the selected quadrants. Listen carefully for bowel sounds, and note their frequency and character; they are heard as clicks and gurgles and usually occur every 5 to 20 seconds. Move the stethoscope in a clockwise manner, assessing all four quadrants systematically. Using the bell of the stethoscope, auscultate over the aorta, renal arteries, and iliac arteries for bruits. Normal findings include increased, decreased, or absent bowel sounds (established after auscultating each quadrant for 5 minutes) and bruits.

Percussion All four quadrants are percussed in a systematic, clockwise manner to identify fluid, masses, or air. The nurse should note the distribution of sounds. Normal sounds are tympany over the abdomen, dullness over the liver, and dullness over a full bladder. The predominate percussion note in abdominal assessment is tympany. Abnormal findings include decreased tympany and increased dullness (possibly caused by fluid or a mass).

Palpation The pads of the fingers are used to palpate with a light, gentle, dipping motion. Watch the client's face for nonverbal signs of pain during palpation. Palpate each quadrant in a systematic manner, noting muscular resistance, tenderness, enlargement of the organs, or masses. The abdomen should normally be soft, relaxed, and free of tenderness. Abnormal findings include involuntary rigidity, spasm, and pain.

Male and Female Genitalia

This section discusses inspection and palpation of the genitalia. A discussion of male and female anatomy is in Chapter 40. A description of an internal pelvic examination is also included in this chapter, although individual health agency policies vary on whether this is included as part of the nursing examination. Equipment required includes a vaginal speculum, a good light source, and disposable gloves. The client should have an empty bladder.

Female Genitalia

The external female genitalia consist of the mons pubis, labia majora and minora, clitoris, vestibular glands, vaginal vestibule, vaginal orifice, and urethral opening (Fig. 24-49). Factors in assessing the female genitalia include menstrual history, sexual history, use of contraceptives, and frequency of pelvic examinations. The woman is placed in the lithotomy position on the examination table, legs in stirrups, and draped so that only the genitalia are exposed. She should be told about the procedure and helped to relax as it is carried out. The nurse wears gloves during this assessment.

Initially, the external genitalia are inspected. The pubic area is inspected for color, size, lesions, and discharge. The vulva normally has more pigmentation than other skin areas, and the mucous membranes will be dark pink and moist. The skin and mucosa should be smooth, without lesions or swelling. There may normally be a small amount of clear or whitish vaginal discharge.

A speculum is used to inspect the cervix and vagina (Fig. 24-50). The nine-step inspection procedure is as follows:
- Explain the procedure to the client.
- Warm the speculum under warm, running water; if cytologic specimens are to be taken, the water serves as

F I G U R E   2 4 - 4 9

External female genitalia.

- Mons pubis
- Prepuce
- Clitoris
- Labia majora
- Urinary meatus
- Labia minora
- Vaginal introitus
- Hymen
- Perineum
- Anus

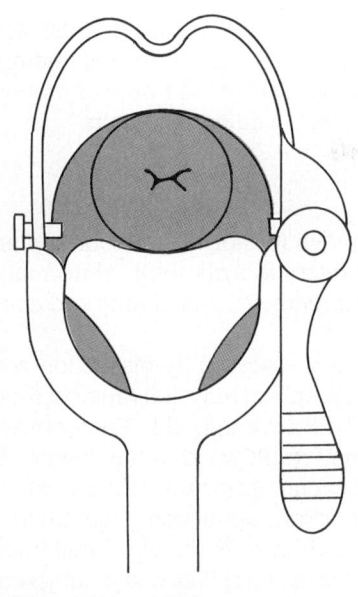

FIGURE 24-50

View of the cervix and cervical os through a vaginal speculum.

the lubricant; if no specimens are needed, a water-soluble lubricant may be used.
- Using two fingers placed just inside the vagina, press down gently on the posterior vaginal wall.
- Insert the speculum blades into the vagina, posterior in direction at a 45-degree angle. Ensure no pubic hair is caught in the speculum.
- Turn the speculum so that the handle is down and the blades are in a horizontal position.
- Open the blades and close the screw that locks the blades open.

- Inspect the cervix and os for size, color, shape, lesions, and discharge.
- Withdraw the blades slowly, observing the vaginal walls.
- When the speculum blades are clear of the cervix, release the screw so that the blades close, and withdraw the speculum from the vagina.

Abnormal findings include redness, swelling of glands, discharge, lesions, and pain. For related assessments, such as the urinary tract and sexually transmitted diseases (STDs), see Chapters 34 and 40, respectively.

Male Genitalia

The male genitalia (Fig. 24-51) include the penis, testicles, epididymis, scrotum, prostate gland, and seminal vesicles. Factors to consider for assessment of male genitalia include the client's employment, sexual history, and testicular self-examination. The client may be standing or in the supine position. Gloves are worn by the nurse during this assessment.

The external male genitalia are inspected for size, placement, contour, appearance of the skin, inflammation, and discharge. The male client may be circumcised or uncircumcised; if uncircumcised, the foreskin is retracted for inspection of the glans penis. The location of the urinary meatus is also assessed. The scrotum is inspected for symmetry; it is not unusual for the left testicle to lie lower in the scrotal sac than the right testicle. The size, shape, and consistency of the scrotal contents should be similar. Abnormal findings are the presence of lesions, pain, discharge, fluid-filled masses in the scrotum, and displacement of the urinary meatus or difficulties with voiding. (See Chapters 34 and 40 for further discussion of the male urinary tract and STDs.)

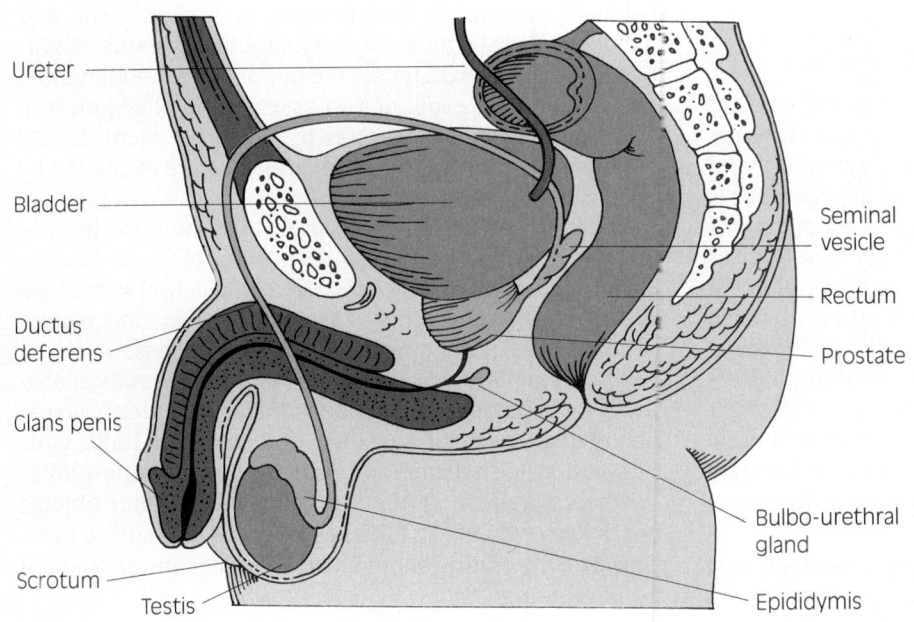

FIGURE 24-51

Organs of the male urogenital system.

Ureter

Bladder

Ductus deferens

Glans penis

Scrotum

Testis

Seminal vesicle

Rectum

Prostate

Bulbo-urethral gland

Epididymis

Rectum and Anus

The rectum and anus form the last portion of the gastrointestinal tract. The anal canal is about 2 to 4 cm in length and opens onto the perineum. Techniques used for examination of the rectum and anus are inspection and palpation. Necessary equipment includes lubricant and good lighting. The nurse wears gloves during this assessment. The client may be in the Sims', knee–chest, or lithotomy position, or may be standing while leaning over the examination table.

Inspection is used to assess the anal area. The area normally has increased pigmentation and some hair growth. Palpation is used to assess the rectum, using a well-lubricated, gloved index finger. Sphincter tone at the anus should be good, and the mucosal lining smooth. (Fecal specimens may be taken at this time, if necessary.) The prostate gland in men can be assessed for size, shape, and consistency through the anterior rectal wall; the gland is normally smooth, firm, and about 1 3/4 inches (4 cm) in size. In women, the cervix may be felt as a small, round mass when palpating the anterior rectal wall. Abnormal findings include relaxed musculature; cracks, nodules, or hemorrhoids at the anal sphincter; bleeding; discharge; and hard or abnormally colored stools.

Musculoskeletal System

The primary structures of the musculoskeletal system are the bones, muscles, cartilage, ligaments, tendons, and joints. The musculoskeletal system provides movement, protection, and support. Assessments are made of muscles, bones, and joints. During the assessment, the client assumes a variety of positions, including standing, sitting, and supine. Assessments of the musculoskeletal system can be integrated into the assessment of other body systems. Factors to consider during this examination include a history of arthritis, trauma, or neurologic disorders; pain; and loss of or altered function.

Muscles

The muscles are examined by inspection and palpation of muscle groups and by testing muscle tone and strength. Muscle groups are observed for bilateral symmetry and palpated for tenderness; normally they are symmetric and are not tender. Muscle *tone* (the normal condition of a muscle at rest) is evaluated by putting each joint and extremity through passive range of motion. Bilateral equal resistance should be present. Muscle strength is assessed by asking the client to move against resistance. Observe muscle contraction and determine muscle strength exerted. An individual's dominant side is normally stronger than the nondominant side. Techniques for testing muscle strength are illustrated in Figure 24-52. Muscle strength should be bilaterally equal with slight increase on the dominant side.

Muscles are normally firm, with good strength and tone. Abnormal findings include *atrophy*, a decrease in size; **tremors**, involuntary movements; and *flaccidity*, weakness of muscles. Other abnormal findings are loss of strength and tone, decreased range of motion, uncoordinated movements, swelling, and pain.

Bones

Bones are palpated for normal contour and prominences, as well as for bilateral symmetry. Abnormal findings include pain, enlargement, and changes in contour.

Joints Joints are assessed by inspection and palpation. Normally, each joint will have full range of motion, will not be tender, and will move smoothly. Each joint is put through full range of motion (ROM), and the degree of ROM is assessed. Joint movements include flexion, extension, hyperextension, abduction, adduction, supination, and pronation. Joints are palpated for the abnormal findings of pain, swelling, nodules, and *crepitation* (a grating sound heard on movement). See Chapter 30 for further discussion and illustration of joint mobility.

Neurologic System

The **neurologic system**, which is responsible for cognitive, behavioral, and involuntary processes, is the most complex of the body systems and integrates all other body systems. The *central nervous system*, comprising the brain and spinal cord, is responsible for receiving sensory stimuli from the environment, using adaptive processes to maintain body functions, controlling cognitive and voluntary behavioral processes, and controlling unconscious and involuntary body functions. The neurologic assessment is conducted by observing the client to detect normal and abnormal findings for cerebral function, cranial nerve function, cerebellar function, motor and sensory function, and reflexes.

Cerebral function is assessed by observing the client's behavior throughout the interview and assessment, and includes mental status, memory, emotional status, cognitive abilities, and behavior. Fine motor skills, coordination, and balance are evaluated to assess cerebellar function. The sensory system is assessed by having the client identify various sensory stimuli, and the reflexes are evaluated by contraction of specific muscles.

Factors for consideration in this examination include environmental hazards (eg, exposure to lead, insecticides, or chemicals); emotional and intellectual status; use of alcohol or other chemicals; medication; and history of seizures, dizziness, weakness, or numbness.

Equipment for this examination includes vials of aromatic substances (eg, peppermint and vanilla); visual acuity devices; penlight; sharp object; cotton balls; vials of solution to test taste (eg, salt or sugar); tuning fork; tongue depressor; reflex hammer; and familiar objects (eg, a key or coin). The client should be in a sitting position, and the environment should be quiet and should not be distracting.

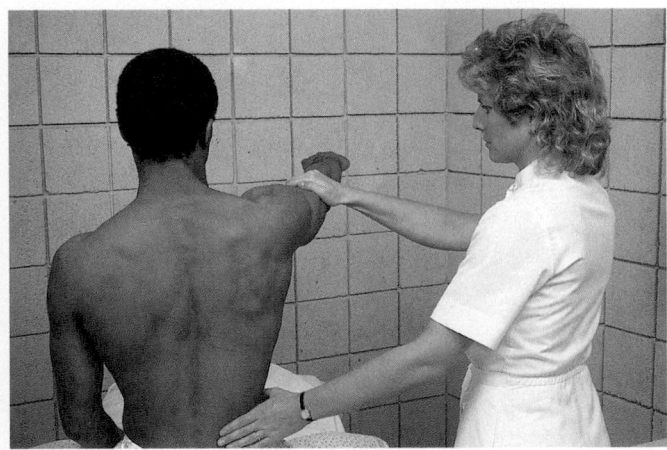

The client flexes shoulder muscle against resistance of examiner's hand.

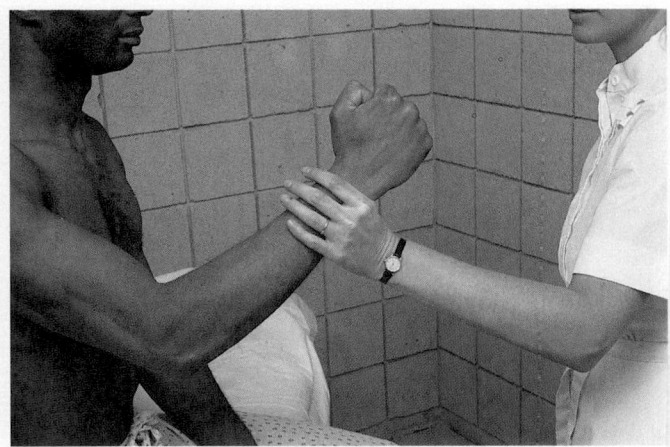

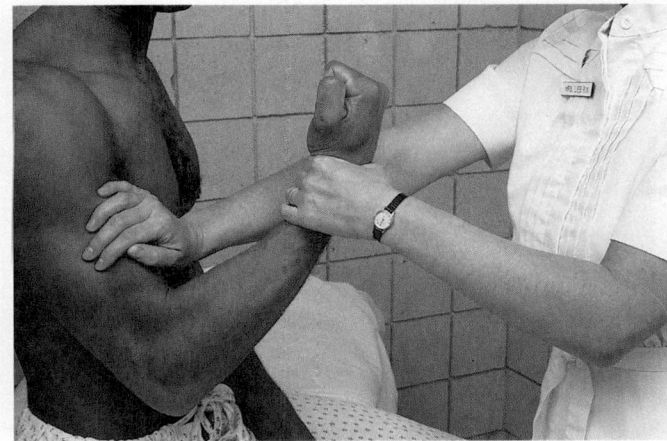

Elbow extension and flexion. The client first extends elbow against resistance by the examiner, then flexes elbow against resistance.

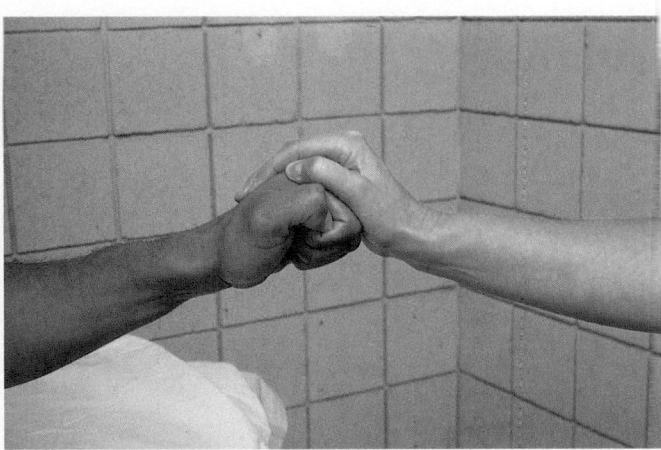

Wrist extension. The client makes a fist and resists the examiner's attempts to pull wrist down.

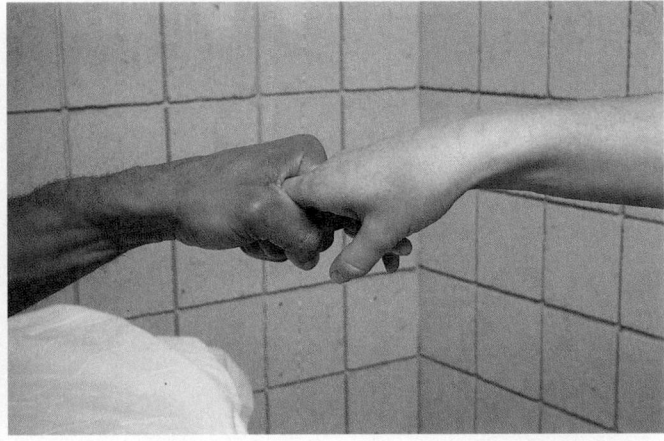

Testing grip. Client squeezes examiner's index and middle fingers.

FIGURE 24-52

Techniques for testing muscle strength. (Photos © Ken Kasper.)

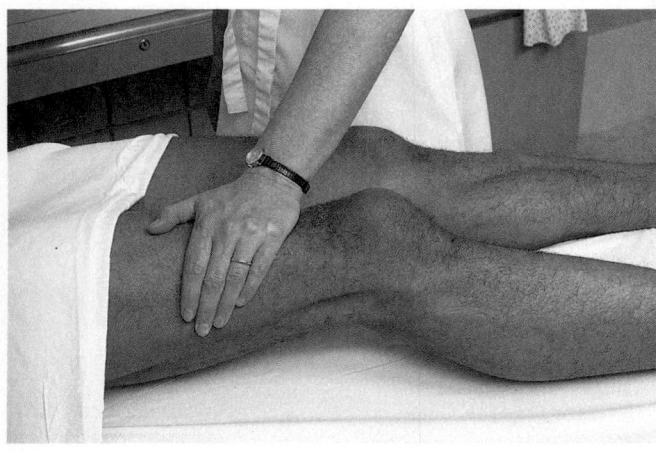

Hip flexion. Client attempts to raise his thigh against examiner's resistance.

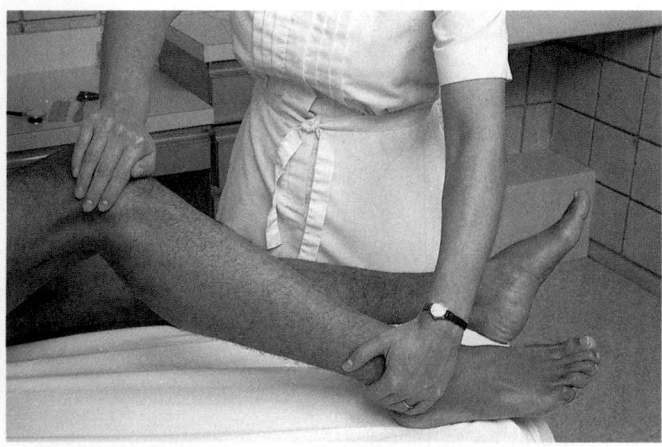
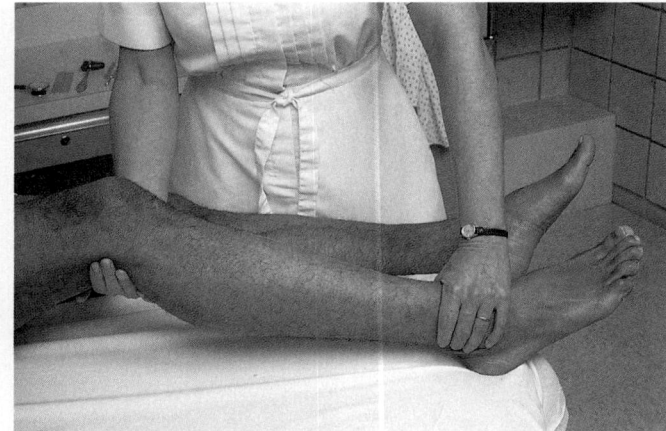

Knee flexion and extension. With the client's knee bent and foot on the examining table, the client attempts to keep foot down while examiner attempts to straighten the client's leg to test flexion. To test extension, the examiner supports client's knee, and the client attempts to straighten his leg against examiner resistance at the ankle.

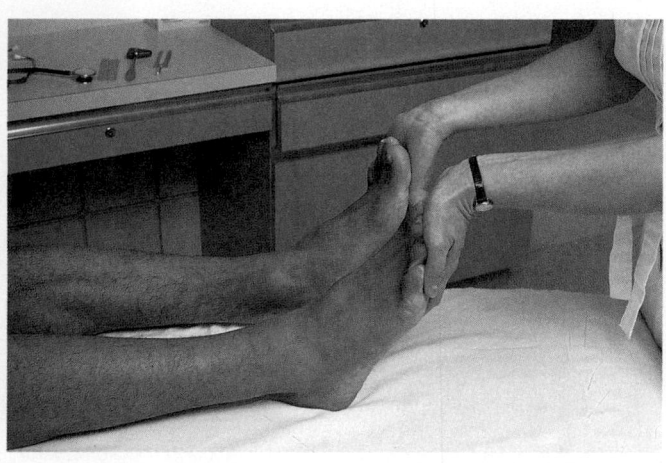
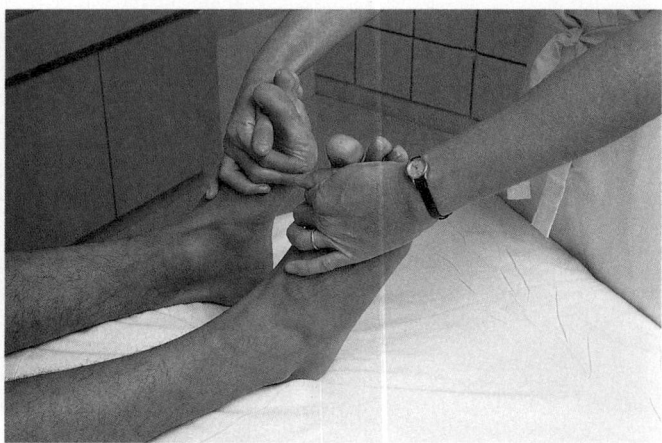

Ankle plantar flexion and dorsiflexion. The client first pushes the balls of the feet against resistance of examiner's hands, then attempts to pull against examiner's resistance.

F I G U R E   2 4 - 5 2 (continued)

FOCUS ON THE OLDER ADULT

Normal Alterations in Physical Examinations With Aging

Integument

- Wrinkles, dryness, scaling
- Decreased turgor
- Raised dark areas (senile keratosis)
- Flat brown age spots (senile lentigines)
- Small, round, red spots (cherry angioma)
- Fine, brittle, gray or white hair
- Loss of hair (alopecia)
- Coarse facial hair in women, decreased body hair in both men and women
- Thick, yellow toenails; may be ingrown

Head and Neck

- Dry mucous membranes of mouth
- Unable to taste or smell as acutely
- White ring around iris (arcus senilis)
- Decreased tear production
- Clouding of lens (cataracts)
- Decrease in near vision (presbyopia), in peripheral vision, and in accommodation
- Decreased hearing acuity (presbycusis)

Thorax and Lungs

- Increase in dorsal spinal curve (kyphosis)
- Decreased breath sounds
- Hyperresonance on percussion
- Systolic murmurs are common

Breasts

- Less firm, pendulous, more nodular

Peripheral Vascular

- Rigid, tortuous veins and arteries
- Increased systolic and diastolic blood pressure
- Increased systolic pressure, widening pulse pressure

Abdomen

- Decreased bowel sounds
- Decreased abdominal tone
- Liver span shorter and liver border more easily palpated

Genitalia

- Decrease in size of labia
- Decreased vaginal secretions
- Shortened vaginal vault
- Decrease in size of penis

Musculoskeletal

- Loss of muscle mass and strength
- Decrease in range of motion
- Decrease in height

Neurologic

- Slower thought processes and verbal responses
- Decreased sensory ability
- Slower coordination and voluntary movements
- Decreased or slower reflex responses

Examination of Mental Status

Components of the mental status examination include assessment of orientation, level of consciousness, behavior and appearance, memory, abstract reasoning, and language. The following discussion of each of these components includes sample questions or specific assessments to use during the assessment.

Orientation   Orientation to time, place, and person are included in this part of the examination, which assesses a person's awareness. The following questions may be used:

Time
- What is today's date?
- What day of the week is it?
- What season of the year is this?
- What was the last holiday?

Place
- Where are you now?
- What is the name of this city?
- What state are we in?

Person
- What is your name?
- How old are you?
- Who came to visit you this morning?

Although exceptions may occur, in most instances, individuals who have impaired awareness first lose time orientation, followed by place orientation, and then person orientation. Remember that it is often difficult to know the exact date when one is ill, in pain, or in unfamiliar surroundings.

Level of Consciousness   Consciousness is the degree of wakefulness or the ability of a person to be aroused. This is not the same as orientation; a client may be conscious but not oriented. The two assessments involve (1) describing level of consciousness and (2) using the Glasgow Coma Scale.

Level of consciousness is described as follows:

Awake and alert—fully awake; oriented to person, place and time; responds to all stimuli including verbal commands

Lethargic—appears drowsy or asleep most of the time but makes spontaneous movements; can be aroused by gentle shaking and saying client's name

Stuporous—unconscious most of the time; no spontaneous movement; must shake or shout to arouse; can make verbal responses, but these are less likely to be appropriate

Comatose—cannot be aroused, even with use of painful stimuli; may have some reflex activity (as gag reflex); if no reflexes present, is in a deep coma

The Glasgow Coma Scale is a standardized assessment tool that assesses level of consciousness. Three parameters are evaluated—eye opening, motor response, and verbal response. Scores are given in each category and a total score is recorded, with higher scores indicating a more normal level of functioning. A score of 7 or less defines coma. This is a more accurate evaluation of mental status over time. The scale is illustrated in Table 24-6.

Memory   Memory is assessed by asking questions that call for answers demonstrating immediate recall and recall for past events. The following may be used:

Immediate

- Ask the client to repeat a series of numbers forward or backward (eg, three, six, nine). Start with three numbers and gradually increase the digits until the client cannot respond correctly. Most adults can repeat a series of five to eight numbers forward and four to six digits backward.
- Ask: What did you eat for your most recent meal?

Past

- Ask: When is your birthday? or When is your wedding anniversary?

Abstract Reasoning   Ask the client to explain a proverb such as, "The early bird catches the worm". If intellectual ability is impaired, the client will usually give a literal explanation or repeat the phrase. Be sure that the phrase is not culture-specific.

Language   The cerebral cortex controls the ability to express self through writing, words, or gestures and to understand the spoken and written word. Injury to the cortex can cause *aphasia*, which is a disorder of language ability. Aphasia may be *expressive* (in which the individual understands written and spoken words but cannot write or speak to communicate effectively) or *receptive* (the individual cannot understand written or spoken words). These aphasias also may be combined. Some simple methods of assessing language capabilities include the following:

- Ask the client to name items in the room (eg, bed, flowers, gown, or pajamas).
- Ask the client to follow simple commands, such as, "Point to your head".
- Ask the client to read a short sentence aloud.
- Ask the client to match printed and spoken words with appropriate pictures.

On initial contact, the nurse begins to evaluate the client's orientation level to person, place, and time, as well as cognitive abilities and affect (eg, does the client know who he or she is, where he or she is, and the day or month or year). The nurse observes the client's appearance, general behavior, and responses to questions. Any variation in responses should be noted. The nurse also assesses the client's ability to speak clearly. The client should have a clean, neat appearance with erect posture; be oriented to person, place, and time; have memory recall (both short-term and long-term memory); and have the ability to demonstrate coherent and logical thought processes. Abnormal findings include poor hygiene, inappropriate dress, disorientation, absent memory recall, and incoherent or illogical thought processes.

Examination of Cranial Nerve Function

The function of the twelve cranial nerves is assessed primarily during the neurologic examination, although parts of cranial nerve function are assessed with other body systems (eg, pupillary response). The cranial nerves are outlined in Table 24-7. Each nerve has a specific function and is evaluated individually.

Olfactory (I) Nerve   The olfactory nerve is a sensory nerve and its function is the sense of smell. Two or three vials of liquids with aromatic odors, such as coffee, vanilla, or peppermint, should be available. The client is asked to close the eyes and occlude one nostril (by pressing a finger against the side of the nose). The client is then asked to take

T A B L E   2 4 - 6

Glasgow Coma Scale		
Component	**Response**	**Score**
Eye opening	Spontaneous	4
	To verbal command	3
	To pain	2
	No response	1
Motor response	To verbal command	6
	To localized pain	5
	Flexes/withdraws	4
	Flexes abnormally	3
	Extends abnormally	2
	No response	1
Verbal response	Oriented/talks	5
	Disoriented/talks	4
	Inappropriate words	3
	Incomprehensible sounds	2
	No response	1

TABLE 24-7

Cranial Nerves			
Nerve (Number)	Type	Functions	Methods for Examining Nerve
Olfactory (I)	Sensory	Sense of smell	Test each nostril for smell reception and interpretation
Optic (II)	Sensory	Sense of vision	Test vision for acuity and visual fields
Oculomotor (III)	Motor	Pupil constriction Raise eyelids	Test pupillary reaction to light and ability to open and close eyelids
Trochlear (IV)	Motor	Downward inward eye movement	Test for downward and inward movement of the eye
Trigeminal (V)	Motor	Jaw movements—chewing and mastication	Ask client to open and clench jaws while palpating the jaw muscles
	Sensory	Sensation on the face and neck	Test face and neck for pain sensations, light touch, temperature
Abducens (VI)	Motor	Lateral movement of the eyes	Test ocular movement in all directions
Facial (VII)	Motor	Muscles of the face	As the client to raise eyebrows, smile, show teeth, puff out cheeks
	Sensory	Sense of taste on the anterior two thirds of the tongue	Test for the taste sensation with various agents
Acoustic (VIII)	Sensory	Sense of hearing	Test hearing ability
Glossopharyngeal (IX)	Motor	Pharyngeal movement and swallowing	Ask the client to say "ah," and have client yawn to observe upward movement of the soft palate; elicit gag response; note ability to swallow
	Sensory	Sense of taste on the posterior one third of the tongue	Test for taste with various agents
Vagus (X)	Motor	Swallowing and speaking	Ask the client to swallow and speak; note hoarseness
Accessory (XI)	Motor	Movement of shoulder muscles	Ask the client to shrug shoulders against your resistance
Hypoglossal (XII)	Motor	Movement of the tongue; strength of the tongue	Ask the client to protrude tongue; ask client to push tongue against cheek

a breath as the vial is placed under the open nostril, and to identify the odor; the process is then repeated for the opposite nostril. Normal findings are equal and bilateral sense of smell; abnormal findings are the inability to identify the odor or absence of smell.

Optic (II) Nerve The optic nerve is a sensory nerve whose function is vision. Vision is tested for acuity and visual fields, as described earlier in the chapter in the discussion on examination of the eye. Abnormal findings include changes in vision, blurring of vision, or inability to identify letters, numbers, or pictures.

Oculomotor (III), Trochlear (IV), and Abducens (VI) Nerves The oculomotor, trochlear, and abducens nerves are motor nerves that control movement of the eyes through the cardinal fields of gaze; pupil size, shape, response to light, and accommodation; and opening of the upper eyelids. These assessments are discussed in the examination of the eye, earlier in the chapter. Normal responses include round pupils that are equal in size, direct

and consensual pupillary response, lid margin flush with the surface of the eyeball, equal and complete bilateral lid closure, and parallel movements of the eyes. Abnormal findings include asymmetric eye position, a portion of the eye not covered by the eyelid, lesions, edema, abnormal eye movements, and inability for one or both eyes to follow the cardinal fields.

Trigeminal (V) Nerve The trigeminal nerve is a sensory and motor (sensorimotor) nerve. Motor function is assessed by observing the facial muscles for deviation of the jaw to one side and by instructing the client to clench the jaw and palpating the tone of the muscles. Sensory status of the nerve is assessed by testing for the ability to discriminate between sharp, dull, and light touch. The client is asked to close the eyes, and as the nurse touches each side of the client's face with a needle or paper clip, to report whether the sensation is sharp or dull. The same procedure is used for light touch, using a wisp of cotton and asking the client to tell you when and where on the face the sensation is felt. Normally, the client will correctly identify sharp, dull, and soft sensation of the face and neck bilaterally. Abnormal findings are decreased or absent sensations unilaterally or bilaterally.

Facial (VII) Nerve The facial nerve is a sensorimotor nerve that innervates the muscles of the face and functions also to provide the taste sensation of the anterior two thirds of the tongue. Motor function is evaluated by observing a series of expressions that you ask the client to make: Raise the eyebrows, smile and show the teeth, and puff out the cheeks. Facial expressions should be symmetric. The taste sensation of the tongue is tested by placing a small amount of various taste solutions (eg, sugar, salt, or lemon) on the anterior two thirds of the tongue as the client, with eyes closed, protrudes the tongue. Various substances should be normally correctly identified; abnormal findings include incorrect identification of substances or the inability to taste.

Acoustic (VIII) Nerve The acoustic nerve is a sensory nerve that is tested by assessing hearing ability, as described previously in assessment of the ear. The client should be able to hear bilaterally; abnormal findings are the inability to hear unilaterally or bilaterally.

Glossopharyngeal (IX) Nerve The glossopharyngeal nerve is a sensorimotor nerve that allows tongue movement and swallowing, as well as taste sensations of the posterior one third of the tongue. The motor function of this nerve is assessed with the vagus (X) nerve, and the taste function is assessed with the facial (VII) nerve. The client should be able to identify various taste substances correctly, have a gag reflex, and be able to move the tongue.

Vagus (X) Nerve The vagus nerve is a motor nerve that is assessed by asking the client to open the mouth and say,

"Ah" as the upward movement of the soft palate is observed. The uvula should remain midline and rise symmetrically. The swallowing reflex can be assessed by having the client sip and swallow water.

Accessory (XI) Nerve The accessory nerve is a motor nerve that controls the movement of the head and shoulders. Ask the client to shrug the shoulders upward and turn the head against the resistance of your hands (Fig. 24-53). There should be equal movement and strength of the muscles of the shoulder and head bilaterally.

Hypoglossal (XII) Nerve The hypoglossal nerve is a motor nerve that affects the movement and strength of the tongue. Ask the client to protrude the tongue forward and to push out the cheek with the tongue. The protrusion should be symmetric, and the cheek should have a puffed-out appearance. Abnormal findings include asymmetry of tongue movements, drooping, weakness, tremors, and loss of strength.

Assessment of Motor, Sensory, and Reflex Abilities

This part of the neurologic assessment includes the motor, sensory, and reflex abilities of the client. Motor ability is assessed by balance, gait, and coordination; sensory function is assessed by sensory discrimination of pain, light touch, and vibrations; and deep tendon reflexes are evaluated to determine the functioning ability of specific spinal segment levels.

Motor Abilities

Balance and Gait Balance and gait are evaluated by having the client walk across the room on the toes, on the heels, and heel-to-toe. The nurse observes posture, balance, and arm and leg movements. The posture should be erect, with slight swaying in the standing position, and the gait even with simultaneous arm movements. Abnormal findings include loss of balance, shuffling, wide-based gait, and abnormal patterns of gait.

Motor Function and Coordination Motor function and coordination are evaluated by having the client rapidly touch each finger with the thumb, rapidly pat the hand on the thigh, and tap the foot against the floor (or against your hand, if the client is supine). Normally, the movements should be coordinated.

Sensory Abilities Sensory perception is tested by evaluating the client's response to pain, light touch, and vibrations. With the client's eyes closed, a sharp object and a soft object are used randomly to touch upper and lower extremities to test sensation. This examination proceeds from distal (ie, hands, arms, feet, or legs) to proximal (ie, trunk). The client should be able to distinguish between sharp (pain) and soft or dull touch. The same process is repeated by

F I G U R E   2 4 - 5 3

Test of the spinal accessory nerve. The client shrugs his shoulders against the resistance of the examiner's hands. (Photo © Ken Kasper.)

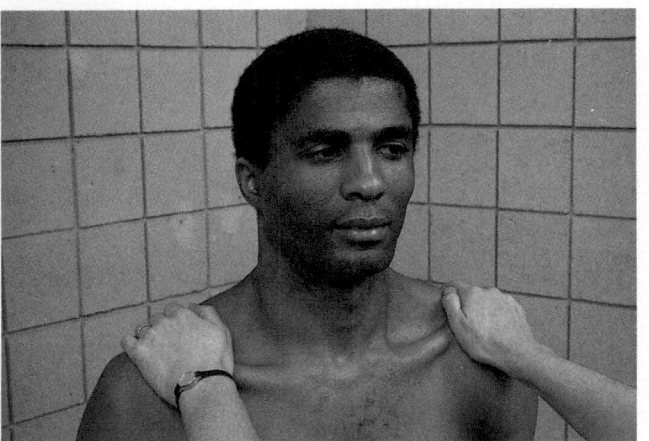

using the tuning fork to test for vibratory sensation and placing the fork on bony prominences. Abnormal findings include inability to perceive pain or light touch, inability to identify the location of touch, and absence of vibratory sensation.

Reflex Function The reflexes are tested to evaluate the function of specific spinal segment levels. The reflex hammer is used to elicit muscle contraction and reflexes. The client may be either sitting or supine. The reflexes are illustrated in Table 24-8.

T A B L E 2 4 - 8

Normal Responses of Commonly Tested Reflexes		
Reflex	**How to Test Reflex**	**Normal Response**
Biceps	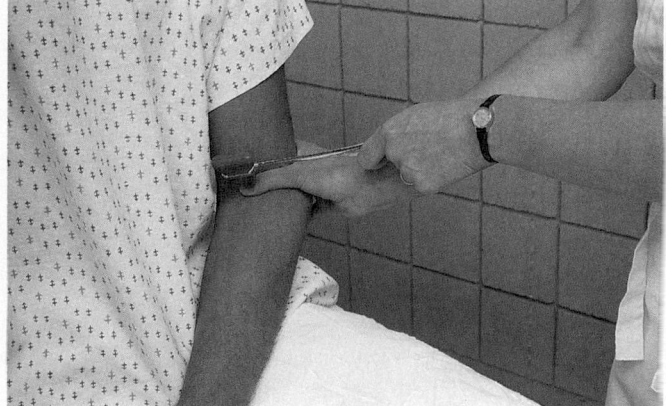	The contraction of the biceps can be seen and felt. To test the biceps reflex, the elbow is slightly bent, and the palm faces downward. The examiner's thumb is placed on the biceps tendon at the bend in the elbow. The percussion hammer strikes the examiner's thumb.
Triceps	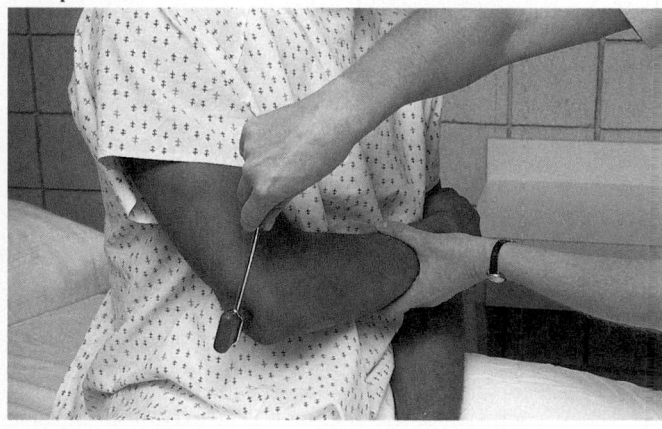	The contraction of the triceps can be seen as the elbow extends. To test the triceps reflex, the client's elbow is sharply bent; the forearm is placed across the chest wall with the palm turned toward the body. The triceps muscle is struck with the percussion hammer just above the elbow.
Knee	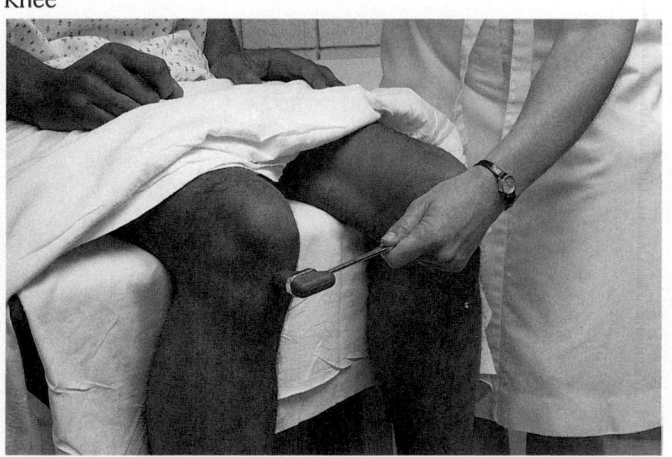	The contraction of the quadriceps causes the knee to extend. To test the knee reflex, the client is in the sitting position. The patellar tendon just below the patella is struck with the percussion hammer. If the client is lying down, the reflex is tested while the examiner's hands are placed under the knees to bend them.

(continued)

T A B L E 2 4 - 8 *(continued)*

Normal Responses of Commonly Tested Reflexes

Reflex	How to Test Reflex	Normal Response
Ankle		The foot jerks and moves downward.

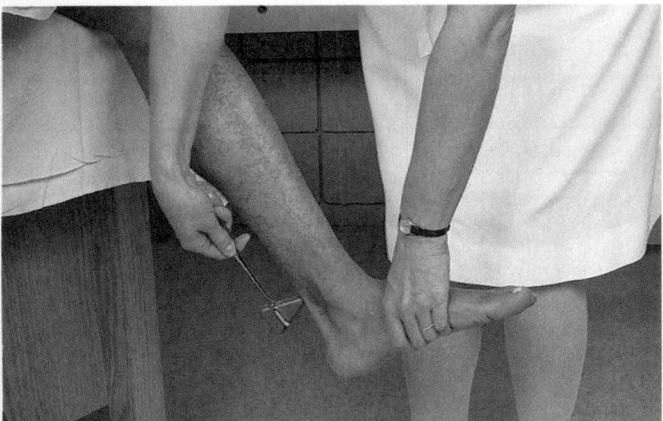

To test the ankle reflex, the leg is bent at the knee and the foot is supported in a walking position. The Achilles tendon is struck with the percussion hammer.

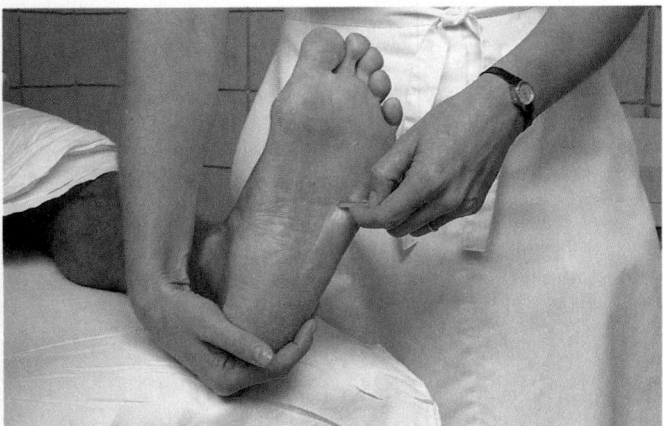

The toes bend or curl.

The lateral aspect of the sole of the foot is stroked with an object, such as a key or a thumbnail, from the heel to the ball of the foot.

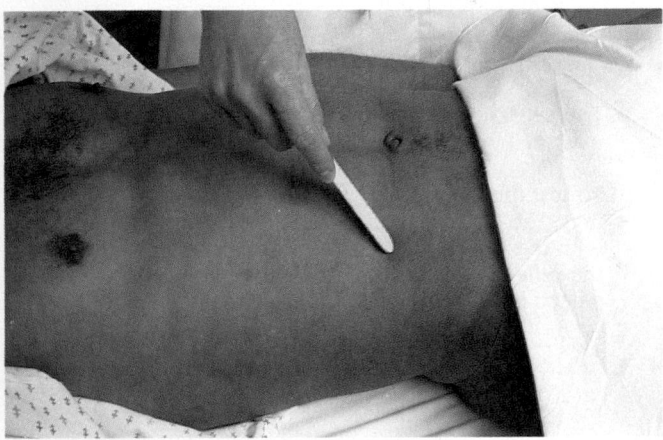

The contraction of abdominal musculature can be seen.

To test the abdominal reflex, with the client lying on the back, each side of the abdomen is stroked from the sides toward the center with a tongue blade or key.

(Photos © Ken Kasper.)

Grading of Reflexes

Reflexes are usually graded on a 0 to 4+ scale:
- 4+ Very brisk, hyperactive; often indicative of disease; often associated with clonus (rhythmic oscillations between flexion and extension)
- 3+ Brisker than average; possibly but not necessarily indicative of disease
- 2+ Average; normal
- i+ Somewhat diminished; low normal
- 0   No response

ward. Strike the client's radius 1 to 2 inches above the wrist. Observe for flexion and supination of the forearm.

Patellar or Knee Reflex The client is placed in a sitting or supine position while the nurse supports the client's knee in a flexed position. Briskly tap the patellar tendon just below the patella and observe for contraction of the quadriceps with knee extension.

Achilles Tendon Reflex or Ankle Reflex The client's leg should be slightly flexed at the knee, with dorsiflexion of the foot at the ankle joint. Strike the Achilles tendon and observe for plantar flexion at the ankle. Reflexes are graded according to their response, with a +2 considered a normal or active response.

Biceps Reflex The client's arms should be partially flexed at the elbow, with the palms down. Place your thumb or finger firmly on the client's biceps muscle, and strike with the reflex hammer, aimed directly toward your finger. Observe for flexion at the elbow, and feel for contraction of the biceps muscle.

Triceps Reflex Flex the client's arm at the elbow, with the client's palm facing the body, and position it across the client's chest. Strike the triceps tendon above the elbow. Observe for contraction of the triceps muscle and extension at the elbow.

Brachioradialis or Supinator Reflex Rest the client's forearm on the abdomen on in the lap, with the palm facing down-

Documenting the Data

After completing the nursing history and examination, the nurse organizes all assessment data accurately and completely for the purpose of identifying actual and potential problems, making nursing diagnoses, planning appropriate care, and evaluating the client's responses to treatment. Often a pattern is established that begins during the history and is confirmed during the physical examination.

The data are documented, with each system recorded individually. Documentation of the nursing examination, using a format based on functional health patterns and integrating the health history and physical assessment, is illustrated in the display entitled Documentation of the Nursing Assessment to demonstrate the application of nursing assessment skills in the clinical setting.

Documentation of the Nursing Assessment

Ms. D comes to a local community outpatient agency for evaluation of her intolerance of fatty foods. The nurse in charge of the agency makes the following assessment, and then refers Mrs. D to her local physician for evaluation.

Health History

Informant Ms. D is a 47-year-old female who lives with her 50-year-old husband on a farm in a rural midwestern area. She graduated from high school and is employed as a secretary for a local insurance company. Baptist religious affiliation. German–English descent. Ms. D is the primary source of information. Client is alert and oriented.

Chief Complaint "I just started having a lot of gas and was sick to my stomach after eating greasy food."

History of Present Illness About 1 month ago, Ms. D noticed that she began having severe gas and was nauseated after eating fried foods and gravy. Has vomited on two occasions. Before this time, has always eaten any type of food without problems. Denies any type of pain. Has taken Tums and used Maalox with little relief of symptoms. Has stopped eating any food that she identified as causing symptoms.

Health History
1. Tonsils removed at age 5 years.
2. Appendectomy at age 22 years.
3. Pregnant ×2 (ages 23 and 27 years) but both pregnancies ended during the fourth month. Decided not to try to have any children.
4. Is allergic to penicillin (rash, difficulty breathing). Has had all immunizations, but last tetanus shot was 10 years ago.

(continued)

Documentation of the Nursing Assessment *(continued)*

Family History
  Maternal grandfather: age 77, "heart problems"
  Maternal grandmother: age 76, diabetes mellitus
  Paternal grandfather: age 70, glaucoma
  Paternal grandmother; age 69, healthy
  Spouse: age 50, chronic back pain
  Sister: age 45, healthy
  Brother: deceased (accident, age 20)

Patient Profile

Developmental Factors   Born in the same community in which she now lives, married at age 21 years. States she has always had a happy life, other than inability to have children. Part of a close-knit extended family and group of friends. Active in church activities, sings in choir. Works one Saturday a month as a volunteer at a local hospital.

Education and Occupation   Expresses satisfaction with her job and educational level, although has at times wished she had gone to college. Has worked at the same insurance agency since she got married, states that her job "feels like a family." Income of the client and her husband is sufficient to maintain a comfortable lifestyle. Has Blue Cross/Blue Shield major medical insurance.

Environment   Lives in a six-room farm house that was totally remodeled 10 years ago. House is on 2 acres of woods. No identified environmental hazards.

Spiritual Factors   Has a deep faith in God; her faith is a strong support system. Attends church twice a week with husband and parents. Sings in choir, is active in church functions.

Interpersonal Factors   Speaks and reads English. Family members supportive. Values include "doing my job well, helping others, being honest."

Life-Style   Sleeps 7–8 hours each night, rarely feels tired. Eats three meals a day, but says she "loves snacks and sweets too much." Smoked cigarettes for 2 years but quit 25 years ago. Does not drink alcohol. Only drugs used are an occasional aspirin for headache and antacids. Recognizes need for a regular exercise program, but "just does not have time."

Self-Concept   Verbalizes strengths, usually feels satisfied with life and self. Has a sense of loss in inability to have children, but has accepted this as God's will. Would like to lose weight. Concerned about current health.

Sexuality   Has a satisfying sexual relationship with husband. Enjoys being a woman and taking care of others.

Stress Response   Eats when she feels stressed. Can talk over worries with husband and parents.

Physical Assessment

General Appearance   Clean, neatly groomed, and appropriately dressed white female who appears younger than stated age. Appears overweight. Walks with erect posture. Does not appear to be in pain or acutely ill. Makes eye contact. Makes appropriate responses.

Vital Signs   Temperature, 98.8°F; pulse, 82; respirations, 16; blood pressure, 130/88.

Height and Weight   Height, 5'4"; weight, 172 lb.

KEY   POINTS

- Data collection during the assessment step of the nursing process includes a nursing history and nursing (physical) assessment. Data from nursing examinations are used to formulate nursing diagnoses.
- Four techniques are used in performing a nursing assessment—inspection, palpation, percussion, and auscultation.
- The nurse should plan the nursing examination at a time that is appropriate for both the client and the nurse. The nurse should prepare the room, gather instruments and equipment, ensure privacy, and meet the client's physical and psychological needs.

- Various positions are used during the nursing examination. The client's privacy and comfort should be considered in each position.
- Each body system is assessed for normal and abnormal findings; included are the integument, the head and neck, the thorax and lungs, the breasts and axilla, the abdomen, the male and female genitalia, the rectum and anus, the musculoskeletal system, and the neurologic system. The techniques of assessment are used to assess the health status of the client systematically.
- The nurse carefully documents normal and abnormal findings.

Integument Skin warm and dry with good turgor. Does not have any abnormal findings other than old appendix scar, RLQ. Nails convex and smooth. Hair shiny and shows normal distribution.

Head and Neck Skull size and shape normal. Facial features are symmetrical. Can raise eyebrows, close eyes, smile, puff out cheeks. External eye structures symmetrical, no pain on palpation of lacrimal glands. Wears contact lenses—states vision is 20/20 with contacts. Sclerae white, conjunctiva without redness. Pupils are equal and reactive to light. Demonstrates accommodation, convergence, and peripheral vision. Lens clear, macula and fovea visualized; no hemorrhages or exudate noted. Hearing tested by use of a clock—heard clearly at 2 feet. External ears symmetric. Canals smooth and pink. Tympanic membranes intact without redness or drainage. Right nostril clear, left nostril occluded. Maxillary sinuses slightly tender to palpation. Teeth in good repair, with three small fillings. Oral mucous membranes smooth and pink. Tonsils absent. Trachea is midline, thyroid nonpalpable. No lymph nodes were palpable.

Thorax and Lungs Chest symmetric with equal expansion and relaxation. Respirations even and unlabored. No tenderness on percussion. Thoracic lung sounds resonant throughout. No visible pulsations noted in neck or precordium. No thrills, lifts, or heaves palpated. S_1 and S_2 heart at pulmonic, aortic, tricuspid, and mitral areas; no extra heart sounds, murmurs, or bruits heard. Apical pulse, 84/min, regular and strong.

Peripheral Vascular Arms and legs equal in size and bilaterally symmetric. Radial pulses equal in rate and strength. Skin pale pink, warm, and dry without edema. Femoral, popliteal, and dorsalis pedis pulses strong and equal. No pedal edema. Toenails thick. Superficial varicose veins on both lower extremities between ankle and knee.

Breasts and Axillae Breasts small, skin pale pink, and dry. No retraction or dimpling noted. Areolae and nipples smooth; no crusting or drainage. Breasts palpated in each quadrant, no massed noted. Axillary lymph nodes nonpalpable.

Abdomen Abdomen rounded, umbilicus midline. No abdominal masses palpable on light palpation. Bowel sounds heard in all four quadrants. No bruits heard over abdominal aorta. Slight pain on palpation of RUQ.

Genitalia Examination deferred until next visit. Currently having menstrual period. Periods occur every 28 days and last 5 or 6 days; has moderate flow with mild abdominal cramping. States she has PMS for a week before start of period.

Rectum and Anus Inspection only with small hemorrhoids visible at the anal sphincter.

Musculoskeletal Stands erect, symmetry noted. Normal concave cervical and lumbar spine; convex thoracic spine. No joint deformities, tenderness or crepitation. Full active range of motion of all extremities. Muscle strength equal bilaterally, slightly stronger on the right (dominant side).

Neurologic System Alert and oriented to person, place, and time. Facial expression symmetric and matches mood. Speech clear and appropriate. Demonstrates short- and long-term memory. All cranial nerves intact. Fine motor movements intact. Gait even. Perceives pain or light touch appropriately. All reflexes 2+.

STUDY QUESTIONS

1. The internal structures of the eye can be visualized by using which of the following instruments?
   a. an otoscope
   b. an ophthalmoscope
   c. a stethoscope
   d. a tuning fork

2. To make accurate assessments during inspection, the nurse must
   a. compare bilateral body parts
   b. have 20/20 vision
   c. focus on selected body systems
   d. use touch judiciously

3. Palpation is a physical assessment technique that uses the sense of
   a. intuition
   b. vision
   c. hearing
   d. touch

4. When percussing over the stomach, the nurse notes the finding of a loud drumlike sound. The term to document this percussion tone is
   a. dullness
   b. flatness
   c. tympany
   d. resonance

5. The bell of the stethoscope is used to hear
   a. tympanic sounds
   b. bowel sounds
   c. lung sounds
   d. heart sounds
6. Skin turgor may be assessed by which of the following techniques
   a. indenting with the finger tips
   b. using special lighting
   c. touching to detect moisture
   d. lightly pinching a skin fold
7. Visual acuity may be assessed by using Snellen's chart. If a client has acuity of 20/40 in both eyes, this means
   a. the client can see twice as well as normal
   b. the client has double vision
   c. the client has less than normal vision
   d. the client has normal vision
8. When using an otoscope to assess the tympanic membrane of an adult, the ear canal is straightened by gently pulling the pinna
   a. up and back
   b. down and forward
   c. away from the examiner
   d. in any direction
9. When percussing the thorax and lungs, a dull sound indicates
   a. an air-filled structure
   b. a bony structure
   c. emphysematous tissue
   d. fluid or a solid mass
10. When auscultating the thorax and lungs, coarse gurgling sounds are heard on expiration. These sounds can be broadly labeled as
   a. adventitious breath sounds
   b. bronchovesicular breath sounds
   c. vesicular breath sounds
   d. bronchial sounds
11. Heart sounds are the result of
   a. blood flow through the heart
   b. movement of blood into the heart from the aorta
   c. closure of the heart valves
   d. contraction of the cardiac muscle
12. When palpating the breast, the examination should be conducted by which division of areas?
   a. quadrants
   b. halves
   c. entire breast tissue
   d. bilateral comparison
13. When assessing the abdomen, which assessment technique should be conducted after inspection?
   a. percussion
   b. palpation
   c. auscultation
   d. sequence does not matter
14. Which of the following assessments of mental status is *not* an assessment of orientation?
   a. time
   b. place
   c. person
   d. consciousness
15. As part of the assessment of cranial nerves, the nurse asks the client to raise the eyebrows, smile, and show the teeth. These actions provide information about which cranial nerve?
   a. olfactory
   b. optic
   c. facial
   d. vagus

Answers With Rationale

1. The correct response is *b*. None of the other instruments can be used to visualize the internal eye.
2. The correct response is *a*. A comparison of bilateral body parts is necessary for recognizing abnormal findings. Perfect vision is unnecessary; the nurse examines all body systems and uses touch during palpation.
3. The correct response is *d*. Palpation is the technique that uses the sense of touch. The other responses are incorrect.
4. The correct response is *c*. Tympany is a loud drum-like sound, heard over an air-filled organ. Dullness has a thud-like quality. Flatness is a flat, high-pitched sound. Resonance is a hollow sound heard over lung tissue.
5. The correct response is *d*. The bell of the stethoscope is used to hear low-pitched sounds, such as those produced by the heart and vascular system.

The diaphragm of the stethoscope is used to hear high-pitched sounds, such as normal lung and bowel sounds.
6. The correct response is *d*. Skin turgor is assessed by lightly pinching a fold of skin and allowing it to return to its shape when released. None of the other techniques would determine skin turgor.
7. The correct response is *c*. Normal vision is 20/20. A finding of 20/40 would mean that a client has less than normal vision.
8. The correct response is *a*. The ear canal of an adult is straightened by gently pulling the pinna of the ear up and back. In children younger than age 3 years, the ear canal is straightened by pulling the pinna gently down and back.
9. The correct response is *d*. A dull sound is heard when percussing over fluid or a solid mass. A flat tone is heard over a bony structure. Tympany is

heard over an air-filled structure. Hyperresonance is heard over emphysematous lung tissue and is an abnormal finding.

10. The correct response is *a*. Adventitious breath sounds are sounds not normally heard in the lungs (such as rales or rhonchi). The other responses are normal breath sounds.

11. The correct response is *c*. Heart sounds are the result of closure of the heart valves. The other responses do not result in heart sounds.

12. The correct response is *a*. The breast is divided into four quadrants—outer upper quadrant, outer lower quadrant, inner upper quadrant, and inner lower quadrant. Each quadrant is systematically palpated in a clockwise direction. Any abnormal findings are recorded by location of the involved quadrant.

13. The correct response is *c*. When assessing the abdomen, the sequence is inspection, auscultation, percussion, and palpation. Auscultation follows inspection because percussion and palpation stimulate bowel sounds.

14. The correct response is *d; a, b,* and *c* are assessments of orientation. Consciousness is the degree of wakefulness or the ability of a person to be aroused, which is not the same as orientation.

15. The correct response is *c*. Motor function of the facial nerve (cranial nerve VII) is assessed by asking the client to raise the eyebrow, smile, and show the teeth. The other responses are also cranial nerves, but have different techniques of assessment.

BIBLIOGRAPHY

Barker, E., & Moore, K. (1992). Neurological assessment. *RN, 55*(4), 28–35.

Bates, B. (1991). *Guide to physical examination and history taking* (5th ed.). Philadelphia: Lippincott.

Becker, K. L. (1988). Get in touch and in tune with cardiac assessment. *Nursing, 18*(3), 51–55.

Becker, K. L., & Stevens, S. A. (1988). Performing in-depth abdominal assessment. *Nursing, 18*(6), 59–63.

Braverman, B. G. (1990). Eliciting assessment data from the patient who is difficult to interview. *Nursing Clinics of North America, 25*(4), 743–750.

Burggraf, V., & Donlon, B. (1985). Assessing the elderly system by system. *American Journal of Nursing, 85,* 974–984.

Dennison, R. (1986). Cardiopulmonary assessment. *Nursing, 16*(4), 34–39.

Fuller, J., & Schaller-Ayers, J. (1990). *Health assessment: A nursing approach.* Philadelphia: Lippincott.

Gallagher, L. P., & Kreidler, M. C. (1987). *Nursing and health. Maximizing human potential throughout the life cycle* Norwalk, CT: Appleton & Lange.

Holgren, C. (1992). Abdominal assessment. *RN, 55*(3) 28–34.

Kain, C. D., Reilly, N., & Schultz, E. D. (1990). The older adult: A comparative assessment. *Nursing Clinics of North America, 25*(4), 833–848.

Malasanos, L., Barkauskas, V., & Stoltenberg-Allen, K. (1990). *Health assessment.* St. Louis: Mosby–Year Book.

McConnell, E. A. (1988). Getting the feel of lymph node assessment. *Nursing, 18*(8), 54–57.

McHugh, J., & McHugh, W. (1990). How to assess deep tendon reflexes. *Nursing, 20*(8), 62–64.

Smeltzer, S., & Bare, B. (1992). *Brunner and Suddarth's textbook of medical–surgical nursing* (7th ed.). Philadelphia: Lippincott.

Smith, C. E. (1988). Assessing bowel sounds: More than just listening. *Nursing, 18*(2), 42–43.

Stevens, S. A., & Becker, K. L. (1988a). A simple step-by-step approach to neurologic assessment. Part I. *Nursing, 18*(9), 53–61.

Stevens, S. A., & Becker, K. L. (1988b). A simple step-by-step approach to neurologic assessment. Part II. *Nursing, 18*(10), 51–58.

Sullivan, J. (1990). Neurologic assessment. *Nursing Clinics of North America, 25*(4), 795–809.

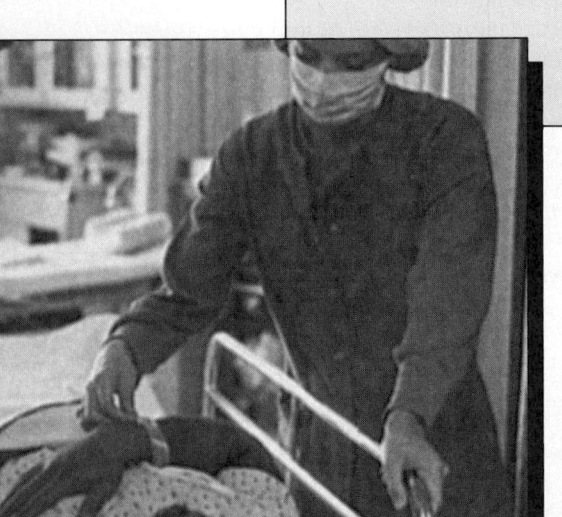

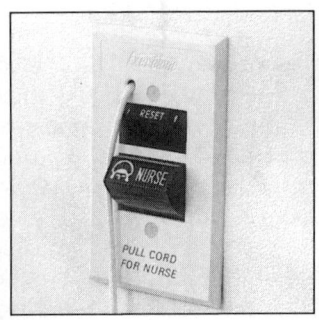

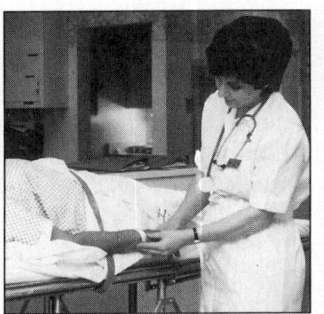

Safety

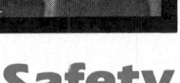

OBJECTIVES

After studying this chapter, the learner should be able to:

Define key terms used in the chapter.

Identify factors that may be safety hazards in the client's environment.

Describe ways in which the client's safety can be promoted in the home and health care setting.

Identify clients at risk of falling.

Describe preventive strategies to decrease the incidence of client falls.

Identify alternatives to using restraints.

Identify nursing diagnoses associated with a client in an unsafe situation.

Describe nursing responsibilities for fire safety.

Identify teaching strategies that should be included in a safety program to prevent poisoning and suffocation.

KEY TERMS

ground
incident report
macroshock
microshock
restraint
suffocation

25

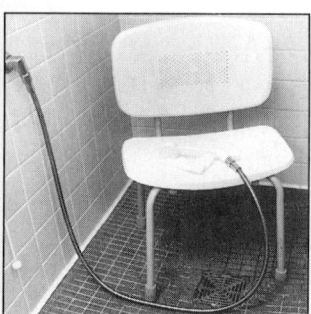

related motor vehicle accidents, sexually transmitted diseases, and suicide is a devastating outcome of these unsafe behaviors. Nurses have become more aware of the growing crisis of elder abuse, which affects about 1 of every 20 older Americans (Roybal, 1991). They have firsthand experience with the specific hazards confronting each age-group and situation.

Study of this chapter provides the student with the problem-solving tools needed to address these safety issues. Use of the nursing process facilitates the nurse's ability to recognize, assess, diagnose, and plan the nursing interventions that will effectively ensure safety for all ages in all environments.

Factors That Affect Safety

Nursing strategies that identify potential hazards and promote wellness evolve from an awareness of the various factors that affect safety in the environment. Table 25-1 lists statistics for the principal causes of accidental death in the United States.

Developmental Considerations

Nurses interact with clients at various developmental levels. Each age has its own particular risks. (See Chapters 11 and 12 for specific age-related safety hazards.) Promoting safety and preventing injury are a dual responsibility. The nurse and client or family cooperate and together strive to eliminate or reduce accident risks in the home, community, or health care setting. Education to promote awareness of potentially dangerous situations must begin as early as possible and continue throughout the life span.

Identification of prenatal high-risk factors allows for appropriate intervention to prevent a developing fetus from being harmed. Infants of mothers who smoke have a lower birth weight. Excessive alcohol consumption and use of addictive drugs may cause adverse effects that are readily apparent in the infant at birth. Pregnant women also should avoid exposure to x-rays in the first trimester, certain pesticides, and anything that is a potential risk for the general population.

The infant or young child has a limited awareness of danger. Parents should be encouraged to teach their children about potential dangers at as early an age as possible. Many childhood accidents are preventable. As motor skills develop, the child's environment expands and potential hazards multiply. Protecting an infant or young child may involve childproofing activities in the home, simple instruction about potentially dangerous situations such as crossing a street, and careful observation during routine activities. Protecting a child also includes a heightened awareness by caregivers of manifestations that indicate child abuse. In 1989, more than 2.4 million cases of child abuse were reported in the United States and countless more went unreported (Jurgrau, 1990). Any suspicion of

Safety and security are basic human needs. Safety is a paramount concern that underlies all nursing care, and the responsibility of all health care providers. The focus on safety encompasses acute and extended-care facilities as well as the home, workplace, and community. All populations are at risk, and there are universal safety concerns common to all as well as unique safety considerations for each age-group.

Injuries and deaths from accidental falls, fire, and poisoning occur with alarming regularity across the life span. Statistics verify the incidence and particular groups at risk:

- Falls are the major safety problem in hospitals and the leading cause of accidental death of elderly people in their homes (Ross, 1991). Although falls can occur at any age, elderly people and young children are particularly at risk.
- Twenty percent of all homes are still not protected by smoke detectors, and such homes are involved in most (60%) house fires (*Accident facts*, 1989). Rarely does a day go by that we do not hear on the evening news of a fire that has swept through a home and resulted in injury or death to family members. The victims often are young children or elderly residents.
- The incidence of childhood poisoning has been dramatically reduced in the past 10 years, but accidental poisoning remains a concern in teenage and adult age-groups (Spencer, 1989). The number of deaths attributed to cocaine abuse nearly doubled in 1988 (Litovitz et al., 1989), and the number of admissions to emergency departments for cocaine abuse is increasing across the country (Levy & Hickey, 1991).

Providing a safe, secure environment requires an awareness of potential hazards for each developmental level. Studies have confirmed that pregnant women who use drugs, consume alcohol, and smoke expose their unborn children to substances that may adversely affect normal growth and development. The nurse frequently is the initial health care provider who has contact with an abused child or a battered woman. Prompt recognition is crucial, and nursing assessment may play a vital role in identifying a harmful environment. Adolescents face great dangers when they choose a pattern of drug or alcohol abuse or high-risk sexual activity. The increasing number of teenagers who become pregnant or are victims of alcohol-

TABLE 25-1

Type	Total Number	Death Rate per 100,000 Population
Motor vehicle	47,865	19.9
Falls	11,444	4.7
Drowning	4777	2.0
Fires, burns	4835	2.0
Poisoning		
Drugs and medicines	4187	1.7
Other solid and liquid substances	544	0.2
Gases and vapors	1009	0.4
Inhalation and ingestion of objects	3692	1.5
Firearms	1452	0.6

Principal Types of Accidental Deaths in the United States for 1986

(Adapted from U.S. Department of Commerce, Bureau of Statistics. [1990]. *National data book and guide to sources: Statistical abstract of the United States.* Washington, DC: Author.)

child abuse deserves immediate investigation and swift intervention, once verified, so that the child can be removed from the dangerous environment and receive treatment.

Adolescents are particularly at risk for becoming involved in motor vehicle accidents. Conflicts with parental values coupled with peer pressure may lead to experimentation with drugs and alcohol, creating an even higher potential for accidents. Young and middle-aged adults are more susceptible to accidents when alcohol is used in response to stressful situations. Many motor vehicle accident fatalities that occur in this age-group are alcohol related. The National Highway Traffic Safety Administration (NHTSA) estimates that in 1989, 48% of teenage motor vehicle fatalities resulted from alcohol-related accidents (American Academy of Pediatrics, 1992). NHTSA also credits the 21-year-old minimum drinking age law for significantly reducing traffic accident deaths in young drivers. Domestic violence is widespread and may represent the most common cause of injury to women (Stark & Flitcraft, 1988). Health care experts estimate that 2 million women each year are battered by their male partners (Bullock et al., 1989). Counseling and education are interventions that promote the safety and well-being of women and interrupt the cycle of violence.

Although elderly people have more experience with their environment, illness or some degree of motor or sensory impairment may increase their risk for accidents. They are vulnerable to falls, exposure to unfavorable environmental conditions, and fire hazards in addition to elder abuse. Realistic concerns exist for elderly clients with slowed reflexes who continue to operate motor vehicles in an overly cautious or inadvertently careless manner. Noncompliance to a medication regimen may be related to failing sight, hearing difficulties, memory lapses, or inadequate communication from the health care provider. Elder abuse, which frequently goes unreported, is more likely to occur when stress and conflict exist in a family situation. It is difficult to identify, and is a sensitive safety issue.

Most hospitalized clients who experience falls are over age 65 (Nelson & Amin, 1990). The mortality rate associated with falls increases with age. More older women fall than men, which may reflect the fact that there are more women than men in this age-group. More than one third of falls in the elderly population are associated with the need to urinate. Checklists that can be used to assess the potential for a fall occurring in the home or health care setting are included in the discussion of nursing assessment later in this chapter.

Life-Style

Certain occupations, recreational activities, and environments place people in more hazardous situations. A worker who operates heavy industrial machinery, functions in perilous settings, or is involved with chemical agents on a consistent basis is at greater risk of accidental injury. Some people, by nature, are more inclined to take risks and place themselves at jeopardy. Failure to wear seat belts or abide by safety precautions is common behavior for some people. Stress may precipitate unhealthful life-styles that involve drug or alcohol abuse. Although much has been done to identify and control environments affected by pollutants, certain areas may statistically prove more hazardous and may expose residents to potentially unhealthy circumstances.

Living in an area where crime is prevalent may pose an additional threat to physical and emotional well-being. Security measures, such as locks and adequate exterior lighting, provide additional safety reassurances.

Mobility

Any limitation in mobility is potentially unsafe. An elderly client with an unsteady gait is prone to falling, and an unfamiliar setting may further aggravate the situation. Someone with paralysis or a spinal cord injury may require assistance with even the simplest movement. Supportive devices, such as canes, walkers, and wheelchairs, may facilitate movement, but they necessitate careful instruction and preparation for safe use. Recent surgery or a prolonged illness can temporarily affect mobility and necessitate special precautions to prevent falls or injuries. Nurses must assess a client's risk for injury with a view toward maintaining independence and fostering self-esteem while providing a safe, predictable environment.

Sensory Perception

Alterations in sensory perception can have a devastating effect on safety. Any impairment in sight, hearing, smell, taste, or sense of touch can reduce sensitivity to the environment. Visual changes may cause a person to stumble, lose his or her balance, and fall. A hearing deficit interferes with normal communication and may result in a client who is insensitive to safety alarms, automobile horns, and sirens and unable to understand instructions relating to health care. A reduction in one's ability to distinguish odors may mean failure to detect leaking gas or smoke. Loss of taste bud receptors can foster unsafe eating habits or result in ingestion of tainted food. A client whose tactile sense is impaired may be unable to perceive extremes in temperature as a threat to safety.

Knowledge

An awareness of safety precautions is crucial in promoting and maintaining wellness. A client needs instruction to adhere accurately to a medical regimen or to follow safety precautions when oxygen is in use. He or she requires a certain amount of knowledge to manage new equipment and unfamiliar procedures. Nursing assessment includes identification and recognition of potentially threatening circumstances. Recommendations for specific safety precautions are included throughout this chapter.

Ability to Communicate

Communication between the environment and the senses is basic to safety. The nurse must be sensitive to any factor that influences the client's ability to receive and send messages. Fatigue, stress, medication, aphasia, and language barriers are examples of factors that can affect any personal interchange and interfere with an accurate perception of events. A valid assessment by the nurse not only identifies the client's level of understanding, but also facilitates a positive communication experience.

Health State

Anything that affects the health state of the client potentially has the ability to impact on the safety of the environment. When a person is chronically ill or in a weakened health state, the focus of health care includes preventing accidents as well as promoting wellness and restoring the client to a healthy state. The nurse caring for a client who is recovering from a stroke identifies the client's neuromuscular impairment, pays particular attention to health teaching concerning the client's maintaining a sense of balance, and carefully assists with ambulation to prevent falls. Many of the clients who fall have a primary or secondary diagnosis of cardiovascular disease. The nurse strives to maximize the client's potential for return to a healthy state by considering safety factors as nursing care plans are developed.

Psychosocial State

Stressful situations tend to narrow a person's attention span and make him more prone to accidents. Stress may be sustained over long periods, but the effects tend to be more devastating in the later years, when there is less adaptive and coping capacity. Depression, when it develops, may result in confusion and disorientation, accompanied by reduced awareness or concern about environmental hazards. Social isolation or lack of social contact may be responsible for a reduced level of concentration, errors in judgment, and a diminished awareness of external stimuli.

Assessing Safety

Environmental safety hazards result in falls, fires, poisoning, suffocation, and accidents involving motor vehicles, equipment, and procedures.

Nursing assessment includes identifying clients at risk and unsafe situations. This requires a knowledge of the various factors mentioned above that influence safety and predispose people to accidents. Recognition of these considerations facilitates development of an individualized plan of care and has implications for nursing interventions aimed at protecting the client. Assessment includes an awareness of risk factors in the home and the health care agency.

The Client

Nursing History In an effort to provide a safe environment, the nurse must be alert for any history of falls or accidents because a person with a history of falling is likely to fall again. Any assistive devices that the client uses (eg, cane, walker) should be noted. The nurse also should attempt to confirm if there is a history of drug or alcohol abuse. Family members or significant others often are valuable resources. Knowledge of family support systems and the home environment is vital as the nurse prepares to plan protective health measures.

Physical Examination The nurse needs to assess the client's mobility status, ability to communicate, level of awareness or orientation, and sensory perception as she completes a nursing examination. Early detection and identification of any potential safety hazard are essential. The nurse's concern for personal safety includes recognition of any manifestations that suggest domestic violence or neglect. Chapters 7 and 11 discuss families who are experiencing violence, neglect, or abuse.

Accident-Prone Behavior Some people seem to be more likely to have accidents. Once an older adult has suffered one fall, it is likely that he or she will fall again. It is not uncommon for some children to be involved in multiple mishaps resulting in fractured bones. Some adolescent drivers repeatedly have motor vehicle accidents. They appear unable to predict situations that may prove hazardous. Opinion varies as to the probable cause of this accident-prone behavior. Some suggest an emotional link, but the consensus is that a client with a history of accidents is likely to have another one.

The Environment

Assessment of the environment requires the same attention to safety risks. The home, community, and health care agency are all settings that have the potential to cause injury. Each must be reviewed on an individual basis with the focus on the client's developmental level and health status. Potential safety hazards in the client's environment that need assessment and appropriate intervention are reviewed in detail later in this chapter in the Implementing section.

Specific Risk Factors

The nurse needs to be aware of those clients who are most at risk for injury as well as specific factors that have consistently been implicated as hazards.

Falls Assessment for risk of falling includes use of the nursing history and nursing examination. The nursing examination includes inspecting for faulty vision and hearing, mobility problems such as alterations in gait or posture, and postural hypotension. Tideiksaar (1989b) suggests the use of the mnemonic *SPLAT* to complete a fall prevention assessment. SPLAT reminds the nurse to gather information about *s*ymptoms, *p*revious falls, *l*ocation, *a*ctivity, and *t*ime.

Falls can occur at any age, but infants and older people are at greater risk for falls. A client is considered a high-risk candidate for a fall if he or she has any of the following characteristics:

- Age greater than 65 years
- Documented history of falls
- Impaired vision or sense of balance
- Altered gait or posture
- Medication regimen includes diuretics, tranquilizers, sedatives or hypnotics, analgesics
- Postural hypotension
- Slowed reaction time
- Confusion or disorientation
- Impaired mobility

Surveillance of environmental hazards in the health care facility and of clients who are at risk for falls must be continuous. Many health care agencies have fall prevention programs. Nurses have the responsibility to identify those clients who are at high risk for falls, document pertinent assessments on the chart, and plan appropriate interventions to ensure their safety. A checklist for preventing falls in a health care facility and modifications to reduce the risk of falls in the home appear in the accompanying displays.

Fires Many fires in the home are started by someone smoking in bed or falling asleep on a sofa or chair while smoking. Kitchen stoves, candles, and electric heaters are other causes of home fires. Faulty wiring and unsafe electrical equipment cause fires in homes and health care facilities. The risk factor for fire in the home can be determined by assessing the knowledge of clients and families. The following questions might be asked:

Do you have smoke detectors in the house?
Are they operable?
How many do you have, and where are they placed?
Do you smoke?
Where in the house do you smoke?
Do you smoke in bed?
Do you smoke while watching television?
Do you remain in the kitchen when you are cooking?
Do you use grease to fry foods, and do you fry foods often?
At what time of the day do you cook?
Do you ever cook late at night when other family members are asleep?
How do you heat your house?
Do you have electricity? gas? oil?
Do you have a kerosene heater, space heater, wood stove, or fireplace?

For clients of limited financial resources, questioning as to how a client heats the house is important, since the electricity or gas may have been turned off and other, unsafe methods may be used. Figure 25-1 is a sample of a fire prevention checklist that may be used in the home.

Fire prevention and emergency response programs in health care facilities often are viewed by staff as time-consuming and unnecessary exercises, but statistics from the National Fire Protection Agency indicate otherwise. An average of 8100 hospital fires and 4300 nursing home fires are reported annually (Collins, 1988).

Hospitals are required by law to establish safety boards and to regularly inspect the facilities for possible hazards. Equipment must be checked periodically, and escape

Checklist for Preventing Falls in the Health Care Facility

Client's name _____ Age _____

Diagnosis _____

Nursing unit and station _____

	Yes	No	Comments
1. Are restraints needed?	☐	☐	_____
If yes, what type?			_____
2. Are side rails up?	☐	☐	_____
3. Is bed in low position?	☐	☐	_____
4. Are bed wheels locked?	☐	☐	_____
Wheelchair brakes on?	☐	☐	_____
5. Is call bell within the client's reach?	☐	☐	_____
6. Does the client understand how to use the call light?	☐	☐	_____
7. Is the night light on?	☐	☐	_____
8. Does the room have any physical hazards (eg, is the floor slippery because of damp mopping)?	☐	☐	_____
9. What type of footwear does the client have on?			_____
10. Are the client's water, tissues, and urinal within reach?	☐	☐	_____
11. If the client is a surgical patient, how many hours or days postoperative is he or she?			_____
12. Does the client have any previously identified limitations?	☐	☐	_____
13. Is the client aware of activity limitations?	☐	☐	_____
14. Is the client showing any physical or mental limitations now?	☐	☐	_____
15. Has the client received any analgesics, hypnotics, sedatives, or relaxants?	☐	☐	_____
If yes, what are they?			_____
16. Is he or she receiving other medications that could cause a fall?	☐	☐	_____
If yes, what are they?			_____

Home Modifications to Prevent Risk of Falls

Exterior	Suggested Improvements
Lighting	Replace burnt-out or dim bulbs. Arrange for lighting along all walking areas.
Walking areas	Surfaces should be even and in good repair.
Steps	Secure hand rails should be available with adequate lighting provided.
General environment	Keep uncluttered and free of debris.

Interior

Bathroom

Floor surface	Apply nonslip adhesive strips on floor in front of toilet, at sink, and in front of and inside shower area.
Toilet	Install raised toilet seat with support arms.
Grab bars	Position secure grab bars next to toilet and in tub or shower area.
Scatter rugs	Eliminate or attach double-faced, nonslip adhesive strips to underneath surface of rug.
Thresholds	Replace with threshold even with floor or plane down existing one.
Lighting	Provide adequate lighting for all areas (toilet, washing areas, medicine cabinet).
Accessories	Use contrasting colors for easier visibility. Use liquid soap in dispenser or bar soap on a rope.
Limited space	Provide grab bars in appropriate locations and modify bathroom fixtures with nonslip adhesive strips to provide nonslippery support area.

Kitchen

Cabinets and shelves	Have secure, sturdy stool with nonslip treads available. Reposition shelves to allow for easier reach.
Lighting	Provide adequate lighting particularly in working areas.
Accessibility of objects	Use hand-held reaching device for inaccessible objects.
Floor area	Install nonslip adhesive strips on floor in front of sink and stove. Remove any scatter rugs.
Chairs	Use sturdy chairs with armrests. Height should be appropriate to allow for easy rising. Avoid chairs with crossbar between front legs because it interferes with placing feet firmly under chair when rising.

Bedrooms and Other Living Areas

Lighting	Provide adequate lighting. Use night lights where appropriate.
Floor area	Avoid scatter rugs. Use nonslip adhesive strips where surface is slippery. Secure raised edges of carpet with tape to prevent catching heel or toe of shoe.
Chairs	Use sturdy chairs with armrests.
Accessory tables	Replace wobbly tables that may be used for support while walking. Keep table surfaces uncluttered. Place colored nonslip adhesive strips on edges of glass tables.

Stairs

Lighting	Provide adequate lighting. Install light switch at top and bottom of stairs.
Steps	Paint or carpet in contrasting color for improved visibility. Install nonslip rubber strips to accentuate stair edges.
Support	Provide secure hand rails on both sides of steps.

How safe is your home from fire? Take a few minutes to walk through your home, looking for these common fire hazards.

YES	NO	**Living room**
☐	☐	Are electrical cords in good condition—not frayed or worn?
☐	☐	Do you avoid threading electrical cords, including extension cords, under carpeting or pinching them behind furniture?
☐	☐	If there are smokers in the house, are ashtrays readily available?
☐	☐	After a party, do you check wastebaskets, ashtrays, furniture, and carpets for carelessly discarded cigarettes? Are all candles extinguished?
☐	☐	Are draperies and furniture more than 3 feet away from the fireplace?

YES	NO	**Fireplace**
☐	☐	Is the fuel for the fireplace—kindling, newspapers, firewood—stacked at least 3 feet from the hearth?
☐	☐	Does a firescreen cover the entire opening of the fireplace?
☐	☐	Is the flue open when a fire is burning in the fireplace?
☐	☐	Are Christmas tree branches or needles properly discarded and not used to start or maintain a fire?
☐	☐	Is a metal pail available to carry out the ashes? Are the ashes cold?
☐	☐	Is the chimney cleaned annually?

☐ ☐ Do you start the fire properly—not with charcoal starter or gasoline?

YES	NO	**Kitchen**
☐	☐	Are all appliances turned off before you go to bed or leave the house?
☐	☐	Do you have a fire extinguisher handy?
☐	☐	When working over the stove, do you wear garments with short or snug sleeves?
☐	☐	Is *baking soda* (not baking powder or flour) handy to snuff out a grease fire?

YES	NO	**Bedroom**
☐	☐	Do you refrain from smoking in bed or in a comfortable chair where you might risk falling asleep?
☐	☐	Have you determined two escape routes out of the bedroom in case there is a fire?
☐	☐	If your house has rooms above the ground floor or if you live in an upper story, have you installed rope or chain ladders to escape from the upper floors quickly?
☐	☐	Do you use an electric space heater? Does it have an automatic shut-off in case it is tipped over? Do you keep the electric heater out of damp or wet areas?
☐	☐	Are smoke detectors installed outside every sleeping area

and are they operable? Do you forbid anyone to "borrow" the batteries from them? Do you resist disconnecting the detectors if they sound because the batteries are weak or because the toast is burning in the kitchen?

YES	NO	**Garage**
☐	☐	Is trash—particularly oily or paint-saturated rags—kept from accumulating in your garage?
☐	☐	Do you store oily rags, gasoline or other flammables away from heating sources or open flames, such as the pilot-lit water heater?
☐	☐	Do you use gasoline or paintbrush cleaner in an open area, where fumes can be dissipated and won't drift toward a source of ignition?
☐	☐	Do you refuse to allow anyone in your home to use gasoline as a cleaner for clothing or furniture?
☐	☐	When a fuse blows, do you replace it with the proper fuse—and not with a penny?

Scoring

A *no* answer to any of these questions indicates that you are not doing all you can to minimize the risk of fires in your home. While no house is fireproof, fires can be prevented. You can and should take all the fire prevention steps suggested in the questions.

F I G U R E 2 5 - 1

Fire prevention checklist for the home. (*Aide Magazine.* [October 1991]. USAA, San Antonio.)

routes must be kept open. Nurses, as part of their daily care procedures, must be aware of equipment and its proper functioning, and assess when and how often drills are performed.

Poisoning Although the incidence of childhood poisoning has been dramatically reduced in the past 10 years, accidental poisoning remains a concern in teenage and adult age-groups (Spencer, 1989). Causes of fatalities from poisoning are listed in Table 25-2. Not all poisons, however, cause death.

Developmental considerations must be taken into account when making assessments. Younger children are more apt to ingest household chemicals, whereas older children may swallow medicines in a suicide attempt. Preschool children also are at risk for ingestion of lead-containing substances. Experimentation with drugs by adolescents and young adults may result in accidental poisoning

TABLE 25-2

Poisoning Deaths by Age and Most Common Cause	
Age (yr)	**Agent or Cause**
5 and under	Carbon monoxide resulting most commonly from improperly vented gas space heaters
10–17	Carbon monoxide from motor vehicle
	Drugs
	Methaqualone
	Alcohol in combination
18–19	Drugs
	Diazepam
	Antidepressants
	Heroin
	Cocaine
	Methadone
	Phencyclidine
	Alcohol in combination
Adults	Drugs
	Alcohol in combination, usually with heroin
	Heroin
	Codeine
	Amitriptyline
	Diazepam
	Propoxyphene
	Phenobarbital
	Cocaine

(Data from Massachusetts Poison Control System. [1983]. Clinical epidemiology of serious poisonings. *Clinical Toxicology Review,* 5:11; printed in Spencer, R. T., et al. [1989]. *Clinical pharmacology and nursing management* [3rd ed.]. Philadelphia: Lippincott.)

and death. The number of deaths attributed to cocaine abuse nearly doubled from 1987 to 1988 (Litovitz et al., 1989). An elderly client may inadvertently consume an overdose of a medication because of confusion or forgetfulness. Poor vision also is a factor in accidental poisoning in the elderly population.

Many poison control centers provide checklists for poison-proofing a home and lists of toxic household items. Reviewing these items will help in assessing and teaching the family about poisonous materials.

Suffocation and Choking **Suffocation**, or asphyxiation, may occur in any age-group, but the incidence is greater in children. It results in a lack of air reaching the lungs and a stoppage of breathing.

Common causes of suffocation include drowning, choking on a foreign substance inhaled into the trachea, and gas or smoke poisoning. An infant may suffocate when a pillow or a piece of plastic inadvertently covers the nose and mouth. A young child may be accidentally strangled by the shoulder harness of a seat belt or become trapped while playing in a discarded refrigerator and suffocate.

Drowning is a form of suffocation. Nearly half of all drowning victims are children under age 5. Most drowning deaths in young children occur because of inadequate supervision in the bathtub and in pools—even small wading pools. Older children are more likely to drown while swimming or boating.

Educating the public about the various causes of suffocation is the strongest factor in promoting wellness in this category. Assessing the knowledge level of clients—especially parents—is vitally important. The following questions might be included in an assessment for hazards that might cause a child to suffocate or choke:

Are plastic bags within reach of young children or infants?

Do you have soft pillows or thick blankets in your infant's crib?

Do you ever place your baby on a water bed to sleep?

Do you cut food into small pieces before giving it to young children?

Do you give peanuts, hard candy, or other small treats to your preschooler?

Are your children playing with toys appropriate for their age?

Do their toys have small or loose parts?

Have you ever left your infant or young child alone in a bathtub—even for a moment?

Does your child have access to a swimming pool?

Is pool rescue equipment nearby?

Is your child closely supervised when near water?

Do you know how to perform cardiopulmonary resuscitation and an abdominal thrust (Heimlich maneuver)?

Diagnosing

Once the nurse has identified a client at risk and an unsafe situation, the nursing diagnosis and care plan should reflect this. The actual or potential statement of the client's health status must be followed by the appropriate contributing or risk factors to individualize the nursing care plan.

Samples of nursing diagnoses pertaining to safety risks include the following:

High Risk for Injury related to visual or auditory sensory deficits; history of falling; unsteady gait; substance abuse; refusal to use seat belt or child safety seat; effects of medication; age greater than 65; generalized weakness

High Risk for Injury related to poisoning as a result of impaired vision; medications stored in unlocked medicine cabinet that is accessible to a child; presence of poisonous plants; excess alcohol intake; use of illicit drugs; knowledge deficit

High Risk for Injury related to suffocation by plastic bag that is accessible to a young child; child left unattended in bathtub; smoking in bed; placing an infant prone in a water bed; lack of safety precautions (door left on discarded refrigerator); unfamiliarity with fire prevention guidelines

High Risk for Injury related to trauma associated with lack of finances necessary for household repairs;

Poison Safety Checklist

Complete the following checklist to see if your home is safe from potential poisons. Check this list to see if all poisons are safely stored out of reach of small children and pets.

Kitchen

- [ ] Cleaners—carpet or upholstery cleaners, furniture polish, soaps or detergents
- [ ] Corrosives—automatic dishwashing detergents, drain cleaners, ammonia, metal cleaners, oven cleaners
- [ ] Medicines—pain relievers such as aspirin and acetaminophen, diet aids, vitamins or iron pills, pet medications
- [ ] Insecticides

Bedroom

- [ ] Cosmetics—nail polish or remover, baby powder
- [ ] Perfumes
- [ ] House plants
- [ ] Jewelry cleaners
- [ ] Medicines

Laundry Room

- [ ] Bleaches
- [ ] Laundry detergents
- [ ] Disinfectants

Bathroom

- [ ] Medicines
- [ ] Aftershave

- [ ] Mouthwashes
- [ ] Cleaners
- [ ] Deodorizers or sanitizers
- [ ] Drain openers
- [ ] Shampoo or hair products
- [ ] Hair removers
- [ ] Fluoride rinses

Garage, Basement, Storage Areas

- [ ] Antifreeze
- [ ] Pesticides
- [ ] Gasoline or kerosene
- [ ] Lighter fluid
- [ ] Paint remover or thinner
- [ ] Paint stripper
- [ ] Weed killer
- [ ] Mothballs

Living Room

- [ ] Cigarette butts, cigarettes
- [ ] Chocolate (hazardous to pets)
- [ ] Plants (check with the poison center to see if they are poisonous)
- [ ] Lamp oil

Miscellaneous

- [ ] Alcoholic beverages
- [ ] Outdoor plants—azalea, rhododendron, poke berry, holly berry

In the event of poisoning, contact the local poison control center.

(Poison Control Center, 1 Children's Center, Philadelphia, PA 19104)

history of previous falls; unsteady gait; presence of unsecured scatter rugs

Impaired Home Maintenance Management related to insufficient finances; substance abuse; physical disability

Planning: Client Goals

Many accidental injuries and deaths are preventable. The nurse considers the varied factors and environment that affect the client's safety and formulates client goals uniquely suited to each situation and circumstance. Nursing interventions focus on meeting these safety needs.

Client goals that promote safety and prevent injury include the following. The client will:

- Identify unsafe situations in his or her environment
- Identify potential hazards in his or her environment
- Demonstrate safety measures to prevent falls and other accidents
- Establish safety priorities with family members or significant others
- Demonstrate familiarity with his or her environment
- Identify resources for safety information
- Remain free of injury during hospitalization

Implementing

Safety measures are an integral part of the nursing care plan. The nurse intervenes to control or modify the environment and promote client safety. These safety recommendations apply to health agency settings, the home, and the community. Nursing implementations are discussed for each developmental level as well as for specific hazards in the environment. Teaching is an important step in accident prevention and health promotion.

Teaching to Prevent Accidents

Many teaching opportunities concerning safety measures arise while the nurse performs regular client care. Careful assessment, diagnosis, and planning prepare the nurse to use these opportunities wisely.

Assessment data and statistical information often prove helpful to health care personnel who are developing a safety program for clients at risk. Safety education classes, in addition to situational health teaching, can be worthwhile for the hospitalized client and his or her family. Recent studies have demonstrated that early assessment of vulnerable clients and preventive education programs can decrease the incidence of falls (Berryman et al., 1989; Easterling, 1990; Nelson & Amin, 1990).

A school nurse has multiple opportunities and a ready audience for health teaching about safety, including screening programs (eg, vision and hearing), fire prevention sessions, drug and alcohol prevention programs, and classes covering various accident prevention techniques. Management of minor accidents that involve children at school provides a forum for teaching additional preventive strategies.

T A B L E   2 5 - 3

Developmental Considerations and Safety Topics to Be Taught		
Developmental Age	**Accidents**	**Safety Topics**
Fetus	Abnormal growth and development	Alcohol consumption Smoking Use of drugs (addicting, prescription, and over the counter) X-ray exposure Pesticides
Neonate	Falls	Neonatal supervision Proper method of caring for neonate Environment—crib, bath, and changing area Infant car seats Use of vitamins, iron medications Feeding
Infant (first 6 mo)	Falls Injuries from toys Burns	Many of above topics Infant supervision Development—rolling over and falls Toy safety—size, construction, lead-free paint Flame-retardant clothes and inflammable toys Smoke alarms Sunburns, bathwater temperature, smoking, hot beverages Kitchen safety Electrical cords and outlets Using medications
Infant (second 6 mo)	Falls Injuries from toys Burns Suffocation or drowning Inhalation or ingestion Foreign bodies	Many of above topics Close supervision for active child Development—crawling, pulling up to stand, and pulling down objects (curiosity) Safety on stairs (gates) Teaching siblings about infant safety Plastic bags Tub and pool safety Child-proofing entire house and any houses the infant visits Poisonous plants Child-resistant packaging of medications and all poisonous substances
Toddler	Falls Cuts from sharp objects Burns Suffocation or drowning	Poison Control Center and instructions for emergencies Many of above topics Toddler supervision Development—inquisitive nature Outdoor safety—cars, driveways, parking lots Safety glass on doors, lock doors and windows, screens

Table 25-3 lists types of accidents according to developmental age, and safety topics that should be discussed with parents and in the school. The material in the remainder of this section on environmental safety is adaptable to teaching.

Considering Developmental Levels

Fetus Consideration for safety begins with an awareness of behaviors that may harm the developing fetus. A pregnant woman's knowledge of the risks associated with excess alcohol consumption, smoking, drug use, and exposure to other dangers in the environment, as listed in Table 25-3, should be reinforced.

Infant The nurse has many opportunities to educate parents about safety and accident prevention for infants and young children. Lack of mobility in early infancy limits opportunities for hazardous activity, but minimal safeguards are vital if accidents are to be prevented.

Safe care entails never leaving the infant unattended, using crib rails, and monitoring objects that the infant could place in the mouth and swallow. As the infant becomes more active, parents and caregivers must be alert to hazards that a curious, mobile infant may encounter. All items within reach must be carefully inspected and, if dangerous, secured in a safe place. Household products, medicines, electric outlets, and sharp instruments may cause injury and death. Because an infant frequently climbs or pulls up on objects, scalding hot liquids must be placed out of reach. Lead-free paint on all furniture and toys ensures that the infant will not be exposed to lead poisoning. All 50 states mandate the need for safe infant car seats and carriers when transporting a child in a motor vehicle. A rear-

Developmental Age	Accidents	Safety Topics
	Inhalation or ingestion Foreign bodies	Animal safety—pets and strange animals Child care seats Storage of hazardous substances (indoors and outdoors) Poisonous plants (indoors and outdoors) Car safety (car seats, unattended children, cars parked in sun) Storage of matches, use of hot liquids Water safety—tubs, jacuzzis, and wading and swimming pools, swimming lessons
Preschooler	Falls Cuts Burns Drowning Inhalation or ingestion Guns and weapons	Many of above topics, plus use of safety equipment when riding bicycles or skateboards Safe play areas (equipment and supervision, streets) Tricycles, scissors, other toys Guns or rifles in the house Begin to teach safety measures to child Fire safety—prevention, emergency measures, fire drills
School-age child	Burns Drowning Broken bones Inhalation or ingestion Guns and weapons Substance abuse	Many of above topics Safety on way to school (traffic, child abuse) Play equipment—bicycles, skateboards, roller skates Competitive sports Use of machinery (farm, lawn, cooking) Teaching safety measures (bicycle, use of phone in emergencies, policeman as helper, substance abuse) Parental role modeling Drug and alcohol abuse education Sexuality education
Adolescent	Drowning Vehicle accidents Guns and weapons Inhalation or ingestion	Many of above topics Responsibilities of new freedoms of being a teenager Driving (driver education, traffic safety, drinking and driving, motorcycles and snowmobiles) Competitive sports (proper equipment, physical examination before beginning sports or going to camp) Safety around water and water sports Emergency procedures, first-aid training Gun safety Substance abuse and role modeling for siblings Stress and coping Sexuality education and discussion of sexually transmitted diseases (including AIDS)

facing safety seat is recommended for infants who weigh less than 20 lb (9.1 kg); a forward-facing car seat may be used for larger infants and toddlers. In December 1991, NHSTA recommended that rear-facing safety seats not be placed in the front seat of a vehicle with passenger-side air bags. The high force of sudden air bag inflation has the potential to cause injury to an infant in the safety seat (American Academy of Pediatrics, 1992). Additional safety counseling measures that focus on tasks and behavior typical for this developmental level are included in Table 25-3.

Toddler and Preschooler To prevent accidental injury and death during the toddler and preschool years, the focus of parental responsibility is on child-proofing the environment. Play areas must allow for exploration but must provide for safety. Vigilant supervision by parents and guardians should anticipate hazardous elements and protect with precautionary devices such as safety locks, guard rails, and electric outlet covers. Child-proofing products are available that help children recognize dangerous items in the home. For example, a parent and child can apply "Ouchy" stickers to hazardous household objects during a safety walk-through (Fig. 25-2).

Ingestion of poisons or medications is a major threat for preschoolers. Their overconfidence and initiative make them more likely to dart into the street while chasing a ball, climb into a discarded refrigerator, or play with matches. When riding in a motor vehicle, children who have outgrown their safety seats should use a booster seat with a shield or harness; older children can use lap and shoulder belts. Nursing measures that safeguard toddlers and preschoolers are included in Table 25-3.

School-Age Child As a child becomes more independent during the school years, accidents continue to be a leading cause of death. Although increasingly independent behavior is typical of this age-group, children need assistance to evaluate activities that are potentially dangerous. The nurse needs to counsel parents of school-age children about specific interventions that provide for safety at home, at school, and in the neighborhood (Fig. 25-3).

Adolescent Nurses and parents must collaborate to reinforce safety behaviors in the adolescent. Much of the adolescent's time is spent away from home, with his or her peer group, or in automobiles. Education must focus on safe driving skills, including wearing a seat belt, discussions about drug and alcohol use, and formulation of a healthful life-style in response to the stress of daily living. Providing safety information is crucial in helping the adolescent to make mature decisions about health hazards peculiar to this age-group.

Adult Young and middle-aged adults need to be reminded about the effects of stress on their life-style. Coping with the demands of raising a family and establishing and promoting a career may lead to the development of unsafe health practices and reliance on drugs or alcohol. Unsafe behaviors can be modified and changed, but this requires considerable effort and commitment on the part of the adult client. The nurse may be directly involved in health education and counseling measures or may suggest resources to contact for additional support.

Older Adult Most accidents that involve elderly clients are preventable. Falls, fires, and motor vehicle accidents are significant hazards for this age-group. Many risk factors for falls (listed earlier in this chapter) apply to the elderly person.

Visual changes and slowed reaction time are realistic concerns that affect the elderly driver. Some become overly cautious, whereas others are prone to careless responses. Interventions aimed at helping the elderly client drive safely include maintaining the automobile in optimum

FIGURE 25-2

"Ouchy" stickers applied to hazardous household objects can help remind children not to touch them.

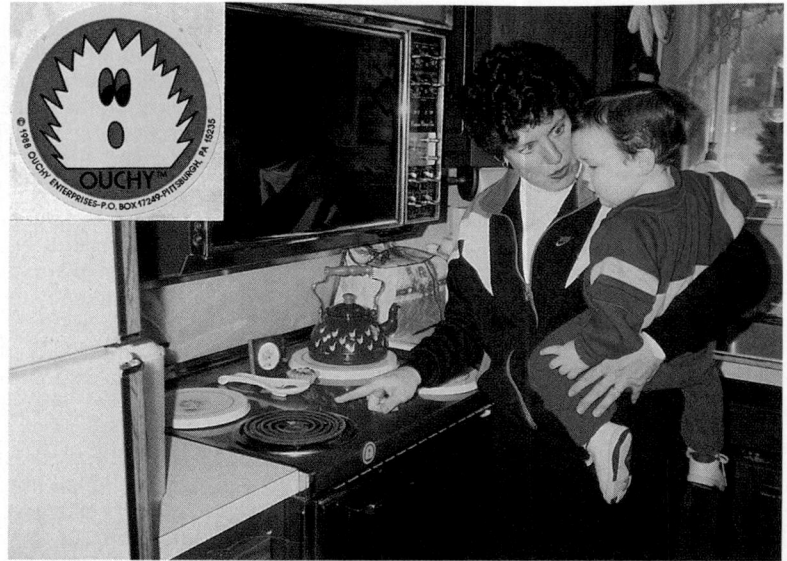

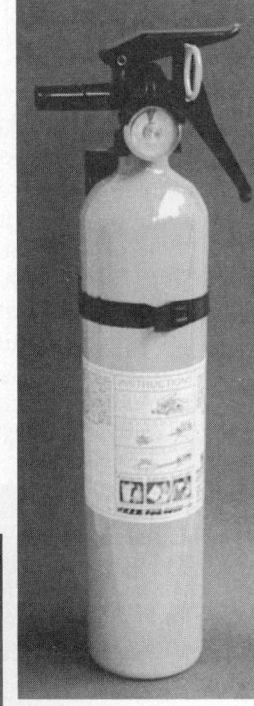

3-prong plug adapters with grounding wire

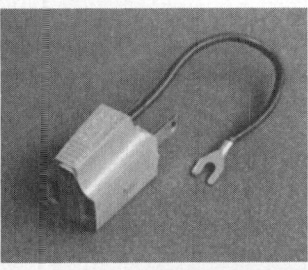

Outlet covers protect curious tots from electrical shock

All-purpose fire extinguishers for the home

Smoke detectors for the home

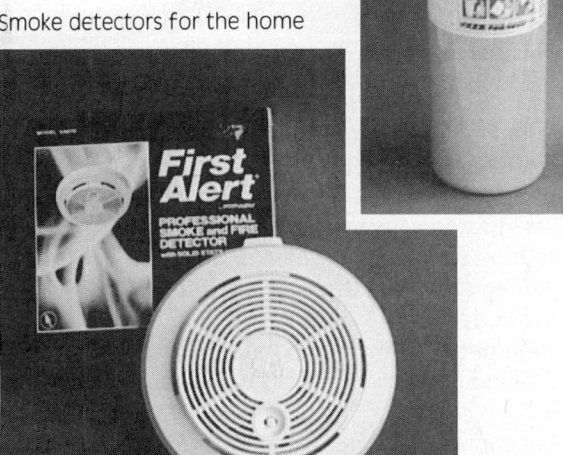

Car seats for infants and small children

Toddler gates at stairs and doors

FIGURE 25-3

The nurse's responsibility in home safety is primarily that of education and counseling, including providing information about home safety devices and sources for additional information.

driving condition, scheduling regular eye examinations, wearing corrective lenses when necessary, and keeping noise from radio and other equipment to a minimum. Some states require additional testing for the elderly client to renew a driving license.

The elderly person is at greater risk for suffering burn injuries. Confusion, forgetfulness, and diminished visual and olfactory senses are factors. More fires occur in the home than in health care facilities, and smoke inhalation frequently is the cause of death. Nursing interventions directed at helping to promote a fire-safe environment for the elderly client at home include admonitions not to smoke in bed, recommendations for installing a smoke-detecting device, and encouragement to wear nonflammable clothing.

Accidental overdosing on medications also is a safety risk. Poor eyesight or confusion may result in dosage errors. Special devices, such as medication trays, can be prefilled, and serve as a reminder to prevent the elderly person from taking additional doses.

Preventing Falls

Major causes of falls in the home include slippery surfaces, poor lighting, clutter, and improperly fitting clothing or slippers. The living room, hall, bedroom, bathroom, and stairs are the areas in the home where most falls occur. Measures as simple as hand rails in bathrooms and on stairs, good lighting, and discarding or repairing broken equipment

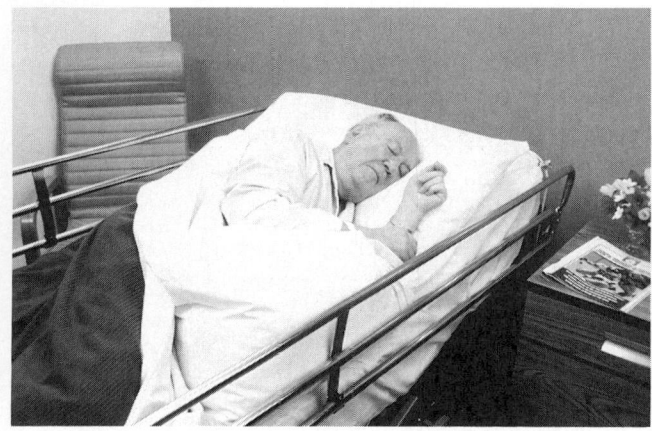

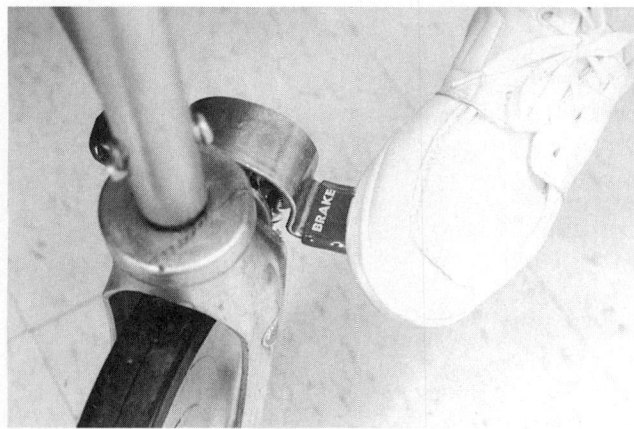

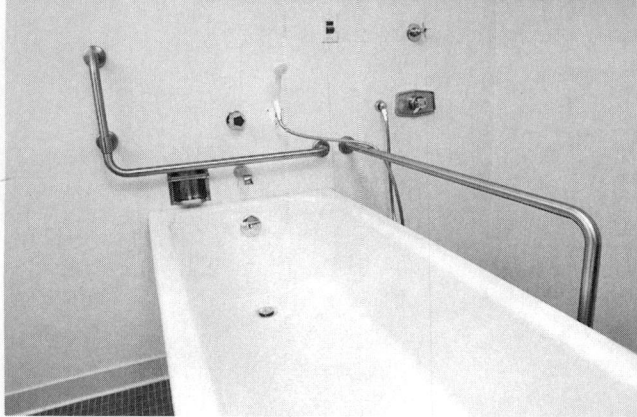

F I G U R E   2 5 - 4

Side rails on beds, locking devices on wheeled equipment, and hand rails in bath facilities are some of the safety devices used in health care agencies to prevent falls.

about the home help prevent accidents. The following safety measures are recommended to reduce the number of falls in acute- and extended-care facilities (Fig. 25-4):

- Thorough orientation to surroundings
- Careful survey of physical surroundings for hazards
- Bed wheels locked and bed in low position
- Call bell and personal articles within client's reach

- Examination of client's footwear
- Appropriate use of restraints when alternative measures have failed

Side rails, common equipment on agency beds, provide support and aid equilibrium but are especially important for the safety of clients who are likely to be disoriented, restless, confused, or unconscious. When in doubt about the client's mental status, it is better to err in the overuse of side rails than to contribute to a situation that results in a client's falling out of bed. A confused client may attempt to climb over side rails or out the foot of the bed. The client may fall out of bed or disturb tubes, equipment, dressings, or wounds. In such cases, restraints may be used with raised side rails to protect the client. An explanation frequently facilitates cooperation with their use.

Using Restraints   Restraints are devices used to limit a client's movement. They may be either physical, or chemical or pharmacologic. Side rails, geriatric chairs with attached trays, and appliances tied at the wrist, ankle, or waist are types of physical restraints. Physical restraints may be used for the following reasons:

- Restricting the movement of an extremity when it is being used for intravenous therapy
- Helping to prevent unconscious or delerious clients from pulling at wound dressings and tubes leading from the body
- Helping to prevent clients who are unsteady and at risk of falling from trying to get out of bed or up from a chair

Nurses consistently cite the risk of injury from falls as the primary reason for applying restraints (Brower, 1991). Chemical or pharmacologic agents, such as sleeping pills, sedatives, and tranquilizers, also may either intentionally or inadvertently restrain activity and behavior. Some clients may require both physical and chemical restraints. Figure 25-5 shows types of physical restraints.

Elderly clients are more likely to be restrained than younger clients. In 1988, in the United States, at least one third of all nursing home residents were regularly restrained (U.S. Health Care Financing Administration, 1988). One in five clients over age 70 in an acute-care hospital is likely to be restrained. A Canadian study examined the use of restraints on a large unit in a teaching hospital and discovered that heavy workloads and unquestioned or vague restraint policies foster the use of restraints for 10% to 15% of their clients (Bock & Schilder, 1988).

Health care providers are concerned about the almost routine use of restraints. Various studies have identified the following hazards as being associated with the immobility and restriction imposed by physically restraining a person (Evans & Strumpf, 1989):

- Danger of suffocation from improperly applied vests
- Impaired circulation
- Altered skin integrity (eg, abrasions, skin tears, bruises)
- Pressure ulcers and contractures
- Dehydration
- Incontinence

RESEARCH IN NURSING Making a Difference

Safety

The increasing number of elderly clients in health care facilities has prompted nurses to investigate methods of identifying people at risk of falling as well as specific nursing interventions that promote safety. Falls are the second leading cause of accidental death, and most falls occur in people over age 65. Extended stays in the hospital frequently result from falls in the elderly population. In the past, restraints have traditionally been one solution nurses used to protect the client and prevent falls. Recent research studies have attempted to focus on alternative safety measures that foster quality care for elderly clients.

Related Research

Garcia R., Cruz, M., Reed, M., Taylor, P., Sloan, G., & Beran, N. (1988). Relationship between falls and patient attempts to satisfy elimination needs. *Nursing Management 19*(7):80V–80X.

Many client falls in the older population are related to the basic need of elimination. Elders reported that a sense of urgency, a fear of incontinence, and a desire to maintain independence made them less likely to wait for the nurse to assist them to the bathroom. A fall alarm monitor and a bedside flow sheet were used to collect data. Recommendations to prevent falls in this population include implementation of a bowel and bladder program and the use of a bedside monitoring device for high-risk clients.

Spellbring, A.M., Gannon, M., Kleckner, T., & Conway, K. (1988). Improving safety for hospitalized elderly. *Journal of Gerontological Nursing 14*(2):31–37.

An increase in the fall rate among geriatric patients at a medical center prompted this research study. Spell-

bring and associates developed a risk assessment tool for the nurse to assist in identifying clients who are likely to fall. A standardized nursing care plan based on the nursing diagnosis High Risk for Injury was developed as well as a safety alert sticker for attachment to the care plan, chart, or bedside. In addition to providing a data base, this study produced an excellent predictor for clients at high risk for falling.

Strumpf, N., & Evans, L. (1988). Physical restraint of the hospitalized elderly: Perceptions of patients and nurses. *Nursing Research 37*(3):132–137.

When restraints are used as a protective measure by the nurse, clients rarely agree that their behavior is potentially unsafe. Instead, they express anger, resistance, discomfort, and fear associated with the application of restraints. As an outcome of this research, the authors reported that a need exists to test alternative safety strategies and limit use of restraints to a last resort used on a short-term basis.

Summary

Safe, effective nursing care requires individualized assessments and interventions. These research studies suggest that planned attention to elimination needs, use of a bedside monitoring device, and implementation of a risk assessment tool can prevent falls in geriatric clients. Alternative nursing strategies should be explored that eliminate routine use of physical restraints without endangering client safety.

- Sensory deprivation
- Emotional distress (fear, anxiety, humiliation, indignation)

In addition, elderly clients may experience a prolonged effect and an increased risk of adverse reactions when a chemical restraint is prescribed.

Nurses frequently have ambivalent feelings about using restraints or protective devices. Their dilemma results when concern about the client's potential risk of injury conflicts with the nurse's awareness of the indignity, anger, and regression an elder person may suffer when placed in restraints. An awareness of the potential harm restraints can cause has prompted nurses to look for alternative methods of ensuring client safety and preventing serious falls. Blakeslee (1988) suggests that a supportive administrator and a staff that is dedicated to finding cre-

ative, resourceful alternatives are critical if a restraint policy is to be changed. Records indicate no greater incidence of injuries from falls in facilities where restraints are not used; in fact, Blakeslee's facility has been restraint-free since its opening almost 20 years ago. One recent study questioned the effectiveness of restraints in preventing falls and observed that restrained elders were three times as likely to sustain fall-related injuries (Tinelti et al., 1992). Alternatives that focus on preserving a client's independence and self-esteem can eliminate the fear, anger, and anxiety that accompany the use of restraints. Careful nursing assessment is the key. Identifying the cause of the problem—although it may require more time and effort than simply applying a restraint or giving a medication—is the critical ingredient in finding a solution. Individualized nursing interventions may effectively reduce confusion or

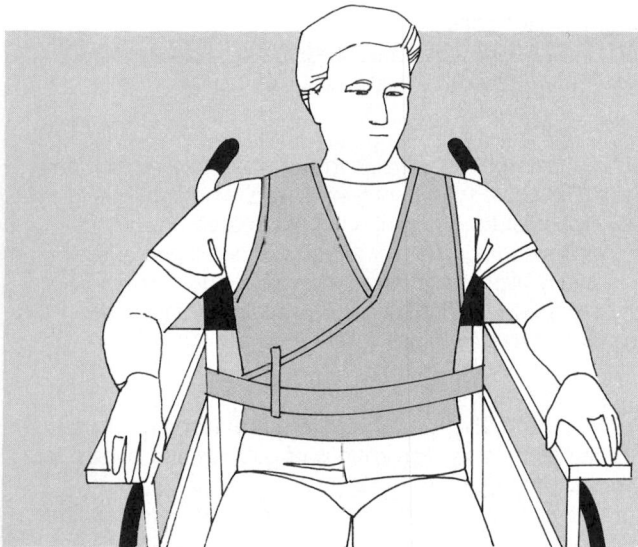

A

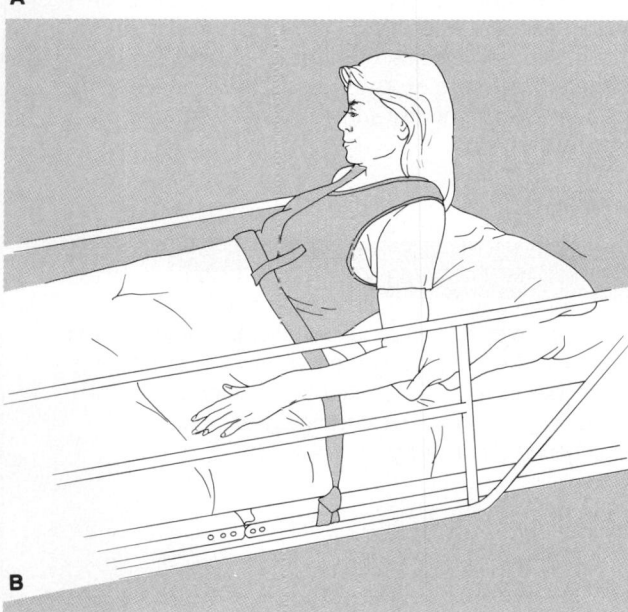

B

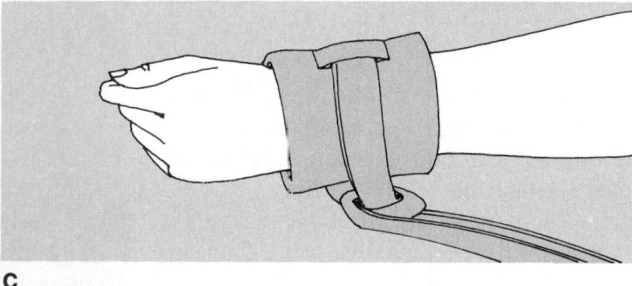

C

FIGURE 25-5

Restraints that can be adjusted to the specific activity limitation desired are more likely to be accepted by the client and his family. The purpose of restraints is to help prevent the client from being harmed. They should not interfere with physiologic functioning, such as impairing circulation, limiting muscular activity to the point of immobilization, or interfering with respiration.

agitation and provide a safe environment. See display entitled Alternatives to Using Restraints.

Despite all efforts, restraints may be the only solution in some situations. It is important to explain to the client and his or her family that the restraints are being applied as a protective device, not as a punishment measure. Documentation should include alternative strategies that were ineffective, the reason for restraining the client, the type of restraint, pertinent nursing assessments, and the regular intervals when restraints were removed. Procedure 25-1 demonstrates the proper method for applying restraints.

A physician's order ordinarily is required to apply restraints, but some agencies allow nurses to apply them in certain emergencies. The nurse is advised to consult with appropriate personnel whenever in doubt and to obtain an order at the earliest opportunity. A clearly stated agency policy assists the nurse in determining when to apply restraints as well as which type to use, and reflects the institution's concern for client safety as well as its respect for the quality of human life. Restraint use can have serious consequences. Thirty-seven deaths directly attributed to restraints were reported in the United States and Canada between 1980 and 1987 (Blakeslee et al., 1991). Most of these deaths resulted from strangulation, but two clients died in fires when they burnt their restraints in an effort to free themselves.

The practice of using restraints as a last resort has received support from the federal government. Guidelines

(Know)

Alternatives to Using Restraints

- Determine if behavior pattern exists.
- Provide pain relief.
- Involve family in care.
- Reduce noise.
- Check environment for hazards.
- Use night light.
- Identify door of room (eg, use of balloon, sign, client's picture, ribbon).
- Use an alarm system.
- Allow restless client to walk after ensuring that environment is safe.
- Use a large plant or piece of furniture as a barrier to limit wandering from designated area.
- Maintain low bed position.
- Use therapeutic touch.
- Play music or video selections of the client's choice.
- Use pillows wedged against the side of the chair to keep client positioned safely.
- Assist with toileting.
- Make the environment as homelike as possible.
- Provide a warm beverage.
- Provide comfortable rocking chairs.
- Allow the client to assist the staff with simple tasks.

PROCEDURE 25-1

Applying Restraints

Equipment

Restraint
Padding, if necessary,
  for bony prominences

Action	Rationale
1 Determine the need for restraints.	Restraints (physical or chemical) should be used only as a last resort when alternative measures have failed.
2 Confirm agency policy for application of restraints. Secure physician's order if required.	Policy protects the client and the nurse and specifies guidelines for application as well as type of restraint to be used.
3 Explain reason for use to client and family. Clarify how care will be given and that use of restraints is a temporary measure.	Explanation to client and family may lessen confusion and anger and provide reassurance.
4 Wash your hands.	Handwashing deters the spread of microorganisms.
5 Apply restraints according to manufacturer's direction:	Proper application ensures that there is no interference with client's respiration and circulation.
a Allow greatest degree of mobility possible.	This provides minimal restriction.
b Pad bony prominences.	Padding prevents skin breakdown.
c For restraint applied to extremity, ensure that two fingers can be inserted between the restraint and client's wrist or ankle.	This prevents impaired circulation to extremity.

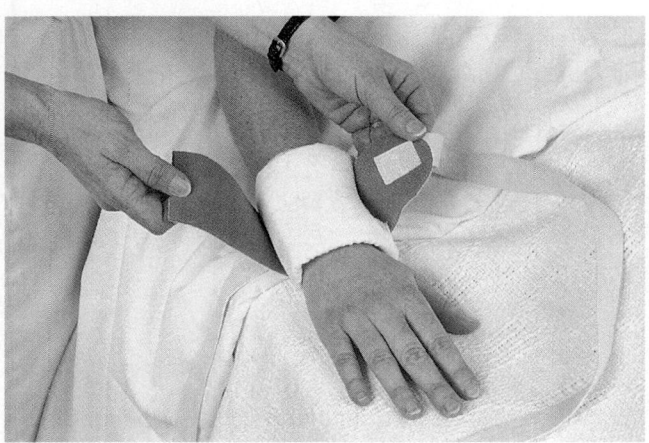

Action 5b: Applying restraint over padded bony prominences.

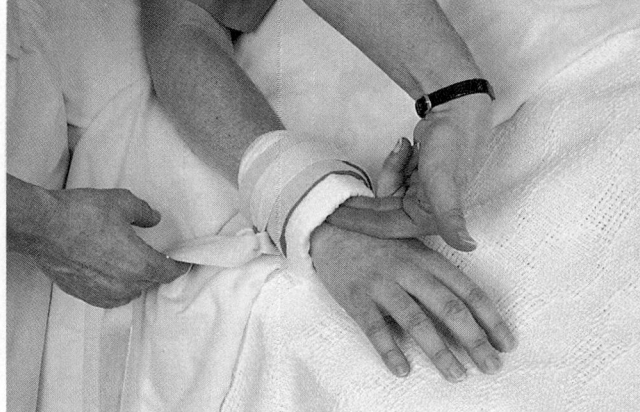

Action 5c: Ensuring that two fingers can be inserted between the restraint and the wrist.

d Maintain restrained extremity in normal anatomic position.	This lessens possibility for development of contracture or musculoskeletal injury.
e Use appropriate knot (see illustration).	Knot ensures that restraint will not tighten when pulled and can be removed quickly in an emergency.
f Fasten restraint to the bed frame and not the side rail. Site should not be readily accessible to the client.	Restraint secured to a side rail may injure the client when side rail is lowered. Tying restraint out of client's reach promotes security.

(continued)

P R O C E D U R E   2 5 - 1 *(continued)*

Applying Restraints

Action

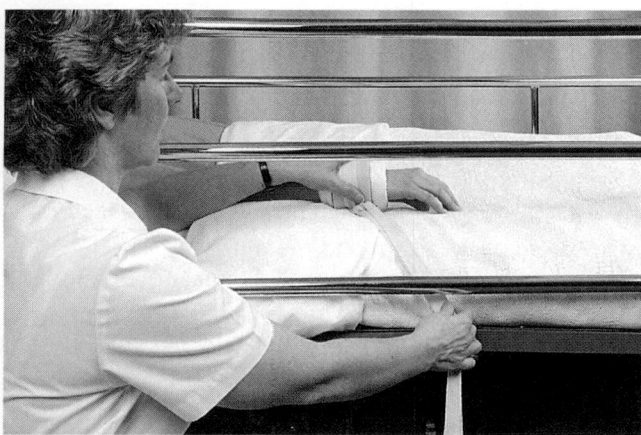

Action 5d: Keeping extremty in normal anatomic position.

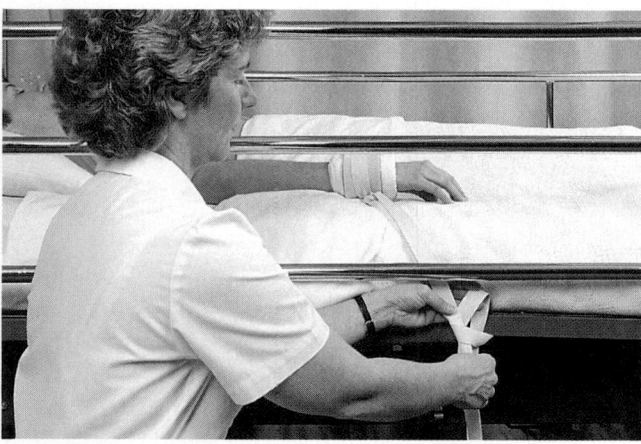

Action 5f: Fastening restraint to bed frame.

6 Remove restraint every 2 to 4 hours for at least 10 minutes according to agency policy and client need.
    a Check for signs of decreased circulation or impaired skin integrity.

    b Perform range-of-motion exercises before reapplying.

7 Reassure client at regular intervals.

8 Assess for signs of sensory deprivation, such as increased sleeping, day-dreaming, anxiety, panic, and hallucinations.

Rationale

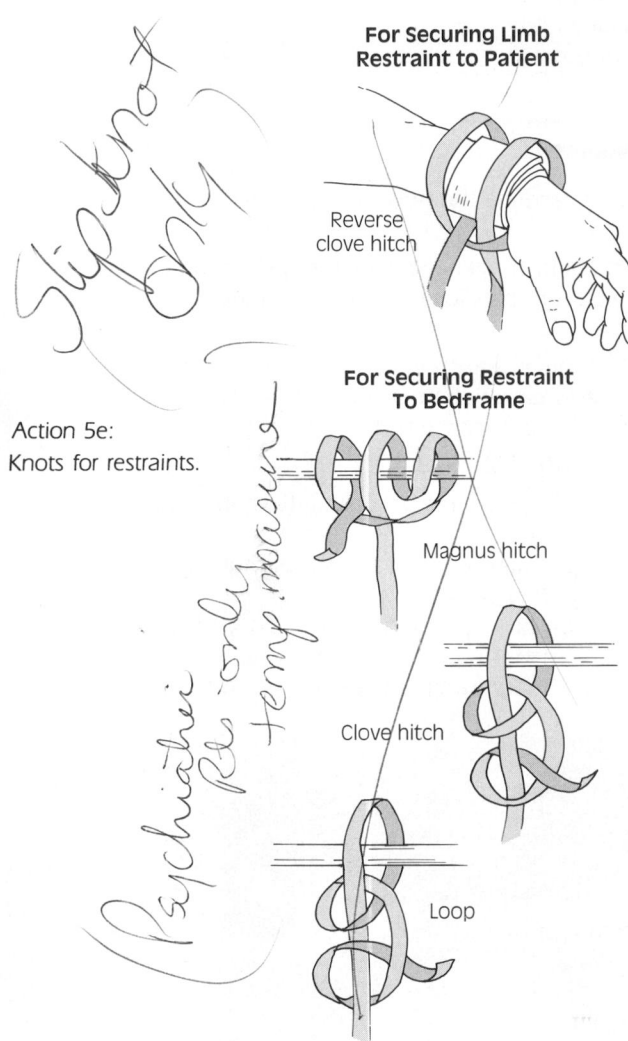

For Securing Limb Restraint to Patient

Reverse clove hitch

For Securing Restraint To Bedframe

Magnus hitch

Clove hitch

Loop

Slipknot only

Psychiatric — Rx only — temp measure

Action 5e:
Knots for restraints.

Removal allows for assessment of client and reevaluation of need for restraint.

Improperly applied restraints may cause skin tears, abrasions, or bruises. Decreased circulation may result in paleness, coolness, decreased sensation, tingling, numbness, or pain in an extremity.

Exercise increases circulation in the restrained extremity.

Reassurance demonstrates caring and provides opportunity for sensory stimulation as well ongoing assessment and evaluation.

Use of restraints may decrease environmental stimulation and result in sensory deprivation.

(continued)

Applying Restraints

Action	Rationale
9 Wash your hands.	Handwashing deters the spread of microorganisms.
10 Document reason for restraining client, type of restraint, times when removed, and result and frequency of nursing assessment for every shift.	Careful documentation supports use of restraints, alternative measures to ensure safety, and assessment data.

formulated by the Health Care Financing Administration as part of the 1987 Omnibus Budget Reconciliation Act emphasize the limited use of restraints in long-term care settings (Strumpf et al., 1990). Regulations prohibit the use of restraints to maintain balance or position and promote the use of the least restrictive device. In 1991, the Food and Drug Administration (FDA) issued a warning about restraints with recommendations for their use in acute and long-term care settings. This FDA directive states that all institutions must publish and communicate protocols for the use of restraints (Tammelleo, 1992). Documentation must verify the use of alternatives to restraints.*

Preventing Fires and Maintaining Fire Safety

Careless smoking in bed and faulty electrical equipment are most frequently implicated as causes of hospital fires; cigarettes, grease, and electric problems are most often responsible for fires in the home.

Home   The focus of nursing education for home fire safety includes a plan of action similar to that used in a health care setting. Priorities and practical suggestions include the following:
- Have emergency numbers near the telephone.
- Rehearse response to fire alarm and fire evacuation routes with family members before an emergency occurs.
- Evacuate family members as soon as smoke or fire is detected.
- Use the stairs to exit; do not use the elevator.
- Use a fire extinguisher if one is available and the fire is small.
- Close the doors to rooms. Open or break a window only if this is necessary to obtain fresh air.
- Remain close to the floor because smoke rises.

*Health care professionals with additional concerns about safe use of restraints should contact the following resource for additional information: Carol Herman, FDA, Center for Devices and Radiological Health, 5600 Fishers Lane, (HS2-250) Rockville, MD 20857.

- Cover your nose and mouth with a wet washcloth to prevent smoke inhalation.
- Do not run if your clothing catches fire. Lie down and roll on the floor to extinguish the flames. Another person may smother the flames with a blanket or coat. Remember: *Stop, drop, and roll.*
- Have approved smoke detectors installed in recommended locations.
- Do not let children play near space heaters, woodburning stoves, or fireplaces.

Health Care Agency   Orientations to health care agencies stress fire prevention information. The nurse is responsible for the client's safety and needs to be familiar with the agency's fire safety plan, exits, location and operation of fire extinguishers, and any special directions to report the fire.

Most hospital procedures emphasize the following priorities:
- Move anyone in immediate danger out of the area first.
- Call for help and activate the fire code system.
- Use the appropriate type of fire extinguisher (Fig. 25-6).

An acronym that may help staff members to remember these steps is *RACE*: *R*escue the client, sound the *a*larm, *c*onfine the fire, and *e*xtinguish it or *e*vacuate (Collins, 1988).

Preventing Poisoning

Concerted efforts by individuals, communities, state governments, and the federal government have reduced the number of accidental deaths by poisoning. Childproof containers are primarily responsible for this reduction.

Nursing intervention involves health education aimed at preventing accidental poisoning in the home. Parents need to be aware of hazardous substances that could result in poisoning if ingested. Plants frequently are implicated as a dangerous poison that is available in or near the home. Products commonly involved in poisonings are listed in the accompanying display. Toxic household substances should

Type of Extinguisher \ Type of Fire	Class "A" Fire in wood, paper, rags and extinguished by reducing the heat.	Class "B" Fire in flammable liquids, etc. Best extinguished by blanketing or smothering action. Fast spreading fire.	Class "C" Fire in energized electrical equipment. Smothering with a nonconducting extinguishing agent is of prime importance. Never use water or solutions with water.
Pressurized Water	**YES** Water soaks burning material and prevents rekindling.	**NO** Water will spread fire. Causes grease to splatter.	**NO** Water conducts electricity.
Carbon Dioxide (CO_2)	**NO** Has limited range. For small surface fires only.	**YES** Carbon dioxide smothers flames. Does not affect equipment or food.	**YES** Carbon dioxide is a non-conductor. Does not damage equipment.
Dry Chemical	**NO** Has limited range. For small surface fires only.	**YES** Chemical absorbs heat and smothers the flames.	**YES** Chemical is a non-conductor.
All Purpose	**YES** Coats material with a fire-retardant blanket to prevent reflash.	**YES** Covers fire with fast, flame-choking smothering action.	**YES** Chemical is a non-conductor.

FIGURE 25-6

Appropriate fire extinguisher usage for specific types of fires.

be removed or stored safely out of a child's reach. Local poison control centers can provide information about poisonous substances found in or near the home. Additional suggestions for childproofing homes are listed in the display.

It is vital that every household have the telephone number of the nearest poison control center readily available. The nurse should emphasize to parents that they should call the poison control center immediately, before they attempt any home remedy. Parents should be instructed to keep syrup of ipecac on hand but not to administer it unless directed to do so by medical authorities to induce vomiting. They may be instructed to bring the child immediately to an emergency facility for treatment. The focus of emergency treatment of poisoning is to stabilize vital body functions, prevent the absorption of the poison, and encourage excretion of the toxic substance.

Preventing Suffocation

Suffocation results almost immediately in unconsciousness, followed by respiratory and cardiac arrest. Emergency measures must be undertaken without delay and involve removing any obstruction and initiating cardiopulmonary resuscitation (see Procedures 36-6, 36-7, and 36-8).

Substances Frequently Implicated in Poisonings

Cleaning products
Analgesics
Cosmetics
Plants
Cough and cold preparations
Pesticides (including rodenticides)
Hydrocarbons
Topicals
Bites (poisonous venoms)
Foreign bodies
Antimicrobials
Chemicals
Sedatives, hypnotics, antipsychotics
Alcohols
Food poisoning
Vitamins

(Data from 1990 statistics compiled by the American Association of Poison Control Center's National Data Collection System.)

The educated, aware parent can reduce the risk of suffocation occurring in the home. The nurse may be involved in child care instruction that emphasizes careful supervision of children when they are drinking from a bottle, eating, bathing, or playing near a swimming pool. When riding in a motor vehicle, a child less than 55 inches (1.4 m) tall needs to be restrained in an appropriate car seat rather than using an adult seat belt and shoulder harness, which can slip with impact and cause neck injury. Other potential hazards include plastic bags, balloons, soft pillows or thick blankets in a crib, and allowing an infant to sleep on a water bed. Health education is a valuable preventive force.

Orienting the Client to the Health Agency

A person who is familiar with his or her surroundings is less likely to suffer an accidental injury. As part of the admission routine, the nurse orients the client to all the safety features and equipment in the room. An explanation and demonstration of the adjustable bed and side rails, call system, telephone, television, and bathroom area facilitate adjustment to the new environment. Application of an identification bracelet and discussion of agency routine further ensure safety and assist the client to adapt to an unfamiliar setting.

Preventing Equipment-Related Accidents

Health Care Agency   With the marked increase in the use of highly sophisticated equipment, it is especially important for health practitioners to learn to use equipment properly

and to recognize the signs that indicate that the equipment is not functioning correctly. For example, failure to use protective belts or side rails on carts and to lock wheelchair wheels can result in client injury. Using suction devices with inadequate vacuum and rate regulators or infusion equipment that delivers erratic amounts of solution also has resulted in equipment-related accidents.

Electrical equipment can present a particular safety hazard to both client and health practitioner when safety measures are ignored. Most electrical equipment used in hospitals is equipped with three-prong plugs. The third prong, when inserted into a properly wired wall outlet, provides a ground for the piece of equipment. A **ground** is a connection from an electricity source to the earth through which electric current leakage can be harmlessly conducted. Current leakage is not uncommon in electrical equipment, but a grounding system renders the equipment safe.

macro shock

Most people have experienced a tingling sensation in the extremities and trunk resulting from an electric current passing through a relatively large area of the body. This is

Household Principles for Prevention of Childhood Poisoning

- Keep all medications and toxic products in original containers
- Keep childproof caps on toxic products if children live in the home or are frequent visitors
- Keep all medications, including vitamins, out of the reach of children, in a locked chest
- Keep household chemical products out of the reach of children
- Do not treat medicines as candy
- Do not take or give medicine in the dark
- Read labels carefully before using drugs or toxic products
- Keep emergency poison control telephone numbers handy
- Have emergency drugs in the home—syrup of ipecac and epsom salts
- Use toxic chemical products in a well-ventilated area
- Do not mix common household cleaning products
- Destroy all old medications
- Destroy unused medications by flushing down toilet or washing down sink rather than by throwing in trash
- Use childproof containers when available
- Identify any poisonous houseplants, and keep seeds, bulbs, leaves, and fruits of such plants away from children

(Spencer, R. T., Nichols, L., Lipkin, G., Sabo, H., & West, F. [1989]. *Clinical pharmacology and nursing management* [3rd ed.]. Philadelphia: Lippincott.)

known as **macroshock**, and although it is unpleasant, it usually is not harmful. Macroshock often results from an ungrounded appliance or one in which the electric wiring has been damaged.

Microshock is the transmission of an electric current through a relatively small area of the body, usually directly into the heart. Because of the sensitivity of the myocardium to electric impulses, microshock can cause serious or even fatal heart irregularities. People with tubes, wires, or electrodes implanted in their chests or hearts are susceptible to microshock dangers because the tubing or wire can conduct leakage electricity directly to the heart muscle. Particularly because of microshock dangers, only equipment with three-prong plugs is recommended for use in health care agencies. Suspicion of ungrounded current leakage, including even a slight tingling sensation when touching a piece of equipment, or any other malfunction of electrical equipment should be reported immediately.

Home Accidents in the home frequently result from the careless use of equipment or from using malfunctioning or poorly maintained equipment. Many injuries and deaths from electric shock can be avoided. Overload of electric circuits, faulty appliances, frayed wires, careless use of electric equipment, and handling of electrical devices and cords when shoes and hands are wet often result in injury and death. The accompanying display lists guidelines to help reduce the number of equipment-related accidents.

Preventing Procedure-Related Accidents

The nurse must always be cautious and alert to prevent a procedure-related accident. The potential for error exists when the nurse is administering medications or intravenous solutions, transferring a client, changing a dress-

---

Guidelines to Help Decrease Equipment-Related Accidents

- Use equipment only for the use for which it was intended.
- Do not operate equipment with which you are unfamiliar.
- Handle equipment with care to prevent damaging it.
- Use three-prong electrical plugs whenever possible.
- Do not twist or bend electrical cords. The wires inside the cord may break.
- Be alert to signs that indicate equipment is faulty, such as breaks in electrical cords, sparks, smoke, electric shocks, loose or missing parts, and unusual noises or odors. Report signs of trouble immediately.
- Make certain that electrical cords are not in a position to be trapped as beds are raised or lowered. This can strip insulation covering the electrical wires.
- Be alert for wet surfaces on areas where electrical cords or connections are present.

---

ing, or applying external heat to a client's extremity. It is vital that the nurse follow correct procedures when administering care. Safeguards to prevent errors include making sure that the client is correctly identified (Fig. 25-7). A system of checking and rechecking further ensures the client's safety. The availability and use of resources further corrob-

---

FIGURE 25-7

Safeguards to prevent procedure-related accidents are based on a system of checking and rechecking. Careful attention should be paid to identifying the patient properly, checking or communicating necessary client records, and preparing the client physically and psychologically for any procedure or transfer. (Photo by Gates Rhodes, courtesy of School of Nursing, University of Pennsylvania.)

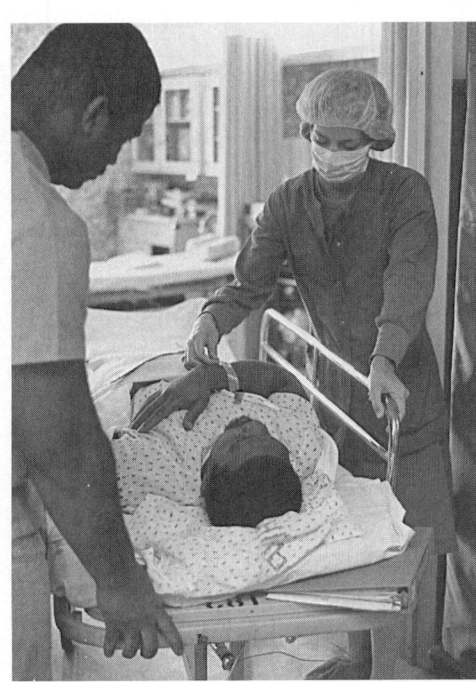 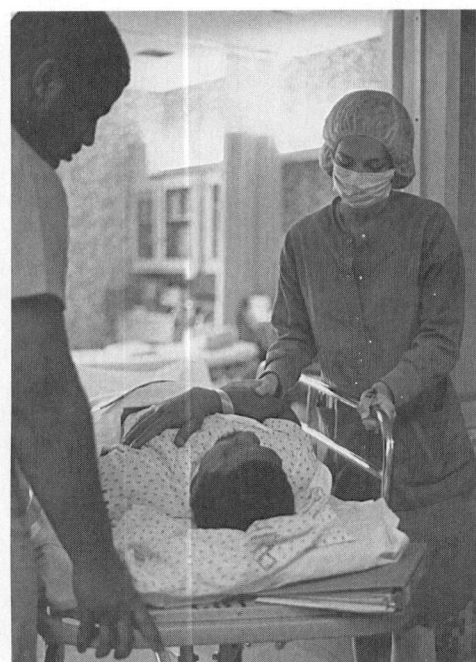

orate any question about correct procedure and prevent procedure-related accidents.

Filing an Incident Report

An accident in a health care agency requires the completion of an incident report, a confidential document that objectively describes the circumstances of the accident. The report also provides detail concerning the client's response and the examination and treatment of the client after the incident. The nurse completes the incident report immediately after an accident and is responsible for recording the occurrence of the accident and its effect on the client in the medical record.

All incident reports are carefully reviewed to detect any potentially threatening situation or pattern. The focus of a conference after the incident report has been filed is prevention of a similar occurrence and continuation of efforts to deliver quality nursing care. Incident reports are discussed in greater detail in Chapter 6.

Evaluating

The nurse must evaluate the effectiveness of interventions to promote environmental safety and prevent injury. If client goals have been met and evaluative criteria have been satisfied, the client will:

- Correctly identify real and potential unsafe environmental situations
- Implement safety measures in the environment
- Use available resources for safety information
- Incorporate accident prevention practices into the activities of daily living
- Remain free of injury

KEY POINTS

- Safety is the responsibility of all health care providers in every environment.
- Falls are the major safety problem in hospitals as well as the leading cause of accidental death for elderly people.
- Clients at high risk of falling include elderly people and those who have previously fallen.
- Careless smoking in bed and faulty electrical equipment are frequently implicated as causes in hospital fires.
- Hazards associated with the use of restraints include suffocation from improperly applied vests, impaired circulation, sensory deprivation, and emotional distress.

- Careful nursing assessment is the critical element in finding creative, resourceful alternatives to using restraints.
- The focus of emergency treatment of poisoning is to stabilize vital body functions, prevent the absorption of the poison, and encourage excretion of the toxic substance.
- Orientation to new surroundings, introduction to staff members, and explanations about equipment and procedures facilitate the client's transfer to a new health care setting.
- An incident report must be filed when an accident occurs in a health care agency. The report should objectively document the circumstances of the accident.

STUDY QUESTIONS

1. The most common cause of injury to women is
   a. motor vehicle accidents
   b. domestic violence
   c. occupational hazards
   d. accidental falls
2. When transporting a toddler in a motor vehicle, car seats are mandatory
   a. in all 50 states
   b. in 36 of the 50 states
   c. if a seat belt is not available
   d. on interstate highways
3. Which child has the greatest risk for choking and suffocating?
   a. a toddler playing with his 9-year-old brother's construction set
   b. a 4-year-old eating yogurt for lunch

   c. an infant covered with a small blanket and asleep in the crib
   d. a 3-year-old drinking a glass of juice
4. A class C electrical fire is appropriately extinguished by
   a. using an all-purpose extinguisher
   b. spraying it with water
   c. smothering it with a blanket
   d. taking the burning item outside
5. The leading cause of accidental death for elderly people at home is
   a. fires
   b. exposure to temperature extremes
   c. drug overdose
   d. falls

6. The nurse applies a vest restraint safely by
   a. securing the straps within the client's reach
   b. crossing the vest on the front side of the chest
   c. securing the knot as tightly as possible
   d. crossing the vest behind the client

7. Nurses most frequently restrain an elderly client because
   a. administration requires it
   b. the family has requested it
   c. they are short-staffed
   d. they fear the client may fall

8. Mr. Kennedy is a disoriented, elderly resident who likes to wander the halls in a long-term care facility. As an alternative to using restraints, the nurse might
   a. seat him in a geriatric chair
   b. use the sheets to secure him snugly in his bed
   c. keep the bed in the high position
   d. identify his door with his picture and a balloon

9. While discussing home safety with the nurse, Mrs. Fuller admits that she always smokes a cigarette in bed before falling asleep at night. An appropriate nursing diagnosis would be
   a. Impaired Gas Exchange related to cigarette smoking
   b. Anxiety related to inability to stop smoking
   c. High Risk for Suffocation related to unfamiliarity with fire prevention guidelines
   d. Knowledge Deficit related to lack of follow-through of recommendation to stop smoking

10. Mr. D'Ambro has weakened knees due to arthritis. The home health care nurse is aware that he understands the need for safety modifications at home because he
   a. uses the towel bar for support to stand up from the commode
   b. leans on the pedestal table in his bedroom when he dresses
   c. sits only in chairs with armrests
   d. uses a small stepladder to reach an item on an upper shelf

11. When a fire occurs in a client's room, the nurse's priority should be
   a. rescue the client
   b. extinguish the fire
   c. sound the alarm
   d. run for help

12. The nurse is planning health teaching for a young mother about responding to a poisoning emergency. She should instruct the mother to first
   a. use salt water to induce vomiting
   b. rush the child to the emergency department
   c. call the poison control center
   d. administer syrup of ipecac

13. After reviewing Mr. Sennett's past history of injuries and completing the assessment, the nurse suspects elder abuse. The nurse is aware that
   a. the client is probably the best source of information about the injuries
   b. the incidence of elder abuse ranges from 20% to 30% of that population
   c. the abuser usually is a paid health care employee
   d. a family in which conflict and stress exist is frequently implicated

14. The nurse orients an elderly client to the safety features in her hospital room. A vital component of this admission routine is to
   a. explain how to use the telephone
   b. introduce the client to her roommate
   c. review the hospital policy on visiting hours
   d. explain how to operate the call bell

15. When completing an incident report, the nurse should
   a. include suggestions to prevent the accident from recurring
   b. provide minimal information about the incident
   c. discuss the details with the client before documenting them
   d. objectively describe the incident in detail

Answers With Rationale

1. The correct response is *b*. Domestic violence is widespread and represents the most common cause of injury to women. Elderly people and young children are particularly at risk of injury from falls; adolescents are injured in motor vehicle accidents more than any other group. The incidence of injury from occupational hazards is relatively low for all groups.

2. The correct response is *a*. All 50, not 36, of the states require safety car seats for infants and toddlers at all times.

3. The correct response is *a*. A young child may place small or loose parts in his or her mouth; thus, a toy that is safe for a 9-year-old could kill a toddler. An infant sleeping in a crib without a pillow or large blanket and a 3- and 4-year-old drinking juice and eating yogurt are not particular safety risks.

4. The correct response is *a*. An all-purpose extinguisher will put out an electrical fire because the chemical used is a nonconductor. Water conducts electricity, and smothering with a blanket or moving a burning item outside are ineffective and dangerous.

5. The correct response is *d*. Falls are the leading cause of accidental death in the elderly population at home. Fires, exposure to temperature extremes, and drug overdose are significant causes of accidental death, but not in this age-group at home.

6. The correct response is *b*. Strangulation deaths have occurred because vest restraints were applied backward. The vest should be crossed in the front with the higher side in the back. Securing the straps within the client's reach allows him or her to undo the restraint, and securing the restraint too tightly may restrict respirations.

7. The correct response is *d*. Nurses most commonly apply restraints to a client because they fear he or she will fall and sustain an injury. Administrators usually say that they do not want clients restrained unless necessary, but may not support the nurse if the client falls. The family also may have ambivalent feelings, but neither their request nor short-staffing is the primary reason for the nurse to apply restraints.

8. The correct response is *d*. Identifying his door with his picture and the balloon may work as an alternative to restraints. Using the geriatric chair and sheets are forms of physical restraint. Leaving the bed in the high position is a safety risk and will probably result in a fall.

9. The correct answer is *c*. Because Mrs. Fuller is not aware that smoking in bed is extremely dangerous, she is at risk of suffocation from fire. The other three nursing diagnoses are correctly stated but not a priority for this situation.

10. The correct response is *c*. Chairs with armrests increase the client's leverage as he attempts to rise. Towel bars are not designed to provide support, the pedestal table is unsteady and unsafe, and standing on a stool and reaching places the client at risk of falling.

11. The correct response is *a*. The patient's safety is always the priority. Sounding the alarm and extinguishing the fire are important once the client is safe. Calling for help, rather than running for assistance, allows you to remain with your clients and is more appropriate, if possible.

12. The correct response is *c*. Always call the poison control center before attempting any home remedies or administering syrup of ipecac. These responses may be dangerous for the victim. The poison control center can supply the doctor or emergency department with specific information to assist in the victim's care.

13. The correct response is *d*. One out of 20 (5%) elder Americans is abused, and most often the abuse involves family members rather than a paid employee. The family situation frequently is a stressful one, with some kind of conflict. For a variety of reasons—fear or shame—the abused elderly person is reluctant to report a family member for abuse.

14. The correct response is *d*. Knowing how to use the call bell is a safety priority, whereas knowing how to use the phone, meeting one's roommate, and an awareness of visiting hours will not necessarily prevent an accidental injury.

15. The correct response is *d*. An incident report is a legal document and must be stated as objectively and completely as possible. It is not a collaborative effort with the client, and any suggestions to prevent this from happening again should be discussed at a postincident conference.

BIBLIOGRAPHY

Accident facts. (1989). Chicago: National Safety Council, p. 96.

American Academy of Pediatrics. (1992). Teen auto safety update. *Safe Ride News, 11*(1), 7.

American Nurses' Association. (1991). *Abuse of prescription drugs: Position statement.* Kansas City, MO: Task Force on Drug and Alcohol Abuse/Addictions.

American Nurses' Association. (1991). *Opposition to criminal prosecution of women for use of drugs while pregnant and support for treatment services for alcohol and drug-dependent women of childbearing age: Position statement.* Kansas City, MO: Task Force on Drug and Alcohol Abuse/Addictions.

Berryman, E., Gaskin, D., Jones, A., Tolley, F., & MacMullen, J. (1989). Point by point: Predicting elder's falls. *Geriatric Nursing, 10*(4), 199–201.

Blakeslee. J. (1988). Untie the elderly. *American Journal of Nursing, 88*(6), 833–834.

Blakeslee, J., Goldman, B., Papougenis, D., & Torell, C. (1991). Making the transition to restraint-free care. *Journal of Gerontological Nursing, 17*(2), 4–8.

Bloom, C., & Braun, J. (1991). Success with wanderers. *Geriatric Nursing, 12*(1), 20.

Bock, K., & Schilder, E. (1988). Physical restraints. *Canadian Nurse, 84*(8), 34–37.

Brains, L., Alexander, K., Grota, P., Chen. R., & Dumas, V. (1991). The development of the RISK tool for fall prevention. *Rehabilitation Nursing, 16*(2), 67–69.

Brannon, P. (1988). Using nursing skills instead of restraints. *Geriatric Nursing, 9*(2), 114–115.

Brower, H. T. (1991). The alternatives to restraints. *Journal of Gerontological Nursing, 17*(2), 18–21.

Bullock, L., McFarlane, J., Bateman. L., & Miller, V. (1989). The prevalence and characteristics of battered women in a primary care setting. *Nurse Practitioner, 14*(6), 47–54.

Carpenito, L. (1992). *Nursing diagnosis: Application to clinical practice* (4th ed.). Philadelphia: Lippincott.

Coberg, A., Lynch, D., & Mavretish, B. (1991). Harnessing ideas to release restraints. *Geriatric Nursing, 12*(3), 133–134.

Collins, H. (1988). Who'd survive a fire on your unit? *RN, 51*(7), 32–36.

Dallaire, L., & Burke, E. (1989). A new program for reducing patient falls. *Nursing, 19*(1), 65.

D'Avanzo, C. (1990). Incest: Break the silence, break the cycle. *RN, 53*(10), 34–36.

Dysart, J. (1990). Rethinking the earth. *Canadian Nurse, 86*(7), 16–17.

Easterling, M. (1990). Which of your patients is headed for a fall? *RN, 53*(1), 56–58.

Evans, L., & Strumpf, N. (1989). Tying down the elderly: A review of the literature on physical restraint. *Journal of American Geriatric Society, 37*(1), 65–74.

Fletcher, K. (1990). Restraints should be a last resort. *RN, 53*(1), 56–58.

Food and Drug Administration. (1991, November 14). Potential hazards with protective restraint devices. (MDA91-3). Rockville, MD: FDA Medical Alert.

Gage, R. (1991). Examining the dynamics of spouse abuse: An alternative view. *Nurse Practitioner, 16*(4), 11–16.

Garcia, R., Cruz, M., Reed, M., Taylor, P., Sloan, G., & Beran, N. (1988). Relationship between falls and patient attempts to satisfy elimination needs. *Nursing Management, 18*(7), 80V–X.

Gross, Y., Shimamoto, Y., Rose, C., & Frank, B. (1990). Why do they fall? Monitoring risk factors. *Journal of Gerontological Nursing, 16*(6), 20–25.

Heischen, S. (1989). Getting a handle on patient mobility. *Geriatric Nursing, 10*(3), 146–147.

Houston, K., & Lach, H. (1990). Restraints: How do you score? *Geriatric Nursing, 11*(5), 231–232.

Jacobson, E. (1990). New hospital hazards: How to protect yourself. *American Journal of Nursing, 90*(2), 36–41.

Jacques, J., & Snyder, N. (1991). Newborn victims of addiction. *RN, 54*(4), 47–52.

Jaffe, E. (1991). Working with troubled teens. *RN, 54*(2), 58–62.

Johnson, D. (1991). Make your own chairbound alternatives. *Geriatric Nursing, 12*(1), 18–19.

Jurgrau, A. (1990). How to spot child abuse. *RN, 53*(10), 26–32.

Ladewig, P., London, M., & Olds, S. (1990). *Essentials of maternal–newborn nursing* (2nd ed.) Redwood City, CA: Addison-Wesley Nursing.

Levy, G., & Hickey, J. (1991). Fighting the battle against drugs. *RN, 54*(4), 44–46.

Litovitz, T., Schmitz, B., & Holm, K. (1989). 1988 Annual Report of the American Association of Poison Control Centers National Data Collection System. *American Journal of Emergency Medicine, 7*(5), 495–525.

McHutchion, E., & Morse, J. (1989). Releasing restraints: A nursing dilemma. *Journal of Gerontological Nursing, 15*(2), 16–21.

Meyer, C. (1992). New evidence in the case against restraints. *American Journal of Nursing, 92*(5), 14.

Mitchell-Pedersen, L., Fingerote, E., Powell, C., & Edmund, L. (1989). Avoiding restraints. *Nursing, 19*(9), 67–72.

Morgan, K. (1991). Motor vehicle-related fatalities: Implications for home healthcare. *Home Healthcare Nurse, 9*(3), 18–22.

Nelson, R., & Amin, M. (1990). Falls in the elderly. *Emergency Medicine Clinics of North America, 8*(2), 309–324.

Press, M. M.: Restraints: Protection or abuse? *Candian Nurse, 87*(11), 29–30.

Rader, J. (1991). Modifying the environment to decrease use of restraints. *Journal of Gerontological Nursing, 17*(2), 9–13.

Rader, J., & Donius, M. (1991). Leveling off restraints. *Geriatric Nursing, 12*(3), 71–73.

Richardson-Jenkins, B. L. (1991) Disaster countdown. *Candian Nurse, 87*(4), 20.

Ross, J. (1991). Iatrogenesis in the elderly. *Journal of Gerontological Nursing, 17*(2), 19–23.

Roybal, E. (1991). Elder abuse: America's hidden crisis. *Caring, 10*(5), 22–24.

Scherer, Y., Janelli, L., Genevieve, W., Kanski, M., Neary, A., & Morth, N. (1991). The nursing dilemma of restraints. *Journal of Gerontological Nursing, 17*(2), 14–17.

Schlapman, N. (1990). Elderly women and falls in the home. *Home Healthcare Nurse, 8*(4), 20–24.

Spellbring, A., Gannon, M., Klecknert, T., & Conway, K. (1988). Improving safety for hospitalized elderly. *Journal of Gerontological Nursing, 14*(2), 31–37.

Spencer, R., Nichols, L., Lipkin, G., Sabo, H., & West, F. (1989). *Clinical pharmacology and nursing management* (3rd ed.). Philadelphia: Lippincott.

Stark, E. & Flitcraft, A. (1988). Violence among intimates: An epidemiological review. In V. Hasselt, et al. (Eds.). *Handbook of family violence*. New York, NY: Plenum, pp. 293–318.

Stilwell, E. (1991). Nurses' education related to the use of restraints. *Journal of Gerontological Nursing, 17*(2), 23–25.

Strumpf, N., & Evans, L. (1988). Physical restraint of the hospitalized elderly: Perceptions of patients and nurses. *Nursing Research, 37*(3), 132–137.

Strumpf, N., Evans, L., & Schwartz, D. (1990). Restraint-free care: From dream to reality. *Geriatric Nursing, 11*(3), 122–124.

Strumpf, N., & Evans, L. (1991). The ethical problems of prolonged physical restraint. *Journal of Gerontological Nursing, 17*(2), 27–30.

Tammelleo, A. (1992). Restaints: A legal catch-22? *RN, 55*(4), 71–74.

Tideiksaar, R. (1989a). Geriatric falls: Assessing the cause, preventing recurrence. *Geriatrics, 44*(7), 57–61.

Tideiksaar, R. (1989b). Home safe home: Practical tips for fall-proofing. *Geriatric Nursing, 10*(6), 280–284.

Tinetti, M., Liu, W., & Ginter S. (1992). Mechanical restraint use and fall-related injuries among residents of skilled nursing facilities. *Annals of Internal Medicine. 116*(5), 369–374.

U.S. Health Care Financing Administration. (1988). *Medicare/Medicaid nursing home information: 1987–1988.* Washington, DC: U.S. Government Printing Office.

Whaley, L., & Wong, D. (1989). *Essentials of pediatric nursing* (3rd ed.). St. Louis: Mosby.

Whedon, M., & Shedd, P. (1989). Prediction and prevention of patient falls. *Image: Journal of Nursing Scholarship, 21*(2), 108–114.

Wolf-Klein, G., Silverstone, F., Basavaraju, N., Foley, C., Pascari, A., & Ma, P. (1988). Prevention of falls in the elderly population. *Archives of Physical Medicine Rehabilitation, 16*, 689–691.

Wright, B., Aizenstein. S., Vogler, G., Rowe, M., & Miller, C. (1990). Frequent fallers. *Journal of Gerontological Nursing, 16*(4), 15–18.

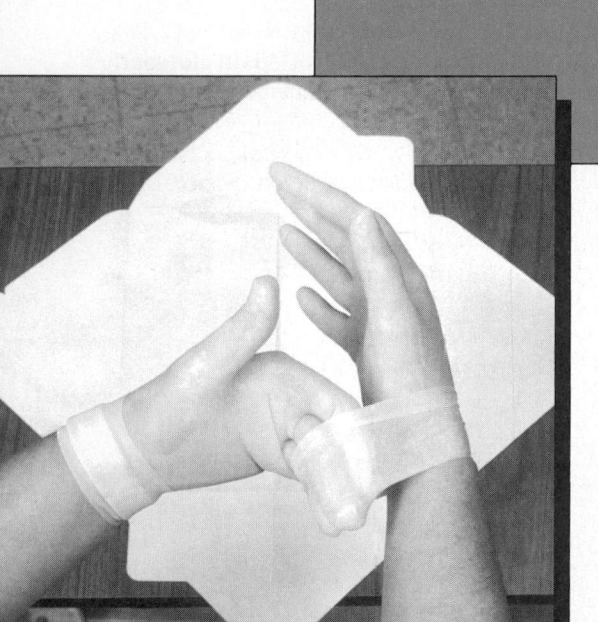
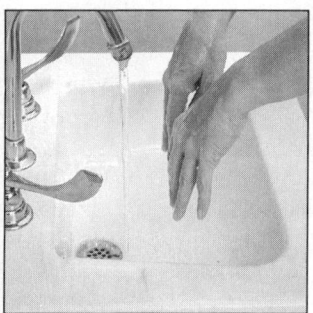

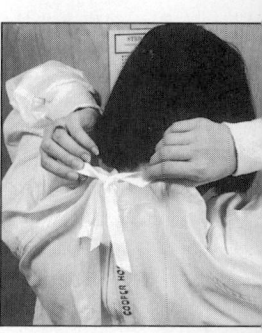

Asepsis

OBJECTIVES

After studying this chapter, the learner should be able to:

Define key terms used in the chapter.

Explain the infection cycle.

Describe nursing interventions used to break the chain of infection.

List the stages of an infection.

Identify clients at risk for developing an infection.

Identify factors that reduce the incidence of nosocomial infection.

Identify situations in which handwashing is indicated.

Identify nursing diagnoses associated with a client who has an infection or is at risk of developing an infection.

Differentiate between category-specific and disease-specific isolation systems.

Differentiate between universal precautions and the body substance isolation system.

Identify protocols for each isolation system.

Describe recommended techniques for medical and surgical asepsis.

KEY TERMS

aerobic
anaerobic
antibacterial
antibody
antigen
antiseptic
asepsis
bacteria
body substance isolation
category-specific isolation system
Centers for Disease Control
convalescent period
disease-specific isolation system
disinfection
endogenous
exogenous
fungi
gram-negative bacteria
gram-positive bacteria
host
iatrogenic infection
immune response
incubation period
infection
inflammatory response
isolation
localized symptoms
medical asepsis
normal flora
nosocomial infection
opportunist
pathogen
prodromal stage
reservoir
resident bacteria or flora
sterilization
surgical asepsis
susceptibility
systemic symptoms
transient bacteria or flora
universal precautions
virulence
virus

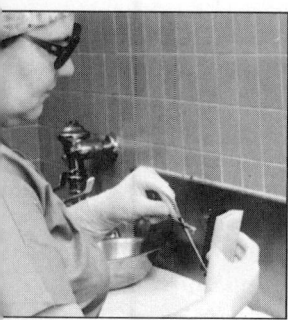

Infectious Agent Some of the more prevalent agents that are capable of causing infection include bacteria, viruses, and fungi. **Bacteria** are the most significant and most commonly observed infection-causing agents in health care institutions. Bacteria can be categorized in various ways. According to shape, they are classified as spherical (cocci), rod-shaped (bacilli), or corkscrew (spirochetes). Based on their reaction to the Gram stain, bacteria may be either gram-positive or gram-negative. **Gram-positive bacteria** have a thick cell wall that resists decolorization (loss of color) and are stained violet. **Gram-negative bacteria** have chemically more complex cell walls and can be decolorized by alcohol. This difference is vital information when

In addition to environmental safety, a major concern of health practitioners is the danger of spreading microorganisms from person to person and from place to place. Microorganisms are naturally present in the environment. Some are beneficial and some are not. Some are harmless to most people, and others are harmful to many people. Still others are harmless, except in certain circumstances.

The efforts of many people are involved in maintaining a microorganism-safe environment. Government agencies at the international, national, state, and local levels; health personnel; citizens from every walk of life; and family members are all involved in making and keeping the environment as free from harmful organisms as possible. Such efforts include mass immunization programs, laws concerning safe sewage disposal, regulations for the control of communicable diseases, and hospital infection-surveillance programs. As medical science continues to grapple with increasingly virulent organisms and immunologically compromised hosts, prevention of infection becomes a major focus for the nurse. As the primary caregiver, the nurse needs to be involved in identifying, preventing, controlling, and teaching the client about infection. Consistent application of the nursing process can prove critical in breaking the chain of infection.

Infection Prevention and Control

Infection Cycle

An **infection** is a disease state that results from the presence of pathogens in or on the body. A **pathogen** is a disease-producing microorganism. An infection occurs as a result of a cyclic process, as shown in Figure 26-1. The six components in the infection cycle are as follows:

- Infectious agent
- Reservoir
- Portal of exit
- Means of transmission
- Portal of entry
- Susceptible host

FIGURE 26-1

Infection process cycle. An infection occurs as a result of interrelated factors. An infection will not develop if the sequence is interrupted. Hence efforts to control infections are directed toward interrupting the sequence.

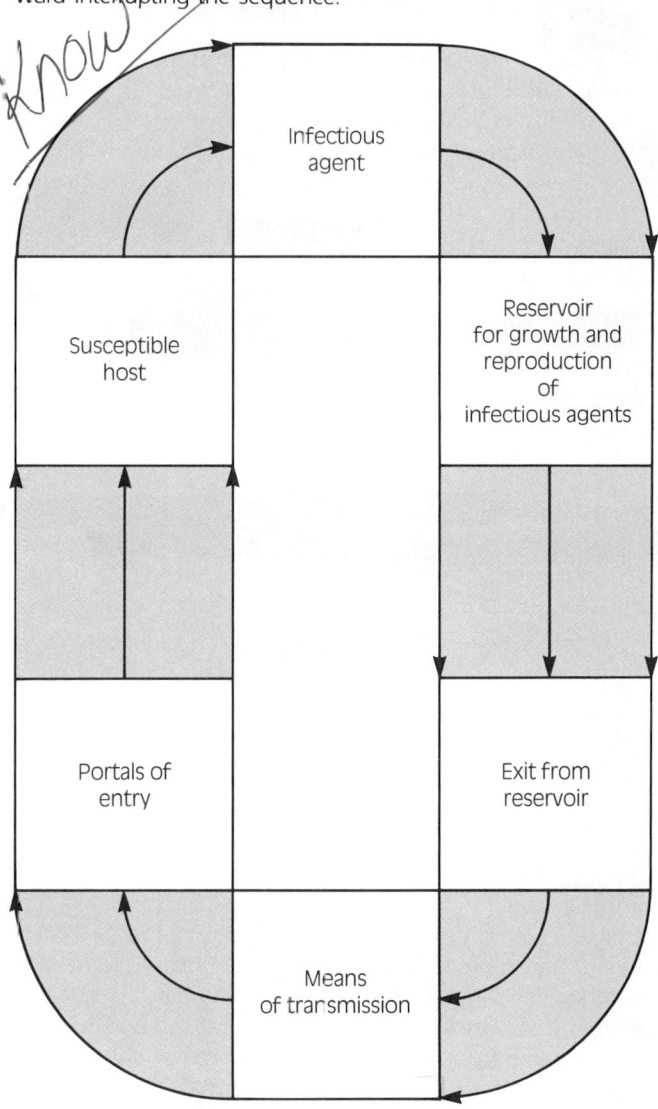

the physician is selecting an antibiotic to prevent or treat an infection. Antibiotics may be either specifically effective against only gram-positive organisms or classified as broad-spectrum and be effective against several groups of microorganisms.

Another distinguishing characteristic of bacteria is their need for oxygen. Most bacteria require oxygen to live and grow and are referred to as **aerobic**. Those that can live without oxygen are **anaerobic** bacteria.

A **virus** is the smallest of all microorganisms and can be seen only by using an electron microscope. Many infections are caused by viruses, including the common cold and the deadly disease acquired immunodeficiency syndrome (AIDS).

Fungi are plantlike organisms (molds and yeasts) that also can cause infection. They are present in the air, soil, and water, and many are resistant to treatment.

An organism's potential to produce disease depends on a variety of factors including the following:

- Number of organisms
- **Virulence** of the organism or its ability to cause disease
- Competence of a person's immune system
- Length and intimacy of the contact between a person and the microorganism

Under normal conditions, an organism may not produce disease. Microorganisms that commonly inhabit various body sites and are part of the body's natural defense system are referred to as **normal flora**. Other factors may intervene and cause this relatively harmless organism to become the source of an infection. Bacteria that may potentially be harmful are referred to as **opportunists**. For example, *Escherichia coli*, which normally resides in the intestinal tract, may produce infection when it migrates into the urinary tract.

Reservoir The **reservoir** for growth and multiplication of microorganisms is the natural habitat of the organism. Possible reservoirs that support organisms pathogenic to humans include other humans and animals, as well as food, water, milk, and inanimate objects.

Other Humans The tubercle bacillus and the spirochete that causes syphilis are examples of pathogens whose reservoirs are inhabited by the infectious agent and exhibit symptoms of disease, whereas others are *carriers* of the disease but do not show any symptoms of illness. For example, a person who has tested positive after a human immunodeficiency virus (HIV) antibody test probably has been infected with HIV. Even though symptoms of AIDS may not be present, the virus may be transmitted by intimate sexual contact, sharing a contaminated needle and syringe, and transfusion with contaminated blood or blood products and from an infected mother to her child during pregnancy or birth. A person's own normal flora can serve as a reservoir of pathogens.

Animals The rabies virus is an example of a pathogen whose reservoir is various animals, notably dogs, squirrels, and raccoons.

Soil Organisms that cause gas gangrene and tetanus are examples of pathogens whose reservoir is soil.

Portal of Exit The *exit from the reservoir* is the point of escape for the organism. The organism cannot extend its influence unless it moves away from its original source. There usually is a primary exit route for each type of microorganism. In humans, common escape routes are the respiratory, gastrointestinal, and genitourinary tracts, as well as breaks in the skin. Blood and tissue also can serve as an exit for pathogens.

Means of Transmission An organism may be transmitted from its reservoir by various means or routes. Some organisms can be transmitted by more than one route. Organisms can enter the body by way of the *contact* route, either directly or indirectly. Direct contact involves proximity between the susceptible host and an infected person or a carrier such as occurs in touching, kissing, or sexual intercourse. The indirect contact route requires personal contact with an inanimate object such as a contaminated instrument. Contaminated blood, food, water, or inanimate objects (fomites) are *vehicle* routes of transmission. *Vectors*, such as mosquitoes, ticks, and lice, are nonhuman carriers that transmit organisms from one host to another. Microorganisms also can be spread by means of the *airborne* route by droplet nuclei when coughing, sneezing, and talking or by becoming attached to dust particles. Table 26-1 presents a summary of the means of transmission and examples of diseases they transmit.

Portal of Entry The organism must find a portal of entry on a host. The *portal of entry* is the point at which organisms enter a host. The entry route often is the same as the exit route. The urinary, respiratory, and gastrointestinal tracts and the skin are common entry points.

Susceptible Host For microorganisms to continue to exist, they must find a source that is acceptable (a **host**) and overcome any resistance mounted by the host's defenses. **Susceptibility** is the degree of resistance the potential host has to the pathogen. It is not uncommon for a person admitted to a hospital to be in a weakened state of health due to illness. Many factors influence a host's susceptibility and are discussed later in the chapter.

Stages of Infection

An understanding of the stages in the development of an infection is necessary if the nurse is to intervene and disrupt the infection cycle. An infection progresses through the following phases:

TABLE 26-1

Means of Disease Transmission

Route	Disease Transmitted
Contact (organisms spread person to person or person to object)	
Direct	Staphylococcal infection
	Herpes simplex
Indirect	Hepatitis B
	Measles
Vehicles (blood, food, water, or inanimate objects contaminated by organisms)	AIDS, hepatitis B and C (blood)
	Cholera, typhoid (water)
	Pseudomonas (infusion product or drug)
	Salmonella, Staphylococcus gastroenteritis (food)
Airborne (organisms contained in droplet nuclei or dust)	Influenza, chickenpox (droplet nuclei)
	Aspergillosis (dust)
Vectors (insects carry organisms)	Malaria, Lyme disease, Rocky Mountain spotted fever (mosquitoes, ticks)
	Brucellosis (domestic animals)

(Adapted from Schabery, D. [1989]. How infections spread in the hospital. *Respiratory Care, 34*[2], 81–84.)

Infection progresses through these phases

1. Incubation period
2. Prodromal stage
3. Full stage of illness
4. Convalescent period

The course and severity of the infection as well as the client's response influence the extent and type of nursing care provided.

Incubation Period The **incubation period** is the interval between the invasion of the body by the pathogen and the appearance of symptoms of infection. During this stage, the organisms are growing and multiplying, and the length of incubation may vary. For example, the common cold develops in 1 to 2 days, whereas tetanus has an incubation period ranging from 2 to 21 days.

Prodromal Stage A person is most infectious during the **prodromal stage**. Early signs and symptoms of disease are present but are vague and nonspecific, ranging from fatigue and malaise to a low-grade fever. This period lasts from several hours to several days.

Full Stage of Illness The presence of specific signs and symptoms indicates the *full stage of illness*. The type of infection determines the length of the illness and the severity of the manifestations. Symptoms that are limited or restricted to a discrete area are referred to as **localized symptoms**, whereas **systemic symptoms** are manifested throughout the entire body.

Convalescent Period The **convalescent period** represents recovery from the infection. The signs and symptoms disappear, and the person returns to a healthy state. Convalescence may vary according to the severity of the infection and the client's general condition.

Body's Defense Against Infection

In addition to the normal flora that inhabit various body sites (see discussion on handwashing later in this chapter), other defense systems help a person combat infection.

The **inflammatory response** is a protective mechanism that eliminates the invading pathogen and allows for tissue repair to occur. The inflammation process is discussed in detail in Chapter 43.

The **immune response** involves specific reactions in the body as it responds to an invading foreign protein such as bacteria or, in some cases, the body's own proteins. The complex mechanisms that constitute the immune response occur as the body attempts to protect and defend itself. The foreign material is called an **antigen**, and the body commonly responds to the antigen by producing an **antibody**. This antigen–antibody reaction is one component of the overall immune response; it also is known as humoral immunity. The cell-mediated defense, or cellular immunity, involves an increase in the number of lymphocytes (white blood cells) for the purpose of destroying or reacting specifically with cells the body recognizes as harmful. Although not completely understood, it is known that these complicated chemical and mechanical responses help to defend the body specifically against bacterial, viral, and fungal infections as well as malignant cells.

Factors That Affect the Risk of Infection

The susceptibility of the host is influenced by various factors, including the following:
- Intact skin and mucous membranes protect the body against microbial invasion.
- The normal pH levels of gastric secretions and of the genitourinary tract help to ward off microbial invasion.
- The body's white blood cells influence resistance to certain pathogens.
- Age, sex, race, and hereditary factors influence susceptibility, although reasons are not always clear. Neonates and elderly people appear to be more vulnerable to infection than the general population.
- Immunization, natural or acquired, acts to resist infection.
- Fatigue, climate, nutritional and general health status, the presence of preexisting illnesses, previous or current treatments, and some kinds of medications may play a part in the susceptibility of a potential host.
- Stress may adversely affect the body's normal defense mechanisms.
- The increasing use of invasive or indwelling medical devices provides more potential sources of disease-producing organisms, particularly in a client whose defenses are already weakened by disease.

Life-style also places a person at risk for developing an infection. Health habits that promote wellness positively influence the susceptibility of a host. Sensible nutrition, adequate rest and exercise, stress reduction techniques, and good personal hygiene habits are examples of activities that can help to maintain optimum bodily function and immune response. Unsafe sex practices and sharing intravenous needles are potentially dangerous and can introduce pathogens that cause infection.

Assessing

The nurse's critical role in controlling infection begins with early detection and surveillance techniques. The extent of the nursing interventions is determined by the susceptibility of the host, the virulence of the organism, and the client's signs and symptoms.

To formulate an individualized nursing care plan, the nurse inquires about the client's immunization status and previous or recurring infections, observes nonverbal cues, and elicits information regarding the history of the current disease process. A review of laboratory data provides further insight into the presence of an infectious process. Any of the following laboratory test results may indicate the presence of an infection:

- An elevated white blood cell (leukocyte) count—normal value is 5000 to 10,000/μL
- An increase in specific types of white blood cells (differential count)
- Presence of pathogen in urine, blood, sputum, or other drainage cultures

This compilation of assessment data constitutes a unique nursing data base that suggests nursing interventions for clients at risk for infection or those clients in whom an infection is already present.

Diagnosing

The potential for infection or the presence of an infection in a client suggests possible nursing diagnoses. The direction or focus of nursing care depends on a nursing diagnosis that accurately reflects the client's condition.

The following are examples of nursing diagnoses that relate to an infectious process:

High Risk for Infection related to presence of chronic disease; altered immune response; effects of medication; altered skin integrity; malnutrition; presence of invasive or indwelling medical device; lack of proper immunization

Social Isolation related to presence of communicable disease (AIDS)

Altered Oral Mucous Membrane related to ineffective dental hygiene; trauma

Diversional Activity Deficit related to lack of visitors; restrictions imposed by airborne isolation precautions

High Risk for Altered Body Temperature related to obstructed urine outflow

Planning: Client Goals

Effective nursing interventions can control or prevent infection. The nurse reviews the assessment data, considers the cycle of events that result in the development of an infection, and incorporates principles of infection control as client goals are formulated. Planning client goals that prevent infection or interfere with the infection cycle provides an exciting challenge for the nurse and an opportunity to see positive results because of these efforts.

The following client goals are appropriate to prevent infection. The client will:
- Demonstrate effective handwashing
- Identify the signs of an infection
- Maintain adequate nutritional intake
- Demonstrate proper disposal of soiled articles
- Use appropriate cleansing and disinfecting techniques
- Demonstrate an awareness of the necessity of proper immunizations
- Demonstrate stress reduction techniques

NURSING TODAY Challenges and Solutions

AIDS

Challenges

- About 1 million Americans are infected with the AIDS virus.
- AIDS has emerged as the ninth leading cause of death among children (1 to 4 years of age) and seventh in young people (15 to 24 years of age).
- Five percent of the hospitals in the United States care for 50% of the nation's cases.
- Median survival time since 1987 for people diagnosed with AIDS and treated with AZT is 770 days. Those not on AZT survive, on the average, 140 days.

Source: Hoyer, R. (August 1991). AIDS: An overview. *Caring Magazine.*

Nursing Solutions

- Two clinical research nurse practitioners in Los Angeles, with a focus on providing information to their AIDS-infected outpatients, have produced a newsletter that is distributed across the country with information on new research. They also are on call for advice, encouragement, and friendship.
- In Cleveland, Ohio, nurses are involved in a project that involves placing computer terminals in the homes of residents with AIDS. In addition to decreasing their sense of isolation, the computer allows their clients to access current information on AIDS.
- Nurse care managers in Raleigh, North Carolina, assess the needs of the county's AIDS patients, arrange for home care, negotiate with insurance companies, and find support groups for them. In 3 years, their caseload has become almost 10 times larger than the original patient group.
- Nurses working at an adult infectious disease clinic in Nashville, Tennessee, conducted a series of sessions designed to educate people and health care providers in rural areas about human immunodeficiency virus.

Source: Selby, T. (1990). HIV/AIDS: America's RNs respond to deepening crisis. *American Nurse, 22*(10), 4–14.

Implementing

Using Medical Asepsis

The nurse uses principles of aseptic technique to halt the spread of microorganisms and minimize the threat of infection. To control the number of organisms, medical and surgical asepsis are vital. The practice of **asepsis** includes any activities that prevent infection or break the chain of infection. It is divided into two types—medical asepsis and surgical asepsis. **Medical asepsis**, or clean technique, involves procedures and practices that reduce the number and transfer of pathogens. **Surgical asepsis**, or sterile technique, includes practices used to render and keep objects and areas free from microorganisms.

Medical asepsis is used continuously both within and outside health agencies because it is always assumed that pathogens are likely to be present. For example, public drinking cups are unsanitary because pathogens may be present on the cup after being used by someone who may be harboring pathogens. In a health care facility, if a specific pathogen is known to be present, special methods of medical asepsis are used to prevent further spread of the organism. Nearly every nursing activity includes practices of medical asepsis. Breaking the chain of infection is the nurse's responsibility. It involves giving safe client care and protecting the client as well as one's self from microorganisms that have at least the potential to cause disease. See the displayed material for basic practices of medical asepsis that nurses should use when giving care to clients.

Teaching Asepsis to Clients   Clients should be taught to use basic principles of asepsis at home and in public facilities. These involve activities of daily living (refer to Chapter 29 for a discussion of personal hygiene). The following are examples of medical asepsis practices recommended in the home:

- Wash hands before preparing food and before eating.
- Prepare foods at temperatures sufficiently high to ensure that they are safe to eat, the most common example being the preparation of fresh pork.
- Use care with cutting boards and utensils, and wash hands before and after handling raw chicken.
- Keep foods refrigerated, especially those containing mayonnaise.
- Wash raw fruits and vegetables before serving them.
- Use pasteurized milk.
- Wash hands after using the bathroom.
- Use individual personal care items, such as washcloths, towels, and toothbrushes.

Observe infection prevention in public facilities by following these guidelines:

- Wash hands after using any public bathroom.
- Use paper towels or hot-air dryers in restrooms.
- Use individually wrapped drinking straws.
- Use tongs to lift food from common service trays in cafeterias, food stores, and salad bars.

The community reinforces medical asepsis practices in various ways, including the following:

- Use of sterilized combs and brushes in barber and beauty shops

---

Basic Practices of Medical Asepsis in Client Care

- Wash hands frequently but especially before handling foods, before eating, after using a handkerchief, after going to the toilet, and before and after each client contact.
- Keep soiled items and equipment from touching the clothing. Carry soiled linens or other used articles so that they do not touch the uniform.
- Do not place soiled bed linen or any other items on the floor, which is grossly contaminated. It increases contamination of both surfaces.
- Avoid having clients cough, sneeze, or breathe directly on others. Provide them with disposable tissues, and instruct them, as indicated, to cover their mouth and nose to prevent spread by airborne droplets.
- Move equipment away from you when brushing, dusting, or scrubbing articles. This helps prevent contaminated particles from settling on the hair, face, and uniform.
- Avoid raising dust. Use a specially treated cloth or a dampened cloth. Do not shake linens. Dust and lint particles constitute a vehicle by which organisms may be transported from one area to another.
- Clean the least soiled areas first and then the more soiled ones. This helps prevent having the cleaner areas soiled by the dirtier areas.

- Dispose of soiled or used items directly into appropriate containers. Wrap items that are moist from body discharge or drainage in waterproof containers, such as plastic bags, before discarding into the refuse holder so that handlers will not come in contact with them.
- Pour liquids that are to be discarded, such as bath water, mouth rinse, and the like, directly into the drain so as to avoid splatterings in the sink and onto you.
- Sterilize items that are suspected of containing pathogens. After sterilization, they can be managed as clean items, if appropriate.
- Use practices of personal grooming that help prevent spreading microorganisms. Examples include shampooing the hair regularly, keeping it short or pinned up to limit the possibility of carrying microorganisms on hair shafts, keeping the fingernails short and free of broken cuticles and ragged nail edges, and avoiding wearing rings with grooves and stones that may harbor microorganisms.
- Follow guidelines conscientiously for isolation or barrier techniques as prescribed by agency.

- Examination of food handlers for evidence of disease
- Enforcement of frequent handwashing by food handlers

Preventing Nosocomial Infections For various reasons and sometimes despite best efforts, certain clients in health agencies develop infections that were not noted to be present on admission. The term **nosocomial** is used to describe a hospital-acquired infection. In its broad meaning, nosocomial means that the infection results while the client is receiving health care, and the source may be either exogenous or endogenous. An **exogenous** infection means that the causative organism is acquired from other people; an **endogenous** infection means that the causative organism comes from microbial life the person himself harbors. An infection is referred to as **iatrogenic** when it occurs as a result of a treatment or diagnostic procedure. Not all nosocomial infections have an iatrogenic component.

Preventing nosocomial infections poses a major challenge for health care providers. At least 6% of all hospital admissions contract a nosocomial infection (Larson et al., 1988; Lynch et al., 1987; Miller & Farr, 1989). Hospital-acquired infections are directly responsible for 20,000 deaths and contribute to another 60,000 deaths per year (Miller & Farr, 1989; Moran, 1990). The $10 million in hospital costs per year is staggering, particularly in light of the

concerted efforts to control spiraling expenses associated with health care.

In 1974 the **Centers for Disease Control** (CDC), a U.S. government agency whose responsibilities include investigation, identification, prevention, and control of disease, began a major project referred to as the Study of the Efficacy of Nosocomial Infection Control. The results of this study were not finalized and reported until 1985 (Larson et al., 1988). The CDC's investigation measured the effects of hospital infection and provided specific information about contributing factors, populations at risk, and approaches aimed at reducing the incidence of nosocomial infection.

Most hospital-acquired infections are caused by bacteria. *Escherichia coli, Staphlococcus aureus, Streptococcus faecalis, Pseudomonas aeruginosa,* and *Klebsiella* species have been implicated as common causative organisms. Gram-negative bacilli are responsible for more than 50% of hospital-acquired infections (Guenthner et al., 1987). Urinary tract infections account for 53% of all nosocomial infections, and indwelling urinary catheters have been implicated in 85% of these (Sawyer, 1989). Surgical wounds are a common site for infections to develop, but the highest mortality rate is associated with hospital-acquired infections that involve the respiratory tract (Hooton, 1989). The increasing use of biomedical equipment frequently is cited as a causative agent. In addition to indwelling urinary catheters, the devices most frequently implicated include central venous pressure monitoring lines, hemodialysis equipment, and respiratory equipment. Often the hands of the health care worker using the instruments are responsible for the contamination.

Nurses, by nature of their role, are in a unique position to prevent the transmission of nosocomial infections. Careful assessment and evaluation of high-risk clients and situations coupled with strict observance of medical and surgical asepsis techniques will minimize infection and reduce the unnecessary suffering imposed on clients. Using nursing diagnoses to generate appropriate nursing interventions makes a significant difference and improves the quality of nursing care.

Health agencies have found the following measures to be successful in reducing the incidence of nosocomial infections:

- Instituting constant surveillance by infection-control committees and nurse epidemiologists. Their work has been noted to reduce infections significantly when better control measures resulting from their findings are initiated.
- Having written infection prevention practices for all agency personnel. The Omnibus Budget Reconciliation Act (OBRA '87), which became effective in October 1990, mandates that all long-term care facilities have formal infection-control programs with emphasis on policies and procedures to prevent the spread of infection (Stolley & Buckwalter, 1991). Adherence to thorough handwashing and barrier precautions or isolation techniques can prevent many nosocomial infections. Typical guidelines are described later in this chapter.
- Using practices to help promote and keep clients in the best possible physical condition. Measures include meeting the client's needs for nutrition, fluids, rest, oxygen, and physical and psychological comfort and security.

Outbreaks of nosocomial infection in either acute-care hospitals or long-term care facilities are costly, frequently difficult to control, and debilitating for clients. Infection-control measures save lives and reduce the risk of transmission of pathogens to clients as well as personnel.

Using Handwashing *Handwashing is, without a doubt, the most effective way to help prevent the spread of organisms.* Differences of opinion persist about proper cleaning agents, length of time for washing, and ideal frequency of adequate handwashing, but everyone agrees that handwashing is the most important procedure in preventing nosocomial, or hospital-acquired, infections. Attention needs to be refocused on this simple procedure that can interrupt the chain of infection.

Bacterial Flora on Hands   Two types of bacterial flora normally are found on the hands—transient bacteria and resident bacteria. **Transient bacteria**, normally picked up by the hands in the usual activities of daily living, are relatively few on clean and exposed areas of the skin. They are attached loosely to the skin, usually in grease, fats, and dirt, and are found in greater numbers under the fingernails. Transient bacteria, pathogenic as well as nonpathogenic, can be removed with relative ease by washing the hands thoroughly and frequently. **Resident bacteria**, normally found in creases in the skin, are relatively stable in number and type. They cling tenaciously to the skin by adhesion and adsorption, and considerable friction with a brush is required to remove them. Also, they are less susceptible than transient bacteria to the action of antiseptics. For practical purposes, it is not considered possible to clean the skin of all bacteria.

Transient bacteria may adjust to the environment of the skin if the flora are present in large numbers over a long enough time. They then become resident bacteria. If pathogenic organisms become resident bacteria on the skin, the hands are then carriers of the particular organism. Therefore, it is important that the hands be cleaned promptly after each contact with contaminated materials to help prevent transient bacteria from becoming resident bacteria on the hands.

Cleansing Agents   Various products are available for handwashing. Soaps and detergents are considered adequate for routine mechanical cleansing of the hands and removal of most transient microorganisms. They help remove soil because they lower surface tension and act as emulsifying agents. Bar, liquid, or other forms of soap are all effective, but the factor that determines selection may be preference of personnel.

Using handwashing products that contain an antiseptic or antibacterial ingredient is recommended for any setting in which there is a high risk for infection. An **antiseptic** is a substance that inhibits the growth of bacteria; an **antibacterial** is an agent that kills bacteria or suppresses their growth. Antibacterial soaps are suggested for intensive care units, emergency departments, and any client-care setting in which exposure to blood and body fluids is likely or clients are immunosuppressed. Using soaps that contain an antimicrobial or antibacterial agent may cause skin dryness and cracking. These irritations defeat the purpose of decreasing the number of surface organisms because damaged skin harbors organisms and is difficult to clean adequately. Products are available that are mild, yet have sufficient antiseptic action. Hand lotion may be used to comfort damaged skin, but it is best applied after client care is completed.

Recommended Techniques   Recommended handwashing techniques for medical asepsis are listed in Procedure 26-1. Handwashing that incorporates surgical asepsis is described in texts that deal with operating and delivery room procedures. Effective handwashing requires at least a 10-second scrub with plain soap or disinfectant and water. Hands that are visibly soiled need a longer scrub. Frequency of handwashing and amount of soap used appear to positively influence the effectiveness of antiseptic prod-

P R O C E D U R E   2 6 - 1

Handwashing

Equipment

Liquid or bar soap   Paper towels
Orangewood stick   Lotion (optional)

Action

1 Stand in front of the sink. Do not allow your uniform to touch the sink during the washing procedure.

2 Remove jewelry, if possible, and secure in a safe place or allow plain wedding band to remain in place.

3 Turn on water and adjust force. Regulate the temperature until the water is warm.

4 Wet the hands and wrist area. Keep hands lower than elbows to allow water to flow toward fingertips.

5 Use about 1 teaspoon liquid soap from dispenser or lather thoroughly with bar soap. Rinse bar and return to soap dish.

6 With firm rubbing and circular motions, wash the palms and backs of the hands, each finger, the areas between the fingers, the knuckles, wrists, and forearms. Wash up the forearms at least as high as contamination is likely to be present.

Rationale

The sink is considered contaminated. Uniforms may carry organisms from place to place.

Removal of jewelry facilitates proper cleansing. Microorganisms may accumulate in settings of jewelry.

Water splashed from the contaminated sink will contaminate your uniform. Warm water is more comfortable and has less tendency to open pores and remove oils from the skin. Organisms can lodge in roughened and broken areas of chapped skin.

Water should flow from the cleaner area toward the more contaminated area. Hands are more contaminated than forearms.

Rinsing the soap removes the lather that may contain microorganisms.

Friction caused by firm rubbing and circular motions helps to loosen dirt and organisms that can lodge between the fingers, in skin crevices of knuckles, on palms and backs of the hands, as well as the wrists and forearms. Cleaning less contaminated areas (forearms and wrists) after hands are clean prevent spreading organisms from the hands to the forearms and wrists.

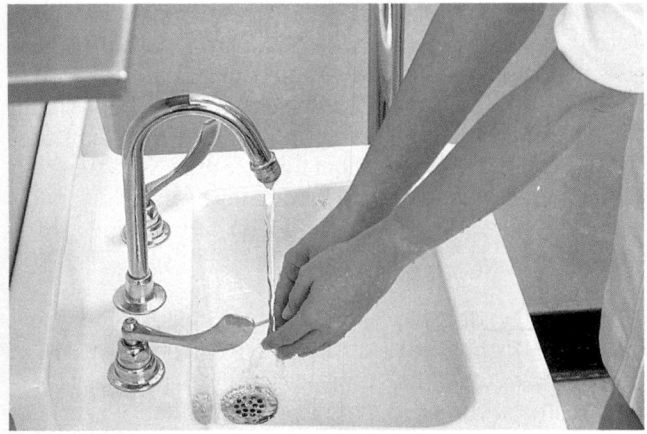

Action 4: Wetting hands and wrists.

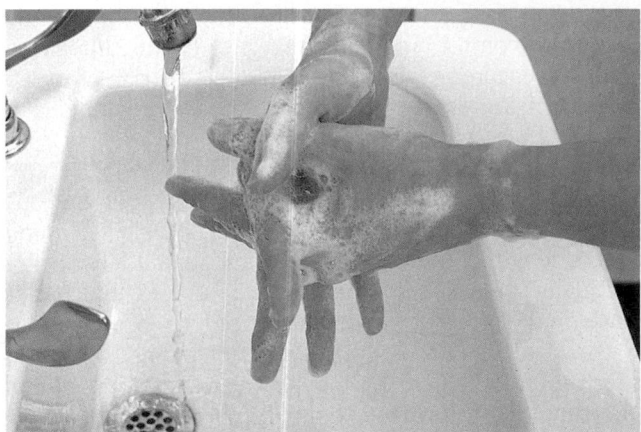

Action 6: Washing hands and forearms with firm rubbing and circular motions.

(continued)

PROCEDURE 26-1 (continued)

Handwashing

Action	Rationale
7 Continue this friction motion for 10 to 30 seconds.	Length of handwashing is determined by degree of contamination.
8 Use fingernails of the other hand or a clean orangewood stick to clean under fingernails.	Organisms can lodge and remain under the nails where they can grow and be spread to others.
9 Rinse thoroughly.	Running water rinses organisms and dirt into the sink.
10 Dry hands and wrists with a paper towel. Use paper towel to turn off faucet.	Drying the skin well prevents chapping. Dry hands first because they are the cleanest and least contaminated area. Turning the faucet off with a paper towel protects the clean hands from contact with a soiled surface.
11 Use lotion on hands if desired.	Lotion helps to keep the skin soft and prevents chapping.

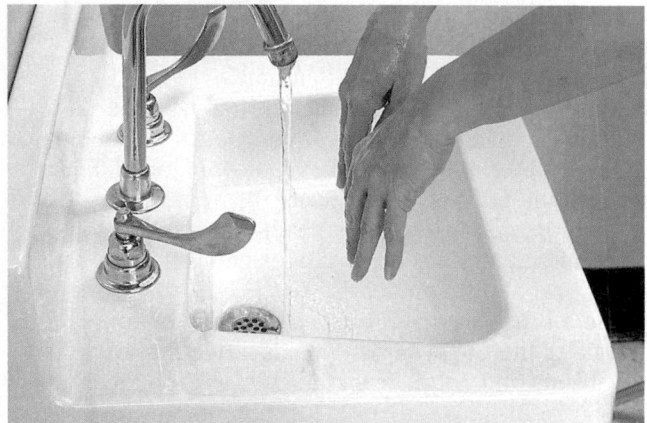

Action 9: Rinsing thoroughly.

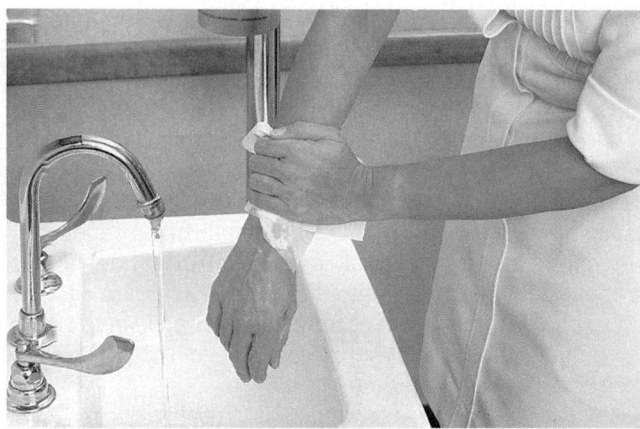

Action 10: Drying with a paper towel.

Age Considerations

Instruct children at early age in proper handwashing techniques.

Special Considerations

Special scrubbing techniques can reduce the risk for nurses who do not remove their rings. Research by Jacobsen and colleagues demonstrated that a 1-minute scrub using liquid soap and a scrub brush, followed by a 1-minute rinse can remove any additional surface bacteria (Jacobsen et al., 1985).

Sinks with various faucet controls are available. In addition to the more common hand faucets, knee- and foot-operated controls may be used. Sinks with elbow controls are generally used in a surgical setting.

ucts; findings are not as conclusive after handwashing with plain soap. One study suggests that a cumulative number of handwashings with nonmedicated soap may be effective in removing gram-negative bacilli from the hands (Guenthner et al., 1987). Most guidelines recommend removal of all jewelry except a wedding band and advise particular attention to the area beneath the fingernails, where bacteria tend to accumulate. A person with polished or artificial nails is less likely to vigorously scrub that area. All researchers agree that handwashing substantially reduces nosocomial transmission of microorganisms.

Even though health care personnel are aware of the importance of handwashing, most studies report that compliance with this simple preventive measure is difficult to achieve (Larson, 1989). Despite intensive educational efforts, handwashing is infrequently practiced. Wearing gloves does not substitute for proper handwashing (CDC, 1988). In reality, the warmth and moisture inside the glove create an ideal environment for bacteria to multiply, making it even more important to wash hands before and after gloves are applied. Research also indicates that gloving does not guarantee complete protection from infectious organisms (Korniewicz et al., 1989). Gloves provide a barrier, but they are not impenetrable and may give the health care worker a false sense of security. Occasional defects in the gloves also reinforce the necessity of washing hands before and after any client contact.

Controlling Infectious Agents by Sterilization and Disinfection

Cleansing, disinfection, and sterilization help to break the chain of infection and prevent nosocomial disease. Most health agencies provide items for client care that are sterile when purchased and disposed of after use. Some items, such as pitchers, water glasses, and thermometers, may be used repeatedly, but by one client only; they are then discarded or sent home with the client on discharge.

Health agencies usually maintain a central supply unit where most reusable equipment is cleaned, kept in good working order, and sterilized as indicated. There are times, especially in homes and in some small health agencies, when the nurse is required to make decisions about how to prepare equipment and supplies so that they are safe for client use. Although nurses may not be directly involved in the actual process, they must be aware of the critical role they play in preventing infection.

Several processes are used to destroy microorganisms. **Disinfection** destroys all pathogenic organisms except spores; **sterilization** is the process by which all microorganisms, including spores, are destroyed. Disinfection and sterilization of contaminated or infected objects and good handwashing diminish and often eliminate microorganisms as potential sources of infection.

Factors in Selecting Method Various factors must be considered when selecting sterilization and disinfection methods. They include the following:

Nature of organisms present: Recommendations from the CDC now state that all supplies, linens, and equipment in a health care setting should be treated as if the client were infectious. Some organisms are easily destroyed, whereas others are able to withstand certain commonly used sterilization and disinfection methods.

Number of organisms present: The more organisms present on an item, the longer it takes to destroy them.

Type of equipment: Equipment with small lumens, crevices, or joints require special care. Certain articles may be damaged by various sterilization and disinfection methods and require special handling.

Intended use of equipment: The need for medical or surgical asepsis influences the preparation and cleaning of equipment. In the home setting, it may be safe to use equipment and supplies that are clean, but most health agencies prefer to use sterilized articles for client care.

Available means for sterilization and disinfection: The choice of chemical or physical means of sterilization and disinfection is made on the basis of the nature and number of organisms, the type and intended use of the equipment, and the availability and practicality of the means.

Time: Time is a key factor when sterilizing or disinfecting articles. Failure to observe recommended time periods is grossly negligent.

Cleaning Supplies and Equipment Proper cleaning of items used in health care before they are sterilized or disinfected is essential to reduce the number of organisms and to dislodge them from crevices and from under layers of contaminating substances. The following techniques are recommended for cleaning equipment:

• Wear waterproof gloves at all times.
• Rinse the articles first with cold running water to remove organic material. Heat coagulates certain organic material, which makes removal more difficult.
• Wash the articles, after rinsing them, in warm water that contains detergent or soap. The combination of warm water and soap facilitates emulsification and removal of dirt and debris.
• Use a brush with stiff bristles as indicated to clean the articles thoroughly. Friction aids in the removal of organisms and debris from difficult to reach areas (Fig. 26-2).
• Rinse and dry the article thoroughly.

FIGURE 26-2

Proper cleaning of items used in health care before sterilization is essential. Items should be rinsed in cold running water, washed in warm water using soap or detergent and a brush, rinsed, and dried in preparation for sterilization or disinfection.

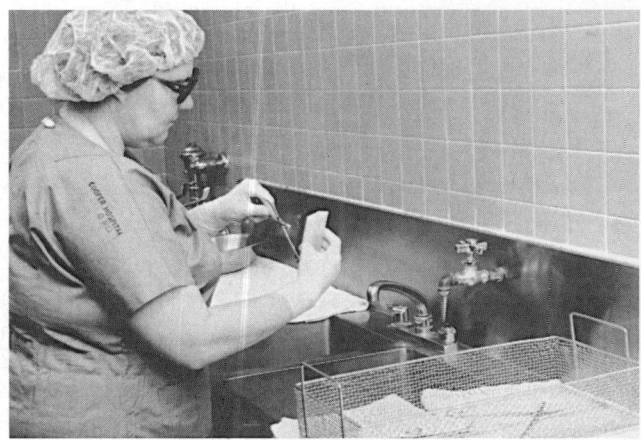

- Prepare the cleaned equipment for sterilization or disinfection.
- Consider the brush, gloves, and the sink or basin in which the articles were cleaned as highly contaminated, and treat or discard them accordingly.

See Table 26-2 for explanation of physical and chemical means of sterilization and disinfection.

Using Surgical Asepsis

Surgical asepsis techniques, used regularly in the operating room, labor and delivery areas, and certain diagnostic testing areas, also are used by the nurse at the client's bedside. Procedures that involve the insertion of a urinary catheter, sterile dressing changes, and preparing an injectable medication are examples of surgical asepsis techniques. An object is considered sterile when all microorganisms, including pathogens and spores, have been destroyed. For example, the needle for an injection is handled so that it is sterile when inserted into a client. A sterile forceps or sterile gloves are used to handle sterile dressings to protect from contamination. The basic principles of surgical asepsis are listed in the accompanying display.

In observing medical asepsis, areas are considered contaminated if they bear, or are suspected of bearing, pathogens. In observing surgical asepsis, areas are considered contaminated if they are touched by any object that is not also sterile. One of the most important aspects of surgical and medical asepsis is that the effectiveness of both depends on the faithfulness and the conscientiousness of those carrying them out. It is far better to err on the side of safety when using surgical asepsis than to take the slightest chance of possible contamination.

Explanation of the surgical asepsis procedure facilitates cooperation of the client. An awareness of which objects and areas may not be touched as well as directions to avoid sudden movements are vital for the client to assist the nurse in maintaining the sterility of the procedure.

Handling Sterile Objects   Sterile gloves or sterile forceps are used for handling items when maintaining sterility is necessary.

Putting on Sterile Gloves   Sterile gloves are donned so that only the inside of the gloves comes in contact with the hands. Procedure 26-2 explains the proper technique for putting on sterile gloves. After the gloves are on, sterile items may be handled with the sterile-gloved hands. Careful removal of the gloves reduces any hand contact with contaminated materials. Good handwashing technique before and after putting on sterile gloves is imperative.

(Text continues on p. 516)

TABLE 26-2

Methods of Sterilization and Disinfection

Method	Discussion	Caution
Physical		
Steam	Higher temperature caused by higher pressure destroys organisms (eg, autoclaving)	Most plastic and rubber devices are damaged by autoclaving
Boiling water	Frequently used in the home—simple and inexpensive; boil item for at least 15 minutes	Spores and some viruses are not destroyed by boiling
Dry heat	Alternative sterilization method for home. Used for metal items. Heat oven to 350°F for 2 or more hours	Insufficient to destroy all microorganisms. Not used in health care agencies
Radiation	Used for pharmaceuticals, foods, plastics, and other heat-sensitive items	Object must be directly exposed to ultraviolet radiation on all surfaces. Poses risk to personnel
Chemical		
Ethylene oxide gas	Destroys microorganisms and spores by interfering with metabolic processes in cells. Gas is released while items (oxygen and suction gauges, blood pressure equipment) are contained in autoclave	Precautions necessary because gas is toxic to humans
Chemical solutions	Generally used for instrument and equipment disinfection and for housekeeping disinfection. Chlorines are useful for disinfecting water and for housekeeping purposes. A solution of sodium hypochlorite (household bleach) in a 1:100 dilution effectively inactivates human immunodeficiency virus. Betadine or alcohol are also used as disinfectants	Method does not destroy all spores and may cause corrosion on metal surfaces

P R O C E D U R E 2 6 - 2

Donning and Removing Sterile Gloves

Equipment

Sterile gloves (size of gloves is indicated on outer wrapping; select appropriate size)

Action	Rationale
To Apply Gloves	
1 Wash and dry hands carefully.	Handwashing deters the spread of microorganisms. Gloves are easier to don when hands are dry.
2 Place sterile glove package on clean, dry surface above your waist.	Moisture could contaminate the sterile gloves. Any sterile object held below the waist is considered contaminated.
3 Open the outside wrapper by carefully peeling the top layer back. Remove inner package, handling only the outside of it.	This maintains sterility of gloves in inner packet.
4 Carefully open the inner package and expose the sterile gloves with the cuff end closest to you.	The inner surface of the package is considered sterile.

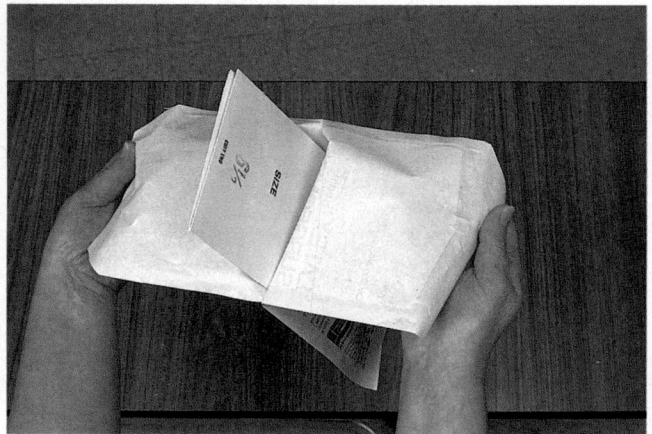

Action 3: Peeling back top layer of outer package.

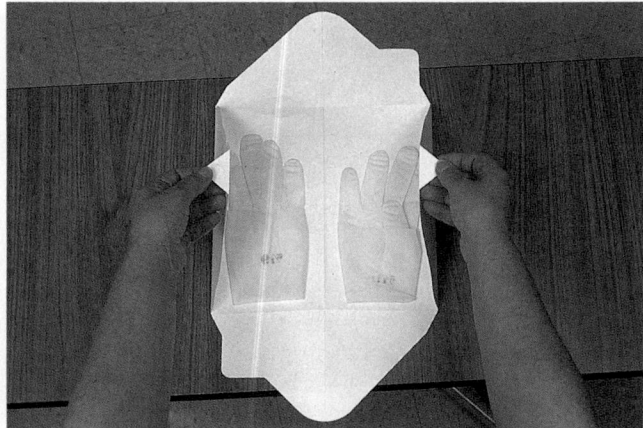

Action 4: Opening inner package.

Action	Rationale
5 With the thumb and forefinger of nondominant hand, grasp the top edge of the folded cuff of the sterile glove for dominant hand.	Unsterile hand only touches inside of glove. Outside remains sterile.
6 Lift and hold glove with fingers down. Be careful it does not touch any unsterile object.	Glove is contaminated if it touches unsterile objects.
7 Carefully insert the dominant hand into glove and pull glove on. Leave cuff folded down until other hand is gloved.	Attempts to turn upward with unsterile hand may result in contamination of sterile glove.
8 Holding thumb outward, slide fingers of gloved hand under cuff of remaining glove and lift glove upward.	Thumb is less likely to become contaminated if held outward.
9 Carefully insert nondominant hand into glove. Adjust gloves on both hands touching only sterile areas.	Sterile surface touching sterile surface prevents contamination.

(continued)

PROCEDURE 26-2 *(continued)*

Donning and Removing Sterile Gloves

Action

Rationale

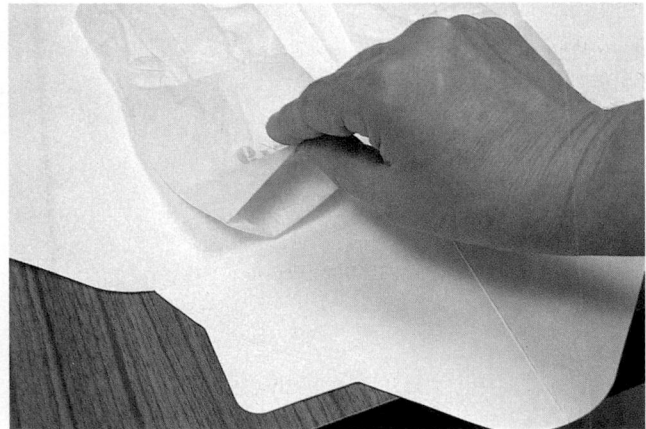

Action 5: Grasping edge of folded cuff.

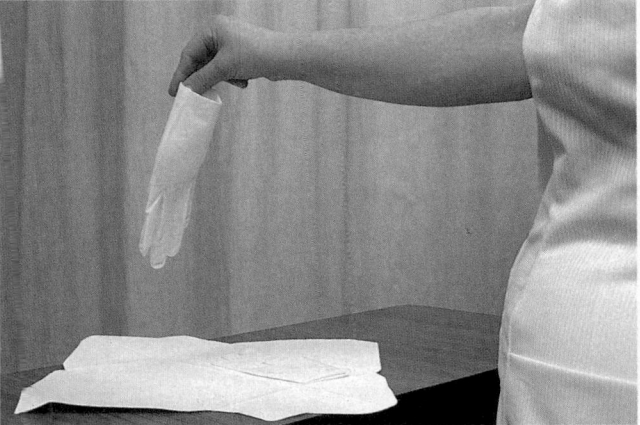

Action 6: Lifting and holding glove with fingers down.

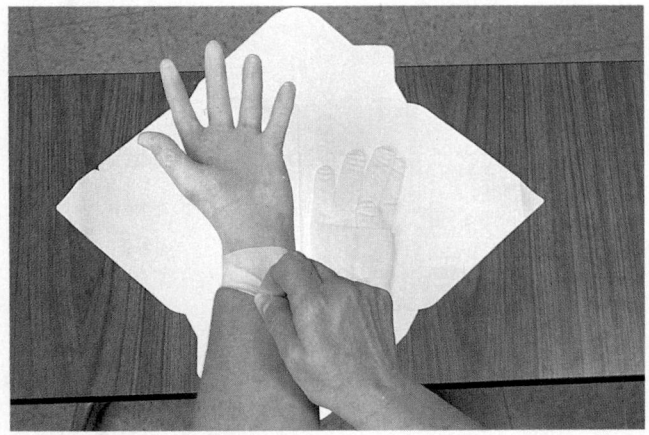

Action 7: Pulling first glove on with cuff folded.

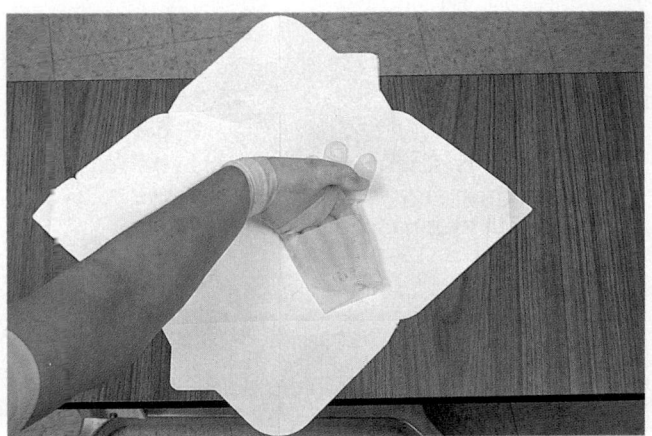

Action 8: Sliding fingers of gloved hand under cuff of second glove.

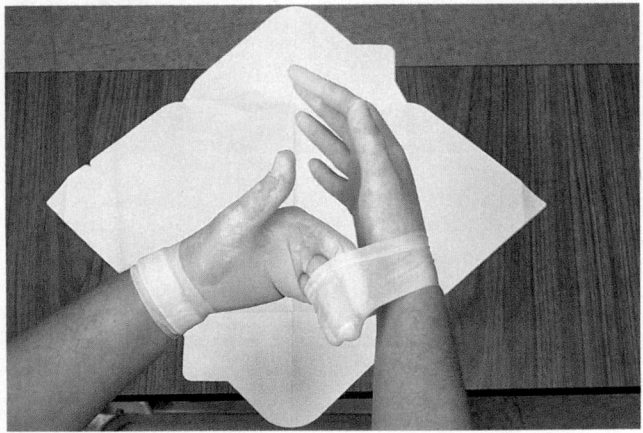

Action 9: Inserting hand with cuff folded.

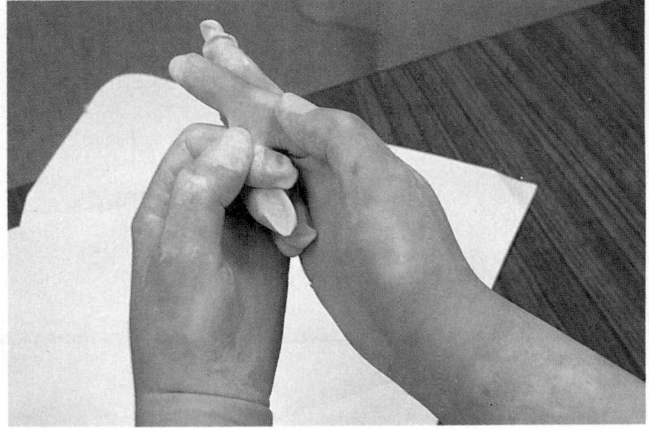

Action 9: Adjusting gloves on both hands.

(continued)

PROCEDURE 26-2 *(continued)*

Donning and Removing Sterile Gloves

Action	**Rationale**

To Remove Gloves

1 Using dominant gloved hand, grasp other glove near cuff end and remove by inverting it, keeping the contaminated area on the inside. Continue to hold onto glove.

Contaminated area does not come in contact with hands or wrists.

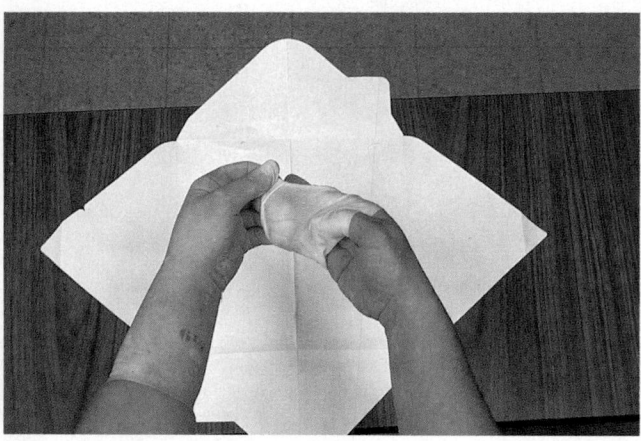

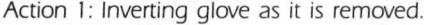

Action 1: Inverting glove as it is removed.

2 Slide fingers of ungloved hand inside the remaining glove. Grasp glove on inside and remove by turning inside out over hand *and other* glove.

Contaminated area does not come in contact with hands or wrists.

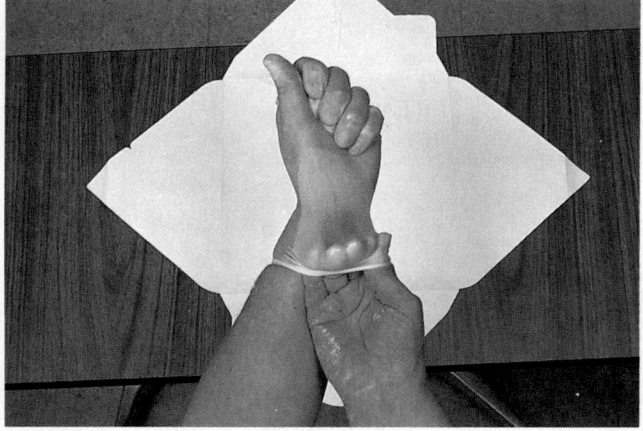

Action 2: Sliding ungloved fingers inside second glove.

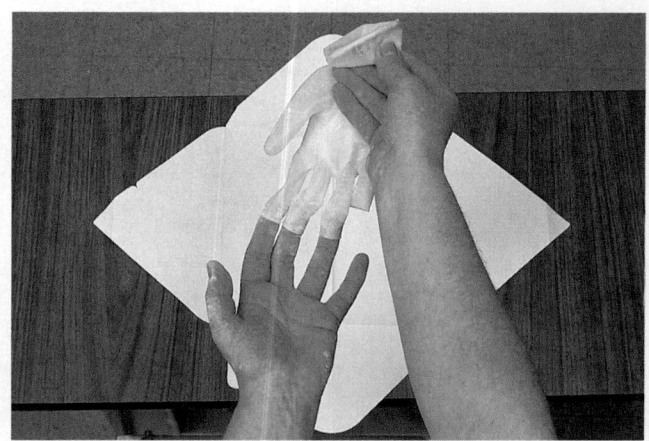

Action 2: Removing second glove inside out.

3 Discard gloves in appropriate container and wash hands.

Handwashing reduces the spread of microorganisms.

Putting on Surgical Cap and Mask For a sterile surgical procedure, the nurse puts on a disposable paper or clean cloth cap. All hair must be covered. The mask, with the rigid strip on the uppermost edge, is held by the upper two strings and tied securely at the back of the head to prevent slipping. The lower two ties are fastened around the neck, making sure that the mouth and chin are completely covered. The mask should be adjusted over the bridge of the nose; if glasses are worn, the upper edge of the mask should be eased under the glasses to minimize fogging. In

Basic Principles of Surgical Asepsis

- Only a sterile object can touch another sterile object. Unsterile touching sterile means contamination has occurred.
- Open sterile packages so that the first edge of the wrapper is directed away from the worker to avoid the possibility of a sterile surface touching unsterile clothing. The outside of the sterile package is considered contaminated. Opening a sterile package is shown and described in Figure 26-3.
- Avoid spilling any solution on a cloth or paper used as a field for a sterile setup. The moisture penetrates through the sterile cloth or paper and carries organisms by capillary action to contaminate the field. A wet field is considered contaminated if the surface immediately below it is not sterile.
- Hold sterile objects above the level of the waist. This will help ensure keeping the object within sight and preventing accidental contamination.
- Avoid talking, coughing, sneezing, or reaching over a sterile field or object. This helps to prevent con-

tamination by droplets from the nose and the mouth or by particles dropping from the worker's arm.
- Never walk away from or turn your back on a sterile field. This prevents possible contamination while the field is out of the worker's view.
- All items brought into contact with broken skin, or used to penetrate the skin in order to inject substances into the body, or to enter normally sterile body cavities, should be sterile. These items include dressings used to cover wounds and incisions, needles for injection, and tubes (catheters) used to drain urine from the bladder.
- Use dry, sterile forceps when necessary. Forceps soaked in disinfectant are not considered sterile.
- Consider the edge (outer 1 inch) of a sterile field to be contaminated.
- Consider an object contaminated if you have any doubt as to its sterility.

the operating room, once the mask becomes moist, it must be covered with a second mask rather than be removed, to avoid its contaminating adjacent objects.

Before removing the mask and cap, the nurse must remove the sterile gloves and wash hands. The mask is then untied, and removed while holding it by the strings. Both cap and mask should be discarded in the proper container (see Procedure 26-4).

Opening a Sterile Package Handwashing is a necessity before opening any sterile item. Sterile packages may be opened after being placed on a flat surface or while hand-held. Opening the flaps in the appropriate sequence eliminates reaching over the sterile field and maintains the sterility of the contents (Fig. 26-3). A sterile item may need to be covered if it is not being used immediately. Reapply the cover by touching only the outside of the wrapper and

FIGURE 26-3

(A) The nurse opens a sterile set or tray by folding the topmost part of the covering wrapper away from him. This leaves sterile equipment and supplies well covered so that they cannot be contaminated by the nurse's reaching across the set or tray to open the wrapper. (B) Next, the nurse opens the second layer of the wrapper to the sides of the set or tray. This still leaves sterile equipment and supplies covered with the last layer of the wrapper. (C) As the last step, the nurse opens the final layer of the wrapper toward himself. The wrapper can now become the sterile field immediately surrounding the sterile set or tray. Note that at no time did the nurse reach across an uncovered sterile field or sterile equipment and supplies.

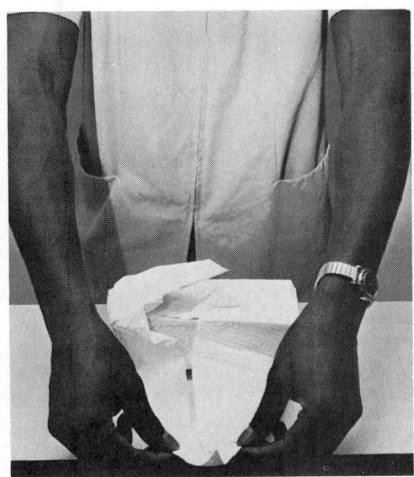

A

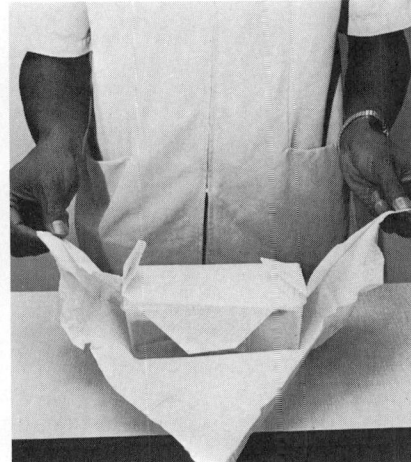

B

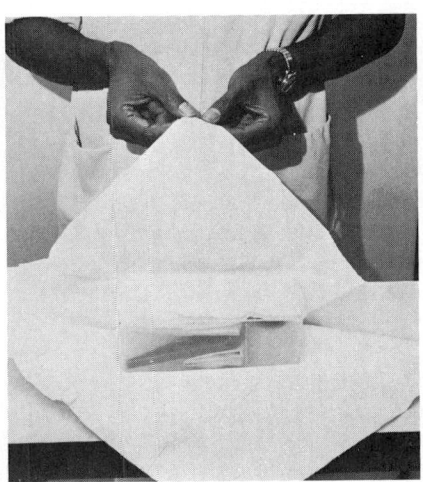

C

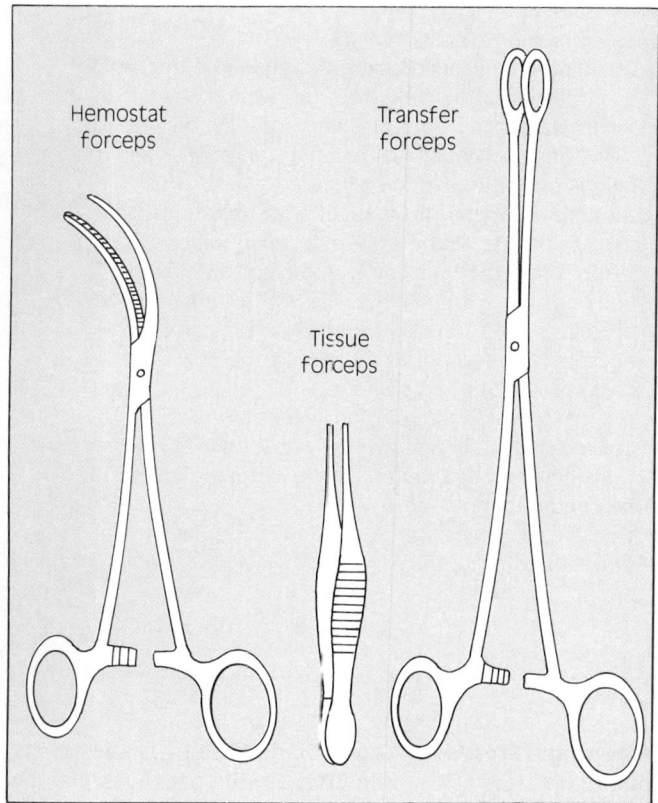

Hemostat
forceps

Transfer
forceps

Tissue
forceps

FIGURE 26-4

Examples of forceps used for sterile procedures.

reversing the opening order. Procedure 26-3 demonstrates the correct method for opening a sterile package.

Using Sterile Forceps Various forceps are available for use in sterile procedures (Fig. 26-4). The practice of consid-

ering forceps sterile that were stored in a germicidal solution and then reused is outdated and unsafe. As with other sterile objects, forceps should be kept above waist level. If handled with the bare hand, only the tips can be considered sterile. Sterile forceps should not touch the edge of a container or sterile wrapper because this outer area is considered unsterile. The forceps' tips need to be held down, particularly if they become wet, so that fluid will not flow from a contaminated area to a sterile one.

Pouring Sterile Solutions Care is necessary when pouring sterile liquids onto a sterile dressing or into a sterile basin. The outer surfaces of the bottle and cap are unsterile. Remove the cap carefully, and do not allow the inner surface of the lid to touch an unsterile area. Pour a small amount of the solution into a sink or waste container to clean the lip of the bottle. Be sure the label side of the container is uppermost when pouring so that the label does not become wet and soiled. Hold the bottle outside the edge of the sterile field and pour carefully, so as not to splash the solution. The tip of the bottle should never touch the sterile container or dressing. Touch only the outside of the cap when recapping (Fig. 26-5).

Once a solution has been opened, the outer bottle should be labeled and dated if it is to be reused. Most solutions are considered sterile for 24 hours after they are opened.

Adding Sterile Supplies to a Sterile Field After establishing a sterile field, it may be necessary to add items to the sterile field (see Procedure 26-3, actions 8 through 10). The nurse should open the sterile item and drop it onto the sterile field from a safe distance, being careful that the outside wrapper does not touch the sterile field. If the item is wrapped in a sterile cloth, the nondominant hand should be used to secure the loose ends away from the item and protect them from contaminating the sterile field.

FIGURE 26-5

Pouring sterile liquids. (*Top*) Working outside the sterile field, the nurse opens the bottle of sterile liquid, being careful to touch only the outside of the cap. (*Bottom left*) The nurse pours a small amount of the liquid into a container that will later be discarded to cleanse the lip of the sterile liquid bottle. (*Bottom right*) The nurse pours the sterile liquid into the graduate, carefully holding the bottle to the outside of the sterile tray and field.

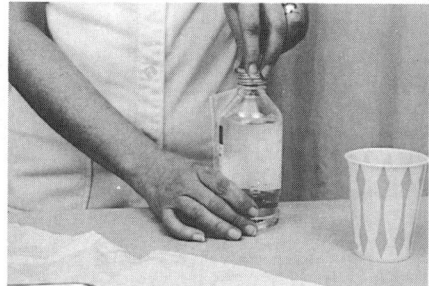

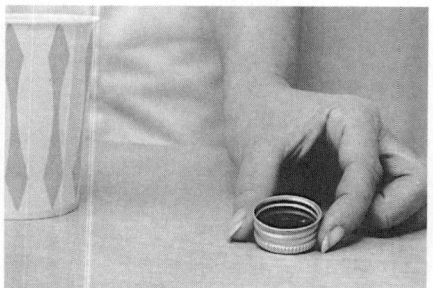

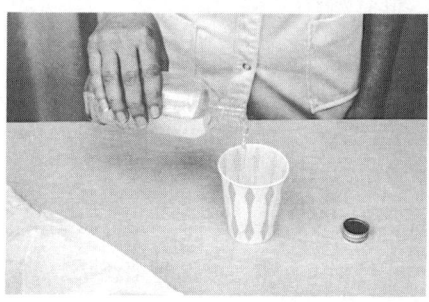

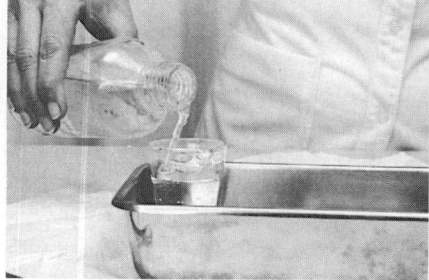

PROCEDURE 26-3

Preparing a Sterile Field

Equipment

Sterile wrapped drape or commercially prepared sterile package

Additional sterile supplies as needed (dressings, container, solution)

Action	Rationale
Initially Preparing the Field	
1 Explain procedure to client.	An explanation encourages client cooperation and reduces apprehension.
2 Gather equipment.	Preparation provides for an organized approach to task.
3 Wash your hands.	Handwashing deters the spread of microorganisms.
4 Check that sterile wrapped drape or package is dry and unopened. Also note expiration date.	Moisture contaminates a sterile package. Expiration date indicates period that package remains sterile.
5 Select a work area that is waist level or higher.	Work area is within sight. Bacteria tend to settle, so there is less contamination above waist level.
6 Open sterile wrapped drape or commercially prepared sterile package.	
a For *sterile wrapped drape*, open outer covering. Remove sterile drape lifting it carefully by its corners. Shake open, hold away from your body, and lay drape on selected work area.	Outer 1 inch (2.5 cm) of drape is considered contaminated. Any item touching this area is also considered contaminated.
b Place *commercially prepared package* in center of work area. Touching outer surface only, carefully reach around item and fold topmost flap of wrapper away from you. Open right and left flap before grasping the nearest flap and opening toward you.	Proper placement prevents contamination by reaching across sterile field. Touching outer side of wrapper maintains sterile field.
7 Place additional sterile items on field as needed.	Sterile field is maintained.

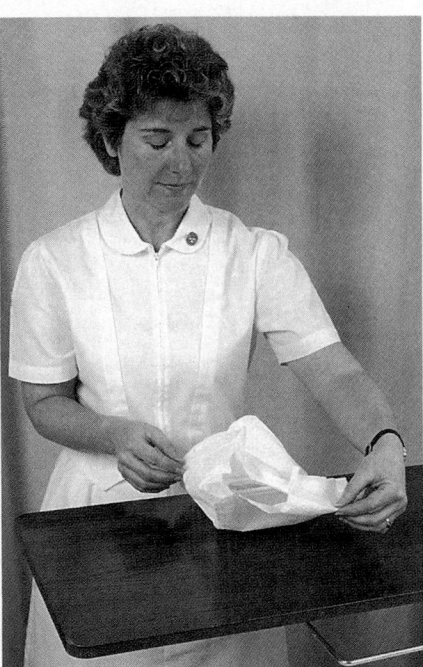

Action 6b: Folding topmost flap of wrapper away from body.

(continued)

PROCEDURE 26-3 *(continued)*

Preparing a Sterile Field

Action	Rationale
Adding a Sterile Item to a Sterile Field	
8 Open agency-prepared item or commercially packaged item:	
a Hold *agency-wrapped item* in one hand with top flap opening away from you. With other hand, unfold top flap and both sides. Keeping a secure hold on item, grasp the corners of the wrapper and pull back toward wrist, covering hand and wrist.	Only sterile surface and item are exposed before dropping onto sterile field.
b If *commercially packaged item* has an unsealed corner, hold package in one hand and pull back on top cover with the other hand. If edge is partially sealed, use both hands to carefully peel apart.	Contents remain uncontaminated by hands.
9 Drop sterile item onto sterile field from a 6-inch (15 cm) height or add item to field from the side. Be careful to avoid 1-inch border.	Wrapper does not contaminate sterile field. Any items landing on 1-inch border are considered contaminated.
10 Discard wrapper.	A neat work area promotes proper technique.

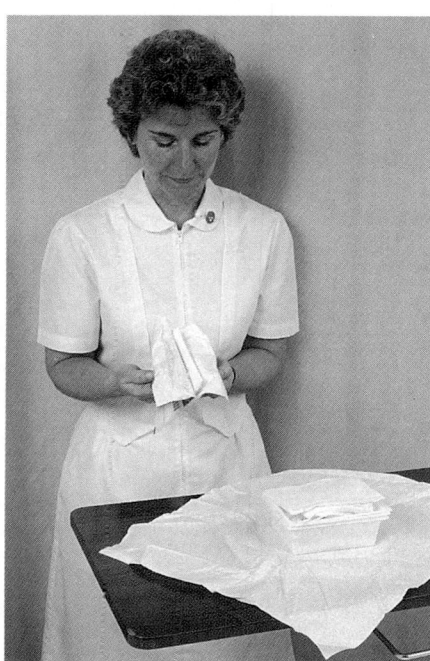

Action 8b: Using both hands to peel apart edges of sterile item packaging.

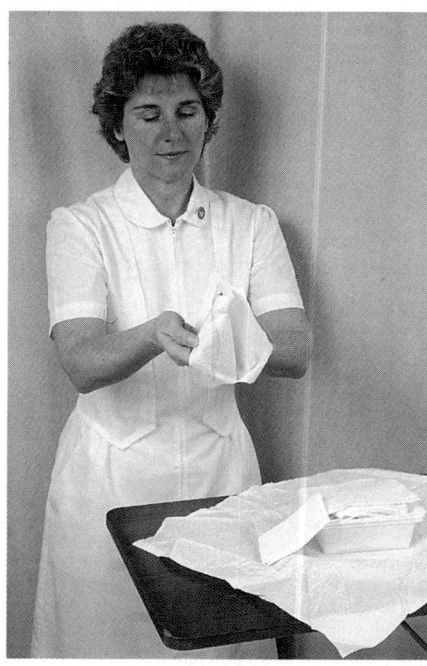

Action 9: Dropping sterile item into sterile field, avoiding 1-inch border.

Pouring a Sterile Solution	
11 Obtain appropriate solution and check expiration date.	Once opened, a bottle should be labeled with date and time. Solution remains sterile for 24 hours.

(continued)

P R O C E D U R E   2 6 - 3 *(continued)*

Preparing a Sterile Field

Action	Rationale
12 Open solution container according to directions and place cap on table with edges up.	Sterility of inside cap is maintained.
13 If bottle has previously been opened, "lip" it by pouring a small amount of solution into waste container.	This cleanses the lip of the bottle.
14 Hold bottle outside the edge of the sterile field with the label side uppermost and prepare to pour from a height of 4 to 6 inches (10 to 15 cm).	Label remains dry and solution may be poured without reaching across sterile field. Minimal splashing occurs from that height.
15 Pour required amount of solution steadily into sterile container positioned at side of sterile field. Avoid splashing any liquid.	Moisture contaminates sterile field.
16 Touch only the outside of the lid when recapping.	Solution remains uncontaminated.

Applying Sterile Drapes   The sterile drape, which ideally is waterproof, may be applied to extend the sterile working area. Using sterile gloves to apply the drape allows the nurse to handle the entire surface. For protection when positioning, the upper edges of the drape should be folded over the sterile-gloved hands (Fig. 26-6). When sterile gloves are not worn, the nurse is allowed to touch only the outer 1 inch (2.5 cm) of the drape. Caution must be used when shaking the drape open, so as not to touch the uni-

form or an unsterile object. Holding the drape by the 1-in upper edge, the nurse positions the drape over the desired area. The nurse must not reach over the drape because this would contaminate a sterile area.

Using Isolation and Barrier Techniques for Infection Prevention and Control   Isolation is a protective procedure that limits the spread of infectious diseases among hospitalized clients, hospital personnel, and visitors. The trans-

F I G U R E   2 6 - 6

Techniques of cuffing a sterile drape over gloved hands.

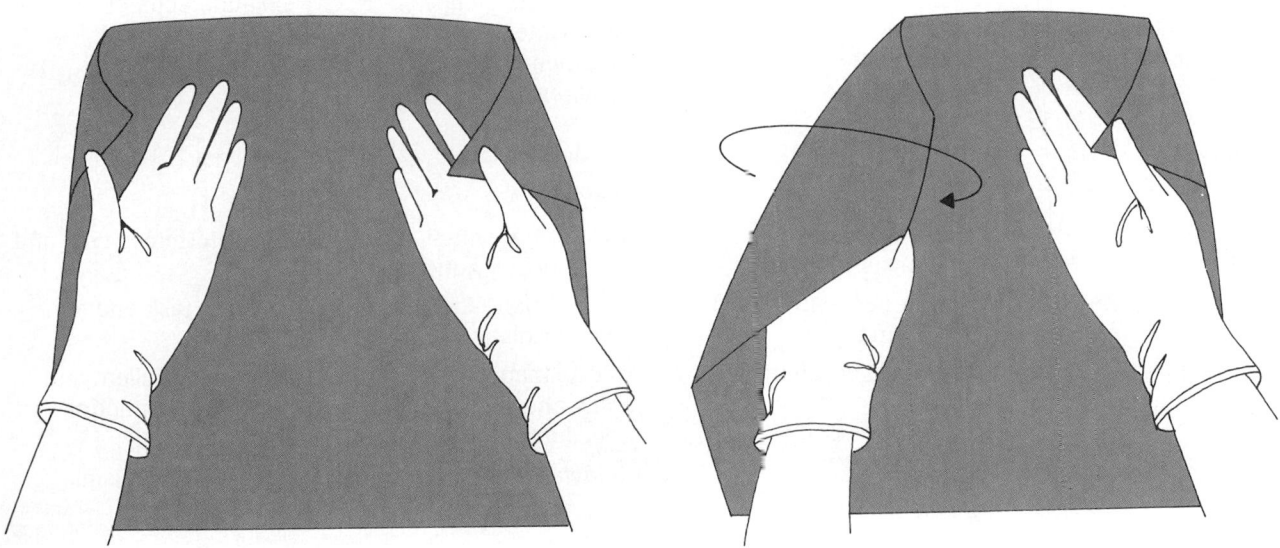

fer of pathogens from person to person can be decreased when dissemination of pathogens is limited. The most practical means of accomplishing this is to develop barriers that prevent common vehicles from transmitting them. Figure 26-7 demonstrates the ability of barriers to break the infection cycle.

The practice of isolation is an extension of the earlier quarantine approach used to track and confine people with communicable diseases. General guidelines for caring for the client on isolation precautions are outlined in Procedure 26-4. Concern about the transmission of blood-borne diseases (eg, AIDS, hepatitis B) and the increasing incidence of nosocomial infections caused a shift in the focus of infection-control programs. Guidelines from the CDC include procedures for category-specific isolation systems, disease-specific isolation categories, and universal precautions (CDC, 1983; CDC, 1988). Body substance isolation systems also are being used in some health care institutions. Nurses need an understanding of the various isolation or barrier techniques if they are to use them correctly and minimize infection risks to clients as well as themselves. Strategies for preventing the spread of infectious disease vary from one institution to another. The traditional practices involve isolating clients with diagnosed communicable diseases. Modifications of CDC guidelines focus on considering all clients potentially infective and using barrier techniques to isolate body substances. Health care institutions may alter CDC guidelines to meet their specific needs, but CDC protocols are viewed as the minimum protection standards. *Handwashing before and after the care of a client with a communicable illness is mandatory for all health personnel in every situation.*

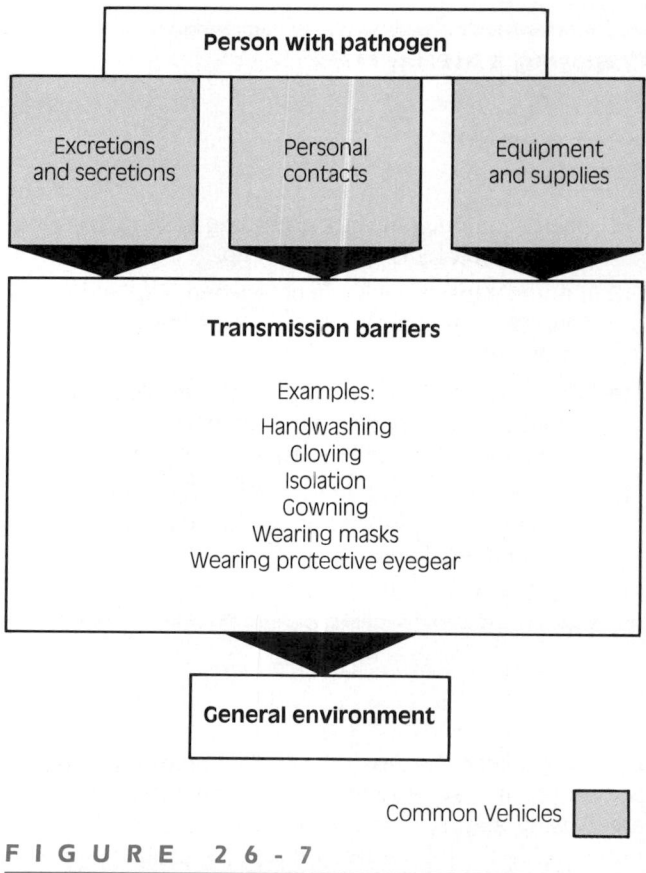

FIGURE 26-7

The transmission barriers prevent common vehicles from transporting pathogens from the infected person to the general environment.

PROCEDURE 26-4

Caring for Client on Isolation Precautions

Equipment (may vary)

Bed linens	Equipment to measure	Water pitcher, cups,	Isolation apparel
Gown and personal	vital signs	and water	Isolation disposal
hygiene items	Medications	Specimen collection	supplies
		equipment	

Action	Rationale
1 Check physician's order for type of isolation and review precautions in Infection Control Manual.	Mode of transmission or organism determines type and degree of precautions.
2 Plan nursing activities and gather necessary equipment prior to entering client's room.	Organization facilitates performance of task and adherence to isolation precautions.
3 Provide instruction about isolation precautions to client, family members, and visitors.	An explanation encourages cooperation of client and family and reduces apprehension about isolation procedures.
4 Wash your hands.	Handwashing deters the spread of microorganisms.

(continued)

Action	Rationale
5 Put on gown, gloves, and mask if recommended as isolation precaution:	Interrupts chain of infection. Protects client and nurse.
a Tie gown securely at neck and waist.	Gown should protect entire uniform.
b Use clean disposable gloves. If worn with gown draw glove cuffs over gown sleeves.	Protect hands and wrists from microorganisms.
c Mask must be securely tied and fitted to face.	Protects nurse from droplet nuclei and large particle aerosols.
6 Enter client's room with necessary equipment. Place on paper towel if necessary to avoid contamination. Leave chart and flow sheets outside room on isolation cart.	Avoids direct contact with infected material.
7 *Measure vital signs* using client's equipment in room (thermometer and sphygmomanometer). Stethoscope and watch should not come into contact with contaminated material. Place them on a clean paper towel. Vital sign recording may also be noted on clean towel placed on top of first paper towel.	Leaving equipment in room prevents spread of microorganisms to other clients. Alcohol may be used to cleanse nurse's equipment prior to being used for another client.
8 *Assist client with care.* Discard his gown and linens in isolation laundry bag and discard paper products in isolation waste container bag.	Identifies need for special precautions with waste disposal and laundry process.
9 *Administer medications* as ordered by physician. Discard uncapped syringes in disposal container kept in room.	Risk of needlestick with contaminated needle is reduced.
10 *Collect specimens* and label appropriately. Place in plastic bag and close securely for transport to laboratory.	Outer wrap protects against spilling and leakage of specimen during transport.
11 *Dispose of linen bags and waste bags* according to agency policy and, usually, at the end of each shift.	Soiled linen is securely transported to laundry facility. If outer bag is soiled, double-bagging is required. Trash or waste is transported in a plastic bag and disposed of according to agency policy or local and state regulations.
12 Remove gloves, gown, and mask before leaving and place in appropriate receptacle.	
a Untie waist strings of gown first. Grasp outside of one glove and turn inside out to remove. Drop in waste container. Insert fingers of ungloved hand inside the cuff of the remaining glove. Grasp glove on inside and remove by turning inside out. Drop in appropriate container.	Ungloved hand is clean and should not touch contaminated areas. Waist strings of gown are considered contaminated. Gloves are always removed first because they are most likely to be contaminated.
b Untie mask and drop by strings into waste container.	Center of mask is contaminated. Strings are considered clean.
c Untie neck strings of gown. Remove gown without touching outside of gown by keeping one hand up and under the gown cuff and using this protected hand to pull the opposite sleeve down and off. Use ungowned arm and hand to grasp the gown from the inside and remove from the remaining arm. Remove gown and turn inside out and drop in appropriate container.	Neck strings are considered clean. Outside of gown is contaminated.

(continued)

523

Caring for Client on Isolation Precautions

Action

Rationale

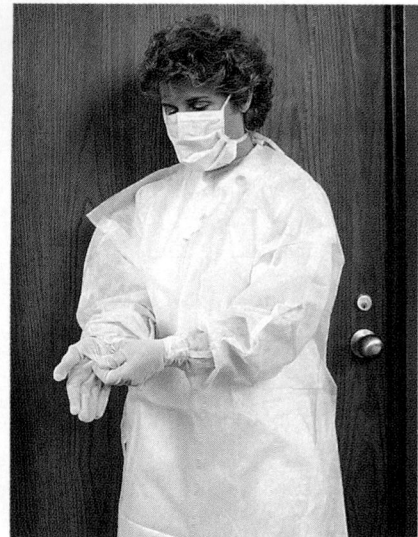

Action 12a: Grasping outside of first glove and pulling it off inside out.

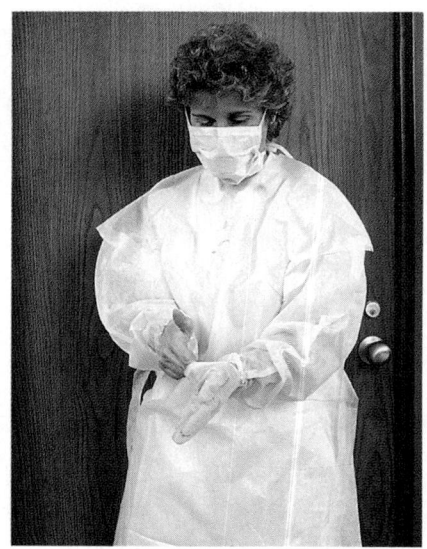

Action 12a: Placing fingers of ungloved hand inside cuff of the remaining glove.

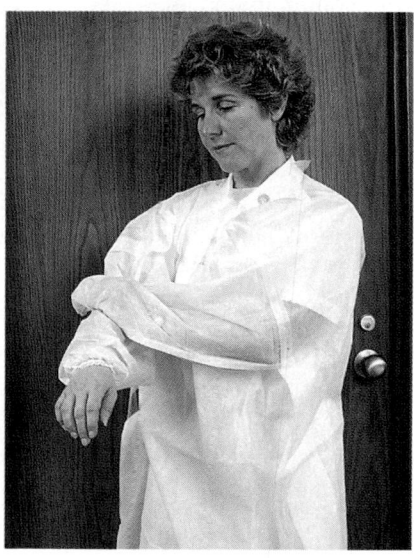

Action 12c: Using protected hand to pull the opposite sleeve down and off.

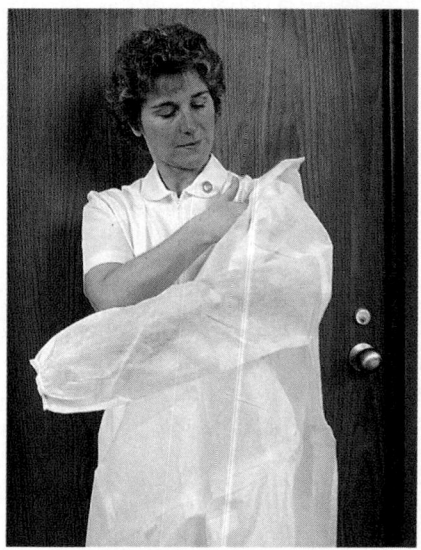

Action 12c: Using ungowned hand to grasp gown from the inside.

13 Wash hands thoroughly.	Prevents spread of microorganisms.
14 Retrieve stethoscope and watch and check notation of vital signs.	Clean hands may touch clean equipment.
15 Close door to room when leaving.	May depend on type of isolation. Check agency policy.
16 Record maintenance of isolation precautions and client's response in chart.	Ensures adequate documentation. Clients may require additional emotional support due to sensory deprivation and feelings associated with being isolated for a disease process.

Category-Specific Isolation Systems In 1970 the CDC recommended the **category-specific isolation systems** in which all infectious diseases that require similar infection-control techniques were grouped together in categories. In 1983 the list of CDC categories was expanded and the protective isolation category was eliminated (Table 26-3 summarizes these categories). Studies revealed that clients who are immunosuppressed more often than not become infected from organisms harbored in their own bodies rather than from pathogens present in the environment or transmitted from other people. Many hospitals still use protective isolation on occasion for an immunosuppressed client (eg, one recovering from transplantation surgery). Clients with diagnosed infectious diseases are assigned to

TABLE 26-3

Category-Specific Isolation System

Type	Purpose	Private Room	Hand-washing	Gowns	Masks	Gloves	Articles	Diseases Requiring Isolation
Strict	Prevents transmission of highly contagious or virulent infections spread by air and contact	X	X	X	X	X	Discard or bag and label and send for decontamination and reprocessing	Diphtheria (pharyngeal) Lassa fever Smallpox Varicella
Contact	Prevents transmission of highly transmissible infections that do not require strict isolation	X	X	Wear if soiling is likely	Wear in close contact with client	Wear if touching infective material	Discard or bag and label and send for decontamination and reprocessing	Acute respiratory tract infections in infants and young children Herpes simplex Impetigo Multiple resistant bacterial infections
Respiratory	Prevents transmission of infectious diseases primarily over short distances by air droplets	X	X	—	Wear in close contact with client	—	Discard or bag and label and send for decontamination and reprocessing	Measles Meningitis Pneumonia, *Haemophilus influenzae* in children Mumps
Tuberculosis	For client with pulmonary tuberculosis who has positive sputuma or chest x-ray that indicates active disease	X	X	Wear if soiling is likely	Wear if client is coughing and does not consistently cover mouth	—	Rarely involved in transmission of tuberculosis. Should still be thoroughly cleaned and disinfected	Tuberculosis
Enteric precautions	To prevent infections that are transmitted by direct or indirect contact with feces	Indicated if client's hygiene is poor and there is risk of contamination with infective materials	X	Wear if soiling is likely	—	Wear if touching infective material	Discard or bag and label and send for decontamination and reprocessing	Hepatitis, viral (type A) Gastroenteritis caused by highly infectious organism Cholera Diarrhea, acute with infectious cause

(continued)

Category-Specific Isolation System *(continued)*

| Type | Purpose | Specifications | | | | | | Diseases Requiring Isolation |
		Private Room	Hand-washing	Gowns	Masks	Gloves	Articles	
Drainage-secretion precautions	To prevent infections that are transmitted by direct or indirect contact with purulent material or drainage from infected site	—	X	Wear if soiling is likely	—	Wear if touching infective material	Discard or bag and label and send for decontamination and reprocessing	Abscess Burn infection Conjunctivitis Pressure ulcer Skin or wound infection
Blood–body fluid precautions	To prevent infections that are transmitted by direct or indirect contact with blood or body fluid	Only if client's hygiene is poor	X	Wear if soiling with blood or body fluids is likely	—	Wear if touching blood or body fluids	Discard or bag and label and send for decontamination and reprocessing	AIDS Hepatitis, viral (type B) Malaria Syphilis, primary and secondary

X = necessary; — = not necessary.

one of the categories based on the mode of transmission of the infecting agent. Specific precautions are indicated for each category. Figure 26-8 is an example of an instruction card for drainage and secretion precautions.

The CDC continues to revise this system as certain precautions are found to be ineffective. Double-bagging of trash and linen is advisable only if the outside of the bag is visibly soiled. Paper trays and plastic eating utensils do not prevent transmission of organisms and are no longer recommended. Special cleaning techniques are no longer considered necessary for a person with a communicable disease. Now, it is recommended that all spills of body fluids or substances be immediately cleaned with the appropriate chemical germicide or disinfectant.

Disease-Specific Isolation Categories   Rather than group similar infectious diseases together, the **disease-specific isolation system** lists each infectious disease separately, along with the individual interventions and barriers that are necessary to prevent transmission of that specific pathogenic organism. This system eliminates unnecessary isolation practices because caregivers respond to specific directions for that disease, and thus individualize care for each client. Because of the many diseases and modes of transmission, this isolation method requires knowledgeable practitioners and accurate medical diagnoses and laboratory reports to facilitate selection of the isolation category. Figure 26-9 is an example of the instruction card placed outside a person's room to indicate the disease-specific isolation category.

Universal Precautions   In 1987, in an effort to protect health care workers from exposure to HIV, hepatitis B virus,

and other blood-borne pathogens, the CDC issued recommendations for **universal precautions**. They recommend that health care workers use gloves, gowns, masks, and protective eyewear when exposure to blood or body fluids is likely and to consider that all clients might be potentially infected.

In 1988 an update from the CDC clarified the specific body fluids affected by universal precautions (see the summary of these universal precautions in the accompanying display). Epidemiologic evidence has implicated only blood, semen, vaginal secretions, and, possibly, breast milk in transmissions. Although the risk is unknown, universal precautions also apply to cerebrospinal fluid, synovial fluid, pleural fluid, peritoneal fluid, pericardial fluid, and amniotic fluid. Universal precautions do not include feces, nasal secretions, sputum, sweat, tears, urine, and vomitus, unless they contain visible blood. The risk of transmitting HIV or the hepatitis B virus from these materials is low to nonexistent.

Universal precautions also recommend the use of puncture-resistant containers for disposing of all needles and sharps. Needles should not be recapped, since most needlestick injuries occur at this time. Research on needle disposal units indicates that the frequency of needlestick injury is probably underestimated, and that educational efforts to prevent needlecapping should continue (Edmond et al., 1988).

The use of universal precaution strategies is not meant to replace other isolation system safeguards. The CDC recommends using universal precautions in conjunction with category-specific or disease-specific isolation systems. Special precautions also have been developed for high-risk professions such as dentistry, for high-risk settings such as

(Front of Card)

Drainage/Secretion Precautions
Visitors—Report to Nurses' Station Before
Entering Room

1. Masks are not indicated.
2. Gowns are indicated if soiling is likely.
3. Gloves are indicated for touching infective material.
4. HANDS MUST BE WASHED AFTER TOUCHING THE PATIENT OR POTENTIALLY CONTAMINATED ARTICLES AND BEFORE TAKING CARE OF ANOTHER PATIENT.
5. Articles contaminated with infective material should be discarded or bagged and labeled before being sent for decontamination and reprocessing.

(Back of Card)

Diseases Requiring Drainage/Secretion Precautions*

Infectious diseases included in this category are those that result in production of infective purulent material, drainage, or secretions, unless the disease is included in another isolation category that requires more rigorous precautions. (If you have questions about a specific disease, see the listing of infectious diseases in Guideline for Isolation Precautions in Hospitals, Table A, Disease-Specific Isolation Precautions.)

The following infections are examples of those included in this category provided they are *not* a) caused by multiply-resistant microorganisms, b) major (draining and not covered by a dressing or dressing does not adequately contain the drainage) skin, wound, or burn infections, including those caused by *Staphylococcus aureus* or group A *Streptococcus,* or c) gonococcal eye infections in newborns. See Contact Isolation if the infection is one of these 3.

Abscess, minor or limited
Burn infection, minor or limited
Conjunctivitis
Decubitus ulcer, infected, minor or limited
Skin infection, minor or limited
Wound infection, minor or limited

_____
*A private room is usually not indicated for Drainage/Secretion Precautions.

FIGURE 26-8

Sample instruction card for drainage and secretion precautions as recommended by the category-specific isolation system.

(Front of Card)

Visitors—Report to Nurses'
Station Before Entering Room

1. Private room indicated? _____ No
   _____ Yes

2. Masks indicated? _____ No
   _____ Yes for those close to patient
   _____ Yes for all persons entering room

3. Gowns indicated? _____ No
   _____ Yes if soiling is likely
   _____ Yes for all persons entering room

4. Gloves indicated? _____ No
   _____ Yes for touching infective material
   _____ Yes for all persons entering room

5. Special precautions _____ No
   indicated for handling blood? _____ Yes

6. Hands must be washed after touching the patient or potentially contaminated article and before taking care of another patient.

7. Articles contaminated with _____ should be
   infective material(s)
   discarded or bagged and labeled before being sent for decontamination and reprocessing.

(Back of Card)

Instructions

1. On Table B, Disease-Specific Precautions, locate the disease for which isolation or cautions are indicated.
2. Write disease in blank space here: _____
3. Determine if a private room is indicated. In general, patients infected with the same organism may share a room. For some diseases or conditions, a private room is indicated if patient hygiene is poor. A patient with poor hygiene does not wash hands after touching infective material (feces, purulent drainage, or secretions), contaminates the environment with infective material, or shares contaminated articles with other patients.
4. Place a check mark beside the indicated precautions on front of card.
5. Cross through precautions that are *not* indicated.
6. Write infective material in blank space in item 7 on front of card.

F I G U R E   2 6 - 9

Instruction card indicating the disease-specific isolation category.

the clinical laboratory, and for invasive procedures. The CDC continues to emphasize that wearing gloves does not eliminate the need for good handwashing technique. Hands should be thoroughly washed before and after care and after any contact with blood or blood-tinged fluids.

Compliance with recommendations for universal precautions has been inconsistent. One study reported that emergency department staff followed CDC precautions to don protective gear only 44% of the time, citing lack of time and reduced dexterity as reasons for noncompliance (Kelen et al., 1989). Because of frequent and extensive involvement in client care, nurses, particularly, need to conscientiously practice risk-reduction behaviors. Universal precautions can prevent contact with blood and body fluids.

The Occupational Safety and Health Administration (OSHA), in December 1991, issued regulations for use of universal precautions in all situations and settings in which occupational exposures to blood and other potentially infectious materials are possible. This OSHA ruling reinforced CDC guidelines for universal precautions and made violations punishable with severe fines. Recognizing that the hepatitis B virus poses the greatest blood-borne risk to health care workers, OSHA also required that employers offer HBV vaccine, free of charge, to employees to prevent transmission of hepatitis B. As many as 300 U.S. health care workers die each year from hepatitis B (Richardson, 1992). The American Nurses' Association is urging OSHA to consider extending this directive to provide immunization and mandate protection against blood-borne diseases for nursing students who practice in these health care facilities.

Body Substance Isolation The **body substance isolation system** is an extension of the CDC guidelines for universal precautions. It was first implemented by Lynch and

Summary of Universal Precautions: Prevention of Transmission of Human Immunodeficiency Virus, Hepatitis B Virus, and Other Blood-Borne Pathogens in Health Care Settings

Under universal precautions, blood and certain body fluids of all clients are considered potentially infectious for human immunodeficiency virus (HIV), hepatitis B virus (HBV), and other blood-borne pathogens. Blood is the single most important source of HIV, HBV, and other blood-borne pathogens in health care settings. Infection-control efforts for HIV, HBV, and other blood-borne pathogens must focus on preventing exposures to blood as well as delivery of HBV immunization.

Epidemiologic evidence has implicated only blood, semen, and vaginal secretions, and, possibly, breast milk in transmissions. Although the risk is unknown, universal precautions also apply to tissues and to the following fluids: cerebrospinal fluid, synovial fluid, pleural fluid, peritoneal fluid, and amniotic fluid. Universal precautions do not apply to feces, nasal secretions, sputum, saliva (except in a situation in which contamination with blood is likely such as a dental setting), sweat, tears, urine, and vomitus unless they contain visible blood. The risk of transmission of HIV and HBV from these materials is extremely low or nonexistent.

Health care workers are at risk for exposure to blood from clients infected with HIV, HBV, and other blood-borne pathogens. Health care workers must consider *all* clients as potentially infected with blood-borne pathogens and must adhere rigorously to infection control precautions for *all* clients.

Precautions to Prevent Transmission of HIV

General Precautions
- Consider *all* clients as potentially infected.
- Wear gloves when touching blood, body fluids containing blood, and body fluids to which universal precautions apply; for handling items or surfaces soiled with blood or applicable fluids; and for performing venipuncture and other vascular access procedures. Change gloves after each contact with a client.
- Use protective barriers (ie, wear masks, protective eyewear or face shields and gowns or aprons) when performing procedures that may produce blood or body fluid droplets or splashes.
- Wash hands and skin surfaces immediately and thoroughly with warm soap and water if contaminated with blood or other body fluids to which universal precautions apply; wash between clients and after removal of gloves even when they are intact.
- Take precautions to prevent injuries from needles, scalpels, and other sharp instruments during procedures, when cleaning instruments, during disposal, or when handling. To prevent needlestick injuries, needles should not be recapped, purposely bent or broken by hand, removed from disposable syringes, or otherwise manipulated. After they are used, dis-

posable syringes and needles, scalpel blades, and other sharp items should be placed in puncture-resistant containers for disposal.
- Use mouthpieces, resuscitation bags, or other ventilation devices when mouth-to-mouth resuscitation is likely to be performed in emergency situations.

Special Considerations
- Health care workers who have exudative lesions or weeping dermatitis should refrain from all direct patient care and from handling patient care equipment until the condition resolves.
- Pregnant health care workers are not known to be at greater risk of contracting HIV infection than health care workers who are not pregnant; however, if a health care worker develops HIV infection during pregnancy, the infant is at risk of infection resulting from perinatal transmission. Because of this risk, pregnant health care workers should be especially familiar with and strictly adhere to precautions to minimize the risk of HIV transmission.

Precautions for Invasive Procedures
(Here an invasive procedure is defined as any surgical entry into tissues, cavities, or organs or repair of major traumatic injuries.) General blood and body fluid precautions listed earlier, combined with the precautions listed below, should be the *minimal precautions for all such invasive procedures*.
- All health care workers who participate in invasive procedures must routinely use appropriate barrier procedures to prevent skin and mucous membrane contact with all patients' blood and other body fluids to which universal precautions apply.
- Gloves and surgical masks must be worn for all invasive procedures.
- Protective eyewear or face shields should be worn for all procedures that commonly result in generation of droplets, splashing of blood, body fluids containing blood, and other applicable body fluids.
- Gowns or aprons made of materials providing an effective barrier should be worn during invasive procedures likely to result in the splashing of blood or other pertinent body fluids.
- All health care workers who perform or assist in vaginal or cesarean delivery should wear gloves and gowns when handling the placenta or the infant until blood and amniotic fluid have been removed from the infant's skin. Gloves should be worn until postdelivery care of the umbilical cord.
- If a glove is torn or a needlestick or other injury occurs, the glove should be removed and a new glove used as promptly as client safety permits; the needle or instrument involved in the incident should also be removed from the sterile field.

(Data from Centers for Disease Control. [1987]. Recommendations for prevention of HIV transmission in health care settings. *Morbidity and Mortality Weekly Report, 36*[Suppl. 25]; Centers for Disease Control. [1988]. Update: Universal precautions for prevention of transmission of human immunodeficiency virus, hepatitis B virus, and other bloodborne pathogens in health care settings. *Morbidity and Mortality Weekly Report, 37*[24]; and [1989] *Morbidity and Mortality Weekly Report, 38*[Suppl. 6], 9–18.)

colleagues (1990) at Harborview Medical Center in Seattle in 1985, and is designed to reduce the risk for cross-transmission of organisms between clients and minimize the risk for infection in health care personnel. Body substance isolation considers *all* body substances as potentially infective, regardless of a person's diagnosis, and advocates consistent use of barriers whenever health care personnel have contact with moist body substances, mucous membranes, and nonintact skin. The more inclusive term body substance extends precautions to include not only blood and blood-tinged fluids, but also feces, urine, wound drainage, oral secretions, vomitus, and any other body substance. The accompanying display lists the elements of the body substance isolation system. Advocates of body substance isolation consider it to be a simple, straightforward approach to infection control.

Using body substance isolation eliminates the need for category-specific or disease-specific systems except for certain airborne diseases that require special precautions. Varicella (chickenpox) and pulmonary tuberculosis are examples of airborne diseases that necessitate a private room with the door closed and a "Stop Sign Alert" on the door. This requests visitors to check with the nurse before entering the room. Masks may be advisable, depending on the organism and the visitor's immune status.

Reminder signs for body substance isolation are strategically placed throughout the unit and near client care areas (Fig. 26-10). Some nurses express concern that not having a sign outside a client's room designating the particular disease and prevention strategy decreases their awareness. By its design, body substance isolation reduces

---

Body Substance Isolation System

The following precautions should be observed by everyone at all times, regardless of the client's diagnosis:

- Wear gloves when contact with body substances, mucous membranes, or nonintact skin is likely.
- Wear a gown or plastic apron to prevent soiling of clothing from body substances.
- Wear masks or eyegear to protect mucous membranes of eyes, nose, and mouth from splattering of body substances.
- Use good handwashing technique before, after, and between each client contact. Pay particular attention to area under fingernails and between fingers.
- Place uncapped needles and sharp instruments in puncture-proof containers.
- Bag soiled linen securely before transporting to laundry area. Dispose of trash in plastic bags according to agency policy.

---

risks for clients and personnel by treating all people in a similar manner, thus minimizing potential infection from unknown, undiagnosed diseases.

Disposable gloves and needle disposal containers are present in every room. Again, every client interaction re-

---

F I G U R E 2 6 - 1 0

Body substance isolation sign.

BODY SUBSTANCE ISOLATION IS FOR ALL PATIENT CARE | BODY SUBSTANCES INCLUDE ORAL SECRETIONS, BLOOD, URINE AND FECES, WOUND OR OTHER DRAINAGE.

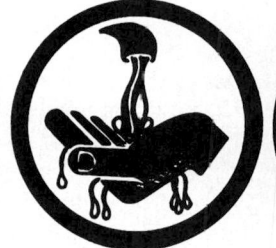 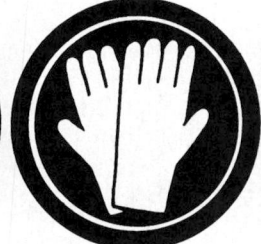  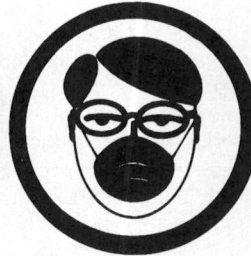 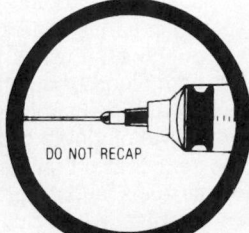

Wash hands.

Wear gloves when likely to touch body substances, mucous membranes or nonintact skin.

Wear plastic apron when clothing is likely to be soiled.

Wear mask/eye protection when likely to be splashed.

Place intact needle/syringe units and sharps in designated disposal container. **Do not** break or bend needles.

© 1987 San Diego Forms

quires good handwashing technique before and after donning gloves. Clean gloves need to be used for each client, and high-stress care situations may demand that gloves be changed several times while caring for one client.

Body substance isolation also provides a consistent approach for soiled linen, trash disposal, and laboratory specimens. Laundry bags are secured and transported in the usual manner. Visible soiling on the outside requires double-bagging. Laundry workers are educated to wear heavy gloves when handling soiled linen and to follow good handwashing technique. Research has indicated that soiled isolation linen is no more contaminated than linen from other clients (Weinstein et al., 1989). Trash is disposed of in securely tied plastic bags according to hospital policy or local and state requirements. All laboratory specimens are placed in plastic bags and sealed to prevent leakage during transportation. No special labels are applied to specimen containers or bags.

The impact of body substance isolation on infection prevention and control is being evaluated. No matter what isolation method the health agency selects, the nurse has responsibility for assessing the client's potential for infection, planning and implementing appropriate isolation techniques, and evaluating the client's reaction and response to the therapy.

Isolation Equipment and Supplies Many health care agencies use isolation carts with all the necessary equipment and supplies placed outside the client's room. This equipment includes sterile gloves, gowns, masks, and protective eye gear. Care must be taken to see that the supplies are replenished as necessary.

Gloves As stated earlier, wearing gloves is not a substitute for good handwashing (CDC, 1988). Gloves are worn only once and then discarded appropriately according to agency policy. Each client interaction requires a clean pair of gloves, and some care activities for an individual client may necessitate changing gloves more than once.

Concern has been expressed about the integrity of the various types of gloves. Korniewicz and colleagues (1991) reported that both latex and vinyl gloves provided some barrier protection, but that latex gloves seemed to be more useful in stressful care situations because they are more flexible and durable, and by nature of the latex composition, tiny glove punctures reseal automatically. Of concern, however, is the recent Food and Drug Administration (FDA) medical alert warning of an increase in the number of allergic reactions caused by gloves and other products that contain latex (Dyer, 1991a). Reactions have ranged from urticaria (hives) to systemic anaphylaxis, an exaggerated allergic reaction that resulted in death for several clients undergoing a barium enema procedure with a latex-cuffed tip on an enema tube. The FDA recommends that client questioning about drug and food allergies should be expanded to include queries about sensitivity to latex products. Health care workers need to be aware of any sensitivity on their part to latex products. Nonlatex gloves may be worn over or under the latex pair, depending on who is sensitive. It also is important to note that long fingernails, rings, and bracelets compromise the effectiveness and safety of gloves by causing punctures and tears.

In high-risk settings such as the operating room, double-gloving may be recommended. A stronger latex surgical glove is being developed that offers more protection and is an alternative to double-gloving.

Gowns In most instances, gowns are worn to prevent soiling of clothing when caring for clients on isolation precautions. They should be stored immediately outside the client's room and should be donned immediately before entering the client's room. Individual gown technique is recommended. This means that gowns are worn only once and then discarded. The recommended practices when gowns are in use for a client on isolation precautions are included in Procedure 26-4.

Masks Masks are intended to prevent the wearer from inhaling large-particle aerosols, which usually travel short distances (about 3 ft [0.9 m]), and small-particle droplet nuclei, which can remain suspended in the air and travel longer distances. Masks also discourage the wearer from touching eyes, nose, and mouth, thus limiting contact of organisms with mucous membrane.

Various practices are observed in the use of masks. In some instances, all personnel and all the client's visitors wear masks; in others, the client wears the mask when transported outside his or her room. Recommended practices when wearing a mask are included in Procedure 26-4.

A mask should be worn only once and should *never* be lowered around the neck and then brought back over the mouth and nose for reuse. The length of time to wear one mask while caring for one client is debatable. It should certainly be changed before it becomes damp from the wearer's exhalations. The recent increase in the number of tuberculosis cases in people who are also HIV-positive has prompted the CDC to recommend a more tightly fitting mask, called a *particulate respirator,* to better protect health care personnel from this particularly virulent drug-resistant form of tuberculosis (O'Brien & Bartlett, 1992).

Protective Eyewear Protective eyewear, such as goggles or a face shield, should be available on the unit anytime there is a risk of contaminating the mucous membranes of the eyes. Situations such as suctioning a tracheostomy or assisting with an invasive procedure may result in splattering of blood or other body fluids, and require protection for the caregiver.

Meeting Psychological Needs of Clients in Isolation The psychological implications of isolation precautions usually are great, whether the client is strictly separated from others or needs only to observe relatively simple precautions. Isolation methods that treat all people in a similar

THROUGH

THE EYES

OF A STUDENT

She was the cutest little girl I have ever known. She was infected with the HIV from birth. Her mother was an IV drug user and engaged in unprotected sex with multiple partners. This little girl, who came into the world with an innocent, fresh, new face full of unconditional love, could not walk, could not talk, could not chew, could not control her urine or bowel movements—but boy could she smile! In the beginning I was so terrified of contracting AIDS that I couldn't walk into her room without a mask, gown, gloves, protective eyewear, and basically a full protective body spacesuit. At the end I wanted to take her into my home and give her all the love, support, and care she needed. I am not saying that I didn't wear gloves when I changed her diapers or when I flushed her heparin lock because I did . . . I was very careful. But I realized that she is a person, a person full of feelings, a person who needed me and from whom I could learn. People with the AIDS virus are just that—people. We need to learn to treat them as such.

I also learned not to fear the person who is diagnosed with HIV infection or AIDS. I know that I will take the proper safety precautions with this person. The person I need to fear is the cute little old man who would never have AIDS because "he's not the type." If I don't use universal precautions, it is possible that one day I'll become infected through contact with someone who is "not the type." If that should ever happen, I hope everyone who cares for me will treat me as a real person and not be afraid.

—Karmi N. Soder, Georgetown University,
Washington, DC

manner greatly minimize the psychological trauma of feeling unclean and undesirable. This feeling is intense for most clients; they feel frightened, lonely, unclean, guilty, and rejected. The likelihood of suffering sensory deprivation and loss of self-esteem is a troublesome accompaniment. Friends and relatives as well as health care personnel may be inclined to spend less time with the client because they are afraid that they will contract the disease or because of the inconvenience of coping with isolation procedures.

Nursing measures to help prevent sensory deprivation and loss of self-esteem are discussed in Chapters 38 and 39.

Teaching and supportive measures are probably the two biggest contributions the nurse can make during this period of a client's illness. The client and family need to have an accurate understanding of the pertinent epidemiologic facts of the situation and of how to carry out the specific precautions. The idea that it is the pathogenic organism that is unwanted, not the person, must be emphasized. The client who resents and ignores precautions also needs help in being accepted as a person and in constructively expressing his or her feelings.

Studies have shown that extensive separation of people from others can be traumatic. Isolation precautions should be discontinued as soon as it is deemed safe. The problem of striking a balance between what is best for both the client and others is a delicate one that often requires the nurse's utmost skill and ingenuity.

A well-informed nurse who understands how to protect self and clients and a well-informed client who is co-operating in his or her care are superior communicable disease precautions.

Educating About Infection Control

Teaching about medical asepsis and infection control is a challenging nursing responsibility. Clients need to be aware of techniques that prevent the spread of infection. Consistent application of the nursing process protects both the client and the nurse.

In the home, medical asepsis techniques are appropriate for most procedures with the exception of self-injection technique. The client frequently must make adjustments and improvise with the resources and supplies available for his or her use. The nurse emphasizes effective handwashing and hygiene practices that interrupt the infection chain.

In the hospital, the infection-control nurse is responsible for educating clients and staff about effective infection-control techniques and for collecting statistics about infections. Many hospitals rely on this specialized practitioner to survey laboratory reports and review records for clients at risk as well as suggest approaches to potentially dangerous situations. Intensive investigative strategies create a positive environment to significantly reduce the incidence of nosocomial infections in health care facilities. The infection-control nurse is aware of the devastating effects of infection and is intent on promoting health and fostering a systematic approach to infection control.

Raising Ethical Concerns About Infection Risks

Isolation and barrier techniques minimize infection risks for clients as well as health care workers. The increasing incidence of HIV- and hepatitis B virus–infected people also has resulted in serious ethical concerns and controversy related to the risk for transmitting these diseases. At issue are the rights of the client versus the rights of the health care worker and the health care agency. The following questions are being discussed and debated:

Should all hospital clients be routinely tested for HIV infections?

Should HIV testing be mandatory for all health care workers?

Should health care workers infected with HIV be permitted to perform exposure-prone invasive procedures?

What procedures should be considered exposure prone?

Will health care facilities be liable if they allow HIV-positive staff to care for clients?

The CDC and various medical and nursing groups are attempting to reach agreement and consensus on these issues based on scientific information and valid statistical evidence. All are in agreement, however, that health care workers who conscientiously adhere to isolation or barrier technique recommendations seriously reduce the risk for infection for clients and themselves.

Evaluating

Nurses, by nature of their role as the primary caregiver, can intervene and impact positively on a client's outcome. By assessing the person at risk, selecting appropriate nursing diagnoses, planning, and intervening to maintain a safe environment, the nurse can reduce a client's potential for developing an infection. Evaluation of the care plan determines whether the individual need for safety is being effectively met. Ongoing systematic evaluation is critical for the nurse who is striving to maintain a secure environment for her clients as well as a safe workplace for herself. If client goals have been met and evaluative criteria have been satisfied, the client will:

- Correctly use techniques of medical asepsis
- Identify health habits and life-style patterns that promote health
- State the signs and symptoms of an infection
- Identify unsafe situations in the home environment

KEY POINTS

- The infeciton chain consists of six components and can be interrupted by measures that halt the spread of disease.
- The stage of an infection and the client's response influence the extent and type of nursing care provided.
- Sterilization and disinfection may be accomplished by physical or chemical means, based on the nature and number of organisms, the type and intended use of equipment, and the availability and practicality of the means.
- Handwashing is the single most effective way to prevent the spread of infection and decrease the incidence of nosocomial infection.
- The most common nosocomial infections are urinary tract infections, surgical wound infections, and pneumonia.
- Medical asepsis, or clean technique, is concerned with reducing the number of pathogens.
- Surgical asepsis, or sterile technique, includes practices that keep objects and areas free of microorganisms.

- Isolation procedures develop barriers that prevent the transmission of pathogens and break the infection cycle.
- The category-specific isolation system groups all infectious diseases that require similar infection-control techniques into categories.
- The disease-specific isolation format lists each infectious disease separately, along with the individual interventions and barriers that are necessary to prevent transmission of that specific pathogenic organism.
- CDC recommendations for universal precautions state that health care workers use gloves, gowns, masks, and protective eyewear when exposure to blood, semen, vaginal secretions, or body fluids is likely. All clients should be considered as potentially infected.
- The body substance isolation system considers all body substances as potentially infective and advocates consistent use of barriers whenever health care personnel have contact with moist body substances, mucous membranes, and nonintact skin.

STUDY QUESTIONS

1. The smallest infectious agents capable of causing an infection are
   a. bacteria
   b. viruses
   c. molds
   d. yeasts

2. Your client has developed a low-grade fever and states that she has felt very tired lately. This phase of an infection is known as the
   a. incubation period
   b. prodromal stage
   c. full stage of illness
   d. convalescent period

3. The highest mortality rate is associated with nosocomial infections that involve the
   a. respiratory tract
   b. integumentary system
   c. urinary tract
   d. intestines

4. A client develops a urinary tract infection after an indwelling urinary catheter has been inserted. This would most accurately be termed
   a. a viral infection
   b. a chronic infection
   c. an iatrogenic infection
   d. an opportunistic infection

5. The nurse has opened his sterile supplies and donned two sterile gloves to complete a sterile dressing change. Maintaining surgical asepsis requires that he
   a. keep splashes on his sterile field to a minimum
   b. cover his nose and mouth as he sneezes with his gloved hands
   c. use the dominant hand to cleanse the incision with a moist saline sponge and then apply the dry dressing
   d. consider the outer 1 inch of the sterile field as contaminated

6. The protective procedure that groups similar diseases according to the infecting agent's mode of transmission is
   a. body substance isolation
   b. universal precautions
   c. disease-specific isolation
   d. category-specific isolation

7. According to the CDC's universal precautions, the risk of transmission is extremely low or nonexistent from
   a. saliva
   b. blood
   c. vaginal secretions
   d. pleural fluid

8. The nurse in a health care agency that uses body substance isolation wears gloves when caring for an incontinent client. She is aware that
   a. gloves can be used between clients if they are intact
   b. long fingernails and rings compromise the safety of gloves
   c. glove use is optional in this situation
   d. gloves protect her when frequent handwashing is not possible

9. The guidelines for minimum protection standards for infection prevention and control were initially developed by
   a. OSHA
   b. individual health care facilities
   c. the state governing body
   d. the CDC

10. When leaving an isolation room, the nurse correctly removes her equipment in the following sequence
    a. mask, gown, and gloves
    b. gloves, mask, and gown
    c. gown, gloves, and mask
    d. gown and mask inside the room and gloves outside the room

11. For the nurse, under normal conditions with unsoiled hands, effective handwashing between clients requires
    a. at least a 10-second scrub
    b. at least a 2-minute scrub
    c. use of an antibacterial product
    d. that a mask be worn when scrubbing

12. Which hospitalized client is most at risk of developing a nosocomial infection?
    a. Mr. Y, a 60-year-old who smokes two packs of cigarettes daily
    b. Mrs. J, a 40-year-old who has a white blood cell count of 6000/μL
    c. Mr. L, a 65-year-old who has an indwelling urinary catheter in place
    d. Mrs. M, a 60-year-old who is a vegetarian and slightly underweight

13. A client develops food poisoning from contaminated potato salad. The means of transmission for the infecting organism is
    a. direct contact
    b. vectors
    c. vehicle
    d. airborne

14. A nurse is caring for an obese 62-year-old client with arthritis who has developed an open reddened area over his sacrum. A priority nursing diagnosis is
    a. Altered Nutrition: More Than Body Requirements, related to immobility
    b. Impaired Physical Mobility related to pain and discomfort
    c. Chronic Pain related to immobility
    d. High Risk for Infection related to altered skin integrity

15. The nurse teaches a client at home to use clean technique when changing a wound dressing. This is
    a. the nurse's preference
    b. safe for the home setting
    c. unethical behavior
    d. grossly negligent

Answers With Rationale

1. The correct response is *b*. A virus is the smallest of all microorganisms and can only be seen with a microscope. Molds and yeasts, which are fungi, and bacteria are larger infectious agents.

2. The correct response is *b*. During the prodromal stage, the person has vague signs and symptoms, such as fatigue and a low-grade fever. There are no obvious symptoms of infection during the incubation period, and they are more specific during the full stage of illness before disappearing by the convalescent period.

3. The correct response is *a*. Urinary tract infections and surgical wounds are common sites for nosocomial infections to develop, but the highest mortality rate is associated with those infections that involve the respiratory tract. The intestine is not particularly prone to nosocomial infections.

4. The correct response is *c*. An infection that develops as a result of the insertion of an indwelling catheter is termed iatrogenic. Because this infection just developed, it is not chronic, nor did it occur because of any altered physiology that may give an opportunistic organism a chance to cause infection. These infections are bacterial, not viral.

5. The correct response is *d*. Considering the outer inch of a sterile field as contaminated is a principle of surgical asepsis. Moisture contaminates the sterile field, and sneezing contaminates the sterile gloves. The sterile hand that cleaned a wound should not be used or should be regloved before applying a sterile dressing.

6. The correct response is *d*. According to the CDC, the category-specific isolation system is based on infectious diseases that require similar infection-control measures being grouped together. Disease-specific isolation lists each disease separately, and universal precautions and body substance isolation recommend barriers based on exposure to blood and body fluids.

7. The correct response is *a*. According to the latest CDC recommendations, only blood, semen, vaginal secretions, and certain body fluids, such as cerebrospinal and pleural fluids, require universal precautions. Universal precautions do not apply to saliva unless it contains visible blood.

8. The correct response is *b*. Long fingernails and rings may cause tears in the gloves, allowing contamination of the nurse's hands. Gloves should never be used for more than one client, and body substance isolation precautions necessitate use of gloves as a barrier for any contact with body substances. Wearing gloves is not a substitute for handwashing.

9. The correct response is *d*. The CDC established the initial minimum requirements for infection prevention and control. OSHA has recently issued and will be monitoring regulations for use of universal precautions in situations and settings in which exposure to blood and other infectious materials is possible.

10. The correct response is *b*. Gloves are always removed first because they are most likely to be contaminated and should not touch the hair or, possibly, the face.

11. The correct response is *a*. Hands that are not visibly soiled can be effectively cleaned with a 10-second scrub. Neither a mask nor an antibacterial product is required in this situation or setting. Hands that are visibly soiled require a longer scrub.

12. The correct response is *c*. Indwelling urinary catheters have been implicated in a majority of nosocomial infections. Cigarette smoking, a normal white blood cell count, and a vegetarian diet have not been implicated as risk factors for developing an infection.

13. The correct response is *c*. Contaminated food is a vehicle for transmitting an infection. Direct contact requires proximity between the susceptible host and an infected person. A vector is a nonhuman carrier, such as an insect, and the airborne means of transmission carries the organism in droplet nuclei or with dust.

14. The correct response is *d*. The priority diagnosis in this situation is the possibility of an infection developing in the open skin area. The others may be potential or probable diagnoses for this client and also may require nursing interventions once the first one is addressed.

15. The correct response is *b*. In the home setting, where the client's environment is more controlled, medical asepsis usually is recommended with the exception of self-injection. This is the appropriate procedure for the home and is neither unethical nor grossly negligent.

BIBLIOGRAPHY

Agency abandons HIV-related list. (1992). *American Nurse* *24*(1), 1.

American Nurses' Association. (1991). *HIV infection and teenagers: Position statement*. Kansas City, MO: HIV Resource Task Force, Congress of Nursing Practice, Congress on Nursing Economics.

Beaufoy, A. (1989). HIV infection: Employee education and infection control measures. *Canadian Journal of Public Health, 80*(Suppl. 1), 31–33.

CDC urges AIDS testing for all hospital patients. (1991). *American Journal of Nursing, 91*(11), 81.

CDC may not get much help from physicians. (1991). *RN, 54*(11), 12.

Centers for Disease Control. (1983). *Guidelines for prevention and control of nosocomial infections*. Atlanta: U.S. Department of Health, Education, and Welfare, Public Health Service.

Centers for Disease Control. (1987). Recommendations for prevention of HIV transmission in health-care settings. *Morbidity and Mortality Weekly Report, 36*(28), Supplement.

Centers for Disease Control. (1988). Update: Universal precautions for prevention of transmission of human immunodeficiency virus, hepatitis B virus, and other blood-borne pathogens in health-care settings. *Morbidity and Mortality Weekly Report, 37*(24), 377–388.

Craft, K. (1990). Do you really know how to handle sharps? *RN, 53*(8), 33–35.

Davey, F. (1991). Glove talk. *Canadian Nurse, 87*(4), 17–18.

Dyer, J. (1991). Life-threatening reactions to latex are increasing, FDA warns. *American Journal of Nursing, 91*(7), 14.

Dyer, J. (1991). Recap on recapping. *American Journal of Nursing, 91*(5), 17.

Edmond, M., Khakoo, R., & McTaggart, B. (1988). Effect of bedside needle disposal units on needle recapping frequency and needlestick injury. *Infection Control Hospital Epidemiology, 9*(3), 114–116.

Flaskerud, J., & Ungvarski, P. (1992). *HIV/AIDS: A guide to nursing care* (2nd ed.). Philadelphia: Saunders.

Gawlikowski, J. (1992). TB plus HIV spells trouble. *American Journal of Nursing, 92*(3), 44–51.

Goldschmidt, R., Gorter, R., & Moran, T. (1989). The care of AIDS patients. *Clinical Advances in Oncology Nursing, 1*(4), 1–9.

Grady, C. (1989). Acquired immunodeficiency syndrome: The impact on professional nursing practice. *Cancer Nursing, 12*(1), 1–9.

Guenthner, S., Hendley, J., & Wenzel, R. (1987). Gram-negative bacilli as nontransient flora on the hands of hospital personnel. *Journal of Clinical Microbiology, 25*(3), 488–490.

Gurevich, I. (1990). How to handle blood and body fluids. *Advancing Clinical Care, 5*(3), 11–13.

Heig, J., & Coleman, D. (1992). Hepatitis kills. *RN, 55*(4), 60–66.

Herrick, C., & Smith, J. (1989). Ethical dilemmas and AIDS: Nursing issues regarding rights and obligations. *Nursing Forum, 24*(3,4), 35–46.

Hooton, T. (1989). Protecting ourselves and our patients from nosocomial infections. *Respiratory Care, 34*(2), 111–115.

Hoyer, R. (1991). AIDS: An overview. *Caring, 10*(8), 4–14.

Jackson, M., & Lynch, P. (1987). An alternative to isolating patients. *Geriatric Nursing, 8*(6), 308–311.

Jackson, M., & Lynch, P. (1989). Infection prevention and control in the era of the AIDS/HIV epidemic. *Seminars in Oncology Nursing, 5*(4), 236–243.

Jacobsen, G., Thiele, J., & McCune, J. (1985). Handwashing: Ring wearing and number of microorganisms. *Nursing Research, 34*(3), 186–188.

Kelen, G., DiGiovanna, T., & Bisson, L. (1989). Human immunodeficiency virus infection in emergency department patients. *Journal of the American Medical Association, 262*(4), 516–522.

Kirkman, M., & Bell, S. (1989). AIDS and confidentiality. *Nursing Forum, 24*(3,4), 47–51.

Korniewicz, D., Laughon, B., Butz, A., & Larson, E. (1989). Integrity of vinyl and latex procedure gloves. *Nursing Research, 38*(3), 144–146.

Korniewicz, D., Kirwin, M., & Larson, E. (1991). Do your gloves fit the task? *American Journal of Nursing, 91*(6), 38–40.

Larson, E. (1988). A causal link between handwashing and risk of infection? Examination of the evidence. *Infection Control Hospital Epidemiology, 9*(1), 28–36.

Larson, E. (1989). Handwashing: It's essential—even when you use gloves. *American Journal of Nursing, 89*, 934–939.

Larson, E., Oram, L., Hedrick, E. (1988). Nosocomial infection rates as an indicator of quality. *Medical Care, 26*(7), 676–683.

Lynch, P., Cummings, M., Roberts, T., Herriott, M., Yates, B., & Stamm, W. (1990). Implementing and evaluating a system of generic infection precautions: Body substance isolation. *American Journal of Infection Control, 18*(1), 1–12.

Lynch, P., Jackson, M., Cummings, M., & Stamm, W. (1987). Rethinking the role of isolation practices in the prevention of nosocomial infections. *Annals of Internal Medicine, 107*, 243–246.

Madsen, L. (1990). Tuberculosis today. *RN, 53*(3), 44–50.

Meisenholder, J., & LaCharite, C. (1989). Fear of contagion: The public response to AIDS. *Image: Journal of Nursing Scholarship, 21*(1), 7–9.

Miller P., & Farr, B. (1989). Survey of patients' knowledge of nosocomial infections. *American Journal of Infection Control, 17*(1), 31–34.

Moran, E. (1990). Infection control investment saves in the long run. *Hospitals, 64*(5), 58.

New definition will swell AIDS population. (1991). *RN, 54*(10), 15.

New guidelines from the CDC on HIV and HBV. (1991). *RN, 54*(9), 12.

New OSHA rules under fire from all angles. (1991). *American Journal of Nursing, 91*(1), 18–22.

O'Brien, L., & Bartlett, K. (1992). TB plus HIV spells trouble. *American Journal of Nursing, 92*(5), 28–32.

OSHA stiffens bloodborne rules: Decrees free hepatitis B vaccine. (1992). *American Journal of Nursing, 92*(1), 82–84.

Pachter, A. (1988). Should nurses receive the Hepatitis B vaccine? *Nursing, 18*(6), 51.

Pritchard, V., & Sanders, N. (1991). Universal precautions: How effective are they against Methicillin-resistant Staphylococcus aureus? *Journal of Gerontological Nursing, 17*(1), 7–11.

Reacting to latex. (1991). *Nursing, 21*(10), 113.

Regs put new legal force behind universal precautions, (1992). *American Journal or Nursing, 92*(1), 82–84.

Richardson, D. (1992). OSHA releases final standard on HIV/hepatitis B exposures. *American Nurse, 24*(1), 1.

Sawyer, D. (1989). Potential for infection: A nursing diagnosis for the patient with an indwelling catheter. *Focus on Critical Care, 16*(1), 46–52.

Schaberg, S. (1989). How infections spread in the hospital. *Respiratory Care, 34*(2), 81–84.

Should hospitals offer HIV testing to all patients? (1991). *RN, 54*(11), 12–13.

Shovein, J. (1989). MRSA: An infection control crisis comes home. *RN, 52*(7), 42–47.

Squires, S. (1992, May 5). Hepatitis B vaccinations. *Washington Post Health*, 9.

Stolley, J., & Buckwalter, K. (1991). Iatrogenesis in the elderly: Nosocomial infections. *Journal of Gerontological Nursing, 17*(9), 30–34.

Tamborlane, T. (1991). Health care professionals with AIDS. *Caring, 10*(8), 50–54.

Tribulski, J. (1988). The true odds of getting AIDS from a patient. *RN, 51*(5), 64–70.

Using personal protective apparel. (1989). *Nursing, 19*(11), 61–64.

Valenti, W. (1988). Universal precautions: The data base emerges. *American Journal of Infection Control, 16*(2), 39–40.

Volk, W., & Wheeler, M. (1988). *Basic microbiology* (6th ed.). Philadelphia: Harper & Row.

Weinstein, S., Gantz, N., Pelletier, C., & Hibert, D. (1989). Bacterial surface contamination of patients' linen: Isolation precautions vs. standard care. *American Journal of Infection Control, 17*, 264–267.

Williamson, K., Selleck, C., Turner, J., Brown, K., Newman, K., & Sirles, A. (1988). Occupational health hazards for nurses: Infection. *Image: Journal of Nursing Scholarship, 20*(1), 48–53.

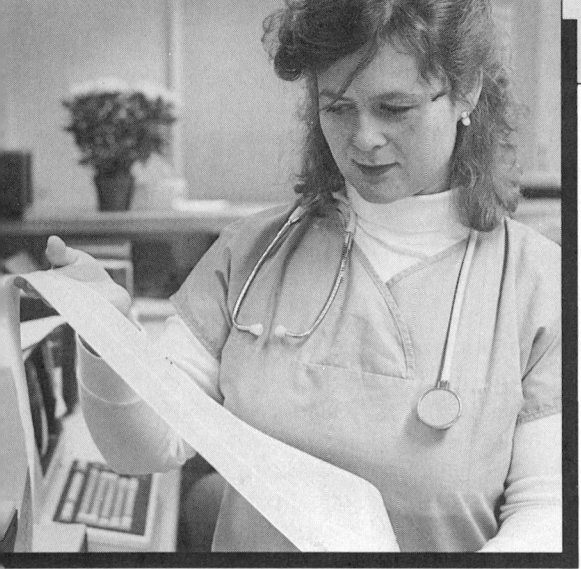

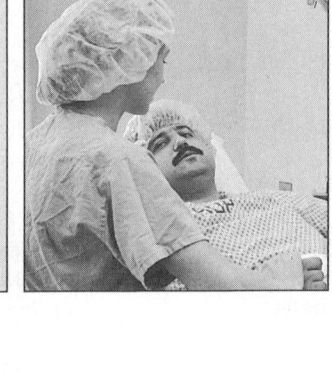

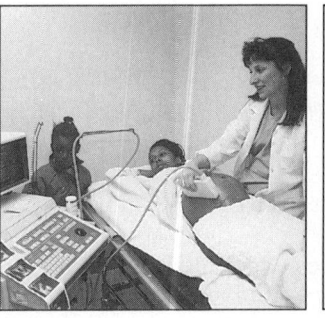

Diagnostic Procedures

OBJECTIVES

After studying this chapter, the learner should be able to:

Define key terms used in the chapter.

Describe various diagnostic tests and their purpose.

Describe nursing responsibilities for a client before, during, and after a diagnostic test.

Discuss the importance of psychological preparation and support to clients having diagnostic tests.

Identify assessment data appropriate for specific diagnostic tests.

Evaluate the client's response after a diagnostic examination.

KEY TERMS

ascites
atrioventricular node
barium enema
biopsy
bronchoscopy
cholecystography
colonoscopy
computed tomography
cystoscopy
depolarize
electrocardiography
electroencephalography
endoscope
endoscopic retrograde
    cholangiopancreatography
esophagogastroduodenoscopy
fasting state
fluoroscopy
intravenous pyelography
leads
liver biopsy
lumbar puncture
magnetic resonance imaging
paracentesis
polarity
proctosigmoidoscopy
Purkinje system
radiography
radioisotope
radiopaque
repolarize
roentgen ray
sinoatrial node
thoracentesis
transducer
ultrasonography
ultrasound waves
upper gastrointestinal series
urinalysis
x-ray

27

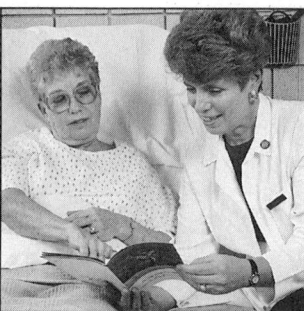

Diagnostic tests are a valuable adjunct to the treatment regimen and provide various information about the client's state of health. Most clients undergo some type of diagnostic evaluation during their lifetime of health care experiences. Decisions concerning which diagnostic tests to schedule are made by the physician when problems are noted during the history or physical examination or because of a problem stated by the client.

In this chapter, basic responsibilities of the nurse assisting with all diagnostic tests are discussed first. Major tests are then summarized. Further information can be obtained from *A Manual of Laboratory Diagnostic Tests* by Frances Fischbach. Some tests mentioned here are fully described in clinical chapters.

Nursing Responsibilities

The nurse assumes a variety of roles and responsibilities when a client requires a diagnostic test. Emphasis on assessing each client's particular needs as well as his or her response to the testing procedure individualizes nursing care and initiates the nursing process. Results of the diagnostic tests add to the knowledge base as the nurse accumulates information, formulates nursing diagnoses, and plans nursing care.

The following section discusses the nurse's basic responsibilities before, during, and after the testing. The definitive protocol may depend on the institution.

Before the Test

Preparing a client for a diagnostic test requires a multifaceted approach by the nurse. Agency policy dictates the need for a permit, the requirements for scheduling the test, necessary equipment that must be available, and the physical preparation of the client for the test. The nurse's responsibility may encompass all these areas but also must focus on the psychological preparation of the client for the examination. Nursing interventions that communicate caring, support, and an awareness of individual needs can ease the client's fear and help immeasurably.

Obtaining Consent   The physician is responsible for obtaining a signed consent form before any diagnostic test. The client has the legal right to know what the test involves, any risks or complications that might directly result from the test, and any other available options. An awareness of all these factors indicates that the client is informed about the procedure, and the client's signature affirms consent. The general consent a client signs on admission to the agency may be sufficient to indicate consent for some diagnostic examinations, whereas other invasive procedures may require that the client sign an additional consent form before the test.

Scheduling Tests   The nurse may be responsible for scheduling diagnostic tests or special procedures with another hospital department. In addition to a thorough understanding of the procedure, it is important for the nurse to know the proper sequence when multiple tests have been ordered. Intravenous pyelography, for example, must be scheduled before any barium studies because barium takes 3 or 4 days to be excreted and may interfere with visualization of the kidneys. Knowledge coupled with practice and experience helps the nurse to collaborate effectively and plan for a diagnostic test. This effort saves the health care consumer time and money, minimizes anxiety and trauma, and may eliminate the need to have a test repeated.

Preparing the Client   The nursing care plan should incorporate physical and psychological preparation of the client before any diagnostic testing. The nurse usually follows written protocols for physical preparation of the client but may feel less confident meeting emotional needs. Both are vital toward promoting cooperation and securing reliable test results.

Physical Preparation   Physical preparation may be simple or extensive, depending on the type of diagnostic study to be performed. Some tests require only a simple explanation beforehand, whereas more involved measures, such as dietary restrictions, enemas, and sedation, may be necessary before other procedures. The preparation may occur in a hospital setting or, if the test is performed on an outpatient basis, in the client's home, in a clinic setting, or in a physician's office. Instruction pamphlets are helpful, particularly if the client is responsible for self-preparation and is probably anxious about the upcoming test and its results.

As a client advocate, the nurse must monitor all test preparations to ensure that the client is not in a prolonged fasting state if tests are scheduled one after the other. It also is important to clarify which, if any, of the client's medications should be continued despite test preparation.

Psychological Preparation   Preparing a client emotionally and intellectually for a diagnostic examination presents a challenging opportunity for the nurse. Uncertainty associated with the preparations for the test, misgivings about pain or the test itself, and anxiety about the results or future treatment are stress-provoking experiences for the client. The nurse needs to recall personal experiences and rely on interpersonal communication skills to help the client deal with these fears.

Explanations by the nurse need to take into account the client's level of understanding and previous experience with the testing situation. Some clients desire explicit information about all facets of the examination and may request details on what they can expect to see, hear, and feel during the study. Simple clarification of the physician's explanation or a brief discussion may be appropriate for other clients. If the client is receptive, any available visual resources, such as pamphlets or films, may provide additional reinforcement (Fig. 27-1).

It is helpful for the nurse to observe as many diagnostic procedures as possible to describe them more accurately to others. A client whose expectations match the actual testing experience is apt to be less anxious, more cooperative, and better able to withstand the demands of any diagnostic procedure.

Assembling Equipment Responsibility for assembling equipment for a diagnostic test varies, depending on the setting. The nurse usually is responsible for gathering supplies and equipment when the examination is performed at

FIGURE 27-1

Preparing a client emotionally and intellectually for a diagnostic procedure may require a simple clarification of the physician's explanation or explicit information about all facets of the test.

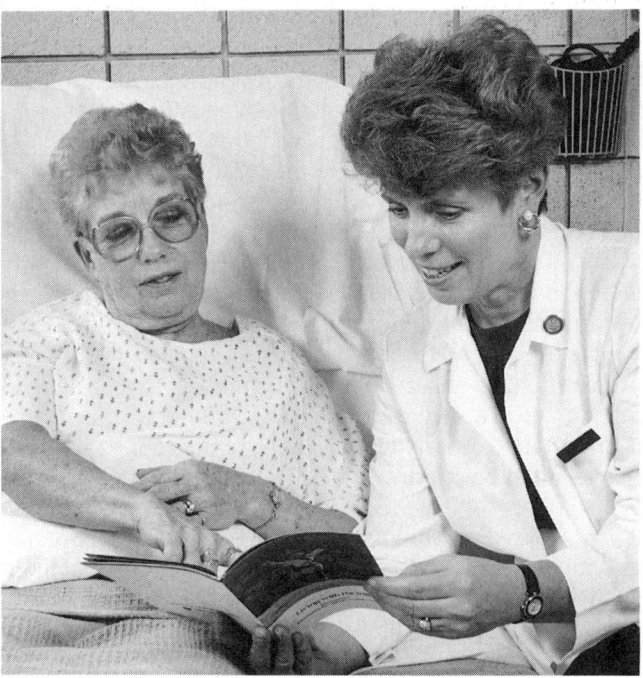

the client's bedside or in a nearby treatment room. It is important for the nurse to take into account the physician's preference for any special instruments as well as the orderly arrangement of all supplies. If the procedure is sterile, the nurse maintains surgical asepsis. It is vital that protective equipment is available (gloves, gown, mask, and goggles) and frequent handwashing done if any contact with blood or body fluids is expected, to prevent transmission of the human immunodeficiency virus, the hepatitis B virus, and other blood-borne organisms.

During the Test

Whether the nurse actually assists with the procedure or evaluates the client's response to it, her primary role during the test is that of client advocate. The client is the focus for nursing assessments and support, and the nurse can communicate concern and support in various ways. Holding the client's hand, helping the client to maintain an awkward position during the test, or reinforcing a direction or explanation demonstrates the compassionate care that belongs uniquely to nursing.

Collecting Baseline Data Baseline data are necessary to evaluate the client's response to the testing process. Any deviation from normal may indicate an unfavorable reaction. The nurse is responsible for informing the physician of any manifestation that may threaten the client's life and that has caused difficulty in the past (eg, hives and itching associated with a previous dye injection). Such reactions may necessitate additional interventions before the test or its postponement and possible cancellation.

Undue anxiety should be noted, so that the physician is aware of the client's fear and may take steps to minimize it before the start of the diagnostic procedure.

Evaluating the Client If the nurse is present during the diagnostic study, assessment of the client is apt to focus on physical reaction and emotional state during the procedure. Any untoward response must be reported immediately to the physician. The nurse needs to be alert for any significant deviation from baseline vital signs, nausea or vomiting, pallor, unusual pain, or excessive anxiety. The physician may opt to intervene medically or to pause to comfort and evaluate the client. It may be that the nurse is most qualified to observe any alteration in the client's condition based on prior knowledge from assessments and interviews.

Supporting the Client Supportive measures are particularly meaningful to the client during a diagnostic test. The nurse respects the client's sense of privacy and provides a drape or cover to ensure warmth. The nurse may have occasion to use touch therapeutically by assisting the client to hold steady in an uncomfortable position. Holding a client's hand may provide comfort during a particularly tense or painful moment. It may be the nurse who reinforces or repeats directions to the client during the test (eg, take a deep breath, cough, hold that position steady) or prepares the client to expect a certain sensation. A nurse who is particularly sensitive to the client's needs is able to support him emotionally as well as physically throughout the test in an individualized, compassionate manner (Fig. 27-2).

Assisting the Examiner The nurse who is assisting with the diagnostic procedure may be responsible for handing equipment to the physician and providing additional supplies as needed in addition to maintaining a sterile field and using whatever protective equipment is required. The client's safety is a paramount concern. If a specimen is obtained, the nurse needs to prepare and label it correctly before it is transported to the laboratory.

After the Test

The nurse's priority after the test is the client's comfort. Assessments may be ordered at regular intervals, and the nurse must be aware of baseline data for comparison with observations and vital signs obtained after the diagnostic study. The type of equipment used and the nature of the laboratory specimen determine the techniques for proper disposal. All nursing assessments and interventions must be documented to ensure that the client's response to the diagnostic procedure is accurately recorded.

Assessing the Client The type of test and the condition of the client determine the interval and type of nursing assessments after a diagnostic test. It is appropriate to assess the client immediately after the procedure. Baseline data should be available for comparison and may indicate the onset of any adverse reactions. Some tests require frequent assessments that are recorded on a flowsheet at the client's bedside. It is imperative that the nurse be familiar with the diagnostic procedure to recognize any clinically significant deviations in the client's health status.

Assisting the Client In addition to being aware of clinical implications after the study, the nurse is concerned about the client's comfort. Supportive measures that provide warmth, relieve pain, or provide direction and explanation are effective nursing interventions. The client may be relieved that the test has been completed but still anxious and apprehensive about test results and future therapy. The client may want to discuss the test experience or may have questions about the results. The physician needs to be notified if the client is unusually apprehensive about the consequences of the test. Specific instructions after the test (eg, concerning position or dietary status) need to be explained clearly to the client and any concerned support people. It is important that the client understand that the frequent nursing assessments are routine rather than an indication of a clinical problem.

Preparing Specimens and Caring for Equipment Any specimens obtained during a test must be properly identified and delivered to the appropriate laboratory. The label

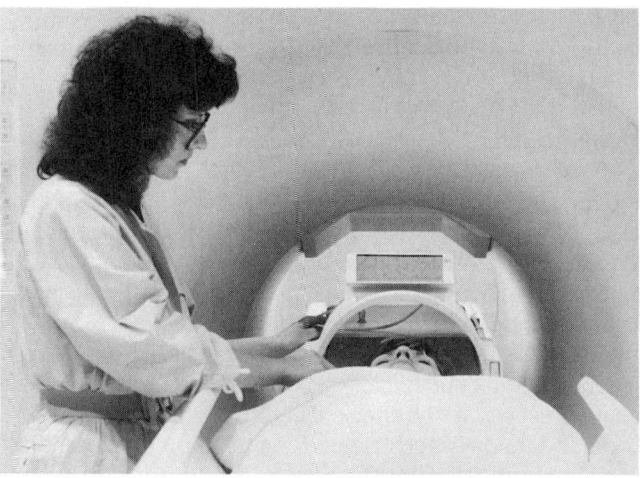

FIGURE 27-2

Diagnostic procedures can be a very uncomfortable and frightening experience for the client. Supportive measures taken by the nurse are particularly meaningful to the client. (Photo by H. Armstrong Roberts.)

should include the client's name and identification number, the date, and the nature of the specimen. Care must be taken to avoid contact with any potentially infective blood or body fluids. Blood and body fluid or substance precautions must be observed. The nurse also needs to be cautious about accidentally discarding the specimen with any used equipment. This action would require that the procedure be repeated.

Equipment that is reusable needs to be rinsed of blood and body fluids and prepared for sterilization. The nurse should wear disposable gloves for protection when handling any used equipment. Disposable equipment needs to be discarded in the proper receptacle. If necessary, replace any supplies and return the room to its former condition.

Documenting the Procedure After a procedure is completed, the nurse needs to record the date and time, the type of diagnostic study, whether a specimen was obtained, and the client's response. Additional documentation may be necessary to record ongoing observations and nursing interventions. The diagnostic testing experience needs to be incorporated into the nursing care plan and used to plan individualized nursing interventions.

Diagnostic Tests

Aspiration Procedures

Certain diagnostic studies involve insertion of a needle or similar instrument into a body organ or cavity. Fluid or tissue may be aspirated, prepared, labeled properly, and sent to the laboratory for examination. The tests may be performed at the client's bedside or in a designated examination area.

Liver Biopsy

A **liver biopsy** is the needle aspiration of a sample of liver tissue. The specimen is then examined to determine if liver disease is present. The procedure is brief and may be performed at the client's bedside. A local anesthetic is administered before the test.

Because liver disease may be associated with some blood-clotting deficiencies, prothrombin time and platelet count must always be checked before the test is performed. Food and fluids are restricted for 4 to 6 hours beforehand. Baseline vital signs must be recorded. Because this is an invasive test, a permit is required.

The client assumes a supine position with the right arm resting near the head or the right hand placed under the head (Fig. 27-3). To immobilize the chest wall and prevent

FIGURE 27-3

Position of the client and site for a liver biopsy.

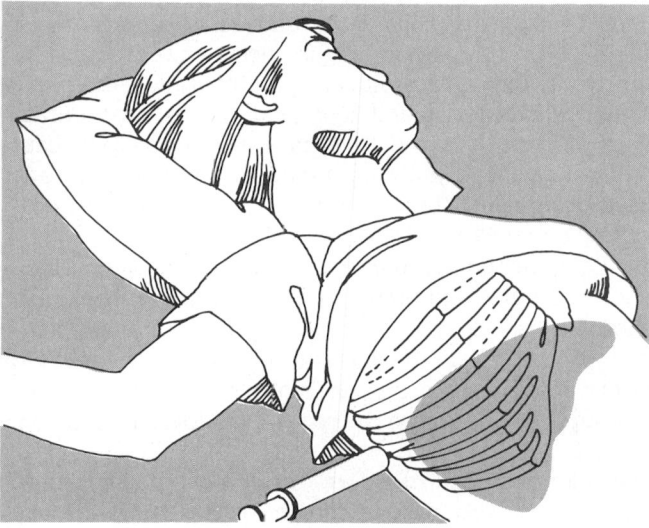

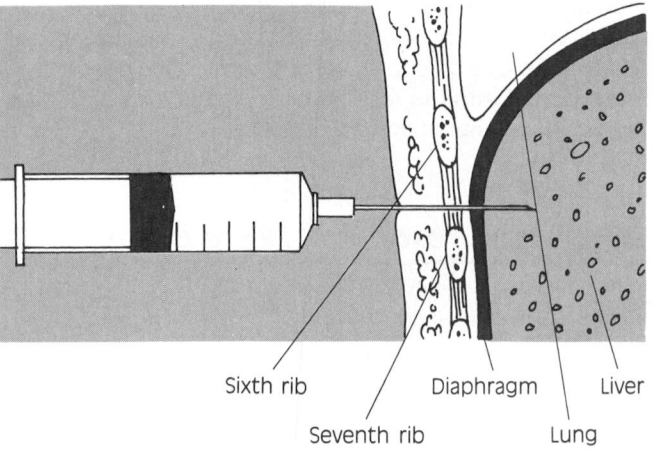

Sixth rib   Diaphragm   Liver

Seventh rib   Lung

injury to the liver, the client is asked to hold his or her breath for about 10 seconds after an exhalation. Using sterile technique, the physician inserts the needle between two of the right lower ribs or below the right rib cage, obtains the biopsy specimen, and removes the needle. Instructions to the client to resume breathing and application of a pressure dressing complete the procedure.

Nursing Responsibilities   The nurse assumes responsibility for collecting baseline data and reviewing pertinent laboratory reports. Any abnormalities must be reported to the physician. Explanations to the client include details of the procedure as well as the instructions and rationale for holding the breath during the needle insertion and biopsy.

After the procedure, the client requires careful assessment and observation. The client is assisted to lie on the right side with a pillow or folded towel under the needle insertion site. This position must be maintained for several hours. Vital signs must be monitored at frequent intervals (eg, every 15 minutes for the first hour, every 30 minutes for the next 2 hours, and then every 4 hours) until they are stable. The nurse needs to be alert for complications such as hemorrhage, peritonitis if bile escapes from the liver, and pneumothorax. Normal diet may be resumed.

If the nurse is responsible for delivery of the specimen, it must be labeled and packaged correctly and quickly transported to the appropriate laboratory.

Lumbar Puncture

A **lumbar puncture**, or spinal tap, is the insertion of a needle into the subarachnoid space in the spinal canal. This test usually is done in the hospital for selected clients and is performed by a physician with the nurse assisting. It is a sterile procedure and requires the use of a local anesthetic. Blood and body fluid or substance precautions must be observed.

Cerebrospinal fluid (CSF), which normally fills the ventricles of the brain, the subarachnoid space, and the central canal of the spinal cord, is clear and transparent. It may be necessary to enter the subarachnoid space for several reasons: to obtain a specimen of the fluid for analysis and for culture; to establish any alterations in the usual pressure of the CSF; to relieve pressure; to inject drugs; or to inject dyes for x-ray visualization. Normal laboratory values for CSF are included in Appendix B.

Before the lumbar puncture, the client needs an explanation of the procedure and reassurance to allay any fears that paralysis may result. The usual site of needle entry is between the third and fourth lumbar vertebrae, which is below the level where the spinal cord ends. A client may express concern about experiencing a postspinal headache, but this is less likely to occur when the client cooperates with instructions during and after the test. Because this is an invasive procedure, a consent form must be signed by the client or a responsible family member.

To spread the vertebrae and to provide the widest possible space for easier insertion of the needle, the client is

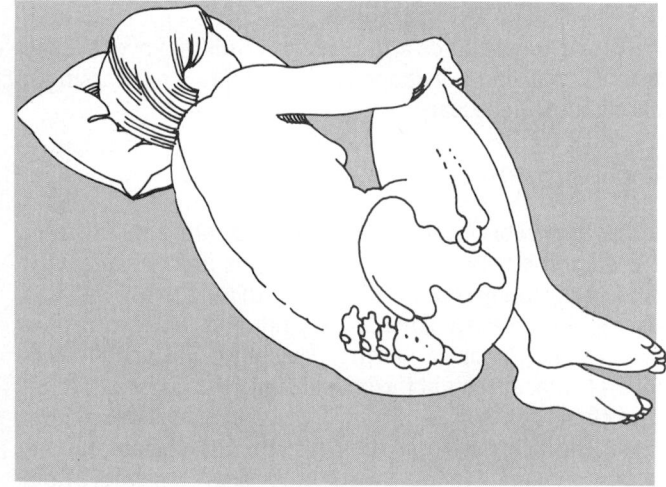

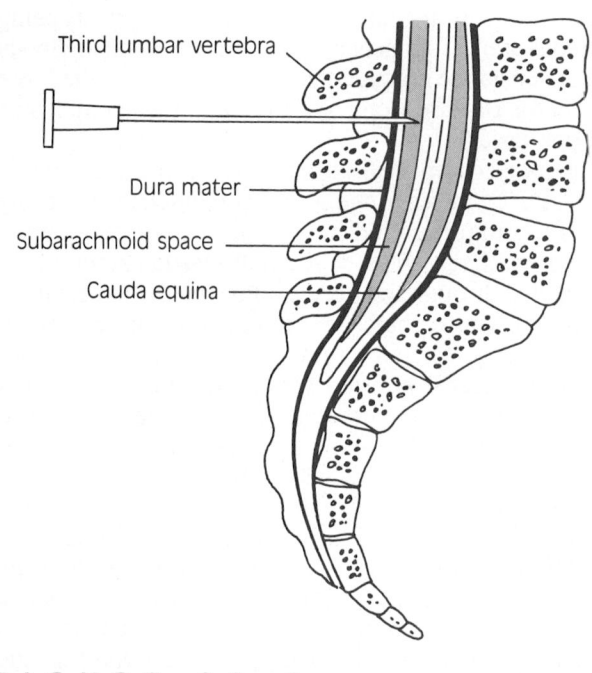

Third lumbar vertebra

Dura mater

Subarachnoid space

Cauda equina

FIGURE 27-4

Position of the client and site for a lumbar puncture.

positioned on the side with the knees flexed and the head bent forward with the chin touching the chest (Fig. 27-4). This hyperextends the spine. A small pillow may be placed under the client's head and between the knees for comfort. Some clients may be unable to assume or maintain this position without assistance. Others may have difficulty in understanding or may be disoriented and require repeated assurances of what is being done. It is important to explain to the client the need to remain motionless and to breathe normally during the procedure. Moving about or hyperventilating makes insertion of the needle more difficult and may interfere with accurate pressure readings.

Nursing Responsibilities During the procedure, the nurse observes the client's reaction carefully. The client's color and pulse and respiratory rates are noted and reported to the physician immediately if they deviate from normal.

The nurse may be asked to assist the physician with Queckenstedt's test. While the lumbar puncture needle is resting freely in the subarachnoid space, pressure is applied to one or both of the client's jugular veins. The nurse assists with this compression. An increase in CSF pressure is the normal response; a blockage in the spinal canal prevents the normal rise in pressure readings. When the procedure is completed, the needle is removed and compression is applied to the site for a short while. A small sterile piece of gauze may be applied to the site and fastened with adhesive.

Immediately after the procedure the client may be placed in the recumbent position, preferably without a pillow. Fluids usually are offered. This is intended to avoid postspinal headache. Some experts believe that the headache is due to the tear in the dura mater made by the needle, which allows for seepage of small amounts of CSF. Differences of opinion exist about the effectiveness of positioning in avoiding the occurrence of the headache. The nurse should follow established agency protocol. If a headache does occur, the client usually is treated symptomatically.

The client's general physical reaction to the procedure is observed. This is of particular importance if the procedure was carried out to relieve pressure. Any unusual reactions, such as twitching, vomiting, or slow pulse rate, are reported to the physician promptly.

Paracentesis

The withdrawal of fluid from the peritoneal cavity is called an *abdominal paracentesis*. The word **paracentesis** means the withdrawal of fluid from any body cavity, but it is common practice to use the term when referring to the removal of fluid from the peritoneal cavity. The technique is used to obtain abdominal fluid for analysis to determine whether or not malignant tumor cells are present. A paracentesis also has therapeutic value because it helps relieve symptoms caused by ascites, which is an accumulation of fluid in the peritoneal cavity.

Because the peritoneal cavity normally is a sterile cavity, surgical asepsis is observed for the procedure. Blood and body fluid or substance precautions also must be observed. The pressure in the peritoneal cavity normally is no greater than atmospheric pressure, but when fluid is present, the pressure is greater. Gravity aids in the removal of fluid, so the fluid drains freely until pressure is equal.

A sterile trocar and cannula are used to enter the peritoneal cavity near the midline of the abdomen, about halfway between the umbilicus and the pubis. The physician anesthetizes the site of entry, incises the skin, and introduces the trocar and the cannula. When the trocar is in place, the physician pulls back on the cannula to see if fluid drains. If it does, the drainage tube is attached. The specimens are obtained and should be carefully labeled. If a plastic catheter is used, it is threaded through at this time.

The nurse places the distal end of the tubing in a clean container for drainage. If fluid is draining too rapidly, the container should be elevated on a stool. Rapid drainage may produce symptoms of shock. No more than 1500 mL should be drained at one time.

Nursing Responsibilities The client is weighed and abdominal girth measured before and after the procedure. Baseline vital signs must be recorded. The client should be encouraged to void before the procedure begins because if the urinary bladder is full, there is danger of puncturing it with the trocar. The physician should be notified if the client is unable to void; the physician may order the client to be catheterized.

Because gravity is used to assist the drainage, the client is placed in a sitting position. The client may be supported in the sitting position in bed or placed at the side of the bed or the treatment table with the feet supported on a chair, or he or she may sit on a chair during the procedure (Fig. 27-5). The client should be covered adequately for warmth and to prevent unnecessary exposure.

During and after the procedure, the nurse observes the client for untoward reactions associated with electrolyte imbalance. The client's color, blood pressure, and pulse and respiratory rates are noted. Fainting may occur. The nurse notes the type and amount of drainage present. After

F I G U R E   2 7 - 5

Position of the client for paracentesis.

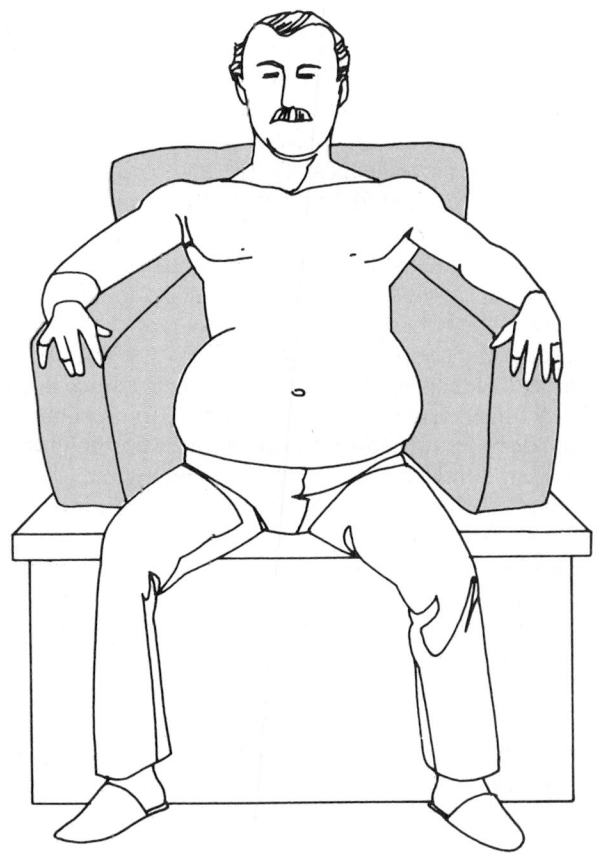

the needle has been withdrawn and the incision sutured, the nurse should place a sterile heavy dressing over the site of incision because leakage usually occurs. The dressing is changed as necessary.

Thoracentesis

A **thoracentesis** is the entering and aspirating of fluid from the pleural cavity. The pleural cavity is a *potential* cavity, since it normally is not distended with fluid or air. Its walls usually are separated by a small amount of lubricating fluid to keep them from adhering. The physician usually performs thoracentesis at the bedside with the nurse assisting. The client is required to sign a permit for this procedure.

A thoracentesis may be performed to obtain and analyze a specimen for diagnostic purposes or to remove fluid that has accumulated in the pleural cavity and caused respiratory difficulty and discomfort. Because the cavity being entered is sterile, surgical asepsis is used. Blood and body fluid or substance precautions also must be observed (see Centers for Disease Control universal precautions inside the book cover).

One way to remove fluid or air from the pleural cavity is to aspirate it with a syringe. Another method for removing fluid is to drain the fluid into a bottle in which a partial vacuum has been created. A small plastic catheter may be threaded through the needle, allowing the needle to be withdrawn. This catheter reduces the possibility of puncturing the lung. When this method is used, the tubing connecting the needle and the bottle should be sterile. It is convenient to use a calibrated bottle for the drainage to readily determine the amount of fluid that has been removed. The upper limit usually is 1000 mL.

The skin is prepared over the area where the physician indicates the needle will be inserted. The exact location depends on the area in which fluid is present and where the physician can best aspirate it. After a local anesthetic is administered, the needle is inserted between the ribs through the intercostal muscles and fascia and into the pleura. When the procedure is completed, the needle or plastic catheter is removed and a small sterile dressing is placed over the entry site.

Nursing Responsibilities The nurse is responsible for the collection of baseline data before the examination. The client must be instructed not to cough or breathe deeply during the test. It is imperative that the client remain as still as possible to diminish the risk of accidental injury to the lung.

This procedure usually is carried out when the client is sitting on a chair or on the edge of a treatment table or bed with the feet supported on a chair. Figure 27-6 shows this position. The client may lie on the side if unable to sit up. The client usually is placed on the affected side with the hand of that side resting on the opposite shoulder.

During the procedure, the nurse observes the client for reactions. The client's color and pulse and respiratory rates are observed, and any deviation from the norm is reported

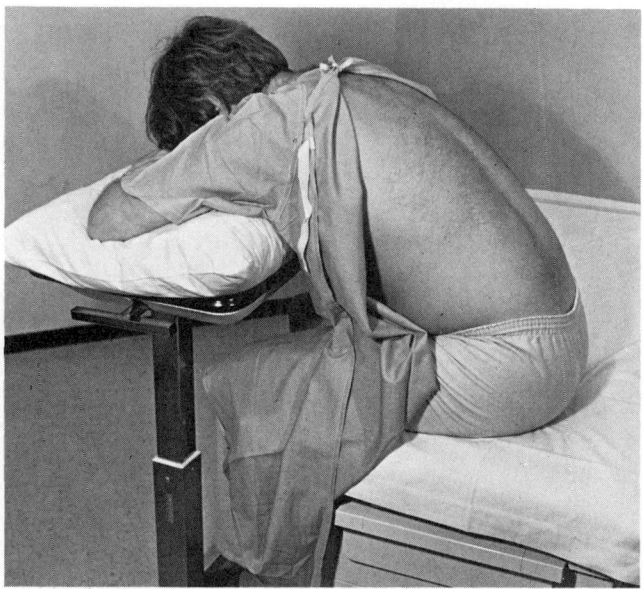

FIGURE 27-6

Position of the client for thoracentesis.

to the physician immediately. Fainting, nausea, and vomiting may occur.

After the procedure, the client should be observed for changes in respirations. If a large amount of fluid is removed, respirations usually are eased. If the lung has been punctured inadvertently, respiratory distress becomes acute. If blood appears in the sputum or the client has severe coughing, the physician should be notified promptly.

Electrical Impulse Procedures

Electrical impulses can be recorded on a graph and displayed on an oscilloscope screen. An **electrocardiogram** is a record of the electrical impulses of the heart and an **electroencephalogram** is a recording of the electrical impulses of the brain. Both studies use a machine with electrodes attached to the body over the appropriate area to monitor electrical activity.

Electrocardiography

Overview The electrocardiographic findings are important for studying heart function. The graphic record produced by the electrocardiograph is called the electrocardiogram, commonly abbreviated ECG or EKG.

The electrical activity in the heart is received through electrodes placed on the skin on various places on the body. The placement patterns of electrodes are called leads. The same cardiac activity is monitored on each lead, but the waves on the ECG look somewhat different, depending on the electrode's placement. The trained observer recognizes normal and abnormal findings for each placement of electrodes. Figure 27-7 shows a client having an ECG.

Heart muscle cells are electrically charged, or polarized, in a state of rest. When cells are electrically stimulated, they **depolarize**, or lose their charge, and contraction occurs. The cells **repolarize**, or regain an electrical charge, during the resting phase that follows contraction. Depolarization and repolarization are electrical happenings that are recorded by the ECG.

The electrical activity that causes the heartbeat originates in the **sinoatrial** (SA) **node** (pacemaker), which is located in the upper part of the right atrium. Electrical currents radiate quickly throughout the atria from the SA node and stimulate contraction. A second node, the **atrioventricular** (AV) **node**, picks up the current. The node is situated at the base of the atrial septum. The AV node divides into two bundle branches, and each in turn gives rise to multiple smaller branches that interlace throughout the ventricles. This interlacing system is called the **Purkinje system**. Figure 27-8 shows the structures through which electric current travels through the heart.

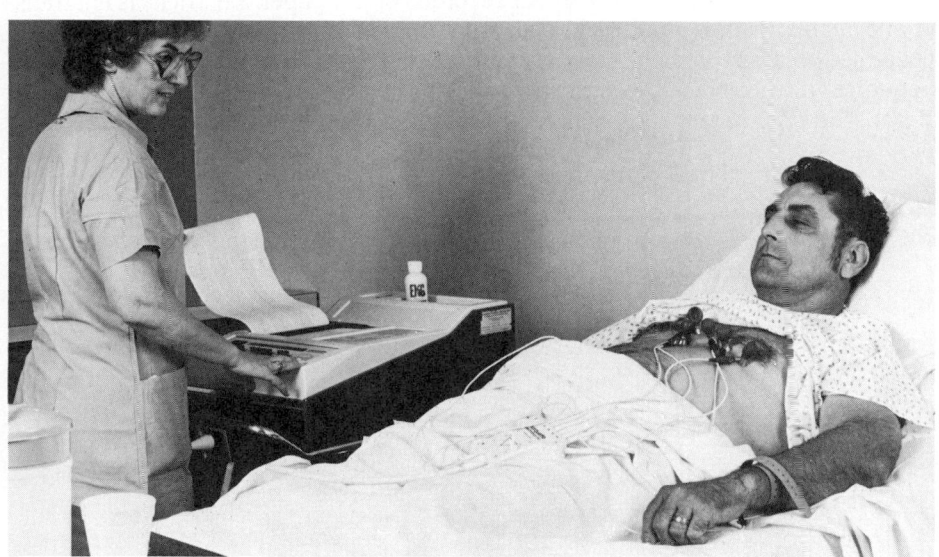

FIGURE 27-7

Electrodes are placed on the arms, legs, and chest of the client undergoing electrocardiography. The nurse operates the electrocardiograph while observing the client.

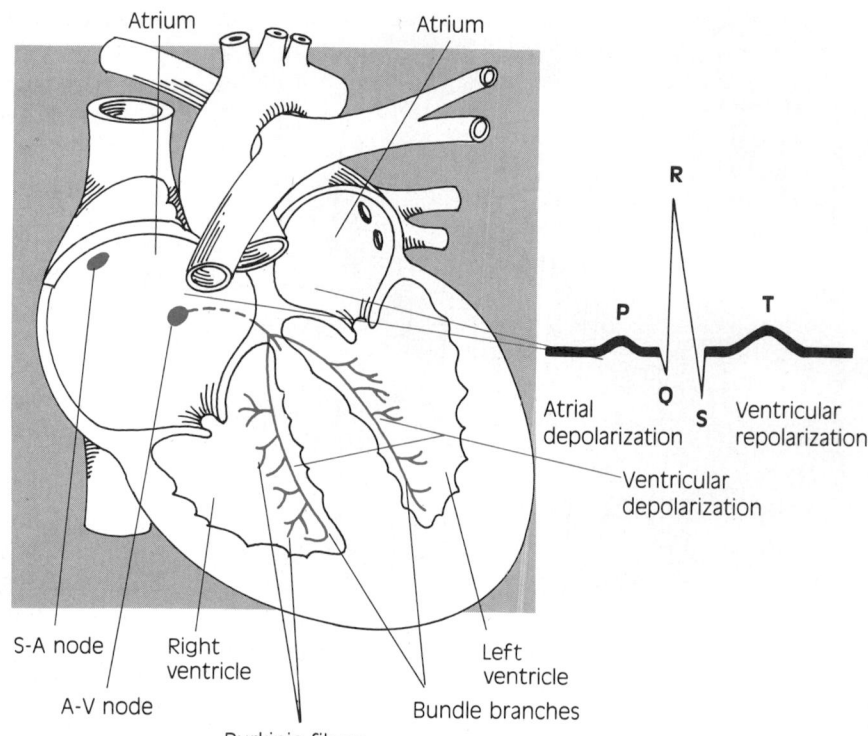

FIGURE 27-8

How electrical phenomena occurring in the normal heart appear on the electrocardiogram.

Figure 27-8 also shows the association between the electrical system in the heart and the waves produced on the ECG. Note that the waves on the ECG are lettered. The P wave occurs when electrical charges, originating in the SA node, cause the atria to depolarize and contract. The QRS complex occurs when the electrical charges result in ventricular depolarization and contraction. The T wave represents relaxation of the ventricles or ventricular repolarization. Repolarization of the atria occurs during the QRS segment, but it is not usually as visible on the electrocardiogram as ventricular repolarization. The sum total of P, QRS, and T waves represents the cardiac cycle. Another way of describing the cardiac cycle is that it consists of atrial and ventricular depolarization and repolarization.

The ruled paper for an ECG is calibrated to assist in reading it. The paper is ruled in 1-mm squares with heavier lines every 5 mm, as Figure 27-9 shows. The horizontal lines represent the measurement of voltage and the vertical lines measure time. When the heart is diseased, the waves may be abnormal in size, form, or position. The time interval between waves also has diagnostic significance.

Nursing Responsibilities The client having an ECG for the first time needs an explanation of the purpose and technique being used. The client should be told that the electrodes are applied to the chest and extremities and that it is necessary to lie quietly while the tracing is being recorded. It should be clearly explained that the electrodes pick up the electrical impulses coming from the heart and that they are recorded on the paper. Electricity is not transferred to the body. Some people misunderstand the use of the word *electrical* and are fearful that they will receive an electrical shock. This fear needs to be allayed. There is no sensation of discomfort from the ECG.

FIGURE 27-9

Calibrated paper used for the electrocardiogram shows time and voltage measures. (Sharp, L.N., & Rabin, B. [1970]. *Nursing in the coronary care unit.* Philadelphia: Lippincott.)

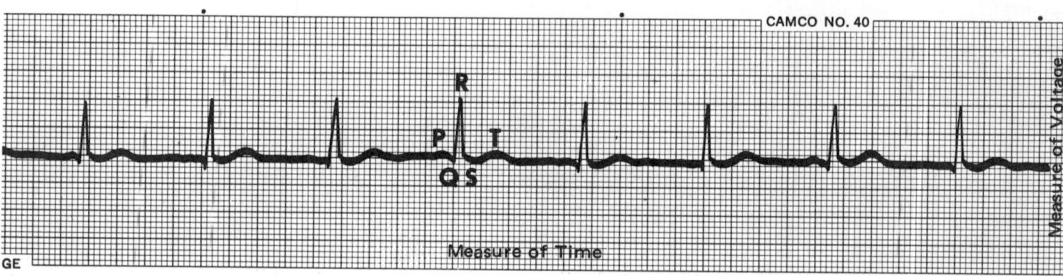

Constant monitoring of the heart action is common in clients who are seriously ill. ECGs are displayed on a video screen, as well as recorded on ECG paper for a permanent record. As the physical condition improves, the client is disconnected from the monitor and attached to a device that permits moving around and allows some activity while still being monitored. A compact recording device, such as a Holter monitor, allows the client a certain amount of mobility but requires that the client record activities during the specified period. These actions are correlated with the events on the ECG. The nurse may need to assist the client with this recording to ensure that all pertinent activities are documented and available for comparison with the ECG tracing. In addition, monitoring is now possible for people not in a health agency who are carrying out normal activities of daily living. The electronic devices extend the health practitioner's ability to secure complete data about the client.

Electroencephalography

Overview The electroencephalograph is an instrument that receives and records electrical currents in the brain. The recording is known as an electroencephalogram, or EEG. From 19 to 25 electrodes in the form of small disks are attached to the scalp with paste. The procedure does not cause any pain or discomfort for the client.

The EEG is a valuable tool that aids in the diagnosis of epilepsy and cerebrovascular diseases. An EEG recording that is flat is an indication of brain death.

During the test, the technician carefully observes the client and notes any activity (eg, talking, blinking, or swallowing) that may cause an artificial movement on the tracing. This provides for a more accurate analysis of the client's brain wave patterns (Fig. 27-10). A baseline recording is standard procedure. As part of the test, the client may be asked to breathe deeply and rapidly for a short period or view a series of flashing lights. These activities may activate a seizure pattern, which is recorded on the EEG tracing.

Nursing Responsibilities The client undergoing an EEG needs a thorough explanation of the procedure and reassurance that no electricity will be transferred to the body. Certain medications may be withheld for 24 to 48 hours before the test. There are no restrictions on food and fluid intake. After the study, the nurse may need to assist the client to shampoo the hair to remove the paste residue from the scalp.

Endoscopic Procedures

Endoscopic studies allow for direct visual examination of various body cavities and organs by means of a hollow, lighted tube, called an **endoscope**. The endoscope may be flexible or rigid. Endoscopic examinations provide valuable diagnostic information and may be used to obtain tissue specimens for **biopsy** or microscopic examination. Another therapeutic reason for endoscopic examination is removal of a foreign body. Common endoscopic studies include the following:

Bronchoscopy—visual examination of the trachea and bronchi

Esophagogastroduodenoscopy—visual examination of the esophagus, stomach, and duodenum (also called *gastroscopy*)

Proctosigmoidoscopy—visual examination of the rectum, rectosigmoid junction, and lower sigmoid colon

Colonscopy—visual examination of the entire large intestine

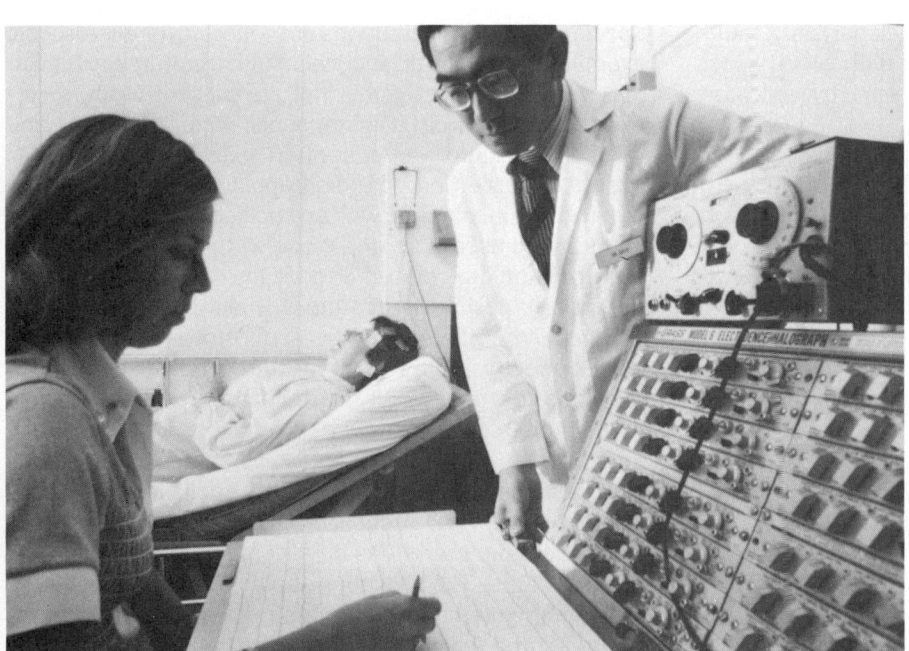

FIGURE 27-10

Neurologist and EEG technician checking the client's electroencephalograph, which is a valuable diagnostic instrument in epilepsy and neurologic disorders. (Courtesy of the National Institute of Neurological and Communication Disorders and Stroke.)

Cystoscopy—visual examination of the bladder, urethra, and urethral orifices

Endoscopic retrograde cholangiopancreatography—visual examination of the esophagus, stomach, and duodenum combined with x-ray visualization, by means of a contrast medium, of the pancreatic ducts and the hepatobiliary tree

Nursing Responsibilities   The client needs an explanation of the procedure and must sign a consent before the procedure. Preparations vary according to the area being studied but may include dietary restrictions and laxatives or enemas. A local anesthetic may be administered as well as an analgesic or a tranquilizer or sedative, which may be given by injection.

After the examination, the client's vital signs need to be checked at frequent intervals. The nurse needs to evaluate the client's gag reflex by checking her ability to cough or swallow if the endoscopic study involved the use of a local anesthetic on the trachea or esophagus. The client needs to be monitored for pain and hemorrhage after the test because perforation with the endoscope is a possible complication (see also Tables 35-3 and 36-2).

Laboratory Procedures

Laboratory test results are invaluable as the physician attempts to diagnose and treat the client. Attention to detail when preparing the client and collecting specimens and transporting them to the laboratory contributes to reliable test results. A vigilant, conscientious approach by the nurse is ultimately beneficial to the client.

Blood Specimens

Blood is one of the most significant body fluids that conveys information about a person's health state. Most physical examinations include some type of blood analysis. A multitude of laboratory tests can be done with blood specimens. Blood specimens usually are collected by laboratory personnel.

Nursing Responsibilities   The role of the nurse is one of explaining to the client what will happen and what preparation is necessary for the examination. Many blood specimens are secured while the client is in the **fasting state** (ie, abstaining from food intake or fluid intake, or both). The period of fasting varies with the tests to be done and laboratory techniques used. Whether in the home or in a health agency, clients need careful explanation about the fasting period.

The nurse should be familiar with the more common normal blood values to be able to recognize deviations. Blood examination results provide data about the client that help plan for effective nursing care. Normal adult values for some of the more common laboratory blood tests are given in Appendix B.

When securing specimens for laboratory examination, the nurse is responsible for the correct labeling of specimens before they are transported to the laboratory. An inaccurate or unmarked specimen can be more hazardous than no specimen. A request for the type of examination desired should accompany the specimen.

Care must be used when handling any blood or body fluids to prevent transmission of human immunodeficiency virus, hepatitis B virus, and other blood-borne infections. Precautions always include thorough handwashing and the use of gloves. Gown, mask, or protective eye covering also may be recommended.

Urine Specimens

A **urinalysis** is the laboratory examination of a urine specimen. Analysis of the urine is another common way of securing data about a person's health state.

Most laboratories prefer a specimen of several hundred milliliters collected soon after arising from sleep. Special urine collection techniques are discussed in Chapter 34.

Nursing Responsibilities   The nurse often is responsible for instructing the client about urine collection techniques or for obtaining a sample of urine from the client. A cooperative client can be instructed to put the specimen into a clean or, in some instances, a sterile container. Care should be taken that the outside of the container is not contaminated. Precautions similar to those used when handling blood are appropriate with all body fluids. (See Chapter 26 for review of safe handling and transportation of specimens.)

As with common blood test results, the nurse should be able to recognize deviations from normal in the urinalysis. Normal adult laboratory analysis values for urine are presented in Appendix B.

Secretion Specimens

Specimens of body secretions are collected for microscopic examination or to introduce them into a culture medium to grow any microorganisms that are present. Body secretions from the throat, vagina, penis, rectum, eye, ear, and wounds or lesions are most often collected for these purposes. A sterile, long-handled applicator or swab and a sterile container or tube with an enclosed ampule of culture medium are used. The sterile cotton-tipped end of the applicator should be placed directly into the area where the specimen is desired, and rotated to make certain secretions adhere to the applicator. The applicator is then carefully placed directly into the test tube and handled according to the laboratory policy. This may involve crushing the ampule of medium to allow the swab tip to be covered by the fluid and carefully capping the container before labeling it. Precautions should be taken so that the applicator is not contaminated before or after securing the secretion specimen. Nor should the secretions be allowed to contaminate the other surfaces. The specimen should be taken to the laboratory immediately for examination. Allowing the specimen to stand for a prolonged period may encourage the overgrowth of other microorganisms.

Nursing Responsibilities The nurse frequently is responsible for the collection of specimens of body secretions. Explanation to the client and careful documentation of the type of specimen, the collection site, and the date and time are vital nursing interventions. Precautions when handling body fluids or secretions must be enforced. Specimens should be packaged and labeled according to agency policy before prompt delivery to the laboratory.

Radiography Procedures

Radiography is the use of x-rays to secure data about health status. An **x-ray** or **roentgen ray** is a high-energy electromagnetic wave capable of penetrating solid matter and acting on photographic film. X-ray films commonly are taken to determine the size, shape, and functioning of some organs, the characteristics of bones, and the detection of masses.

A radiopaque contrast substance may be used to secure more detailed viewing of some organs. **Radiopaque** means impenetrable by x-rays. The radiopaque substance, which usually contains barium or iodine, produces a contrasting shadow on x-ray films as compared with tissues, which are penetrated by the x-rays.

Radiology procedures are performed in various health care settings and on many of the body systems. Certain procedures, such as ultrasonography, frequently are used in conjunction with radiography or nuclear medicine studies and are discussed with these procedures.

Contrast Radiologic Studies

An **upper gastrointestinal** (GI) **series** is the x-ray visualization of the esophagus, stomach, and duodenum. The client usually is in a fasting state and is asked to drink a radiopaque barium preparation immediately before the x-ray examination. The radiopaque substance outlines the organs for visualization. Fluoroscopy, which is the radiologic visualization of the motion of an organ as the radiopaque substance moves through it, also may be used. An upper GI series with fluoroscopy is not uncomfortable, although the radiopaque substance does not taste particularly good. Many people say that it tastes like flavored chalk. An upper GI study usually is completed in 1 hour. After the test, a mild laxative frequently is ordered to allow for evacuation of any residual barium. More details of this test and the following are given in Chapter 35.

A **barium enema** allows for the x-ray visualization of the large intestine. A barium solution is instilled through the anus to distend the rectum and colon. In addition to fasting, preparation for the barium enema includes cleansing of the colon with laxatives and enemas. The technique for giving enemas is discussed in Chapter 35. Laxatives and enemas also may be used to cleanse the intestine of residual barium after the examination. The client should be prepared for the fact that a barium enema is a rather uncomfortable and tiring procedure and also told to expect that fecal material may be white from the barium for several days after the examination.

Oral **cholecystography** is the x-ray visualization of the gallbladder. An iodine radiopaque substance is taken orally, absorbed by the liver, and concentrated in the gallbladder. Preparations usually include some dietary modification on the day preceding the examination, followed by taking pills containing the contrast material during the evening. Cholecystography should be scheduled before any barium studies because barium may interfere with visualization.

The procedure should cause no discomfort, although some people may experience adverse reactions to the contrast material. Any history of allergic reactions to dye must be clearly noted on the chart on admission. Intravenous cholangiography uses contrast material given intravenously. The procedure is similar to that for oral cholecystography. At many hospitals, the ultrasound study has replaced oral cholecystography.

Intravenous pyelography (IVP), or *excretory urography*, is the x-ray visualization of the kidney's ability to excrete urine. IVP should be scheduled before any barium studies because barium takes 3 or 4 days to be excreted and may interfere with visualization of the kidneys. A radiopaque dye is injected intravenously, and films are taken at timed intervals to determine the amount of dye excreted by the kidneys. Preparations for an IVP usually include a laxative or enema and having the person urinate before the examination. There should be no discomfort. Some people, however, are sensitive to the dye and may have allergic reactions to it. This information must be clearly noted on the chart on admission.

Endoscopic retrograde cholangiopancreatography (ERCP) is the x-ray visualization of the pancreatic ducts as well as the liver and biliary tree by means of injection of a contrast medium. This procedure involves passage of an endoscope into the duodenum so that contrast material can be directly introduced through the endoscope and into the pancreatic duct and hepatobiliary tree (Fig. 27-11). ERCP aids diagnosis of pancreatic disease and helps evaluate the cause of a type of jaundice. It is an invasive procedure and requires that the client sign a permit. The client must be in a fasting state. A local anesthetic is used to assist in passage of the endoscope. Any previous allergic reaction to a contrast medium needs to be reported to the physician.

Nursing Responsibilities The role of the nurse in the diagnostic use of x-rays is to teach and to prepare clients as necessary. The physician's order for the specific study and agency protocol determines the type of preparation before the procedure. Food and fluid restrictions vary and must be communicated and reinforced with the client and concerned support people. The nurse is responsible for monitoring the client's condition and recording observations when the diagnostic procedure is completed.

Computed Tomography

Computed tomography, or *CT scanning*, is a noninvasive x-ray procedure. It is a method by which a body part can be scanned from different angles with an x-ray beam and a

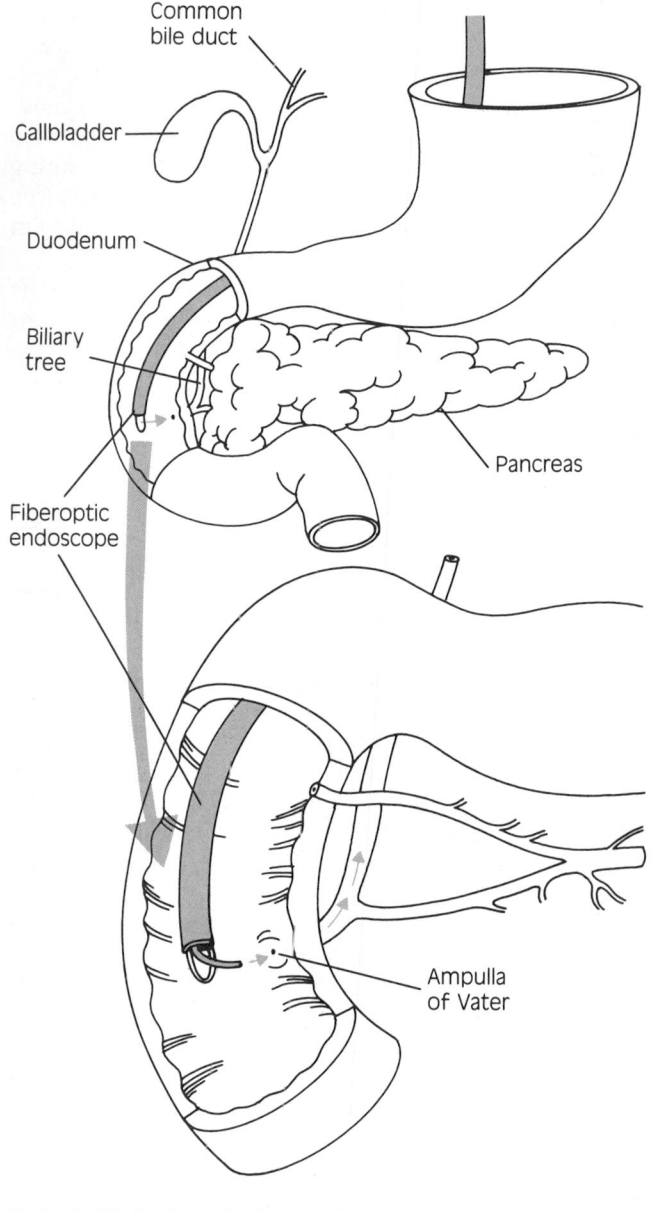

FIGURE 27-11

Endoscopic retrograde cholangiopancreatography uses both radiography and endoscopy to examine the pancreatic ducts and hepatobiliary tree. An endoscope is passed through the esophagus, stomach, and duodenum to the ampulla of Vater. A contrast medium is introduced by inserting a cannula through the endoscope.

computer that calculates varying tissue densities and records a cross-sectional image on paper. The radiologist can distinguish structures by their shape, size, symmetry, color, and position. An iodine contrast dye may need to be given intravenously during the test to enhance tissue contrast. Because iodine preparations may cause nausea and vomiting, food and fluids usually are withheld for 3 to 4 hours before the test. The client must lie absolutely still during the examination. Some people experience a claustrophobic sensation when the head or body is placed inside the CT scanner.

Nursing Responsibilities The client requires an explanation of any reactions that may occur related to the dye injection (warm sensation and flushing of the face, nausea, vomiting, salty taste in the mouth). Any history of allergic reaction or hypersensitivity to shellfish, iodine, or any contrast dye is vital information and needs to be reported to the physician. An antihistamine or steroid preparation may be prescribed, or the physician may decide to use newer non-ionic contrast agents that produce minimal adverse reactions. All metal objects need to be removed from the body area being scanned. The nurse should explain that the test itself is brief (15 to 30 minutes) and reassure the client that exposure to radiation is no more than that experienced in conventional x-ray studies.

Magnetic Resonance Imaging

Magnetic resonance imaging (MRI) is an advanced scanning technique that uses magnetism and radiofrequency waves to produce cross-sectional images of body tissues on a computer screen. This diagnostic tool can provide unique information about the chemical makeup of tissues without the risks associated with radiation. It can show deviations between normal and diseased blood vessels, clearly display the heart's pumping action, and distinguish lesions or masses in fluid-filled soft tissues. MRI is being used increasingly to evaluate central nervous system anatomy, particularly the brain.

MRI is a noninvasive procedure that requires the client to be placed head first in the supine position into a narrow tunnel-like machine (Fig. 27-12). All metal objects must be removed, and because the MRI uses magnetism, any client with a surgically implanted metal device, such as a pacemaker or implanted insulin pump, may not undergo the study. Other contraindications to MRI include marked obesity, claustrophobia, and pregnancy, since long-term effects are unknown. Only clients in stable physical condition are eligible because the confined structure does not allow for recording of vital signs or monitoring of cardiac rhythms. Continuous intravenous infusions require manual regulation because infusion pumps cannot be used in the scanning room.

Nursing Responsibilities A well-prepared client is better able to withstand the claustrophobic experience of an MRI scan. Suggestions to keep the eyes closed during the test sometimes prove helpful. The client also needs to be aware of the necessity to lie still while enclosed in the machine. It is important that the client empty the bladder beforehand to be comfortable during the procedure.

The technician maintains communication with the client during the test through nonmetallic earphones. The client also should be told that the machine makes a monotonous, steady noise when operating. No special observations are necessary when the test is completed.

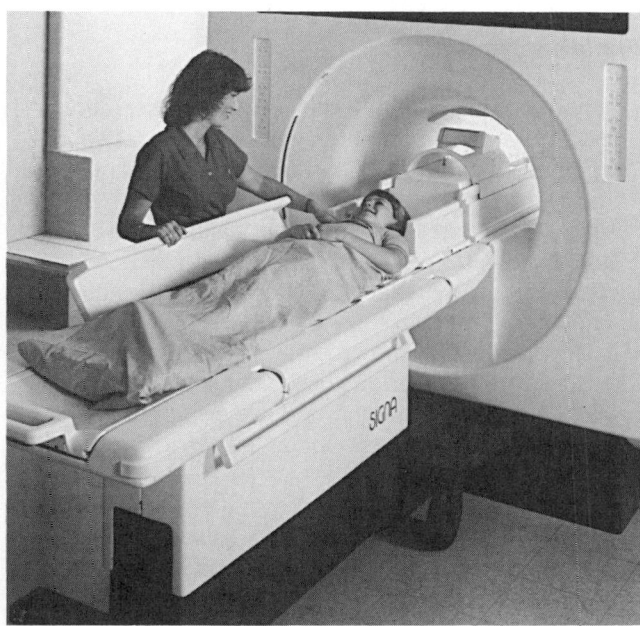

FIGURE 27-12

The magnetic resonance imaging scanning machine can provide unique diagnostic information in a noninvasive technique but requires that the client be placed head first in the supine position into a narrow tunnel-like space within the machine. The nurse must prepare the client with the knowledge that the procedure may be a claustrophobic experience. Keeping eyes closed during the procedure sometimes lessens the discomforting sensation. (Courtesy of GE Medical Systems.)

Radioisotope Scanning

A **radioisotope** is a radioactive chemical used in nuclear medicine procedures. When used for diagnostic examination, a substance containing a small amount of radioisotope is administered orally or by injection. The particular substance is selected according to its ability to localize in the target organ. Blocking agents are sometimes given to prevent its absorption by other organs. The heart, vessels, brain, spinal canal, lungs, thyroid, and abdominal organs are examined in this way. The size, shape, and function of organs and the presence of abnormal masses can be determined. A mechanism called a *scanner* detects emission of the radioactive waves and records them on a photographic plate. The lungs are commonly studied using radioisotope scanning, as discussed in Table 36-2.

Nursing Responsibilities Preparation for radioisotope scanning should include reassurance that the amount of radioisotope normally used is minute and produces no more radiation than that of a single x-ray. Some people fear that they will become dangerously radioactive. The client also should be prepared for the fact that lengthy placement in an awkward position may be necessary during the test. No discomfort should be experienced except for that caused by injection and the positioning.

Ultrasonography

Ultrasonography is a noninvasive procedure that involves the use of ultrasound to produce an image or photograph of an organ or tissue. This procedure also is referred to as echography. The kidneys, liver, spleen, pancreas, gallbladder, thyroid, heart, eyes, lymph nodes, peripheral blood vessels, and female reproductive organs can be examined in this way. **Ultrasound waves** are extremely high-frequency and inaudible sound waves. The ultrasound waves penetrate and bounce back, or echo, according to the density of the tissue. A **transducer** or probe, an instrument that converts energy from one form to another, produces the ultrasound waves and converts the reflected waves into electrical energy. The electrical energy then produces an image on a viewing screen that may be recorded on film, videotape, slides, or chart paper. The person is asked to remain quiet while the probe, which is about 1 inch (2.5 cm) in diameter, is applied to the lubricated skin and moved about over the area to be examined.

Nursing Responsibilities No special preparations are necessary, except for abdominal ultrasonography, which requires food and fluid restrictions. An ultrasound examination should be scheduled before barium studies, since barium interferes with visualization. There is no discomfort with this procedure. It is helpful if the client is aware of the need to remain motionless during the test.

Genetic Testing and Screening

Genetic testing and screening is a rapidly developing science. Prenatal test results are used to identify genetic and biochemical defects, thus allowing treatment to be initiated (Fischbach, 1992). Chromosomal analysis can assist in the diagnosis of certain common disorders, such as Down syndrome and Tay-Sachs disease. Researchers have identified a previously unknown chromosomal disorder, referred to as the fragile-X syndrome, that affects the central nervous system. Genetic predispositions also are known to exist for adult disorders, such as certain cancers, diabetes, heart disease, and alcoholism. Genetic testing and screening procedures will make it possible in the future to clearly identify those people who are likely to develop one of these diseases.

As this science develops, nurses are positioned to play a key leadership role. With their multiple client contacts and focus on promoting wellness and preventing disease, nurses can reach people at risk to make referrals and direct clients to appropriate resources. Many controversial ethical issues will surface. Will parents decide to abort a child who may be handicapped? Can employers use genetic testing to screen and possibly reject prospective employees who may be at risk for developing cancer or having a heart attack? The consequences and implications associated with these particular diagnostic tests are far-reaching, and nurses will need to have a working knowledge of genetic testing to effectively influence the health and well-being of their clients.

KEY POINTS

- Diagnostic tests ordered by the physician provide valuable information about the client's state of health.
- Nursing responsibilities associated with diagnostic tests may include witnessing a client's consent, scheduling the test, physical and emotional preparation of the client, nursing care after the test, disposal of equipment, and proper care of any specimen.
- A liver biopsy involves the needle aspiration of a sample of liver tissue to determine the presence of a disease process.
- A lumbar puncture involves withdrawal of fluid from the subarachnoid space in the spinal canal to obtain a specimen for culture and analysis, to relieve pressure or check for alterations in the usual pressure of CSF, or to inject drugs or dyes for x-ray visualization.
- In thoracentesis, fluid is aspirated from the pleural cavity; in paracentesis, fluid is aspirated from the peritoneal cavity.
- An ECG is a recording of the electrical impulses of the heart; an EEG is a recording of the electrical activity of the brain.
- An endoscopic study provides valuable diagnostic information obtained by direct visual examination of an organ or cavity and allows for microscopic examination of tissue specimens taken from the site.

- Laboratory analysis of blood, urine, and secretion specimens is a common way of securing data about a person's health state. Minimal client preparation is involved.
- Radiologic studies, or x-rays, are valuable diagnostic tests for determining size, shape, and functioning of some organs, the characteristics of bones, and the detection of masses.
- A CT scan produces a cross-sectional image of a body part that reflects various tissue densities.
- MRI uses magnetism and radiowaves to produce cross-sectional images of body tissues on a computer screen.
- Radioisotope scanning requires the oral intake or the injection of a small amount of radioisotope that, when localized in a target organ, aids in the determination of the size, shape, and function of the organ and the presence of an abnormal mass.
- An ultrasound study is a recording of the pattern of sound waves as they are reflected off body tissues.

STUDY QUESTIONS

1. Nursing responsibilities before a diagnostic test may include all the following *except*
   a. scheduling the test
   b. physical preparation of the client
   c. obtaining the consent
   d. psychological preparation of the client
2. The nurse's priority after the client has a diagnostic test is
   a. documentation of the test
   b. the client's comfort
   c. delivery of the specimen to the laboratory
   d. collecting baseline data
3. What laboratory testing must be completed before a client is scheduled for a liver biopsy?
   a. prothrombin time and platelet count
   b. hemoglobin and hematocrit
   c. serum electrolytes
   d. differential white blood cell count
4. Immediately after a liver biopsy, a priority nursing intervention is
   a. relieving pain
   b. resuming the client's diet
   c. encouraging the client to void
   d. positioning the client

5. The term paracentesis commonly refers to aspiration of fluid from the
   a. peritoneal cavity
   b. pleural cavity
   c. subarachnoid space
   d. synovial joints
6. The maximum amount of fluid that should be aspirated during thoracentesis is
   a. 250 mL
   b. 500 mL
   c. 1000 mL
   d. 2000 mL
7. The nurse prepares the client for an EEG by telling her that
   a. the test is painful
   b. it is a record of the electrical activity of the heart
   c. during the test, she may receive a slight electrical shock
   d. food and fluids will not be restricted before the test
8. A client has just returned from a bronchoscopy and requests a glass of juice. The first nursing response is to

a. check that the client's gag reflex has returned
b. administer a glass of ice water first
c. administer an analgesic
d. inform the client he must remain NPO for 4 more hours

9. Mr. Byers is scheduled for an upper GI series tomorrow morning. Preparation for the test includes
a. cleansing the bowel with laxatives and enemas
b. instruction about taking pills containing contrast material the evening before
c. administration of a sedative
d. fasting the night before the test

10. Which study frequently is performed instead of oral cholecystography?
a. an x-ray of the abdomen
b. a barium enema
c. an ultrasound study
d. a colonoscopy

11. While hospitalized, Mrs. Baxter is scheduled for a barium enema and IVP. The nurse would
a. schedule IVP before the barium enema
b. schedule the barium enema first followed by IVP
c. determine which study is first based on availability of appointments
d. allow the client to decide which test should be first

12. A CT scan is
a. an ultrasound study
b. a noninvasive x-ray procedure
c. an electrical impulse study
d. a venipuncture procedure

13. Mr. Kelly is scheduled for a CT scan with contrast dye. The nurse informs him that with the dye injection he may experience
a. chills and tremors
b. a warm sensation or flushing of the face
c. severe posttest headaches
d. cherry-colored urine

14. Which client would *not* be a candidate for MRI?
a. Mr. M, who has a reddened sacral area
b. Mrs. R, who has a hearing deficit
c. Mrs. W, who has a pacemaker
d. Mr. Z, who is 20 lb underweight

15. Instruction for a client scheduled for an ultrasound study of peripheral blood vessels would include which of the following?
a. no special preparation is required
b. fasting is required the night before the study
c. shave prep of the area is required
d. an analgesic is given immediately before the study

Answers With Rationale

1. The correct response is *c*. The physician is responsible for obtaining a signed consent before the diagnostic test. The remaining items may all be nursing responsibilities.
2. The correct response is *b*. The client's comfort is the priority after the test. Documentation and delivery of a specimen are secondary to the client's needs. Baseline data is collected before the test for comparison afterward.
3. The correct response is *a*. Liver disease frequently is associated with blood-clotting deficiencies. The other tests are not required before a liver biopsy.
4. The correct response is *d*. After the procedure, the client is assisted to lie on the right side with a pillow under the needle insertion site to apply pressure to the area. The other nursing actions are not priorities.
5. The correct response is *a*. Paracentesis is the aspiration of fluid from the peritoneal cavity.
6. The correct response is *c*. The upper limit usually is 1000 mL, so as not to cause any cardiac or pulmonary distress when the fluid is shifted or aspirated from the pleural cavity.
7. The correct response is *d*. Dietary and fluid restrictions are not required before an EEG. The test is not painful, records electrical currents in the brain, and does not cause the client to receive even a small amount of electrical current.
8. The correct response is *a*. Before resuming fluid intake, the gag or cough reflex must be checked so that the client will not aspirate whatever he drinks. Providing the gag reflex is present, the normal diet can be resumed after the test.
9. The correct response is *d*. Preparation for an upper GI series only requires fasting the night before the test.
10. The correct response is *c*. An ultrasound study can provide accurate results in situations where oral cholecystography is not accurate or effective. Preparation for the ultrasound does not require the ingestion of an oral contrast agent.
11. The correct response is *a*. Barium takes several days to be expelled and interferes with visualization of the kidneys during IVP.
12. The correct response is *b*. A CT scan is a noninvasive x-ray procedure.
13. The correct response is *b*. The injection of the dye during the study causes a temporary warm sensation or flushing of the face. It does not cause any of the other manifestations.
14. The correct response is *c*. Because the MRI study uses magnetism, which interferes with the action of a pacemaker, any person with one should not have the study. The other situations are not contraindications to the study.
15. The correct response is *a*. An ultrasound study of an area other than the abdomen does not require any special preparation.

BIBLIOGRAPHY

Barkett, P. (1988). Cardiac M.U.G.A. scan: Taking first-pictures of the heart. *Nursing, 18*(10), 76–78.

Brown, S. (1990). Behind the numbers on the CBC. *RN, 53*(2), 46–50.

Cella, J., & Watson, J. (1989). *Nurse's manual of laboratory tests*. Philadelphia: Lippincott.

Clinical laboratory tests: Values and implications. (1991). Springhouse, PA: Springhouse Corp.

Corbett, J. (1992). *Laboratory tests and diagnostic procedures with nursing diagnoses* (3rd ed.). Norwalk, CT: Appleton & Lange.

Drew, B. J. (1992). Using cardiac leads: The right way. *Nursing, 22*(5), 50–54.

Fischbach, F. (1992). *A manual of laboratory diagnostic tests* (4th ed.). Philadelphia: Lippincott.

Garner, B. (1989). Guide to changing lab values in elders. *Geriatric Nursing, 10*(3), 144–145.

Gawlikowski, J. (1992). White cells at war. *American Journal of Nursing.* 92(3), 44–51.

Hahn, K. (1989). When a patient's scheduled for G.I. series. *Nursing, 19*(3), 88.

Kee, J. (1991). *Laboratory and diagnostic tests with nursing applications* (3rd ed.). Norwalk, CT: Appleton & Lange.

Monroe, D. (1989). Patient teaching for X-ray and other diagnostics (upper GI, barium enema). *RN, 51*(12), 36–40.

Monroe, D. (1989). Will your patient survive that trip to X-ray? *RN, 52*(3), 24–29.

Monroe, D. (1990). Patient teaching for X-ray and other diagnostics (ERCP, oral cholecystogram). *RN, 52*(4), 52–56.

Monroe, D. (1990). Patient teaching for X-ray and other diagnostics (IVP). *RN, 53*(9), 42–44.

Monroe, D. (1991). Patient teaching for X-ray and other diagnostics. *RN, 54*(2), 44–46.

Morrison D., Seiger, L., & Totty, W. (1990). MRI's current role in joint imaging. *Patient Care, 24*(14), 18–24.

Phillips, P. (1990). Ultrasound taking venogram role. *Medical World News, 31*(2), 22.

Plankey, E., & Knauf, J. (1990). What patients need to know about magnetic resonance imaging. *American Journal of Nursing, 90*(1), 27–28.

Rudolphi, D. (1990). Duplex scanning. *American Journal of Nursing, 90*(4), 123–124.

Thrasher, S. (1989). What I didn't know really hurt me. *RN, 52*(9), 49–56.

Tomky, D. (1989). A three-pronged approach to monitoring. *RN, 52*(3), 24–29.

Wilkinson, M. (1990). Your role in needle biopsy of the liver. *RN, 53*(8), 62–66.

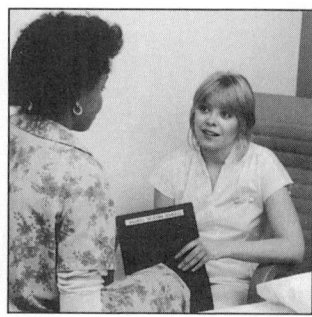
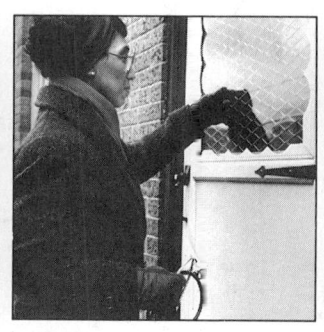
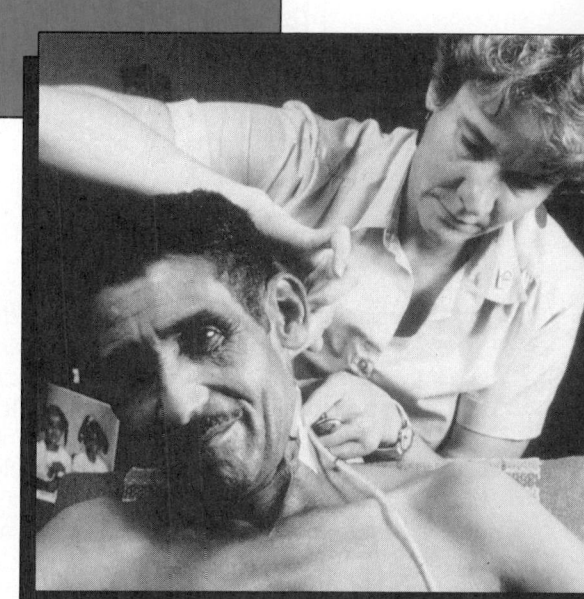

OBJECTIVES

After studying this chapter, the learner should be able to:

Define key terms used in the chapter.

Describe the role of the nurse in ensuring continuity of care.

Discuss considerations for establishing an effective nurse–client relationship when admitting a client to a health care setting.

Compare and contrast admission of a client to an ambulatory setting and a hospital setting.

Discuss transfer of clients within and among health care settings.

Describe the components of discharge planning in providing continuity of care.

KEY TERMS

ambulatory facilities
continuity of care
discharge planning

Continuity of Care

28

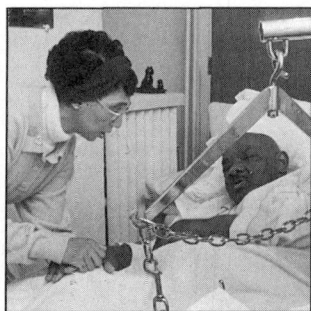

Entering and leaving a health care setting are experiences that produce anxiety for the client and for family members. Equally anxiety producing is the care that must be given at home or in a different location after the client leaves the health care setting. The nurse is the person who most often is responsible for helping the client make a smooth transition from one type of setting to another or to home. This chapter discusses admission and dismissal from the hospital setting, transfer from one type of setting to another, and discharge planning in preparation for home care. The focus of the discussion is on the client's needs and the nurse's role in providing continuity of care.

Nurse's Role in Providing Continuity of Care

At some point in their lives, all people require health care, whether for wellness promotion, health maintenance, or health restoration. Most individuals were born in a hospital; thus, they became consumers of health care from the first day of life and continue to require services of some type until they die. Although many different health care providers and settings will be a part of that care (see Chapter 3), the nurse is often the primary person responsible for communicating needs; teaching self-care; and, in many instances, providing needed care. As a result, one of the primary responsibilities of the nurse as caregiver is ensuring continuity of care.

Continuity of care is the coordination of services provided to clients before they enter a health care setting, during the time they are in the setting, and after they leave the setting (Zarle, 1989). Continuity of care ensures a smooth transition between ambulatory or hospital care and home care or other types of community-based care, thus reducing anxiety and facilitating the client in reaching optimal functioning or wellness.

The philosophy of continuity of care is essential in the current health care delivery system. The emphasis on wellness and prevention of illness makes individualized teaching for individuals of all ages critical components of client care. In addition, economic constraints on health care financing have resulted in shorter hospital stays, increased use of ambulatory services, and a trend toward care at home. To provide continuity of care, the nurse must do the following:

- Include discharge planning in the care of any person admitted to any type of health care setting
- Collaborate with other members of the health care team in meeting physical, psychological, sociocultural, and spiritual needs of the client and family in all settings and in all levels of health
- Involve the client and the client's family in the planning process

The purpose of planning for continuity of care, which is more commonly referred to as *discharge planning*, is to ensure that client and family needs are consistently met as the client moves from one level of care to another. Discharge planning is described in detail later in the chapter, but it basically involves the following:

- Assessing the strengths and limitations of a client; those strengths and limitations encompass all dimensions of the client that affect wellness
- Planning for continuity in health care from one setting to another, including the home
- Implementing and coordinating the care plan, considering individual client needs as well as individual, family, and community resources
- Evaluating the effectiveness of care

This chapter is intended to be only an introduction to the different ways in which clients enter a health care setting and move from one type of setting to another. Discharge planning is discussed primarily in relation to the care of the client at home; this aspect of care will become increasingly common as the nursing profession moves into the 21st century.

Admission to a Health Care Agency

People enter the health care setting to become clients (consumers of health care services) for many different reasons. Consider the following examples:

Joe Sol, aged 5 years, has been having increasing numbers of throat infections, and his tonsils are badly infected. Joe's pediatrician has decided that Joe must have a *tonsillectomy* (removal of tonsils) in a hospital, entering the morning of surgery and going home that afternoon.

Jane Yee, aged 38 years, has had heavy menstrual periods. As a diagnostic procedure, her doctor schedules her for a dilation of the cervix and curettage of the uterus (*D & C*) at a community ambulatory surgery center.

Tom Valiz, aged 28 years, injured his back while working at his construction job. After diagnostic studies, he has been going to a community health center each day for heat therapy and exercises.

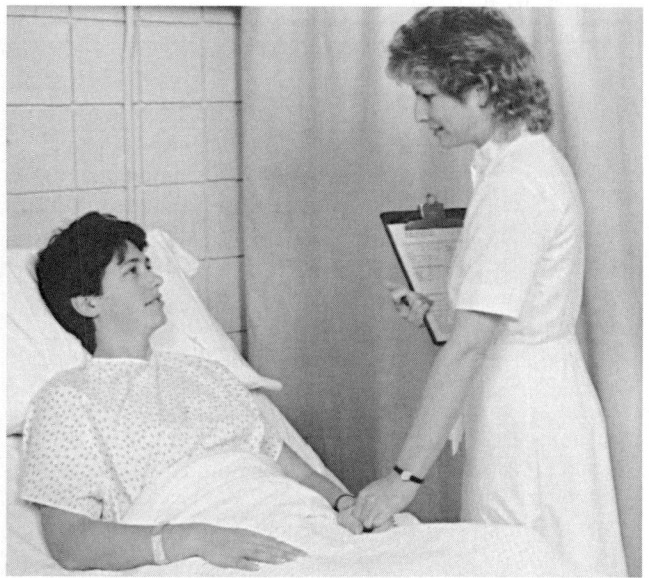

FIGURE 28-1

Admission to the hospital can be a traumatic experience. The matter in which the client is admitted can help diminish some of the fear and anxiety. Establishing rapport and a trusting nurse–client relationship is important. (Photo © Ken Kasper.)

Sarah Hale, aged 16 years, has been brought to the hospital emergency room for acute alcohol intoxication. After treatment, she is admitted to the hospital's chemical dependency unit for observation.

Sadie Aird, aged 78 years, has had congestive heart failure for the past 10 years. She is cared for at home by her daughter, with the help of a community health nurse.

Jim Zamba, aged 28 years, is admitted to the hospital through the emergency room, sent to surgery, and then placed in the intensive care unit (ICU) for treatment of severe head injuries following a motorcycle accident. After recovery from the acute phase of care, Jim will go to a special rehabilitation center.

Although all of these individuals require care, they will not all have the same kind of needs nor will they be alike as clients. Some of them will be admitted and discharged on the same day, some of them will remain in the acute-care setting only as long as acute care is needed, and some will require long-term care.

For years, hospitals have been the primary method of delivering care to people who were too ill to be cared for at home or required surgery. However, because of increasing costs and a health care cost reimbursement program that is prospective instead of retrospective, hospital admissions for many surgical procedures and lengths of hospital stay are decreasing. Increasing numbers of clients are having surgery, diagnostic tests, and emergency care in ambula-

tory-care settings or on an outpatient basis. Even clients who are admitted may stay for fewer than 24 hours, may be admitted the morning of the surgery, or may go home during an interim period between diagnosis and care.

All people who enter a health care setting must take on a new role. They must add to their already established roles (eg, spouse, parent, sibling, police officer, student) the role of client. In addition to adding a new role, they also enter an environment in which they are surrounded by strangers and in which they encounter different sounds, sights, and smells.

All people who become health care clients have needs that require attention (Fig. 28-1). In meeting these needs during admission of the client, the nurse is providing holistic care while establishing the base for the way in which the client will respond to and evaluate the remainder of the client's stay. The accompanying display describes nursing guidelines for establishing an effective nurse–client relationship to ensure that each client is considered as an individual in any type of setting.

During the admission process, the nurse acts not only as a practitioner but also as a person concerned about the welfare of client and family. The admission period corresponds to the orientation phase of the helping relationship described in Chapter 20.

Admission to an Ambulatory Health Care Facility

An individual may require care in many different kinds of ambulatory facilities, including physician offices, clinics, outpatient services, emergency rooms, and same-day surgery centers. **Ambulatory facilities** are those in which the client receives health care services but does not remain overnight. The goal of such facilities is to keep ambulatory those clients under care or to enable those clients who are able to provide self-care at home with assistance as necessary from health care providers. Individuals go to ambulatory settings for wellness promotion, health maintenance, or for medical or surgical treatment.

In most ambulatory settings, clients enter a reception area, where they are asked to complete a short health history. They then go to an examination room and a physical assessment is completed. Depending on their needs, diagnostic tests may be done, immunizations given, medications prescribed, or minor surgery performed. All clients require teaching, which should include written instructions about care at home, health promotion activities, and how to contact someone for further questions. Referrals to community agencies, support groups, or other types of health care settings may be necessary.

Admission to ambulatory or same-day surgery facilities is somewhat different. Screening tests, teaching, and admission procedures usually are completed before clients enter the setting. They arrive at the setting, have the procedure, and go home when recovery is satisfactory (see Chapter 4?). If clients have surgery in the hospital setting,

G U I D E L I N E S   F O R   N U R S I N G   C A R E

Establishing an Effective Nurse–Client Relationship Respectful of Client Individuality

- Recognize and take necessary steps to reduce anxiety. Anxiety is a natural reaction to the unknown. Anxiety reduction can be facilitated through therapeutic communications, teaching, and acceptance. Some common concerns that cause anxiety follow:
  Will I have pain?
  Who will take care of my family if I die?
  Will strangers be looking at my body?
  How much will this cost?
  What if I can't keep my job?
- Remember that the medical or surgical condition for which the client is being treated is only one part of the client's life. Although it may be the primary concern for the client, other concerns include family needs, financial status, and the future.

- Communicate with the client as an individual so that he or she can maintain his or her own identity. Ask clients how you should address them—some people would prefer Mr. or Mrs., Ms.   ; others would rather be called by their first name. Do not lump all older adults as "Grandma" or "Grandpa." Be sure that you do not refer to Mr. Jones, admitted to room 2218 for treatment of a ruptured appendix, as "the appendix in 2218."
- Take time to learn *who* the client being admitted is, including the client's cultural and religious background. Respect the client's values and beliefs even though they may differ from yours.
- Provide for client–family participation and decision making in all aspects of care.

the regular admission procedures are completed on arrival; in most instances, screening tests and teaching are done before the day of surgery. It is the nurse's responsibility to assess what has been done and individualize the care plan to clients' needs.

Admission to the Hospital Setting

In most hospitals, admission begins in the admitting office. Staff obtain information about clients and print that information on an admission sheet. This admission sheet becomes part of a client's permanent record, and includes the following information:

Full name
Address
Date of birth
Name of admitting physician
Gender
Marital status
Nearest relative
Occupation and employer
Financial status for health care payment
Religious preference
Date and time of admission
Identification number
Admitting diagnosis

The identification number, as well as the client's name and physician's name (and any other information required by a specific institution), becomes a part of the identification bracelet that is placed on the client's wrist. This bracelet is an important safety component during the client's treatment because it is the means of accurate identification for

many procedures and treatments, including medication administration, diagnostic tests, and surgery. The bracelet is essential for identifying clients who are irrational, comatose, or young.

After the necessary forms have been completed in the admitting office, clients are usually taken to the unit to which they have been assigned. Because of cost-containment measures, laboratory studies and x-rays as well as the admitting office procedures may be completed on an outpatient basis before the day of admission.

Preparing the Room for Admission

The admitting office should notify the unit before the client's arrival so the room can be prepared. The following activities should be carried out by the nurse in anticipation of the client's arrival:

- Position the bed. For the ambulatory client, the bed should be in its lowest position. Place the bed in its highest position if the client will arrive on a stretcher. Ensure furniture in the room has been arranged to allow easy access to the bed (Fig. 28-2).
- Open the bed. Fold back the bedspread, top blanket, and top sheet.
- Assemble necessary equipment and supplies. A hospital admission pack (which contains such items as a bath basin, water pitcher, drinking glass, tissues, soap, and lotion) is placed in the room. A hospital gown or pajamas should be in the room, although the client may choose to wear personal pajamas or gowns. Equipment for taking vital signs (ie, stethoscope, sphygmomanometer, or thermometer) and

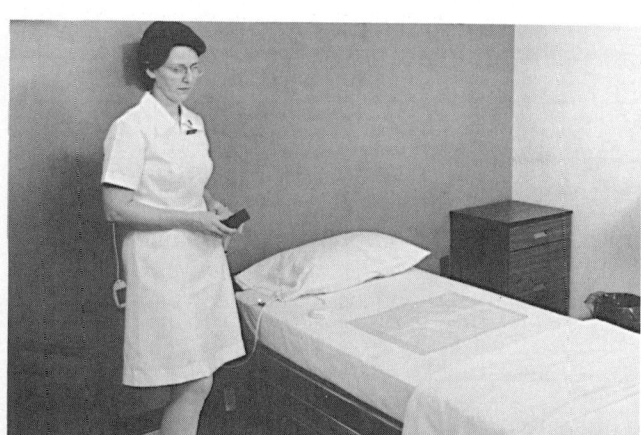

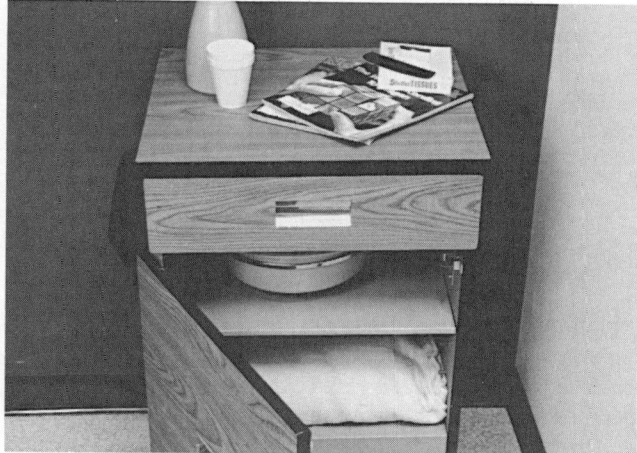

FIGURE 28-2

In anticipation of the client's arrival, the nurse should open the bed, position the bed, and assemble necessary equipment and supplies.

client on arrival to the unit. The nurse makes the admission assessment and documents the information on the admission data base. A sample form illustrates typical information that is collected and documented. Each agency has its own form (Fig. 28-3). The information on the form is used to develop the nursing care plan for the client and also is used as a data base for discharge planning and home care (see Chapter 15).

The client should be welcomed to the unit in the same courteous manner that would be used in welcoming a guest into one's own home. In most instances, the client is accompanied by family members who may either remain with the client to provide support and information or be asked to wait in the waiting room during the admission procedure. The nurse needs to assess the needs of the client and family and decide which should be done.

Transfer Within and Between Settings

Although little has been written about the transfer of clients, it is common for some type of move to be made within settings as well as among settings. For example:

- Clients often are moved within the hospital setting from emergency room to hospital room; from ICU to hospital room (and vice versa); from one floor to another; or from one room to another room on the same floor.
- Clients are transferred to and from acute-care settings to long-term settings.
- Clients are transferred from acute-care settings to rehabilitation centers.
- Clients are transferred from ambulatory-care settings to acute-care settings.

height and weight should be in the room or readily available. If lab work has not been done previously, a container for a clean urine specimen should also be available.
- Assemble special equipment and supplies. The client may require oxygen therapy, cardiac monitoring, or suction equipment. The nurse ensures equipment is functioning properly and is ready for the client's use on arrival.
- Adjust the physical environment of the room. This may include turning on lights and setting the room temperature.

Arrival of the Client on the Unit

Although other members of the health care team may assist in the admitting procedure (Procedure 28-1), it is the nurse who is responsible for the comfort and well-being of the

FIGURE 28-3

The admission data base is used for the present hospitalization and for discharge and home care planning. (Photo © Ken Kasper.)

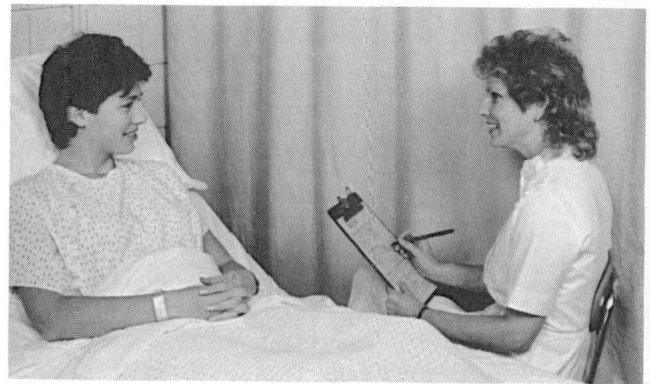

PROCEDURE 28-1

Admitting a Client to the Unit

Action	Rationale
1 Check the client's identification band. Greet the client and relatives by name. Introduce yourself to the client and the client to his or her roommate.	Calling the client by name, extending common courtesies, and welcoming the client and relatives often helps them to feel at ease and less frightened.

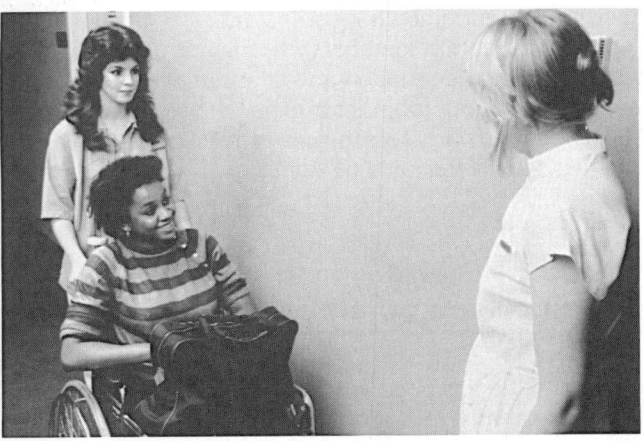

Action 1: Greeting the client.

Action	Rationale
2 Explain use of the bathroom and equipment, such as the call system, bed controls, television, telephone, and lights. Explain agency routines, such as meal times, visiting hours, and so on. Explain what space and territory belongs to the client.	Explaining agency routines and how to use equipment helps put the client at ease. Knowing how to use equipment also decreases the risk of accidents. Explaining space and territory allows the client a sense of control over the environment.
3 Place the signal device and other equipment so that they will be convenient for the client to use.	Being unable to call for help is unsafe and can result in accidents. When equipment is handy for clients, accidents, such as falling, are less likely to occur.
4 Obtain the client's temperature, pulse and respiratory rates, and blood pressure. Obtain a urine specimen at a convenient time during the admission procedure.	Obtaining these signs and a specimen is an important part of the client's physical examination on admission and is the nurse's responsibility.
5 Provide for privacy. Ask relatives to leave unless they will assist with undressing the client.	Providing privacy shows respect and interest in the client.
6 Help the client to undress, if indicated, and assist the client into a comfortable position in bed.	Assisting the client to undress and get into bed conserves strength, helps prevent accidents, and prepares the client for care. If he or she does not have any functional limitations, it is important to allow the client the opportunity to change alone.

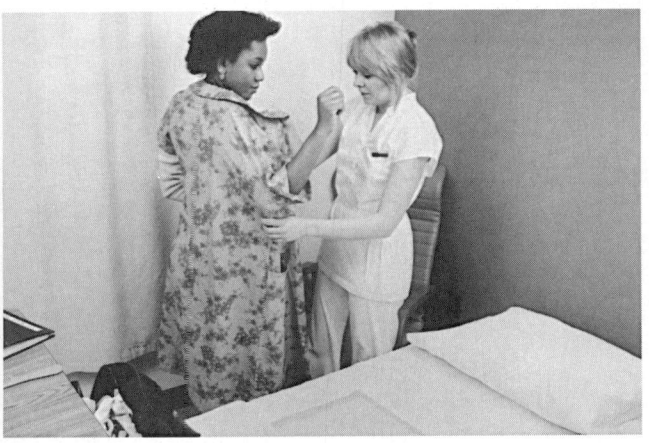

Action 6: Helping the client change into sleepwear.

(continued)

PROCEDURE 28-1 *(continued)*
Admitting a Client to the Unit

Action	**Rationale**
7 Take care of the client's clothing and valuables. Follow agency procedure.	Losing items is upsetting to the client and can result in legal problems.
8 Indicate to family members that they may return to the client's bedside. Ask if there are any questions or concerns, and answer questions or make referrals as appropriate.	The worries and fears of family and significant others should be considered during the admission process.
9 Carefully explain to the client what will be happening and what to expect. Elicit questions about the admission process and answer questions honestly.	Not knowing what will happen is stressful. This explanation may help decrease anxiety. Therapeutic communications help to establish a sense of trust and rapport.

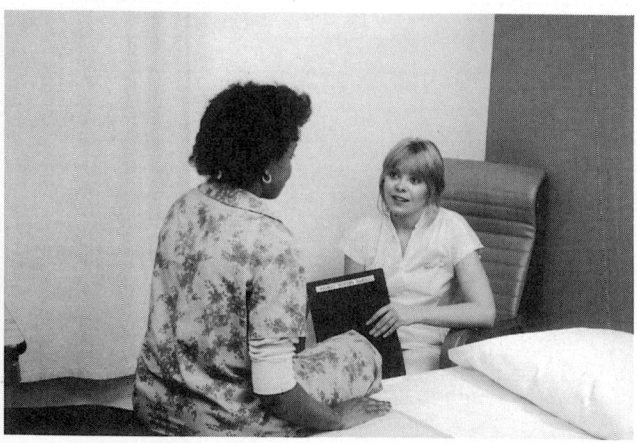

Action 9: *Talking to the client about what to expect.*

10 Do necessary recording on client's record, following agency policy. Begin the nursing history and assessment—it may or may not be advisable to have the family in the room.	The information is an important part of the client's permanent record. Presence of family may inhibit the responses of the client.
11 If the client is an adult, continue the history and assessment. If the client is an infant, child, elderly person, or is confused, collect necessary data from family or significant others before they leave.	The client may divulge important information that is not shared with family members. If the client cannot provide information, consultation with secondary sources may be necessary.

All of these examples demonstrate how often a client may be transferred (moved), often to meet the needs of the setting rather than to meet the needs of the client.

When a transfer occurs, the client must readjust to new surroundings, new roommates, new routines, and new people providing care. If the transfer is to a higher level of care, as in a move to ICU, the client experiences unfamiliar sights and sounds. A transfer to a long-term facility may be one that is not desired but has become necessary if family members cannot provide care at home or if no other support people are available. All of these factors cause stress and anxiety.

The nurse may not be responsible for the actual physical move but is responsible for ensuring that the comfort, safety, and knowledge needs of the client and family are met. Although documentation and procedures differ depending on the institution and type of transfer, client needs are always a priority in ensuring a smooth transition and ensuring continuity of care. In general, considerations for transfer include the following:

Transfer Within the Hospital Setting
- In some situations in which a client moves from room to room on the same floor, the furniture (eg, bed or bedside table) is moved as well.

(Text continues on p. 564)

Admission Data Base

NURSING ADMISSION DATA

CURRENT MEDICATIONS, SUPPLEMENTS, NON-PRESCRIPTION DRUGS:

NAME	DOSE/FREQUENCY	LAST DOSE
Aspirin	2 prn	1 month
Maalox	prn	this Am

□ MEDICATION TO PHARMACY □ MEDICATION SENT HOME

ALLERGEN: (DRUGS, FOOD, TAPES, DYES, OTHERS)

ALLERGEN	SYMPTOMS
Penicillin	rash

DATE __1-16-93__ TIME ____0900____

ADMISSION   □ OBSERVATION

☒ AMBULATORY □ WHEELCHAIR □ STRETCHER
□ CORRECT INDENTIFICATION BAND
ADMITTED FROM: ☒ HOME □ NURSING FACILITY
        □ EMERGENCY ROOM □ OTHER_____
INFORMATION GIVEN BY: □ FAMILY MEMBER □ FRIEND ☒ PATIENT
    □ UNABLE TO TAKE HISTORY - PATIENT UNRESPONSIVE/CONFUSED/
        NOT ACCOMPANIED BY FAMILY OR FRIEND
    □ PREVIOUS MEDICAL RECORD

ORIENTATION TO ROOM
☒ VISITING HOURS ☒ CALL LIGHT IN REACH: ☒ EXPLAINED
☒ OPERATION OF BED AND SIDE RAILS ☒ USE OF PHONE
☒ VALUABLES SENT HOME □ IN SAFE □ IN POSSESSION
    SPECIFY_____
☒ PATIENT HANDBOOK   ☒ INTRODUCED TO ROOMMATE

LEGAL GUARDIAN (NAME/PHONE)_____
CONTACT PERSON (NAME/PHONE) Mrs. Solle, 335-4001
PHYSICIAN NOTIFIED ✓ TIME 0830
PRIMARY CARE PHYSICIAN Dr. Wills

MEDICAL HISTORY
ADMITTED MEDICAL DIAGNOSIS Peptic Ulcer

PAST HOSPITALIZATIONS AND/OR ILLNESS: (MEDICAL, SURGICAL, EMOTIONAL PROBLEMS) 1986 - Apperdectomy

WHAT IS REASON FOR ADMISSION? (PATIENT'S OWN WORDS)
"My doctor says I have An ulcer"

*OBJECTIVE DATA:
1. CLINICAL DATA
AGE 36 HEIGHT 5'6"
WEIGHT 122 ☒ BEDSCALE □ STANDING APPROXIMATE____
TEMP: 98.4 PULSE: 118 RESPIRATIONS 16
BLOOD PRESSURE (RIGHT ARM) 120/68 (LEFT ARM) 122/70
            ☒ SITTING □ LYING
N.T./N.A. INITIALS O.B.

2. NUTRITIONAL/METABOLIC PATTERN
ORAL MUCOSA: ☒ HEALTHY COLOR_____
    □ MOIST □ DRY □ LESIONS_____
TEETH: ☒ NO PROBLEM CONDITION:_____
    □ DENTURES □ UPPER □ LOWER □ PARTIAL
    □ MISSING TEETH □ CAPS/CROWNS
☒ WELL NOURISHED □ OBESE □ EMACIATED
SKIN: ☒ TURGOR NORMAL □ OTHER_____
    ☒ INTACT □ OTHER_____
    TEMP Warm COLOR brown □ DIAPHORESIS
□ TUBES

3. RESPIRATION/CIRCULATION PATTERN
BREATH SOUNDS Clear
LIP COLOR Pink □ USE OF ACCESSORY MUSCLES
COUGH: □ NON-PRODUCTIVE □ PRODUCTIVE SPUTUM COLOR____
APICAL RATE 120 RHYTHM: ☒ REGULAR □ IRREGULAR
ABNORMAL HEART SOUNDS NOTED NO
NECK VEIN DISTENTION AT 45 DEGREES: □ PRESENT ☒ ABSENT
□ EDEMA: LOCATION
RIGHT DORSALIS PEDAL PULSE: ☒ STRONG □ WEAK □ ABSENT
LEFT DORSALIS PEDAL PULSE: ☒ STRONG □ WEAK □ ABSENT
CALF TENDERNESS ☒ NO □ YES □ N/A
EXTREMITIES COLOR brown
    TEMP Warm

4. ELIMINATION PATTERN
ABDOMEN: ☒ SOFT   □ FIRM
    □ NON-TENDER   □ TENDER
    □ NON-DISTENDED □ DISTENDED _____Girth
□ OSTOMIES/TUBES: TYPE_____
□ NORMAL BOWEL SOUNDS □ HYPOACTIVE ☒ HYPERACTIVE □ ABSENT

*SUBJECTIVE DATA:
1. HEALTH PERCEPTIONS/HEALTH MANAGEMENT PATTERN
GENERAL HEALTH Excellent
USE OF: □ TOBACCO: HOW MUCH/HOW LONG? No
    □ ALCOHOL: HOW MUCH/HOW LONG? No
    □ OTHER DRUGS TYPE(s) None

2. NUTRITIONAL/METABOLIC PATTERN
DIET/RESTRICTIONS/SUPPLEMENTS: Regular diet

□ INSTRUCTED IN DIET PREVIOUSLY BY:_____
TIME OF LAST P.O. INTAKE: 0700
FLUID INTAKE (AMOUNT/DAY) 5-6 glasses
WEIGHT: □ NO PROBLEMS_____
□ GAIN ☒ LOSS/HOW MUCH/HOW LONG 10 lbs/1 month
☒ SKIN NORMAL □ HEALING PROBLEMS
    □ COLOR CHANGE OF SKIN
    □ SKIN LESIONS/RASH_____

3. RESPIRATION/CIRCULATION PATTERN
HISTORY OF: □ COUGH □ SPUTUM _____
□ SHORTNESS OF BREATH □ WITHOUT EXERCISE □ WITH EXERCISE

HISTORY OF: □ PACEMAKER □ RATE_____
    □ BLOOD CLOTS □ CHEST PAIN □ PEDAL EDEMA

☒ CHECK BOX IF DATA IS PERTINENT
*SEE NURSES NOTES FOR FURTHER NOTATIONS OR ANY CHANGES.

(Courtesy of Southeast Missouri Hospital, Cape Girardeau, Missouri.)   (continued)

Admission Data Base (*continued*)

*SUBJECTIVE DATA (Cont'd) LBM_____

4. ELIMINATION PATTERN

BOWEL HABITS: STOOLS/DAY _2_ COLOR _dk. brown_ ☒ SOFT/FORMED

☐ CONSTIPATION: ☐ LAXATIVE ☐ ENEMA

☐ DIARRHEA ☐ INCONTINENCE

BLADDER HABITS: URINATES/DAY _5-6_ ☒ NO PROBLEM ☐ SELF-CATH

☐ URGENCY ☐ FREQUENCY ☐ NOCTURIA

☐ DYSURIA ☐ HEMATURIA ☐ INCONTINENCE

5. SEXUALITY/REPRODUCTIVE PATTERN
(IF APPROPRIATE)

LAST MENSTRUAL PERIOD _1-10-93_ MENSTRUAL PROBLEMS ☐ YES ☒ NO

BIRTH CONTROL MEASURES _None_ #PREGNANCIES _2_

COMPLICATIONS OF PREGNANCIES _None_

HX VENEREAL DISEASE _No_

SEXUAL CONCERNS: _None_

6. ACTIVITY/EXERCISE PATTERN

ENERGY LEVEL: ☐ TIRES EASILY ☐ AVERAGE ☒ HIGH/ENERGY

ABLE TO: ☒ FEED SELF ☒ BATHE SELF

☐ BATHE/FEED SELF WITH ASSISTANCE

☒ AMBULATE ☒ CLIMB STAIRS

☒ CAN DO HOUSEHOLD CHORES

AIDS: ☐ CANE ☐ WALKER ☐ WHEELCHAIR ☐ OTHER _____

GAIT: ☐ STEADY ☐ UNSTEADY ☐ LIMP ☐ UNABLE TO WALK

PROTHESIS_____

7. SLEEP/REST PATTERN

DO YOU FEEL RESTED AFTER SLEEP? ☒ YES ☐ NO ☐ NO PROBLEM

SLEEP PROBLEMS: ☐ TROUBLE FALLING ASLEEP ☐ EARLY AM WAKING

☐ OTHER_____

8. COGNITIVE/PERCEPTUAL PATTERN

HEARING: ☒ NORMAL ☐ IMPAIRED: ☐ LEFT EAR ☐ RIGHT EAR ☐ AID

VISION: ☐ NORMAL ☐ IMPAIRED ☒ GLASSES ☐ PROTHESIS

☐ FARSIGHTED ☐ NEARSIGHTED

OTHER PROBLEMS_____

COMMUNICATION: LANGUAGE SPOKEN _English_

UNDERSTANDS_____UNABLE TO: ☐ READ ☐ WRITE

ABLE TO: ☒ READ ☒ WRITE ☐ LIP READ

COGNITION: ☒ NO PROBLEMS ☐ RECENT MEMORY CHANGE

☐ DIFFICULTY LEARNING

DISCOMFORT/PAIN: ☐ NO ☒ YES DESCRIBE _Epigastric_

HOW DO YOU MANAGE YOUR PAIN? _Bland food, Maalox_

9. COPING/STRESS TOLERANCE PATTERN

SPECIAL CONCERNS REGARDING HOSPITALIZATION? ☐ NO ☒ YES

Care of children

10. SELF-PERCEPTION/SELF-CONCEPT PATTERN

CONCERNS ABOUT HOW YOUR ILLNESS AFFECTS YOU? ☐ NO ☒ YES

Concerned about health

11. ROLE/RELATIONSHIP PATTERN

MARITAL STATUS: ☐ MARRIED ☐ SINGLE ☐ WIDOWED ☒ DIVORCED

CHILDREN (#) _2_ OTHER DEPENDENT(S) _0_

OCCUPATION _Secretary_

RESIDENCY (TYPE) _Apartment_

WHO LIVES AT HOME WITH YOU? _Children_

SUPPORT SYSTEM (CLOSE FRIEND/FAMILY MEMBER) _Yes_

FAMILY CONCERNS ABOUT HOSPITALIZATION? _Yes_

12. VALUE/BELIEF PATTERN

RELIGIOUS AFFILIATION _Baptist_

RELIGIOUS RESTRICTIONS _0_

☐ WOULD LIKE CHAPLAIN TO VISIT (IF YES, NOTIFY CHAPLAIN)

☒ WOULD LIKE FAMILY MINISTER TO VISIT

NAME _Mr. Ame_ PHONE _314-6000_

RELIGIOUS ACTIVITIES IMPORTANT TO YOU _Bible_

SUBJECTIVE DATA SIGNATURE _P. LeMone, RN_ _____ (Nurse)

E. ACTIVITY/EXERCISE PATTERN

ROM: ☒ FULL ☐ OTHER_____

BALANCE AND GAIT: ☒ STEADY ☐ UNSTEADY ☐ LIMP_____

HAND GRASPS: ☒ EQUAL ☒ STRONG

☐ WEAKNESS/PARALYSIS ☐ RIGHT ☐ LEFT

LEG MUSCLES: ☒ EQUAL ☒ STRONG

☐ WEAKNESS/PARALYSIS ☐ RIGHT ☐ LEFT

8. COGNITIVE/PERCEPTUAL PATTERN

LEVEL OF CONSCIOUSNESS: ☒ ALERT ☒ RESPONDS TO PAIN

ORIENTED TO: ☒ TIME ☒ PLACE ☒ PERSON

MOOD: ☒ CALM ☐ SAD ☐ ANGRY

☐ WITHDRAWN ☐ OTHER_____

PUPILS: ☒ EQUAL ☒ REACTIVE ☐ OTHER_____

COGNITION: ☒ ABLE TO FOLLOW SIMPLE COMMANDS

☒ RESPONDS APPROPRIATELY TO QUESTIONS

☐ UNABLE TO FOLLOW COMMANDS

☐ OTHER_____

HEARING: ☒ NORMAL ☐ OTHER_____

VISION: ☒ NORMAL ☐ OTHER_____

MANIFESTATIONS OF PAIN_____

10. SELF-PERCEPTION/SELF-CONCEPT PATTERN

EYE CONTACT: ☒ APPROPRIATE ☐ DOWNCAST ☐ STARING

BODY POSTURE: ☒ RELAXED ☐ STOOPED ☐ RIGID

BEHAVIOR: _____ 1 ② 3 4 5 (CIRCLE)

RELAXED NERVOUS

OTHER_____

11. ROLE/RELATIONSHIP PATTERN

BEHAVIOR: ① 2 3 4 5 (CIRCLE)

PASSIVE ASSERTIVE AGGRESSIVE

INTERACTION WITH FAMILY/SIGNIFICANT OTHER: ☐ N/A

☒ RELAXED ☐ TENSE ☐ ANGRY ☐ WITHDRAWN ☐ OTHER_____

COMMENTS: _____

_Worried about effect of
illness and possible surgery
on care of children, job,
and income. Has strong
support of family._

SIGNATURE _P. LeMone, RN_ _____ (Nurse)

- The client's personal belongings must be moved and put up in the new room. Every effort must be made to ensure that belongings are not misplaced or lost.
- If the client is moved to ICU, it may be necessary for family members to take home personal belongings and flowers.
- The client's chart, Kardex, care plan, and medications must be correctly labeled for the new room, and other hospital departments (eg, dietary, pharmacy, or physical therapy) must be notified as appropriate.
- If the client is transferred to another floor or to (or from) ICU, the nurse at the original area gives a verbal report about the client to the nurse at the new area. Care priorities are identified and the existence of advance directives is noted. Accurate and complete communications are essential in ensuring continuity of care.

Transfer to a Long-Term Facility
- All of the client's belongings are carefully packed and sent to the facility with the client. Prescriptions and appointment cards for return visits to the physician's office also may be sent with the client.
- The client is discharged from the hospital setting, but a copy of the chart may be sent to the long-term facility (depending on physician preference and agency protocol). The original chart, being a legal document, remains at the hospital.
- In most instances, a detailed assessment and care plan is sent from the hospital to the long-term facility. In addition, verbal communications from the nurse at the hospital to the nurse at the long-term facility are used to ensure continuity of care.

Discharge From a Health Care Setting

In meeting the needs of the client on discharge from a health care agency, the nurse must consider that the person is changing from a dependent role to a more independent self-care role. Although discharge is almost always a welcome event, it can also be one that causes anxiety and fear. The procedure for discharge is outlined in Procedure 28-2.

Discharge Planning

Planning for the discharge of a client from a health care institution actually begins on admission, when information about the client is collected and documented. **Discharge planning** is a systematic process of preparing the client to leave the health care agency and for maintaining continuity of care. The key to successful discharge planning is an exchange of information among the client, the caregivers, and those responsible for care both while the client is in the institution and after the client returns home. The coordination of care is usually the nurse's responsibility, with some hospitals having a nurse whose primary responsibility is discharge planning.

With earlier discharge, clients often are still acutely ill when they go home, and they require complicated treatment and care by family members. It is no longer unusual for family members to change sterile dressings, monitor intravenous medications, give complete physical care, and prepare special diets. If they are unprepared for these interventions, the client may have an exacerbation of the illness or experience complications that would require readmission to the hospital. The nurse must ensure that family members are taught the necessary knowledge and skills and that referrals are made to such agencies as home health care or social services to provide support and assistance during the recovery period.

Discharge planning is virtually the same as the nursing process. It is a process by which a multidisciplinary team anticipates and plans for the needs of a client and family after discharge from a health care facility. The ultimate goal in assisting the client and family is the achievement of an optimal level of wellness. Effective discharge planning also guarantees continuity of care in the least stressful manner.

Discharge planning can occur in a number of ways. Each institution has its own organizational structure to which it must adhere. Discharge planning must:
- Be coordinated
- Be interdisciplinary
- Be initiated as early as possible
- Be carefully planned
- Involve the client, family, or significant others who are caregivers

Initiation of the process involves identifying clients who need discharge planning. All clients need this service, but certain clients are at higher risk for specific needs and services. The nurse who conducts the initial nursing assessment is in the best position to determine these special needs. Burgess and Ragland (1983) have described the following characteristics that indicate the need for a formal discharge plan and referral to another agency:
- Lack of knowledge of treatment plan
- Social isolation
- Newly diagnosed chronic disease
- Major surgery
- Radical surgery
- Prolonged recuperation from major surgery or illness
- Emotional or mental instability
- Complex home-care regimen
- Financial difficulties
- Lack of available or approximate referral sources
- Terminal illness

Discharge planning is also indicated when a client is to be placed in a nursing home or other continued care setting. The American Nurses' Association (1975) has published the following in support of discharge planning:

Continuity of care planning in an organized health care system establishes a process designed to meet the needs of the client during every phase of care.

P R O C E D U R E   2 8 - 2

Discharging a Client From a Health Care Agency

Action	**Rationale**
1 Check to see that the client has a discharge order.	It is the physician's responsibility to discharge a client.
2 Make sure the client or support person has had discharge instructions (ie, regarding diet, medications) and signs that he or she understands these instructions.	The client or a support person should be able to continue with necessary care after discharge when properly instructed.
3 Have all necessary equipment and supplies ready for the client.	Having equipment and supplies ready saves time and the annoyance of having to wait for them when the client is ready to leave.
4 Check to see that proper financial arrangements have been made by the client or support person. Obtain valuables. Observe agency policies.	These actions help to avoid legal problems.
5 Assist the client to dress and pack belongings. Make sure the client has all personal belongings.	Assisting the client conserves client strength. Time and trouble are saved when the client leaves with all belongings.
6 If the client needs reimbursement for future home visits, be sure the physician has given a written order for all services.	There must be a physician's order for reimbursement by Medicare and other third-party payers.
7 Transport the client and belongings to a car and assist the client into the car as necessary.	Assisting the client conserves client strength. Such assistance is courteous and helps the client feel that personnel are interested in the client's welfare.
8 Make necessary recordings on the client's records and complete the discharge summary.	It is important legally and for hospital records to complete the client's permanent record.

Special Considerations

If the client is leaving without a physician's consent, check to see that the proper form has been completed. If the client refuses to sign the form, document your explanation to the client and consequent refusal to sign release form; notify the physician. Because a person cannot be held legally in an institution against one's wishes, a properly signed form releases the agency and physician from responsibility should problems arise because the client refused further care.

The process involves admission planning, discharge planning, referral and follow-up.

Assessing

Assessment involves collecting and organizing data about a client. (Assessment and interviewing are covered in detail in Chapters 15 and 20.) When assessing the client for discharge, the family is included as the unit of care. The client and family must be actively involved in the discharge process if the transition from hospital to home is to be effective.

The sample data base form, including information for discharge planning (see Fig. 28-3), follows Gordon's (1982)

organizing framework based on functional health patterns (see Chapter 15). Important elements of a discharge planning assessment are listed in the accompanying display. Whatever assessment tool is used, it must be a holistic assessment that encompasses all aspects of the client or family life. The medical record and physician orders must also be consulted for the exact medication and treatment plan before a nursing care plan can be developed.

Diagnosing

Nursing diagnoses, based on the discharge planning assessment, are developed that recognize the needs of both the client and the family. The family, the unit of care, is

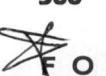

FOCUSED ASSESSMENT GUIDE

Discharge Planning

Factors to Assess	Questions and Approaches
Health data	Establish the following data base: age; sex; height; weight; medical diagnosis; past medical history; current health problems; surgery; and functional limitations (eg, amputations, wheelchair or walker use, impaired hearing or sight).
Personal data	"How do you feel about being discharged?" (Note specifically if client appears anxious or frightened.) "What are your expectations for recovery?" (Unrealistic expectations require additional teaching.) "What personal coping methods do you use? Are these effective or ineffective? What language do you speak and understand?"
Caregivers	Establish who the caregivers are and ask the following of them: "What are your expectations and fears about providing care at home? What do you believe about health and illness? Do you live with the client?"
	Establish the caregivers' age, sex, relationship to the client, past experience with this treatment or illness, and values, beliefs, and cultural practices that may affect client care.
Environment	Assess both the home and the community: Are there barriers that will inhibit function (eg, narrow stairs if the client requires a wheelchair)? Are there assistive devices in the bathroom? Are hot water, heat, and space needed for supplies available? Is the community rural or urban? Is health care accessible and readily available? Is transportation available? Are there any known hazards in the environment?
Financial and support services	Complete a financial profile, to include expenses for care after discharge (consider medications, special foods, equipment, supplies).
	What resources are available to assist in caring for the client? (Consider all available resources, including Medicaid, food stamps, meal services to the home.) If the client will be living alone, what support services are available and how can they be obtained?

affected by the health status of the member requiring care. Examples of nursing diagnoses for a client being discharged from the health care setting are as follows:

- Self-Care Deficit related to inability to bathe or dress self secondary to right-sided weakness following a left-brain cerebrovascular accident (ie, stroke).
- Anxiety related to uncertain outcome of treatment of cancer by chemotherapy.
- Ineffective Family Coping related to lack of financial or personal support systems.
- Impaired Home Maintenance Management related to chronic respiratory illness (emphysema) that limits ability to shop for food and clean the home.

It is important to determine whether the problems are actual or potential. For example, the client with chronic respiratory problems may have assistance from a member of the family who has come to stay for 1 month, but the client will be alone at home after that time. In this case,

the problem is not currently an actual problem but has the potential to become one unless planning is done to meet needs in 1 month.

Planning: Client Goals

Client goals must be mutually set and realistic if they are to be met. When goals are established with the client, *compliance* (the act of completing what is expected of one) with the treatment regimen is more likely. Goals that are not mutually agreed on or not based on a complete assessment of the client's needs most often result in noncompliance. For example, a client may have been taught about a special diet but does not follow the diet after discharge because of financial problems, lack of transportation, and lack of refrigeration for food storage.

There are important elements of teaching that must be included in the nursing care plan for the client and must be implemented before discharge (Fig. 28-4). (The teaching plan is discussed in detail in Chapter 21.) These elements include the following:

Medications: Drug name, dosage, purpose, effects, times to be taken, and possible side effects. The information specific to medications should be given both verbally and in writing. It is often helpful to make a large clock face and write the names of the medications in the correct time slot.

Procedures and treatments: All steps of the procedure (eg, dressing changes) should be demonstrated, practiced, and given in writing. The caregiver should then demonstrate the procedure or treatment. It is important that caregivers understand the purpose of what is being done and have information about how to get supplies.

Diet: The purpose of the diet as well as expected outcomes should be clearly described. Examples of written diet plans and meals are helpful. It is also helpful for the caregiver to plan diets while the client is in the hospital and to save any menu or meal forms to use as a reference at home.

Referrals: Often appointments are made from the hospital for the first visit to a physician or agency. Whether this is done or not, the client and family members should be instructed on how to make contact with providers of follow-up care, as well as who to call if they have questions or problems. Information about referrals should be based on knowledge of the client's economic situation, access to transportation, support systems, and home environment.

Health promotion: All aspects of the illness or effects of treatment should be clearly described with verbal and written materials. Many sources of written information are available to give to clients; these sources range from printed organizational literature (eg, from the American Heart Association) to teaching materials developed by the institution. The client not only should be able to verbally discuss the physical and emotional effects of the illness but should also be able to describe what will be done to achieve the highest level of wellness possible.

The following example demonstrates consideration of all dimensions of the person in planning and coordinating discharge planning. Mr. Smith is a 55-year-old married man with a diagnosis of cerebrovascular accident (stroke) with left hemiparesis (weakness). He also has difficulty communicating verbally and has a history of hypertension for 10 years. He is to be discharged from the hospital in 3 days if his blood pressure remains stable. He will be going home with four new medications, an indwelling urinary catheter, and feeding tube. After reviewing the medical record, the nurse interviews Mr. and Mrs. Smith. The assessment reveals Mr. Smith is limited in his ability to transfer from bed to chair. Both Mr. and Mrs. Smith are fearful of discharge, but Mr. Smith believes he will be able to return to work as an accountant in 3 weeks, and Mrs. Smith thinks he'll never

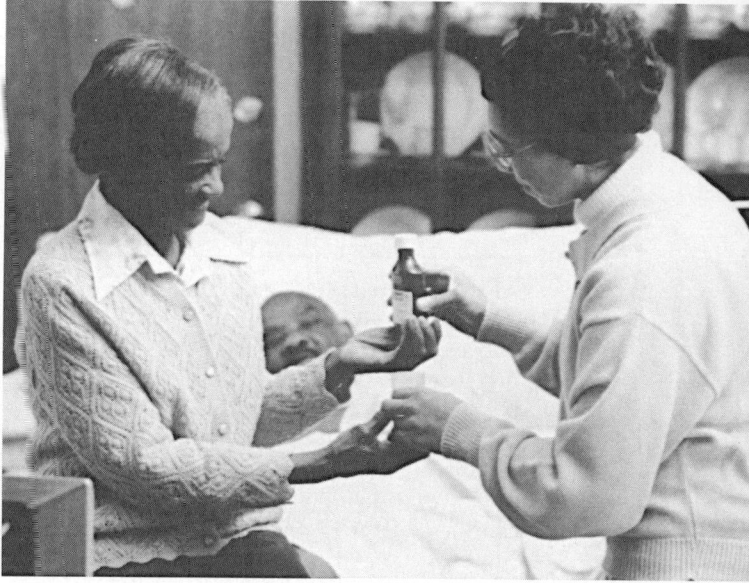

FIGURE 28-4

Clients or caregivers must be taught special skills such as medication administration, diet planning, or feeding so that they can care for themselves when nursing services are no longer provided. (Photo by Robert Coldwell, courtesy of Community Home Health Services of Philadelphia.)

work again. They have never faced a life-threatening illness in the past, but he has had severe hypertension and has not complied with diet or medication regimen. Mr. Smith believes he will be fine soon and hates the thought of being an invalid at his age. The Smiths are both Roman Catholic. They have no strong cultural preferences in terms of diet. They have two adult children who live out of state with their own families. Mrs. Smith does have a younger sister who lives nearby. They are both college educated. The Smiths live in a suburban area in a two-story home with narrow stairs leading to two baths and three bedrooms on the second floor. They have adequate plumbing but no assistive devices. Their doctor's office is about 1 mile away, and shopping is nearby.

Mrs. Smith does not believe she can manage care of the feeding tube and indwelling catheter. She also needs instruction in the new medication and diet regimen. She is terrified that she may be unable to handle an emergency in the middle of the night. Financially, this two-income family has quickly become one and will shortly have no income. Mr. Smith is not 65 years old, and thus is not yet eligible for Medicare.

How would the nurse coordinate this discharge plan? The physician must be consulted for diet, medication, and other treatment orders. Physical therapy has already been initiated at the hospital. Occupational therapy also needs to evaluate Mr. Smith's ability to perform activities of daily

Discharge Summary

Nursing Services
DISCHARGE SUMMARY
(This side to be filled out by nursing staff)

1) HEALTH MANAGEMENT PATTERN
Follow-up Care, Appointments:
Physician: _____Dr. Wills_____ Date __1-29-93__ Time __13 00__
_____ Date _____ Time _____
Outpatient Appt: _____ Date _____ Time _____

2) NUTRITIONAL/METABOLIC PATTERN
Diet - Order at Discharge _____Soft - Regular as tolerated_____
Dressings ☒ Not Applicable ☐ Reach to Recovery Referral
Wound Care _____
_____
_____
_____

Written Instructions given ☒ _Diet_____ Instructor Signature _P LeMone RN_

4) ELIMINATION PATTERN: ☐ Incontinent: Management _____
LBM __1-28-93_____.
Urinary - Catheter Care: _____
Written instructions given ☐ Instructor Signature _____

6) ACTIVITY/EXERCISE PATTERN
Activity at Discharge:☒ as tolerated ☐ with assist ☐ bed rest
Pt ☐ Significant other ☐ Instructed on: _____
  ☐ surgical limitation (explain) _____
  ☐ other limitation (explain) _____

8) COGNITIVE/PERCEPTUAL PATTERN
Medications - Instructions: ☒ Pt ☒ Significant other
Preadmission meds returned ☐ initials _____

Continued Home Meds	Instruct. Sheet #	New Prescriptions	Instruct. Sheet #
		Tagamet 150mg BID	

Discharge Assessment _Discharged to home with family members._
States pain is relieved and verbalizes reduction of
concerns. Understands diet (to avoid foods that cause distress)
and importance of continuing medications.

Date __1-29-93__ Departure Time __11 00__ Transported by _WC / Volunteer_
Via: ☒ w/c ☐ ambulatory ☐ ambulance ☐ child carried by _____ ☐ AMA
Signature of Discharging Nurse _P. LeMone, RN_

(Courtesy of Southeast Missouri Hospital, Cape Girardeau, Missouri.)

living and to fit him with assistive devices. The nutritionist needs to counsel the Smiths on the low-sodium diet (1 g) and on creative ways to prepare low-salt meals. The social worker has been called for financial assessment to determine exactly what services the Smiths can expect to have reimbursed by their insurance carrier, and how they will manage their out-of-pocket expenses. The nurse begins to formulate a teaching plan for medications and treatment. Mrs. Smith must learn about the Foley catheter and feeding tube before discharge to feel more in control. It is hoped some of the Smiths' fears are addressed and new coping strategies develop. The nurse also makes a referral to the local visiting nurses association to continue physical therapy and nursing care and to evaluate if any more teaching is necessary at home.

Teaching Plan The teaching plan is discussed in great detail in Chapter 21. Review of the sample teaching plan in Chapter 21 aids in understanding the steps and strategies of discharge planning. All aspects of teaching may not be completed in the hospital, and referral to a home care agency may be necessary for follow-up care and teaching.

Implementing

Implementation is the actual carrying out of the teaching plan and referrals. All teaching should be documented in the nurse's notes and the discharge summary. Written instructions are given to the client (Fig. 28-5). Return demon-

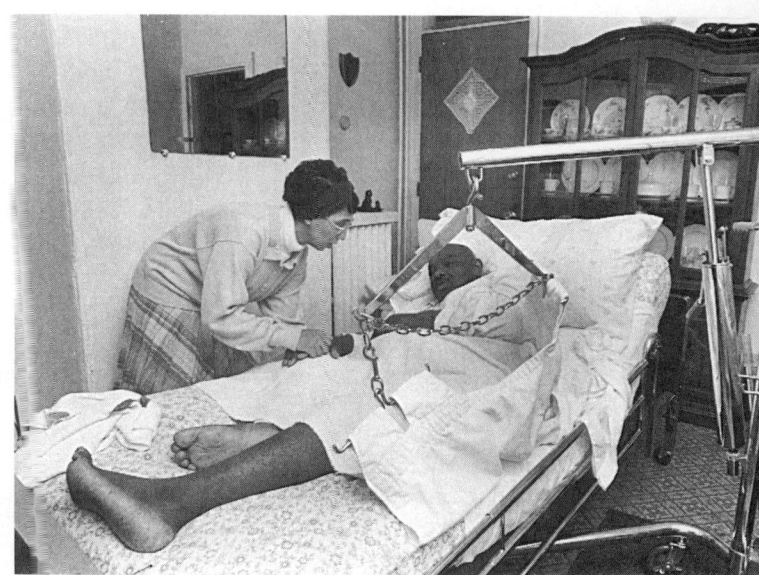

F I G U R E 2 8 - 6

Caring for the sick at home is not new but has become a highly specialized area of health care and a major component of a continuum of comprehensive health care. (Photo by Robert Coldwell, courtesy of Community Home Health Services of Philadelphia.)

F I G U R E 2 8 - 5

Written instructions for continuing self-care at home should be given to the client. The nurse should review the instructions with the client to ensure that the client clearly understands the instructions. (Photo © Ken Kasper.)

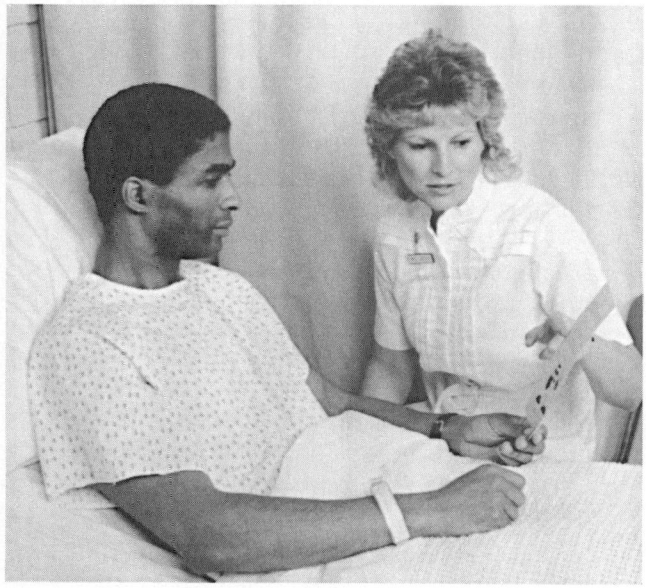

strations must be satisfactory. The client and caregiver must have exposure to and practice with the equipment they will be using at home.

The home-care referral is made before the client is actually discharged. As much information as possible about the client and the hospitalization should be given to the agency. Such information includes the kind of surgery; medication (including need for intravenous fluids at home); the client's physical and mental status; significant social factors (eg, frail caregiver with health problem, no caregiver); and expected needs of the family. Transportation should be arranged at this time (Fig. 28-6).

For a home-care referral to be made and subsequent home visits to be reimbursed, there must be a written order by the physician for all services. Clients must meet certain criteria to have home-care services reimbursed by Medicare and other third-party payers.

Discharging a Client Against Advice The client who is leaving the hospital against medical advice (sometimes abbreviated *AMA*) must sign a form releasing the hospital and physician from responsibility and any ill effects that may result from such action. The client has the right to terminate health care, but the nurse has an obligation to discuss with the client the possible outcomes of this decision. Each agency has its own form for clients who choose to leave against medical advice. It is required that the client's signature on the form be witnessed and that financial arrangements be completed through the business office.

Evaluating

Evaluation of the discharge plan is crucial in making the discharge planning process work. Planning and referrals must be scrutinized to ensure quality and appropriateness of services. Evaluation is ongoing, and the need for revision of plans also changes.

Further evaluation of the discharge process is usually conducted a few weeks after the client has been home. It may be carried out by way of a telephone call, a questionnaire, or a home visit.

KEY POINTS

- The nurse is the primary person responsible for ensuring continuity of care as clients move from one type of health care setting to another.
- Continuity of care is the coordination of services provided to clients; it ensures a smooth transition between ambulatory or hospital care and home care or other types of community-based care.
- Continuity of care is provided by including discharge planning as a part of the care plan from admission, collaborating with other members of the health care team, and involving the client and family in planning.
- Anxiety about the unknown can be reduced by establishing a therapeutic nurse–client relationship on admission to a setting that provides health care.
- Although admission and dismissal from ambulatory and hospital settings differ, the focus is on meeting client needs and providing individualized care. The nurse is responsible for assessments, teaching, and developing a care plan with the client and family.
- Transfer of a client from one level of care or setting to another is common. The nurse provides care to meet comfort, safety, and knowledge needs of the client and family, ensuring continuity of care.
- Discharge planning is a systematic process of preparing the client to leave a health care agency and for maintaining continuity of care. This process is coordinated and multidisciplinary and is carried out with consideration of each client's needs when moving to a different level of care or setting. Information about medications, diet, procedures and treatments, referrals, and health promotion activities may be included in the teaching plan for discharge.

BIBLIOGRAPHY

American Nurses' Association. (1975). Continuity of care and discharge planning programs in institutions and community agencies: A statement of the American Nurses' Association Division of Medical–Surgical Nursing Practice and the Division on Community Health Nursing Practice. Kansas City, MO: Author.

Bagis-Smith, J., & McKeehan, K. M. (1990). Continuity of care across hospital-community boundaries. In J. C. McCloskey & H. K. Grace (Eds.), *Current issues in nursing* (pp. 131–186). St. Louis: Mosby.

Bulachek, G. M., & McClosky, J. C. (1985). *Nursing interventions: Treatments for nursing diagnoses.* Philadelphia: Saunders.

Burgess, W., & Ragland, E. C. (1983). *Community health nursing: Philosophy, process, practice.* Norwalk, CT: Appleton-Century-Crofts.

Carpenito, L. J. (1992). *Nursing diagnoses: Application to clinical practice* (4th ed.). Philadelphia: Lippincott.

Christopher, M. A. (1986). Home care for the elderly—in three part harmony: Assessment of the patient's health, home and community. *Nursing, 16*(7), 50–55.

Clemen-Stone, S., Eigsti, D. G., & McGuire, S. L. (1987). *Comprehensive family and community health nursing.* New York: McGraw-Hill.

Eggland, E. T. (1987). Nurse's guide to home health care. *Nursing, 17*(10), 75–81.

Eliopolos, C. (1990). *Caring for the elderly in diverse care settings.* Philadelphia: Lippincott.

Esper, P. S. (1988). Discharge planning: A quality assurance program. *Nursing Management, 19*(10), 66–68.

Gordon, M. (1982). *Nursing diagnosis: Process and application.* New York: McGraw-Hill.

Gordon, M. (1982). Historical perspective: The national group for classification of nursing diagnoses. In M. J. Kim & D. A. Moritz (Eds.), *Classification of nursing diagnoses* (p. 3). New York: McGraw-Hill.

Haddock, K. S. (1991). Characteristics of effective discharge planning programs for the frail elderly. *Journal of Gerontological Nursing, 17*(7), 10–14.

Jackson, M. F. (1990). Use of community support services by elderly patients discharged from general medical and geriatric medical wards. *Journal of Advanced Nursing, 15,* 167–175.

Koch, M. W. (1991). Synergy. *Continuing Care, 10*(6), 12, 14–15.

Kowlsen, T. (1991). The balancing act. *Continuing Care, 10*(7), 18–20.

LeNoble, E. (1991). Pre-admission possible. *Canadian Nurse, 87*(2), 18–20.

Mezzanotte, E. T. (1987). A checklist for better discharge planning. *Nursing, 17*(10), 55.

Stanhope, M., & Lancaster, J. (1992). *Community health nursing: Process and practice for promoting health* (3rd ed.). St. Louis: Mosby–Year Book.

Zarle, N. C. (1989). Continuity of care: Balancing care of elders between health care settings. *Nursing Clinics of North America, 24*(3), 697–705.

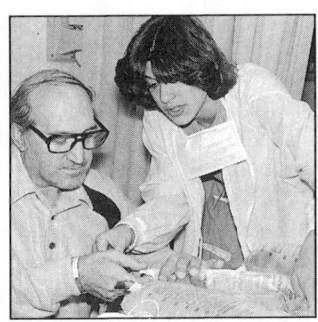  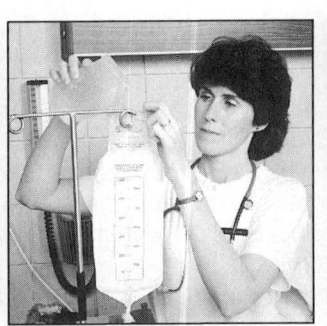 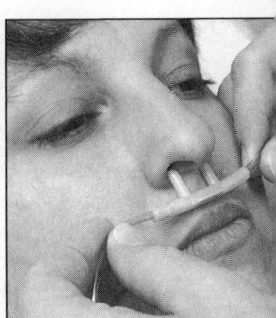

Promoting Healthy Physiologic Responses

The art and science of caring are blended when nurses implement actions to meet basic human needs and to promote healthy physiologic responses. The chapters in Unit VII focus on information and guidelines essential to nursing practice in a wide variety of clinical settings and involving both healthy and ill clients of all ages. Included are nursing interventions to promote safety and comfort and to meet basic physiologic needs—hygiene, activity and rest, nutrition, elimination, oxygenation, and fluid–electrolyte balance.

Each basic physiologic need is discussed first by reviewing concepts pertinent to the specific area of human function and response and then by presenting factors that affect need satisfaction. The steps of the nursing process are used to provide guidelines and information necessary for making accurate assessments, establishing goals, and planning, implementing, and evaluating specific nursing interventions to meet needs and promote wellness. A section entitled Nursing Process in Clinical Practice at the end of each chapter provides application of knowledge by providing a case study, selected nursing diagnoses, and a care plan, illustrating how skilled nursing interventions and caring are combined to resolve problems and meet ends.

The content of Unit VII enables the beginning nurse caregiver to integrate the knowledge and skills necessary to promote healthy physiologic responses in clients in any practice setting. Nursing process skills are further refined to ensure that care is holistic, comprehensive, and individualized.

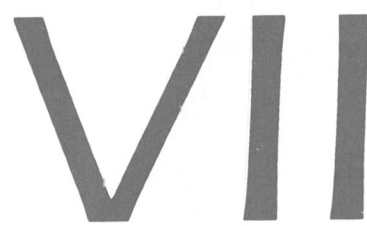

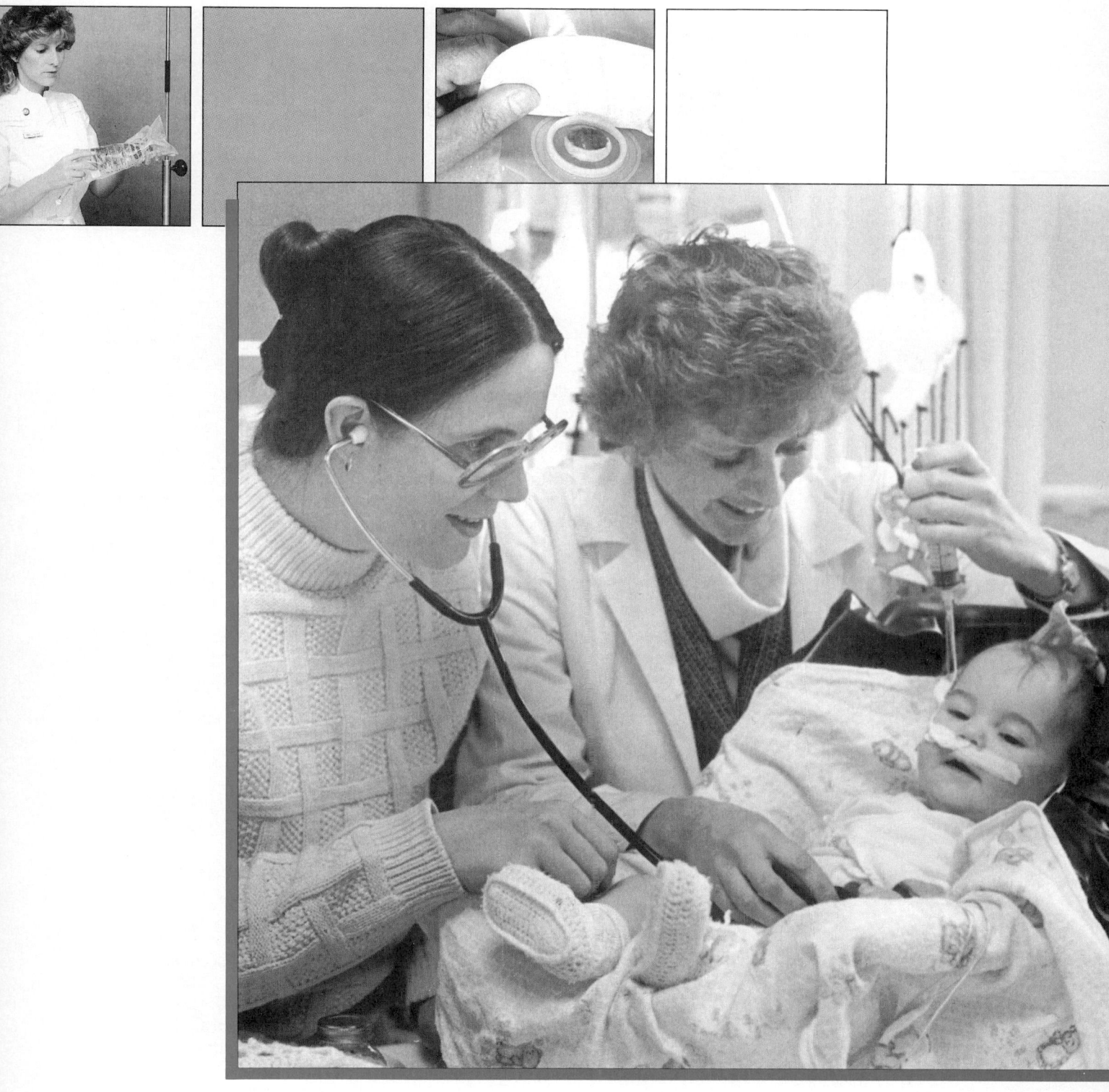

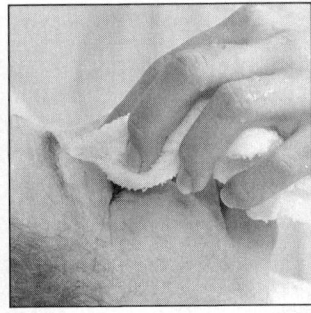

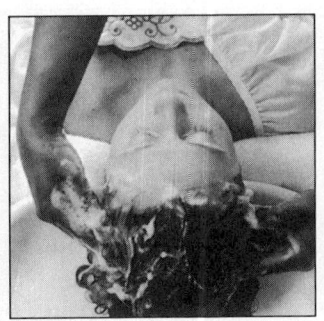

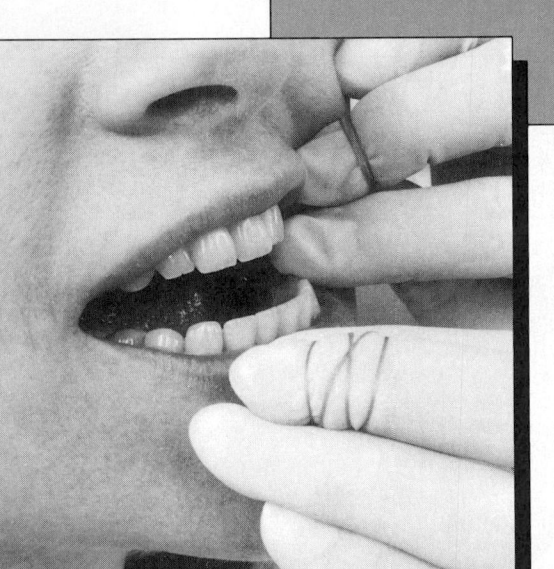

Hygiene

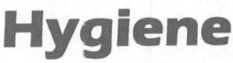

29

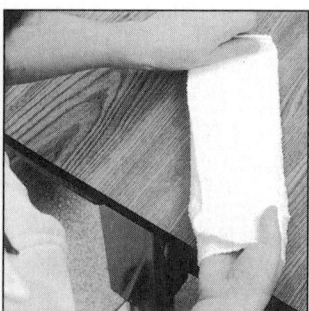

Ordinarily, the well person is responsible for self-hygiene. Through teaching, the nurse may assist the well person to develop personal hygiene habits the person may lack.

Illness, hospitalization, and institutionalization may demand modifications in hygiene practices. In these situations, the nurse helps the client to continue sound hygienic practices and has an opportunity to teach the client and family members regarding hygiene. The nurse who assists a client with basic hygiene respects individual client preferences and administers only that amount of care the client cannot or should not provide for himself or herself.

Personal Hygiene

Measures for personal cleanliness and grooming that promote physical and psychologic well-being are called **personal hygiene**. Personal hygiene practices vary widely from one person to another. The time of day for bathing or the frequency of shampooing the hair and changing the bed linens and sleeping garments is relatively unimportant. What is important is that personal care be carried out conveniently and often enough to promote personal hygiene.

This chapter provides the nurse with knowledge of the multiple factors that affect personal hygiene and of nursing measures that promote personal hygiene. A practical guide for assessing the adequacy of personal hygiene behaviors is presented. Because the data the nurse collects when assisting with hygiene may lead to the identification of multiple nursing diagnoses and collaborative problems, samples of these are provided. Client goals are presented, as are descriptions of specific nursing strategies used when performing care of the skin; mouth; eyes, ears, and nose; feet; and perineal and vaginal areas.

In the section Nursing Process in Clinical Practice, focused assessment, diagnosis, planning, implementation, and evaluation guides are offered for caring for clients with pressure ulcers. These guides and the concluding case study (on feminine hygiene) illustrate how the nurse's knowledge of personal hygiene practices and the integumentary system is combined with specific nursing interventions to successfully resolve nursing diagnoses and promote the client's general sense of well-being.

Physiology of the Skin

Integument refers to the skin. The **integumentary system** comprises the skin and its appendages, that is, the hair, glands in the skin, and the nails. The skin is one of the body's vital organs and is essential for maintaining life.

The skin consists of three layers. The superficial portion, the **epidermis**, comprises layers of stratified epithelial cells. These cells are fused to form a protective, waterproof layer of keratin material. Epithelial cells have no blood vessels of their own and depend on underlying tissues for nourishment and waste removal. When well nourished, epithelium regenerates relatively easily and quickly.

The next layer of skin, the **dermis**, consists of smooth, muscular tissue; nerves; hair follicles; certain glands and their ducts; arteries; veins and capillaries; and fibrous, elastic tissue. Each hair consists of the shaft, which projects through the dermis beyond the surface of the skin, and the hair follicle, which lies in the dermis. The *hypodermis* consists of a subcutaneous fatty tissue layer that anchors the other skin layers and serves as a heat insulator for the body. This fatty tissue layer contains blood and lymph vessels, nerves, and fat cells.

The skin covers the entire body and is continuous with the mucous membrane at normal body orifices. A cross section of normal skin is illustrated in Figure 29-1. Glands in the skin include the sebaceous glands, the sweat glands, and the ceruminal glands. The **sebaceous glands** secrete an oily substance called **sebum**, which lubricates the skin and hair and keeps the skin and scalp pliant. The sweat glands secrete perspiration. The **cerumen** in the external ear canals, consisting of a heavy oil and brown pigment, is secreted by **ceruminal glands**.

Functions of Skin and Mucous Membranes

The skin serves six major functions:
- Protects the body
- Regulates body temperature
- Senses stimuli from the environment and transmits these sensations (ie, pain, temperature, touch, and pressure)
- Excretes waste products
- Helps maintain water and electrolyte balance
- Produces and absorbs vitamin D

These functions are described further in Table 29-1.

Mucous membranes line body cavities that open to the outside of the body and can also be found in the digestive tract, the respiratory passages, and the urinary and reproductive tracts. Epithelium covers the mucous membrane surfaces and contains cells that secrete mucus. Connective tissue lies beneath the epithelium. Mucous membranes have receptors that offer the body protection; for example, an irritating substance in the upper respiratory tract causes a person to sneeze, and food caught in the larynx or trachea causes a person to cough. Sneezing and coughing are protective mechanisms that help rid the body of foreign mate-

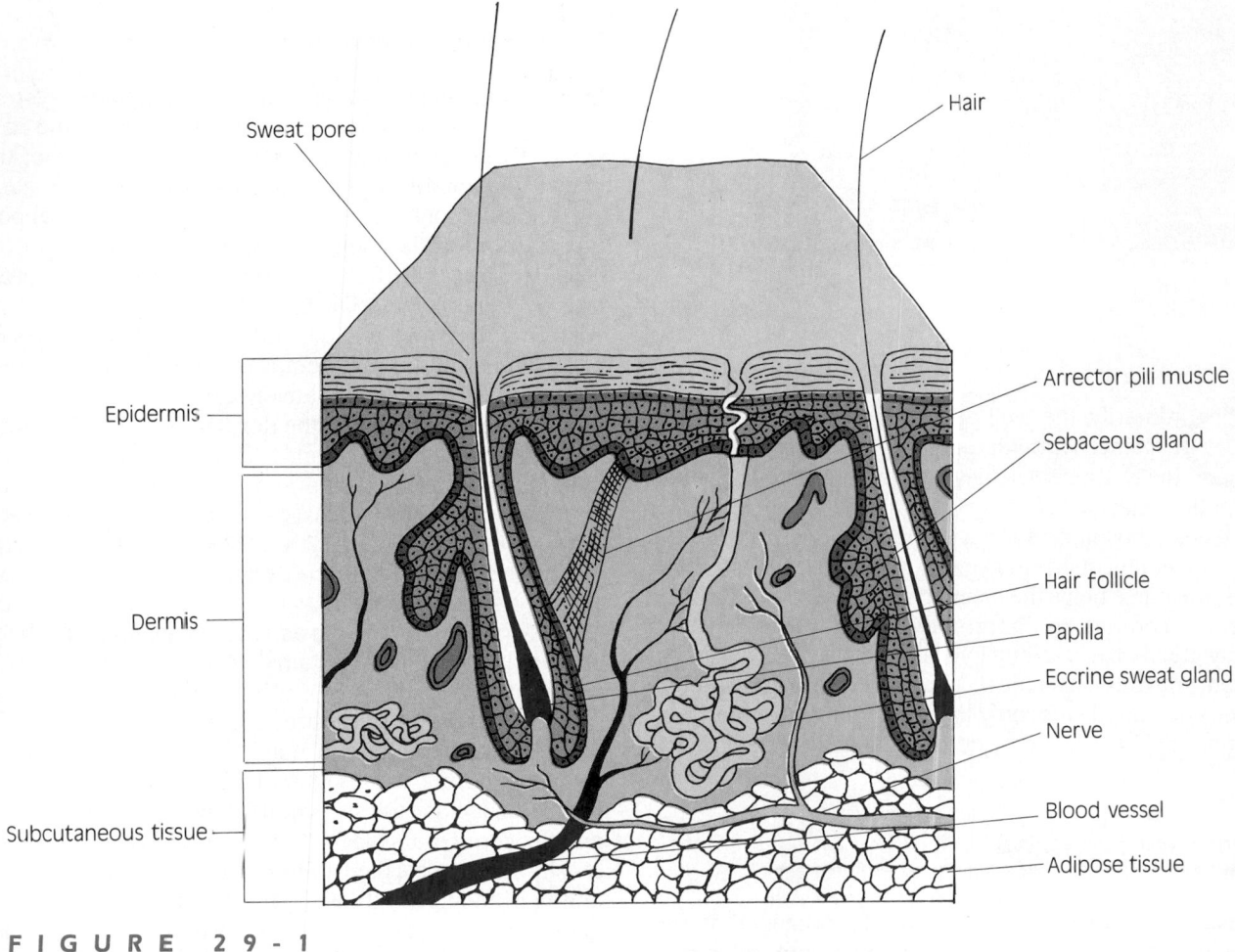

Sweat pore

Epidermis

Dermis

Subcutaneous tissue

Hair

Arrector pili muscle

Sebaceous gland

Hair follicle

Papilla

Eccrine sweat gland

Nerve

Blood vessel

Adipose tissue

F I G U R E   2 9 - 1

A cross section of normal skin.

rials. Mucous membranes are insensitive to temperature, except in the mouth and rectum, but are sensitive to pressure. Mucous membranes also function to absorb substances from their surface; for example, digested food is absorbed through the mucous membrane in the small intestine.

Principles of Skin Care

Knowledge of the functions of the skin and mucous membranes and of factors affecting them includes an understanding of certain basic principles that become important in the care of the skin and mucous membranes:

Unbroken and healthy skin and mucous membranes serve as the first lines of defense against harmful agents.

Resistance to injury of the skin and mucous membranes varies among people. Factors influencing resistance include a person's age, the amount of underlying tissues, and illness conditions.

Adequately nourished and hydrated body cells are resistant to injury. The better nourished the cell, the better its ability to resist injury and disease.

Adequate circulation is necessary to maintain cell life. The cells are inadequately nourished and wastes are poorly removed when circulation is impaired for any reason.

Factors Affecting Skin Condition and Personal Hygiene

Skin Condition

A person's developmental stage and health condition influence the skin in various ways.

Developmental Considerations
• An infant's skin and mucous membranes are easily injured and subject to infection. Careful handling of infants is required to prevent injury and infection of the skin and mucous membranes.

TABLE 29-1

Functions of the Skin

Function	Mechanisms
The skin protects the body	Invasion of the body by bacteria is prevented by intact skin. Injury to underlying tissues and organs is decreased by intact skin.
The skin helps regulate body temperature	The production of perspiration and its loss by evaporation help cool the body.
	Much heat is lost from the body by radiation and by conduction when the blood supply to the skin is increased by vasodilatation.
	Lack of perspiration and vasoconstriction help the body retain heat.
	The phenomenon of producing gooseflesh, which is caused by contraction of pilomotor muscles in the skin, helps conserve body heat because the hair standing on end forms a layer of air on the body for insulation.
The skin is a sense organ	There are receptors for pain, touch, pressure, and temperature in the skin that help the body receive stimuli from the environment.
The skin is an excretory organ	Water, salts, and nitrogenous wastes are lost from the skin, although in much smaller quantities than are lost from the kidneys.
The skin helps maintain water and electrolyte balance	The escape of excess water and electrolytes from the body is prevented by the skin.
The skin produces and absorbs vitamin D	A precursor for vitamin D is present in the skin, which in conjunction with ultraviolet rays from the sun produces vitamin D.

- A child's skin becomes increasingly resistant to injury and infection. However, the skin requires special care because of the toilet and play habits of children.
- An adolescent's skin ordinarily has enlarged sebaceous glands and increased glandular secretions, caused by hormonal changes in the body. These characteristics predispose to acne, which is discussed later in this chapter.
- Secretions from the skin glands are at their maximum during adolescence and up to around age 50 years.
- Changes that occur in the skin with aging are irreversible. The skin becomes thinner and less elastic and less supple with aging. Subcutaneous fat that normally helps absorb injury to the skin decreases. Wrinkles appear, most of which are deep in the dermis.

The skin becomes dry, often scaly, and rough in appearance because less oil is secreted from sebaceous glands. Brown spots, called *liver spots*, often appear. They may begin appearing as early as age 35 years and tend to become more numerous and larger with aging. These spots result from exposure to the wind and sun and are not caused by liver disease.

Illness

- Very thin and very obese people tend to be more susceptible to skin irritation and injury.
- Fluid loss through fever, vomiting, or diarrhea reduces the fluid volume of the body and is called *dehydration*. Dehydration makes the skin appear loose and flabby.
- Excessive perspiration, often associated with being ill, predisposes to skin breakdown, especially in areas where the skin folds.
- *Jaundice*, a condition caused by excessive bile pigments in the skin, results in a yellowish skin color. The skin is often itchy and dry in the presence of jaundice.
- Diseases of the skin are usually characterized by various lesions that require special care to promote personal hygiene and to carry out therapeutic regimens.

Personal Hygiene

The nurse caring for clients from diverse backgrounds quickly learns that hygiene practices vary widely among individuals. The following factors may influence personal hygiene behaviors.

Culture Many people in North America place a high value on personal cleanliness and feel unclean unless they shower or bathe at least once daily. They consider bathing incomplete without the use of multiple products to reduce or mask normal body odors. People from other cultures often find a weekly bath sufficient and feel no need to mask normal body odors. Culture may also dictate whether bathing is a private or communal activity.

Socioeconomic Class Financial resources often define the hygiene options available to individuals. A single person renting one room in a boarding house may have limited or no access to tubs or showers and limited finances for the purchase of soap, shampoo, shaving cream, and deodorants. Homeless people, who often carry all their belongings in a car or shopping cart, may welcome the warm running water and soap available in a roadside or other public restroom. Other people may refrain from using public restrooms because they are perceived as being dirty.

Religion Religion may dictate ceremonial washings and purifications, which may be a prelude to prayer or eating. For example, in the orthodox Jewish tradition, ritual baths are required for women after childbirth and menstruation. In some religions, contact with a deceased person or a deceased rodent may make a person "unclean."

Developmental Level and Knowledge Level Children learn different hygiene practices while growing up. Family practices may dictate morning or evening baths, the frequency of shampooing, feelings about nudity, frequency of clothing changes, and so on. A teenager may experience the need to change hygiene measures practiced throughout childhood and begin to take long, frequent hot showers. The elderly often experience the need to decrease bathing times and the use of deodorant soaps to avoid excessively drying the skin.

Health State Disease or injury may adversely affect an individual's ability to perform hygiene measures or motivation to follow usual hygiene habits. Weakness, dizziness, and fear of falling may prevent an individual from entering a tub or shower or from bending to wash the lower extremities. Illness may also create a demand for new or modified hygiene measures.

Personal Preferences Different people have different personal preferences with regard to hygiene practices. Showers versus tub baths, bar soap versus liquid soap, washing to wake oneself or to relax before sleep are personal preferences. One's self-concept and sexuality are also personal influences on hygiene.

Nurse as Role Model

Nurses consistently serve as role models for clients in regard to personal hygiene. Before attempting to teach clients healthy hygiene practices, it is important that nurses evaluate their own practices. If unable to meet the following goals, you may wish to take the time now to examine your own hygiene practices.
- The nurse's physical appearance and body scents give evidence of adequate hygiene practices:
  - Hair is clean and neatly styled.
  - Skin is clean.
  - Mouth evidences satisfactory oral hygiene.
  - Nails are neatly manicured.
  - Body is free of unpleasant odors.
- The nurse's diet and exercise habits contribute to clean and intact skin.
- The nurse brushes teeth after each meal, flosses daily, and goes to the dentist for a checkup at least annually.
- The nurse's care of clients demonstrates an appreciation for the relationship between hygiene and overall well-being.
- The nurse consistently uses appropriate aseptic safeguards (ie, handwashing, use of gloves) to prevent the transmission of microorganisms.

Assessing

A comprehensive assessment of the skin and mucous membranes includes the following:
- Collection of data about usual hygiene practices:

- Showering or bathing practices
- Skin, hair, and scalp care
- Eye, ear, nose, and mouth care
- Nail and foot care
- Perineal care
- Assessment of any sensory, cognitive, endurance, mobility, or motivation deficit that interferes with the individual's hygiene practices
- Identification of any existing problems of the skin or mucous membranes, as well as associated care and its effectiveness
- Nursing examination of the skin and mucous membranes

Skin and basic hygiene assessment guidelines follow. Focused assessment criteria for select body parts appear later in the chapter.

Nursing History

While assessing hygiene practices, it is important to remember that different individuals and families possess different ideas regarding personal cleanliness. Bathing practices and cleansing habits and rituals vary widely. Before a nurse decides that an individual's hygiene practices are inadequate, a clear threat to health must exist. The nurse assessing the adequacy of hygiene practices evaluates whether the individual possesses the knowledge, attitude, skills, and resources to care for the skin and mucous membranes. See the Focused Assessment Guide in the accompanying display.

The nursing history also includes data about problems of the integumentary system. The client should be questioned about any past or current problems such as rashes, lumps, itching, dryness, lesions, ecchymoses, masses, or specific changes in the hair or nails. When skin problems are present, the client should be asked,

"How long have you had this problem?"
"Does it itch or bother you?"
"How does it bother you?"
"Have you found any care helpful in relieving these symptoms?"
Sample entries in a nursing history follow:
Hygiene: "Showers twice daily, once in the AM and after working out in the evening. Skin tends to be very dry, and moisturizing creams are used daily. Aveeno Oilated baths prn. Allergic to deodorant soaps."
Integument: "History of athlete's foot since high school days with outbreaks every 2 to 3 months. Knowledgeable about appropriate foot care. Uses Tinactin cream [topical fungicidal agent] and Mexsana medicated powder [topical protectant]."

Physical Assessment

The inspection and palpation skills used to assess the integumentary system are described in detail in Chapter 24. The nurse who assists a client with basic hygiene measures has an excellent opportunity to examine the client's skin

FOCUSED ASSESSMENT GUIDE

Hygiene Practices

Factors to Assess	Questions and Approaches
Daily and weekly bathing habits	Tell me about your daily and weekly bathing habits.
	Are there special bathing or hygiene products you routinely use or cannot use?
	How can nurses best help you to meet your hygiene needs?
Factors interfering with hygiene practices (sensory, cognitive, endurance, mobility, or motivation)	What recently or in the past has interfered with your hygiene practices?
	Does anything interfere with your ability to be as clean as you would like?
History of skin or mucous membrane problems (nature, onset of problem and frequency, causes, severity, symptoms, interventions attempted, and results)	Describe any skin problems with rashes, lumps, itching, dryness, lesions, ecchymosis, or masses.
	Are you allergic to any cleansing or cosmetic products?
Special hygiene practices (eg, inflamed gums or menstruation)	I notice that your gums look inflamed. How do you clean your teeth and gums? Have you seen a dentist about this problem?
	Do you follow any special hygiene practices during menstruation? What type of feminine hygiene products (eg, pads, tampons, douches) do you use?

carefully. Many individuals are unaware of skin lesions such as precancerous moles, which, if untreated, could prove fatal. Early detection and treatment of skin problems are important nursing functions.

In examining the skin, the nurse pays careful attention to cleanliness, color, texture, temperature, turgor, moisture, sensation, vascularity, and the presence of lesions. If a lesion is detected, the nurse documents the type, color, size, distribution and grouping, location, and consistency. Terminology helpful in describing these findings is presented in Chapter 24. General guidelines for assessing the skin are as follows:

- Proceed systematically in head-to-toe fashion.
- Use a good source of light, preferably daylight.
- Compare bilateral parts for symmetry.
- Use standard terminology to report and record findings.
- Allow data obtained in the nursing history to direct the skin assessment.
- Identify any variables known to cause skin problems, such as deficient self-care abilities; immobility; malnutrition; decreased hydration; decreased sensation; vascular problems (altered tissue perfusion or venous return); or presence of irritants (body secretions or excretions on the skin, other chemicals, mechanical devices).

Because life-style factors, changes in health state, illness, and certain diagnostic and therapeutic measures may

adversely affect the skin, the nurse needs to identify high-risk populations and perform the appropriate skin assessment. Knowing *when* to perform the skin assessment and incorporating this into the client's care plan is as important as knowing *how* to do this well. Table 29-2 identifies sample factors that place an individual at high risk for skin alterations.

Sample entries under integumentary system in the nursing examination follow:

"Skin is pink, warm, dry, and elastic; no petechiae, lesions, or excoriation; multiple moles of small size and regular border and surface."

"Red, macular rash generalized over trunk and thighs; semiconfluent lesions measure 1 to 2 mm; abrupt onset."

Diagnosing

A careful assessment of the skin and mucous membranes may lead to the identification of numerous client problems that can be classified as nursing diagnoses. Problems concerning deficient hygiene are categorized as self-care deficits. Self-Care Deficit diagnoses address four specific activities necessary to meet daily needs—feeding, bathing and hygiene, dressing and grooming, and toileting. It is important to identify the etiology of these problems correctly. If hygiene is deficient because of insufficient knowledge, health education can quickly remedy the problem. If, how-

T A B L E   2 9 - 2

Factors Placing an Individual at High Risk for Skin Alterations

Factor	Nursing Implications
Life-Style Variables	
Homosexual male, with a history of multiple sexual partners; drug users; hemophiliacs; bisexual male; partners of the above	• High-risk profile for acquired immunodeficiency syndrome (AIDS). • Assessment needs to include careful examination of the skin for purple blotches that may be indicative of Kaposi's sarcoma.
Occupation that gives a fair thin-skinned individual prolonged exposure to the sun	• Places individual at high risk for developing skin cancer, which has an excellent prognosis if detected and treated in its early stages but which may be fatal if treatment is delayed. • Assessment needs to include careful examination for a sore that does not heal or a change in size or color of a wart or mole.
Changes in Health State	
Dehydration or malnutrition	• If fluid, protein, and vitamin C intake is deficient, skin loses elasticity and becomes prone to breakdown. • Nursing care is directed toward preventing skin breakdown: frequent changes of client's position with skin assessment at each change, special mattresses and protection of bony prominences, use of lotions, attention to fluid and nutritional status.
Reduced sensation (paralysis, local nerve damage, circulatory insufficiency)	• Client's inability to sense temperature extremes, pressure, friction, and other such factors can easily result in injury. • Nursing care incorporates special attention to safety.
Illness	
Diabetes mellitus	• Numerous factors combine to cause skin problems in diabetics: cuts and sores that do not heal, lesions on the lower extremities that ulcerate and become necrotic, recurrent bacterial and fungal infections. • The diabetic must be taught special hygiene measures to prevent trauma to the skin and learn to assess the skin carefully to detect any alteration.
Diagnostic Measures	
Gastrointestinal (GI) series	• The GI cleansing preparations administered to clients having GI studies done may result in diarrhea, which irritates the sensitive skin in the perianal area—especially if the client had bouts of diarrhea before the studies; anticipating the problem, noting redness and inflammation, and beginning warm baths and ointments are welcome nursing measures that clients may be too embarrassed to seek.
Therapeutic Measures	
Bed rest	• Bedrest predisposes clients to skin breakdown; the harsh detergents used on hospital laundry compound this problem. • Pressure points need to be examined frequently and protected.
Casts	• Casts easily irritate the skin; careful assessment, covering the rough edges of the cast, and skin care are indicated.
K-thermia unit	• Moist wet heat has therapeutic benefit but if applied to the skin too long may macerate the skin; follow protocol in length of application, examine skin carefully between treatments, and allow to dry.
Medications	• Medications may cause allergic skin reactions, such as rashes. • When evaluating the client's response to a new drug, examine the skin for redness and itching.

ever, the individual attaches low priority to hygiene, or lacks the physical ability to perform hygiene measures, these problems must be addressed before health education can be effective.

Sample nursing diagnoses related to hygiene and skin problems follow:

Bathing/Hygiene Self-Care Deficit related to sensory, cognitive, endurance, mobility, or motivation deficits

Pain related to skin or mucous membrane alterations

Ineffective Individual Coping related to chronic skin problems

Altered Health Maintenance (eg, dental caries, periodontal disease, halitosis) related to deficient oral hygiene practices

Knowledge Deficit related to new therapeutic regimen to manage skin or mucous membrane alteration

Impaired Physical Mobility related to painful foot condition (calluses, corns, plantar warts)

Altered Oral Mucous Membrane related to inadequate oral hygiene, stomatitis, malnutrition, or dehydration

High Risk for Infection related to broken skin or traumatized tissue

Body Image Disturbance related to visible integumentary problems, body odors

Altered Sexuality Patterns related to fear of transmitting or acquiring sexually transmitted disease, painful genital lesions

Impaired Skin Integrity related to altered circulation, nutritional and fluid deficit or excess, impaired mobility, irritants (chemical, thermal, mechanical, radiation)

Impaired Social Interaction related to negative body image (eg, acne, alopecia)

Impaired Swallowing related to reddened, irritated oropharyngeal cavity

Impaired Tissue Integrity (eg, cornea, mucous membrane, integumentary, or subcutaneous) related to altered circulation, nutritional or fluid deficit or excess, impaired mobility, irritants (chemical, thermal, mechanical, radiation)

In certain situations, a wellness nursing diagnosis may be appropriate as the client progresses toward an increased level of health awareness and wellness. An example of a wellness diagnosis is as follows:

Potential for Enhanced Oral Hygiene Practices

Additional diagnoses related to specific body parts are discussed later in this chapter.

Data collected during the nursing assessment may also lead to the identification of a collaborative problem. A nurse caring for a client receiving intravenous chemotherapy should carefully check the infusion site every shift, realizing that phlebitis commonly occurs with certain chemotherapeutic agents. Careful preparation and administration of the drug according to the manufacturer's instructions, adherence to nursing protocols for the maintenance of intravenous infusions, and ongoing nursing assessment may decrease the likelihood of phlebitis. If redness, warmth, tenderness, or swelling is noted with any intra-

venous infusion, immediate collaborative intervention is indicated.

Similarly, a nurse may notice a 1.5-cm mole with an irregular border on a client's back during a bath. Prompt reporting of this finding to the physician may lead to the detection and early, successful treatment of the medical diagnosis—malignant melanoma.

Planning: Client Goals

Each plan of nursing care identifies nursing measures to assist the client to develop or maintain hygiene practices that contribute to a sense of well-being. Appropriate client goals include the following. The client will:

- Verbalize feeling comfortable and clean
- Participate fully in necessary hygiene measures according to cognitive, sensory, mobility, and endurance abilities
- Maintain intact skin and mucous membranes
- Demonstrate correct skin care measures (when indicated)
- Demonstrate signs of healing in existing lesions

Client goals related to specific body parts are presented later in this chapter.

Implementing

The nurse, in performing general personal hygiene skills, respects the client's personal preferences in hygiene measures, allows and encourages as much self-care as the client can perform, meets the client's needs for privacy, and promotes physiologic and psychologic wellness. In the following sections, general hygiene measures are discussed, including providing scheduled care, helping with bathing, massaging, bedmaking, and providing environmental care. Nursing care related to specific body parts is discussed later in this chapter.

Providing Scheduled Hygienic Care

When clients require nursing assistance with personal hygiene, it is important to schedule this care at regular intervals. In most hospitals and long-term care settings, the following types of hygienic care are provided. These are individualized to clients according to their personal and cultural preferences.

Early Morning Care Shortly after awakening, the client is assisted with toileting if necessary and then provided comfort measures designed to refresh the client and prepare the client for breakfast (or diagnostic tests). Nursing measures include washing the face and hands and providing mouth care. Agency policy dictates whether the nurses on night shift or day shift are responsible for early morning care. This is an excellent time to note if the supplies needed for morning care are available and to order any that are lacking.

Morning Care (AM Care)   After breakfast, the nurse completes morning care. Depending on the client's self-care abilities, the nurse offers assistance with toileting; oral care; bathing; back massage; special skin care measures (eg, pressure ulcer); hair care (includes shaving if indicated); cosmetics (if desired); dressing; and positioning for comfort. Agency policies are followed in refreshing or changing bed linens, and the client's bedside area is tidied. When morning care is completed, the client should feel refreshed and be in a comfortable and safe environment. For some clients, this may mean positioning the call light within reach and using protective devices such as bed rails or restraints.

   Morning care is often characterized as self-care, partial care, or complete care. *Self-care* clients are capable of managing their personal hygiene independently once oriented to the bathroom. These clients should still be offered a back massage and receive quality nursing time directed to assessing their day-to-day needs. *Partial care* clients most often receive morning hygiene care at the bedside or seated near the sink in the bathroom. Because of weakness, these clients may be able to wash only the parts of their bodies that are within easy reach. The nurse washes the back and legs and sometimes the axillae and perineum because these body parts have the most secretions and are difficult to reach. *Complete care* clients require nursing assistance with all aspects of personal hygiene. A complete bed bath is done or the client is taken to the shower or tub.

Afternoon Care (PM Care)   Because hospitalized clients frequently receive visitors in the afternoon or evening, or use this time to rest when not scheduled for tests, the nurse should ensure the client's comfort after lunch and offer assistance to nonambulatory clients with toileting, handwashing, and oral care. Straightening bed linens and helping clients with mobility problems to reposition themselves comfortably are other welcome nursing measures.

Hour of Sleep Care (hs Care)   Shortly before the client retires, the nurse again offers assistance with toileting, washing of face and hands, and oral care. Many clients find that a back massage helps them to relax and fall asleep and this should be offered routinely. Soiled bed linens or clothing should be changed and the client positioned comfortably. If protective devices are indicated for night hours (ie, side rails or restraints) these are applied at this time. The call light and any other objects the client desires (eg, urinal, radio, or water glass) should be within easy reach.

As Needed Care (prn Care)   In addition to scheduled care, the nurse offers individual hygiene measures as needed. Some clients require oral care every 2 hours. Clients who are *diaphoretic* (sweating profusely) may need their clothing and bed linens changed several times a shift. At other times, a nurse may decide to forego hygienic measures because the client's need for undisturbed rest may take precedence.

Helping With Bathing

Purposes of Bathing   Bathing serves a variety of purposes, including the following:
- It cleanses the skin.
- It acts as a skin conditioner.
- It helps relax a restless person.
- It promotes circulation by stimulating the skin's peripheral nerve endings and underlying tissues.
- It serves as a musculoskeletal exercise through activity involved with bathing and thus improves joint mobility and muscle tonus.
- It stimulates the rate and depth of respirations.
- It promotes comfort through muscle relaxation and skin stimulation.
- It provides the person with sensory input.
- It helps improve self-image.
- It gives the nurse an excellent opportunity to strengthen the nurse–client relationship, to observe the client's physiologic and emotional status closely, to teach the client as indicated, and to demonstrate that the nurse cares for the client and is interested in the client's general welfare.

Shower and Tub Baths   Using a shower or a tub is the preferred method of bathing for hospitalized people who are ambulatory. Even though clients can, for the most part, do this on their own, the nurse still has responsibilities:
- Check to see that the bathroom is available, clean, and safe. Showers and tubs should have mats or non-skid strips to prevent the client from slipping and falling.
- Ensure that necessary articles, such as soap, a washcloth, a towel, and a gown, are available for the client.
- Provide for a place for a weak or physically disabled client to sit in a shower. Most health agencies have a stool or chair that can be used in a shower, and hand-held shower heads may facilitate the process. Some nurses have reported that a commode chair with the pan removed serves effectively as a shower chair, and it offers the client more support than a stool or chair.
- Assist the client to the shower or bathroom, as indicated. Clients who are beginning ambulation need assistance to help prevent falling and fainting.
- Check to see that the water temperature is safe and comfortable, 43° to 46°C (110° to 115°F).
- Help the client get in and out of a bathtub, as indicated. Have the client grasp handrails at the side of the tub, or place a chair at the side of the tub. The client sits on the chair and eases to the edge of the tub. After putting both feet into the tub, it is then relatively easy for the client to reach the opposite side and ease down into the tub. The client may kneel first in the tub and then sit in it, and the client can leave the tub in the same manner. Use a hydraulic lift, when available, to lower and lift a helpless and heavy client in and out of a tub.
- Ensure privacy for the client who is safe to shower or

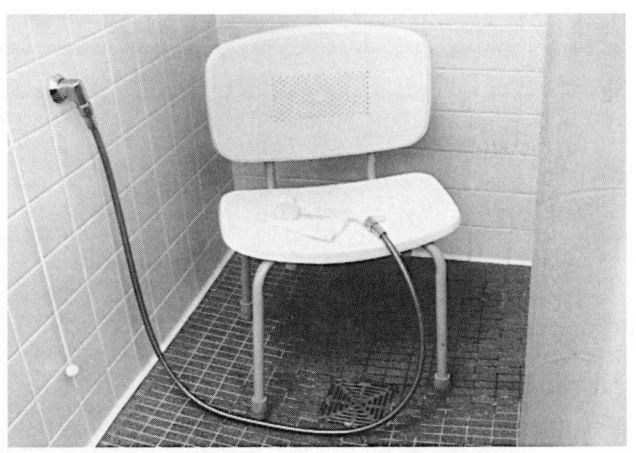

A chair placed in the shower with a hand-held shower head.

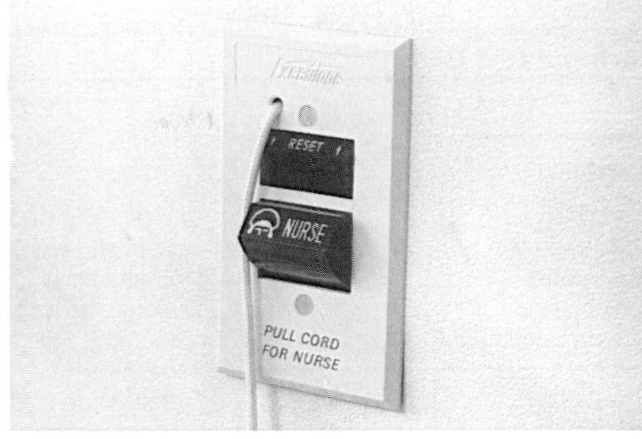

A call bell equiped with a pull cord.

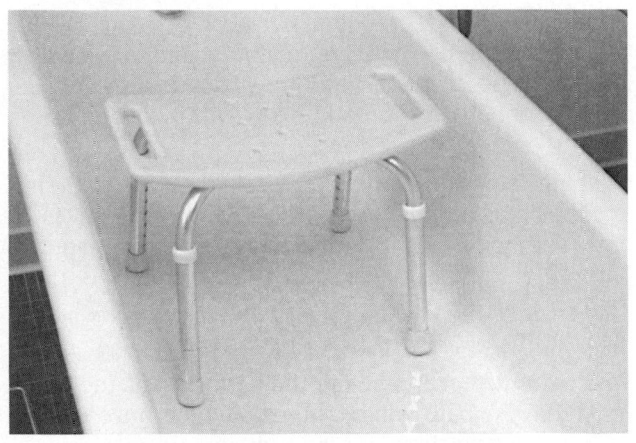

A stool in the bath tub to facilitate getting in and out of the tub and nonslip strips adhered to the bottom of the tub.

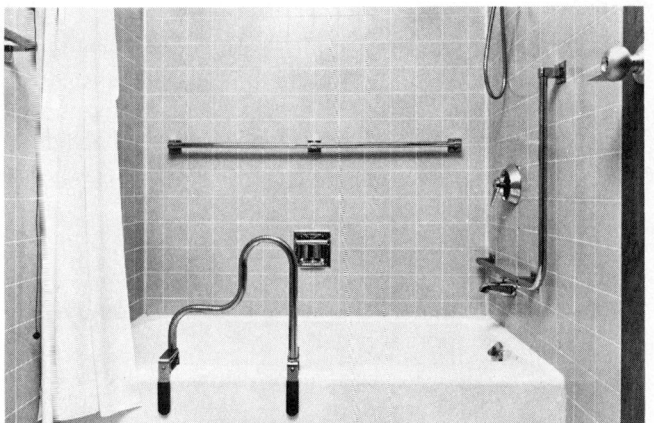

A bath equipped with safety hand rails.

FIGURE 29-2

Examples of features that add to the safety of a client in the bath.

bathe independently. See to it that a call device is handy so that the client can obtain help if necessary.

- Keep the bathroom door unlocked. Health personnel should be able to enter with ease if the client needs help. A sign hung on the door ensures privacy. Children should never be left alone in bathrooms.
- Help wash and dry areas of the body that the client cannot reach, such as the back.

Figure 29-2 illustrates several features that add to the safety of a client who takes a shower or tub bath.

Bed Baths Some clients must remain in bed as a part of their therapeutic regimen, but they are able to bathe themselves. The nurse helps the client who takes a bath in bed in several ways:

- Provide the client with articles for bathing. Provide a basin of water that is of a comfortable and safe temperature. Place these items conveniently for the client on a bedside stand or overbed table.

- Provide privacy for the client. See to it that the call device is within reach.
- Remove top linens on the client's bed while replacing them with a bath blanket.
- Place cosmetics in a convenient place for the client's use. Provide a mirror, a good light, and hot water for the client who wishes to shave with a razor.
- Assist clients who cannot bathe themselves completely. For example, some clients are able to wash only the upper parts of the body. The remainder of the bath is then completed by nursing personnel.

Bathing procedures for the client who requires total nursing assistance vary among health agencies. The one described in Procedure 29-1 is offered as a guide. It assumes that the client is able to be raised or lowered in bed and that, although the client may have limited movement, it is possible for the nurse to manage the client alone.

(*Text continues on p. 590*)

P R O C E D U R E   2 9 - 1

Giving a Bed Bath

Equipment

Wash basin
Soap and dish
Washcloths
Bath blanket
Gown or pajamas
Bed linen
Towels (2)

Disposable gloves—for anal and
  perineal care (optional for
  remainder of bath)
Personal hygiene supplies—deodorant, lotion, and others
Bedpan or urinal
Laundry bag or cart

Action	Rationale
1 Discuss procedure with the client and assess the client's ability to assist in the bathing process as well as personal hygiene preferences. Review the client's chart for any limitations in physical activity.	This discussion promotes reassurance and provides knowledge about the procedure. Dialogue also encourages client participation and allows for individualized nursing care.
2 Bring necessary equipment to the bedside stand or overbed table.	Bringing everything to the bedside conserves time and energy. Arranging items nearby is convenient, saves time, and helps prevent unnecessary stretching and twisting of muscles on the part of the nurse.
3 Close the curtains around the bed and close the door to the room if possible.	This ensures the client's privacy and lessens the possibility of loss of body heat during the bath.
4 Offer the client the bedpan or urinal.	Voiding or defecating before the bath lessens the likelihood that the bath will be interrupted, because warm bath water may stimulate the urge to void.
5 Wash your hands.	Handwashing deters the spread of microorganisms.
6 Raise the client's bed to the high position.	Having the bed in a high position prevents strain on the nurse's back.
7 Lower the side rail nearer to you and assist the client to the side of the bed where you will work. Have the client lie on his or her back.	Having the client positioned near the nurse and lowering the side rail help prevent unnecessary stretching and twisting of muscles on the part of the nurse.
8 Loosen top covers and remove all except the top sheet. Place bath blanket over the client and then remove the top sheet while the client holds the bath blanket in place. If linen is to be reused, fold it over a chair. Place soiled linen in the laundry bag.	The client is not exposed unnecessarily and warmth is maintained. If a bath blanket is unavailable, the top sheet may be used in place of the bath blanket.
9 Assist the client with oral hygiene, as necessary, and as described in Procedure 29-5.	This helps maintain teeth and gums in good condition, alleviates unpleasant odor and taste, and may improve appetite. Some clients may prefer oral care after the bath is completed.
10 Remove the client's gown and keep the bath blanket in place. If client has an intravenous line, remove the gown from the other arm first. Lower the intravenous container and pass the gown over the tubing and the container. Rehang the container and check the drip rate.	This provides uncluttered access during the bath and maintains warmth of the client. Intravenous fluids must be maintained at the prescribed rate.

(continued)

P R O C E D U R E   2 9 - 1 *(continued)*

Giving a Bed Bath

Action	Rationale
11 Raise the side rail. Fill the basin with a sufficient amount of comfortably warm water (between 43° and 46°C [110° to 115°F]). Change as necessary throughout the bath. Lower the side rail closer to you when you return to the bedside to begin the bath.	Warm water is comfortable and relaxing for the client. It also stimulates circulation and provides for more effective cleansing. Side rails maintain client safety.
12 Fold the washcloth like a mitt on your hand so there are no loose ends, as illustrated.	Having loose ends of cloth drag across the client's skin is uncomfortable. Loose ends cool quickly and will feel cold to the client.

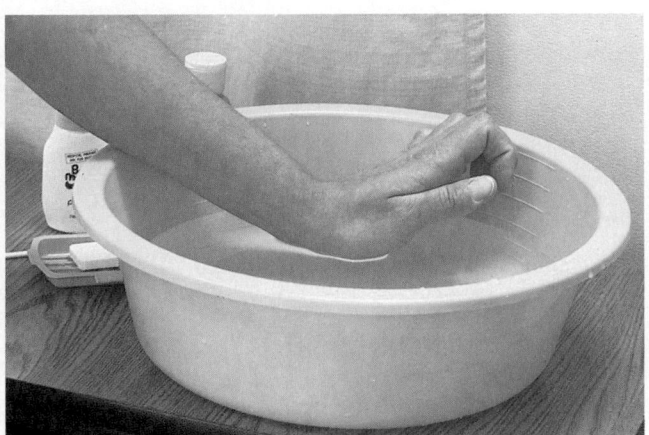

Action 11: Testing water temperature.

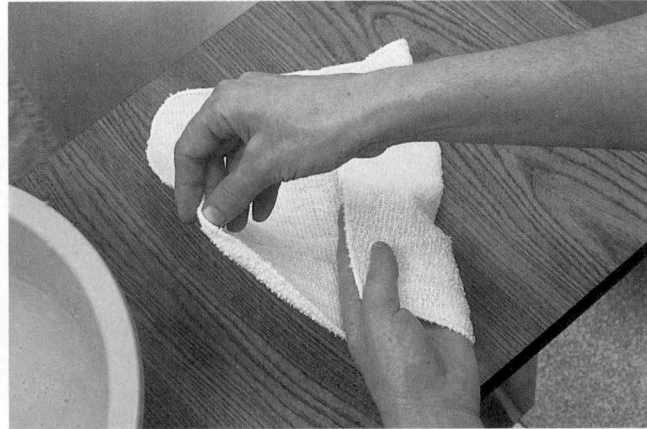

Action 12: Folding washcloth in thirds around hand to make a bath mitt.

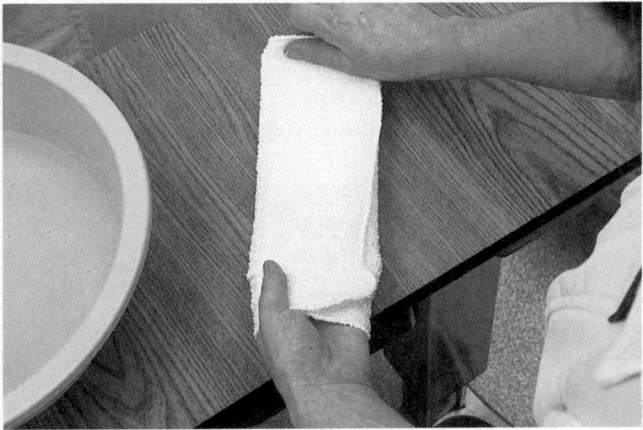

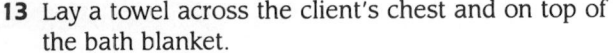

Action 12: Straightening washcloth before folding into mitt.

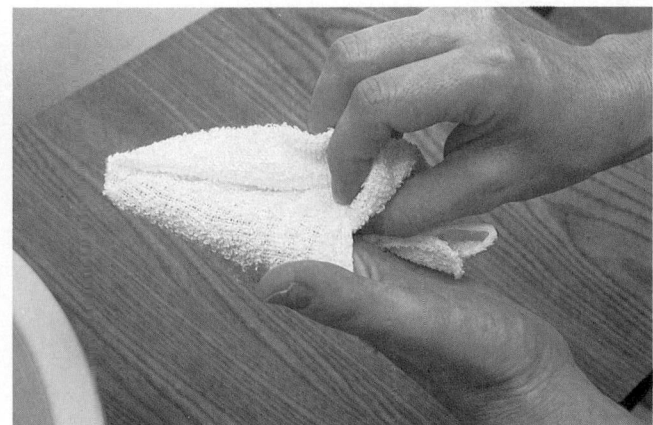

Action 12: Folding ends over and tucking ends under folded washcloth over palm.

Action	Rationale
13 Lay a towel across the client's chest and on top of the bath blanket.	This prevents chilling and keeps the bath blanket dry.

(continued)

PROCEDURE 29-1 *(continued)*

Giving a Bed Bath

Action

Rationale

14 With no soap on the washcloth, wipe one eye from the inner part of the eye, near the nose, to the outer part. Rinse or turn the cloth before washing the other eye.

Rinsing or turning the washcloth prevents spreading organisms from one eye to the other. Soap is irritating to the eyes. Moving from the inner to the outer aspect of the eye prevents carrying debris toward the nasolacrimal duct.

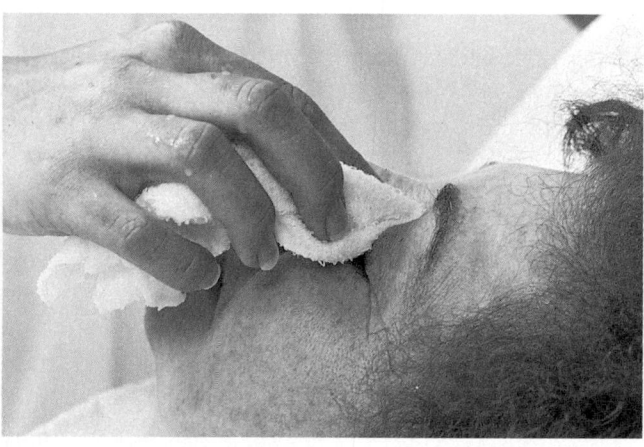

Action 14: Washing from the inner corner of the eye outward.

15 Bathe the client's face, neck, and ears, avoiding soap on the face if the client prefers.

Soap can be drying and may be avoided as a matter of personal preference.

16 Expose the far arm of the client and place the towel lengthwise under it. Using firm strokes, wash the arm and axilla, rinse, and dry.

The towel helps to keep the bed dry. Washing the far side first eliminates contaminating a clean area once it is washed. Gentle friction stimulates circulation and muscles and helps remove dirt, oil, and organisms. Long, firm strokes are relaxing and more comfortable than short, uneven strokes.

17 Place a folded towel on the bed next to the client's hand and put the basin on it. Soak the client's hand in the basin. Wash, rinse, and dry the hand.

Placing the hands in the basin of water is comfortable and relaxing for the client, allows for a thorough washing of the hands and between the fingers, and facilitates removal of debris from under the nails.

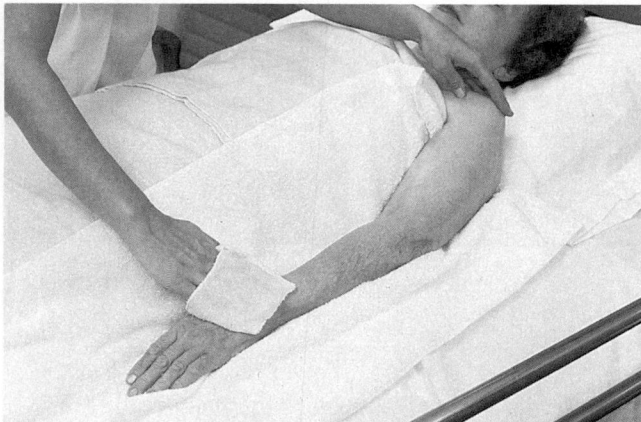

Action 16: Exposing the far arm and washing.

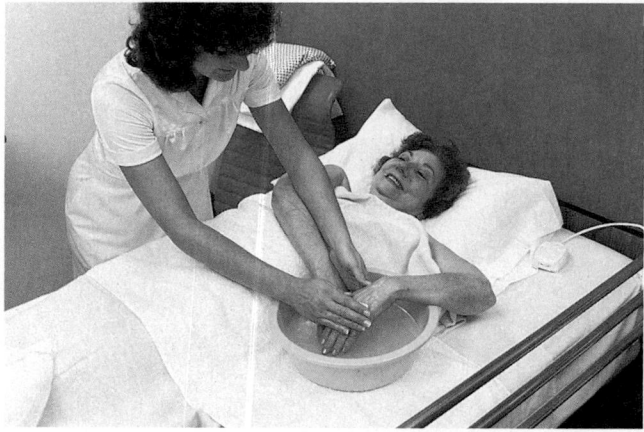

Action 17: Soaking hand in basin.

(continued)

PROCEDURE 29-1 *(continued)*

Giving a Bed Bath

Action

Rationale

18 Repeat actions 16 and 17 for the arm nearer to you. (An option for the shorter nurse or one prone to back strain might be to bathe one side of the client and move to the other side of the bed to complete the bath.)

19 Spread a towel across the client's chest. Lower the bath blanket to the client's umbilical area. Wash, rinse, and dry the client's chest. Keep the client's chest covered with the towel between the wash and rinse. Pay special attention to skin folds under the breasts of clients.

Exposing, washing, rinsing, and drying one part of the body at a time avoids unnecessary exposure and chilling. Skin fold areas may be sources of odor and skin breakdown if not cleansed and dried properly.

20 Lower the bath blanket to the client's perineal area. Place a towel over the client's chest.

Keeping the bath blanket and towel in place avoids exposure and chilling.

21 Wash, rinse, and dry the client's abdomen. Carefully inspect and cleanse the umbilical area and any abdominal folds or creases.

Skin-fold areas may be sources of odor and skin breakdown if not cleansed and dried properly.

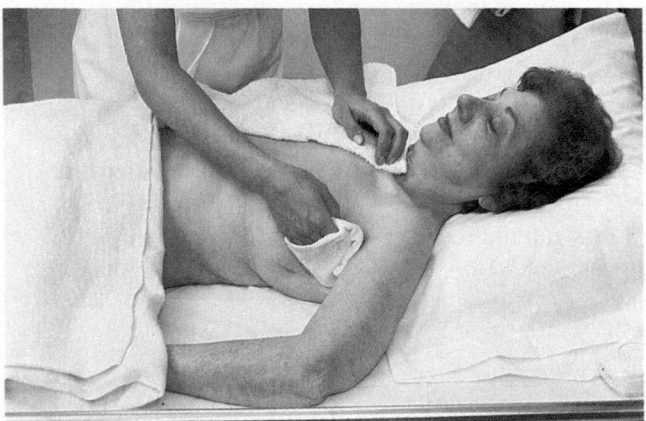

Action 19: Washing the chest area, including the axillae.

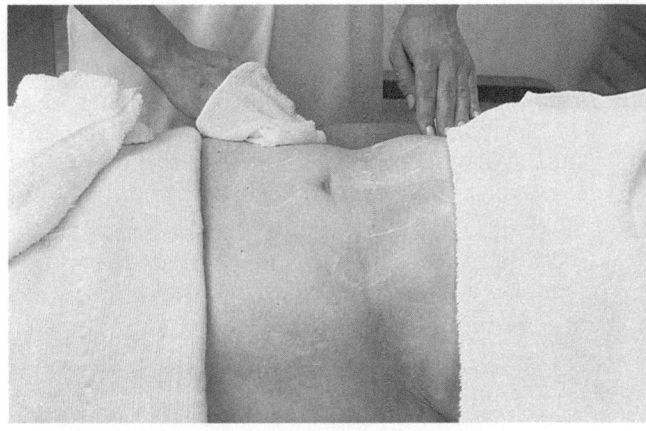

Action 21: Washing the abdomen, with perineal and chest areas covered.

22 Return the bath blanket to its original position and expose the far leg of the client. Place the towel under the far leg. Using firm strokes, wash, rinse, and dry the client's leg from ankle to knee and knee to groin.

The towel protects linens and prevents the client from feeling uncomfortable from a damp or wet bed. Washing from ankle to groin with firm strokes promotes venous return.

23 Fold a towel near the client's foot area and place the basin on it. Place the client's foot in the basin while supporting the client's ankle and heel in your hand and the leg on your arm. Wash, rinse, and dry, paying particular attention to the area between the toes.

Supporting the client's foot and leg helps reduce strain and discomfort for the client. Placing the feet in a basin of water is comfortable and relaxing and allows for a thorough cleaning of the feet and the areas between the toes and under the nails.

24 Repeat actions 22 and 23 for the other leg and foot.

25 Make sure the client is covered with the bath blanket. Change water at this point or earlier if necessary. Assist the client onto his or her side.

The bath blanket maintains warmth and privacy. Clean, warm water prevents chilling and maintains the client's comfort.

(continued)

P R O C E D U R E   2 9 - 1 *(continued)*

Giving a Bed Bath

Action

Rationale

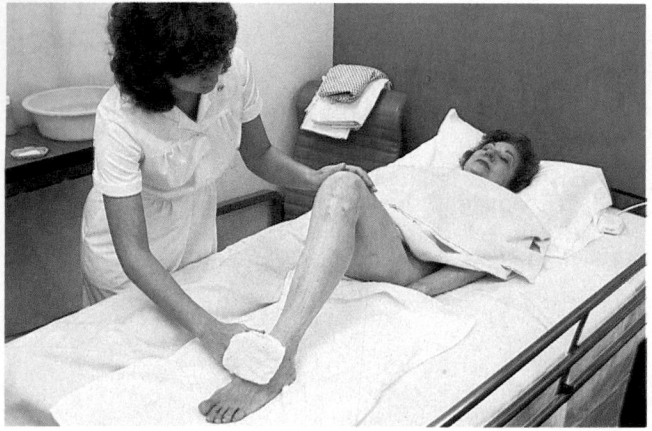

Action 22: Washing and drying far leg, keeping other leg covered.

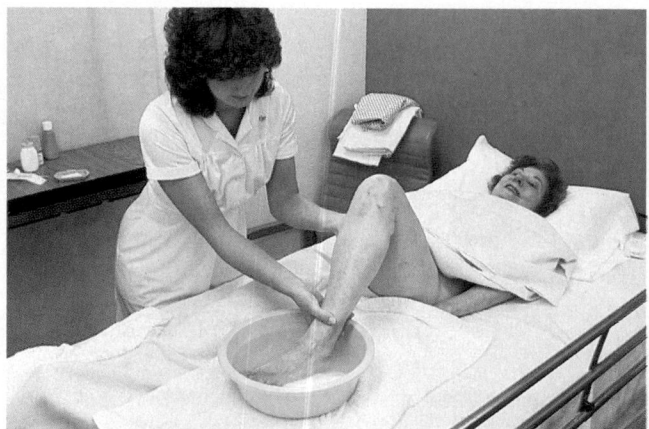

Action 23: Soaking the foot in basin.

26 Assist the client to a prone or side-lying position. Position the bath blanket and towel to expose only the back and buttocks.

27 Wash, rinse, and dry the client's back and buttocks area. Pay particular attention to cleansing between gluteal folds and observe for any indication of redness or skin breakdown in the sacral area.

28 If not contraindicated, give the client a back rub, as described in Procedure 32-1. Back massage may be given also after perineal care.

Positioning of the towel and bath blanket protects the client's privacy and provides warmth.

Fecal material near the anus may be a source of microorganisms. Prolonged pressure on the sacral area or other bony prominences may compromise circulation and lead to development of decubitus ulcer.

A back rub improves circulation to the tissues and is an aid to relaxation. A back rub may be contraindicated in clients with cardiovascular disease or musculoskeletal injuries.

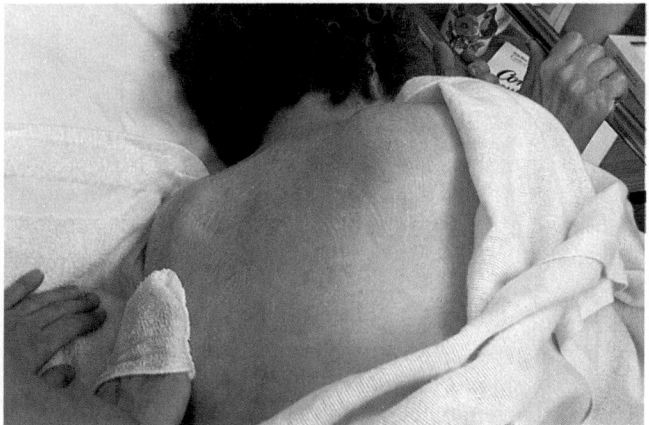

Action 27: Washing the upper back.

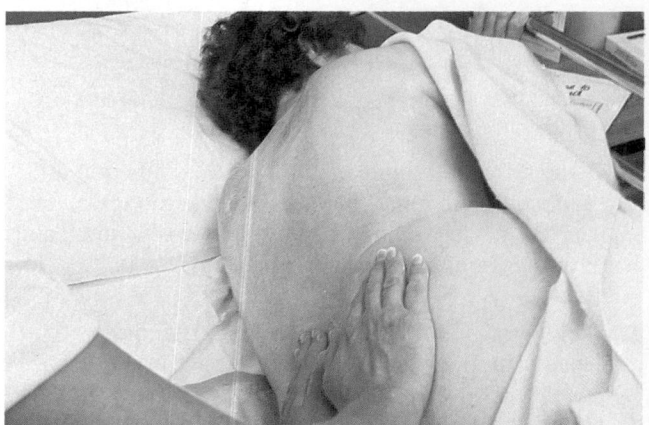

Action 28: Giving a backrub, after washing lower back.

29 Refill basin with clean water. Discard washcloth and towel.

The washcloth, towel, and water are contaminated after washing the client's gluteal area. Changing to clean supplies decreases the spread of organisms from the anal area to the genitals.

(continued)

PROCEDURE 29-1 *(continued)*

Giving a Bed Bath

Action	Rationale
30 Clean the client's perineal area or set up the client so he or she can complete perineal self-care.	Providing perineal self-care may decrease embarrassment for the client. Effective perineal care reduces odor and decreases the chance of infection through contamination.

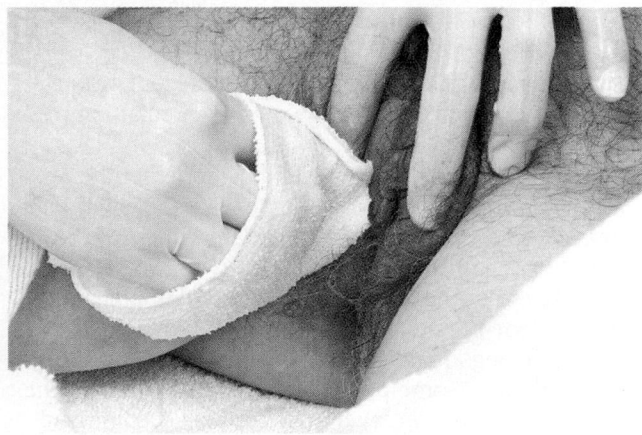

Action 30: Cleansing the perineal area.

Action	Rationale
31 Help the client put on a clean gown and attend to personal hygiene needs.	This provides for the client's warmth and comfort.
32 Protect the pillow with a towel, and groom the client's hair, as described in the text.	
33 Change bed linens, as described in Procedures 29-3 and 29-4.	
34 Record any significant observations and communication on the client's chart.	A careful record is important for planning and individualizing the client's care.

Age Considerations

When bathing an infant or young child, have all supplies within easy reach and support or hold the child securely at all times to ensure safety. Never leave the child alone.

Check temperature of water, particularly before bathing an older client because sensitivity to temperature may be impaired.

An elderly client who is not incontinent may not require a full bed bath with soap and water every day. If dry skin is a problem, water and skin lotion or bath oil may be used on alternate days.

Special Considerations

Removal of gown if client has an intravenous line necessitates taking the gown off, uninvolved arm first, and then threading the intravenous tubing and bottle or bag through the arm of the gown after the affected arm has been removed from the gown. To replace the gown, reverse the procedure. Place the clean gown on the unaffected arm first and thread intravenous tubing and bottle or bag from inside the arm of the gown on the involved side. *Never* disconnect intravenous tubing to change a gown because this causes a break in a sterile system and is a potential for infection.

Certain clients may not be able to tolerate lying flat in bed during the bed bath. Position may have to be modified to accommodate needs of such clients.

Change water as often as necessary to maintain at a comfortable temperature. Always change the water after performing perineal care or when the water is soiled.

Home Care Considerations

Evaluate the safety of the bathing area in the home. Tub mats, adhesive strips, grab bars, and shower stools are helpful accessories to prevent falls.

Towel Baths   The in-bed towel bath, or lotion bath, uses a quick-drying solution containing a cleaning agent, a disinfectant, and a softening agent mixed with water that is 43.3° to 48.9°C (110° to 120°F). A commonly used solution developed cooperatively by a nurse and Vestal Laboratories is called Septi-Soft. A recommended procedure for giving the towel bath follows:

- Place a terry cloth towel, about 3 × 7 feet, in a plastic bag, and saturate it with the warmed cleaning solution.
- Wring out the towel well and unroll it over the client while simultaneously removing the upper bed linens.
- Fold an extra amount of the towel under the client's chin for later use.
- Use a massaging motion to clean the body, beginning with the client's feet and working up the body.
- Fold the towel upward as the bath proceeds while a clean sheet is unfolded over the client.
- Cleanse the client's face, neck, and ears with the part of the towel that is folded under the chin.
- Fold the towel into quarters, soiled side turned in, and turn the client to the side. The folded towel is used to wash the back and buttocks.
- Remove the towel after finishing the bath. The back may then be rubbed.
- Place clean linen on the bed, and dress and position the client.
- The client need not be dried because the cleaning solution dries in a matter of seconds.

According to reports, the towel bath can be accomplished with little fatigue to the client; the towel remains warm during the short procedure; clients state they feel clean and refreshed; and the oil in the bathing solution eliminates dry, itchy skin. The bathing procedure and linen change take about 10 minutes. The brevity of the bath may be its greatest disadvantage. The nurse has less time with his or her clients than when giving the traditional bath in bed, which is especially important for developing a helping relationship.

Assisting With Antiembolism Stockings

Antiembolism stockings are often used for clients with limited activity to help prevent phlebitis and thrombi formation (these conditions are described in Chapter 30). They are made of elastic material and are manufactured by several companies. Antiembolism stockings help force blood in superficial veins of the legs to deeper veins and prevent stagnation of blood in the veins of the legs.

Antiembolism stockings should always be removed during morning care, the legs inspected, and the stockings reapplied before the client is out of bed, as shown in Procedure 29-2. General nursing guidelines for assisting with antiembolism stockings follow:

- Measure the client's leg to ensure that a proper size stocking is used. The manufacturer whose stockings are being used gives directions for measuring. Some

stockings fit either leg; others are designated right or left. An improperly fitting stocking is uncomfortable, ineffective, and may even harm the client.
- Be prepared to apply the stockings in the morning before the client is out of bed and while the client is supine. If the client is sitting or has been up and about, have the client lie down with legs and feet well elevated for at least 15 minutes before applying the stockings. After the leg vessels are congested with blood, the effectiveness of using the stockings is defeated.
- Do not massage the legs. If a clot is present, it may break away from the vessel wall and circulate in the bloodstream.
- Be sure the client's heel is well positioned in the stocking. The purpose of the stocking is likely to be defeated if the stocking is applied improperly.
- Pull the toes of the stockings slightly to relieve pressure on the toes after the stockings are in place if they have no toe openings.
- Check the legs regularly for redness, blistering, swelling, and pain. Some people recommend checking the legs at least once every 8 hours; others recommend twice a day. The stockings should be removed completely once a day to bathe the legs and feet.
- Launder the stockings as necessary but at least every 3 days. Soiled stockings irritate the skin. The stockings should be dried on a flat surface to prevent them from stretching.

Several manufacturers produce men's and women's hose that are capable of applying pressure to the legs from the foot to mid-thigh or higher. Some apply mild pressure whereas others are capable of applying pressure equivalent to an elastic bandage. The stockings are available in a variety of colors so that other stockings are not needed to cover them for the ambulatory person. Many people who are on their feet or remain in one position a great deal, such as homemakers, nurses, salespeople, and businesspeople, find them useful. The stockings should be fitted correctly to the person's measurements. Also, they should be applied immediately on awakening, before getting out of bed and before the legs are in a dependent position.

Massaging the Back

A back rub generally follows the client's bath. This acts as a general body conditioner. It can be used as a stimulant or a relaxant, or both. Giving a back rub provides an opportunity for the nurse to observe the skin for signs of breakdown. It improves circulation and provides a means of communication with the client through the use of touch.

Because some clients may consider the back rub a luxury and be reluctant to accept it, the nurse should simply say to the client, "Now it is time for your back massage." An effective back rub should take 4 to 6 minutes to complete. A lotion for massaging the back is usually used. Alcohol is used infrequently because of its drying effect. For the com-

PROCEDURE 29-2

Applying Antiembolism Stockings

Equipment

Elastic stockings (in correct size)
For knee-high stockings
- Measure from heel to popliteal space

- Measure circumference of calf at widest point
Measuring tape
Talcum powder (optional)

For thigh-high stockings
- Measure from heel to gluteal fold
- Measure circumference of calf and thigh at widest point

Action	Rationale
1 Explain the rationale for use of elastic stockings to the client.	Explanation encourages the client's cooperation.
2 Wash your hands.	Handwashing deters the spread of microorganisms.
3 Assist the client to the supine position. If the client has been sitting or walking, it is necessary to have him or her lie down with the legs and feet well elevated for at least 15 minutes before applying the stockings.	Dependent position of legs encourages blood to pool in the veins.
4 Provide privacy. Expose legs one at a time, and powder lightly unless client has dry skin. If the skin is dry, a lotion may be used. Powders and lotions are not recommended by some manufacturers.	Powder and lotion reduce friction and make application of stockings easier.
5 Place hand inside stocking and grasp heel area securely. Turn stocking inside out to the heel area.	Inside-out technique provides for easier application and less compromising of circulation to the extremity from bunched elastic material.
6 Ease the foot of the stocking over the client's foot and heel. Check that client's heel is centered in heel pocket of stocking.	Wrinkles or improper fit interfere with circulation.
7 Using your fingers and thumbs carefully grasp the edge of the stocking and pull it up smoothly over the ankle and calf until entire stocking is turned right side out. Pull forward slightly on toe section. Repeat for the other leg. Caution the client not to roll stockings partially down.	Easing the stocking carefully into position ensures proper fit of the stocking to the contour of the leg. Rolling stockings may have a constricting effect on veins. Loosening the toe section provides for comfort in that area.

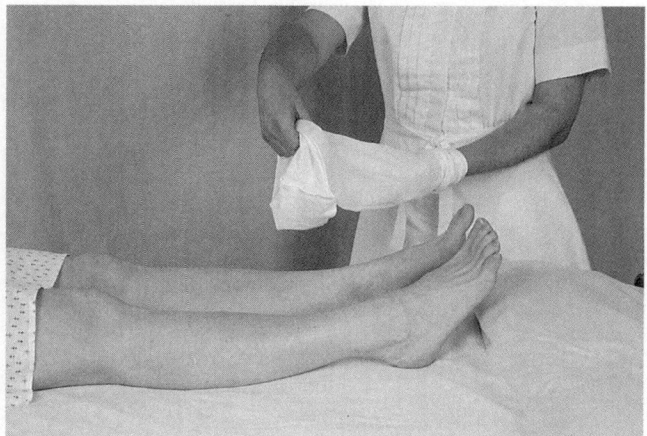

Action 5: Turning stocking inside out while grasping heel area of stocking.

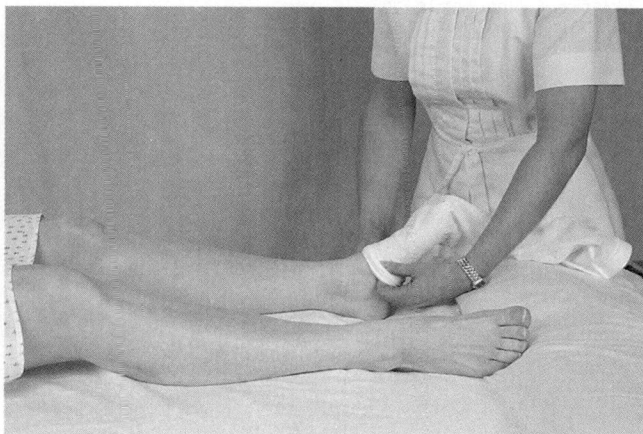

Action 6: Easing the foot of the stocking over the client's foot.

(continued)

P R O C E D U R E   2 9 - 2 *(continued)*

Applying Antiembolism Stockings

Action	Rationale

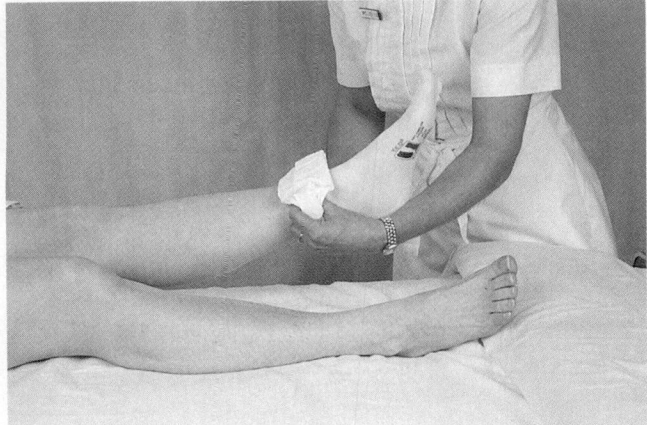

Action 6: *Easing the foot of the stocking over the client's heel.*

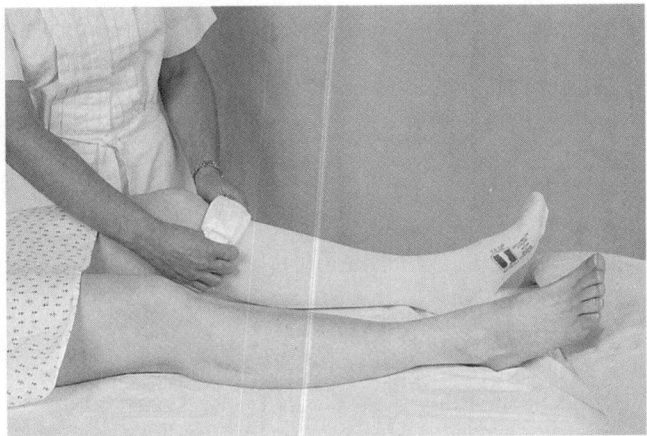

Action 7: *Pulling stocking smoothly over calf.*

8 Wash your hands.

9 To remove stocking, grasp the top of the stocking with your thumb and fingers and smoothly pull the stocking off inside out to heel. Support the client's foot and ease stocking over it.

10 Remove stockings once every shift for 20 to 30 minutes. Wash and air dry as necessary (according to manufacturer's directions).

11 Record the application of elastic stockings as well as assessment of the client's circulatory status and skin condition.

Handwashing deters the spread of infection.

This preserves elasticity and contour of the stocking.

This allows observation of the client's circulatory status and condition of the skin on the lower extremity.

This provides accurate documentation of the procedure.

Home Care Considerations

Make sure that the client has an extra pair of stockings ordered during the hospitalization before discharge (for payment and convenience purposes).

Special Considerations

At times, despite the use of elastic stockings, a client may develop thrombophlebitis. A positive Homans' sign (pain on dorsiflexion of the foot) may be an indication of a deep thrombosis or development of a blood clot in the calf.

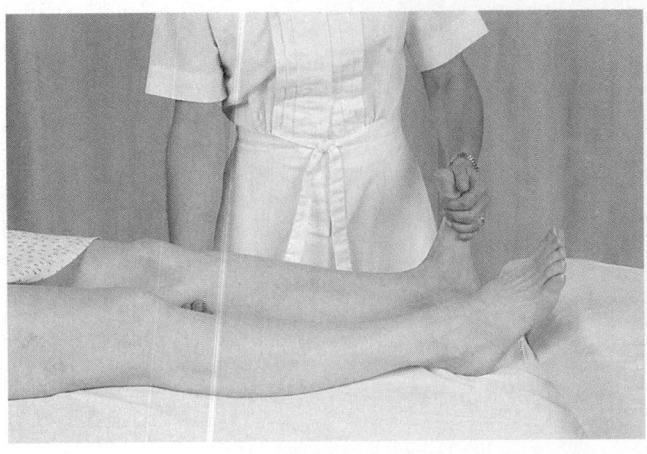

Special consideration: *Checking for Homans' sign.*

fort of the client, the lotion or alcohol should be warmed before applying it to the back. The nurse should be aware of the client's diagnosis when a back rub is being considered. A back rub is contraindicated, for example, when the client has had back surgery or has fractured ribs. Position the client on the abdomen or, if this is contraindicated, on the side for a back rub. Recommended techniques for administering a back rub are outlined in Procedure 32-1.

Bedmaking

It is usual procedure to change bed linens after the bath. The bed is made for the client who is up and about in the manner described in Procedure 29-3. If the client is bedridden, the occupied bed is made according to Procedure 29-4.

There are minor variations in the procedure for making the occupied bed. However, these small differences have no real effect on the client's comfort. In some instances, it is necessary for nurses to devise unique ways to change the linens on a client's bed because of the nature of the client's condition, orthopedic appliances on the bed, or treatments that may be in progress.

Providing Environmental Care

Bedside Unit   Because the client's environment contributes positively or negatively to the sense of well-being, it is important for the nurse to ensure that the *bedside unit*, the furnishings and equipment in the space surrounding the client's bed, is clean, safe, and pleasant. Basic furniture includes the bed, overbed table, bedside stand, and chairs.

Standard equipment in the hospital environment includes the call light, oxygen, suction, and electrical outlets; light fixtures; bath basin; emesis basin; bedpan or urinal; water pitcher and glass; and bed linens. A nursing responsibility is ensuring that necessary equipment and items are in their proper place and functioning properly.

Because the client's personal items are generally stored in the bedside stand, the nurse should request permission of the alert client before opening the stand to obtain the bath basin, lotion, or other items. When assisting with hygiene, respecting the client's right to privacy and ownership of personal goods decreases the client's sense of powerlessness.

Before leaving the bedside unit, it is good nursing practice to say to the client, "Is there anything else I can do to make you more comfortable?" Checking with the client compensates for any oversight on the nurse's part and communicates genuine caring. Limits may need to be set for manipulative clients as to what comfort and hygiene measures the nurse is able to perform.

Elements of a safe bedside unit include the following:
- Client call light functioning and always within reach
- Bed positioned properly and at the appropriate height
- Side rails and restraints safely used when indicated
- Principles of medical asepsis followed
- Electrical equipment safely grounded
- Uncluttered walk space

Elements of providing a comfortable bedside unit include attention to ventilation, odors, room temperature, lighting, and noise.

(*Text continues on p. 602*)

THROUGH THE EYES OF A STUDENT

One of my first clients was a man in his late sixties who had suffered a stroke. I was assigned to care for him and his care included a bed bath and complete linen change—with him *in the bed*. I was determined to complete this task totally on my own, without asking anyone for help. This was my first mistake.

The client yelled obscenities at me and had very rough mannerisms. I kept thinking to myself, "I must treat him with gentle care and not show any fear." Inside I was shaking furiously.

I managed to complete his bath and then began to change the sheets. I helped the client to turn to one side, tucking the dirty linens close to him. I applied the fitted sheets to the upper portion of the bed . . . so far so good. Immediately going to the foot of the bed, I applied the bottom portion. The top portion popped off—I ran to the top of the bed, reapplied the top portion—the bottom portion popped off—I reapplied it . . . . I must have spent 15 minutes running back and forth trying to get both ends to stay on. By this time sweat was pouring off my face.

When I finally cried "Uncle," I discovered that certain fitted sheets just didn't fit all the mattresses. The usual routine in this case is to walk to the linen closet and get another fitted sheet. That probably takes about 15 seconds!

—Linda A. Keough, Delaware County Community College, Media, Pennsylvania

P R O C E D U R E   2 9 - 3

Making an Unoccupied Bed

Equipment

Two large sheets (or one large
  sheet and one fitted sheet)
Drawsheet
Blankets
Bedspread

Pillowcases
Linen hamper or bag
Bedside chair
Waterproof sheet or protective pad
  (optional)

Action

1 Wash your hands.

2 Assemble equipment and arrange on a bedside
   chair in the order in which items will be used.

3 Adjust the client's bed to the high position, and
   drop the bed side rails.

4 Check bed linens for the client's personal items and
   disconnect call bell or any tubes from bed linens.

5 Loosen all linen as you move around the bed from
   the head of the bed on the far side to the head of
   the bed on the near side.

6 Fold reusable linens, such as blankets or spread, in
   place on the bed in fourths and hang them over a
   clean chair.

7 Snugly roll all of the soiled linen inside of the bottom sheet and place directly into the laundry hamper. Do not place them on the floor or on furniture.
   Do not hold soiled linens against your uniform.

Rationale

Handwashing deters the spread of microorganisms.

Organization facilitates performance of task.

Having the bed in the high position and the side rails
down reduces strain on the nurse while working.

It is costly and inconvenient when personal belongings
are lost.

Loosening linen helps prevent tugging and tearing on
linen. Loosening the linen and moving around the bed
systematically reduce strain caused by reaching across
the bed.

Folding saves times and energy when reusable linen is
replaced on the bed. Folding linens while they are on
the bed reduces strain on the nurse's arms.

Rolling soiled linens snugly and placing them directly
into the hamper helps prevent the spread of organisms.
The floor is heavily contaminated; soiled linen will further contaminate furniture. Soiled linen contaminates
the nurse's uniform, and this may spread organisms to
another client.

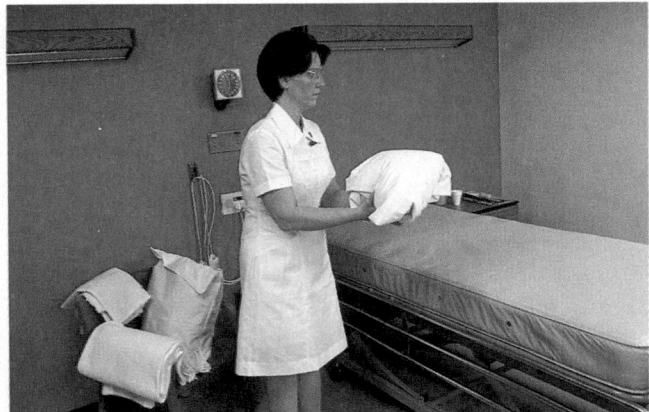

Action 7: Bundling soiled linens in bottom sheet and holding
away from body.

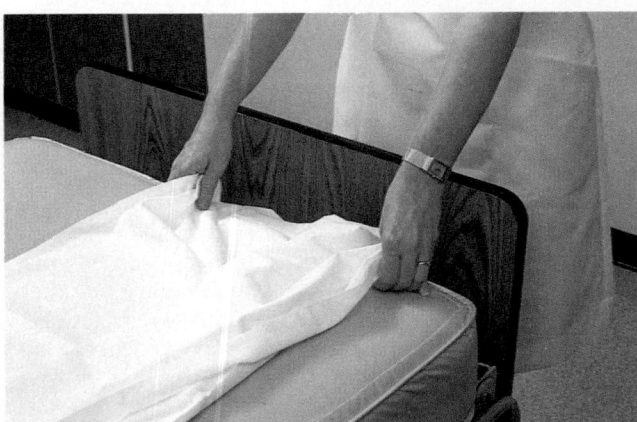

Action 9: Placing clean linens to begin bed making.

(continued)

PROCEDURE 29-3 (continued)

Making an Unoccupied Bed

Action

8 Grasp mattress securely and shift up to the head of the bed.

9 Place the bottom sheet with its center fold in the center of the bed and high enough to have a sufficient amount of the sheet to tuck under the head of the mattress.

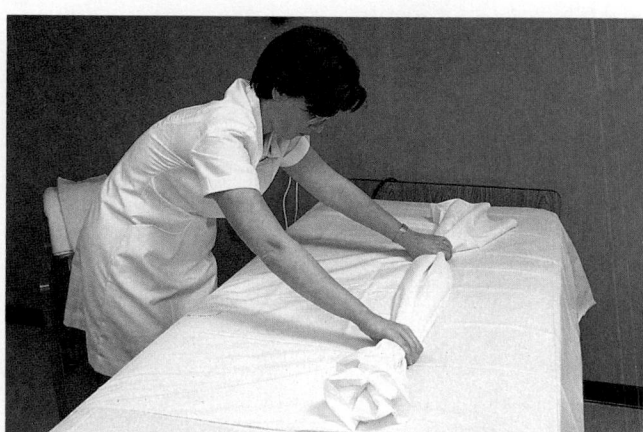

Action 10: Placing the drawsheet on the bed.

10 If a waterproof sheet or protective pad is used, place it over the bottom sheet in the proper area. Place the cotton drawsheet in the same manner over the waterproof covering. Not all agencies use drawsheets routinely. The nurse may decide to use one.

11 Tuck the bottom sheet securely under the head of the mattress on one side of the bed, making a corner according to agency policy. A mitered corner is shown in the illustrations. Using a fitted bottom sheet eliminates the need to miter corners. Tuck the remaining bottom sheet and drawsheet securely under the mattress. (At this point, before moving to the other side of the bed, top linens may be placed on the bed, unfolded, and secured, allowing the entire side of the bed to be completed at one time as shown in the illustrations.)

12 Move to the other side of the bed to secure bottom linens. Secure top of sheet under the head of the mattress and miter the corner. Pull remainder of sheet tightly and tuck under mattress. Do the same for the drawsheet.

Rationale

This allows more foot room for the client and moves the mattress against the head of the bed.

Opening linens on the bed reduces strain on the nurse's arms and diminishes the spread of organisms.

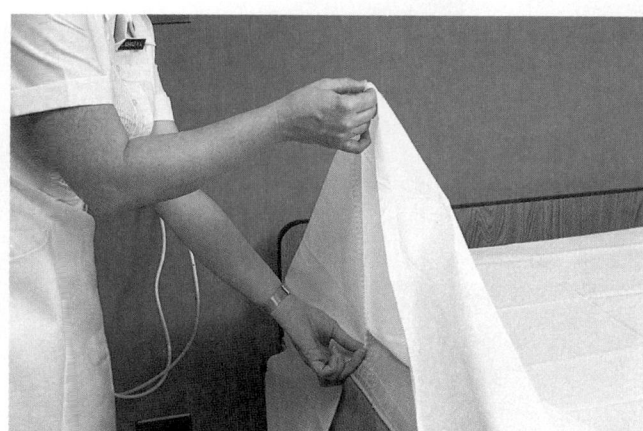

Action 11: Beginning to make mitered corner by creating a triangular fold.

When a client soils the bed, drawsheets can be changed without the bottom and top linens on the bed. Having all bottom linens in place before tucking them under the mattress avoids unnecessary moving about the bed. A drawsheet also is an aid when moving the client in bed.

Making the bed on one side and then completing the bed on the other side saves time. Having bottom linens free of wrinkles reduces discomfort to the bedridden client.

This rids bottom linens of any wrinkles that can cause discomfort for the client.

(continued)

Making an Unoccupied Bed

Action	Rationale

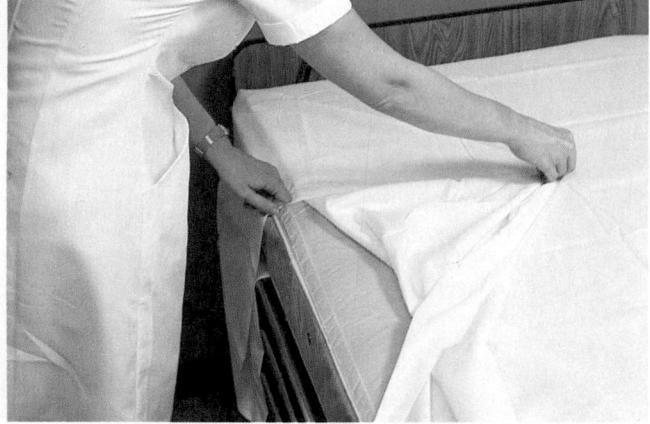

Action 11: Laying triangular fold on top of bed.

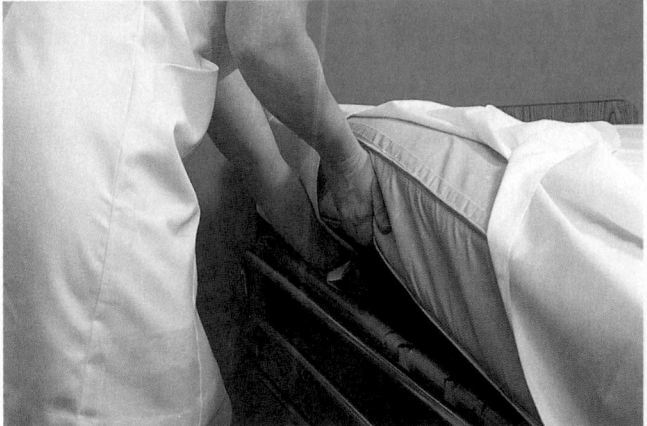

Action 11: Tucking end of sheet under mattress.

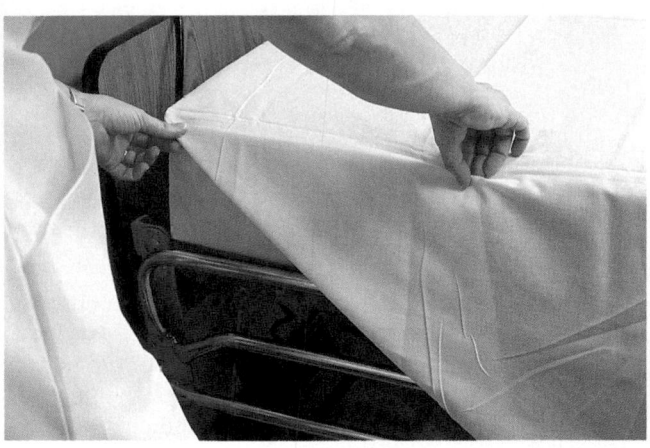

Action 11: Folding triangular linen fold down over side of mattress.

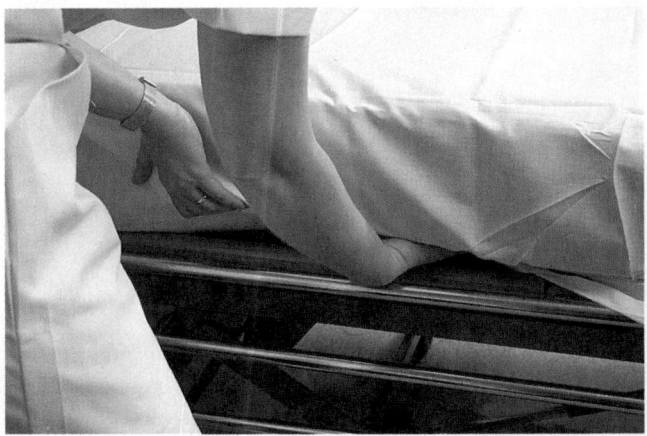

Action 11: Tucking end of triangular linen fold under mattress to complete mitered corner.

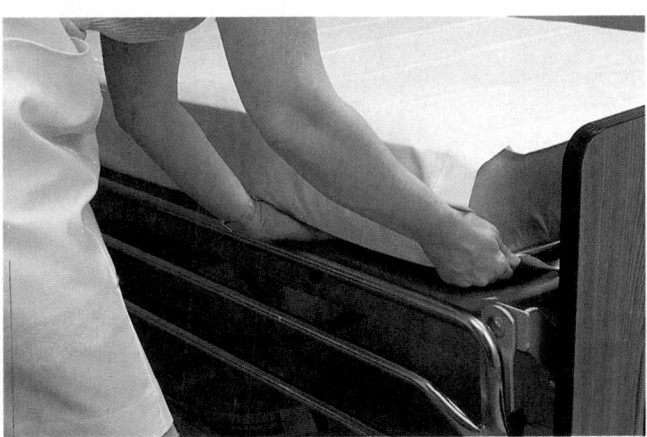

Action 11: Tucking sheet snugly under foot of mattress.

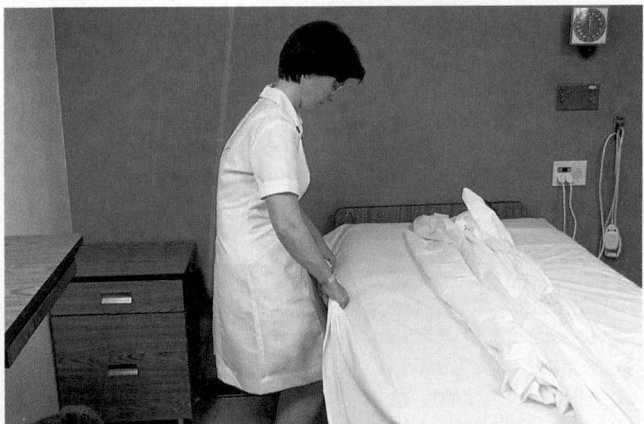

Action 12: Pulling bottom sheet tightly on opposite side of bed.

(continued)

PROCEDURE 29-3 *(continued)*

Making an Unoccupied Bed

Action	Rationale
13 Place the top sheet on the bed with its center fold in the center of the bed and with the top of the sheet placed so that the hem is even with the head of the mattress. Unfold the top sheet in place, as illustrated. Follow same procedure with top blanket or spread, placing the upper edge about 6 inches below the top of the sheet.	Opening linens by shaking them spreads organisms into the air. Holding linens overhead to open them causes strain on the nurse's arms.

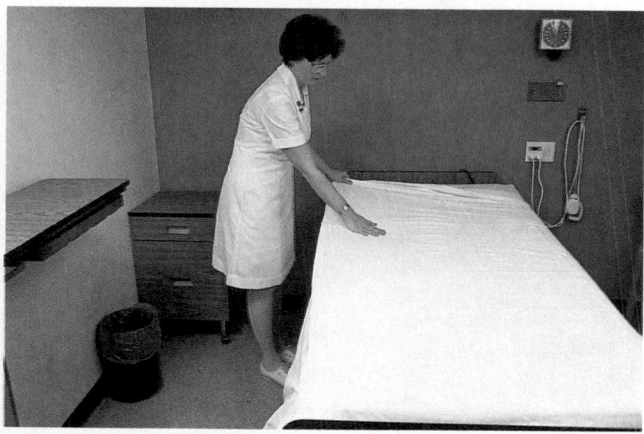

Action 13: Smoothing linens.

Action	Rationale
14 Tuck the top sheet and blanket under the foot of the bed on the near side. Miter the corners.	This saves time and energy and keeps the top linen in place.
15 Fold the upper 6 inches of the top sheet down over the spread and make a cuff.	This makes it easier for the client to get into bed and pull the covers up.

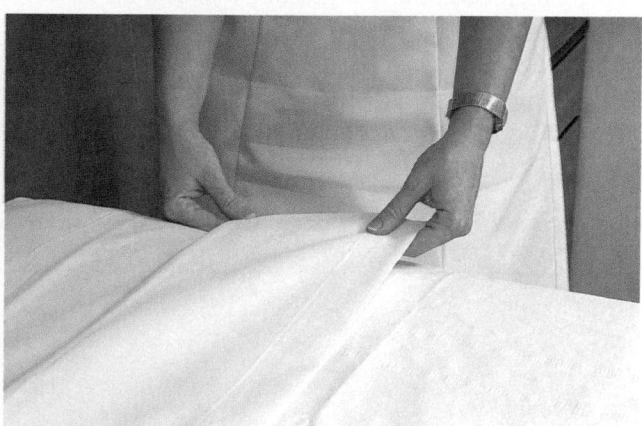

Action 15: Cuffing top linens.

Action	Rationale
16 Move to the other side of the bed and follow the same procedure for securing top sheets under the foot of the bed and making a cuff.	Working on one side of the bed at a time saves energy and is more efficient.
17 Place the pillows on the bed. Open each pillowcase in the same manner as opening other linens. Gather the pillowcase over one hand toward the closed end. Grasp the pillow with the hand inside the pillowcase. Keeping a firm hold on the top of the pillow, pull the cover onto the pillow.	Opening linens by shaking them causes organisms to be carried about on air currents. Covering the pillow while it rests on the bed reduces strain on the nurse's arms and back.

(continued)

P R O C E D U R E   2 9 - 3   *(continued)*

Making an Unoccupied Bed

Action	Rationale
18 Place the pillow at the head of the bed with the open end facing toward the window.	This provides for a neater appearance.
19 Fan-fold or pie-fold the top linens.	Having linens opened makes it more convenient for the client to get into bed.
20 Secure the signal device on the bed according to agency policy.	Having the signal device handy for the client makes it possible for the client to call for assistance as necessary.

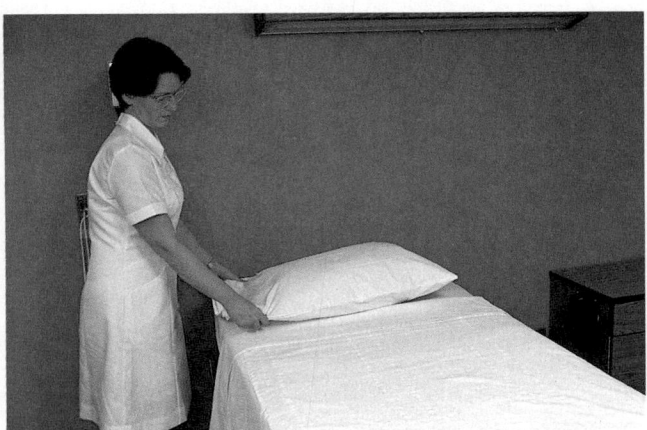

Action 18: Placing pillow with fresh pillowcase.

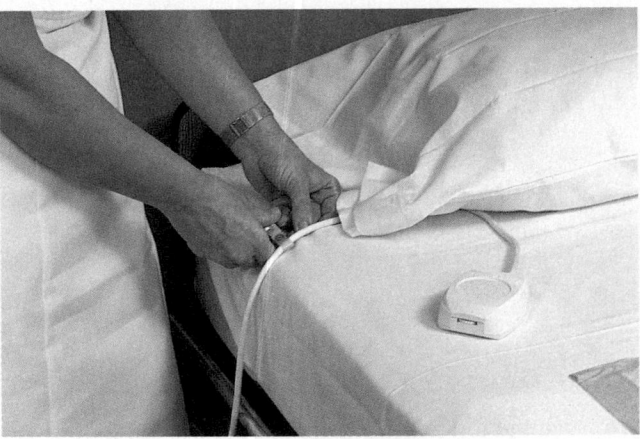

Action 20: Securing the signal device on bed.

Action	Rationale
21 Adjust the bed to the low position.	Having the bed in the low position makes it easier and safer for the client to get into bed.
22 Dispose of soiled linen according to agency policy. Wash your hands.	This deters the spread of microorganisms.

P R O C E D U R E   2 9 - 4

Making an Occupied Bed

Equipment

Two large sheets (or one large sheet and one fitted sheet)
Drawsheet
Blanket (optional)
Bedspread
Pillowcases

Linen hamper or bag (optional)
Bedside chair
Waterproof sheet or protective pad (optional)
Bath blanket (optional)

Action	Rationale
1 Explain the procedure to the client. Check the client's chart for limitations on the client's physical activity.	This facilitates client cooperation and determines level of activity.

(continued)

PROCEDURE 2 9 - 4 *(continued)*

Making an Occupied Bed

Action	Rationale
2 Wash your hands.	Handwashing deters the spread of microorganisms.
3 Assemble equipment and arrange on the bedside chair in the order the items will be used.	Organization facilitates performance of task.
4 Close door or curtain.	This provides for privacy.
5 Adjust the client's bed to the high position. Lower the side rail nearest you, leaving the opposite side rail up. Place the bed in the flat position if the client can tolerate it.	Having the bed in the high position reduces strain on the nurse while working. Having the mattress flat facilitates making a wrinkle-free bed.
6 Check bed linens for client's personal items and disconnect the call bell or any tubes from bed linens.	It is costly and inconvenient when personal items are lost. Disconnecting tubes from linens prevents discomfort and accidental dislodging of the tubes.
7 Place a bath blanket, if available, over the client. Have the client hold onto the bath blanket while you reach under it and remove top linens. Leave the top sheet in place if a bath blanket is not used. Fold linen that is to be reused over the back of a chair. Discard soiled linen in a laundry bag or hamper.	This provides warmth and privacy.

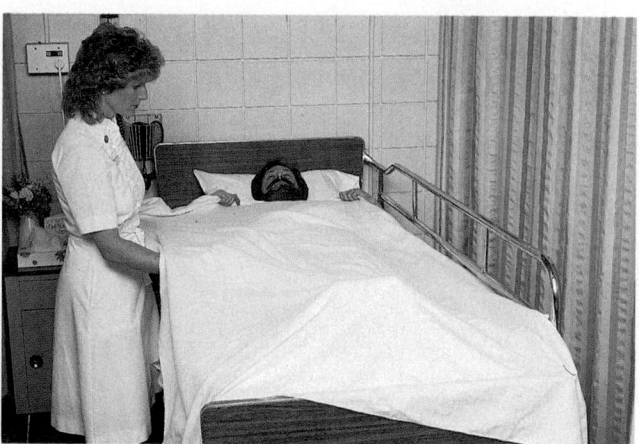

Action 7: Removing top linens from under bath blanket.

Action	Rationale
8 Grasp mattress securely and shift it up to the head of the bed (you may require the assistance of another person).	This allows more foot room for the client and positions the mattress against the head of the bed.
9 Assist the client to turn toward the opposite side of the bed and reposition the pillow under the client's head.	This allows the bed to be made on the vacant side.
10 Loosen all bottom linens from the head and sides of the bed.	This facilitates removal of linens.
11 Fan-fold soiled linens as close to the client as possible.	This facilitates removal of linens when the client turns to the other side.
12 Use clean linen and make near side of bed following actions 9, 10, and 11 of Procedure 29-3. Fan-fold the clean linen as close to the client as possible.	This positions clean linen to make the side of the bed.

(continued)

P R O C E D U R E 2 9 - 4 (continued)

Making an Occupied Bed

Action	Rationale

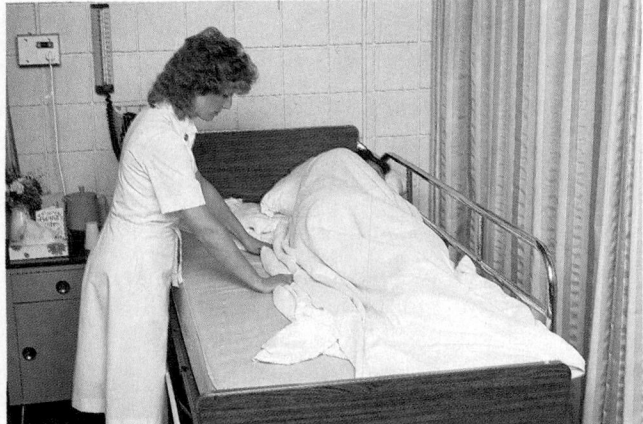

Action 11: Fanfolding soiled linen close to client.

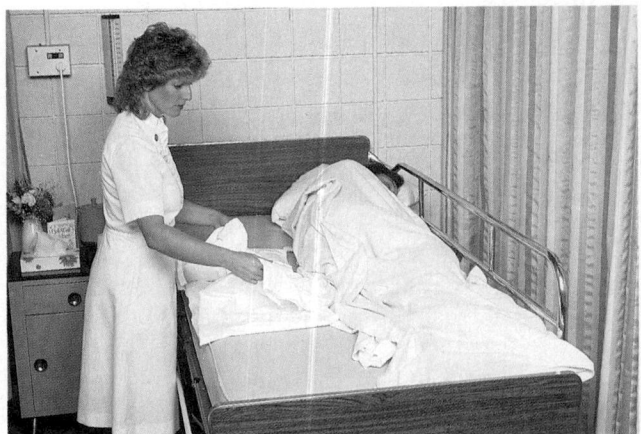

Action 12: Unfolding clean linens.

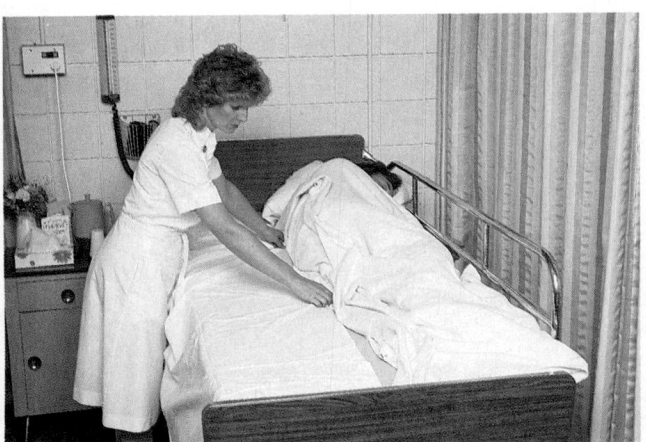

Action 12: Aligning clean bottom sheet on half of bed.

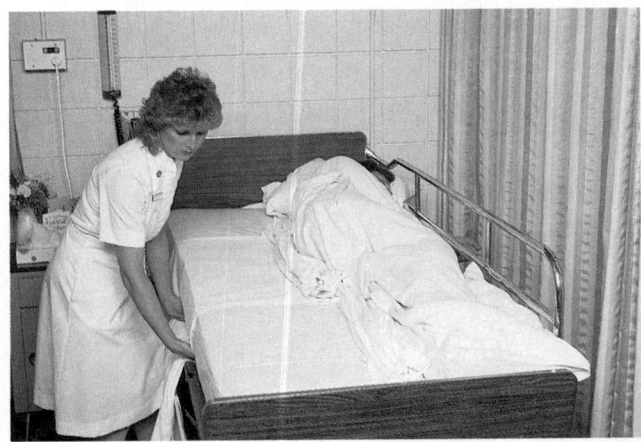

Action 12: Tucking bottom sheet and drawsheet tightly.

13 Raise the side rail. Move to the other side of the bed and lower the side rail. Assist the client to roll over the folded linen in the middle of the bed and toward the other side. Reposition the pillow and bath blanket or top sheet.

This ensures client safety. The movement allows the bed to be made on the other side. The bath blanket provides warmth and privacy.

14 Loosen and remove all bottom linen. Place these in a linen bag or hamper. Hold soiled linen away from your uniform.

Proper disposal of soiled linen prevents spread of micro-organisms.

15 Ease the clean linen from under the client. Pull taut and secure the bottom sheet under the head of the mattress. Miter corners. Pull the side of the sheet taut and tuck under the side of the mattress. Repeat this with the drawsheet.

This removes wrinkles and creases in the linens, which are uncomfortable to lie on.

16 Assist the client to return to the center of the bed. Remove the pillow and change the pillowcase before replacing, with open end facing toward the window.

This provides for a neater appearance.

(continued)

PROCEDURE 29-4 *(continued)*

Making an Occupied Bed

Action	**Rationale**

17 Apply top linen so that it is centered and top hems are even with the head of the mattress. Have the client hold onto the top linen so the bath blanket can be removed.

This allows bottom hems to be tucked securely under the mattress and provides for privacy.

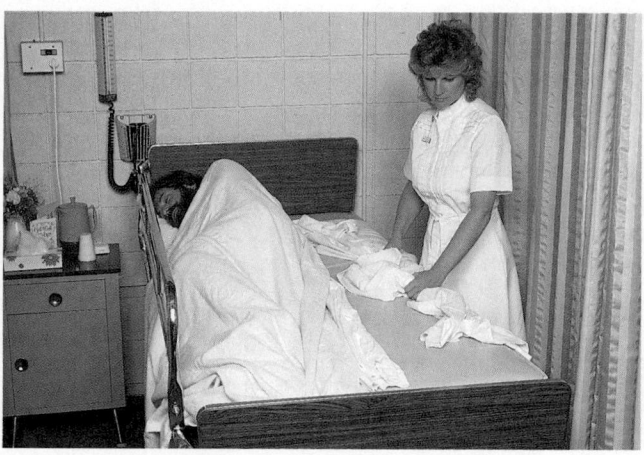

Action 14: Removing soiled bottom linens from other side of bed.

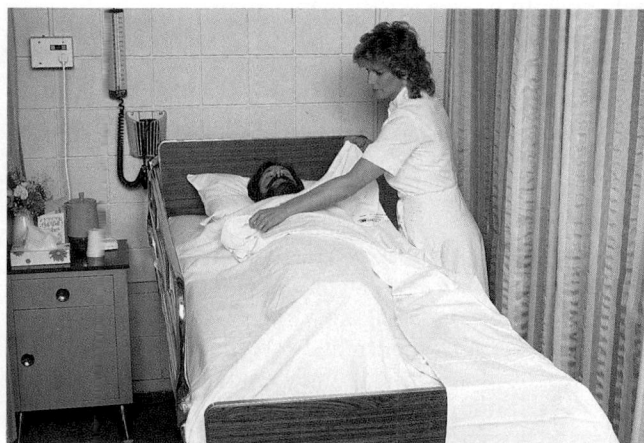

Action 17: Applying top linen over bath blanket.

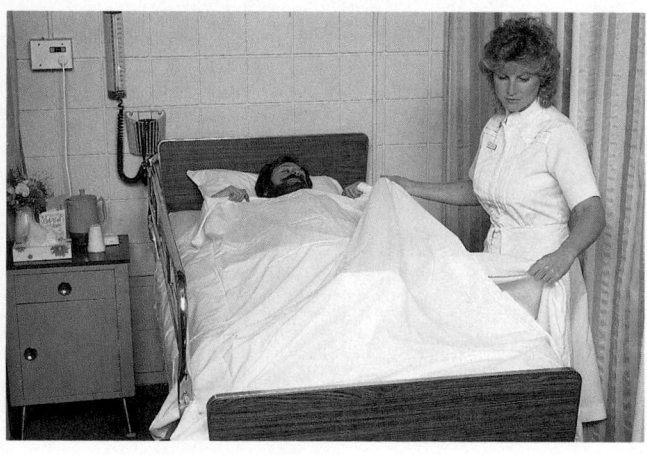

Action 17: Removing the bath blanket from under the top linens.

18 Secure top linens under the foot of the mattress and miter corners. Loosen top linens over the client's feet by grasping them in the area of the feet and pulling gently toward the foot of the bed.

This provides for a neat appearance. Loosening linens over the client's feet gives more room for movement.

19 Raise the side rail. Lower bed height and adjust the head of the bed to a comfortable position. Reattach call bell and drainage tubes.

This provides for the client's safety.

20 Dispose of soiled linens according to agency policy. Wash your hands.

This prevents spread of microorganisms.

Age Considerations

Use of a synthetic sheepskin, a soft bath blanket, or flannelette blanket as a bottom sheet may solve the problem of "coldness" for elderly clients with vascular problems or arthritis.

Ventilation and Odors   Because of all the pathogens in hospitals and unpleasant odors associated with body secretions and excretions (ie, urine, stool, vomitus, draining wounds, or body odors), good ventilation in client rooms is imperative. Because many clients are sensitive to drafts, it is often wise to air the room during times when clients are out of their rooms for diagnostic or therapeutic procedures. Odors may be decreased by promptly emptying bedpans, urinals, and emesis basins, and by being careful not to dispose of soiled dressings or anything with a strong odor in the waste receptacle in the client's room. Deodorizers may need to be used.

Room Temperature   Whenever possible, client preferences (which may vary widely) should be followed regarding room temperature. In general, the room temperature should fall between 20° and 23°C (68° and 74°F).

Lighting and Noise   Because many clients find it difficult to sleep in a hospital and may need to be disturbed frequently for assessment or treatment purposes, the nurse should be careful to reduce harsh lighting and noises whenever possible. However, adequate lighting should be provided for all nursing procedures. Clients may enjoy sunlight or find it disturbing, and drapes may be arranged accordingly. Whenever possible, conversations should not be carried on immediately outside the client's room. Many clients find this stressful both because the noise disturbs them and because they believe whatever is being said involves them.

Beds   Because many people who are ill spend a large portion of the day—if not the entire day—in bed, the bed is an important part of the client's environment. Nursing responsibilities include ensuring both a safe and comfortable bed.

Bed Safety   The typical hospital bed has a motorized metal frame in three sections, which allows the height of the bed to be raised or lowered as well as the head and foot of the bed to be adjusted. It is important that the nurse know how to operate the bed and explain this to the client. Bed positions are described in Chapter 30. Because certain positions may actually be harmful to some clients, the client and family should be instructed about advisable bed positions and use of the bed controls. Hospital beds are generally 66 cm (26 inches) from the floor. This is higher than most beds at home and enables the nurse to reach the client without undue musculoskeletal strain.

Whenever the client's condition indicates the need for upper or lower side rails, these should be used to prevent dangerous falls. The wheels (or casters) on the hospital bed should be locked whenever the bed is stationary to prevent the bed from slipping away from a client who is transferring from the bed to an upright position or to a stretcher. The headboard of most hospital beds is removable to allow close client contact in an emergency situation. Before leaving the client's bedside, ensure the following:

- The bed is in its lowest position
- The bed position is safe for the client
- The bed controls are functioning (bed is electrically safe)
- Side rails (upper and lower) are raised if indicated
- The wheels or casters are locked

Bed Comfort   The hospital mattress is firm and generally covered with a water-repellent material that can be easily wiped down with a bactericidal solution between clients. Many clients find it uncomfortable to rest with just a sheet between them and the rubberized mattress; thus, the nurse may need to find creative solutions—especially for clients at high risk for impaired skin integrity. The egg-crate mattress (Fig. 29-3, *top*) is often an acceptable solution. Clients with arthritis and vascular problems often find the rubberized mattress cold; the use of sheepskin (Fig. 29-3, *bottom*) or a soft bath blanket or flannelette blanket used under or as a substitute for the bottom sheet may solve this problem. Pillows covered with water-repellent material can be especially uncomfortable to clients. Clients spend-

F I G U R E   2 9 - 3

The egg-crate mattress (top) adds to comfort and helps distribute body weight evenly to reduce the risk of pressure sores. Sheepskin (bottom) placed over the bottom sheet is softer and warmer than just a bottom sheet over the rubberized mattress.

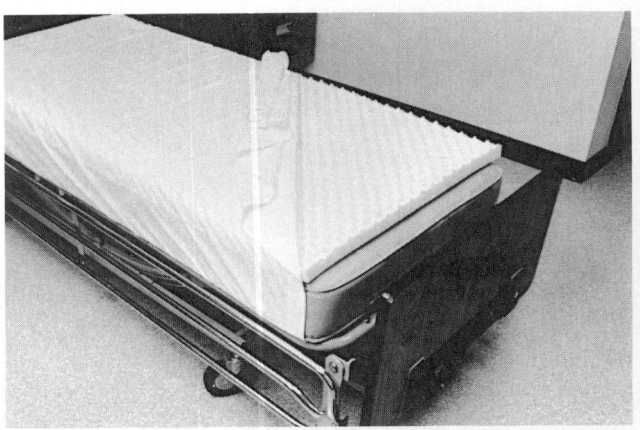

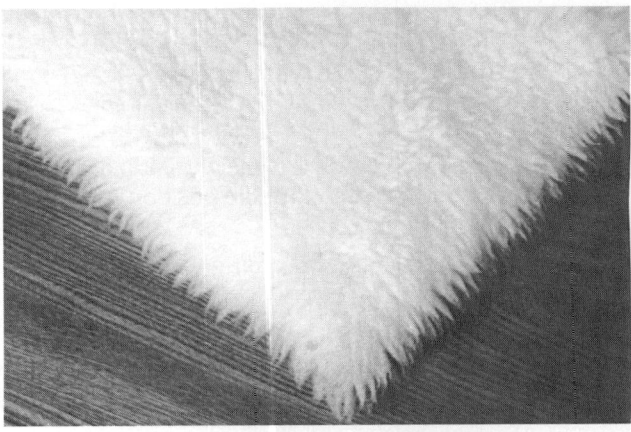

ing many days in bed may find that having a pillow from home greatly aids their rest.

Agency policies usually dictate the availability and use of bed linens. Bed linens include mattress covers, sheets, drawsheets, incontinent pads, pillow cases, blankets, bedspreads, and bath blankets. Towels, washcloths, and client gowns are often included in linen packs. Devices to support and protect the client confined to bed are described in Chapter 30. In some settings, making the bed is not nursing's responsibility. However, ensuring client comfort is always a priority in nursing, and this often involves creating a comfortable bed environment. Before leaving a client, the nurse should ensure the following:

- Linens are clean and wrinkle free
- The client feels comfortably warm
- Pressure points on the client at High Risk for Impaired Skin Integrity are protected from rough sheets, hem edges, and water-repellent materials

Teaching Clients About Skin Problems and Skin Care

The nurse can share information with the client during assessment and care procedures. Occasionally, clients ask for specific information. The following section concerns skin problems and skin care.

Skin Problems

Dry Skin Dry skin is characteristically flaky and is easily susceptible to injury and irritation. Suggestions for people whose skin is dry and injured easily are the following:

- Bathe less frequently, especially when the outdoor temperature and humidity are low.
- Rinse off soaps or detergents well when they are used for cleansing the skin. Residue left on the skin predisposes to skin irritation and breakdown.
- Avoid defatting agents, such as alcohol, on dry and easily injured skin.
- Avoid wearing garments made of woolen fabrics because wool tends to irritate dry skin.
- Wash garments made of wrinkle-resistant fabrics once or twice before wearing them. The chemical impregnated in the fabric tends to irritate dry skin.
- Add moisture to the air through a humidifier when the skin is dry.
- Increase fluid intake when the skin is dry.
- Try using a bath oil when the skin is dry. These oils make bathtubs slippery, and care should be used to prevent falls. Bubble bath preparations, which often contain oil, should be mixed well in the bath water before the person sits in the tub. Urinary tract infections have been correlated with the use of bubble bath preparations.
- Use an **emollient**, an agent used to soften, soothe, and protect dry skin, after cleansing the skin. Emollient or moisturizing creams do not add moisture to the skin. Rather, the film they leave on the skin retards normal moisture evaporation and helps to hold down the scaly skin surfaces. Cocoa butter, petroleum

jelly, and lanolin are examples of effective emollients that are used in many emollient creams.

- Use creams to clean skin that is dry or allergic to soaps and detergents.

Acne Oily skin is especially bothersome during adolescence, when hormones cause enlargement of the sebaceous glands and increased glandular secretions. Blackheads and pustules appear when these secretions become dammed up in the sebaceous ducts, and inflammation with infection occurs. The condition is referred to as **acne** and most often appears on the face, neck, shoulders, and back. From a health standpoint, acne is not a serious condition, although it can lead to permanent scarring and psychological problems for the person suffering from it. There are various recommended ways to help control acne and minimize scarring:

- The infected areas should not be squeezed or picked. This tends to cause a spread of the infection and scarring of the skin.
- The person with acne should wash the skin and shampoo hair with soap or detergent and hot water frequently to remove oil and debris.
- Oily cosmetics, cleansing creams, and emollients should be avoided. They tend to make the condition worse.
- Cosmetics should be used sparingly to avoid further blocking of sebaceous gland ducts.
- Exposure to an ultraviolet lamp may occasionally be prescribed to help keep acne under control. However, caution should be exercised to prevent burning the skin.
- Foods that are found to aggravate the condition should be eliminated from the diet. Chocolate, nuts, cola beverages, and foods containing iodine tend to make acne worse for some people.

In severe cases, the services of a physician are recommended. Treatment modalities vary.

Prescribed combination therapies that control the clinical manifestations of acne may result in **erythema** (redness) and skin peeling. Sun exposure during some of these treatments may be dangerous and cause an exaggerated sunburn.

Skin Rashes Rashes are eruptions or inflammations of the skin that may be found anywhere on the body. Rashes may be precipitated by the skin's contact with an allergen (eg, chemicals in cleansers and soaps) or by overexposure to the sun or to moisture. They may also result from systemic causes such as the body's response to medications or to certain diseases. Rashes may be described as flat or raised, pruritic or nonpruritic, localized or systemic, dry or wet. Scratching a rash may result in inflammation and infection. Interventions include the following:

- Wash the area thoroughly with a mild cleansing agent and rinse well.
- Use a moisturizing lotion on a dry rash to prevent itching and to promote healing.

- Use a drying agent on a wet rash.
- Tepid baths or soaks may relieve inflammation and itching.
- Antiseptic sprays or lotions may be useful in lessening itching, promoting healing, and preventing skin breakdown.
- A number of over-the-counter products such as Caladryl (benedryl hydrochloride) lotion and hydrocortisone creams may be useful, depending on the nature of the rash. Read the manufacturer's recommendations and cautions before testing a new product.
- If the causative agent is known, avoid exposure to it.
- Refer to a physician if symptoms do not respond to treatment.

Pressure Ulcers **Pressure ulcers** are areas of cellular necrosis caused by the lack of blood circulation to the involved area. At best, they are extremely painful and debilitating to clients and at worst they may be life-threatening. They offer a persistent challenge to even the most experienced nurse. Preventing pressure ulcers whenever possible and identifying and treating them at the earliest stage possible are critical nursing responsibilities. This topic is explored in detail at the end of this chapter.

Skin Care

Soaps, Detergents, and Creams A great variety of soaps and detergents are available. Expensive cleansing agents have not been found to be superior to the less expensive ones. For most people, the best way to cleanse the skin is with soap or detergent and water. Soaps are often made from vegetable and animal fats. Most detergents are made from petroleum derivatives and are especially satisfactory when the water is hard, cold, or salty. People who

R E S E A R C H   I N   N U R S I N G   Making a Difference

Personal Hygiene

An integral component of self-esteem and comfort in clients who are unable to carry out self-care activities is nursing intervention aimed at maintaining skin integrity to prevent skin breakdown and facilitating healing when breakdown has occurred. Nursing research has been carried out to examine this problem from various perspectives.

Related Research

Neal, M. (1990). A cost-effective alternative to specialty beds for pressure relief. *Rehabilitation Nursing, 15*(4), 202–204.

The study examined the ability of an inflatable air mattress overlay to reduce pressure exerted on a client's trochanter area. Two types of inflatable mattresses had a positive effect on diminishing tissue pressures for clients on bedrest. The author reported that use of the air mattresses rather than the more costly specialty beds significantly decreased client charges and proved beneficial for clients at risk of developing pressure ulcers.

Neander, K., & Birkenfeld, A. (1990). Alternating-pressure mattresses for the prevention of decubitus ulcers: a study of healthy subjects and patients. *Intensive Care Nursing, 6*(2), 67–73.

These authors addressed the effectiveness of using alternating-pressure mattresses for intensive care clients at risk of developing a decubitus or pressure ulcer. Measurement of sacral tissue pressure on healthy test subjects confirmed that mechanical pressure on the skin does cause a decrease in tissue oxygen pressures and blood supply to the skin.

Though duration of pressure may be significant, more than 20% of clients on an alternating-pressure mattress while in an intensive care unit developed a pressure ulcer. Results of this study did not support the continued use of this prophylactic device.

Kemp, M., Keithley, J., Smith, D., & Morreale, B. (1990). Factors that contribute to pressure sores in surgical patients. *Research in Nursing and Health, 13,* 293–301.

The study focused on identifying clients at risk for developing a decubitus ulcer while undergoing surgery. Statistics indicate that figure at between 13% and 17%. Compromised tissue perfusion was indirectly measured using a formula that related to the number of times during surgery that the client's diastolic blood pressure was below 60 mm Hg. As a result of this research the authors identified age, time on the operating table, and extracorporeal circulation (process of circulating blood outside the body through a hemodializer or heart–lung machine) as significant risk factors leading to pressure ulcer formation in surgical clients.

Summary

Nursing care is often implemented to maintain skin integrity in clients on bedrest for any extended time. The use of these findings can help nurses discover which therapeutic devices (special mattresses) are more beneficial in preventing the development of pressure ulcers and help identify clients undergoing surgery who are more at risk for developing pressure ulcers. This research and future research can assist nurses to recognize and manage clients with altered skin integrity.

are sensitive to soap often find they can use detergents without difficulty.

Cold creams usually consist of an oil or wax, water, and perfume. The cream feels cold because the water evaporates, producing a feeling of coolness. The oil and wax liquify on the skin and loosen and suspend dirt, oily secretions, perspiration, bacteria, cosmetics, dead cells, and other foreign material. They are then removed with a tissue or a soft cloth. Cleansing creams are similar to cold creams except they contain little or no water.

Deodorants and Antiperspirants Perspiration is essentially odorless, although it contains some waste products, such as uric acid and ammonia. The odor of perspiration occurs when bacteria, normally present on everyone's skin, act on the skin's normal secretions.

Keeping the body and clothing clean is the prime requisite for preventing body odors. Deodorants and antiperspirants may be used *after* the skin is clean. Antiperspirants are intended to reduce the amount of perspiration. They act as astringents and tend to close the exits of the sweat glands. Antiperspirants and deodorants should be used with care and according to directions to prevent irritation of the skin.

Cosmetics Cosmetics frequently enhance the appearance of clean and healthy skin, although certain cultural and religious groups may not believe so. Cosmetics used judiciously help disguise blemishes, improve skin coloring, and make wrinkles appear less obvious. Creams and lotions made by reputable concerns are safe to use.

Periodically, cosmetics containing harmful ingredients, such as various dyes used to color cosmetics, have appeared on the market. The nurse should be alert to such agents and help consumers avoid their use. The U.S. Department of Health and Human Services, Food and Drug Administration (FDA), enforces federal laws on the purity of foods, drugs, and cosmetics and on the advertising claims of their manufacturers. The FDA is a good source of information about these products. Similar agencies exist in Canada.

Cosmetics often become contaminated with bacteria and fungus. It is best to discard cosmetics after they are about 4 months old, especially those applied near the eyes. Make-up applicators and puffs should be kept immaculately clean. Cosmetics should not be shared.

Evaluating

Daily contacts with the client while hygiene measures are being performed enable the nurse to frequently evaluate whether the client is meeting hygiene goals. Evaluative criteria include the following:

- Level of client's participation in hygiene program
- Elimination, reduction in or compensation for factors interfering with the client's independent execution of hygiene measures (eg, weakness, decreased motivation, lack of knowledge)

- Client's achievement of goals related to specific skin problems, by giving attention to the healing of skin lesions, the elimination or reduction of causative factors, and the client's ability to manage the prescribed treatment program independently

Oral Care

The mouth is the first part of the alimentary canal and is an adjunct of the respiratory system. The ducts of the salivary glands open into the vestibule of the mouth. The teeth and the tongue are accessory organs in the mouth and play an important role in beginning digestion by breaking up food particles and mixing them with saliva. Saliva is also important as a mechanical cleaner of the mouth.

General good health is as essential as cleanliness for maintaining a healthy mouth and teeth. The relationship, for example, between good teeth and a diet sufficient in calcium and phosphorus along with vitamin D, which is necessary for the body to use these minerals, is well established.

There are several benefits for maintaining good oral hygiene and dental care. There is aesthetic value in having a clean and healthy mouth. Having one's own teeth contributes to an intact body image. The beginning of the digestive process and gustatory pleasure are enhanced when the mouth and teeth are in good condition.

Assessing

Nursing History Identify the client's normal oral hygiene practices—brushing, flossing, use of rinses, presence and care of dentures or other orthodontic devices, frequency of dental examinations, and variables influencing these practices. Note the history of any oral problems and related treatments.

Physical Assessment Examine the lips for color, moisture, lumps, ulcers, lesions, and edema. Examine the buccal mucosa for color, moisture, lesions, nodules, and bleeding. Examine the color of the gums and surface of the gums for lesions, bleeding, edema, and exudate. Examine for loose, missing, or carious (decayed) teeth. Note the presence of dentures or other orthodontic devices. Examine the tongue for color, symmetry, movement, texture, and lesions. Examine the hard and soft palates for intactness, color, patches, lesions, and petechiae. Examine the oropharynx for movement of the uvula and condition of tonsils, if present. Note unusual mouth odors. Assess adequacy of mastication and swallowing.

High-Risk Variables Identify any variables known to cause oral problems, such as deficient self-care abilities, poor nutrition and excessive intake of refined sugars, family history of periodontal disease, or ingestion of chemotherapeutic agents that produce oral lesions. Clients at high risk for oral problems include those who are seriously ill, comatose, dehydrated, confused, depressed, or paralyzed. Clients who are mouth breathers, who can have no oral intake of nutrition or fluids, who have nasogastric tubes or oral airways in place, and who have had oral surgery are also at increased risk.

Common Oral Problems

When inspecting the oral cavity, the nurse frequently observes oral problems that at best are benign and only mildly annoying to clients but that may also be life threatening. It is imperative to identify the problem and its cause and to initiate the appropriate treatment. This may require consultation with a dentist or physician.

Dental Caries   The decay of teeth with the formation of cavities is called **caries**. Caries result from the failure to remove **plaque**, an invisible, destructive, bacterial film that builds up on everyone's teeth and eventually leads to the destruction of tooth enamel. A successful plaque-fighting program includes elimination of sweet snacks between meals, such as soft drinks, candy, gum, jams, and jellies; thorough cleansing; and regular dental checkups. The use of antiplaque, fluoride toothpastes and mouth rinses helps prevent dental caries.

Periodontal Disease   The major cause of tooth loss in adults older than age 35 years is gum disease. **Gingivitis** is an inflammation of the **gingiva**, the tissue that surrounds the teeth.

Pyorrhea, or **periodontal disease**, is a marked inflammation of the gums and also involves the alveolar tissues. Symptoms include bleeding gums; swollen, red, painful gum tissues; receding gum lines with the formation of pockets between the teeth and gums; pus that appears when gums are pressed; and loose teeth. If unchecked, plaque builds up and, along with dead bacteria, forms hard deposits called **tartar** at the gum lines. The tartar attacks the fibers that fasten teeth to the gums and eventually attacks bone tissue also. The teeth then loosen and fall out. A strong mouth odor (**halitosis**) or persistent bad taste in the mouth may be the first indication of periodontal disease. Regular dental treatment by a dentist is imperative.

Other Oral Problems   Other oral problems that the nurse may observe when inspecting the oral cavity include the following:

Stomatitis is an inflammation of the oral mucosa with numerous causes, such as bacteria, virus, mechanical trauma, irritants, nutritional deficiencies, and systemic infection. Symptoms may include heat, pain, increased flow of saliva, and halitosis. Manifestations include such diverse problems as aphthous ulcers; herpetic ulcers (fever blisters); fungal ulcers (*Candida albicans*—induced thrush); and chemotherapy-induced stomatitis.

Glossitis is an inflammation of the tongue.

Cheilosis is an ulceration of the lips (reddened fissures at the angles of the mouth) most often caused by vitamin B complex deficiencies (especially riboflavin).

Dry oral mucosa may simply be related to dehydration or may be caused by mouth breathing, an alteration in salivary functioning, or by certain medications (eg, anticholinergic drugs).

Oral malignancies appear as lumps or ulcers; it is critical that these be distinguished from benign mouth problems because early detection may be the difference between cure and radical dissecting surgery and death. Teach clients if they notice white or red patches, persistent sores, swelling, bleeding, numbness, or pain in the mouth to see their dentist immediately.

Diagnosing

Make a judgment about the adequacy of the client's oral hygiene practices, identifying any factors contributing to deficiencies. An example is as follows:

Self-Care Deficit: Oral Hygiene, related to low value attached to regular brushing, flossing, and dental examinations

Identify actual or potential oral problems that nurses can treat, noting contributing factors. Identify unhealthy client responses to oral problems. Examples include:

Pain related to chemotherapy-induced oral ulceration

High Risk for Infection related to breaks in oral mucosa and inadequate secondary defenses

Altered Nutrition: Less Than Body Requirements, related to painful oral lesions (ill-fitting dentures, gingivitis)

Altered Oral Mucous Membrane related to dehydration (ineffective oral hygiene, medication)

Impaired Swallowing related to neuromuscular impairment

Body Image Disturbance related to loss of teeth, halitosis, or dental caries

Planning: Client Goals

Identify nursing measures that will assist the client to develop or maintain oral hygiene practices to promote oral health and general well-being and resolve identified nursing diagnoses. Plan to achieve the following client goals. The client will:

- Have lips, oral mucosa, gums, and tongue that are intact, moist, and free of inflammation and lesions
- Have clean teeth (or dentures)
- Demonstrate the ability to masticate and swallow food
- Demonstrate signs of healing of oral lesions
- Demonstrate correct oral hygiene measures—brushing and flossing
- Verbalize importance of fluoride use and regular dental examinations

Pertinent nursing measures to include in the care plan are the following:

- Teach proper brushing and flossing techniques; instruct clients about fluoride use and the importance of regular dental examinations.
- Teach correct denture care or provide this when necessary.
- Perform mouth care for the unconscious client (clean the mouth with swabs dipped in dilute mouth rinse or in a solution of one part hydrogen peroxide to one to three parts water; suction as necessary to prevent aspiration; apply a petroleum jelly to the lips).
- Perform mouth care for clients with oral lesions (cleanse to prevent infection and numbing if indicated to encourage eating).

In the care plan, identify any supplies needed to carry out the specified oral care and the timing and frequency of oral hygiene measures.

Implementing

While carrying out the care plan, the nurse uses each nurse–client interaction for ongoing assessment of the client's oral cavity and evaluation of the adequacy of the care plan. Techniques for administering and teaching oral care are described in this section. See the accompanying display for sample documentation of oral hygiene care.

Administering Oral Hygiene

The mouth must be cared for even during illness. However, there are times when care must be modified to meet the specific needs of a client. If the client is able to assist with mouth care while bedridden, the nurse provides necessary materials (Procedure 29-5). If the client is helpless, the nurse needs to make certain that attention is given to the client's mouth as often as necessary to keep it clean and moist, as often as every hour or two, if necessary. This is especially true for clients who are unable or are not permitted fluids by mouth. Procedure 29-6 gives techniques for administering oral hygiene to the dependent client. The nurse should wear disposable gloves when giving oral care to prevent exposure to blood and blood-borne infections such as AIDS and hepatitis B. Moisten the mouth with water, if allowed, and lubricate the lips sufficiently frequently to keep the membranes well moistened.

Sample Documentation of Oral Hygiene

10/20/93   Client generally breathes with mouth open. Sordes present on palate, teeth, gums, and oral mucosa. Toothettes dipped in 1 part hydrogen peroxide to 3 parts water solution used for cleansing every 4 hours. Lubricating jelly to lips.

C. Moser, RN

The procedure of cleaning the mouth thoroughly is more important than the agent used. This supports the personal experience of many people that no mouthwash, breath freshener, ointment, or paste replaces a thorough mechanical cleaning of the oral cavity.

Denture Care   Keeping dentures out for long periods permits the gum line to change, thus affecting their fit. If the client has been instructed to remove dentures while sleeping, a disposable denture cup is convenient and easy to use. Dentures should not be wrapped in toilet tissue or disposable wipes because these are likely to be thrown away. It is recommended that dentures be stored in water to prevent drying and warping of plastic materials (Fig. 29-4). A deodorant solution of water and a few drops of ammonia or white vinegar can be used. A few drops of essence of peppermint may be added also. Dentures made of vulcanite, which is a porous material, are especially prone to develop unpleasant odors.

The person with dentures is more likely to keep them in the mouth when dentures are kept clean. When the client is unable to care for them, the nurse is responsible for ensuring that dentures are clean. Care should be exercised when handling a client's dentures. They represent a considerable financial investment, and damage or loss becomes expensive. When cleaning dentures, the nurse should don gloves and hold them over a basin of water or over a soft towel so that if they slip from the nurse's grasp, they will not fall onto a hard surface and break. Warm water should be used to cleanse them. Hot water may warp the plastic material from which most dentures are made. The use of a brush and a nonabrasive powder or paste is also recommended.

(*Text continues on p. 611*)

FIGURE 29-4

Dentures should be stored in water to prevent warping. Many health care agencies provide denture cups for storage and cleaning. Soaking dentures in special cleaning preparations helps remove stains and hardened particles.

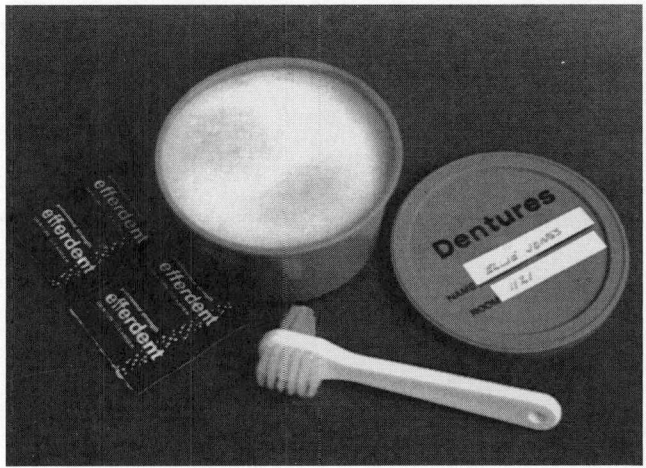

P R O C E D U R E 2 9 - 5

Assisting the Client With Oral Care

Equipment

Toothbrush
Toothpaste
Emesis basin
Glass with cool water
Disposable gloves
Towel
Mouthwash (optional)
Dental floss (optional)

Denture-cleansing equipment (if
necessary)
Denture cup
Denture cleaner
4 × 4 gauze
Washcloth or paper towel
Petroleum jelly (optional)

Action	Rationale
1 Explain the procedure to the client.	Explanation facilitates cooperation.
2 Wash your hands. Don disposable gloves if assisting with oral care.	Handwashing deters the spread of microorganisms. Gloves protect the nurse from exposure to blood and blood-borne infections.
3 Assemble equipment on an overbed table within the client's reach.	Organization facilitates performance of task.
4 Provide privacy for the client.	Client may be embarrassed if cleansing involves removal of dentures.
5 Lower side rail and assist client to sitting position if permitted, or turn the client onto the side. Place the towel across the client's chest. Raise the bed to a comfortable working position.	The sitting or side-lying position prevents aspiration of fluids into the lungs. The towel protects the client from dampness.
6 Encourage the client to brush own teeth or assist if necessary:	
a Moisten the toothbrush and apply toothpaste to bristles.	Water softens the bristles.
b Place brush at a 45-degree angle to gum line and brush from gum line to crown of each tooth. Brush outer and inner surfaces. Brush back and forth across biting surface of each tooth.	This facilitates removal of plaque and tartar. The 45-degree angle of brushing permits cleansing of all surface areas of the tooth.

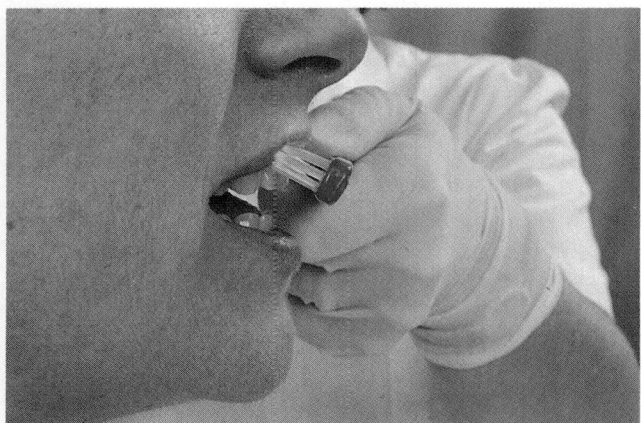

Action 6b: Placing brush at a 45-degree angle to the gum line.

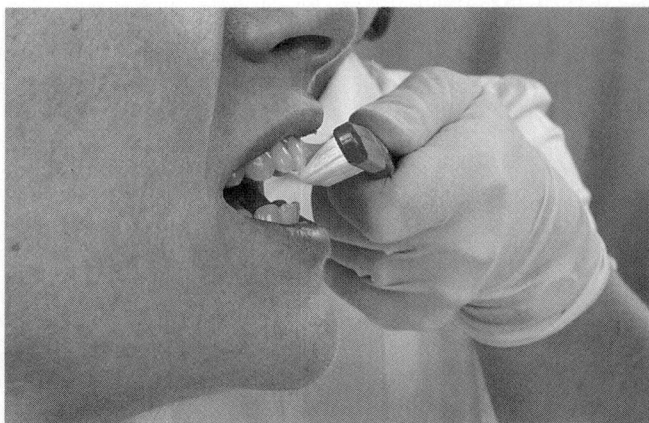

Action 6b: Brushing from the gum line to the crown of each tooth.

(continued)

Assisting the Client With Oral Care

Action	Rationale
c Brush tongue gently with toothbrush.	This removes coating on the tongue. Gentle motion does not stimulate gag reflex.
d Have the client rinse vigorously with water and spit into emesis basin. Repeat until clear.	The vigorous swishing motion helps to remove debris.
e Assist the client to floss teeth if necessary.	Flossing aids in removal of plaque and promotes healthy gum tissue.
f Offer mouthwash if the client prefers.	Mouthwash leaves a pleasant taste in the mouth.
7 Assist the client with removal and cleansing of dentures if necessary:	
a Apply gentle pressure with 4 × 4 gauze to grasp upper denture plate and remove. Place it immediately in the denture cup. Lift the lower denture using slight rocking motion, remove, and place in the denture cup.	Rocking motion breaks suction between the denture and gum. Using 4 × 4 gauze prevents slippage and discourages spread of microorganisms.
b If the client prefers, add denture cleanser to the cup with water and follow directions on preparation or brush all areas thoroughly with toothbrush and paste. Place paper towels or washcloth in sink while brushing.	Dentures collect food and microorganisms and require daily cleansing. Paper towels or washcloth in the sink protects against breakage.
c Rinse thoroughly with water and return dentures to the client.	Water aids in removal of debris and acts as a cleansing agent.
d Offer mouthwash so client can rinse his or her mouth before replacing dentures.	Mouthwash leaves a pleasant taste in the mouth and removes food particles, thus permitting proper fit of dentures.
e Apply petroleum jelly to lips if needed.	Petroleum jelly prevents cracking and drying of lips.
8 Remove equipment and assist the client to a position of comfort. Record any unusual bleeding or inflammation. Raise side rail and lower the bed.	This promotes oral hygiene and provides for oral assessment. Elevated side rails and lowered bed position maintain safety for bedridden clients.
9 Remove disposable gloves from inside out and discard appropriately. Wash your hands.	This protects the nurse from contact with any microorganism. Handwashing deters spread of microorganisms.

PROCEDURE 29-6

Providing Oral Care for the Dependent Client

Equipment

Toothbrush
Toothpaste
Emesis basin
Disposable gloves
Cup with cool water
Towel
Mouthwash

Denture-cleansing equipment (if necessary)
    Denture cup
    Washcloth or paper towel
Sponge toothette or tongue blades padded with 4 × 4 gauze sponges

Irrigating syringe with rubber tip (optional)
Cleansing agent (hydrogen peroxide to one to three parts water)
Petroleum jelly
Suction catheter with suction apparatus (optional)

(continued)

P R O C E D U R E 2 9 - 6 *(continued)*

Providing Oral Care for the Dependent Client

Action

1 Explain the procedure to the client.

2 Wash your hands and don disposable gloves.

3 Assemble equipment on overbed table within reach.

4 Provide privacy for the client. Adjust the height of the bed to a comfortable position. Lower one side rail and position the client on the side with head turned toward you and tilted toward the mattress. Place the towel across the client's chest and emesis basin in position under the chin.

5 Open the client's mouth and gently insert a padded tongue blade between the back molars if necessary.

Rationale

Explanation facilitates cooperation.

Handwashing and disposable gloves deter the spread of microorganisms.

Organization facilitates performance of task.

The side-lying position with head turned down prevents aspiration of fluid into lungs. Towel and emesis basin protect client from dampness.

Padded tongue blade keeps mouth open for easier cleaning and prevents the client from biting the nurse's fingers.

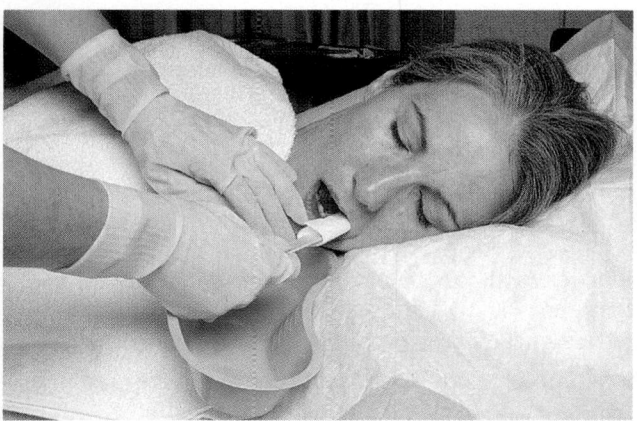

Action 5: Gently inserting padded tongue blade between back molars.

6 If teeth are present, brush carefully with toothbrush and paste. Remove dentures if present and clean before replacing (see action 7 of Procedure 29-5). Use toothette or gauze-padded tongue blade moistened with hydrogen peroxide gently to cleanse gums, mucous membranes, and tongue.

Toothbrush or padded tongue blade provides friction necessary to clean areas where plaque and tartar accumulate. Hydrogen peroxide solution effectively cleans and removes encrustations from the oral cavity.

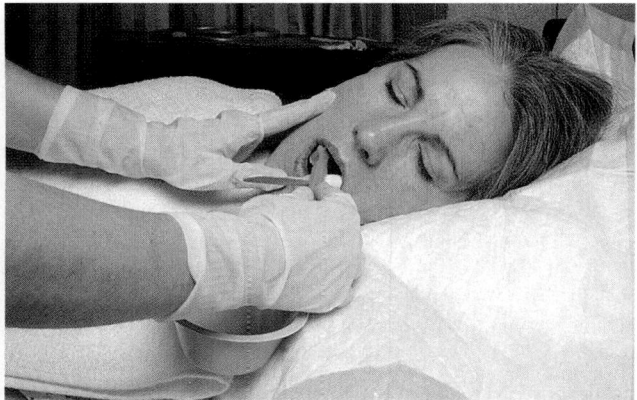

Action 6: Carefully brushing client's teeth.

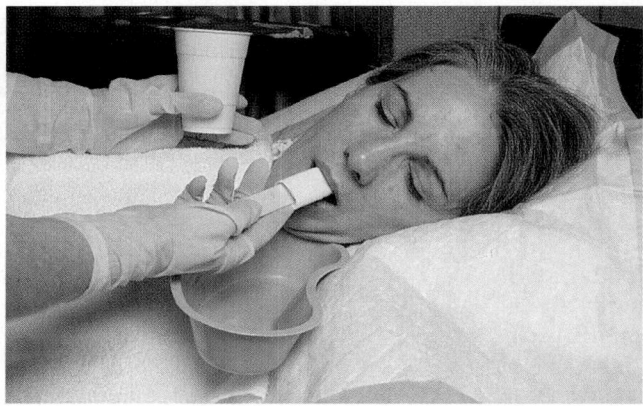

Action 6: Using moistened padded tongue blade to cleanse gums, mucous membranes, and tongue.

(continued)

Providing Oral Care for the Dependent Client

Action	Rationale
7 Use gauze-padded tongue blade dipped in mouthwash solution to rinse the oral cavity. If desired, insert the rubber tip of the irrigating syringe into the client's mouth and rinse gently with a small amount of water. Position the client's head to allow for return of water or use suction apparatus to remove the water from oral cavity.	Rinsing helps to cleanse debris from the mouth. Solution that is forcefully irrigated may cause aspiration.

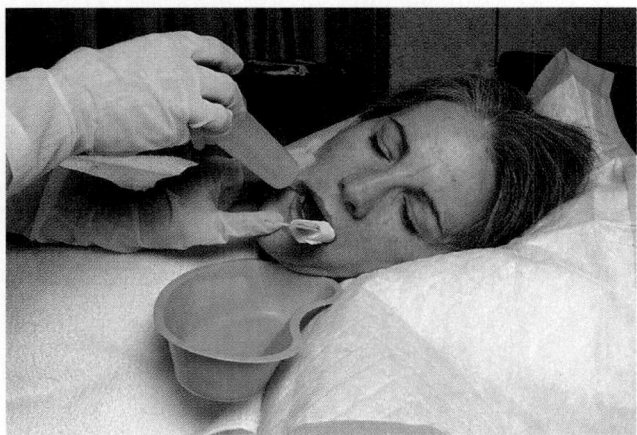

Action 7: Using irrigating syringe and a small amount of water to rinse mouth.

Action	Rationale
8 Apply petroleum jelly to the client's lips.	This prevents drying and cracking of lips.
9 Remove equipment and return the client to a position of comfort. Raise the side rail and lower the bed. Record any unusual bleeding or inflammation.	This promotes oral hygiene and provides for oral assessment. Raised side rail and lowered bed maintain client safety.
10 Wash your hands.	Handwashing deters spread of microorganisms.

Special Considerations

A client receiving chemotherapy medication may have bleeding gums and extremely sensitive mucous membranes. Use a soft sponge toothette for cleaning or substitute a salt water rinse (1/2 teaspoon salt in 1 cup of warm water) for brushing of teeth.

There are also preparations in which to soak dentures to help remove stain and hardened particles. The dentures are rinsed well in warm water after cleaning. The client should be given the opportunity to rinse his or her mouth before the dentures are replaced.

Teaching Oral Hygiene

Toothbrushing and Flossing A toothbrush should be small enough to reach all teeth. The bristles should be sufficiently firm to clean but not so firm that they are likely to injure tooth enamel and gum tissue. Brushes should be cleaned and dried between uses. There is a difference of opinion as to the best way to brush teeth. When assisting and teaching a client, the nurse should follow the preference of the client's

dentist. One recommended brushing regimen is illustrated in Figure 29-5. Most damage is done by bacteria directly after eating. Therefore, it is ideal practice to brush the teeth immediately after eating or drinking. The tongue also should be cleaned with the brush.

Automatic toothbrushes, electric or battery operated, have been found to be simple to use and as good as hand brushes in removing debris and plaque. Waterspray units are available to assist with oral hygiene. However, if an undue amount of water pressure is used, particles of debris may be forced into tissue pockets and damage may occur to gum tissue. Therefore, it is recommended that their use be discussed with a dentist.

The toothbrush cannot effectively reach areas between the teeth where food lodges; hence, flossing once a day is

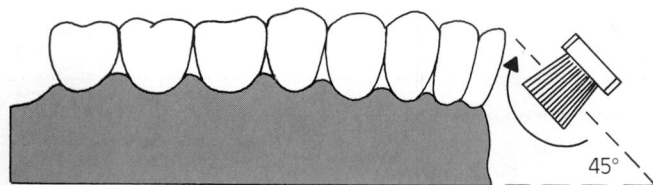

To clean gum line, surfaces, and between teeth, hold the tooth-brush with the bristles at a 45° angle to the gum line and brush from the gum line to the crown of each tooth with a short, semi-circular wrist action.

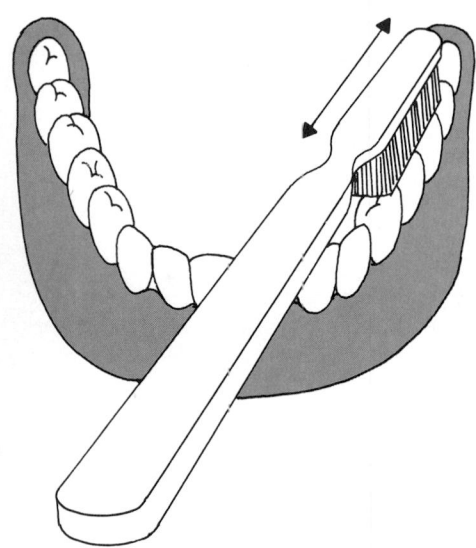

To clean biting and chewing surfaces of the teeth, hold the top of the bristles parallel to the tooth surface and brush back and forth.

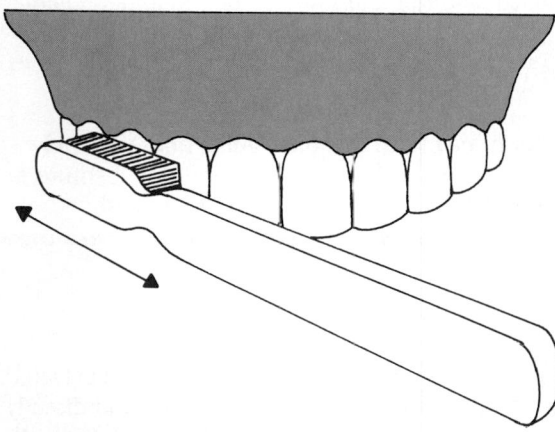

To polish the sides of the teeth, hold the brush bristles parallel to the surface of the teeth and gently brush back and forth.

F I G U R E   2 9 - 5

Techniques for brushing teeth.

recommended. The practice not only removes what the brush cannot but also helps to break up colonies of bacteria. Figure 29-6 illustrates a flossing technique. The following are additional recommended techniques for flossing the teeth:

- Wear gloves when flossing a client's teeth.
- Keep about 1 to 1½ inches of floss held taut between the fingers.
- Do not force the floss between the teeth, but insert it gently by moving it back and forth where teeth touch each other.
- Move the floss up and down while using both fingers, first on the side of one tooth and then on the side of the other tooth, until the surfaces are squeaky clean.
- Go to the gum tissue with the floss but not into the gum, because this may result in discomfort, soreness, or bleeding.

F I G U R E   2 9 - 6

Dental flossing is necessary for removal of plaque and tartar between teeth. Flossing helps prevent gum disease as well as tooth decay by removing debris just below the gum line.

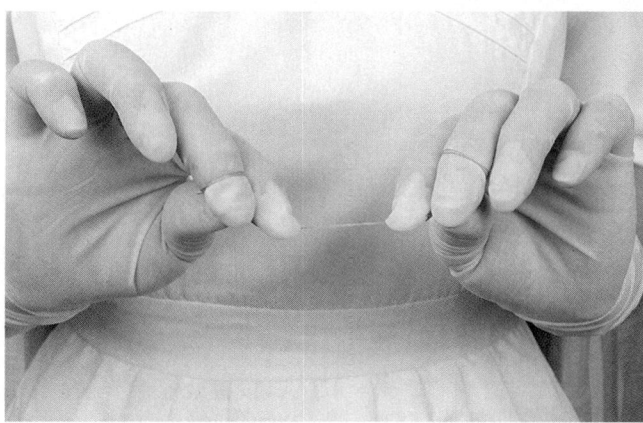

Floss may be wrapped around the middle fingers of each hand or simply grasped in each hand in such a way that it can be stretched and held taut between the controlling fingers.

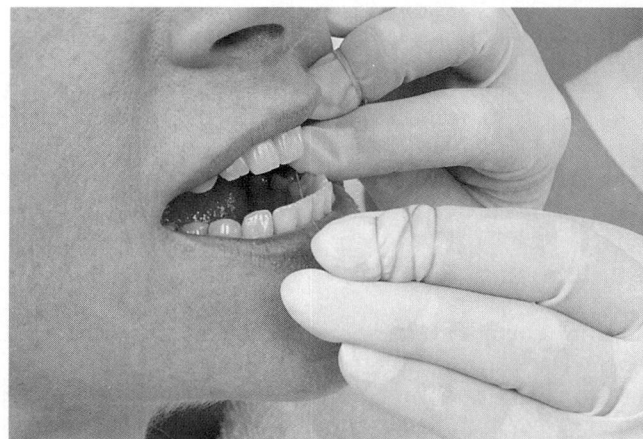

Gently insert the floss between the teeth and move it with a sawing motion up from the gum line along the side of each tooth.

- Advance the floss from one hand to the other to bring up a fresh section of floss when it has become frayed or soiled.
- Rinse the mouth well with water after flossing to remove food particles and plaque that have been loosened. Also, rinse after eating when flossing or brushing is impossible.

Toothpastes and powders aid the brushing process, usually have a pleasant taste, and often encourage brushing, especially among children. Most dentifrices are safe to use, but those containing harsh abrasives may scratch the enamel of the teeth and therefore are not recommended. Salt, sodium bicarbonate, or precipitated chalk are just as effective for cleaning the mouth and the teeth and are far less expensive than proprietary products on the market. Dentifrices containing stannous fluoride and antiplaque rinses have proven to be effective in helping to decrease dental caries and hence are recommended by many dentists.

Mouthwashes An offensive breath or halitosis is often systemic in nature. For example, the odor of onions and garlic on the breath comes from the lungs, where the oils are being removed from the bloodstream and eliminated with respiration. A mouthwash cannot remove halitosis when odors are being eliminated by respiration.

If the cause of halitosis is poor oral hygiene, cleaning reduces the odor. Commercial mouthwashes may be helpful and many people enjoy their fresh aftertaste. If concentrated mouthwashes are used frequently for debilitated clients, they may injure oral tissue, and infection and additional odor may result.

Evaluating

At designated intervals, evaluate whether the client has met the goals established during planning and revise the care plan if indicated. An example follows:

> 10/26/93 Goal partially met. Client's oral mucosa is intact, but thick, dry secretions continue to build on oral mucosa and gums despite q [every] 4 hour care.
> *Revision*: Increase frequency of oral hygiene to q 2 hours. Instruct family.
>
> *N. Glynn, RN*

Care of the Eyes, Ears, and Nose

Assessing

Nursing History Identify any special eye, ear, or nose care the client performs. Include the use and care of visual aids or prostheses (glasses, contact lenses, artificial eye) and hearing aids. Note any history of eye, ear, and nose problems and related treatments.

Physical Assessment In the eye examination, note the position, alignment, and general appearance of the eye. Check that eyelashes are equally distributed and curl outward. Note the presence of lesions, nodules, redness, swelling, crusting, flaking, excessive tearing, or discharge of eyelids. Check the color of the conjunctivae, presence of blink reflex, and visual acuity (ability to read newsprint).

In the ear examination, note the position, alignment, and general appearance of the ear. Pay particular attention to a buildup of wax in the canal, dryness, crusting, or the presence of any discharge or foreign body. Check hearing acuity.

During examination of the nose, note its position and general appearance, patency of nostrils, and presence of tenderness, dryness, edema, bleeding, discharge, or secretions.

Diagnosing

Make a judgment about the adequacy of the client's self-care practices related to eye, ear, and nose care, identifying any factors that contribute to deficiencies. For example,

> Self-Care Deficit: Artificial Eye Care, related to knowledge deficit

Identify actual or potential eye, ear, and nose problems that nurses can treat, noting contributing factors. Identify unhealthy client responses to eye, ear, and nose problems, for example,

> Sensory/Perceptual Alterations (Visual, Auditory, or Olfactory) related to psychologic stress
> Altered Health Maintenance related to perceptual impairment (visual or auditory)
> Impaired Social Interaction related to visual or auditory impairment
> Fear related to sudden loss of vision or hearing
> Anticipatory Grieving related to increasing visual or auditory impairment
> High Risk for Injury related to visual impairment

Planning: Client Goals

Identify nursing measures that will assist the client to develop or maintain eye, ear, and nose care measures that will contribute to healthy eye, ear, and nose functioning and to the client's general sense of well-being. Plan to achieve the following client goals. The client will:

- Demonstrate healthy functioning of eyes, ears, and nose
- Have eyes, ears, and nose that appear clean
- Show signs of healing (if realistic, specify these signs) of sensory impairment (visual, auditory, olfactory), or seek aids appropriate to impairment
- Demonstrate correct eye, ear, and nose care measures, including the proper use and care of visual or auditory aids

Pertinent nursing measures to include in the care plan are as follows:

Eye

- Clean the eye from the **inner canthus** (angle of the eye closest to the nose where the upper and lower lids meet) to the **outer canthus** (lateral angle of the eye where the upper and lower lids meet) using a wet, warm washcloth, cotton ball, or compress to soften crusted secretions. Carefully avoid cross contamination.
- When the blink (corneal) reflex is decreased or absent (eg, in the comatose client), use artificial tear solution or normal saline at least every 4 hours to keep the eyes moist and protected from drying; a protective shield may be necessary to keep the lids closed.
- Offer correct eyeglasses, contact lens, or artificial eye teaching and care.

Ear

- Clean the external ear with a washcloth-covered finger, instructing the client never to insert objects into the ear for cleaning purposes. Use of cotton-tipped swabs is discouraged because they may impact cerumen.
- Assist with the softening and removal of excessive wax deposits.
- Offer hearing aid teaching and care.

Nose

- Clean the nose by instructing the client to blow the nose while both nares are patent (nasal suctioning with a bulb syringe may be indicated) unless contraindicated (eg, following brain surgery or head trauma).
- Remove crusted secretions around the nose and keep this tissue intact by applying a non–water-soluble ointment (eg, petroleum jelly).

In the care plan, identify any supplies needed to carry out the specified eye, ear, and nose care and the timing of these measures.

Implementing

Carry out the care plan, remembering to use each nurse–client interaction for ongoing assessment of the client's eyes, ears, and nose and for evaluation of the adequacy of the care plan. The following sections describe select nursing measures related to eye, ear, and nose care. See accompanying display for sample documentation of eye care.

Cleaning the Eyes

Normally, the eyes are clear and kept clean with lacrimal secretions. During illness, the eyes may produce more secretions than they normally do and appear glasslike. The following techniques are recommended when secretions adhere to the eyelashes and become dry and crusty, or when there is discharge present:
- Wear gloves during the cleaning procedure.
- Use water or normal saline and cotton balls or a clean washcloth or compress to clean the eyes. Boric acid solution, once popular for cleaning the eyes, is no

---

Sample Documentation of Eye Care

10/20/93, nursing
#1 Self-Care Deficit: Care of Artificial Eye, related to knowledge deficit, fear, and nonacceptance

S: "I can't believe they expect me to take care of this eye. I don't even want to touch it."
O: One week postenucleation; to date has not participated in care.
A: Fear, nonacceptance of loss of eye, and lack of knowledge are all limiting client's ability to develop new eye care skills.
P: Encourage client to verbalize feelings about the artificial eye.

Begin to implement the prepared teaching plan for care of an artificial eye.

Demonstrate artificial eye care every morning and encourage a return demonstration until client performs this independently.

N. Glynn, RN

---

longer recommended because of its toxicity when absorbed from mucous membrane. The eyes are never cleaned with soap because of its irritating effects on eye tissues.
- Position the client on the same side as the eye to be cleaned so that solution and debris do not run across the bridge of the nose and contaminate the other eye.
- Dampen a cotton ball with the solution of choice and wipe once while moving the cotton ball from the inner canthus to the outer canthus of the eye. This technique minimizes forcing debris into the area drained by the nasolacrimal duct. Discard the used cotton ball.
- Continue this technique, using one cotton ball for each stroke, until the eye is clean.
- Turn the client to the opposite side and clean the other eye in the same manner.
- Wipe the lashes dry with a paper tissue or a clean washcloth, exposing a clean area of the tissue or cloth with each stroke.

Caring for the Unconscious Client's Eyes

Clients with diminished or absent blink (corneal) reflexes and clients whose eyelids remain open require frequent eye care (at least every 4 hours). If the eye is not kept moist, corneal ulceration may result from excessive drying of the eye. Nursing measures include using saline or artificial tears to lubricate the eye and a protective eye shield to keep the eye closed.

Providing Eyeglasses Care

Eyeglasses are essential for many people and represent a considerable financial investment. The nurse should take precautions to prevent their breakage or loss. Clients needing glasses should be encouraged to wear them to avoid eye strain.

Plastic lenses are popular because they are considerably lighter in weight than glass lenses and as accurate in correction as glass. One disadvantage of plastic is that the material scratches easily.

Eyeglasses should be cleaned over a terry towel so that if they slip they will not become scratched or broken. Glasses are cleaned with warm water and soap, or using a special cleansing preparation. Hot water may warp plastic lenses and frames. The glasses should be rinsed well when cleansed with soap and water. They should be dried with a clean, soft cloth, such as a cotton handkerchief or cotton napkin. Paper products are made of wood pulp and are likely to scratch the lenses. Eyeglasses should not be cleaned with a dry paper tissue or cloth.

Providing Care of Contact Lenses

A contact lens is a small disc worn directly on the eyeball. It stays in place by surface tension of the eye's tears. Contact lenses are either hard or soft. The older hard lenses are not gas permeable whereas newer hard lenses are gas permeable and more comfortable because they allow oxygen to pass directly through the lens to the cornea. Soft lenses are of a plastic material that absorbs water to become soft and pliable. They are brittle when dehydrated and absorb water when placed in solution, usually normal saline, or when in contact with tears. Soft lenses may be used for daily wear or extended wear. Newer disposable soft lenses currently are available.

People wearing contact lenses need to take special precautions to keep them free of microorganisms that may lead to eye infections and to use them in a manner that does not injure or scratch the surface of the eye. Hands must always be washed before touching eye surfaces and lenses. Lens wearers need to be cautious about eye irritation in the presence of noxious vapors or smoke. The lenses should not be in contact with cosmetics, soaps, or hair sprays because eye irritation may result. It is recommended that any adverse reaction to their use be reported to the prescribing physician immediately.

The cornea, which consists of dense connective tissue, does not have its own blood supply. It is nourished primarily by oxygen from the atmosphere and from tears. When wearing contact lenses, the cornea requires more than its normal supply of oxygen because its metabolic rate increases. To allow the cornea to receive a maximal supply of oxygen, hard lenses should be removed before sleeping and should not be worn more than 12 to 16 hours. Extended-wear soft lenses can be left in place for 1 to 30 days, depending on the manufacturer. It is recommended that extended-wear lenses be cleansed at least once weekly.

Excessive tearing, pain, and redness signal the need to remove lenses.

There may be times when the nurse may be required to remove lenses if a client cannot do so. To leave them in place for long periods could result in permanent eye damage. This may occur, for example, when the nurse is attending an unconscious client. Figure 29-7 illustrates and describes how to remove hard and soft contact lenses when the person is unable to do so independently.

Soft lenses are removed by gently grasping the lens near the lower edge, between the forefinger and thumb. Each lens folds up with this technique and is then lifted from the eye. Soft lenses are cleaned, rinsed, and placed in a container of solution for storage. The lenses should be identified as being for the right or left eye because the two lenses are not necessarily identical. The nurse should not try to remove lenses, however, if an eye injury is present, because of the danger of additional injury.

Providing Care of an Artificial Eye

Most clients who wear an artificial eye prefer to take care of it themselves, and they should be encouraged to do so when possible. The necessary equipment includes a small basin, soap and water for washing, and solution for rinsing the prosthesis. Normal saline or tap water can be used for rinsing. Most people have their own method for cleaning the eye socket and the area around it. The nurse should ask the client how he or she does this and make it possible for the client to continue with the usual practice. The client should be lying down so that the eye does not accidentally fall to the floor. The socket is ordinarily flushed with normal saline before replacing the eye.

Providing Ear Care

Other than cleaning the outer ears, little more is needed for routine hygiene of the ear. After the ears are washed, they should be dried carefully with a soft towel so that water and cerumen (wax) are removed by capillary action. Forcing the towel into the ear for drying may aid in the formation of wax plugs.

If a wax plug is present in the auditory canal, it is removed by gentle irrigation of the ear. The stream of water should be directed toward the side of the canal to prevent injury to the drum (see Chapter 42 for the procedure for ear irrigations). Using bobby pins, hairpins, paper clips, or fingernails to remove wax from the ear is extremely dangerous because these may injure or puncture the eardrum.

Hearing Aids If the client uses a hearing aid, batteries should be checked routinely and the earpieces cleaned daily with mild soap and water.

Providing Nose Care

The best way to clean the nose is to blow it gently. Both nostrils should be open while doing this. Closing one nostril adds to the danger of forcing debris into the eustachian

Removing hard contact lenses

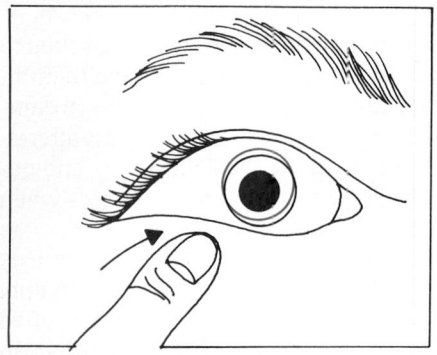

If the lens is not centered over the cornea, apply gentle pressure on the lower eyelid to center the lens.

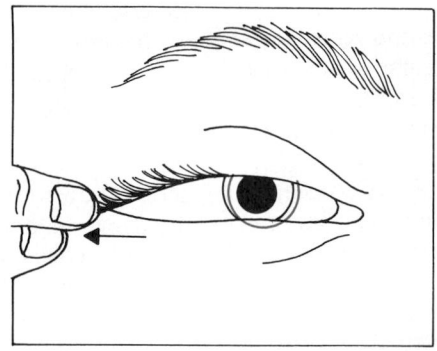

Gently pull the outer corner of the eye toward the ear.

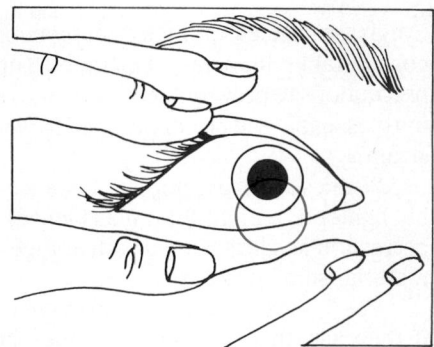

Position the other hand below the lens to receive it and ask the client to blink.

or

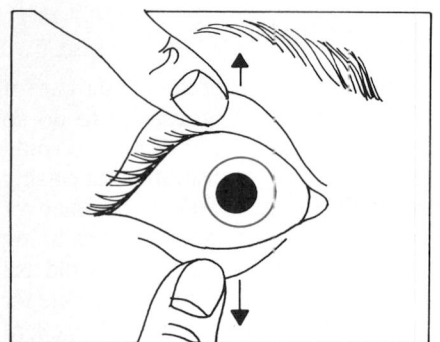

Gently spread the eyelids beyond the top and bottom edges of the lens.

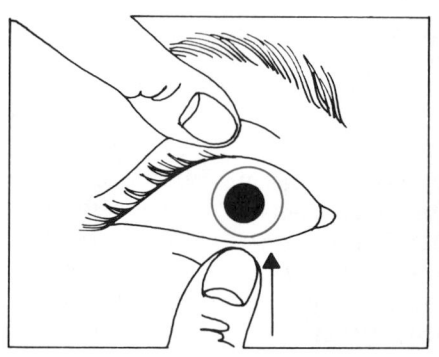

Gently press the lower eyelid up against the bottom of the lens.

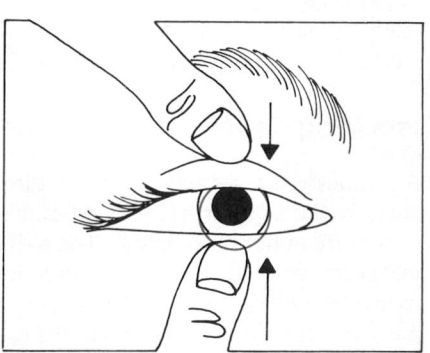

After the lens is tipped slightly, move the eyelids toward one another to cause the lens to slide out between the eyelids.

Removing soft contact lenses

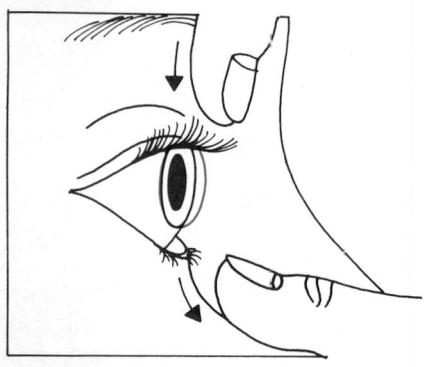

Have the client look forward. Retract the lower lid with one hand. Using the pad of the index finger of the other hand, move the lens down to the sclera.

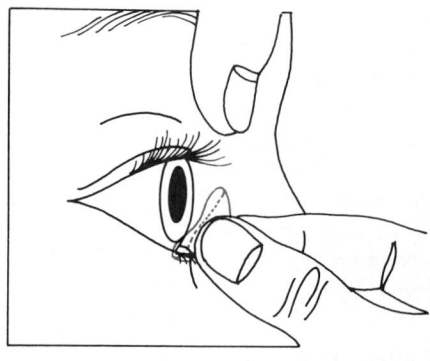

Using the pads of the thumb and index fingers grasp the lens with a gentle pinching motion and remove.

Storing lenses

Because lenses may be different for each eye, storage cases are marked L and R designating left and right lenses. It is important to place the first lens in its designated cup in the storage case before removing the second lens to avoid mixing them up.

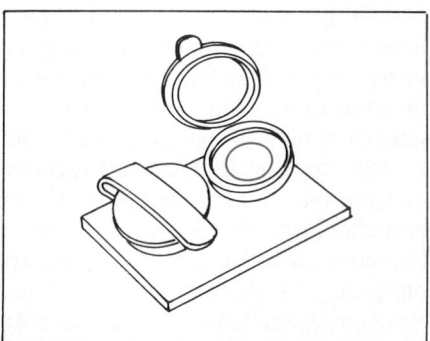

F I G U R E   2 9 - 7

Removing contact lenses.

tubes. Irrigations are usually contraindicated because of the possible danger of forcing material into the sinuses.

If the external nares are crusted, applying mineral or cottonseed oil helps to soften and remove the crusts. Disposable paper tissues are recommended for nasal secretions. A cotton applicator may be used to clean the nares but with great care to avoid injury. The applicator should never be introduced into the nares.

Evaluating

At designated intervals, evaluate whether the client has achieved the goals established during planning. Revise the care plan if indicated. An example follows:

> 10/24/93   Goal met. Client demonstrated correct care (cleaning) of artificial eye for the past two mornings. States, "I guess I should be happy to be alive and still able to see."
>
> *N. Glynn, RN*

Hair Care

Hair is an accessory structure of the skin. Good general health is essential for attractive hair and skin, and cleanliness helps in keeping hair and skin attractive. Illness affects the hair, especially when endocrine abnormalities, increased body temperature, poor nutrition, or anxiety and worry are present. Changes in the color or condition of the hair shaft are related to changes in hormonal activity or to changes in the blood supply to hair follicles.

Assessing

Nursing History   Identify the client's usual hair and scalp care practices, including styling preferences. Note any history of hair or scalp problems, possible etiologies for changes in the distribution, texture, or amount of hair, and related treatments.

Physical Assessment   Assess the condition of the hair (texture, cleanliness, oiliness) and scalp (scaling, lesions, inflammation, infection).

Risk Factors   Identify any factors known to cause hair or scalp problems or that require special care—deficient self-care abilities, immobility, malnutrition, treatments known to result in hair loss (eg, irradiation of the head, certain chemotherapeutic agents).

Common Scalp and Hair Problems

Dandruff   Dandruff is a condition characterized by itching and flaking of the scalp that may be further complicated by the embarrassment it causes. Persistent severe cases usually require medical attention. Daily brushing and shampooing with a medicated shampoo may be all that is needed to keep the scalp free of dandruff.

Hair Loss   Hair growth and hair loss are ongoing, daily processes. Hair loss from plaiting, excessive back combing and teasing, or the use of hair rollers is usually temporary, and hair returns when the tension on the hair shaft is halted. Some people experience hair loss owing to illness with high fever, certain medications, x-ray therapy of the head, childbirth, and general anesthesia. There appears to be no evidence that hair loss occurs as a result of wearing wigs or excessive shampooing. It is believed by some that an excessive intake of vitamin A may play a role in hair loss. Some permanent thinning of hair normally accompanies aging.

Baldness is called **alopecia**. It is common in men but rare in women, and it is believed to be hereditary. There is no known cure for baldness, although some external medications are currently in use and others are being developed. Their long-term efficacy is unknown. Hairpieces, frequently worn by people who are bald, require the same care as normal hair but less frequent washing.

A surgical procedure for baldness is the hair transplant. Hair is taken from donor sites, usually from the back or sides of the scalp, and transplanted to areas with no hair. The procedure is long and expensive but reportedly has decided benefits for people who find baldness psychologically unpleasant. Complications include serious scalp infections.

Pediculosis   Infestation with lice is called **pediculosis**. There are three common types of lice—*Pediculus humanus capitis*, which infests hair and scalp; *P. humanus corporis*, which infests the body; and *Phthirus pubis*, which infests the shorter hairs on the body, usually the pubic hair and the axillary hair. Lice lay eggs, called nits, on the hair shafts. **Nits** are white or light gray and look like dandruff, but they cannot be brushed or shaken off the hair. Frequent scratching and scratch marks on the body and the scalp suggest the presence of pediculosis. Although anyone may become infested with lice, the continued presence of pediculosis is usually a result of uncleanliness. Pediculosis can be spread directly by contact with infested areas or indirectly through clothing, bed linen, brushes, and combs. Teaching clients, especially children, not to share personal items is a good way to prevent transmission. The linen and personal-care items of a client with pediculosis require separate and careful handling to prevent spreading from person to person.

There are any number of preparations, called **pediculicides**, for the treatment of pediculosis, some of which destroy the nits as well as the lice. Several treatments are usually necessary before all the nits are destroyed. The procedures and the medications used for the treatment of pediculosis vary among health agencies. Shaving off the infested hair may be done, especially when pubic hair and axillary hair are infested. Sexual partners must be notified if the lice were sexually transmitted.

Ticks Ticks are small, gray-brown, blood-sucking parasites important because of their ability to transmit serious diseases such as Lyme disease, Rocky Mountain spotted fever, and tularemia. Ticks should never be forcibly pulled out of the skin. Because oil suffocates the tick, covering the tick with mineral oil or a lubricating jelly such as petroleum jelly facilitates its removal.

Diagnosing

Make a judgment about the adequacy of the client's self-care practices. Identify factors contributing to deficiencies, for example,

Self-Care Deficit: Hair Care, related to continuous bed rest

Identify actual or potential hair or scalp problems that nurses can treat, noting contributing factors. Identify unhealthy client responses to these problems, for example,

High Risk for Infection related to hair transplant

Body Image Disturbance related to baldness

Impaired Skin Integrity related to scalp laceration (head bandages), pruritus

Planning: Client Goals

Identify nursing measures that will assist the client to develop or maintain needed hair and scalp care practices or that otherwise resolve nursing diagnoses. Specify any special products needed for hair care. Plan to achieve the following client goals. The client will:
- Have clean and neatly styled hair
- Demonstrate decreased or absent scalp lesions (or infestation)
- Verbalize satisfaction with appearance
- Participate in hair and scalp care as able

Implementing

Carry out the care plan remembering to use scheduled hygienic care interactions for ongoing assessment of the client's hair and scalp and for evaluating the adequacy of the care plan. The following discussions give suggestions for grooming hair, shampooing hair, caring for beards and mustaches, and assisting with unwanted hair removal.

Grooming the Hair

There are many cultural overtones associated with hair; however, styles also change within a culture from decade to decade. The nurse shows consideration when hair is groomed in the style preferred by the client. Daily brushing of the hair helps to keep it clean and distributes oil along the shaft of each hair. Brushing also stimulates the circulation of blood in the scalp. Hair that becomes entangled is difficult to comb. Combing of tiny sections of hair at a time may be necessary if a client's hair has not been combed for even 1 day. The best way to protect long hair from matting and tangling is to ask the client for permission to braid it. Clients usually consent to the procedure if it provides them with more comfort. Parting the hair in the middle on the back of the head and making two braids, one on either side, prevents the discomfort of lying on one heavy braid on the back of the head.

Occasionally, a client's hair is almost hopelessly matted, and cutting the hair may be necessary. Before a client's hair is cut, it is usual procedure to have the client sign a written consent. It is also recommended that the nurse discuss the necessity for cutting the hair with an immediate member of the client's family.

The care of a person with kinky hair usually requires special attention. The hair is normally dry, curly, and becomes easily matted and tangled. The comb used for arranging the hair should have widely spaced teeth. Oil should be used, and white petrolatum or mineral oil is often recommended. However, a skin lotion has been used effectively also. Braiding the hair of a person with kinky hair is usually the best way to prevent matting and tangling.

Shampooing the Hair

The hair is exposed to the same dirt and oil as the skin. It should be washed as often as necessary to keep it clean. The comb and the brush should be washed each time the hair is washed and as frequently as necessary between shampoos. Many health agencies have beauticians and barbers to assist with the care of the client's hair, including shampooing it. However, the convenience does not relieve the nurse of responsibility.

Before shampooing the hair, it is recommended that the nurse, or the client, if able, brush and comb the hair well to stimulate the scalp and undo tangled hair. The client may then shampoo the hair while showering, if able. In some hospitals, a physician's order is required for shampooing a client's hair.

The following techniques are recommended for shampooing the hair of a client on bed rest (Fig. 29-8):
- Prepare several pitchers of water of a suitably warm temperature for a thorough washing and rinsing, shampoo soap, one or two towels for drying, and a receptacle to receive wash and rinse water.
- Place a protective pad under the head.
- Place the client in a position over the pad so that there is constant drainage of water directed into the receptacle.
- Wet the hair, apply soap, and massage the scalp well while washing the hair.
- Rinse the hair and apply soap for a second washing, if indicated.
- Rinse the hair thoroughly after washing it with soap and water.
- Apply conditioner if requested.
- Dry the hair as quickly as possible to prevent the client from becoming chilled, and arrange the hair according to the client's preference.

Dry Shampoo Dry shampoos cannot replace the cleaning benefits of regular shampoos, but they are helpful in removing at least some of the dirt, oils, and odors from the

I entered the room with a feeling of dread. How could I possibly bathe the sick, elderly, helpless woman lying in this hospital bed? I had never bathed anyone older than age 2 years, other than myself, of course. How would I be able to move her limp, seemingly lifeless old body? What would an 85 year old body look like? I could not imagine. I've read all the manuals that describe this procedure, I know what to do, so why am I so nervous? I must be worried that I will hurt her in some way. Maybe she has not been cared for properly before and her hygiene is poor. Well, I might as well get this over with because I'll be doing it the rest of my life. I've got to learn sometime.

I've mustered up enough courage to enter my client's room. Michelle, her primary nurse, offers to help me because the client is so difficult to move. Boy, am I relieved! Right before Michelle and I are about to begin, my client, Mrs. Ash, asks for her teeth. I assume this must mean her dentures and reassure her that I have not seen them but will be happy to look for them as soon as we have completed her bath. Michelle and I each take a side and begin to bathe her. It's truly amazing how those range-of-motion exercises come to mind so easily. I had thought they were long forgotten with the rest of the past semester. Wouldn't my instructors love to hear me now! Suddenly Mrs. Ash yells, "I need the bed pan!" "Oh no!" I thought, as I rushed to the bathroom with soapy gloved hands trying frantically to locate her bed pan before there could be an accident. Michelle, who remained calm during my frenzy, simply stated, "Don't worry, she has an indwelling catheter. She says that every time I bathe her." I knew she had a catheter, how did I forget? Somewhat humbled, I returned to the procedure. I really wanted to put some lotion on her skin because it was so dry. We are ready to do her back so we prepare to lift her. I pull her toward me and Michelle was to continue the bath. We were not prepared for what we saw underneath. Firmly cushioned in Mrs. Ash's lower left buttock were none other than her dentures! On removing them, Michelle and I had to smile at the periodontal grin implanted on Mrs. Ash's bottom. Michelle then asked her how her teeth had gotten to the location where we found them. All she seemed to know was that she needed those teeth back in her mouth STAT! She snatched the dentures from Michelle's hand and attempted to insert them. Michelle and I in unison blurted out, "No, Mrs. Ash, please wait until we clean your teeth before you put them back in your mouth!" Mrs. Ash, somewhat confused, begrudgingly handed over her teeth to be cleaned. Michelle had the honors while I finished the last touches of good hygiene for Mrs. Ash.

What a difference cleanliness can make, not only for the client but also for me, the student nurse. I felt better knowing that Mrs. Ash was clean and that this procedure was behind me. And to think that I was apprehensive! This was definitely an interesting learning experience.

—Marilyn Johnson, Holy Family College,
Philadelphia

hair of clients too ill or incapacitated to have a wet shampoo. Dry shampoos or powders are not recommended for people with kinky hair because of their normally dry hair and scalp. The dry shampoo or powder is applied and then combed or brushed from the hair. The teeth of a comb can be pulled through gauze, which helps remove and capture the powder.

Caring for Beards and Mustaches

Most clients with beards or mustaches are able to groom them independently. Dependent clients require nursing assistance to keep the beard and mustache clean, especially after eating. For no reason should a nurse trim or shave off a client's beard or mustache without the client's consent.

Shaving

Individual preferences for shaving methods are based on such factors as the type of skin, the quality of the beard, the frequency with which one shaves, the presence of skin problems, and convenience. An electric shaver is usually recommended when the client is on anticoagulant therapy or has a bleeding disorder. Blade razors tend to give a closer shave than electric razors, but many clients find electric razors convenient and practical. They are especially conve-

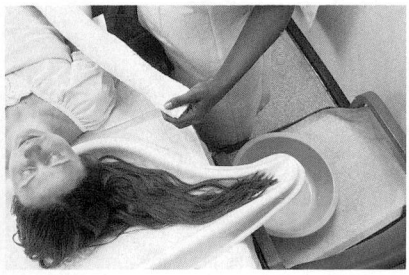

Place a waterproof pad under the client's shoulders, neck, and head. Position the shampooing trough under the client's head with the drainage spout extending over the edge of the bed. Place a recepticle below the spout to catch the water. Place a rolled towel under the client's neck at the edge of the trough.

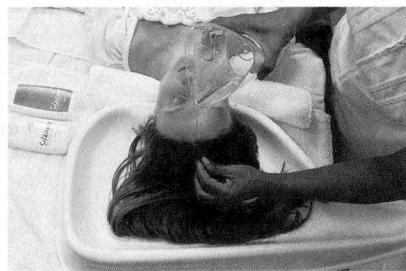

Using a pitcher of comfortably warm water, wet the client's hair completely.

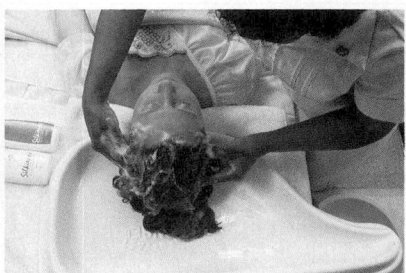

Apply shampoo and lather using both hands and working from the front to the back of the head.

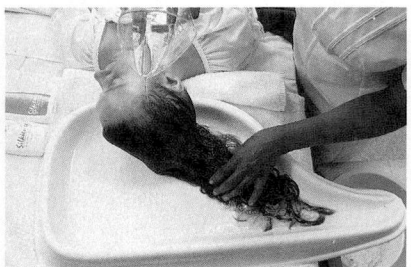

Rinse hair completely. Repeat shampooing and rinsing if necessary. Apply conditioner if requested and rinse again.

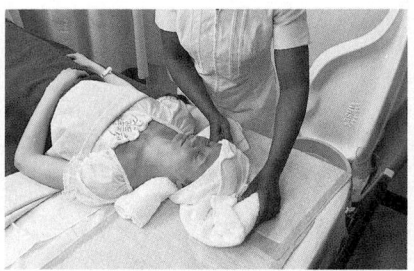

Wrap the client's head in towels to remove as much moisture as possible from the scalp and hair. Dry the client's face and neck.

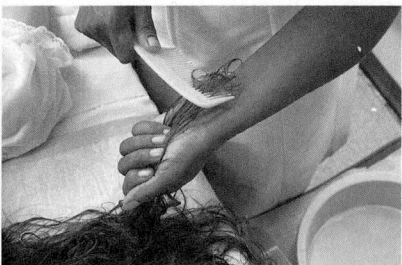

Comb gently to remove tangles. Complete drying of the hair using a dryer or towel according to agency policy.

F I G U R E   2 9 - 8

Technique for shampooing a client's hair in bed.

nient for the ill and bedridden client. The technique for shaving clients who are unable to shave themselves is described here and illustrated in Figure 29-9.

- Glove use is optional but recommended because contact with blood is possible should any skin nicks occur.
- Shaving cream or a warm soap lather is first applied to the skin to soften the facial hair and prevent pulling.
- The skin of the face is pulled taut.
- Short, firm strokes in the direction of hair growth are used. Clients often can give suggestions on how they shave.
- Wash the client's face of residual lather and dry.
- Aftershave lotion may be applied. Aftershave preparations tend to make the face feel good and have a cosmetic rather than a therapeutic effect.

Evaluating

At designated intervals, evaluate whether the client has achieved the goals established during planning and revise the care plan if indicated. An example follows:

F I G U R E   2 9 - 9

To shave a client's face with a razor, first apply shaving cream or warm soap lather to soften the beard. Shave the face by gently pulling the skin taut and using short, firm strokes in the direction of hair growth. After shaving, wash off any residual lather and dry the client's face. Aftershave lotion may be applied if requested.

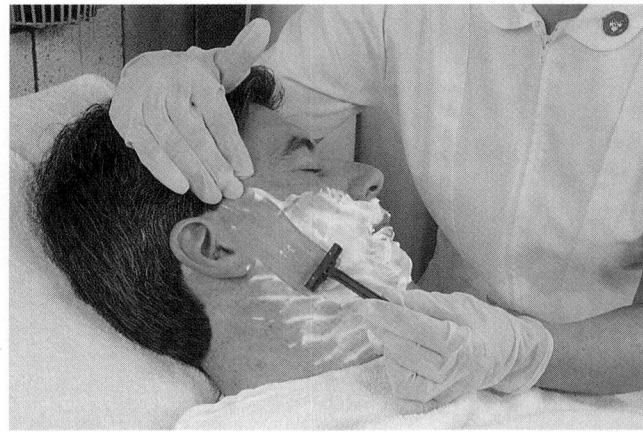

10/27/93 Goal partially met. Client reports that she is uncomfortable wearing a wig yet but feels better since its purchase.
Revision: Because client still has many questions about effects of chemotherapy, continue teaching and use opportunities to build self-esteem.

C. Moser, RN

Nail and Foot Care

The nails are an accessory structure of the skin and comprise epithelial tissue. The body of the nail is the exposed portion; the root lies in the skin in the nail groove where the nail grows and is nourished. Healthy nails have a pink color and are convex and evenly curved. With certain pathologic conditions, and to some extent with aging also, the nails become ridged and areas become concave.

Assessing

Nursing History Identify the client's normal nail and foot care practices, the type of footwear worn, and any history of nail or foot problems and their related treatments.

Physical Assessment Examine nails for intactness and cleanliness; note capillary refill and the contour of the nailbed; observe the nail base for redness, swelling, bleeding, discharge, and tenderness. Examine the feet for cleanliness and intactness of skin, and note the presence of swelling, inflammation, lesions, tenderness, or orthopedic problems. Examine carefully the skin between the toes.

High-Risk Factors Identify any variables known to cause nail and foot problems, such as deficient self-care abilities, vascular disease, arthritis, diabetes mellitus, history of biting nails or trimming them improperly, frequent or prolonged exposure to chemicals or water, trauma, ill-fitting shoes, or obesity.

Diagnosing

Make a judgment about the adequacy of the client's self-care practices related to nail and foot care, identifying any factors that contribute to deficiencies. An example is as follows:

Self-Care Deficit: Diabetic Foot Care, related to knowledge deficit and weakened physical state

Identify actual or potential nail or foot problems that nurses can treat, noting contributing factors. Identify unhealthy client responses to these problems. For example,

Pain related to corns (calluses, plantar warts, ingrown nails) in foot

Impaired Physical Mobility related to painful foot condition [specify]

High Risk for Infection related to traumatized nail base or deficient nail or foot care

Impaired Skin Integrity related to altered circulation to feet

Planning: Client Goals

Identify nursing measures that will assist the client to develop or maintain healthy nail and foot care practices. Plan to achieve the following client goals. The client will:

- Have intact, clean, and manicured nails
- Have intact, clean, and lesion-free foot skin
- Have reduced or absent nail and foot problems (specify: calluses, corns, plantar warts, ingrown nails, athlete's foot)
- Demonstrate correct nail and foot care measures
- Verbalize nails and feet contribute to general sense of comfort and well-being

Pertinent nursing measures to include in the care plan are as follows:

- Soaking nails and feet and assisting with cleaning of nails and trimming nails (if not contraindicated)
- Massaging the feet to promote relaxation and comfort
- Teaching correct nail and foot care

In the care plan, identify any supplies needed to carry out the specified nail and foot care and the timing of these measures.

Implementing

Carry out the care plan remembering to use bath times to continually assess the status of the client's nails and feet and to evaluate the adequacy of the care plan. Techniques for providing fingernail and foot care are described in this section. See the accompanying display for sample documentation of foot care.

Providing Care of Fingernails

The following are recommended techniques for the care of fingernails:

- File the nails to form an oval at the ends. Do not trim so far down on the sides that injury to the skin and cuticles occurs.
- Remove hangnails, which are broken pieces of cuticle, by cutting them off. Take special care to avoid injury to tissue with the cuticle scissors.
- *Gently* push cuticles back off the nail after they are soft and pliable following a soaking in warm water.
- Push back cuticles with a blunt instrument or a terry cloth.
- Apply an emollient to the cuticle to help prevent hangnails.
- Clean under the nails with a blunt instrument or the large end of a toothpick, being careful to prevent injuring the area where the nail is attached to the underlying tissue.

Splitting and peeling of the nails are usually caused by dryness. It is helpful to avoid contact with soap and water as much as possible, use a good hand cream frequently,

Sample Documentation of Foot Care

10/20/93, nursing
#7 Impaired Skin Integrity: Right toe related to altered circulation

S: "I guess I cut that nail too short . . . that toe's been hurting for 2 months now." History of adult-onset diabetes since 1975.

O: Great toe on right foot is swollen, red, and painful; skin at base of nail is white; limps when walking.

A: Healing of traumatized tissue right toe delayed because of altered circulation (diabetes mellitus).

P: Soak feet after each bath and dry carefully afterward. Consult with physician.

C. Moser, RN

and avoid the use of nail polish and polish remover, both of which have a tendency to dry the nails.

Providing Foot Care

Proper foot care is important at any age. It becomes even more so with aging and when such conditions as circulatory disturbances or diabetes mellitus are present. Techniques for foot care follow:
• Bathe the feet thoroughly in a basin of soap or detergent and water solution. Be sure to clean the interdigital areas.
• Rinse the feet to remove soap or detergent residue, which irritates the skin if improperly removed.
• Continue to soak the feet in a basin of warm water if the toenails are brittle, thick, and striated before attempting to trim them. Or, wrap the feet in damp cloths and place them in plastic bags to soften the nails, if this is more convenient.
• Trim the nails straight across and not so short that tender areas of skin are exposed to the normal friction from shoes and stockings when the client is walking. In many institutions, a physician's order is necessary for cutting nails.
• When trimming the nails, avoid digging into or cutting the toenails at the lateral corners. These practices predispose to ingrown nails. Clients with ingrown toenails, especially older people and clients with circulatory disorders or diabetes mellitus, may require the services of a physician or podiatrist.
• Clean under the nails with a blunt instrument or the large end of a toothpick, being careful to prevent injury to the area where the nail is attached to the underlying tissue.
• Apply powder to the feet and interdigital areas. If the skin is dry, use a lanolin cream instead.
• Bathe the feet at least daily but more often if they tend

to perspire freely. Using a foot powder containing a nonirritating deodorant is helpful when foot odor is due to excessive perspiration. Foot powders are more absorbent than regular bath powders and often contain menthol, which makes the skin feel cool.
Improperly fitting and extremely worn or soiled hosiery contributes to foot problems. For some people with allergies or skin infections, nylon hosiery is contraindicated.

The nurse should be alert to any signs of foot problems, including infection, inflammation, ingrown nails, breaks in the skin in the interdigital areas, corns, calluses, bunions, and pressure areas, that may result in ulcerations. This is especially important for the client with diabetes.

Providing Foot Care for the Diabetic Client

A diabetic client is especially prone to foot problems owing to skin irritation, infection, and ulcers, which, without proper precautions, can result in gangrene. There are certain additional precautions that should be observed and taught to the client with diabetes:
• File the toenails. Scissors are too likely to slip and injure tissues.
• Do not cut off corns or calluses. Also, do not use commercial removers because they contain ingredients that often lead to irritation, infection, and ulcers.
A physician who treats foot disorders, or **podiatrist**, should be consulted when corns and calluses are present.
• Do not use nonprescription preparations to treat athlete's foot and ingrown toenails because they may contain ingredients that lead to infection and ulcers. A physician or podiatrist should be consulted when athlete's foot or ingrown nails are present. The causative fungi of athlete's foot are species of *Trichophyton* or *Epidermophyton floccosum* and are capable of attacking the hair and nails as well as the skin.
• Avoid using heating pads and hot-water bottles applied to the feet because of the danger of blistering and burning the feet.
• Teach the client to avoid wearing round garters and stockings with elastic tops and not to sit with the knees crossed to prevent obstruction of circulation to the lower extremities and feet.
• Prop the feet up above the level of the hips a few minutes several times a day if the feet swell.
• Explain the dangers of going barefoot. The client may injure the skin of the feet or acquire athlete's foot in such places as public showers.
• Keep the feet dry and warm in shoes and stockings that provide plenty of room.
• Break in new shoes gradually; begin with a half hour of wear the first day and increase the time by about 1 hour a day. Improperly fitting shoes are a major cause of foot problems and can lead to corns, calluses, bunions, and blisters. The back of the shoe, or the counter, should fit snugly but not tightly. A heel offering safe support is recommended. When standing, there should be about 3/4 inch of space in the shoe beyond

the great toe and also at the widest part of the shoe. In a shoe that fits well, the arch of the foot lies comfortably over the arch in the shoes. The soles should be flexible and nonslippery. Shoes with rough ridges, wrinkles, or tears in the linings should be discarded or repaired.

Evaluating

At designated intervals, evaluate whether the client has achieved the goals established during planning and revise the care plan if indicated. An example follows:

> 10/24/93 Goal met. Client correctly verbalized rationale for diabetic foot care program and expressed interest in attending the diabetic classes.
>
> *C. Moser, RN*

Perineal and Vaginal Care

The perineal area is dark, warm, and often moist, which favors bacterial growth. The client who is unable to clean the perineal area needs the nurse's assistance for this important part of personal hygiene. Neglecting cleaning the perineal area of the client who is unable to provide self-care often results in physical and psychologic discomfort for the client, a breakdown in the skin, and offensive odors.

Assessing

Nursing History Identify any special perineal and vaginal hygiene practices the client performs, products used, and variables influencing these practices. Note any history of perineal or vaginal problems and related treatments.

Physical Assessment Examine the male genitalia (penis, scrotum, and perineum) for lesions, swelling, inflammation, excoriation, tenderness, and discharge (amount, color, odor, and source); examine the female genitalia (pubic area, labia, clitoris, urinary meatus, and perineum) for color, size, lesions, masses, swelling, inflammation, excoriation, tenderness, and discharge (amount, color, odor, and source). Examine the anal area for cracks, nodules, distended veins, masses, or polyps; note strong perineal odors.

Risk Factors Identify any variables known to cause perineal or vaginal problems or to create a need for special care: urinary or fecal incontinence, indwelling Foley catheters, childbirth, rectal or genital surgery, diseases such as urinary tract infection, diabetes mellitus, and certain sexually transmitted diseases (STDs such as, herpes).

Diagnosing

Make a judgment about the adequacy of the client's perineal (vaginal) self-care practices, identifying any factors that contribute to deficiencies. An example is

Self-Care Deficit: Perineal Care, related to cognitive impairment

Next, identify actual or potential perineal and vaginal problems that nurses can treat, noting contributing factors, and identify unhealthy client responses to these problems. Examples of these are

Pain related to excoriated perineal area

High Risk for Infection related to client's deficient perineal hygiene

Knowledge Deficit: Advisability of Using Deodorized Feminine Hygiene Products related to inexperience and a desire to "be clean"

Disturbance in Body Image related to genital lesions

Altered Sexuality Patterns related to painful genital lesions

High Risk for Impaired Skin Integrity related to urinary and fecal incontinence

Planning: Client Goals

Identify nursing measures that will assist the client to develop or maintain healthy perineal (vaginal) care practices that will contribute to the client's general sense of well-being. Plan to achieve the following client goals. The client will:

• Demonstrate clean perineal area with skin intact
• Demonstrate signs of healing of perineal lesions or excoriations (discharge is decreased or absent)
• Demonstrate correct perineal and vaginal hygiene measures

Pertinent nursing measures to include in the care plan include the following:

• Cleaning the male genitalia (penis, scrotum, perineum, and rectal area) or the female genitalia (pubic area, labia, clitoris, urinary meatus, perineum, and rectal area)
• Instructing the client on perineal hygiene practices

Implementing

Carry out the care plan, remembering to use bath time, when appropriate, for ongoing assessment of the client's perineum and for evaluation of the adequacy of the care plan. Procedures for perineal and vaginal care are described in this section. See the accompanying display for sample documentation of teaching care of genitalia.

Providing Perineal Care

It is not always possible for male nurses to attend to male clients and female nurses to attend to female clients. When the perineal cleaning is carried out in a matter-of-fact and dignified manner, clients generally do not find care by a person of the opposite gender to be offensive or embarrassing.

Some nurses use a sitz tub to clean the client's perineal and anal areas. The portable type is especially handy when it is cumbersome to move a client to a stationary sitz tub.

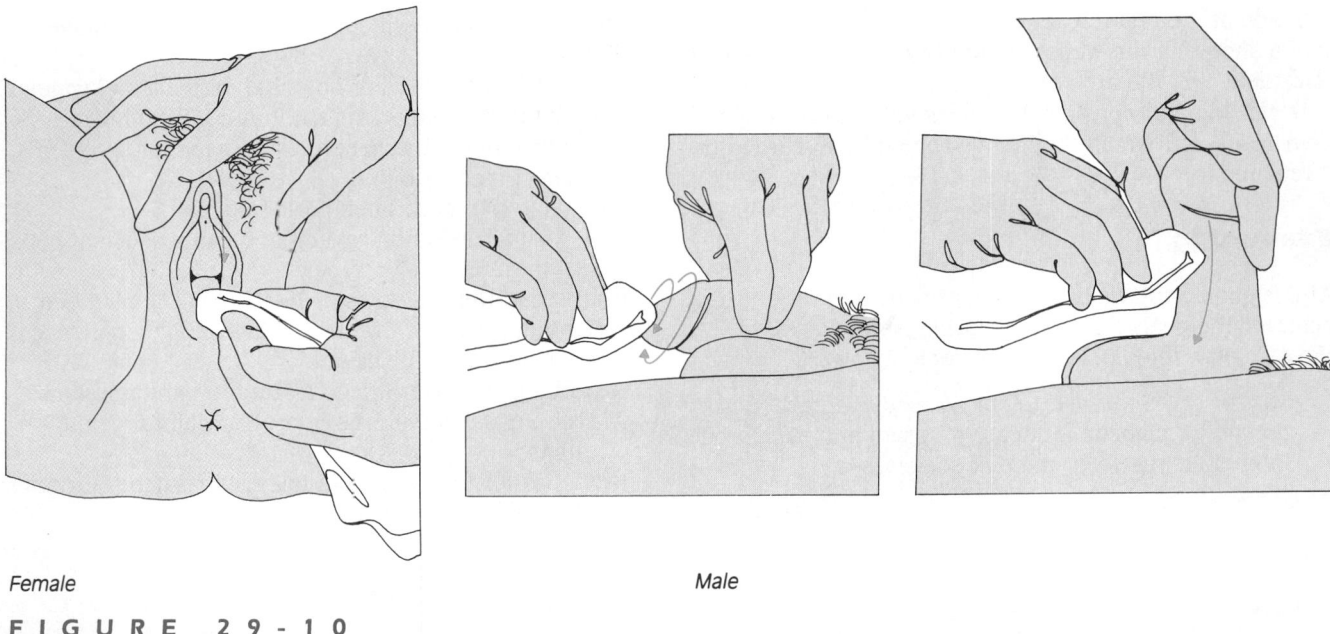

Female   Male

FIGURE 29-10

Performing normal perineal care.

The procedure may be carried out while the client remains in bed. The following techniques are recommended to administer perineal care to clients (Fig. 29-10):

- Assemble supplies and provide for privacy.
- Explain the procedure to the client and don disposable gloves.
- Wash and rinse the groin area for both the male and female client.
- Always proceed from the least contaminated area to the most contaminated area. For a female client, spread the labia and move the washcloth from the pubic area toward the anal area to prevent carrying organisms from the anal area back over the genital area. Use a clean portion of the washcloth for each stroke. For a male client, move the washcloth in a spiral motion from the tip of the penis down its length toward the pubic area.
- In an uncircumcised male client, retract the foreskin (prepuce) while washing the penis. Rinse well with plain water.
- Rinse the washed areas well with plain water.
- Pull the uncircumcised male client's foreskin back into place over the glans penis to prevent constriction of the penis, which may result in edema and tissue injury.
- Wash and rinse the male client's scrotum. Handle the scrotum, which houses the testicles, with care because the area is sensitive.
- Dry the cleaned areas, and apply an emollient as indicated. Powder the area only if the client requests it. For the female client, powder may become a medium

for the growth of bacteria, and studies currently are linking use of powder with increased risk of cervical cancer.

- Turn the client on his or her side and continue with cleansing the anal area. Continue in the direction of least contaminated to most contaminated area. In the female, cleanse from the vagina toward the anus. In both female and male clients, change the washcloth with each stroke until the area is clean. Rinse and dry the area.

Providing Vaginal Care

In normal, healthy women, regular daily internal douching is believed to be both unnecessary and unwise. The practice tends to remove normal bacterial flora from the vagina,

---

Sample Documentation

Teaching Care of Genitalia

10/20/93   Child presented with large amount of smegma under the foreskin and painful urination. Mother and child were instructed in the need and correct technique for cleansing the uncircumcised penis. Child correctly returned the demonstration.

C. Moser, RN

and if the solution is high in acid content, it may irritate or injure normal cells. Many women use douches for personal hygiene reasons after intercourse. The practice is satisfactory when the solution is nonirritating. There are many products on the market that can be used safely in douching solutions. Many gynecologists apparently believe that a mild white-vinegar solution, using 1 or 2 tablespoons in 1 quart of warm water, or normal saline, is just as satisfactory. Douching more often than twice a week is not recommended for normal personal hygiene purposes.

The following are recommended techniques for administering a vaginal douche for therapeutic reasons:

- Fill a douche bag with 1 or 2 quarts of the warmed solution of choice, and allow the tubing and tip to fill with solution. Bulb syringes are available for douching but are less frequently recommended because of the danger of injecting solution with too much force and forcing it into the cervix.
- Place the client on a bedpan. The client may lie in a bathtub if she is able to administer the douche herself. Standing up in the tub is not recommended because it requires too much force to carry solution to the vagina for thorough cleaning.
- Hold the bag or hang it on a standard so that it is about 24 to 36 inches (60 to 90 cm) above the level of the hips.
- Separate the labia with gloved fingers, and insert the douche tip by directing it downward and backward to follow the normal contour of the vagina. Allow the solution to begin flowing.
- Hold the vulva snugly to close the vaginal orifice or ask the client to contract her muscles around the orifice to allow solution to collect and distend the vagina; then allow the solution to escape. Repeat this procedure during the douche until all of the solution is used. This technique distends the vagina and permits better cleaning of its convoluted walls.
- Do not raise the level of the bag containing the solution during the douche because this may cause undue force that may result in the introduction of organisms into the cervix.

Medical attention is recommended when a discharge or irritation and itching about the vaginal orifice persist. Douching to relieve the symptoms may only tend to aggravate the cause of the problem. Before a vaginal examination, a douche is contraindicated because it removes secretions and discharge needed for specimens necessary for diagnostic procedures. Most authorities recommend not having a vaginal douche for 24 to 48 hours before a vaginal examination.

Deodorants to control odor around the vaginal orifice may be applied directly to the area or placed on sanitary napkins. Although these deodorants do not contain aluminum salts, which are irritating to the mucous membrane, they are intended for external use only. They should not be used on tampons. Some have been reported as possibly harmful when sprayed into the vagina. Repeated use is not generally recommended because of reported irritation and rashes, nor should they be used on broken skin areas. No therapeutic benefit from their use has been proven to date. These special deodorants cannot replace cleanliness of the area.

Evaluating

At designated intervals, evaluate whether the client has achieved the goals established during planning, and revise the care plan if indicated. An example follows:

> 11/20/93 Goal partially met. Child returned to clinic with clean perineal area and relief of painful urination. Mother reports child spends half the time with her and half with father (parents separated) and that father is uncommitted to hygiene practices. *Revision:* Stress again to child importance of retracting foreskin during perineal care.
>
> C. Moser, RN

 NURSING PROCESS

In Clinical Practice

Some 3% to 14% of hospitalized clients in the United States develop pressure ulcers (Hoff, 1989; Kelley & Mobily, 1991), and the statistics in Canada are similar. Estimates of treatment costs range from $5000 to $30,000 per case (Colburn, 1990). The threat these ulcers pose to the client's physical and mental well-being and the amount of nursing energy they consume make them one of nursing's persistent top-priority challenges. For this reason, the nursing diagnosis Impairment of Skin Integrity related to pressure ulcer is explored.

Impaired Skin Integrity Related to Pressure Ulcer

Description

A pressure ulcer is an area of cellular necrosis that is caused by the lack of blood circulation to the involved area. **Necrosis** means that there is death of cells. The terms *pressure ulcer, decubitus ulcer,* and *bedsore* are used synonymously.

The term *decubitus* derives from a Latin word meaning lying down. However, lying down does not cause a decubitus ulcer, and a client need not be bedridden to develop one. Therefore, some people prefer the term *pressure ulcer* because pressure is the most prominent underlying cause of a decubitus ulcer.

Pathologic changes at the site of a pressure ulcer are caused by the collapse of blood vessels in the area of the ulcer, especially the arterioles and capillaries. The damage to vessels is a result of pressure, usually from body weight. When the blood supply is occluded owing to the pressure on vessels, cells are inadequately nourished, and cell wastes accumulate. Death of cells eventually occurs, leading to the characteristic ulcer of a pressure sore. The steps of this process are as follows: pressure → compression of small nutrient vessels of skin and underlying tissue → tissue anoxia and ischemia → necrosis of tissue cells → sloughing and ulceration → invasion by microorganisms → infection → sepsis → involvement of underlying fascia, muscle, and bone → rapidly irreversible condition (Smeltzer & Bare, 1992, pp. 236–237).

The first sign that a pressure ulcer may be developing is a blanching of the skin over the area under pressure. Instead of a healthy, pink color, the skin becomes pale and white. In nonwhite clients, this blanching is more difficult to see. However, insufficient blood circulation in the capillaries makes the skin appear pale when compared with areas where circulation is good. Local anemia owing to poor circulation in the area is called **ischemia**, which means containing little blood.

When pressure is relieved, ischemia is rapidly followed by hyperemia. The area appears red and feels warm. In nonwhites, hyperemia may best be detected by touch. The skin feels warm. Hyperemia is a compensatory mechanism. The body literally floods the area with blood to nourish and remove wastes from the cells. This phenomenon is called **reactive hyperemia**. If pressure is not relieved, the area remains red, but circulation cannot occur to the extent necessary for cell survival, and the tissue cells eventually die. The skin breaks, and a shallow crater or ulcer develops. The pressure sore then is often called superficial and with proper care ordinarily heals with relative ease.

A pressure ulcer is usually described as deep when a superficial pressure sore extends and involves underlying tissues. Shearing forces are often responsible for deep decubitus ulcers. A **shearing force** results when layers of tissue move on each other. Small blood vessels and capillaries are stretched and may even tear, thus resulting in poor circulation to tissue cells under the skin. The area of skin over an area damaged by a shearing force usually appears bluish in color, and sometimes a lump can be felt under the skin. A small break in the skin, which leads to necrotic tissue in the underlying area, eventually appears. Figure 29-11 illustrates how shearing forces occur.

The skin can tolerate considerable pressure without cell death but for short periods only. Duration is more im-

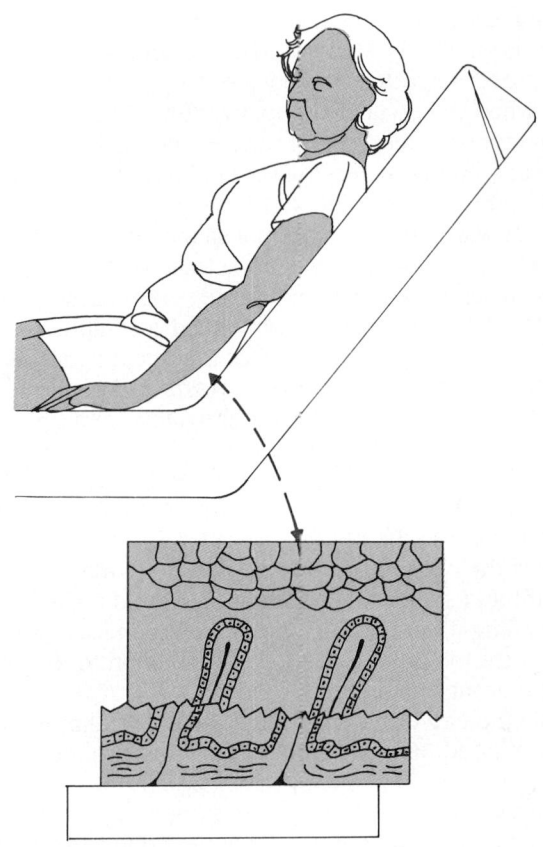

F I G U R E 2 9 - 1 1

Shearing force can occur when a client is moved carelessly or slides down in bed. Friction causes resistance on the surface layers of the skin, while underlying tissue moves in the direction of the body movement. Capillaries in underlying tissue are stretched and torn in pressure areas by opposing forces of movements.

portant than the amount of pressure in the formation of a pressure ulcer. Most pressure ulcers develop within 2 weeks of admission to a health care facility.

Common Sites for Pressure Ulcers

Pressure ulcers usually occur over bony prominences where body weight is distributed over a small area that does not have many subcutaneous tissues to cushion damage to the skin. Common sites for pressure ulcers are illustrated in Figure 29-12. Of the susceptible areas, most pressure ulcers occur over the sacrum and coccyx followed by the trochanter.

Risk Factors

Numerous factors predispose to pressure ulcers. Usually a combination of factors cause their development.

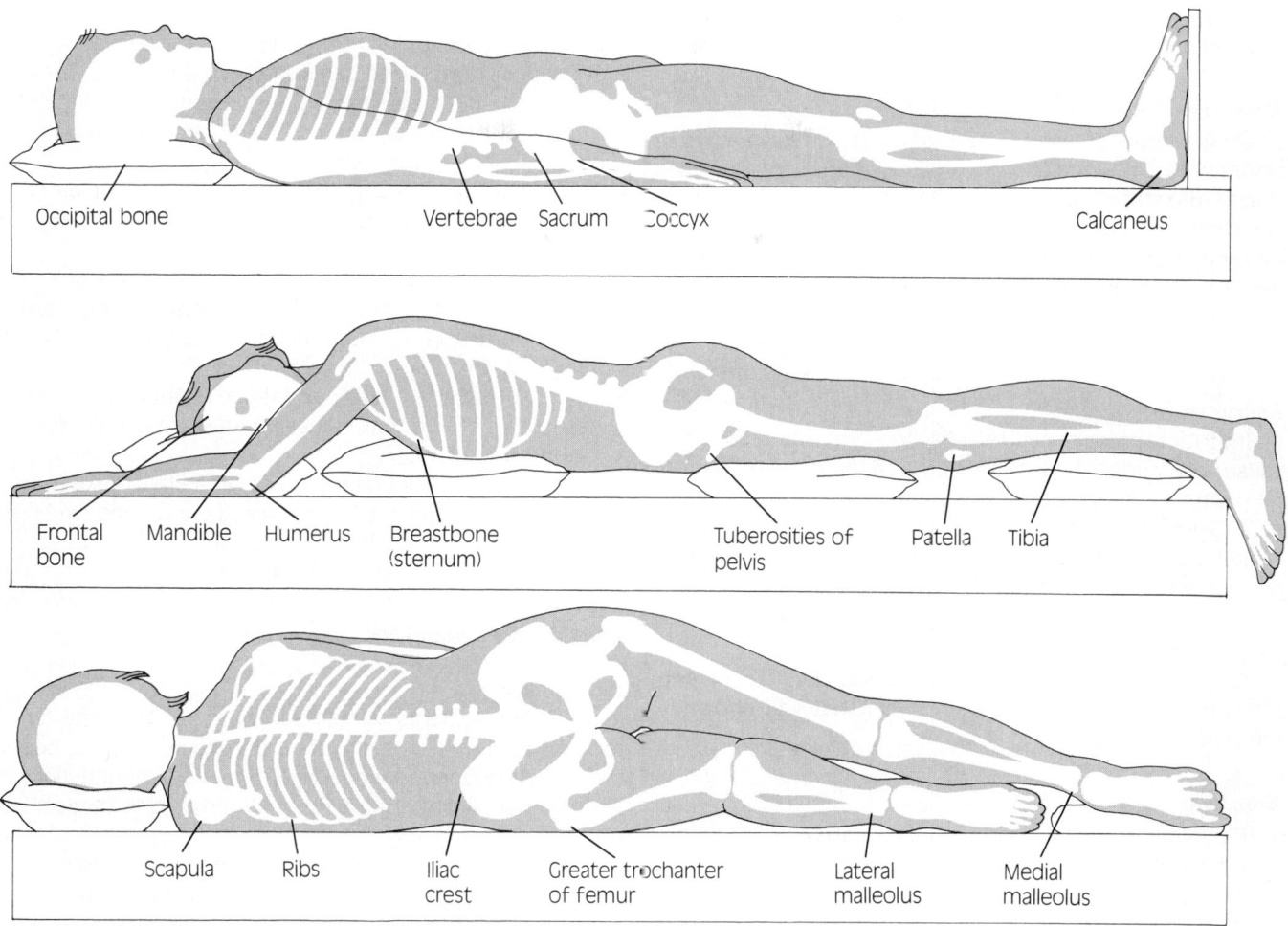

FIGURE 29-12

Common sites for development of pressure ulcers.

Pressure

The most formidable predisposing factor for a decubitus ulcer is pressure over an area, which results in occluded blood capillaries and poor blood circulation to tissues. This lack of sufficient circulation causes cell death and ulcer formation.

Immobility

The person who sits or lies most of the time is a candidate for a pressure sore because immobility predisposes to prolonged pressure on body areas. The up-and-about person does not develop pressure ulcers because no part of the body suffers from prolonged pressure. During sleep, the well person tends to move about in bed freely. Unconscious and paralyzed clients are subject to pressure sores if allowed to remain in one position in bed. So also are emotionally depressed people who do not ordinarily tend to move much. Additional factors that cause immobility and

may result in development of a pressure ulcer are lengthy surgery and the use of tranquilizers or sedatives.

Shearing Forces

Clients who are carelessly moved in bed or from beds to stretchers or chairs suffer from shearing forces as skin and underlying tissues are pulled over each other. A client who is partially sitting up in bed is susceptible when skin sticks to the sheet and underlying tissues move downward with the body. This may occur also in the client who sits in a chair but slides down while skin sticks to clothing and the back of the chair.

Friction

The client who lies on wrinkled sheets is likely to suffer tissue damage due to friction. The skin over the elbows and heels often suffers when clients lift and help move themselves in bed with the use of their arms and feet. Friction burns also occur on the back when clients are pulled or slid over sheets in bed or on a stretcher.

Moisture

Prolonged moisture on the skin reduces its resistance to trauma. Warmth increases the cells' demands for oxygen. Hence, moisture and warmth eventually lead to cell destruction, especially when pressure is present. If personal hygiene is poor, the skin contains many organisms that thrive in the warm, moist environment. This adds to the danger of developing a pressure ulcer that will become infected.

Malnutrition

Malnutrition predisposes to pressure sore formation because poorly nourished cells are easily damaged. For example, vitamin C deficiency causes capillaries to become fragile, and poor circulation to the area results when they break. Negative nitrogen balance and electrolyte imbalances also predispose to pressure sore formation.

Incontinence

Urinary or fecal incontinence increases the risk of an individual developing a pressure ulcer that will become infected.

Edema

Water imbalances and the accumulation of excessive fluid in tissues interfere with proper cell nourishment.

Mental Status

The more alert an individual is the more likely he or she is to protect skin integrity by relieving pressure periodically and managing adequate skin hygiene. Apathy, confusion, or a comatose state can diminish these self-care abilities and increase the likelihood of skin breakdown.

Miscellaneous Factors

Additional factors predispose to pressure ulcers:

- Older people are good candidates for developing pressure ulcers because the skin is susceptible to injury. See the display Focus on the Older Adult, which outlines risk factors for elderly people.
- People with debilitating diseases are likely candidates for developing pressure ulcers because skin nourishment ordinarily becomes poor.
- Destruction of tissues leading to pressure sores becomes relatively easy when illness causes an elevated temperature and normal functioning of body cells is altered in any way.
- Clients whose skin is dry and those clients whose skin has been irritated with adhesive tape are candidates for pressure ulcers.
- Various kinds of debris in bed or on a chair, such as crumbs, hairpins, buttons, pencils and pens, and pieces of silverware, irritate and damage the skin so that a pressure ulcer is likely to develop.

Nursing Management

Assessment

Identify those clients at risk and note predisposing factors—pressure, immobility, shearing forces, friction, edema, moisture, incontinence, health management deficits, malnutrition, debilitating disease. When a pressure ulcer is noted,

- Describe the pressure ulcer in terms of site, size, edema, warmth, color, odor, eschar, slough, drainage, and surrounding skin. Description of the ulcer must be ongoing. Many agencies use a special pressure ulcer assessment form. See Figure 29-13 for a sample assessment tool.
- Describe the skin in general: turgor, dryness or moisture, sensation in pressure areas, and warmth.

F O C U S   O N   T H E   O L D E R   A D U L T

Risk Factors That Predispose Elderly Clients to a Pressure Ulcer

Risk Factor	Implication
Decrease in subcutaneous tissue and thinning and wrinkling of skin	↑ Susceptibility to injury
Decrease in vascular supply	↓ In tissue profusion
Presence of chronic illnesses	↓ Energy and awareness of need to be active
Decrease in sensitivity of nerve endings in the skin	↓ Awareness of discomfort
Inadequate nutrition	↑ Risk of tissue breakdown
Depression and apathy	↓ Motivation and energy needed for self-care
Incontinence of bladder and bowels	↑ Susceptibility for breakdown of warm, moist skin

Nursing Services
Nursing Care Plan

Page 1 of 1

Potential for Alteration in Skin Integrity

Date	Problem Nursing Diagnosis	Date of Resolution	Expected Patient Outcome	Date	Plan of Care	Signature
	P: Potential for Alteration in Skin Integrity E: Select level per assessment _____ Low risk _____ Moderate risk _____ High risk S:		Patient's skin will remain intact.		I. LOW RISK 1. Pressure relief A. Encourage patient to turn in bed, OOB _____ 2. Local skin care A. Moisturize dry areas q _____ II. MODERATE RISK/HIGH RISK Interventions as above plus 1. Pressure relief A. Initiate turning schedule B. Obtain bioguard (pink) mattress. C. Cushion chairseat when OOB. D. Pad susceptible areas (ie., heels, elbows between knees). E. Use devices to assist patient to move trapeze. 2. Local skin care A. Keep skin clean and dry. B. Use Sween Kit for incontinent patients. C. Limit use of blue pads directly against patient's skin. 3. Nutritional care A. Consult dietitian for nutritional assessment.	

F I G U R E   2 9 - 1 3

Assessment form for assessing potential for pressure ulcers.

(continued)

Assessment of Potential for Pressure Sores

Directions: Complete this form on admission for all patients. Use to reassess patients at risk. If patient has actual breakdown on admission, DO NOT use this form for reassessment.

RISK	% BREAKDOWN	REASSESS	INITIATE CARE PLAN ENTITLED:
Low	None	q Monday	Potential for Alteration in Skin Integrity
Moderate/High	None	M-W-F	Potential for Alteration in Skin Integrity
	Present		Actual Alteration in Skin Integrity

CLINICAL CONDITION PARAMETERS		Date/Initials	Date/Initials	Date/Initials	Date/Initials	Date/Initials	Date/Initials	Date/Initials
GENERAL PHYSICAL CONDITION								
Good—Usually free of major health problems	0							
Fair—Major health problems are controlled	1							
Poor—Chronic serious health problems	2							
LEVEL OF CONSCIOUSNESS								
Alert—Responds readily to commands	0							
Lethargic—Slow response to commands/sleeps most of 24 hours	1							
Semicomatose—Responds only to verbal or painful stimuli	2							
Comatose—No response to stimuli	3							
ACTIVITY								
Ambulant without assistance	0							
Ambulant with assistance/crutch/walker	1							
Chairfast—Confined to chair/wheelchair	4							
Bedfast—Unable to sit in chair	6							
MOBILITY								
Full active range of motions	0							
Restricted movement—Limited assistance to move/pain/cast	1							
Moves only with assistance—Severe pain on movement	4							
Immobile—Never voluntarily changes position	6							
INCONTINENCE								
None	0							
Occasional loss of bladder control in times of stress	1							
Usually no bladder control/occasional fecal soiling	4							
Total—No control	6							
NUTRITION								
Good—Eats/drinks 50% or more of meal/weight appropriate	0							
Fair—Underweight/overweight/urine output low	1							
Poor—Weight loss/tube feeding/skin dry or flaking/TPN	2							
None—Inadequate oral intake/unable to swallow	3							
EXISTING BREAKDOWN								
None—No skin breakdown noted on assessment	0							
Stage I	4							
Stage II, III, IV	8							

TOTAL SCORE
Low risk = 0–12
Moderate risk = 12–25
High risk = 26+

Stage I   Reddened area
Stage II   Blister, skin break
Stage III   Skin break exposing subcutaneous tissue
Stage IV   Skin break exposing muscle and bone

INITIALS	SIGNATURE	INITIALS	SIGNATURE

F I G U R E   29-13 (continued)

- Describe contractures or any predisposing environmental factors (eg, casts, wrinkled linen, rubber drawsheet).
- Describe the client's self-care abilities: hygiene, mobility, nutrition, and continence.
- Describe the current nursing care: special skin care, pressure-relief measures, nutritional support, and incontinence management or devices.

Diagnosis

Unless the institution specifies a different classification system, diagnose the pressure ulcer according to the four-stage classification system commonly used by rehabilitation specialists (Braun et al., 1988; National Pressure Ulcer Advisory Panel, 1989) that is shown in Figure 29-14.

Stage 1: The primary sign is redness. The skin does not return to a normal color when the pressure is relieved, but there is no induration (area of hardened tissue); the skin and underlying tissues remain soft.

Stage 2: Redness persists, usually accompanied by edema and induration. The epidermis may blister or erode.

Stage 3: There is an open lesion and a crater, exposing subcutaneous tissue. You may be able to see fascia at the base of the ulcer.

Stage 4: Necrosis extends through the fascia and may even involve the bone. *Eschar* (crusty, black nonviable tissue) is a common finding. Bone destruction can lead to periostitis, osteitis, and osteomyelitis.

Sample nursing diagnoses are as follows:

Impaired Skin Integrity: Stage 2 Sacral Pressure Ulcer related to incontinence and malnutrition as manifested by persistent redness and edema in sacral area

Impaired Skin Integrity: Stage 4 Heel Pressure Ulcer related to immobility as manifested by 3-cm black necrotic area on the left heel involving fascia

Planning: Client Goals

The client will:

- Demonstrate signs of pressure ulcer healing
- Eliminate predisposing factors or reduce their effects
- Demonstrate appropriate self-care behaviors (if able):
  - Demonstrate satisfactory hygiene
  - Shift weight and change position every 1 to 2 hours
  - Eat nutritious diet (high in protein, iron, vitamin C; zinc supplements; sufficient fluids)
  - State rationale for treatment measures
- Develop no new areas of skin breakdown

Interventions

Nurses are really the first line of defense to prevent the development of pressure ulcers. An awareness of risk factors coupled with assessments made while bathing and caring for the client are of critical importance in preventing skin breakdown. The variety of nursing measures and skin-care interventions are addressed in the display Guidelines for Nursing Care.

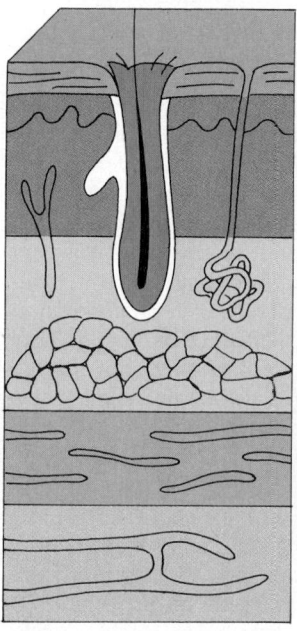
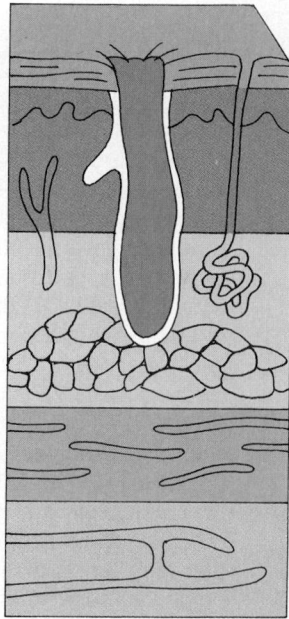

Stage 1
The primary sign is redness. The skin doesn't return to a normal color when the pressure is relieved, but there is no induration—the skin and underlying tissues remain soft.

Stage 2
Redness persists, usually accompanied by edema and induration. The epidermis may blister or erode.

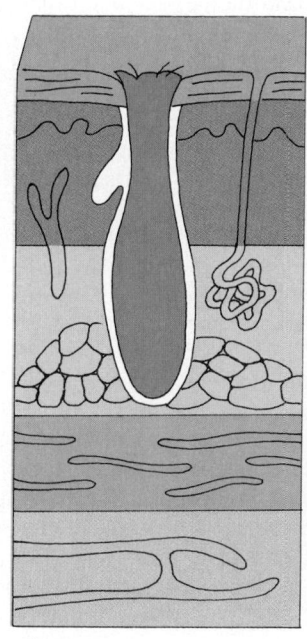
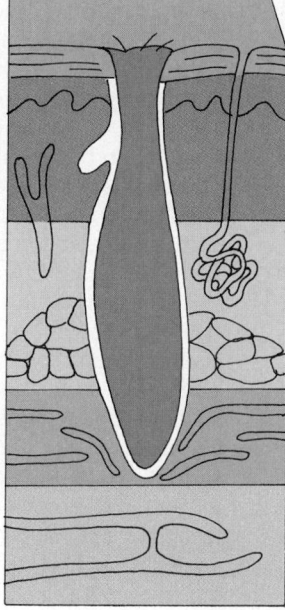

Stage 3
There is an open lesion and a crater exposing subcutaneous tissue. You may be able to see fascia at the base of the ulcer.

Stage 4
Necrosis will extend through the fascia and may even involve the bone. Eschar is a common finding. Bone destruction can lead to periosteitis, osteitis, and osteomyelitis.

FIGURE 29-14

Stages of development of pressure ulcers.

Preventing Pressure Ulcers

- Change the client's position *frequently* to relieve pressure, which if unrelieved, is the most important cause of a pressure ulcer. This should be done every 1 to 2 hours or on an individualized schedule based on the client's meals and activities. The back-lying position should be used as infrequently as possible because it causes the greatest amount of pressure to many vulnerable areas of the body. A turn of only 30 degrees to an oblique position is an effective alternative (refer to Chapter 30). It reduces pressure over bony prominences and can be managed by one nurse using several pillows to support the client. The right and left side-lying positions and lying on the abdomen are preferred.

- Do everything possible to keep the client in the best possible physical condition. This includes seeing to it that the client eats nutritious meals, takes plenty of fluids, has sufficient rest, and receives active and passive activity, including ambulation. Healthy, well-nourished cells are less likely to deteriorate.

- Keep the skin dry and clean. Dampness and uncleanliness predispose to skin breakdown and infection.

- Use a mild soap or detergent and water when cleaning the skin, and rinse soap or detergent from the skin. Soap and detergent residues are irritating and predispose to skin breakdown. Blot tender skin dry to prevent friction. Some agencies use a special skin care program for high-risk clients that includes a water-repellant ointment for the perineal area.

- Avoid using waterproof material on the client's bed. It tends to cause the client to perspire and prevents evaporation of moisture. Pads made of synthetic fibers or closely cropped wool may be placed under pressure-prone areas. The spaces between the tufts allow air circulation and help keep the area dry. The use of diapers is discouraged because they increase skin temperature in the area and are likely to lead to skin breakdown.

- Massage areas carefully and frequently where there is pressure on the body *except when redness is already present*. Redness, or erythema, that does not disappear within 30 minutes is recognized as a stage 1 ulcer. Massaging normally stimulates circulation to the area but may worsen the soft tissue damage already present. Alcohol for massaging is drying but tends to toughen the skin. A lotion or cream adds moisture, but if it is not allowed to dry well, it may soften the skin and predispose to breaks in the skin.

- Protect areas especially prone to pressure, such as the coccyx, heels, and elbows. There are various devices on the market to protect such areas as the heel and elbow. Also, consider using packs filled with gelatinous material under parts of the body where pressure is present. They are available in various sizes and shapes to fit different parts of the body.

- Prevent friction on the skin when moving the client. Avoid sliding the client on bed linens or on a chair. Friction burns predispose to pressure-sore formation.

- Support clients in bed and in a chair securely so that they do not slip down and cause a shearing force to occur. It is recommended that an ulcer-prone patient not have the head of the bed elevated more than 30 degrees to prevent sliding down in bed.

- Avoid using air-inflated rings, or use them only with the greatest care. They may relieve pressure over an area, but they restrict circulation where the body part rests on the ring. This pressure may cause more problems than the ring may prevent.

- Keep bed linens free of wrinkles, and dry and clean to prevent friction and irritation to the skin.

- Avoid applying top linens on the client's bed so that they restrict freedom of movement. Also, avoid pressure and irritation from casts, adhesive, tubing, arm boards, and the like.

- Protect areas of the skin especially susceptible to pressure sores. A silicone and zinc oxide mixture dispensed in aerosol has been used effectively. So also has tincture of benzoin.

- Use pressure-relieving devices such as synthetic sheepskin, air mattresses, egg-crate mattresses, air–fluid support systems, and low air-loss bed systems. The Clinitron bed minimizes pressure and eliminates shear, friction, and maceration by means of the fluidization principle. The client floats on a dry fluid created by forcing a gentle flow of temperature-controlled air upward through a mass of fine ceramic microspheres. The client's body fluids pass downward through a specially designed filter shell. This elimination of moisture and the desiccating effect on the warm, dry air flow provide a clean immediate environment hostile to bacterial growth. Maceration is virtually eliminated so there is reduced need for dressings, topicals, and antibiotics. A low air-loss system such as the Mediscus bed consists of the bed and an air-supply system. The frame provides ease in position changes, allowing the client's head and trunk to be elevated, the feet and thighs to be raised, and the knees flexed. Other systems allow for side-to-side rotation. The client lies directly on vapor-permeable air sacs, controlled by preset dials determined by client size and comfort. The sacs are machine washable, and drawsheets may be used for the incontinent client.

- Use topical agents or wound treatments as ordered by the physician to treat pressure ulcers. The stage of the ulcer determines the type of dressing. A moist environment appears to facilitate healing of stage 1 and 2 ulcers. Polyurethane films or hydrocolloid dressings are occlusive, maintain a moist environment, and allow epithelial cells to more easily bridge

(continued)

Preventing Pressure Ulcers *(continued)*

the open surface of the wound and close it. The presence of drainage may necessitate irrigation of the wound before the occlusive dressing is applied. Stage 3 and 4 ulcers are larger wounds that are frequently infected and have necrotic tissue. They may require débridement or removal of the necrotic tissue and additional surgical procedures to close the wound. Many products are currently available to treat pressure ulcers but selection of the appropriate dressing often proves difficult. Researchers continue to test and evaluate these various methods in an effort to identify the treatment of choice for the various stages of pressure ulcers.

- Irrigate a decubitus ulcer only if ordered by the physician. Normal saline is frequently prescribed because it is less traumatizing than other solutions to tissues and does not destroy the newly formed granulation tissue. Hydrogen peroxide, povidone-iodine (Betadine), and Dakin's antiseptic solution are currently being discouraged for treatment of open pressure ulcers because they delay healing (Wound Care Update 91, 1991). The traditional method of using a bulb syringe may not produce enough pressure to

cleanse the wound and a large syringe (35 mL or larger) with a 19-gauge needle is recommended by some researchers (Rogness, 1985).

- Avoid the use of a heat lamp. Heat is no longer recommended because it destroys the moist environment necessary for wound healing. Using a heat lamp also increases the tissue requirement for oxygen in an area that is already ischemic (Maklebust, 1991).
- Use wet-to-damp dressings rather than wet-to-dry for packing open wounds. The wet-to-dry technique removes drainage and necrotic tissue but also interferes with formation of fragile granulation tissue. The wet-to-damp dressing continues the moist environment necessary for effective wound healing without disrupting new tissue (Wound Care Update 91, 1991).
- Use a risk assessment scale if one is available in the health care facility to predict which clients are likely to develop a decubitus ulcer and require nursing intervention. Items that are assessed may include physical and mental condition, activity level, mobility, and incontinence. A sample risk assessment tool can be found on pages 629 and 630.

Because of the lack of consensus on pressure ulcer management, it is generally recommended that the nurse follow agency guidelines for the treatment of pressure ulcers in each of their four stages. Débridement guidelines (stage 3 and 4 ulcers); cleansing and rinsing solutions; and dressing treatment should be specified. Wound irrigations are described in Chapter 43. Aggressive intervention can

spare the client unnecessary pain and discomfort, prevent further tissue deterioration, hasten wound healing, and save millions of health care dollars.

Evaluative Criteria
The client meets the previously stated goals.

 C A S E   S T U D Y

Glenda Davis is a nurse practitioner who works in a campus health clinic at a state university. She is frequently approached by women who ask questions about feminine hygiene. Realizing that each woman who presents with a question probably represents many other women with similar unvoiced questions, she decides to develop an insert titled *Self-Care: Feminine Hygiene* for the campus newspaper.

Assessment Findings

- Heterogeneous female population is of various ages, cultures, religions, sexual orientation, and family and life-style backgrounds.
- Knowledge about feminine hygiene varies widely from almost no knowledge to students who are well read or members of women's health professions.
- Students who present with questions are mostly con-

cerned about dangers of certain products (eg, tampons and toxic shock syndrome) or have questions related to intercourse (eg, advisability of douching, how to avoid getting an STD, and so forth).

- Numerous students report to the clinic with vaginal infections and urinary tract infections.
- Interest is high; ability to comprehend written material is high.

Nursing Diagnosis

Self-Care Deficit: Feminine Hygiene, related to knowledge deficit

Planning: Client Goals

Ms. Davis talks with other nurses at the campus health clinic and together they decide to make education about

▼ PROMOTING WELLNESS

Self-Care: Feminine Hygiene

Many women have concerns about feminine hygiene. Personal health care practices are influenced by past experiences, cultural knowledge, and societal expectations. It is important for women to feel comfortable with their bodies and to be knowledgeable about self-care practices that promote health and well-being and prevent infection and disease. If this is a concern for you, take a few minutes to respond to the questions below and read the accompanying information.

Assessment Guide (Check the phrase that best describes you)	Self-Care Knowledge, Attitude, Skills
☐ I feel comfortable with my body. I accept its uniqueness. ☐ My body often makes me feel uncomfortable (fearful, anxious, guilty).	A woman's health and sense of self can be uniquely influenced by her sexuality and its expression and by several changes in her physiology: the onset of menstruation, pregnancy, interruption of pregnancy, childbirth, postpartum, nursing, and menopause. By virtue of ownership, women have the right to control their own bodies. This includes *knowing* their bodies, accepting their uniqueness, and caring for their bodies appropriately. Distorted ideas that the genital area is somehow "dirty" and needs special deodorizing and scenting or that it is shameful to discuss problems in this area or to talk about related concerns need to be replaced by healthier attitudes. Often these ideas are deep-seated and reinforced by culture, religion, and society (advertising world).
☐ I am knowledgeable about feminine hygiene practices and products. I value preventive measures that promote health and reduce the likelihood of infection. ☐ I have never thought much about feminine hygiene nor discussed this with anyone.	Each woman can be an expert in the care of her own body. Feminine hygiene practices that promote health and prevent infection include the following: • Wash the perineal area at least once daily to remove perspiration and smegma accumulations; pat rather than rub the area dry; towels and washcloths should be clean and never shared. • Always wipe from front to back after voiding and defecation to avoid introducing bacteria into the vagina or urethra. • Sprays, soaps, powders, deodorants, and tampons and pads that are perfumed or irritating in any way should not be used; any chemicals that irritate the skin or vaginal mucosa or alter the vaginal environment should be avoided. • Avoid clothing that is too tight, does not allow free air flow to the

feminine hygiene a priority for the year. Ms. Davis volunteers to develop a standardized care plan as well as a feminine hygiene health education handout for publication in the campus newspaper and distribution at the clinic. After discussion, the staff agrees on the following goals.

Long-Term Goals
• Female students consistently demonstrate positive ownership of their bodies and practice good personal hygiene.

Short-Term Goals
• Students will express positive body image, valuing their uniqueness.
• Students will correctly describe feminine hygiene self-care behaviors that they are willing to incorporate into their daily life-styles.
• Campus health clinic records will demonstrate a

reduction in both new and recurrent genitourinary infections.

The short-term goals may be evaluated at each client visit or at periodic intervals, for example, 6 months after development and use of handout on feminine hygiene.

Implementation

To develop better feminine hygiene self-care abilities successfully, the nurse needs the following specialized abilities:
• Strong interpersonal skills—the ability to communicate to women of many different backgrounds concern for their health questions and fears and the commitment to work with women to develop healthier self-care behaviors
• Attentive listening and other interviewing skills to assess the health care needs of this population correctly

perineum, or traps moisture; underpants and pantyhose should always have a cotton crotch.
- Douching should be avoided or kept to a minimum; douching can strip the vagina of its normal flora, introduce bacteria, and aggravate inflammation.
- If tampons are used during menstruation, choose the smallest absorbency needed to absorb flow; change regularly (every 3 to 4 hours), and use good handwashing techniques before insertion; women who have had toxic shock syndrome should not use tampons until *Staphylococcus aureus* is no longer present in the vaginal flora.
- Sexual partners should be clean: it is okay to discuss this with partners before intercourse; advise use of condoms; if any doubts exist about partner, refrain from contact; void before and after intercourse; if lubricant is needed during intercourse, a sterile, water-soluble type should be used. A final cautionary note: "Don't put anything in your vagina you wouldn't put in your mouth."

☐ I understand that changes in vaginal discharge, pain, and bleeding may indicate pathology or disease or may be a normal variation of the menstrual cycle.

☐ I know when to seek help.

☐ Changes in my body make me feel uncomfortable. I would probably delay seeking help with discomforting symptoms because of my anxieties.

Throughout her life, the average woman will experience bleeding, pain, or discharge associated with her reproductive organs or functions. These may cause discomfort, interference with life-style, and cause both physical and emotional distress. At times, professional assistance may be required to distinguish the normal from the abnormal, to identify pathology, and to explore the meaning of the symptom or illness.

Symptoms frequently experienced that may require the assistance of a health-care professional include abnormal vaginal discharge and itching of the vulva and vagina, gynecologic pain, differences in cyclic bleeding patterns or bleeding that is perceived as abnormal, and problems with urinary elimination.

Every woman should have a health care professional she trusts with whom she can discuss gynecologic problems. The nurses at the campus health clinic are committed to helping women with gynecologic problems.

(Adapted from Fogel, C. I., & Woods, N. F. [1981]. *Health care of women: A nursing perspective* [pp. 220–255]. St. Louis: Mosby.)

- Knowledge of feminine hygiene and advantages and disadvantages of various women's health care practices and products
- The ability to communicate to women acceptance and understanding of the female body—body parts (appearance, odor) and cycles
- Teaching and counseling skills to work one-on-one with women who come to the campus health clinic
- Written communication skills to develop a self-care feature on feminine hygiene for campus publication
- Accountability; self-direction

Documentation

This is a sample documentation of a nursing intervention written after a teaching session with a client who presented at the campus clinic.

SOAP Format

6/15/93, 3 PM, nursing

#1 Self-Care Deficit: Feminine Hygiene, related to knowledge deficit

S: Became sexually active this year; sexual intercourse once or twice weekly
"Many of my friends use douches . . . are there any douche products you particularly recommend?"
Expresses concern about contracting an STD from partners
O: —
A: Lacks knowledge about feminine hygiene practices related to intercourse
P: *Diagnostic*: Assess accuracy of what she has learned about feminine hygiene in general and specifically re-

lated to intercourse; explore her knowledge and feelings about her body.

Educative: Using the *Self-Care: Feminine Hygiene* handout, instruct regarding self-care practices. Clarify misconception regarding the advisability of douching. Counsel about her right to talk with a sexual partner about STDs and previous contacts with infected individuals; advise refraining from contact or to use condom when she has any doubts about partner.

I: Above were carried out.

E: Client reports feeling more "in charge" of body and better able to care for it.

Evaluation

Goal achievement is ongoing, once the nursing staff in the campus health clinic is committed to improving the self-care feminine hygiene behaviors of students and identifies this as a priority. Using the standardized care plan, short-term goal achievement may be evaluated at the conclusion of each client visit or at designated time intervals (eg, 6-month evaluation). See the care plan for related evaluative statements.

NURSING CARE PLAN

for Female University Students

Nursing Diagnosis:	Self-Care Deficit: Feminine Hygiene, related to knowledge deficit
Signs and Symptoms:	Female students present to the campus clinic with questions about feminine hygiene; high incidence of vaginal and urinary tract infections; negative attitudes about feminine body frequently expressed.
Long-Term Goal:	Female students consistently demonstrate positive ownership of their bodies, practicing good personal hygiene.

Goal: Students will:
- Express positive body image, valuing their uniqueness

Nursing Actions	**Rationale**	**Evaluative Statement**
With each student who presents at the clinic for help with a gynecologic concern or problem, take the time to assess her knowledge of the female body, and her acceptance of her body and comfort with it.	The women's health movement has encouraged women to feel ownership of their bodies, to appreciate their uniqueness as women, and to increase their awareness of their physical bodies and the feelings associated with them. Many women still feel that the genital area and cyclic phenomena such as the menstrual cycle and the female sexual response cycle are "dirty" and symptoms in this area may evoke fear, guilt, anxiety, and shame.	*Six-month evaluation:* 6/30/93 Goal partially met: students are beginning to discuss gynecologic concerns more freely yet great hesitancy persists. *Revision*: Continue to help women to know, understand, and accept their bodies and to talk about their bodies. Make this a priority of the nursing staff at the clinic. *G. Davis, RN*
Counsel appropriately.	It is important for nurses to provide women with information about their bodies.	

(continued)

NURSING CARE PLAN (continued)

for Female University Students

Students will:
- Correctly describe feminine hygiene self-care behaviors they are willing to incorporate into their daily life-styles

Nursing Actions	**Rationale**	**Evaluative Statement**
Assess with each client her knowledge of feminine hygiene practices (correct any misconceptions) and motivation to use them consistently.	Many women have never been instructed about feminine hygiene and harmful practices may be "picked up" from the media and other sources (eg, the use of frequent douching and deodorants to eliminate normal body odors).	6/30/93 Goal met. Following publication of the *Self-Care: Feminine Hygiene* feature and one-on-one counseling using this printed handout, clients are knowledgeable about preventive hygiene measures.
Address specific concerns related to menstruation, intercourse, other maturational events.	Maturational events, such as menstruation, becoming sexually active, and pregnancy, may result in a need for new or modified hygiene practices.	*G. Davis, RN*
Teach the importance of using preventive hygiene measures to reduce the likelihood of acquiring a urinary tract or vaginal infection. Distribute the *Self-Care: Feminine Hygiene* handout and discuss this with the client.	It is better to prevent a genitourinary infection than to treat it.	

Campus health clinic records will:
- Demonstrate a reduction in both new and recurrent genitourinary infections

Nursing Actions	**Rationale**	**Evaluative Statement**
Educate women regarding preventive hygiene measures (refer to the *Self-Care* handout).	It is better to prevent a genitourinary infection than to treat it.	6/30/93 Goal met. Six months after publication and use of the *Self-Care: Feminine Hygiene* handout, the incidence of genitourinary infections is reduced 10%. Will continue to keep education in this regard a priority.
Educate women to distinguish normal from abnormal findings (vaginal discharge, pain, bleeding, problems with urination) and to seek help when appropriate. Nursing measures include teaching preventive measures, instructing in recognition of symptoms, and assisting with self-care activities to prevent and teach infections, including the securing of assistance when indicated.	Early treatment of genitourinary infections reduces the likelihood of residual problems.	*G. Davis, RN*
Document new and recurrent genitourinary infections; identify predisposing factors.	Documentation facilitates ongoing management of a recurring problem.	

KEY POINTS

- Personal hygiene refers to measures of personal cleanliness and grooming that promote physical and psychological well-being.
- People differ in personal hygiene practices, which may be affected by culture, socioeconomic class, religion, developmental level, knowledge level, health state, and personal preferences.
- A comprehensive assessment of the skin and mucous membranes includes the collection of data about usual hygiene practices (showering or bathing practices; skin, hair, and scalp care; eye, ear, nose, and mouth care; nail and foot care; and perineal care); an assessment of any sensory, cognitive, endurance, mobility, or motivational deficit that interferes with the individual's hygiene practices; the identification of any existing problems of the skin or mucous membranes and associated care and its effectiveness; and a physical examination of the skin and mucous membranes.
- Because life-style factors, changes in health state, illness, and certain diagnostic and therapeutic measures may adversely affect the skin, the nurse needs to identify high-risk populations and perform the appropriate skin assessment, teach the client how to examine and care for the skin, and institute preventive skin care measures.

- Nursing diagnoses may be written that specifically address problems of deficient hygiene (Self-Care Deficit: Personal Hygiene) or that identify the effects problems of the skin, hair, scalp, eye, ear, nose, mouth, nail, feet, or perineum have on other areas of human functioning (comfort, mobility, nutrition).
- The individual with cognitive, sensory, endurance, mobility, or motivational deficits may require nursing assistance with any or all aspects of personal hygiene. The nurse promotes independence in these measures consistently. Whenever possible, the nurse offers assistance compatible with the individual's preferences and usual routines. When indicated, the client and family are taught necessary hygiene measures.
- Hospitalized clients receive scheduled hygienic care. This care includes careful attention to ensuring the safety and comfort of the client's bedside unit. Because of the long hours many ill clients spend in bed, the condition of bed linens is checked periodically throughout the day.
- Pressure ulcers continue to be a priority nursing problem. Identifying high-risk clients and immediately initiating a plan of preventive care are nursing's first concerns. When a pressure ulcer develops, ongoing assessment, diagnosis (staging), planning, treatment, and evaluation are imperative. The numerous treatment strategies available and absence of any one clearly successful modality underscore the need for preventive care.

STUDY QUESTIONS

1. An elderly client's skin requires special care because
   a. subcutaneous fat increases
   b. sebaceous glands secrete more oil
   c. the skin becomes increasingly dry
   d. the skin thickens
2. An appropriate nursing intervention for a client wearing antiembolic stockings is
   a. measure legs before applying stockings to assure proper fit
   b. apply stockings while the client is sitting in a chair
   c. massage the legs when the stockings are removed
   d. leave stockings in place for 1-week intervals
3. During a bath, the nurse observes that a client has dry skin. The nurse's best action is to
   a. bathe the client more frequently
   b. use an emollient on the dry skin
   c. massage the skin with alcohol
   d. discourage fluid intake

4. An adolescent client discusses her acne condition with the nurse. The nurse recommends that the client
   a. wash the skin frequently using soap
   b. use cosmetics liberally to cover blackheads
   c. use emollients on the area
   d. squeeze blackheads as they appear
5. A marked inflammation of the gums involving the alveolar tissue is referred to as
   a. glossitis
   b. caries
   c. cheilosis
   d. pyorrhea
6. A priority nursing action when administering oral care to a dependent client is
   a. assist the client to the dorsal recumbent position
   b. wear disposable gloves
   c. use a firm toothbrush to cleanse teeth and gums
   d. irrigate forcefully with hydrogen peroxide

7. Mr. James has an eye infection with a moderate amount of discharge. To clean his eyes, the nurse should
   a. use hydrogen peroxide
   b. wipe from the outer canthus to the inner canthus
   c. position on the same side as the eye to be cleansed
   d. use only one cotton ball per eye

8. The nurse's responsibility when giving foot care to an elderly client includes
   a. using scissors to correct an ingrown toenail situation
   b. trimming toenails as short as possible
   c. using an alcohol rub if the feet are dry
   d. bathing the feet at least daily

9. Providing perineal care to a client requires that the nurse
   a. use a clean portion of the washcloth for each stroke
   b. proceed from most contaminated to least contaminated area
   c. use sterile gloves
   d. leave the foreskin undisturbed in an uncircumcised male

10. An elderly invalid client sits and slumps in her chair most of the day. She is most likely to develop a pressure ulcer because of
    a. malnutrition
    b. shearing forces
    c. edema
    d. a chronic disease

11. The nurse assesses a stage 3 pressure ulcer. The nurse has observed
    a. redness that persists when pressure is relieved
    b. an open lesion with subcutaneous tissue exposed
    c. a necrotic area extending through the fascia to bone
    d. a reddened area that has blistered

12. A nurse assesses that a bedridden client is at risk for developing a pressure ulcer. As the nurse plans to change the client's position, the nurse is aware that
    a. a 30-degree turn to an oblique position is effective
    b. position should be changed once a shift
    c. the back-lying position should be used most frequently
    d. including position change in a care plan requires a physician's order

13. A priority nursing action to prevent a client from developing a pressure ulcer is
    a. use waterproof material on the bed
    b. massage any reddened area frequently
    c. use an air-inflated ring to relieve pressure on areas
    d. use a mild soap when cleansing the skin

14. Usual treatment for a stage 2 pressure ulcer is
    a. an occlusive hydrocolloid dressing
    b. surgical débridement
    c. exposure to a heat lamp four times daily
    d. irrigation with povidone-iodine (Betadine)

15. When making an occupied bed, it is important for the nurse to
    a. keep the bed in the low position
    b. use a bath blanket or top sheet for warmth and privacy
    c. constantly keep side rails raised on both sides
    d. move back and forth from one side to the other when adjusting the linens

Answers With Rationale

1. The correct response is *c*. With age the skin becomes increasingly dry, subcutaneous fat decreases, sebaceous glands secrete less oil, and the skin becomes thinner.

2. The correct response is *a*. The legs should always be measured according to manufacturer's directions before ordering antiembolism stockings. Stockings may be uncomfortable if applied while the client is sitting because leg veins are apt to be congested. Massage is dangerous because it may cause a clot to break away and circulate in the bloodstream. Stockings should always be removed once daily.

3. The correct response is *b*. An emollient soothes dry skin, whereas frequent bathing increases dryness, as does alcohol. Discouraging fluid intake leads to dehydration and, subsequently, dry skin.

4. The correct response is *a*. Washing the skin frequently with soap removes oil and debris, whereas liberal use of cosmetics and emollients can clog the pores. Squeezing blackheads is always discouraged because it may lead to infection.

5. The correct response is *d*. Pyorrhea is a marked inflammation of the gums, whereas caries refers to the presence of tooth decay. Cheilosis is ulceration of the lips and glossitis is an inflammation of the tongue.

6. The correct response is *b*. Disposable gloves provide a barrier to protect the nurse and client. The dorsal recumbent position is unsafe because the client may easily aspirate any secretions or fluids. A soft toothbrush is recommended to avoid causing irritation and bleeding, and forceful irrigation is never safe. Water would be the choice for any gentle irrigation.

7. The correct response is *c*. Positioning on the same side as the involved eye discourages any contamination of the other eye. Water or normal saline should

be used for cleansing the eye of any discharge and one cotton ball should be used for each stroke. Always cleanse from the inner canthus to the outer canthus to avoid forcing debris into the nasolacrimal duct.

8. The correct response is *d*. An elderly client should have foot care once daily. Correcting an ingrown toenail situation should be done by a podiatrist and trimming the toenails may require a physician's order. Additionally, cutting the toenails as short as possible exposes tender areas to friction and may lead to the skin being cut during trimming. Alcohol is drying and should not be used when dry skin is usually already a problem.

9. The correct response is *a*. Using a clean portion of the washcloth for each stroke prevents contamination of other areas. Cleansing should always proceed from the least contaminated to the most contaminated area. Clean gloves, not sterile gloves, are used to provide perineal care, and the foreskin in an uncircumcised male should be pulled back to allow cleansing underneath and then gently returned to its former position.

10. The correct response is *b*. Sitting slumped in a chair for an extended period can easily result in shearing force causing a pressure ulcer. Malnutrition, edema, and the presence of a chronic disease may certainly be risk factors for the development of a pressure ulcer, but the most likely cause in this situation is shearing force.

11. The correct response is *b*. A stage 3 pressure sore is an open lesion that exposes subcutaneous tissue. Redness that persists is stage 1, a reddened area that has blistered is stage 2, and stage 4 would involve a necrotic area extending through the fascia to the bone.

12. The correct response is *a*. A 30-degree turn to the oblique position relieves pressure on vulnerable areas. Position needs to be changed at least every 2 hours and is an independent nursing action. The back-lying position should be avoided as much as possible because it places pressure on many vulnerable sites.

13. The correct response is *d*. A mild soap is less irritating and the skin should be rinsed and dried thoroughly. Waterproof materials may cause the client to perspire, massage is not recommended for areas that are already traumatized, and air-inflated rings place additional pressure and compromise circulation to the area where they are used.

14. The correct response is *a*. An occlusive hydrocolloid dressing provides a moist environment for wound healing. A heat lamp or irrigation with Betadine are no longer recommended, and surgical débridement is used for stage 3 and 4 pressure ulcers.

15. The correct response is *b*. Using the bath blanket or top sheet keeps the client warm and provides privacy. Keeping the bed in the low position and working over raised siderails may strain the nurse's back. Continually moving back and forth to tuck and arrange linen is time-consuming and disorganized.

BIBLIOGRAPHY

Auld, E. (1988). Oral health. *Geriatric Nursing, 9*(6), 340–341.

Braden, B., & Bryant, R. (1990). Innovations to prevent and treat pressure ulcers. *Geriatric Nursing, 11*(4), 182–186.

Braun, J., Silvetti, A., & Xakellis, G. (1988). Decubitus ulcers: What really works? *Patient Care, 22*(16), 22–28.

Carnevali, D., & Patrick, M. (1986). *Nursing management for the elderly* (2nd ed.). Philadelphia: Lippincott.

Celia, L., & Wind, S. (1988). About pressure sores. *Nursing, 18*(5), 97.

Chovaz, C. (1989). Nursing the hearing impaired patient. *Canadian Nurse, 85*(3), 34–36.

Colburn, L. (1990). Preventing pressure ulcers: How to recognize and care for patients at risk. *Nursing, 20*(12), 60–63.

Conforti, C. (1989). Pressure sores: Dressed for successful healing. *Nursing, 19*(3), 58–61.

Echevarria, K., Bezon, J., Black, J., & Ross, V. (1988). A team approach to foot care. *Geriatric Nursing, 9*(6), 338–340.

Fowler, E., Cuzzel, J., & Papen, J. (1991). Healing with thin-film dressings. *American Journal of Nursing, 91*(3), 36–38.

Greifzu, S., Radjeski, D., & Winnick, B. (1990). Oral care is part of cancer care. *RN, 52*(6), 43–46.

Hoff, J. (1989). Effecting a change in nursing practice: Pressure ulcer prevention. *Journal of Nursing Quality Assurance, 3*(4), 56–63.

Irvine, A., & Black, C. (1990). Pressure sore practices. *Nursing Times, 86*(38), 74–78.

Iverson-Carpenter, M. (1988). Impaired skin integrity. *Journal of Gerontological Nursing, 14*(3), 25–29.

Kelley, L., & Mobily, P. (1991). Iatrogenesis in the elderly: Impaired skin integrity. *Journal of Gerontological Nursing, 17*(9), 24–29.

Kemp, M., Keithley, J., Smith, D., & Morreale, B. (1990). Factors that contribute to pressure sores in surgical patients. *Research in Nursing and Health, 13*(5), 293–301.

Kennedy, J. (1989). Ring cushions—An outmoded treatment. *Nursing Times, 85*(48), 34–35.

Lovell, H., & Anderson, C. (1990). Put your patient on the right bed. *RN, 52*(5), 66–72.

Maklebust, J. (1991). Pulling the plug on heat lamps. *RN, 51*(12), 79.

Maklebust, J. (1991). Pressure ulcer update. *RN, 53*(12), 56–62.

McCord, F., & Stalker, A. (1988). Brushing up on oral care. *Nursing Times, 84*(13), 40–41.

McDowell, S. (1991). Are we using too much Betadine? *RN, 53*(7), 43–45.

Meckstroth, R. (1989). Improving quality and efficiency in oral hygiene. *Journal of Gerontological Nursing, 15*(6), 38–42.

Miller, R., & Rubinstein, L. (1987). Oral health care for hospitalized patients: The nurse's role. *Journal of Nursing Education, 26*(9), 362–366.

Murray, S., & Thompson, R. (1991). We've organized our approach to pressure sores. *RN, 53*(1), 42–44.

National Pressure Ulcer Advisory Panel. (1989). *Pressure ulcers: Incidence, economics, risk assessment* (Consensus Development Conference Statement). West Dundee, IL: S-N Publications.

Neal, M. (1990). A cost-effective alternative to specialty beds for pressure relief. *Rehabilitation Nursing, 15*(4), 202–204.

Neander, K., & Birkenfeld, R. (1990). Alternating-pressure mattresses for the prevention of decubitus ulcers: A study of healthy subjects and patients. *Intensive Care Nursing, 6*(2), 67–73.

Olson, B. (1989). Effects of massage for prevention of pressure ulcers. *Decubitus, 2*(4), 32–37.

Palumbo, M. (1990). Hearing Access 2000: Increasing awareness of the hearing impaired. *Journal of Gerontological Nursing, 16*(9), 26–30.

Rodeheaver, G. (1988). Topical wound management. *Ostomy/Wound Management, 20*, 58.

Rogness, H. (1985). High pressure wound irrigation. *Journal of Enterostomal Therapy, 12*, 27.

Smeltzer, S., & Bare, B. (1992). *Brunner and Suddarth's textbook of medical–surgical nursing* (7th ed.). Philadelphia: Lippincott.

Staab, A., & Lyles, M. (1990). *Manual of geriatric nursing.* Glenview, IL: Scott, Foresman.

Travis, S. (1990). Personalizing self-care. *Geriatric Nursing, 11*(2), 72–73.

U.S. Department of Health and Human Services, Agency for Health Care Policy and Research. (May 1992). *Pressure ulcers in adults: Prediction and prevention.* Rockville, MD: Author.

Wound care update 91. (1991). *Nursing, 21*(4), 47–50.

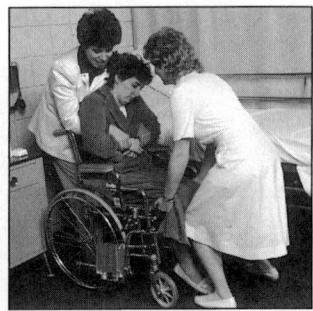
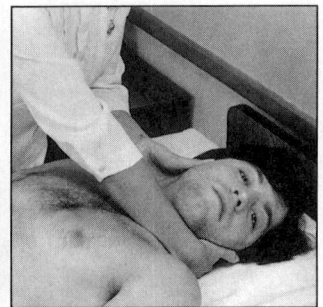
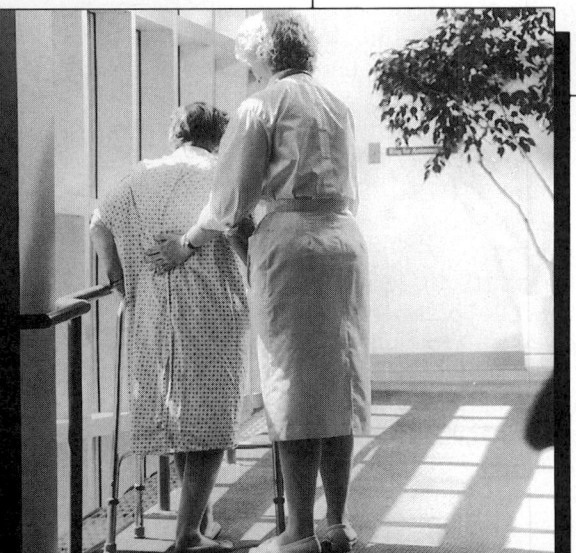

Activity

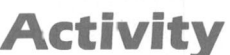

30

OBJECTIVES

After studying this chapter, the learner should be able to:

Define key terms used in this chapter.

Describe the role of the skeletal, muscular, and nervous systems in the physiology of movement.

Identify seven variables that influence body alignment and mobility.

Differentiate isotonic, isometric, and isokinetic exercise.

Describe the effects of exercise and immobility on major body systems.

Assess body alignment, mobility, and activity tolerance, using appropriate interview questions and physical assessment skills.

Develop nursing diagnoses that correctly identify mobility problems amenable to nursing therapy.

Use proper body mechanics when positioning, moving, lifting, and ambulating clients.

Design exercise programs.

Plan, implement, and evaluate nursing care related to select nursing diagnoses involving mobility problems.

KEY TERMS

abduction
active-assistive exercise
active exercise
adduction
aerobic exercise
ankylosis
atelectasis
atrophy
cartilage
circumduction
contractures
dorsiflexion
eversion
extension
external rotation
flaccidity
flexibility
flexion
footdrop
Fowler's position
hemiplegia
hyperextension
internal rotation
inversion
isokinetic exercise
isometric exercise
isotonic exercise
ligaments
osteoporosis
paraplegia
passive exercise
plantar flexion
pronation
prone position
range of motion
rotation
semi-Fowler's position
spasticity
supination
supine position
Sims' position
synovial joints
tendons

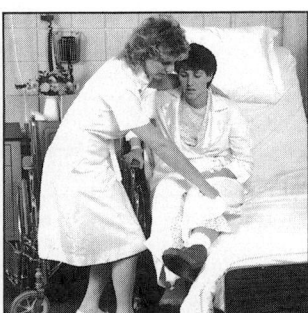

For most healthy individuals, the ability for movement is taken for granted. People simply expect our amazingly complex skeletal, skeletal muscle, and nervous systems to work together smoothly and on command to enable us to stand upright, to walk, and to reach for and grasp what we want. Often little thought is given to the need to care for the systems that promote and coordinate healthy movement until disuse, trauma, or illness cripples some aspect of movement. Although exercise and fitness are valued by some, many people live overwhelmingly inactive life-styles that limit their ability to experience and enjoy life to its fullest and that openly invite degenerative and chronic diseases such as hypertension, ischemic heart disease, or diabetes.

The ability to move is closely related to the fulfillment of other basic human needs. Although breathing continues during rest, movement facilitates pulmonary functioning and increases peripheral blood flow. Because regular exercise contributes to the healthy functioning of each body system and, conversely, immobility negatively affects each body system, nurses actively promote exercise to promote wellness, prevent illness, and restore health. It currently is generally accepted that there are more serious health consequences related to a sedentary life-style than there are risks related to exercise.

Study of this chapter provides the student with knowledge of the physiology of movement, the principles of body mechanics, and factors affecting body alignment and mobility. A comprehensive section on exercise differentiates types of exercise, explores the role of exercise in disease prevention and health promotion, notes risks related to exercise, and allows the design of individualized exercise programs. The effects of immobility on body systems are presented with a full discussion of related nursing interventions. A practical guide to assessing body alignment and mobility states is offered with pertinent interview questions and physical assessment techniques. Analysis of mobility data may lead to the nursing diagnoses of Impaired Physical Mobility or Activity Intolerance or to diagnoses identifying the effect of mobility problems on other areas of human functioning. Examples of nursing diagnoses are included. Client goals are identified and specific nursing strategies are presented. In the section entitled Nursing Process in Clinical Practice, focused assessment, planning, implementation, and evaluation guides are offered for select nursing diagnoses of common mobility problems: Ac-

tivity Intolerance; Impaired Physical Mobility; High Risk for Injury: Complications of Immobility; and Altered Health Maintenance: Lack of Exercise Program. These guides and the concluding case study illustrate how the nurse's knowledge of body mechanics and mobility is combined with specific nursing interventions and caring to successfully promote fitness and to resolve mobility problems.

Physiology of Movement

Purposeful coordinated movement of the body requires the integrated functioning of the skeletal, skeletal muscle, and nervous systems of the body. The following is a review of the physiology of movement.

Skeletal System

The framework of bones and cartilage that protects our organs and allows us to move is called the *skeletal system*. Functions of this system include the following:

- It supports the soft tissues of the body (maintains body form and posture).
- It protects the delicate structures of the body (brain, lung, heart, spinal cord).
- It furnishes surfaces for the attachments of muscles, tendons, and ligaments, which in turn pull on the individual bones and produce movement.
- It serves as storage areas for mineral salts and fat.
- It produces blood cells (hematopoiesis).

The 206 bones in the human body are classified on the basis of their shape. *Long bones*, which are found in the upper and lower extremities, contribute to height and length. *Short bones*, located in the wrist and ankle, contribute to movement. *Flat bones* are relatively thin (eg, ribs and several of the skull bones) and contribute to shape (structural contour). *Irregular bones* are all those bones not included in the preceding classifications (eg, bones of the spinal column and jaw).

Because bones are too rigid to bend without damage, all movements that change the positions of the bony parts of the body occur at joints. The terms *articulation* and *joint* refer to the area where bones come into close contact with one another. Joints are classified according to the amount of movement they permit. Of concern are the freely movable joints called *diarthroses* or **synovial joints**, in which there is a space between the articulating bones. Movements possible at diarthric joints include abduction, adduction, flexion, extension, and rotation. Special movements of the forearm, ankle, and clavicle include supination, pronation, inversion, and eversion. These movements are defined in Table 30-1 and illustrated in Figure 30-1. Types of freely movable joints include the following:

Ball-and-socket joint: Rounded head of one bone fits into a cuplike cavity in the other; flexion–extension, abduction–adduction, and rotation are permitted (eg, shoulder and hip joints).

T A B L E   3 0 - 1

Terms Commonly Used to Describe Body Positions and Movements

Term	Definition and Example
Abduction	Lateral movement of a body part away from the midline of the body. *Example:* A person's arm is abducted when it is moved away from the body.
Adduction	Lateral movement of a body part toward the midline of the body. *Example:* A person's arm is adducted when it is moved from an outstretched position to a position alongside the body.
Circumduction	Movement of the distal part of the limb to trace a complete circle while the proximal end of the bone remains fixed. *Example:* The leg is outstretched and moved in a circle.
Flexion	The state of being bent. *Example:* A person's cervical spine is flexed when the head is bent forward chin to chest.
Extension	The state of being in a straight line. *Example:* A person's cervical spine is extended when the head is held straight on the spinal column.
Hyperextension	The state of exaggerated extension. It often results in an angle greater than 180 degrees. *Example:* A person's cervical spine is hyperextended when looking overhead, toward the ceiling.
Dorsiflexion	Backward bending of the hand or foot. *Example:* A person's foot is in dorsiflexion when the toes are brought up as though to point them at the knee.
Plantar flexion	Flexion of the foot. *Example:* A person's foot is in plantar flexion in the footdrop position.
Rotation	Turning on an axis; the turning of a body part on the axis provided by its joint. *Example:* A thumb is rotated when it is moved to make a circle.
Internal rotation	A body part turning on its axis toward the midline of the body. *Example:* A leg is rotated internally when it turns inward at the hip and the toes point toward the midline of the body.
External rotation	A body part turning on its axis away from the midline of the body. *Example:* A leg is rotated externally when it turns outward at the hip and the toes point away from the midline of the body.
Special Movements	
Pronation	The assumption of the prone position. *Examples:* A person is in the prone position when lying on the abdomen; a person's palm is prone when the forearm is turned so that the palm faces downward.
Supination	The assumption of the supine position. *Examples:* A person is in the supine position when lying on the back; a person's palm is supine when the forearm is turned so that the palm faces upward.
Inversion	Movement of the sole of the foot inward (occurs at the ankle)
Eversion	Movement of the sole of the foot outward (occurs at the ankle)

Condyloid joint: Oval head of one bone fits into a shallow cavity of another bone; flexion–extension and abduction–adduction are permitted (eg, wrist joint).

Gliding joint: Articular surfaces are flat; flexion–extension and abduction–adduction are permitted (eg, carpal bones of wrist and tarsal bones of feet).

Hinge joint: Spool-like surface fits into a concave surface; only flexion–extension is permitted (eg, elbow, knee, and ankle joints).

Pivot joint: Ringlike structure that turns on a pivot; movement is limited to rotation, for example, turning a doorknob (eg, joints between the atlas and axis and between the proximal ends of the radius and the ulna).

Saddle joint: Bone surfaces are convex on one side and concave on the other; movements are side to side and back and forth (eg, joint between the trapezium and metacarpal of the thumb).

The strength and flexibility of the skeletal system also depend on ligaments, tendons, and cartilage. **Ligaments** are tough, fibrous bands that bind joints together and connect bones and cartilage. **Tendons** are strong, flexible, inelastic fibrous bands that attach muscle to bone. **Cartilage** is nonvascular connective tissue found in the joints as well as in the nose, ear, thorax, trachea, and larynx.

Muscular System

Bones and joints provide form to the body and serve as the levers and fulcrums that make body movement possible. It is the contraction and relaxation of skeletal muscles, however, that actually produce movement by pulling on bones. The excitability, contractility, extensibility, and elasticity of muscles enable them to perform three important functions for the body through contraction:

- Motion
- Maintenance of posture (skeletal muscle contractions hold the body in stationary positions)
- Heat production (skeletal muscle contractions produce heat and help maintain body temperature)

There are actually three types of muscles: (1) skeletal, (2) cardiac, and (3) smooth or visceral. The skeletal muscle

Neck

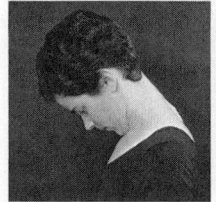
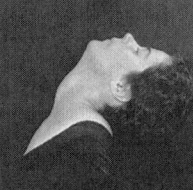
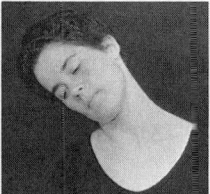
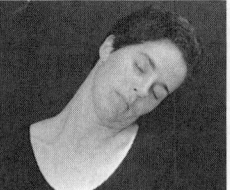
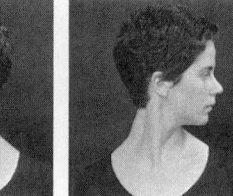

Flexion   Hyperextension   Lateral flexion   Rotation

Shoulder

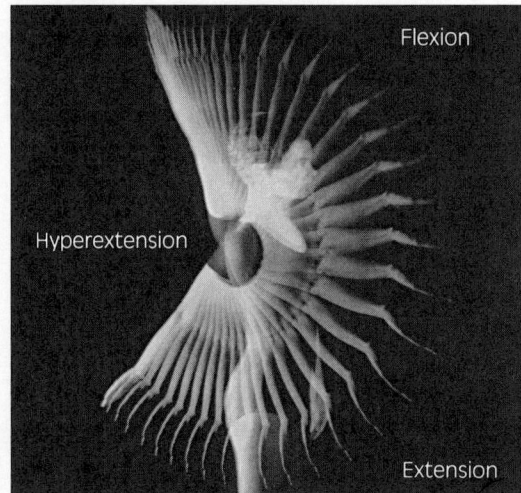
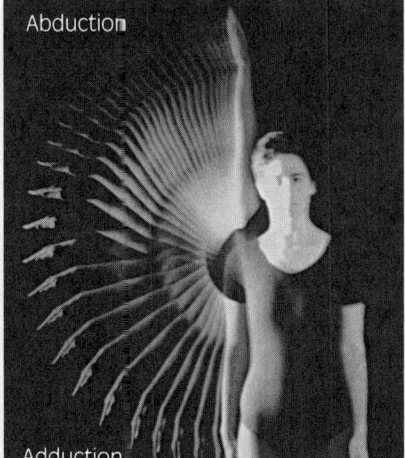
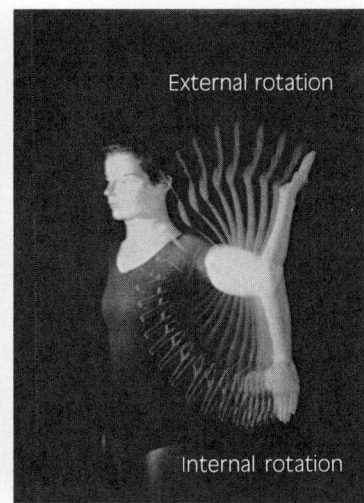

Elbow

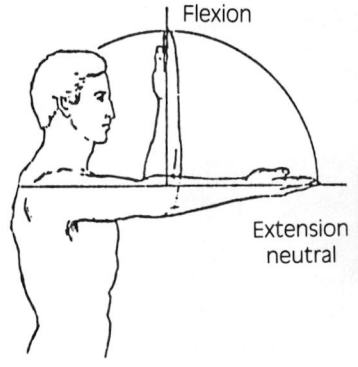
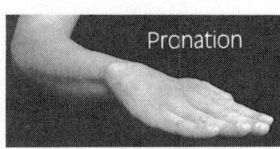
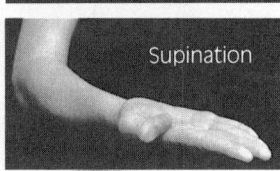

Flexion

Extension
neutral

Pronation

Supination

Wrist

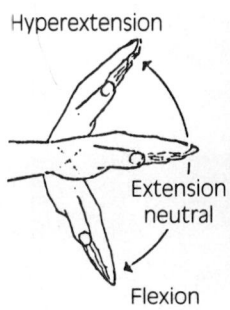
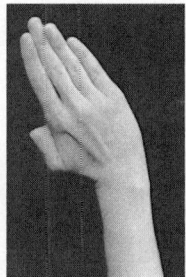
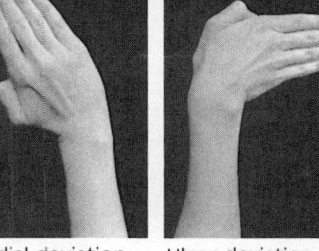

Hyperextension

Extension
neutral

Flexion

Radial deviation   Ulnar deviation

Fingers

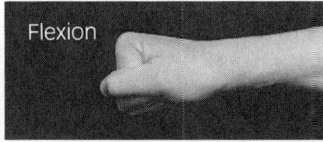
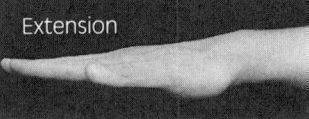
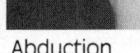
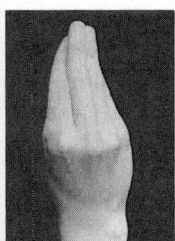
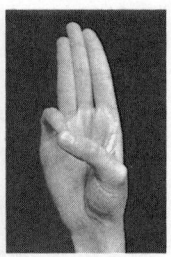

Flexion

Extension

Abduction   Adduction   Apposition of
thumb to finger

FIGURE 30-1

Normal range of motion of selected joints.

Hip

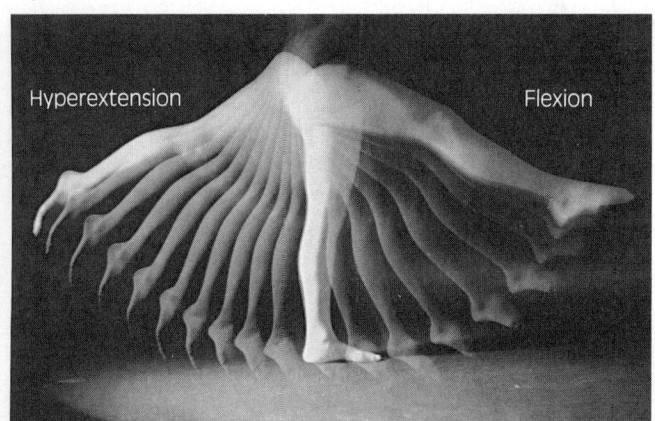

Extensicn

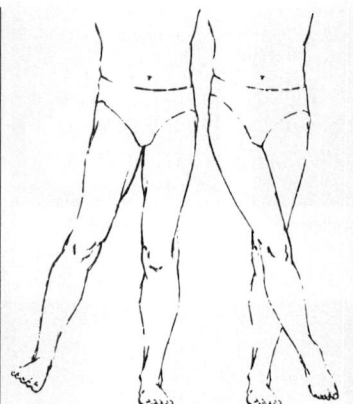

Abduction   Adduction

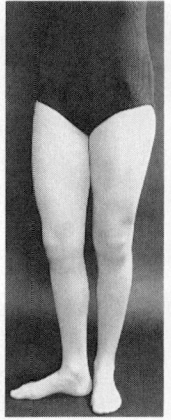

External rotation

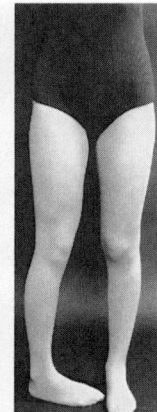

Internal rotation

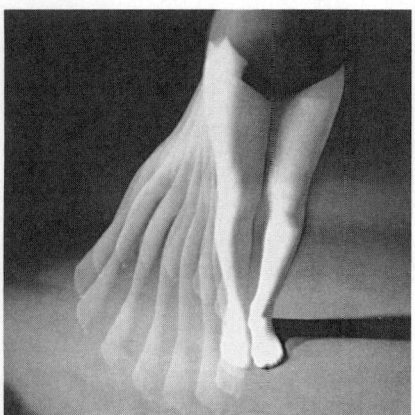

Rotation

Knee

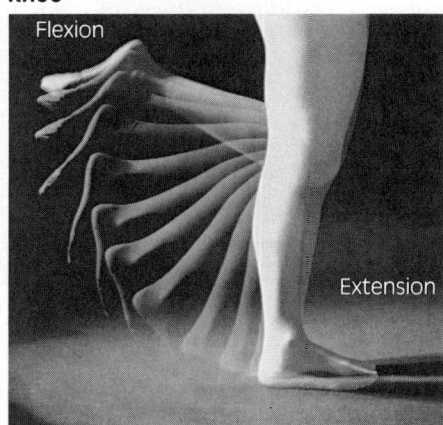

Flexion

Extension

Ankle

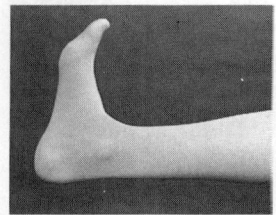

Dorsiflexion

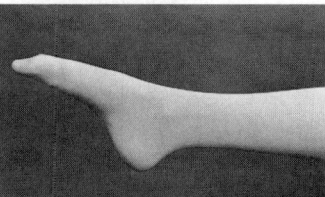

Plantar flexion

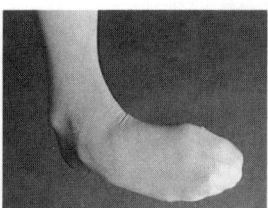

Inversion

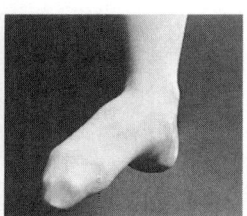

Eversion

Toes

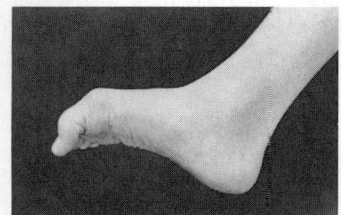

Flexion

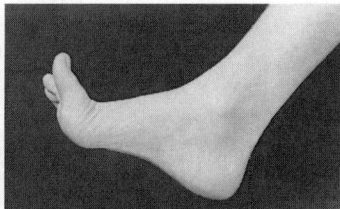

Extension

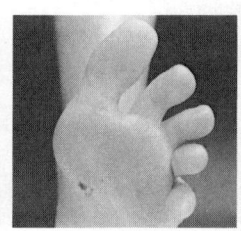

Abduction

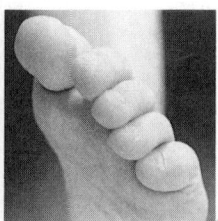

Adduction

F I G U R E   3 0 - 1 *(continued)*

system includes the skeletal muscle tissue and connective tissue that compose individual muscle organs, such as the biceps. Movement is the result of a skeletal muscle contracting and exerting force on a tendon, which in turn pulls on a bone. Muscles have two differing points of attachment: (1) attachment of a muscle to the more stationary bone is called the *point of origin* and (2) attachment to the more movable bone is the *point of insertion*. Between these two points is the fleshy "belly" of the muscle. Figure 30-2 illustrates the relationship of skeletal muscles to bones and the use of bones as levers and joints as fulcrums to produce body movement.

Nervous System

The skeletal and muscular systems cannot produce purposeful movement without a functioning nervous system. It is a nerve impulse that stimulates muscles to contract. More specifically,

- The afferent nervous system conveys information from receptors in the periphery of the body to the central nervous system (eg, light pressure on nose).
- Nerve cells called *neurons* are responsible for conducting impulses from one part of the body to another.
- This information is processed by the central nervous system (CNS) and a response is decided on (eg, "There is a fly on my nose. I want to brush it off").
- The efferent system conveys the desired response from the CNS to skeletal muscles by way of the somatic nervous system (eg, muscles in the arm, wrist, and hand contract and the fingers brush the fly from the face).

Body Mechanics

Body mechanics is the efficient use of the body as a machine and as a means of locomotion. Body mechanics is directly related to the effective functioning of the body. The correct use of body mechanics should be evident in every activity and even during rest periods.

Because correct use of the body is another phase of illness prevention and health promotion, the nurse has a major responsibility to teach both directly and indirectly by example. To be able to evaluate the client's musculoskeletal needs, the nurse must understand and use correct body mechanics. Every activity in which the nurse engages requires understanding and use of these principles, from as simple an activity as moving a chair to lifting a client out of bed.

Orthopedics means the correction or the prevention of disorders of the body's structures for locomotion. Nurses have long recognized that basic orthopedic principles apply to all areas of nursing, not just to the client who has a bone fracture or some other pathologic skeletal change. For example, the person who has a sedentary occupation and engages in little physical activity may have poorly developed muscles. The client who is on complete bed rest is in danger of losing muscle tonus. *Tonus* is the term used to

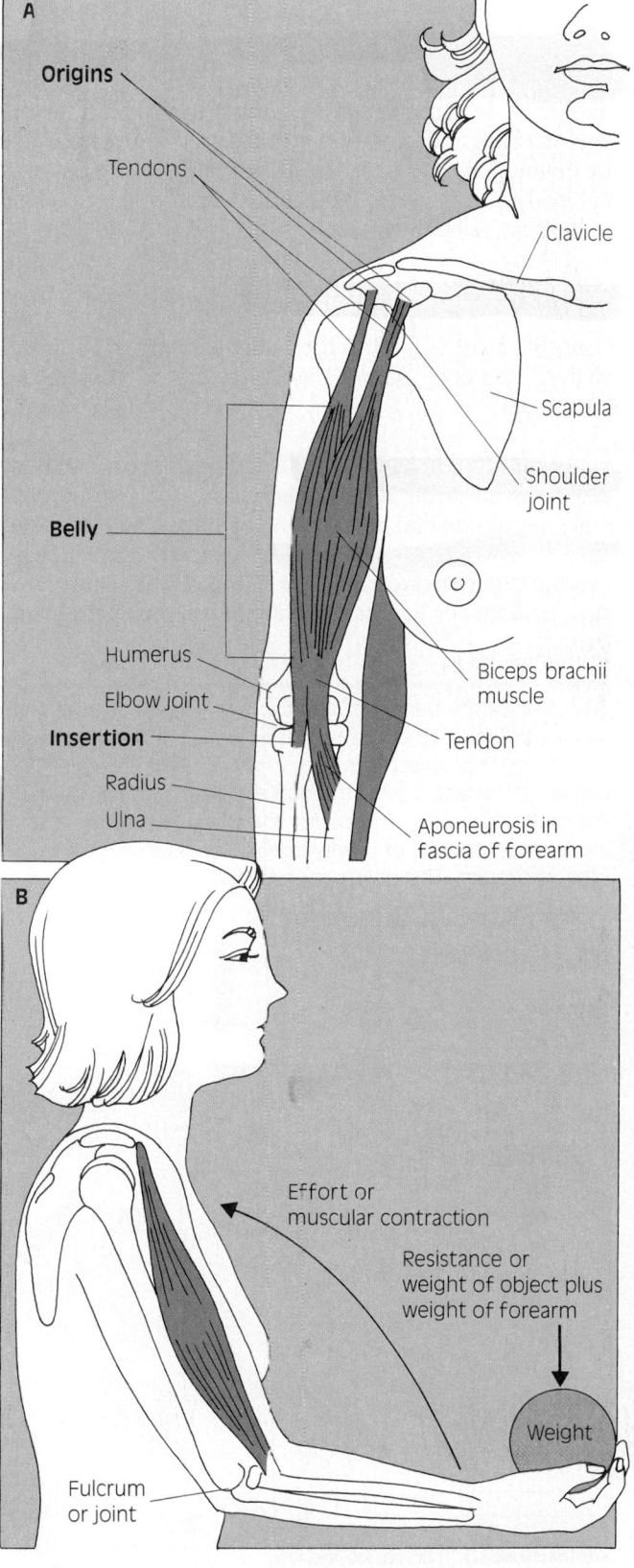

F I G U R E   3 0 - 2

Relationship of skeletal muscles to bones. (*Top*) Skeletal muscles produce movements by pulling on bones. (*Bottom*) Bones serve as levers, and joints act as fulcrums for the levers. The lever and fulcrum principle is illustrated by the movement of the forearm lifting a weight.

describe the state of slight contraction—the usual state of skeletal muscles. Should bed rest be prolonged, there is danger of developing contractures if the client does not have exercise and joint motion and if provision is not made for maintaining good posture. Functioning of various internal body processes is also influenced by position and movement or by their absence.

Concepts of Body Mechanics

Concepts most helpful to the understanding of body mechanics are body alignment, balance, and coordinated movement.

Body Alignment or Posture   Good posture or good body alignment is that alignment of body parts that permits optimal musculoskeletal balance and operation and promotes healthy physiologic functioning. A person in correct alignment is experiencing no undue strain on the joints, muscles, tendons, or ligaments while balance is maintained.

F I G U R E   3 0 - 3

The effect of the base of support and gravity on balance is shown. (A) The line of gravity passes through the wide base of support. This object is the most stable of the three. (B) The line of gravity also passes through the base support, although the base is narrower. This object is less stable than the one on the left. (C) The line of gravity does not pass through the base of support. This object is unstable.

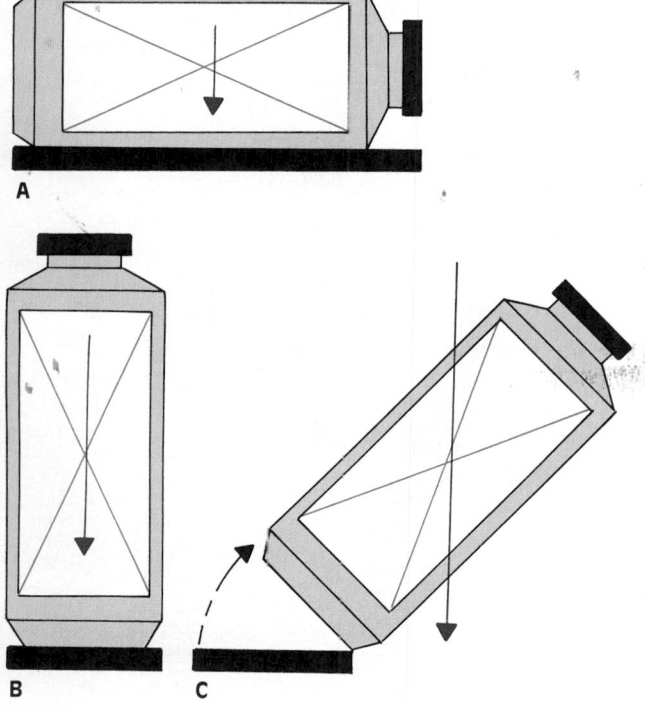

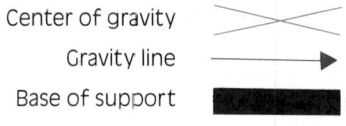

Center of gravity

Gravity line

Base of support

Criteria for correct alignment in the standing, sitting, and reclining positions are presented in the assessment section later in this chapter.

Balance   A body in correct alignment is balanced. An object is balanced when its center of gravity is close to its base of support, the line of gravity goes through the base of support, and the object has a wide base of support. The *center of gravity* of an object is the point at which its mass is centered. In humans, the center of gravity when standing is located in the center of the pelvis about midway between the umbilicus and the symphysis pubis. The *line of gravity* is a vertical line that passes through the center of gravity. The *base of support* is the foundation that provides for an object's stability. The wider the base of support and the lower the center of gravity, the greater the stability of the object. Figure 30-3 illustrates body balance.

Nurses can increase body balance when working by spreading their feet farther apart (broadening the base of support) and by flexing their hips and knees (lowering the center of gravity). These two simple maneuvers are important principles in body mechanics by which nurses can decrease musculoskeletal strain.

Coordinated Body Movement   Because the nurse providing direct client care must frequently use the body to assist in positioning, turning, and lifting both clients and equipment, it is important to do this knowledgeably to avoid musculoskeletal strain and injury. This work is facilitated when the nurse uses major muscle groups rather than weaker ones and takes advantage of the body's natural levers and fulcrums. For example, rather than attempt to push a client to the opposite side of the bed, the nurse flexes the knees, positions the forearms above and below the client's buttocks (preferably under a pull sheet), and rocks backward sliding the client toward self. This one coordinated movement illustrates the following principles:

- The nurse is using major muscle groups—flexors, extensors, and abductors of the thighs; flexors and extensors of the knees; flexors and extensors of the upper and lower arms—rather than weaker ones.
- Use of the arm bones as levers and the elbows as fulcrums facilitates lifting a weight against resistance (force of gravity)—the lever and fulcrum principle.
- Using a pull sheet and smooth, dry, firm bed foundation decreases the effects of friction, which increases the amount of effort required to move an object. Rough, wet, or soiled surfaces contribute to friction's effect.
- By positioning the arms under the client's center of gravity (hips) and sliding the body back toward himself or herself, the nurse is working close to the object to be moved and decreasing the effort involved.

Postural Reflexes

Integrated functioning of the musculoskeletal and nervous systems is essential for body alignment and balance. Postural tonus, the sustained contraction of select skeletal

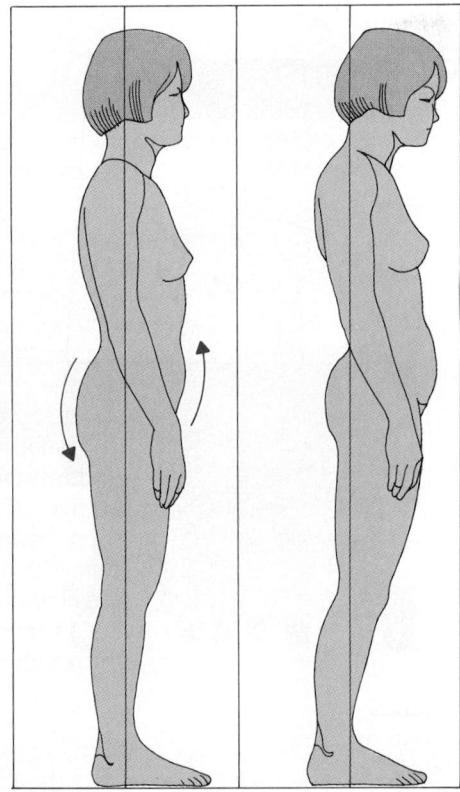

FIGURE 30-4

(*Left*) Internal girdle "on." Abdominal muscles contracted, giving a feeling of upward pull, and gluteal muscles contracted, giving a downward pull. (*Right*) Slouch position, showing abdominal muscles relaxed and body out of good alignment.

muscles that keeps the human body in an upright position against the force of gravity, depends on the functioning of several postural reflexes:

Labyrinthine sense: This is provided by the sensory organs in the inner ear, which are stimulated by body movement (changes in head position) and transmit these impulses to the cerebellum.

Proprioceptor or kinesthetic sense: This informs the brain of the location of a limb or body part as a result of joint movements stimulating special nerve endings in muscles, tendons, and fascia.

Visual or optic reflexes: Visual impressions contribute to posture by alerting the person to spatial relationships with the environment (nearness of ceilings, walls, furniture, condition of floor, and so on).

Extensor or stretch reflexes: Conceivably, the force of gravity could exert enough force to flex the body at the hip and knees; when extensor muscles are stretched beyond a certain point (eg, when knees buckle under), their stimulation causes a reflex contraction that reestablishes erect posture.

Body Mechanics Used for Work

The following guidelines are offered for the use of body mechanics when the person is at work:

- Develop a habit of erect posture (correct alignment) and, whenever necessary, begin activities by broadening the base of support and lowering the center of gravity.
- Use the longest and the strongest muscles of the arms and the legs to help provide the power needed in strenuous activities. The muscles of the back are less strong and are easily injured when used improperly.
- Use the internal girdle and a long midriff to stabilize the pelvis and to protect the abdominal viscera when stooping, reaching, lifting, or pulling. The internal girdle is made by contracting the gluteal muscles in the buttocks downward and the abdominal muscles upward. It is helped further by making a long midriff. This is done by stretching the muscles in the waist. Figure 30-4 illustrates the internal girdle.
- Work as closely as possible to an object that is to be lifted or moved. This brings the body's center of gravity close to that of the object being moved, thereby permitting most of the burden to be borne by the leg and arm muscles. Figure 30-5 illustrates a proper and an improper way to pick up an object.
- Use the weight of the body as a force for pulling or pushing, by rocking on the feet or leaning forward or

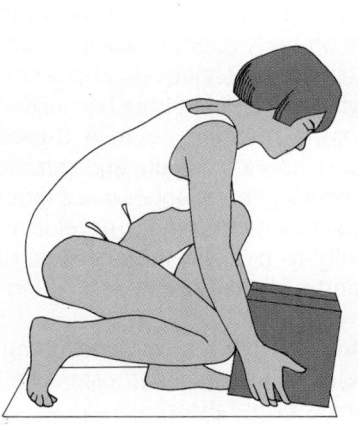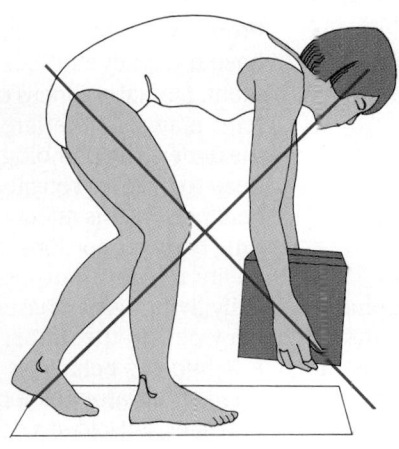

FIGURE 30-5

(*Left*) A good position for lifting is illustrated. This person is using the long and strong muscles of the arms and legs and holding the object so that the line of gravity falls within the base of support. (*Right*) This is an incorrect position for lifting because pull is exerted on the back muscles and leaning causes the line of gravity to fall outside the base.

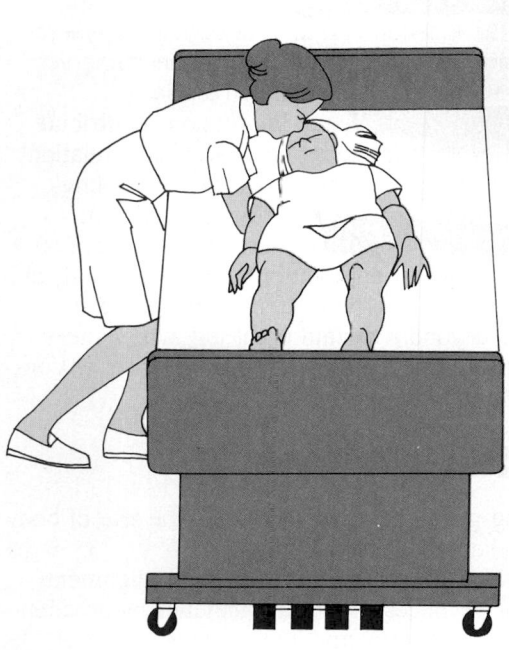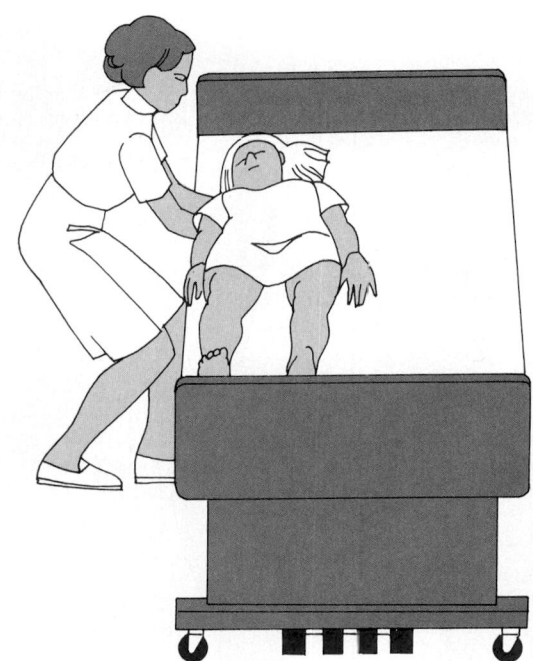

FIGURE 30-6

Before sliding a client to the edge of the bed, establish a wide base of support with one knee near the edge of the bed and both knees flexed. Place arms under the client as far as possible while close to and leaning over the client. Rock backward, using your own body weight to assist in moving the client toward you.

backward. This reduces the amount of strain placed on the arms and the back.

- Slide, roll, push, or pull an object rather than lift it to reduce the energy needed to lift the weight against the pull of gravity.
- Use the weight of the body to push an object by falling or rocking forward, and to pull an object by falling or rocking backward. Sliding a client in bed while rocking backward is illustrated in Figure 30-6.
- Place the feet apart to provide a wider base of support when increased stability of the body is necessary.
- Flex the knees, put on the internal girdle, and come down close to an object that is to be lifted.

The nurse can demonstrate to others the proper way of using the musculoskeletal system if good habits are consciously developed in the use of the musculoskeletal system.

Factors Affecting Body Alignment and Mobility

Numerous factors, including growth and development, physical health, mental health, life-style variables, attitude and values, fatigue and stress, and external factors, such as weather, influence an individual's posture, movement, and daily activity level.

Developmental Considerations

A person's age and degree of neuromuscular development markedly influence body proportions, posture, body mass, movements, and reflexes. To promote neuromuscular development in clients of all ages and to facilitate each client's use of the body to perform self-care actions, the nurse needs to be familiar with developmental variations in body proportions and neuromuscular development. These variations are presented in Table 30-2 with related nursing assessment priorities and nursing interventions.

Physical Health

Problems in the musculoskeletal or nervous systems can have a negative influence on body alignment and movement. Similarly, illness or trauma involving other body systems may also interfere with movement either because of the underlying pathology or the treatment regimen. Nurses need to develop sensitivity to how both acute and chronic health problems affect a client's general appearance (posture, body proportions, and movements) and to develop an ability to move purposefully to perform the activities of daily living. When assessing a client's response to a mobility deficit, the nurse:

- Reinforces behaviors that promote healthy functioning (eg, congratulates a client who manages transfers well despite left-sided weakness or paralysis)

TABLE 30-2

Structural and Functional Developmental Changes in Body Alignment and Mobility With Related Nursing Assessment and Intervention Priorities

Developmental Changes	Assessment Priorities	Nursing Interventions
Infant		
Structure: The newborn term infant usually lies with extremities flexed and hands closed; the spine is flexed and lacks the anteroposterior curves of the adult. *Function*: The infant's spontaneous activity varies greatly. Periods of activity and alertness alternate with quiet periods and sleep. • By age 3 months, the infant in the prone position is generally able to raise the chest and head from the floor. • By 5 months, head control is usually achieved in both the sitting position and when being held erect.	Newborn assessments should include attention to structure of spine and extremities (deformities); muscle tone and strength (abnormal movements and tremors); reflex responses; and activity level and alertness (jitteriness, lethargy, paresis). *3- to 6-month assessment* • Head control • Ability to sit *6- to 9-month assessment* *Gross motor* Ability to: • Sit steadily • Roll over adeptly • Creep on all fours • Pull to a standing position *Fine motor* • Improved hand–eye coordination *9- to 12-month assessment* *Gross motor* • Progress toward unassisted walking *Fine motor* • Skill in using hands—ability to pick up even tiny objects	Parents may need the nurse's help in "examining" their baby (eg, counting fingers and toes). This is an excellent time for the nurse to respond to any concerns parents have about minor variations in their newborn's appearance or behavior. Nurses may need to explain to parents that there is great individual variation in total activity patterns and neuromuscular development among infants and children.
Toddler		
Structure: The young toddler's long trunk, short legs, and undeveloped abdominal musculature (potbelly) give the toddler a top-heavy, sway-backed appearance. Growth during this period is rapid and faster in the legs than in the trunk. The young toddler walks on a broad base with flat feet that tend to toe in or out. Balance is achieved slowly. *Function*: Both gross and fine motor development continue rapidly. By 15 months, most toddlers can walk unassisted; they are running at age 18 months and jumping by 2 years. By age 3 years, most toddlers can stack blocks, string large beads, work simple puzzles, and dress themselves.	Assess progress in walking, running, and jumping. Assess small muscle coordination as evidenced in everyday skills: ability to dress themselves, wash hands, brush teeth. Distinguish slow developers who fall within normal ranges from those whose developmental lags may indicate deprivation of environmental stimulation or retardation.	Because individual differences in motor activity, balance, and grace become evident during this period, help parents to learn and accept their child's uniqueness. Teach parents the importance of providing a safe environment in which the toddler is free to explore, to satisfy curiosity, and to develop skill in motor control; that reinforcement, enthusiasm, and praise for progress stimulate the toddler's mastery of new skills; and that limits need to be set so the toddler does not overextend himself or herself in his or her newfound drive for mastery. The sense of mastery achieved through safe exploration and the practice of motor skills lays the foundation for all later physical, social, and intellectual pursuits.
Child		
Structure: Between ages 3 and 6 years, the child's arms and legs continue to grow rapidly relative to the trunk and the child develops better balance. By	Use developmental charts to assess gross and fine motor development.	Because important attitudes about the body and exercise are developed during childhood, parents should be questioned about these during the

(continued)

T A B L E   3 0 - 2 (continued)

Structural and Functional Developmental Changes in Body Alignment and Mobility With Related Nursing Assessment and Intervention Priorities		
Developmental Changes	**Assessment Priorities**	**Nursing Interventions**
Child		
age 6 years, the child has replaced "baby fat" with muscle, developed increased tone in abdominal muscles (loss of potbelly), and developed a more prominent chest. *Function:* Muscles, bones, and the nervous system are developing a harmony that allows greater gross and fine motor control. • By age 4 years, most children can negotiate stairs without using a hand rail, walk backward, and hop on one foot. • By age 5 years, most children have learned to skip, to play in running games, to jump rope, and to jump off heights of several steps. • Progress in fine motor development is reflected in the child's manipulation of writing materials. • By the time children enter school they have acquired all the basic mechanisms for physical locomotion they will use later in life.		nursing history. Teach or counsel as appropriate.
Adolescent		
Structure: There is considerable increase and change of the musculoskeletal system, resulting in increased size as well as the appearance of secondary sex characteristics. The adolescent growth spurt gives the adolescent an awkward, gangling appearance, and there is an increase in muscle mass and a decrease in fat, especially in boys. *Function:* For the physically fit adolescent this can be a time of boundless energy and great athletic performance. Life-style factors (inactivity, poor nutrition) may begin a lifelong unhealthy pattern of immobility and disuse.	Interview the client to determine current activity level and type of regular exercise. Evaluate safety of recreational choices. Note history of any musculoskeletal or neurologic problems. During the physical assessment, note posture and alignment. Screening for scoliosis (lateral curvature of the spine) should be made before the adolescent's peak growth velocity and a referral made when there is more than a 15-degree curvature of the spine. Examine muscle mass, tone, and strength and joint mobility.	Adolescents have many questions about their changing bodies and will often value nursing input, although they seldom seek professional advice. Life-style counseling regarding the importance of exercise and fitness is critical. Adolescents may need encouragement to exercise regularly or help in gauging their physical limits and a caution not to "push too hard."
Adult		
Structure: The healthy adult stands and sits erect and is capable of balanced and coordinated purposeful movement. During pregnancy, the developing fetus shifts the mother's center of gravity forward and she compensates by leaning backward and walking with a broader base of support. *Function:* Activity levels vary greatly among adults and are influenced by numerous factors explained in this chapter.	Assess the balance between activity and rest in the client's life-style and note any life-style factors or illnesses that interfere with the client's mobility or ability to carry out activities of daily living.	For most adults, the most important nursing intervention is fitness counseling, which includes clarifying misconceptions about exercise and designing and monitoring safe exercise programs. Clients with mobility alterations require special care.

(continued)

Structural and Functional Developmental Changes in Body Alignment and Mobility With Related Nursing Assessment and Intervention Priorities

Developmental Changes	Assessment Priorities	Nursing Interventions
Older Adult		
Structure: There is increased convexity in the thoracic spine (kyphosis) from disc shrinkage and decreased height, flexed posture, loss of muscle tone, and increased prominence of bony structure because of subcutaneous fat loss. Arthritic joint changes are often present. *Function*: General slowness of movement with progressive decrease in activity tolerance.	Assess general ease of movement and gait; alignment; joint structure and function; and muscle mass, tone, and strength.	Teach and counsel clients about: • Importance of regular exercise • Need to maintain appropriate weight to reduce stress on joints • Need for high-protein, calcium and vitamin D–enriched diet • To pace activities to compensate for decreased strength • To use assistive devices safely when needed • To safety-proof homes to reduce likelihood of falls

• Corrects behaviors that compound the mobility deficit over time (eg, client with arthritis who severely restricts movement because of joint stiffness and tenderness learns successful adaptive strategies that can be shared with other clients and families; or energy conservation measures used by clients with emphysema who have greatly decreased activity tolerance)

Musculoskeletal Problems

Congenital or Acquired Postural Abnormalities The newborn with congenital hip dysplasia or a clubfoot; the teenager with scoliosis (lateral curvature of the spine); and the elderly person with kyphosis (increased convexity in the curvature of the thoracic spine) are all experiencing postural abnormalities that affect appearance and mobility. Nursing responsibilities may include the following:
• Early detection and referral of these problems
• Exploration and selection of client education, counseling, and support as treatment options
• Careful attention to positioning, transfers, and exercise
• Education of the client and family regarding safe self-care activities

Problems With Bone Formation or Muscle Development Problems with bone formation may be any of the following:
• *Congenital*, such as achondroplasia, in which premature bone ossification leads to dwarfism, or osteogenesis imperfecta, which is characterized by excessively brittle bones and multiple fractures both at birth and later in life
• *Dietary related*, for example, vitamin D deficiency, which results in deformities of the growing skeleton (rickets)
• *Disease related*, such as in Paget disease, in which excessive bone destruction and abnormal regeneration

result in skeletal pain, deformities, and pathologic fractures
• *Age related*, such as osteoporosis, in which bone destruction exceeds bone formation; the resultant thin, porous bones fracture easily

The muscular dystrophies are a group of genetically transmitted disorders that have in common progressive degeneration and weakness of skeletal muscles. They vary in terms of the muscle groups involved and their clinical course. Myasthenia gravis is a weakness of the skeletal muscles caused by an abnormality at the neuromuscular junction that prevents muscle fibers from contracting.

Nursing responsibilities with problems of bone formation and muscle development and functioning include the following:
• Careful collaboration with the physician and health care team to determine the motor capacities of the individual
• Client and family education aimed at developing optional mobility
The nurse must be knowledgeable about the underlying disease process and be able to position, lift, transfer, and exercise the client safely, with attention to client comfort.

Problems Affecting Joint Mobility Inflammation, degeneration, and trauma can all interfere with joint mobility. The term *arthritis* describes more than 20 diseases, all characterized by inflammation in one or more joints and possibly pain and stiffness in adjacent body parts. *Degenerative joint disease*, also termed *osteoarthritis*, is a noninflammatory, progressive disorder of movable joints, particularly weight-bearing joints, characterized by the deterioration of articular cartilage and pain with motion. Spurs form, which restrict joint movement. Trauma to a joint may result in either a *sprain*, in which the wrenching or twisting of a joint results in a partial tear or rupture to its attachments or a *dislocation*, that is, the displacement of a bone from a joint with tearing of ligaments, tendons, and capsules. Any condition restricting joint mobility has potentially crippling effects.

The nurse caring for clients with joint problems works collaboratively with the physician and physical therapist to maintain joint mobility. Client education is directed to the client's mastery of an exercise and care program, which fosters tissue repair and maximal independence in activities of daily living.

Problems Affecting the Central Nervous System

A problem in any of the principal parts of the brain or spinal cord concerned with skeletal muscle control can affect mobility:

Cerebral motor cortex: Assumes the major role of controlling precise, discrete movements. A cerebrovascular accident (stroke) or head trauma may damage the motor cortex and produce temporary or permanent voluntary motor impairment.

Basal ganglia: Integrate semivoluntary movements such as walking, swimming, and laughing. In Parkinson's disease, there is progressive degeneration of the basal ganglia of the cerebrum. Unnecessary skeletal movements result in tremors and muscle rigidity, which interfere with voluntary movement.

Cerebellum: Assists the motor cortex and basal ganglia by making body movements smooth and coordinated. In multiple sclerosis, the myelin sheaths of neurons in the CNS deteriorate to hardened scars or plaques. Plaque formation in the cerebellum may produce lack of coordination of one hand.

Pyramidal pathways: Voluntary motor impulses are conveyed from the brain through the spinal cord by way of two major pathways: (1) the pyramidal pathway and (2) the extrapyramidal pathway. With trauma to the spinal cord, transection of these motor pathways results in complete bilateral loss of voluntary movement below the level of the trauma.

The overwhelming complaint of clients with injury to the CNS is that no one talks with them (or with their families) about how the disease will progress and affect their functioning. Nurses caring for these clients need knowledge about the pathology and clinical course of these diseases so that appropriate client education and counseling can occur.

Trauma to the Musculoskeletal System

Injury to the musculoskeletal system can result in fractures and soft tissue injuries. A *fracture* is a break in the continuity of the structure of bone or cartilage. It may result from a traumatic injury or occur as a result of some underlying disease process. Healing requires realignment of the bone fragment, immobilization, and restoration of the bone's function. Soft tissue injuries include sprains, strains, and dislocations. (Dislocations and sprains are discussed under Problems Affecting Joint Mobility.) A *strain*, the least serious

of these injuries, is a stretching of a muscle. Nurses need to be knowledgeable in first-aid measures for musculoskeletal trauma as well as in acute and rehabilitative care.

Problems Involving Other Body Systems

The pathology of numerous other acute and chronic illnesses may also affect mobility. Chronic obstructive lung disease and conditions such as ascites may alter posture. Any illnesses that interfere with oxygenation at the cellular level decrease the amount of oxygen available to the muscles for work and thus decrease activity tolerance. These illnesses include anemia, angina, cardiac dysrhythmias, congestive heart failure, and chronic obstructive pulmonary disease. Diseases characterized by negative nitrogen balance (eg, anorexia nervosa and certain cancers) result in muscle wasting and decreased physical energy for movement and work. Symptoms accompanying many illnesses such as fatigue, muscle aches, and pain may also immobilize clients. Bed rest is an important component of the treatment regimen for many diseases or trauma states such as myocardial infarction, surgery, and fractures. Although rest is integral to the healing process, immobility may cause its own problems (Table 30-3). Nurses need to be vigilant in determining the effect any injury or illness will have on mobility and in providing care that facilitates optimal mobility.

Mental Health

Just as an individual's physical health influences body appearance and movement, so also does mental health. Bodily processes tend to slow down in depression and there is a lack of visible energy and enthusiasm. The depressed person often sits with the head bowed and shoulders slumped and may lack the energy to feed or even to toilet. Even facial movement may be decreased to the point where the individual's face registers no emotion (termed a *flat affect*). On the other hand, high-energy individuals have erect posture and animated facial features.

Life-Style Variables

Whether an individual opts for an active or sedentary life-style is influenced by many factors. Among the most important are an individual's occupation, leisure activity preferences, and cultural influences. Because most professional occupations as well as many blue-collar jobs are sedentary in nature, individuals wishing to exercise regularly need to plan leisure activities that give the body a workout. Cultural influences may encourage or discourage exercise. For example, currently in North America it is popular for both male and female professionals to engage in some form of aerobic exercise. In the not-so-distant past, it was considered unladylike for women to be involved in most sports activities. Other life-style variables that influence mobility include a person's diet and smoking history.

(*Text continues on p. 660*)

TABLE 30-3

Problems of Immobility With Related Etiologies, Assessment Priorities, Client Goals, and Nursing Interventions

Problems Related to Immobility	Etiologies	Assessment Priorities	Client Goals	Nursing Interventions
Cardiovascular				

Activity Intolerance: Increased Cardiac Workload	Supine position contributes to greater volume of circulating blood, which must be pumped by the heart; decreased vascular resistance	• Assess apical and peripheral pulses.
		 • Note increased heart rate; presence of third heart sound; weakened peripheral pulses.
		 • Note the presence of edema (check sacrum, legs, feet).
			Client will maintain baseline vital signs.	• When possible, encourage the client to sit in the Fowler position; avoid lying supine for prolonged intervals.
				 • Avoid any activities that increase intrathoracic pressure:
				    • Discourage straining while moving or defecating (Valsalva maneuver).
				    • Exhale through mouth while exercising.

Altered Tissue Perfusion; Thrombus Formation	Venous stasis secondary to a lack of muscular contraction in the legs Calcium leaving bones and entering blood increases its coagulability External pressure on the veins (eg, that exerted by the knee gatch of the hospital bed) (Note: poor positioning can result in partial or total occlusion of the blood vessels.)	• Assess for complaints of pain, especially calf pain; signs of warmth, redness, swelling, tenderness—compare one extremity to the other. • Daily calf or thigh circumference measurements may be indicated (mark spot to be measured).	Client will show signs of adequate venous return (absence of dependent edema, thrombi, emboli).	• Encourage active exercise of legs (range of motion and quadriceps settings) three or four times daily. • Elevate legs periodically. • Position clients carefully, following agency guidelines; avoid prolonged knee and hip flexion. • Apply antiembolism stockings if ordered. • Assess for signs of thrombosis. *Never* rub or massage the legs—especially if the client complains of pain.
High Risk for Injury: Orthostatic Hypotension	Skeletal muscle weakness and decreased vessel tone (failure of arteriole vasoconstriction on assuming an erect position) Hypovolemia	• Assess for complaints of light-headedness, dizziness, seeing spots, or fainting. • Compare blood pressure before position change with that taken immediately afterward.	Client will change from a lying to a sitting or standing position safely without injury.	• If not contraindicated, have client sleep sitting up or in an elevated position. • Encourage client to change position gradually and with support if needed: supine to Fowler's to sitting at edge of bed to standing (each change may require 15 to 20 minutes of stabilization time); instruct client never to jump to his or her feet and begin walking.

(continued)

TABLE 30-3 *(continued)*

Problems of Immobility With Related Etiologies, Assessment Priorities, Client Goals, and Nursing Interventions

Problems Related to Immobility	Etiologies	Assessment Priorities	Client Goals	Nursing Interventions
Cardiovascular				• Use waist-high anti-embolism stockings. • Encourage leg exercises. • Encourage client to increase time out of bed as condition allows; gradually increase the frequency and duration of ambulation. • Remind client to get out of a hot bath slowly. • Teach the client to avoid the Valsalva maneuver or any activity involving holding the breath. • Encourage client to use a rocking chair to improve lower extremity circulation.
Respiratory				
Ineffective Breathing Pattern	Limited chest expansion: Prolonged sitting or lying position Muscle disuse— atrophy Loss of muscle coordination Depressant pharmacologic agents: analgesics, sedatives, anesthetics	• Assess rate, rhythm, and quality of respirations; note a decrease in the depth and rate of respirations. • Assess the symmetry of chest wall movements.	Client will maintain baseline respiratory rate and depth. Client coughs and deep breathes every 1 to 2 hours.	• Adhere to every-2-hour position change schedule. • If the client is allowed out of bed, encourage deep breathing when the client stands and ambulates. • Teach the client to cough and deep breathe every 1 to 2 hours. • If abdominal binders or rib supports are in place, remove them every 2 hours and encourage deep breathing.
Ineffective Airway Clearance	Altered function of mucous membranes and cilia Decreased position changes Ineffective coughing secondary to weakness, incisional pain, depressant pharmacologic action	• Auscultate the entire lung region and note regions of diminished breath sounds, rales, rhonchi, or wheezes. • Percuss the chest and note any dull area. • Assess sputum (color, texture, odor);	Client's lungs will be clear to auscultation. Client will remain free of signs of respiratory tract infection (fever, productive cough, chest pain)	• See nursing interventions for Ineffective Breathing Pattern. • Keep client well hydrated. • Initiate chest physiotherapy. • Suction as needed.

(continued)

T A B L E 3 0 - 3 *(continued)*

Problems of Immobility With Related Etiologies, Assessment Priorities, Client Goals, and Nursing Interventions

Problems Related to Immobility	Etiologies	Assessment Priorities	Client Goals	Nursing Interventions
Respiratory				
	Dehydration Stasis of secretions	culture and sensitivity test may be ordered.		
Impaired Gas Exchange (O_2/CO_2 ratio)	Decreased respiratory movement Pooling of secretions	• Note any changes in the client's behavior, mental status. • Compare clinical picture with changes in arterial blood gas values, pulmonary function test values, or pulse oximetry.	Client will maintain an adequate O_2/CO_2 ratio.	• See nursing interventions for Ineffective Breathing Pattern and Ineffective Airway Clearance.
Musculoskeletal				
High Risk for Activity Intolerance (self-care deficits) Impaired Physical Mobility	Decreased muscle mass, tone, and strength (atrophy) Contractures Stiffness and pain in the joints Limited range of motion Joint degeneration (ankylosis) Decreased stability Bone demineralization (disuse osteoporosis) Decreased endurance	• Assess for weakness, fatigue, complaints of muscle pain or joint pain or tenderness. • Assess for decreased muscle mass (anthropometric measurements, tape measurements); decreased muscle tone; and strength test joint flexibility; note any contractures or ankyloses.	Client will maintain adequate muscle strength and joint mobility to perform basic self-care activities.	• Incorporate range-of-motion exercises (as client's condition permits) and isometric setting exercises into client's daily routine (at least three to four times daily).
High Risk for Injury: Pathologic Fractures	Excessive bone demineralization (disuse osteoporosis)	• Bone demineralization is not detectable through physical assessment. • Relate clinical picture to blood chemistries (note elevated serum calcium and phosphorus levels).	Client will remain free of contractures, ankyloses, pathologic fractures.	• Increase client's activity tolerance gradually: • Participates in positioning in bed • Transfer from bed to chair • Ambulates • Gradually increases frequency and duration of sitting out of bed and frequency and distance of walks • Progresses to independence in all self-care activities
Metabolic				
Altered Nutrition: Less Than Body Requirements	Negative nitrogen balance Anorexia	• Assess diet history and note problems with anorexia, digestion, or elimination.	Client will maintain appropriate weight for height.	• Provide client with high-protein, high-calorie diet; explore parenteral and en-

(continued)

T A B L E   3 0 - 3 (continued)

Problems of Immobility With Related Etiologies, Assessment Priorities, Client Goals, and Nursing Interventions

Problems Related to Immobility	Etiologies	Assessment Priorities	Client Goals	Nursing Interventions
Metabolic				
Altered Nutrition: More Than Body Requirements Fluid Volume Excess: Dependent Edema	Imbalance between calories ingested and burned off Fluid shifts secondary to negative nitrogen balance	• Monitor intake and output and correlate client's clinical picture with laboratory studies that evaluate fluid and electrolyte status. • Evaluate muscle atrophy by way of anthropometric measurements (height, weight, mid-upper arm circumference, and triceps skin-fold measurements). • Assess skin turgor and wound healing.	Client's fluid output will approximately equal intake. Client's electrolyte values and serum protein will fall within normal range. Client's skin will demonstrate adequate turgor.	teral (nasogastric, gastrostomy, or jejunostomy tubes) alternatives if the client is unable to eat. • Serve small, frequent feedings in a pleasant environment. • Monitor intake and output.
Gastrointestinal				
Constipation	Decreased gastric motility and muscle tone Decreased fluid intake	• Assess frequency and consistency of bowel movements (use of elimination aids). • Examine for bowel sounds, abdominal tone, and anal sphincter tone.	Client will have a formed, semisolid stool every 1 to 3 days. Client will be free of signs of fecal impaction (distended abdomen, no bowel movement for several days or liquid bowel movement, lethargy)	• Respect client's usual elimination schedule. • Offer assistance with the bedpan or commode if needed and provide privacy. • Increase fluid intake and roughage. • Caution about Valsalva's maneuver (straining with mouth closed).
Urinary				
Altered Urinary Elimination Urinary Retention High Risk for Infection: Urinary Tract	Renal calculi Urinary stasis	• Assess voiding patterns—time and amount (note history of small, frequent voidings); question about urgency, dysuria, pain. • Monitor fluid output. • Examine for bladder distention. • Examine urine for cloudiness or odor (culture urine if indicated).	Client will maintain usual voiding pattern (frequency and amount). Client will be free of renal calculi. Client will be free of signs of urinary tract infection (urgency, burning, flank pain, fever).	• Keep the client well hydrated (aim is for client to void large amounts of dilute urine). • Maintain usual voiding pattern. • If needed, provide assistance with bedpan or urinal—respect client's privacy.
Skin				
Impaired Skin Integrity (pressure ulcer)	Decreased local blood circulation to the tissues	• Examine skin, especially pressure points, for beginning	Client's skin will show no sign of breakdown.	• Reposition client in correct alignment at least every 1 hour to

(continued)

T A B L E   3 0 - 3 (continued)

Problems of Immobility With Related Etiologies, Assessment Priorities, Client Goals, and Nursing Interventions

Problems Related to Immobility	Etiologies	Assessment Priorities	Client Goals	Nursing Interventions
Skin				
	Prolonged pressure on the skin	signs of breakdown with each position change (at least every 2 hours). • Assess for factors that place client at high risk for breakdown (malnutrition, incontinence, and so on).		2 hours and ensure protection of pressure points where possible (eg, heel and elbow protectors). • Decrease effects of shearing forces. • Massage pressure points and keep skin clean and dry. • Keep bed linens dry and free of wrinkles.
Psychological and Social				
Self-Esteem Disturbance Powerlessness Impaired Social Interaction Altered Thought Processes Knowledge Deficit Ineffective Individual Coping Ineffective Family Coping Sleep Pattern Disturbance	Inability to move body voluntarily Dependency on others Inability to fulfill role expectations Pain experience Skeletal deformities Exaggerated emotional and behavioral responses Loss of mobility to contact friends Decreased stimuli to maintain orientation Immobility-induced depression Decreased motivation to learn Decreased ability to learn and decreased retention Decreased motivation to solve problems Increased need for assistance with self-care abilities Exaggerated emotional responses Decreased physical exercise Increased bedtime and napping	• Assess client for changes in behavior, emotional status, and mental abilities. • Explore with the client and family possible reasons for these changes. • Assess the adequacy of the client's and family's coping strategies. • Assess sleep–wake patterns.	Client will identify personal strengths. Client will verbalize positive body image. Client will describe successful coping strategies. Client will demonstrate ability to problem solve.	• Use care contacts with client to explore immobility's effects on the client's mental status and behavior. • Explore means to meet client's needs for socialization. • Increase stimuli to maintain client's orientation. • Encourage client to be as independent as possible and to structure daily activities and schedule as closely as possible to preimmobilization; encourage wearing of personal clothes, use of cosmetics, and so on. • Challenge client intellectually. Communicate that you expect the client to reason, to problem solve. • Explore impact of client's illness on family and counsel appropriately.

Attitude and Values

In some families, such as those that hike together, swim together, and play ball together, children learn early to value regular exercise. As these children mature, they often continue to value exercise and find new ways to incorporate regular exercise into their daily routine. Similarly, children may be raised in sedentary families where watching sports is the closest anyone comes to exercise. This attitude may also be internalized for a lifetime. Many individual values also explain the exercise options people make. Elderly people who integrate a planned exercise regimen into their daily routine benefit physiologically and report improved self-esteem.

Individuals who place a high value on physical attractiveness may be highly committed to regular exercise because it produces the body they want. Another individual may exercise because of the desire for physical strength, relating strength with power. Someone more disposed to intellectual pursuits may perceive body development as simply wasting time that could be better used to develop the mind.

Fatigue and Stress

Chronic stress may deplete body energy to the point that fatigue makes even the thought of exercise overwhelming. Ironically, regular exercise is energizing and can better equip a person to deal with daily stresses. At the same time, excessive exercise may stress the body and lead to injury as well as to fatigue.

External Factors

Many external factors can influence mobility. Among these, weather probably exerts the greatest influence. A brisk, clear day is invigorating and invites increased activity. High humidity and high temperatures, on the other hand, discourage any extra movement. Sufficient financial resources for exercise memberships and equipment, safe outdoor parks and sports areas, the availability of malls for early morning walkers, support people, and occupational or insurance rewards for exercise can all encourage regular exercise. Detractors include insufficient funds, air pollution, unsafe neighborhoods, and lack of support and reinforcement.

Exercise

Active exertion of muscles involving the contraction and relaxation of muscle groups is termed *exercise*. Each of the many different types of exercise has the potential to produce different physiologic and psychological benefits.

Types of Exercise

Muscle Contraction Exercise may be categorized according to the type of muscle contraction involved as being isotonic, isometric, or isokinetic (Fig. 30-7).

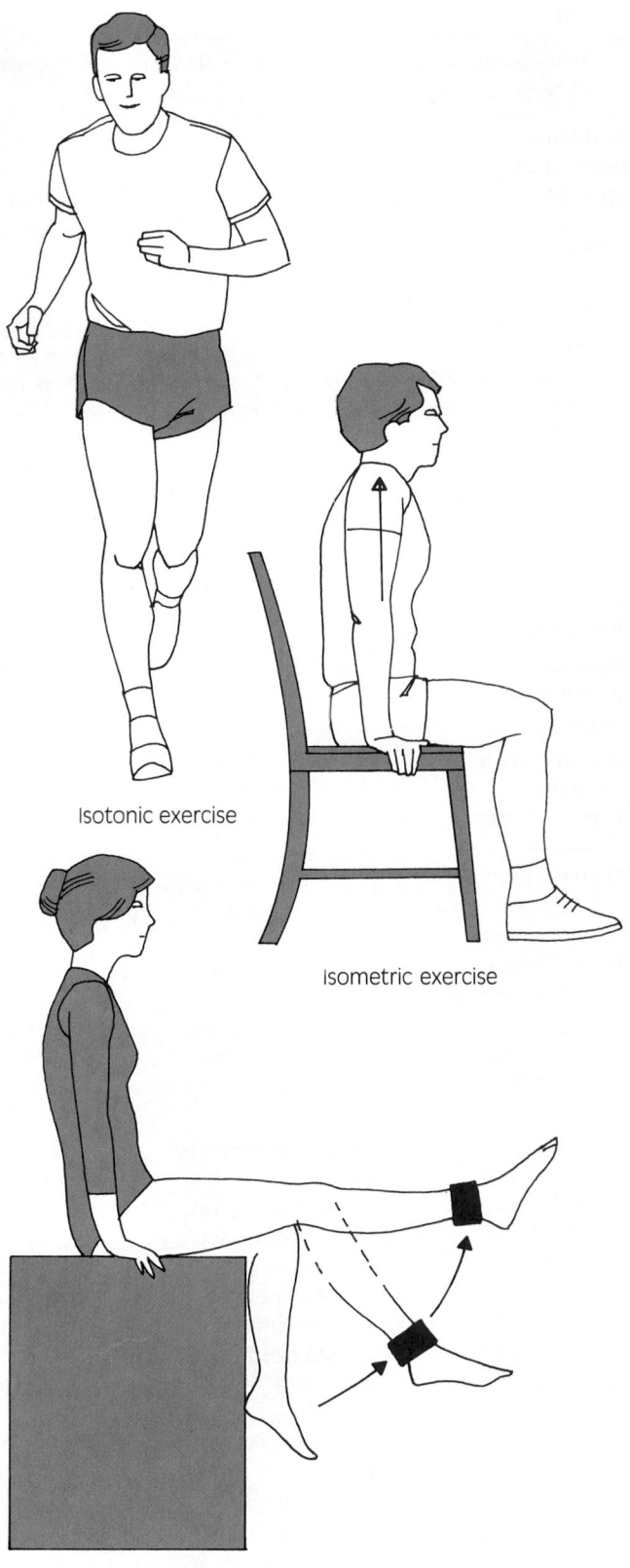

Isotonic exercise

Isometric exercise

Isokinetic exercise

F I G U R E   3 0 - 7

Three types of exercise: (1) isotonic, which involves muscle shortening and active movement; (2) isometric, which involves muscle contraction without shortening; and (3) isokinetic, which involves muscle contraction with resistance.

Isotonic exercise involves muscle shortening and active movement. Examples include carrying out activities of daily living, independently performing range-of-motion exercises, and swimming, walking, jogging, and bicycling. Potential benefits include increased muscle mass, tone, and strength; improved joint mobility; increased cardiac and respiratory function; increased circulation; and increased osteoblastic activity. When the nurse or family member performs passive range-of-motion exercises for a client, the client's muscles do not exert effort and potential benefits are reduced to improved joint mobility and increased circulation.

Isometric exercise involves muscle contraction without shortening (ie, there is no movement or a minimum shortening of muscle fibers). Examples include contractions of the quadriceps and gluteal muscles. Potential benefits are increased muscle mass, tone, and strength; increased circulation to the exercised body part; and increased osteoblastic activity. Nurses encourage both isotonic and isometric exercises for hospitalized clients with limited mobility.

Isokinetic exercise involves muscle contractions with resistance, varying at a constant rate produced by a device with a capacity for variable resistance. Examples include rehabilitative exercises for knee and elbow injuries. Using the isokinetic device, the muscles and joint are taken through a complete range of motion without stopping with resistance at every point.

Body Movement Exercise activities may also be categorized according to the type of body movement involved and the health benefits they produce. Fuller and Schaller-Ayres (1991) offer the following breakdown:

Aerobic exercise: Sustained (often rhythmic) muscle movements that increase blood flow, heart rate, and metabolic demand for oxygen over time, promoting cardiovascular conditioning. Activities that may be aerobic are swimming, walking, jogging, cross-country skiing, aerobic dance, bicycling, jumping rope, and racquetball. (Aerobic exercise may be further distinguished as having high versus low impact. The number of injuries, such as shin splints, related to high-impact aerobic workouts led to the development of low-impact workouts that place less stress on the musculoskeletal system.)

Stretching exercises: Movements that allow muscles and joints to be stretched gently through their full range of motion increase flexibility. Specific warm-up and cool-down exercises, hatha yoga, and some forms of dance are examples. Benefits include increased range of joint movements, improved circulation and posture, and relaxation.

Strength and endurance exercises: A variety of muscle-building programs fall into this category. Weight training, calisthenics, and specific isometric exercises can build both strength and endurance, increasing the power of the musculoskeletal system and generally improving the whole body. They may or may not have aerobic benefit.

Movement and activities of daily living: Housecleaning, running after playful toddlers, climbing stairs instead of riding in elevators, all have an effect on health. Increased fitness does not require a gym.

Effects of Exercise and Immobility on Major Body Systems

The human body was designed for motion, and regular exercise is necessary for its healthy functioning. Individuals who choose inactive life-styles or who are forced to inactivity by illness or injury place themselves at high risk for serious health problems. The effects of both regular exercise and immobility on major body systems are explored in this section. Just as individuals differ in the benefits they receive from exercise, complications resulting from immobility differ in their occurrence and severity according to the client's age and overall health state.

Cardiovascular System

Effects of Exercise To meet the demand for oxygen created by the rhythmic contraction and relaxation of skeletal muscle groups, the supply of oxygenated blood to skeletal muscle needs to be increased. The cardiovascular system meets this challenge by increasing the heart rate, increasing the contractile strength of the myocardium, and increasing stroke volume (volume of blood ejected), thus increasing cardiac output. Arterial (systolic) blood pressure is increased and blood is shunted from the nonexercising tissues to the heart and muscles. Exercise also improves venous return because the contracting muscles compress superficial veins and push blood back to the heart against gravity. Over time, with cardiovascular conditioning, regular exercise produces the following benefits:

- Increased efficiency of the heart
- Decreased heart rate and blood pressure
- Increased blood flow to all body parts
- Increased circulating fibrinolysin (substance that breaks up small clots)

Effects of Immobility The primary and serious effects of immobility on the cardiovascular system include increased cardiac workload, orthostatic hypotension, and venous thrombosis. Immobility results in an increased workload for the heart. It has been demonstrated that the heart works more when the person is resting, probably because there is less resistance offered by the blood vessels and because there is a change in the distribution of blood in the immobile person. As a result, the heart rate, cardiac output, and stroke volume increase.

Immobility predisposes to thrombi formation because of venous stasis, especially in the legs, where normal muscular activity helps move blood toward the central circulatory system. Thrombus formation is also caused by an increased rate in the coagulation of blood, one reason being that during periods of immobility, calcium leaves bones and enters the blood, where it has an influence on blood coagulation.

The immobile person is more susceptible to developing orthostatic hypotension. The person tends to feel weak and faint when the condition occurs. The phenomenon is probably due to a decrease in the neurovascular reflexes, which normally cause vasoconstriction, and to a loss of muscle tone. The result is that blood pools and does not squeeze from veins in the lower part of the body to the central circulatory system.

Pertinent nursing diagnoses and collaborative problems related to immobility include the following:

Altered Tissue Perfusion related to prolonged bed rest

High Risk for Injury: Deep Vein Thrombosis related to venous stasis, hypercoagulability, and decreased muscle activity

High Risk for Injury: Falls related to orthostatic hypotension

Activity Intolerance related to fatigue and inadequate tissue oxygenation

Impaired Tissue Integrity related to shearing force and prolonged bed rest

Several collaborative problems related to the effect of immobility on the cardiovascular system include the following:

Potential complication: hemostasis or thrombus formation

Potential complication: hypoxemia

Respiratory System

Effects of Exercise The respiratory and cardiovascular systems work together to make increased oxygen available to the muscles. During exercise, the depth of respiration, respiratory rate, gas exchange at the alveolar level, and rate of carbon dioxide excretion are increased. Over time, regular exercise leads to improved pulmonary functioning.

Effects of Immobility The effects of immobility on the respiratory system are related to decreased ventilatory effort and increased respiratory secretions. Immobility causes a decrease in the depth and rate of respirations owing at least partially to a reduced need for oxygen by body cells. When areas of lung tissues are not used over time, atelectasis may occur. **Atelectasis** is an incomplete expansion or collapse of lung tissue. Immobility results in a poor exchange of carbon dioxide and oxygen, upsets their balance in the body, and results eventually in an acid–base imbalance.

When a person is immobile, the movement of secretions in the respiratory tract is decreased, resulting in the pooling of secretions and in respiratory tract congestion. These conditions predispose to respiratory tract infections. *Hypostatic pneumonia* is a type of pneumonia that results from inactivity and immobility. The situation worsens when the person is dehydrated or using pharmaceutical agents that increase the tenacity of secretions, depress the coughing mechanism, and depress respirations.

Decreased movement in the thoracic cage during respirations also results from immobility. This decrease may be due to loss of tonus in muscles involved with respirations, to pressure on the chest wall owing to the client's position in bed, and to depression of the respiratory apparatus by various pharmaceutical agents.

Pertinent nursing diagnoses related to immobility include the following:

Ineffective Breathing Pattern related to limited chest expansion

Ineffective Airway Clearance related to decreased position changes, ineffective coughing, and stasis of secretions

Impaired Gas Exchange related to decreased respiratory movement (loss of muscle tonus)

High Risk for Infection related to accumulation of secretions

A collaborative problem related to the effect of immobility on the respiratory system is the following:

Potential complication: hypoxemia secondary to pneumonia

Musculoskeletal System

Effects of Exercise The rhythmic contraction and relaxation of muscle groups during exercise result in increased muscle mass, tone, and strength and increased joint mobility. The more a person exercises, the more strength he or she has to exercise or work in the future. Regular exercise produces the following benefits:

• Increased muscle efficiency (strength) and flexibility
• Increased coordination
• Increased efficiency of nerve impulse transmission

Regular exercise is also believed to slow the effects of aging (ie, it helps prevent osteoporosis associated with aging).

Effects of Immobility Effects of immobility on the musculoskeletal system are rapidly seen in clients confined to bed. People attempting to walk after several days of bed rest are often surprised to find how weak their legs have become. Immobility (musculoskeletal disuse) leads to decreased muscle size (**atrophy**), tone, and strength; decreased joint mobility and flexibility; bone demineralization; and limited endurance, resulting in problems with activities of daily living.

Immobility is often the cause of **contractures**, which are permanent contraction states of muscle (muscle shortening), and **ankylosis**, which is a consolidation and immobilization of a joint. Contractures result from atrophy of muscles with resulting incompetence, and from a decrease in the muscle's strength, coordination, and endurance. A joint can be permanently fixed when ankylosed.

The process of bone demineralization (**osteoporosis**) is also increased in the immobile client. Normally the stress and strain of weight-bearing activity stimulate bone formation and balance destruction. With immobility, however, bone formation slows while breakdown increases, with a net loss of bone calcium, phosphorus, and matrix. This condition, **disuse osteoporosis**, is characterized by bones that may be either spongy or brittle. Bone demineralization may result in pathologic fractures related to the bone's brittleness; bone deformities related to the bone's sponginess; arthropathy (joint disease) related to calcium depletion in the joints; and renal calculi (stones) related to the excessive excretion of calcium through the kidneys and urinary tract.

Pertinent nursing diagnoses and collaborative problems related to immobility include the following:

Activity Intolerance related to decreased muscle mass, tone, and strength

Impaired Physical Mobility related to muscle atrophy (contractures) and limited joint mobility (ankylosis)

High Risk for Injury: Pathologic Fracture related to excessive bone demineralization (disuse osteoporosis)

Self-Care Deficit related to decreased muscle strength and decreased flexibility

Fatigue related to increased energy needed to perform activities of daily living

Metabolic System

Effects of Exercise The metabolic rate increases during exercise so that sufficient glucose and fatty acids can be converted to provide the energy needed for increased muscle function. During strenuous exercise, the metabolic rate can increase to up to 20 times normal. Increased body heat and waste products are also produced. With regular exercise the body develops:

- Increased efficiency of metabolic system
- Increased efficiency of body temperature regulation

Effects of Immobility Because the resting body requires less energy, the cellular demand for oxygen is decreased and this is reflected by a decreased metabolic rate. In many immobilized clients, however, factors such as fever, trauma, chronic illness, or poor nutrition can actually increase the body's metabolic demands and increase *catabolism* (the breakdown of the body's protein stores to provide energy to meet the body's energy requirements). If unchecked, this process results in muscle wasting. When more protein is being broken down than manufactured, the body excretes more nitrogen than it takes in and *negative nitrogen balance* occurs. Anorexia, or decreased appetite, often accompanies and compounds this problem. Negative nitrogen balance and poor nutrition thus worsen the muscle atrophy and weakness already resulting from immobility. Numerous fluid and electrolyte imbalances, alterations in the exchange of nutrients and gases at the cellular level, and gastrointestinal problems can all result from metabolic disturbances.

Pertinent nursing diagnoses related to immobility include the following:

Altered Nutrition: Less Than Body Requirements, related to negative nitrogen balance and anorexia

Altered Nutrition: More Than Body Requirements, related to imbalance between calories ingested and burned off

Fluid Volume Excess: Dependent Edema related to fluid shifts (intravascular to interstitial compartments) secondary to negative nitrogen balance

Figure 30-8 summarizes the effects of exercise and immobility by body system.

Gastrointestinal System

Effects of Exercise During exercise, blood is shunted away from the stomach and intestines to the exercising muscles—hence the advice never to exercise on a full stomach. With regular exercise:

- Appetite is increased
- Intestinal tone is increased, which improves digestion and elimination

Effects of Immobility Immobility leads to disturbances in appetite, decreased food intake, altered protein metabolism, and poor digestion and utilization of food. If individuals increase food intake while decreasing energy expenditure, weight gain will result.

Normal muscular activity in the gastrointestinal tract also slows down in the immobile person, which often results in constipation, poor defecation reflexes, and an inability to expel feces and gas adequately.

Pertinent nursing diagnoses related to immobility include the following:

Constipation related to decreased gastric motility and muscle tone

Altered Nutrition: More Than Body Requirements, related to imbalance between food intake and activity (decreased energy expenditure)

Altered Nutrition: Less Than Body Requirements, related to anorexia and difficulty swallowing

Urinary System

Effects of Exercise Regular exercise increases blood circulation, including improved blood flow to the kidneys. This allows the kidneys to more efficiently maintain the body's fluid balance and acid–base balance and excrete body wastes.

Effects of Immobility In the nonerect client, the kidneys and ureters are level and urine stays longer in the renal pelvis before being expressed against gravity into the ureters and bladder. Urinary stasis favors the growth of bacteria that, when present in sufficient quantities, may cause urinary tract infections. Poor perineal hygiene, incontinence, decreased fluid intake, or an indwelling Foley catheter can increase the risk of urinary tract infection for an immobile client.

Immobility also predisposes to renal calculi, or kidney stones, which are a consequence of high levels of urinary calcium; urinary retention and incontinence resulting from decreased bladder muscle tone; the formation of alkaline urine, which facilitates growth of urinary bacteria; and decreased urinary volume.

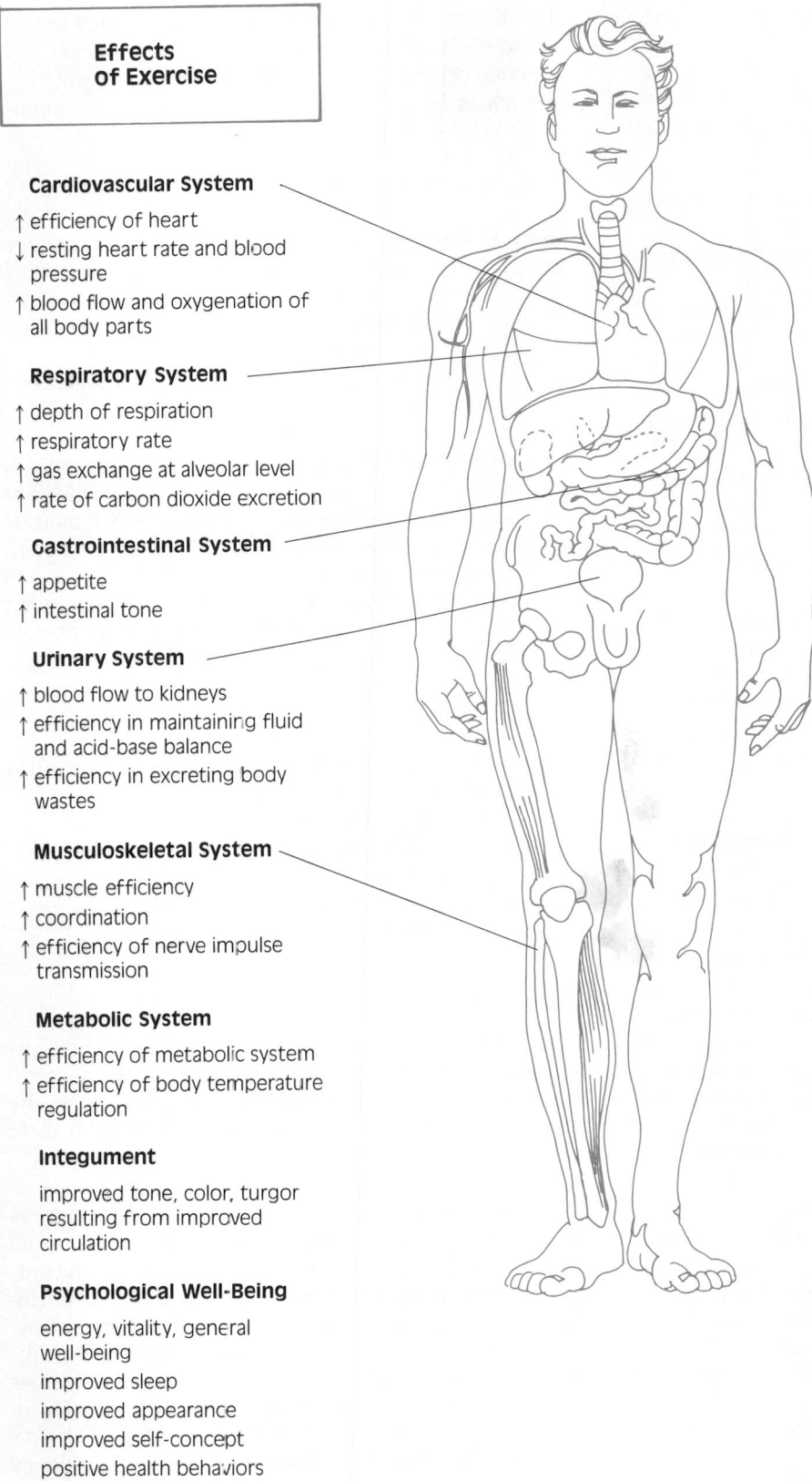

Effects of Exercise

Cardiovascular System

↑ efficiency of heart
↓ resting heart rate and blood pressure
↑ blood flow and oxygenation of all body parts

Respiratory System

↑ depth of respiration
↑ respiratory rate
↑ gas exchange at alveolar level
↑ rate of carbon dioxide excretion

Gastrointestinal System

↑ appetite
↑ intestinal tone

Urinary System

↑ blood flow to kidneys
↑ efficiency in maintaining fluid and acid-base balance
↑ efficiency in excreting body wastes

Musculoskeletal System

↑ muscle efficiency
↑ coordination
↑ efficiency of nerve impulse transmission

Metabolic System

↑ efficiency of metabolic system
↑ efficiency of body temperature regulation

Integument

improved tone, color, turgor resulting from improved circulation

Psychological Well-Being

energy, vitality, general well-being
improved sleep
improved appearance
improved self-concept
positive health behaviors

Effects of Immobility

Cardiovascular System

↑ cardiac workload
↑ risk of orthostatic hypotension
↑ risk of venous thrombosis

Respiratory System

↓ depth of respiration
↓ rate of respiration
pooling of secretions
impaired gas exchange

Gastrointestinal System

disturbance in appetite
altered protein metabolism
altered digestion and utilization of nutrients

Urinary System

↑ urinary stasis
↑ risk of renal calculi
↓ bladder muscle tone

Musculoskeletal System

↓ muscle size, tone and strength
↓ joint mobility, flexibility
bone demineralization
↓ endurance, stability
↑ risk of contracture formation

Metabolic System

↑ risk of electrolyte imbalance
altered exchange of nutrients and gases

Integument

↑ risk of skin breakdown and formation of decubitus ulcers

Psychological Well-Being

↑ sense of powerlessness
↓ self-concept
↓ social interaction
↓ sensory stimulation
altered sleep-wake pattern
↑ risk of depression

F I G U R E 3 0 - 8

A summary and comparison of the effects of exercise and immobility by body system.

Pertinent nursing diagnoses related to immobility include the following:

Pain related to inability to pass renal calculi

Urinary Retention related to prolonged immobility

High Risk for Infection: Urinary Tract, related to urinary stasis and increased urine alkalinity

Skin

Effects of Exercise Increased circulation resulting from regular exercises nourishes the skin and promotes its general health.

Effects of Immobility In elderly or debilitated immobile clients, the impaired circulation that accompanies immobility may result in serious skin breakdown. Prolonged pressure over bony prominences produces areas of breakdown, or pressure ulcers, which can progress from stage 1, redness, to stage 4, destruction of subcutaneous tissue and muscle. Pressure ulcers are described in detail in Chapter 29.

Pertinent nursing diagnoses related to immobility include the following:

Impaired Skin Integrity (specify stage of pressure ulcer) related to decreased circulation and pressure on skin overlying bony prominences

Psychological and Social

Effects of Exercise Some of the most important benefits of regular exercise are psychological:

- Increased energy, vitality, and general well-being
- Improved sleep
- Improved appearance (body image)
- Improved self-concept
- Increased positive health behaviors

Effects of Immobility When a person can no longer move the body purposefully and needs to depend on someone else for assistance with simple self-care activities, the sense of self is often threatened. Skeletal deformities can influence body image; an inability to meet role expectations can decrease self-concept; and a prolonged period of lying dependent in bed can lead to feelings of worthlessness and diminished self-esteem.

Immobility can produce exaggerated emotional responses to the stresses of everyday living. People who become apathetic, possibly because of decreased sensory stimulation, often exhibit altered thought processes. Lack of mobility can also diminish an individual's opportunities to interact socially and deprive that person of normal support systems. Coping difficulties are common in both the immobilized client and the client's family. Furthermore, the amount of time the immobilized client spends resting often disrupts usual sleep–wakefulness patterns and may interfere with both the quantity and quality of sleep.

Pertinent nursing diagnoses related to immobility include the following:

Self-Esteem Disturbance related to immobility and need to depend on others (and other variables)

Powerlessness related to increasing dependency in basic self-care activities

Impaired Social Interaction related to immobility

Altered Thought Processes: Disorientation related to decreased stimulation to maintain orientation

Knowledge Deficit (specify) related to decreased motivation to learn

Ineffective Individual Coping related to prolonged bed rest and increasing activity intolerance

Sleep Pattern Disturbance related to increased bedtime or napping and decreased physical exercise

Role of Exercise in Preventing Illness and Promoting Wellness

Promoting exercise and emphasizing wellness behaviors are challenging opportunities for nurses. Nurses are committed to assisting and supporting clients to make life-style changes that improve the clients' health and well-being. As researchers focus on the potential of regular exercise activities to slow the aging process, nurses intervene to prevent the deleterious effects associated with decreased physical activity.

Positive physical benefits of exercise include the following:

- Improved cardiopulmonary function
- Decreased blood pressure
- Increased bone mineral content
- Increased muscle strength, coordination, and joint range of motion
- Improved fat and carbohydrate metabolism

Data also indicate that psychological benefits of exercise can be identified:

- Improved sense of well-being
- A greater sense of control over life
- A decrease in fear, among elderly clients, of falling
- An improved body image

Although there is no evidence that exercise prevents the occurrence of chronic disease, clinical improvement has been noted when clients participate in regular exercise activities.

Risks Related to Exercise

Among the reasons many people offer for not exercising is fear of causing some personal harm. Nurses need to respond to these fears with realistic knowledge of the risks associated with exercise and specific prevention strategies.

Avoiding Exercise The greatest risk associated with exercise is viewing it as too much of a chore and avoiding it.

Precipitating a Cardiac Event Although the risk of exercise precipitating a major cardiac event in a healthy individual is minimal, the risk is much higher for individuals with known or documentable cardiovascular disease. Thus, a preexercise medical examination, medical supervision dur-

R E S E A R C H   I N   N U R S I N G   Making a Difference

Exercise

Exercise is an essential component in improving circulation and maintaining muscle strength and joint mobility. Nursing interventions traditionally have been carried out to prevent the complications associated with immobility, but nursing research has expanded the scope of nursing in this area by analyzing exercise and performance of activities of daily living as therapy in maximizing the health status of clients at all levels of wellness.

Related Research

Gueldner, S., & Spradley, J. (1988). Outdoor walking lowers fatigue. *Journal of Gerontological Nursing, 14*(10), 6–12.

Nursing home residents who participated in a short outdoor walk (0.1 mile) three times a week for 3 weeks reported significantly lower fatigue than nonwalking residents. The study indicated that regular outdoor walking for ambulatory clients contributes to an improved state of health and encourages increased social interaction among residents. Societal attitudes that restrict institutionalized elderly clients to an indoor setting limit their opportunity to continue to actively exercise in a varied, stimulating outdoor environment.

MacVicar, M., Winningham, M., & Nickel, J. (1989). Effects of aerobic interval training on cancer patients' functional capacity. *Nursing Research, 38*(6), 348–351.

A 10-week aerobic exercise training protocol for women with breast cancer who are undergoing chemotherapy was effective in improving their physical ability to engage in activity. The study suggests that similar interventions could successfully improve the ability of clients with cancer or other chronic diseases to perform self-care activities and thus maintain a higher level of independence.

Medhat, A., Huber, P., & Medhat, M. (1990). Factors that influence the level of activities in persons with lower extremity amputation. *Rehabilitation Nursing, 15*(1), 13–18.

The study identified specific problems that people with amputations of the lower extremity experience as they attempt to perform activities of daily living and maintain their independence. Yard care, shower bathing, and gardening proved most difficult for the amputees because these tasks required considerable skill in balance, gross motor movement, and maneuverability. The rehabilitation nurse is uniquely situated not only to monitor the client's progress but also to help the amputee fulfill his or her basic needs and creatively modify the client's activities and role so he or she can reach a maximum level of functioning.

Summary

Nursing research in the area of exercise, physical fitness, and daily activities has important implications for promoting wellness and preventing illness. Life-style changes to behaviors that promote normal physiologic functioning have lifelong effects, and exercises to improve alterations in tissue function are beneficial in improving self-care and independence.

---

ing exercise, and an individually designed exercise plan are recommended for sedentary people older than age 35 years and for any person with a past or current cardiovascular condition.

Orthopedic Discomfort and Disability The most common injuries associated with exercise are orthopedic in nature and are caused by irritation of bones, tendons, ligaments, and sometimes muscles. This irritation may result from added weight-bearing stress or from collision with the ground, an object, or another person. Teach clients when injured to rely on the acronym RICE—rest, *ice*, compression, and elevation. A physician should be contacted immediately to diagnose the extent of the injury. Exercise should not be continued until the injury is healed, or further damage may be done.

Other Health Problems Many other types of health problems may be associated with different types of exercise, depending to a large extent on external factors (temperature on a given day, humidity, pollution index, safety of the neighborhood) as well as internal factors (age, history of previous injury, overuse, obesity, health history).

Nurse as Role Model

Nurses who wish to role model healthy mobility behaviors to clients demonstrate a commitment to using the principles of body mechanics in both their leisure and work activities and to exercising regularly to promote fitness. Use the self-assessment checklist for exercise in the accompanying display to determine how well you are meeting your need for exercise. Because nurses who work closely with clients providing physical care are at high risk for developing musculoskeletal problems if they do not use their bodies properly, they also have a personal reason for being attentive to the use of good body mechanics. Similarly, the work of nursing places heavy demands on a nurse's psychic and physical energy; the nurse who is physically fit is better able to respond to these challenges. Nurses who are effective role models easily meet the following goals:

- Consistently use sound principles of body mechanics in both leisure and work activities
- Incorporate regular periods of physical exercise into life-style (minimum of three 30- to 45-minute exercise sessions weekly)
- Demonstrate a preference for an active versus a sedentary life-style (eg, uses stairs in preference to elevators, walks rather than drives short distances, balances active leisure alternatives with sedentary options)
- Appear physically fit to clients and colleagues (appropriate weight for height; adequate muscle mass, tone, and strength; performs work activities without becoming short of breath or excessively fatigued)

It is not uncommon to hear nurses who are retiring or leaving the profession cite back injuries as an influencing factor. Nurses may incur back injuries as a result of poor body mechanics or become injured when a client falls. Statistics indicate that, in Canada, the average time lost by a nurse due to a back injury is 35.5 days. In an effort to significantly decrease the injury rate among staff nurses, nursing researchers in Canada have developed and marketed the *Patient Transfer Assessment Program* (Haley & Colgate, 1990). This innovative format includes an assessment of the client's transfer ability, criteria for determining the proper transfer method, and colorful communication decals to reinforce good lifting techniques.

Videman and colleagues (1989) have concluded that many back injuries are preventable and have identified student nurses and recent graduate nurses as a group particularly at risk. They recommend additional emphasis in the nursing curriculum on principles of body mechanics and client-lifting techniques as an initial preventive measure to improve the nursing environment.

Assessing

The nurse performing a comprehensive nursing assessment uses both interview and physical assessment skills to elicit data about the client's mobility status. When alterations in a client's physical or mental health state result in impaired mobility, more detailed assessment skills are needed.

▽ PROMOTING WELLNESS

Exercise

Use the following assessment checklist to determine how well you are meeting your need for exercise. Then develop a prescription for self-care by choosing appropriate behaviors from the list of suggestions.

Assessment Checklist

almost never / sometimes / almost always

1. My life-style demonstrates that I place a high value on exercise as a component of wellness (eg, I walk stairs instead of using elevators).

2. I exercise for 30 to 45 minutes three or four times per week.

3. I have sufficient energy for each day's tasks.

4. I maintain my target weight.

Self-Care Behaviors

1. Decide to make the most of everyday opportunities for exercise: use stairs instead of elevators, walk instead of ride, park your car farther from your destination than usual and walk the distance briskly, and so forth.
2. Choose exercise activities you enjoy and plan three or four 30- to 45-minute exercise sessions weekly.
3. Obtain medical clearance for exercise if you fall in a high-risk group. Learn and observe the appropriate exercise safeguards (eg, wear running shoes with the proper support).
4. Alternate types of exercise to avoid boredom.
5. Use part of your lunchtime for brisk walking or other exercise.
6. Invite a friend to exercise with you so you have the added support of a buddy.
7. Join a spa, health club, or exercise group.
8. Build up exercise sessions gradually to avoid overexertion and injury to muscles.
9. Evaluate your life-style to see what prevents you from exercising regularly and address these factors (low value attached to health or exercise, low motivation, lack of time, lack of rest, or faulty nutrition).

Nursing History

During the nursing history the nurse interviews the client regarding daily activity level, endurance, exercise and fitness goals, mobility problems, physical or mental health alterations that affect mobility, and external factors affecting mobility. It is important to question clients about their fitness goals. This interviewing strategy communicates to clients that you expect them to be exercising and is itself a powerful teaching tool.

The history of a client's mobility status is brief if initial questioning reveals no problems. The accompanying display illustrates elements common to a mobility status history. When a problem exists (eg, loss of joint mobility or decreased tolerance for physical activity), the nurse assesses the nature of the problem, onset and frequency, known causes, severity, symptoms, effect of problem on everyday functioning, and interventions attempted by the client and results obtained.

FOCUSED ASSESSMENT GUIDE

Mobility and Exercise

Factors to Assess	Questions and Approaches
Daily activity level	Describe the activities you normally carry out during a routine day.
	What type of physical exercise is a part of your daily life-style?
	• Activities of daily living
	• Type, frequency, duration of physical exercise
	• Past history of activity and exercise; recent changes
Endurance	Describe how much and what type of activity makes you tired.
	• History of dizziness, dyspnea, frequent pauses in activity to rest, or marked increase in respiratory rate after moderate activity
Exercise/fitness goals	What exercise or fitness goals are you currently working on?
	• Attitudes about exercise and physical fitness
	• Knowledge of the benefits of exercise
	• Motivation to exercise
	• Current exercise and fitness goals
Mobility problems	Do you experience any problems with movement or with more vigorous activity or exercise? If yes, please describe these problems.
	• Nature of the problem
	• Onset of disturbance and frequency
	• Known causes
	• Severity
	• Symptoms
	• Effect of problem on everyday functioning
	• Interventions attempted and results
Physical or mental health alterations	Are there any physical or mental health problems that may be affecting your mobility? Tell me about them.
	• Decrease of strength or endurance (eg, myocardial infarction, congestive heart failure, cardiomyopathy, chronic obstructive pulmonary disease, cancer, gastrointestinal disorders)
	• Neuromuscular impairment (multiple sclerosis, Parkinson's disease, spinal injuries)
	• Musculoskeletal impairment (arthritis, fractures, muscular dystrophy)
	• Perceptual or cognitive impairment (cerebrovascular accident, brain tumor or trauma, vision disorders)
	• Pain or discomfort (burns, rheumatoid arthritis, chronic pain syndrome, postoperative pain)
	• Depression or severe anxiety (neurosis, schizophrenia)
External factors affecting mobility	Is there anything else you can think of that limits your ability to get around?
	• Environmental factors (stairs, lack of railings or other assistive devices, unsafe neighborhood)
	• Financial resources

Physical Assessment

Physical assessment of mobility status includes an assessment of general ease of movement and gait; alignment, joint structure, and function; muscle mass, tone, and strength; and endurance. Table 30-4 provides normal findings and significant alterations. The nurse performing this assessment directs attention to both structure and function. The client's ability to stand, walk, sit up, and grasp are important because these enable the client to wash, dress, and feed himself or herself, and perform other basic activities of daily living.

General Ease of Movement and Gait

The nurse begins the examination of the ambulatory client the moment the client walks into the room. Voluntarily controlled, fluid, and coordinated body movements are

TABLE 30-4

Overview of the Physical Assessment of Mobility Status

Component	Normal Finding	Significant Alterations
General ease of movement	Body movements are: • Voluntarily controlled (purposeful) • Fluid • Coordinated	Involuntary movements: • Tremors • Tics • Chorea • Athetosis • Dystonia • Fasciculations • Myoclonus • Oral–facial dyskinesias
Gait and posture	• Head erect, vertebrae are straight • Knees and feet point forward • Arms at side with elbows flexed • Arms swing freely in alternation with leg swings • While one leg is in the stance phase the other is in the swing phase	Abnormalities of gait and posture: • Spastic hemiparesis • Scissors gait • Steppage gait • Sensory ataxia • Cerebellar ataxia • Parkinsonian gait • Gait of old age • Use of assistive devices for ambulation
Alignment	Independent maintenance of correct alignment: • In the standing and sitting position, a straight line can be drawn from the ear through the shoulder and hip • In bed, the head, shoulders, and hips are aligned	• Abnormal spinal curvatures • Inability to maintain correct alignment independently
Joint structure and function	Absence of joint deformities Full range of motion	• Limitation in the normal range of motion • Increased joint mobility • Swelling or tenderness in or around the joint • Heat or redness • Crepitation • Deformities • Muscle atrophy, nodules, skin changes • Asymmetry of involvement
Muscle mass, tone, and strength	Adequate muscle mass, tone, and strength to accomplish movement and work	• Atrophy, hypertrophy • Hypotonicity (flaccidity), spasticity • Paresis or paralysis
Endurance	Ability to turn in bed, maintain correct alignment when sitting and standing, ambulate, and perform self-care activities	Physiologic or psychological inability to tolerate an increase in activity: • Significantly increased pulse, respirations, blood pressure after rest • Shortness of breath, dyspnea • Weakness • Pallor • Confusion • Vertigo

keys to the integrated functioning of the skeletal, skeletal muscle, and nervous systems. Significant findings include the presence of any of the following involuntary movements (Bates, 1991, pp. 554–556):

Tremors—relatively rhythmic oscillatory movements

> *Resting tremors*—most prominent at rest and may decrease or disappear with voluntary movement
>
> *Intention tremors*—appear with activity and may increase in severity as the target is neared
>
> *Postural tremors*—appear when the affected part is maintaining a posture; may be aggravated by anxiety or fatigue

Tics—brief, repetitive, stereotyped, coordinated movements occurring at regular intervals (eg, repetitive winking, grimacing)

Chorea—brief, rapid, jerky, irregular, and unpredictable movements that occur at rest or interrupt normal, coordinated movements; seldom repeat themselves

Athetosis—movements that are slower, more twisting and writhing than chorea movements and have a larger amplitude; commonly involve the face and distal extremities

Dystonia—movements similar to athetosis but that involve larger portions of the body, including the trunk; may result in grotesque, twisted postures

Fasciculations—fine, rapid, flickering, or twitching movements originating in relatively small groups of muscle fibers; vary irregularly in frequency and extent, but rarely move a joint

Myoclonus—sudden, brief, rapid, unpredictable jerks, usually involving the limbs or trunk; may be single or repetitive

Orofacial dyskinesias—repetitive, bizarre movements that chiefly involve the face, mouth, jaw, and tongue

The nurse also notes if the body movements are quick and sure or slow and deliberate. These observations communicate both a sense of the person's emotional status and self-care abilities.

The gait of the ambulatory client is also noted. The client's movements while walking should be coordinated and the posture well balanced. The arms should swing freely in alternation with leg swings. Figure 30-9 illustrates stance and swing, the two phases of the normal gait. The heel of the right foot strikes the ground (stance) while the toe of the left foot pushes off and leaves the ground, moving the leg from behind to in front of the body (swing). While one leg is in the stance phase the other is in the swing phase.

Gait abnormalities should be noted because they may place the individual at risk for injury and also because they may be indicative of intoxication or a neuromuscular disorder. Common abnormalities of gait and posture are illustrated in Figure 30-10.

If a client uses a brace, cane, walker, or crutches to assist with ambulation, this should be noted. The nurse also determines if this aid is meeting the client's needs and is being used safely. The use of a wheelchair is also noted.

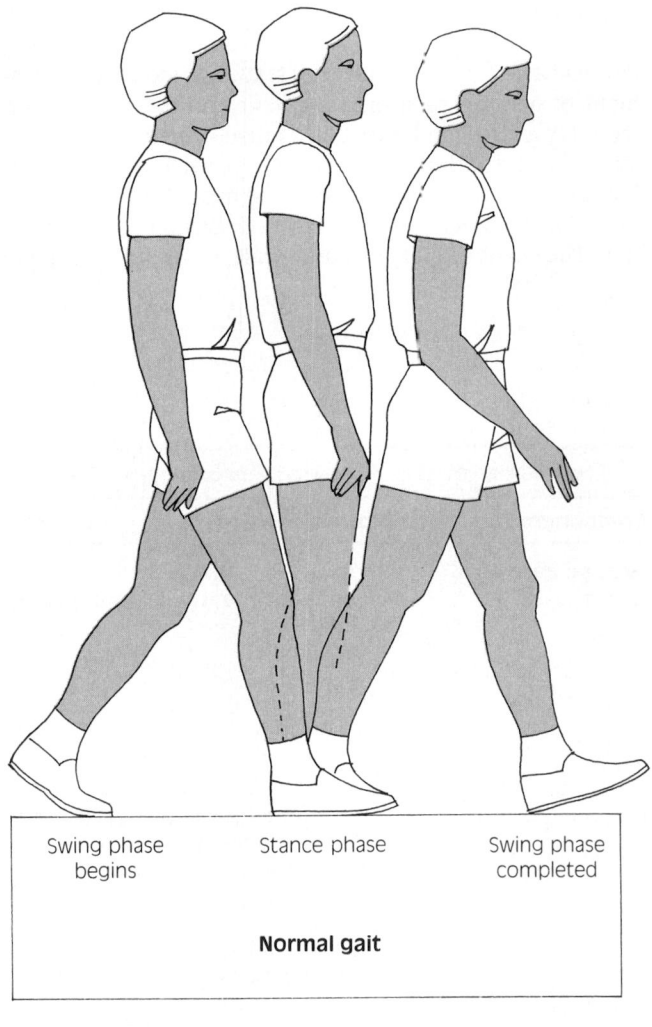

| Swing phase begins | Stance phase | Swing phase completed |

Normal gait

F I G U R E   3 0 - 9

The stance and swing phases of normal gait.

Alignment

Correct body alignment permits optimal musculoskeletal balance and operation and promotes good physiologic functioning. Deviations in body alignment may result from chronic poor posture, trauma, muscle damage, or nerve dysfunction. Fatigue and a person's mental and emotional status may also influence alignment. Alignment may be observed when a client is standing, sitting, or lying (Fig. 30-11). The nurse notes whether the client is able to maintain correct alignment independently.

Correct body alignment when standing is as follows:
- The head is held erect.
- The face is in the forward position, in the same direction as the feet.
- The chest is held upward and forward.
- The spinal column is elongated, and the curves of the spine are within normal limits.

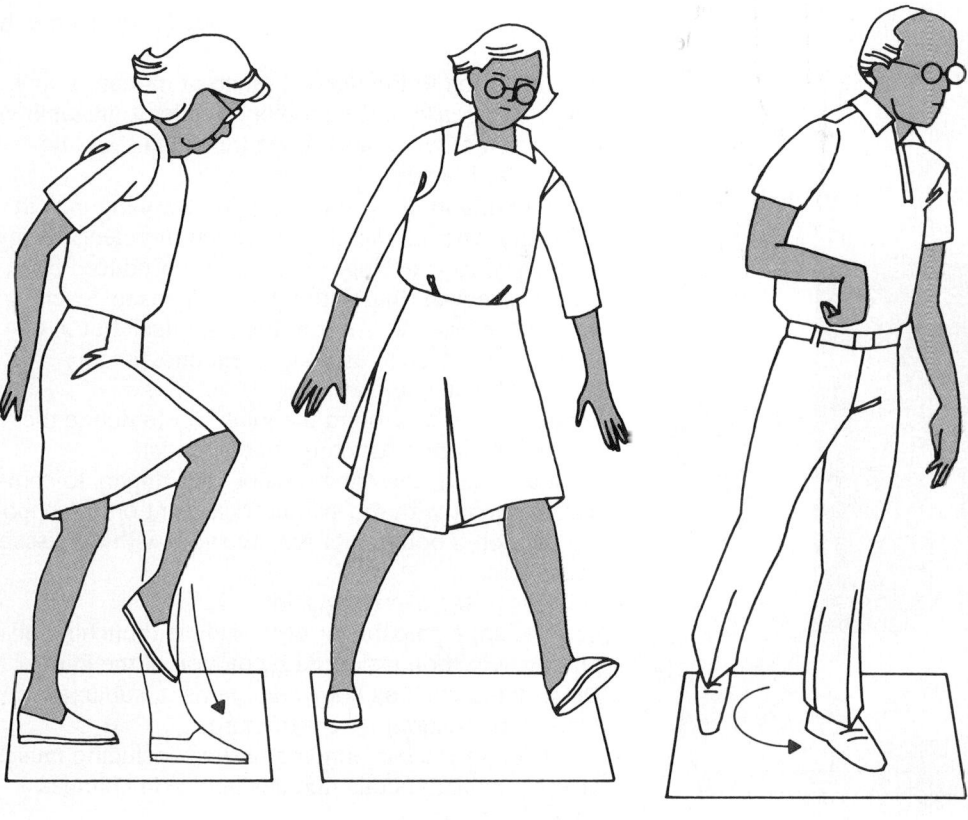

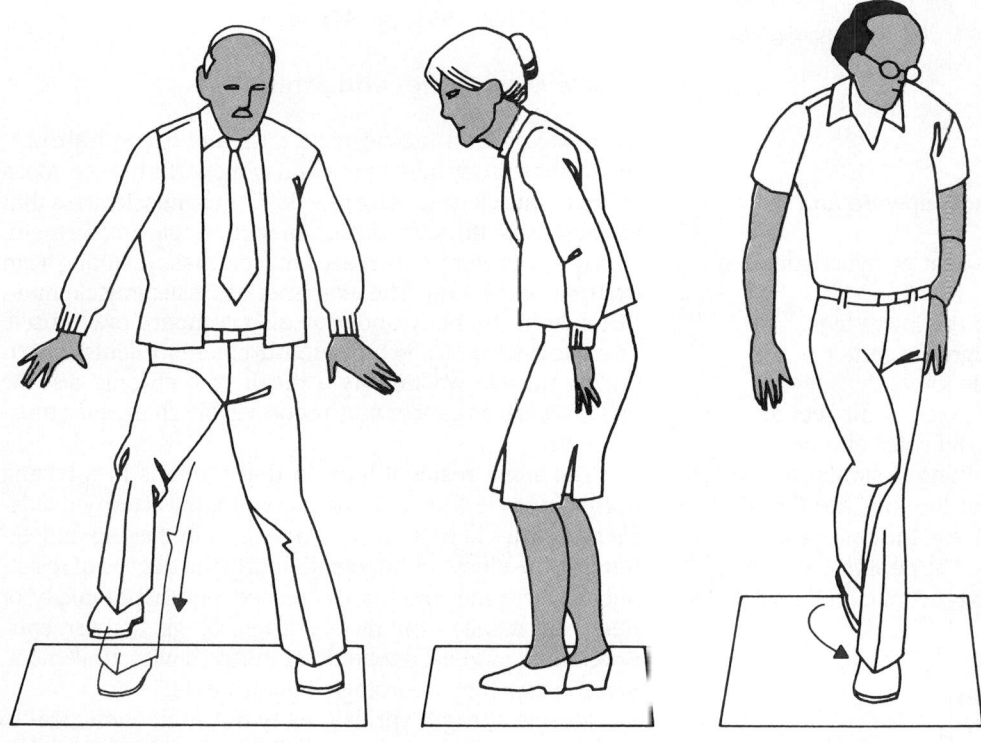

FIGURE 30-10

Gait abnormalities. (Adapted from Bates, B. [1980]. *A guide to physical examination.* Philadelphia: Lippincott.)

(*Top left*) Steppage gait is associated with footdrop, usually secondary to lower motor neuron disease. The feet are lifted high, with knees flexed, and then brought down with a slap on the floor. The client looks as if he were walking up stairs.

(*Top middle*) Cerebellar ataxia is associated with disease of the cerebellum or associated tracts. The gait is staggering, unsteady, and wide based, with exaggerated difficulty on the turns. The client cannot stand steadily with feet together, whether eyes are open or closed.

(*Top right*) Spastic hemiparesis is associated with unilateral upper motor neuron disease. One arm is flexed, close to the side, and immobile; the leg is circled stiffly outward and forward (circumducted), often with dragging of the toe.

(*Bottom left*) Sensory ataxia is associated with loss of position sense in the legs. The gait is unsteady and widebased (the feet are far apart). The feet are lifted high and brought down with a slap. The client watches the ground to guide his or her steps. He or she cannot stand steadily with feet together when the eyes are closed (positive Romberg's sign).

(*Bottom middle*) Parkinsonian gait is associated with the basal ganglia defects of Parkinson's disease. The posture is stooped, the hips and knees slightly flexed. Steps are short and often shuffling. Arm swings are decreased and the client turns around stiffly—"all in one piece."

(*Bottom right*) Scissors gait is associated with bilateral spastic paresis of the legs. Each leg is advanced slowly and the thighs tend to cross forward on each other at each step. The steps are short. The client looks as if he or she were walking through water.

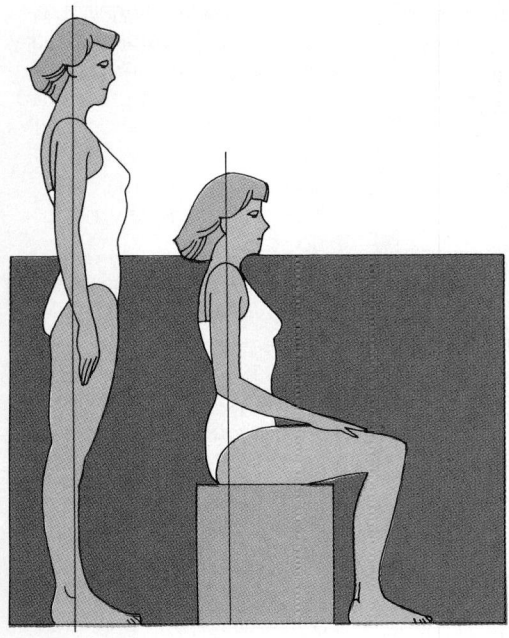

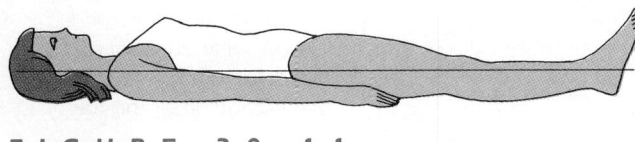

FIGURE 30-11

Adequate posture. In the sitting and standing positions, a straight line can be drawn from the ear through the shoulder and hip. In bed, the head, shoulders, and hips are aligned.

- The abdominal muscles are held upward and the buttocks downward.
- The knees are extended—not bent or hyperextended in the knee-locked position.
- The feet are at right angles to the lower legs.
- The line of gravity goes through the center of the knees and in front of the ankle joints.
- The base of support is on the soles of the feet and weight is distributed through the soles and heels.

Correct body alignment when sitting is similar to correct alignment when standing except the hips are flexed, the knees are flexed and not crossed, and the base of support is on the buttocks and upper thighs. The popliteal area should be free of the edge of the chair to prevent circulatory stasis and possible nerve injury.

Joint Structure and Function

The nurse uses inspection and palpation to examine joints, their range of motion, and the surrounding tissue. **Range of motion** is the complete extent of movement of which a joint is normally capable. See Figure 30-1, which illustrates the range of motion of selected joints. When assessing joint

mobility, Bates (1991) has recommended nurses note the following:

- Any limitation in the normal range of motion or any unusual increase in the mobility of a joint (instability). Range of motion varies among individuals and decreases with aging.
- Any swelling in or around the joint. Swelling may involve the synovial membrane, which then feels boggy, or doughy, to your fingers, or may be produced by excessive synovial fluid within the joint space. Swelling sometimes originates not in the joint itself but in tissues around it, such as bones, tendons, tendon sheaths, bursae, and fat.
- Tenderness in or around the joint. Try to define the specific anatomic structure that is tender.
- Increased heat. Use the backs of your fingers to compare the joint with the symmetrical joint on the opposite side or, if both joints are involved, with the tissues near them.
- Redness of the overlying skin
- Crepitation, a palpable or even audible crunching or grating sensation produced by motion of the joint
- Deformities, such as bony enlargement, subluxation (partial dislocation), or contracture
- Condition of the surrounding tissues, including muscle atrophy, subcutaneous nodules, and skin changes
- Muscular strength
- Symmetry of involvement. Note whether arthritic changes involve several joints symmetrically on both sides of the body or affect only one or perhaps two joints (Bates, 1991, pp. 475–476)

Muscle Mass, Tone, and Strength

Adequate skeletal muscle mass, tone, and strength are prerequisites to body movement and work performance. Mass refers to muscle size. **Atrophy** describes muscle mass that is decreased through disuse or neurologic impairment. *Hypertrophy* refers to increased muscle mass resulting from exercise or training. The examiner assesses muscle mass throughout the body and may also compare one muscle group to another using tape measurements. Clients experiencing muscle wasting as a result of a chronic disease process such as cancer may report visible changes in muscle mass.

The slight residual tension that remains in a resting normal muscle with an intact nerve supply is termed *muscle tone*. Muscle tone may be assessed by flexing and extending the elbow or knee and noting the degree of resistance to these movements. Decreased tone, hypotonicity, or **flaccidity** results from disuse or neurologic impairments. **Spasticity**, increased tone that interferes with movement, is also caused by neurologic impairments.

Muscle *strength* varies greatly from one individual to another and within the same individual, and is affected by muscle use. Muscle strength is tested by asking the client to move actively against resistance. For example, the client may be instructed to push the examiner's palms apart or to push the foot against the examiner's palm. When comparing muscle groups it is important to remember that a person's dominant side tends to be stronger.

Impaired muscle strength or weakness is termed *paresis*. Absence of strength secondary to nervous impairment is *paralysis*. *Hemiparesis* refers to weakness of one half of the body, and **hemiplegia** to paralysis of one half of the body. **Paraplegia** is paralysis of the legs, and *quadriplegia* is paralysis of the arms and legs.

Nursing's concern is that the client's muscle strength is adequate for the performance of tasks the client deems necessary. For example, a client whose primary means of ambulation is a wheelchair requires upper body strength.

Endurance

When assessing *endurance*, the nurse evaluates the client's ability to turn in bed, maintain correct alignment when sitting or standing, ambulate, and perform self-care abilities. When a physical or psychologic factor is believed to be affecting endurance, the nurse:

* Takes the vital signs while the client is at rest
* Instructs the client to perform the activity (eg, ambulation)
* Observes the client's response during and after the activity
* Takes the vital signs immediately after the activity
* Reassesses the vital signs after the client has rested for 3 minutes

Significant findings include significantly increased pulse, respirations, and blood pressure; shortness of breath; dyspnea; weakness; pallor; confusion; and vertigo.

Diagnosing

The nurse must recognize cues that indicate both potential and actual problems when analyzing data about a client's mobility status. Because the problems accompanying immobility can seriously undermine well-being and often require complex and costly treatment, nursing energies are directed to preventing these problems whenever possible. The care plan for the client with an alteration in mobility should contain nursing diagnoses that identify the complications of immobility for which the client is at greatest risk.

Nursing diagnoses specifically addressing problems of mobility include Activity Intolerance and Impaired Physical Mobility. Examples of pertinent etiologies and defining characteristics may be found in the accompanying display.

Examples of nursing diagnoses that describe the effect of mobility alterations on other areas of human functioning follow. This list is by no means exhaustive—multiple etiologies are possible for many of these problem statements.

Ineffective Airway Clearance related to prolonged bed rest, decreased position changes, ineffective coughing related to weakness

NURSING DIAGNOSES FOR COMMON PROBLEMS

Mobility

Problem	Related Factors		Sample Defining Characteristics
Activity Intolerance	Any condition that interferes with the transport of oxygenated blood to tissue (eg, cardiac problems such as congestive heart failure and arrhythmias; respiratory problems, especially chronic obstructive pulmonary disease; circulatory problems; diabetes mellitus)		Decreased ability to perform basic self-care activities: turning in bed, changing position, ambulating, washing, dressing, eating, and so on
	Any condition that causes fatigue (depression, pain, sleep disturbances, prolonged bed rest, sedentary life-style)		Altered response to activity: • Dyspnea, shortness of breath, excessive increase in respiratory rate • Weak pulse, excessive increase in pulse rate, change in rhythm • Blood pressure that fails to increase with activity or that decreases • Weakness, pallor, confusion, vertigo
Impaired Physical Mobility	• Neuromuscular impairment (arthritis, stroke, Parkinson's disease) • Musculoskeletal impairment • Decreased strength and endurance • Pain or discomfort • Depression		• Physical inability to move purposefully or a reluctance to move • Limited range of motion • Decreased muscle mass, tone, or strength • Therapy-related restrictions on movement (eg, an order for bed rest, traction, cast, or splints)

Constipation related to inactivity, decreased muscle tone

Ineffective Breathing Pattern related to limited chest expansion (prolonged bed rest, muscle disuse, atrophy, loss of muscle coordination)

Pain related to inability to change body position independently

Pain: Joint, related to limited range of motion and muscle atrophy

Ineffective Individual Coping [or Ineffective Family Coping] related to loss of ability to move purposefully in environment, spouse's need for assistance with all self-care activities

Fluid Volume Excess related to prolonged bed rest

Impaired Gas Exchange related to decreased respiratory movement

Altered Health Maintenance related to lack of mobility to procure needed services—no support people

Impaired Home Maintenance Management related to immobility

High Risk for Infection: Urinary Tract, related to urinary retention secondary to immobility

High Risk for Injury: Falls related to orthostatic hypotension secondary to immobility

High Risk for Injury: Venous Thrombosis related to immobility

High Risk for Injury: Musculoskeletal Problems related to infrequent, excessive exercise

Knowledge Deficit: Exercise Program, related to having no previous experience with regular exercise

Noncompliance With Exercise Prescription related to decreased endurance, decreased motivation

Powerlessness related to inability to move self

Self-Care Deficit: Bathing/Hygiene, Feeding, Dressing/Grooming, Toileting, related to physical weakness (decreased muscle mass and strength), altered mobility (upper or lower extremities)

Self-Esteem Disturbance related to postural deviation, inability to perform self-care activities, inability to meet role expectations

Sexual Dysfunction related to neuromuscular impairment

Impaired Skin Integrity related to inability to change positions independently, prolonged bed rest

Sleep Pattern Disturbance related to lack of exercise (sedentary life-style)

Impaired Social Interaction related to decreased activity tolerance

Urinary Retention related to prolonged bed rest

Altered Tissue Perfusion (Cardiopulmonary) related to prolonged supine position and greater volume of circulating blood

For clients who are incorporating some form of exercise in their daily routine, the following wellness diagnoses may be appropriate:

Potential for Enhanced Activity Level

Potential for Enhanced Compliance With Exercise Regimen

Planning: Client Goals

If the client is not experiencing any mobility problems, client goals are directed toward the promotion of physical fitness. For example, the client will:

- Follow a program of regular physical exercise that improves cardiovascular function, endurance, flexibility, and strength

To achieve this long-term goal, numerous short-term goals may be needed. Examples of these follow.

By the next visit, 2/20/93, the client will:

- Identify four personal benefits of regular exercise
- Describe an exercise program (activities, frequency, duration) client is willing to follow
- Identify the target heart range
- Obtain medical clearance for the exercise program if at high risk for complications
- List support systems that will reinforce exercise efforts

Clients at high risk for developing specific mobility problems require different goals. The client will:

- Demonstrate correct body alignment whenever observed (alignment)
- Adhere to an every-2-hour positioning schedule (alignment)
- Demonstrate full range of joint motion (joint mobility)
- Demonstrate adequate muscle mass, tone, and strength to perform functional activities of daily living (muscle mass, tone, and strength)

Specific goals for the client at risk of developing complications related to immobility may be found in Table 30-3. Goals for more specific problems, for example, for the client learning to walk with crutches or needing to master transfer techniques with only upper body mobility, need to be individualized to the client.

Implementing

Nursing strategies designed to promote correct body alignment, mobility, and fitness are described in this section. Techniques for positioning clients; performing range-of-motion exercises; moving, lifting, and ambulating clients; and designing exercise programs are highlighted.

Positioning Clients

Positioning that maintains correct body alignment and facilitates physiologic functioning contributes to the client's psychological and physical well-being. The force of gravity pulls parts of the body out of alignment unless adequate support is provided. Various positions are therefore protective in nature only when the client is positioned properly.

Common Devices to Promote Correct Alignment

Many devices can help maintain good body alignment and muscle tonus while the client is in bed and alleviate discomfort or pressure on various parts of the body.

Pillows Pillows are used primarily to provide support or to provide elevation of a part. Pillows of different sizes are useful for different body parts. Those intended for the head are usually full- or large-sized pillows. Small pillows are ideal for support or elevation of the extremities, shoulders, or incisional wounds. Specially designed heavy pillows are useful to elevate the upper part of the body when an adjustable bed is unavailable, such as in a home situation.

Mattresses For a mattress to be comfortable and supportive, it must be firm but have sufficient "give" to permit good body alignment. A client who must remain in a bed with a nonsupportive mattress might well complain of backache and other discomforts.

A well-made and well-supported foam-rubber mattress retains a uniform firmness. This mattress is made of natural or synthetic rubber, or both in combination. A large volume of air is incorporated. The foam-rubber mattress conforms to the contours of the body and supplies support at all points. Its greatest advantage is that it does not form slopes and valleys as the innerspring mattresses are likely to do. Moreover, the foam-rubber mattress does not create as much pressure against bony prominences, such as the ankles, the elbows, the scapulae, and the coccyx. Special mattresses and pads used to help prevent decubitus ulcers are discussed in Chapter 29.

Bed Board If the mattress does not provide sufficient support, a bed board may help to keep the client in better alignment. Bed boards usually are made of plywood or some other firm composition. The size varies with the needs of the situation. For home use, full bed boards are available commercially or can easily be made at home from available materials.

Adjustable Bed The head of an adjustable bed can be elevated to the desired degree. This positioning is discussed later in this chapter. The foot of an adjustable bed can also be elevated to the desired degree. Some adjustable beds allow the bed to be "broken," or gatched, so that the client can rest the knees over an elevated portion of the mattress. This position is rarely recommended or is used only for brief periods because it may cause nerve injury and decreased circulation.

The adjustable bed can also be changed so that the distance of the bed to the floor can be altered. The client can get in and out of bed easier when the bed is in the lowest position. The higher positions are used by health care workers so they do not strain their backs while giving bed care.

Rocking Bed The rocking bed, although used primarily in the care of clients with vascular or respiratory diseases, is also of great value in the care of immobile clients. This bed is mounted on a frame that can be made to rock rhythmically up and down. The bed is adjusted to rock at the frequency of the client's respirations. The rocking aids respiration by shifting the abdominal viscera, which in turn helps move the diaphragm up and down, helping air to be forced out and into the lungs. The constant changing of position also helps blood flow.

Chair Bed Another type of bed used in the care of clients requiring bed rest is one that can be placed into a chair position. These beds were designed primarily for clients with heart ailments. They permit the client to be in a semi-sitting position, which may aid the client's cardiac output.

Circular Bed The electric circular bed is a 6- or 7-foot metal frame with a diameter support for the client. The direction of the support can be changed so the client can be placed in a variety of positions. This bed is especially useful for the client who will be completely helpless for an extended period. Other therapeutic beds used to prevent complications of immobility are discussed in Chapter 29.

Stryker Frame The Stryker frame is a narrow support that can be turned 360 degrees. The client can be alternated between the supine and prone positions without changing alignment. This bed is particularly useful for the totally immobilized client, such as one who is paralyzed.

Footboards The greatest danger to the feet occurs when they are unsupported in the dorsal flexion position. The toes drop downward, and the feet are in plantar flexion. Because of the pull of gravity, this position of the feet occurs naturally when the body is at rest. If maintained for extended periods, plantar flexion can cause an alteration in the length of muscles, and the client may develop a complication called **footdrop**. In this position, the foot is unable to maintain itself in the perpendicular position, heel-toe gait is impossible, and the client will experience extreme difficulty in walking. The use of a foot support, such as the footboard, helps avoid this complication. The footboard also provides a firm surface against which the feet of the bedfast client can be placed for proprioceptor stimulation.

Commercial footboards, such as the one pictured in Figure 30-12, are available. They are generally adjustable

F I G U R E 3 0 - 1 2

Adjustable footboard, used to keep the client's feet in dorsal flexion. (Courtesy of J. T. Posey Company, Arcadia, CA.)

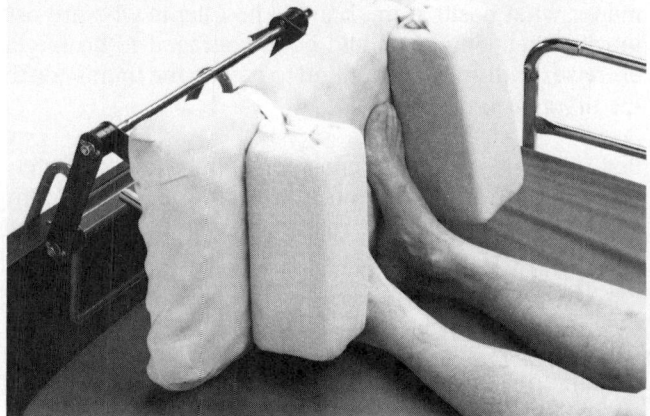

for clients of different heights. The footboard must come far enough up from the foot of the bed so that the client's feet rest firmly against it without the client sliding down in bed. Also, the footboard should not be so far from the foot of the bed that the client's knees are flexed when the feet are against it.

If the client is in a sitting position while in bed, the footboard must be placed at an angle. This prevents hyperextension of the knees, which would result if the feet were kept in dorsiflexion while the trunk was flexed forward. Some clients at risk for developing footdrop are also being advised to wear high-top canvas sneakers while on bed rest in conjunction with the footboard.

Cradle If top bedding must be kept off the client's lower extremities, a device called a cradle is used. A *cradle* is usually a metal frame that supports the bed linens away from the client while providing privacy and warmth. Some cradles are equipped with light bulbs, which provide extra heat. There are any number of sizes and shapes of cradles. If used, the cradle should be fastened securely to the bed so that it does not slide or fall on the client.

Sandbags Sandbags immobilize an extremity and support body alignment. Their value is enhanced if they are available in various sizes. When properly filled, they are not hard or firmly packed. They should be pliable enough to be shaped to body contours and to give support. They should be placed so they do not create pressure on a bony prominence.

Trochanter Rolls Trochanter rolls are used to support the hips and legs so that the femurs do not rotate outward. Figure 30-13 illustrates and describes how to use trochanter rolls. Properly placed pillows can also be used to help prevent the thighs from turning outward, but they tend to slip out of place and require frequent adjusting to be effective.

Hand–Wrist Splints If a client is paralyzed or unconscious, it may be necessary to provide a means for keeping the thumb in the correct position, that is, slightly adducted and in apposition to the fingers. A commercial plastic or aluminum splint may be used to hold the thumb in place no matter what position the hand is in. Clients who are not moving their fingers should be encouraged to do finger exercises with special attention to having the thumb touch the tip of each finger.

Bed Side Rails One of nursing personnel's greatest safety concerns is to prevent clients from falling out of bed. Many hospitals require that side rails be present on all beds and used except when the client is receiving care or is ambulating. The use of side rails requires explanation to clients and their families. Clients should be helped to understand how the side rails offer protection if they are weak or receiving certain drugs and cannot prevent themselves from falling should they roll to the edge of the bed. They also help to remind clients that they are not in their usual environment,

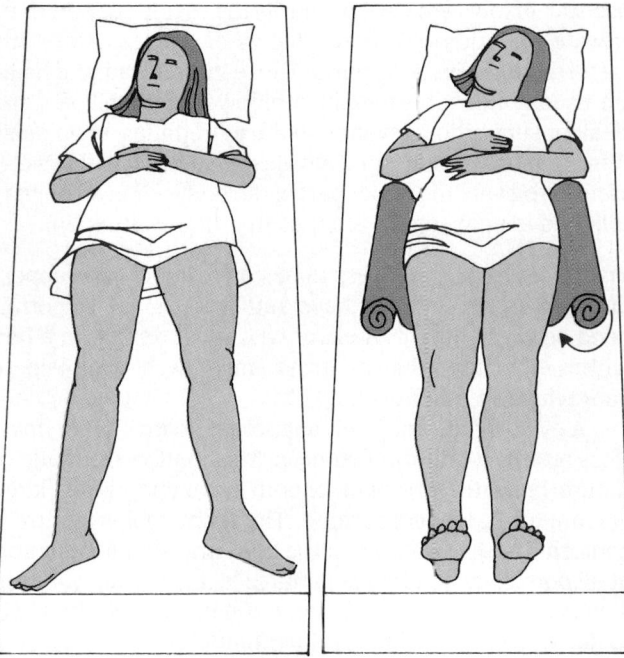

F I G U R E   3 0 - 1 3

Trochanter rolls prevent the external rotation of the hips of a bedridden client. The client is placed on a folded sheet so that the top edge is at the hips and the lower edge is about one third of the way down the thighs. Towels or a bath blanket is rolled under each side until the roll is snugly against the client's hips and thighs. The support cannot unroll, and the weight of the client keeps it secure.

should they awaken during the night and wish to get out of bed.

Side rails make it possible for a client to roll from one side to the other or to sit up without calling for assistance. This in itself is a good activity: it helps the client retain or regain muscle efficiency.

Bed side rails may not deter some clients from getting out of bed. Many a client has crawled over the foot of the bed. It currently is recommended that side rails extend only for three fourths of the length of the mattress. Then, if clients do attempt to get out of bed, they do not have to climb over the side rail or the foot of the bed and further increase the danger of falling. When a client sleeps restlessly or has frequent involuntary movements of the extremities and is in danger of harming himself or herself against the side rails, protective padding may be ordered.

Trapeze Bar A *trapeze bar* is a handgrip suspended from a frame near the head of the bed. The client can grasp the bar with one or both hands and then raise the trunk from the bed. The trapeze makes moving and turning considerably easier for many clients and facilitates transfers into and out of bed. It can also be used to perform exercises that strengthen some muscles of the upper extremities (eg, biceps).

Protective Positioning

Clients accustomed to an active life-style who generally only use a bed for sleep are often unaware of the importance of correct body alignment and regular position changes when on prescribed bed rest. Whenever possible, nurses should teach both the client and family the following:

- Correct positioning techniques
- The need to change positions frequently, at least every 2 hours
- The importance of using the time allotted to position changes to exercise the extremities and to assess and massage pressure area (Reddened areas should not be massaged.)

When the client is unable to change position independently, a turn schedule should be posted at the bedside so that nurses assist with and document the rotation of positions. Table 30-5 describes nursing measures to prevent complications associated with common bed positions.

Fowler's Position   The semisitting position is called *Fowler's position* and calls for the head of the bed to be elevated 45 to 60 degrees. This position is often used to promote cardiac and respiratory functioning because abdominal organs drop in this position and thereby provide maximal space in the thoracic cavity. This is also the position of choice for eating, conversation, vision, and urinary and intestinal elimination.

Variations of Fowler's position include high Fowler's and low Fowler's or semi-Fowler's position. In the high Fowler's position, the head of the bed is elevated 90 degrees. When a bedside table with a pillow on top of it is placed in front of the client in high Fowler's position, the client can lean forward and rest the arms on the pillow, assuming a posture that allows for maximal lung expansion. In the **low** or semi-Fowler's position, the head of the bed is elevated 30 degrees. In Fowler's position, the buttocks bear the main weight of the body. Other skin areas that require assessment and massage include the heels, the sacrum, and the scapulae.

The arms and feet need particular attention when the client is in a semisitting position. Unless properly supported, the arms fall to the bed and pull on the shoulders, and the feet fall into a footdrop position. Supportive devices may be necessary, including pillows supporting the upper back and head, the elbows and wrist joints, the lower back, the thighs, and the ankles; trochanter rolls; and a footboard. The correct positioning and nursing actions to prevent complications associated with the Fowler's position are presented in Table 30-5.

Supine or Dorsal Recumbent Position   In the supine position, the client lies flat on the back with the head and shoulders slightly elevated with a pillow unless contraindicated. The pillow under the head and upper shoulders may not be allowed following a spinal anesthetic or surgery on the spinal vertebrae.

The body areas in need of attention when in the supine position are the feet and neck. Pillows are almost always used to support the head to tilt it forward so that the person's vision is improved. This causes flexion of the cervical spine. The feet will fall into a plantar flexion position unless support is provided. Table 30-5 describes nursing actions to prevent complications associated with this position and illustrates correct alignment in the supine position.

Side-Lying or Lateral Position   In the side-lying position, the client lies on the side and the main weight of the body is borne by the lateral aspect of the lower scapula and the lateral aspect of the lower ilium. Because many people routinely fall asleep in the side-lying position, this is a comfortable alternate to the supine position for the client on bed rest. Although it relieves pressure on the scapulae, sacrum, and heels and allows the legs and feet to be comfortably flexed, support pillows are needed for correct positioning. Areas of the body in need of particular attention when in the side-lying position are the arm and leg on the side opposite the one on which the person is lying. Unless properly supported, the arm will interfere with proper breathing and will be adducted, and the leg adducts and rotates internally. Table 30-5 describes and illustrates the protective side-lying position.

The *oblique position* is recommended as an alternative to the side-lying position because it places significantly less pressure on the trochanter region. The client turns toward the side with the hip on the top leg flexed at a 30-degree angle and the knee flexed at 35 degrees. The calf of the upper leg is positioned slightly behind the body's midline. Pillows support the client's back and calf of the top leg (Fig. 30-14).

A variation of the lateral position is the *Sims' position*. In this position, the client again lies on the side but the lower

(*Text continues on p. 680*)

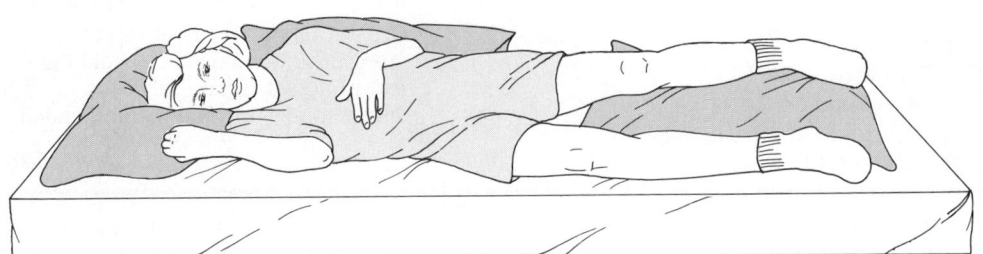

Modified lateral position (oblique position) is an alternative to the side-lying position and results in significantly less pressure on the trochanter area.

T A B L E   3 0 - 5

Common Bed Positions and Protective Nursing Actions		
Position	**Complication to Be Prevented**	**Suggested Preventive Actions**
Fowler's Position		
	Flexion contracture of the neck	Allow the head to rest against the mattress or be supported by a small pillow only.
	Exaggerated curvature of the spine	Use a firm support for the back; position the client so the angle of elevation starts at the hips.
	Dislocation of the shoulder	Support the forearms on pillows to elevate them sufficiently so that no pull is exerted on the shoulders.
	Flexion contracture of the wrist	Support the hand on pillows so it is in natural alignment with the forearm.
	Edema of the hand	Support the hand so it is slightly elevated in relation to the elbow.
	Flexion contractures of the fingers and abduction of the thumbs	Provide hand–wrist splints if necessary.
	Impaired lower extremity circulation and knee contracture, pressure on heels	Elevate the knees for only brief periods; place one or two pillows under the lower legs from below the knees to the ankles; avoid pressure on the popliteal vessels; avoid using the knee gatch.
	External rotation of the hips	Use trochanter roll.
	Footdrop	Support the feet in dorsal flexion. Use footboard; high-top sneakers can also be used.
Protective Supine Position		
	Exaggerated curvature of the spine and flexion of the hips	Provide a firm supportive mattress; use a bed board if necessary.
	Flexion contracture of the neck	Place pillows under the upper shoulders, the neck, and the head so that the head and the neck are held in the correct position.
	Internal rotation of the shoulders and extension of the elbows (hunch shoulders)	Place pillows or arm supports under the forearms so that the upper arms are alongside the body and the forearms are pronated slightly.
	Flexion of the lumbar curvature	Place rolled towel or small pillow under lumbar curvature if needed.
	Extension of the fingers and abduction of the thumbs (clawhand deformities)	Use hand–wrist splints if appropriate.
	External rotation of the femurs	Place sandbags or a trochanter roll alongside the hips and the upper half of the thighs.
	Hyperextension of the knees	Place a pillow under the lower legs from below the knees to the ankles.
	Footdrop	Use a footboard or make an improvised firm foot support to hold the feet in dorsal flexion; high-top sneakers may also be recommended.

(continued)

TABLE 30-5 (continued)

Common Bed Positions and Protective Nursing Actions

Position	Complication to Be Prevented	Suggested Preventive Actions
Protective Side-Lying or Lateral Position		
	Lateral flexion of the neck	Place a pillow under the head and the neck.
	Inward rotation of the arm and interference with respiration	Place a pillow under the upper arm; lower arm should be flexed and positioned comfortably.
	Extension of the finger and abduction of the thumbs	Provide hand–wrist splint if necessary.
	Internal rotation and adduction of the femur	Use one or two pillows as needed to support the leg from the groin to the foot.
	Twisting of the spine	Ensure that the two shoulders are aligned with the two hips.
Protective Sims' Position		
	Lateral flexion of the neck	Place a small pillow under the head unless the drainage of oral secretions is desired.
	Damage to nerves and blood vessels in the axillae of the lower arm	Carefully position lower arm behind and away from the client's back.
	Internal shoulder rotation and adduction	Abduct the upper shoulder slightly so that shoulder and elbow are flexed; place a pillow between the chest and upper arm.
	Internal rotation and adduction of the hip; lumbar lordosis	Place a pillow under the upper flexed leg from the groin to the foot.
	Twisting of the spine	Ensure that the two shoulders are aligned with the two hips.
	Footdrop	Support the lower foot in dorsal flexion with a sandbag.
Protective Prone Position		
	Flexion on the cervical spine	Place a small pillow under the head.
	Hyperextension of the spine; impaired respirations	Place some suitable support under the client between the end of the rib cage and the upper abdomen if this facilitates breathing and if there is space there.
	Footdrop	Move the client down in bed so that the feet are over the mattress, or support the lower legs on a pillow just high enough to keep the toes from touching the bed.

arm is behind the client and the upper arm is flexed at both the shoulder and the elbow. Because in this position the main body weight is borne by the anterior aspects of the humerus, clavicle, and ilium, the major pressure points differ from those in the lateral and other bed-lying positions (see Table 30-5).

Prone Position   In the *prone position*, the person lies on the abdomen with the head turned to the side. The body is straightened out in the prone position because the shoulders, head, and neck are in an erect position, the arms are easily placed in correct alignment with the shoulder girdle, the hips are extended, and the knees can be prevented from flexing or hyperextending. When clients on bed rest use this position periodically, it helps to prevent flexion contractures of the hips and knees. However, the pull of gravity on the trunk when the client lies prone produces a marked lordosis. The position is thus contraindicated for people with spinal problems. The pull of gravity on the feet may result in plantar flexion unless the legs and feet are positioned carefully. Table 30-5 illustrates correct alignment in the prone position and describes nursing activities to prevent complications.

Turning the Client in Bed

Frequently, the client is unable to turn in bed without assistance. Nurses need to use correct body mechanics and knowledge of correct alignment to turn the client from the back onto the side, from the back onto the abdomen, and from the abdomen onto the back. The technique for turning a client in bed is described and illustrated in Procedure 30-1. Mastering this turning technique will help the nurse to adhere to an every-2-hour turn schedule for an immobile client.

Assisting With Range-of-Motion Exercises

Range of motion is the complete extent of movement of which a joint is normally capable. Engaging in routine tasks, such as bathing, eating, dressing, and writing, helps use muscle groups that keep many joints in effective range of motion. When all or some of normal activities of daily living are impossible, attention should be given to the joints not being used at all or to those that are limited in their use.

Unless contraindicated, active, active-assistive, or passive range-of-motion exercises should be encouraged regularly and included in the client's care plan. In **active exercise**, the client independently moves joints through their full range of motion (isotonic exercise). In **active–assistive exercise**, the nurse may provide minimal support, whereas in **passive exercise**, the client is unable to move independently and the nurse moves each joint through its range of motion. Both active and passive exercises improve joint mobility and increase circulation to the affected part, but only active exercise increases muscle mass, tone, and strength and improves cardiac and respiratory functioning. Thus, exercises should be as active as the client's physical

condition permits. It is also helpful to teach isometric exercises to clients to increase muscle mass, tone, and strength.

Directives should be included in the nursing care plan for range-of-motion exercises. The nursing orders should explain what, how, and when, so that all who care for the client observe the same routine. In some institutions, nurses work closely with physiotherapists in designing and implementing exercise programs. The following are basic guidelines for the nurse when helping to put the client's joints through range of motion:

- Teach the client what exercising is being undertaken, why, and how it will be done. Using a show-and-tell technique is often helpful.
- Avoid overexertion and using exercises to the point that the client develops fatigue. The exercises are not to exhaust or tax the client. Certain exercises may need to be delayed until the client's condition allows.
- Avoid neck hyperextension and attempts to achieve full range of motion in all joints with the elderly client. These movements may prove painful. Encourage adequate range of motion in those joints necessary to perform activities of daily living.
- Start gradually and work slowly. All movements should be smooth and rhythmic. Irregular and jerky movements are uncomfortable for the client.
- Move each joint until there is resistance but not pain. Uncomfortable reactions should be reported and exercises halted until further instructions are obtained.
- While exercising joints, use a variety of support measures to prevent muscle strain or injury to the client (Fig. 30-15):
  - *Cupping*—placing a cupped hand under the joint to support it (eg, under the ankle)
  - *Cradling*—supporting the joint with one hand while cradling the distal portion of the extremity with the remaining arm (eg, the calf or forearm might be cradled while the knee or elbow is supported)
  - Supporting the joint by holding the adjacent distal and proximal muscular areas (indicated when a joint is painful); grasping muscle groups or major tendons is likely to cause injury to the tissues.
- Return the joint to a neutral position, that is, its normal position of alignment, when finishing each exercise.
- Keep friction at a minimum when moving extremities to avoid injuring the skin.
- Use range-of-motion exercises twice a day, and do the exercises regularly to build up muscle and joint capabilities. Each exercise is carried out two to five times. Many of the exercises can be carried out when the client is being bathed and become part of that procedure. Routine tasks, such as eating, dressing, self-bathing, and writing, also help to put certain joints through range of motion and should be encouraged.
- Expect the client's respiratory and heart rate to increase during exercising, which is good. These rates should return to normal within a few minutes. If they do not, the exercises are probably too strenuous for the client.

PROCEDURE 30-1

Turning a Client in Bed

Action	Rationale
1 Explain the procedure to the client.	This facilitates the cooperation of the client.
2 Wash your hands.	Handwashing deters the spread of microorganisms.
3 Raise the bed to your waist level. Adjust to flat position or as low as the client can tolerate. Lower side rail nearest you and raise the opposite side.	This position facilitates the turning maneuver and minimizes strain on the nurse yet keeps the client safe.
4 Position the client closer to the far side of the bed in the supine position.	The client will be in the center of the bed after turning is accomplished.
5 Place the client's arms across the chest and cross the client's far leg over the near one.	This facilitates the turning motion and protects the client's arms during the turn.
6 Stand opposite the client's center with your feet spread and one foot ahead of the other. Tighten your gluteal and abdominal muscles and flex your knees.	This positions the turner opposite the center of the body mass. It places the nurse in a stable position with good body alignment and prepared to use large muscle masses to turn the client.

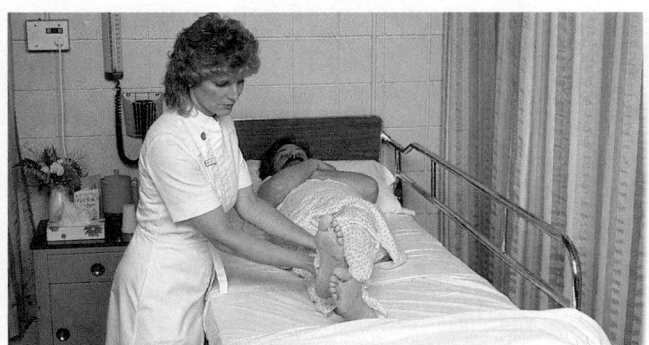

Action 5: Positioning client's arms and legs.

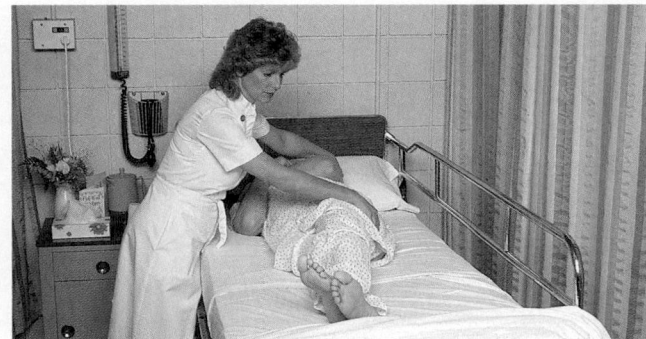

Action 6: Preparing to turn client.

Action	Rationale
7 Position your hands on the client's far shoulder and hip and roll the client toward you.	This maneuver supports the client's body and makes use of the nurse's weight to assist with turning.
8 Make the client comfortable and position in proper alignment.	This ensures that the client will be able to maintain desired position.

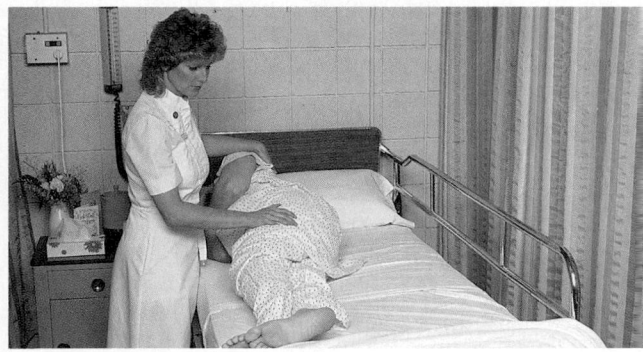

Action 7: Turning client.

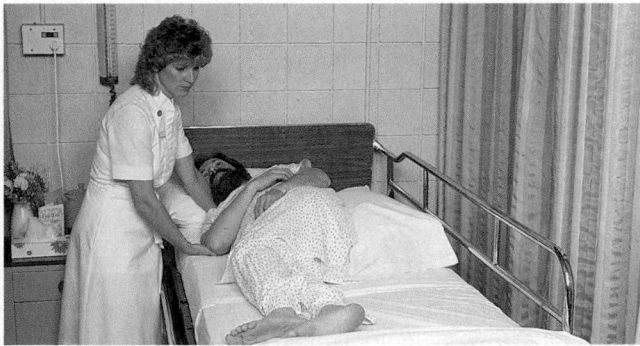

Action 8: Making client comfortable.

Action	Rationale
9 Readjust the bed height and position and raise side rail if appropriate.	This ensures the client's safety.
10 Wash your hands.	Handwashing deters the spread of microorganisms.

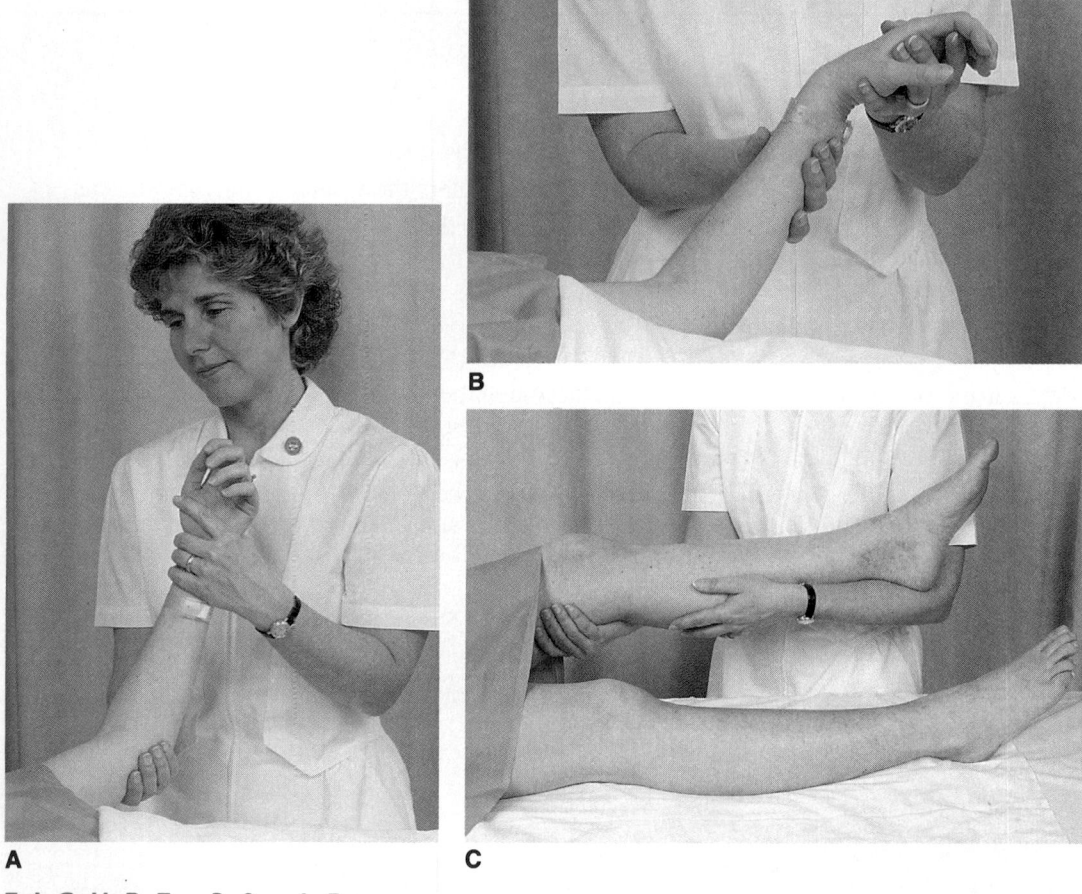

F I G U R E 3 0 - 1 5

Support measures used to prevent muscle strain or injury to the client during range-of-motion exercises (A) using a cupped hand to support a joint; (B) cradling the distal portion of an extremity; and (C) supporting the joint by holding the distal and proximal areas adjacent to the joint.

• Use passive exercises as necessary, but encourage active exercises of the same kind when the client is able to do so independently. Exercises should continue at home after a period of hospitalization, as necessary.

The goal of range-of-motion exercises is to keep the client in the best possible physical state while bed rest is necessary. When range-of-motion exercises are not considered as routine measures, the client's physician should be consulted. Figure 30-16 illustrates a series of passive range-of-motion exercises.

Moving and Lifting the Client

Frequently it is necessary to move a helpless client. The client must be kept in good alignment and protected from injury while being moved. There are certain recommended guidelines the nurse should follow when moving and lifting clients:

• Know the client's diagnosis, capabilities, and any movement not allowed. Place braces or any device the client wears before helping from bed.

• Plan carefully what you will do before moving or lifting a client. Assess mobility of attached equipment. You may injure the client or yourself if you have not planned well. If necessary, enlist the support of another nurse. This reduces the strain on all involved.

• Explain to the client what you plan to do. Then, use what abilities the client has to assist you. This technique often decreases work and possible injury to yourself.

• If the client is in pain, administer the prescribed analgesic sufficiently in advance of the transfer to allow the client to participate in the move comfortably.

• Remove obstacles that may make moving and lifting inconvenient.

• Elevate the bed as necessary so that you are working at a height that is comfortable and safe for you.

• Lock the wheels of the bed, wheelchair, or stretcher so that they do not slide about while you are moving the client.

(*Text continues on p. 687*)

FIGURE 30-16

In this example of a passive range-of-motion exercise, the nurse begins with the neck and works down to the toes on one side of the client's body then up the opposite side. Prone or lateral position is necessary to hyperextend the neck, shoulders, and hips. All exercises should be done slowly, evenly, smoothly, and gently. Joints should be moved to the point where resistance is felt, but never to the point of pain. Each exercise should be repeated the prescribed number of times. When supporting a body part, the nurse grasps firmly above and below the joint with fingers together. After each movement, the body part is returned to its normal anatomical position.

Neck

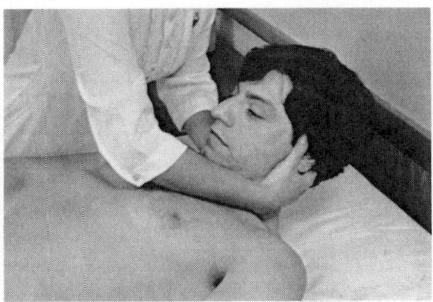

Flexion
Flex the head forward trying to place the chin to the chest.

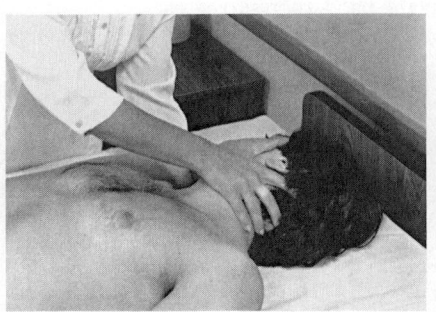

Rotation
Rotate the head to each side trying to place the chin on the shoulder.

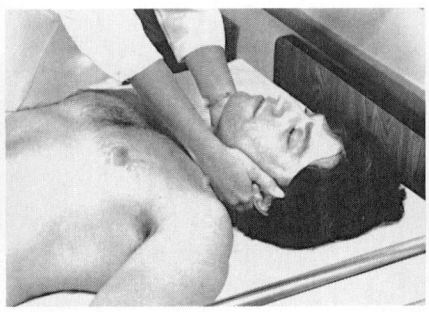

Lateral flexion
Tilt the head to each side trying to place the ear on the shoulder.

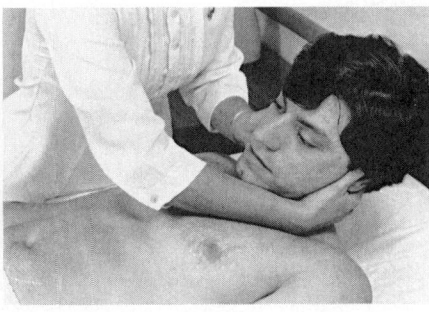

Rotation
Flex the neck and circumduct the head from side to side in as wide a semi-circle as possible.

Shoulder

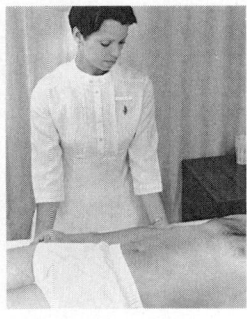

Flexion
Support the arm above the elbow with one hand. With the other hand grasp the client's hand. Extend the arm upward above the head.

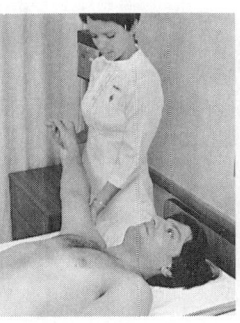

Abduction, Adduction
Abduct the shoulder by moving arm away from body to the side. Adduct the shoulder by returning the arm to the neutral position.

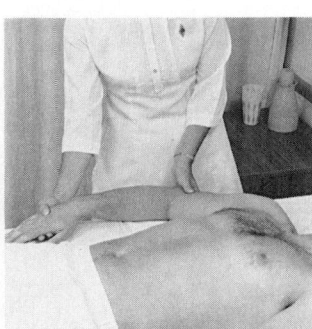

External/Internal rotation
Position the arm with the upper arm perpendicular to the body and the lower arm parallel to the body. Rotate the shoulder

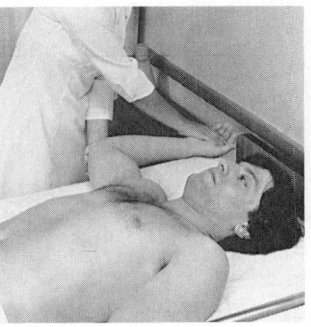

through a 180 degree arc and return to neutral position. With the elbow extended and the arm supported above the elbow, circumduct the shoulder in as wide a semi-circle as possible.

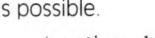

(continued)

Elbow

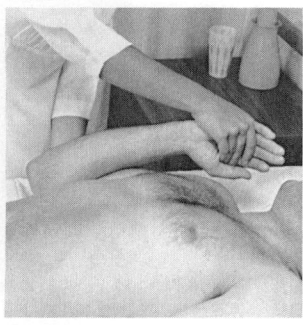

Forearm

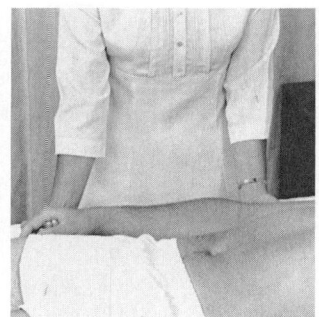
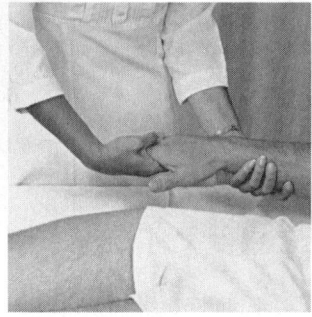

Flexion and Extension
With the client's upper arm at his side, flex and extend the elbow.

Pronation and Supination
Support the forearm with one hand. With the other, grasp the client's hand. Pronate the hand, then supinate it.

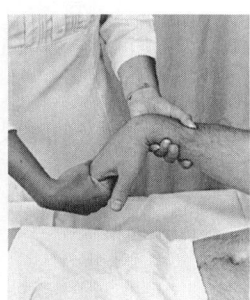
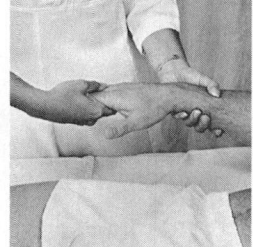
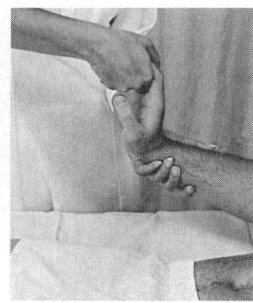

Flexion and Extension
Flex the wrist, extend the wrist and hyperextend the wrist.

Radial and Ulnar deviation
With the palm down, perform a radial deviation of the wrist and an ulnar deviation of the wrist.

Fingers and Thumb

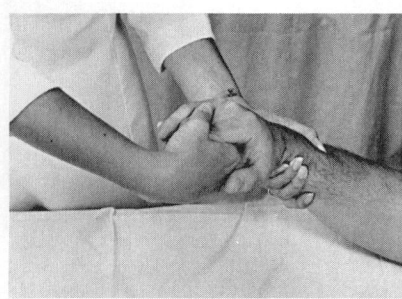
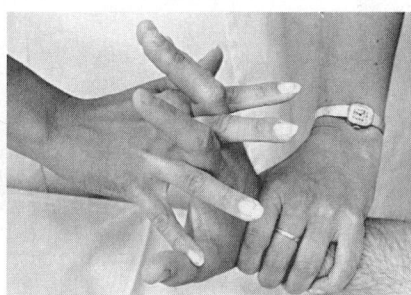

Rotation
Slowly and gently move the wrist in as wide a circle as possible, first in one direction and then the other.

Abduction/Adduction
Abduct the fingers by interlacing your fingers with the client's. Then adduct them moving the thumb across the palm as far as possible.

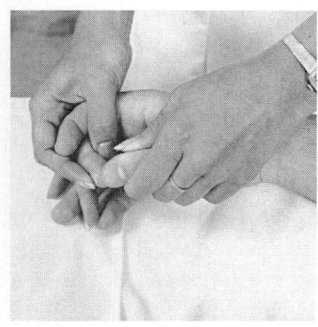
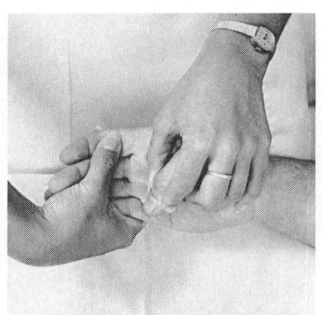
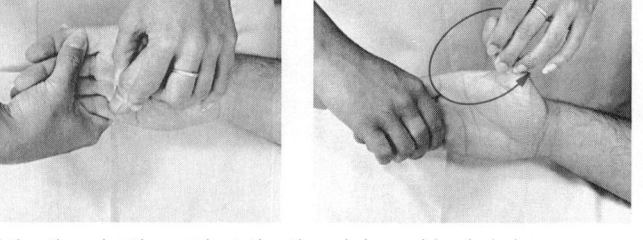

Flexion/Extension and Opposition
Flex fingers individually by touching each fingertip with the tip

of the thumb. Circumduct the thumb in a wide circle in one direction and then the other.

Trunk

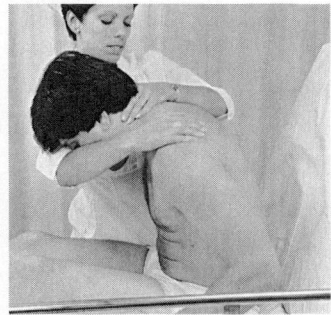 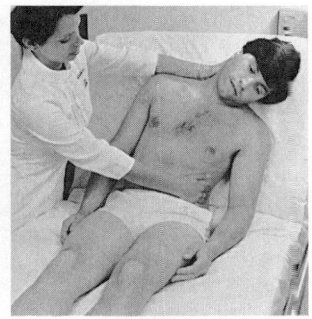 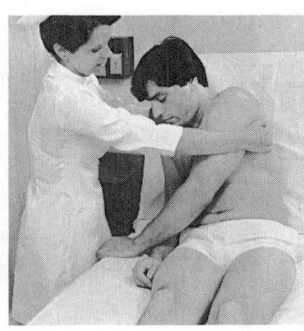 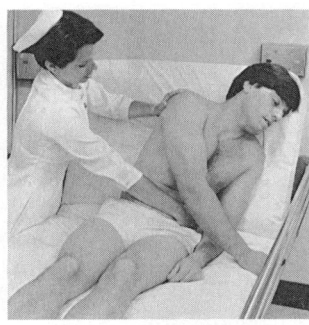

Flexion
With the head of the bed raised and the client in a sitting position, flex the trunk by bending the client forward. Lateral flexion occurs as you pull the client's waist toward you while pushing his neck and shoulders away from you.

Rotation
Rotate the trunk by placing the client's forearm across waist, grasping the upper body just below the shoulders and rocking backward, pulling the client toward you.

Hip and Knee

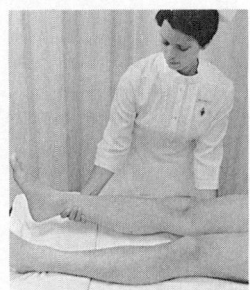 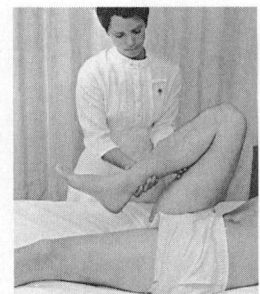 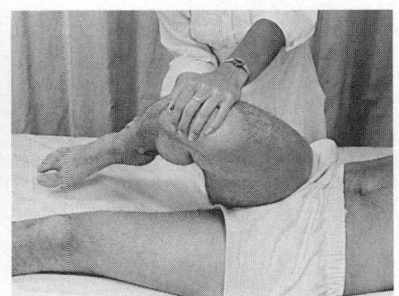

Flexion/Extension
With the client in a supine position and bed flat, combine flexion of hip and knee. Supporting the upper leg and the heel, lift the leg as far as possible while flexing the knee. Extend the leg.

Internal/External Rotation
Flex the knee and place the client's foot on the bed next to the other knee. Lift the foot just off the sheet and swing the knee toward you maintaining flexed postion. This motion produces external rotation of the hip. Internal rotation is effected by moving the foot away from the midline while moving knee across the midline and down.

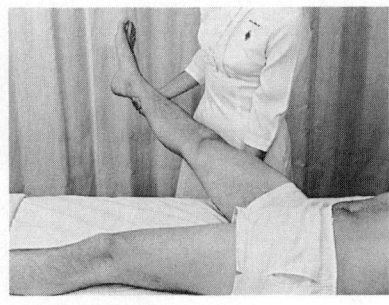 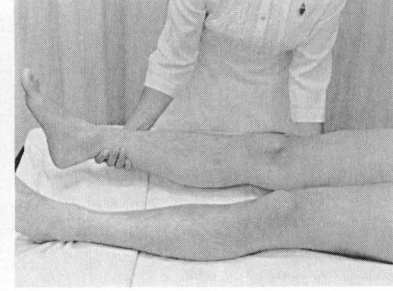 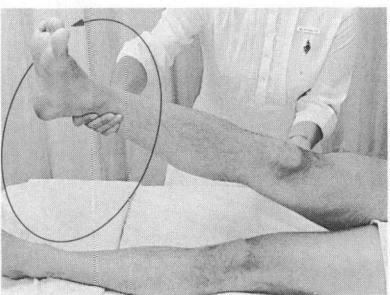

Abduction/Adduction
Abduct and adduct the hip as for the shoulder.

Rotation
Rotate the hip in as large a semi-circle as possible.

F I G U R E   3 0 - 1 6 (continued)

Ankle

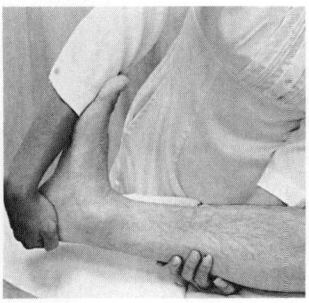 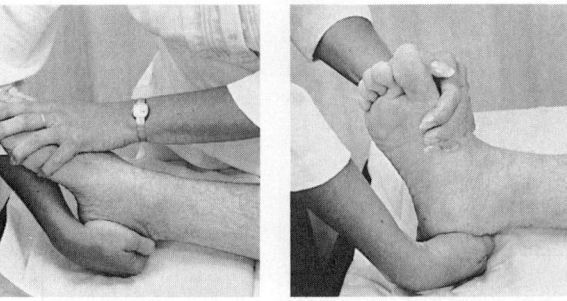 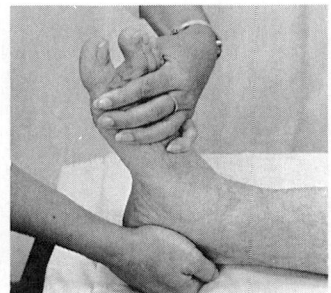

Dorsiflexion/Plantarflexion
Cupping the heel and resting the sole of the foot on your forearm, produce dorsiflexion by pressing against the ball of the foot with your forearm.

Inversion/Eversion
Cupping the heel and grasping the distal portion of the foot, turn the foot to point the sole toward the midline, then away form the midline to effect inversion and eversion of the ankle.

Toes

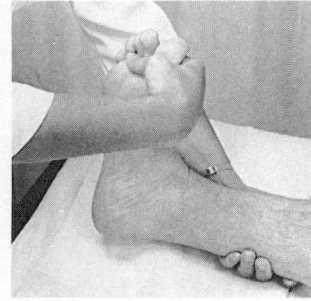 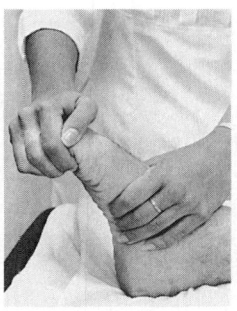 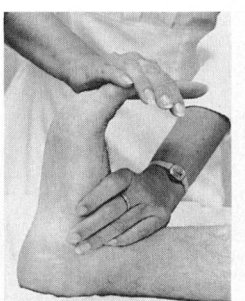 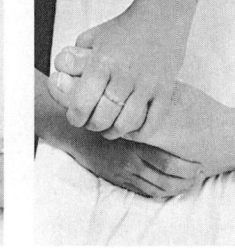

Rotation
Rotate the ankle in as wide a circle as possible, first in one direction and then the other.

Flexion/Hyperextension
Manually flex and hyperextend the toes as shown.

Abduction/Adduction
Abduct and adduct the toes as for the fingers.

Having completed exercises on both sides of the client in the supine position, turn the client over.

Neck   **Shoulder**

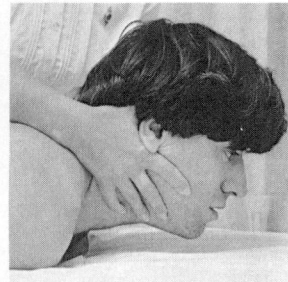 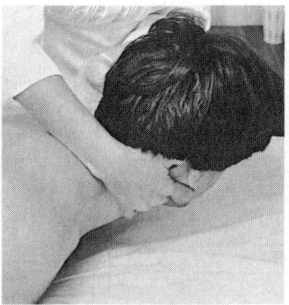 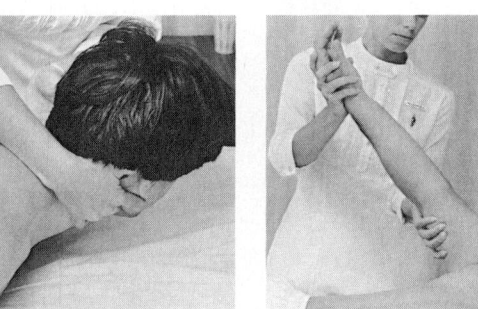 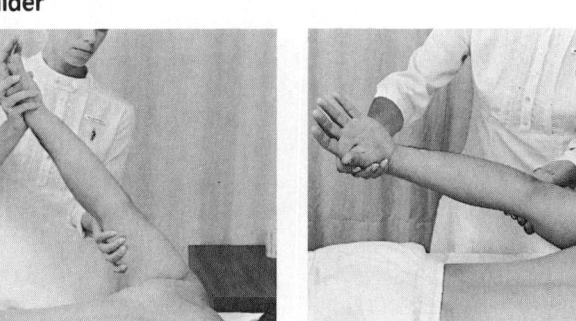

Hyperextension
Hyperextend the neck gently.

Rotation
Rotate the neck in as large a semi-circle as possible.

Hyperextension
Hyperextend the shoulder.

Rotation
Rotate the shoulder in as large a semi-circle as possible.

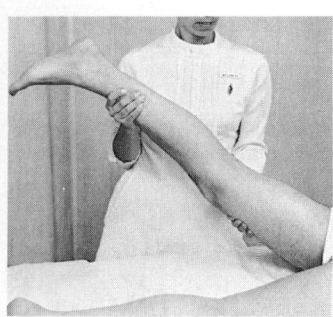 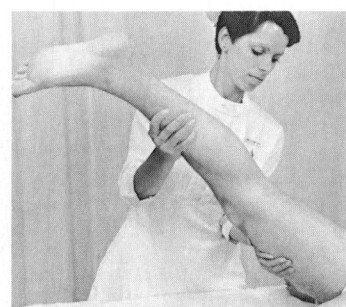

Hip

Hyperextension
Hyperextend the hip by lifting the leg with the knee extended.

Rotation
Rotate the hip in as large a semi-circle as possible.

F I G U R E   3 0 - 1 6 *(continued)*

- Observe principles of body mechanics while you work to prevent injuring yourself.
- Be sure the client is in good body alignment while being moved and lifted to protect the client from strain and muscle injury.
- Support the client's body well. Avoid grabbing and holding an extremity by its muscles.
- Avoid causing friction on the client's skin during moving. Friction can be reduced by sprinkling powder or cornstarch on bed linens and on the client's skin.
- Move your body and the client in a smooth, rhythmic motion. Jerky movements tend to put extra strain on muscles and joints and are uncomfortable for the client.
- Use mechanical devices such as a Hoyer lift or turning board when they are available for moving clients. Be sure that you understand how the device operates and that the client is properly secured and informed of what will occur. Clients who do not understand or are afraid may be unable to cooperate and may suffer injury as a result.
- Be realistic about how much you can safely do without injury. Two small people cannot lift or move an obese client without risking muscle strain and injury.

Moving the Client Up in Bed

Children and lightweight adults are relatively easy to slide toward the head of the bed without the assistance of a second person. A technique used to move a client up in bed when the client is able to assist is described and illustrated in Procedure 30-2. The procedure also describes and illustrates how two nurses can move the client up in bed.

Using a Sheet to Move the Client Up in Bed   Although the methods described may be convenient, the amount of effort expended by the nurse can be reduced when moving a client up in bed. A drawsheet or a large sheet may be placed under the client so that it extends from the client's head to below the buttocks, and can be used to lift the client. When using the sheet lift, the friction that must be overcome is between the lift sheet and the bed linen. Therefore, the client's skin is spared the effects of abrasion and friction.

Moving the Client From Bed to Stretcher

Considerable care must be taken when moving a client from a bed to a stretcher, or vice versa, to prevent injury to the client. If the client is unconscious or helpless, additional nurses are needed to support the extremities and the head. The skills are explained in Procedure 30-3. For clients who are obese, use of a transfer board or roller board will facilitate the move from stretcher to bed and ensure that the client's body is properly aligned during the transfer. When returning the client to the bed from the stretcher, the same techniques are observed. However, the carriers should first move the client from the stretcher onto the edge of the bed. Then, one member of the team supports the client on the edge of the bed to prevent falling off while the other two team members go around to the opposite side of the bed and place their arms underneath the client. After the two people on the opposite side of the bed have a good grip on the client, the third person is able to join them and assist in sliding the client to the center of the bed.

Sometimes clients must be lifted and carried. This can be done by means of a three-carrier lift. If done properly, the client will feel secure, and those lifting will not suffer strain. The three-carrier lift is described and illustrated in Procedure 30-4. The three-carrier lift is used in various other situations, such as lifting a client who has fallen to the floor and is unable to get up independently or lifting a client out of a chair into the bed.

For clients who present special problems because of their excessive weight or a cast, it may be necessary to have an additional person to support the heaviest or most cumbersome part of the client. The people distribute their arms while carrying so that the heaviest part is well supported.

Moving the Client From Bed to Chair

Safety and comfort are paramount concerns when the nurse assists the client out of bed. Preliminary assessment of vital signs provides baseline data and subsequent recordings can be used to determine the effect of this activity on the client. The position of the nurse as he or she prepares to move the client and placement of the chair are critical elements in the transfer. Client's apparel should be sufficient to prevent embarrassment and provide warmth yet not impede movement. The techniques for assisting a client to transfer from bed to chair is described in Procedure 30-5.

It is possible for only one person to get a helpless client from a bed to a chair, although two people simplify matters. The one-person technique is valuable for nurses to know for the home care of invalids and for emergency use. More than one person should be available if the bed and chair seat are not the same height. The technique for transferring a client by two nurses is described in Procedure 30-6.

Helping Clients Ambulate

Fortunately for most clients, prolonged periods of bed rest are no longer considered necessary during most illnesses. Activity, even as mild as a stroll around the room, down the hall, from the bedroom to the living room, or out into the yard, is a protective measure for the body.

Physical Conditioning

Clients who are not confined to bed for long periods, who sleep well, and who experience possibly short periods of rest during the day may not require special considerations for increased physical activity in preparation for ambulation. However, there are others who will have to be prepared for the day when ambulation is resumed. Certain exercises that strengthen the overall efficiency of the musculoskeletal system can be done in bed.

(Text continues on p. 696)

PROCEDURE 30-2

Moving a Client Up in Bed (One Nurse)

Action

1 Explain the procedure to the client.

2 Wash your hands.

3 Raise the bed to a comfortable position for you. Adjust the bed to flat position if the client can tolerate it. Lower the side rail nearest you.

4 Remove the pillow and place it at the head of the bed.

5 If able to assist, have the client flex the knees with the feet flat on the bed.

6 Assist the client to grasp the overhead trapeze bar or, if unable to assist, fold the client's arms across the chest.

7 Instruct the client to flex the neck with the chin on the chest.

8 Stand opposite the client's center with your feet spread and turned toward the head of the bed. Position one foot slightly forward.

Rationale

This facilitates cooperation of the client.

Handwashing deters spread of microorganisms.

This position facilitates moving the client upward and minimizes strain on the nurse.

This reduces friction and protects the client's head from striking the top of the bed.

The client is prepared to push upward by using a major muscle group.

This provides assistance and reduces friction.

This prevents hyperextension of the neck.

This positions the mover opposite the center of the body mass. It places the nurse in a stable position, with good alignment.

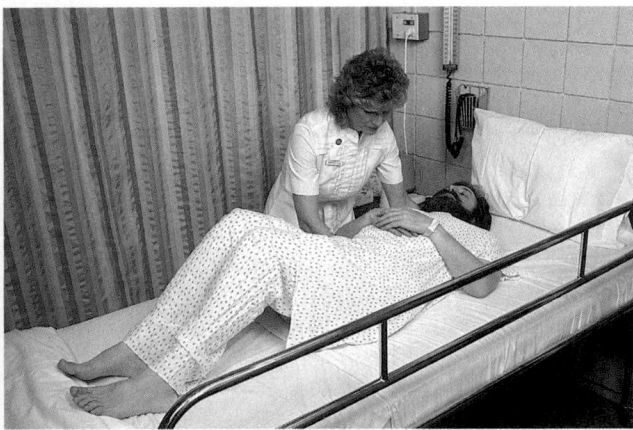

Action 5: Preparing client for move.

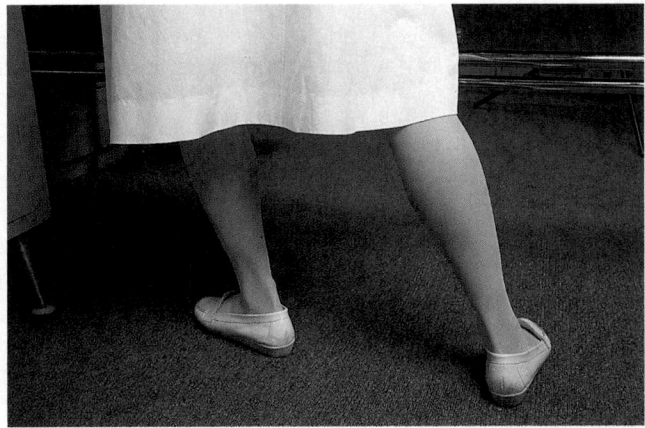

Action 8: Placing legs and feet for stable position.

9 Flex your knees and hips. Place one arm under the client's neck and shoulders, grasping the far shoulder with your hand. Place your other arm under the client's upper thighs. Pull the client closer to your side of the bed. Move the client's head and legs into alignment.

10 Review the plan of movement with the client. Tighten your abdominal and gluteal muscles. Assume the position to move the client (see action 9).

11 Shift your weight back and forth from back leg to front leg, and on count of three, move the client upward in bed. If possible, the client should push with the legs and assist movement upward by grasping the trapeze. Repeat if necessary.

This prepares the nurse to use a large muscle mass to aid in lifting. The placement of the arms supports and evenly distributes the weight of the client.

These muscles stabilize the pelvis before the lifting maneuver.

The rocking motion uses your weight to counteract the client's weight when moving the client up in bed. If the client assists, less effort is required by the nurse.

(continued)

PROCEDURE 30-2 *(continued)*

Moving a Client Up in Bed (One Nurse)

Action	**Rationale**
12 Assist the client to a comfortable position in the center of the bed. Reposition the pillow. Raise the side rail and adjust the bed position, if necessary.	This ensures the client's safety.

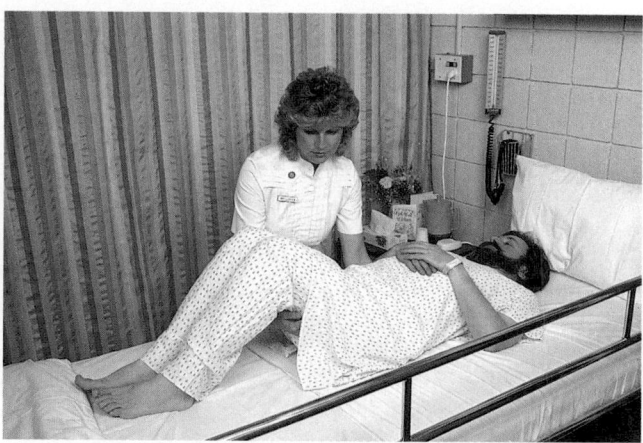

Action 11: Moving client.

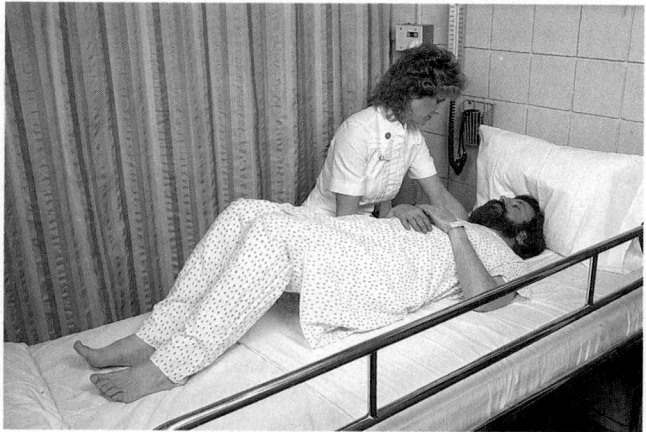

Action 12: Assisting client in new position.

13 Wash your hands.	Handwashing deters the spread of microorganisms.

Special Considerations

Two nurses on opposite sides of the bed may move a client up in bed by interlocking their arms under the client's shoulders and thighs and lifting as described previously.

Two nurses on opposite sides of the bed may move a client up in bed by using a draw-sheet placed under the client from shoulder to thigh area. Fold or bunch the drawsheet close to the client and lift as described previously.

PROCEDURE 30-3

Transferring a Client From Bed to Stretcher

Action	**Rationale**
1 Explain the procedure to the client.	This facilitates the cooperation of the client.
2 Wash your hands.	Handwashing deters the spread of microorganisms.
3 Move the bed and equipment in the room to make room for the stretcher. Make sure that assistants are available. Close the door or curtain.	This facilitates transfer movement and provides for privacy.
4 Raise the bed to the same height as the stretcher and adjust the head of the bed to the flat position if the client can tolerate it. Lower side rails.	Pushing and pulling require less effort than lifting. This position facilitates moving the client.
5 Place a drawsheet under the client if one is not already there. Use the drawsheet to move the client to the side of the bed where the stretcher will be placed.	This facilitates movement of the client to the stretcher.

(continued)

P R O C E D U R E 3 0 - 3 *(continued)*

Transferring a Client From Bed to Stretcher

Action	Rationale
6 Position stretcher next to the bed and parallel to it. Lock wheels on the stretcher and bed. Remove the pillow from the bed and place it on the stretcher.	Positioning of the stretcher and locking the wheels facilitate safe transfer of client.
7 To move the client:	
a The first nurse should kneel on far side of the bed away from the stretcher. Position the knee at the upper torso closer to the client than the other knee. Grasp the drawsheet securely.	The nurse uses a major muscle group to assist in movement. The nurse's flexed hips help avoid back injury.
b The second nurse should reach across the stretcher and grasp the drawsheet at the head and chest areas of the client.	This promotes safe transfer by supporting the client's head and upper body.
c The third nurse should reach across the stretcher and grasp the drawsheet at the client's waist and thigh area. Ask the client to fold arms across the chest.	This supports the lower part of the client's body for safe transfer.
d At a signal given by the first nurse, the second and third nurses pull while the first nurse lifts the client from the bed to the stretcher.	Working in unison distributes the work of moving the client and facilitates the transfer.

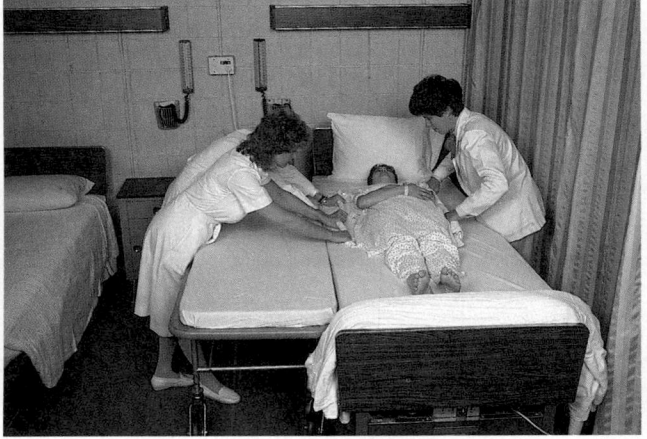

Action 5: Using drawsheet to move client to side of bed.

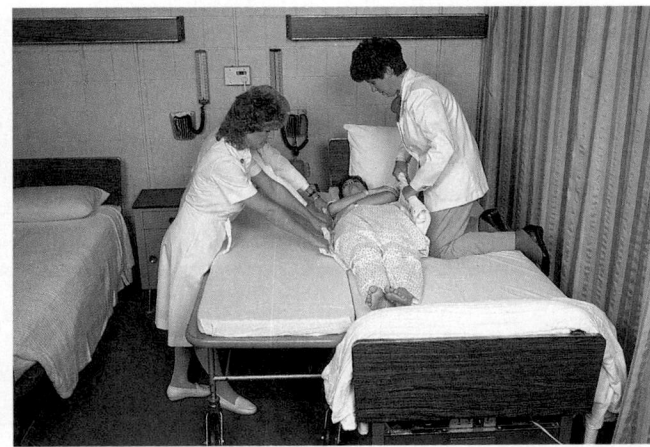

Action 7: Moving client to stretcher.

8 Secure the client on the stretcher until side rails are raised. Assist the client to a comfortable position with the covering in place. Leave the drawsheet in place for transfer back to bed.	This ensures client safety and comfort.
9 Wash your hands.	Handwashing deters the spread of microorganisms.

Special Considerations

A long polyethylene board with handgrips on the edges may be used to assist with the transfer:

- Turn the client on his or her side with the back toward the stretcher.
- Position the transfer board lengthwise and midway between the bed and stretcher.
- Return the client to his or her back with a bottom sheet or drawsheet between the client and the board.

(continued)

P R O C E D U R E   3 0 - 3 *(continued)*

Transferring a Client From Bed to Stretcher

Special Considerations

- Using the sheet, slide the client across the transfer board and onto the stretcher.
- Reposition the client on the stretcher, remove the board, and secure with safety belts and side rails.

P R O C E D U R E   3 0 - 4

Transferring a Client From Bed to Stretcher (Three-Carrier Lift)

Action	Rationale
1 Explain the procedure to the client.	This facilitates the cooperation of the client.
2 Wash your hands.	Handwashing deters the spread of microorganisms.
3 Place the stretcher at a right angle to the foot of the bed. Lock the wheels of the bed and the wheels of the stretcher. Raise the bed to the height of the stretcher.	The stretcher will be in position for the carriers after they pivot away from the bed.

4 Decide on responsibility for the lift. Each person must support one section of the body:
  a Head, shoulders, and chest
  b Hips
  c Thighs and legs
	Opinions differ about how to determine who lifts which area. The recommendations are that the strongest helper should support the heaviest body area or that the tallest person with the longest reach should support the client's head and shoulders.

5 In preparation for the lift, flex your knees and separate your feet, with the foot closest to the stretcher slightly forward.	Broad-based stance improves balance and lowers the lifter's center of gravity.
6 Slide your arms under the client as far as possible and, on signal, all helpers should simultaneously roll the client toward their chests.	"Logrolling" the client onto the carriers brings the centers of gravity of all objects closer, thereby increasing the stability of the group and reducing strain on the carriers.
7 On signal, the helpers should stand up and steady the client securely against their chests.	Flexed knees and body position allow workers to lift with strong leg muscles.

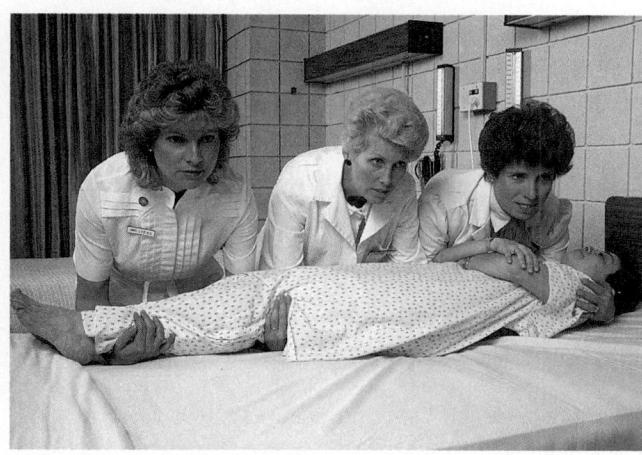

Action 6: Positioning client close to lifters.

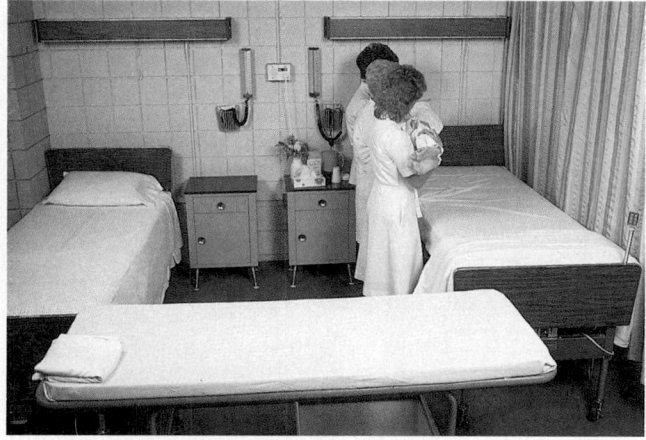

Action 7: Standing with client held to chest.

(continued)

P R O C E D U R E   3 0 - 4 *(continued)*

Transferring a Client From Bed to Stretcher (Three-Carrier Lift)

Action	Rationale
8 Helpers should step back together, pivot around to the stretcher, and, on signal, lower the client onto the stretcher.	This lets the large leg and arm muscles do the work of lowering the client.

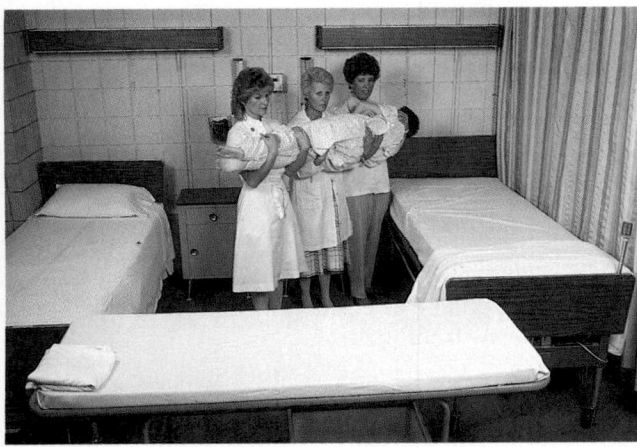

Action 8: Pivoting to stretcher.

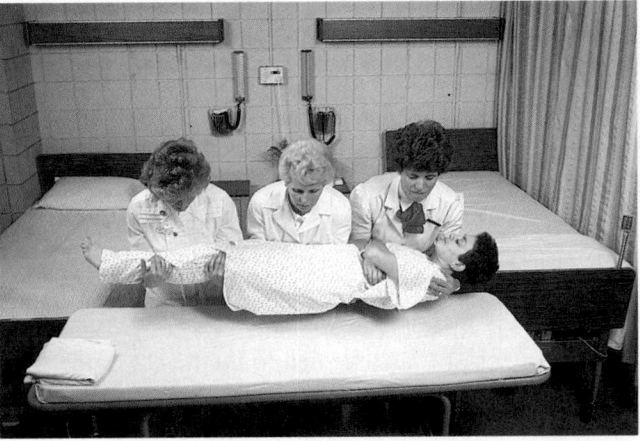

Action 8: Lowering client to stretcher.

Action	Rationale
9 The client should be covered with a sheet or blanket and positioned as necessary. Stretcher side rails should be raised.	This ensures comfort and safety of the client.
10 Wash your hands.	Handwashing deters the spread of microorganisms.

P R O C E D U R E   3 0 - 5

Assisting a Client to Transfer From Bed to Chair

Action	Rationale
1 Explain the procedure to the client. Offer bedpan.	This facilitates cooperation of the client. Empty bladder will increase client comfort.
2 Wash your hands.	Handwashing deters the spread of microorganisms.
3 Assess the client's ability to assist with transfer. Move equipment as necessary to make room for the chair. Close the door or curtain.	This ensures client safety and facilitates the transfer. Closing the door or curtain provides for privacy.
4 Place the bed in the low position.	This facilitates transfer to chair.
5 Assist the client to put on a robe and slippers with nonskid soles.	These provide warmth. Slippers provide protection and stability.
6 Position the chair at the bedside: **a** *For a client with unimpaired mobility*: Bring chair close to the bedside facing the foot of the bed and, if possible, brace the back of the chair against a bedside table.	This increases stability and ensures client safety during the transfer.

(continued)

PROCEDURE 30-5 *(continued)*

Assisting a Client to Transfer From Bed to Chair

Action	Rationale
b *For a client with impaired mobility*: Position the chair facing the head or foot of the bed. When sitting on the side of the bed, the client should be able to steady self by using the hand on the unaffected side to grasp the arm of the chair.	This uses the strong side to provide balance and improve stability during the transfer.

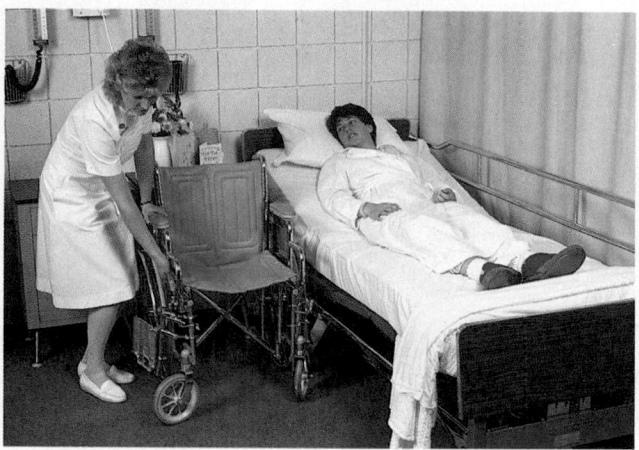

Action 6: Placing chair at bedside.

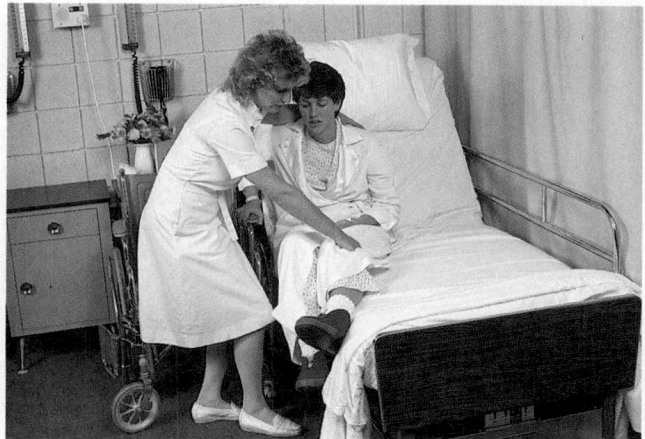

Action 9: Supporting client while moving legs off bed.

Action	Rationale
7 Lock the wheels on the chair and bed if appropriate. Raise the foot pedals on the wheelchair to the up position.	This ensures client safety.
8 Raise the head of the bed to the highest position.	Moving from the sitting to the standing position requires less energy.
9 Assist the client to sit on the side of the bed by supporting the client's head and neck while moving the client's legs off the bed to dangle. Steady the client in that position for a few minutes.	The sitting position facilitates transfer to the chair and allows the circulatory system to adjust to a change in position.
10 Assist the client to the standing position:	
a *For a client with unimpaired mobility*: Face the client and brace your feet and knees against the client. Place your hands around the client's waist while the client holds onto you between the shoulders and the waist. Use your legs to help you raise the client to the standing position.	This provides for stability and for use of major muscle groups to facilitate movement. Allowing the client to grasp the nurse around the neck could injure the nurse if the client should fall.
b *For a client with impaired mobility*: Face the client and brace your feet and knees against the client, especially against the affected extremity. Place your hands around the client's waist. The client may place the unaffected arm around your shoulder or use the unaffected arm to reach for the arm of the chair and to push up while raising to the standing position.	This provides for stability and makes use of the unaffected extremities to facilitate movement.

(continued)

PROCEDURE   30 - 5 *(continued)*

Assisting a Client to Transfer From Bed to Chair

Action

Rationale

11 Pivot the client (on the unaffected limb if applicable) into position in front of the chair with legs positioned against the chair.

This provides security and proper position before sitting.

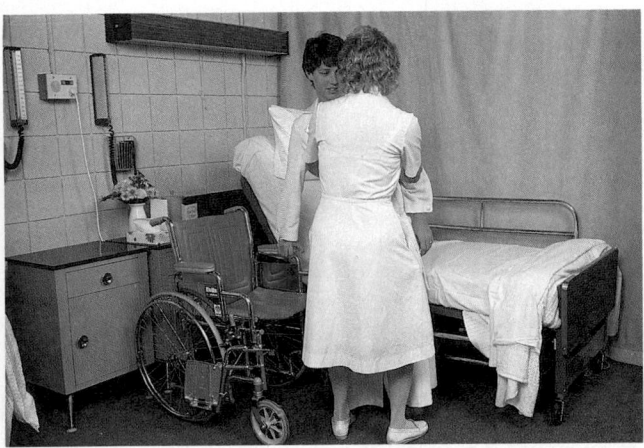

Action 10b: Assisting client to stand.

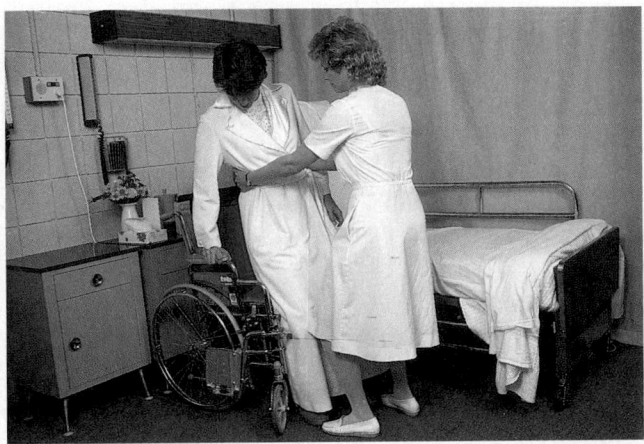

Action 12: Bracing client's knees while lowering client to chair.

12 The client may use one arm (the unaffected limb if applicable) to place on the arm of the chair and steady self while slowly lowering to the sitting position. Continue to brace the client's knees with your knees and flex your own hips and knees when seating the client.

The client uses own arm for support and stability. The nurse flexes the knees and hips to use a major muscle group to aid in movement and reduce strain on the back.

13 Adjust the client's position using pillows where necessary. Cover the client and use restraint if necessary. Position the call bell so it is available for use.

This maintains proper body alignment and provides for comfort and safety.

14 Wash your hands.

Handwashing deters the spread of microorganisms.

15 Document the client's tolerance of the procedure and length of time in the chair.

This provides accurate documentation and ensures continuity of care.

Special Considerations

- A walking or transfer belt may be used to assist the transfer. With the belt secure around the client's waist, the nurse can grasp the belt on both sides (or use handles if they are available) and assist the client to stand and move to the chair.
- A sliding board may also be used to ease the client who cannot stand into a chair.

PROCEDURE 30-6

Transferring a Dependent Client From Bed to Chair (Two Nurses)

Action	Rationale
1 Explain the procedure to the client.	This facilitates cooperation of the client.
2 Wash your hands.	Handwashing deters the spread of microorganisms.
3 Move equipment as necessary to make room for the chair. Close the door or curtain. Assist the client to put on a robe and slippers.	This ensures client safety and facilitates transfer. It provides for privacy and warmth.
4 Move the client to the near side of the bed and cross the client's arms across the chest if possible. Lock the wheels of the bed.	This requires less effort to move the client. Locked wheels will prevent the bed from moving if the client leans against it.
5 Position the chair next to the bed near the upper end and with the back of the chair parallel to the head of the bed. (If wheelchair, remove the armrest closer to the bed if possible). Lock the wheels if appropriate.	Positioning the chair next to the bed facilitates easier movement into the chair.
6 Adjust the bed to a comfortable level for nurses or at the level of the armrest if one is present on the chair.	This facilitates transfer with minimal muscle strain on the nurses.

7 Prepare to lift the client from the bed to the chair:
  a The first nurse should stand behind the chair. Slip the arms under the client's axillae and grasp the client's wrists securely.
  b The second nurse should face the wheelchair and support the client's knees by placing the arms under them.
  c On a predetermined signal, both nurses flex their hips and knees and simultaneously lift the client gently to the chair.
	Two people lifting the client distributes weight and decreases the effort needed for transfer.

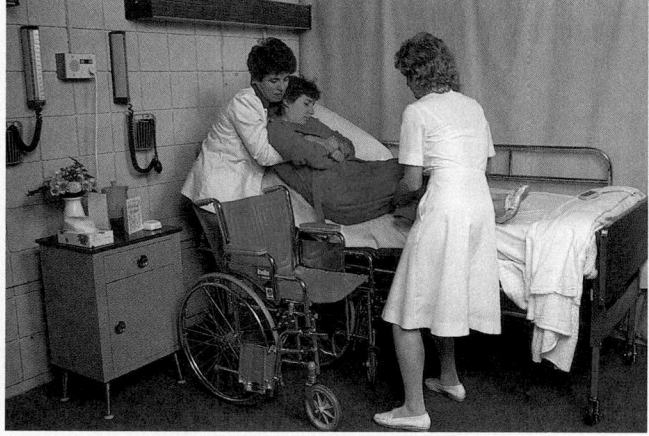

Actions 7a & b: First nurse slips arms under client's axillae and grasps wrists; second nurse supports client's knees.

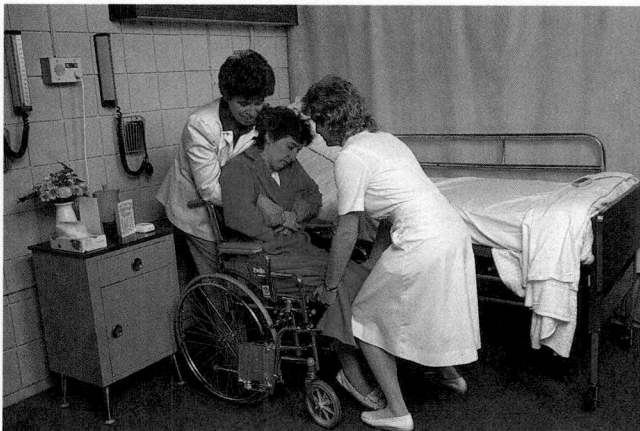

Action 7c: Lowering client into chair.

Action	Rationale
8 Adjust the client's position using pillows where necessary. Cover the client and use restraint if necessary. Position the call bell so it is available for use.	This maintains proper body alignment and provides for comfort and safety.
9 Wash your hands.	Handwashing deters the spread of microorganisms.
10 Document the client's tolerance of the procedure and length of time in the chair.	This provides accurate documentation and ensures continuity of care.

Quadriceps Drills (Sets) Quadriceps drills are an isometric exercise, an exercise in which muscle tension occurs without a significant change in the length of the muscle. One of the most important muscle groups used in walking is the quadriceps femoris. This muscle group helps extend the leg and flexes the thigh. To help reduce weakness and make first attempts at walking easier, bedridden clients should be encouraged to contract this muscle group frequently. The following are techniques for quadriceps drills:

- Have the client contract the muscles on the front of the thighs by pulling the kneecaps toward the hips. The client has the feeling of pushing the knees downward into the mattress and pulling the feet upward.
- Have the client hold the position just described while counting slowly to four, and then relax the muscles for an equal amount of time. Emphasize that relaxation is important to prevent muscle fatigue.
- Caution the client not to hold his or her breath during these exercises to avoid straining the heart.
- Teach the client to do quadriceps drills two or three times each hour, four to six times a day.
- Instruct the client to stop the exercise short of muscle fatigue.

The muscles in the buttocks can be exercised in the same way by pinching the buttocks together and then relaxing them. This is called gluteal settings. Tightening and holding the abdominal muscles for 6 seconds and then relaxing them also strengths this muscle group and facilitates walking.

Push-Ups The muscle strength of the arms and shoulders also may need to be improved before the client is ready to be out of bed. Exercises should improve the strength needed to hold onto or get into a chair and to move about better. They are part of the preparation for clients who must learn to walk on crutches.

A trapeze attached to the bed of a client who has limited use of the lower part of the body helps the client to move about in bed and strengthens muscles in the upper part of the body. However, this does not strengthen the triceps, which is the muscle group necessary for crutch walking or for moving from a bed to a chair. More suitable exercises are push-ups, which are done as follows:

- Sitting up in bed without support is one type of push-up exercise. Instruct the client to lift the hips off the bed by pushing down with the hands on the mattress. If the mattress is too soft, a block of books can be placed on the bed under the client's hands.
- Push-ups may also be done with the client lying in bed on the abdomen. Instruct the client to place the hands near the outstretched body at about shoulder level, with palms down on the mattress and elbows bent sharply. Then have the client straighten the elbows while lifting the head and shoulders off the bed.
- Push-ups may also be done when the client sits in an armchair or wheelchair. The client places the hands on the arms of the chair and then raises the body out of the seat.

Push-ups are usually done three or four times a day, with the number increased as upper body strength is increased.

Dangling *Dangling* refers to the position in which the person sits on the edge of the bed with legs and feet over the side of the bed. This exercise helps prepare the client for being out of bed also. It is carried out as follows:

- Place the client in the sitting position in bed for a few minutes. This will accustom the client to this position and help prevent feelings of faintness.
- Place the bed in the low position or have a footstool handy on which the client can rest the feet while dangling.
- Move the client toward the side of the bed near you so that you do not stretch and strain while turning the client.
- Pivot the client a quarter of a turn by supporting the shoulders and legs. Swing the client's legs over the side of the bed. The client may place his or her hands on your shoulders.
- Rest the client's feet on the floor or on a footstool. This gives a sense of security, and the client is less likely to slide from the bed.
- Have the client pick up and put down the feet alternately in a marching motion. This promotes circulation in the legs.
- Remain with the client, and be ready to put the client in a lying position if feeling faint so that the client does not fall out of bed.

Daily Activities for Purposeful Exercise Many activities can be carried out with benefit to the client. These include placing the bedside stand so that the client must use shoulder and arm muscles to reach what is needed instead of placing it so that little effort is required to take things from it; placing the signal cord so that the client must engage in either arm or shoulder action to reach it; encouraging the client to sit up and reach for the overbed table, to pull it close, and then to push it back in place; encouraging a client to try to wash the back; and having the client put on socks while still in bed. There are innumerable ways in which clients can be helped to exercise, and when they understand the purpose, they often adopt other exercises for themselves.

Assisting the Client to Walk

Many clients who have been confined to bed for a long time find that they must almost learn to walk all over again. Often, it is the nurse who plays a major role in the client's recovery and mental outlook, hope and faith, especially when the client must adhere to a rigid and often difficult schedule of reeducating muscle groups. A client able to raise the leg only 2.5 cm (1 inch) from the bed possesses sufficient power to permit walking.

When the major problem of muscle reeducation presents itself, the client will need the assistance of experts in physical medicine. However, nurses assist clients out of bed and help them to walk when a physical therapist is not present. The nurse should also plan to walk with a client who is using this activity for the first few times after a period of bed rest.

Before getting the client out of bed, the nurse does the following:

- Assesses the client's ability to walk and need for assistance (one nurse, two nurses, walker, cane, walking belt, or crutches)
- Explains to the client exactly what is to be done: transfer technique from bed to erect position, projected distance to be ambulated, assistance available and the correct manner of using it; the client is instructed to alert the nurse immediately if feeling dizzy or weak
- Ensures that the client has a clear path for ambulation

The nurse then slowly assists the client to an erect position and ambulation, pausing after the client is seated at the edge of the bed and again after the client first stands to ensure that the client feels steady. The nurse reminds the client to take deep breaths to promote good aeration of the lungs while walking. Clients who are fearful of walking often tend to look at their feet and may need to be reminded to stand erect and to hold the head high to achieve the full benefits of walking. Because it is not unusual for clients who are walking for the first time after prolonged bed rest to feel faint or weak, a short distance should be planned. As this distance is increased, it is helpful to have chairs readily available should the client need to rest. Should a client faint or begin to fall while walking, the nurse stands with feet apart to create a wide base of support and rocks the pelvis out on the side facing the client. With arms under the client's axillae and encircling the client, the nurse slides the client down the nurse's own body to the floor, carefully protecting the client's head. If the client is wearing a walking belt, the nurse can use the belt to ease the client backward against her own body and gently ease the client to the floor while protecting the client's head. This maneuver should be practiced before it is needed in an emergency situation.

One-Nurse Assist   The client who requires minimal nursing assistance may ambulate well with the nurse walking alongside. The nurse best supports the client by standing at the client's side and placing both hands at the client's waist. By supporting the client at the waist, the nurse helps the client maintain an erect posture and is prevented from pulling the client unintentionally to one side. Use of a walking belt snugly secured around the client's waist also facilitates this type of support. The nurse grasps the belt securely in the back and walks behind and slightly to the side of the client (Fig. 30-17).

Frequently it is necessary to assist the client to ambulate with intravenous (IV) therapy equipment. The nurse should secure a portable IV pole that moves easily. The client ambulates with the assistance of the nurse and the portable IV pole. The nurse needs to secure all the equipment before ambulating and be alert for any tension or

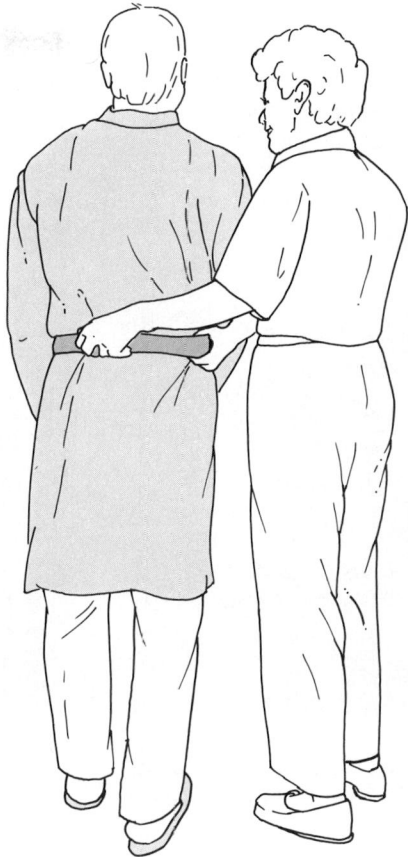

FIGURE   30-17

The nurse using a walking belt to support a client while walking.

sudden action that might dislodge or interfere with the infusion (Fig. 30-18).

When a client has weakness or paralysis on one side, the nurse usually stands on the weaker or affected side and stabilizes the client by putting one arm around the client's waist. Support for the client's weak arm can be accomplished by placing the nurse's other arm around the inner aspect of the client's upper arm in the axilla area or using the nurse's hand to support the client's forearm and hand (Fig. 30-19). Supporting the client's weak arm in the axillary area allows the nurse to more easily support the client's weight and ease him or her to the floor should the client feel faint. A transfer belt should always be used with clients who are unstable. A two-nurse assist is the safer method when the nurse is uncertain of the client's ability to ambulate.

Two-Nurse Assist   There are two methods of ambulation that two nurses can safely use to support a client. In the first, the nurses stand at the client's sides with their near hands grasping the inferior aspect of the client's near upper arm and their far hands holding the client's lower arm or hand. The second position provides more support to the

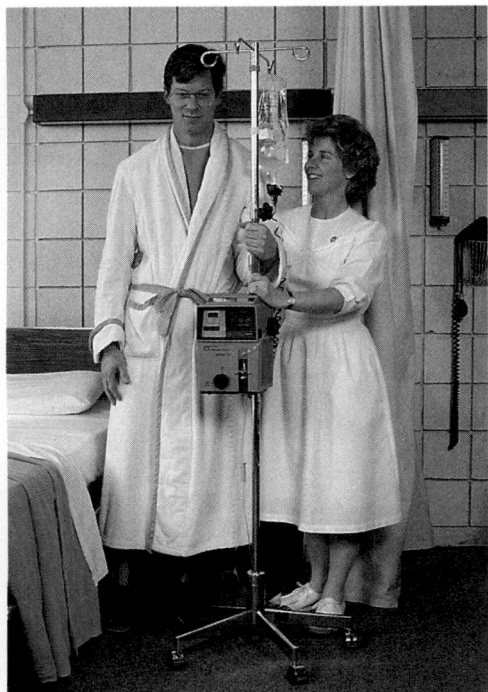

F I G U R E   3 0 - 1 8

The nurse assists the client to ambulate with a portable IV pole. (Photo © B. Proud.)

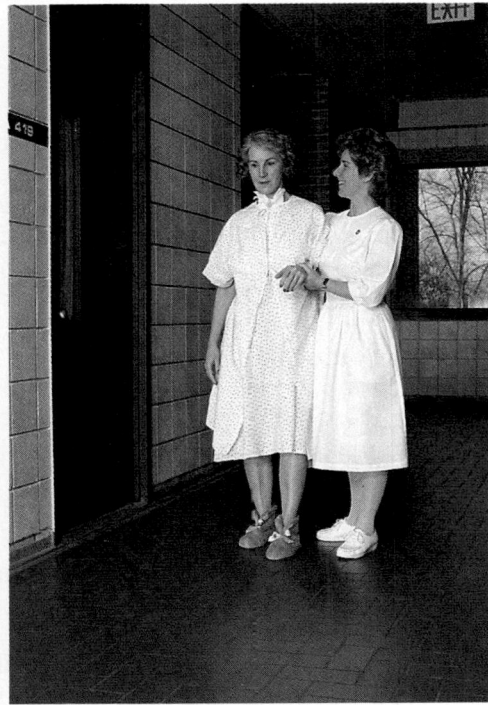

F I G U R E   3 0 - 1 9

The nurse assists the client with weakness or paralysis on one side to ambulate by supporting the client on the affected side. (Photo © B. Proud.)

client but requires the three people involved to be of similar heights. The nurses again position themselves at the client's sides, slipping their near arms under the client's arms and around the client's back, grasping one another's wrists. The client stretches the arms around the nurses' shoulders and the nurses grasp the client's hands with their far hands. In both these positions, the nurses and the client step in unison (Fig. 30-20).

Using Mechanical Aids for Walking

Various devices can assist a client with walking. The most common are walkers, canes, braces, and crutches. Most often a client is fitted for these devices and instructed in their use in a department of physical medicine or physical therapy. In this instance, nursing's concern is chiefly to reinforce the teaching the client has received and to ensure the client continues to use the device properly to assist in safe ambulation. However, in some work settings, nurses may be responsible for fitting clients for these devices. Whenever a nurse assesses a client who has been using a walker, cane, brace, or crutches over time, it is important to determine if the device is still needed, if it continues to meet the client's needs, and if the client continues to use it properly.

General guidelines for helping clients who need the assistance of a walker, cane, brace, or crutches are the following:

- Whenever possible, instruct the client and family members in the correct use of the device before it is needed (eg, before surgery). If family members are knowledgeable, they can reinforce the teaching as needed.
- When ready to begin ambulation with the new device, make sure the client is wearing rubber-soled, well-fitting shoes and that there is a clear path for ambulation (clean, flat, dry, and well lighted). If the client is at high risk for falls, use a walking belt for added support.
- Before moving, make sure the client is steady on the feet when standing; instruct the client to stand erect, looking straight ahead, and walk behind and slightly to one side of the client (in cases of hemiparesis or hemiparalysis, walk on the client's affected side). Should the client lose balance, be prepared to grasp the client's shoulder and the transfer belt to steady the client.

Walker A walker is a lightweight metal frame (usually aluminum) with four legs (Fig. 30-21). The walker provides a sense of security and support. There are several variations of walkers, and they are specified according to the arm strength and balance of the client.

When the client stands between the back legs of the walker, the walker should extend from the floor to the client's hip joint; the client's elbows should be flexed about 30 degrees. Rubber tips should be intact to prevent slipping.

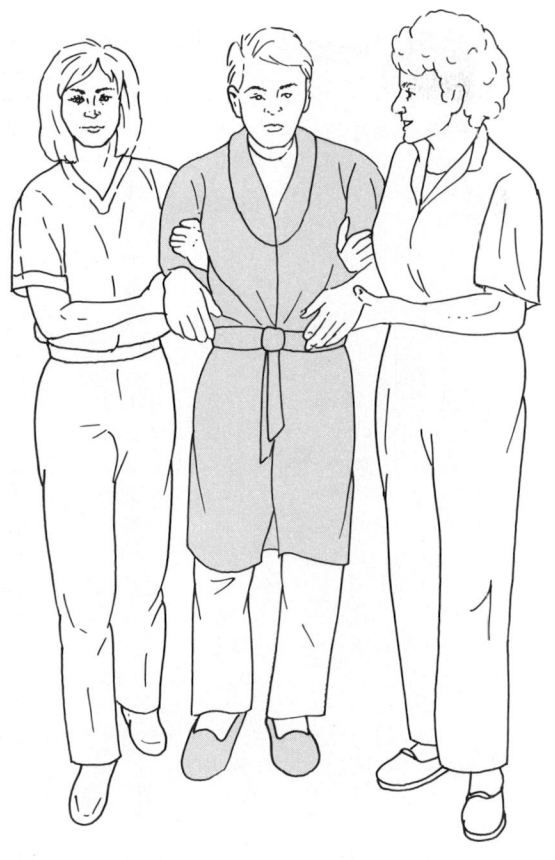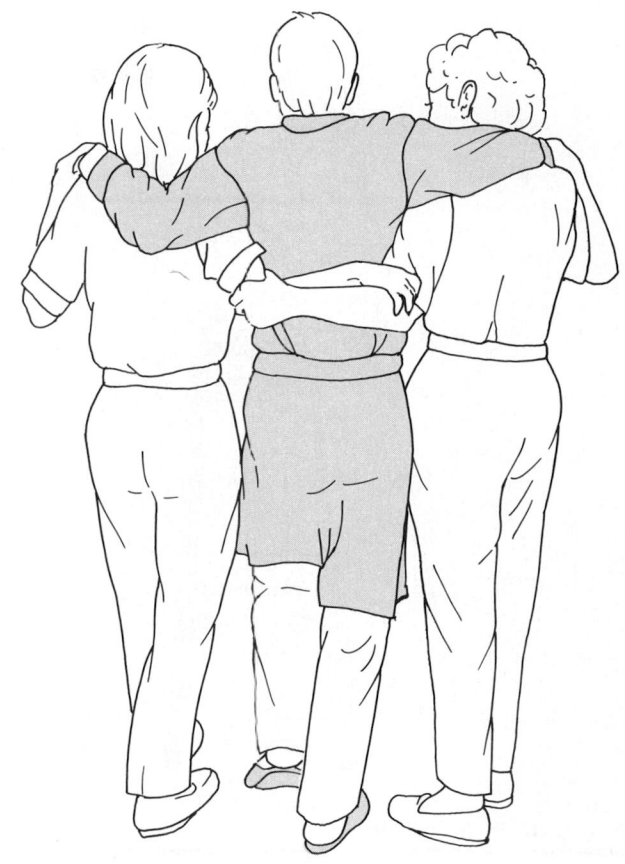

FIGURE 30-20

Two techniques for two nurses to safely assist a client to ambulate.

Generally the client lifts the walker ahead of himself or herself and steps into it. However, the gaits may be specified. Elderly clients frequently develop dangerous walking patterns with a walker and may require close observation.

Canes   Canes come in basically three variations (Fig. 30-22):

- Single-ended canes with half-circle handles are recommended for clients requiring minimal support and if the client will be using stairs frequently.
- Single-ended canes with straight handles are recommended for clients with hand weakness because their handgrips are easier to hold; they are not recommended for clients with poor balance.
- Canes with three or four prongs or legs to provide a wide base of support (tripod or quad cane) are recommended for clients with poor balance. Instruct the client to use a cane with as small a base as possible, and eventually to progress to a single-ended cane if possible. The smaller the base, the less the client relies on the cane for support.

Many canes are adjustable and should be fitted so that when the client stands with the cane's tip 4 inches (10 cm)

to the side of the foot, the cane extends from the floor to the client's hip joint. The elbow should be flexed at a 30-degree angle when holding the cane. Rubber tips on the cane prevent slipping and accidents. They should be inspected regularly for this reason. Clients should be taught to stand erect when walking with a cane and not to lean out over the cane.

When walking with a cane, clients are generally instructed to hold the cane on the unaffected side to provide additional support for the weaker leg. Ambulation proceeds in the following fashion:

- The client stands with weight evenly distributed between the feet and the cane.
- The cane is held on the client's stronger side and is advanced 4 to 12 inches (10 to 30 cm).
- Supporting weight on the stronger leg and the cane, the client advances the weaker foot forward, parallel with the cane.
- Supporting weight on the weaker leg and the cane, the client next advances the stronger leg forward ahead of the cane (heel slightly beyond the tip of the cane).
- The weaker leg is moved forward until even with the stronger leg and the cane is once again advanced as in step 2.

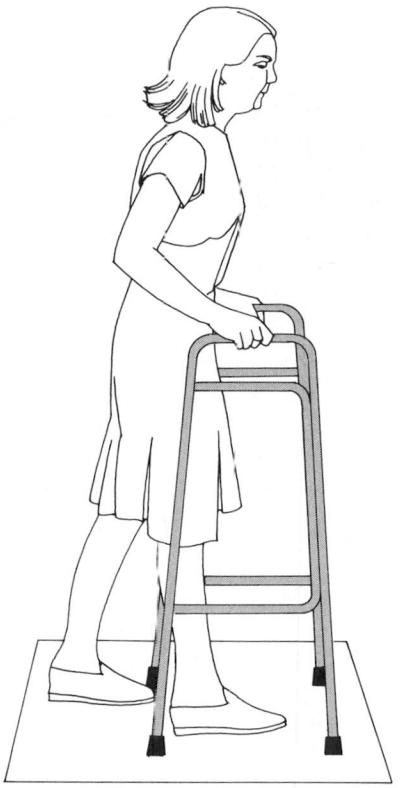

A walker is a lightweight metal frame with a broad, four-point base of support. The walker should be adjusted to the height of the client's hip joint so that the client's elbows are flexed about 30 degrees.

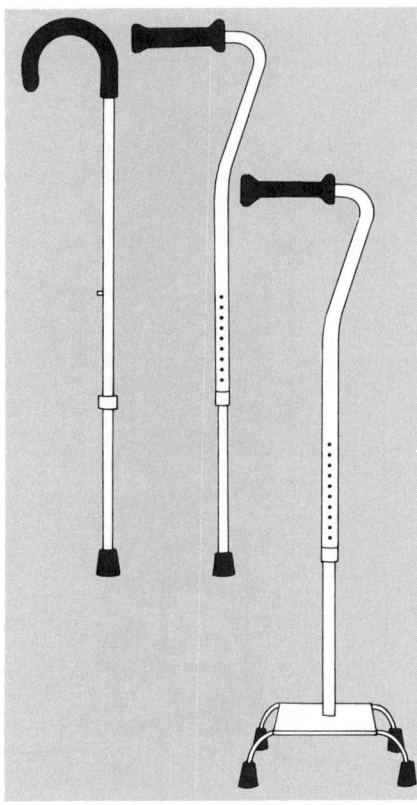

Three types of canes. Single-ended canes with half-circle handles are recommended for clients requiring minimal support. Single-ended canes with straight handles are recommended for clients with hand weakness. Three- or four-prong canes are recommended for clients with poor balance.

When less support is required from the cane the client can advance the cane and stronger leg forward while the cane and weaker leg support the client's weight. Clients should be taught to position their canes within easy reach when they sit down so that they can rise easily.

Braces Braces that support weakened leg muscles are available in many variations. Nursing responsibilities include learning with the client when the brace is to be worn and the correct technique for applying the brace; monitoring the client's correct use of the brace; and observing for any untoward problems the brace might be causing (eg, skin irritation). Muscle changes such as those occurring with growth and development or brought about by illness (atrophy) may result in the brace needing to be refitted to maintain its effectiveness.

Crutches Sometimes, it is necessary for clients to use crutches for a time to avoid using one leg or to help strengthen one or both legs. This procedure is taught best by a physical therapist; however, there are numerous instances when the nurse is called on to measure clients for

crutches and to teach them to use them. Even if a client is being taught to crutch walk by a physical therapist, it is necessary for the nurse to understand the client's progress and the gait being taught. The nurse must often guide the client at home or in the hospital after the initial teaching is completed. The two types of crutches most commonly used are the underarm or axillary crutches and the forearm support crutches (Fig. 30-23).

Measuring for Axillary Crutches The following techniques are used to measure the client for axillary crutches:
- Have the client lie flat in bed on the back while wearing shoes to be used when walking.
- Measure the distance from the anterior fold of the axilla straight down to the heel, and then add 2 inches (5 cm). Or, measure the distance from the anterior fold of the axilla diagonally out to a point 6 inches (15 cm) away from the heel.
- Use the client's height and subtract 16 inches (40 cm) to obtain an approximate crutch length.
- After proper crutches are obtained, have the client stand to adjust the handgrips. Secure the handgrips

Also, the crutches should not be forced into the axillae each time the body moves forward.

It is important that axillary crutches are properly fitted and used correctly to prevent damage to nerves and circulation in the axillae from being cut off, and to provide well-balanced support. There are crutches available that have no axillary support. A supportive frame extends beyond the handgrip for the lower arm to help guide the crutch. These crutches are more likely to be used by clients who have permanent limitations and will always need crutch assistance for ambulation.

Exercises to Prepare for Crutch Walking   Before being asked to use the crutches, several exercises will help the client to be more confident and skillful. The client begins by strengthening the arm and the shoulder muscles. The push-up exercise is most helpful. The muscles of the hand must also be strengthened. Squeezing a rubber ball 50 times a day by flexing and extending the fingers helps to do this.

The client should be assisted into a chair that is close to the wall and then helped to stand against the wall and the crutches placed in the client's hands. Next, standing slightly away from the wall, the client should sway on the crutches from side to side. This accustoms the hands and the arms to weight-bearing.

After this, the client should be asked to lean against the wall and pick one crutch up about 15 cm (6 inches) from the floor and then place it down. This should be repeated with the other crutch, and the whole exercise should be done six to eight times. Then, still leaning against the wall, the client should be asked to pick up both crutches from the floor and place them down. This too should be repeated several times.

After these exercises, it will be possible to judge the client's ability to hold and manage the crutches without the added concern for movement. If judged capable, the client proceeds to the practice of a gait. If possible, it is recommended that the client begin with the four-point gait.

Nurses also need to be aware that a high degree of cardiovascular stress has been associated with axillary crutch walking (Bhambhani et al., 1990). This is due primarily to the isometric contraction required of the upper extremities. Clients using axillary crutches need to be carefully screened for cardiovascular problems and advised to ambulate slowly to reduce cardiovascular stress.

Crutch Gaits   There are four crutch gaits—four-point, three-point, two-point, and swing-through. These gaits are described in Table 30-6.

The swing-through gait is used by some clients when they become accustomed to the use of crutches and wish to get about quickly. The gait is also used by clients who have had a leg amputated. A disadvantage of this gait is that it does not simulate normal walking. Its extended use will lead to atrophy of the muscles in the lower extremity that is not being used, or in both legs if they both swing through.

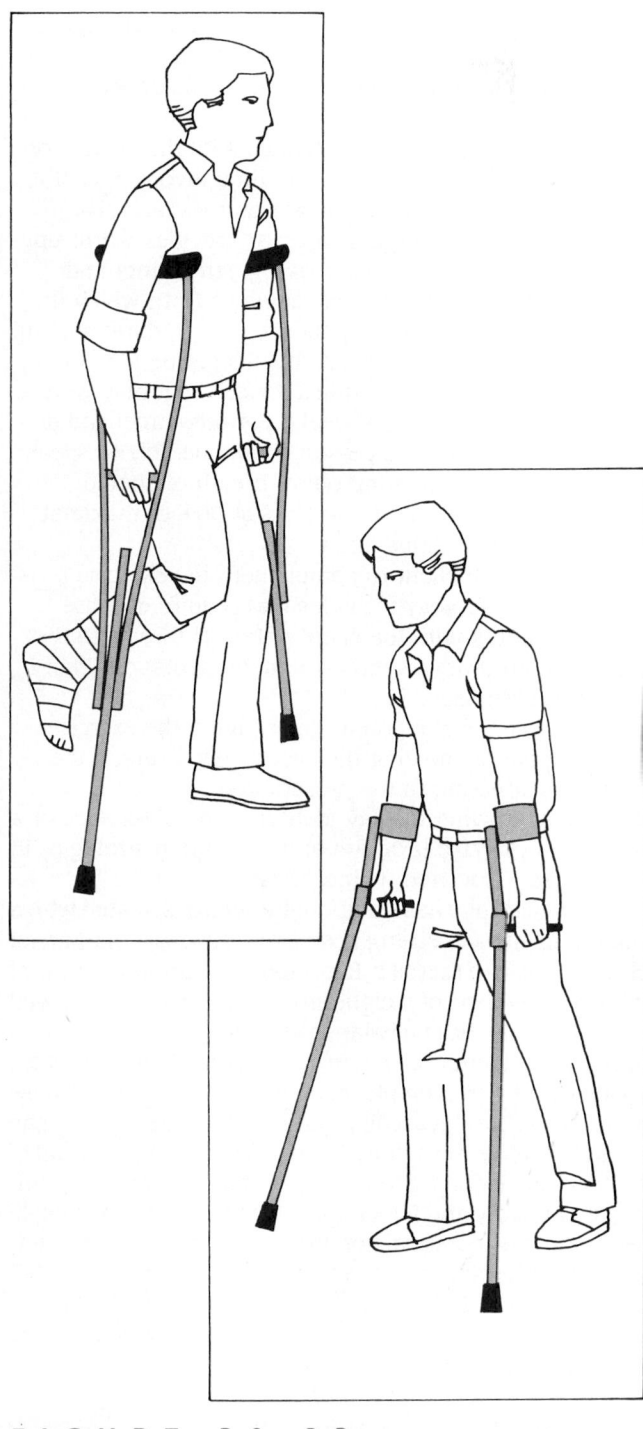

F I G U R E   3 0 - 2 3

Axillary and forearm support crutches.

while the client grasps them in the hands with elbows slightly bent and wrists bent backward.

• Teach the client that the support of body weight should come primarily on the hands and arms while using the crutches, not in the axillary areas, where pressure may damage nerves and cut off circulation.

T A B L E   3 0 - 6

Crutch-Walking Gaits

Gait	Walking Pattern
Four-point	Weight-bearing is permitted on both legs. *Pattern:* Right crutch forward, left foot forward, left crutch forward, right foot forward.
Two-point	Weight-bearing is permitted on both feet. The pattern is a speed-up of the four-point gait. *Pattern:* Right crutch and left foot forward at the same time, left crutch and right foot forward at the same time.
Three-point	Weight-bearing is permitted on only one foot; the other foot cannot support, but acts as a balance. *Pattern:* Both crutches and the nonsupportive leg go forward, then the weight-bearing leg comes through; the crutches are brought forward immediately, and the pattern is repeated.
Swing-through	Weight-bearing is permitted only on one foot. *Pattern:* Unaffected foot bears weight while both crutches are brought forward; then both legs swing through between the crutches, and weight-bearing returns to the unaffected leg. Swing-through gait can also be used by the paraplegic client with weight-bearing on both feet.

Designing Exercise Programs

The benefits of exercise on each of the major body systems are so important that designing individualized exercise programs for clients is an important nursing responsibility. These programs incorporate activities of daily living and planned exercise sessions. Depending on the physical condition of the client, exercise is designed to promote optimal fitness.

An individual's commitment to a program of regular exercise rests on the following:

- Knowledge of the benefits of exercise and problems related to immobility
- Appreciation of the fact that in society, sedentary lifestyles are common and most people must consciously choose to exercise
- Belief that each person is responsible for self-health and that exercise is essential to well-being

Nurses can foster a commitment to regular exercise by teaching and counseling clients about exercise. To do this, the nurse needs knowledge of the types and benefits of exercise as well as of the risks associated with exercise.

The nurse working with a client to develop an individualized exercise prescription completes the following process:

- Explore the client's fitness goals, interests, skills, exercise opportunities, and exercise capacity.
- Assist the client in obtaining medical clearance for exercise.
- Explore feasible exercise activities with the client, considering health benefits sought, time involved, cost, need for special equipment, precautions, and risk.
- Develop an exercise program that specifies warm-up and cool-down activities (walking, stretching) and three or four major exercise activities from which the client can choose. Specify the frequency, duration, and intensity of the exercise activity. Recommended frequency is at least three times a week (but may work up to five or six times a week). For recommended duration and intensity, a person should be able to speak normally without getting out of breath or should maintain a *target heart rate* (60% to 90% of maximal heart rate [220 minus age]).
- Encourage the client to complement the exercise program with everyday activities that require exercise.
- Try to identify with the client potential threats to the exercise program's successful implementation. Plan support strategies.
- Use ongoing evaluation to determine if the exercise prescription is meeting the client's needs and if the client is adhering to the prescription.

The accompanying display identifies characteristics of a successful exercise program and prevention strategies to avoid risks associated with exercise.

Advanced age has traditionally been associated with a decline in muscle strength and reticence on the part of elderly people to exercise. Research has demonstrated that a limited regimen of weight lifting significantly improved strength, mobility, and balance in a selected group of nursing home residents older than age 80 years (Fiatarone et al., 1990). Evans (1992) emphasizes that while aerobic exercise benefits the cardiovascular system, strength training can actually reverse the aging process. An ongoing program of exercise for elderly clients may effectively promote improved mobility and foster continued independence while lessening the potential for falls and nursing home admissions. The National Academy of Science reported that prolonging institutionalization of elderly clients by just 1 month could result in a $3 billion savings in Medicare and Medicaid benefits (Evans; 1992).

Teaching Exercise Benefits to Populations at Risk

Health promotion and wellness are areas where the nurse can significantly contribute to the well-being of all populations. The emphasis remains on prevention. Assessment and intervention priorities that promote positive health behaviors for each developmental stage are outlined in Table 30-2. As life expectancy increases, nursing activities will particularly focus on teaching that regular exercise is a positive factor contributing to longevity. Interviews with healthy elders older than age 85 years consistently identified activity and exercise as one of the most important

---

Characteristics of a Successful Exercise Program

- The program is individually designed (considers the individual's fitness goals, interests, skills, exercise opportunities, and exercise capacity).
- The program specifies warm-up and cool-down activities and a variety of major exercise activities—variety is preferable to a single-exercise activity.
- The program specifies frequency, intensity, and duration of exercise.
- The program is convenient to perform, compatible with the individual's life-style, and fun!
- The individual in such a program should understand the program and feel confident that exercise will result in definite health benefits.

Prevention Strategies to Avoid Risks Associated With Exercise

People beginning exercise programs should be familiar with the following guidelines:

- Obtain a preexercise medical examination and medical supervision during exercise if older than age 35 years and sedentary or if there is any past or current cardiovascular condition.
- Begin a new exercise program slowly and allow your body's support structure time to accommodate to the new stress.
- Know your body and respect its limitations. Never force a joint beyond its natural range of motion.
- Respect fatigue. Whenever you feel tingling, pain, or burning in a muscle stop and rest the muscle for 15 minutes before continuing to exercise.
- Follow the safety guidelines for specific exercises; for example, joggers are recommended to run on soft surfaces as opposed to cement or asphalt, to wear well-constructed shoes with thick soles and arch supports, and to run in a safe environment with a low pollution index.

---

factors contributing to their long life (Hogstel & Kashka, 1989). In addition to improving the quality of life, exercise plays an important role in the prevention or slowing of osteoporosis. Nurses can help elderly clients use physical exercise to avert or alleviate the effects of this debilitating aging process.

Evaluating

When evaluating the effectiveness of a care plan designed to help clients enhance, maintain, or regain mobility and fitness goals, the nurse uses each nurse–client interaction to evaluate the client in the following respects:
- General ease of movement and gait
- Alignment
- Joint structure and function
- Muscle mass, tone, and strength
- Endurance

An excellent time to assess these essential ingredients of well-being is when the client is performing simple everyday tasks such as ambulating, undertaking hygiene measures, dressing, and eating. Because illness and enforced inactivity can affect these tasks negatively, ongoing evaluation is necessary if serious problems are to be avoided. Specific criteria for evaluating individualized plans of care follow.

 NURSING PROCESS

In Clinical Practice

Once a mobility problem is detected, the nurse implements each phase of the nursing process to ensure correct identification and treatment of the problem. The nurse who wishes to identify and manage the mobility problem correctly and to prevent complications related to immobility must possess the knowledge and clinical skills described earlier in this chapter. The following discussion outlines the assessment priorities, client goals, nursing interventions, and evaluative criteria for the following nursing diagnoses:
  Activity Intolerance
  Impaired Physical Mobility
  High Risk for Injury: Complications of Immobility
  Altered Health Maintenance: Lack of Exercise Program

In the case study that follows, a care plan is developed to address the mobility needs of a client with left-sided hemiplegia following a cerebrovascular accident (stroke).

Activity Intolerance

Nurses working with clients with chronic illnesses that affect oxygen transport or with immobilized clients will frequently observe in these clients a reduced ability to perform the activities of daily living. Activity intolerance is the diagnostic label describing the physical or psychological inability to tolerate an increase in activity. For one client, this may translate into an inability to climb the four sets of stairs leading to an apartment, whereas for another client, it may mean the inability to walk the few steps from the bed to the bathroom without becoming winded.

Any factor causing fatigue or interfering with the amount of oxygen being delivered to the muscles for the work of contraction and relaxation can produce activity intolerance. Common etiologies include the following:

- Developmental factors (decreased strength in an older person)
- Pathophysiologic factors (illnesses altering oxygen transport: cardiac—congestive heart failure, arrhythmias, angina, myocardial infarction; respiratory—chronic obstructive pulmonary disease; circulatory—anemia, peripheral arterial disease; other chronic diseases; malnourishment)
- Situational (prolonged bed rest or inactivity, depression, decreased motivation, pain, anything causing fatigue)

Assessment

- Note complaints of fatigue, weakness, or an inability to perform usual tasks without dizziness, dyspnea, or frequent pauses to rest.
- Identify any contributing factors that increase fatigue or compromise oxygen transport.
- Assess the client's response to activity:
  - Take resting vital signs and note the client's mental status and skin characteristics.
  - Have the client perform an activity (eg, ambulation) and take the vital signs immediately after the activity and after the client rests for 3 to 5 minutes. Although it is customary for the pulse, blood pressure, and respiratory rate to rise with exercise, they should return to the baseline rate after rest. Weakness, pallor, diaphoresis, confusion, and vertigo may all signal activity intolerance.

Planning: Client Goals

The client will:
- Identify factors contributing to activity intolerance
- Reduce or eliminate these factors to the extent possible
- Increase endurance to the point of being able to perform key activities of daily living (specify)
- Demonstrate energy conservation measures
- Demonstrate decreased signs of anoxia (sustained increases in pulse rate, blood pressure, respiratory rate, dyspnea, pallor)

Interventions

- Set daily realistic activity goals with the client and offer immediate reinforcement if the goal is met. Explore the client's motivation to increase the activity level.
- Assist the client to reduce or eliminate factors contributing to the decreased tolerance (eg, improve quantity and quality of sleep, offer pain medication before the client's activity, inspire client with a sincere "can do" mentality).
- Pace the activities according to the client's strength and intersperse activities with periods of rest.
- Teach the client and family how to progress activities gradually and how to conserve energy for priority activities.

Evaluative Criteria

The client meets the previously stated goals.

Impaired Physical Mobility

Because impaired physical mobility may interfere with an individual's ability to meet other human needs (eg, obtain, prepare, and eat food; bathe and dress self; toilet self) as well as with self-concept, it is important that problems affecting physical mobility be correctly identified and worked up in the care plan. Mobility impairments may affect the upper or lower limbs, or both. Possible etiologies include the following:

- Developmental factors (muscle weakness or painful movement of joints in elderly clients)
- Pathophysiologic factors (neuromuscular or musculoskeletal impairment)
- Situational factors (need for bed rest; devices such as casts, splints, and braces; pain; nonfunctioning or missing limbs; effects of medications)

Assessment

- Observe the client to determine the precise nature of the mobility impairment:
  - Inability to maintain body alignment
  - Inability to execute coordinated, purposeful movements (includes bed mobility, transfers, ambulation—gait)
  - Decreased muscle strength or control (motor function in all four extremities—strong, weak, absent, spastic; weight-bearing potential)
  - Limited joint mobility
  - Impaired perception of position or presence of body parts
- Identify all etiologic factors. Carefully assess the client's motivation to be mobile and the effect of any secondary gains being derived from the immobility.
- When illness or trauma is causing the mobility problems, consult with the physician to determine both the immediate and future effects of the mobility deficit on human functioning so that realistic client counseling can be planned.

Planning: Client Goals

Depending on the nature of the mobility impairment, the following goals need to be individualized. The client will:
- Maintain (or increase) muscle strength and control in the upper/lower/right/left extremities

- Demonstrate correct execution of isometric or isotonic exercise program
- Independently (or with the correct use of adaptive devices) demonstrate correct alignment, transfers, and ambulation
- Demonstrate correct use of safety measures to prevent injury
- Perform activities of daily living with greatest degree of independence possible

Interventions

- Whenever possible, reduce or eliminate factors contributing to immobility (fear of falling, apathy, effects of nonessential medications).
- If pain is contributing to immobility, administer the prescribed analgesic before the client's activity.
- Ensure that the client is positioned in correct alignment and changes position every 2 hours.
- Develop an exercise program that includes complete range-of-motion exercises, isometric setting exercises, and ambulation (as possible).
- Encourage maximal participation in activities of daily living.
- Provide the appropriate nursing care for casts, traction devices, slings, braces, and prosthetic devices.
- Teach the client how to transfer and ambulate safely using a cane, walker, crutches, or wheelchair.
- Be vigilant for the development of any of the complications of immobility. Identify high-risk clients and include preventive care in the care plan (see Table 30-3).

Evaluative Criteria

The client meets the previously stated goals.

High Risk for Injury: Complications of Immobility

The effects of immobility on major body systems as well as on an individual's psychosocial functioning are presented earlier in this chapter. Nursing's challenge is to identify clients at high risk for developing problems related to immobility and to institute nursing measures immediately to prevent these problems. Because the problems are multiple, they are presented in table format according to body system with specific etiologies, assessment priorities, client goals, and related nursing interventions (see Table 30-3). Nursing care plans for immobilized clients should reflect nursing's concern to prevent immobility problems.

Altered Health Maintenance: Lack of Exercise Program

Although in recent years a fitness craze has prompted many individuals to develop more active life-styles, many people still live overwhelmingly sedentary lives. Reasons for the lack of regular physical exercise are many:

- Science and technology have developed complex machines and services to aid in the performance of the activities of daily living, which formerly required an expenditure of physical energy. In the past, people who wished to survive had no choice but to be active. Currently, an individual must consciously choose to be active.
- Convenience (reduced energy expenditure) has come to be valued over activities requiring more effort.
- Children are quickly socialized into valuing sedentary activities such as watching television or listening to the radio.
- Society's fetish for cleanliness leads some people to abhor any activities that produce sweat.
- There is still lack of knowledge and much confusion about the benefits of regular exercise.
- Some individuals become discouraged from being more active following unsuccessful attempts.
- Physical injury or discomfort resulting from a poorly designed exercise program may cause a person to discontinue the activity.
- Some people believe that exercise is simply too much bother.
- Some people are unable to find the time for regular exercise.
- Embarrassment may be related to an individual's appearance, ability, or physical condition.
- Some people erroneously believe that the need for exercise decreases with age and eventually disappears.
- Some people overrate the benefits of light, sporadic exercise.
- Some people underrate their own abilities and exercise capacity.

Assessment

- Interview the client to determine past and present history of exercise; knowledge about the benefits of exercise; motivation to adhere to a regular program of exercise; exercise preferences; feasibility of these preferences (time involved, cost, need for special equipment, presence of support systems, safety concerns); any contraindications for beginning to exercise without medical supervision (eg, history of chest pain or pressure with activity, past or current cardiovascular or respiratory problems, degenerative joint diseases or other orthopedic problems); and ability to design and follow safe exercise program.
- Identify factors likely to sabotage the client's efforts to exercise (decreased motivation, multiple demands on time, lack of funds for child care, and so on).
- Perform a physical examination to rule out any physical contraindications (eg, obesity, high blood pressure, musculoskeletal problems) to exercising without medical clearance. (Stress testing is mandatory for sedentary people older than age 35 years and for anyone with a past or current cardiovascular condition.)

Planning: Client Goals

Long-Term
The client will:
- Adhere to a regular program of exercise that promotes cardiovascular function, endurance, flexibility, and strength

Short-Term
The client will:
- Identify four personal benefits of exercise
- Identify personal factors that tend to prevent regular exercise
- Develop a feasible and safe exercise program, including specifics for the following:
  - Warm-up activities
  - A variety of exercise activities including aerobic and stretch exercises (type, frequency, duration)
  - Cool-down activities
- Identify the risks inherent in this program and the precautions that will be taken
- Obtain medical clearance for exercise program if needed
- Describe three means to reinforce exercise goals (reward system, exercise partner, use of other supports)

Interventions

- Teach the client:
  - Four components of fitness: (1) cardiovascular function; (2) endurance, (3) **flexibility** (ability to use a muscle through its entire range of motion); and (4) strength)
  - Benefits of regular exercise
  - Types of exercise
- Assist the client to determine exercise preferences by comparing and contrasting different types of exercise: time required, place, equipment needed, cost, aerobic versus anaerobic value, advantages, disadvantages, and precautions and risks.
- Assist the client in developing an individualized exercise program:
  - Choose warm-up, major, and cool-down activities.
  - Set objectives for duration, intensity, and frequency.
  - Teach the client how to take a radial pulse and how to determine his or her target heart rate if necessary.
  - Consider the best setting for the activity and the equipment and money needed to perform the exercise safely.
  - Identify risks and safety factors.
  - Explore with the client potential threats to the exercise program and existing supports.
- Help the client to develop a strategy to evaluate the attainment of the exercise goals. A self-contract with or without additional nursing intervention may be sufficient.

Evaluative Criteria

The client meets the previously stated goals.

C A S E   S T U D Y

Quan Hong Nguyen is an alert 57-year-old married man who was admitted to the hospital with a diagnosis of right cerebrovascular accident secondary to thrombosis. He has a history of hypertension. This is his fifth hospital day and the attending physicians have termed the stroke a *completed stroke*, that is, Mr. Nguyen's neurologic deficits have been unchanged for 2 days and he is believed to be ready for more aggressive rehabilitative treatment.

Assessment Findings

On hospital day 5, an assessment of Mr. Nguyen's mobility status and ability to participate in activities of daily living revealed the following data:
- *Mental status*—basically alert and able to follow simple commands; expresses his needs verbally when encouraged but speech is slow; seems forgetful of usual routine for basic self-care activities
- *Neuromuscular status*—hemiplegia; severe motor and sensory deficits of the left side of the face and the left arm and leg
  - *Muscle mass, tone, and strength*—well-developed muscles in all extremities; history of a lifetime of sports, most recently played tennis two to four times weekly; decreased muscle tone (hypotonicity, flaccidity) in left arm and leg; motor function is absent in left arm and very weak in left leg; strong motor function on right extremities; incapable of weight-bearing on left side; incapable of independent turning, sitting, standing, transferring, or ambulation
- *Joint mobility*—decreased on left side; otherwise full range of motion; no contractures
- *Endurance*—fatigues quickly (eg, during complete bath)
- Some deficit in spatial–perceptual orientation (eg, ignores objects on his left side) but difficult to assess this completely yet

Nursing Diagnoses

Impaired Physical Mobility (turning in bed, sitting, standing, transferring, and ambulating) related to left hemiplegia and weakness
Self-Care Deficit related to decreased alertness and left-sided motor and sensory deficits

Planning: Client Goals

Because it is unknown to what extent Mr. Nguyen is able to comprehend his illness, the nurse operates on the assumption that he is able to understand a simple explanation of how the stroke is affecting his motor function and how he can best work together with his family and the nurse to regain motor function. After assessing both his past and current motor abilities, the nurse shares with Mr. Nguyen and his wife and son the following short-term goals:

- Whenever observed, the client will be in correct body alignment with each joint on the left side higher than the joint proximal to it and supportive devices appropriately in place (bed board, footboard, trochanter roll, hand–wrist splint, shoulder sling, pillows).
- By hospital day 10, the client will:
  - Replace the passive range-of-motion exercises the nurse is performing four times daily to all joints with active exercise of his left arm and leg and active range of motion of all other joints
  - Perform quadriceps settings, gluteal settings, and abdominal settings five times daily
  - Participate in the every-2-hour positioning schedule by assisting with turning to the degree he is able
  - Use a sling on the left arm when upright so long as the arm muscles are hypotonic
  - Keep the left arm and hand elevated with a pillow to prevent dependent edema
  - Demonstrate a safe pivot transfer from bed to chair and chair to bed
  - Demonstrate standing balance
  - Show beginning ability to resume self-care activities despite motor and sensory deficits on left side
- On discharge from the acute-care hospital to the rehabilitation center, the client will:
  - Be free of contractures
  - Show signs of physical and mental readiness to acquire increasing independence in self-care

Both the client and family express great willingness to work to achieve these goals. Later the wife confides to the nurse, "It's been so awful just sitting here not knowing what was going to happen. At least now I feel like we have something to work for."

See the Nursing Care Plan for Mr. Nguyen for details of the nursing strategies used to achieve these goals.

Implementation

In implementing the care plan, the nurse needs the following specialized abilities:

- The belief that nursing can make a difference in the quality of this family's present and future life and the commitment of nursing energies to help Mr. Nguyen reach his full rehabilitative potential
- Strong assessment skills (interviewing and primarily physical assessment) to determine how the neurologic dysfunction is influencing the client's mobility and coordination
- Knowledge of how the skeletal, muscular, and nervous systems function to produce purposeful and coordinated movement
- Interpersonal skills to communicate to Mr. Nguyen and his family empathy for their situation and to mobilize their energies for the long process of rehabilitation
- Excellent use of body mechanics when positioning Mr. Nguyen and assisting him with transfers (and when teaching these techniques to the family)
- Vigilant caregiver skills directed to preventing complications and maintaining muscle strength and joint mobility to facilitate an optimal return of function.
- Teaching and counseling skills to enable Mr. Nguyen to regain independence in self-care activities
- Interpersonal and leadership skills to motivate the entire nursing staff to value Mr. Nguyen's rehabilitation
- Ability to work collaboratively with many other members of the health care team while coordinating all their efforts into a comprehensive care plan
- Accountability and patience

Documentation

Sample documentation of nursing interventions follows.

Traditional Note Format

1/25/93, 3 PM, nursing

Dr. Steel examined the client at 1 PM and noted he is now in "completed stroke stage and ready for more aggressive rehabilitative treatment." This was explained to client, his wife, and his son. The client smiled and seemed to understand that he is out of immediate danger. Initial instructions given to the client on how he can assist with position changes and actively exercise his left arm and leg. Correctly demonstrated these maneuvers with verbal cuing. Motor function still absent in left arm and weak in left leg. Care plan revised to incorporate new exercise goals.

Susan Beecker, RN

SOAP Format

1/27/93, nursing
#2 Self-Care Deficit related to decreased alertness and left-sided motor and sensory deficits

S: "Get out of here."
O: Client threw washcloth at nurse during bath and refused to assist with bathing; later observed crying.
A: Temporary setback influenced by frustration with absent motor function in left arm and emotional lability.
P: *Educative:* Explain to client that most people in his position get frustrated and that his behavior is normal. Reinforce the importance of his continued efforts to regain independence in self-care activities.
Therapeutic: Make determined effort to compliment his progress to date (assistance with turning, range-of-motion exercises, feeding). Communicate warm acceptance of client and understanding of his anger and frustration.

NURSING CARE PLAN

for Quan Hong Nguyen

Nursing Diagnosis: Impaired Physical Mobility (turning in bed, sitting, standing, transferring, and ambulating) related to left hemiplegia and weakness

Signs and Symptoms: Motor function is absent in left arm and very weak in left leg; muscles are well developed but hypotonic; decreased joint mobility in left extremities; fatigues quickly

Long-Term Goal: Client will regain independence in turning, sitting, standing, transferring, and ambulating.

Goal: 1/25/93 Whenever observed, the client will:
- Be in correct body alignment with (1) each joint on the left side higher than the joint proximal to it and (2) supportive devices in place (bed board, footboard, trochanter roll, hand–wrist splint, shoulder sling, pillows)

Nursing Actions

At each position change (as dictated by every-2-hour turn schedule posted at the bedside), make sure that the client is in correct alignment. Follow agency positioning guidelines for the supine, side-lying (lies on unaffected side), and prone positions.

Use the following supportive devices: firm mattress, footboard, trochanter roll, shoulder sling when client is in upright position, volar resting splint, and pillows.

Teach both the client and family the importance of correct positioning.

Allow the family to participate in helping the client to get comfortable in the different positions.

Rationale

Correct positioning prevents contractures, relieves pressures, and maintains alignment.
- Positioning each joint higher than the preceding one prevents edema and its resulting fibrosis.
- Placing the client in the prone position for 30 minutes two or three times daily helps prevent knee and hip flexion contractures.

Support devices aid in maintaining the client in correct positioning.
- Firm mattress provides skeletal support.
- Footboard during flaccid period prevents footdrop, heel cord shortening, and plantar flexion.
- Trochanter roll prevents external rotation of hip when client is in dorsal position.
- Shoulder sling during flaccid period prevents shoulder subluxation and shoulder–hand syndrome.
- Volar resting splint supports the wrist and hand in a functional position.
- A pillow in the axilla of the left side prevents adduction of the affected side.

Teaching promotes self-care and lays the foundation for successful rehabilitation.

Involving the family in the client's care facilitates the coping process.

Evaluative Statement

1/27/93 Goal being met. Every 2-hour positioning schedule being followed with client in correct body alignment to prevent contractures.

S. Beecher, RN

(continued)

NURSING CARE PLAN *(continued)*

for Quan Hong Nguyen

Goal: By hospital day 10, 1/30/93, the client will:
- Replace the passive range-of-motion exercises the nurse is now performing four times daily to all joints with (1) the client's active exercise of the left arm and left leg and (2) the client's active range-of-motion exercises for all other joints

Nursing Actions	Rationale	Evaluative Statement
Assess the client's knowledge of the importance of exercise and ability and motivation to exercise.	Unless the client understands the reason for exercise and is physically, mentally, and attitudinally capable of exercise, he will not follow through.	1/30/93 Goal partially met. Client has successfully demonstrated complete set of range-of-motion exercises (to both left and right sides); however, he tires during the exercises and stops unless verbally encouraged.
Teach the client how to exercise his left arm and leg by using his unaffected (right) extremities.	Active exercise maintains joint mobility, prevents contracture development in the paralyzed extremity, prevents further deterioration of the neuromuscular system, helps to regain motor control, and increases circulation.	*Revision:* Monitor client's exercise four times daily; continue to enlist family's support.

S. Beecher, RN |
| Demonstrate a complete set of range-of-motion exercises to the client and family and have the client return the demonstrations. | Involving the family helps ensure the success of the exercise program because it requires a big time and effort commitment. | |

Goal: By hospital day 10, 1/30/93, the client will:
- Perform quadriceps, gluteal, and abdominal settings five times daily

Nursing Actions	Rationale	Evaluative Statement
Teach the client and family how to tighten the quadriceps, gluteal, and abdominal muscles and hold them for 6 seconds (slow count to 4) before relaxing. A 2-minute rest should be allowed between contractions and the client cautioned not to hold his breath during these exercises because this places strain on the heart. The exercises should be stopped short of muscle fatigue.	These exercises will maintain muscle mass; tone; and strength (while the client is on bed rest); and prevent atrophy. They also increase circulation to the exercised body parts.	1/30/93 Goal partially met. Client has demonstrated exercises correctly; however, he needs to be reminded to perform them. Family is effective in this regard. *Revision:* Compliment family on excellent job they are doing and reinforce importance of exercise to maximize rehabilitative potential.

S. Beecher, RN |

Goal: By hospital day 10, 1/30/93, the client will:
- Participate in the every-2-hour positioning schedule by assisting with turning to the degree he is able

Nursing Actions	Rationale	Evaluative Statement
Teach the client how he can help to reposition himself by grabbing onto the side rail with his right hand and also by placing his unaffected leg under the left one to move himself.	The more the client can do independently, the more in control he will feel. These activities will pave the way to increasing independence in self-care activities.	1/27/93 Goal met. Client consistently assists in repositioning. Seems pleased to be able to help the nurses in this way.

S. Beecher, RN |

(continued)

NURSING CARE PLAN *(continued)*

for Quan Hong Nguyen

Goal: By hospital day 10, 1/30/93, the client will:
* Demonstrate a safe pivot transfer from bed to chair and chair to bed

Nursing Actions	Rationale	Evaluative Statement
Assess the stage of recovery of muscle function.	Most clients will begin to show signs of spasticity with exaggerated reflexes within 48 hours—this denotes progress. If muscles are still flaccid after several weeks, prognosis for regaining function is poor.	1/30/93 Goal met. Client can safely transfer from bed to chair and chair to bed but requires nursing assistance. *S. Beecher, RN*

Goal: By hospital day 10, 1/30/93, the client will:
* Demonstrate standing balance

Nursing Actions	Rationale	Evaluative Statement
Assess activity tolerance by taking vital signs before attempting balance training and transfers.	Vital signs and the client's physical condition should be assessed before a new activity, during the activity, and shortly afterward to assess activity tolerance.	1/30/93 Goal not met. Client has not demonstrated standing balance; falls to left side without nursing support. *Revision:* Allow more time for goal achievement. *S. Beecher, RN*
Precede transfers with balance training. Assist the client to a sitting position at the edge of the bed and observe for steadiness and the ability to maintain an erect posture.	The client needs sitting and standing balance before progressing to harder tasks. Dizziness or syncope may signal vasomotor instability.	
Place the chair by the bed on the client's unaffected side and assist the client to dress. Initially the nurse helps the client to stand by placing his or her right knee against the client's strong knee, grasping the client around the waist with both arms, and pulling the client forward while rocking back on the left leg (nurse's knees are slightly flexed).	This prevents the client's knees from buckling and the pressure of the nurse's knee forces the client to straighten the strong knee and bear weight on it. In this position the client's feet cannot slip forward. In this position, the nurse is using good principles of body mechanics.	
Once the client is standing, assess standing balance and observe for signs of activity intolerance (pallor, shortness of breath, excessive increase in pulse rate, perspiration). Direct the client to (1) grab the far arm of the chair with his strong arm, (2) turn on his strong foot, and (3) sit down. The nurse's right leg and the client's strong leg are used as a pivot.	Using the unaffected extremity facilitates movement and provides stability.	

(continued)

NURSING CARE PLAN (continued)

for Quan Hong Nguyen

Pivot client out of bed to chair three times a day (may pivot out of bed to bedside commode). Gradually increase time in chair based on client's tolerance. Correctly align client in chair using supportive devices as necessary.

Increasing exercise to the client's tolerance level promotes improved muscle strength and maintenance of range of motion.

Goal: On discharge to rehabilitation center, the client will:
  • Be free of contractures

Nursing Actions	Rationale	Evaluative Statement
Implement previously stated nursing actions.	These actions promote independence and return to activities of daily living.	1/31/93 Goal met. Client has no contractures. *S. Beecher, RN*

Nursing Diagnosis: Self-Care Deficit (all basic self-care activities) related to decreased alertness and left-sided motor and sensory deficits

Signs and Symptoms: Unable to use left arm for any activities; client's right side is dominant; incapable of ambulation at present; basically alert but seems forgetful of usual routine for self-care activities; tires quickly

Long-Term Goal: Client demonstrates increasing independence in self-care abilities.

Goal: By hospital day 10, 1/30/93, the client will:
  • Demonstrate beginning ability to resume self-care activities despite motor and sensory deficits of left side; use right arm to (1) assist in morning hygiene; (2) feed himself (finger foods, beverages); and (3) exercise

Nursing Actions	Rationale	Evaluative Statement
Continue to assess extent of client's motor and sensory deficits and ability to perform self-care activities.	This facilitates recognition of any recovery of function and allows setting of appropriate goals.	1/29/93 Goal met. For the past 2 days, client has washed his left arm, abdomen, and legs; combed his hair; fed himself; and performed range-of-motion exercises. *S. Beecker, RN*
Set realistic short-term goals for each session with client and reward progress: "This morning we'll see how much of your bath you are able to manage yourself!" "It must feel good to be able to do this for yourself again."	Adding *realistic* new tasks for each day gives the client a goal to work toward; a pattern of *noticed* success encourages continued efforts.	
Approach client from his unaffected side and place call light, bedside table, phone, and so on, on this side.	This helps the client to compensate for alterations in sensory perception.	

(continued)

NURSING CARE PLAN (continued)

for Quan Hong Nguyen

Teach client how to transfer all self-care activities to the un-affected side and how to use one-handed techniques and adaptive equipment.	There is never only one way to do anything.
Encourage client to brush his teeth, comb his hair, bathe and feed himself, and to assist in toileting. Explain to the family why it is critical to allow him to do these things himself, even if movements are tiring, clumsy, and initially frustrating.	This improves the client's sense of control of his own activities of daily living and improves morale.
Continually reevaluate the client's need for gentle care versus firm, directive encouragement. Involve the family in this process.	Emotional lability is common after stroke. Clients fluctuate between heroic efforts toward independent self-care and whining demands to be totally cared for. The appropri-ate nursing response varies from moment to moment and runs the range of tender care to unrelent-ing firm direction. All nursing re-sponses need to communicate the nurse's sincere care for the client and commitment to developing his best potential.

Goal: On discharge to rehabilitation center, the client will:
- Show signs of physical and mental readiness to acquire increasing independence in self-care

Nursing Actions	Rationale	Evaluative Statement
Implement previously stated nurs-ing actions.	These actions help the client to-ward regaining control of his daily living and improve moral.	1/31/93 Goal met. Client's mus-cle strength and joint mobility maintained during hospitalization. Client is now participating in self-care activities and is eager to learn skills to become more independent.

S. Beecher, RN

KEY POINTS

- The fulfillment of most human needs depends, at least partially, on the body's ability to move. Purposeful, coordinated movement of the body requires the inte-grated functioning of the skeletal, muscular, and ner-vous systems of the body.

- Bones and joints provide form for the body and serve as the levers and fulcrums that make body movement possible. It is the contraction and relaxation of skeletal muscles, however, that actually produce movement by pulling on bones, and it is nerve impulses that stimu-late the muscles to contract.

- Good body mechanics is the efficient use of the body as a machine and as a means of locomotion. To role model healthy body mechanics, the nurse pays special attention to body alignment, balance, and coordinated body movement during work and leisure activities.
- Factors that influence body alignment and mobility include developmental considerations, physical health, mental health, life-style variables, attitudes and values, fatigue and stress level, and external factors.
- The active exertion of muscles involving the contraction and relaxation of muscle groups is termed exercise. Isotonic exercise involves muscle shortening and active movement, and its potential benefits include increased muscle mass, tone, and strength; improved joint mobility; increased cardiac and respiratory function; increased circulation; and increased osteoblastic activity. Isometric exercise involves contraction without movement, and potential benefits are increased muscle mass, tone, and strength; increased circulation to the exercised body part; and increased osteoblastic activity.
- Individuals who choose to live inactive life-styles place themselves at high risk for serious health problems. Problems of immobility include increased cardiac workload, thrombus formation, orthostatic hypotension, ineffective breathing patterns, ineffective airway clearance, impaired gas exchange, activity intolerance, pathologic fractures, nutritional alterations, fluid volume excesses, constipation, alteration in urinary elimination, potential for urinary tract infection, impairment of skin integrity, disturbances in self-esteem, powerlessness, impaired social interaction, altered thought processes, ineffective coping, and sleep pattern disturbances.
- People beginning exercise programs should be familiar with the following guidelines: Begin program slowly and allow the body time to adjust to the new stress, know your body and respect its limitations, and follow the safety guidelines for specific exercises.
- When assessing mobility status, interview the client regarding daily activity level, endurance, exercise and fitness goals, mobility problems, physical or mental problems that affect mobility, and external factors that affect mobility. The physical assessment of mobility status includes an assessment of general ease of movement and gait; alignment; joint structure and function; muscle mass, tone, and strength; and endurance.
- Nursing diagnoses for mobility problems include Activity Intolerance and Impaired Physical Mobility. Both problem statements have multiple etiologies. Because mobility influences so many other areas of human functioning, many nursing diagnoses have as their etiology a problem with mobility.
- The aim of nursing care for both well and ill clients is that the client follow a program of regular physical exercise that improves cardiovascular function, endurance, flexibility, and strength.
- Nursing strategies that promote mobility for clients on bed rest include careful attention to positioning that maintains correct alignment and facilitates physiologic functioning, safe transfer of client from bed to chair or stretcher, and the early and safe ambulation of clients. The nurse may also play a key role in teaching clients to use mechanical aids for walking.
- Clients require specialized nursing care if they have the following mobility diagnoses: Activity Intolerance, Impaired Physical Mobility, High Risk for Injury related to complications for immobility, and Altered Health Maintenance related to lack of exercise program.

STUDY QUESTIONS

1. The strong, flexible inelastic fibrous bands that attach muscle to bone are
   a. tendons
   b. ligaments
   c. cartilage
   d. joints
2. The nurse spreads her feet apart as he or she prepares to help raise a client from a chair. The most important reason for doing this is to
   a. use the body's weight to assist movement
   b. make a long midriff
   c. provide a wide base of support
   d. facilitate use of the stronger back muscles
3. A client performs rehabilitative exercises with resistance after a knee injury. This type of exercise is referred to as
   a. isotonic
   b. isokinetic
   c. isometric
   d. aerobic
4. The expected result when more protein is broken down than is manufactured is
   a. fluid volume excess
   b. a contracture
   c. osteoporosis
   d. negative nitrogen balance
5. An immobile client experiences multiple urinary tract infections. Urinary bacteria are more likely to grow when urine is
   a. alkaline
   b. dilute
   c. aromatic
   d. acidic
6. Mr. Brown is experiencing some difficulty breathing. The nurse most appropriately assists him into the
   a. dorsal recumbent position

b. lateral position

c. Fowler's position

d. Sims' position

7. While doing range of motion exercises with a bed-ridden client, the nurse is aware that

a. neck hyperextension should be encouraged particularly in elderly people

b. exercises should be continued until the client is fatigued

c. exercises should be done frequently so as to lessen pain for the client

d. each joint is exercised to the point of resistance but not pain

8. The nurse is assisting a client with conditioning exercises to prepare for ambulation. The nurse correctly instructs the client to

a. do full-body push-ups in bed six to eight times daily

b. breathe in and out smoothly during quadriceps drills

c. dangle on the side of the bed for 30 to 60 minutes

d. allow the nurse to completely bathe the client to prevent fatigue

9. In many situations, a client has sufficient strength to walk if he or she can

a. lie prone for 1 hour

b. bathe himself or herself

c. raise the foot off the bed 1 inch

d. sit up in bed for 1 hour

10. Mrs. Eden tells the nurse she feels faint while walking in the corridor with the nurse. The nurse

a. instructs the client to quicken her pace so they can return to her room

b. leaves her momentarily to find another nurse to help

c. advises her to look down at her feet to help maintain her balance

d. guides her to a chair in the corridor and eases her onto it to rest

11. When using a cane for assistance the nurse is aware the client should

a. hold the cane on the weaker side

b. distribute weight evenly between the feet and the cane

c. keep the elbow straight and stiff that is holding the cane

d. advance the weaker foot ahead of the cane

12. When measuring a client for axillary crutches, the nurse should

a. have the client lie flat on the back in bed while wearing walking shoes

b. have the client stand with feet separated 12 inches and arms extended at shoulder height

c. measure the distance from the shoulder to the heel and add 4 inches

d. measure the distance from the anterior fold of axilla diagonally to a point 12 inches from the heel

13. When using the swing-through crutch gait, the client should

a. bear weight on the unaffected foot

b. bear weight on both feet

c. simulate normal walking as closely as possible

d. move the right crutch and left foot forward at the same time

14. When working with an older client to develop an exercise program, the nurse would recommend

a. a frequency of six times a week

b. exercising to the point of breathlessness when trying to speak

c. maintaining a target heart rate of 220 plus age

d. medical clearance before beginning the program

15. A bedridden client who is blind is admitted to a health care facility from his or her home with pressure ulcers on the sacral area. A priority nursing diagnosis is

a. High Risk for Altered Body Temperature related to stage 2 pressure ulcer

b. Impaired Skin Integrity related to immobility

c. Feeding Self-Care Deficit related to blindness

d. Activity Intolerance related to prolonged bed rest

Answers With Rationale

1. The correct response is *a*. Tendons are the strong fibrous bands that attach muscle to bone. Ligaments bind joints together and connect bones and cartilage, whereas cartilage is nonvascular connective tissue found in the joints as well as in the nose, ear, thorax, trachea, and larynx.

2. The correct response is *c*. Spreading the feet apart broadens the base of support and lowers the center of gravity. The muscles of the back are not as strong as the long muscles of the arms and legs and making a long midriff is accomplished by stretching the muscles in the waist. Rocking on the feet or leaning forward or backward uses the weight of the body as a moving force.

3. The correct response is *b*. Isokinetic exercise involves muscle contraction with resistance, whereas isotonic exercise involves muscle shortening and active movement. Isometric exercise involves muscle contraction without shortening and aerobic exercise is sustained muscle movements that increase

blood flow, heart rate, and metabolic demand for oxygen over time, promoting cardiovascular conditioning.

4. The correct response is *d*. Negative nitrogen balance results when the body excretes more nitrogen than it takes in. Contractures are permanent contraction states of muscles and osteoporosis involves bone demineralization. Fluid volume excess is indirectly related to protein manufacture or breakdown.

5. The correct response is *a*. Bacteria grow more easily in alkaline urine than acidic urine. Whether urine is dilute or aromatic is not a factor in bacteria growth.

6. The correct response is *c*. The Fowler's position promotes maximal breathing space in the thoracic cavity and is the position of choice when someone is having difficulty breathing. Lying flat on the back or side or Sims' position would not facilitate respiration and would be difficult for the client to maintain.

7. The correct response is *d*. Joints should never be exercised to the point of pain or fatigue. Joints should be exercised slowly, smoothly, and rhythmically. Neck hyperextension should be avoided in elderly clients and may prove painful.

8. The correct response is *b*. The client should never hold his or her breath during exercise drills because this places a strain on the heart. Push-ups are usually done three or four times a day and involve only the upper body. Dangling for 30 to 60 minutes is unsafe. The nurse encourages the client to be as independent as possible to prepare for return to normal ambulation and activities of daily living.

9. The correct response is *c*. Being able to raise the foot 1 inch off the bed frequently indicates sufficient strength for walking. Lying prone, bathing himself or herself, or sitting up in in bed do not necessarily indicate the muscle coordination and strength necessary in the lower limbs for walking.

10. The correct response is *d*. Guiding the client to a chair in the hall and easing her into it is the safest action. Asking her to walk faster or leaving her alone are definitely unsafe actions. If the client looks down at her feet, she may become dizzy and unbalanced.

11. The correct response is *b*. The client's weight should be evenly distributed between his or her feet and the cane. Holding the cane on the weaker side is difficult and unsafe. The elbow should be flexed at a 30-degree angle when holding the cane.

12. The correct response is *a*. Axillary crutches should be measured when the client is lying flat in bed with his or her walking shoes on. The distance is measured from the anterior fold of the axilla straight down to the heel, and then add 5 cm (2 inches). Or, measure the distance from the anterior fold of the axilla diagonally out to a point 15 cm (6 inches) away from the heel.

13. The correct response is *a*. With the swing-through gait, weight-bearing is permitted only on one foot. A disadvantage of this gait is that is does not simulate normal walking. Both crutches are brought forward at the same time and then both legs swing through and between the crutches with weight-bearing returning to the unaffected leg.

14. The correct response is *d*. Clients older than 35 years should always get medical clearance before initiating an exercise program. Frequency is initially three times a week and exercise should be maintained so that the client is able to talk without becoming breathless. The target heart rate is calculated as 60% to 90% of maximal heart rate (220 minus age).

15. The correct response is *b*. The priority nursing diagnosis for this client at this moment is Impaired Skin Integrity related to the pressure ulcer. The other nursing diagnoses may be appropriate but are not the priority on admission to the health care facility.

BIBLIOGRAPHY

Aaronson, L., Carlon-Wolf, W., & Schoener, S. (1991). Pressures that fall on rising. *Geriatric Nursing, 12*(12), 67.

Allison, M. (1991), Aging and exercise: Improving the odds. *Harvard Health Letter, 16*(4), 4–6.

Anderson, S. (1990). The health club. *Canadian Nurse, 86*(6), 34–35.

Bates, B. (1991). *A guide to physical examination and history taking* (5th ed.). Philadelphia: Lippincott.

Bhambhani, Y., Clarkson, H., & Gomes, P. (1990). Axillary crutch walking: Effects of three training programs. *Archives of Physical Medicine and Rehabilitation, 71*(6), 484–488.

Carnevali, D., & Patrick, M. (1986). *Nursing management for the elderly* (2nd ed.). Philadelphia: Lippincott.

Carpenito, L. J. (1991). *Nursing care plans and documentation.* Philadelphia: Lippincott.

Carpenito, L. J. (1992). *Nursing diagnosis: Application to clinical practice* (4th ed.). Philadelphia: Lippincott.

Cirullo, J. (1989). Osteoporosis. *Clinical Management in Physical Therapy, 9*(3), 14–19.

Eustace, C. (1991). Back up and wait. *RN, 54*(6), 49–51.

Evans, W. (1992). Give me strength: No rest for the aging. *Nutrition Action Health Letter, 19*(5), 1–7.

Fiatarone, M., Marks, E., Ryan, N., Meredith, C., Lipsitz, L., & Evans, W. (1990). High-intensity strength training in nonagenarians. *Journal of the American Medical Association, 263*(11), 3029–3034.

Fuller, J., & Schaller-Ayers, J. (1991). *Health assessment: A nursing approach.* Philadelphia: Lippincott.

Haley, E., & Colgate, W. (1990). Standing up for your back. *Canadian Nurse, 86*(11), 26–27.

Heeschen, S. (1989). Getting a handle on patient mobility. *Geriatric Nursing, 10*(3), 146–147.

Hogstel, M., & Kashka, M. (1989). Staying healthy after 85. *Geriatric Nursing, 10*(1), 16–18.

Holm, K., & Walker, J. (1990). Osteoporosis: Treatment and prevention update. *Geriatric Nursing, 11*(3), 140–142.

Kisner, C., & Colby, L. (1990). *Therapeutic exercise: Foundations and techniques* (2nd ed.). Philadelphia: Davis.

Kolanowski, A., & Gunter, L. (1988). Do retired career women exercise? *Geriatric Nursing, 9*(6), 350–352.

Lake, F., Henderson, K., Briffa, T., Openshaw, J., & Musk, W. (1990). Upper-limb and lower-limb exercise training in patients with chronic airflow obstruction. *Chest, 97*(5), 1077–1081.

Lovell, H., & Anderson, C. (1990). Put your patient on the right bed. *RN, 53*(5), 66–72.

Madson, S. (1989). How to reduce the risk of post-menopausal osteoporosis. *Journal of Gerontological Nursing, 15*(9), 20–23.

McConnell, E. (1990). Placing your patient in the lateral position. *Nursing, 20*(7), 65.

Milde, F. (1988). Impaired physical mobility. *Journal of Gerontological Nursing, 14*(3), 20–24.

Mobily, P., & Kelly, L. (1991). Iatrogenesis in the elderly: Factors of immobility. *Journal of Gerontological Nursing, 17*(9), 5–11.

Moore, S. (1989). Walking for health: A nurse-managed activity. *Journal of Gerontological Nursing, 15*(7), 26–28.

Morissey, M., & Baldwin, J. (1987). Exercise and chronic heart disease. *Geriatric Nursing, 8*(3), 138–140.

Neville, K. (1988). Promoting health for seniors. *Geriatric Nursing, 9*(1), 42–43.

Norman, G., & Gibbs, A. (1991). Why walk when you can ride? *Journal of Gerontological Nursing, 17*(8), 28–33.

North American Nursing Diagnosis Association. (1989). *Taxonomy I revised—1990.* St. Louis: Author.

Olsen, E., Johnson, B., & Thompson, L. (1967). The hazards of immobility. *American Journal of Nursing, 67*(4), 780–797.

Owen, B. (1989). The magnitude of low-back problem in nursing. *Western Journal of Nursing Research, 11*(2), 234–242.

Perry, G. (1988). Living with osteoporosis. *Geriatric Nursing, 9*(3), 174–176.

Ryan, S. (1988). Exercise to reduce cardiovascular risk. *Cardiovascular Nursing, 97*(5), 1077–1082.

Schilke, J. (1991). Slowing the aging process with physical activity. *Journal of Gerontological Nursing, 17*(6), 4–8.

Sparling, P., Cantwell, J., Dolan, C., & Niederman, R. (1990). Strength training in a cardiac rehabilitation program: A six-month follow-up. *Archives of Physical Medicine and Rehabilitation, 71*, 148–151.

Staab, A., & Lyles, M. (1990). *Manual of geriatric nursing.* Glenview, IL: Scott, Foresman.

Thomas, G. (1989). Swimming: An alternative form of therapy. *Clinical Management in Physical Therapy, 9*(3), 24–26.

Urrows, S., Freston, M., & Pryor, D. (1991). Profiles in osteoporosis. *American Journal of Nursing, 91*(12), 33–37.

Van Oteghen, S. (1987). An exercise program for those with Parkinson's disease. *Geriatric Nursing, 8*(4), 183–184.

Videman, T., Ravhala, H., Asp, S., Lindstrom, K., Cedercreatz, G., Kamppi, M., Tola, S., & Troup, J. (1989). Patient-handling skill, back injuries, and back pain: An intervention study in nursing. *Spine, 14*(2), 148–155.

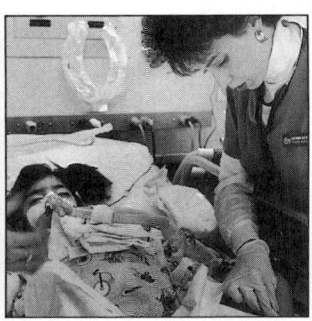
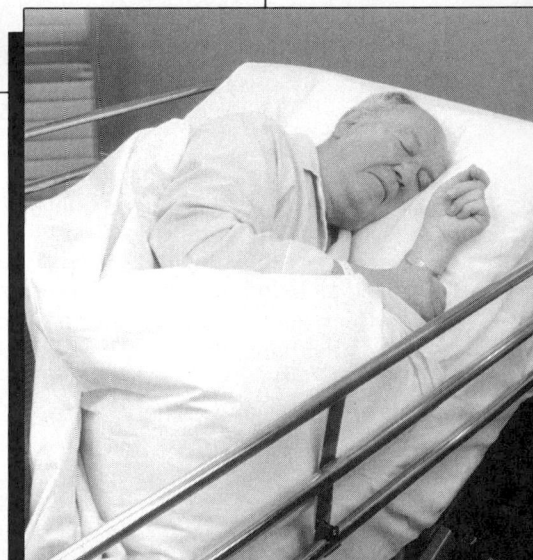

Rest and Sleep

OBJECTIVES

After studying this chapter, the learner should be able to:

Define key terms used in this chapter.

Describe the functions and physiology of sleep.

Identify 12 variables that influence rest and sleep.

Describe nursing implications for age-related differences in the sleep–wakefulness cycle.

Perform a comprehensive sleep assessment using appropriate interview questions, a sleep diary when indicated, and physical assessment skills.

Describe common sleep disorders, noting key assessment criteria.

Develop nursing diagnoses that correctly identify sleep problems that may be treated through independent nursing intervention.

Describe nine nursing strategies to promote rest and sleep, and identify their rationale.

Plan, implement, and evaluate nursing care related to select nursing diagnoses involving sleep problems.

KEY TERMS

circadian rhythm
circadian synchronization
delta sleep
electroencephalograph
electromyograph
electrooculogram
enuresis
hypersomnia
insomnia
narcolepsy
nocturnal myoclonus
non–rapid eye movement
 sleep
parasomnias
polysomnography
rapid eye movement sleep
rest
sleep
sleep apnea
sleep cycle
sleep deprivation
somnambulism

31

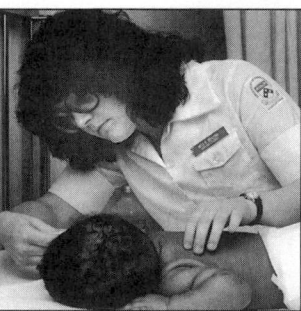

Physiology of Sleep

Two systems in the brain stem, the reticular activating system and the bulbar synchronizing region, are believed to work together to control the cyclic nature of sleep. The reticular formation (Fig. 31-1) is found in the brain stem. It extends upward through the medulla, the pons, the midbrain, and then into the hypothalamus. It comprises many nerve cells and fibers. The fibers have connections that relay impulses into the cerebral cortex and into the spinal cord. The reticular formation facilitates reflex and voluntary movements, as well as cortical activities related to a state of alertness. During sleep, the reticular system experiences few stimuli from the cerebral cortex and the periphery of the body. Wakefulness occurs when the reticular system is activated with stimuli from the cerebral cortex and from periphery sensory organs and cells. For example, an alarm clock awakens us from sleep to a state of consciousness when we realize that we must prepare ourselves for the day. Sensations such as pain, pressure, and noise produce wakefulness by means of periphery organs and cells. Wakefulness is activated by the cerebral cortex and body sensations. During sleep, stimuli from the cortex are minimal.

The hypothalamus has control centers for several involuntary activities of the body, one of which concerns

On the average, people spend one third of their lives asleep. Although the exact purpose of sleep is unclear, the functions of sleep are usually characterized as being protective and restorative. The advice "everything will look better after a good night's sleep" is based on the belief that sleep:

- Restores physical well-being
- Relieves stress and anxiety
- Restores the ability to cope and to concentrate on activities of daily living

In this chapter, **rest** connotes a condition in which the body is in a decreased state of activity with the consequent feeling of being refreshed, and **sleep** means a state of altered consciousness throughout which varying degrees of stimuli produce wakefulness. Sleep is an active and complex rhythmic state involving a progression of repeated cycles, each representing different phases of body and brain activity.

Most people can fall asleep easily and remain asleep until the desired waking time; on the other hand, some individuals rarely fall asleep without a struggle and, even then, their sleep is fragmented. Many people have sleep disturbances that go undetected for years, progressively undermining energy and destroying their sense of self. The discomfort produced by physical and mental illness and the need for hospitalization and treatment may interfere dramatically with a client's ability to sleep. Consequently, nurses need to be vigilant in both detecting and treating sleep disturbances.

Study of this chapter provides the nurse with knowledge of the functions and physiology of sleep, dreams and dream theories, and factors affecting sleep. Practical suggestions for performing a comprehensive sleep assessment are given. Sample interview questions for both a general and focused sleep history are presented along with information on sleep diaries and pertinent physical assessment data. The importance of analyzing these data is noted and numerous examples of nursing diagnoses are offered. Client goals and specific nursing strategies for promoting rest and sleep are described. In the section Nursing Process in Clinical Practice, guides to focused assessment, diagnosis, planning, implementation, and evaluation are offered for select nursing diagnoses related to the sleep disturbances insomnia and sleep deprivation. These guides and the concluding case study illustrate how the nurse's knowledge of rest and sleep, combined with skilled nursing interventions and caring, can successfully resolve sleep problems.

FIGURE 31-1

Reticular formation in brain stem and diencephalon with radiations to the cerebral cortex.

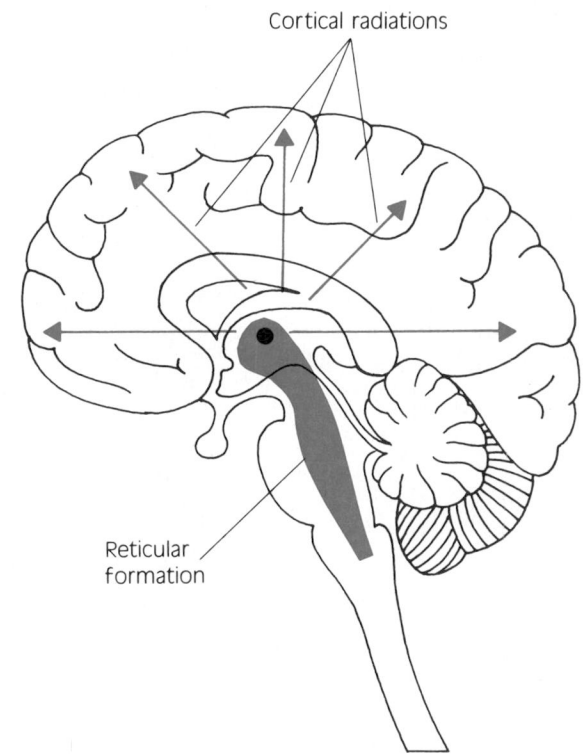

Cortical radiations

Reticular formation

sleeping and waking. Injury to the hypothalamus may cause a person to sleep for abnormally long periods.

It has been shown that some compounds play a role as neurotransmitters and are involved with the sleeping process. Norepinephrine and acetylcholine, followed by dopamine, serotonin, and histamine, are involved with excitation. Gamma-aminobutyric acid (GABA) appears to be necessary for inhibition. However, research has yet to prove exactly how biochemical changes and hormones function in sleep.

Circadian Rhythms

Rhythmic biologic clocks are currently known to exist in plants, animals, and humans. Influenced by both internal and external factors, they regulate select biologic and behavioral functions in humans. Some cycles are monthly, such as a woman's menstrual cycle. **Circadian rhythms** complete a full cycle every 24 hours. Fluctuations in heart rate, blood pressure, body temperature, hormone secretions, metabolism, and in an individual's performance and mood depend in part on circadian rhythm.

Sleep is one of the body's most complex biologic rhythms. **Circadian synchronization** exists when an individual's sleep–wake patterns follow the inner biologic clock. That is, when physiologic and psychologic rhythms are high or most active, the person is awake, and when these rhythms are low, the person is asleep. Although light and dark appear to be powerful regulators of the sleep–wake circadian rhythm, they do not exert primary control. The regulating mechanism is an individualized biologic clock subject to occupational demands, social pressures, and so forth. The nurse who works the night shift may routinely sleep from 2 to 8 PM and peak physiologic activity may occur between 10 PM and 6 AM during work. Problems of desynchronization occur when sleep–wake patterns are frequently altered and an individual attempts to sleep during high activity rhythms and to work when the body is physiologically prepared to rest.

Stages of Sleep

Research illustrates that there are two major stages of sleep: **non–rapid eye movement** (NREM) and **rapid eye movement** (REM). These stages have been studied and analyzed with the help of the **electroencephalograph** (EEG), which receives and records electrical currents from the brain; the **electrooculogram** (EOG), which is a recording of eye movements; and the **electromyograph** (EMG), which records muscle tone.

NREM Sleep   NREM sleep consists of four stages. Stages I and II, consuming about 5% to 50%, respectively, of a person's sleep, are light sleep, and the person can be aroused with relative ease. Stages III and IV, each composing about 10% of total sleep time, are deep-sleep states termed **delta sleep**, or slow-wave sleep (SWS). The arousal threshold (intensity of stimulus required to awaken) is usu-

ally greatest in stage IV NREM. Throughout the stages of NREM sleep, the parasympathetic branch of the autonomic nervous system dominates, and decreases in pulse, respiratory rate, blood pressure, metabolic rate, and body temperature are observed. Characteristics of the four stages of NREM sleep are summarized in Table 31-1.

REM Sleep   It is more difficult to arouse a person during REM sleep than during NREM sleep. In normal adults, the REM state consumes 20% to 25% of a person's nightly sleep. If people are awakened during the REM state, they almost always report that they have been dreaming. Many researchers state that everyone dreams; those people who say they do not simply are unable to recall their dreams.

During REM sleep, the pulse, respiratory rate, blood pressure, metabolic rate, and body temperature increase whereas general skeletal muscle tone and deep tendon reflexes are depressed. REM sleep is believed to be essential to mental emotional equilibrium and to play a role in learning, memory, and adaptation.

When a person is deprived of REM sleep for several nights, he or she generally spends more time in REM sleep on successive nights. This phenomenon is termed REM

T A B L E   3 1 - 1

Characteristics of NREM Sleep	
Stage	**Characteristics**
I	Is transitional stage between wakefulness and sleep
	The person is in a relaxed state but still somewhat aware of the surroundings.
	Involuntary muscle jerking may occur and waken the person.
	The stage normally lasts only for minutes.
	The person can be aroused easily.
	Constitutes only about 5% of total sleep.
II	The person falls into a stage of sleep.
	The person can be aroused with relative ease.
	Constitutes 50% to 55% of sleep.
III	The depth of sleep increases and arousal becomes increasingly difficult.
	Composes about 10% of sleep.
IV	The person reaches the greatest depth of sleep, which is called *delta sleep*.
	Arousal from sleep is difficult.
	Physiologic changes in the body include the following: Slow brain waves are recorded on an EEG. Pulse and respiratory rates decrease. Blood pressure decreases. Muscles are relaxed. Metabolism slows and the body temperature is low.
	Constitutes about 10% of sleep.

rebound and allows the total amount of REM sleep to remain fairly constant over time. Characteristics of REM sleep are summarized in Table 31-2.

Sleep Cycle

During a **sleep cycle**, a person normally passes consecutively through the four stages of NREM sleep. Then, the person reverses this pattern and returns from stage IV to stage III to stage II. Instead of reentering stage I and awakening, the person enters into the stage of REM sleep, after which he or she reenters NREM sleep at stage II and returns to stages III and IV. If a person is awakened from sleep at any time, he or she returns to sleep again by starting at stage I of NREM sleep.

It is typical to go through four or five cycles of sleep each night. On the average, each cycle lasts about 90 to 100 minutes. The cycles tend to become longer as morning approaches. Ordinarily, more sleep occurs in the delta stage in the first half of the night, especially if one is tired or has lost sleep.

Figure 31-2 illustrates the normal sleep pattern of young adults. Variations in the sleep cycle are observed according to age, as Figure 31-3 illustrates.

Sleep Requirements and Patterns

For no known reason, 8 hours of sleep every night has been the accepted standard, despite obvious variances shown in the general population. There is no rigid formula for normal periodicity and duration of sleep. It is important, however, that each person follow a pattern of rest that maintains well-being.

Despite variations, some generalities can be stated. On the average, infants sleep from 14 to 20 hours each day. Growing children require from 10 to 14 hours of sleep.

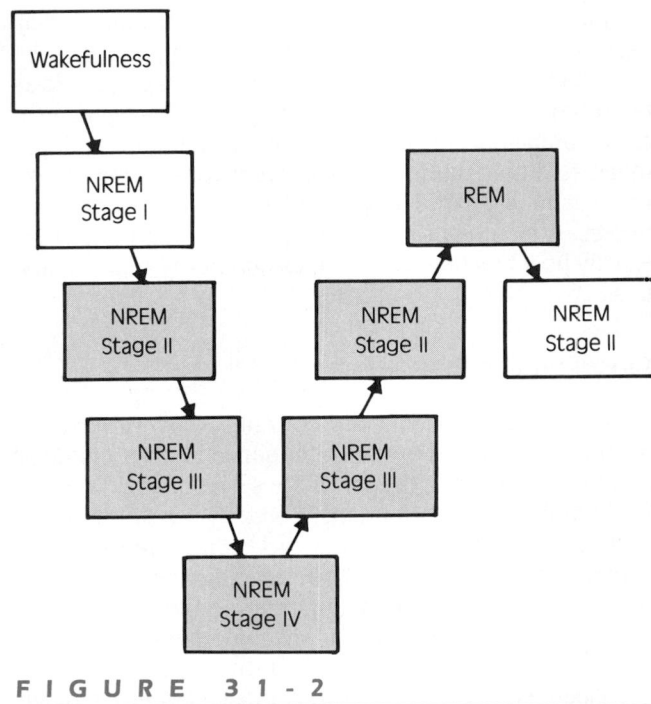

F I G U R E   3 1 - 2

A single normal sleep cycle. In the normal nocturnal pattern, the shaded cycle is repeated four or five times. Periods of REM sleep generally increase in duration, and periods of deep sleep (stage IV) progressively decrease as morning approaches.

Adults average 7 to 9 hours, although a 4-hour range has been observed in many normal adults. Those who are able to relax and rest easily, even while awake, often find that less sleep is needed, whereas others may find that more sleep is required to overcome fatigue. Fatigue can be considered a normal, protective body mechanism and nature's warning that sleep is necessary. Chronic fatigue is abnormal and is often a symptom of illness.

Sleep patterns of elderly people vary. However, elderly people are characterized by requiring a longer time to go to sleep, waking earlier, and being less able to cope with changes in their usual sleep patterns than younger people. Elderly people tend to nap during the day, which often results in sleeping fewer hours at night.

Patterns of sleep periodicity appear to be learned. For example, most people learn to sleep at night and to be awake and work during the day. However, many night workers learn to sleep equally well during the day.

Factors Affecting Sleep

A variety of factors influence both the quality and quantity of sleep.

Developmental Considerations   Age variations also exist in sleep–wakefulness cycles. These are presented with related nursing interventions in Table 31-3.

T A B L E   3 1 - 2

Characteristics of REM Sleep	
Item	**Characteristics**
Eyes	Dart back and forth quickly
Muscles	Small-muscle twitching, such as on the face
	Large-muscle immobility, resembling paralysis
Respirations	Irregular; sometimes interspersed with apnea
Pulse	Rapid or irregular
Blood pressure	Increases or fluctuates
Gastric secretions	Increase
Metabolism	Increases; body temperature increases
Brain waves	Encephalogram tracings active
Sleep cycle	REM sleep enters from stage II of NREM sleep and reenters NREM sleep at stage II: arousal from sleep difficult

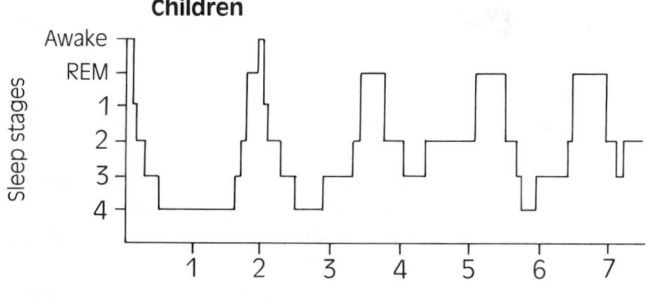

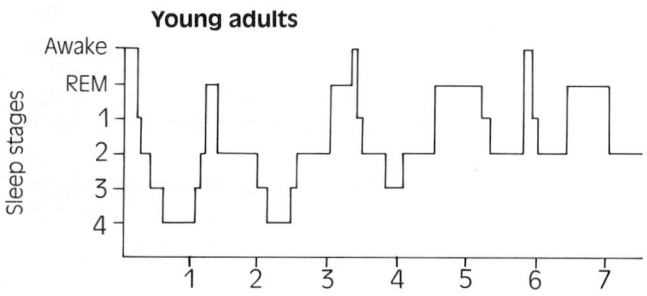

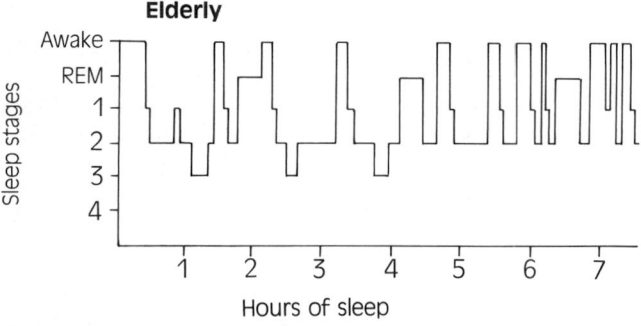

Hours of sleep

FIGURE 31-3

A comparison of developmental differences in NREM and REM cycles during nocturnal sleep for children, young adults, and elderly people.

Physical Activity Activity and exercise influence sleep by increasing fatigue and, in many instances, by promoting relaxation that is followed by sleep. It appears that physical activity increases both REM and NREM sleep.

Psychological Stress Illness and situations in daily living that cause psychological stress tend to disturb sleep. Generally, psychological stress affects sleep in two ways: (1) the person experiencing stress tends to find it difficult to obtain the amount of sleep he or she needs, and (2) REM sleep decreases in amount, which tends to add to anxiety and stress.

Motivation A desire to be wakeful and alert helps overcome sleepiness and sleep. For example, a tired person may be wakeful and alert when at a party or when attending an interesting play or concert. The opposite is also true—when there is minimal motivation to be awake, sleep generally follows.

Diet It is believed that the dietary amino acid L-tryptophan acts to promote sleep. It is a precursor of serotonin, a neurotransmitter. A diet containing adequate protein enhances normal sleep whereas a diet lacking in essential protein may well interfere with it. It has been theorized that elderly people who have difficulty falling asleep and remaining asleep may have diets lacking in sufficient protein or may be absorbing protein poorly.

Alcohol Intake Alcoholic beverages, when used in moderation, seem to help induce sleep in some people. However, large quantities have been found to limit REM and delta sleep. This effect may partially explain the phenomenon of hangover after excessive alcohol consumption.

Caffeine-Containing Beverages Caffeine is a central nervous system stimulant. For many people, beverages containing caffeine interfere with the ability to fall asleep. Examples of beverages containing caffeine include coffee, tea, most cola drinks, and chocolate.

Smoking Nicotine has a stimulating effect and smokers usually have a more difficult time falling asleep. They are more easily aroused once asleep and may describe themselves as light sleepers. Eliminating cigarette smoking after the evening meal seems to improve the smoker's ability to fall asleep, and they usually report improved sleep patterns once nicotine use is discontinued.

Environmental Factors Most people sleep best in their usual home environments. Sleeping in a strange or new environment tends to influence both REM and NREM sleep for most.

Life-Style Various life-styles affect the ability to sleep well. People working a shift other than the day shift must reorganize their priorities. Developing a sleep pattern is especially difficult if the shift changes periodically. The type of television watched in the evening, involvement in emotionally stirring outside activities, and the amount of activity or exercise in which one participates can all affect sleep. Moderate exercise is a healthy way to promote sleep, but excessive exercise can defeat sleep. One's ability to relax from work-related pressures or to regard or disregard conflict in the home are important factors in the ability to fall asleep.

Illness Illness acts as a physiologic and psychologic stressor and, as a result, influences sleep. Certain illnesses are more closely related to sleep disturbances than others. Several examples follow.

Gastric secretions increase during REM sleep. Many people with peptic ulcers awaken at night with pain. They find that eating a snack to help neutralize stomach acidity is often helpful to relieve discomfort and promote sleep.

The pain associated with diseases of the coronary arteries and the occurrence of myocardial infarctions is often

(Text continues on p. 725)

TABLE 31-3

Developmental Variation in the Sleep–Wakefulness Cycle

Sleep–Wakefulness Cycle	Nursing Implications

Infants

The infant exhibits six states or levels of arousal
1. *Regular sleep*—Muscle tonus is low, eyelids are closed and still, respirations are about 36 breaths per minute, even, and of regular rhythm.
2. *Irregular sleep*—Muscle tonus is greater; movements follow no sequence, grimaces are frequent; there is intermittent gross mouthing (ie, chomping, chewing, and licking); respirations are irregular; and the mean rate is greater than during regular sleep.
3. *Periodic sleep* (intermediate between regular and irregular sleep)—Respiratory rates are periodic (ie, bursts of rapid shallow breathing alternate with bursts of deep, slow respirations similar to Cheyne-Stokes respiration).
4. *Drowsiness*—Less activity than in irregular or periodic but more activity than in regular sleep; the eyes have a dull glazed appearance, open and close intermittently, and just before closing may roll upward; generally regular respirations may become tachypneic; there may be a high-pitched squeal.
5. *Alert inactivity*—The eyes are open and bright and make conjugate movements in the vertical and horizontal plane, the face is relaxed, respirations are more variable and faster than in regular sleep; not seen before 3½ weeks of age.
6. *Crying*—Vocalization accompanied by gross motor activity, open or closed eyes, tears can been seen as early as 24 hours after birth; characteristic patterns of crying identifiable as early as the first 5 days of life.

In older infants, a state of active wakefulness is seen, during which they explore their world. This becomes increasingly evident as they mature. Each infant has a unique sleep pattern. Generally, by 8 to 16 weeks, the infant's biologic rhythms coincide with daytime and nighttime hours, and he or she will sleep through the night. The younger infant may sleep 17 to 20 hours a day. The 12- to 16-week-old infant will sleep 14 to 18 hours and by the end of the first year the infant may sleep from 12 to 16 hours a day. Young infants spend much time in irregular or REM sleep. This is believed to furnish great quantities of functional excitement to the higher brain centers.

Nurses may need to help parents understand the infant's sleep and wakefulness patterns. The eye movements, groaning, moving, grimacing, and irregular breathing and gasping are normal and require no attention.

Most infants are content to sleep on their abdomens, and this position prevents the aspiration of mucous or regurgitated milk.

During waking hours, infants enjoy stimulation and play. The nurse should determine if the parents provide visual, auditory, and tactile stimulation for the infant when the child is awake.

The parents' perception of the amount of sleep and activity the infant needs and the type of schedule provided should also be assessed. Guide and counsel as needed.

Toddlers

The toddler averages from 10 to 15 hours of sleep in a 24-hour period. Two naps a day are more common in the early toddler period; the number and length of naps generally decline as the child approaches the preschool years.

Awakening two or three times during the night occurs with most toddlers. This may be due to separation anxiety, loneliness, teething pains, illness, nightmares, or a stressful family situation. Often the toddler is able to fall back to sleep, but some toddlers may need attention and comfort from a parent.

A circadian sleep–wakefulness rhythm can be identified by age 3 months, and a gradual maturation of this cycle occurs between the ages of 2 and 10 years in children. Thus, the toddler should manifest an individual pattern of night sleep, naps, and awake time in a 24-hour period.

Establishing a regular bedtime routine with the toddler will facilitate sleep. Routines can include a parent reciting or reading a story, singing a lullaby, rocking the child, or giving the child a bottle of water to suck on. Such activities provide the toddler with love and security and time to settle down after a busy day.

To avoid behavioral or emotional disruptions caused by alterations in the toddler's cycle, it is important that parents learn to allow the child to follow a routine sleep pattern, with only occasional interruptions in the pattern.

(continued)

T A B L E 3 1 - 3 *(continued)*

Developmental Variation in the Sleep–Wakefulness Cycle

Sleep–Wakefulness Cycle	Nursing Implications

Preschoolers

Most authorities agree that by the age of 2 to 3 years, the child's sleep–wakefulness cycle, physiologic rhythms, and hormonal cycles are established. The sleep–wakefulness cycle is fully developed by age 2 years; the REM sleep pattern is like an adult pattern by the preschool era. In children, naps represent about 12% of sleep for toddlers, 5% for 4-year-olds, and 0% for 5-year-olds. It is estimated that children from age 2 to 5 years need about 9 to 16 hours of sleep per day, which decreases as the child gets older.

When assessing the sleep–wakefulness cycle, it is essential that the nurse explore the parents' perception of the amount of sleep the child needs and elicit information regarding the schedule the parents use for the child's sleep and rest times. Also, the sleeping patterns of the family should be determined so that congruency or conflict with the preschooler's pattern can be identified. If the child's primary caregiver is unable to obtain sufficient rest, the nurse needs to explore alternative ways to help her or him to get more rest so that health and caretaking responsibilities are not jeopardized.

The nurse should determine if there are any external factors that might interfere with the child's sleep. Some significant factors include noise, heat, light, and disturbance from siblings. The nurse should offer the parents suggestions on how to change or eliminate any problem-causing environmental conditions.

School-Aged Children

Normally children require an average of 8 to 10 hours of sleep, but this will vary with each individual. During periods of increased physical growth, the need for sleep may increase.

Parents may need reassurance that it is not uncommon for interruptions in sleep–rest patterns to occur at this age. Frequently, sleep disturbances are the result of increasing awareness of the concept of death. This knowledge, usually gained through television and books, can be frightening to the child, who views himself or herself as powerless in face of the perceived danger. Preparing the child for sleep in a relaxed manner (eg, through quiet talking or reading sessions) and establishing bedtime routines (eg, prayers) may help diminish anxiety. Adults, through their presence and support, can increase the child's own coping resources and help alleviate fears.

Adolescents

Adolescent clients may have an unusual sleep–wakefulness cycle, especially if they live outside the family. Older adolescents tend to prefer sleeping late in the morning and going to bed late at night whenever possible. The sleep needs of different teenagers vary widely.

It is important to assess the amount of sleep the teenager needs and is able to obtain during each 24-hour period. Because adolescents may be sensitive about their personal habits, the nurse should always be careful to ask questions about these subjects in a nonjudgmental manner. Questions such as "Do you feel rested when you wake after sleeping?" or "Do you feel you get enough sleep?" or "How would you describe the way you sleep?" allow the client to describe personal perceptions (questions about dreams and waking during the sleep period should be included). A teenager may often have complaints about fatigue or inability to do well in school because of poor sleeping patterns.

Young Adults

Of all the rhythmic patterns, the most important for the young adult is the sleep–wakefulness cycle. Many factors influence the need for rest and sleep, including physical health, type of occupation, and amount of daily exercise. The young adult is generally full of energy and participates in many activities—attending school, participating in family responsibilities and working. All of these activities present new and exciting frontiers to explore as an adult, with minimal or no parental influence.

If there is a problem in sleep habits, the nurse needs to explore the client's current life-style to see if adequate time is being allocated for sleep. If stress is hindering sleep, means other than medication should be established for handling and decreasing the problem. The client might be encouraged to take a brief rest period during the day or to participate in stress-reduction exercises. Such activities may prevent sleepless nights. Brief periods of watching television, reading, or sewing may be just enough to bring easy rest at the end of the day.

(continued)

T A B L E   3 1 - 3 *(continued)*

Developmental Variation in the Sleep–Wakefulness Cycle

Sleep–Wakefulness Cycle	Nursing Implications

Young Adults

The young adult often maintains an active life-style, interrupting sleep patterns along the way. Traditionally, it has been thought that the young adult requires 7 to 8 hours of sleep per night, but some members of this age group seem to do well with less.

The percentage of time spent in each stage of sleep decreases with age; however, interestingly enough, the percentage of time spent in stage I REM sleep does not change throughout life, consistently composing 20% to 25% of total sleep time. This particular biologic rhythm is thought to be very important for maintaining a stable psychologic balance in each individual, no matter what age.

Frequently, the young adult will take medication to alter sleep patterns. Because of significant stress (eg, trying to achieve, to maintain a family, to establish meaningful relationships, to participate in extracurricular activities), the young adult may have difficulty falling asleep. He or she becomes overtired and increasingly worried about the inability to sleep. Medications may seem a logical way to get some rest quickly. All too often, the potential hazards of sleep medications are overlooked, and the young adult may become a prime target for some specific health problems.

Sleep medications significantly decrease REM sleep. If these medications are taken consistently, there is a gradual return to the normal amount of REM sleep. However, when the medication is stopped, the individual may undergo withdrawal symptoms, including insomnia, nightmares, fatigue, and increased sensitivity to pain. These symptoms may last up to 5 weeks.

Whatever the prescription, the young adult needs to know the impact that a sustained, frantic, exhausting schedule will have over time. Good sleep habits established during the young adult years will not only have a significant impact on sustaining current health but on maintaining long-term wellness as the client ages.

Middle Adults

For the middle adult, gradual changes in the sleep patterns develop in earlier life and continue through middle adulthood. Specifically, total sleep time decreases, with a particular decrease in the amount of stage IV sleep. The number of sleep arousals increases, and the percentage of time in bed spent awake begins to increase. This will be exaggerated in people who follow previously established sleep patterns after their sleep requirements have decreased.

Because of the multiple changes and stresses in middle age, sleep disturbances are common. However, any sleep aberration should be investigated to exclude the possibility of underlying anxiety or depression that can be reflected by difficulty in falling asleep, early morning awakening, or alternatively, hypersomnia. Sleeping pills or other aids may be used by middle adults, and such use should be determined during the health history.

Older Adults

Sleep–wakefulness patterns are altered in the aged. Older people know they no longer sleep deeply. Many elders report that they have difficulty falling asleep and are more easily awakened once asleep. They are more likely to be disturbed by noise despite the fact that their sense of hearing is less acute. Even though older adults may spend more actual time in bed, they frequently comment that they feel less refreshed upon awakening in the morning. The proportion of REM and NREM sleep time changes with age. In elderly adults, stage I time increases, and less time is spent in stages III and IV. Some elder adults have no stage IV sleep—this decrease or loss of restorative sleep may result in signs and symptoms of sleep deprivation such as fatigue, daytime sleepiness, headaches, and poor concentration.

Sleep disturbances in elderly clients, although common, are not trivial. Age-related changes in sleep–wake patterns, concurrent medical or psychiatric disorders, and environmental changes may produce an array of sleep-related complaints. Comprehensive assessment and individualized intervention can be effective in the long-term care of these individuals.

(continued)

T A B L E 3 1 - 3 *(continued)*

Developmental Variation in the Sleep–Wakefulness Cycle

Sleep–Wakefulness Cycle	Nursing Implications
Older Adults	
The amount of REM sleep decreases because the length of each episode shortens. Roberts (1990) summarized the possible reasons for abnormal sleep patterns in elder adults: • Decline in physical health that may result in pain or signs and symptoms of chronic disease • Psychologic factors such as depressive disorders, mourning for a loved person or pet, or change in body image • Undesirable effects of drug therapy such as nocturia • Environmental factors (noise, temperature, familiarity of setting)	

(Data from Murray, R., & Zentner, J. [1989]. *Nursing assessment & health promotion strategies through the life span* [4th ed.]. Norwalk, CT: Appleton & Lange.)

associated with REM sleep. Seizure attacks owing to epilepsy are most likely to occur during NREM sleep and appear to be depressed by REM sleep. Liver failure and encephalitis tend to cause a reversal in day–night sleeping habits. Hypothyroidism tends to decrease the amount of NREM sleep, especially stages II and IV.

Some research, especially when children were studied, has demonstrated that asthma attacks appear to occur less frequently during stage IV sleep, and efforts to increase this stage of sleep are recommended. One method is to increase exercise to assist in promoting extended periods of deep sleep; the type of exercise should be one the client can tolerate.

Most people suffering from infectious diseases require more than normal amounts of sleep to overcome fatigue. Infectious hepatitis requires marked increases in the quantity of sleep. The fatigue associated with this disease extends well into the convalescing period.

Medications Sleep quality is also influenced by certain drugs. Some examples of drugs that decrease REM sleep are barbiturates, amphetamines, and antidepressants. Chloral hydrate and flurazepam (Dalmane) appear to influence the quality of sleep least and promote normal sleep.

Common Sleep Disorders

The nurse interviewing a client to obtain a sleep history needs to be knowledgeable about common sleep disturbances to recognize significant data. A brief description of these disturbances follows. Specific interview questions may be found in Table 31-4.

Primary Sleep Disorders Primary sleep disorders are those in which the sleep disturbance is the main symptom or sign of the problem. Examples include insomnia, hypersomnia, narcolepsy, and sleep apnea.

Insomnia is characterized by difficulty in falling asleep, intermittent sleep, or early awakening from sleep. Usually, people complaining of insomnia have been observed to fall asleep more quickly and sleep more than they report they do. However, the condition can lead to such distress that further wakefulness results. It is the most common of all sleep disorders.

Hypersomnia is a condition characterized by excessive sleep, particularly sleep during the day. Although this condition may result from medical conditions, it is frequently used as a coping mechanism when someone has no desire or energy to face a new day.

Narcolepsy is a condition characterized by an uncontrollable desire to sleep. The person with narcolepsy can literally fall asleep standing up, while driving a car, in the middle of a conversation, or while swimming. It is considered to be a neurologic disorder. The condition usually begins in susceptible people during adolescence or early adulthood and continues through life. Agrypnotic drugs that cause wakefulness are used to control narcolepsy. People using such drugs should take them faithfully because if they are discontinued, the uncontrollable desire to sleep returns.

Sleep apnea refers to periods of no breathing between snoring intervals. The person may not breathe for periods of 15 seconds to as long as 2 minutes. During long periods of apnea, there is a drop in the oxygen level of the blood, the pulse usually becomes irregular, and the blood pressure

(Text continues on p. 728)

Common Sleep Problems: Description and Pertinent Interview Questions

Sleep Problem	Description	Sample Interview Techniques and Questions
Primary Sleep Disorders (sleep alteration is the only symptom or sign of a problem)		
Insomnia	Shortened sleep period; may be characterized by difficulty in falling asleep (*initial insomnia*), frequent or prolonged awakening (*maintenance or intermittent insomnia*), or early morning awakening (*terminal insomnia*). In imaginary or subjective insomnia, the client has actually slept but claims he or she has not.	*Initial insomnia* • Are you able to fall asleep easily? • How long does it ordinarily take you to fall asleep? • What are you doing, thinking about, feeling, before you fall asleep? *Maintenance insomnia* • Do you find yourself waking up in the night after you have fallen asleep? • Tell me how often this happens on a usual night. • What do you do once you are awake? *Terminal insomnia* • What time do you normally wake up? • What might be causing you to wake up so early? • How often does this happen? • How does this affect the rest of your day?
Hypersomnia	Excessive sleep—in particular, sleep during the day. May occur from medical conditions (diabetic acidosis, increased intracranial pressure, hypothyroidism), but is more often a coping mechanism used when the individual has no desire or ability to face the day (depression, hysteria).	• Tell me again how many hours you sleep per day. • Is this all at one time or does it include naps? • What are you thinking when you first wake up in the morning? • Do you get out of bed as soon as you wake up? If no, what do you do? • Do you know of any medical conditions that might be causing you to sleep more?
Narcolepsy	A condition characterized by an uncontrolled and abrupt onset of "sleep attacks" during normally alert activities (eg, while eating, driving a car, talking. Undiagnosed, the narcoleptic is potentially dangerous to himself or herself and others. Clients with narcolepsy tend to fall asleep quickly, find it difficult to wake up, sleep fewer hours than others, and sleep restlessly. Common symptoms include sleep attacks, *cataplexy* (abrupt weakness or paralysis of voluntary muscles), *hypnagogic hallucinations* (frightening "dream attack" that occurs while the person is falling asleep), and *sleep paralysis* (skeletal muscle paralysis while falling asleep or waking up).	• Do you ever fall asleep suddenly during the day? If yes, tell me more about that. • Has anyone ever teased you about falling asleep on them, right in the middle of your work, a conversation, or a meal? • Have you ever had an attack of muscle weakness or paralysis? Wanted to move and couldn't? If yes, what were you doing when this occurred? How often does it happen? • Do you ever experience dreams right as you are falling asleep? What are they like? • Does sleep pose any particular problems for you?

Sleep apnea	Period of no breathing during sleep—may last for periods of 15 seconds to as long as 2 minutes; during periods of apnea, there is a drop in the oxygen level of the blood, the pulse may become irregular, and the blood pressure may increase. Many people experience sleep apnea without symptoms. At high risk for complications are middle-aged men in whom repeated episodes may cause anginal attacks, cardiac arrhythmias, and pulmonary hypertension. It is currently postulated that sleep apneas are related to mortality, which occurs during sleep.
	   Obstructive apnea—Caused by pharyngeal obstruction in the upper airway (see Fig. 31-4)
	   Central apnea—Stoppage of all attempts to breathe; may be related to defects in the respiratory center in the brain
	   Mixed apnea—Combination of central sleep apnea followed by an obstructive apnea
	   Hypopnea—Reduction in the amplitude of ventilation
		• Has anyone ever told you that there are times during sleep when you stop breathing for awhile and then start back up again?
		• If yes, tell me what this means to you. Do you have any concerns about this habit?
		• Do you snore? Is there someone who can describe your snoring?
		• Any recent problems with headache and nausea (related to low oxygen levels)?
		• Do you have a history of any heart or lung problems? Chest pain?
		• Are you aware of any changes in your mental abilities or any emotional changes?
		• Inspect body build.
		• Observe for airway deformities (short neck, thick tongue, deviated nasal septum).
		• In the hospitalized client, compare vital signs during apnea with baseline signs.
		• A report from a bed partner or a tape recording of the client's sleep may be helpful in establishing a diagnosis.

(continued)

Common Sleep Problems: Description and Pertinent Interview Questions

Sleep Problem	Description	Sample Interview Techniques and Questions
Sleep apnea	*Hypersomnia–sleep apnea*—Obesity and airway deformities place both men and women at risk for this syndrome in which sleep is restless and interrupted by snoring and periods of apnea; daytime sleepiness is common. Sleep deprivation affects the mental and emotional functioning of these individuals in whom anxiety, depression, and jealousy are common.	

Secondary Sleep Disorders (sleep alterations caused by another clinical disorder)

Numerous clinical problems can cause sleep alterations. Among the most common are

- Hypothyroidism—Decreased stages III and IV sleep time
- Hyperthyroidism—Increased stages III and IV sleep time
- Chronic renal insufficiency—Sleep disturbances just before dialysis
- Depression—Difficulty falling asleep, more rapid transition from stage to stage, more frequent awakening, less slow-wave sleep, less total sleep time, and more REM activity
- Schizophrenia—Reduction in REM sleep, reduced stages III and IV
- Alcoholism—REM deprivation
- Anorexia nervosa—Reduction of deeper sleep, stages III and IV, as well as of REM sleep increased stage I sleep but reduction of total sleep time.

- Are there any medical or psychiatric illnesses that might be affecting your sleep? (These may be unknown to the client but present on the client record.) Have you noticed any changes in your sleep since this disease began? Or since you started treatment for this illness? If yes, please describe these for me.

Parasomnias (patterns of waking behavior that appear during sleep)

Somnambulism (sleep walking)—Occurs during stages III and IV of NREM sleep; danger is that somnambulist may hurt himself or herself; protective environment is required

Sleep talking—Occurs before REM sleep; rarely presents a problem unless annoying to others

Nocturnal erections—Occur during REM sleep

Bruxism (grinding of teeth during sleep)—Usually occurs during stage II sleep

Enuresis—Bedwetting during sleep (see Chapter 34)

The questions may be directed to the client:
- Has anyone ever told you that you walk in your sleep, talk in your sleep, and so forth?

Or the questions may be directed to a child's parent:
- Have you ever noticed your child walking in his or her sleep? Talking while asleep?

With yes to any of these questions:
- Are you aware of any stressful event or emotional conflict before these sleep events?
- Describe a typical day and what you might have been feeling before one of these events.
- Does this sleep activity pose any problems for you? Tell me how you are dealing with it.

Sleep Deprivation

There are basically three types of sleep deprivation:

- REM deprivation (absence of dreaming) characterized by irritableness, insecurity, impaired concentration, and anxiousness. Increased sensitivity to pain and increased appetite may result.
- NREM deprivation (slow-wave sleep deprivation) characterized by fatigue, lethargy, depression, and difficulty in executing repetitive tasks of everyday living
- Total sleep deprivation—Rarely occurs except in laboratory setting; characterized by weariness progressing to total disintegration of personality

In what way is your sleep shortened?
What might be causing this?
How do you feel when you get up?
In what ways do you think your lack of sleep is affecting you?

(Data from Malasonas, L., Barkauskas, V., & Stoltenberg-Allen, K. [1986]. *Health assessment* [3rd ed.]. St. Louis: Mosby.)

Normal Unoccluded Airway

Occluded Airway

Occlusion

F I G U R E   3 1 - 4

Obstructive sleep apnea occurs when the airway is occluded due to collapse of the hypopharynx. Normally the airway remains open during sleep (*see inset*).

often increases. Although most commonly seen in middle-aged men, women and people of other ages may also experience it. Obstructive sleep apnea results when the airway is occluded due to collapse of the hypopharynx (Fig. 31-4). Fortunately, sleep apnea is not particularly common. Some investigators have theorized that sleep apnea possibly may explain certain cases of death that occur during sleep. **Polysomnography** is the only certain method of diagnosing sleep apnea. This sleep study consists of an EEG recording of the stages of sleep and any episodes of apnea, continuous monitoring of arterial oxygen saturation, and an electrocardiogram (ECG) to detect any cardiac dysrhythmias.

Parasomnias   Parasomnias refers to patterns of waking behavior that appear during sleep. Common examples include **somnambulism** (sleepwalking); sleeptalking; nocturnal erections; bruxism (grinding of teeth during sleep); and **enuresis** (bedwetting during sleep).

Sleep Deprivation   **Sleep deprivation** may result from decreased REM sleep, NREM sleep, or from total sleep deprivation. Causes are multiple, and manifestations progress from irritability and impaired mental abilities to a total disintegration of personality. The strange environment of the hospital, physical discomfort and pain, the effects of medications, and the need for 24-hour nursing care may all contribute to sleep deprivation in the hospitalized client.

Nurse as Role Model

It is difficult for clients to work collaboratively with a nurse to achieve sleep and rest goals when the nurse's appearance and behavior demonstrate inadequate rest and sleep.

Because professional, personal, and family demands can all outrank sleep on a nurse's list of priorities, nurses often find themselves showing up for work with inadequate rest and energy. Nurses who value their own well-being and who wish to be role models of healthy sleep self-care behaviors must develop life-styles supportive of the following nurse goals. The nurse will do the following:

- Routinely obtain the amount of sleep necessary to provide energy for the next day's work (specify number of hours)
- Incorporate three to four periods of regular exercise into each week
- Perform some relaxing activity 1 hour before retiring
- Evaluate the use of nicotine, caffeine, alcohol, and any pharmacologic sleep aids
- When possible, limit shift rotations and working two shifts back-to-back to prevent disrupting usual circadian rhythm

Use the self-assessment checklist in the accompanying display to monitor how well you are achieving sleep and rest goals for yourself.

Assessing Rest and Sleep

Sleep History

Because rest and sleep are important components of general health, a sleep history should be included in each comprehensive nursing history. Interview questions are used to identify the client's sleep–wakefulness patterns, the effect of these patterns on everyday functioning, sleep aids, and the presence of sleep disturbances and contributing factors. The sleep history may be brief (four questions) if the client's sleep is adequate and posing no problems, or it may

PROMOTING WELLNESS

Rest and Sleep

Use the assessment checklist to determine how well you are meeting needs for rest and sleep. Then develop a prescription for self-care by choosing appropriate behaviors from the list of suggestions.

Assessment Checklist

almost always | sometimes | almost never

☐ ☐ ☐ 1. I feel rested and refreshed when I get up in the morning.

☐ ☐ ☐ 2. I have energy to carry out normal activities of daily living.

☐ ☐ ☐ 3. I understand the normal changes in sleep and rest requirements and patterns that occur with aging.

☐ ☐ ☐ 4. I set aside time for quiet recreation and restful activities each day.

Self-Care Behaviors

1. Follow a regular routine for bedtime and morning awakening.
2. Accept individual differences in need for sleep.
3. Use relaxation exercises to relax before bedtime, especially if feeling stressed.
4. Avoid caffeine, smoking, and alcohol before bedtime.
5. Adjust bedcoverings, room temperature, and lighting to your preferences.
6. Drink a glass of milk before going to bed.
7. Am aware of the potential dangers of sleeping pills.
8. Use some part of each day for quiet, enjoyable activities, such as crafts, hobbies, reading, watching television, listening to music, visiting with friends.

---

be detailed. When the client's response to any of the interview questions indicates a potential problem, open-ended questions may be used to gather more data (see the accompanying display entitled Focused Assessment Guide).

If the client is being admitted to a care facility it is important to assess the client's usual times for retiring and waking, bedtime rituals, and client preferences regarding sleep environment so that these can be incorporated into the care plan, if possible. Sensitivity to small matters can make the difference between a good night's sleep and no sleep.

When a sleep disturbance is noted, the history should determine the following:
- The nature of the problem
- Its cause
- The related signs and symptoms
- When it first began and how often it occurs
- How it affects everyday living
- The severity of the problem and whether it can be treated independently by nursing or needs to be referred to another professional
- How the client is coping with the problem and the success of any treatments attempted

Interview questions may be directed to the client, to his or her bed partner, or to a caregiver. The client record may also contain pertinent information (eg, a history of illnesses that influence sleep or a history of drug dependency or withdrawal).

Sample recordings of a sleep history in a comprehensive nursing assessment are as follows:

Reports needs 8 to 9 hours of sleep to feel his best and usually gets this without problem. Generally retires at 11:30 PM and rises at 7:30 AM. No special sleep rituals.

Mother reports toddler has erratic sleep patterns. May nap at anytime in the afternoon or evening and sleep from 1 to 3 hours. Depending on nap, goes to bed anywhere from 7 to 11 PM and sleeps about 11 to 13 hours. Resists falling asleep and wants "water, story, snack, kisses, etc." Parents' life-style is constantly changing—little consistency for the child regarding sleep expectations.

Sleep Diary

A sleep diary or log provides more specific data of the client's sleep–wakefulness patterns over a prolonged period. The diary generally is kept for 14 days and includes the following:

1. A graph of the total number of hours of sleep per day. Depending on the nature of the problem, graphs may be made of the number of undisturbed hours of sleep, number of awakenings, and so forth.
2. A daily record of the following:
   - Time client decided to retire
   - Time client actually tries to fall asleep

F O C U S E D   A S S E S S M E N T   G U I D E

Rest and Sleep

Factors to Assess	Questions and Approaches
Usual sleep–wakefulness pattern: Recent changes	
• Usual sleeping and waking times	How many hours of sleep to you usually get in a day?
	Do you wake up earlier in the morning than you would like and find it difficult to fall back asleep?
	Have there been any recent changes in your usual sleep–wake patterns? If yes, describe them and tell me if they are causing any problems for you.
	Do you usually go to bed and wake up about the same time each day?
• Number of hours of undisturbed sleep	How have you been sleeping?
	Do you have any difficulty falling asleep?
	Do you wake up frequently during the night?
	Do you dream at night?
	Are your dreams frightening?
• Quality of sleep	How much sleep do you think you need to feel rested?
• Number and duration of naps	Do you take naps throughout the day?
Effect of sleep pattern on everyday functioning	In what way does the sleep you get each day affect your everyday living?
	Has this sleep disturbance caused any change in your sex life?
• Energy level (ability to perform activities of daily living)	Do you feel rested and ready to start the day when you wake up?
	Are there times during the day or certain activities when you feel especially tired?
	What happens when you don't get enough sleep?
	Are you having difficulty concentrating?
Sleep aids	
• Means of relaxing before bedtime	What do you do to relax before you get ready for bed?
• Bedtime rituals	Describe what you usually do to help yourself fall asleep.
• Sleep environment	Tell me how you like your room (lights, noises, ventilation, position of door, temperature) and bed (mattress, pillows, blankets) when you are sleeping.
• Pharmacologic aids	Do you take any medications to help you sleep?
	Are you taking any medicine at all?
Sleep disturbances and contributing factors	
• Nature of the sleep disturbance	Tell me about your sleep problem.
• Onset of disturbance	How often does it occur?
• Causes (physical, psychosocial, medicine related)	Are you doing anything differently now that might be causing the problem?
• Severity	Do you wake up gasping for air?
• Symptoms	Do you snore?
	Do you recall changing your position frequently during the night?
• Interventions attempted and results	What have you been doing to deal with the problem?

- Approximate time client falls asleep
- Time of any awakenings during the night and when sleep was resumed
- Time of awakening in the morning
- Presence of any stressors client believes are affecting his or her sleep
- A record of any food, drink, or medication client believes has positively or negatively influenced his or her sleep (include time of ingestion)
- Record of physical activities—type, duration, and time
- Record of mental activities—type, duration, and time
- Record of activities performed 2 to 3 hours before bedtime, bedtime rituals, changes in sleep environment
- Presence of any worries or anxieties client believes are affecting his or her sleep

It is helpful if the client has a bed partner who can assist with the diary. It should be stressed to the client that the diary is simply a diagnostic tool. If keeping the diary causes too much stress for the client and further interferes with his or her ability to sleep restfully, it should be discontinued.

Physical Assessment

Physical findings during the nursing examination should either confirm that the client is getting sufficient rest to provide energy for the day's activities or validate the existence of a sleep disturbance that is decreasing the quantity or quality of sleep. Key findings include energy level (presence of physical weakness, fatigue, lethargy); facial characteristics (narrowing or glazing of eyes, swelling of eyelids, decreased animation); behavioral characteristics (yawning, rubbing eyes, slow speech, slumped posture). Data suggestive of potential sleep problems (eg, obesity, enlarged neck, deviated nasal septum) may also be noted.

If the nurse or a bed partner is able to observe the client sleeping, other sleep characteristics to assess include restlessness, sleep postures, and sleep activities such as snoring or leg jerking (nocturnal myoclonus).

Snoring Snoring is caused by an obstruction to the air flow through the nose and mouth. Other than disturbing people sharing the same bedroom, snoring is ordinarily not considered to be a sleeping disorder. However, snoring accompanied by apnea can present a problem. When snoring changes from the characteristic "sawing wood" sound to a more irregular silence followed by a snorting, this is indicative of obstructive apnea.

Nocturnal Myoclonus Observed in 10% to 20% of chronic insomniacs, **nocturnal myoclonus** involves marked muscle contraction that results in the jerking of one or both legs during sleep. The jerking lasts about 28 seconds and may arouse the sleeper. *Restless leg syndrome* is a different condition in which the awake individual is unable to lie with his or her body, and especially his or her legs, still long enough to fall asleep. Both conditions may contribute to insomnia.

Diagnosing

Sleep Pattern Disturbance as the Problem When assessment data point to a sleep problem that is amenable to nursing therapy, it receives the label Sleep Pattern Disturbance and may then be further specified:

Insomnia: Difficulty falling asleep
Insomnia: Difficulty remaining asleep
Insomnia: Premature awakening
Hypersomnia: Excessive daytime sleeping
Sleep deprivation
Altered sleep–wake patterns

Common etiologies for sleep pattern disturbances include the following:

Physical discomfort or pain
Emotional discomfort or pain caused by anxiety and stress
Changes in bedtime rituals or sleep environments
Disruption of circadian rhythm
Exercise just before sleep
Caffeine, nicotine, or alcohol after dinner
Drug dependency and withdrawal
Symptoms of physical illness

Sample nursing diagnoses in which the sleep disturbance is the primary problem are presented in the accompanying display.

Sleep Pattern Disturbance as the Etiology Sleep pattern disturbances may affect many other areas of human functioning. In the nursing diagnoses that follow, the sleep pattern disturbance is the etiology of another problem:

Anxiety related to inability to fall asleep, inability to control behavior while asleep, sleep apnea—threat of death
Activity Intolerance related to sleep deprivation
Ineffective Individual Coping related to insomnia: Insufficient quantity and quality of sleep
Fear related to narcoleptic's potential to harm himself or herself, or others
Impaired Gas Exchange related to sleep apnea (oxygen saturation of the blood)
High Risk for Injury related to somnambulism, narcolepsy, sleep apnea
Knowledge Deficit (specify: eg, nonpharmacologic remedies for insomnia) related to misinformation, lack of interest in learning, cognitive limitation
Self-Esteem Disturbance related to effects of sleep deprivation (hypersomnia or sleep apnea syndrome)
Anxiety related to nocturnal enuresis
Impaired Social Interaction related to excessive daytime sleeping, sleep deprivation
Altered Thought Processes related to chronic insomnia, sleep deprivation

Important Distinctions Because the *problem statement* of the nursing diagnosis identifies what is wrong with the client and suggests the client goals and the *etiology* of the problem directs nursing interventions, it is important for

N U R S I N G   D I A G N O S E S   F O R   C O M M O N   P R O B L E M S

Sleep

Problem	Related Factors	Sample Defining Characteristics
Sleep Pattern Disturbance: Difficulty Falling Asleep	Worries about family and lack of destressing rituals	• "At least four of five nights a week I lay in bed awake for 3 or 4 hours before I finally fall asleep. Sometimes it is two or three in the morning and I'm still awake worrying about the kids. I've tried getting up and reading or paying my bills, but even that doesn't make me sleepy." • Reports problem falling asleep for past 6 months; is widowed and very concerned about two teenage sons. Never sleeps until both sons are home. States she does nothing special to relax. Feels her worries are "her business"—no support person with whom she shares these.
Sleep Pattern Disturbance: Difficulty Remaining Asleep	Noise of hospital environment and need for periodic treatments	• Admitted to hospital 3/6/93; cholecystectomy 3/7/93 • "I don't think I've had one decent night's sleep since my surgery. I've been falling asleep about 9 PM and then someone wakes me up for my medicine. I just about get back to sleep and someone's putting the light on to poke at my dressing or to check this tube. I know I'm getting grouchy." • Orders include every-4-hour vital signs; nursing assessment of the incision, nasogastric tube, intravenous therapy; and medication for pain and for sleep.
Sleep Pattern Disturbance: Premature Awakening	Barbiturate dependency and lack of knowledge of nonpharmacologic aids for insomnia	• Client has history of mild to moderate depression, related to loss of job and perceived role inadequacy, for the past 3 years; has been taking secobarbital (Seconal), a barbiturate hypnotic, 100 mg by mouth nightly for the past year and a half.

the nurse analyzing the assessment data to decide if the sleep data are indicative of the problem, are contributing to a different problem, or are signs or symptoms of the problem. For some reason, sleep data seem to fit well in all three categories. For example, when altered sleep–wake patterns are noted in the graduate nurse who is getting adjusted to a new full-time job, shift work, and increased independence, three different diagnoses might be written.

Sleep Pattern Disturbance: Altered Sleep–Wake Pattern (Insomnia) related to shift work and stress of new job as manifested by complaints of always feeling tired and never getting enough sleep

Altered sleep–wake patterns are the problem statement; priority nursing energies are directed to changing these patterns and to helping the client achieve both the necessary quantity and quality of sleep.

Ineffective Individual Coping related to multiple stresses of new job and altered sleep–wake patterns (→ sleep deprivation) as manifested by statements like "I don't know how much longer I can do this." "I'm always tired anymore and all I want to do is sleep." "I'm so grouchy—people must hate me!"

Here, the altered sleep–wake patterns is just one of the factors contributing to the client's problem of ineffective coping; priority nursing energies are directed toward improving the client's coping skills; by teaching the client how to increase the quantity and quality of sleep.

Ineffective Individual Coping related to multiple stressors and lack of destressing rituals as manifested by inability to fall asleep (altered sleep–wake patterns); excessive fatigue; and feelings that personality is changing

In this instance, altered sleep–wake patterns are merely a symptom of the client's actual problem—ineffective coping; it is expected that when the coping problem is resolved, the symptom will disappear.

None of the preceding diagnoses is more correct than the others. With each client, the nurse must make a deci-

Problem	Related Factors	Sample Defining Characteristics
		• "I seem to be waking up earlier and earlier, can't fall back asleep, and I start each day feeling like I have a hangover."
		• "I'd like to get off these drugs, but I'm terrified that without them I won't sleep at all."
Sleep Pattern Disturbance: Excessive Daytime Sleeping	Altered sleep cycle and inability to cope with multiple stresses	• Only child, first-year college student who is living away from home for the first time. Shares a dormitory room with a roommate. Sleep patterns are erratic and depend on school and social demands. Has recently broken up with high school boyfriend. Fears she is failing three courses. Has no desire to do anything but sleep. "When I get up my only thought is: When can I go back to bed? I often sleep through class."
Sleep Pattern Disturbance: Excessive Daytime Sleeping	Effects of biologic aging (moderate increase in stage I and II sleep; slow-wave sleep, stages III and IV, decreases by 50% or more)	• Male client, aged 74, complains during his annual physical that he seems to be napping more during the day, yet when he tries to fall asleep at night he often cannot.
		• "I'm spending more time in bed, but I'm less rested. Worst of all is not knowing whether or not I'll be awake enough to drive my car or enjoy a good card game."
Sleep Pattern Disturbance: Altered Sleep–Wake Patterns	Frequent rotations of shift and overtime	• Graduate nurse, 24 years old, who has been working on a busy medical floor for 6 months; rotates 11–7 and 7–3 shifts; recently a problem with staffing has necessitated frequent rotations. Client often volunteers (two or three times a week) for overtime.
		• "I don't know what is wrong with me. I'm so tired anymore and don't feel at all like myself. All I want to do when I'm off is to sleep—but often I can't fall asleep when I lay down. Please help!"

sion with each cluster of significant data and pull out the key problem, contributing factors, and related signs and symptoms. How the diagnosis is developed directs the nursing interventions.

Planning: Client Goals

Rest and sleep are essential components of well-being. Planning for client care, especially in the hospital, involves planning with the client suitable measures to promote rest and sleep. Whenever nurses care for a client, nursing measures support the following client goals. The client will:

• Maintain a sleep–wake pattern that provides sufficient energy for the day's tasks
• Demonstrate self-care behaviors that provide a healthy balance between rest and activity

When the client's physical, psychosocial, or spiritual condition contributes to sleep disturbances, individualized client goals are developed. For example,

• By 1/10/94, the client will identify two stress relieving rituals that will enable him or her to fall asleep more easily.
• The client will demonstrate decreased signs of sleep deprivation by 3/8/94,
  Is attentive to conversation
  Has ability to concentrate on complex task (eg, learning about new medication)
  Verbalizes feeling less fatigued and more in control of situation

Implementing

Because sleep problems are often not the primary reason for a client's interaction with the health care system, the key to their detection is often the attitude the nurse communicates to the client. Clients who believe the nurse is generally concerned about their well-being are not reluctant to discuss insomnia or voice concern about a child who is a bedwetter. Fundamental to the success of any nursing measure to correct a sleep problem is the client's belief that the nurse cares and is readily available for extra help to promote rest and sleep.

Preparing a Restful Environment

Having a comfortable bed helps promote rest and sleep. The bottom linen should be tight and clean. The upper linen, while secure, should allow freedom of movement and should not exert pressure, especially over the legs and feet. Having the body in good alignment is conducive to relaxation. For clients who must assume unusual positions because of their illness, ingenuity and skill are necessary to keep muscle strain and discomfort at a minimum. For example, the client who must remain in the orthopneic position to aid breathing should be well supported in a manner that relieves muscle strain.

A quiet and darkened room, with privacy, is relaxing for nearly everyone. In a strange environment, unfamiliar noises, such as people walking or entering and leaving the room, and the closing of elevator doors, bring complaints from most hospitalized clients. Although some of these sources are difficult for the nurse to control, every effort should be made toward reducing disturbances to promote relaxation and sleep.

The temperature of the room, the amount of ventilation, and the quantity of bed covering are matters of individual choice. The client's wishes should be met when at all possible.

Promoting Bedtime Rituals

Most people have bedtime rituals to help relaxation and promote sleep. Reading, listening to the radio, watching television, talking to a family member, and praying are common before-sleep activities. Children may search out a favorite doll, stuffed toy, or blanket before going to bed; insist on a bedtime story; kiss everyone goodnight; and say prayers before bed. Readiness for sleep is preceded by a personal hygiene routine for many people, such as brushing teeth, washing hands and face, voiding, or taking a bath or shower. Snacks are important elements in the bedtime rituals of many children and adults. Whereas it is true that eating the wrong foods may produce a bad night's sleep, going to bed hungry may also interfere with sleep.

The nurse should be alert to the client's bedtime rituals and make every effort to observe them as far as possible to aid in promoting relaxation and sleep. These rituals should appear in the client's care plan so that all health personnel can observe them.

Offering Appropriate Bedtime Snacks and Beverages

Because the dietary amino acid L-tryptophan helps promote sleep, there currently appears to be justification for offering a high-protein beverage, such as milk, or high-protein snacks, such as cheese or nuts, before bedtime when this is allowed in the client's regimen. An alcoholic beverage helps to promote sleep for some people, but, generally, alcohol after dinner should be avoided. For most, beverages containing caffeine should be avoided for at least 4 to 5 hours before bedtime. It is best that the client take fluids during the day and avoid excessive fluid intake before bedtime to help prevent the necessity of using the bathroom during sleeping hours.

Promoting Relaxation

One can relax without sleeping, but sleep rarely occurs until one is relaxed. Stress and anxiety-producing situations tend to interfere with a person's ability to relax, rest, and sleep. Effective means for dealing with worries include dealing with problems as they arise; conditioning oneself to worry only during preset times; teaching oneself that worrying never solves problems and is counterproductive; and giving the worries over to another (eg, a trusted family member or friend, caregiver, or God). The distraction and relaxation techniques described in Chapters 9 and 32 may be beneficial when counseling a client whose worries are contributing to a sleep disturbance. Back rubs, warm baths, and face washing if the client is bedridden are typical nursing measures to help the client relax. The technique for back massage is given in Procedure 32-1.

Promoting Comfort

One of the greatest deterrents to rest and sleep is pain; it is often a realistic experience when illness is present. Depending on the cause and severity of the discomfort or pain, appropriate nursing measures include remaining with a lonely and frightened child or adult, using the simple strategy of caring presence and touch, offering a back massage, obtaining an extra blanket, or administering an analgesic. These and other nursing techniques to promote comfort are described in Chapter 32. However, the nurse must be sensitive to the client's discomfort before he or she can relieve it.

Respecting Normal Sleep–Wake Patterns

Every effort should be made to observe the client's normal periods of sleep. In many instances, it is hardly necessary to insist that all clients retire and awaken at specific times. For example, is there a good reason to wake a client at 7 AM when the client ordinarily sleeps until 9 AM? It is also recommended that a client's normal napping habits be followed when possible. It has been observed that REM sleep is common during morning naps whereas NREM sleep is common during naps later in the day. With this knowledge, the nurse can help the client plan napping periods that best fit individual needs and that interfere least with nighttime sleeping.

Scheduling Nursing Care to Avoid Unnecessary Disturbance

Common client complaints are that they are awakened to take sleeping pills and are aroused at early morning hours to prepare for breakfast long before it is served. These common observations should be considered when planning care that will help most to promote rest and sleep.

Every effort should be made to time care during periods when the client is normally awake. When this cannot be done, it is preferable to avoid awakening the client during REM sleep, when the rapid eye movements can be observed. Because a client's need for sleep is important, priorities should be examined. For example, the nurse should ask if checking a vital sign or carrying out a particular nursing measure is more important than the client's sleep.

Using Medications to Produce Sleep

Medications for sleep are often ordered for clients. Sedative-hypnotics induce sleep; antianxiety drugs reduce anxiety and tension. The sleep produced by sedative-hypnotics is an unnatural sleep. All these drugs disturb either REM or NREM sleep to some degree. Although most sedative-hypnotics provide several nights of excellent sleep, the medication often loses its effect after a week or two. At this point, many people increase the dosage of the medication or complement the drug with alcohol. Vigorous nursing intervention is needed to prevent a client from developing a pattern of drug dependency and alcohol abuse.

Nurses also need to be alert to the dangers of withdrawal symptoms that can accompany the abrupt cessation of barbiturate sedative-hypnotics. Progressive withdrawal symptoms include weakness, tremulousness, restlessness, insomnia, increased pulse and heart rates, anxiety, convulsions, psychosis, continued seizures, and death.

Flurazepam (Dalmane), a popular nonbarbiturate sedative-hypnotic, disturbs NREM slow-wave sleep, which results in daytime drowsiness and the morning hangover effect. Some people counteract this side effect by taking amphetamines, or uppers. The antianxiety medications, once hoped to be the answer to the sleeping pill dilemma, are increasingly implicated in physical and psychologic dependence.

Many times these medications are ordered on a prn (as needed) basis. The nurse should administer these medications only when indicated and always with full knowledge of their limitations. Thorough client teaching should accompany their use. Nurses should aid clients in developing other self-care strategies, including developing healthy sleep and life-style behaviors.

Teaching the Client About Rest and Sleep

A well-informed person is better able to cope with distressing situations. Helping clients and their families understand the nature of rest and sleep and their importance to well-being through teaching is an important nursing function. Teaching should include aspects of normal variations in sleep patterns and common measures to promote relaxation and sleep. Also, the care plan should be discussed with the client for acceptability. When sleep disorders become a problem and common nursing measures are inadequate, the nurse can assist and teach by recommending the services of health practitioners especially prepared to deal with them.

NURSING PROCESS

In Clinical Practice

When identifying and treating sleep disturbances categorized as nursing diagnoses, the nurse uses each phase of the nursing process. Quality care depends on the nurse's possession of the knowledge and clinical skills described earlier in this chapter. What follows are the assessment priorities, client goals, nursing interventions, and evaluative criteria for two common types of sleep problems treated by nurses: (1) insomnia and (2) sleep deprivation.

Sleep Pattern Disturbance: Insomnia (difficulty falling asleep, difficulty remaining asleep, or premature awakening)

Sleep Pattern Disturbance: Sleep Deprivation

Sleep Pattern Disturbance: Insomnia

Sleep Pattern Disturbance: Insomnia

An inability to obtain the quantity or quality of sleep that is essential for an individual's healthy functioning is insomnia. The knowledge base for insomnia was discussed in Table 31-4. Insomnias may also be classified as transient or chronic (Morton, 1989). Transient insomnia is a difficulty in falling asleep or staying asleep, which has existed for 3 weeks or less and is associated with significant life change. Nursing intervention is directed to helping the client understand the relationship between the sleep problem and the stressor. Chronic insomnias last for longer than 3 weeks and may continue throughout life. They are the most common complaint reported by clients seen in sleep disorder centers. Morton (1989) identified advanced age, and medical, behavioral, and psychiatric problems as causes of chronic insomnia. Other sleep disorders such as sleep apnea may also produce chronic insomnia.

Assessment

- Use interview questions directed to the client and his or her bed partner and direct observation when possible to determine if the insomnia is caused by difficulty falling asleep, periodic awakenings, or early morning awakenings. Determine if the client's perception of his or her sleep–wakefulness pattern corresponds to reality.

- Explore the client's life-style and physical and mental health for contributing factors. Because problems in sexual adjustment or functioning may contribute to insomnia, a sexual history may be indicated.
- Instruct the client to keep a sleep diary that may include a graph of undisturbed hours of sleep per night. Use the diary to relate factors causing or correcting the insomnia to sleep–wakefulness patterns.
- Assess for signs of sleep deprivation.
- Assess the actual and perceived degree of control the client has over his or her insomnia.
- Assess the safety and effectiveness of aids client has used to deal with insomnia.

Planning: Client Goals

The client will:
- Report that his or her regular pattern is reestablished or that a new pattern characterized by ease in falling asleep and diminished or absent nighttime and early morning awakenings is established
- Identify the reversible causes of the insomnia
- Institute life-style changes to eliminate factors contributing to insomnia (eg, decrease caffeine intake)
- Incorporate appropriate destressing rituals into pre-bedtime activities (eg, listening to soothing music, progressive relaxation, prayer)

Interventions

Interventions for insomnia vary according to its cause and severity. Life-style counseling includes the recommendation, when appropriate, for the following:
- Eating high-protein food before bedtime, such as cheese or milk; it is thought that tryptophan from digested protein helps to induce sleep
- Eliminating caffeine and alcohol in the evening because both are known to disrupt the normal sleep cycle
- Decreasing or stopping smoking because nicotine withdrawal can occur 3 hours after the last cigarette and cause sleep restlessness, altered sleep cycle, and early awakening to obtain a cigarette
- Incorporating a period of regular exercise into each day—but not before bedtime; avoiding any stimulating activity before attempting to fall asleep
- Setting aside time for destressing rituals (relaxation exercises, music, conversation, prayer) immediately before retiring; having someone with whom one can share fears, worries, and anxieties is often helpful
- Trying to sleep only when sleepy and not when wakeful

- Observing a regular bedtime hour and awakening hour because biologic clocks are affected by staying up later or rising later in the day
- Avoiding naps during the day and evening because, for some people, the ability to fall asleep is related to the time interval since the last sleep period
- Leaving the bed and bedroom when awake; even if this occurs during the night, the client should take up a quiet, nonstimulating activity (reading, television, music) in another room—so that the bed remains firmly associated with sleep

Independent nursing measures for insomnia may include all those described earlier in the chapter. The nurse may also need to collaborate with the physician in determining the best course of action if the client's insomnia is drug related. Clients who have used hypnotic medications for a long time will probably benefit most from a gradual program of withdrawal and will value nursing support throughout this process. On the other hand, a short course of treatment with a sedative-hypnotic or antianxiety agent may be indicated, in which case the nurse works collaboratively with the prescribing physician and teaches the client the action of the drug, the reason it is being used, safe administration particulars, side-effects to watch for and to report, and potential dangers of overreliance on medication.

For severe problems of insomnia, referral for psychiatric evaluation and treatment may be necessary. Clients may also be referred to a sleep disorder clinic (for listings, write: The Association of Sleep Disorders Centers, P.O. Box 2604, Del Mar, CA 92014; phone: 619-755-6566).

Evaluative Criteria

- The client meets the previously stated goals.

Sleep Pattern Disturbance: Sleep Deprivation

Shortchanging one's sleep rarely results in any serious problems, but a prolonged pattern of sleep deprivation produces symptoms progressing from irritability and fatigue to generalized personality disintegration. There are basically three types of sleep deprivation:

REM deprivation (absence of dreaming): Caused by certain drugs (especially alcohol and barbiturates), general sleep disturbances (eg, shift work, travel, or hospitalization—especially in intensive care setting). When people are denied dreaming during normal REM sleep, they become irritable, insecure, and anxious. Also, their sensitivity to pain increases, they are unable to concentrate, and they exercise poor judgment. Relationships with other people suffer. Depression is a common mental symptom, and in extreme cases, a person's ethical standards have been known to deteriorate. Symptoms of psychoses have appeared in rational people after prolonged REM sleep deprivation. These same subjects, when allowed to sleep uninterrupted, experience more frequent REM periods, as if the body were trying to make up for losses. It has been observed that when people are denied REM sleep for whatever reason, REM sleep with dreaming, often including nightmares, increases. Similarly, when stage IV NREM sleep is denied, the person tries to catch up on lost NREM sleep. If both REM and NREM sleep are insufficient, stage IV NREM sleep increases.

NREM deprivation (delta sleep or SWS deprivation): Causes may be the same as for REM deprivation, and also may include continual interruption of the sleep cycle (eg, with frequent treatments); certain medications (eg, diazepam [Valium]; flurozepam [Dalmane]; and morphine); and conditions such as sleep apnea, hypothyroidism, and diseases causing respiratory distress. Elderly people frequently experience lack of NREM sleep. Symptoms include fatigue, lethargy, depression, and difficulty in executing the repetitive tasks of everyday living.

Total sleep deprivation: Rarely occurs except in controlled laboratory situations. Symptoms of total sleep loss occur in a relatively slow but predictable pattern, mounting as time goes on. As weariness begins, normal performance fades off with lapses in attention and concentration. Unpleasant sensations, such as blurred vision, glazed and itching eyes, nausea, and headache are common symptoms of fatigue. Hallucinations and illusions eventually become vivid, and mental confusion and inability to determine reality occur. There may be a lack of memory, a decrease in intellectual effort, and an attitude of not caring what happens.

Exactly why sleeplessness leads to ill effects is unknown. It is unknown whether irreversible damage to body tissue results from prolonged or chronic sleep deprivation. However, that sleep deprivation produces changes in physical and mental functioning supports observations that sleep is essential for well-being.

RESEARCH IN NURSING Making a Difference

Strategies to Promote Sleep in Elderly Clients

The human body uses sleep for rest, recuperation, and adaptation to physical and emotional stress. Although sleep disturbances may occur at any age, it has been documented that the older adult often experiences difficulty in achieving restful sleep. Sleep disturbances in this age group have been the topic of nursing research, with the goal of developing nursing interventions to promote rest and sleep.

Related Research

Young, S., Muir-Nash, J., & Ninos, M. (1988). Managing nocturnal wandering behavior. *Journal of Gerontological Nursing 14*(5), 7–11.

These authors studied the pattern of night wandering behavior in inpatient geriatric clients with Alzheimer's disease. The use of "modified white noise," which consists of low-intensity, slow, continuous, monotonous sounds such as the whirl of a fan or the sound of the surf did decrease nocturnal restlessness in one fourth of the subjects. This suggests that a noninvasive intervention rather than chemical means or physical restraints also may be effective in managing the nocturnal agitation commonly observed with Alzheimer's disease.

Walgenbach, J. (1990). Lullaby and not a good night? *Geriatric Nursing 11*(6), 278–279.

This study examined the effects of high noise levels (anything louder than 35 decibels) on sleep deprivation in residents of a long-term care facility. Symptoms accompanying alteration in the depth and duration of sleep in elders frequently lead to misdiagnosis. Sleep disrupted by environmental sound was not statistically correlated in this study to diminished well-being in these elder adults but nursing interventions to decrease noise pollution were identified.

Gall, K., Petersen, T., & Riesch, S. (1990). Night life: Nocturnal behavior patterns among hospitalized elderly. *Journal of Gerontological Nursing 16*(10), 31–35.

This investigation examined the nocturnal activity patterns of hospitalized geriatric clients and determined that medications, treatments, and assessments regularly interrupt their sleep pattern. As a client advocate, the nurse can positively influence the sleep cycle by integrating the client's treatment regimen with the client's usual pattern of nocturnal behavior. Providing adequate pain relief and eliminating unnecessary noise and interruptions further promote a healthy sleep environment.

Summary

Implications from nursing research about sleep in elderly clients include creating a physical environment that is conducive to a restful night, assessing for symptoms of sleep deprivation, and incorporating measures for a healthy sleep cycle into the nursing care plan.

Assessment

- Use interview questions directed to the client and family and observation skills to determine the type of sleep deprivation, its probable causes, its effect on everyday functioning, and the severity of the problem.
- Instruct the client to keep a sleep diary and note increases or decreases in quality sleep and the factors that contribute to or detract from quality sleep.
- Assess the actual and perceived amount of control the client has over his or her sleep–wakefulness patterns.

Planning: Client Goals

The client will:
- Keep a sleep diary (if feasible) until factors causing sleep deprivation and factors that facilitate sleep are identified
- If indicated, change or eliminate life-style behavior contributing to sleep deprivation
- Increase REM and NREM sleep until usual sleep cycle is reestablished (specify)
- Increase REM and NREM sleep until behaviors indicating sleep deprivation (specify) are no longer present

Interventions

As soon as the cause of the sleep deprivation has been identified, nursing measures are instituted to eliminate the cause or to modify either it or the client's response:
- If insomnia is the cause, the nurse institutes the interventions for insomnia described earlier.
- If hospitalization is the cause, appropriate nursing measures include the following:
  - Familiarizing the client with the hospital environment
  - Recreating the client's usual sleep environment as much as possible: favorite pillow, dim light or darkness, ventilation, door open or closed, child's favorite toy

- Respecting the client's presleep habits and rituals when these are sleep producing—eating an evening snack of milk, watching the 11 PM news, listening to music, taking a warm shower or bath, using relaxation exercises, praying
- Using good nursing care measures to ensure the client's comfort before he or she falls asleep: body is repositioned and in good alignment, supported if necessary; bed linens are clean and straightened; client is free of pain; tubes are patent and draining; equipment is functioning optimally (if frequent checks are needed throughout the night [eg, with an intravenous line] keeping a soft night light on continuously may be less distressing than having each nurse fumble for a light); finally, if pharmacologic aids are to be used to promote sleep, a determination should first be made that they are not negatively interfering with REM or NREM sleep
- Carefully evaluating the need for nursing interventions throughout the night that are likely to awaken the client and to schedule nursing care to allow the client the longest periods of undisturbed rest; careful assessment of the sleeping client also allows the nurse to determine when a sleep cycle is completed and when it might be best to awaken the client
- If medications are contributing to sleep deprivation, the nurse needs to consult with the physician regarding the advisability of their use and possible substitutes.
- When alcohol is contributing to sleep deprivation, the nurse needs to teach the client about alcohol's effects in the body and counsel the client about decreasing or eliminating alcohol intake.
- When sleep deprivation results from shift work, travel, and so forth, the nurse must explore with the client the need for this activity and suggest means to compensate if the activity is necessary.

Evaluative Criteria

- The client meets the previously stated goals.

C A S E   S T U D Y

Mr. Bitner is an 86-year-old alert, black, widowed man who was admitted to a nursing home 2 months ago. He is ambulatory and performs most of his self-care. Admitting medical diagnoses included diabetes mellitus and hypertension. He adds to this list "a touch of arthritis." His daughter complains to the charge nurse that her dad seems to be spending more and more time during the day napping and that he says he does not sleep well at night.

Assessment Findings

A comprehensive sleep assessment of Mr. Bitner following his daughter's expression of concern revealed the following data.

Sleep–Wakefulness Pattern
- Client goes to bed between 8 and 9 PM and gets out of bed between 7 and 8 AM because the staff are getting

his roommate out of bed at this time. He states he never falls asleep before midnight because he always watched the late news at home. He usually wakens twice during the night to void and often cannot fall back asleep.

- During the day, client is frequently observed dozing in his chair. If not discouraged, he returns to his room midmorning and afternoon for a 1-hour nap.

Effect of Sleep Pattern on Everyday Living

- Client states: "I'm always tired. I don't seem to have much energy anymore."
- Client has not socialized yet with other residents, and without strong encouragement does not participate in group activities.
- From his point of view, life holds little reason for him to be awake. "I worked for the railroad for almost 50 years and I never overslept once."

Sleep Aids

- Client denies ever using medication to fall asleep. States he often relaxed at home in the evening with a couple of beers.
- Client likes a dim light on during the night so he can find the bathroom easily and likes his bedroom door ajar.
- Client sleeps with two blankets and is often still cold.

Sleep Disturbances and Contributing Factors

- Client states: "Ever since my wife died, I'm just not getting enough sleep and since I came here it's worse. I don't know why I don't fall asleep when I go to bed or why I wake up so much. It sure makes the nights long."
- Client has no regular periods of exercise and drinks black coffee with every meal and one or two diet colas in the evening.

Nursing Diagnosis

Sleep Pattern Disturbance: Difficulty Falling Asleep and Remaining Asleep related to new sleep environment and schedule, evening caffeine intake, and insufficient meaningful daytime activity

Planning: Client Goals

Mr. Bitner is eager to do anything that will help him to get a better night's sleep, and his daughter is supportive. During the planning process, it is important to communicate to Mr. Bitner and his daughter that some of his sleep disturbance may be an unavoidable result of aging. It is not that less sleep is needed, but that the ability to sleep well seems to diminish with age. Planning will be directed toward strengthening the sleep–wake cycle rhythm and combating the age-related tendency to develop several brief sleep episodes in a 24-hour period (see the Nursing Care Plan).

During a family conference attended by Mr. Bitner, his daughter, the primary nurse, the unit's social worker, and the activity director, Mr. Bitner endorsed the following goals.

Short-Term Goals

By the next monthly assessment, 1/20/94, the client will:

- Retire after viewing the 11 PM news in the TV room with Mr. Sparter
- Report that he falls asleep within 1 hour of getting into bed
- Decrease nighttime awakenings to one, after which he returns to a sound sleep
- Attend the center's exercise sessions Monday through Friday at 10 AM
- Substitute noncaffeine beverages for coffee and cola at supper and evening snack
- Report obtaining a minimum of 6 hours of quality sleep nightly

To assist him in achieving these short-term goals, Mr. Bitner's daughter will bring her father noncaffeine cola and include a walk in her visits to her father.

Long-Term Goals

Mr. Bitner establishes a new sleep–wakefulness pattern that provides sufficient energy for daytime activities:

- Six to 7 hours of quality sleep nightly
- Daytime napping decreased to one nap anytime before evening meal

Implementation

In implementing the care plan, the nurse needs the following specialized abilities:

- Strong assessment skills and knowledge of how aging affects sleep–wakefulness patterns. The following common sleep complaints of older adults are related to changes in the proportion of REM and NREM sleep and to alterations in the quality of sleep that are consistent signs of biologic aging: spending more time in bed, taking longer to fall asleep, awakening more often, being sleepy in the daytime, and needing longer to adjust to changes in the usual sleep–wake schedule (Emra & O'Herrerra, 1989).
- Knowledge of the multiple factors that contribute to insomnia and its severity; knowledge of which insomnias can be independently treated by nursing.
- Interpersonal skills to communicate to both Mr. Bitner and his daughter that something can be done to improve the duration and quality of his sleep and that nursing is committed to helping.
- Teaching and counseling skills to help Mr. Bitner understand the relationship between life-style factors (eg, decreased exercise, caffeine, lack of meaningful activity) and his sleep difficulty and to initiate the necessary changes.
- Interpersonal and leadership skills to motivate the

nursing staff to value Mr. Bitner's goals and to work collaboratively with the social worker and activities director.

Documentation

Sample documentation of the family conference follows.

Traditional Note Format

12/20/93, nursing

Family conference to discuss Mr. Bitner's sleep disturbance—initiated by daughter's concern. Present were Mr. Bitner and his daughter (A. Jelner); K. Behner (social worker); W. Quing (activity director); and M. LeBon (primary nurse). Primary nurse presented findings from comprehensive sleep assessment; Nursing diagnosis: Sleep Pattern Disturbance: Difficulty Falling Asleep and Remaining Asleep related to new sleep environment and schedule, evening caffeine intake, and insufficient meaningful daytime activity. Discussion centered on strategies to help Mr. Bitner develop interests in the center including possibilities for increased physical exercise; decrease his evening caffeine intake (daughter to bring noncaffeine colas); and reestablish usual retiring and waking times. See care plan. Client's progress will be evaluated at next monthly assessment, 1/20/94.

M. LeBon, RN

SOAP Format

12/20/93, 2 PM, nursing
#3 Difficulty falling asleep and remaining asleep

S: "Ever since my wife died I'm just not getting enough sleep and since I came here, it's worse."
 Reports fewer than 5 hours sleep nightly with frequent awakenings.
 Reports drinking coffee at every meal and cola in the evening.
O: Frequently observed to be awake at night; often found asleep in chair during the day; rarely observed at center's activities.
A: Sleep Pattern Disturbance related to new sleep environment and schedule, evening caffeine intake, and insufficient meaningful daytime activity (exercise)
P: 1. Attempt to reestablish his usual retiring and waking times
 2. Decrease caffeine intake, especially in the evening
 3. Increase his participation in center activities, especially exercise program
 Reevaluate sleep status at next monthly assessment, 1/20/94.

M. LeBon, RN

Evaluation

Short-term goal achievement is evaluated at next monthly assessment. See the care plan for related evaluative statements and revisions of the care plan. Long-term goal achievement is an ongoing evaluation.

 N U R S I N G C A R E P L A N

for Mr. Bitner

Nursing Diagnosis:	Sleep Pattern Disturbance: Difficulty Falling Asleep and Remaining Asleep related to new sleep environment and schedule, evening caffeine intake, and insufficient meaningful daytime activity
Long-Term Goal:	Client establishes a new sleep–wakefulness pattern that provides sufficient energy for daytime activities: (1) 6 to 7 hours of quality sleep nightly, (2) daytime napping decreased to one consistent nap time anytime before evening meals
Goal:	By the next monthly assessment, 1/20/94, the client will: • Retire after viewing the 11 PM news in the TV room with Mr. Sparter

Nursing Actions	**Rationale**	**Evaluative Statement**
Assess advisability of reestablishing Mr. Bitner's usual retiring pattern of going to bed after the 11 PM news. Assess how client spends the time from the evening meal to 11 PM—explore relaxing alternatives with him. Investigate possibility that he and Mr. Sparter might become social partners.	Strengthens the natural rhythm of his sleep–wake cycle. Elimination of evening naps will facilitate his falling asleep more easily.	1/18/94 Goal met. Client does not go to bed until after the news and has been observed talking with Mr. Sparter. *Recommendation:* Continue to develop evening activities with him—he finds that the time after supper "drags."

M. LeBon, RN

for Mr. Bitner

Goal: By the next monthly assessment, 1/20/94, the client will:
• Report that he falls asleep within 1 hour of getting into bed

Nursing Actions	Rationale	Evaluative Statement
Continue to assess how long it takes client to fall asleep after getting into bed.	In elderly clients, stage I time is increased.	1/18/94 Goal partially met. Three or four nights a week he falls asleep within 30 minutes of going to bed. States he really misses comfort of his wife.
Explore with client means to relax before falling asleep—deep breathing, imagery, prayer.	Activities that calm and relax the person prepare the body for sleep.	
Teach the importance of using the bed only as a place to sleep. Advise client when he cannot sleep to get out of bed and to go to another room where he can perform some monotonous activity (watching television, listening to radio).	This maintains the bed as a powerful stimulus for sleep and helps to prevent "conditioned" insomnia ("Well, here I am in bed now and I know sleep won't come").	*Revision:* Investigate client's sense of loss and need for touch. May be a good candidate for pet therapy program. *M. LeBon, RN*

Goal: By the next monthly assessment, 1/20/94, the client will:
• Decrease nighttime awakenings to one after which he returns to a sound sleep

Nursing Actions	Rationale	Evaluative Statement
Assess and manipulate factors that contribute to nighttime awakenings: • Need to void (time of day diuretic is taken, amounts of fluid intake in the evening) • Roommate's wakefulness, snoring, or need for care • Uncomfortableness in strange environment • Comfort (eg, temperature)	Individualizing the client's bedtime environment and meeting comfort needs (warmth, soft light, and so forth) promote sleep onset and maintenance	1/18/94 Goal partially met. Nighttime awakenings vary from none to three nightly. See previous revision. *M. LeBon, RN*
Teach client how, on awakening, to concentrate on breathing until he falls back to sleep.	This uses the power of positive thinking to facilitate return to sleep.	

Goal: By the next monthly assessment, 1/20/94, the client will:
• Attend the center's exercise sessions Monday through Friday at 10 AM

Nursing Actions	Rationale	Evaluative Statement
Assess whether client understands the relation between daily exercise and his ability to sleep.	Regular exercise throughout the day is known to increase physical fatigue and to promote sleep. Exercise or stimulating activities immediately before retiring interfere with sleep's onset.	1/20/94 Goal met. Client has become an enthusiastic participant in exercise sessions—attends daily. *L. Fox, RN*

(continued)

N U R S I N G C A R E P L A N (continued)

for Mr. Bitner

Determine how his exercise needs can best be met (ie, through a group program or an individualized program of walking, or other program)

Exercise program must be individualized based on physical state and interests of client.

Use positive verbal reinforcement to communicate to client that someone cares that he is using positive means to remedy his sleep disturbance and increase his well-being.

Activity provides the opportunity for socialization and improvement of a self-image.

Encourage client's daughter to go for walks with him when she visits and to question him about his exercise program.

Communication and interaction with family members helps the elderly client to maintain self-esteem and to feel valuable and loved.

Goal: By the next monthly assessment, 1/20/94, the client will:
• Substitute caffeine-free beverages for coffee and cola at supper and evening snack

Nursing Actions

Assess client's willingness to substitute caffeine-free beverages for coffee and cola.

Consult with dietary department and his daughter about options. Experiment with options until his preferences are determined.

Gradually reduce his caffeine intake, especially from evening meal onward. Offer a high-protein evening snack.

Rationale

Caffeine is a stimulant that can cause difficulty sleeping.

Caffeine-free versions of beverages are often available and can be used based on client acceptance.

High-protein snack appears to promote sleep.

Evaluative Statement

1/20/94 Goal met. Client now drinks decaffeinated coffee with meals and milk in the evening. Dislikes caffeine-free sodas.

M. LeBon, RN

Goal: By the next monthly assessment, 1/20/94, the client will:
• Report obtaining a minimum of 6 hours of quality sleep nightly

Nursing Actions

Assess Mr. Bitner's progress weekly. Continue to identify factors that contribute to better sleep or interfere with his sleep.

Rationale

Because multiple factors influence sleep-wakefulness cycles in elderly clients, ongoing assessment is needed.

Evaluative Statement

1/20/94 Goal partially met. Mr. Bitner is pleased he is sleeping better but still reports "two or three bad nights" a week. Continue to implement plan and reassess 2/20/94.

M. LeBon, RN

KEY POINTS

- Most people spend about one third of their lives asleep; sleep of some quality and duration is an essential component of well-being.
- Sleep is a state of altered consciousness throughout which varying degrees of stimuli produce wakefulness. It is an active and complex rhythmic state, a progression of repeated cycles.
- The cyclic nature of sleep is controlled by the reticular activating system and bulbar synchronizing region in the brain stem. Biochemical changes and hormones also influence the sleep process.
- Circadian synchronization occurs when an individual's sleep–wake patterns follow the inner biologic clock. Shift work, traveling across time zones, and irregular sleep–wake patterns can easily lead to desynchronization and poor quality sleep and decreased work performance.
- There is both NREM sleep and REM sleep. During a sleep cycle, a person passes through the four stages of NREM sleep and through REM sleep. The average person has four or five complete sleep cycles each night.
- Factors affecting sleep include age, physical activity, psychologic stress, motivation, diet, alcohol intake, caffeine intake, nicotine use, environment, life-style, illness, and medications. Most people with sleep disturbances can initiate life-style changes that will improve sleep.
- Nurses should explore parents' perceptions about the amount of sleep their infant or child needs and the schedule the parent uses for sleep and rest times. Development variations and the need for consistent sleep–wake patterns and bedtime rituals may need to be taught.
- For the young adult, the sleep–wakefulness cycle is the most important of all the rhythmic patterns and the one most likely to be abused. Multiple stressors can interfere with the young adult obtaining sufficient rest and sleep and can encourage the use of alcohol or sleep medications. Teaching needs to include the importance of developing good sleep habits to promote long-term wellness.
- The nurse who wishes to be an effective role model in promoting rest and sleep uses appearance and energy level to communicate to clients the value of proper rest and sleep self-care behaviors.
- A comprehensive sleep history includes data on sleep–wakefulness pattern, the effect of the sleep pattern on everyday functioning, sleep aids, sleep disturbance, and contributing factors.
- When a sleep disturbance exists, the assessment attempts to identify the nature of the problem, its cause, related signs and symptoms, onset and frequency, effect on everyday living, severity, if the problem can be treated independently by nursing, and the coping means the client has used and their success. A sleep diary and information from a bed partner may be needed to establish a diagnosis.
- Common sleep problems include insomnia; hypersomnia; narcolepsy; sleep apnea; parasomnias (sleep walking, sleep talking, enuresis); and sleep deprivation.
- Nursing diagnoses may be written to specifically address sleep pattern disturbances (insomnia: difficulty falling asleep, difficulty remaining asleep, or premature awakening; hypersomnia) or to identify the effect sleep pattern disturbances have on other areas of human functioning (eg, anxiety, comfort, coping, alteration in thought process).
- Nursing interventions to promote rest and sleep include establishing a trusting relationship, preparing a restful sleep environment, attending to bedtime rituals, offering appropriate bedtime snacks, promoting relaxation and comfort, respecting normal sleep–wake patterns, scheduling nursing care to avoid disturbances, using medications to promote sleep, and teaching the client about rest and sleep.

STUDY QUESTIONS

1. A client's body temperature is 99°F (37.2°C) in the late afternoon. This is most likely
   a. a sign of an infection
   b. normal circadian rhythm
   c. hyperpyrexia
   d. due to a warm environment
2. Muscle tone is recorded by the
   a. electroencephalograph (EEG)
   b. electrocardiogram (ECG)
   c. electrooculogram (EOG)
   d. electromyograph (EMG)

3. The nurse observes some involuntary muscle jerking in her sleeping client. The client is most likely in
   a. stage I NREM sleep
   b. stage II NREM sleep
   c. stage IV NREM sleep
   d. REM sleep
4. The nurse observes a slight increase in her client's vital signs when she assesses them while the client is sleeping during the night. According to his stage of sleep, the nurse expects that

a. he is aware of his surroundings at this point
b. he is in delta sleep at this time
c. it would be most difficult to awaken him at this time
d. this is most likely an NREM stage

5. How many cycles of sleep does a person typically go through each night?
   a. 2
   b. 4 or 5
   c. 10
   d. 20 to 25

6. While discussing factors that induce sleep with an elderly client, the nurse teaches her that
   a. dietary protein may interfere with sleep
   b. large quantities of alcohol promote a deep sleep
   c. the amount of REM sleep decreases with age
   d. physical activity decreases REM and NREM sleep

7. A client falls asleep in the middle of a conversation. This disorder is called
   a. hypersomnia
   b. narcolepsy
   c. somnambulism
   d. sleep apnea

8. It is recommended that a sleep diary include all the following *except*
   a. the time the client falls asleep at night
   b. bedtime rituals
   c. a record of daily physical activity
   d. a record of body temperature each evening

9. To help Mr. Yang get to sleep, the nurse suggests that he
   a. follow his usual bedtime routine if possible
   b. drink two or three glasses of water at bedtime
   c. have a large snack at bedtime
   d. take a sedative-hypnotic every night at bedtime

10. The most common complaint of clients visiting sleep disorder clinics is
    a. hypersomnia
    b. narcolepsy

c. chronic insomnia
d. enuresis

11. A prolonged pattern of REM deprivation may result in
    a. symptoms of psychosis
    b. increased episodes of dreaming
    c. decreased sensitivity to pain
    d. increased mental alertness

12. Active dreaming occurs during
    a. stage II NREM
    b. stage III NREM
    c. stage IV NREM
    d. REM sleep

13. Illness is a stressor and can influence sleep during various stages. An example is
    a. asthma attacks appear to occur less frequently during stage IV NREM sleep
    b. a person with heart disease is more likely to have chest pain during NREM sleep
    c. an epileptic is more likely to have seizures during REM sleep
    d. an increase in gastric secretion in a person with an ulcer will most likely occur in NREM sleep

14. Caffeine is a known stimulant and intake should be
    a. avoided at least 30 minutes before bedtime
    b. combined with milk to counteract its effect
    c. avoided at least 4 to 5 hours before bedtime
    d. encouraged during waking hours to counteract effects of sleeplessness

15. Medications that induce sleep (sedative-hypnotics) may disturb REM or NREM sleep. The nurse should be aware that
    a. they should be taken with alcohol for increased effect
    b. these medications usually become ineffective after several weeks
    c. they can usually be given at intervals during the night
    d. they should be combined with daytime use of amphetamines to counteract any hangover effect

Answers With Rationale

1. The correct response is *b*. A slight increase in body temperature in the late afternoon is a normal circadian rhythm. This slight variation from normal does not necessarily mean an infection is present nor is it hyperpyrexia (high fever). A warm environment might possibly cause an elevation in body temperature but the most likely cause is normal circadian rhythm.

2. The correct response is *d*. An EMG measures muscle tone whereas an EEG records electrical currents from the brain. An EOG is a recording of eye movements and an ECG records cardiac activity.

3. The correct response is *a*. Involuntary muscle jerking occurs in stage I NREM sleep. In the other

stages, the muscles proceed from a relaxed state to large muscle immobility.

4. The correct response is *c*. During REM sleep, it is difficult to arouse a person and the vital signs increase. Delta sleep is NREM stage III and IV.

5. The correct response is *b*. A person goes through probably four or five cycles of sleep each night with each cycle lasting 90 to 100 minutes.

6. The correct response is *c*. Dietary protein intake promotes sleep and large quantities of alcohol limit REM and delta sleep. Physical activity increases both REM and NREM sleep.

7. The correct response is *b*. Narcolepsy is an uncontrollable desire to sleep. Hypersomnia refers to ex-

cessive sleep, somnambulism is sleepwalking, and sleep apnea is a period where breathing ceases between snoring.

8. The correct response is *d*. All of the other choices should be included in a sleep diary but a record of the body temperature is insignificant.

9. The correct response is *a*. Drinking two or three glasses of water at bedtime will probably awaken the client during the night to void. A large snack may be uncomfortable right before bedtime and taking a sedative-hypnotic every night disturbs REM and NREM sleep. The sedative also loses its effectiveness shortly.

10. The correct response is *c*. Chronic insomnia is the most common reason why people visit a sleep disorder clinic.

11. The correct response is *a*. Prolonged episodes of REM deprivation may cause symptoms of psychosis. REM deprivation results in an absence of episodes

of dreaming, sensitivity to pain increases, and the person is less mentally alert.

12. The correct response is *d*. Active dreaming occurs during REM sleep.

13. The correct response is *a*. Chest pain occurs more frequently during REM sleep. Epileptic seizures occur more frequently during NREM sleep and gastric secretions increase during REM sleep.

14. The correct response is *c*. Caffeine should be avoided at least 4 to 5 hours before bedtime. Milk does not counteract its effect, and caffeine use is never recommended, even during waking hours.

15. The correct response is *b*. Sedative-hypnotics should never be taken with alcohol because it potentiates their effect. They are usually ordered only at bedtime and may have one repeat order if the client cannot fall asleep. However, they are not given at intervals during the night. Amphetamine use is never recommended.

BIBLIOGRAPHY

Ancoli-Israel, S., Klauber, M., Kripke, D., Parker, L., & Cobarrubias, M. (1989). Sleep apnea in female patients in a nursing home. *Chest, 96*(5), 1055–1058.

Bahr, S., & Mitchell, C. (1987). Response to sleep apnea in Alzheimer's patients and the healthy elderly. *Scholarly Inquiry for Nursing Practice: An International Journal, 1*(3), 237–240.

Balsmeyer, B. (1990). Sleep disturbances of the infant and toddler. *Pediatric Nursing, 16*(5), 447–452.

Barker, J., & Mitteness, L. (1989). Shedding light on nocturia. *Geriatric Nursing, 10*(5), 239–240.

Berman, T. (1990). Sleep disorders: Take them seriously. *Patient Care, 24*(11), 85–88.

Carpenito, L. (1992). *Nursing diagnoses: Application to clinical practice* (4th ed.). Philadelphia: Lippincott.

Childs-Clarke, A. (1990). Stimulus control techniques for sleep onset insomnia. *Nursing Times, 86*(35), 52–53.

Cohen, F. (1988). Narcolepsy: A review of a common lifelong sleep disorders. *Journal of Advanced Nursing, 13*(5), 546–555.

Davis-Sharts, J. (1989). The elder and critical care: Sleep and mobility issues. *Nursing Clinics of North America, 24*(3), 755–764.

Dootson, S. (1990). Sensory imbalance and sleep loss. *Nursing Times, 86*(35), 26–29.

Emra, K., & O'Herrerra, C. (1989). When your patient tells you he can't sleep. *RN, 52*(9), 79–84.

Fossey, E. (1990). Shiftwork can seriously damage your health. *Professional Nurse, 5*(9), 476–480.

Fuller, J., & Schaller-Ayers, J. (1990). *Health assessment: A nursing approach*. Philadelphia: Lippincott.

Jaquis, J. (1987). Obstructive sleep apnea syndrome. *Nurse Practitioner, 12*(6), 51–56.

Klein, L., & Bruce, N. (1989). Night shift work in nursing and biorhythms. *Imprint, 36*(4), 112–115.

Kolcaba, K., & Miller, C. (1989). Geropharmacology treatment. *Journal of Gerontological Nursing, 15*(5), 29–35.

Littrell, K., & Schumann, L. (1989). Sleep in the C.C.U. The impossible dream? *Nursing, 19*(11), 32.

Malasanos L., Barkauskas, V., & Stoltenberg-Allen, K. (1989). *Health assessment* (4th ed.). St. Louis: Mosby.

Mead-Bennett, E. (1990). The relationship of primigravid sleep experience and select moods on the first postpartum day. *Journal of Obstetric, Gynecologic and Neonatal Nursing, 19*(2), 146–151.

Metzler, D., & Finesilver, C. (1990). When to worry if your patient can't sleep. *RN, 53*(3), 52–57.

Morton, P. (1989). *Health assessment in nursing*. Springhouse, PA: Springhouse Corporation.

Murray, R., & Zentner, J. (1989). *Nursing assessment & health promotion strategies through the life span* (4th ed.). Norwalk, CT: Appleton & Lange.

North, A. (1990). The effect of sleep on wound healing. *Ostomy/Wound Management, 27*(2), 56–58.

Oesting, H., & Manza, R. (1988). Sleep apnea. *Geriatric Nursing, 9*(4), 232–233.

Pollack, C., Perlick, D., Linsner, J., Wenston, J., & Hsien, F. (1990). Sleep problems in the community elderly as predictors of death and nursing home placement. *Journal of Community Health, 15*(2), 123–135.

Roberts, A. (1990). Senior systems: Older patients and their medication. *Nursing Times, 86*(11), 14–20.

Skipper, J., Jung, F., & Coffey, L. (1990). Nurses and shiftwork: Effects on physical health and mental depression. *Journal of Advanced Nursing, 15*(7), 835–842.

Stewart, A. (1991). The sleep apnea/hypopnea syndrome. *Canadian Nurse, 87*(10), 25–27.

Walsleben, J., & Baer, L. (1989). Disorders of excessive daytime sleepiness. *Nurse Practitioner, 14*(3), 11–16.

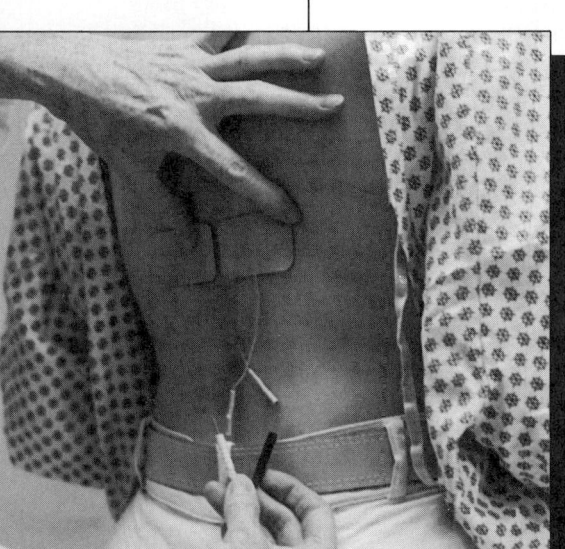

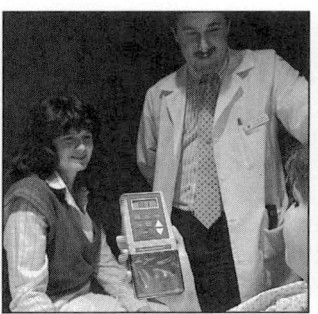
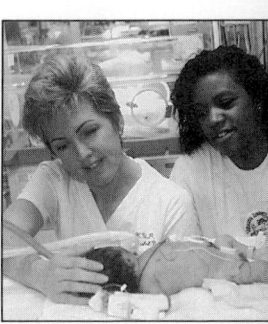

Comfort

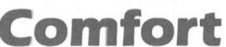

O B J E C T I V E S

After studying this chapter, the learner should be able to:

Define key terms used in the chapter.

Describe specific elements in the pain experience.

Compare and contrast acute and chronic pain.

Identify factors that may affect an individual's pain experience.

Obtain a complete pain assessment using appropriate interviewing and physical assessment skills.

Develop nursing diagnoses that correctly identify pain problems and demonstrate the relation between pain and other areas of human functioning.

Demonstrate the correct use of noninvasive pain-relief measures—distraction, relaxation, cutaneous stimulation.

Administer analgesic agents safely to produce the desired level of analgesia without causing undesirable side effects.

Collaborate with the members of other health disciplines using different treatment modalities to promote pain relief.

Plan, implement, and evaluate nursing care related to select nursing diagnoses for pain problems.

Use teaching and counseling skills to empower clients to direct their own pain management programs.

K E Y   T E R M S

acupressure
acupuncture
acute pain
analgesic drug
chronic pain
continuous subcutaneous
    infusion
contralateral stimulation
cutaneous pain
cutaneous stimulation
dynorphins
endorphins
enkephalins
epidural analgesia
gate control theory
hypnosis
imagery
neuromodulators
nociceptors
opioid
pain
pain threshold
pain tolerance
patient-controlled analgesia
phantom limb pain
placebo
psychogenic pain
referred pain
relaxation
somatic pain
visceral pain

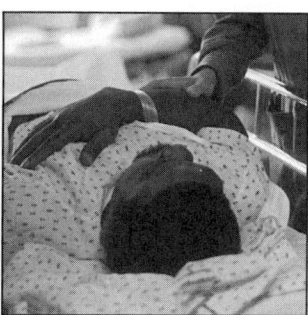

A person in pain often experiences pain as an all-consuming reality and wants only one nursing intervention—pain relief. If pain relief were as simple as rubbing a back or administering a prescribed analgesic, nursing's task would be easy. However, no two people experience pain exactly the same way. Differences in individual pain perception and response to pain as well as the multiple and diverse etiologies of pain require highly specialized abilities of the nurse seeking to promote comfort and relieve pain. The most essential of these are the nurse's belief that the client's pain is real, willingness to become involved in the client's pain experience, and competence in developing effective pain management regimens. Nursing studies repeatedly indicate that although pain is often an all-consuming priority for clients, it is frequently a low priority for nurses because it is an intangible commodity. Unfortunately, it is easier to ignore a client's poorly communicated pain than it is to ignore a dressing that needs to be changed, a client who requires assistance with ambulation, or a prescribed medication. Nurses who somehow manage to practice nursing while remaining insensitive to the comfort needs of their clients do a grave disservice to these clients and to the nursing profession itself.

Nurses are not alone in undervaluing the need for pain management. Although pain is the single most common reason for seeing a physician and the number one reason why people take medication, medical science is still ill equipped to deal with this widespread occurrence. A comprehensive study of pain conducted in 1985 (Donovan, 1990) revealed that most of those interviewed had experienced pain within the past year, with headache, backache, and joint pain occurring with the greatest frequency.

Study of this chapter will provide the student with knowledge of the pain experience and factors that influence it. A detailed guide to assessing alterations in comfort is presented, including specific questions and approaches to use when assessing various pain factors. Numerous examples of nursing diagnoses are offered that either identify specific alterations in comfort or the effects of these alterations on other areas of human functioning. Specific nursing strategies for promoting comfort and assisting clients to achieve pain management goals are detailed. These include establishing a trusting nurse–client relationship; teaching the client about pain; manipulating factors that affect the pain experience; initiating noninvasive pain-relief measures (distraction, relaxation, cutaneous stimu-

lation); assisting with the pain therapies of other disciplines (analgesic administration, hypnosis, acupuncture, biofeedback, local anesthesia, neurosurgery, and electrical nerve stimulation); and evaluating the effects of the care plan. The recently published acute pain management guideline developed by the Agency for Health Care Policy and Research is presented as a standard for effective pain management by nurses (Acute Pain Management Guideline Panel, 1992).

In the section Nursing Process in Clinical Practice, focused assessment, planning, implementation, and evaluation guides are offered for nursing diagnoses of acute and chronic pain problems. These guides and the concluding case study illustrate how the nurse's knowledge of and sensitivity to the client's pain experience may be combined with specific nursing interventions to resolve pain problems successfully.

The Pain Experience

Definition

Pain is an elusive and complex phenomenon, and despite its universality, its exact nature remains a mystery. It is one of the human body's defense mechanisms that indicates the person is experiencing a problem. Aristotle defined pain as well as anyone when he wrote that it is the antithesis of pleasure, the epitome of unpleasantness. Richard Sternback (1968), a psychologist, is credited with the classic definition of pain, which expresses both its sensory and reactive components: "Pain is an abstract concept which refers to (1) a personal, private sensation of hurt; (2) a harmful stimulus which signals current or impending tissue damage; (3) a pattern of responses which operate to protect the organism from harm" (p. 12). The definition of pain that is probably of greatest benefit to nurses and their clients is that offered by Margo McCaffery (1979): "Pain is whatever the experiencing person says it is, existing whenever he (or she) says it does" (p. 11). This definition rests on the belief that the only one who can be a real authority on whether an individual is experiencing pain is that individual.

Pain is present whenever a person says it is, even when no specific cause of the pain can be found. Health practitioners must rely on the client's description of the pain because it is a subjective symptom that only the client can identify and describe.

Origins of Pain

Pain is categorized as cutaneous, deep somatic, or visceral in origin. **Cutaneous** (or superficial) **pain** usually involves the skin or subcutaneous tissue. A paper cut that produces sharp pain with a burning sensation is an example of cutaneous pain. Deep **somatic pain** is diffuse or scattered and originates in tendons, ligaments, bones, blood vessels, and nerves. Strong pressure on a bone or damage to tissue that occurs with a sprain causes deep somatic pain. **Visceral pain** is poorly localized and originates in body organs in the thorax, cranium, and abdomen. This pain may be **referred** or perceived in an area that is distant from its point of origin. Pain associated with a myocardial infarction, or heart attack, is frequently referred to the neck, shoulder, or arms (usually the left arm).

Pain may originate from physical causes, that is, a physical cause for the pain can be identified. Pain may also have a psychogenic origin (**psychogenic pain**), that is, a physical cause for the pain cannot be identified. However, it has been observed that a pure origin is probably rare, and pain usually has both physical and psychogenic components. Furthermore, pain that results from a mental event can be just as intense as pain that results from a physical event.

When the threshold of perception for pain has been reached and when there is injured tissue, it is believed that the injured tissue releases chemicals that excite nerve endings. A damaged cell releases histamine, which excites nerve endings. Lactic acid accumulates in tissues injured by lack of blood supply and is believed to excite nerve endings and cause pain or to lower the threshold of nerve endings to other stimuli (eg, heat or pressure).

Recent research has indicated that other substances are released that also stimulate **nociceptors** or pain receptors. These include bradykinin, prostaglandins, and substance P.

- *Bradykinin*, a powerful vasodilator that increases capillary permeability and constricts smooth muscle, plays an important role in the chemistry of pain at the site of an injury even before the pain message gets to the brain. It also triggers the release of histamine, and in combination with histamine, produces the redness, swelling, and pain typically observed when an inflammation is present.
- *Prostaglandins* are hormonelike substances that send additional pain stimuli to the central nervous system.
- *Substance P* is believed to act as a stimulant at pain receptor sites and may also be involved in the inflammatory response in local tissues (Fuller & Schaller-Ayers, 1990).

T A B L E   3 2 - 1

Common Pain Syndromes

Pain Syndrome	Description
Peripheral Pain Syndromes	
Causalgia	Pain occurs in the area of a partially injured peripheral nerve (the most common lesions are of the brachial plexus or median or sciatic nerve). The pain is described as burning, severe, diffuse, and persistent, and occurs most commonly on the palms of the hands, soles of the feet, and in the digits. Hyperalgesia (excessive sensitivity to pain) and hyperesthesia (excessive sensitivity to stimuli) are often so severe that any stimuli (eg, contact with clothing) can trigger the dreaded pain.
Postherpetic neuralgia	Pain syndrome that follows an acute central nervous system infection primarily of the dorsal root ganglia by the varicella zoster (herpes) virus. The herpes syndrome is characterized by a vesicular eruption and neuralgic pain, which is usually unilateral and encircles the body in bandlike clusters. The severity of the pain may be mild to severe and the quality may be burning, sharp, or dull. In the postherpetic syndrome, severe, intractable pain persists for months and years, with episodes of lightning-like pain in the area of the original eruption.
Phantom limb pain	May occur in any person who has had a body part amputated either surgically or traumatically. Pain varies and may be a severe, burning, fiery sensation; crushing; cramping; a sense that the limb is edematous; or a sensation that the limb is being twisted and distorted. It may be triggered by the sensation of touching the stump, the occurrence of another illness, fatigue, atmospheric changes, and emotional stress.
Central Pain Syndromes	
Thalamic syndrome	Syndrome characterized by severe, spontaneous, and often continuous pain and hyperesthesia on the contralateral side of the lesion in the thalamus. This pain syndrome is often accompanied by a myriad of symptoms resulting from a disturbance in the major relay function of the thalamus.
Trigeminal neuralgia	Paroxysms of lightning-like stabs of intense pain in the distribution of one or more divisions of the trigeminal nerve, the fifth cranial nerve. Pain is usually experienced in the mouth, gums, lips, nose, cheek, chin, and surface of the head, and may be triggered by everyday activities like talking, eating, shaving, or brushing one's teeth. Serious consequences of this syndrome are dehydration, wasting, and exhaustion because clients will refrain from anything that triggers the pain.

Receptors in the skin and superficial organs, although incapable of responding selectively, are stimulated by mechanical, thermal, chemical, and electrical agents. Friction from bed linens and pressure from a cast are mechanical stimulants. Sunburn and cold water on a tooth with caries are thermal stimulants. An acid burn is the result of a chemical stimulant. The jolt of a static charge is an electrical stimulant.

Stretching of the hollow viscera, pulling on the omentum, and muscle spasms result in pain. Some investigators believe that at least some of the deep-lying organs have their own individual pain receptors, the uterus being an example. Some organs, such as the lungs, are insensitive to pain.

It has been observed that pain may be present without injury and may not be present with injury. Therefore, tissue injury does not necessarily accompany pain in all instances. For example, tissue injury is present when the client experiences pain because of a first- or second-degree burn. On the other hand, although physiologic changes do occur, tissue injury or destruction is not necessarily present when the client has a headache owing to psychologic tension. In addition, intensity of pain may not accurately relate to the seriousness of a particular condition giving rise to the pain. Thus, the client may not experience pain until the ravages of a malignancy are beyond control, whereas the severe pain that usually accompanies a bunion is not in keeping with the degree of pathology involved.

Pain Syndromes Although the causes of pain are many, certain major pathologic pain syndromes have been identified to describe the conditions most frequently associated with producing severe or prolonged pain. Common pain syndromes highlighted in Table 32-1 include peripheral pain syndromes (causalgia, postherpetic neuralgia, and phantom limb pain); central pain syndromes (thalamic syndrome, trigeminal neuralgia); and pain with underlying pathology syndromes (musculoskeletal pain syndromes, headache, cancer pain syndrome). Because appropriate treatment of these syndromes is often delayed because of misdiagnosis, nursing can play an important role in their early detection.

Pain Syndrome	Description
Pain With Underlying Pathology Syndromes	
Musculoskeletal pain syndromes	Many conditions are capable of causing severe pain in the musculoskeletal structures—the bones, joints, cartilage, synovial membranes, fibrous sheath, muscles, and tendons. Clients may present with pain that is acute or chronic and local or referred, and that varies in intensity.
Myofascial pain syndrome	Pain in the muscles and fascia; these syndromes are among the most frequent causes of severe disabling pain; characterized by the presence of trigger points in muscles or connective tissue together with a specific syndrome of pain: muscle spasm, tenderness, stiffness, limitation of motion, weakness, and occasionally autonomic dysfunction. Pain is described as dull and aching and its intensity varies from mild to severe and disabling.
Intervertebral disc syndrome	Pain syndrome caused by ruptured, herniated, or prolapsed intervertebral discs; most often occurs in the lower back or cervical area. Pain and limitation are the most frequent symptoms.
Arthritis	Chronic, systemic, often painful disease of connective tissue; one of the major disabling chronic diseases in North America. Rheumatoid arthritis (joint and muscle involvement) is characterized by pain, inflammation, swelling, tenderness, and stiffness in the involved joints. In contrast, osteoarthritis occurs primarily in weight-bearing joints and is benign and slowly progressive.
Headache	The most common type of deep, somatic pain; experienced by about 90% of the population in some form or another. Headaches have multiple intracranial and extracranial causes. A careful analysis of the quality of the pain (dull, deep aching; sharp, throbbing; pressure, tightness): its location; its onset, duration, frequency, and time course; and prodromal signs and symptoms is important in accurately diagnosing the headache.
Cancer pain syndrome	Pain syndromes in cancer patients may develop due to the progression of the disease, as a result of the therapy directed at the control or cure of the disease, or unrelated to the disease.

All of these pain syndromes are capable of causing severe pain.

(Adapted from Meinhart, N.T., & McCaffery, M. [1983]. *Pain: A nursing approach to assessment and analysis.* Norwalk, CT: Appleton-Century-Crofts.)

Transmission of Pain Stimuli

Pain sensations are conducted along pathways that have been rather clearly defined in certain areas but are still somewhat questionable in other areas. There are no specific pain organs or cells in the body. Rather, an interlacing network of undifferentiated free nerve endings receive painful stimuli. Free nerve ending pain receptors include *A delta-fibers*, for fast-conducting, acute, well-localized pain, and *C fibers*, for slow-conducting, diffuse, chronic pain. It is estimated that there are several million of these nerve endings in the body. They are numerous in the layers of the skin and in some internal tissues, such as the joint surfaces. In the deeper tissues of the body, the pain receptors are diffusely but unevenly spread.

Somatic sensation is carried to the dorsal gray horn cells of the spinal cord, then to the spinothalamic tract, and eventually to the cerebral cortex. Although the autonomic nervous system is an efferent system—that is, it carries impulses from the central nervous system—pain sensations from the viscera apparently course along the autonomic system. Through that system, these sensations from deep-lying structures reach the spinal cord by way of the dorsal roots and then continue along the same pathways as sensations from the skin and superficial body structures. Pain impulses are also carried by the cranial nerve to the central nervous system. There is integration of the sensory impulses of pain along its entire central nervous system route, but the highest level of integration occurs in the cortex. Figure 32-1 illustrates the transmission of the pain sensation and the initiation of response.

Referred pain is transmitted to a cutaneous (skin) site different from where it originated. This is possible because *afferent neurons*, or those carrying impulses from the pain receptors toward the brain, enter the spinal cord at the same level as the cutaneous site to which the pain has been referred. Figure 32-2 illustrates cutaneous areas to which pain from various organs is usually referred.

Stimulation of sensory receptors and intactness of their nerve supply are neither necessary nor sufficient conditions for pain. It would seem that a receptor for pain and a nerve route that eventually carries the impulse to the brain are necessary when pain is present, yet it is well-known that this is not always necessary. The pain that is often referred to an amputated leg where receptors and nerves are clearly absent is a real experience for the client. This type of pain is called **phantom limb pain** and is without demonstrated physiologic or pathologic substance.

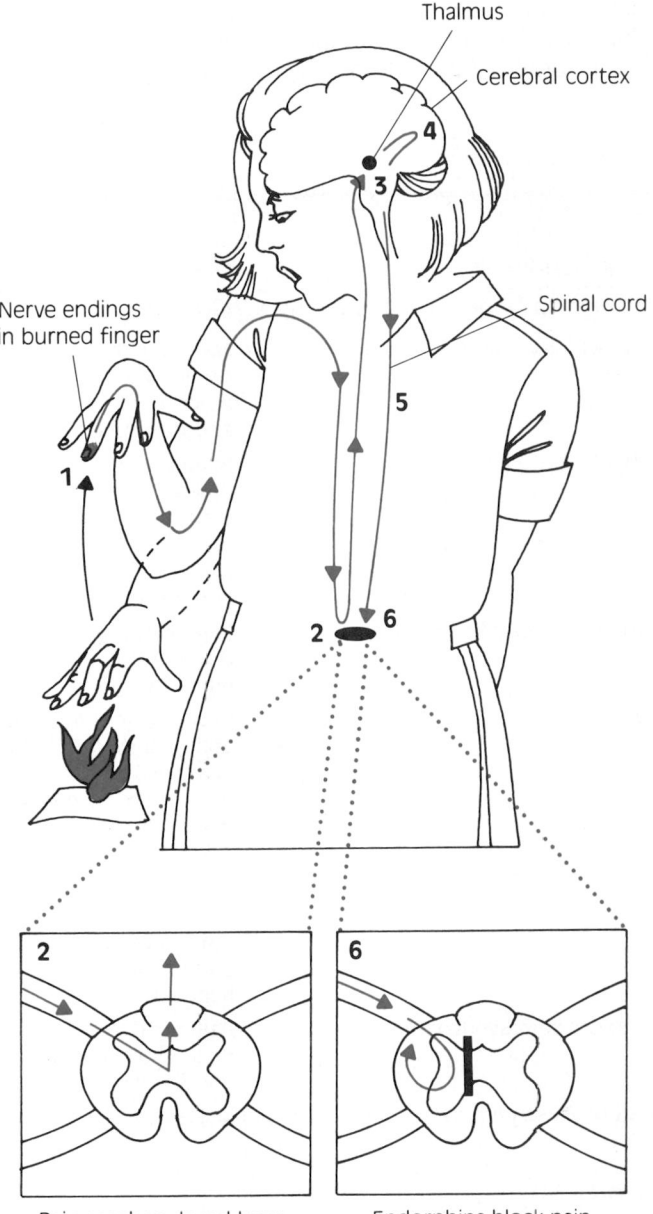

FIGURE 32-1

Pain sensation and relief. (1) Pain's path begins as a message is received by nerve endings in a burned finger. Potent chemicals (substance P, bradykinin, prostaglandins) are released, sensitizing the nerve endings, helping to transmit the pain message from the injured finger toward the brain, and setting the stage for healing (inflammatory response). (2) The pain signal from the burned finger travels as an electrochemical impulse along the length of the nerve to the dorsal horn on the spinal cord (a region that runs the length of the spine and receives signals from all over the body). (3) The message is relayed to the thalamus, a sensory center in the brain where sensations like heat, cold, pain, and touch first become conscious. (4) It then travels on to the cortex, where the intensity and location of pain are perceived. Little is known about factors that influence the individual's perception of pain at this point, the meaning attributed to the pain, and the voluntary responses elicited. (5) Pain relief begins as a signal from the brain descends by way of the spinal cord. (6) In the dorsal horn, chemicals like endorphin S are released to diminish the pain message from the injured finger. (Adapted from [1984, June 11]. Unlocking pain's secrets. *Time*, pp. 58–66.)

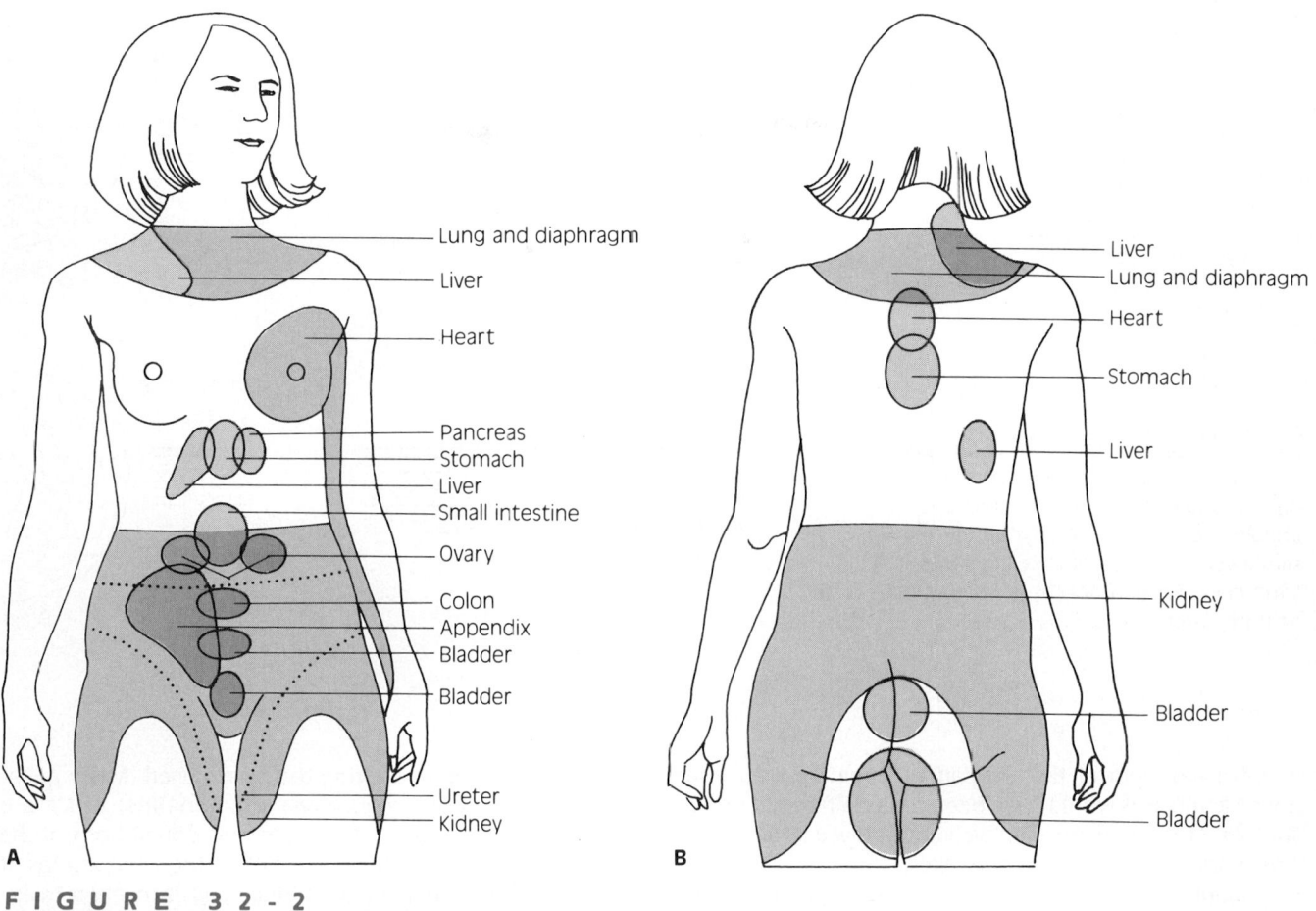

FIGURE 32-2

These drawings representing the anterior (A) and posterior (B) views of the body illustrate areas to which various organs refer pain. (Redrawn from Chaffee, E. E. & Lytle, M. M. [1980]. *Basic physiology and anatomy* [4th ed.]. Philadelphia: Lippincott.)

Gate Control Theory of Pain The **gate control theory** of pain is related to the transmission of painful stimuli and recognizes a relation between pain and emotions. The theory states that certain nerve fibers, those of small diameter, conduct excitatory pain stimuli toward the brain, but nerve fibers of a large diameter appear to inhibit the transmission of pain impulses from the spinal cord to the brain. There is a gating mechanism that is believed by some to be located in substantia gelatinosa cells in the dorsal horn of the spinal cord. The exciting and inhibiting signals at the gate in the spinal cord determine the impulses that eventually reach the brain. Thus, only a limited amount of sensory information can be processed by the nervous system at any given moment. When too much information is sent through, certain cells in the spinal column interrupt the signal as if closing a gate. The brain also appears to influence the gating mechanism. Past experiences and learned behaviors, which are interpreted by the brain, have the effect of regulating or adjusting the eventual behavioral responses to pain. This helps explain why similar painful stimuli are

interpreted differently by different people. Although not everyone accepts the gate control theory, it appears to explain why mechanical and electrical interventions or heat and pressure may effectively relieve pain. Nursing measures such as a massage or a warm compress to a painful lower back area stimulate large nerve fibers to close the gate, thus blocking pain impulses from that area. Figure 32-3 outlines the gate control theory of pain.

Perception of Pain

The perception of pain involves the sensory process when a stimulus for pain is present. It includes the person's interpretation of the pain. The threshold of perception is the lowest intensity of a stimulus that causes the subject to recognize pain. This threshold is remarkably similar for everyone. Still, it is theorized by at least some authorities that phenomenon of adaptation does occur; that is, the **pain threshold** can be changed within certain ranges. This phenomenon has been studied, for example, when pris-

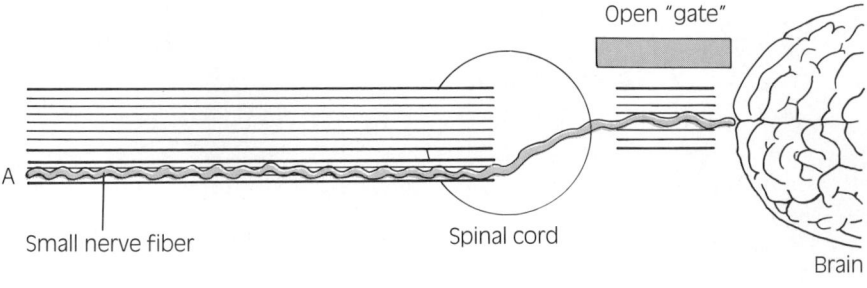

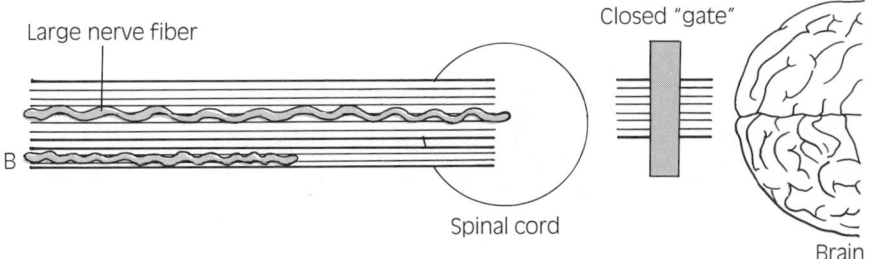

FIGURE 32-3

Diagrammatic sketch of gate control theory (A) Small nerve fibers conduct pain impulses to the brain. (B) Synapses are stimulated by impulses traveling across large nerve fibers acting as gates to block pain impulses.

oners of war reported that the pain of repeated torture was not as acute as it would have been under different circumstances. Many factors might well have played a role, but at least some adaptation appears likely.

Adaptation may also be present when a person's hand is immersed in warm water. A sensation of pain eventually occurs as the water is heated. However, the person can tolerate a higher temperature as water is gradually heated to the pain level than if the hand had been plunged into hot water without any preparation.

Modulation of Pain

The sensation of pain appears to be regulated or modified by substances called neuromodulators. **Neuromodulators** are endogenous opioid compounds, meaning they are naturally present morphinelike chemical regulators that are found in the spinal cord and brain. They appear to have analgesic activity and alter the perception of pain. It is believed that these endogenous opioid compounds produce their analgesic effects by binding to specific opioid receptor sites throughout the central nervous system and blocking release or production of pain transmitting substances. Both pain and stress seem capable of activating the endogenous opiate system.

To date, three groups of opioids have been identified—endorphins, enkephalins, and dynorphins. **Endorphins** are produced at neural synapses at various points in the central nervous system pathway, They are powerful pain-blocking chemicals that have prolonged analgesic effects and produce euphoria. It is suggested that endorphins may be released when certain measures are used to relieve pain, such as skin stimulation and relaxation techniques, and

when certain pain-relieving drugs are used. Many questions remain about endorphins. **Enkephalins,** which are widespread throughout the brain and dorsal horn of the spinal cord, are considered less potent then endorphins. It is believed that enkephalins reduce pain sensation by inhibiting the release of substance P from the terminals of afferent neurons. Little is known about the analgesic activity of **dynorphins**, which have recently been discovered. Initial research seems to indicate they are potent pain relievers.

Pain is a highly personal experience. A person learns to know what causes unpleasantness and what to interpret as pain. Each person's interpretation is influenced by background, such as how he or she has experienced and dealt with pain in the past and what cultural factors have taught about pain. Through past experiences, each person also learns to differentiate among the various types of pain and to associate pain with certain descriptive words.

Duration, Severity, Quality, and Periodicity of Pain

Pain is a mixed sensation and occurs in varying degrees. It is also associated with other sensations, such as the sensations of stretching, pulling, pressure, squeezing, heat, or cold. Terms commonly used to describe the duration, severity, quality, and periodicity of pain are listed in Table 32-2. Usually, the more intense the stimulation, the more likely it will produce pain and the more likely the pain will be severe. For example, there normally is pressure from a cast on the body part to which it has been applied but the sensation of the pressure is not painful. However, if there is abnormal swelling of the body part within the cast, the

TABLE 32-2

Terms Used to Describe the Duration, Severity, Quality, and Periodicity of Pain

Duration

Acute	An episode that lasts for seconds to fewer than about 6 months
Chronic	An episode of pain that lasts for 6 months or longer. The pain may be intermittent or continuous.

Quality

Sharp	Pain that is sticking in nature and that is intense
Dull	Pain that is not as intense or acute as sharp pain, possibly more annoying than painful. It is usually more diffuse than sharp pain.
Diffuse	Pain that covers a large area. Usually the client is unable to point to a specific area without moving the hand over a large surface, such as the entire abdomen.
Shifting	Pain that moves from one area to another, such as from the lower abdomen to the area over the stomach.

Other terms used to describe the quality of pain include sore, stinging, pinching, cramping, gnawing, cutting, throbbing, shooting, viselike pressure.

Severity

Severe or excruciating Moderate Slight or mild	These terms depend on the client's interpretation of pain. Behavioral and physiologic signs help assess the severity of pain. On a scale of 1 to 10, slight pain could be described as being between about 1 and 3; moderate pain, between about 4 and 7; and severe pain, between about 8 and 10.

Periodicity

Continuous	Pain that does not stop
Intermittent	Pain that stops and starts again
Brief or transient	Pain that passes quickly

pressure may exceed the pain threshold and be perceived as pain. Pain perception is sharply increased if tissue injury results from unrelieved cast pressure.

Responses to Pain

The three types of responses to pain are physiologic, behavioral, and affective. These responses are summarized in Table 32-3.

The severity of pain and its duration affect responses to pain. Mild pain experienced briefly may produce little or no behavioral responses, whereas intense pain experienced briefly usually results in reflex action to escape the cause. Pain that continues for a relatively short time, such as for a few days or a week, is often accepted by the client without its being all-consuming. The client expects relief and believes the cause is self-limiting. However, anxiety is ordinarily present. On the other hand, chronic pain tends to consume the entire person. It demands total attention so that the client has limited resources to take care of other matters of daily living. It is physically and emotionally exhausting and tends to result in depression and irritability. Chronic fatigue usually accompanies chronic pain.

Lack of an obvious response to pain does not mean the client is without pain. Careful assessment is especially important to understand what the client is experiencing.

Acute Versus Chronic Pain

Pain is classified in many ways. Perhaps the most common distinction is between acute and chronic pain. **Acute pain** is generally rapid in onset, varies in intensity from mild to severe, and may last from a brief period up to any period less than 6 months. Acute pain is protective in nature, that is, it warns the individual of tissue damage or organic disease. Once its underlying cause is resolved, acute pain disappears. Causes of acute pain include a pricked finger, sore throat, or surgery.

Chronic pain is pain that may be limited, intermittent, or persistent, but that lasts for 6 months or longer and interferes with normal functioning. Pain associated with cancer or other progressive disorders is termed *chronic malignant pain* and pain in people whose tissue injury is nonprogressive or healed is termed *chronic nonmalignant pain*. Clients have difficulty describing chronic pain because it may be poorly localized and health care personnel have difficulty assessing it accurately due to the unique responses of individual clients to persistent pain. Most pain researchers agree that as much as one third of the population may have persistent or recurrent chronic pain. Chronic pain currently is the third largest health problem in the United States (Simon, 1989). According to Ferrel, Ferrel, and Osterweil (1990), about 70% of elder clients residing in nursing homes have significant pain and one third of these are in constant pain. Unlike acute pain, chronic pain is often perceived as meaningless and may lead its host to withdrawal, depression, anger, frustration, and dependency.

Management of clients with chronic pain can be adversely affected by the misconceptions and personal biases of caregivers. Individuals with chronic pain may be perceived more negatively by nurses (Taylor, Skelton, & Butcher, 1984) and viewed in general by health care personnel as hysterical personalities, malingerers, or hypochondriacs. On the other hand, nurses who have experienced chronic pain or struggled through the experience with a loved one have a special awareness of its debilitating, destructive nature. Holm and colleagues (1989) reported that nurses who have experienced intense pain tend to be more sympathetic to clients in pain. Nurses need an

TABLE 32-3

Common Responses to Pain	
Response	**Comments**
Behavioral (Voluntary) Responses	
Moving away from painful stimuli	The person moves self or a part of the body away from the source of pain. It is one of the body's protective mechanisms.
Grimacing, moaning, and crying	These responses are normal in many cultures when they are in keeping with the amount of pain the client experiences.
Restlessness	Restlessness keeps the person alert and probably also serves as a distraction from pain (eg, pacing the floor).
Protecting the painful area and refusing to move	The person assumes a posture to protect the painful area, such as holding a painful hand or drawing the knees up when abdominal pain is present. The client may assume a posture and then refuse to move.
Physiologic (Involuntary) Responses	
Typical sympathetic responses when pain is moderate and superficial Increased blood pressure Increased pulse and respiratory rates Pupil dilation Muscle tension and rigidity Pallor (peripheral vasoconstriction) Increased adrenalin output Increased blood glucose	These signs are the body's responses to promote homeostasis; the body is preparing for emergency action, or the fight-or-flight phenomenon, as described in Chapter 9.
Typical parasympathetic responses when pain is severe and deep Nausea and vomiting Fainting or unconsciousness Decreased blood pressure Decreased pulse rate Prostration Rapid and irregular breathing	The body shows signs of being unable to cope with the stressor of pain.
Affective (Psychologic) Responses	
Exaggerated weeping and restlessness Withdrawal Stoicism Anxiety Depression Fear Anger Anorexia Fatigue Hopelessness Powerlessness	A person's previous experience with pain and sociocultural background play an important role in the emotional responses to pain. Emotional responses differ according to whether pain is acute or chronic. Anxiety is most often associated with acute pain and is frequently present when pain is anticipated. Depression is most often associated with chronic pain. Emotional responses tend to intensify the reactions to pain, causing a vicious cycle that may be difficult to break. Emotional responses help explain why some people experience pain that seems to be without physiologic cause or why some tend to complain of pain more than others when circumstances are similar. Pain is real as reported by the person, but for some, pain may help relieve feelings of guilt or serve as a way to gain attention and relieve loneliness.

awareness of their own personal feelings toward pain and the factors that affect pain if they are to assess and manage their client's pain creatively and effectively.

Factors Affecting the Pain Experience

Many factors influence the comfort status of a person at any given moment. When an individual experiences pain, almost anything can influence how the painful stimulus is transmitted to the brain, how it is perceived, and the response that is made to it.

Culture

Because cultural norms dictate much of our daily behavior, attitudes, and values, it is natural to assume that culture influences the individual's response to pain. It is important for nurses to understand that there are ways other than their own of responding to pain. A form of pain expression that is frowned on in one culture may be desirable in another cultural group. The nurse studies cultural variations not to stereotype clients of different cultural backgrounds but to develop an understanding of cultural influences on the following:

- The meaning of the pain event
- Ways in which clients may choose to demonstrate and cope with the pain experience
- Responsibilities in pain relief (Ludwig-Beymer, 1989).

Ethnic Variables Much research has been done on cultural influences on pain. The classic study on behavioral responses to pain present in groups of people of similar ethnic origin was done by Zborowski (1969). He studied males in four cultural groups—Old American (American-born, white, Protestant, and without identification with any foreign group); Jewish, Italian; and Irish. A summary of his findings follows.

Old American A man of this background describes his pain efficiently to health care practitioners, minimizes his pain when with family and friends, carefully controls his expression of pain, and tends to withdraw when his pain is severe—he wants to be alone. The Old American finds little value in pain and expects to have it relieved.

Jewish A man of Jewish background tends to be more vocal about his pain and uses pain to elicit sympathy and support from others. Like the Old American, he is future oriented and concerned with the significance of his pain but he is less confident that modern medicine can cure the cause of the pain. He often seeks the advice of several physicians, including specialists.

Italian The Italian man finds it natural to respond to pain with cries, moans, complaints, gestures, and body movements. Unlike the Old American and Jewish men, the Italian man is oriented to the present and is concerned with the sensation of pain itself rather than with its significance. The Italian wants quick pain relief and willingly accepts pain-relief measures.

Irish Like the Old American, the Irish man is calm and unemotional about pain, believing that complaining serves no purpose; he wants to be alone with his pain. He takes pride in his ability to handle pain, generally using two strategies—relaxing and fighting. The Irish male may struggle with his pain for a long time before consulting a physician.

Other The nurse working with other ethnic groups can find pertinent studies in the literature. Additional information on cultural influences on pain can be found in Chapter 8.

Family, Gender, and Age Variables Variables related to culture are family, gender, and age. Snelling (1990) studied the role of the family in relation to chronic pain and reported the following:

- There is a tendency for individuals with chronic pain to come from families that include a member suffering from pain.

- Spouses may reinforce pain behavior in their partners.
- Family size and birth order are not significant in distinguishing chronic pain sufferers.

Children growing up in different families may quickly learn to ignore pain, to exploit pain as a means to secure the attention and services of family members, or to value pain as a means the body uses to teach important truths. Similarly, children may learn that there are gender differences in pain expression; whereas it may be acceptable for a little girl to run home crying with a scraped knee, a little boy may be told that he should be brave and not cry. Adult men and women may hold onto gender expectations regarding pain communication and incorrectly interpret the presence or absence of pain expressions in others. In addition, different age groups have different beliefs and norms regarding pain sensation and response. At one time, the infant's inability to communicate pain led health care practitioners to the erroneous assumption that pain sensation was diminished or absent. It is now generally believed that infants and small children are sensitive to pain.

Among elderly people, pain has often been viewed as a natural component of the aging process and is often ignored when present as an indicator of a treatable condition. On the other hand, conditions normally painful in young adults (eg, myocardial infarction) may present minimal pain complaints in elderly people. That an elderly person does not complain of pain may indicate that he or she fears the treatment for the pain or just refuses to give in to the pain (Ferrell & Ferrell, 1990). These variables, which influence pain sensation, perception, and response, make pain assessment a complex task for the nurse.

Religion

Religious beliefs may powerfully influence the individual's experience of pain. In some religions, individuals view pain and suffering not as good in themselves but as a means of purification or as a means of making up for individual and community sin. This meaning helps the individual to cope with pain and becomes a source of strength. Clients with this belief may refuse analgesics and other pain-relief measures, feeling that this lessens their offering. On the other hand, illness and pain may also be viewed as punishment from a vengeful God. Individuals may find their faith shaken and question the existence of a loving God. How can belief in a loving God be compatible with their present experience of pain? Anger, resentment, and depression may then compound the pain experience. Clients may find it helpful to confer with a spiritual adviser about their pain experience.

Environment and Support People

An individual's environment and the presence or absence of caring support people may also influence the experience of pain. Many people find that the strangeness of the hospital environment, and especially the lights, noise, and constant activity of a critical care unit, compound the experience of pain. The sense of powerlessness that accompanies admission to an institution may decrease the individual's ability to cope with pain. Depersonalization, separation from a favorite pillow, pet, or source of music, may further decrease the person's sense of comfort. For some, the presence of a loved family member or friend is essential to their sense of well-being. Others prefer to be alone when in pain and may become agitated in the presence of a family member.

Some clients may use their pain to acquire secondary gains, such as special attention and services from their families. Because this tendency, if unchecked, usually leads to resentment and anger in family members and their eventual avoidance of the client, the nurse should intervene and attempt an honest discussion of this problem when noting its occurrence.

Anxiety and Other Stressors

Anxiety, which is almost always present when pain is anticipated or being experienced, tends to increase the perceived intensity of pain. The threat of the unknown is ordinarily more devastating and anxiety producing than a threat for which one has been prepared. Studies have indicated that clients who were taught preoperatively about what to expect postoperatively did not require as much medication for pain as those who had similar operative procedures but were not taught preoperatively.

Pain is ordinarily aggravated when anxiety, muscular tension, and fatigue are present. A vicious circle can easily develop when pain interferes with rest and relaxation, and tension and fatigue almost always aggravate the discomfort. The rested and relaxed person can often cope with great discomfort.

The individual who is greatly fatigued and who has no competing demands requiring attention may experience pain acutely. For example, many people have discovered that the pain of a footache or ingrown toenail that was only mildly annoying during the day's work became unbearable at night when there was nothing else to distract the mind from the pain. Similarly, athletes can be so determined to win a game that they are oblivious to the pain of a serious sports injury. After the game and particularly if the game was lost and the effort seemingly useless, the pain becomes overpowering.

Past Pain Experience

Whether an individual has experienced pain in the past and the qualities of that experience profoundly affect new pain experiences.
- Some clients have never known severe pain and have no fear of pain, not realizing how intense the sensation can be.
- Some clients have experienced severe acute or chronic pain in the past but received immediate and adequate pain relief. These clients are generally unafraid of pain and initiate appropriate requests for assistance.
- Some clients have known severe pain in the past and were unable to secure relief. Even the suggestion of

new pain can throw these clients into a frenzy of fear and feelings of despair and hopelessness.
- The individual whose past pain experience led to correction of unhealthy behavior and produced a greater sense of health and well-being may respect and value pain and study the meaning and significance of a new pain carefully.
- In general, people who have experienced more pain than usual in their lifetimes tend to anticipate more pain and to exhibit increased sensitivity to pain.
- Some pain memories are virtually unerasable and new contact with conditions similar to those that caused the earlier pain can provoke a violent response.

Nurse as Role Model

The nurse who wishes to role model healthy pain management behaviors to clients does the following:
- Balances work and leisure activities to promote optimal personal well-being (consistently communicates to self "I care about you!")
- Respects pain as the body's means of signaling that all is not well
- Treats what is producing pain as opposed to simply trying to eradicate pain
- Uses an effective coping model (pain view and view of self) when responding to personal pain
- Routinely incorporates comfort measures into nursing care
- Practices nursing sensitive to the pain needs of clients and is committed to pain relief:
  - Communicates to clients the belief that their pain experience is real and that help is available
  - Assigns high nursing priority to assisting clients (and family members) to develop effective pain management strategies compatible with their belief systems
  - Designs varied pain management programs that incorporate noninvasive and invasive interventions; works collaboratively with other health professionals
  - Supports pain management programs with attention to the client's overall nutrition, hydration, elimination, rest, activity, and stimulation
- Continuously updates knowledge of pain theories, assessment strategies, and treatment modalities

Use the self-assessment checklist in the accompanying display to monitor your progress in learning to meet comfort needs.

Assessing the Pain Experience

Because the pain experience is unique to each individual, the nurse who wants to understand a client's pain to help the client achieve pain control needs sophisticated pain

PROMOTING WELLNESS

Comfort

Use the assessment checklist to determine how well you are meeting comfort needs. Then develop a prescription for self-care by choosing appropriate behaviors from the list of suggestions.

Assessment Checklist

almost always	sometimes	almost never	
□	□	□	1. I seek medical attention when pain persists.
□	□	□	2. I am aware of my usual behavioral responses to pain.
□	□	□	3. I use stress reduction techniques regularly.
□	□	□	4. I am able to have a restful sleep at night
□	□	□	5. I have a positive outlook about my present situation.
□	□	□	6. I am aware of how to use distraction strategies to deal with pain

Self-Care Behaviors

1. Obtain a medical evaluation when acute or chronic pain is present.
2. Control stress in the environment.
3. Avoid excessive fatigue.
4. Practice stress reduction or diversionary behaviors when pain is present.
5. Become aware of personal preconceived notions that affect your perception of pain in others.

---

assessment skills. It is necessary to assess all factors that affect the pain experience—psychologic, emotional, and sociocultural as well as physiologic. Pain is complex and difficult to interpret and requires a reliable assessment tool.

Misconceptions

Many client misconceptions interfere with the client's ability to communicate pain:

- The nurse will know when I am in pain and will do something to relieve it if possible.
- The doctor has ordered pain-relieving medication for me, which I will be given routinely.
- If I ask for something for my pain, I may become addicted to the medication.
- I should somehow be able to control my pain. It is immature to talk about pain.
- It is better to wait until the pain gets really bad before asking for help.

Misconceptions and prejudices about pain and pain relief that hamper the nurse's assessment of the client with pain have been summarized by McCaffery and Beebe (1989) and are presented in Table 32-4.

Components of Pain Assessment

Various forms used to help guide the assessment of pain have been described in the nursing literature. The primary purposes of using a guide to assess pain are to eliminate guesswork and biases when dealing with the client's pain, to understand what the person is experiencing, and to analyze findings that will help prepare an appropriate nursing care plan for the client.

Characteristics of pain generally assessed include the following:

- The client's verbalization and description of the pain
- Duration of the pain
- The location of the pain
- The quantity and intensity of the pain
- The quality of the pain
- Chronology of the pain
- Aggravating factors
- Physiologic indicators of pain
- Behavioral responses
- The effect of the pain experience on activities and lifestyle.

Christoph (1991) suggests that accurate assessment and effective management of acute pain in seriously ill clients positively influences the sense of trust vital to a therapeutic nurse–client relationship, whereas Burckhardt (1990) emphasizes the importance of using verbal and nonverbal methods to ensure a comprehensive assessment of the client with chronic pain. See the accompanying Focused Assessment Guide for the pain experience that suggests questions or approaches helpful in assessing the various pain factors.

Some pain centers ask clients to complete a self-questionnaire. The McGill-Melzack Pain Questionnaire is an

TABLE 32-4

Misconceptions About Assessment of Patients Who Indicate They Have Pain	
Misconception	**Correction**
The health team is the authority about the existence and nature of client's pain sensation.	The person with pain is the only authority about the existence and nature of that pain, because the sensation of pain can be felt only by the person who has it.
Our personal values and intuition about the trustworthiness of others is a valuable tool in identifying whether a person is lying about pain.	Personal values and intuition do not constitute a professional approach to the patient with pain. The client's credibility is not on trial.
Pain is largely an emotional or psychological problem, especially in the patient who is highly anxious or depressed.	Having an emotional reaction to pain does not mean that pain is caused by an emotional problem. If anxiety or depression is alleviated, the intensity of pain will not necessarily be any less.
Lying about the existence of pain, malingering, is common.	Few people who say they have pain are lying about it. Outright fabrication of pain is considered rare.
The client who obtains benefits or preferential treatment because of pain is receiving secondary gain and does not hurt as much as he or she says or may not hurt at all.	The client who uses pain to his or her advantage is not the same as a malingerer and may still hurt as much as the client says he or she does. Also, secondary gain may be an inaccurate diagnosis.
All real pain has an identifiable physical cause.	All pain is real, regardless of its cause. Almost all pain has both physical and mental components. Pure psychogenic pain is rare.
Visible signs, either physiologic or behavioral, accompany pain and can be used to verify its existence and severity.	Even with severe pain, periods of physiologic and behavioral adaptation occur, leading to periods of minimal or no signs of pain. Lack of pain expression does not necessarily mean lack of pain. How must the client act for us to believe he or she has pain?
Comparable physical stimuli produce comparable pain in different people. The severity and duration of pain can be predicted accurately for everyone on the basis of the stimuli for pain.	Comparable stimuli in different people do not produce the same intensities of pain. Comparable stimuli in different people will produce different intensities of pain that last different periods. There is no direct and invariant relation between any stimulus and the perception of pain.
People with pain should be taught to have a high tolerance for pain. The more prolonged the pain or the more experience a person has with pain, the better is his or her tolerance for pain.	Pain tolerance is the individual's unique response, varying among clients and varying in the same client from one situation to another. People with prolonged pain tend to have an increasingly low pain tolerance. Respect for the client's pain tolerance is crucial for adequate pain control.
When the client reports pain relief following a placebo, this means that the patient is a malingerer or that the pain is psychogenic.	There is not a shred of evidence anywhere in the literature to justify using a placebo to diagnose malingering or psychogenic pain.

(McCaffery, M., & Beebe, A. [1989]. *Pain: Clinical manual for nursing practice.* St. Louis: Mosby.)

example of such a questionnaire (see the accompanying display). Using this questionnaire, an individual checks words that fit the description of the pain experience. Marks can be made on the figure to show pain location. Comparison of changes on subsequent questionnaires aids in determining an individual's improvement or regression. When a client presents with severe pain, the pain requires quick assessment and relief. The comprehensive pain assessment should be performed when the client is more comfortable and better able to respond to questions. A McGill Comprehensive Pain Questionnaire can be used in such instances.

Assessment in the Cognitively Impaired Client Assessment of pain in children and in people who are cognitively impaired presents special challenges to nurses. It currently is generally recognized that children and cognitively impaired adults are frequently undertreated. Special efforts are needed to identify accurate means of assessing pain in individuals in early or altered stages of cognitive development who are unable to express concepts such as pain magnitude.

Little is known about pain expression and measurement in confused, nonverbal elderly clients. Because most pain assessments rely on verbal reports, this group is most

The Pain Experience

Factors to Assess	Questions and Approaches
Characteristics of the pain	
Location	"Where is your pain? Is it external or internal?" (Asking the client with acute pain to point to the painful area with one finger may help to localize the pain. Clients with chronic pain may have difficulty trying to localize their pain, however.)
Duration	"How long have you been experiencing pain? How long does a pain episode last? How often does a pain episode occur?"
Quantity	Ask the client to indicate the degree (amount) of pain currently experienced on the scale below:

0   1   2   3   4   5   6   7   8   9   10

No pain   Mild   Moderate   Severe   Pain as bad as it can be

It is also helpful to ask how much pain the client has (on the same scale) when the pain is at its least and at its worst:

Least _____ Worst _____

Quality	"What words would you use to describe your pain?" (Useful in research, this characteristic is least useful in day-to-day clinical practice.)
Chronology	"How does the pain develop and progress?" (If pattern can be identified, interventions early in a pain sequence will often be far more effective than those used after the pain is well established.) "Has the pain changed since it first began? If so, how?"
Aggravating factors	"What makes the pain occur or increase in intensity?"
Alleviating factors	"What makes the pain go away or lessen? What methods of relief have you tried in the past? How long were they used? How effective were they?" (Methods of relief currently in effect for hospitalized clients should be apparent from the chart. It is important to verify the use of current orders and their effectiveness with the client. Outpatients may need to be asked to record a medication profile, a thorough and accurate account of all medications they are taking.)
Associated phenomena	"Are there any other factors that seem to relate consistently to your pain? Any other symptoms that occur just before, during, or after your pain?"
Physiologic responses	Signs of sympathetic stimulation commonly occur with acute pain. Signs of parasympathetic stimulation (decreased blood pressure and pulse, rapid and irregular respirations, pupil constriction, nausea and vomiting, and warm, dry skin) may be present, especially in prolonged, severe pain, visceral, or deep pain.
Vital signs (blood pressure, pulse, respirations) Skin color Perspiration Pupil size Nausea	
Muscle tension	Observe. Ask the client if he or she is aware of any tight, tense muscles.
Anxiety	Are signs of anxiety evident? (May include decreased attention span or ability to follow directions, frequent asking of questions, shifting of topics of conversation, avoidance of discussion of feelings, acting out, somatizing.)
Behavioral responses	
Posture, gross motor activities	Does client rub or support a particular area? Make frequent position changes? Walk, pace, kneel, or assume a rolled-up position? Does client rest a particular body part? Protect an area from stimulation? Lie quietly? (In acute pain, postural and gross motor activities are often altered; in chronic pain, the only signs of change may be postures characteristic of withdrawal.)

(continued)

F O C U S E D A S S E S S M E N T G U I D E

The Pain Experience (continued)

Facial features	Does the client have a pinched look? Are there facial grimaces? Knotted brow? Overall taut, anxious appearance? (A look of fatigue is more characteristic of chronic pain.)
Verbal expressions	Does the client sigh, moan, scream, cry, repetitively use the same words?
Affective responses	
Anxiety	"Do you feel anxious? Are you afraid? If so, how bad are these feelings?"
Depression	"Do you feel depressed, down, or low? If so, how bad are these feelings? Are your feelings about yourself mostly good or bad? Do you have feelings of failure? Do you see yourself or your illness as a burden to those you care about?"
Interactions with others	How does the client act when he or she is in pain in the presence of others? How does the client respond to others when he or she is not in pain? How do significant others and caregivers respond to the client when the client is in pain? When the client is not in pain?
Degree to which pain interferes with client's life (use past performance as baseline)	"Does the pain interfere with sleep? If so, to what extent? Is fatigue a major factor in the pain experience? Is the conduct of intimate or peer relationships affected by the pain? Is work function affected? Participation in recreational–diversional activities?" (An activity diary is often helpful—sometimes crucial. One to several weeks of hourly activity recorded by the client may be necessary. Levels of pain, intake of food, and sleep–rest periods are noted along with activities performed. Separate diaries for inpatient and outpatient episodes may be necessary, because hospitalization markedly affects the nature and type of activities performed.)
Perception of pain and meaning to client	"Are you worried about your illness? Do you see any connection between your pain and the nature or course of illness? If so, how do you see them as related? Do you find any meaning in your pain? If so, is this beneficial or detrimental to you? Are you struggling to find some meaning for your pain?"
Adaptive mechanisms used to cope with pain	"What do you usually do to relieve stress? How well do these things work? What techniques do you use at home to help cope with the pain? How well have they worked? Do you use these in the hospital? If not, why not?"
Goals	"What would you like to be doing right now, this week, this month, if the pain were better controlled? How much would the pain have to decrease (on the 0 to 10 scale) for you to begin to accomplish these goals?"

(Adapted from Donovan, M.I., & Girton, S.E. [1984]. *Cancer care nursing* [2nd ed.]. Norwalk, CT: Appleton-Century-Crofts.)

likely ignored and undertreated. Marzinski (1991) conducted pain assessments on an Alzheimer's unit in a nursing home and expressed concern about the lack of an operational definition of pain and reliable assessment tools for use with this population. Although these tools are being developed, nurses must rely on careful assessments and their empathetic qualities as a guide to pain management.

Pain Assessment in the Child

In recent years, health care personnel have become more concerned about children and their response to pain. It was formerly believed that young children lacked the neurologic development to sense pain the way adults do and pain relief was not a priority when children were hospitalized. Young

children frequently received no treatment for pain during entire hospital stays. New methods of assessing and measuring children's pain involve simple observation of facial expressions, body positions, and whether children cry. Physiologic responses also provide additional information. In a summary of pediatric pain assessment techniques, Goldstein (1991) mentioned psychologic tests in which children are asked to describe or draw a cartoon about the color or shape of their pain and various scales in which children are asked to compare their pain to a series of faces ranging from a broad smile to a tearful grimace. (Figure 32-4 is an example of a pediatric pain assessment scale.) Children may also be asked to record their pain experiences in a daily diary. Detecting and accurately assessing pediatric pain has resulted in new and innovative approaches toward pain control in children.

McGill - Melzack Pain Questionnaire

Patient's Name _____ Date _____ Time _____ am/pm

Analgesic(s) _____ Dosage _____ Time Given _____ am/pm

_____ Dosage _____ Time Given _____ am/pm

Analgesic Time Difference (hours): +4 +1 +2 +3

PRI: S _____ A _____ E _____ M(S) _____ M(AE) _____ M(T) _____ PRT(T) _____
(1-10)   (11-15)   (16)   (17-19)   (20)   (17-20)   (1-20)

PPI _____ COMMENTS:

1 FLICKERING	11 TIRING
QUIVERING	EXHAUSTING
PULSING	12 SICKENING
THROBBING	SUFFOCATING
BEATING	13 FEARFUL
POUNDING	FRIGHTFUL
2 JUMPING	TERRIFYING
FLASHING	14 PUNISHING
SHOOTING	GRUELLING
3 PRICKING	CRUEL
BORING	VICIOUS
DRILLING	KILLING
STABBING	15 WRETCHED
LANCINATING	BLINDING
4 SHARP	16 ANNOYING
CUTTING	TROUBLESOME
LACERATING	MISERABLE
5 PINCHING	INTENSE
PRESSING	UNBEARABLE
GNAWING	17 SPREADING
CRAMPING	RADIATING
CRUSHING	PENETRATING
6 TUGGING	PIERCING
PULLING	18 TIGHT
WRENCHING	NUMB
7 HOT	DRAWING
BURNING	SQUEEZING
SCALDING	TEARING
SEARING	19 COOL
8 TINGLING	COLD
ITCHY	FREEZING
SMARTING	20 NAGGING
STINGING	NAUSEATING
9 DULL	AGONIZING
SORE	DREADFUL
HURTING	TORTURING
ACHING	PPI
HEAVY	0 No pain
10 TENDER	1 MILD
TAUT	2 DISCOMFORTING
RASPING	3 DISTRESSING
SPLITTING	4 HORRIBLE
	5 EXCRUCIATING

CONSTANT
PERIODIC
BRIEF

ACCOMPANYING SYMPTOMS:
NAUSEA
HEADACHE
DIZZINESS
DROWSINESS
CONSTIPATION
DIARRHEA
COMMENTS:

SLEEP:
GOOD
FITFUL
CAN'T SLEEP
COMMENTS:

ACTIVITY:
GOOD
SOME
LITTLE
NONE

FOOD INTAKE:
GOOD
SOME
LITTLE
NONE
COMMENTS:

COMMENTS:

Key:
PPI = present pain intensity
PRI = pain rating index
 S = sensory components of pain
 A = affective, or emotional, components of pain
 E = evaluative terms
 M = miscellaneous terms

Combinations of words can be identified: M(S) and M(AE) and the entire number totaled: PRI(T). (Copyright 1970. Ronald Melzack)

Assessment in the Elderly Client Because many elderly people have chronic disease, pain is a prevalent occurrence. Visual or hearing impairments may influence the assessment format. Multiple drug regimens that are common in elderly people can also affect reliable reporting of pain. Herr and Mobily (1991) suggest some reasons why pain assessment is more complex in elderly people:

- There is a common belief that pain is an expected outcome as one ages.
- There is a fear that the admission of pain may limit independence.
- Pain is frequently considered an ominous sign—a forecast of serious illness or death.
- Terminology describing pain may vary significantly.
- The expression and interpretation of pain varies according to culture or ethnic group.
- Changing patterns or presentations of pain have been observed in elderly people.

F I G U R E   3 2 - 4

Wong/Baker Faces Rating Scale. (Wong, D., & Whaley, L. [1986]. *Clinical handbook of pediatric nursing* [2nd ed.]. St. Louis: Mosby.)

1. Explain to the child that each face is for a person who feels happy because he or she has no pain (hurt, or whatever word the child uses) or feels sad because he or she has some or a lot of pain.

2. Point to the appropriate face and state, "This face . . . ":
0—"is very happy because he [or she] doesn't hurt at all."
1—"hurts just a little bit."
2—"hurts a little more."
3—"hurts even more."
4—"hurts a whole lot."
5—"hurts as much as you can imagine, although you don't have to be crying to feel this bad."

3. Ask the child to choose the face that best describes how he or she feels. Be specific about which pain (eg, "shot" or incision) and what time (eg, Now? Earlier before lunch?)

- Boredom, loneliness, and depression may affect an elder's perception and report of pain.

Special attention and consideration of an elderly client's pain can positively affect the nurse's ability to accurately assess pain.

Diagnosing

Pain is such a complex phenomenon that its analysis often requires the collaboration of different members of the health team. Although nursing has much to offer individuals experiencing both acute and chronic pain, the data collected by the nurse during the comprehensive pain assessment will most benefit the client when shared with physicians and other members of the health care team.

Initially, pain must be viewed as a symptom and its physical etiology pursued. Interventions for pain done before an accurate assessment may mask the true cause of the client s pain, thus causing further suffering and possibly even death by allowing the progression of signs, symptoms, and the disease process. A thorough assessment provides the opportunity of ascribing the accurate meaning to a given set of behaviors and variables such as a pain pattern.

Only after all physiologic causes that are treatable by traditional medical and surgical techniques are ruled out does one treat pain as a disease entity. Even when pain becomes a treatable disease, vigilance must be maintained for *any changes and new symptoms*. Additional information may provide a more accurate diagnosis; therefore, a different treatment plan may be devised. (Meinhart & McCaffery, 1983, pp. 27–28)

The nurse who notes a pattern of headaches in a client and relates this to the client's description of recent stress (divorce, relocation, new job) may erroneously assume that the headaches are merely stress related and devise and implement a plan of relaxation exercises. A more careful analysis of client data, however, may reveal that the headaches are of vascular origin; migraine in nature, and medical intervention is indicated. The headaches may also be symptomatic of intracranial disease such as a brain tumor and delay in diagnosis may decrease the possibility of treatment and cure.

When a nursing diagnosis of acute or chronic pain is developed, the diagnostic statement and care plan should identify the following:
- Type of pain
- Etiologic factors, to the extent that they are known and understood
- The client's behavioral, physiologic, and affective responses
- Other factors affecting pain stimulus, transmission, perception, and response

Pain or Chronic Pain as the Problem   Many diagnoses could be developed for pain problems. The importance of the nurse identifying these problems and including them as priorities in the care plan cannot be overstated. Examples of two-part nursing diagnoses follow. See the accompanying display for examples of defining characteristics for

NURSING DIAGNOSES FOR COMMON PROBLEMS

Pain

Problem	Related Factors	Sample Defining Characteristics
Pain: Acute Postoperative	Fear of taking prescribed analgesics	• Recent cholecystectomy • Face is pale and drawn; vital sings elevated from baseline. • States, "I don't like to ask for anything for pain because I know people often get addicted."
Pain: Left Leg	Fractured femur and multiple lacerations; unsuccessful attempts to determine effective analgesic	• Recent motor vehicle accident • Grimaces whenever left leg is moved • Directs abusive language to anyone who touches left leg • Refused to have dressing changed on left leg • Reports analgesic "only takes the edge off" the pain
Pain	Prolonged labor (dystocia) and commitment to natural childbirth	• Admitted to labor unit 18 hours ago with moderate contractions 2 minutes apart • Strength of contractions weakening; progress of dilatation and effacement slow; failure to progress • "I'll feel like a failure if I take anything for pain. I want to 'go natural.' I know I can do it. Besides, the drugs would only hurt my baby."
Pain: Heightened Anticipation	Child's history of undergoing frequent painful procedures	• Child diagnosed at age 3 years with acute nonlymphoid leukemia • History of bone marrow aspirations, spinal taps, platelet transfusions, chemotherapy, and other such procedures • Child "freezes" when unfamiliar health care worker enters room
Pain: Chest	Decreased blood supply to myocardium (angina) and fear	• "I never know when it will grab me next. I get this crushing pain in my chest and can't do anything. Usually one or two of those nitro tablets bring me relief. I'm always scared, though, that the pain won't go away."
Chronic Pain: Headaches	Inadequate pain management secondary to belief that somehow client "deserves this pain"	• Reports history of migraine headaches for past 5 years • Never sought treatment • "My mother told me that we all get the pain in life that we deserve—and goodness, I've been no saint." • "I can't help feeling, though, that no one is meant to live like this."
Chronic Pain	Inadequate pain management of metastatic cancer involving bone	• Diagnosed with cancer of bladder 2 years ago; presently metastic spread to spine • Rates pain 10 on a scale of 1 (minimal) to 10 (greatest) • "I haven't been taking as much of this pain medicine as the doctor said I could because if I get used to it now nothing will work when the pain gets even worse later." • "When I told the nurse in the hospital about my pain she said I'd have to get used to it." • "I don't want to burden my wife and kids with my pain."
Chronic Pain	Rheumatoid arthritis and inappropriate activity during exacerbations	• Stiffness of joints, limitation of motion, heat, swelling, and tenderness • States pain is often intense after activity • "I can't accept not being able to do all I want to do for my husband and children."

these diagnoses. In general, it is not recommended that the medical diagnosis be used as the etiology of the problem statement in the nursing diagnosis. However, when stating nursing problems of pain, it may be difficult to avoid this without sacrificing the specificity desired. Remember that the purpose of the etiology is to direct the nursing interventions.

Pain: Postoperative related to fear of taking prescribed analgesics

Pain related to fractured femur and multiple lacerations and unsuccessful attempts to determine effective analgesic

Pain related to prolonged labor (dystocia) and commitment to natural childbirth

Anxiety related to heightened pain anticipation from child's history of undergoing frequent painful procedures

Pain related to decreased blood supply to myocardium (angina)

Chronic Pain: Headache related to inadequate pain management secondary to belief that client somehow "deserves" this pain

Chronic Pain related to inadequate pain management of metastatic cancer involving bone

Chronic Pain related to rheumatoid arthritis

Pain or Chronic Pain as the Etiology   Because the experience of pain affects so many other aspects of human functioning, pain may be the etiology of numerous other nursing diagnosis statements:

Ineffective Airway Clearance related to postoperative incisional pain

Anxiety related to pain anticipation and inadequate pain management in the past

Constipation related to chronic use of narcotic analgesics

Ineffective Family Coping: Disabling, related to father's inability to allow family to share his pain experience

Ineffective Individual Coping related to failure of chronic pain management strategies to date

Altered Health Maintenance related to loss of will to live secondary to prolonged chronic pain

Hopelessness related to belief that present pain means imminent death

High Risk for Injury related to decreased pain sensation

Knowledge Deficit: Angina Pain Management, related to belief that nothing will help the pain

Fatigue related to lack of relief from chronic pain

Fear related to possible significance of pain

Impaired Physical Mobility related to arthritic pain

Altered Nutrition: Less Than Body Requirements, related to gastrointestinal distress

Self-Care Deficit: Dressing/Grooming, related to painful movement of joints

Altered Sexuality Patterns related to painful intercourse

Sleep Pattern Disturbance: Inability to Fall Asleep related to pain's worsening at night

Spiritual Distress related to belief that God is unfairly causing this pain as some sort of undeserved punishment

Altered Thought Processes related to effects of chronic pain and overmedication

High Risk for Self-Directed Violence related to loss of will to live with unrelieved chronic pain

Planning: Client Goals

Once the diagnosis of a pain problem is made, it is critical for nurses to develop a care plan that, when implemented, demonstrates nursing's commitment to assist the client to develop effective pain management strategies. Table 32-5 illustrates possible outcomes of two different nursing responses to a client with low back pain.

Nursing measures are directed toward the achievement of the following client goals for the client whose pain is acute in nature (ie, it is expected that with healing the pain will subside and eventually disappear).

Long-Term Goal
The client will:
- Verbalize that pain is eliminated (if client is nonverbal, the absence of the signs that indicated the presence of pain is sought)

Short-Term Goals
The client will:
- Describe a gradual reduction of pain using a scale ranging from 0 (no pain) to 10 (pain as bad as it can be)
- Demonstrate competent execution of successful pain management program (specify)

Chronic Pain

For the client whose pain is chronic in nature, the long-term goals differ somewhat.

Long-Term Goals
The client will:
- Verbalize (demonstrate) the ability to control pain to the point of being able to manage and enjoy key elements of everyday living
- Family and significant others will relate feeling better able to share and to cope with the pain experience of the client

Short-Term Goal
An important short-term goal for the client with chronic pain may be contacting a hospice or a pain clinic.

Implementing

Once the care plan is developed, the nurse implements the nursing strategies that are most likely to assist the client to achieve pain-relief goals. Nursing interventions described in this chapter include establishing a trusting nurse–client

TABLE 32-5

Different Outcomes for a Client With Low Back Pain

Client

A 32-year-old married man, father of two, presents to the hospital with complaints of dull and aching low back pain, weakness, and stiffness. Pelvic traction, heat treatments, and antiinflammatory medication are ordered.

Situation A	Situation B
Nursing Priorities During Client's Hospitalizations	
• Administer medications. • Set up pelvic traction and instruct client in its use. • Inquire how heat treatments are going. • No detailed pain assessment is performed.	• Nursing and medicine collaborate in detailed pain assessment. • Once a diagnosis of degenerative disc disease is made the nurses teach the client about the disease and related self-care measures (eg, alternate methods of pain control, including use of heat, activity, massage, and progressive relaxation). • Intensive inhospital care includes use of pelvic traction, administration of medications, and heat treatments.
Typical Nursing Comments	
• "Did you injure your back to get a couple of days off? I've often thought of doing that myself." (Some nurses are upset about understaffing and angry with two nurses claiming work-related back injuries.)	• "Gee, it must be awfully hard for someone as healthy as you've been to suddenly find yourself in bed with all this pain. How's it going?" • "How do you think your back problem will affect you once you get home?"
Client's Discharge and Evaluation of Care	
• Client withdrawn during hospitalization; discharged after 5 days of treatment reporting relief of symptoms. • Tells family: "No one in there believed I had pain—or if they did, they sure didn't care. I wish someone would have wanted to help me. I won't go that route again!"	• While hospitalized, client experiences an increased sense of self-respect and worth as well as hope that relief from pain will be found. • Many years later when the disc herniates, the client returns to the hospital confident in the health care team's ability and willingness to help him.
Aftermath of Hospitalization	
• Client tries to ignore pain when it recurs. • Irreversible musculoskeletal damage occurs from prolonged muscle spasm. • Weakness, endocrine imbalance (loss of weight), and sleep disturbance are frequent. • Client experiences irritability, depression, feelings of worthlessness, powerlessness, personality changes, decreased motivation, suicidal ideation. • Client is unable to meet role expectations as spouse, father, friend, and employee—results in divorce, unemployment, and destruction of the quality of his life and that of his family.	• Early treatment and lifelong care of back complemented by general health behaviors (eg, good nutrition, regular exercise, stress management), prevent the development of symptoms related to the gradual buildup of paravertebral spasms. • Health status and quality of life are actually improved following client's hospitalization.

relationship; teaching the client about pain; manipulating factors that affect the pain experience; initiating the appropriate noninvasive pain-relief measures (distraction, relaxation, cutaneous stimulation); and assisting with the pain therapies of other disciplines.

Establishing a Trusting Nurse–Client Relationship

Most clients with pain feel better, suffer less, and experience less anxiety when they believe that a competent nurse cares about their experience of pain and is available for help and support. Without the confidence developed in a good nurse–client relationship, nothing seems to work. With it, often amazing results have been obtained by using measures that ordinarily are only modestly effective. Measures that help strengthen the nurse–client relationship and promote pain relief include discussing pain with the client, allowing the client to help decide on a method of pain relief, and visiting and remaining with the client in pain. These measures promote a collaborative relationship in which the client's pain is treated with respect.

R E S E A R C H   I N   N U R S I N G   Making a Difference

Effective Assessment and Understanding of Pain Promotes Effective Intervention

The relief of pain has long been a subject of study. Pain is a physical response to malfunction of an organism but can also occur in the absence of an organic cause. Despite the cause, the person still responds with alterations in comfort (pain). Increased anxiety also interferes with the benefits of rest and thus prevents comfort. Nursing research in these areas continues to explore appropriate interventions.

Related Research

Walker, J., Akinsanya, J., Davis, B., & Marcer, D. (1990). The nursing management of elderly patients with pain in the community: Study and recommendations. *Journal of Advanced Nursing, 15,* 1154–1161.

 Walker and colleagues conducted this study to determine the factors that influence pain and affect the quality of life of elderly people living in the community. They discovered that pain assessment tools, although infrequently used by nurses in this setting, can help to identify triggers for pain and determine the effectiveness of various treatment options. In addition, for pain control to become a reality, nurses need to assess the elderly client's past regrets, occupation, the presence of other stressful problems, and how well informed the client feels about his or her condition as elements that affect his or her ability to deal effectively with persistent pain.

Dalton, J. (1989). Nurses' perceptions of their pain assessment skills, pain management practices, and attitudes toward pain. *Oncology Nursing Forum, 16*(2), 225–231.

 This study suggests that nurses who are aware of their own feelings about the pain experience and have additional professional experience and continuing education more frequently assess and comprehensively evaluate the cancer pain experienced by their clients. Recommendations to improve pain management and aid in selecting appropriate treatment strategies include emphasizing the importance of assessing the pain coping skills of client and family and determining which clients might benefit from an understanding of the use of behavioral methods to control pain.

Closs, S. (1990). An exploratory analysis of nurses' provision of postoperative analgesic drugs. *Journal of Advanced Nursing, 15,* 42–49.

 The purpose of this study was to examine the pattern of delivery of analgesics to postoperative clients during the nighttime hours. Considerably fewer analgesic doses were given during the night compared with doses during the day, and the frequency of medications used for pain control during the postoperative period was considerably less than that prescribed. This suggests that additional nursing research is needed to understand the nurse's role in the assessment and control of pain at night during the postoperative period.

Summary

These studies demonstrate several implications for clinical nursing practice including the importance of using assessment tools for pain; the more nurses understand the pain experience, the better equipped they are to assess and evaluate pain in their clients; and more study is needed to determine why clients tend to require less postoperative analgesic medication at night than in the day. It is the responsibility of the nurse to promote maximum well-being for all clients and to accept that pain is a unique and individual response deserving appropriate therapeutic interventions.

Teaching the Client About Pain

The well-informed person can often cope better with the distress of pain and tends to experience less anxiety about pain. In many situations, teaching about pain should include family members so that they understand and may help the person in pain.

 The following are examples of information to share with the client and family when pain is present:
- Function of pain
- Cause of pain
- When pain can be anticipated and when it need not be anticipated
- Quality and duration of pain to expect
- Assurance that it is acceptable to express feelings about pain
- What pain-control measures can and will be used
- Assurance that the client's complaints about pain are believed
- Knowledge that it is easier to control pain before it is allowed to become severe

 Play may often be used effectively to discover a child's experience of pain and to teach the child how to cope with pain. Children are usually receptive to using dolls to act out pain experiences.

Manipulating Factors Affecting the Pain Experience

Removing or Altering the Cause of Pain   Removing or altering the cause of the pain is ideal and sometimes possible. Ways of doing this include removing or loosening a tight binder, if permissible; seeing to it that a distended bladder is emptied; taking steps to relieve constipation and flatus; changing body positions and ensuring correct body alignment; and changing soiled linens and dressings that may be irritating the skin. The hungry or thirsty client may need a snack or a drink to feel more comfortable.

Certain drugs are useful for removing or altering the intensity of painful stimuli. For example, drugs that decrease smooth muscle spasms in the gastrointestinal tract and those that decrease contractions of skeletal muscles reduce discomfort.

Altering Factors Affecting Pain Tolerance   As a result of the pain assessment and the trusting relationship he or she has established, the nurse is better able to identify those factors that are increasing the client's pain experience and decreasing his or her pain tolerance. **Pain tolerance** is the point beyond which a person is no longer willing to endure pain. These factors should be alleviated whenever possible. For example, clients whose families have never acknowledged their pain and who have repeatedly been told that their pain is all in their head may experience a greater ability to deal with their pain when someone finally takes the pain seriously. Nursing measures include communication to the client that responses to pain are acceptable as well as education of the client's family.

Fatigue tends to increase pain, and promoting rest is then helpful. The client in pain usually feels more comfortable when the environment is quiet and restful. Although sensory restrictions such as eliminating unnecessary noise, bright lights, and so on are usually indicated, it is rarely helpful to leave the client alone in an environment with little sensory input. The client then is more likely to focus on self and the discomfort.

Lack of knowledge, finding no meaning in the pain, being pessimistic about its relief, and fear may also interfere with the client's ability to deal with pain. Common fears include a fear of losing control and embarrassing oneself by being unable to deal with the pain maturely, and the fear of taking pain-relief medication because this may be viewed as a sign of weakness, may become addictive, or will lose its effectiveness later. Elderly clients, in particular, are frequently frustrated by similar concerns about pain management. See the Focus on the Older Adult display for specific nursing strategies for this rapidly growing segment of the population.

Initiating Noninvasive Relief Measures

Distraction

Conscious attention often appears to be necessary to experience pain, whereas preoccupation with other things has been observed to distract the client from pain. Distraction requires the client to focus attention on something other than the pain. It is not entirely clear whether distraction raises the threshold of pain or increases pain tolerance. Many clients whose pain is relieved by distraction report being able to place pain in the periphery of awareness. This is compatible with the theory that if the reticular formation in the brain stem receives sufficient sensory input it can ignore or block out select sensations such as pain. The Lamaze method of childbirth illustrates one common use of distraction.

Distraction is best used before pain begins or soon thereafter. People in mild to severe pain can successfully use distraction, but distraction cannot generally be practiced for long periods and may result in an increased sense

---

F O C U S   O N   T H E   O L D E R   A D U L T

Nursing Strategies for Pain Affecting Older Adults

Communication Difficulties

- Observe carefully for any behavioral manifestations or indications of pain (eg, change in activity level or grimacing with movement).
- Use open-ended questions to solicit information about pain.
- Rely on family or caregiver to assist with information gathering process.
- Monitor for any behavior changes or confusion after medication has been taken.

Denial of Pain

- Clarify terms used to describe pain or discomfort.
- Emphasize importance of reporting pain to caregivers.

- Express concern about pain and willingness to help.
- Explain that pain is not a normal consequence of aging.

Altered Physiologic Response to Analgesics

- Be aware of dosage and frequency to avoid oversedation and toxicity.
- Monitor carefully for oversedation and respiratory depression.
- Explain side effects of analgesics to client.
- Use memory aid if necessary to avoid overdosing.
- Discourage self-medication.
- Caution about use of alcohol with analgesics.
- Caution about driving when taking analgesics.

of pain and fatigue at its completion. In general, clients who are experiencing chronic pain need a greater variety of distractions than clients with pain of short duration.

Distraction may be successfully used with children. For distraction to be effective, the individual must be aware of activities or situations that are the most exciting, interesting, or absorbing. Distractions may be visual, auditory, tactile, kinesthetic, or "project" (see the accompanying display, Techniques That Distract Attention).

Imagery

The client who uses **imagery**, an example of mind–body interaction, to decrease pain sensation imagines something that involves one or all of the senses, concentrates on that image, and gradually becomes less aware of the pain. Imagery may be as simple as a child thinking of "happy things" (a beloved pet, lollipops, Christmas morning, grandmom's lap) or as involved as an adult recreating a favorite place and then experiencing the healing presence or touch of a loved person or the healing energies of nature in that setting. Imagery has also been used to create an image in which the cause of the pain is visualized and then overcome, counteracted, by some more powerful image.

Imagery has been found to be more effective for the client with chronic pain than for the client with acute, severe pain. The nurse can teach a client to use imagery by performing guided imagery. The nurse sits close to the client but not touching the client and in a gentle voice invites the client to use all five senses to recreate a favorite restful scene. This scene would have been previously de-

scribed to the nurse by the client. If the client becomes restless or upset, the imagery experience is terminated and attempted later when the client seems better disposed. Guided imagery is discussed in Chapter 9.

Relaxation

Relaxation techniques reduce skeletal muscle tension and lessen anxiety. By assisting the client with relaxation techniques, the nurse acknowledges the client's pain and expresses a willingness to help the client relieve the distress caused by his or her pain. The positive effects of relaxation for the person with pain include the following:

* Improved quality of sleep
* Improved problem-solving ability
* Decreased fatigue
* Increased confidence and sense of self-control in coping with pain
* Lessening of the detrimental physiologic effects of continued or repeated stress from pain
* Distraction from pain
* Increased effectiveness of other pain relief measures
* Improved ability to tolerate pain
* Decreased distress or fear during anticipation of pain
* Reassurance that the nurse is aware of his or her problem and wants to help (McCaffery & Beebe, 1989)

Most relaxation techniques can be learned with little practice and with relative ease. Some require the help and guidance of a person experienced in the technique, such as Zen or yoga. Practices producing relaxation generally have four elements in common:

* Assuming a comfortable position with the body in good alignment
* Being in quiet surroundings
* Repeating a certain word, sound, phrase, or prayer
* Adopting a passive attitude when distracting thoughts enter the individual's consciousness

Relaxation is most effective as a pain alleviator when combined with slow, deep, easy breathing from the abdomen or diaphragm while the eyelids are closed or with the individual focusing on a real or imagined fixed spot. Relaxation techniques are discussed in Chapter 9. Many tapes currently are available to direct this process. A free catalog of tapes on relaxation and imagery may be obtained from:
Psychology Today Tapes
Dept. 728, P.O. Box 059073
Brooklyn, NY 11205-9061
Phone: Toll free 1-800-345-8112

Other techniques that promote relaxation include listening to restful music or nature sounds while concentrating or relaxing; thinking about something that is relaxing, such as lying on a beach while listening to the roar of the waves, meditation, yoga, Zen, biofeedback, systematic desensitization, and operant conditioning. Relaxation strategies appear to be more effective in chronic pain situations.

Cutaneous Stimulation

The success of techniques that stimulate the skin's surface in relieving pain is often explained on the basis of the gate

---

Techniques That Distract Attention

Visual Distractions

* Staring at an object or spot and describing it in detail
* Counting objects
* Reading or watching television

Auditory Distractions

* Listening to music

Tactile Kinesthetic Distractions

* Holding or stroking a loved person, pet, or toy
* Rocking
* Slow, rhythmic breathing

Project Distractions

* Playing a challenging game (puzzles, card game, computer game)
* Performing meaningful play or work (hobby, vocational work, creative work, such as writing a journal, taping memoirs, and other such projects)

PROCEDURE 32-1

Giving a Back Massage

Equipment

Massage lubricant or lotion	Bath blanket
Powder	Towel

Action	Rationale
1 Explain the procedure and offer back massage to the client.	Back massage can facilitate circulation and promote relaxation.
2 Wash your hands.	Handwashing deters the spread of microorganisms.
3 Close the curtain or door.	Privacy increases relaxation.
4 Assist the client to the prone position or side-lying position with the back exposed from the shoulders to the sacral area. Use the bath blanket to drape the client. Raise the bed to the high position and lower the side rail closest to you.	This position exposes an adequate area for massage with privacy and warmth maintained. Having the bed in the high position reduces back strain for the nurse.
5 Warm the lubricant or lotion in the palm of your hand or place the container in warm water.	Cold lotion causes chilling and uncomfortable sensation.
6 Using light strokes (*effleurage*), apply lotion to client's shoulders, back, and sacral area.	Effleurage relaxes the client and lessens tension.
7 Place your hands beside each other at the base of the client's spine and stroke upward to the shoulders and back downward to the buttocks in slow, continuous strokes. Continue for several minutes.	Continuous contact is soothing and stimulates circulation and muscle relaxation.
8 Massage the client's shoulders, entire back, areas over iliac crests, and sacrum with circular stroking motion. Keep your hands in contact with the client's skin. Continue for several minutes, applying additional lotion as necessary.	A firmer stroke with continuous contact promotes relaxation.
9 Knead the client's skin by gently alternating grasping and compression motions (*pétrissage*).	Kneading increases blood circulation to areas.
10 Complete the massage with additional long stroking movements.	Long stroking motion is soothing and promotes relaxation.
11 During massage, observe the client's skin for reddened or open areas. Pay particular attention to the skin over bony prominences.	Pressure may interfere with circulation and lead to development of decubitus ulcers. Back rub stimulates circulation to these areas.
12 Use the towel to pat the client dry and to remove excess lotion. Apply powder if the client requests it.	This provides additional comfort for the client.
13 Wash your hands.	Handwashing deters the spread of microorganisms.
14 Assess the client's response and record your observations on the client's chart.	This provides accurate documentation of the procedure and condition of the client's skin.

control theory. The gate control theory of pain postulates that cutaneous nerve fibers are large-diameter fibers carrying impulses to the central nervous system. When the skin is stimulated, pain is believed to be controlled by closing the gating mechanism in the spinal cord. This decreases the number of pain impulses that reach the brain for perception.

Cutaneous stimulation techniques include the following:

• Massage (with or without stimulants such as liniments or menthol ointments; see Procedure 32-1
• Application of heat or cold, or both intermittently
• Vibration
• Pressure

One example of pressure is myotherapy, which is a modern-day Western descendant of acupuncture. Using this technique, the therapist applies pressure for 4 to 7 seconds on select trigger points, starving the area of needed oxygen and thus relieving the pain. Trigger points are highly irritable, painful muscle spots at which the pain from various body pathologies is registered.

Contralateral stimulation is a technique that involves stimulating an area opposite the painful area. For example, if the left arm is painful, skin stimulation is used on the right arm. The reason contralateral stimulation works is not understood.

Cutaneous stimulation is limited in that unless the pain can be localized it is most likely too diffuse to benefit from these techniques and most individuals cannot tolerate stimulation of the painful area but may be helped by stimulation of the surrounding or contralateral area.

Assisting With Pain Therapies of Other Disciplines

A team of health care professionals is often involved in the client's care and nurses work collaboratively with other team members to secure pain relief for the client. One of nursing's important functions is to assist the client to explore pain-relief alternatives by providing or securing information about different treatment modalities. These modalities may range from simple folk remedies to complex surgical treatments. The nurse's role is not to make decisions for the client but to provide the support and knowledge that enable the person in pain to secure helpful assistance. Depending on the nature of the person's pain, this assistance may be provided by a family member, a member of the clergy, a folk healer, a clinical psychologist, a nurse, or a physician. Nursing interventions may include referral assistance as well as support and protection during the treatment.

Analgesic Administration

An **analgesic drug** is a pharmaceutical agent that relieves pain. Analgesics function to reduce the person's perception of pain and to alter the person's responses to discomfort. There are three general classes of drugs used for pain relief:
- Nonnarcotic analgesics (eg, aspirin, acetaminophen, nonsteroidal antiinflammatory agents)
- Narcotic analgesics or opioids (all controlled substances; eg, morphine, codeine, meperidine, methadone); **opioid** is the more correct term for narcotic analgesics because these drugs act by binding to opiate receptor sites in the central nervous system (McCaffery & Ferrell, 1990)
- Adjuvant analgesics (anticonvulsants, antidepressants, and others)

These classes are compared in Table 32-6.

The nurse administering analgesics needs to combine a healthy respect for the drug being administered with thorough knowledge of its mechanism of action, side effects, and administration guidelines. This respect for the drug

should result in analgesics being used wisely to produce their desired effect. McCaffery and Beebe (1989, pp. 78–79) offer an equianalgesic drug chart illustrating how different drugs relate to the traditional analgesic standard (10 mg of subcutaneous morphine). Comparative knowledge of common analgesics enables the nurse to tailor the client's regimen and communicate professionally with physicians about a client who is being undermedicated or who needs a different drug or route of administration.

At no time should analgesics be used as a substitute for good nursing care that includes other measures to relieve discomfort. If the administration of painkillers is the only treatment strategy a nurse consistently uses to deal with pain, then care is grossly deficient. On the other hand, nurses should not refrain from using analgesics or reduce their doses because of an unrealistic fear of their potency and side effects. A recent position statement was issued by the American Nurses' Association (ANA) Task Force on End of Life Decisions (see the accompanying display) supported effective pain management for dying clients (*American Nurse*, p. 8).

Repeated studies have demonstrated that pain is usually undertreated in hospitalized individuals. Physician, nurse, and client variables all contribute to this outcome. Physicians often prescribe insufficient analgesic doses because of a tendency to overestimate the efficacy and duration of analgesics, underestimate the pain experience, and worry excessively about the possibility of respiratory problems and addiction. Nurses who ideally spend the most time with the client and who are supposed experts in human responses, for example, such as the response to pain, often compound this problem by further reducing the insufficient analgesic dose or by not administering the medication at all. Nurse variables include the low priority nurses give to pain management; arbitrary pain assessments and erroneous judgments about a client's pain and need for analgesia; and fear of being the person who administers the drug that causes respiratory depression or another serious side effect. The inability of many clients to discuss their pain and to request pain assistance perpetuates this problem.

McCaffery and associates (1992) surveyed nurses and reported that a client's life-style may influence a nurse's

---

Position Statement

ANA Task Force on End of Life Decisions

- "Nurses should not hesitate to use full and effective doses of pain medication for the proper management of pain in the dying patient."
- "The increasing titration of medication to achieve adequate symptom control, even at the expense of life, thus hastening death secondarily, is ethically justified."

(American Nurses' Association. [1991]. *Position statement on promotion of comfort and relief of pain in dying patients.* Kansas City, MO: Author.)

T A B L E   3 2 - 6

Comparison of Narcotic and Nonnarcotic Analgesic Agents

Agents	Development of Tolerance and Physical Dependency	Analgesic Efficacy	Site and Mechanisms of Analgesic Effect	Common Side Effects
Narcotic analgesics or opioids (morphinelike)	Yes; discontinuance of narcotic administration or administration of a narcotic antagonist (ie, precipitated withdrawal after prolonged use) causes withdrawal syndrome	Greater efficacy—can relieve pain of a more severe nature In sufficient dosage are considered capable of relieving pain of virtually every nature	Produce analgesia by central nervous system (ie, brain and spinal cord) mechanisms	Nausea, vomiting, dizziness, mental clouding, sedation, constipation, respiratory depression
Nonnarcotic analgesics (aspirinlike, anti-inflammatory)	No	Less efficacy—limited to relief of mild to moderate pain (eg, headache, muscle and joint pain) regardless of the dose administered	Chiefly produce analgesia by peripheral mechanisms outside of the central nervous system (eg, by way of interference with the biosynthesis of prostaglandins)	Nausea, vomiting, dyspepsia, gastric ulceration, decreased blood clotting
Adjuvant analgesics (antidepressants, anticonvulsants, and others)	No	May relieve pain in specific situations when used alone or in combination with opioids	Exact mechanism of antidepressants is unknown—may block pain transmission and decrease the perception of pain. Anticonvulsants appear to suppress abnormal nerve firings resulting from injury to nerve tissue	Drowsiness and sedation, constipation, dry mouth, hypotension, nausea, double vision, rashes, decreased blood clotting

decision to administer pain medication. For example, suspicion of a substance abuse problem may result in undertreatment of pain. Recognition of the level of pain as reported by the client and discussion and support from colleagues help to prevent negative feelings from interfering with proper management of pain.

General Principles for Administering Analgesics

Goals for Pain Relief   When using medications for pain relief the nurse must first assess the client's pain and understand the client's goals for pain relief. McCaffery and Beebe (1989) recommend the following guidelines for effective, individualized pain management:

- Try various pain control measures
- Use pain control measures before pain increases in severity
- Ask the client what has proved effective for pain relief in the past
- Select and modify pain control measures based on the client's response
- Encourage the client to try the pain treatment several times before labeling it ineffective
- Be open-minded about pain relief strategies

- Be persistent
- Be a safe practitioner

Various organizations and groups have made recommendations for pain control in a variety of settings. These include the American Pain Society, the NIH National Center for Nursing Research, and the previously mentioned ANA. The Agency for Health Care Policy is the major federal agency responsible for health services research and has issued guidelines for management of acute pain accompanied by a pain control plan that facilitates participation of clients and their families as members of the health care team (see accompanying displays). This guideline will be updated regularly to reflect the most current information on pain control. Quality assurance techniques have also been recommended to monitor the effectiveness of pain management by health care agencies (Jacox et al., 1992).

Ongoing Assessment   Just as the pain experience of each client is unique, so is the response of each client to a prescribed analgesic. The nurse needs continually to evaluate whether the medication is producing the desired analgesic effect; identify changes in the client's condition (correction or worsening of pathology, increased drug tolerance) that necessitate changes in the analgesic agent, dose, or route

Clinical Practice Guideline for Acute Pain Management: Operative or Medical Procedures and Trauma

Summary Recommendations

1. *Promise patients attentive analgesic care.* Patients should be informed before surgery, verbally and in printed format, that effective pain relief is an important part of their treatment, that talking about unrelieved pain is essential, and that health professionals will respond quickly to their reports of pain. It should be made clear to patients and families, however, that the total absence of any postoperative discomfort is normally not a realistic or even a desirable goal.

2. *Chart and display assessment of pain and relief.* A simple assessment of pain intensity and pain relief should be recorded on the bedside vital sign chart or a similar record that encourages easy, regular review by members of the health care team and is incorporated in the patient's permanent record. The intensity of pain should be assessed and documented at regular intervals (depending on the severity of pain) and with each new report of pain. The degree of pain relief should be determined after each pain management intervention, once a sufficient time has elapsed for the treatment to reach peak effect. A simple, valid measure of intensity and relief should be selected by each clinical unit. For children, age-appropriate measures should be used.

3. *Define pain and relief levels to trigger a review.* Each institution should identify pain intensity and pain relief levels that will elicit a review of the current pain therapy, documentation of the proposed modifications in treatment, and subsequent review of its efficacy. This process of treatment review and followup should include participation by physicians and nurses involved in the patient's care.

4. *Survey patient satisfaction.* At regular intervals defined by the clinical unit and quality assurance committee, each clinical unit should assess a randomly selected sample of patients who have had surgery within 72 hours. Patients should be asked their current pain intensity, the worst pain intensity in the past 24 hours, the degree of relief obtained from pain management interventions, satisfaction with relief, and their satisfaction with the staff's responsiveness.

5. *Analgesic drug treatment should comply with several basic principles:*
   a. *Non-opioid "peripherally acting" analgesics.* Unless contraindicated, every patient should receive an around-the-clock postoperative regimen of an NSAID. For patients unable to take medications by mouth, it may be necessary to use the parenteral or rectal route.
   b. *Opioid analgesics.* Analgesic orders should allow for the great variation in individual opioid requirements, including a regularly scheduled dose and "rescue" doses for instances in which the usual regimen is insufficient.

6. *Specialized analgesic technologies,* including systemic or intraspinal, continuous or intermittent opioid administration or patient controlled dosing, local anesthetic infusion, and inhalational analgesia (e.g., nitrous oxide) should be governed by policies and standard procedures that define the acceptable level of patient monitoring and appropriate roles and limits of practice for all groups of health care providers involved. The policy should include definitions of physician and nurse accountability, physician and nurse responsibility to the patient, and the role of pharmacy.

7. *Nonpharmacological interventions:* Cognitive and behaviorally based interventions include a number of methods to help patients understand more about their pain and to take an active part in its assessment and control. These interventions are intended to supplement, not replace, pharmacological interventions. Staff should give patients information about these interventions and support patients in using them.

8. *Monitor the efficacy of pain treatment:* Periodically review pain treatment procedures as defined in summary recommendations 1–4 above, using the institution's quality assurance procedures.

(Acute Pain Management Guideline Panel. [February 1992]. *Acute pain management: Operative or medical procedures and trauma–Clinical practice guideline* [pp. 75–76]. [AHCPR Publication No. 92-0032]. Rockville, MD: Agency for Health Care Policy and Research, Public Health Service, U.S. Department of Health and Human Services.)

of administration; and identify the development of side effects of the analgesic that may warrant its discontinuance. As long as the client's pain exists, the need for ongoing assessment is imperative. The flow sheet in Figure 32-5 facilitates this assessment. Basic to this assessment is the knowledge of the basic action, doses, routes of administration, side effects, and administration guidelines of the analgesic being administered.

Timing Timing is an important consideration when administering analgesics. Their effect is usually greatest when administered before pain occurs or becomes severe.

Pain Control Plan

Pain control plan for

_____
Your name

Before surgery, I will take

_____
Name of medicine

Instructions for use

_____

_____

_____

_____

_____

After surgery, I will take

_____
Name of medicine

in the hospital.

The medicine will be given to me

_____ as a pill

_____ through a vein

_____ as a shot

_____ through a tube in my back

I will receive the medicine

_____ at regularly scheduled times

_____ every _____ hours for

_____ days:

_____ around the clock

_____ when I call the nurse

I will also use these nondrug pain control methods in the hospital and at home (*list methods*)

_____

_____

_____

_____

_____

At home, I will take

_____
Name of medicine

Instructions for use

_____

_____

_____

_____

_____

(Acute Pain Management Guideline Panel. [February 1992]. *Acute pain management: Operative or medical procedures and trauma—Clinical practice guideline* [AHCPR Publication No. 92-0032]. Rockville, MD: Agency for Health Care Policy and Research, Public Health Service, U.S. Department of Health and Human Services.)

To time analgesics appropriately, the nurse needs to know the average duration of action for the drug and time administration so that the peak analgesic effect occurs when the pain is expected to be most intense. For example, an analgesic would be offered before ambulating a client postoperatively.

A prn (as-needed) drug regimen may meet the needs of many people experiencing acute pain. However, with a prn protocol, the client usually has to request the pain medication and has no guarantee that the nurse will administer it promptly. Often there is a long delay between the client's request for pain medication and the nurse's administration of the drug, which is a source of frustration for both clients and nurses.

The prn protocol is totally inadequate for clients experiencing chronic pain. Regular administration of analgesics

Pain Flow Sheet

Patient _____ Date _____

Pain rating scale used* _____

Purpose: To evaluate the safety and effectiveness of the analgesic(s).

Analgesic(s) prescribed: _____

Time	Pain Rating	Analgesic	R	P	BP	Level of Arousal	Other[1]	Plan & Comments

* *Pain rating: A number of different scales may be used. Indicate which scale is used and use the same one each time. For example, 0 to 10 (0 = no pain, 10 = worst pain).*

[1] *Possibilities for column: bowel function, activities, nausea and vomiting, other pain relief measures. Identify the side effects of greatest concern to the patient, family, physician, and nurses.*

F I G U R E   3 2 - 5

Flow sheet for pain. (McCaffery, M. & Beebe, A. [1989]. *Pain: Clinical manual for nursing practice.* St. Louis: Mosby.)

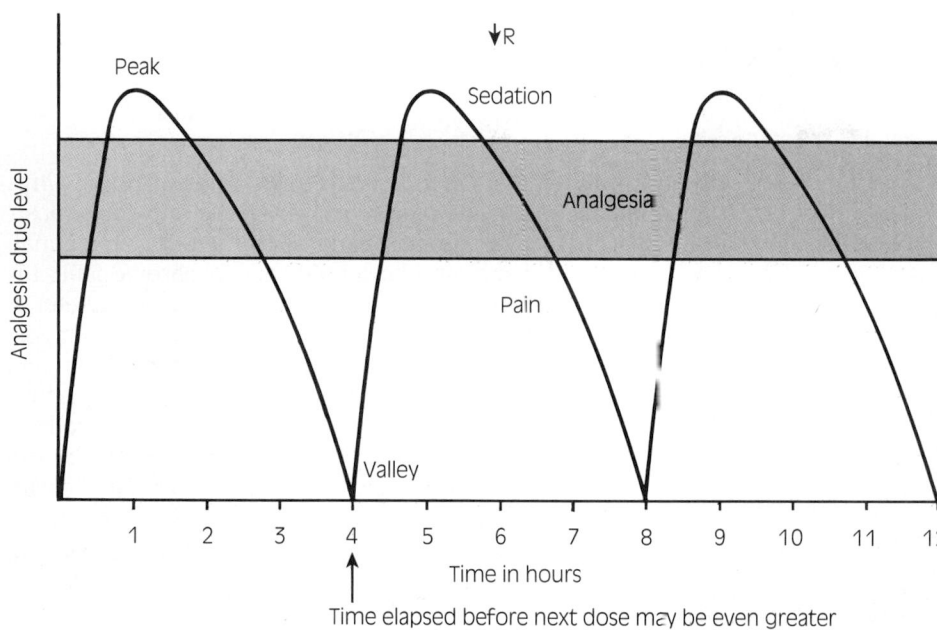

F I G U R E   3 2 - 6

Illustration of the peaks and valleys that often occur when analgesia by the oral, intramuscular, or subcutaneous route is given in the traditional prn manner that requires the patient to wait for the return of pain before requesting or obtaining the next dose of analgesic. The top line indicates toxic drug levels, the middle therapeutic, and the bottom ineffective drug levels.

or ATC administration (around the clock at regularly scheduled intervals) has been shown to offer superior pain management for chronic pain. Figure 32-6 illustrates the deficiencies in chronic pain treatment with a prn medication whose schedule is insufficient to control pain. A comparison of Figures 32-6 and 32-7 quickly demonstrates the superiority of a regularly administered effective analgesic.

Patient-Controlled Analgesia

Patient-controlled analgesia (PCA) is an increasingly popular technique developed to provide effective individualized, client-controlled analgesia and comfort. The PCA unit is an infusion pump that holds a vial of an intravenous analgesic that allows the client to regulate the intravenous infusion of small amounts of a narcotic at short intervals (Jones & Brooks, 1990). This approach has many advantages:

- Consistent analgesia is maintained rather than the inconsistent analgesia obtained with periodic intramuscular injections, which results in sharp rises and falls of serum narcotic levels.
- The narcotic is delivered intravenously so that absorption is faster and more predictable than with the intramuscular route.
- The client is in charge of the pain management program.

The PCA unit has two settings (appropriate dose and lock-out interval), which, once set, limit the amount of narcotic the client can receive. Built-in safety features help

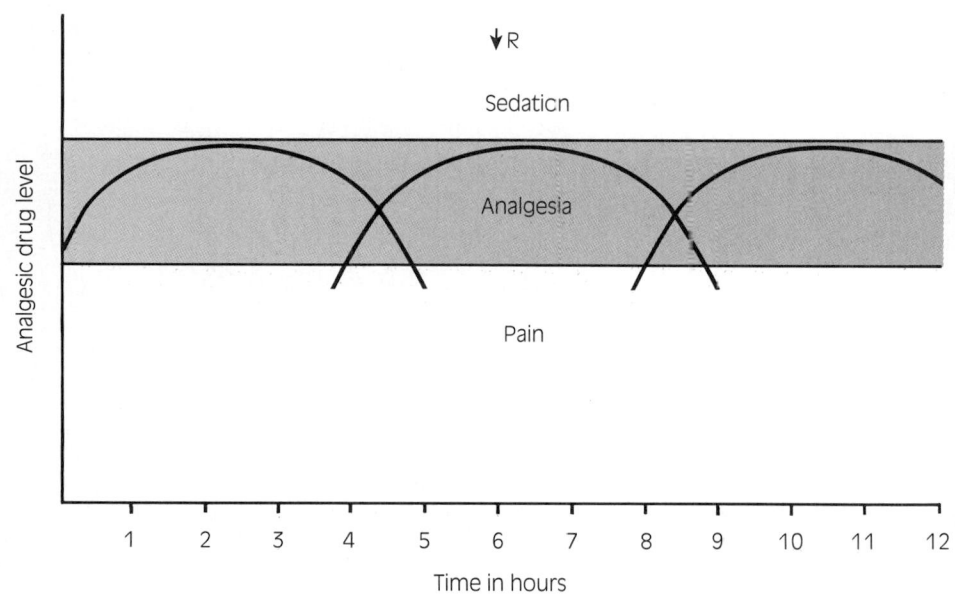

F I G U R E   3 2 - 7

Illustration of the relatively smooth analgesic level that can be obtained by individualizing the dose and using an around-the-clock approach with oral, intramuscular, or subcutaneous analgesics. Analgesics are administered before the pain returns; ideally, no noticeable peaks and valleys occur. That is, the drug level does not rise above what is required for analgesia, causing side effects such as sedation and respiratory depression; and the drug level does not fall below what is required for analgesia, causing increasing pain. The top line indicates toxic drug levels, the middle therapeutic, and the bottom ineffective drug levels.

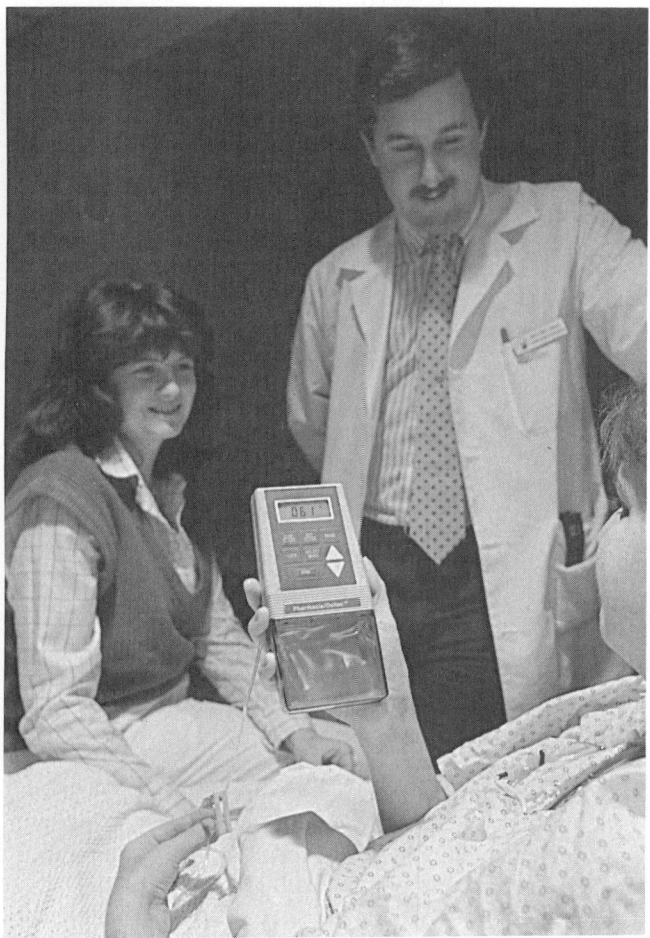

A patient-controlled analgesia unit allows the client to regulate the intravenous infusion of small amounts of analgesic as needed. (Photo by Don Walker, courtesy of Thomas Jefferson University, Philadelphia.)

client is able and willing to participate and safe limits are set.

Epidural Analgesia

Epidural analgesia is being used with increasing frequency to provide pain relief during the immediate postoperative phase (particularly after thoracic, abdominal, orthopedic, and vascular surgery) and for chronic pain situations. The anesthesiologist usually inserts the catheter in the mid-lumbar region into the epidural space. For temporary therapy, the catheter exits directly over the spine, whereas for long-term therapy, the catheter usually is tunneled subcutaneously and exits on the side of the body or on the abdomen (Fig. 32-9). The narcotic or opioid acts directly on the opiate receptors in the spinal cord and pain relief is achieved with smaller doses and less severe side effects. Morphine is frequently the drug of choice. Nursing responsibilities vary at each institution but must include careful monitoring of the client's response to therapy with particular attention to the respiratory rate and pattern. Too much narcotic or a displaced catheter may allow the medication to exert its depressant effect on the brainstem center, causing life-threatening respiratory depression. Other potential side effects include infection or contamination, pruritus, urinary retention, and nausea and vomiting (Dunajcik, 1988). Research has yet to determine the ideal client and specialized situation that is most appropriate for this type of analgesia.

to prevent narcotic theft and overdose. Nursing responsibilities include the following:

- Identifying clients who are good candidates for PCA (alert and capable of controlling the unit; no prior history of drug or alcohol abuse)
- Setting up the PCA unit and ensuring that it is functioning properly
- Educating clients in the use of PCA
- Evaluating the effectiveness of this type of pain management control for the client
- Assessing carefully for side effects of the medication

Figure 32-8 demonstrates a PCA device.

A broader definition of PCA is advocated by McCaffery and Beebe (1989), for whom PCA encompasses any drug administration method (oral, PCA pump, intravenous, subcutaneous, or spinal route) that allows the client to exercise control. They recommend that all analgesics be given on the basis of this concept, provided the

Placement of an epidural catheter for long-term use.

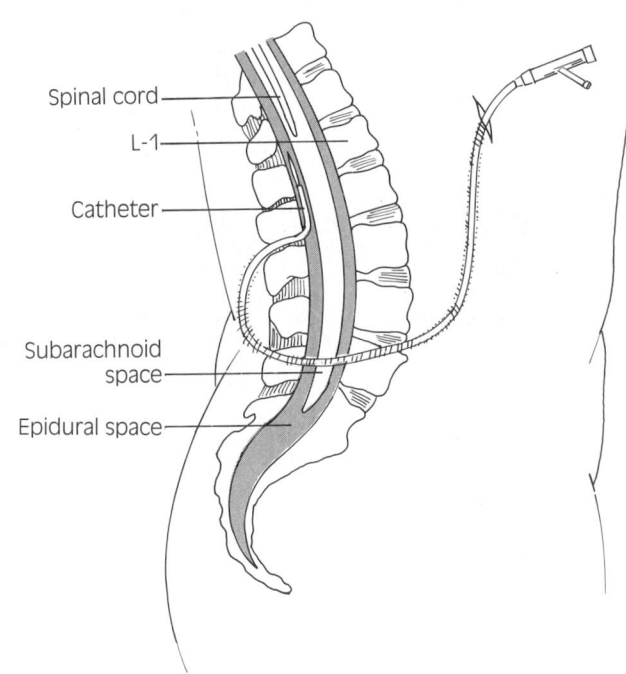

Continuous Subcutaneous Infusions

Continuous subcutaneous infusion (CSI) has resurfaced as an alternative means of controlling pain. Formerly used specifically for hydration purposes, this route can effectively deliver small doses of narcotics or opioids that are controlled by an infusion pump and absorbed from subcutaneous tissue. Candidates for CSI include clients who

- Cannot take oral opioids
- Have not experienced relief from oral opioids
- Require prolonged use of parenteral opioids
- Have difficulty with intravenous access
- Are experiencing dysphagia or gastrointestinal obstruction (Logan & Fothergill-Bourbonnais, 1990; McLaughlin-Hagan, 1991)

Nursing responsibilities include careful monitoring of the volume of the infusion (should not exceed 1 mL/hr to limit local irritation), assessing for infection, documenting pain relief, and checking for adverse effects from the narcotic or opioid.

Other Pain-Control Methods

The Placebo Controversy

The term **placebo** is a Latin word meaning "I shall please." It consists of an inactive substance often given to satisfy a person's demand for a drug. The person, unaware of the placebo's properties, may find it to be effective for the relief of pain because of the perception that it will provide comfort and because of belief in the person administering it. It is an injustice to judge a person experiencing relief from pain after the use of a placebo as a malingerer or as mentally ill. If the pain is relieved, the placebo has served its purpose. Various researchers have reported that a positive placebo effect may be related to a physiologic response (release of endorphins) or the client's cultural expectations, attitudes, health beliefs, or anticipation of a positive response (Shlafer & Marieb, 1989). Many believe that the placebo has its place in health care to help prevent addiction to certain drugs, to offer relief when an analgesic is contraindicated, and to substitute an innocuous agent when a person seems dependent on drug therapies that are deemed unnecessary.

The use of placebos, however, raises serious ethical questions. Can the good done by the placebo justify lying to a client? The nurse who administers a placebo must be willing to risk the possible consequence of the client becoming aware of the duplicity and then refusing to trust the nurse or any other health care professional again. Clients who feel themselves to be in pain are vulnerable. If such a client discovers a seeming plot to trick him or her into feeling better, it is unlikely that the client will respect or appreciate the good intentions of the physicians and nurses involved. The long-term effects of this practice would seem to outweigh its benefits. It is recommended that nurses decide their stand on placebos before encountering a situation in practice in which they are expected to administer one. The nurse has firm legal and ethical grounds for refusing to administer a placebo but must also communicate the basis for refusal to the appropriate authorities.

Hypnosis

Hypnosis, a technique that produces a subconscious condition accomplished by suggestions made by a hypnotist, has been used successfully in many instances to control pain. The person's state of consciousness is altered by suggestions so that pain is not perceived as it normally would be. According to many hypnotists, it also alters the physical signs of pain. Many people can be taught autohypnosis, that is, self-induced hypnosis, for the control of pain. It is generally believed that a successful response to hypnosis is related to the individual's openness to suggestion, belief that hypnosis will work, and emotional readiness.

Acupuncture

Acupuncture is a technique that uses needles of various lengths to prick specific parts of the body to produce insensitivity to pain. After the needles are inserted into the body, they are twirled or used to conduct a mild electrical current. The technique was developed in China and has been used for centuries in many Asian countries. It is beginning to gain acceptance in the Western world and is being investigated as a possible tool to help control discomfort. The relief of pain by acupuncture is generally explained on the basis of the gate control theory. The needles are believed to stimulate large-diameter nerve fibers and thereby the gating mechanism is closed and pain impulses do not reach the brain for perception. Self-hypnosis may also account for some of acupuncture's success. Repeated treatments are often needed.

Acupressure is the application of pressure or massage, or both, to usual acupuncture sites. It is usually applied with the thumb, a finger, the palm of the hand, or a fingernail. Its effectiveness may be explained on the basis of the gate control theory.

Biofeedback

Biofeedback is a technique that uses a teaching machine with a feedback signal to help a client learn by trial and error to control the supposedly involuntary body mechanisms (eg, poor circulation, muscle spasms) that may cause pain. The technique decreases the individual's pain by reducing the anxiety associated with lack of control over bodily functions, by distracting the person's attention from the pain to concentration on the person's inner state and the feedback signal, and by reducing the cause of the pain. Limitations for this method include the high degree of motivation needed and difficulty of maintaining control at the end of the training program.

Local Anesthesia

Anesthetic agents may be applied topically to the skin or mucous membranes or injected into the body to produce a temporary loss of sensation and motor and autonomic function in a localized area. The agents work by chemically blocking the nerve pathways involved in pain sensation and response and are sometimes called *nerve blocks*. Many people have experienced nerve blocks during dental work. Nursing measures include noting any allergic responses the client has had in the past to anesthetic agents, alerting the client to the pain the initial injection of the anesthetic may cause if the physician does not numb the area first, offering emotional support to the client during the procedure and observing for any untoward effects, and protecting the client from injury until sensory and motor functions return.

Neurosurgery

Transmission of pain may be interrupted permanently by surgical (or thermocoagulation) neural destruction. Because the destruction is permanent, it is usually used only as a last resort for intractable pain. In people for whom psychologic elements contribute heavily to the pain experience, the pain may persist after nerve transection. These procedures require highly skilled neurosurgeons and anesthesiologists and their execution varies from medical center to medical center.

Neurectomy Neurectomy is a partial or total excision of a peripheral or cranial nerve to relieve localized pain. It may result in total loss of sensation and some paralysis of the affected area.

Rhizotomy Rhizotomy is an interruption (by surgical resection) of the posterior root just outside the posterior horn cells of the spinal cord. This procedure offers the benefit of relief of both localized acute pain and deep visceral pain (interrupts sensory function) while preserving motor function. A surgical rhizotomy is indicated for localized pain in the neck, chest, back, and perineum if the client is in good physical condition.

Cordotomy Cordotomy is a surgical resection of the spinal and cerebral tracts carrying painful impulses and is used for advanced disease and intractable pain. Ideally, pain and temperature sensation below the level severed are obliterated whereas the sense of touch and awareness of position are retained. This procedure carries a heavy risk of complications, and permanent paralysis may result from accidental resection of the motor nerves. This open surgical procedure has been largely replaced by percutaneous thermoregulation.

Sympathectomy Sympathectomy is a severing of the sympathetic afferent nerve pathways that is used primarily for causalgias, phantom pain, and pain due to vascular disorders.

Electrical Nerve Stimulation

Selective electrical stimulation of large-diameter fibers has been used successfully to inhibit transmission of painful impulses carried over small-diameter fibers. All the electroanalgesia methods use electrodes attached to or im-

planted in the area to be stimulated. The gate control theory is used to explain the success of these methods as is the theory that the analgesia is produced through the release of endorphins both in the spinal cord and centrally.

Types of nerve fiber stimulation include the following:
- Transcutaneous nerve stimulation (TNS) or transcutaneous electrical nerve stimulation (TENS)
- Dorsal column stimulation (DCS)
- Percutaneously implanted spinal cord epidural stimulation (PICES)
- Central gray stimulation

Specific indications, application and care procedures, and cautions exist for each of these types.

Evaluating

As soon as a pain problem is identified and a treatment plan developed and implemented, evaluation becomes ongoing. Evaluation is directed toward the changing nature of the pain experience; the treatment modalities (pain management program); and the client and family's response to the care plan, all of which overlap.

The Pain Experience

The pain the client is experiencing may change in many ways and the nurse must be careful not to make a judgment about this too quickly. For example, if the pain lessens in intensity or disappears, it may mean that the underlying cause of the pain is diminished or absent and that treatment should be stopped, or it may mean that the pain management program is effective and should be continued. When pain intensity is increased, it may simply indicate the need for more aggressive therapy, or it may be a warning that the underlying pathology has changed or worsened and that new medical intervention is required. Often a new problem amenable to treatment is masked by "old pain" and its detection may be delayed to the point that treatment is useless.

Treatment Modalities

The use of both noninvasive and invasive therapies must be continually evaluated to determine if they are the best possible means the client could use to obtain pain relief and if they are effective with only minimal risk to the client. Too often a client stays with the first analgesic prescribed without questioning if it is the most effective drug for the particular pain, if the dosage and timing guidelines are correct for the client, and if the analgesic is perhaps producing annoying or even harmful side effects that another drug would not produce. Similarly, one client may take to progressive relaxation exercises and find them helpful, whereas another client may obtain similar benefits from a daily walking program. Nursing time spent evaluating the effectiveness of each pain-relief therapy is well spent and results in a pain management program that is truly individualized to the client.

Client and Family Response

Ultimately, the care plan is unsuccessful unless the client and family are satisfied with the results. A successful care plan results in the achievement of specified client goals that the client values. Whenever possible, nursing care should terminate when the client and family can independently direct the pain management program with the assistance of appropriate resources.

 # NURSING PROCESS

In Clinical Practice

Once a pain problem is suspected, the nurse implements each phase of the nursing process to ensure its correct identification and treatment. The knowledge and clinical skills described in this chapter will enable the nurse to manage these problems successfully. The following outlines specific assessment priorities, client goals, nursing interventions, and evaluative criteria for nursing diagnoses representative of the two major classifications of pain—acute and chronic:

Pain: Acute Postoperative
Chronic Pain: Malignant

The case study that follows the discussion of these diagnoses presents a woman suffering from the discomforts of premenstrual syndrome (PMS). Although her symptoms considered individually hardly constitute a pain problem, together they afford the client sufficient discomfort to interfere with her everyday functioning. This case illustrates the close relation between an individual's comfort level and functional abilities.

Pain: Acute Postoperative

Once the anesthesia administered during surgery begins to wear off, the surgical client generally experiences pain. Etiologies for the preceding diagnoses vary. The nature and degree of surgical trauma, the physical and mental health of the client, and the presence of other discomforting conditions (eg, nausea and vomiting, flatulence, drains and dressings, multiple tubes and equipment) contribute to the client's pain experience. The client's lack of knowledge of pain-relief measures and self-imposed restrictions on pain expression or use of relief measures, as well as deficient pain management skills of health care professionals, may compound the client's pain.

Assessment

Initiate this assessment preoperatively and continue postoperatively.
- Conduct a thorough assessment of the client's pain experience (see the Focused Assessment Guide for the pain experience). Note in particular the accuracy of the client's knowledge about pain (ie, its protective function) and assess the client's ability to manage pain appropriately by using both invasive (drug) and noninvasive treatment modalities.
- Never rely on the client to communicate the need for pain medication or assistance with pain relief. Anticipate the client's need for help and initiate a pain assessment during times when pain is probable. Communicate that the client's pain responses are "okay."

Planning: Client Goals

The client will:
- Identify pain as the body's means to protect itself
- Request prescribed analgesic or initiate appropriate noninvasive relief modalities before pain becomes severe and before beginning a painful activity
- Report a gradual reduction in pain and its eventual elimination

Interventions

- Teach the client preoperatively about the purpose of pain and its value in alerting us to certain body conditions. Inform the client that pain-relieving medications will be available (on request if prn protocol is in place) and that they are most effective when taken before the pain becomes severe. Review the management of patient-controlled analgesia (PCA) if that will be used or discuss expectations and assessments necessary when epidural analgesia is ordered by the physician for control of postoperative pain. Correct any misconceptions the client has and counsel regarding fears.
- During the immediate postoperative period, carefully assess the lessening of anesthetic effect and the need for pharmacologic analgesia. Initial doses of narcotics may need to be reduced if the client is hypotensive; however, the pain may also be causing the hypotension.
- Use good nursing care to keep the client as comfortable as possible. This includes assistance with turning, positioning, and ambulation (as ordered); assistance with coughing and deep breathing; assistance with hydration and nutrition (mouth care for the client who is allowed no oral intake of nutrition or fluids); wound care; massage; help with bathing; and attention to bed linens and elimination needs. Family members may be shown how to comfort clients through massage, repositioning, feeding, and other comfort measures.

- Administer analgesic medications as needed, carefully assessing whether they are producing the desired analgesia without producing undesired side effects. Collaborate with physicians, noting when doses need to be increased or decreased or when a different medication is needed. Use the power of suggestion to enhance the analgesic effect: "Here is your Demerol. You should be feeling good relief shortly. . . . Let me know."
- Assist the client to develop a repertoire of noninvasive pain-relief modalities (distraction, relaxation, cutaneous stimulation) that he or she can use both during hospitalization and at home.

Evaluative Criteria

The client meets the previously stated goals.

Chronic Pain: Malignant

Clients frequently describe chronic malignant pain as hopeless, cyclical, all consuming, meaningless, and as leading to fear, anxiety, depression, and helplessness. Common causes include cancers involving infiltration of nerves, blood vessels, or lymphatic channels; pathologic fractures; and obstruction of hollow organs. The untoward side effects of the treatment for cancer may contribute to the severity of this chronic pain. The client's inability to effectively communicate the severity of the pain or the need for analgesia coupled with possible insensitivity to the pain by health care personnel may compound the problem. Managing this type of pain most often involves the energies of a multidiscipline health care team and the active involvement of the client and family. Many nursing interventions are collaborative in nature.

Assessment

- Conduct a thorough assessment of the client's pain experience and update this as necessary. Note any difficulty the client has in communicating or expressing pain or the need for pain relief.
- Assess:
  - Characteristics of the pain (location, duration, quantity, quality, chronology, aggravating and alleviating factors, associated phenomena)
  - Physiologic responses
  - Behavioral responses
  - Affective responses
  - Interactions with others
  - Degree to which pain interferes with the client's life
  - Perception of pain and its meaning to the client
  - Adequacy of adaptive mechanisms used to cope with pain
- Collaborate with the medical team to identify the physiologic reasons for the client's pain.
- Continually assess the client's response to treatment modalities and note any changes in the client that would necessitate a change in the care plan; be especially sensitive to the development of discomforting or harmful side effects.
- Assess the effect of the client's pain on the family and note the family's coping strategies.

Planning: Client Goals

The client will:
- Relate ability to draw strength (sense of control) from the conviction that the pain will be treated
- Identify people and resources that can be used to secure assistance with pain relief
- Describe a gradual reduction of the pain using a scale ranging from 0 (no pain) to 10 (pain as bad as it can be)
- Demonstrate competent execution of pain management program
  - Analgesics (produce desired pain relief with minimal side effects—sedation, respiratory depression, gastrointestinal problems)
  - Noninvasive pain-relief measures
- Demonstrate the ability to control pain by managing and enjoying key elements of everyday living

The family will report feeling better able to deal with the client's pain.

Interventions

- Establish a trusting nurse–client-family relationship within which the client can freely express pain, fears, and concerns. Be alert to misconceptions about pain and specific fears (fear of losing control, of being abandoned, of addiction; the family's fear that the client will use pain for secondary gains). Whenever possible, assure the client that he or she need never (or never again) feel overwhelmed by pain, and then work to make this promise real.
- Work closely with the physician to develop effective pain control with narcotic analgesics or opioids. Realize that addiction is generally not a problem with this type of pain. Continual experimentation with drug dosage is usually necessary to keep the dose in the zone between oversedation and recurrence of pain. Use of the pain flow sheet (see Fig. 32-5) is helpful. The client in severe pain needs relief with narcotic analgesics or opioids before noninvasive treatment modalities can be helpful. When in severe pain, the client does not have sufficient psychic energy for hypnosis, imagery, or progressive relaxation.

  Analgesic options are varied. For rapid and flexible control initially, intramuscular or subcutaneous morphine has been unsurpassed and around-the-clock (ATC) administration has proved most effective. Because the goal for maintenance management is an oral drug, opiate cocktail mixtures were used for years. More recently, a sustained-release oral morphine and analgesia administration via percutaneous absorption (patch) have been used quite successfully. Severe, intractable cancer pain has also been treated with morphine administered by continuous intravenous drip and epidural analgesia is used with increasing frequency for long-term therapy. With the continuous drip route, more uniform pain control is achieved with lower doses of the drug. Safe administration is facilitated with use of an infusion pump and requires close monitoring of vital signs. A narcotic antagonist, for example, naloxone (Narcan), should be readily available to reverse respiratory depression if needed. Depending on the client, other narcotic and nonnarcotic analgesics may become the drug of choice. Nursing responsibilities with all drug therapy include client education, safe administration, and the reduction or elimination of drug side effects:

- Identify other factors that compound the client's pain experience and work with the health care team to resolve these problems. Common disturbances include the following:
  - *Anxiety and depression*: Interventions include simple psychologic support; attention to social, financial, and legal problems; and administration of low doses of tricyclic antidepressants or anxiolytic agents
  - *Gastrointestinal symptoms*: Common problems include anorexia and dysphagia, mouth problems, nausea and vomiting, intestinal obstruction, constipation and diarrhea, and ascites; because each of these problems can cause discomfort to the client, nursing needs to identify them quickly and initiate measures for their management and control
  - *Skin problems*—decubitus ulcers, other open lesions, pruritus
  - *Fever*

- *Weakness*
- *Respiratory symptoms*
- Collaborate with the client and family in initiating appropriate noninvasive pain-relief measures—distraction, relaxation, cutaneous stimulation; remember that these may have little effect on severe, intractable pain.
- Work with the client and family to improve the self-care abilities that promote the life-style they desire.
- Assist the family to respond optimally to the client's pain experience.
- If necessary, refer the client and family to a hospice or a pain clinic for assistance.

Resources

American Pain Society
340 Kingsland Street
Nutley, NJ 07110
Phone: (201) 235–0587

National Hospice Organization
1311 Dolly Madison Boulevard
McLean, VA 22101
Phone: (703) 356–6770

Palliative Care Foundation
288 Bloor Street West
Toronto, Ontario, Canada M5S/V8

For directions on pain clinics:

Committee on Pain Therapy
American Society of Anesthesiologists
515 Busse Highway
Park Ridge, IL 60068

CASE STUDY *

Patti Potter is a 26-year-old white woman. She is unmarried and has no children. She is employed at a large company as a computer programmer. During the past 7 months, Patti has been experiencing periodic fatigue, anxiety, irritability, depression, and mood swings. Her general health is excellent. The nurse practitioner at the gynecologist's office believes Ms. Potter may be suffering from PMS.

Assessment Findings

The nurse practitioner who interviewed Ms. Potter noted the following data:
- Client has generalized discomfort—fatigue, anxiety, irritability, depression, and mood swings—about 1 week before her menses; discomfort subsides after onset of menses.

*Case study and accompanying nursing care plan contributed by Ruth E. Gordon, RNC, MSN, CRNP (doctoral candidate), Assistant Professor, Department of Nursing, Millersville University, Millersville, PA.

- Discomforts are believed to be heightened by stress at work but do not depend on this. Client denies any new or unusual stress in life currently but believes symptoms are affecting her job performance and relationships.
- Client relates history of "bad cramps" ever since periods started. Client lacks knowledge of appropriate dietary and stress management techniques.
- Client relates she has occasionally taken some of her friend's "tranquilizers" to ease her through a bad day—but she prefers not to take medication.

Nursing Diagnosis

Ineffective Individual Coping related to irritability, anxiety, depression, and mood swings

Planning: Client Goals

The nurse practitioner collaborates with Ms. Potter in establishing a two-step care plan. The client first needs to establish a daily record of her symptoms to identify if they are directly related to her menstrual cycle. If so, Ms. Potter and the nurse practitioner will outline a care plan to relieve the symptoms of PMS.

Ms. Potter has provided positive feedback and has accepted the following client goals. By the completion of one menstrual cycle, the client will:

- List all symptoms that cause her the most difficulty
- Complete a daily record of all symptoms from her list as they occur
- Return for office visit with her daily record at the completion of one menstrual cycle

Documentation

Traditional Note Format

8/13/93, nursing

Consultation with client regarding apparent symptoms of PMS. She states she experiences fatigue, anxiety, irritability, depression, and mood swings about 1 week before her menses. She states these symptoms interfere with her job performance and relationships. She also states that these symptoms seem to subside after onset of her menses. Client admits to use of tranquilizers but prefers not to use medication. Advised client to keep daily record of symptoms for one complete menstrual cycle. Client indicated understanding of all instructions. She will return to office after completion of daily record for its analysis and to begin treatment, if indicated.

R. Gordon, RNC

SOAP Format

8/13/93, nursing

#2 Ineffective Individual Coping related to irritability, anxiety, depression, and mood swings

S: "I'm really flaky before I get my period and it's starting to affect my job."
O: 26-year-old white woman, no history of pregnancy
A: General health excellent, eager to collaborate on care plan
P: Keep daily record of all symptoms for one menstrual cycle and return to office for analysis and treatment if indicated.

R. Gordon, RNC

Ms. Potter returned to the office with her daily record of symptoms complete after one menstrual cycle. Her record revealed that her symptoms were occurring largely from 10 days before her menses to the day her menses began. She experienced 1 full week of no symptoms after her menses. This information validates that she is suffering from PMS.

Revised Nursing Diagnosis

Ineffective Individual Coping related to discomforts of premenstrual symptoms

Planning: Client Goals

The nurse practitioner outlined a treatment plan for Ms. Potter to alleviate her premenstrual symptoms. The plan includes the general areas of relaxation, diet, exercise, and vitamin supplements.

Long-Term Goal
The client will:
- Verbalize symptom-free menses that will enable her to work at optimal effectiveness

Short-Term Goals
See the care plan.

Implementation
The nurse needs to possess the following specialized abilities to implement the care plan:
- Assessment skills—interviewing and physical assessment skills
- Knowledge of women's health and of current modes of treatment of PMS
- Interpersonal skills to collaborate with client for a care plan that will work for her
- Teaching skills to provide client with the knowledge she needs to control discomforts of PMS
- Counseling skills to listen and empathize with client regarding her symptoms and how they are affecting her job performance and relationships

Evaluation

Short-term goals will be evaluated monthly. Long-term goal will be evaluated at 6 months.

 N U R S I N G   C A R E   P L A N

for Ms. Potter

Nursing Diagnosis:	Ineffective Individual Coping related to discomforts of premenstrual symptoms
Signs and Symptoms:	Client complains of fatigue, anxiety, irritability, depression, and mood swings.
Long-Term Goal:	Client will report symptom-free menses that will enable her to work at optimal effectiveness.

(continued)

NURSING CARE PLAN (continued)

for Ms. Potter

Goal: By the next monthly assessment, 10/30/93, client will:
- Use relaxation techniques during periods of anxiety

Nursing Actions	Rationale	Evaluative Statement
Assess client's knowledge of relaxation techniques and motivation to use them.	Effective use of relaxation techniques requires a motivated client.	10/30/93 Goal partially met, client used relaxation techniques during two periods of anxiety. Was driving on expressway during another period of anxiety, which made relaxation difficult.
Instruct client regarding the use of progressive relaxation exercises and controlled breathing during periods of anxiety. For example, "Find a quiet, comfortable place and sit down. Consciously contract and relax the muscles of the whole body starting at the head and neck and working down to the feet until completely relaxed. At the same time, take slow, rhythmic breaths. Continue until anxiety passes."	Relaxation and controlled breathing are used to decrease anxiety and increase coping mechanisms.	*R. Gordon, RNC*

Goal: By the next monthly assessment, 10/30/93, the client will:
- Use a meal plan that includes three balanced meals per day and excludes caffeine, sugar, and sodium

Nursing Actions	Rationale	Evaluative Statement
Assess client's nutritional intake. Have client identify current food preferences high in caffeine, sugar, and sodium and discuss substitutes. Teach client rationale for decreasing intake of caffeine, sugar, and sodium.	Refined sugar and caffeine contribute to feelings of tension and irritability. Sodium contributes to water retention in the body.	10/30/93 Goal met. Client used meal plan for three balanced meals per day and alleviated all sugar, caffeine, and sodium from diet.
Instruct client in developing a meal plan that includes three balanced meals per day.	Balanced meals provide optimal nutrition.	*R. Gordon, RNC*

Goal: By the next monthly assessment, 10/30/93, the client will:
- Incorporate exercise into routine

Nursing Actions	Rationale	Evaluative Statement
Assess value client attaches to physical fitness and regular periods of aerobic exercise; explore preferences.	Exercise can alleviate symptoms of depression, tension, anxiety, fatigue, and irritability. Exercise also serves as a distraction from discomforts.	10/30/93 Goal met. Client includes daily brisk walk around her neighborhood in her routine.
Instruct client in use of regular daily exercise; design exercise prescription.	The fitness produced by regular exercise contributes to self-esteem.	*R. Gordon, RNC*

(continued)

NURSING CARE PLAN (continued)

for Ms. Potter

Goal: By the next monthly assessment, 10/30/93, the client will:
• Supplement her diet with 50 mg of vitamin B₆ daily

Nursing Actions	Rationale	Evaluative Statement
Instruct client on daily use of vitamin B₆.	Vitamin B₆ may be effective in relieving symptoms of irritability, fatigue, and depression.	10/30/93 Goal met. Client supplements her diet daily with 50 mg of vitamin B₆. *R. Gordon, RNC*

Goal: By the next monthly assessment, 10/30/93, the client will:
• Continue use of daily record of PMS symptoms

Nursing Actions	Rationale	Evaluative Statement
Instruct client to continue use of daily record of PMS symptoms throughout the menstrual cycle.	Record keeping allows evaluation of the effectiveness of care plan.	10/30/93 Goal met. Client continued daily record, which illustrated drastic reduction in occurrence of PMS symptoms. Client expressed delight in greater feeling of control she now has over how she feels. "I never realized that so many things affect my comfort level and health." *R. Gordon, RNC*

KEY POINTS

• Pain is a universal human experience, yet no two individuals experience and respond to pain exactly the same way. The most important services nurses offer a client experiencing pain are belief that the client's pain is real, willingness to become involved in the client's pain experience, and competence in developing effective pain management regimens.

• Pain may originate from physical (cutaneous, somatic or visceral) causes or mental or emotional (psychogenic) causes. Most often pain is a blend of both. There is no direct and constant relation between a stimulus for pain and its perception. Little is understood about what causes individuals to perceive pain differently.

• The transmission of pain stimuli is a complex process involving the release of potent chemicals that sensitize the nerve endings, help transmit the pain message, and set the stage for healing; transmission of the pain signal as an electrochemical impulse along the length of the nerve to the dorsal horn of the spinal cord; and relay of the pain signal to the thalamus and eventually to the cortex.

• The gate control theory of pain transmission postulates that only a limited amount of sensory information can be processed by the nervous system at any given moment. The effectiveness of many nursing measures to relieve pain (cutaneous stimulation, imagery) may result from their overstimulation of nerve fibers and the "closing of the gate" to pain stimuli.

• Pain is a mixed sensation and occurs in varying degrees. Pain characteristics include duration, severity, quality, and periodicity. Pain responses may be physiologic, behavioral, or affective.

• Many factors influence the pain experience. Among these are culture, religion, environment, support people, anxiety and other stressors, and past experience with pain.

• Numerous misconceptions about pain by both clients and health care professionals interfere with the client's communication of pain and relief needs and with pain assessment and management.

• It is helpful for nurses to assume that all clients are experiencing some degree of discomfort or pain and to initiate a pain assessment rather than waiting for the client to indicate experiencing pain.

- Pain flow sheets clearly demonstrate the effectiveness of treatment modalities and the development of undesirable side effects.
- Multiple nursing diagnoses may be written that specifically address pain problems or identify the effect of pain problems on other areas of human functioning. Nursing diagnoses developed for pain problems should identify type of pain; etiologic factors; client responses; and other factors affecting pain stimulus and transmission, perception, and response.
- Client goals regarding pain are directed toward the reduction and elimination of discomfort and pain and, whenever possible, to the client's management of a pain-relief program that makes possible the client's desired life-style patterns.
- Nurses are often reluctant to become involved in pain management because of a natural tendency to avoid pain and because pain in the past has evoked in them feelings of fear, frustration, inadequacy, uselessness, and incompetence.
- The unique relationship that can be developed between a client, the family, and the nurse makes the nurse a critical member of the pain management team. Nursing skills are ideal for developing in the client and family the needed self-care behavior to direct an effective pain management program.

- Nursing interventions for pain relief include education, empowerment, manipulating factors that affect the pain experience, initiation of noninvasive treatment modalities (distraction, relaxation, cutaneous stimulation), safe and effective administration of analgesics, and participation in the treatment modalities of other health care professionals.
- Cancer pain requires specialized nursing skills. The chief objective with severe cancer pain is to prevent rather than treat the pain and this most often involves regular doses of narcotic analgesics. Until the client with cancer pain trusts that the pain can be effectively managed, he or she has little psychic energy for other life activities. The nurse's vigilant control of newly developing symptoms can contribute greatly to the client's comfort.
- Evaluation of the care plan necessitates the nurse's ongoing attention to the client's pain experience and the continual modification of pain therapies as needed. Integral to evaluation is feedback from the client and family regarding their feelings about themselves and their current ability to deal with pain.

STUDY QUESTIONS

1. Abdominal pain that is difficult to localize is most likely categorized as
   a. causalgia
   b. visceral
   c. superficial
   d. psychogenic
2. Pain that is transmitted to a cutaneous site different from where it originates is termed
   a. transient pain
   b. superficial pain
   c. phantom pain
   d. referred pain
3. A client who has fallen and injured his or her wrist carefully cradles it with the other hand. This response to pain is referred to as
   a. behavioral
   b. affective
   c. physiologic
   d. involuntary
4. To help relieve her pain, Ann concentrates on a favorite vacation setting. This is known as
   a. distraction
   b. relaxation
   c. recall
   d. imagery

5. Intractable pain is best described as being
   a. intermittent in nature
   b. resistant to treatment
   c. excruciating
   d. widespread
6. According to the gate control theory of pain, an effective nursing intervention for a client with lower back pain is
   a. encouraging regular use of analgesics
   b. applying a K-pad to the area at prescribed intervals
   c. reviewing the pain experience with the client
   d. ambulating the client after medicating him or her
7. A physiologic response to moderate pain is
   a. increased blood pressure
   b. restlessness
   c. decreased pulse rate
   d. protection of the painful area
8. The nurse medicates Mr. Kim, an Oriental client, for pain. Her assessment that he required an analgesic was most likely based on
   a. nonverbal manifestations of pain
   b. verbal expressions of pain
   c. his previous history of pain
   d. exaggerated weeping

9. When assessing pain in a child, the nurse needs to be aware that
   a. immature neurologic development results in reduced sensation of pain
   b. inadequate or inconsistent relief of pain is widespread
   c. reliable assessment tools are currently unavailable
   d. narcotic analgesic use should be avoided

10. Mr. Wright is recovering from abdominal surgery. When the nurse assists him to ambulate, she observes that he grimaces, moves stiffly, and becomes pale. She is aware that he has consistently refused his pain medication. A priority nursing diagnosis would be
    a. Acute Postoperative Pain related to fear of taking prescribed medications
    b. Impaired Physical Mobility related to surgical procedure
    c. Anxiety related to outcome of surgery
    d. High Risk for Infection related to surgical incision

11. When planning strategies for pain control in elderly clients, the nurse should be aware that
    a. pain is a natural outcome of the aging process
    b. sensitivity to pain increases with age
    c. narcotic use should be avoided
    d. denial of pain may occur

12. Chronic pain is most effectively relieved when analgesics are administered
    a. on a prn (as-needed) basis
    b. conservatively
    c. at regularly scheduled intervals
    d. intramuscularly

13. Candidates for continuous subcutaneous infusion as a pain control measure include
    a. clients requiring large doses of opioids for pain relief
    b. clients requiring prolonged use of parenteral opioids
    c. clients requiring rapid control of severe pain
    d. clients requiring frequent dosage alteration of analgesic

14. Using a placebo for pain control is
    a. a widespread practice
    b. consistently effective
    c. an ethical dilemma for the nurse
    d. justified to determine if the pain is real

15. The client receiving epidural analgesia requires careful monitoring to prevent the occurrence of
    a. pruritus
    b. urinary retention
    c. nausea and vomiting
    d. respiratory depression

Answers With Rationale

1. The correct response is *b*. Visceral pain is poorly localized and can originate in body organs in the abdomen. Causalgia is pain that occurs in the area of injured peripheral nerves whereas cutaneous pain is superficial and usually involves the skin or subcutaneous tissue. When a physical cause for the pain cannot be identified, it is known as psychogenic pain.

2. The correct response is *d*. Referred pain is perceived in an area distant from its point of origin whereas transient pain is brief and passes quickly. Superficial pain originates in the skin or subcutaneous tissue. Phantom pain may occur in a person who has had a body part amputated, either surgically or traumatically.

3. The correct response is *a*. Protecting or guarding a painful area is a behavioral response. Affective responses are psychologic ones and examples of a physiologic or involuntary response would be increased blood pressure and dilation of the pupils.

4. The correct response is *d*. Imagery is a mind–body interaction that decreases pain sensation by focusing on pleasurable images. Distraction involves preoccupation with other things to relieve pain and relaxation is a technique that reduces skeletal muscle tension and lessens anxiety. Recall is not a noninvasive relief measure.

5. The correct response is *b*. Intractable pain is severe pain that is resistant to relief measures. The other terms do not describe this resistance to treatment.

6. The correct response is *b*. Nursing measures such as applying warmth to the lower back stimulate the large nerve fibers to close the gate and block the pain. The other choices do not involve attempts to stimulate large nerve fibers that interfere with pain transmission as explained by the gate control theory.

7. The correct response is *a*. Increased blood pressure is a physiologic or involuntary response to moderate pain whereas decreased pulse rate occurs when pain is severe and deep. Restlessness and protection of the painful area are behavioral responses.

8. The correct response is *a*. Members of the Asian culture rarely complain about what is bothering them. The nurse must rely on nonverbal cues that indicate pain is present. Exaggerated weeping is also atypical of this culture and a previous history of pain does not necessarily affect this current experience.

9. The correct response is *b*. Health care personnel are only now becoming aware of pain relief as a priority for children in pain. There currently is more evidence to support the belief that children do indeed

feel pain and reliable assessment tools are available specifically for use with children. Narcotic analgesics may be safely used with children as long as they are carefully observed.

10. The correct response is *a*. Mr. Wright's immediate problem is his pain that is unrelieved because he refuses to take his pain medication for an unknown reason. The other nursing diagnoses are plausible but not a priority in this situation.

11. The correct response is *d*. Elderly people frequently deny pain because they view it as an ominous sign that may interfere with their independence. Pain sensitivity may decrease with age but even this assumption is unsafe and it is not a natural outcome of the aging process. Narcotic medications can be used if the elderly client's response is carefully monitored and evaluated.

12. The correct response is *c*. The prn protocol is totally inadequate for clients experiencing chronic pain. Regularly scheduled doses of analgesic are more effective whereas conservative pain management for whatever reason may also prove ineffective. Intra-

muscular administration is not practical on a long-range basis for a client with chronic pain.

13. The correct response is *b*. Candidates for continuous subcutaneous infusion to control pain must require prolonged use of a parenteral opioid. This route can effectively deliver only small doses of narcotics that are delivered at a slow rate, thus having a slow onset.

14. The correct response is *c*. Using a placebo to control pain poses an ethical dilemma for nurses who are attempting to form a trusting relationship. It is not a widespread practice, may be ineffective, and is never used to determine if pain is real. Pain exists when the client says it does.

15. The correct response is *d*. Too much narcotic given by way of an epidural catheter or a displaced catheter may result in the occurrence of respiratory depression. Pruritus, urinary retention, and nausea and vomiting may occur but are not life-threatening.

BIBLIOGRAPHY

American Nurses' Association. (1991). Position statement on promotion of comfort and relief of pain in dying patients. Kansas City, MO: Author.

American Nurses' Association Task Force on End of Life Decisions. (1991). Board approves position on pain management. *American Nurse, 10*(10), 8.

American Pain Society. (1990). *Principles of analgesic use in the treatment of acute pain or chronic cancer pain* (3rd ed.). Skokie, IL: Author.

Baquie, L. (1989). What matters most in chronic pain management. *RN, 52*(3), 46–50.

Berker, M., & Hughes, B. (1990). Using a tool for pain assessment. *Nursing Times, 86*(24), 50–52.

Bilderback, B. (1991). Playing pain games. *American Journal of Nursing, 91*(5), 19–20.

Burckhardt, C. (1990). Chronic pain. *Nursing Clinics of North America, 25*(4), 863–869.

Camp, L. (1988). A comparison of nurses' recorded assessments of pain with perceptions of pain as described by cancer patients. *Cancer Nursing, 11*(4), 237–243.

Carpenito, L. (1992). *Nursing diagnosis: Application to clinical practice* (4th ed.). Philadelphia: Lippincott.

Chalupka, S., & Gillon-Allard, B. (1989). When your patient has an epidural catheter. *RN, 52*(12), 70–77.

Christoph, S. (1991). Pain assessment: The problem of pain in the critically ill patient. *Critical Care Nursing Clinics of North America, 3*(1), 11–16.

Clark, J., Queener, S., & Karb, V. (1990). *Pharmacological basis of nursing practice* (3rd ed.). St. Louis: Mosby.

Cushing, M. (1992). Pain management on trial. *American Journal of Nursing, 92*(2), 21–23.

Dalton, J. (1989). Nurses' perception of their pain assess-

ment skills, pain management practices, and attitudes toward pain. *Oncology Nursing Forum, 16*(2), 225–231.

Donovan, M. (1990). Acute pain relief. *Nursing Clinics of North America, 25*(4), 851–861.

Doody, S., Smith, C., & Webb, J. (1991). Nonpharmacologic interventions for pain management. *Critical Care Nursing Clinics of North America, 3*(1), 69–74.

Dunajcik, L. (1988). Controlling the dangers of epidural analgesia. *RN, 51*(1), 40–45.

Eland, J. (1988). Pain management and comfort. *Journal of Gerontological Nursing, 14*(4), 10–15.

Ferrell, B. (1991). Managing pain with long-acting morphine. *Nursing 91, 21*(10), 34–39.

Ferrell, B., & Ferrell, B. (1990). Easing the pain. *Geriatric Nursing, 11*(4), 175–178.

Ferrell, B. A., Ferrel, B. R., & Osterweil, D. (1990). Pain in the nursing home. *Journal of American Geriatric Society, 38*(4), 1–5.

Fuller, J., & Schaller-Ayers, J. (1990). *Health assessment: A nursing approach.* Philadelphia: Lippincott.

Goldstein, A. (1991, March 26). Telling the doctor where it hurts. *Washington Post Health,* p. 9.

Halfens, R., Evers, G., & Abu-Saad, H. (1990). Determinants of pain assessment by nurses. *International Journal of Nursing Studies, 27*(1), 43–48.

Hansberry, J., Bannick, K., & Durkan, M. (1990). Managing chronic pain with a permanent epidural catheter. *Nursing, 20*(10), 53–55.

Herr, K., & Mobily, P. (1991). Complexities of pain assessment in the elderly. *Journal of Gerontological Nursing, 17*(4), 12–19.

Holm, K., Cohen, F., Dudas, S., Medema, P., & Allen, B.

(1989). Effect of personal pain experience on pain assessment. *Image: Journal of Nursing Scholarship, 21*(2), 72–75.

Ignatavicius, D., & Bayne, M. (1991). *Medical–surgical nursing*. Philadelphia: Saunders.

Jackson, D. (1989). A study of pain management: Patient controlled analgesia versus intramuscular analgesia. *Journal of Intravenous Nursing, 12*(1), 42–51.

Jacox, A., Heidrich, G., Hester, N., & Miaskowski, C. (1992). Managing acute pain: A guideline for the nation. *American Journal of Nursing, 92*(5), 49–55.

Jaros, J. (1991). The concept of pain. *Critical Care Nursing Clinics of North America, 3*(1), 1–9.

Jones, L., & Brooks, J. (1990). The ABCs of PCA. *RN, 53*(5), 54–63.

Lea, P. (1992). Delivering women from labor pain. *Canadian Nurse, 88*(3), 17–19.

Lindley, C., Dalton, J., & Fields, S. (1990). Narcotic analgesics: Clinical pharmacology and therapeutics. *Cancer Nursing, 13*(1), 28–38.

Logan, M., & Fothergill-Bourbonnais, F. (1990). Continuous subcutaneous infusion of narcotics. *Canadian Nurse, 86*(4), 31–32.

Lubenow, T., & Ivankovich, A. (1991). Patient-controlled analgesia for postoperative pain. *Critical Care Nursing Clinics of North America, 3*(1), 35–41.

Ludwig-Beymer, P. (1989). Transcultural aspects of pain. In J. Boyle & M. Andrews (Eds.), *Transcultural concepts in nursing care* (pp. 283–302). Glenview, IL: Scott, Foresman/Little, Brown College Division.

Marzinski, L. (1991). The tragedy of dementia: Clinically assessing pain in the confused, nonverbal elderly. *Journal of Gerontological Nursing, 17*(6), 25–28.

McCaffery, M. (1979). *Nursing management of the patient with pain* (2nd ed.). Philadelphia: Lippincott.

McCaffery, M., & Beebe, A. (1989), *Pain: Clinical manual for nursing practice*. St. Louis: Mosby.

McCaffery, M., & Ferrell, B. (1990). Do you know a narcotic when you see one? *Nursing 90, 20*(6), 62–63.

McCaffery, M., Ferrell, B., & O'Neill-Page, E. (1992). Does life-style affect your pain-control decisions? *Nursing, 22*(4), 58–61.

McGuire, L. (1990). The power of non-narcotic pain relievers. *RN, 53*(4), 28–35.

McLaughlin-Hagan, M. (1991). Continuous subcutaneous infusions: New use for an old route. *Nursing, 21*(7), 58–59.

Meinhart, N., & McCaffery, M. (1983). *Pain: A nursing approach to assessment and analysis*. Norwalk, CT: Appleton-Century-Crofts.

Melzack, R. (1990). The tragedy of needless pain. *Scientific American, 262*(2), 27–33.

Mueller, R. (1992). Cancer pain: Which drugs for which patients? *RN, 55*(5), 38–46.

Oberle, K., Wry, J., Paul, P., & Grace, M. (1990). Environment, anxiety, and postoperative pain. *Western Journal of Nursing Research, 12*(6), 745–757.

Olsson, G., Leddo, C., & Wild, L. (1989). Nursing management of patients receiving epidural narcotics. *Heart & Lung, 18*(2), 130–137.

Porth, C. (1986). *Pathophysiology: Concepts of altered health states* (2nd ed.). Philadelphia: Lippincott.

Seidel, H., Ball, J., Dains, J., & Benedict, G. (1991). *Mosby's guide to physical examination* (2nd ed.). St. Louis: Mosby/Year Book.

Shannon, M., & Wilson, B. (1992). *Govoni and Hayes' Drugs and Nursing Implications* (7th ed.). Norwalk, CT: Appleton & Lange.

Shlafer, M., & Marieb, E. (1989). *The nurse, pharmacology, and drug therapy*. Redwood City, CA: Addison-Wesley.

Simon, J. (1989). A multidisciplinary approach to chronic pain. *Rehabilitation Nursing, 14*(1), 23–28.

Snelling, J. (1990). The role of the family in relation to chronic pain: Review of the literature. *Journal of Advanced Nursing, 15*(7), 771–776.

Southern, J. (1990). How to access an epidural implanted port. *Nursing 90, 20*(7), 48–51.

Staab, A., & Lyles, M. (1990). *Manual of geriatric nursing*. Glenview, IL: Scott, Foresman/Little Brown Higher Education.

Sternback, R. (1968). *Pain: A psychophysiological analysis*. New York: Academic Press.

Taylor, A., Skelton, J., & Butcher, J. (1984). Duration of pain condition and physical pathology as determinants of nurses' assessment of patients in pain. *Nursing Research, 33*(1), 4–8.

Thiederman, S. (1989). Stoic or shouter, the pain is real. *RN, 52*(6), 49–51.

Tigges, K., & Matthew, W. (1989). Pain assessment: An interdisciplinary perspective. *Home Healthcare Nurse, 7*(6), 18–22.

Uram, M. (1992). A new delivery system makes pain control easier. *RN, 55*(5), 46–51.

Vissering, T. (1991). Pharmacologic agents for pain management. *Critical Care Nursing Clinics of North America, 3*(1), 17–22.

Walker, M., & Wong, D. (1991). A battle plan for patients in pain. *American Journal of Nursing, 91*(6), 32–36.

Wild, L., & Coyne, C. (1992). The basics and beyond: Epidural analgesia. *American Journal of Nursing, 92*(4), 26–34.

Willens, J. (1991). Disconnected epidural catheter. *Nursing, 21*(8), 33.

Williams, A., Beaulavrier, K., & Seal, D. (1990). Chronic cancer pain management with the Du Pen epidural catheter. *Cancer Nursing, 13*(3), 176–182.

Yasko, J. (1983). *Guidelines for cancer care: Symptom management*. Reston, VA: Prentice-Hall.

Zborowski, M. (1969). *People in pain*. San Francisco: Jossey-Bass.

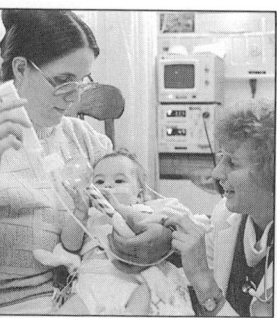
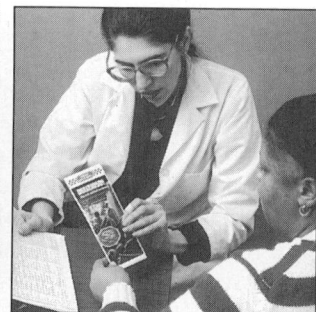

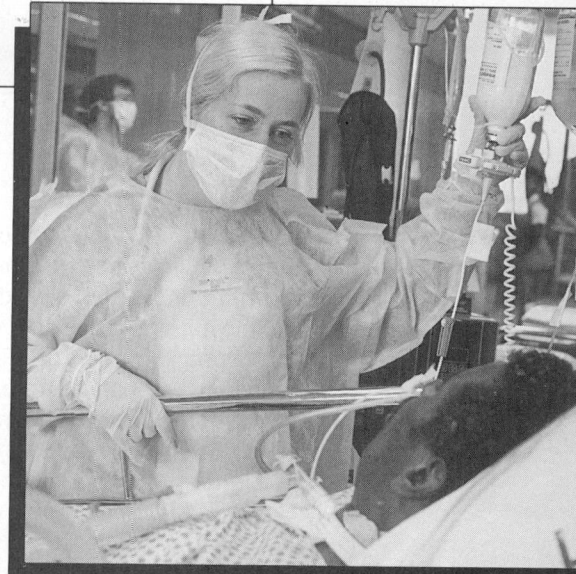

OBJECTIVES

After studying this chapter, the learner should be able to:

Define key terms used in the chapter.

List the six classes of nutrients and explain the significance of each, including variables that affect nutrient requirements.

Evaluate a diet using the food group approach.

Identify dietary, medical–socioeconomic, anthropometric, clinical, and biochemical risk factors for poor nutritional status.

Describe nutritional implications of growth and development throughout the life cycle.

Perform a nutritional assessment using appropriate interview questions, a 24-hour food recall when indicated, and a nursing examination.

Describe common nutritional problems, noting key assessment criteria.

Develop nursing diagnoses that correctly identify nutritional problems that may be treated by independent nursing intervention.

Describe nursing interventions to help clients achieve their nutritional goals.

Plan, implement, and evaluate nursing care related to selected nursing diagnoses that involve nutritional problems.

Differentiate between the various types of enteral tubes.

KEY TERMS

amino acid
anorexia
anorexia nervosa
anthropometric
basal metabolism
bulimia
calorie
cholesterol
complete proteins
disaccharides
enteral nutrition
fatty acid
Food and Drug Administration
incomplete proteins
lipid
macromineral
macronutrient
micromineral
micronutrient
minerals
monosaccharides
nitrogen balance
nutrient
nutrition
obesity
parenteral nutrition
polysaccharides
recommended dietary allowance
saturated fatty acids
triglycerides
unsaturated fatty acids
vitamins

Nutrition

33

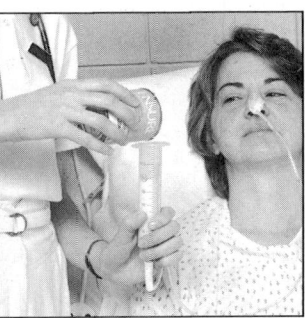

Nutrition is a basic human need that changes throughout the life cycle and along the wellness–illness continuum. Food provides nutrition for both the body and the mind. Eating has evolved from being simply a necessity; it may be a source of pleasure, a pasttime, a social happening, a political statement, a religious symbol, a cultural emblem, or an integral component of medical treatment. As such, food, eating, and nutrition take on different meanings to different people, and changing a person's eating behaviors may be a difficult and slow process. Because nutrition is vital for life and health, and because poor nutrition can seriously decrease one's level of wellness, it is a vital component of nursing.

This chapter provides a knowledge base of basic nutrition theory, focusing on the six classes of nutrients, energy balance, choosing an adequate diet, food patterns and habits, and factors that affect nutrition. Components of simple screening and in-depth nutritional assessments are outlined. Two sets of nursing diagnoses are provided, and client goals for healthy nutrition are discussed. In the section titled Nursing Process in Clinical Practice, focused assessment, diagnosis, planning, implementation, and evaluation guides are offered for select nursing diagnoses related to Altered Nutrition: More Than Body Requirements or Less Than Body Requirements, and Knowledge Deficit related to a new medical diet. These guides and the concluding case study illustrate the significance of nutrition in nursing care.

Principles of Nutrition

The science of **nutrition** encompasses the study of nutrients and how they are handled by the body, as well as the impact of human behavior and environment on the process of nourishment. As such, this discipline includes physiology, psychology, and socioeconomics.

Nutrients are specific biochemical substances used by the body for growth, development, activity, reproduction, lactation, health maintenance, and recovery from illness or injury. Because the metabolic processes involved in these functions are complex, most nutrients work better together than they do alone. Also, nutrient needs change throughout the life cycle in response to changes in body size, activity, growth, development, and state of health.

Some nutrients are considered essential because they are either not synthesized in the body or made in insufficient amounts; essential nutrients must be provided in the diet or through supplements. Essential nutrients that supply energy and build tissue (such as carbohydrates, fats, and protein) are referred to as **macronutrients. Micronutrients**, such as vitamins and minerals, are required in much smaller amounts to regulate and control body processes.

Nonessential nutrients do not have to be supplied through exogenous sources because they are either not required for body functioning or synthesized in the body in adequate amounts. Some nutrients can be converted to others in the body. For instance, the body converts excess carbohydrates and protein into fat, and stores them as triglycerides.

Of the six classes of nutrients, three supply energy (carbohydrates, protein, and lipids) and three regulate body processes (vitamins, minerals, and water).

Energy Balance

Energy in the diet is measured in the form of kilocalories, commonly abbreviated as **calories** or cal (kilojoule [KJ] in Canada). Only carbohydrates, protein, and fat (and alcohol) provide energy; vitamins and minerals are needed for the metabolism of energy but do not provide calories. Total energy intake for a meal, a day, or longer can be calculated by using food composition tables: The values given for total calories for each food eaten can simply be added, or the grams of carbohydrate, protein, and fat for each food eaten can be added and multiplied by the appropriate calorie level (4, 4, and 9 cal, respectively).

Energy in the body is used to carry on any kind of activity, whether voluntary or involuntary. A person's total daily energy expenditure is the sum of all the calories used to perform physical activity, maintain basal metabolism, and digest, absorb, and metabolize food.

Basic Metabolic Requirements **Basal metabolism** is the amount of energy required to carry on the involuntary activities of the body at rest, such as maintaining body temperature and muscle tone, producing and releasing secretions, propelling food through the gastrointestinal tract, inflating the lungs, and beating the heart. As the amount of energy used on physical activity declines, the proportion of calories used for basal metabolism increases; it accounts for more than half of most people's total energy requirements. Because of their larger muscle mass, males have a higher basal metabolic rate (BMR) than females. Other factors that increase BMR include growth, infections, fever, emotional tension, extreme environmental temperatures, and elevated levels of certain hormones, especially epinephrine and thyroid hormones. Aging, prolonged fasting, and sleep all decrease BMR. Most nutritionists agree that fasting or following a very low-calorie diet (VLCD) defeats a weight loss plan because the body interprets this eating pattern as starvation and compensates by slowing down the resting metabolic rate, making it even more difficult to lose weight. BMR is about 1 cal/kg of body weight per hour for men and 0.9 cal/kg/hr for women.

T A B L E   3 3 - 1

1983 Metropolitan Life Insurance Company Height and Weight Table

Height	Weight (lb)		
	Small frame	Medium frame	Large frame
Men*			
5' 2"	128–134	131–141	138–150
5' 3"	130–136	133–143	140–153
5' 4"	132–138	135–145	142–156
5' 5"	134–140	137–148	144–160
5' 6"	136–142	139–151	146–164
5' 7"	138–145	142–154	149–168
5' 8"	140–148	145–157	152–172
5' 9"	142–151	148–160	155–176
5' 10"	144–154	151–163	158–180
5' 11"	146–157	154–166	161–184
6' 0"	149–160	157–170	164–188
6' 1"	152–164	160–174	168–192
6' 2"	155–168	164–178	172–197
6' 3"	158–172	167–182	176–202
6' 4"	162–176	171–187	181–207
Women†			
4' 10"	102–111	109–121	118–131
4' 11"	103–113	111–123	120–134
5' 0"	104–115	113–126	122–137
5' 1"	106–118	115–129	125–140
5' 2"	108–121	118–132	128–143
5' 3"	111–124	121–135	131–147
5' 4"	114–127	124–138	134–151
5' 5"	117–130	127–141	137–155
5' 6"	120–133	130–144	140–159
5' 7"	123–136	133–147	143–163
5' 8"	126–139	136–150	146–167
5' 9"	129–142	139–153	149–170
5' 10"	132–145	142–156	152–173
5' 11"	135–148	145–159	155–176
6' 0"	138–151	148–162	158–179

*Weights at ages 25 to 59 are based on lowest mortality. Weight in pounds are according to frame (in indoor clothing weighing 5 lb, shoes with 1-inch heels).

†Weights at ages 25 to 59 are based on lowest mortality. Weight in pounds are according to frame (in indoor clothing weighing 3 lb, shoes with 1-inch heels).

(Courtesy of Statistical Bulletin, Metropolitan Life Insurance Company.)

Body Weight Standards Ideal body weight (IBW) is an estimate of optimal weight for optimal health. A general guideline for adult women is to allow 100 lb (45.4 kg) for the first 5 ft (152.4 cm) of height and add 5 lb (2.3 kg) for each additional inch (2.54 cm). A range spanning 10% below and above is considered normal, depending on body frame size. For men, the guidelines suggest 106 lb (48.1 kg) for the first 5 ft (152.4 cm) of height, with an additional 6 lb (2.7 kg) for each additional inch (2.54 cm). Again, this weight can be adjusted up or down by 10%, depending on body frame. (Height and weight tables commonly are used for infants and children.)

The 1983 Metropolitan Life Insurance Company height and weight table has consistently been the standard reference that nurses use for IBW (Table 33-1). The weight standards on the chart represent survey results of Americans who purchased life insurance, and are adjusted according to height and frame size for the 25- to 59-year age bracket. The height range may be limiting for some, and the calculated weights do not reflect body fat stores. A person usually is considered overweight if he or she weighs 10% to 20% more than ideal, and obese if he or she weighs more than 20% above ideal weight for his or her height.

Although numerous tables and approaches have been devised for determining ideal weight, many health experts now consider the body mass index (BMI) to be the most precise parameter. The BMI is a ratio of height to weight, and more accurately reflects total body fat stores in the general population. The BMI does not differentiate according to sex, and is calculated in the following manner:

$$BMI = \frac{\text{weight in kilograms}}{\text{height}^2 \text{ in meters}} \quad \begin{array}{l} (2.2 \text{ lb} = 1 \text{ kg}) \\ (39.37 \text{ inches} = 1 \text{ m}) \end{array}$$

The desirable BMIs for various age-groups are listed in Table 33-2. Many health practitioners use this more accurate weight calculation as an initial assessment of nutritional status.

T A B L E   3 3 - 2

Desirable Body Mass Index in Relation to Age

Age Group (yr)	BMI (kg/m²)
19–24	19–24
25–34	20–25
35–44	21–26
45–54	22–27
55–65	23–28
>65	24–29

(National Academy of Sciences. [1989]. *Diet and health*. Washington, D.C.: National Academy Press.)

Caloric Requirements Just like IBW can be determined in a variety of ways, so can a person's calorie requirements (Table 33-3). The Food and Nutrition Board, National Research Council, has published recommended energy intake ranges based on age and sex (see Appendix C-2). The Bureau of Nutritional Sciences of the Department of National Health and Welfare (Canada) has developed a similar energy requirement table (see Appendix D-1). (All tables referring to nutrition for Canada have been placed together in Appendix D.) After calorie requirements have been determined, adjustments can be made for weight gain or loss as needed. For instance, 1 lb (0.45 kg) of body fat equals about 3500 cal. Therefore, to gain or lose 1 lb (0.45 kg) in a week, daily calorie intake should be increased or decreased, respectively, by 500 cal (3500 cal divided by 7 days = 500 cal/d). Similarly, a weight gain or loss of 2 lb (0.9 kg) per week would require an adjustment of 1000 cal/d. Because it becomes increasingly difficult to plan an adequate diet as the calorie level drops, diets that result in more than a 2-lb (0.9-kg) weight loss per week are not recommended.

Energy Nutrients

Carbohydrates

Significance Carbohydrates, commonly known as sugars and starches, are organic compounds composed of carbon, hydrogen, and oxygen. They serve as the structural framework of plants; the only animal source of carbohydrate in the diet is lactose, or "milk sugar."

The significance of carbohydrates cannot be overstated. Because they are relatively easy to produce and store, carbohydrates are the most abundant and least expensive source of calories in the diet worldwide. In fact, carbohydrate intake is correlated to income: as income increases, carbohydrate intake decreases and protein intake, a more expensive form of energy, increases. In countries where grains are the dietary staple, carbohydrates may contribute as much as 90% of total calories. In the United States, the average person consumes about half of his or her total calories from carbohydrates, an amount many health care professionals think should be higher. In Canada, the recommended amount is 55% (Murray & Beare-Rogers, 1990).

Classification Depending on the number of molecules within the structure, carbohydrates are classified as either simple sugars (monosaccharides and disaccharides) or complex (polysaccharides). **Monosaccharides** are composed of only one sugar molecule; as the simplest sugar, they are absorbed without undergoing digestion. Monosaccharides with nutritional significance include glucose (dextrose), fructose, and galactose.

Disaccharides are double sugars composed of glucose and one other monosaccharide. Disaccharides (ie, sucrose, lactose, and maltose) must be broken down by enzymes within the intestinal tract before they can be absorbed.

Polysaccharides, such as starch, glycogen, cellulose, and other types of fiber, are complex molecules composed of hundreds to thousands of glucose units. They are not sweet, and vary in their degree of digestibility. Table 33-4 summarizes the sources, functions, and significance of dietary carbohydrates.

Metabolism Carbohydrates are more easily and quickly digested than protein and fat. Ninety percent of carbohydrate intake is digested; the percentage decreases as fiber intake increases.

Although a small amount of cooked starch may begin to be digested in the mouth, the primary site of chemical digestion is the small intestine. Polysaccharides and disaccharides are broken down into monosaccharides through the action of pancreatic and intestinal enzymes, which are

---

T A B L E 3 3 - 3

Three Methods of Calculating Caloric Requirements

Method 1

Adults
Multiply ideal body weight (IBW) by 10 to determine basal body requirements. Depending on activity level, multiply IBW by the appropriate number indicated below and add to the basal body requirement.

Activity	Calories
Sedentary	Basal calorie needs × 3
Moderate	Basal calorie needs × 5
Heavy	Basal calorie needs × 10

Children (under 12 years old)
Generally allow 100 calories plus 100 calories per year of age. For example, a 4-year-old child needs about 1000 + (100 calories × 4) = 1400 calories.

Method II

Depending on activity level, multiply IBW in pounds by the appropriate number of calories.

Activity	Cal/lb of IBW
Sedentary	11–12
Light	13–14
Moderate	15–16
Heavy	18–19

Method III: USDA Guidelines for Calculating Caloric Requirements

Based on activity level, multiply IBW in pounds by the appropriate number of calories per pound according to sex.

Activity	Cal/lb of IBW	
	Males	Females
Sedentary	16	14
Moderate	21	18
Heavy	28	22

(Adapted from Dudek, S. G. [1993]. *Nutrition handbook for nursing practice.* [2nd ed.]. Philadelphia: Lippincott.)

TABLE 33-4

Sources, Functions, and Significance of Carbohydrates, Protein, and Fat

Nutrient	Sources	Functions	Significance
Carbohydrates			
Simple sugars and starch	Fruits Vegetables Grains: rice, pasta, breads, cereals Dried peas and beans Milk (lactose) Sugars: white and brown sugar, honey, molasses, syrup	Provide energy Spare protein so it can be used for other functions Prevent ketosis from inefficient fat metabolism	Provide about 46% of the calories in the typical American diet (40% in Canadian); many believe carbohydrate intake should be increased to 50%–60% of total calories Low carbohydrate intake can cause ketosis; high simple sugar intake increases the risk of dental caries
Cellulose and other water-insoluble fibers	Whole wheat flour and wheat bran Vegetables: cabbage, peas, green beans, wax beans, broccoli, brussels sprouts, cucumber skins, peppers, carrots Apples	Absorbs water to increase fecal bulk Decreases intestinal transit time	Is nondigestible; therefore, it is excreted Helps relieve constipation North Americans are urged to eat more of all types of fiber Excess intake can cause gas, distention, and diarrhea
Water-soluble fibers	Oat bran and oatmeal Dried peas and beans Vegetables Prunes, pears, apples, bananas, oranges	Slow gastric emptying Lower serum cholesterol level Delay glucose absorption	Help improve glucose tolerance in diabetics
Protein	Milk and milk products Meat, poultry, fish Eggs Dried peas and beans Nuts	Tissue growth and repair Component of body framework: bones, muscles, tendons, blood vessels, skin, hair, nails Component of body fluids: hormones, enzymes, plasma proteins neurotransmitters, mucus Help regulate fluid balance through oncotic pressure Help regulate acid–base balance Detoxify harmful substances Form antibodies Transport fat and other substances through the blood Provide energy when carbohydrate intake is inadequate	Most North Americans consume twice the RDA (RNI) for protein Experts recommend that we eat less animal protein and more vegetable protein. Protein deficiency is characterized by edema, retarded growth and maturation, muscle wasting, changes in the hair and skin, permanent damage to physical and mental development (in children), diarrhea, malabsorption, numerous secondary nutrient deficiencies, fatty infiltration of the liver, increased risk of infections, and high mortality Except for elderly people, fad dieters, hospitalized clients, and people of low income, protein deficiency is rare in the United States and Canada
Fat	Butter, oils, margarine, lard, salt pork, salad dressings, mayonnaise, bacon Whole milk and whole milk products High-fat meats Nuts	Provides energy Provides structure Insulates the body Cushions internal organs Necessary for the absorption of fat-soluble vitamins	Fat supplies about 37% of total calories in the typical North American diet; experts suggest a reduction to 30% or less of total calories High-fat diets increase the risk of heart disease and obesity, and are correlated with an increased risk of colon and breast cancers

(Dudek, S. G. [1993]. *Nutrition handbook for nursing practice* [2nd ed.]. Philadelphia: Lippincott.)

complex protein molecules that facilitate chemical reactions without undergoing change themselves. Monosaccharides are absorbed through the intestinal mucosa and transported to the liver through the portal blood circulation. Cellulose and other undigestible fibers cannot be digested by human enzymes and are, therefore, excreted in the feces unchanged.

In the liver, monosaccharides are converted to glucose, which may then be released into the bloodstream to keep serum glucose levels within a normal range (Fig. 33-1). Under normal conditions, certain tissues, particularly the central nervous system, rely on glucose as their sole source of fuel; therefore, a constant supply of glucose is necessary. Hormones, especially insulin and glucagon, are responsible for keeping serum glucose levels fairly constant during both feasting and fasting.

Through a series of steps, cells oxidize (burn) glucose to provide energy, carbon dioxide, and water. Depending on a person's state of energy balance, the period between carbohydrate consumption and when it is used for energy may vary from minutes to months or longer. Unlike protein and fat, glucose is burned efficiently and completely, and does not leave a toxic product for the kidneys to excrete.

When the supply of glucose exceeds what is needed for energy and to maintain serum levels, it is stored. If muscle or liver glycogen stores are deficient, glucose is converted to glycogen and stored (glycogenesis). Conversely, glycogen is broken down in time of need to supply a ready source of glucose (glycogenolysis). When glycogen stores are adequate, the body converts excess glucose to fat and stores it as triglycerides in adipose tissue.

Functions and Recommended Dietary Allowance   The primary function of carbohydrates is to supply energy. Except for undigestible fiber, all carbohydrates provide 4 cal/g, regardless of the source. Carbohydrates also function to spare protein (ie, using carbohydrates for energy spares protein so it can be used to carry on functions specific for protein, such as building and repairing tissue). Carbohydrates also are needed to efficiently burn fat for energy and thereby prevent ketosis. Research has indicated that carbohydrate intake may also affect a person's mood resulting in increased fatigue and relaxation or mood elevation and lessening of depression depending on individual sensitivities to this nutrient (Cerrato, 1992).

The recommended daily allowance (RDA) of essential nutrients refers to recommendations for average daily amounts that healthy population groups should consume over time. Although an exact requirement for carbohydrates has not been established, at least 50 to 100 g is needed daily to prevent ketosis. In terms of an optimal diet, most health experts recommend that carbohydrates provide 50% to 60% of the diet's total calories, mostly in the form of complex carbohydrates.

Protein

Significance   Protein is a vital component of every living cell. Within the human body, more than a thousand different proteins are made by combining various amounts and

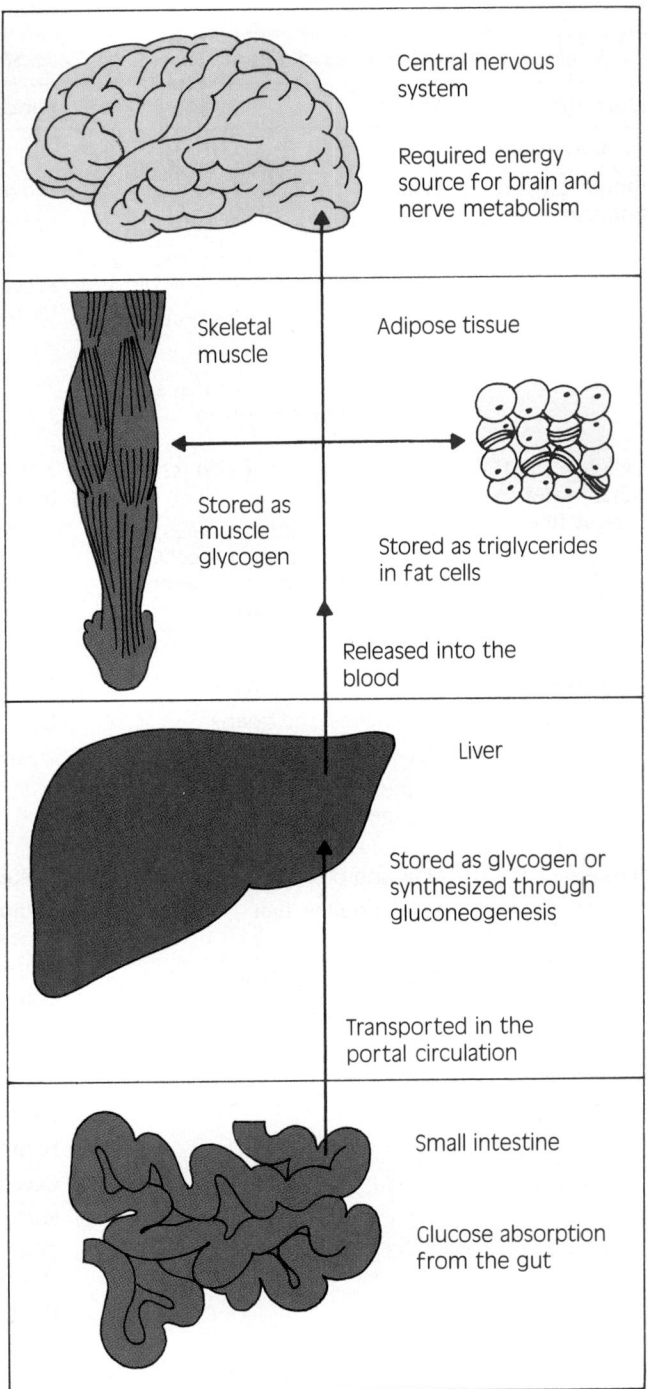

F I G U R E   3 3 - 1

Glucose is an efficient fuel on which certain tissues, particularly the central nervous system, rely almost exclusively as an energy source. Glucose ingested in the diet is transported from the gastrointestinal tract, through the portal vein, to the liver. The liver stores glucose and regulates its entry into the blood. (Adapted from Porth, C. M. [1986]. *Pathophysiology: Concepts of altered health states* [2nd ed., p. 604]. Philadelphia: Lippincott.)

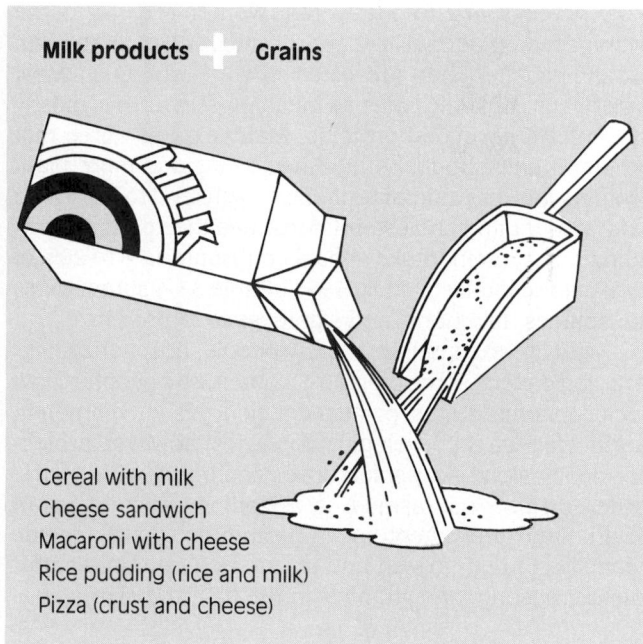

Milk products ✚ Grains

Cereal with milk
Cheese sandwich
Macaroni with cheese
Rice pudding (rice and milk)
Pizza (crust and cheese)

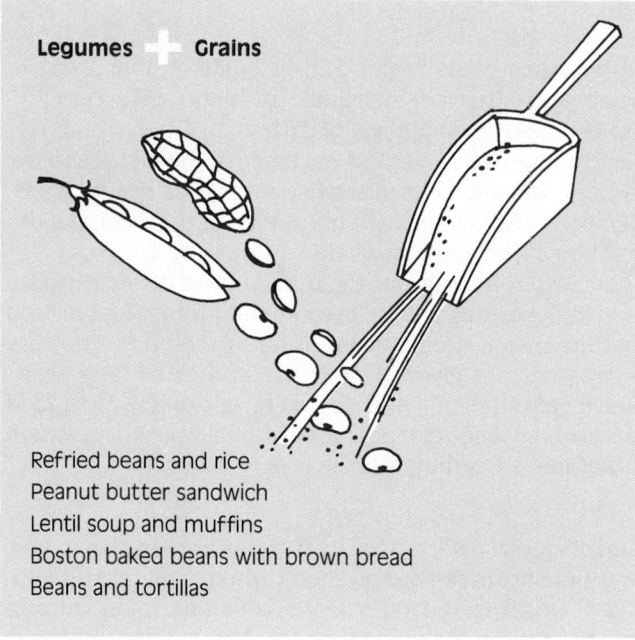

Legumes ✚ Grains

Refried beans and rice
Peanut butter sandwich
Lentil soup and muffins
Boston baked beans with brown bread
Beans and tortillas

FIGURE 33-2

Combinations of legumes and grains, and milk products and grains in appropriate quantities at the same meal provide high-quality proteins in complement.

proportions of the 22 basic building blocks known as **amino acids**. Although amino acids, like carbohydrates, contain carbon, hydrogen, and oxygen, they differ in that amino acids also contain nitrogen. Nine amino acids are classified as essential because they cannot be synthesized in the body; the remaining amino acids are no less important, but because the body can make them if a supply of nitrogen is available, they are termed nonessential.

Classification Dietary proteins may be labeled complete (high quality) or incomplete (low quality), based on their amino acid composition. **Complete proteins** contain sufficient amounts and proportions of all the essential amino acids to support growth, whereas **incomplete proteins** are deficient in one or more essential amino acids. Generally, animal proteins (eggs, dairy products, and meats) are complete, and plant proteins (grains, legumes, and vegetables) are incomplete. Because different sources of plant proteins lack different amino acids, a plant protein can be complemented and its quality made high by combining it with a different plant protein or by adding a small amount of an animal protein. Examples of complementary vegetable proteins include corn tortilla and refried beans and lentil rice soup (Fig. 33-2). Complementary proteins that use a small amount of animal protein are cereal with milk, rice pudding, and a cheese sandwich.

Metabolism Chemical digestion of protein begins in the acid medium of the stomach; however, most protein digestion occurs in the small intestine through the action of pancreatic and intestinal proteases. Amino acids are absorbed through the intestinal mucosa into the portal blood circulation for transport to the liver. Neonates are uniquely able to absorb whole proteins—antibodies from breast milk—which affords them a certain degree of immunity from infections. Only a small amount of ingested protein normally remains undigested and is excreted in the feces.

Once in the liver, amino acids can then be recombined to form new proteins, or may be released into the bloodstream and carried to tissues and cells for protein synthesis (Fig. 33-3). The body's protein tissues are in a constant state of flux: tissues are continuously being broken down (catabolism) and replaced (anabolism). **Nitrogen balance**, a comparison between catabolism and anabolism, can be measured by comparing nitrogen intake (protein intake) and nitrogen excretion (nitrogen lost in urine, urea, feces, hair, nails, and skin). When catabolism and anabolism are occurring at the same rate, as in healthy adults, the body is in a state of neutral nitrogen balance (ie, nitrogen intake equals nitrogen excretion). A positive nitrogen balance occurs when nitrogen intake is greater than excretion—for example, during periods of growth, pregnancy, lactation, and recovery from illness. A negative nitrogen balance, an undesirable state such as starvation and the catabolism that immediately follows surgery, illness, trauma, and stress, indicates that more nitrogen is being excreted than consumed.

Functions The major function of protein is to maintain body tissues that break down from normal wear and tear and to support the growth of new tissue. Protein also is a component of the body's framework (bones, muscles, tendons, blood vessels, skin, nails, and hair), many essential secretions and fluids (hormones, enzymes, neurotransmitters, breast milk, mucus, sperm, and bile acids), and body compounds, such as the blood-clotting factor thrombin. Protein plays a role in fluid and acid–base balance, helps to detoxify harmful foreign substances, and forms antibodies

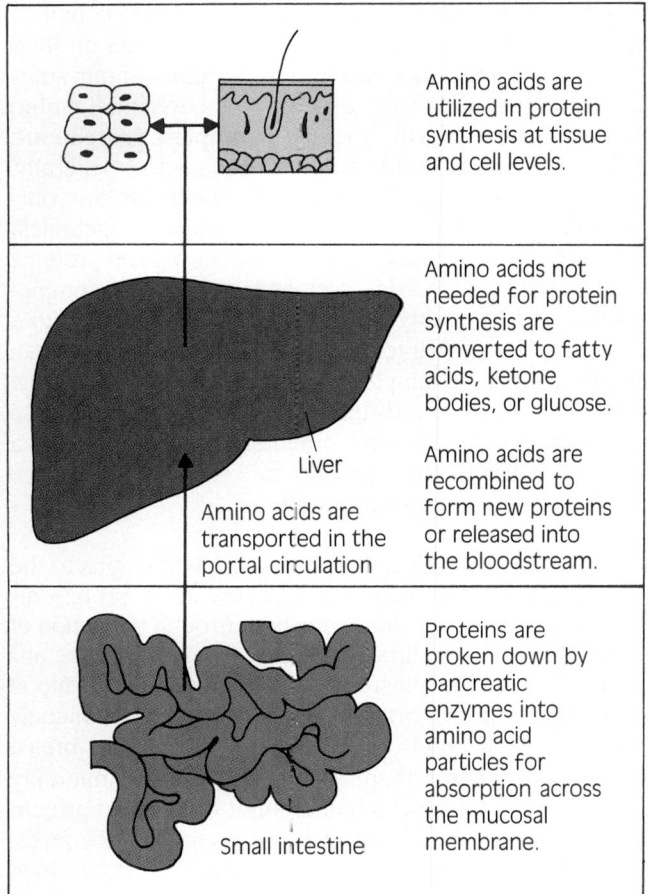

Amino acids are utilized in protein synthesis at tissue and cell levels.

Amino acids not needed for protein synthesis are converted to fatty acids, ketone bodies, or glucose.

Liver

Amino acids are transported in the portal circulation

Amino acids are recombined to form new proteins or released into the bloodstream.

Small intestine

Proteins are broken down by pancreatic enzymes into amino acid particles for absorption across the mucosal membrane.

F I G U R E   3 3 - 3

Dietary protein is broken down into amino acid particles by pancreatic enzymes in the small intestine and absorbed through the intestinal mucosa for transportation to the liver. In the liver, amino acids are recombined into new proteins or are released into the bloodstream for use in protein synthesis by tissues and cells. Excess amino acids are converted to fatty acids, ketone bodies, or glucose, and stored or used as metabolic fuel. Proteins are essential for the formation of all body structures, including genes, enzymes, muscle, bone matrix, and hemoglobin. Amino acids are the building blocks of protein.

to help the body resist infection and certain diseases. It helps move fat, fat-soluble vitamins, minerals, and other substances through the blood. Lastly, protein can be oxidized to provide 4 cal/g. Using protein for energy is more expensive both financially and physiologically than using carbohydrates; the nitrogen remaining after protein is metabolized burdens the kidneys and requires energy to be excreted. Like carbohydrates, protein consumed in excess of need can be converted to and stored as fat.

Recommended Dietary Allowance   The recommended daily dietary allowance (RDA) for protein for adults is 0.8 g/kg, or about 44 g, for the average woman and 56 g for the average man (National Research Council, 1980). (Canadian protein requirements are listed in Appendix D-2.) Most Americans consume twice as much protein as this, mostly in the form of animal proteins. Many experts agree that protein intake should be modified to include more plant proteins and less animal proteins, which tend to be high in saturated fat and cholesterol. Most health experts recommend that protein intake should contribute 10% to 20% of total caloric intake (Dudek, 1993). Table 33-4 summarizes the sources, functions, and significance of protein.

With the exception of elderly people, hospitalized clients, fad dieters, some pregnant women, and people of low socioeconomic status, protein deficiency is uncommon in North America. In developing countries, however, protein deficiency alone (kwashiorkor) or combined with calorie undernutrition (marasmus) is a leading cause of infant death. Signs and symptoms of protein deficiency include edema, retarded growth and maturation, mental apathy, muscle wasting, and changes in the hair and skin.

Fats

Significance   Fats in the diet, or **lipids**, are insoluble in water and, therefore, insoluble in blood. Like carbohydrates, they are composed of carbon, hydrogen, and oxygen. Ninety-five percent of the lipids in the diet are in the form of fats and oils, otherwise known as simple lipids. Compound lipids (such as phospholipids, in which a lipid is combined with another substance) and derived lipids (such as cholesterol) constitute the remainder of the lipid intake.

Triglycerides are the predominant form of fat in food and the major storage form of fat in the body. They are composed of a glycerol molecule and three fatty acids, which vary in length and degree of saturation. Most food fats are composed of long-chain fatty acids (ie, they contain more than 12 carbon atoms).

Classification   **Saturated fatty acids** are not able to hold any more hydrogen atoms; their carbon bonds are all saturated. **Unsaturated fatty acids** have one (monounsaturated) or more (polyunsaturated) double bonds between carbon atoms; therefore, they have the potential to hold more hydrogen atoms if the double bonds are broken. Food fats contain mixtures of saturated and unsaturated fatty acids. Most animal fats are considered saturated because they contain proportionately more saturated fatty acids and have a solid consistency at room temperature. Conversely, most vegetable fats are considered unsaturated because they contain more unsaturated than saturated fatty acids. Unsaturated fats are liquid at room temperature and referred to as oils. Commercially, the addition of hydrogen atoms to unsaturated fats (hydrogenation) makes a fat more saturated and thereby increases its shelf life and stability. Saturated fats tend to raise serum cholesterol levels, whereas unsaturated fats lower serum cholesterol levels.

Cholesterol is a fatlike substance found only in animal products. It is not essential that cholesterol be provided in the diet because the body synthesizes about twice as much cholesterol as most people in North America eat. Cholesterol is an important component of cell membranes and is especially abundant in brain and nerve cells. It also is used to synthesize bile acids and is a precursor of the steroid hormones and vitamin D. Although cholesterol serves many important functions in the body, high serum levels are clearly associated with an increased risk of atherosclerosis. To help lower serum cholesterol levels, researchers recommend limiting cholesterol intake, eating less total fat—especially saturated fat—eating more unsaturated fat, and increasing fiber intake, which increases fecal excretion of cholesterol.

Linoleic acid is the only fatty acid the body cannot synthesize; therefore, it is labeled essential. Linoleic acid is important for capillary strength and cell membrane structure, is a precursor of prostaglandins, and helps decrease serum cholesterol levels. Because the requirement for linoleic acid is so small (about 2% to 3% of total calories), a deficiency is rare. The best sources of linoleic acid are polyunsaturated vegetable oils, such as sunflower, soybean, and corn.

Metabolism Fat digestion largely occurs in the small intestine. Bile, secreted by the gallbladder, emulsifies fat to increase the surface area so that pancreatic lipase can break down fat more effectively. Through a complex series of events, most fats are absorbed into the lymphatic circulation with the help of a protein carrier and are transported to the liver (Fig. 33-4). Of 100 g eaten, only about 3 g is excreted in the feces.

Functions Fats are the most concentrated source of energy in the diet, providing 9 cal for every gram. Fat increases the palatability of the diet (eg, to most people, filet mignon tastes better than flank steak) and has a high satiety value because it delays gastric emptying time. In the body, fat aids in the absorption of the fat-soluble vitamins and provides insulation, structure, and temperature control. Table 33-4 summarizes the source, functions, and significance of fat.

Recommended Dietary Allowance Because fat can be synthesized in the body from carbohydrates and protein, an RDA for fat has not been established. Americans consume about 37% of their total caloric intake in the form of fat. Most experts agree that fat should not contribute more than 30% of the day's caloric intake, and saturated fat intake should be limited to 10% or less of total fat calories (Dudek, 1993).

Regulatory Nutrients

Vitamins, minerals, and water are regulatory nutrients because they are needed by the body for the metabolism of energy nutrients.

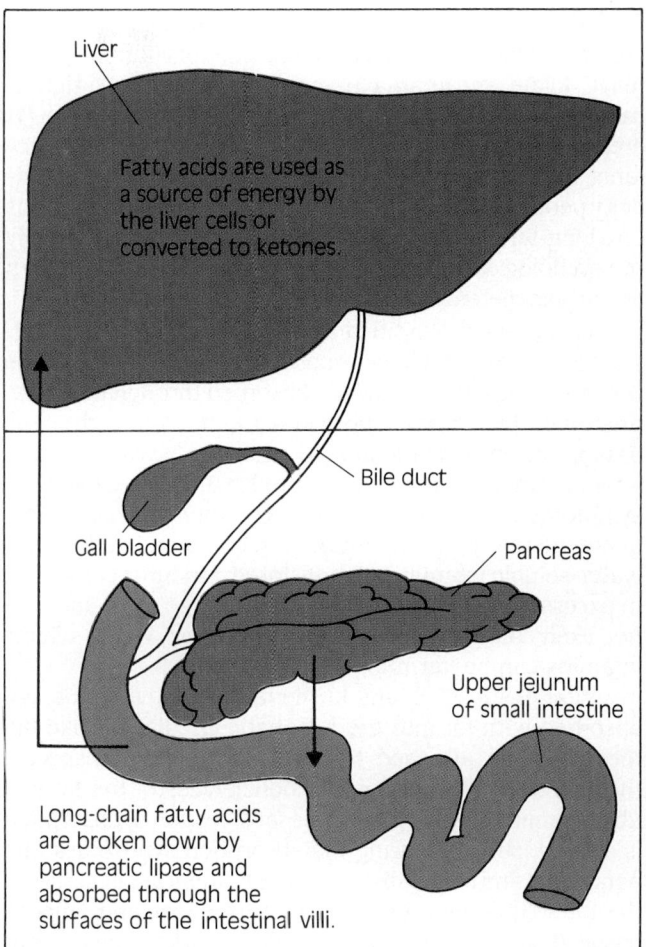

FIGURE 33-4

The average adult consumes 60 to 100 g of fat daily, mostly as triglycerides. These triglycerides are broken down by pancreatic lipase and are absorbed primarily in the upper jejunum. Fatty acids transported to the liver are used by the liver cells as a source of energy or are converted to ketones.

Vitamins

Vitamins are organic compounds needed by the body in small amounts. Most vitamins are active in the form of a coenzyme, which together with enzymes facilitate thousands of chemical reactions in the body. Although vitamins do not provide energy (calories), they are needed for the metabolism of carbohydrates, protein, and fat. Because most vitamins are either not synthesized in the body or made in insufficient quantities, they are essential in the diet.

Vitamins are present in foods in only small amounts. Because vitamins may be destroyed by light, heat, and air and during preparation, fresh foods are higher in vitamins than processed foods. The exception is in the case of fortification, when vitamins that do not naturally occur in a food are added (eg, vitamin D–fortified milk).

In North America, severe vitamin deficiencies are uncommon. Mild or subclinical deficiencies of vitamin A, vitamin C, folate, and vitamin B$_6$, however, may affect a significant proportion of the population, especially those who (1) are members of certain age-groups or client groups (infants, adolescents, pregnant and lactating women, and elderly people); (2) smoke, abuse alcohol, or use medications on a long-term basis; (3) are chronically ill, either physically or psychologically; and (4) are poor or finicky eaters, such as chronic dieters, strict vegetarians, and food faddists.

Vitamins are classified as either water-soluble or fat-soluble. Water-soluble vitamins include vitamin C and the B-complex vitamins. They are absorbed through the intestinal wall directly into the bloodstream. Although some tissues are able to hold limited amounts of water-soluble vitamins, they usually are not stored in the body. Deficiency symptoms are apt to develop quickly when intake is inadequate; therefore, a daily intake is recommended. Because water-soluble vitamins are not stored, amounts consumed in excess of need are excreted in the urine. Toxicities are not likely, although megadoses of certain water-soluble vitamins can be harmful.

Vitamins A, D, E, and K, the fat-soluble vitamins, are absorbed with fat into the lymphatic circulation; like fat, they must be attached to a protein to be transported through the blood. Secondary deficiencies of the fat-soluble vitamins can occur anytime fat digestion or absorption is altered, such as during malabsorption syndromes and pancreatic and biliary diseases. The body stores excesses of the fat-soluble vitamins mostly in the liver and adipose tissue. Because they are stored, a daily intake is not imperative, and deficiency symptoms may take weeks to months to years to develop. Excessive intakes, particularly of vitamins A and D, are toxic.

Table 33-5 summarizes water- and fat-soluble vitamins. (Canadian Recommended Nutrient Intakes [RNI] are listed in Appendix D-2.)

Minerals

Minerals are inorganic elements found in all body fluids and tissues in the form of salts (eg, sodium chloride) or combined with organic compounds (eg, iron in hemoglobin). Some minerals function to provide structure within the body, whereas others help to regulate body processes. Because they are elements, minerals are not broken down or rearranged in the body but are contained in the ash that remains after digestion. Although excessive soaking and cooking in water can cause loss of minerals from food, minerals commonly are not destroyed by food processing. Calcium, phosphorus, and magnesium are considered **macrominerals** because they are needed by the body in amounts greater than 100 mg/day. Required intake of **microminerals** or trace elements is less than 100 mg/day. Iron, zinc, manganese, and iodine are examples of microminerals. Trace elements with an established RDA or RNI (Canada) include iron, iodine, and zinc. Ranges of estimated safe and adequate daily intakes have been suggested for copper, manganese, fluorine, chromium, selenium, molybdenum; no recommendations have been made for cobalt, nickel, vanadium, arsenic, and silicon. Macrominerals and microminerals are summarized in Table 33-6. (Canadian RNIs are listed in Appendix D-2.)

Water

As the major body constituent present in every body cell, water accounts for between 50% and 60% of the adult's total weight; infants have proportionately more water. About two-thirds of the body's water is contained within the cells (intracellular fluid [ICF]); the remainder is called extracellular fluid (ECF), and includes all other body fluids, such as plasma and interstitial fluid. Total body water and ECF decreases with age; ICF increases with an increase in body mass.

Water is more vital to life than food because it provides the fluid medium necessary for all chemical reactions, it participates in many reactions, and it is not stored in the body. Water acts as a solvent that dissolves many solutes, thereby aiding digestion, absorption, circulation, and excretion. Through evaporation from the skin, water helps to regulate body temperature. As a lubricant, water is needed for mucous secretions and between moving joints.

Sources of water in the diet include not only beverages but also solid foods, which contain from 10% to 98% water. Water also is produced through the metabolism of carbohydrates, protein, and fat. It leaves the body through urine, feces, expired air, and perspiration. Water intake (an average of 1500 to 3000 mL/day) usually equals water output. Water balance may be seriously affected when either intake (eg, in comatose states) or output (eg, in altered renal function, profuse perspiration, diarrhea, vomiting, fistulas, drainage tubes, hemorrhage, and severe burns) is altered.

How to Choose an Adequate Diet

An adequate diet provides a balanced intake of all essential nutrients in appropriate amounts; what constitutes an adequate diet is less obvious. Although a major problem in developing countries, malnutrition related to poor dietary intake is uncommon in North America. Rather, nutritional concerns focus more on problems of overnutrition. Tools for planning or evaluating a diet for adequacy include food groups, the RDA or RNI, dietary recommendations and guidelines issued from health and U.S. governmental agencies, Nutrition Recommendations for Canadians, and Canada's Food Guide.

Food Groups The food group approach to diet planning suggests how many servings of food, not the quantity of particular nutrients, a person should consume daily from each of four or more food groups. Food groupings are made on the basis of vitamin and mineral content; the calorie, fat,

(*Text continues on page 804*)

TABLE 33-5

Summary of Water- and Fat-Soluble Vitamins*

Nutrient and Adult RDA	Sources	Functions	Signs and Symptoms of Deficiency	Signs and Symptoms of Excess	Pharmacologic Uses
Water-Soluble Vitamins					
Vitamin C (ascorbic acid) 60 mg (60–100 mg for smokers)	Citrus fruits and juices, guava, broccoli, brussels sprouts, green pepper, strawberries, greens, tomatoes, cabbage	Collagen formation, protects other nutrients from oxidation, enhances iron absorption, converts folic acid to its active form, involved in the metabolism of certain amino acids	Scurvy, characterized by bleeding gums; hemorrhaging; muscle degeneration; delayed wound healing; softening of the bones; soft, loose teeth; anemia; increased susceptibility to infection, hysteria, and depression	Kidney stones, scurvy on withdrawal, nausea, abdominal cramps, diarrhea, false-positive test for urinary glucose	Treatment of scurvy only proven effective use; no evidence that it cures or prevents colds, cures cancer, or improves breathing in asthmatics
Vitamin B complex B₁ (thiamine) 1–1.4 mg	Pork, liver, organ meats, whole grain and enriched grains, nuts, dried peas and beans, eggs	Energy metabolism, especially the metabolism of carbohydrates, normal nervous system functioning	Beriberi, mental confusion, fatigue, peripheral paralysis, muscle weakness, painful calf muscles, anorexia, edema, enlarged heart, heart failure	None known	Treatment of thiamine deficiency only
B₂ (riboflavin) 1.2–1.7 mg	Milk and dairy products, organ meats, eggs, enriched grains, green leafy vegetables	Carbohydrate, protein, and fat metabolism; other metabolic functions	Ariboflavinosis, dermatitis, cheilosis, glossitis, photophobia, reddening of the cornea	None known	Treatment of riboflavin deficiency only
Niacin 13–19 mg	Kidney, liver, poultry, lean meat, fish, yeast, peanut butter, enriched and whole grains, dried peas and beans, nuts	Carbohydrate, protein, and fat metabolism	Pellagra, dermatitis, diarrhea, dementia, death	Flushing and itching, nausea, vomiting, diarrhea, hypotension, tachycardia, hypoglycemia, and liver damage	Treatment of niacin deficiency and pellagra; megadoses of nicotinic acid used to lower serum cholesterol levels in people who do not respond adequately to diet and weight loss
B₆ 2–2.2 mg	Yeast, wheat germ, pork, organ meats, egg yolk, whole-grain cereals, potatoes	Amino acid metabolism, blood formation, maintenance of nervous tissue, conversion of tryptophan to niacin	Dermatitis, cheilosis, glossitis, abnormal brain wave pattern, convulsions, anemia	Difficulty walking, numbness of the feet and hands, sensations of shock	Treatment of vitamin B₆ deficiency; used experimentally to relieve malaise and depression in women using oral contraceptives; used with some success to relieve nausea and vomiting during pregnancy and after radiation therapy

(continued)

T A B L E 3 3 - 5 *(continued)*

Summary of Water- and Fat-Soluble Vitamins*

Nutrient and Adult RDA	Sources	Functions	Signs and Symptoms of Deficiency	Signs and Symptoms of Excess	Pharmacologic Uses
Water-Soluble Vitamins					
Folic acid (folacin) 180–200 μg	Green leafy vegetables, asparagus, broccoli, liver, organ meats, milk, eggs, yeast, wheat germ	RNA and DNA synthesis, formation and maturation of RBC, amino acid metabolism	Macrocytic anemia: fatigue, weakness, pallor, diarrhea, weight loss, glossitis	None known	Treatment of folic acid deficiency; used prophylactically to prevent anemia during pregnancy
B$_{12}$ (cobalamin) 2 μg	Only foods of animal origin: meat, fish, seafood, poultry, eggs, milk, dairy products	RNA and DNA synthesis, myelin formation: carbohydrate, protein, and fat metabolism; folic acid metabolism	Pernicious anemia (B$_{12}$ deficiency related to impaired absorption related to lack of intrinsic factor): macrocytic anemia, pallor, dyspnea, weakness, fatigue, palpitations, glossitis, anorexia, indigestion, recurring diarrhea or constipation, weight loss, paresthesia of the hands and feet, poor muscle coordination, poor memory, irritability, depression, paranoia, delirium, hallucinations	None known	Treatment of B$_{12}$ deficiency only; no evidence exists to support claims that B$_{12}$ relieves infectious hepatitis, multiple sclerosis, poor appetite, poor growth, aging, or fatigue
Pantothenic acid 4–7 mg	Liver, kidney, salmon, egg yolk, fresh vegetables, yeast, whole-grain cereals	Carbohydrate, protein, and fat metabolism	None known	None known	Credited with improving the burning-food syndrome
Biotin 30–100 μg	Liver, organ meats, peanuts, mushrooms, egg yolk, milk, yeast	Carbohydrate, protein, and fat metabolism; conversion of tryptophan to niacin	Produced by adding large amounts of raw egg white to a biotin-deficient diet. Raw egg white contains avidin, which prevents biotin absorption. Symptoms include dry, scaly dermatitis, anorexia, nausea, vomiting, glossitis, and depression	None known	None known

(continued)

TABLE 33-5 (continued)

Summary of Water- and Fat-Soluble Vitamins*

Nutrient and Adult RDA	Sources	Functions	Signs and Symptoms of Deficiency	Signs and Symptoms of Excess	Pharmacologic Uses
Fat-Soluble Vitamins					
Vitamin A (retinol, retinal, retinoic acid) 800–1000 RE	Liver; egg yolk; fortified milk, dairy products, margarine, breakfast cereals; dark green and yellow vegetables, such as sweet potatoes, winter squash, carrots, broccoli, spinach, greens; peaches; apricots; cantaloupe	Visual acuity in dim light, formation and maintenance of skin and mucous membranes, normal growth and development of bones and teeth	Night blindness; dry, rough skin; dry mucous membranes; dry eyes (xerosis); decreased saliva secretion leading to difficulty chewing and swallowing, impaired digestion and absorption, diarrhea; increased susceptibility to respiratory tract, urinary tract, and vaginal infections; impaired bone and teeth development	Anorexia, nausea, vomiting, abdominal pain, diarrhea, weight loss, irritability, fatigue, ascites and portal hypertension, loss of hair, dry skin, bone pain and fragility, spleen enlargement, extensive liver damage, hydrocephalus (in infants and children)	Treatment of vitamin A deficiency; treatment of severe, resistant forms of acne
Vitamin D (cholecalciferol, ergosterol) 5–10 μg	Sunlight; fortified milk, margarine, and breakfast cereals; butter; egg yolk; liver; fish liver oils	Calcium and phosphorus metabolism, stimulates calcium absorption, mobilizes calcium and phosphorus from the bone, stimulates reabsorption of calcium and phosphorus by the kidney	Rickets in infants and children: retarded bone growth, bone malformation, enlargement of ends of long bones, malformed teeth, tooth decay; osteomalacia in adults: bone deformities, pain, easy fracture, involuntary muscle twitching and spasms	Excessive calcification of the bones, renal calculi, nausea, vomiting, headache, weakness, weight loss, constipation, polyuria, polydipsia. Mental and physical growth retardation and failure to thrive in children. Drowsiness and coma in severe cases	Treatment of hypocalcemic diseases: rickets, renal osteodystrophy, postoperative tetany, idiopathic tetany, hypoparathyroidism
Vitamin E (tocopherol) 8–10 mg	Vegetable oils, wheat germ, whole-grain products	Protects vitamin A and polyunsaturated fatty acids from oxidation, helps maintain cell membrane integrity, heme synthesis	Increased RBC hemolysis and macrocytic anemia in premature infants	Relatively nontoxic, although large doses can cause depression, fatigue, diarrhea, cramps, blurred vision, and headaches; also interferes with normal blood clotting and vitamin A metabolism	Treatment of vitamin E deficiency only. Claims that vitamin E treats coronary heart diseases, infertility, cancer, diabetes, ulcers, skin disorders, burns, shortness of breath, and muscular dystrophy are unfounded, as are claims that it increases physical performance and sexual potency and slows the aging process

(continued)

T A B L E   3 3 - 5 *(continued)*

Summary of Water- and Fat-Soluble Vitamins*

Nutrient and Adult RDA	Sources	Functions	Signs and Symptoms of Deficiency	Signs and Symptoms of Excess	Pharmacologic Uses
Fat-Soluble Vitamins					
Vitamin K 65–80 µg	Dark green leafy vegetables, vegetables of cabbage family; synthesized in the intestines from gut bacteria	Synthesis of certain proteins necessary for blood clotting	Hemorrhagic disease of the newborn, delayed blood clotting	Hemolytic anemia and liver damage with synthetic vitamin K	Treatment of coagulation disorders related to impaired vitamin K synthesis or absorption; used prophylactically to treat hemorrhagic disease of the newborn; used to treat oral anticoagulant–induced prothrombin deficiency

*See Appendix D for Canadian RNIs.

(Dudek, S. G. [1993]. *Nutrition Handbook for nursing practice* [2nd ed.] Philadelphia: Lippincott.)

T A B L E   3 3 - 6

Summary of Macrominerals and Microminerals*

Nutrient and Adult RDA	Sources	Functions	Signs and Symptoms of Deficiency	Signs and Symptoms of Excess
Macrominerals				
Calcium 800 mg (18–24 yr: 1200 mg)	Milk and dairy products, canned fish with bones, green leafy vegetables	Bone and tooth formation, blood clotting, nerve transmission, muscle contraction, cell membrane permeability, activation of certain enzymes	Osteomalacia; osteoporosis; hypocalcemia leads to tetany: intermittent, tonic contractions of the extremities, muscle cramps, uncontrolled seizures, possible convulsions. Hypocalcemia, in combination with other factors, may promote hypertension.	Hypercalcemia can cause nausea, vomiting, anorexia, abdominal pain, constipation, polyuria, polydipsia, renal calculi, excessive calcification of the bones and soft tissues. Coma and death result if not treated
Phosphorus 800–1200 mg	Milk and milk products, meat, poultry, fish, eggs, dried peas and beans, nuts, soft drinks, processed foods	Bone and tooth formation, acid–base balance, energy metabolism, cell membrane structure, component of nucleic acids, regulates activity of hormones and coenzymes, fat absorption and transportation, glucose absorption	Hypophosphatemia: anorexia, weakness, circumoral paresthesia, hyperventilation	Hyperphosphatemia: symptoms of hypocalcemic tetany
Magnesium 280–350 mg	Green leafy vegetables, nuts, dried peas and beans, grains, seafood, cocoa, chocolate	Bone and tooth formation, smooth-muscle relaxation, protein synthesis, carbohydrate metabolism, cell reproduction and growth, hormonal activity	Hypomagnesemia: increased neuromuscular and CNS irritability, loss of muscle control, tremors, disorientation, tetany, convulsions	Hypermagnesemia: CNS depression, coma, hypotension

(continued)

T A B L E   3 3 - 6 (continued)

Summary of Macrominerals and Microminerals*

Nutrient and Adult RDA	Sources	Functions	Signs and Symptoms of Deficiency	Signs and Symptoms of Excess
Sulfur (provided by adequate amounts of protein)	Meat, fish, poultry, eggs, milk, dried peas and beans, nuts	Store and release energy; structural component of nucleic acids, some vitamins, some amino acids, insulin, and heparin; promotes certain enzyme reactions; detoxification	None known	None known
Sodium 1100–3300 mg†	Salt, sodium-containing preservatives and additives, processed foods, canned meats and vegetables, condiments, pickled foods, soft water, ham, foods prepared in brine solutions, milk, meat, carrots, celery, beets, spinach	Fluid balance, acid–base balance, muscle irritability, cell permeability, nerve impulse transmission	Hyponatremia: cold and clammy skin, decreased skin turgor, apprehension, confusion, irritability, anxiety, hypotension, tachycardia, headache, tremors, convulsions, abdominal cramps, nausea, vomiting, diarrhea	Edema, weight gain; hot, flushed, dry skin; dry red tongue; intense thirst; restless agitation; oliguria or anuria
Potassium 1875–5625 mg†	Whole grains, legumes, fruits, leafy vegetables, broccoli, sweet potatoes, potatoes, meat, tomatoes	Fluid balance, acid–base balance, nerve impulse transmission, striated skeletal and cardiac muscle activity, carbohydrate metabolism, protein synthesis, catalyst for many metabolic reactions	Hypokalemia: muscle cramps and weakness, including cardiac muscle weakness, anorexia, nausea, vomiting, mental depression, confusion, drowsiness, abdominal distention, increased urine output, shallow respiration, irregular pulse	Hyperkalemia: irritability, anxiety, listlessness, mental confusion, nausea, diarrhea, poor respirations, GI hyperactivity, muscle weakness, numbness of the extremities, hypotension, cardiac arrhythmia, heart block, cardiac arrest
Chlorine 1700–5100 mg†	Salt	Component of hydrochloride in the stomach, fluid balance, acid–base balance	Hypochloremia: muscle spasms, alkalosis, depressed respiration, possible coma	Hyperchloremia: acidosis

Microminerals

Iron 10–15 mg	Liver, lean meats, enriched and whole-grain breads and cereals	Oxygen transport by way of hemoglobin and myoglobin, constituent of enzyme systems	Microcytic anemia, pallor, decreased work capacity, fatigue, weakness, spoon-shaped nails	Hemosiderosis, acute iron poisoning from accidental overdose leads to GI cramping, nausea, vomiting, possible shock, convulsions, coma
Iodine 150 mg	Iodized salt, seafood, food additives, dough conditioners, daily disinfectants	Component of thyroid hormones	Goiter	Acne-like skin lesions, iodine goiter
Zinc 12–15 mg	Oysters, liver, meats, poultry, dried peas and beans, nuts	Tissue growth, development, and healing; sexual maturation and reproduction; enzyme formation; immune response	Impaired growth, sexual maturation, and immune system functioning; skin lesions; decreased sense of taste and smell	Anorexia, nausea, vomiting, diarrhea, muscle pain, lethargy, drowsiness, bleeding gastric ulcers, decreased serum levels of high-density lipoproteins

(continued)

T A B L E   3 3 - 6 (continued)

Summary of Macrominerals and Microminerals*

Nutrient and Adult RDA	Sources	Functions	Signs and Symptoms of Deficiency	Signs and Symptoms of Excess
Microminerals				
Copper 1.5–3 mg†	Liver, kidney, shellfish, grains, dried peas and beans, dried fruit, fresh fruit	Bone and blood formation, formation and activity of some enzymes, integrity of heart and large arteries	Anemia, altered bone formation, hyper-cholesterolemia	Nausea, vomiting, headache, dizziness, heartburn, weakness, diarrhea
Manganese 2–5 mg	Whole grains, nuts, dried peas and beans, fruit	Needed for bone formation, reproduction, and blood clotting; protein and energy metabolism	Poor reproductive performance, growth retardation, abnormal bone and cartilage formation, impaired glucose tolerance	None known
Fluorine 1.5–4 mg†	Fluoridated water, fish, tea	Tooth formation and integrity, bone formation and integrity	Tooth decay, may increase the risk of osteoporosis	Mottling and discoloration of tooth enamel
Chromium 0.05–0.2 mg†	Whole grains, meat	Cofactor for insulin, proper glucose metabolism	Impaired glucose tolerance, insulin resistance	None known
Selenium 40–70 µg	Wheat (if grown in high-selenium soil), organ meats, other meat, seafood	Antioxidant	None known	Loss of hair, brittle fingernails, fatigue
Molybdenum 75–250 µg†	Liver, whole grains, dried peas and beans, organ meats	Oxidizes sulfur and products of sulfur and nucleic acid metabolism	None known	Interferes with copper metabolism
Cobalt Unknown—apparently minute	Organ meats	Essential component of vitamin B_{12}	None known	None known

*See Appendix D for Canadian RNIs.

†Estimated safe and adequate intake.

(Dudek, S. G. [1993]. *Nutrition handbook for nursing practice.* [2nd ed.]. Philadelphia: Lippincott.)

sodium, and fiber content of foods usually are not addressed. Portion sizes are suggested, and the recommended number of servings per day varies according to age. The plan provides only about 1200 cal (4000 to 6000 kJ) for adults; therefore, additional servings may be added, depending on a person's caloric requirements and appetite. A variety of foods is encouraged; however, the food group guide does not address the issue of fluid intake or the use of popular convenience or fast foods.

In 1979, with the addition of a fifth group comprising fats, sweets, and alcohol, the Basic Four Food Groups became the *Hassle-Free Guide* or *Modified Food Guide.* Confusion about this fifth group being recommended rather than restricted led to the return of the Basic Four Food Groups, which is shown in Figure 33-5.

Food Guide Pyramid   In response to the concerns of nutritionists and health officials, the U.S. Department of Agriculture has replaced the Basic Four Food Group wheel with the Food Guide Pyramid (Fig. 33-6). This graphic device places the grain and cereal group at the base of the pyramid followed by the fruit and vegetable group, the meat and dairy groups, and a fat, oil; and sweets group at the peak. The intent of the pyramid is to emphasize the grain and cereal group as the basic food in the diet with the less desirable foods playing a much smaller nutritional role. Representatives of the meat and dairy industries were critical of the food pyramid, and temporarily stalled its adoption. After minor design changes, the Food Guide Pyramid was adopted in April 1992.

Recommended Dietary Allowance and Recommended Nutrient Intakes   The RDA, prepared by the Committee on Dietary Allowances of the Food and Nutrition Board, and the RNI, prepared by the Health Promotion Directorate, National Health and Welfare in Canada, are recommenda-

Fruits and vegetables 4 to 5 servings
Meat, poultry, and fish 2 servings
Grains 3 to 5 servings
Milk and milk products 2 to 4 servings
Canada
Bread and cereals 4 or more servings
Meat, poultry, and fish 2 or more servings
Fruits and vegetables 4 or more servings
Milk and milk products 2 to 4 servings
USA

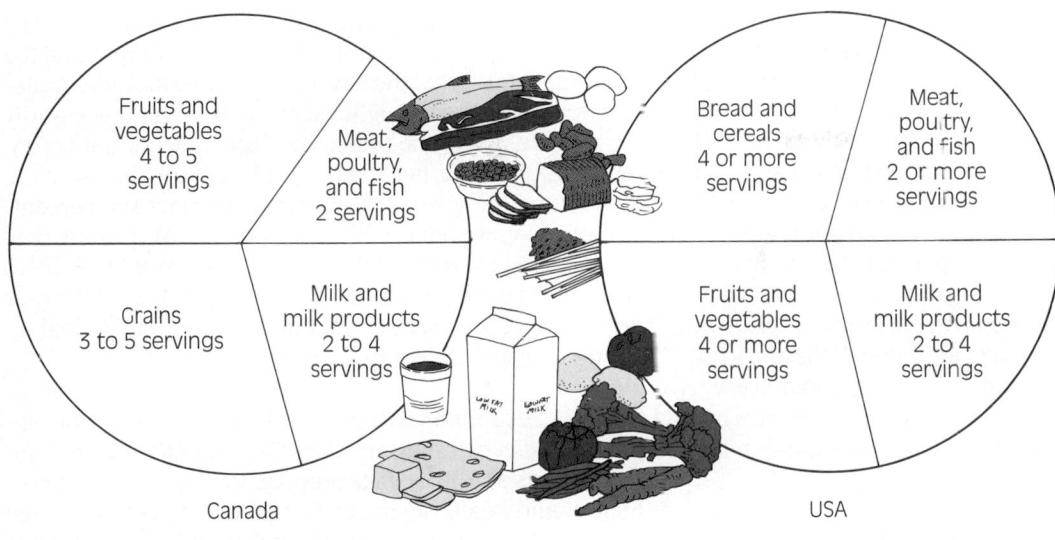

FIGURE 33-5

U.S. and Canadian recommendations for daily dietary intake by food groups.

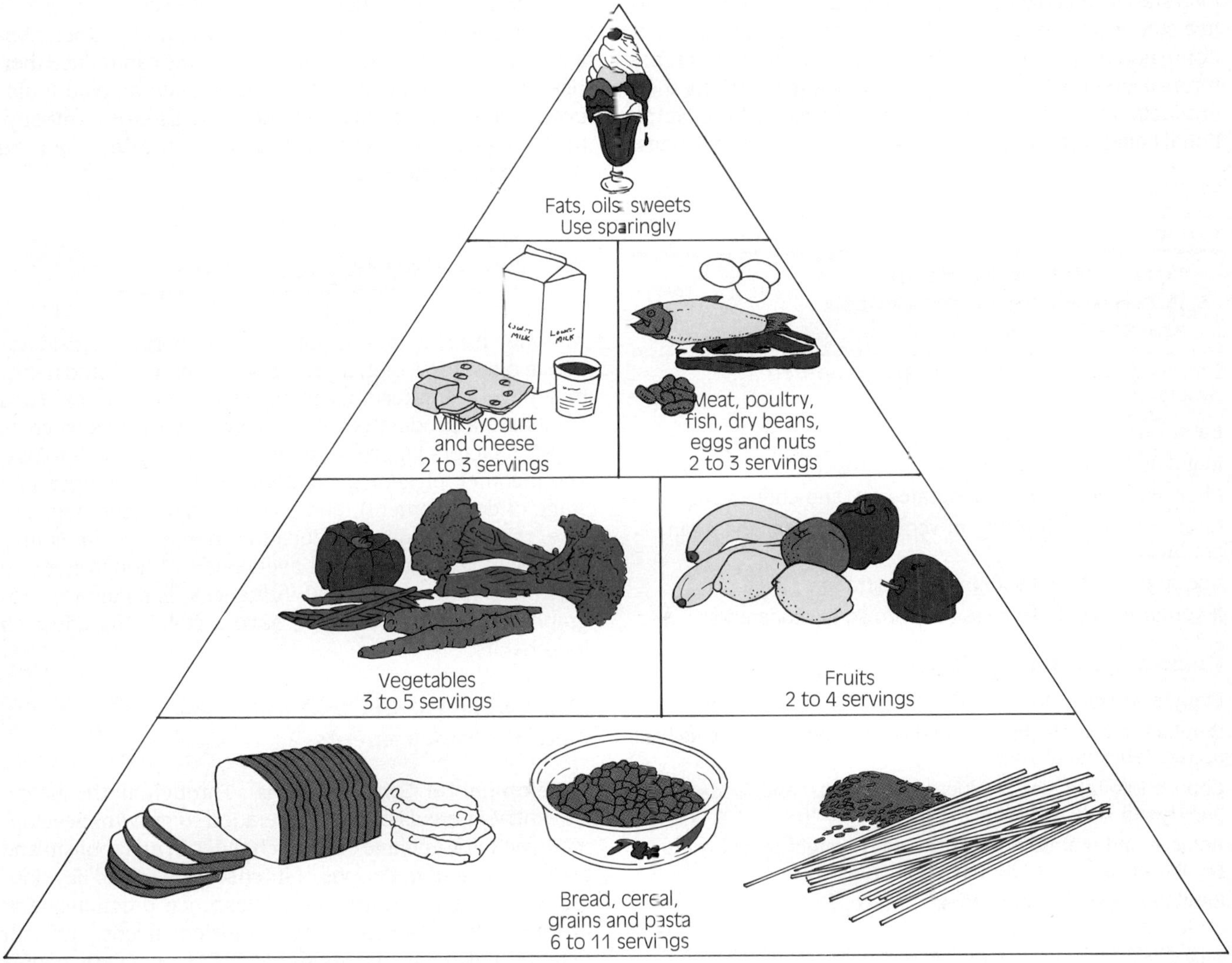

Fats, oils, sweets Use sparingly
Milk, yogurt and cheese 2 to 3 servings
Meat, poultry, fish, dry beans, eggs and nuts 2 to 3 servings
Vegetables 3 to 5 servings
Fruits 2 to 4 servings
Bread, cereal, grains and pasta 6 to 11 servings

FIGURE 33-6

The Food Guide Pyramid that replaced the Basic Four Food Group Wheel in 1992.

tions for average daily amounts of nutrients considered to be adequate to meet the known nutritional needs of practically all healthy people (Appendix C-1). (A summary of Canadian RNIs can be found in Appendix D-2.) Unlike a requirement, which is the amount of a nutrient needed to prevent a deficiency, an allowance has a safety factor built in to account for individual variations. Because the RDA and the RNI are intended for populations and not individuals, some people may not be able to meet their individual requirements, despite consuming the RDA or RNI. Likewise, it is possible for some people to eat less than the RDA or RNI and still avoid deficiencies. Although RDAs and RNIs are defined for age and sex and are revised about every 5 years as new information becomes available, they have not been established for all nutrients. Like the food group approach, variety is recommended.

Food Labeling Regulations that control food labels have always been controversial. In 1975, the **Food and Drug Administration** (FDA), a federal agency charged with protecting the U.S. food and drug supply, enacted legislation for a standardized label format that was considered a positive step toward educating the consumer about nutrition. Confusion and misinformation resulted as food manufacturers oversimplified or exaggerated health claims for their products. In the fall of 1990, Congress passed the Nutritional Labeling and Education Act, which requires all foods, including fruits and vegetables, to be clearly labeled. The food industry was given until May 1993 to comply, and the FDA is debating what the new labels should look like. Canadian food products are labeled by content (not necessarily the amounts), and the breakdown lists the amount of protein, carbohydrate, fat, sugar, starch, dietary fiber, sodium, and potassium (given in milligrams or grams and percentage of recommended daily allowances). All professional organizations agree that the food label is primarily a tool to educate the public about nutrition, and they expect the new law to go a long way toward ensuring that nutritional labeling is responsible and accurate.

Dietary Recommendations Unlike the food group approach to diet planning and the RDAs and RNIs, diet recommendations and guidelines proposed by numerous governmental and health agencies focus not on getting enough nutrition but on avoiding nutritional excesses. The FDA has proposed replacement of the U.S. RDAs for vitamins and minerals with daily values (DVs) that reflect the lowered recommended intakes for some vitamins and minerals (Liebman, 1992). Although these diet recommendations are not guaranteed to prevent diseases, many experts believe that most Americans and Canadians can reduce their risk of chronic diet-related diseases, such as type II diabetes, certain types of cancer, and heart disease, by modifying the typical diet. Table 33-7 compares the Canadian and American recommendations.

T A B L E   3 3 - 7

Comparison of Nutrition Recommendations for Canada and the United States

Dietary Guidelines for Americans (proposed new version)

Eat a variety of foods.

Maintain healthy weight.

Choose a diet low in fat, saturated fat, and cholesterol.

Choose a diet with plenty of vegetables, fruits, and grain products.

Use sugar, salt, and sodium in moderation.

If you drink alcoholic beverages, do so in moderation.

Canada's Guidelines for Healthy Eating

Enjoy a *variety* of foods.

Emphasize cereals, breads, and other grain products as well as vegetables and fruits.

Choose low-fat dairy products, lean meats, and foods prepared with little or no fat.

Achieve and maintain a healthy body weight by enjoying regular physical activity and healthy eating.

Limit salt, alcohol, and caffeine intake.

(Langserth, L. [ed.] [1990] Proposed revisions in dietary guidelines for Americans and new Canadian nutrition recommendations. *Nutrition Research Newsletter, 9*[11], 126–127.)

Factors Affecting Nutrition

Although nutritional adequacy is an important consideration in planning a diet, a person's food patterns and habits may have a greater impact on overall food intake. Food habits are a product of many evolving variables, such as physical factors (eg, geographic location, food technology, and income), physiologic factors (eg, health, hunger, and stage of development), and psychosocial factors (eg, culture, religion, tradition, education, politics, social status, food ideology, and learned aversions). Although not static, conservative traditional influences, like culture, geographic region, and religion, have a stabilizing effect on food habits.

Physiologic Factors That Influence Nutrient Requirements

Developmental Considerations Throughout the life cycle, nutrient needs change in relation to growth, development, activity, and age-related changes in metabolism and body composition. Periods of intense growth and development, such as during infancy, adolescence, pregnancy, and lactation, cause an increase in nutrient needs. Nutrient needs stabilize during adulthood, although elderly people may need more or less of some nutrients. Refer to the display for nutritional problems that affect older adults.

FOCUS ON THE OLDER ADULT

Nursing Strategies for Nutritional Problems Affecting Older Adults

Altered Ability to Chew Related to Loss of Teeth, Ill-Fitting Dentures, and Gingivitis

- Encourage and instruct client to care for and retain own teeth and dentures.
- Encourage proper tooth-brushing and use of special toothpaste if gums and teeth are sensitive.
- Chop, shred, or puree foods that are difficult to chew.
- Select ground meat, fish, or poultry as protein sources more easily chewed.

Loss of Senses of Smell and Taste

- Serve food that is attractive and at proper temperature.
- Eat one food at a time rather than mixing foods.
- Serve foods with different textures and aromas.

Decreased Peristalsis in the Esophagus

- Avoid cold liquids.
- Avoid emotional upsets and stress-producing situations.
- Take anticholinergic drugs as ordered by physician.

Gastroesophageal Reflux

- Avoid overeating.
- Avoid juices, chocolate, and fat.
- Avoid alcohol and smoking.
- Elevate the head of the bed 30 to 40 degrees when sleeping.
- Lose weight if necessary.
- Avoid bending over.
- Take antacids or other medications as ordered by physician.

Decreased Gastric Secretions

- Chew food thoroughly.
- Eat meals on a regular schedule.
- Use antacids or other medications as prescribed by physician.
- Be alert for symptoms of deficiency of nutrients, particularly iron, calcium, fat, protein, and vitamin B_{12}.
- Ensure adequate intake of vitamin D for calcium absorption.

Slowed Intestinal Peristalsis

- Eat a high-fiber diet.
- Remain as active as possible.
- Increase fluid intake.
- Avoid laxative use.
- Eat meals at a regular time.
- Drink prune juice or eat prunes every morning.

Lowered Glucose Tolerance

- Eat more complex carbohydrates.
- Avoid sugar-rich foods.

Reduction in Appetite and Thirst Sensation

- Offer fluids at regular intervals and at preferred temperature.
- Be alert for symptoms of dehydration and electrolyte imbalance.
- Offer small meals at frequent intervals.

Nutritional Deficiencies Related to Alcohol Intake

- Encourage diet high in protein and carbohydrates.
- Offer small, frequent meals to maintain caloric intake.
- Restrict sodium and fluids if edema is present.
- Take multivitamin supplements as ordered by physician.

Loss of Appetite Associated with Depression and Loneliness

- Promote mealtime as a social event.
- Set an attractive table in a pleasant setting.
- Eat outdoors whenever possible.
- Invite guests as often as possible.
- Participate in special programs for senior citizens.

Physical Handicaps

- Open cartons and assist with setup of meal.
- Arrange for home-delivered meals.
- Conserve energy when preparing meals (sit on a stool, and so forth).
- Provide transportation and assistance to obtain food.

Low Income

- Buy specials when available at food store.
- Use generic brands.
- Use coupons.
- Cook larger quantities than necessary and freeze the leftovers for future use.
- Substitute eggs, skim milk powder, and beans for meat.

Malnutrition

- Eat essential foods first.
- Select nutrient-dense foods.
- Monitor for signs of nutritional deficiencies.
- Encourage eating by planning special events.

Drug–Nutrient Interactions

- Avoid unnecessary drugs.
- Be aware of drug actions and interactions.
- Check with pharmacist to determine if medication may or may not be taken with food.
- Assess for confusion and inability to manage medication regimen.

Age influences not only nutrient requirements but also food intake. The consistency of food, eating patterns, and the significance of food change with physical and psychosocial development. Nutrient needs and developmental landmarks are summarized in Table 33-8.

Sex   Men have somewhat different nutrient requirements than women related to differences in body composition and reproductive function. Their larger muscle mass translates into higher caloric and protein requirements (and therefore slightly higher needs for B vitamins that metabolize calories and protein) because it is more metabolically active than adipose tissue, of which women proportionally have more. Women of childbearing age have higher iron requirements related to menstruation.

State of Health   The alteration in nutrient requirements that results from illness and trauma varies with the intensity and duration of the stress. For instance, fevers increase the need for calories and water. However, unlike fevers related to septicemia, fevers caused by a mild case of the flu require few dietary adjustments.

Trauma, like major surgery, burns, and crush injuries, is followed by hormonal changes that profoundly affect the body's use of nutrients. To preserve or replenish body nutrient stores and to promote healing and recovery, nutrient requirements increase dramatically in the adaptive phase after stress. In some cases of severe trauma, such as major burns, the rehabilitative phase of recovery, characterized by the gradual normalization of nutrient needs, may last for years.

Chronic disorders, like diabetes mellitus, renal disease, hypertension, heart disease, gastrointestinal disorders, and cancer, can alter nutrient requirements by influencing nutrient intake, digestion, absorption, metabolism, utilization, or excretion.

Alcohol Abuse   Alcohol can alter the body's use of nutrients, and thereby its nutrient requirements, by numerous mechanisms. The toxic effect of alcohol on the intestinal mucosa interferes with normal nutrient absorption: thus, requirements increase as the efficiency of absorption decreases. Need for B vitamins increases because they are used to metabolize alcohol. Alcohol also can influence nutrient metabolism by impairing nutrient storage, increasing nutrient catabolism, and increasing nutrient excretion. Alcohol abuse that results in liver damage has profound effects on the body's nutrient metabolism and requirements.

Medication   Many drugs have the potential to influence nutrient requirements. *Nutrient absorption* may be altered by drugs that (1) change the pH of the gastrointestinal tract, (2) increase gastrointestinal motility, (3) damage the intestinal mucosa, or (4) bind with nutrients, rendering them unavailable to the body. *Nutrient metabolism* can be altered by drugs that (1) act as nutrient antagonists, (2) alter the enzyme systems that metabolize nutrients, or (3) alter nutrient degradation. Some drugs alter the renal reabsorption of nutrients, and therefore may increase or decrease *nutrient excretion.*

Megadoses of Nutrient Supplements   Because some nutrients compete against each other for absorption, an excess of one nutrient can lead to a deficiency (or increase the requirement) of another, especially if one is absorbed preferentially. For instance, a delicate balance exists between zinc and copper. People who take therapeutic levels of zinc run the risk of developing a copper deficiency—which is otherwise rare—unless they also increase their intake of copper.

Sociocultural and Psychological Factors

Religion   Nurses need to be aware of dietary restrictions associated with the various religions that might affect a client's nutritional requirements. During the lenten season, Roman Catholics, for example, fast on Ash Wednesday and Good Friday in addition to abstaining from meat on every Friday, and the nurse may recommend alternative food choices or meal patterns. Kosher dietary laws require special food preparation techniques and prohibit intake of pork and shellfish. The nurse must be conscious of the client's religious affiliation and its impact on his or her nutritional regimen. Kosher diets and other special diets are available in Canadian hospitals, nursing homes, homes for the aged, and Meals on Wheels programs.

Economics   The adequacy of the food budget affects dietary choices and patterns. The increasing cost of food coupled with limited purchasing power may result in a decrease in the nutritional quality of the diet. Many variables influence the types of foods that are purchased. Creative use of the food dollar means using unit pricing to determine cost per serving (eg, comparing the unit price of $.39 per serving with another similar product's $.42 per serving), selecting foods that contain adequate nutrients, and buying seasonal foods that are more economical and can be prepared easily at home. Avoiding convenience foods and meals purchased away from home saves food dollars.

Psychosocial Factors   Food plays multiple roles in the lives of most people. In addition to satisfying hunger and providing nutrition, food may signify a celebration, a social gathering, or a reward. Some people use various foods to indicate caring or to give comfort and reassurance during times of stress or unhappiness. Mealtime may evoke memories of family discussions, laughter, and enjoyable times. Some may remember conflicts associated with eating or avoid eating because it reminds them of their loneliness and isolation. Others, because of society's emphasis on being thin, may resort to fad or crash-reducing diets to resolve eating conflicts and lose weight rapidly. This initial weight reduction seldom is sustained for an extended period, and a cycle of yo-yo dieting frequently results. Drastic weight loss is followed by an eating binge that causes the

TABLE 33-8

Nutritional Implications of Characteristic Developmental Landmarks Throughout the Life Cycle

Age and Characteristic Development	Nutritional Implications
Infants (birth to 1 year)	
• Most rapid period of growth after birth; birth weight doubles in 4 to 6 months and triples by age 1 year; length increases 50% in first year.	• Nutritional needs per unit of body weight are greater than at any other time in life cycle.
• Inborn reflexes, such as rooting, sucking, swallowing, and gagging, disappear between 4 and 6 months.	• Milk feedings are most appropriate for the first 4 to 6 months. • Breastfeeding is recommended as the major source of nutrition for the first 6 months; supplements of vitamins C and D, fluoride, and iron may be prescribed.* • A variety of routine and special infant formulas are available if mothers choose not to breastfeed or if breastfeeding is contraindicated because of medical problems in the infant or mother.
• Muscle control of the head, neck, jaw, and tongue develops, as does hand–eye coordination and the ability to sit and self-feed.	• Spoon-feeding becomes possible. Solids may be introduced between ages 4 and 6 months. • Common progression is iron-fortified infant cereals followed by strained vegetables, noncitrus fruits, noncitrus fruit juices. • Texture increases gradually to table food at 1 year. • Finger foods and drinking from a cup may begin around 6 months.
• Stomach capacity is limited at birth, peristalsis is rapid. • Pancreatic amylase (starch-digesting enzyme) is limited at birth until age 3 months. • Iron stores present at birth start to become depleted between 3 and 4 months. • Immune system matures between 4 and 6 months.	• Initially, small frequent feedings are necessary. • Starch digestion (ie, cooked cereal) does not develop until age 3 months. • Exogenous iron is necessary. Cow's milk given too early (ie, before the infant is eating the equivalent of 1½ jars of baby food a day) contributes to iron deficiency anemia. • Solid foods given too early may trigger allergic reactions. • New foods should be introduced one at a time for 5 to 7 days so that allergic reactions can be noted. • Egg whites should not be given until age 1.
Toddlers and Preschoolers	
• Decrease in growth rate is dramatic.	• Appetite dramatically decreases and becomes erratic; caloric needs per unit of body weight decline.
• Maturation of biting, chewing, and swallowing continues. • Mobility, autonomy, and coordination increase.	• A variety of textures are eaten. • Self-feeding is complete by age 2 years. Food is sought independently. Food may be used to manipulate parents; food jags begin around 15 months.
• Muscle mass and bone density increase.	• Adequate amounts of protein, calcium, and phosphorus are needed.
• Language skills increase.	• Food is associated with name; food likes and dislikes are verbalized.
• Food attitudes develop between ages 3 and 5.	• Inappropriate use of food (ie, to punish, reward, bribe, or convey love) may lead to inappropriate food attitudes.
School-Aged Children (6- to 12-year-olds)	
• Erratic, uneven growth pattern; wide variations in growth rate among individuals.	• Appetite improves but may still be irregular; caloric needs per unit of body weight gradually decline.
• Digestive system matures. Permanent teeth erupt.	• Can eat larger meals and eat less frequently. • Fluoride, vitamins A and D, calcium, and phosphorus are important for dental health.
• Socialization and independence increase.	• Parents' role as primary gate keepers of what their children eat diminishes; advertising impacts on food choices; variety of food eaten increases.

(continued)

T A B L E   3 3 - 8 *(continued)*

Nutritional Implications of Characteristic Developmental Landmarks Throughout the Life Cycle	
Age and Characteristic Development	**Nutritional Implications**

Infants (birth to 1 year)

- Reserves are laid down for upcoming adolescent growth spurt.

- Nutrient needs increase toward the end of school-aged period in preparation for growth spurt.

Adolescents

- Period of rapid physical emotional, social, and sexual maturation.
- Growth spurt begins at different ages among individuals, begins earlier for girls than boys.
- Boys experience an increase in muscle mass, lean body tissue, and bones.
- Girls begin menstruation and experience fat deposition.

- Nutrient needs, especially for calories, protein, calcium, and iron, increase to support growth.
- Physiologic age is a more valid indicator of need than chronologic age.
- Iron needs increase; boys have higher caloric needs than girls to maintain larger muscle mass.
- Iron needs increase; body fat requires fewer calories to be maintained, so girls need fewer calories than boys.
- Weight consciousness becomes compulsive in 1 of 100 teenaged girls and results in **anorexia nervosa**, an eating disorder characterized by extreme weight loss, muscle wasting, arrested sexual development, refusal to eat, and bizarre eating habits.
- An estimated one in five teenage girls suffers from **bulimia**, an eating disorder characterized by gorging followed by purging with self-induced vomiting, diuretics, or laxatives.
- Teenage pregnancy occurring within 3 to 4 years after menstruation begins places mother and fetus at increased nutritional risk.

- Period of intense psychosocial growth, family conflict, social and peer pressure.

- Nutritional needs may be hard to meet because fewer meals are eaten at home, peer influence, busy schedules, and because independence may be expressed through diet.

Adults

- Growth ceases.
- Basal metabolic rate (BMR) declines each decade.

- Physical activity may decline.

- Nutrient needs level off.
- Fewer calories are required for BMR; weight gain occurs if adjustments in intake are not made.
- Also contributes to weight gain if caloric intake does not decrease.

Pregnant Women

- Fetus, maternal tissues, and placenta grow dramatically.

- Nutrient needs increase to support growth and maintain maternal homeostasis.
- Key nutrients include protein, calories, iron, folic acid, calcium, and iodine. Iron and folic acid supplements are necessary to meet needs.
- Actual nutrient needs increase little during the first trimester in a well-nourished mother but increase steadily throughout the remainder of pregnancy.

- Weight gain occurs.

- Recommended pattern: 2 to 4 lb (1 to 3 kg) during the first trimester; 0.8 to 0.9 lb (0.45 kg) per week during second and third trimesters; underweight women may need more, overweight women less.
- Pattern of weight gain is more significant than total amount.

- GI changes occur that may cause nausea, vomiting, heartburn, or constipation.

- Dietary changes may help relieve unpleasant symptoms.

(continued)

T A B L E   3 3 - 8 *(continued)*

Nutritional Implications of Characteristic Developmental Landmarks Throughout the Life Cycle	
Age and Characteristic Development	**Nutritional Implications**

Lactating Women

- The quantity of milk produced is dependent on an adequate supply of nutrients.

- Caloric needs are higher for lactation than pregnancy, as are the requirements for vitamin A, niacin, riboflavin, iodine, zinc, and fluid. Calcium and protein also are important.
- Calories may come from diet or fat mobilized from adipose tissue.

- The quality of milk is not affected by maternal diet, with the exception of vitamin C, riboflavin, thiamine, and fat.

- The nutritional quality of breast milk is maintained at the expense of maternal nutrition if the diet is inadequate.

Elderly People

- Energy expenditure decreases related to a decrease in BMR, decrease in physical activity, and loss of lean body mass.

- Caloric needs decrease.

- Loss of teeth, periodontal disease, and jaw bone disease may result in difficulty chewing.

- Food intake may be limited to soft, easy-to-chew foods; meat is the food most commonly eliminated.

- Constipation is a common problem related to decreased activity, decreased peristalsis due to a loss of abdominal muscle tone, inadequate fluid and fiber intake, or secondary to drug therapy.

- Increasing fiber and fluid may help relieve constipation.

- Digestive disorders may occur related to normal changes in GI function.

- Diet modifications may be necessary to relieve discomfort.

- Loss of taste begins between ages 55 and 59; people lose tastes of sweet and salt; bitter and sour remain.

- Taste threshold increases, which may lead to an increase in sugar and salt intake or anorexia.

- Sensation of thirst decreases.
- Physical disabilities related to arthritis or strokes may develop.
- Income becomes fixed.

- Elderly people are prone to dehydration.
- Food preparation may be difficult or impossible.
- Most sacrificed items on a limited food budget are milk and meats.

- Degenerative diseases and the use of medications are more common with aging.

- Nutrient intake, digestion, absorption, metabolism, or excretion may be altered.

- Social isolation, poor self-esteem, or being institutionalized may affect intake.

- Lack of interest in eating is common.

* In Canada, vitamin B_{12} may be prescribed if mothers are strict vegetarians.

(Dudek, S. G. [1993]. *Nutrition handbook for nursing practice* [2nd ed.]. Philadelphia: Lippincott.)

dieter to regain all the lost weight and, possibly, some additional weight each time the sequence occurs. Nutritional deficiencies may occur and place them at risk for other diseases. Losing weight and keeping it off require a change in eating habits as part of the overall commitment to health. Nurses can help by being aware of the multitudes of meanings that food has for people.

Cultural Factors   Nutritional diversity is common among cultural or ethnic groups. The variety and selections are unique to each group and represent their personal beliefs and customs. Culture determines what is eaten, how it is prepared, and what combinations of food are permitted. The variations in food choices within a culture also are dependent on income levels and availability of foods. Table

33-9 summarizes the food preferences for common ethnic groups.

Decreased Food Intake

Food intake may decrease for various reasons. **Anorexia**, or the lack of appetite, may be related to systemic and local diseases; numerous psychosocial causes, such as fear, anxiety, and depression; pain; and impaired ability to smell and taste. Or it may occur secondary to drug therapy or medical treatments. Others who may have limited food intake include those who have difficulty chewing and swallowing, those who experience chronic gastrointestinal problems or undergo certain surgeries, and those on inadequate food budgets.

TABLE 33-9

Cultural Variations on Nutrition

Culture	Milk	Meat	Bread and Cereals	Fruits and Vegetables	Additional Variations
Italian	Seldom use milk; cheese is calcium source	Chicken, beef, veal, fish—baked, simmered, or browned in olive oil	Bread and pasta basic foods	Squash, tomatoes, salad; fruit used as dessert	Drink red or white wine with dinner; use garlic for seasoning
Chinese	Use little milk or cheese	Pork, lamb, chicken, fish—cooked in combination with vegetables	Rice with most meals	Cabbage, snow peas, squashes, mushrooms; fruit usually eaten fresh	Fresh foods prepared by stir-frying; unsweetened green tea
Japanese	Little milk or cheese	Seafood main protein source, especially raw fish	Rice is basic grain; white and wheat bread being increasingly used	Steamed and served with soy sauce; tray of fruit served at main meal	Soy sauce main seasoning; soybean oil main cooking fat; traditionally, dinners follow specific sequence of courses; tea is main beverage
Greek	Little milk; yogurt popular; cheese a favorite food	Lamb favorite meat; little beef eaten	Bread center of every meal; rice commonly served	Large amounts of vegetables, cooked and seasoned, preferably fresh; large quantities of fresh fruit	Meal is family ritual; holidays are special occasions with great variety of foods
Puerto Rican	Little milk	Most cannot afford meat; may use dried codfish; legumes good protein source	Rice	Almost all eat viandas, which are starchy vegetables and fruits, such as plantain and green bananas; other fruits and vegetables used in limited quantity	Simple daily diet that contrasts with holiday meal; economy major factor in food selection
Mexican	Little milk	Little meat used	Corn basic grain used in bread and cereal; oatmeal popular cereal	Corn, fresh or canned, and chili peppers; fruit use depends on availability	Drink large amounts of coffee; common seasonings chili pepper, onions, and garlic; lard basic cooking fat
African American	Low intake of milk and dairy foods	Diet usually high in protein; favorite meats pork and chicken; most meats fried or barbecued	Sweet potatoes and hominy grits	High intake of dark, leafy green vegetables; fruits used in limited quantity	Diet high in fat and sodium because of methods of preparation

Nurse as Role Model

A nurse's credibility as a health practitioner may be severely questioned if he or she appears badly nourished, or displays poor eating habits, weight problems, or other clinical signs of nutritional deficiencies. As a role model for health behaviors, the nurse should adopt the following goals:

• Attain and maintain ideal body weight.
• Use RDA guidelines for adequate nutrient intake.
• Maintain appropriate balance between food intake and exercise.

PROMOTING WELLNESS

Nutrition

Use the assessment checklist to determine how well you are meeting your nutritional needs. Then develop a prescription for self-care by choosing appropriate behaviors from the list of suggestions.

Assessment Checklist

almost always | sometimes | almost never

☐ ☐ ☐ 1. I know and use the recommended dietary guidelines and servings.

☐ ☐ ☐ 2. My weight is within 10% of the ideal for my height and body frame.

☐ ☐ ☐ 3. I maintain an appropriate balance between exercise and food intake.

☐ ☐ ☐ 4. I limit my fat, sugar, salt, and red meat intake.

☐ ☐ ☐ 5. I limit my caffeine intake.

☐ ☐ ☐ 6. I use alcoholic beverages in moderation.

Self-Care Behaviors

1. Maintain desirable weight, eating a variety of foods in adequate amounts from each of the four food groups.
2. Eat slowly, take smaller portions, and avoid second helpings if trying to control overeating.
3. Eat a variety of foods low in calories and high in nutrients to lose weight.
4. Obtain medical clearance before starting a weight-loss program.
5. Avoid too many foods high in cholesterol (milk, egg yolk, organ meats, fats, oils); instead choose lean meat, fish, poultry, and beans.
6. Eat foods high in fiber: whole-grain breads and cereals, fruits, vegetables, dry beans.
7. Avoid excess use of salt and sugar.
8. Begin an exercise program, and maintain it.
9. Learn healthy eating habits; read labels, become familiar with healthy fast-food and restaurant menus, drink alcohol moderately (if at all).
10. Substitute healthy rewards for yourself that do not include high-calorie, low-nutrition snacks and beverages.

- Limit intake of alcohol, fats, sugar, salt, caffeine, and red meats.
- Eat foods high in fiber.

Assessing Nutritional Status

Nutritional status has a significant impact on both health and disease. For well clients, good nutritional status can help to maintain health, promote normal growth and development, and protect against disease. During illness, good nutritional status can reduce the risk of complications and speed recovery time. Conversely, poor nutritional status can increase the risk of illness or death.

The nature of the nurse–client relationship affords nurses the opportunity to incorporate nutritional assessment in the nursing process. Like other aspects of nursing care, nutritional assessment is a systematic approach used to identify the client's actual or potential needs, formulate a plan to meet those needs, initiate the plan or assign others to implement it, and evaluate the effectiveness of the plan. As such, nutritional assessment is appropriate for all clients, although the level of assessment may range from simple screening to a comprehensive, in-depth assessment, depending on individual circumstances (see display). Nurses can collect assessment data through history taking (dietary and medical–socioeconomic data), physical assessments (anthropometric and clinical data), and laboratory data.

Discussion continues among health experts about determining what is the most effective method to assess for risk of developing nutritionally related complications. After extensive research at the University of Toronto and Toronto General Hospital, workers have concluded that clinical assessment and the serum albumin level provide the best estimate of risk (Detsky, 1987). Nurses, by nature of their caring role and personal encounters, are ideally situated to identify nutritional needs and assess and monitor for nutritional risks. An awareness of specific changes in elderly people that may reflect on the accuracy of the assessment process is necessary (see display).

Dietary Data

Dietary data may be collected from the client or family and can be evaluated according to the food group approach, dietary guidelines, or the RDA (RNI in Canada), depending on the purpose of the assessment.

24-Hour Recall Method The easiest way to collect dietary data is to obtain a 24-hour recall of all food and

Elements of a Nutritional Assessment

Dietary Data

Screen
  24-hour food recall
  Food frequency record
In-depth
  Food diary
  Diet history

Medical–Socioeconomic Data

Screen
  Brief personal and family history
In-depth
  Sequential history, including current and past
  health status, social history, and family history

Anthropometric Data

Screen
  Height
  Weight
  Ideal body weight (IBN)
  Usual body weight (UBN)
In-depth
  Triceps skinfold (TSF)
  Midarm circumference (MAC)
  Midarm muscle circumference (MAMC)
  Body mass index (BMI)

Clinical Data

Screen and in-depth
  Observe for signs and symptoms of malnutrition

Biochemical Data

Screen
  Serum hemoglobin and albumin levels and
  hematocrit
  Total lymphocyte count (TLC)
In-depth
  Serum transferrin level
  Antigen skin testing
  24-hour urinary creatinine excretion
  Urinary urea nitrogen (UUN)

Nutritional Assessment Considerations for Older Adults*

Biochemical Data

- Low serum albumin level (below 3.5 mg/dL) may be a reflection of the aging process rather than a nutritional risk factor. Albumin synthesis declines with age.
- Hemoglobin levels that are lower than normal may only reflect anemia observed in elderly people as part of the aging process.

Anthropometric Data

- Because of age-related changes in body composition, skin fold measurements should be taken from several body sites.

Dietary Data

- Dietary recall may be inaccurate because of vision and memory problems.
- Question use of vitamin and mineral supplements.
- Gather information concerning medication regimen (prescribed and over-the-counter) to assess for food–drug interactions and adverse effects of medications.

  *Specific clinical data for elderly people may be found in the Focus on the Older Adult display.

beverages the client normally consumes during an average day. It includes the client's usual portion sizes, meal and snack patterns, meal timing, and the place where food is eaten. Because this method relies on memory and accurate interpretation of portion sizes, the information may not be reliable.

Food Diaries Food frequency questionnaires or food diaries may provide a better overall picture of nutrient intake because the client records all food and beverages consumed in a specified period, usually 3 to 7 days.

Diet History A more comprehensive approach to diet assessment is taking a full diet history. In addition to a 24-hour food recall and food frequency record, interview questions are geared to provide information on past and present food intake and habits. Sample questions are included in the Focused Assessment Guide (see display).

The following findings are considered dietary risk factors for poor nutritional status:

- Inadequate food intake, fad dieting, numerous food intolerances or allergies
- Use of inadequate modified diet (ie, clear liquid) for more than 3 days without adequate supplementation
- NPO with simple IV therapy for longer than 3 days
- Inadequate tube feedings
- Difficulty chewing or swallowing
- Changes in taste, smell, or appetite

Medical–Socioeconomic Data

Medical, social, and economic factors, as well as cultural and psychological influences, should be evaluated for their impact on nutritional requirements and food choices.

FOCUSED ASSESSMENT GUIDE

Nutrition

Factors to Assess	Questions and Approaches
Usual dietary intake	Does your current intake differ from your usual intake?
	If so, is the reason a loss of appetite, changes in smell or taste, difficulty chewing and swallowing, hospitalization, a modified diet?
Food allergies or intolerances	Do you have any food allergies or intolerances?
Food preparation and storage	Who does the food shopping?
	Who prepares the meals?
	How is the food normally prepared? For instance, is food usually fried, baked, or broiled?
	Do you have adequate food storage space and preparation equipment?
Type of diet	Do you now or have you in the past followed a modified diet prescribed by a physician?
Dietary practices	Do you now or have you in the past used a fad diet, health foods, or self-prescribed supplements?
Eating disorder patterns	Do you view yourself as overweight?
	Do you weigh yourself frequently during one day?
	How is your appetite?
	Do you binge on large amounts of food in a short period?
	Have you ever caused yourself to vomit after eating a meal?
	Have you used laxatives, diuretics, or over-the-counter weight loss pills to lose weight?

Table 33-10 outlines medical–socioeconomic data for assessment.

The following findings are considered medical–socioeconomic risk factors for poor nutritional status:
- Medical conditions that alter intake or nutrient requirements—cancer, malabsorption, diarrhea, hyperthyroidism, severe infection, recent surgery, hemorrhage, physical or mental disabilities, multiple wounds or fractures, extensive burns
- Persistent fever above 37°C (98.6°F) for more than 2 days
- Chronic use of drugs that affect nutritional status
- Alcohol abuse
- Inadequate food budget

Anthropometric Data

Anthropometric measurements are used to determine body dimensions. In children, anthropometric measurements are used to assess growth rate; in adults, they can give indirect measurements of body protein and fat stores. For the data to be accurate and reliable, standardized equipment and procedures must be used and the data must be compared with the appropriate reference standards for the client's age and sex.

Height and weight, the most common anthropometric measurements, should be determined when the client is admitted to the hospital and periodically thereafter. A client should be weighed on the same scale each time and at the same time of day, preferably before breakfast. Weight should be compared with IBW and usual body weight. Because actual weight may be inflated if the client has edema, hydration status should be considered. Although self-reported weight may be recorded when actual weight is unobtainable, it is highly inaccurate and should be duly noted.

In-depth anthropometric measurements include triceps skin fold measurements, a measure of subcutaneous fat stores (Fig. 33-7); midarm circumference, a measure of skeletal muscle mass; and midarm muscle circumference, a measure of both skeletal muscle mass and fat stores.* Reference standards have been determined for men and women for all three measures, as have figures representing 90%, 80%, 70%, and 60% of standard.

*In Canada, the Quetelet, or body mass, index:

$$BMI = \frac{weight\ (kg)}{height\ m^2}$$

T A B L E   3 3 - 1 0

Medical—Socioeconomic Data for Nutritional Assessment	
Collect	**Evaluate**
Medical Data	
Medical history: type of disorder, treatment (including diet and drug)	Effect on intake, digestion, absorption, metabolism, and excretion of nutrients
Current illness or chief complaint	Need for diet modifications
Family medical history	
Surgical history: type, date, length of hospitalization, development of complications	
Past and current drug history: name of prescription and nonprescription drugs used on a regular basis, purpose, dosage, duration of use	Potential or actual effects on nutritional status; need for diet modification
History of drug dependence; drug abuse	
Ability to chew and swallow (Does the client have missing teeth? Full or partial dentures? Do the dentures fit?)	Impact on food intake
Appetite, food intolerances and allergies, bowel habits	Normal pattern, recent changes, impact on intake and nutritional status, need for diet modification
Social Data	
Age, gender	Effect on nutritional requirements
Position in family; number in family; life-style	Outside support systems; social aspects of eating
Occupation; frequency and intensity of physical exercise; usual number of hours of sleep per day	Effect on caloric requirements and meal timing
Religious affiliation, cultural and ethnic background	Effect on food choices and aversions
Educational background	Ability to comprehend diet instruction; appropriate teaching materials and methods
Use of alcohol and tobacco	Effect on food intake, food budget, and nutrient requirements
Economic Data	
Source of income	Reliability and adequacy; eligibility for social assistance
Food budget	Adequacy

(Dudek, S. G. [1993]. *Nutrition handbook for nursing practice.* [2nd ed.]. Philadelphia: Lippincott.)

The following findings are considered anthropometric risk factors for poor nutritional status:
- Weight 20% greater or 10% less than ideal
- Recent unintentional weight loss greater than 10% of weight
- Arm muscle circumference or triceps skin fold less than 85% of standard
- Inconsistent growth rates in children or abnormal weight for height

Clinical Data

Although signs and symptoms of malnutrition may be observed during a physical assessment (Table 33-11), they usually do not appear until malnutrition is advanced. In addition, further investigation is necessary to determine whether abnormal findings are actually caused by a nu-

tritional deficiency, possibly related to a nutritional deficiency, or unrelated to nutritional status.

Biochemical Data

Laboratory tests, which measure blood and urine levels of nutrients or biochemical functions that are dependent on an adequate supply of nutrients, can objectively detect nutritional problems in their early stages. Most routine biochemical tests measure protein status; measures of body vitamin, mineral, and trace element status also are available.

Hemoglobin, the oxygen-carrying protein of the red blood cells, and hematocrit, the volume of red blood cells packed by centrifugation in a given volume of blood, are measures of plasma protein also used to assess iron status. Protein status also can be determined by measuring serum

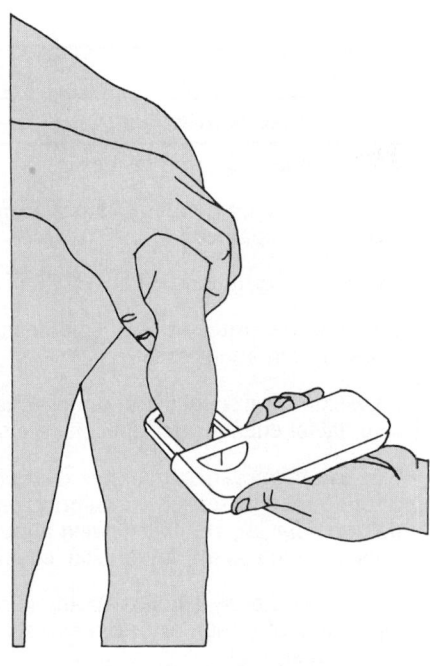

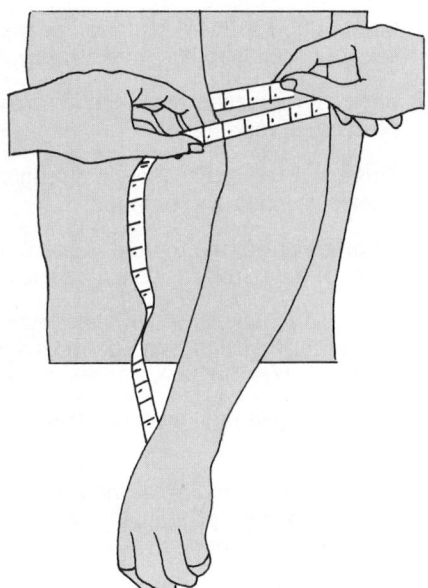

FIGURE 33-7

Two anthropometric measurements to assess nutritional status—triceps skin fold measurement (*top*) and midarm muscle circumference (*bottom*).

albumin and transferrin levels and by a total lymphocyte count. Twenty-four-hour urine tests used to measure protein metabolism are urine creatinine excretion and urine urea nitrogen.

The following findings are considered biochemical risk factors for poor nutritional status:

- Low hemoglobin level and hematocrit
- Decreased lymphocyte count
- Serum albumin level less than 3.5 g/dL
- Elevated or decreased cholesterol level

Diagnosing

Assessment data may reveal actual or potential nutritional problems.

Altered Nutrition as the Problem

Altered Nutrition: Less Than Body Requirements, related to NPO, inadequate tube feeding, prolonged use of a clear liquid diet, numerous food intolerances or allergies, excessive dieting, anorexia, chewing or swallowing difficulties, nausea, vomiting, chronic diarrhea; malabsorption, psychological eating disorders (anorexia nervosa, bulimia), alcoholism, metabolic and endocrine disorders, inappropriate use of supplements

Altered Nutrition: More Than Body Requirements, related to overeating, inactivity, metabolic and endocrine disorders, inappropriate use of supplements

Altered Nutrition: High Risk for More Than Body Requirements, related to inappropriate eating, closely spaced pregnancies, metabolic and endocrine disorders, inappropriate use of supplements

Samples of three of these diagnoses are given in the adjoining display.

Altered Nutrition as the Etiology
Nutritional problems may affect other areas of human functioning. In the following nursing diagnoses, the nutritional problem is the cause of another problem.

Activity Intolerance related to inadequate caloric intake, obesity, iron deficiency anemia

Altered Health Maintenance related to lack of knowledge about adequate nutrition

Anxiety related to obesity

Constipation related to inadequate fluid or fiber intake

Diarrhea related to overeating, excessive fiber intake, excessive sorbitol intake (sugar alcohol)

Fluid Volume Deficit related to inadequate fluid intake

High Risk for Infection related to inadequate calorie intake, inadequate protein intake

Impaired Home Maintenance Management related to inability to purchase, store, or prepare food for family

Impaired Skin Integrity related to protein malnutrition, vitamin A deficiency

Knowledge Deficit related to new medical diet, nutrition misinformation, lack of interest in nutrition, intellectual deficit

Noncompliance to a particular diet order related to lack of motivation, misinformation

Self-Esteem Disturbance related to obesity

Sleep Pattern Disturbance related to excessive caffeine intake

Social Isolation related to obesity

T A B L E   3 3 - 1 1

Clinical Observations for Nutritional Assessment

Body Area	Signs of Good Nutritional Status	Signs of Poor Nutritional Status
General appearance	Alert, responsive	Listless, apathetic, and cachexic
General vitality	Endurance, energetic, sleeps well, vigorous	Easily fatigued, no energy, falls asleep easily, looks tired, apathetic
Weight	Normal for height, age, body build	Overweight or underweight
Hair	Shiny, lustrous, firm, not easily plucked, healthy scalp	Dull and dry, brittle, loss of color, easily plucked, thin and sparse
Face	Uniform skin color; healthy appearance, not swollen	Dark skin over cheeks and under eyes, flaky skin, facial edema (moon face), pale skin color
Eyes	Bright, clear, moist, no sores at corners of eyelids, membranes moist and healthy pink color, no prominent blood vessels	Pale eye membranes, dry eyes (xerophthalmia); Bitot's spots, increased vascularity, cornea soft (keratomalacia), small yellowish lumps around eyes (xanthelasma), dull or scarred cornea
Lips	Good pink color, smooth, moist, not chapped or swollen	Swollen and puffy (cheilosis), angular lesion at corners of mouth or fissures or scars (stomatitis)
Tongue	Deep red, surface papillae present	Smooth appearance, beefy red or magenta colored, swollen, papillae, hypertrophy or atrophy
Teeth	Straight, no crowding, no cavities, no pain, bright, no discoloration, well-shaped jaw	Cavities, mottled appearance (fluorosis), malpositioned, missing teeth
Gums	Firm, good pink color, no swelling or bleeding	Spongy, bleed easily, marginal redness, recessed, swollen and inflamed
Glands	No enlargement of the thyroid, face not swollen	Enlargement of the thyroid (goiter), enlargement of the parotid (swollen cheeks)
Skin	Smooth, good color, slightly moist, no signs of rashes, swelling, or color irregularities	Rough, dry, flaky, swollen, pale, pigmented, lack of fat under the skin, fat deposits around the joints (xanthomas), bruises, petechiae
Nails	Firm, pink	Spoon shaped (koilonychia), brittle, pale, ridged
Skeleton	Good posture, no malformations	Poor posture, beading of the ribs, bowed legs or knock-knees, prominent scapulas, chest deformity at diaphragm
Muscles	Well developed, firm, good tone, some fat under the skin	Flaccid, poor tone, wasted, underdeveloped, difficulty walking
Extremities	No tenderness	Weak and tender, presence of edema
Abdomen	Flat	Swollen
Nervous system	Normal reflexes, psychological stability	Decrease in or loss of ankle and knee reflexes, psychomotor changes, mental confusion, depression, sensory loss, motor weakness, loss of sense of position, loss of vibration, burning and tingling of the hands and feet (paresthesia)
Cardiovascular system	Normal heart rate and rhythm, no murmurs, normal blood pressure for age	Cardiac enlargement, tachycardia, elevated blood pressure
GI system	No palpable organs or masses (liver edge may be palpable in children)	Hepatosplenomegaly

(Adapted from Christakis, G. [Ed.]. [1973]. *Nutritional assessment in health programs.* Washington, D. C.: American Public Health Association; and Williams, S. R. [1990]. Essentials of nutrition and diet therapy [5th ed.]. St. Louis: Times Mirror/Mosby.)

NURSING DIAGNOSES FOR COMMON PROBLEMS

Nutrition

Problem	Related Factors	Sample Defining Characteristics
Altered Nutrition: Less Than Body Requirements	Malabsorption	• "I seem to eat all day long and yet I keep losing weight." - Reports losing 15 lb within the past 3 weeks. Has 8 to 10 bowel movements daily of frothy, odorous stools that float. Fecal fat excretion test indicates steatorrhea. Client appears fatigued and undernourished; muscle wasting is evident. Laboratory data reveal low serum albumin level (protein deficiency) and iron deficiency anemia.
Altered Nutrition: More Than Body Requirements	Decreased thyroid function leading to a decrease in metabolism	• I don't eat enough to keep a bird alive, but I just keep getting fatter and fatter. I don't know what else to do unless I stop eating altogether." • Client reports a 10-lb weight gain within the past month despite following a 1200-calorie diet. Other symptoms noted include fatigue, amenorrhea, and dry skin. Laboratory data indicate low serum thyroxine (T_4) level and protein-bound iodine and elevated serum thyroid-stimulating hormone and cholesterol levels. Radioactive iodine uptake was low.
Altered Nutrition: High Risk for More Than Body Requirements	Inappropriate use of supplements	• "I sent a sample of my hair away for a nutritional analysis, and the report came back saying that I should take supplements of zinc, iron, potassium, and magnesium." • For the past week, client has been taking supplements of 500% of the RDA for zinc and magnesium. She takes twice as much iron as recommended, and large doses of potassium ad lib.

Wellness Diagnosis

For clients who are incorporating sound nutritional practices in their daily routine, the following wellness diagnosis may be appropriate:
    Potential for enhanced compliance with low-fat diet
    regimen

Planning: Client Goals

Client goals evolve from the actual or potential nutritional problems diagnosed. General client goals follow. The client will:
• Attain and maintain ideal body weight
• Eat a diet adequate but not excessive in all nutrients
• Eat a variety of food in each of three or more meals
• Follow the appropriate modified diet, when necessary, to restore health, avoid disease recurrences, and prevent or delay potential complications

Implementing

Providing proper and adequate nourishment to the hospitalized client is a team effort: Diet orders are written by the physician, confirmed by the dietitian, and usually delivered by the nurse. The nurse also may be responsible for observing intake and appetite, evaluating the client's tolerance, assisting the client with eating, administering tube and parenteral feedings, consulting with the dietitian and physician when dietary problems arise, obtaining more food or snacks for the client when appropriate, monitoring food brought by visitors, and conducting or reinforcing diet instructions.

Stimulating Appetite

To the hospitalized client, food and eating may take on much greater meaning. Loss of control over food choices, the way food is prepared, and when and how food is served, and eating alone may do little to encourage normal eating.

Pain, illness, anxiety, and medications can contribute to anorexia and poor intake. Every effort must be made to ensure that the proper food is not only served but also eaten. The following measures may help to stimulate appetite:

- Serve small, frequent meals to avoid overwhelming the client with large amounts of food.
- Solicit food preferences and encourage food from home, if possible.
- Provide encouragement and a pleasant eating environment.
- Be sure the client's tray looks attractive.
- Schedule procedures and medications at times when they are least likely to interfere with appetite.
- Control pain, nausea, or depression with medications.
- Offer alternatives for items the client cannot or will not eat.
- Encourage or provide good oral hygiene.
- Remove clutter from area in which client is eating.
- Keep eating area free from irritating odors.
- Arrange food tray so that client can easily reach food.
- Provide a comfortable position.

Providing Special Diets

A variety of normal and modified diets are available in the hospital setting. Normal or house diets are designed to maintain a client's good nutritional status by providing adequate amounts of all nutrients. The diet's actual composition varies with the quantity and types of food selected; the average calorie content ranges from 1400 to 2500 cal.

Liquid diets are used most often as transitional diets when eating resumes after acute illness, surgery, or parenteral nutrition. *Clear liquid diets* contain only foods that are clear liquids at room or body temperature—gelatin, fat-free broth, bouillon, ice pops, clear juices, carbonated beverages, regular and decaffeinated coffee, and tea. Because clear liquid diets are inadequate in calories, protein, and most nutrients, they should be progressed as soon as possible.

Full liquid diets contain milk, plain frozen desserts, pasteurized eggs, cereal gruels, and milk and egg substitutes in addition to clear liquids. High-calorie, high-protein supplements are recommended if the diet is used for more than 3 days.

Soft diets usually are regular diets that have been modified to eliminate foods that are hard to digest and to chew, including those that are high in fiber, high in fat, and highly seasoned. Soft diets are adequate in calories and nutrients and may be used on a long-term basis.

Assisting With Eating

The loss of independence that comes with the inability to self-feed can be a severe blow to a client's self-esteem. The following nursing measures may help a client maintain dignity while being fed:

- Involve the client as much as possible. Solicit his or her preferences with regard to the order of items eaten and the eating pace.
- Engage the client in pleasant conversation to ease tension.
- Place a napkin, not a bib, over the client's clothes for protection.
- Use straws or special eating utensils whenever possible.

Food Restriction

Hospitalized clients may be ordered NPO (nothing by mouth) for several reasons. Food is prohibited before surgery to prevent aspiration related to anesthesia, and after surgery until bowel sounds return. NPO also may be necessary for clients undergoing certain medical tests and for clients experiencing severe nausea and vomiting, an inability to chew or swallow, coma, various acute or chronic gastrointestinal abnormalities, and labor and delivery.

Well-nourished clients can easily withstand the stress of NPO for a short period. Clients with increased nutritional requirements or those who will be NPO for more than 2 days may require nutritional support from tube feedings or parenteral nutrition.

The following measures may provide comfort to clients who are NPO:

- Encourage or provide good oral hygiene.
- Provide the client with ice chips, sips of water, hard candies, or gum, as allowed.
- Let the client chew favorite foods without swallowing.
- Urge the client to avoid watching others eat. Suggest alternate activities at mealtimes.

Enteral and Parenteral Nutrition

The preferred and most effective method of feeding clients is orally. When clients cannot receive food orally, they can receive the required nutrients through enteral or parenteral methods. **Enteral nutrition** involves passing a tube into the gastrointestinal tract to administer a formula containing adequate nutrients. **Parenteral nutrition** bypasses the gastrointestinal tract, and the client's nutritional needs are met by way of nutrient-filled solutions administered intravenously.

After the oral method of feeding, the next best method is the enteral route. For clients whose gastrointestinal tract is functional but who are unable or unwilling to consume adequate amounts of food, enteral tube feeding is used to deliver total or supplemental nutrition.

Enteral Nutrition or Tube Feedings

Enteral nutrition is by tube feedings directly into the gastrointestinal tract either by way of a tube inserted through the nose and into the stomach (nasogastric feeding) or by way of a tube surgically inserted directly into the stomach (gastrostomy tube). Another method is to insert the tube directly into the intestine either by way of a tube through the nose (nasoduodenal or nasojejunal) or by way of a tube surgically inserted into the small intestine (jejunostomy)

There are risks and advantages of both the stomach route and the intestinal route. Nasogastric feedings have the advantage of allowing the stomach to be used as a natural reservoir, regulating the amount of foods and liquids released into the small intestine. Nasogastric tubes do carry the risk of becoming dislodged or of the client aspirating formula into the lungs if vomiting occurs.

When the feeding tube bypasses the stomach and delivers formula directly into the intestine, a type of dumping syndrome may result with associated complications such as gas, bloating, pain, diarrhea, and, subsequently, hypoglycemia. Mild hypoglycemia results when a high-carbohydrate meal is rapidly absorbed, causing a rise in the blood glucose level. The increased blood glucose level triggers an overproduction of insulin, leading to a drop in the blood sugar and manifestations of hypoglycemia. Continuous feedings, rather than bolus feedings, are given to help avoid triggering the adverse effects of the dumping syndrome. There also is greater risk of infection because the tube bypasses the stomach and the influence of antiinfective gastric acids. The advantage of using the intestinal route is that it eliminates the risk of food being aspirated into the lungs in the client with a dysfunctional gag reflex.

Parenteral Nutrition

Clients who have nonfunctional gastrointestinal tracts, who are comatose, or who cannot consume a nutritionally adequate diet enterally (eg, clients undergoing aggressive cancer therapy, or those recovering from extensive burns, sepsis, or multiple fractures) may require parenteral nutrition. Sterile infusions of nutrients normally found in the blood may be delivered peripherally (isotonic solutions) or through the central vein (hypertonic solutions) if nutrient needs are great. Although all the client's nutritional needs can be met through total parenteral nutrition (TPN), this therapy is expensive, requires constant monitoring, and has the potential for causing infectious, metabolic, and mechanical complications (Table 33-12). TPN should be used only when an enteral intake is inadequate or contraindicated, and should be gradually discontinued as soon as possible. Research supports the use of enteral feeding instead of TPN whenever possible (Mobarhan & Trumbore, 1991).

Inserting Tubes Nasogastric or nasointestinal tubes are inserted nonsurgically through the nose and into the stomach or small intestine. The nasal method of insertion commonly is used; it requires a smaller tube and skill in insertion. Gastrostomy tubes or jejunostomy tubes are surgically implanted, not easily dislodged, and avoid any upper gastrointestinal obstructions that may be present, such as tumors. Insertion of a nasogastric tube is discussed in Procedure 33-1.

TABLE 33-12

Potential Complications of Total Parenteral Nutrition

Infection and Sepsis Related to

Catheter contamination during insertion
Long-term indwelling catheter
Catheter seeding from blood-borne or distant infection
Contaminated solution

Metabolic Complications

Dehydration
Hyperglycemia
Rebound hypoglycemia
Hyperosmolar, hyperglycemic nonketotic coma
Azotemia
Electrolyte disturbances
   Hypocalcemia
   Hypophosphatemia, hyperphosphatemia
   Hypokalemia
   Hypomagnesemia
High serum ammonia levels
Deficiencies of
   Essential fatty acid
   Trace elements
   Altered acid–base balance
   Elevated liver enzymes

Mechanical Complications Related to Catheterization

Catheter misplacement
Hemothorax (blood in the chest)
Pneumothorax (air or gas in the chest)
Hydrothorax (fluid in the chest)
Hemomediastinum (blood in the mediastinal spaces)
Subcutaneous emphysema
Hematoma
Arterial puncture
Myocardial perforation
Catheter embolism
Air embolism
Endocarditis
Nerve damage at the insertion site
Laceration of lymphatic duct
Chylothorax
Lymphatic fistula
Thrombosis

(Dudek, S. G. [1993]. *Nutrition handbook for nursing practice.* [2nd ed.]. Philadelphia: Lippincott.)

Irrigating the Tube Irrigate the client's gastric tube at regular intervals to determine and maintain patency. Irrigation of the nasogastric tube is done on the physician's orders. Nasogastric tubes used for *decompression* or removal of stomach contents or flatus usually are connected to an intermittent gastric suction device. They require irrigation with normal saline solution (0.9% sodium chloride solution) to compensate for electrolytes that are lost in the

(Text continues on page 824)

PROCEDURE 33-1

Inserting a Nasogastric Tube

Equipment

Nasogastric tube of appropriate size (8 to 18 French)
Small basin filled with ice or warm water (optional)
Water-soluble lubricant
Tongue blade
Flashlight

Stethoscope
Normal saline solution (for irrigation only)
Asepto bulb syringe or Toomey syringe (20 to 50 mL)
Tape (1 inch wide)
Tissues

Glass of water with straw
Suction apparatus
Bath towel or disposable pad
Safety pin and rubber band
Clamp
Emesis basin
Disposable gloves (optional)

Action	Rationale
1 Check physician's order for insertion of nasogastric tube.	This clarifies procedure and type of equipment required.
2 Explain procedure to client.	Explanation facilitates client cooperation.
3 Gather equipment.	This provides for organized approach to task.
4 If nasogastric tube is rubber, place it in a basin with ice for 5 to 10 minutes or place a plastic tube in a basin of warm water.	Cold stiffens the rubber tube, making it easier to insert. Plastic tube may be placed in warm water to make it more flexible.
5 Assess client's abdomen.	Assessment determines presence of bowel sounds and amount of abdominal distention.
6 Wash your hands. Don disposable gloves.	Handwashing deters the spread of microorganisms.
7 Assist the client to high Fowler's position, and drape his chest with bath towel or disposable pad. Have emesis basin and tissues handy.	Upright position is more natural for swallowing and protects against aspiration, if the client should vomit. Passage of tube may stimulate gagging and tearing of eyes.
8 Check the nares for patency by asking the client to occlude one nostril and breathe normally through the other. Select the nostril through which air passes more easily.	Tube passes more easily through the nostril with the largest opening.
9 Measure the distance to insert the tube by placing tip of tube at client's nostril and extending to tip of earlobe and then to tip of xiphoid process. Mark tube with a piece of tape.	Measurement ensures that the tube will be long enough to enter the client's stomach.

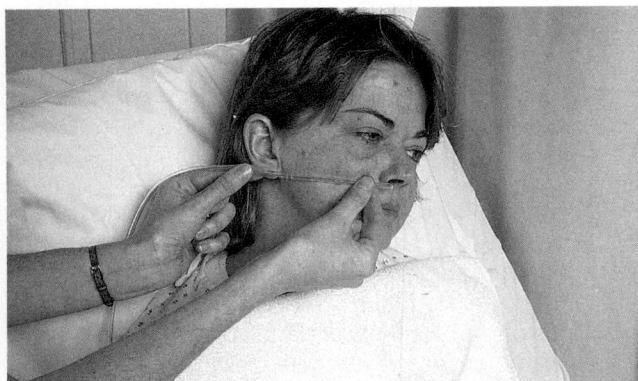

Action 9a: Measuring distance from nostril to tip of earlobe.

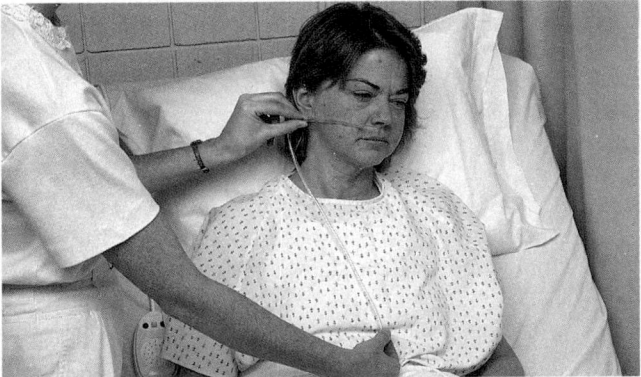

Action 9b: Measuring distance from earlobe to tip of xiphoid process.

(continued)

Inserting a Nasogastric Tube

Action	Rationale

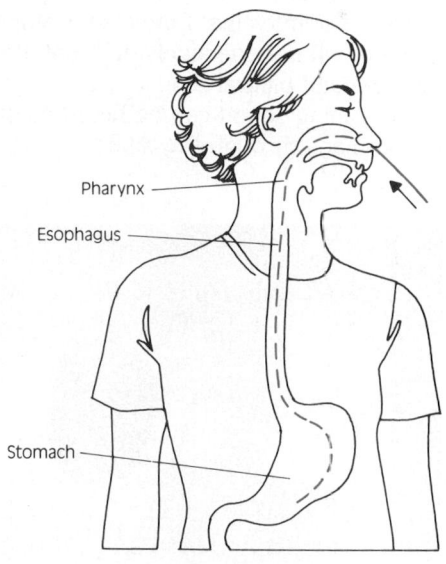

Pharynx

Esophagus

Stomach

Path of the tube.

10 Lubricate the first 10 to 20 cm (4 to 8 inches) of the tube with a water-soluble lubricant.

Lubrication reduces friction and facilitates passage of the tube into the stomach. Water-soluble lubricant will not cause pneumonia if tube accidentally enters the lungs.

11 Ask the client to lift his head, and insert the tube into the nostril while directing the tube downward and backward. The client may gag when the tube reaches the pharynx.

Following the normal contour of the nasal passage while inserting the tube reduces irritation and the likelihood of mucosal injury. The gag reflex is readily stimulated by the tube.

12 Instruct the client to keep head in upright or normal eating position. Encourage him or her to swallow even if no fluids are permitted. Advance the tube in a downward and backward direction when the client swallows. Stop when the client breathes. Provide tissues for tearing or watering of eyes. If gagging and coughing persist, check placement of tube with a tongue blade and flashlight. Keep advancing the tube until the tape marking is reached. Do not use force. Rotate the tube if it meets resistance.

Bringing the head forward helps close the trachea and open the esophagus. Swallowing helps advance the tube, causes the epiglottis to cover the opening of the trachea, and helps to eliminate gagging and coughing. Tears are a natural response as the tube passes into the nasopharynx. Excessive coughing and gagging may occur if the tube has curled in the back of throat. Forcing the tube may injure mucous membranes.

13 Discontinue the procedure and remove the tube if there are signs of distress, such as gasping, coughing, cyanosis, and the inability to speak or hum.

The tube is not in the esophagus if the client shows signs of distress and is unable to speak or hum.

14 Determine that the tube is in the client's stomach (these methods are appropriate for large-bore tubes but may be ineffective to check placement of small-bore, pliable tubes):

   a Attach the syringe to the end of the tube and aspirate 10 to 20 mL of stomach contents.

The tube is in the stomach if its contents can be aspirated.

(continued)

P R O C E D U R E   3 3 - 1 *(continued)*

Inserting a Nasogastric Tube

Action	Rationale
b Measure the pH of aspirated fluid.	The pH of gastric contents is acidic, compared with an average pH of 7.0 or greater for respiratory fluid. Because pH of intestinal fluid also is slightly basic, this method will not effectively differentiate between intestinal fluid and pleural fluid.
c Place 10 to 20 mL of air in syringe and inject air into the tube. Simultaneously auscultate over the epigastric area with a stethoscope.	A whooshing sound can be heard when the air enters the stomach through the tube.

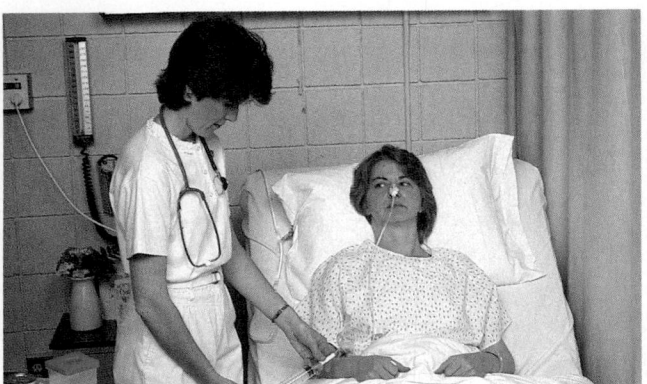

Action 14a: Aspirating gastric contents.

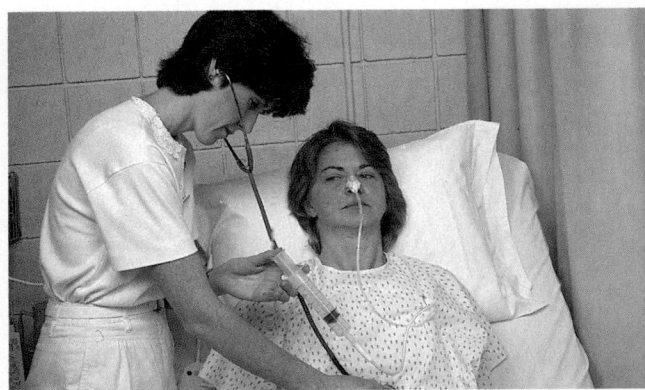

Action 14c: Listening for sound of air entering stomach.

15 Secure the tube with tape to the client's face. Be careful not to pull the tube too tightly against the nose: 　**a** Cut a 4-inch piece of tape and split bottom 2 inches. 　**b** Place unsplit end over bridge of client's nose. 　**c** Wrap split ends under the tubing and up and over onto the nose.	Constant pressure of the tube against the skin and mucous membranes causes tissue injury.
16 Attach tube to suction or clamp the tube with a screw-type clamp, according to the physician's orders.	Suction provides for decompression of stomach and drainage of gastric contents.
17 Secure tube to the client's gown by using a rubber band or tape and a safety pin. If double-lumen tube is used, secure vent above stomach level. Attach at shoulder level.	This prevents tension and tugging on the tube. Securing the double-lumen tube above stomach level prevents seepage of gastric contents and keeps the lumen clear for venting air.
18 Wash hands. Remove all equipment and make client comfortable.	Handwashing deters the spread of microorganisms.
19 Record the insertion procedure, type and size of tube, description of gastric contents, and client's response.	This facilitates documentation and provides for comprehensive care.

gastric fluids removed by the suction. Tubes used for feeding purposes usually are cleared before and after use, or according to the physician's order, with tap water. The actions and rationale for irrigation are discussed in Procedure 33-2.

Types of Tubes   Short tubes, used for placement in the stomach, are about 127 cm long. Single-lumen tubes (the lumen is the inner open space) without air vents are available in several sizes. A Levin tube is an example of a single-lumen tube. Single-lumen tubes lack a venting system;

Irrigating a Nasogastric Tube

Equipment

Nasogastric tube connected to continuous or intermittent suction
Irrigation set (Asepto or Toomey syringe and container for irrigating solution)
Normal saline solution (0.9% sodium chloride solution) for irrigation

Stethoscope
Disposable pad or bath towel
Clamp
Disposable gloves (optional)

Action	Rationale
1 Check physician's order for irrigation. Explain procedure to client.	This clarifies schedule and irrigating solution. An explanation encourages client cooperation and reduces apprehension.
2 Gather necessary equipment. Check expiration dates on irrigating saline solution and irrigation set.	This provides for organized approach to task. Agency policy dictates safe interval for reuse of equipment.
3 Wash your hands.	Handwashing deters the spread of microorganisms.
4 Assist client to semi-Fowler's position, unless this is contraindicated.	This position minimizes risk of aspiration.
5 Check placement of nasogastric tube (refer to Procedure 33-1, action 14).	
6 Clamp suction tubing near connection site. Disconnect tube from suction apparatus and lay on disposable pad or towel.	This protects client from leakage of nasogastric drainage.
7 Pour irrigating solution into container. Draw up 30 mL of saline solution (or amount ordered by physician) into syringe.	This delivers measured amount of irrigant through tube. Saline solution compensates for electrolytes lost through nasogastric drainage.
8 Place tip of syringe in tube. If Salem sump or double-lumen tube is used, make sure that syringe tip is placed in drainage port and not in air vent. Hold syringe upright and gently insert the irrigant (or allow solution to flow in by gravity if agency or physician indicates). Do not force solution into tube.	Position of syringe prevents entry of air into stomach. Gentle insertion of saline solution (or gravity insertion) is less traumatic to gastric mucosa.

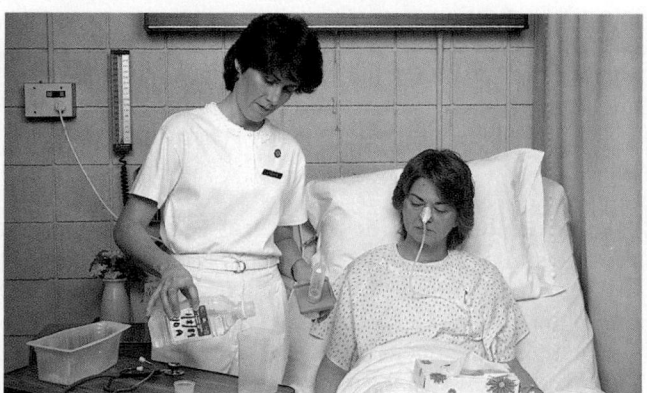

Action 7: Preparing irrigant.

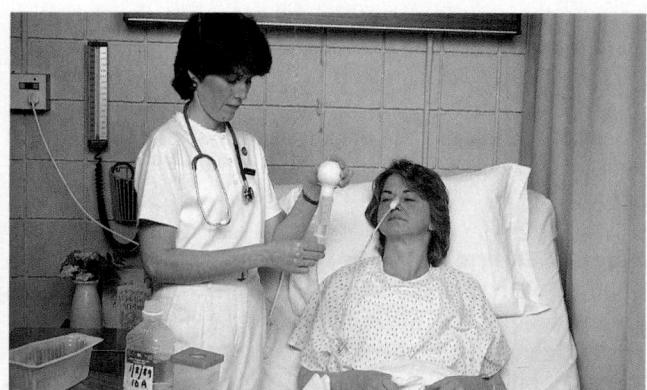

Action 8: Introducing irrigant into tube.

(continued)

P R O C E D U R E 3 3 - 2 *(continued)*

Irrigating a Nasogastric Tube

Action	Rationale
9 If unable to irrigate tube, reposition client and attempt irrigation again. Check with physician if repeated attempts to irrigate tube fail.	Tube may be positioned against gastric mucosa, making it difficult to irrigate.
10 Withdraw or aspirate fluid into syringe. If no return, inject 20 cc of air and aspirate again.	Injection of air may reposition the end of tube.
11 Reconnect tube to suction. Observe movement of solution or drainage.	Observation determines patency of tube and correct operation of suction apparatus.
12 Measure and record amount and description of irrigant and returned solution.	Irrigant placed in tube is considered intake; solution returned is recorded as output.
13 Rinse equipment if it will be reused.	This promotes cleanliness and prepares equipment for next irrigation.
14 Wash your hands.	Handwashing deters the spread of microorganisms.
15 Record irrigation procedure, description of drainage, and client's response.	This facilitates documentation of procedure and provides for comprehensive care.

therefore, mucosal damage may result if they are suctioned for decompression. Double-lumen sump tubes are a tube-within-a-tube. One lumen empties the stomach while the second lumen provides for a continuous flow of air. The airflow lumen controls suction by preventing the drainage lumen from pulling stomach mucosa into the tube's eyes and irritating the stomach lining. Suction can be continuous rather than intermittent, as is required when a single-lumen tube is used. Salem and Ventrol sump tubes are examples. Newer tubes for nasoenteral therapy (ie, Dobbhoff tubes) are smaller, softer, and more pliable, and can be placed in the stomach or the small intestine. The advantage of increased client comfort may be offset by difficulty checking tube placement. Initial and interval placement of these tubes is verified by x-ray examination. Percutaneous endoscopic gastrostomy (PEG) or jejunostomy tubes have become the standard method for accessing the gastrointestinal tract when long-term nutritional support is necessary (Mobarhan & Trumbore, 1991). A PEG tube is threaded by means of an endoscope through the esophagus into the stomach and then pulled through a stab wound made in the abdominal wall. The complication rate for this procedure is low.

Types of Enteral Feedings The nutritional composition of tube feedings depends on the feeding route, the client's ability to digest and absorb nutrients, and his or her nutrient and fluid requirements. Other considerations include the availability and cost of the formula, medical conditions that require diet modifications, food intolerances and allergies, and "taste." Even though the client cannot truly taste a tube feeding, its appearance and aroma influence palatability and acceptance. Many types of enteral feeding formulas are available. Detailed information on their composition and caloric value (most formulas contain 1 kcal/mL) can be obtained from the product label.

Enteral tube feedings can be given on an intermittent or a continual basis. Intermittent feedings have the following advantages:

- Residual (amount of formula remaining in the stomach) can be checked without interrupting the feeding.
- Client has greater flexibility, and mobility is not restricted.
- Feeding schedule may continue supplementally as client is reintroduced to oral feedings.

An intermittent feeding may range from 300 to 500 mL of formula and usually is administered in less than 1 hour. An intermittent gravity drip is used frequently in the home setting (Young & White, 1992). Continuous feedings facilitate administration of smaller volumes that are more easily tolerated by the client. An infusion pump commonly is used and has the advantage of maintaining accuracy in the administration of the feeding. The basic method for administering a tube feeding is outlined in Procedure 33-3.

Nursing Responsibilities in Enteral Feedings Agency protocols may differ and should be followed, but nursing actions that contribute to successful tube feedings include the following:

- Check the placement of a nasogastric tube before beginning a new or intermittent feeding (see display for techniques).
- For intermittent feedings, check the amount of residual; if it is more than 100 mL, investigate reasons for

(Text continues on p. 830)

PROCEDURE 33-3

Administering a Tube Feeding

Equipment

Tube feeding at room temperature
Stethoscope
Asepto or Toomey syringe, feeding
  bag, or prefilled tube feeding set

Clamp (Hoffman or butterfly)
Disposable pad or towel
Water
Sterile gauze

Rubber band
Enteral feeding pump
  (if ordered)
IV pole

Action	Rationale
1 Explain procedure to client.	This facilitates cooperation and provides reassurance for client.
2 Assemble equipment. Check amount, concentration, type, and frequency of tube feeding on client's chart.	This provides for organized approach to task. Ensures that correct feeding will be administered.
3 Wash your hands.	Handwashing deters the spread of microorganisms.
4 Position client with head of bed elevated at least 30 degrees or as near normal position for eating as possible.	This position minimizes possibility of aspiration into trachea.
5 Unpin tube from client's gown and check to see that the nasogastric tube is properly located in the stomach, as described in Procedure 33-1, action 14.	Even when initially positioned correctly, a nasogastric tube left in place can become dislodged between feedings. The instillation of water or nourishment could lead to serious respiratory problems if a gastric tube is in the trachea or a bronchus, rather than in the stomach.
6 Aspirate all gastric contents with a syringe and measure. Return immediately through tube and proceed with feeding if amount of residual does not exceed policy of agency or physician's guideline. Disconnect syringe from tubing.	This indicates gastric emptying time. A residual more than half of the previous hour's intake is significant and must be reported to physician. Fluid should be returned to stomach so as not to cause any fluid or electrolyte losses.

For Intermittent Feedings

7 When using Asepto or Toomey syringe:
   a Remove plunger or bulb from syringe and attach syringe to tube that has been pinched with finger and introduce the prescribed amount slowly.

The syringe acts to receive the nourishment. Introducing the nourishment slowly gives the stomach time to accommodate the fluid and decreases gastrointestinal distress.

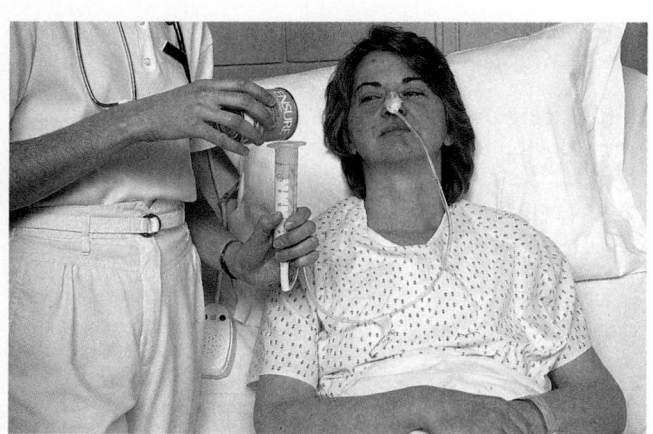

Action 7a: Introducing nourishment slowly.

(continued)

P R O C E D U R E 3 3 - 3 *(continued)*

Administering a Tube Feeding

Action	Rationale
b Hold the syringe about 12 inches above the stomach. Allow solution to run in by gravity. Raise the syringe to increase the rate of flow, and lower the syringe to decrease the rate of flow.	Nourishment enters the stomach by gravity when gastric gavage is used.
c Do not let the syringe empty while introducing the nourishment.	This technique prevents air from being forced into the stomach when the syringe is refilled.
d Introduce 30 to 60 mL (1 to 2 oz) of water into the tube after the nourishment is introduced.	Washing the tube with water forces remaining nourishment in the tube into the stomach and prevents nourishment from adhering to the tube and souring.
e Clamp the tube immediately after the nourishment and water are instilled. Disconnect the syringe and cover end of tubing with gauze secured with rubber band.	Clamping the tube prevents nourishment from draining back into the tube and air from entering the stomach. Cover on end of tube deters entry of microorganisms and protects client and linens from fluid leakage from tube.

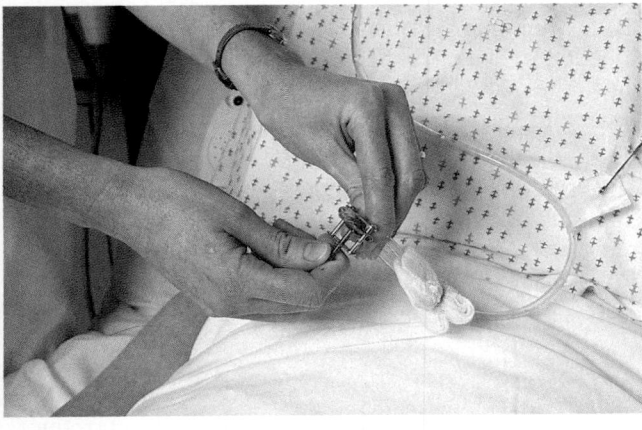

Action 7e: Clamping the tube after feeding.

8 When using a feeding bag:	
a Hang bag on IV pole and adjust to about 12 inches above the stomach. Clamp tubing and pour formula into the bag. Release clamp enough to allow formula to run through tubing. Close clamp.	Formula displaces air in the tubing.
b Attach tubing to feeding tube, open clamp, and regulate drip according to physician's order.	Introducing the formula at a slow, regular rate allows the stomach to accommodate to the feeding and decreases gastrointestinal distress.
c Add 30 to 60 mL (1 to 2 oz) of water to feeding bag when feeding is almost completed and allow it to run through tube.	Water rinses the feeding from the tube and helps to keep it patent.
d Clamp the tubing immediately after water has been instilled. Disconnect from tube. Clamp tube and cover end with gauze secured with a rubber band.	Clamping the tube prevents air from entering the stomach. Cover on end of tube deters entry of microorganisms and protects client and linens from fluid leakage from tube.

(continued)

PROCEDURE 33-3 *(continued)*

Administering a Tube Feeding

Action	Rationale

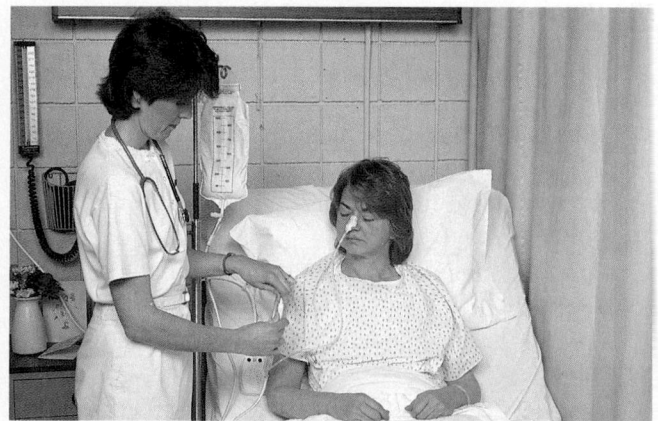

Action 8b: Attaching feeding-bag tubing to tube.

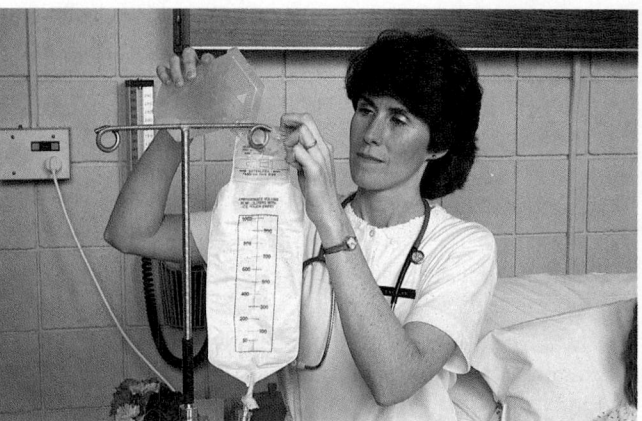

Action 8c: Adding water to rinse feeding tube.

9 When using prefilled tube feeding setup:

   a Remove screw-on cap and attach administration setup with drip chamber and tubing. Hang set on IV pole and adjust to about 12 inches above the stomach. Clamp tubing and squeeze drip chamber to fill one third to one half of capacity. Release clamp and run formula through tubing. Close clamp.

   b Follow Actions 8b, 8c, and 8d. Feeding pump may be used with tube feeding setup to regulate drip.

Formula displaces air in tubing.

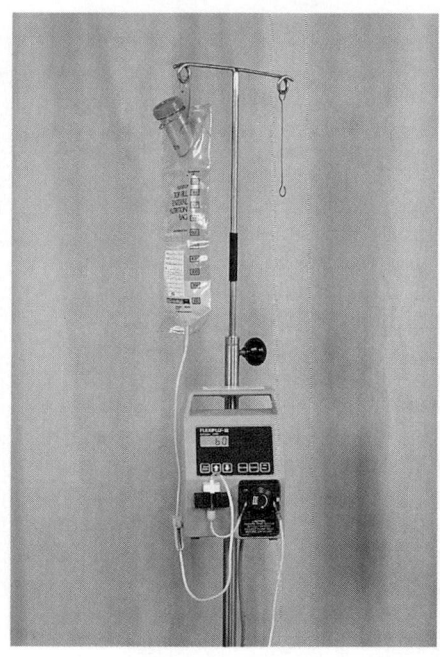

Action 9b: Feeding pump with feeding.

For Continuous Feedings

10 When using a feeding pump:

   a Close flow regulator clamp on tubing and fill feeding bag with prescribed formula. The amount used depends on agency policy. Place label on container.

Feeding intolerance is less likely to occur with smaller volumes. Hanging smaller amounts of feeding also reduces risk of bacteria growth and contamination of feeding at room temperature.

(continued)

P R O C E D U R E   3 3 - 3 *(continued)*

Administering a Tube Feeding

Action	Rationale
b Hang feeding container on IV pole and allow solution to flow through tubing.	This prevents air from being forced into the stomach or intestines.
c Connect to feeding pump following manufacturer's directions. Set rate.	Smaller volume of feeding is infused continuously and is more easily tolerated by the client.
d Check residual every 4 to 6 hours.	Checking verifies placement of the tube and proper absorption of the feeding.
11 Observe client's response during and after tube feeding.	Pain may indicate stomach distention, which may lead to vomiting.
12 Have client remain in upright position for at least 30 minutes after feeding.	This position minimizes risk of backflow and discourages aspiration, if any vomiting should occur.
13 Wash and clean equipment or replace according to agency policy. Wash your hands.	This prevents contamination and deters spread of microorganisms.
14 Record type and amount of feeding and client's response. Monitor urine or blood glucose, if ordered by physician.	This provides accurate documentation of procedure. Many feedings contain high amounts of carbohydrates.

Methods to Check Placement of a Feeding Tube

Methods of checking placement of feeding tubes vary according to tube size. It is difficult to verify correct placement of a small-bore, pliable enteral tube using the standard techniques. Methods may have to be tried several times, and if any coughing or choking is observed, the tube position may need to be verified by x-ray visualization. Common methods include the following:

1. Aspirate 10 to 20 mL of gastrointestinal fluid.
2. Measure the pH of aspirated gastrointestinal fluid. Gastric fluid is acidic, whereas intestinal fluid and pleural fluid usually are slightly basic (pleural fluid usually is 7.4; intestinal fluid ranges from 7.5 to 8.0).
3. Inject 10 to 20 cc of air into the tube (insufflation) while simultaneously auscultating over the epigastric area with a stethoscope. A whooshing or gurgling sound may indicate that the tube is in the stomach, but it is difficult to distinguish exact placement in the gastrointestinal tract by interpreting varying sounds.
4. Ask the client to talk or hum. A large-bore tube in the trachea would prohibit the client from speaking, but a smaller tube does not usually interfere with speech.

delayed emptying and follow physician's order or agency policy before proceeding. For continual feedings, the residual should be checked every 4 to 6 hours and should not exceed the hourly rate or volume (Murphy, 1990).

- Feeding solution and equipment (tubing and bag) need to be changed every 24 hours to prevent contamination (Murphy, 1990).
- Irrigate the tube before and after medication administration to prevent clogging of the feeding tube. Chapter 42 has additional information on medication administration by way of a nasogastric tube.
- Enteral feeding tubes occasionally become clogged, particularly the smaller tubes. Methods for declogging tubes are controversial and include instillation of carbonated colas, cranberry juice, meat tenderizer in a solution prepared by the pharmacist, and Viokase (a pancreatic enzyme) into the tube. Caution should always be taken to ascertain that a feeding tube is properly positioned (by means of a chest or an abdominal radiograph) and whether agency policy requires a physician's order before any attempt is made to declog a tube. Preventive maintenance measures are still the best option (Webber-Jones, et al., 1992).
- Administer oral hygiene frequently to prevent drying of tissues and to relieve thirst. Lubricate the lips generously.
- Keep the nares clean, especially around the tube where secretions tend to accumulate. Using a lubricant after cleaning the nares is recommended.
- Help control local irritation from the tube in the

throat. Analgesic throat lozenges or local anesthetic sprays may be effective.

- Allow the client to verbalize feelings.

The nurse has the responsibility of assessing a client receiving nourishment by gastric gavage for indications of the following complications:

Dehydration, diarrhea, and intestinal cramping. These symptoms often are present when the nourishment being used is highly concentrated and high in carbohydrate content. They usually can be controlled by reducing the strength of the formula and by introducing it more slowly. Diarrhea is a common complication of enteral feedings and according to Young and White (1992) is defined as more than five stools in 24 hours.

Spilling of glucose in the urine (glycosuria) and frequent urination. These signs are due to a high carbohydrate load from the nourishment. They can usually be relieved by reducing the strength of the formula and by introducing it more slowly. Insulin may need to be used in some instances.

Nausea. Nausea usually is the result of delayed emptying of the stomach. The feedings should be stopped and the client examined for gastric residual. Slowing the administration rate of the nourishment is ordinarily indicated.

Aspiration of nourishment. This complication is serious! It usually can be prevented by keeping the client in a semisitting position, so that the nourishment is less likely to enter the esophagus and be aspirated.

Vomiting. Vomiting tends to occur when the nourishment does not leave the stomach. The gastric residue should be checked and the amount of feedings reassessed.

Procedure 33-4 gives additional nursing actions in monitoring the client with a nasogastric tube in place.

Removing the Tube The tube must be removed as carefully as it is inserted to provide as much comfort as possible to the client. Oral hygiene follows removal of the tube. This is especially important to remove disagreeable tastes and odors, and should be done thoroughly when the tube has been in the intestinal tract and in contact with intestinal contents. Directions for removing the nasogastric tube are given in Procedure 33-5.

PROCEDURE 33-4

Monitoring a Nasogastric Tube

Action	Rationale
1 Confirm physician's order for nasogastric tube, type of suction, and directions for irrigation.	This ensures correct implementation of physician's order.
2 Observe drainage from tube. Check amount, color, consistency, and odor. Hematest drainage to confirm presence of blood in drainage.	Normal color of gastric drainage is light yellow to green because of the presence of bile. Bloody drainage may be expected after gastric surgery but must be closely monitored. Presence of coffee ground–type drainage may indicate bleeding.
3 Inspect suction apparatus if it is in use. Check that setting is correct for type of suction (continuous or intermittent) and range of suction (low, medium, high), and that drainage is moving through tubing.	Checking ensures correct implementation of physician's order and that suction is present and correctly adjusted. Loose connections or a kink or blockage in tube may interfere with suction.
4 Assess placement of tube (see Procedure 33-1, action 14).	Tube may be displaced into trachea through movement or manipulation.
5 Assess comfort of client. Check for presence of nausea and vomiting, feeling of fullness, or pain.	Discomfort may indicate incorrect operation of nasogastric suction or blockage in tube.
6 Assess client's abdomen for distention, and auscultate for presence of bowel sounds.	Abdominal distention may be related to the accumulation of gas or internal bleeding. Presence of bowel sounds indicates the return of peristalsis.
7 Assess mobility of client and respiratory status.	Turning from side to side in bed and ambulation when permitted encourage the return of peristalsis and facilitate drainage. Presence of tube may discourage client from coughing and deep breathing necessary for adequate respiratory exchange.

(continued)

PROCEDURE 33 - 4 (continued)

Monitoring a Nasogastric Tube

Action	Rationale
8 Observe condition of client's nostrils and oral cavity.	Nostrils need cleansing and lubrication with water-soluble lubricant, and tape must be changed when necessary to minimize irritation from tube. Frequent mouth care (at 2-hour intervals) improves comfort and maintains moisture in oral mucosa.
9 Monitor overall safety of client with tube. Check for proper placement of tape on nose and correct attachment of tube to gown.	Tube that is secured to client's nose with tape and pinned to gown allows easier movement. Call bell within reach allows client ready access to nursing assistance. Any kinks or obstruction interferes with patency of tube. A semi-Fowler's position facilitates drainage and minimizes any risk of aspiration.
10 Monitor tube and suction apparatus at least every 2 hours. Irrigate at interval ordered by physician (see Procedure 33-2).	These procedures promote safe operation of system. Any change in client's condition or type of drainage necessitates more frequent observation and notification of physician.
11 Record and measure nasogastric irrigations and drainage on intake/output chart according to schedule and agency protocol. Document description of drainage and client's response on chart.	Irrigations are recorded as intake. Drainage from tube is measured as output every 8 hours. If drainage is copious, more frequent emptying of collection container will be necessary. Documentation provides accurate record of client's response to nasogastric drainage.
12 Replenish supplies and maintain equipment according to agency policy and manufacturer's recommendations.	This ensures availability of necessary supplies. Provides for safe operation of equipment and efficient drainage of client's gastric contents.

PROCEDURE 33 - 5

Removing a Nasogastric Tube

Equipment

Tissues
Bath towel or disposable pad
Disposable plastic bag
50-mL syringe (optional)

Normal saline solution for irrigation (optional)
Clean disposable gloves

Action	Rationale
1 Check physician's order for removal of nasogastric tube.	This ensures correct implementation of physician's order.
2 Explain procedure to client and assist to semi-Fowler's position.	Explanation facilitates client cooperation. Sitting position decreases risk of aspiration, if vomiting should occur.
3 Gather equipment.	This provides for organized approach to task.
4 Wash your hands. Don clean disposable gloves.	Handwashing deters the spread of microorganisms. Gloves protect hands from contact with abdominal secretions.

(continued)

PROCEDURE 3 3 - 5 *(continued)*

Removing a Nasogastric Tube

Action	Rationale
5 Place towel or disposable pad across client's chest. Give tissues to client.	Precautions protect client from contact with gastric secretions. Tissues are necessary if client wants to blow his nose when tube is removed.
6 Discontinue suction and separate tube from suction. Unpin tube from client's gown and carefully remove adhesive tape from client's nose.	Unconnecting tube allows for its unrestricted removal.
7 Attach syringe and flush with 10 mL normal saline solution or clear with 30 to 50 cc of air (optional).	Air or saline solution clears the tube of feeding or debris.
8 Instruct client to take a deep breath and hold it.	This prevents accidental aspiration of gastric secretions in tube.
9 Clamp tube with fingers by doubling tube on itself. Quickly and carefully remove tube while client holds breath.	Careful removal minimizes trauma and discomfort for client. clamping prevents drainage of gastric contents in tube.
10 Place tube in disposable plastic bag. Remove gloves and place in bag.	This prevents contamination with microorganisms.
11 Offer mouth care to client and make client comfortable.	Provides for comfort.
12 Measure nasogastric drainage. Remove all equipment and dispose according to agency policy. Wash your hands.	Measuring nasogastric drainage provides for accurate recording of output. Proper disposal deters spread of microorganisms.
13 Record removal of tube, client's response, and measurement of drainage.	Facilitates documentation and provides for comprehensive care.

Teaching Nutritional Information

For the greatest chance of success, diet instructions should be individually tailored to the client's life-style, intellectual ability, and level of motivation. Although strict guidelines and printed handouts may be viewed as the ideal, in practice, simplicity and compromise often are the keys to client compliance. Although specific instructions vary according to the diet order, the following guidelines are applicable for all types of diets:

- Provide simple verbal instructions. When appropriate, include family members and provide written teaching aids (Fig. 33-8).
- Advise the client to eliminate any foods not tolerated.
- Advise the client to alert the physician if the diet conflicts with religious beliefs, if adverse effects develop, or if special foods required are too costly or difficult to locate.
- Offer support and encouragement.
- If possible, spread diet instructions out over a period of days or weeks, so as not to overwhelm the client with too much information at one time and to allow

FIGURE 3 3 - 8

Diet instructions should be individually tailored to the client's life-style, abilities, and level of maturation. Printed information is ideal.

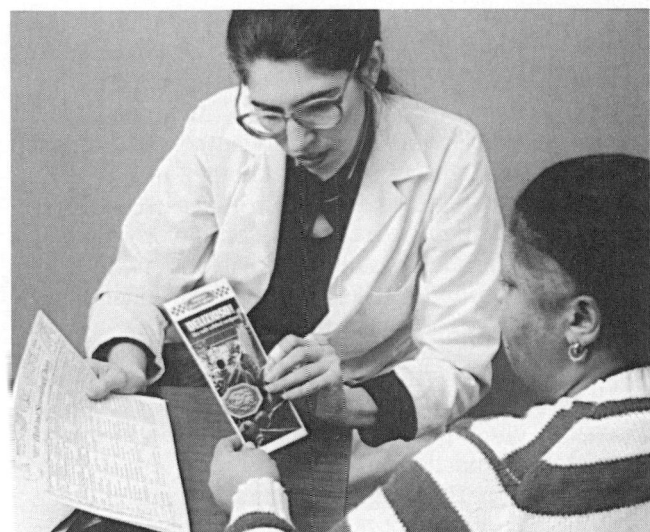

the client time to internalize the information and form questions.
• Evaluate the client's level of understanding; assess the need for reinforcement or elaboration.

Evaluating

The effectiveness of the plan of care is evaluated as the last step in the nursing care process. On an ongoing basis, the nurse should:

• Evaluate the client's progress toward meeting nutritional goals
• Evaluate the client's tolerance and adherence to the diet, when appropriate
• Assess the client's level of understanding of the diet and the need for further diet instruction or reinforcement
• Communicate findings to other members of the health care team
• Revise the plan of care, as needed, or terminate nursing care

 # N U R S I N G   P R O C E S S

In Clinical Practice

Nursing diagnoses related to the client's nutritional status can be made after assessment data have been collected and analyzed. Nursing diagnoses may cite actual or potential nutritional problems, deal with how nutritional problems affect other areas of human functioning, or be related to nutritional knowledge deficits. The following three examples of nutritional diagnoses include assessment priorities, client goals, nursing interventions, and evaluative criteria.

Altered Nutrition: More Than Body Requirements—Obesity

Obesity is defined as body weight 20% or more above ideal weight (Fuller & Schaller-Ayers, 1990). A positive caloric balance, resulting from an excess caloric intake or a decrease in energy expenditure, leads to the gradual accumulation of weight. Although society assumes that obese people gorge themselves with food, studies have shown that obese people actually eat less than their thin counterparts. The cascading effect of increased weight gain leading to a decrease in activity and social isolation perpetuates the problem of obesity.

About 30% to 40% of adult Americans are obese (Burrel, 1992). A recent Canadian fitness study indicated that almost 24% of the participants had BMIs above 27 (obesity) and 16% fell into the overweight BMI range of 25 to 27 (Report of the Scientific Review Committee, 1990). Obesity strikes all segments of society, although an increase in socioeconomic status is related to an increased risk of obesity in men and a decreased risk of obesity in women.

Obesity is probably multifactorial in origin, with different factors contributing to its development in different people. Numerous theories have been proposed.

Genetic Theories
   Metabolism: Faulty adenosine triphosphate production causes obese people to use less energy performing metabolic functions.
   Familial traits: The weight of natural children is highly correlated to that of their natural parents, whereas

there is only a slight correlation between the weight of adopted children and their adopted parents.

Physiologic Theories
   Fat cell theory: Obese people have more fat cells in their body, which have the propensity to store fat.
   Set-point theory: The hypothalamus determines the body's ideal biologic weight (set point) and struggles to maintain that weight—even when caloric intake is restricted—by lowering metabolic rate. As the metabolic rate decreases, losing weight becomes increasingly difficult without further reducing calories, which in turn further reduces the metabolic rate.
   Brown fat: Obese people have less brown fat, and thus use less energy producing heat through nonshivering or diet-induced thermogenesis.
   Insulin response: Obese people respond more readily to external cues (the sight, sound, or smell of food), which stimulate insulin release and lead to a decreased serum glucose level and the sensation of hunger accompanied by an increase in fat formation.
   Hormonal imbalances: An undersecretion of thyroid hormones causes a decrease in metabolic rate and, therefore, a decrease in energy expenditure.

Environmental Theories
   Food environment: Some people may be lured into overeating because of the abundance of food.
   Family environment: Obesity tends to run in families. For instance, a child with no obese parents has a 10% chance of becoming obese. The risk increases to 40% if one parent is obese, and children who have two obese parents have an 80% chance of becoming obese.
   Work environment: Since the turn of the century, mechanization, shorter work days, and shorter work weeks have led to a decrease in energy expenditure.

Psychological Theories
   Compulsiveness: People overeat because they suffer from a compulsive behavioral disorder similar to that in alcoholics and drug abusers.

Nutrition

Current interest in nutrition and fitness has created a focus on the dietary behavior of our society. Despite emphasis on developing healthy eating habits, obesity continues to be a widespread problem. Nurses need an awareness of causative factors, familiarity with successful weight management programs, and a nonjudgmental approach to have a positive impact on this prevalent health problem.

Related Research

Sherman, J. B., & Alexander, M. (1990). Obesity in children: A research update. *Journal of Pediatric Nursing, 5*(3), 161–166.

Many obese children become obese adults. Recent research has identified factors in the environment as well as individual characteristics that are associated with obesity in children. Because of their unique role, nurses can provide the preventive counseling and parental education at critical periods of development that is necessary to prevent obesity in children.

Allan, J. (1989). Women who successfully manage their weight. *Western Journal of Nursing Research, 11*(6), 657–675.

This study explores the characteristics that were predictive of successful weight loss and maintenance in a group of women who managed their own weight reduction regimen. The author found that experimentation with self-initiated life-style changes enabled this group to experience success and positively influence their weight loss efforts. Nursing strategies that reinforce the client's self-focused reasons for weight loss may be more effective than emphasis on the negative aspects of obesity as a risk factor.

Paternelj-Taylor, C. A. (1989). The effects of patient weight and sex on nurses' perceptions: A proposed model of nurse withdrawal. *Journal of Advanced Nursing, 14,* 744–754.

This study examined the impact of obesity on the nurse–client relationship. Nurses negatively evaluated obese clients using the Nurse Evaluation of Patient Scale but did not demonstrate withdrawal in any aspect of client care. More research needs to be done to explore whether conditioned attitudes held by nurses toward obese clients might impact on the quality of care and a therapeutic environment.

Summary

Nursing research about obesity is valuable as nurses intervene to improve the health prospects of their clients. Linking theory to the practice setting may positively affect the ability to predict the behavior of the client and the nurse's response.

Emotional crutch: People use food to satisfy various emotional needs.

Compensation: People overeat to compensate for lack of affection and companionship.

Release: People overeat to relieve boredom, tension, anxiety, frustration, and feelings of inadequacy

Obesity presents a serious health problem physically, socially, and emotionally. It increases the risk of numerous medical problems, such as hypertension, hyperlipidemia, cardiovascular and respiratory disorders, diabetes mellitus, and osteoarthritis; increases the risks associated with surgery; increases the risk of complications during pregnancy, labor, and delivery; and increases morbidity and mortality. Socially, obese people often are discriminated against in social, educational, and employment settings. And in a society that values thinness, obesity can cause one to feel desperate, frustrated, and rejected and to feel like a failure.

Obesity is resistant to treatment, and weight loss usually is temporary at best. Only about 5% of dieters are able to maintain their weight loss (Williams, 1990)

The following assessment criteria, client goals, nursing interventions, and evaluative criteria are for a client diagnosed with obesity related to overeating.

Assessment

A thorough assessment to determine not only the degree of obesity but also whether the client is likely to succeed in a weight loss program must be performed before a plan of care can be devised. Although all obese clients have the potential to benefit from weight loss, not all clients are motivated enough to lose weight and to keep it off. In addition, static obesity may be less harmful than frequent weight loss and regain. Thrusting weight loss diets on unmotivated clients also may cause "negative contagion," which may spread to others in a group setting; failure, which can have devastating consequences that preclude later attempts at dieting when the client may have had a better chance of success; and loss of morale among the health care professionals (Brownell, 1984).

To determine the severity of the obesity and the client's level of motivation:

- Use interview questions to assess pertinent dietary factors, such as the pattern and frequency of eating; the social environment surrounding eating; the client's actual and perceived reasons for eating; the client's previous use of weight loss diets; cultural, familial, religious, and ethnic influences on eating habits and their relative importance to the client; and nutritional knowledge.
- Explore the client's life-style and physical and mental health for factors that contribute to obesity.
- Instruct the client to keep a food diary for 3 to 7 days to determine his or her level of motivation as well as to gain knowledge about his or her eating habits.
- Compare the client's current weight and IBW and determine the percentage of excess body weight.
- Obtain body measurements, such as bust or chest, waist, hips, and thighs, for use in ongoing evaluation. Skin fold measurements also may be helpful in determining body fatness and measuring weight loss progress.
- Assess for complications—hypertension, diabetes, heart disease, osteoarthritis.
- Assess the duration of obesity—age of onset, family history.
- Assess activity patterns and how activity is affected by obesity.
- Assess the actual and perceived degree of control the client has over food.
- Assess the client's feelings about obesity and weight loss diets, his or her sense of body image and self-esteem.
- Determine if outside support systems are present.
- Assess the safety and effectiveness of weight loss aids the client has used in the past.

Planning: Client Goals

The client who undertakes a weight control program will:
- Identify eating attitudes and behaviors that contribute to obesity
- Practice behavior modification techniques to control factors that contribute to overeating
- Incorporate some type of physical activity into his or her daily routine, gradually increasing the intensity and duration of activity
- Enlist the support of family and friends, and attend group weight loss sessions, if possible

Interventions

Interventions for obesity vary according to its cause and severity. Weight loss programs should combine dietary changes, social support, exercise, and behavior modification.

Dietary Interventions
- Decrease calories for a gradual, weekly weight loss of about 1 to 2 lb (about 0.5 to 1 kg/wk).

Low caloric intake can be achieved by several methods, depending on the amount of weight the client has to lose and his or her level of motivation. For clients who do not have a lot of weight to lose, simply eliminating second helpings and snacks may be adequate. Counting total calories consumed throughout the day may work, but it does not ensure nutritional adequacy. A more effective and realistic approach uses exchange lists that state the size and number of servings allowed daily from each of six or more food group lists.

Traditional low-calorie diets may produce too gradual a weight loss for clients who are moderately to morbidly obese (ie, greater than 40% and 100% above ideal weight, respectively). In such cases, a medically supervised VLCD—otherwise known as a protein-sparing modified fast—may be indicated. A VLCD provides 1.5 g of high biologic value protein per kilogram of body weight in the form of meat, fish, poultry, or a powdered supplement. Supplemental vitamins and minerals are given, based on the client's laboratory data, and the client is closely monitored for tolerance, weight loss, and complications. Although the average weight loss in a 12-week period is about 45 lb (20.4 kg), the loss tends to be poorly maintained after the diet is discontinued.

Social Support
- Enlist the support of family and friends.
- Encourage the client to enroll in a group weight loss program. Such programs usually are more successful than individual programs.

Exercise
- Incorporate an exercise period into each day, gradually increasing its intensity and duration.

Behavior Modification Techniques
(which suggest how to and how not to, as opposed to stipulating dos and don'ts)
- Think thin by listing reasons why the client wants to lose weight, setting long-term weight loss goals, rewarding successes periodically with nonfood items, and avoiding talk about food.
- Plan strategies: Keep food only in the kitchen and avoid the kitchen except for mealtime. Cook only as much food as is needed for each meal, avoid tasting food while cooking. Position low-calorie food in the front of the refrigerator and higher-calorie items in the back. Keep tempting items out of sight, preferably out of the house. Limit the list of forbidden foods.
- Change eating habits: Wait 10 minutes after feeling the urge to eat. Eat slowly. Never skip meals. Eat only in one designated place, and do not do anything else while eating. Eat low-calorie foods first. Use a small plate, and leave some food on your plate. Chew food thoroughly and eat slowly.
- Modify shopping habits: Never shop while hungry. Always shop from a list. Buy only as much food as needed. Do not buy items that you know are your weakness.

- Incorporate life-style changes: Keep busy with projects and hobbies. Accept changes in eating as a way of life, not a short-term hurdle to overcome. Trim recipes of extra fat and sugar. Do not weigh yourself too frequently. Accept setbacks or infrequent cheating without giving up on the plan—they are inevitable.

Although numerous prescription and over-the-counter drugs are promoted as diet aids, they are inappropriate and ineffective when used alone. At best, some drugs may be useful on a short-term basis when combined with other weight loss measures. If drugs are prescribed, the nurse instructs the client about the action of the drug, the reason for its use, adverse effects to be aware of and to report, and the potential dangers of the drug.

Surgical intervention, such as gastric stapling, may be used as a last resort in clients who cannot lose weight by nonsurgical methods or are at increased risk of illness because of obesity and in those whose obesity poses a greater risk than the risk of surgery. A row of staples across the stomach forms a small pouch that initially holds 1 to 2 oz (28.4 to 56.7 g) of food. Because the pouch can eventually expand to hold more food, and because the staples can burst under too much pressure, it also is imperative that a low-calorie diet of small, frequent meals be followed.

Clients who suffer from compulsive overeating may benefit from Overeaters Anonymous, a self-help program designed to identify and cope with feelings that lead to overeating. Other options include referral for psychiatric evaluation.

Evaluative Criteria

The client meets the previously stated goals.

Altered Nutrition: Less Than Body Requirements—Iron Deficiency Anemia

One of iron's major functions in the body is to form heme, the pigment that combines with the protein globin in the blood to form hemoglobin. Hemoglobin is responsible for carrying oxygen from the lungs to the tissues, and therefore it is needed by all body cells for the release of energy.

Iron deficiency anemia, characterized by small (microcytic), pale (hypochromic) red blood cells, is a nutritional deficiency disorder that is found worldwide. Without sufficient iron, the body cannot produce enough hemoglobin, which hinders oxygen transport and leads to fatigue, weakness, and pallor.

The incidence rate in the United States for iron deficiency anemia is 10% to 50% (10% to 60% in Canada) among those in high-risk groups who simply do not consume enough dietary iron to meet their requirements—infants and children under age 2, menstruating women, elderly people, people in low-income groups, and vegetarians. Iron deficiency anemia commonly is related to an inadequate intake for two reasons. First, iron is not plentiful in the diet, and there are few excellent sources—liver and other organ meats, muscle meats, clams, liver sausage, oysters, pork loin, sardines, shrimp, and dark poultry meat.

These animal sources are known as heme iron. Nonheme sources of iron include enriched and fortified grains and cereals, dried fruit, dried peas and beans, nuts, and green, leafy vegetables. Second, only about 10% of dietary iron is absorbed, with a 15% to 35% absorption rate for heme iron and a 3% to 8% absorption rate for nonheme iron. Unlike heme iron, nonheme iron absorption is greatly influenced by other dietary factors. For instance, vitamin C, heme iron, and certain animal proteins enhance nonheme iron absorption, whereas tea, coffee, bran, phosphates, oxalates, phytates, and antacids inhibit its absorption.

Iron deficiency anemia also may occur secondary to an increase in iron requirement related to the following:
- Chronic blood loss—bleeding ulcers, gastritis, cancer, parasites, closely spaced pregnancies
- Inadequate absorption—chronic diarrhea, malabsorption syndrome, partial or total gastrectomy, pica, poor iron bioavailability of foods consumed
- Accelerated growth—pregnancy, infancy, and puberty

The following assessment criteria, client goals, nursing interventions, and evaluative criteria are for a toddler diagnosed with iron deficiency anemia related to inadequate intake.

Assessment

To determine the severity of the iron deficiency anemia and contributing factors:
- Observe for signs and symptoms of iron deficiency anemia, which vary with severity and chronicity— fatigue, weakness, pallor, sensitivity to cold, anorexia, dizziness, headaches, thin and spoon-shaped fingernails, sore tongue and mouth, and pica (ingestion of nonfood substances, such as dirt, clay, or laundry starch).
- Interview the primary caregiver to determine the amount and sources of iron normally consumed. Be aware that toddlers who consume more than a quart of milk daily are at risk of iron deficiency anemia because milk displaces the intake of foods rich in iron.
- Assess intake for the influence of nonheme iron inhibitors and enhancers.
- Assess medical–socioeconomic data to determine whether the child's inadequate intake is related to low socioeconomic status or compounded by another medical problem.
- Interview the primary caregiver to determine whether the client has ever or is currently taking iron supplements; symptoms of iron overload may mimic iron deficiency anemia.

Planning: Client Goals

The client will:
- Increase iron intake, especially heme iron
- Eat a source of heme iron at every meal
- Include a rich source of vitamin C at each meal (ie, citrus fruits and juices, broccoli, tomatoes, strawberries, cantaloupe, green pepper, brussels sprouts)

- Avoid tea and coffee immediately before and after eating because of their inhibitory effect on nonheme iron absorption

Interventions

- Instruct the family on ways to increase the iron content of the diet:
  - Use iron-fortified infant cereals until the child is 18 months old, if possible, because the iron in these cereals is absorbed more readily than the iron in other cereals.
  - Eat more organ meats, muscle meats, and poultry dark meat.
  - Eat meat at every meal, if possible.
  - Limit milk intake to less than 1 qt (0.95 L) a day to avoid displacing other iron-rich foods.
  - Add dried fruits to cereals and cookies; use as a snack or dessert.
  - Use crushed iron-fortified cereals as a breading for meat, fish, poultry, and vegetables; mixed with butter for a casserole topping; as a meat extender in meatloaf, meatballs, and burgers; sprinkled on ice cream, fruit salad, yogurt, pudding.
  - Substitute whole grains for refined products.
  - Cook in iron pots whenever possible, especially acidic foods (tomatoes, foods with vinegar or lemon).
- Instruct the family on ways to increase iron absorption:
  - Eat meat at every meal, if possible.
  - Include a rich source of vitamin C at every meal.
  - Do not give a child tea or coffee.
- Instruct the family that if the client is anorexic or a finicky eater, small, frequent meals may be better tolerated.
- Advise the family to avoid giving the client acidic and salty foods, strong spices, coarse breads, raw vegetables, and hot foods and beverages if the oral mucosa is inflamed.
- If an inadequate food budget is contributing to poor iron intake, refer the family to the appropriate social service.
- If iron supplements are prescribed, teach the family when they should be taken, possible adverse effects to watch for, and the dangers of overuse.

Evaluative Criteria

The client meets the previously stated goals.

Knowledge Deficit—New Medical Diet

The following assessment criteria, client goals, nursing interventions, and evaluative criteria may be used for a client who is being discharged from the hospital on a high-fiber diet (for diverticulum) that he has been receiving for 3 days.

Assessment

Through interview questions, obtain a diet history to determine the following:

- Quantity and sources of fiber in the client's usual diet
- Client's tolerance of a high-fiber diet while in the hospital. Potential adverse effects of initiating a high-fiber diet too quickly include flatus, distention, cramping, and diarrhea.
- Client's willingness to make the appropriate dietary changes
- Who shops and prepares the client's meals

Planning: Client Goals

The client will:

- Eat a variety of high-fiber foods daily
- Substitute high-fiber foods for foods of lower fiber content
- Add bran to the diet slowly to decrease the likelihood of developing flatus and distention
- Drink six to eight glasses of water daily
- Recognize the signs and symptoms of eating too much fiber

Interventions

- Instruct the client that a high-fiber diet will increase stool bulk, stimulate peristalsis, and reduce pressure within the bowel to avoid aggravating the diverticulum.
- Instruct the client that many types of fiber exist in the diet; some are effective as laxatives, and others tend to lower serum cholesterol levels and may lower glucose levels in diabetics.
- Advise the client and family that the following dietary changes should be incorporated gradually:
  - Eat more raw vegetables and fresh fruit, preferably with the skin on.
  - Substitute whole-grain breads and cereals for those that contain refined grains.
  - Add up to 3 tbsp of coarse bran to the diet. The fiber in bran is the type most effective as a laxative. Bran can be sprinkled over cereal, applesauce, or eggs; added to muffins, quick breads, casseroles, and meatloaves before baking; and mixed with fruit juice or milk.
  - Drink six to eight glasses of water daily; fiber absorbs water in the gut to increase fecal bulk.
- Inform the client about the potential adverse effects of eating too much fiber too quickly—flatus, distention, cramping, and diarrhea. Advise the client to reduce fiber intake if symptoms appear.

Evaluative Criteria

The client meets the previously stated goals.

CASE STUDY

Susan Oakland, a 21-year-old student, was seen at the prenatal clinic for her first pregnancy at 5 weeks' gestation. On her next visit, 4 weeks later, she complained of nausea and vomiting and had lost 3 lb (1.4 kg).

Assessment Findings

A comprehensive nutritional assessment revealed the following data:

Anthropometric Data

Usual body weight: 112 lb (50.8 kg)
Weight at 9 weeks' gestation: 109 lb (49.4 kg)
Height: 5 feet 5 inches (165.1 cm)
Ideal body weight: 125 lb (56.7 kg; range is 113 to 137 lb [51.3 to 62.1 kg])
Expected weight gain for 9 weeks' gestation: 1 to 2 lb (0.45 to 0.9 kg)

Biochemical Data

• Laboratory data revealed low hemoglobin level and hematocrit.

Medical–Socioeconomic Data

• Client complains of nausea and vomiting, which begin in the morning and continue until midafternoon. Her appetite is poor. She also states, "I'm always tired."
• Client and her husband are first-semester graduate students; their source of income is graduate assistantships, so their food budget is limited.
• Client states that she did not intend to become pregnant, but both she and her husband are excited about becoming parents. She plans to take a leave of absence from school for one semester when the baby is born; she wants to breastfeed.

Clinical Data

Client appears pale. No other abnormal physical findings were noted.

Dietary Data

• Client's 24-hour recall revealed an inadequate intake from the milk group and a marginal intake from the grain and meat groups. She skips breakfast because of a hurried schedule, which is now complicated by nausea; lunch comprises soup, salad, and fruit; dinner usually is composed of chicken; cooked vegetables; pasta, rice, or potatoes; and fruit. Client dislikes red meat and eats it only once or twice a month. She also dislikes milk, and substitutes sugar-free soft drinks and water. Before becoming pregnant, she drank five or six cups of black coffee a day, but now she avoids it. Her snacks usually consist of fresh fruit and vegetables.

• Client is very weight conscious; she periodically crash diets to maintain her weight at 112 lb (50.8 kg).
• Client does not take vitamins, medications, or drugs; she drinks socially.
• Nutritional problems and contributing factors include the following:
  • Inadequate intake of milk and calories contributed to by nausea and vomiting, dislike for milk, limited food budget, weight consciousness
  • Poor iron intake contributed to by lack of good sources of iron in her diet, no supplemental iron intake
  • Meal-skipping contributed to by nausea and vomiting, hurried schedule
  • Underweight or weight loss contributed to by weight consciousness, nausea and vomiting

Nursing Diagnosis

Altered Nutrition: Less Than Body Requirements, related to increased requirements imposed by pregnancy, nausea and vomiting, weight consciousness, hurried schedule, and food dislikes

Planning: Client Goals

Mrs. Oakland is concerned about her pregnancy and willing to make dietary changes for the sake of the baby. Her husband is supportive. Planning will focus on maintaining good dietary habits, improving overall intake and meal patterns to meet the demands of pregnancy and subsequent lactation, initiating dietary changes aimed at avoiding nausea and vomiting, and increasing iron intake.

Short-Term Goals

Short-term goals agreed on by the client follow. By the next monthly assessment, the client will:
• Eat three or more small meals a day
• Eat dry crackers, bread sticks, or dry cereal 30 minutes before getting up in the morning to help prevent nausea
• Drink water between meals instead of with meals
• Avoid diet soft drinks
• Eat the recommended number of servings from each of the food groups suggested by the daily food guide for pregnancy
• Gain 1 to 2 lb (0.45 to 0.9 kg); realize that weight gain during pregnancy is necessary and that excess weight can be lost during lactation after the baby is born
• Take prenatal vitamins as prescribed

Long-Term Goals

Susan Oakland establishes new dietary habits and patterns that provide adequate nourishment for herself, the baby, and subsequent lactation, such as the following:

- Eats an adequate serving from each of the food groups, according to the daily food guide for pregnancy
- Gradually gains 25 to 35 lb (11.5 to 16 kg)
- Avoids hunger by eating three meals and two or three snacks daily
- Drinks six to eight glasses of fluid daily
- Takes supplements as prescribed by the physician
- Avoids the use of sugar substitutes, alcohol, and caffeine

Implementation

- Instruct the client and her husband:
  - On the importance of nutrition for maternal and infant health
  - On the optimal amount and rate of weight gain
  - How to modify her diet to avoid nausea and vomiting: Eat dry crackers, bread sticks, or cereal before rising; do not drink fluid with meals; eat small, frequent meals to avoid hunger; avoid high-fat foods and foods the client does not tolerate. Assure the client that nausea and vomiting usually subside by the end of the first trimester.
  - How to modify her diet to meet the increased nutritional requirements: Eat more whole-grain breads and cereals; use yogurt, cheese, and puddings as substitutes for milk; eat at least three meals a day
  - To take supplements as prescribed by the physician
  - To avoid alcohol during pregnancy
  - To avoid all drugs and medications unless approved by the physician
- Investigate the client's eligibility for the WIC Program, a federally funded supplemental food program for women, infants, and children. In Canada, the program is called Nutrition and Financial Support Systems for a Pregnant Woman.
- Conduct an assessment and evaluation at each visit. Provide dietary instructions as needed to reinforce previous instructions or to meet the client's changing needs.

Documentation

Sample documentation of the prenatal visit follows.

Traditional Note Format

5/22/93, nursing
    Mrs. Oakland was seen for routine prenatal checkup at 9 weeks' gestation. Assessment findings reveal that the client is underweight, has lost 3 lb (1.4 kg) in the past 4 weeks, is experiencing nausea and vomiting, has a deficient hemoglobin and hematocrit, and is fatigued. Nursing diagnosis: Altered Nutrition: Less Than Body Requirements, related to increased requirements imposed by pregnancy, nausea and vomiting, weight consciousness, hurried schedule, food dislikes. Discussion centered on maintaining good dietary habits, improving overall intake and meal patterns to meet the demands of pregnancy and subsequent lactation, initiating dietary changes aimed at avoiding nausea and vomiting, and increasing iron intake. See care plan. Client's progress will be evaluated at the next monthly visit, 6/26/93.

L. Swift, RN

SOAP Format

5/22/93, nursing
    #2 Altered Nutrition: Less Than Body Requirements

S: "Who can eat with nausea and vomiting? And anyway, I'm often too tired to cook and eat nowadays."
    "I don't really like red meat. Besides, its too expensive when you're on a limited food budget like we are. I don't care for milk either."
    "I've always tried to stay slim, but with the baby coming, I guess that will have to change."
O: Underweight; 3-lb (1.4 kg) weight loss within 4 weeks, deficient hemoglobin and hematocrit
A: Altered nutrition is related to the increase in nutritional requirements imposed by pregnancy, nausea and vomiting, weight consciousness, hurried schedule, and food dislikes.
P: 1. Increase overall intake to meet the daily food guide recommendations for pregnancy.
   2. Modify meal patterns and intake to avoid nausea and vomiting.
   3. Recognize the importance of adequate weight gain during pregnancy.
   4. Alter schedule to allow for regular meals and snacks.
   5. Substitute acceptable alternatives to red meat (for iron) and milk (for calcium) in the diet.
   6. Reevaluate nutritional status at the next monthly checkup.

L. Swift, RN

Evaluation

Short-term goal achievement is evaluated at next monthly assessment. See the nursing care plan for related evaluative statements and revisions of the care plan. Long-term goal achievement is an ongoing evaluation.

NURSING CARE PLAN

for Susan Oakland

Nursing Diagnosis:	Altered Nutrition: Less Than Body Requirements, related to increased requirements imposed by pregnancy, nausea and vomiting, weight consciousness, hurried schedule, food dislikes
Long-Term Goals:	Client meets the increased nutritional requirements imposed by pregnancy by (1) adequate intake from each of the food groups as recommended by the daily food guide for pregnancy, (2) gradually gaining 25 to 35 lb, (3) eating three meals a day with two to three small snacks, (4) drinking six to eight glasses of fluid daily, (5) taking prenatal supplements as prescribed by the physician, (6) avoiding sugar substitutes, alcohol, and caffeine

---

Goal: By the next monthly assessment, 6/26/93, the client will:
- Eat three or more small meals a day

Nursing Actions	**Rationale**	**Evaluative Statement**
Determine how the client's schedule may be altered to allow time for meals. Encourage the client to have easy-to-eat foods available for quick snacks, like cartons of yogurt, cheese and crackers, muffins, and fresh fruit.	Client complained that her current schedule prevents regular meals. Easy-to-eat foods may be more acceptable and can be nutritionally comparable to traditional meals.	6/26/93 Goal met. Client eats three meals daily. Tries snacking on easy-to-eat foods when possible.
Advise the client that nausea may be lessened by avoiding periods of hunger, and that later in the pregnancy, avoiding hunger will help ensure a steady supply of nutrients to the fetus.	Low blood glucose may contribute to nausea early in pregnancy; later in pregnancy, low blood glucose and resultant ketosis may be harmful to the fetus.	*Recommendation:* Encourage more snacking to increase overall food intake. *L. Swift, RN*

Goal: By the next monthly assessment, 6/26/93, the client will:
- Eat dry crackers, bread sticks, or dry cereal 30 minutes before rising

Nursing Actions	**Rationale**	**Evaluative Statement**
Advise the client to eat a source of dry carbohydrates before getting up in the morning.	Eating dry carbohydrates 30 minutes before rising helps avoid nausea.	6/26/93 Goal met. Client eats dry crackers every morning 30 minutes before getting out of bed. Reports that it prevents morning nausea. *L. Swift, RN*

Goal: By the next monthly assessment, 6/26/93, the client will:
- Drink water between meals

Nursing Actions	**Rationale**	**Evaluative Statement**
Advise the client to avoid fluid with meals. Recommend fluids be consumed 1 hour before or 2 hours after eating.	Fluid with meals may contribute to nausea.	6/26/93 Goal met. Client avoids liquids with meals. Nausea is occurring less frequently throughout the day. *L. Swift, RN*

(continued)

N U R S I N G   C A R E   P L A N (continued)

for Susan Oakland

Goal: By the next monthly assessment, 6/26/93, the client will:
- Avoid diet soft drinks

Nursing Actions
Advise the client to avoid diet soft drinks. Recommend acceptable nutritional alternatives to the client.

Rationale
The effects of saccharin and aspartame on the fetus have not been proven safe.

Evaluative Statement
6/26/93   Goal partially met. Client reports that she drinks two or three cans of diet soft drinks a week at school to relieve thirst because nothing else is available.

Recommendation:
Encourage the client to bring something to drink during the day from home, such as frozen drink boxes of 100% fruit juice, which will thaw at room temperature, or an insulated container of ice water or milk flavored with vanilla (dislikes plain milk).

L. Swift, RN

Goal: By the next monthly assessment, 6/26/93, the client will:
- Eat the recommended number of servings from each food group as suggested by the daily food guide for pregnancy

Nursing Actions
Provide the client with a daily food guide for pregnancy, and explain the rationale for the increased recommendations. Investigate acceptable alternatives for red meat and milk, which the client normally does not consume.

Rationale
Because this is the client's first pregnancy, she is not aware of the recommendations for eating during pregnancy. Although no one particular food is essential during pregnancy, red meat is essential during pregnancy and an excellent source of iron, and milk is an excellent source of calcium, two minerals important for the developing fetus. If the client is not provided with nutritionally equivalent alternatives, her diet may not be optimal, even if she consumes the recommended number of servings from the meat and milk groups (ie, client may not be getting as much iron as she can from her diet if she relies on fish, cheese, and white-meat poultry to satisfy the meat group recommendations).

Evaluative Statement
6/26/93   Goal partially met. Client's intake is improved: intake from the grain and meat groups is adequate instead of marginal. However, the client still has difficulty consuming enough items from the milk group.

Recommendation:
Continue encouraging the client to consume more items from the milk group, such as cheese, yogurt, and pudding. Will advise the client to add skim milk powder whenever possible to fortify home-cooked and home-baked products. Will recommend that the client increase her intake of nondairy sources of calcium, such as broccoli, spinach, and greens.

L. Swift, RN

(continued)

NURSING CARE PLAN (continued)

for Susan Oakland

Goal: By the next monthly assessment, 6/26/93, the client will:
- Gain 1 to 2 lb

Nursing Actions	**Rationale**	**Evaluative Statement**
Advise the client on the recommended rate and amount of weight gain. Stress the importance of quality weight gain.	Client needs to understand that a 25- to 35-lb gradual weight gain is considered optimal for fetal development, and results in little gain in maternal fat tissue. However, because the fetus and maternal tissues require nutrients along with calories, it is essential that the weight gain comes from eating nutrient-dense calories instead of empty calories.	6/26/93 Goal met. Noting a relief from nausea and an increase in the number of daily meals, the client gained 2 lb. *L. Swift, RN*

Goal: By the next monthly assessment, the client will:
- Take prenatal vitamins as prescribed by the physician

Nursing Actions	**Rationale**	**Evaluative Statement**
Advise the client to take the supplement as prescribed and that the supplements are not a substitute for an adequate diet.	Supplements are intended to be used in conjunction with an optimal diet, not in place of one, because they do not provide optimal amounts of all required nutrients. Because the requirements for folic acid and iron during pregnancy are usually not met through diet alone, supplements of these two nutrients in particular are necessary.	6/26/93 Goal met. Client reports taking supplement as prescribed. No adverse effects noted. *Recommendation:* Will continue to monitor client's tolerance of supplement. Will continue to implement plan and reassess at next monthly appointment, 7/28/93. *L. Swift, RN*
Advise the client that the iron content in the supplements may cause constipation and the stools to become black.	Common adverse effects of large iron doses are constipation and black stools.	

KEY POINTS

- A person's state of energy balance can be determined by comparing caloric intake with caloric expenditure, which is the sum of calories used during physical activity, for basal metabolism, and for specific dynamic action.
- The six classes of nutrients needed by the body are carbohydrates, protein, fats, vitamins, minerals, and water.
- Carbohydrates provide most of the calories in the diet. Glucose, the only carbohydrate present in systemic circulation, may be burned for energy, stored as glycogen, or converted to fat and stored as adipose.
- Protein is broken down by the body into amino acids, which are then recombined to form proteins. Eight or nine amino acids are considered essential because they cannot be made in the body and must be supplied in the diet. Protein is used in the body for tissue growth and repair, as well as for the production of enzymes, hormones, antibodies, blood and other substances, and secretions; it also may be oxidized for energy. Excess protein is converted to fat and stored as adipose.

- Lipids provide more than twice the calories per unit as either carbohydrates or protein. Essential fatty acids cannot be made by the body, and therefore must be supplied through the diet. Dietary fat not used for immediate energy is stored as adipose.
- Vitamins and minerals do not provide calories but are needed for the metabolism of energy.
- Water provides the medium for all chemical reactions within the body; it is more vital to life than food.
- Tools used to evaluate a diet for adequacy include food groups and RDAs or RNIs. Dietary guidelines issued by health and governmental agencies focus on avoiding excesses rather than on obtaining sufficient quantities of nutrients. Most experts recommend that Americans and Canadians eat a variety of food; maintain their ideal weight; reduce their intake of fat, saturated fat, cholesterol, salt, and alcohol; and eat more complex carbohydrates and fiber.
- A person's food habits are a product of many variables, such as physical factors (eg, geographic location, food technology, income), physiologic factors (state of health, hunger, stage of development), and psychosocial factors (culture, religion, tradition, education, politics, social status, food ideology).

- Factors that influence nutrient requirements include age, sex, state of health, alcohol abuse, the use of medications, and megadoses of nutrient supplements. Nutrient intake can be affected by numerous physiologic and psychological factors.
- A systematic approach is used to identify the client's actual or potential needs, formulate a plan to meet those needs, initiate the plan or assign others to implement it, and evaluate the effectiveness of the plan.
- Nutritional assessment data can be collected through history taking (dietary data and medical–socio-economic data), physical examination (anthropometric data and clinical data), and laboratory data.
- Nursing diagnoses may be written to specifically address nutritional problems (Altered Nutrition: Less Than Body Requirements, More Than Body Requirements, Potential for More Than Body Requirements) or to identify the effect nutritional problems have on other areas of human functioning (eg, Activity Intolerance, Anxiety, Constipation, Diarrhea).
- Implementing a plan of care may involve nursing actions that are concerned with stimulating appetite, providing special diets, assisting with eating, withholding food, feeding by tube, feeding by vein, and conducting diet instructions.

STUDY QUESTIONS

1. The most concentrated source of energy in the body is
   a. protein
   b. carbohydrates
   c. fat
   d. macrominerals
2. The Food Guide Pyramid that is a replacement for the food group wheel
   a. puts meat and dairy products at the peak
   b. was approved in April 1991
   c. initially met with resistance from the meat and dairy industries
   d. focuses on deficiencies in our diet
3. Which laboratory test result indicates that a client is at risk for poor nutritional status?
   a. decreased serum albumin level
   b. increased lymphocyte count
   c. decreased blood urea nitrogen level
   d. increased platelet count
4. Mr. Yow is refusing to eat. What nursing action may stimulate his appetite?
   a. administer pain medication after meals
   b. encourage food from home when possible
   c. schedule his respiratory therapy before each meal
   d. reinforce the importance of his eating exactly what is delivered to him

5. Mrs. James has progressed to a full liquid diet. The nurse expects to see what items on her tray?
   a. apple juice and bouillon
   b. water ice and ginger ale
   c. pureed beef and cream of broccoli soup
   d. custard and a glass of milk
6. Parenteral nutrition provides nutrients to the client by way of the
   a. gastrostomy tube
   b. intravenous route
   c. nasoduodenal route
   d. jejunostomy tube
7. Anthropometric measurements that indicate fat and muscle stores include all the following *except*
   a. height and weight
   b. triceps skin fold measurement
   c. midarm muscle circumference
   d. intake and output
8. The nurse and Mrs. Young discuss a weight reduction plan. The nurse teaches Mrs. Young that 1 lb of body fat is equal to about
   a. 1500 cal
   b. 2400 cal
   c. 3500 cal
   d. 5000 cal
9. Mr. White has been admitted to the alcoholic referral unit in the local hospital. Nutritionally, he will most commonly be prone to

a. vitamin B malnutrition
b. obesity
c. dehydration
d. vitamin C deficiency

10. A client has a nasogastric tube inserted for feeding purposes. Using the stomach as a reservoir for food is advantageous in preventing what complication?
    a. dumping syndrome
    b. duodenal ulcers
    c. hyperglycemia
    d. gastric ulcers

11. Intermittent suction is used in the client with a single-lumen nasogastric tube for the purpose of
    a. draining the stomach more effectively
    b. preventing electrolyte losses
    c. helping to prevent dumping syndrome
    d. helping to prevent the tube from suctioning the mucosa

12. Mr. Lang is receiving tube feedings every 4 hours by way of a nasogastric tube. The nurse checks the tube's placement each time because
    a. the physician ordered it to be done
    b. the tube could be misplaced in the ileum

c. the tube should be in the esophagus for feeding
d. the tube can become dislodged and enter the trachea

13. Saline solution is used to irrigate the nasogastric tube. The rationale for this is
    a. irrigating with water is a contaminated procedure
    b. saline solution is a hypertonic solution
    c. saline solution replaces electrolytes lost through nasogastric suction
    d. saline solution is less irritating to the gastric mucosa

14. Gorging followed by purging with self-induced vomiting describes the disorder of
    a. anorexia
    b. morbid obesity
    c. bulimia
    d. cachexia

15. Protein helps to regulate fluid balance by
    a. oncotic pressure
    b. hydrostatic pressure
    c. secretion of antidiuretic hormone
    d. retention of sodium

Answers With Rationale

1. The correct response is *c*. Fat provides 9 cal for every gram compared with 4 cal/g of protein and carbohydrates. Macrominerals are regulatory nutrients, not energy nutrients.

2. The correct response is *c*. The meat and dairy industries believed that their products were deemphasized in the Food Guide Pyramid and exerted pressure that blocked initial acceptance of it in April 1991. Fats are at the peak of the pyramid, which focuses on grains and cereals as the basic food group.

3. The correct response is *a*. A decreased serum protein level places a client at nutritional risk. The other test results do not pose a nutritional risk.

4. The correct response is *b*. Food from home that the client enjoys may stimulate him to eat. Pain medication should be given before meals, respiratory therapy should be scheduled after meals, and telling the client what he must eat is no guarantee that he will comply.

5. The correct response is *d*. Custard and milk are items found in a full liquid diet. Apple juice, bouillon, water ice, and ginger ale are clear liquids, and pureed beef and cream of broccoli soup are more likely to be found in a soft diet.

6. The correct response is *b*. Parenteral nutrition is given intravenously. Gastrostomy tube, nasoduodenal route, and jejunostomy tube are routes for enteral feedings.

7. The correct response is *d*. Intake and output measurements indicate fluid balance. The other three measurements indicate body dimensions.

8. The correct response is *c*. One pound of body fat is equal to about 3500 cal.

9. The correct response is *a*. The need for B vitamins is increased in alcoholics because they are used to metabolize alcohol.

10. The correct response is *a*. When the stomach is used as a reservoir, the formula is released at a controlled rate, preventing the occurrence of the dumping syndrome.

11. The correct response is *d*. Intermittent suction prevents damage to the mucosa of the stomach, and that is the primary purpose for using it with a single-lumen tube.

12. The correct response is *d*. Checking tube placement verifies that the tube is in the stomach and has not slipped into the trachea. The nurse's concern is to prevent aspiration of the feeding, leading to severe respiratory problems.

13. The correct response is *c*. Saline solution compensates for electrolytes lost during nasogastric drainage and is, therefore, the irrigant of choice.

14. The correct response is *c*. Bulimia is the only eating disorder mentioned that involves the cycle of gorging and purging.

15. The correct response is *a*. Serum proteins are responsible for maintaining oncotic pressure, which exerts a "pull" pressure.

BIBLIOGRAPHY

Alltop, S. (1988). Teaching for discharge: Gastrostomy tubes. *RN, 51*(11), 42–46.

American Institute of Nutrition and the American society for Clinical Nutrition. Nutrient labeling of food products under consideration. (1990). *Nutrition Today, 25*(3), 32–34.

Andresen, G. (1989). A fresh look at assessing the elderly. *RN, 52*(6), 28–39.

Aronson, V., Fitzgerald, B., & Hewes, L. (1990). *Guidebook for nutrition counselors* (2nd ed.). Englewood Cliffs, NJ: Prentice-Hall.

Beare, P., & Myers, J. (1990). *Adult health nursing.* St. Louis: Mosby.

Beck, M. (1989). Percutaneous endoscopic gastrostomy. *Nursing, 19*(4), 76–77.

Bockus, S. (1991). Troubleshooting your tube feedings. *American Journal of Nursing, 91*(5), 24–30.

Brownell, K. (1984). The psychology and physiology of obesity: Implications for screening and treatment. *Journal of the American Dietetic Association, 84*, 406.

Burrell, L. (1992). *Adult nursing in hospital and community settings.* East Norwalk, CT: Appleton & Lange.

Camp, D., & Otten, N. (1990). How to insert and remove nasogastric tubes quickly and easily. *Nursing, 20*(9), 59–64.

Carnevali, D., & Patrick, M. (1986). *Nursing management for the elderly.* Philadelphia: Lippincott.

Carpenito, L. (1992). *Nursing diagnosis: Application to clinical practice* (4th ed.). Philadelphia: Lippincott.

Castiglia, P. (1989). Obesity in adolescence. *Journal of Pediatric Health Care, 3*(4), 221–223.

Cerrato, P. (1989). Food poisoning makes a dangerous comeback. *RN, 52*(10), 73–78.

Cerrato, P. (1989). Spotting the patient who looks healthy but isn't. *RN, 52*(3), 81–83.

Cerrato, P. (1990). Does diet affect the immune system? *RN, 53*(6), 67–70.

Cerrato, P. (1990). Piecing together the osteoporosis puzzle. *RN, 53*(4), 77–82.

Cerrato, P. (1991). The low-fat approach to weight loss. *RN, 54*(11), 69–71.

Cerrato, P. (1992). The patient's eating—why is he losing weight? *RN, 55*(4), 77–80.

Cerrato, P. (1992). Pasta: The perfect pick-me-up? *RN, 55*(5), 79–92.

Collinsworth, R., & Boyle, K. (1989). Nutritional assessment of the elderly. *Journal of Gerontological Nursing, 15*(12), 17–21.

The confusion in obesity research standards. (1990). *Western Journal of Nursing Research, 12*(5), 584–585.

Detsky, A. (1987). What is subjective global assessment of nutritional status? *Journal of Parenteral Enteral Nutrition, 11*, 8.

Dudek, S. (1993). *Nutrition Handbook for Nursing Practice,* 2nd ed. Philadelphia: Lippincott.

Esberger, K. (1991). Guide to gastrointestinal problems of elders. *Geriatric Nursing, 12*(2), 74–75.

Fuller, J., & Schuller-Ayers, J. (1990). *Health assessment: A nursing approach.* Philadelphia: Lippincott.

Fullmer, S., Geiger, C., & Parent, C. R. (1991). Consumers' knowledge, understanding, and attitudes toward health claims on food labels. *Journal of the American Association, 91*(2), 166–171.

Gallagher Allred, C. (1991). Nutrition and the elderly. *Caring, 10*(5), 68–72.

Gibson, R., & Deveny, K. (1991). Americans' ignorance about nutrition hinders efforts to improve nation's diet. *Wall Street Journal,* CCXVII(96), November 13.

Gorman, C. (1991, July 15). The fight over food labels. *Time,* pp. 52–56.

Groth, K. (1988). Age-related changes in the gastrointestinal tract. *Geriatric Nursing, 9*(5), 278–280.

Guenter, P., Jones, S., Jacobs, D., & Rombeau, J. (1990). Administration and delivery of enteral nutrition. *Enteral and tube feeding* (2nd ed.). Philadelphia: Saunders.

Henderson, C. (1991). Safe and effective tube feeding of bedridden elderly. *Geriatrics, 46*(8), 56–66.

Jansen, R., Kendall, P., & Jansen, C. (1990). *Diet evaluation: A guide to planning a healthy diet.* San Diego: Academic Press.

Jeejeebhoy, K. (1990). Assessment of nutritional status (chap. 6). *Enteral and tube feeding* (2nd ed.). Philadelphia: Saunders.

Lan, S., & Justice, C. (1991). Use of modified diets in nursing homes. *Journal of the American Dietetic Association, 91*(1), 46–51.

Langseth, L. (ed.). (1990). *Nutrition research newsletter, 9*(11), 126–127.

Laquatra, I., & Gerlach, M. (1990). *Nutrition in clinical nursing.* New York: Delmar.

Lehmann, S., & Barber, J. (1991). Giving medications by feeding tube. *Nursing, 21*(11), 58–61.

Liebman, B. (1992). Fix that label. *Nutrition Action Health Letter, 19*(1), 8–9.

Mahan, L., & Arlin, M. (1992). *Krause's Food, Nutrition, and Diet Therapy,* 8th ed. Philadelphia: Saunders.

McGinnis, J., & Nestle, M. (1989). The Surgeon General's report on nutrition and health: Policy implications and implementation strategies. *American Journal of Clinical Nutrition, 49*(1), 23–28.

Mobarhan, S., & Trumbore, L. (1991). Enteral tube feeding: A clinical perspective on recent advances. *Nutrition Reviews, 49*(5), 129–138.

Murphy, J. (1990). Tube feeding problems and solutions. *Advancing Clinical Care, 5*(2), 7–10.

Murray, R., & Zenter, J. (1989). *Nursing assessment and*

health promotion strategies through the life span. East Norwalk, CT: Appleton & Lange.

Murray, T., & Beare-Rogers, J. (1990). Nutrition recommendations, 1990. *Journal of the Canadian Dietetic Association, 51*(3), 391–395.

National Research Council: *Recommended Dietary Allowances,* 9th ed. Washington, DC: National Academy of Sciences, 1980.

Nutrition recommendations: Report of the Scientific Review Committee. (1990). Minister of Supply and Services Canada, Cat. No. H49-42/1990E.

Russell, R. (1992). Nutrition and aging. *Nutrition Action Health Letter, 19*(4), 5–7.

Sherman, J., & Alexander, M. (1990). Obesity in children: A research update. *Journal of Pediatric Nursing, 5*(3), 161–166.

Stephen, A., & Deneer, M. (1990). The effect of dietary fat reduction on intake of major nutrients and fat soluble vitamins. *Canadian Dietetic Association, 51*(1), 281–284.

Van Daalen, C., & Marko, T. L. (1991). Eating disorders: A guide for community health nurses. *Canadian Nurse, 87*(5), 28–29.

Walker, D., & Beauchene, R. (1991). The relationship of loneliness, social isolation, and physical health to dietary adequacy of independent living elderly. *Journal of the American Dietetic Association, 91*(3), 300–304.

Webber-Jones, J., Sweeney, K., Winterbottom, A., Fontneau, L., Johnson, K., & Fradette, M. (1992). How to declog a feeding tube. *Nursing 92, 22*(4), 63–64.

Williams, P. (1989). How do you keep medicines from clogging feeding tubes? *American Journal of Nursing, 91*(2), 181–182.

Williams, S. (1990). *Essentials of nutrition and diet therapy* (5th ed.). St. Louis: Times Mirror/Mosby College Publishing.

Woolcott, D. (1990). Importance of a nutrition monitoring and surveillance system for research and practice in Canada. *Journal of the Canadian Dietetic Association, 51*(4), 469–471.

Young, C., & White, S. (1992). Tube feeding at home. *American Journal of Nursing, 92*(4), 46–53.

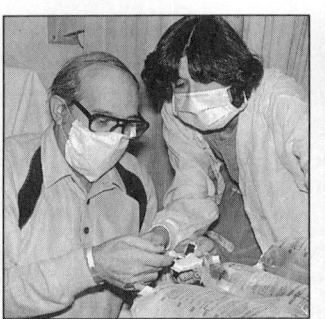
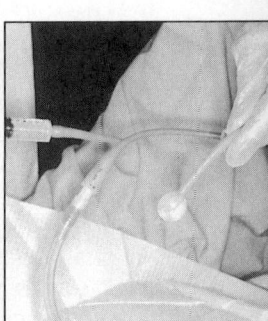

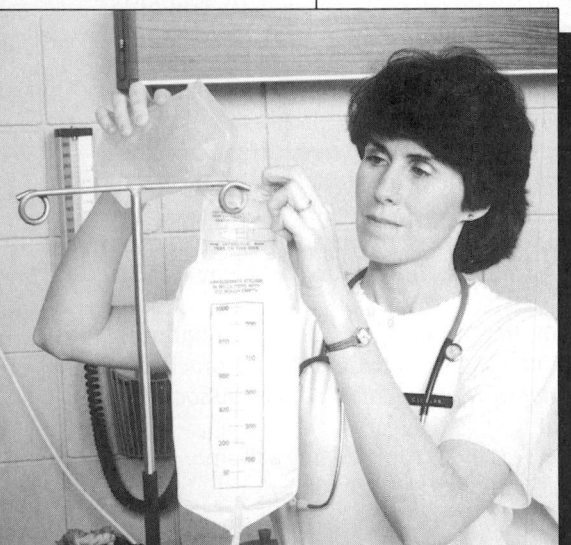

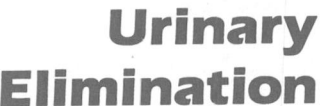

Urinary Elimination

34

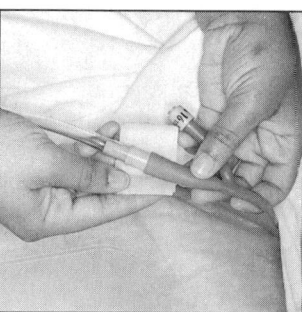

Elimination from the urinary tract helps to rid the body of waste products and materials that exceed bodily needs. The proper functioning of the urinary system is essential to the body's physical well-being, to life itself, and to a person's general sense of well-being. The nurse assisting a client with urination or intervening to resolve health problems related to urination needs many specialized abilities.

This chapter provides the student with knowledge of the physiology of the urinary system and the multiple factors that affect urination. A practical guide to assessing urinary elimination is presented, including detailed information on specific assessment measures, such as monitoring fluid intake, collecting urine specimens, testing urine, and assisting with other diagnostic procedures. Analysis of urinary data may lead to the identification of multiple nursing diagnoses or, when reported to the physician, to the early detection of a medical problem. Numerous examples of nursing diagnoses are offered. Client goals are established in planning care, and specific nursing strategies are presented. The section Nursing Process in Clinical Practice offers focused assessment, diagnosis, planning, implementation, and evaluation guides for select nursing diagnoses of common urinary problems (Altered Urinary Elimination related to dysuria and maturational enuresis; Urinary Incontinence: Stress Incontinence, Reflex Incontinence, Urge Incontinence, Functional Incontinence, Total Incontinence; Urinary Retention; High Risk for Infection related to indwelling urinary catheter). These guides and the concluding case study illustrate how the nurse's knowledge of the urinary system and urinary pathology is combined with specific nursing interventions to successfully resolve urinary problems.

Physiology

Kidneys and Ureters

The kidneys are located on either side of the vertebral column behind the peritoneum and in the posterior portion of the abdominal cavity. One of the more significant functions of the kidneys is to maintain the composition and volume of body fluids. They perform this function in a selective manner by filtering and excreting blood constituents that are not needed and retaining those that are. It is estimated that the total blood volume passes through the kidneys for waste removal about every half hour. Despite varying kinds and amounts of food and fluids ingested, body fluids remain relatively stable if there is proper kidney functioning. The waste product that the kidneys excrete, called *urine*, contains organic, inorganic, and liquid wastes.

The nephron is the basic unit of kidney structure. There are about 1 million nephrons in each kidney. Urine from the nephrons empties into the pelvis of each kidney. From each kidney, urine is transported by rhythmic peristalsis through the ureters to the urinary bladder. The ureters enter the bladder obliquely, and a fold of membrane in the bladder closes the entrance to the ureters so that urine is not forced up the ureters to the kidneys when pressure exists in the bladder. Figure 34-1 shows views of the male and female urinary systems and shows the position of the kidneys and ureters in the abdominal cavity.

Bladder

The urinary bladder is a smooth muscle sac that serves as a reservoir for urine. There are three layers of muscle tissue in the bladder—the inner longitudinal layer, the middle circular layer, and the outer longitudinal layer. These three layers are called the *detrusor muscle*. At the base of the bladder, the middle circular layer of muscle tissue forms the internal, or involuntary, sphincter, which guards the opening between the urinary bladder and the urethra. The urethra conveys urine from the bladder to the exterior of the body.

The urinary bladder muscle is innervated by the autonomic nervous system. The sympathetic system carries inhibitory impulses to the bladder and motor impulses to the internal sphincter. These impulses cause the detrusor muscle to relax and the internal sphincter to constrict. This, in turn, causes urine to be retained in the bladder. The parasympathetic system carries motor impulses to the bladder and inhibitory impulses to the internal sphincter. These impulses cause the detrusor muscle to contract and the sphincter to relax. The male and female urinary bladders are shown in Figure 34-1.

The bladder normally contains urine under very little pressure, and as the volume of urine increases, the pressure increases only slightly. This adaptability of the bladder wall to pressure is believed to be due to the characteristics of muscle tissue in the bladder, and makes it possible for urine to continue to enter the bladder from the ureters against low pressure. When the pressure becomes sufficient to stimulate stretch receptors located in the bladder wall, the desire to empty the bladder becomes apparent.

Urethra

The urethra differs in males and females. The male urethra is common to both the excretory system and the reproductive system. It is about 13.7 to 16.2 cm (5½ to 6¼ inches) long and consists of three parts—the prostatic, the mem-

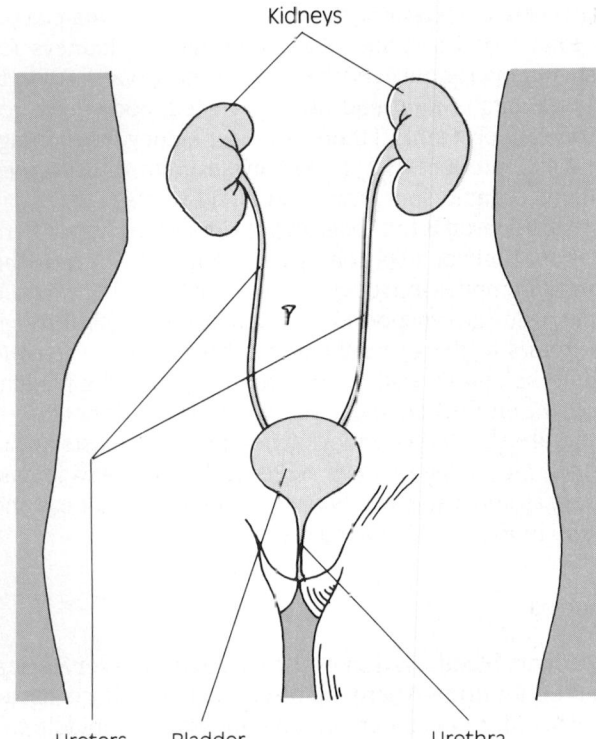

Kidneys

Ureters   Bladder   Urethra

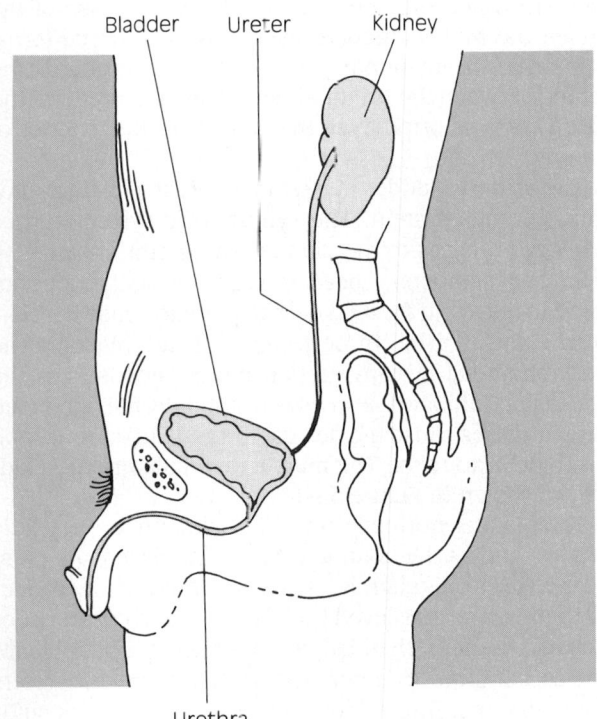

Bladder   Ureter   Kidney

Urethra

F I G U R E   3 4 - 1

Frontal view of the female urinary tract (*top*) and lateral view of the male urinary tract (*bottom*).

branous, and the cavernous portions. The external urethral sphincter consists of striated muscle, and is located just beyond the prostatic portion of the urethra. The external sphincter is under voluntary control.

The female urethra is about 3.7 to 6.2 cm (1½ to 2½ inches) long. Its function is to convey urine from the bladder to the exterior. The external, or voluntary, sphincter is located about midurethra. No portion of the female urethra is external to the body, as is true in the male. Most literature refers to muscle at the meatus in the female as the external sphincter.

Act of Micturition

The process of emptying the bladder is known as **micturition**; it also is called **voiding** or **urination**. Nerve centers for micturition are situated in the brain and the spinal cord. Voiding is largely an involuntary reflex act, but its control can be learned.

After stimulation of the stretch receptors in the bladder as the urine collects, the desire to void is experienced. Usually this occurs when about 100 to 200 mL for the child and 200 to 300 mL for the adult has collected. If micturition is initiated, the detrusor muscle contracts, the internal sphincter relaxes, and urine enters the posterior urethra. The muscles of the perineum and the external sphincter relax, and micturition occurs. The act consists of relaxation of the internal sphincter, contraction of the detrusor muscle, slight contraction of the muscle of the abdominal wall, and lowering of the diaphragm. The act of micturition normally is painless. During micturition, the pressure within the bladder is many times greater than it is during the time the bladder is filling. The voluntary control of voiding is limited to initiating, restraining, and interrupting the act.

Restraint of voiding is believed to be subconscious when the volume of urine in the bladder is small. But when voiding is delayed, the bladder continues to fill. Discomfort may then be felt when undue distention occurs, and the urgency to void becomes paramount.

Sometimes increased abdominal pressure, as occurs with coughing and sneezing, forces the escape of urine involuntarily, especially in the female, since the urethra is shorter. Strong psychic factors, such as marked fear, also may result in involuntary urination. Under certain conditions, it may be difficult to relax the restraining muscles sufficiently to void, such as when a urine specimen is requested from a shy or an embarrassed person.

When the higher nerve centers develop after infancy, the voluntary control of micturition develops also. Until that time, voiding is purely reflex. People whose bladders are isolated from control of the brain because of injury or disease also void by reflex only. This is called *autonomic bladder*.

Frequency of Micturition

The frequency of micturition depends on the amount of urine being produced. The more urine produced, the more often voiding is necessary, and vice versa. Unless the fluid intake is very large, most healthy people do not void during normal sleeping hours. The first voided urine of the day usually is more concentrated than urine excreted during the remainder of the day. The nurse should remember that because the first voiding of the day is not fresh, but rather an accumulation of a number of hours of kidney output, this urine may or may not be used as a specimen for certain tests.

Some people normally void small amounts at frequent intervals because they habitually respond to the first early urge to void. This habit is insignificant and not necessarily an indication of disease. Conversely, if this pattern is not a habit but a change in urination routine, it can be an indication of illness.

Other people have habits that result in infrequent voiding. For example, some people go 8 to 12 waking hours or longer without urinating. Factors such as a habitual low fluid intake owing to environmental conditions or age may be the reason. The inaccessibility of toilet facilities owing to travel, work circumstances, or illness, and limitations of mobility also can be the cause of infrequent urination. People who habitually urinate infrequently develop more urinary tract infections and kidney disorders than those who urinate at least every 3 to 4 hours. The reason is believed to be stagnation of urine in the bladder, which serves as a good medium for bacterial growth. Infrequent voiding that is a change in one's urination pattern also can be indicative of a decreased production of urine owing to kidney or circulatory disorders.

Factors Affecting Micturition

Numerous factors affect the amount and quality of urine produced by the body and the manner in which it is excreted.

Developmental Considerations

Infants are born without voluntary control of micturition and with little ability to concentrate urine. Most children develop urinary control between ages 2 and 5 years. Daytime control precedes nighttime control, and most girls develop control earlier than boys. Older children and adults control urination voluntarily and seldom wake to void at night because their kidneys are able to concentrate urine and produce less urine at night because of decreased renal blood flow.

Toilet Training Most children begin to control urination voluntarily at age 18 to 24 months. Toilet training should not begin until the child is able to (1) hold urine for 1 to 2 hours, (2) recognize bladder fullness, and (3) communicate the need to void and control urination until seated on the toilet. The child's desire to gain control also is important. Wanting to be like a parent or older sibling often provides adequate motivation. Lifelong attitudes toward urination, the body, and cleanliness may develop during the time of toilet training. (Enuresis, involuntary urination, is discussed later in the section Nursing Process in Clinical Practice.)

Aging Physiologic changes that accompany normal aging may affect urination in elderly people:
- Diminished ability of the kidneys to concentrate urine may result in nocturia.
- Decreased bladder muscle tone may reduce the capacity of the bladder to hold urine and increase frequency.
- Decreased bladder contractility may lead to urine retention and stasis, which increase the likelihood of urinary tract infection.
- Neuromuscular problems, degenerative joint problems, alterations in thought processes, and weakness may interfere with voluntary control and the ability to reach a toilet in time.

Elderly people who view themselves as old, powerless, and neglected may cease to value voluntary control over urination and simply find toileting too much bother. Incontinence often is the result.

Food and Fluid

When the body is functioning well, the kidneys preserve a careful balance of fluid intake and output, which should be about equal. When the body is dehydrated, the kidneys will reabsorb fluid and the urine produced will be more concentrated and decreased in amount. Conversely, with fluid overload, the kidneys will excrete a large quantity of dilute urine.

Caffeine-containing beverages (cola, coffee, tea) have a diuretic effect and increase urine production. Alcohol produces the same effect by inhibiting the release of antidiuretic hormone. Foods high in water content may increase urine production. Foods and beverages with high sodium content cause sodium and water reabsorption and retention, thereby decreasing urine formation. Also, certain foods may affect the odor of the urine (asparagus, onions) or its color (beets).

Life-Style

Many individual, family, and sociocultural variables influence a person's normal voiding habits. For some people, voiding is a personal and private act, something one does not talk about. Needing assistance with a bedpan or urinal thus provokes great embarrassment and anxiety, which can be compounded when the bedpan is offered by a nurse of the opposite sex. For others, voiding is a natural act, and these people readily excuse themselves to void whenever the urge presents.

Psychological Variables

Many people who experience stress void smaller amounts of urine at more frequent intervals. Stress also can interfere with the ability to relax perineal muscles and the external urethral sphincter. When this happens, the urge to void is present, but emptying the bladder completely becomes difficult or impossible.

Activity and Muscle Tone

Among the many benefits of regular exercise are increased metabolism and optimal urine production and elimination. With prolonged periods of immobility, decreased bladder and sphincter tone can result in poor urinary control and urinary stasis. People with indwelling urinary catheters lose bladder tone because the bladder muscle is not being stretched as the bladder fills with urine. Other causes of decreased muscle tone include childbearing, menopausal muscle atrophy, and damage to muscles from trauma.

Pathologic Conditions

Certain renal or urologic problems can affect both the quantity and the quality of urine produced. Diseases known to be associated with renal problems include congenital urinary tract abnormalities, polycystic kidney disease, urinary tract infection, urinary calculi (kidney stones), hypertension, diabetes mellitus, gout, and certain connective tissue disorders.

Diseases that reduce physical activity or lead to generalized weakness, such as arthritis, Parkinson's disease, and degenerative joint disease, may interfere with toileting. Cognitive deficits and certain psychiatric problems can interfere with a person's ability or desire to control urination voluntarily. Fever and diaphoresis (profuse perspiration) result in the kidney's conservation of body fluids. Urine production is decreased, and the urine is highly concentrated. Other pathologic conditions, such as those present in congestive heart failure, may lead to fluid retention and decreased urine output.

Medications

Medications have numerous effects on urine production and elimination. Of gravest concern are the many prescription and nonprescription drugs known to be nephrotoxic (capable of causing kidney damage). Abuse of analgesics, such as aspirin, has resulted in nephrotoxicity; some antibiotics, such as kanamycin, can be nephrotoxic.

Diuretics (water pills), which commonly are used in the treatment of hypertension and other disorders, prevent the reabsorption of water and certain electrolytes in the tubules. Depending on their strength, they cause moderate to severe increases in production and excretion of dilute urine. *Cholinergic* medications stimulate contraction of the detrusor muscle and produce urination. Some *analgesics* and *tranquilizers* that suppress the central nervous system interfere with urination by diminishing the effectiveness of the neural reflex.

Certain drugs cause urine to change color (see display). Anticoagulants may cause hematuria (blood in the urine).

Nurse as Role Model

Before intervening to help clients develop healthy urinary elimination patterns, it is important for nurses to assess the adequacy of their own urinary elimination habits and patterns. If you are unable to meet the following goals, you may want to take the time now to revise your own health practices, so that you will be an effective role model for clients. The nurse:

- Empties the bladder completely at regular intervals
- Responds to the urge to void (ie, does not routinely postpone voiding because of being too busy)
- Drinks 8 to 10 glasses of water daily
- Responds to changes in urinary characteristics (or frequency) by seeking their cause and getting medical assistance when necessary

Assessing

A comprehensive nursing assessment of the functioning of the urinary system includes the following:

- Collection of data about voiding patterns, habits, and difficulties and a history of current or past urinary problems
- Physical examination of the kidneys, bladder, and urethral meatus; assessment of skin integrity and hydration; and examination of the urine
- Correlation of these findings with the results of diagnostic tests and procedures for examining urine and the urinary tract

Nursing History

In the initial nursing history, the nurse questions the client (or the caregiver) about usual voiding habits and the current or past occurrence of voiding difficulties. Terminology should be used that the client understands. Elements of

---

Urine Color Changes Commonly Seen With Medications

Urine Color	Medication
Pale yellow	Diuretics
Orange, orange-red, or pink	Pyridium (urinary tract analgesic)
	Sulfonamides (antiinfectives)
	Dilantin (anticonvulsant)
	Rifampin (antitubercular)
Green or blue-green	Elavil (antidepressant)
	B complex vitamins
Brown or black	Levodopa (antiparkinsonian)
	Injectable iron compounds

Urine Elimination

Use the assessment checklist to determine how well you are meeting your need for urine elimination. Then develop a prescription for self-care by choosing appropriate behaviors from the list of suggestions.

Assessment Checklist

almost always / sometimes / almost never

1. I urinate at regular intervals throughout the day.
2. I have an adequate fluid intake.
3. I limit my sodium intake.
4. My urine volume remains relatively constant.

Self-Care Behaviors

1. Maintain a normal voiding pattern and volume.
2. Respond as soon as possible to the urge to void.
3. Drink 8 to 10 glasses of water daily.
4. Avoid foods that contain excess sodium.
5. Monitor use of caffeine, alcohol, or medication schedules that promote voiding and may interfere with sleep.
6. Seek medical assistance for any change in the characteristics of urine or presence of pain on urination.

a urinary elimination history are suggested in the accompanying display.

With infants and young children, it is important to assess whether the child has achieved bladder control and if a toileting schedule has been established. The nursing history and plan also should note the words the child uses to indicate the need to void.

With older adults, decreased bladder tone may be a problem, and the nursing history should note any problems, how the person normally handles these problems, and nursing judgments about the adequacy of the solution.

People with limited or no bladder control as well as those with urinary diversions usually have well-established routines for emptying the bladder. The procedures and

FOCUSED ASSESSMENT GUIDE

Urinary Elimination

Factors to Assess	Questions and Approaches
Usual patterns of urinary elimination	How often do you urinate (pass your water) during the day?
	Do you awaken at night to empty your bladder?
	How would you describe your urine?
Recent changes in urinary elimination	Have you noticed any changes in your usual voiding patterns (frequency, amount, force of stream, difficulty, comfort)?
Aids to elimination	Is there anything you do that helps you to urinate?
Present or past occurrence of voiding difficulties (nature of problem, onset, frequency, causes, severity, symptoms, intervention attempted, and results)	Tell me about any problems you are having now when you urinate (urgency, pain or burning, difficulty starting or stopping stream, dribbling, incontinence).
	If there is a problem, describe what you feel like before you urinate and while you are urinating.
	Have you had any urinary problems in the past (any history of urinary tract infections, kidney or bladder disease or problems)?
Presence of artificial orifices (normal routine, history of problems)	Tell me about your usual routine with your ureterostomy.

equipment used should be assessed to make sure they follow accepted guidelines and are not predisposing the person to infection or other risk. Any special routine, equipment, or supplies used for urinary elimination should be noted in both the history and the nursing care plan.

When a problem with voiding is reported, its duration, severity, and precipitating factors should be explored. See the display titled Common Urinary Problems for definitions of terms used to describe such problems. It also is important to note the client's perception of the problem and the adequacy of the client's self-care behaviors.

Common Urinary Problems

Anuria: Technically, no urine voided; 24-hour urine output is less than 100 mL; synonyms are complete *kidney shutdown* or *renal failure*

Dysuria: Difficulty in voiding; may or may not be associated with pain; a feeling of warm local irritation occurring during voiding is called *burning*

Enuresis: Most often used to refer to the child who involuntarily urinates during the night

Frequency: Increased incidence of voiding

Glycosuria: Presence of sugar in the urine; if due to an unusually large intake of sugar or to marked emotional disturbances and is temporary, there is little cause for alarm

Hematuria: Blood in the urine; if present in large enough quantities, urine may be bright red or reddish brown

Hesitancy: Delay or difficulty in initiating voiding

Incontinence: Inability voluntarily to control the discharge of urine

Nocturia: Frequency of urination during the night

Oliguria: Scanty or greatly diminished amount of urine voided in a given time; 24-hour urine output is 100 to 400 mL

Orthostatic albuminuria: Presence of albumin in urine that is voided after periods of standing, walking, or running; phenomenon of the circulatory system and not necessarily a symptom of kidney disorders

Pneumaturia: Passage of urine containing gas

Polyuria: Excessive output of urine (diuresis)

Proteinuria: Albumin in the urine; indication of kidney disease

Pyuria: Pus in the urine; urine appears cloudy

Retention: Inability to void although urine is produced by the kidneys and enters the bladder; excessive storage of urine in the bladder

Suppression: Stoppage of urine production; normally the adult kidneys produce urine continuously at the rate of 60 to 120 mL/h

Urgency: Strong desire to void

Physical Assessment

Physical assessment of urinary functioning includes an examination of the kidneys, urinary bladder, urethral meatus, skin, and urine.

Kidneys

In the normal adult, the kidneys are well protected by a considerable amount of fat and connective tissue and are difficult to palpate. The right kidney is at the level of the 12th rib and is lower than the left kidney. The right kidney may at times be palpated by the nurse if pushed down by the diaphragm when the client inhales. The nurse stands to the right of the supine client and places the left hand under the client's flank while the right hand palpates the abdominal wall. This technique requires deep palpation and should be practiced under supervision. The left kidney is palpated similarly. The contour and size of the kidneys are noted, as is any tenderness or lumps.

An examination of the kidneys includes checking for costovertebral tenderness. The costovertebral angle is formed by the 12th rib and the spine. When the kidneys are inflamed, the client experiences pain when this angle is percussed or struck. The nurse places one palm flat over the costovertebral angle and strikes the back of this hand with the other fist.

Bladder

The bladder normally is positioned below the symphysis pubis and cannot be assessed by the nurse when it is empty. Once the bladder becomes distended, it rises above the symphysis pubis and may reach to just below the umbilicus. At this point, the nurse observes the lower abdominal wall, noting any swelling, and palpates this area for tenderness, also noting the smoothness and roundness of the bladder. The height of the edge of the bladder above the symphysis pubis may be measured, and the bladder also may be percussed. A full bladder produces a dull sound.

Urethral Orifice

The urethral orifice is inspected for any signs of inflammation or discharge. In the female, the urethral meatus is a pink slitlike opening below the clitoris and above the vaginal orifice. The female needs to be in the dorsal recumbent position with the inner labia retracted for good visualization of the meatus. In the male, the meatus is at the tip of the penis. If the male is uncircumcised, the foreskin may need to be retracted for visualization of the meatus. Foul odors should be noted.

Skin Integrity and Hydration

Because problems with urinary functioning may result in disturbances in hydration and excretion of body wastes, the skin should be carefully assessed for color, texture, turgor, and the excretion of any wastes. The integrity of the skin in the perineal area also should be assessed. Problems with continence may result in severe excoriation.

Urine

Each time a client's urine is handled it should be assessed for color, odor, clarity, and the presence of any sediment. Abnormalities should be noted. In select clients, the pH and specific gravity of the urine will be monitored as well as the presence of abnormal constituents, such as protein, blood, glucose, ketone bodies, and bacteria. Normal characteristics of urine and special considerations for observation are detailed in Table 34-1.

Assessment Measures

In addition to interviewing the client and performing the physical examination, the nurse gathers data about urinary elimination by carrying out the following assessment measures: measuring urine output, collecting urine specimens, determining the presence of abnormal constituents in the urine, and assisting with diagnostic procedures. Discussions of the nursing responsibilities related to each of these measures follow.

Measuring Urine Output Measuring the client's intake and output is an important nursing responsibility. Accuracy of the total fluid intake and output from all sources is essen-

TABLE 34-1

Characteristics of Urine

Characteristic	Normal Findings	Special Considerations
Color	A freshly voided specimen is pale yellow, straw-colored, or amber, depending on its concentration.	Urine is darker than normal when it is scanty and concentrated. Urine is lighter than normal when it is excessive and diluted.
		Certain drugs, such as cascara, L-dopa, and sulfonamides, alter the color of urine.
Odor	Normal urine smell is aromatic. As urine stands, it often develops an ammonia odor because of bacterial action.	Some foods cause urine to have a characteristic odor; for example, asparagus causes urine to have a strong, musty odor.
		Urine high in glucose content has a sweet odor.
		Urine that is heavily infected has a fetid odor.
Turbidity	Fresh urine should be clear or translucent; as urine stands and cools, it becomes cloudy.	Cloudiness observed in freshly voided urine is abnormal and may be due to the presence of red blood cells, white blood cells, bacteria, vaginal discharge, sperm, or prostatic fluid.
pH	The normal pH is about 6.0, with a range of 4.6 to 8. (Urine alkalinity or acidity may be promoted through diet to inhibit bacterial growth or urinary stone development or to facilitate the therapeutic activity of certain medications.) Urine becomes alkaline on standing when carbon dioxide diffuses into the air.	A high-protein diet causes urine to become excessively acid.
		Certain foods tend to produce alkaline urine, such as citrus fruits, dairy products, and vegetables, especially legumes.
		Certain foods tend to produce acidic urine, for example, meat and cranberry juice.
		Certain drugs influence the acidity or alkalinity of urine; for example, ammonium chloride produces acidic urine, and potassium citrate and sodium bicarbonate produce alkaline urine.
Specific gravity	This is a measure of the concentration of dissolved solids in the urine. The normal range is 1.010 to 1.025.	Concentrated urine will have a higher than normal specific gravity and diluted urine will have a lower than normal specific gravity. In the absence of kidney disease, a high specific gravity usually indicates dehydration and a low specific gravity indicates overhydration.
Constituents	*Organic* constituents of urine include urea, uric acid, creatinine, hippuric acid, indican, urene pigments, and undetermined nitrogen. *Inorganic* constituents are ammonia, sodium, chloride, traces of iron, phosphorus, sulfur, potassium, and calcium.	*Abnormal constituents* of urine include blood, pus, albumin, glucose, ketone bodies, casts, gross bacteria, and bile.

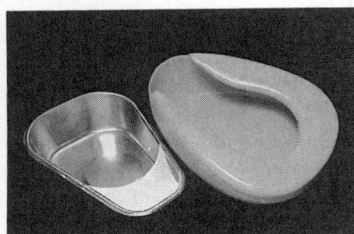

Bedpan and fracture pan
Containers used to collect urine
from nonambulatory clients

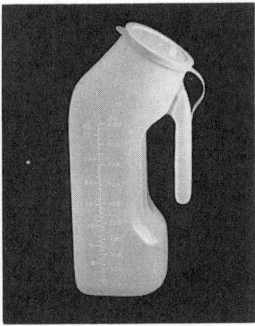

Urinal
Container used to collect
urine from nonambulatory
male clients

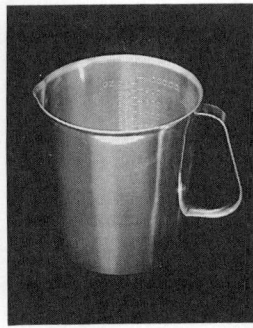

Calibrated measuring
device
Device which makes possi-
ble the recording of an
accurate urine output

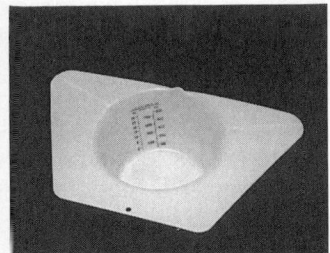

Specimen hat
Container which when placed
anteriorly in the toilet, underneath the seat, collects urine for
measurement or study

Straight catheter and specimen
container
Single lumen catheter which
drains urine from the bladder—
here into a sterile urine specimen
container

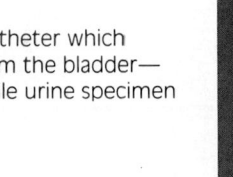

Small urine collection bag well-
suited to ambulatory clients; may
be easily emptied in the toilet;
easily concealed in pants or a
skirt

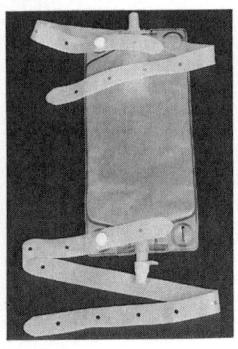

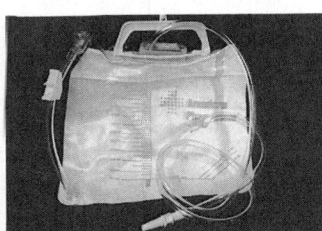

Large urine collection bag—
generally emptied once each
eight-hour shift; provides an
approximate measure of urine

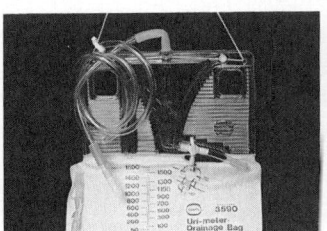

Large urine collection bag with
accurately callibrated small chamber for determining precise
hourly urine outputs

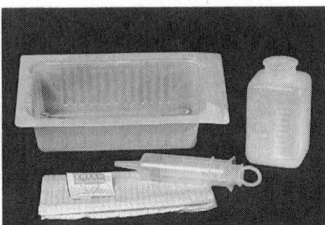

Irrigation tray containing a sterile
piston syringe, a sterile container
for holding the irrigation fluid,
and a sterile tray for collecting
the solution which returns from
the catheter

3000 cc bag of irrigation fluid for
continuous bladder irrigation

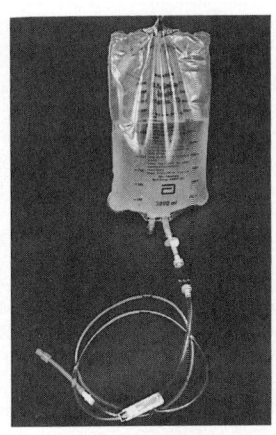

F I G U R E   3 4 - 2

Devices for collecting and measuring urine.

tial for the planning of the client's nursing and medical care. The measurement of intake and output is described further in Chapter 37. Wearing gloves when handling urine is recommended because they protect the nurse from possible exposure to pathogenic microorganisms or blood that may be present in the urine.

The procedure for measuring the urine output of the client who is voiding is as follows:

- Have the client void into a bedpan or urinal, either in bed or in the bathroom. Urinary devices used to collect or measure urine are shown in Figure 34-2.
- Pour urine voided into a bedpan or urinal into the appropriate measuring device provided by the agency. The devices are calibrated in milliliters.
- Place the calibrated container on a flat surface, such as a shelf, for an accurate reading. Note the amount of urine voided, read at eye level, and record it on the appropriate form. Figure 34-3 shows a form commonly used for recording urine output. The form is kept at the client's bedside or may be taped to the bathroom door. The total amount voided during each

shift and 24-hour period is recorded on the client's permanent record.

- Do *not* discard the urine if a specimen is required. Otherwise, the urine is discarded in the toilet.
- Tell clients who are ambulatory when their urine output is to be measured and recorded, so that they do not use the bathroom without measuring output. Clients who are willing and able can be taught to measure and record their own output.

When a client has an indwelling urinary catheter, the procedure for measuring urine output is as follows:

- Bring a calibrated measuring device to the bedside and place it beneath the collection bag.
- Place the drainage spout from the collection bag above, but not touching, the calibrated measuring device and open the clamp.
- Allow urine to flow from the collection bag into the measuring device. Then proceed as described above.

For catheterized clients who are acutely ill, urine may need to be measured hourly. This is facilitated by using a special collection bag with a built-in calibrated measuring

FIGURE 34-3

An example of a form commonly used for recording intake and output.

Intake and Output Chart

7:00 AM _11-18_ to 7:00 AM _11-19_

	Oral	I.V.		Blood	Other	Comments	Urine	Stool	Gastric tube	Drainage tubes		Vomitus	Other	Comments
7-8	250					Force fluids to 1100cc/shift	300							
8-9														
9-10	120													
10-11	60													
11-12	100						250							
12-1	300													
1-2	240													
2-3	100						200							
8 hr Tot	1170						750							voiding 5 discomfort
3-4														
4-5														
5-6														
6-7														
7-8														
8-9														
9-10														
10-11														
8 hr Tot														
11-12														
12-1														
1-2														
2-3														
3-4														
4-5														
5-6														
6-7														
8 hr Tot														
24 hr Tot														

Total intake	Total output

chamber. After the nurse assesses and records the amount of urine produced hourly, the measuring chamber is tilted, and this urine empties into the general collection bag. The measuring chamber is now ready to collect the next hour's urine.

Collecting Urine Specimens General nursing responsibilities for diagnostic tests are discussed in Chapter 27. Details are explained here.

Routine Urinalysis The collection of urine specimens for urinalysis is a nursing responsibility. A sterile urine specimen is not required for a routine urinalysis. Urine is collected by having the client void into a clean bedpan, urinal, or receptacle in the toilet bowl. Care must be taken to avoid contamination with feces. If a woman is menstruating when a urine sample is obtained, this must be noted on the laboratory slip because red blood cells may appear in the urine. The urine is poured into an appropriate container; labeled with the client's name, date, and time of collection; and sent to the laboratory for examination. Urine should not be left standing at room temperature for a long period before being sent to the laboratory because this may alter both the appearance and chemistry of the urine.

Specimens From Infants and Children Plastic disposable collection bags are available for infants and young children who have not yet achieved voluntary bladder control. The manufacturer's instructions should be followed and care taken in application and removal so as not to irritate the sensitive perineal skin.

Clean-Catch or Midstream Specimen A clean-catch specimen of urine is required in some situations. Most health agencies specify that a clean-catch specimen be collected during midstream. This means that the client voids a little urine, which is discarded; the specimen is then collected during midstream; and the last urine in the bladder also is discarded. The first voided urine helps to flush away organisms that may be near the meatus. The urinalysis findings may be inaccurate if these organisms enter the specimen. Also, it is generally thought that urine voided at midstream is most characteristic of the urine the body is producing. A clean-catch midstream specimen from a male is sterile. The female may be catheterized if a sterile specimen is required. Catheterization is discussed later in this chapter.

The client who can carry out proper techniques may collect his or her own clean-catch midstream urine specimen and often prefers to do so. The nurse should provide the appropriate equipment and instructions to carry out the procedure.

Guidelines for obtaining a clean-catch midstream urine specimen from a female client and from a male client are as follows:

Female Client
- Wear sterile gloves.
- Spread the labia well, and keep them apart until the specimen is obtained.

- Clean the area at the external meatus with sterile gauze or cotton balls and antiseptic soap and water. Move the gauze or cotton balls from the meatus toward the anus, and use one piece of gauze or one cotton ball for each stroke.
- Have the client void about 30 mL and discard this urine.
- Position the sterile specimen container near, but not touching, the meatus, and ask the client to void forcibly if she is lying down. This prevents collecting a specimen that has dribbled down and across the perineal area.
- Stop collecting urine before the client empties her bladder. Release the labia. Allow the client to continue emptying her bladder, and discard the urine not needed for the specimen.
- Use a sterilized bedpan to collect the midstream specimen if the client has difficulty voiding into the container, and then transfer the urine into the sterile specimen container.
- Label the specimen container appropriately and send the specimen to the laboratory.

Male Client
- Wear sterile gloves.
- Retract the foreskin to expose the glans penis in the uncircumcised male client.
- Clean the area of the external meatus with sterile gauze or cotton balls and antiseptic soap and water. Move gauze or cotton balls in a circular manner at the meatus, and move down the shaft of the penis a few inches.
- Have the client void about 30 mL and discard this urine.
- Have the client void directly into the sterile container.
- Stop collecting urine before the client empties his bladder. Allow the client to empty his bladder, and discard this urine. Return the foreskin to its normal position to prevent swelling and irritation of the glans penis.
- Use a sterilized urinal to collect the midstream specimen if the client has difficulty voiding into the container, and then transfer the urine into the sterile specimen container.
- Label the specimen container appropriately and send the specimen to the laboratory.

Sterile Specimen From an Indwelling Catheter Sterile urine specimens may be obtained by catheterizing the client's bladder (see Procedures 34-1 and 34-2) or by withdrawing the specimen from an indwelling catheter already in place.

When it is necessary to collect a urine specimen from a client with an indwelling catheter, it should be done from the catheter itself. A specimen from the collecting receptacle (drainage bag) may not be fresh urine, and its use could result in an inaccurate analysis. Sterile technique must be observed.

The size of the syringe is determined by the specific

laboratory test. A urine culture requires about 3 mL, whereas routine urinalysis necessitates the collection of at least 10 mL of urine. A sterile 21- to 25-gauge needle, an antiseptic swab, a specimen container, and, possibly, a clamp complete the list of necessary equipment. Wearing gloves protects the nurse from any accidental contact with the specimen.

If urine is not present in the tube, it may be necessary to clamp the tube below the collection port briefly (not to exceed 30 minutes) to allow urine to accumulate. Most catheters have a self-sealing area that tolerates a needle puncture. It is unsafe to puncture a Silastic or plastic catheter, as leakage will probably occur. Clean the entry port with an antiseptic swab, and carefully insert the sterile needle into the catheter. Aspirate urine into the syringe, remove the syringe, release the clamp if one was used, and transfer the specimen into the appropriate container. The specimen is then packaged and transported according to agency policy.

Care must be taken not to aspirate urine above the Y-junction of the catheter. It is possible for the needle of the syringe to lodge in the lumen of the tube leading to the balloon. In this case, the water inflating the balloon holding the catheter in place will be aspirated instead of urine.

Figure 34-4 shows how urine is removed from an indwelling catheter.

Collecting 24-Hour Urine Specimens For some types of laboratory studies, 24-hour specimens are required. It is critical that the client and the entire nursing team understand the importance of collecting *all* the urine voided in a 24-hour period. A sign posted on the client's bathroom door is a helpful reminder not to discard urine. The collection is initiated at a specific time (which is recorded) by having the client empty his bladder. This urine is discarded. All urine excreted for the next 24 hours is collected.

Depending on the type of examination used, the urine from each voiding may be kept in a separately marked container and the time of each voiding recorded. Or, all voidings may be collected in a common receptacle. The laboratory should be contacted to determine whether or not a preservative is needed to retard decomposition and if the specimens are to be refrigerated or kept on ice.

Determining Abnormal Constituents in the Urine In some situations, the nurse may perform tests on urine specimens, especially when specimens are being tested repeatedly for known abnormalities, when screening tests are being used, or when laboratory facilities are not readily available. For example, a nurse may test urine for the presence of glucose, protein, bilirubin, and blood. The results of the test are recorded on the client's record. Many types of commercially prepared diagnostic kits are available for determining the presence of abnormal substances in the urine. Although the performance of these tests is economical and fast, laboratory analysis is recommended when more precise results are needed.

Most diagnostic kits contain needed equipment and the appropriate reagent, a substance used in a chemical reaction to detect another substance. Reagents are pre-

FIGURE 34-4

The nurse is obtaining a urine specimen from a patient using an indwelling catheter. (A) She first uses a swab moistened with an antiseptic to clean the area where she will introduce a sterile needle. (B) She then inserts the needle and withdraws a specimen of urine. Body substance precautions require that gloves be used when contact with urine is probable.

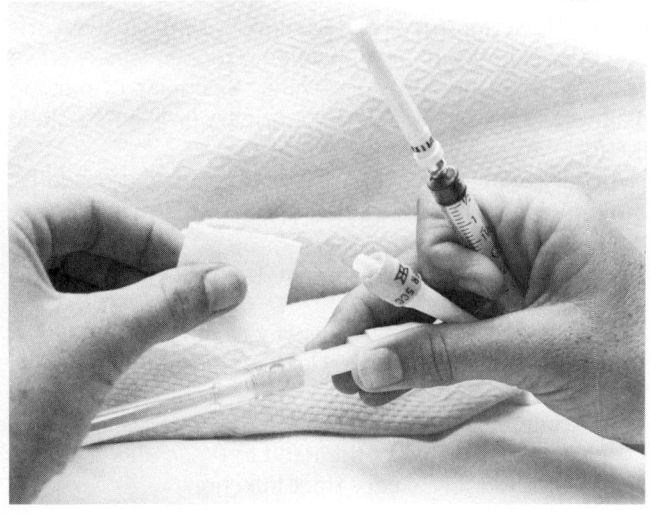

A

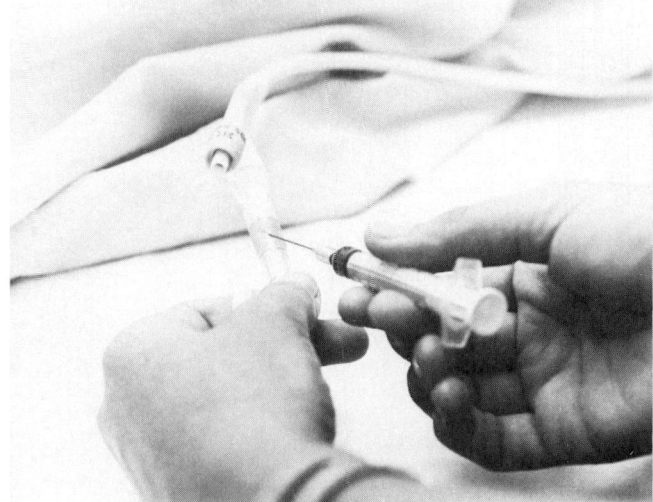

B

pared in the form of tablets, fluids, impregnated paper, and plastic strips with a special coating. When the reagent is brought in contact with urine, a chemical reaction occurs, which causes a color change. The reaction is then compared with an accompanying chart that describes the significance of the color.

The precise directions for the amount of the specimen, the time allowance for the chemical reaction, and the significance of the colors vary with the manufacturer. Therefore, it is important to read the directions accompanying the diagnostic kit carefully and to follow them exactly.

Determining Specific Gravity Determining the specific gravity of urine requires an instrument called a **urinometer**, or a **hydrometer**. The urinometer has a calibrated scale for the measurement of specific gravity. Urine is placed in a cylindrical container, and the urinometer is inserted in a circular motion without touching the bottom or side of the container. The reading on a urinometer should be made at eye level at the bottom of the meniscus formed by the urine (Fig. 34-5). The density of the urine supports the urinometer. If the urine is concentrated, the urinometer will be buoyed up high in the urine container and will register high on the measurement scale. If the urine is diluted, the urinometer will be supported low in the urine, and a low specific gravity reading will result.

FIGURE 34-5

To determine specific gravity, the urinometer should be read at eye level at the base of the meniscus formed by the urine.

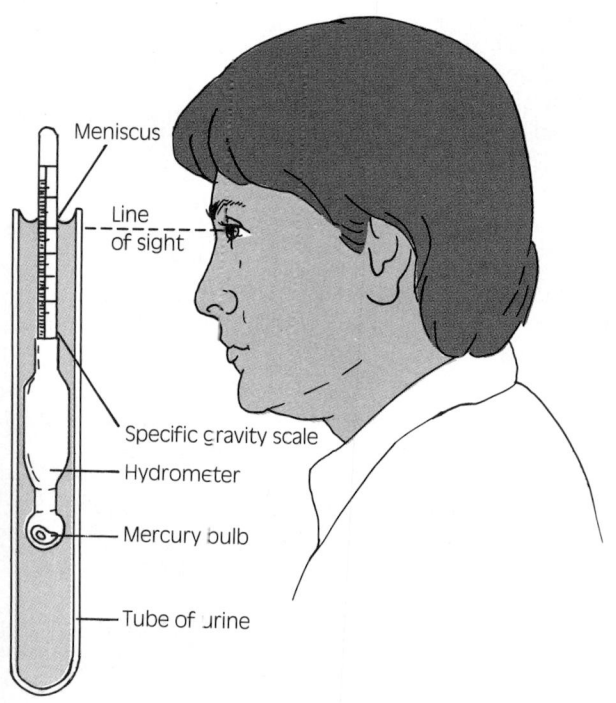

Assisting With Diagnostic Procedures Various diagnostic procedures, ordinarily performed in an operating room, are used to study the urinary system. The nurse is responsible for preparing the client and giving appropriate aftercare. Anxieties the client may have tend to be reduced when the nurse explains the procedure. Three common diagnostic procedures used to study the urinary system include cystoscopies, intravenous pyelograms, and retrograde pyelograms. A **cystoscopy** provides a direct visualization of the bladder, the ureteral orifices, and the urethra. The instrument used is a cystoscope. **Intravenous pyelography,** or **excretory urography,** involves the injection of a contrast material intravenously, followed by x-ray examination of the kidney and urethra. In a **retrograde pyelogram**, x-ray films are taken of the kidney and ureters after a contrast material is injected into the renal pelvis through the ureter. Descriptions of the preparation and aftercare of the client for each of these procedures are presented in Table 34-2.

Diagnosing

The data the nurse collects about the client's urinary functioning may lead to the development of one or several nursing diagnoses. Some data are appropriately reported to the physician and may contribute to the physician's identification of a medical diagnosis. It is important that nurses detect significant urinary findings, record these appropriately, and report them to the proper people.

Urinary Functioning as the Problem Nursing diagnoses that specifically address problems in urinary functioning include problems of incontinence, pattern alteration, and urinary retention. Sample defining characteristics for these diagnoses appear in the display Nursing Diagnoses for Common Urinary Problems.

Urinary Functioning as the Etiology Difficulty with urination or changes in normal voiding problems may affect other areas of human functioning. Examples of nursing diagnoses that may be related to urinary problems include the following:

Anxiety related to incontinence, diagnostic procedures

High Risk for Infection related to indwelling urinary catheter

Impaired Skin Integrity (Actual, High Risk for) related to incontinence

Knowledge Deficit related to any existing or new urinary disease or disorder, lack of information about personal hygiene

Noncompliance with Medication Regimen related to misunderstanding of the need to finish all doses of medication for urinary tract infection

TABLE 34-2

Common Diagnostic Procedures Used to Study the Urinary Tract

Preparation	Aftercare
Cystoscopy: The direct visual examination of the bladder, ureteral orifices, and urethra with a cystoscope	
The client is allowed liquids on the morning of the examination.	Tissue swelling, dysuria, and hematuria may occur owing to trauma from the procedure.
Sedation and analgesics are usually prescribed before the procedure.	Encourage a generous fluid intake, and observe and measure urine output for at least 24 hours.
A signed consent form is required for the procedure.	Observe the client for urinary retention and for signs of infection; nosocomial infection after a cystoscopy is common.
The procedure is ordinarily painless.	
Intravenous Pyelography (excretory urography): The x-ray examination of the kidney and ureter after a contrast material is injected intravenously	
No fluids or food are given for at least 12 hours before the examination so that contrast material will concentrate in the urinary system. Elderly, debilitated, or young clients may not tolerate this dehydration, and compromises may need to be made.	Fluids and food may be given immediately after the examination.
A laxative the evening before the examination and an enema the morning of the examination are given so that stool and gas do not interfere with visualization.	Observe the client for signs of a reaction to the contrast material, such as a rash, nausea, and hives.
The client should void before the examination.	
Retrograde Pyelography: The x-ray examination of the kidney and ureters after a contrast material is injected into the renal pelvis through the ureter	
No fluids and food are given after midnight before the examination.	Foods and fluids may be given, but if anesthesia has been used, this is delayed for several hours.
A laxative the evening before the examination and an enema the morning of the examination are given so that stool and gas do not interfere with visualization.	Check the vital signs regularly if anesthesia has been used.
The client should void before the examination.	Observe the client for signs of a reaction to the contrast material, such as a rash, nausea, and hives.
A signed consent form is recommended for the procedure.	Ureteral catheters may be in place and should be connected to drainage receptacles so that the amount and character of drainage from each catheter can be noted.

Pain related to bladder spasms, dysuria, urinary retention, cancer of the bladder, diagnostic procedures

Self-Esteem Disturbance related to urinary incontinence, urinary diversion

Sexual Dysfunction related to urinary incontinence, urinary diversion

Sleep Pattern Disturbance related to nocturia

Toileting Self-Care Deficit related to parent's lack of knowledge or motivation to toilet-train child, neuromuscular impairment or musculoskeletal disorders, immobility, trauma or surgical procedures, confusion, disorientation

The nurse's challenge is to correctly identify human responses to alterations in urinary elimination that pose specific health problems for the client and his or her family.

Planning: Client Goals

When the client is ambulatory and not experiencing difficulties with the urinary system, the promotion of normal voiding is not a problem. Trauma or illness may result in the client's need for nursing assistance with voiding. Nursing interventions (which follow) should be supportive of planned client goals.

The client will:
- Produce urine output about equal to fluid intake
- Maintain fluid and electrolyte balance
- Empty the bladder completely at regular intervals
- Report ease of voiding
- Maintain skin integrity

Client goals for specific urinary problems follow later in this chapter.

NURSING DIAGNOSES FOR COMMON PROBLEMS

Urinary Elimination

Problem	Related Factors	Sample Defining Characteristics
Altered Urinary Elimination	Enuresis (maturational) Dysuria	Parents report 6-year-old son wets bed three or four times a week. Small bladder capacity, less than 300 mL "It hurts when I pass my water." Urinalysis reveals hematuria and proteinuria.
Functional Incontinence	Altered environment Sensory, cognitive, or mobility deficits	"I don't know why Johnny started wetting since he's been hospitalized. He has been toilet-trained for 6 months now." "When I remember to take mother to the toilet she urinates fine. But if I don't remember, I find her wet."
Reflex Incontinence	Neurologic impairment	Client with spinal cord lesion reports no awareness of bladder filling, no urge to void or feelings of bladder fullness, involuntary loss of urine at somewhat regular intervals.
Stress Incontinence	Age-related degenerative changes High intraabdominal pressure Incompetent bladder outlet Overdistention between voidings Weak pelvic muscles and structural supports	Obese mother of four reports involuntary dribbling of urine with coughs, sneezes, hearty laughter. Client "too busy to void" during day reports involuntary leakage of urine with sudden movement, cough, and so on.
Total Incontinence	Neurologic impairment Trauma or disease affecting spinal cord nerves	Constant flow of urine at unpredictable times without distention or uninhibited bladder contractions. Nocturia
Urge Incontinence	Decreased bladder capacity Bladder spasms Increased intake of caffeine or alcohol Increased urine concentration Overdistention of bladder	"I can never make it to the bathroom in time." Urgency, frequency, nocturia, bladder contracture or spasm
Urinary Retention	High urethral pressure caused by weak detrusor Inhibition of reflex arc Strong sphincter Blockage	Elderly male diagnosed with benign prostatic hypertrophy complains of inability to urinate despite feeling bladder is full. Woman 6 hours after delivery has had no urine output since labor; 800 mL IV fluids infused; fundus of uterus is displaced to the right by a full bladder.

Implementing

Promoting Normal Urination

Maintaining Normal Voiding Habits

If the client's voiding habits are adequate, the nurse takes care to maintain these habits to ensure comfort and satisfactory urine output. Attention to the following variables is helpful:

Schedule: Some clients will report voiding on demand in no apparent pattern. Others have inflexible patterns that have developed over the years, and become anxious if these are interrupted. Some clients need assistance voiding and may experience urgency. Adhering to the client's normal voiding patterns as much as possible is recommended.

Privacy: Many adults and children cannot void in the presence of another person. Unless the extreme weakness of the client demands the nurse's assistance, privacy should be offered to the client.

Position: Assisting clients to assume *normal* voiding positions may be all that is necessary to resolve an inability to void. Some males cannot use a urinal while lying down or sitting; the nurse should then assist them to void while standing at the bedside unless this is contraindicated. Similarly, some females cannot void easily on a bedpan and respond favorably to the use of a bedside commode.

Hygiene: Clients who are confined to bed will find it difficult to perform their usual genital hygiene. Careful cleansing of the perineal and genital areas is needed to promote client comfort and prevent infection. This is easily accomplished for clients on bed rest by placing them on a bedpan and then pouring warm soapy water over the perineal area followed by clear water. Families providing care for ill members at home also may be taught this technique.

Because many people customarily wash their hands after toileting, clients confined to bed should be offered a moistened towelette or soap and water to wipe their hands after the nurse removes the bedpan. Specific recommendations for urinary elimination problems that affect elderly people are listed in the display Focus on the Older Adult.

Promoting Fluid Intake

Many people routinely drink less fluid than is optimal to promote healthy urinary functioning. The adult who has no disease-related fluid restrictions should drink 2000 to 2400 mL (8 to 10 8-oz glasses) of fluid daily. A common misper-

FOCUS ON THE OLDER ADULT

Nursing Strategies for Urinary Elimination Problems Affecting Older Adults

Nocturia, Frequency, and Urgency

- Ensure easy access to the bathroom or commode.
- Discourage fluid intake at bedtime.
- Discourage alcohol use before bedtime.
- Evaluate medication regimen and schedule, particularly diuretics and drugs that produce sedation or confusion.
- Use a night light.
- Use clothing that is easily removed for voiding.
- Keep assistive ambulatory devices (walkers, canes, etc.) readily available.
- Provide call bell if assistance is necessary.
- Evaluate gait and ability to ambulate safely.
- Assess for urinary tract infection.

Incontinence

- Maintain a fluid intake of 1500 to 2000 mL/day.
- Discourage use of alcohol, NutraSweet, and caffeine.
- Provide easy access to the bathroom.
- Assess factors that influence voiding.
- Use assistive devices when necessary (raised toilet seat, grab bars, walker).
- Use collection devices when necessary (urinal or bed pan).

- Ensure safety when ambulating (eg, skid-proof slippers).
- Encourage use of whole, unprocessed, coarse wheat bran to prevent constipation and fecal impaction.
- Perform Kegel exercises several times daily.
- Encourage participation in a bladder retraining program.
- Consider insertion of an indwelling catheter as the *last resort.*

Urinary Tract Infections

- Maintain a liberal fluid intake.
- Encourage shower instead of tub bath to decrease opportunity for bacteria in bath water to enter urethra.
- Void at frequent intervals.
- Void immediately after sexual intercourse.
- Assess for signs of urinary tract infection (may be nonspecific in elderly client).
- Use dipstick (Microstix) if recommended to monitor bacteria count in urine.
- Continue antimicrobial therapy as ordered.

ception is that drinking this much fluid causes water retention and contributes to weight gain. This is false. If a good proportion of the daily fluid intake is water, the kidneys and urinary structures will be well flushed and waste products will be removed, including potentially harmful bacteria. Fluid intake should be monitored for potentially harmful excesses of caffeine-containing beverages, high-sodium beverages such as diet sodas, and high-sugar beverages.

Fluids of preference, fresh water and juices, should be made available to clients confined to bed. Also, children and confused clients may need to be reminded to drink. With certain diseases, fluid restrictions may be ordered by the physician. In others, forced fluids (above-average intake of fluids) are prescribed. This needs to be incorporated in the plan of care.

Strengthening Muscle Tone

Strengthening muscle tone in the perineal and abdominal muscles can facilitate voluntary control of urination. Clients should be instructed to exercise perineal muscles by voluntarily starting and stopping the stream of urine (**Kegel exercises**) and by tightening the muscles around the anus. Once the client is familiar with these sensations, these muscles should be contracted and relaxed several times each waking hour for 2 to 3 months. The exercises can be done anywhere, and clients should be assisted to incorporate them into their daily activities.

Stimulating Urination

Urinary retention, the inability to void even though the bladder is full, is discussed later in this chapter. Many people experience hesitancy, a delay, or difficulty in initiating voiding. This problem may be resolved by resorting to simple nursing measures:

- Assist the client to void when the urge to void is first experienced. Routine delaying of urination may result in difficulty initiating a stream.
- Make use of the factors noted earlier to provide a natural environment for voiding—relaxed and private setting and normal position. Squatting or leaning forward may assist by putting pressure on the suprapubic area.
- Run tap water within the client's hearing.
- Use a warm bedpan.
- Pour warm water over the perineal area. Measure the amount of water if the voided specimen needs to be measured.
- Pour warm water over the client's fingers.
- Stroke the client's leg or thigh.
- Exert gentle downward pressure over the bladder to facilitate bladder emptying. This technique differs from Credé's maneuver, in which manual bladder compression is used to stimulate urination by creating a sensation of bladder fullness and relaxing the urethral sphincter. The nurse places one hand on top of the other over the client's bladder (between the umbilicus and the symphysis pubis, fingers pointing downward) and exerts downward pressure to com-

press the bladder walls and forcefully expel urine. This maneuver should be performed only when bladder flaccidity exists and the client is not expected to regain voluntary control. It usually requires a physician's order.

- If urination is being stimulated for the purposes of obtaining a urine specimen and the client is cooperative, sometimes having the client forcefully cough will create sufficient intra-abdominal pressure to stimulate the micturition reflex.
- Ask the client to blow bubbles through a straw in a glass of water.

Assisting With Toileting

Toilet Despite the client's ability to use the bathroom toilet, the nurse is responsible for noting any abnormalities of elimination. In some instances, clients may need to be taught to report abnormalities to the nurse and instructed not to flush the toilet until the nurse checks the urine. In other instances, when the urine volume is to be calculated, the client may need to urinate in a bedpan or some other receptacle placed on the toilet so the urine can be measured before it is discarded. Although many clients can easily be taught to measure their urine output, the nurse should observe the urine at least once during a work shift and more frequently if warranted.

A weak client should be assisted to the bathroom. Someone should remain in attendance if there is any danger of the client's falling. Bathrooms should not be locked, and, especially in hospitals, a signal bell should be within easy reach of the client so that help can be summoned easily if the client feels weak and needs assistance. A hand rail near the toilet is helpful.

Commode Commodes can be used for clients who are able to be out of bed but unable to use the bathroom toilet. Commodes are chairs, straight-back chairs, or wheelchairs with open seats under which there is a shelf or a holder on which a bedpan is placed. The commode can be placed adjacent to the bed, and the client can be assisted to it with minimal exertion.

Bedpan and Urinal Male clients confined to bed usually use the urinal for voiding and the bedpan for defecation; female clients use the bedpan for both. When a female client is unable to sit up in bed—for example, when she is in a body cast—a female urinal may be used. The bedpan and the urinal are difficult to use and embarrassing to many clients. Privacy is important to almost all clients when they use a bedpan or urinal.

A special bedpan called a fracture bedpan is frequently used by people with fractures of the femur or lower spine. Smaller and flatter than the ordinary bedpan, it is helpful for clients who cannot easily raise themselves to use the regular bedpan.

Figure 34-2 displays the types of bedpans and urinals and Procedure 35-1 shows how to help a client use a bedpan or urinal.

Safety Considerations Many dangerous situations have been created in the absence of a signal bell or bedpan. Clients confined to bed have gotten up to go to the bathroom to void, sometimes climbing over or around bed side rails or removing oxygen masks or infusion tubings. Offering a bedpan or urinal frequently can save clients from fracturing their hips, dislodging an intravenous infusion, or being embarrassed by soiled linen. A very ill or sedated client may not think to ask in time. As a precaution, family members of clients at home may need to be made aware of this. The nurse is responsible for the client's safety.

Teaching Feminine Hygiene Female clients often need to be taught the proper technique for perineal care after urination. Drying or washing of the perineal area should be from the front to the back, or from the urethra toward the rectum. A reverse cleaning motion can result in fecal organisms being introduced into the urethra or vagina. This type of contamination is a common cause of urinary tract and vaginal infections.

Catheterizing the Client's Bladder

Urinary catheterization is the introduction of a catheter through the urethra into the bladder for the purpose of withdrawing urine. A **catheter** is a tube for injecting or removing fluids. Catheterization is considered the most prominent cause of nosocomial infections, that is, an infection acquired in a hospital. Whenever possible, it is recommended that catheterization be avoided. When deemed necessary, it should be performed with careful technique. (See Nursing Process in Clinical Practice, later in this chapter.)

Types of Catheters If a catheter is to remain in place for continuous drainage, an **indwelling urethral catheter** is used. Indwelling catheters also are called **retention** and **Foley catheters**. The indwelling urethral catheter is designed so that it does not slip out of the bladder. These catheters are used for the gradual decompression of an overdistended bladder, for intermittent bladder drainage and irrigation, and for continuous bladder drainage.

An indwelling catheter has a balloon, which is inflated after the catheter is inserted into the bladder. Several types of indwelling catheters are available, but the principles on which they operate are similar.

The indwelling catheter has more than one lumen. In a double-lumen catheter, one lumen is connected directly with the balloon, which is distended with solution, and the other is the lumen through which the urine drains. The triple-lumen catheter provides an additional lumen for the instillation of irrigating solution. Figure 34-6 shows a triple-lumen, a double-lumen, and a straight catheter. Wear gloves to protect against possible exposure to blood and body substances.

Intermittent or **straight catheters** are used to drain the bladder for shorter periods (5 to 10 minutes). Clients can be taught to insert and remove intermittent catheters them-

FIGURE 34-6

(A) Triple-lumen indwelling catheter. (B) Double-lumen indwelling catheter. (C) Straight catheter.

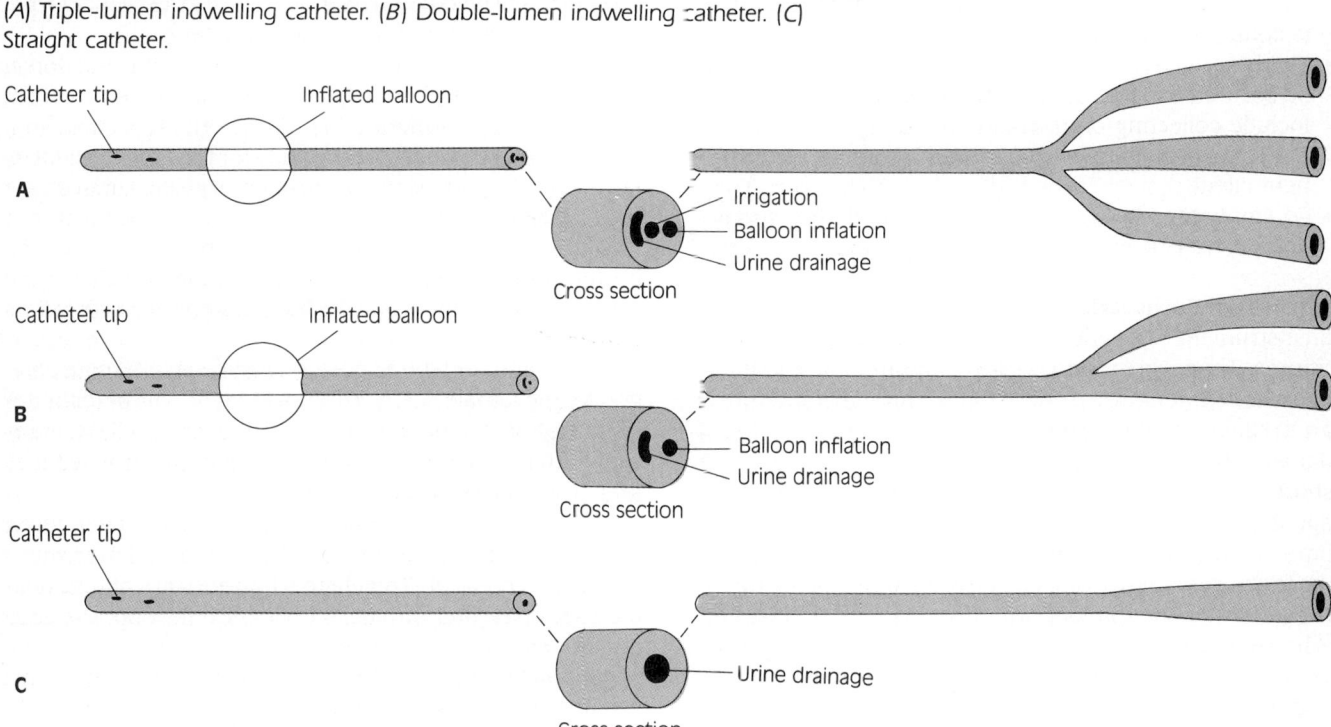

selves. Intermittent catheters are discussed later in this section.

A **suprapubic catheter** occasionally is used for continuous drainage. This type of catheter is inserted through a small incision above the pubic area. Care of the client with a suprapubic catheter is more appropriately discussed in clinical texts.

Facts About the Lower Urinary Tract System The following basic facts about the lower urinary tract system should be borne in mind when considering catheterization:
- The bladder normally is a sterile cavity.
- The external opening to the urethra can never be sterilized.
- The bladder has defense mechanisms. It empties itself of urine regularly and maintains an acidic environment, which has antibacterial advantages. These help to maintain a sterile bladder under normal circumstances and also help in clearing an infection if it occurs.
- Pathogens introduced into the bladder can ascend the ureters and lead to bladder and kidney infection.
- A normal bladder is not as susceptible to infection as an injured one. A client's lowered resistance, present in many diseases and stressful situations, predisposes to urinary infection.

Reasons for Catheterization The following are common reasons for performing a urinary catheterization:
- To relieve urinary retention
- To obtain a sterile urine specimen from a woman
- To measure the amount of **residual urine** in the bladder. The client is first asked to void and is then catheterized to determine how much urine stays in the bladder after normal voiding. An amount over 50 mL is considered abnormal.
- To obtain a urine specimen when a specimen cannot be secured satisfactorily by other means. Examples include collecting an uncontaminated specimen from a woman who is menstruating and from an incontinent client.
- To empty the bladder before, during, and after surgery and before certain diagnostic examinations.

Hazards of Catheterization The hazards of introducing an instrument or a catheter into the bladder are sepsis and trauma. The male urethra is especially vulnerable to injury because of its length. An object forced through a stricture or an irregular opening from the wrong angle can seriously damage the urethra. Although the urethra in the female is shorter than that in the male, it also is susceptible to damage if a catheter is forced through it. The mucous membrane lining the urethra is delicate and easily damaged by the friction resulting from the insertion of a catheter. Bacteria can enter the bladder when the catheter is inserted. When the catheter is left in place, the organisms may move up the catheter lumen or the space between the catheter and the urethral wall.

Intermittent catheterization may be necessary for clients with spinal cord injuries or other neurologic conditions. It may be done by the client or a caregiver in the home setting. Although the risk of developing a urinary tract infection is always present, most research supports the use of clean rather than sterile technique in this environment. Moore (1991) reports that antibiotic use or more frequent catheterization (every 4 hours) may effectively reduce bacterial count in the urine. Because bladder irrigations with antibiotics are difficult when done at home and frequent use of oral antibiotics may lead to the development of resistant strains of bacteria, their use is not recommended.

Equipment The equipment used during a catheterization usually is prepackaged in a sterile, disposable tray. Most kits already contain a standard-size catheter. The trays used for catheterizing male and female clients are the same. Catheters are graded on the French scale according to lumen size. For the female adult, 14 and 16 French catheters commonly are used. Smaller catheters usually are not necessary, and the size of the lumen is so small that it increases the length of time necessary for emptying the bladder. Larger catheters distend the urethra and increase the discomfort of the procedure. For the male adult, 18 and 20 French catheters commonly are used, but if these are too large, a smaller catheter should be used. Size 8 and 10 French catheters commonly are used for children.

Client Preparation Before the catheterization, the client should be given an adequate explanation of the procedure and the reason for it. A catheter being inserted produces a sensation of pressure and some discomfort, and this should be explained to the client. In addition, the client should be assured that every measure to avoid exposure and embarrassment will be taken. The more relaxed the client can be, the easier it will be to insert the catheter.

The most common position for the client is the dorsal recumbent, preferably on a solid surface, such as a firm mattress or a treatment table. Catheterizing a client in a bed with a soft mattress, especially for the female client, is not as satisfactory because the client's pelvic surfaces are not firmly supported, and visualization of the meatus is difficult. Also, the client may sink into the bed, causing the bladder to be lower than the outlet of the catheter. If the client is in bed, supporting the buttocks on a firm cushion is helpful.

The Sims', or lateral, position can be an alternate position for the female client. This position may allow for better visualization and be more comfortable for the client, especially if hip and knee movements are difficult. A reduced area of exposure also can result in less psychic discomfort for the client. The client may lie on either side, depending on which position is easiest for the nurse and best in terms of the client's comfort. The client's buttocks are placed near the edge of the bed with her shoulders at the opposite edge and her knees drawn toward her chest. The nurse lifts the upper buttock and labia to expose the urinary meatus. This positioning is shown in Figure 34-7.

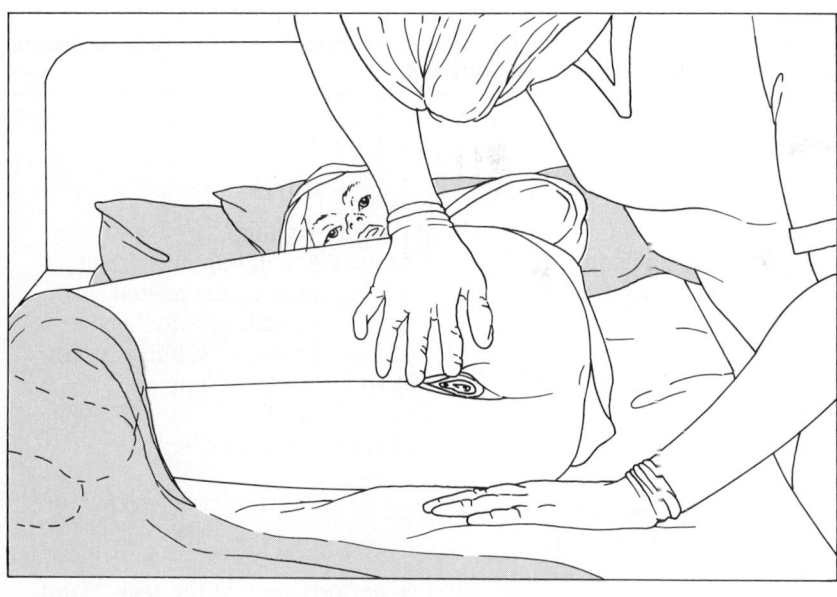

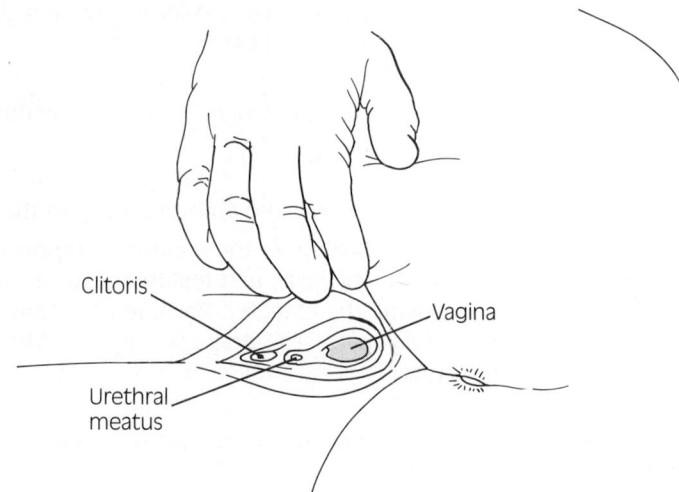

Clitoris

Vagina

Urethral meatus

Demonstration of the side-lying position (*top*) and of how to expose the urinary meatus when catheterizing a female patient (*bottom*).

Procedure Catheterization of the urinary bladder for female and male clients is described in Procedures 34-1 and 34-2. Techniques of surgical asepsis are of extraordinary importance when catheterizing a client to help prevent urinary tract infection.

Indwelling Catheters

Inserting and Connecting to the Drainage System The procedure for inserting an indwelling catheter is the same as for inserting a straight, single-lumen catheter with the following differences:

• Inflate the balloon with the prefilled syringe before inserting the catheter, to check for balloon patency. Aspirate the fluid back into the syringe when it is determined that the balloon is patent.

• Hold the catheter with one hand, and inflate the balloon, according to the manufacturer's instructions, as soon as the catheter is in the bladder and urine has begun to drain from the bladder. Usually 4 to 5 mL

more sterile water than the size of the balloon is used. This additional water remains in the tube leading to the balloon.

• If the client complains of pain after the balloon is inflated, allow it to empty and replace the catheter with another one. The balloon is probably located in the urethra and is causing discomfort owing to distention of the urethra.

Technique to Complete Closed Urinary Drainage System The following technique is used to complete the closed urinary drainage system:

- Check to see that the drainage tubing is not kinked. Do not place it under the leg, where it may be compressed. Also, do not place it in a manner so that it moves above the level of the bladder. This may cause the client's bladder to drain by suction rather than by gravity, risking injury to the bladder mucosa.

(Text continues on p. 875)

P R O C E D U R E 3 4 - 1

Catheterizing the Female Urinary Bladder (Straight and Indwelling)

Equipment

Sterile catheterization kit that
  contains:
  Sterile gloves
  Sterile drapes (one of which is
    fenestrated)
  Antiseptic solution
  Lubricant
  Cotton balls or gauze squares

Forceps
Straight or indwelling catheter
  (size must be appropriate for
  client)
Prefilled syringe
Basin (base of kit usually serves
  as this)
Specimen container

Flashlight or lamp
Urine collection bag and drainage
  tubing (may be connected to
  sterile indwelling catheter if a
  closed drainage system is used)
Velcro leg strap or tape
Disposal bag
Waterproof pad or Chux

Action	Rationale
1 Assemble equipment. Wash your hands. Explain the procedure and its purpose to the client.	Organization facilitates performance of the task. Hand-washing deters spread of microorganisms. An explanation encourages client cooperation and reduces apprehension.
2 Provide for good light. Artificial light is recommended (use of a flashlight requires an assistant to hold and position it).	Good lighting is necessary to see the meatus clearly.
3 Provide for privacy by closing the curtains or door.	The procedure may be embarrassing for the client.
4 Assist the client to the dorsal recumbent position with the knees flexed and the feet about 2 feet apart and drape the client. Or, if preferable, the client can be placed in the side-lying position as shown in Figure 34-7. Slide the waterproof drape under the client.	Good visualization of the meatus is important. Embarrassment, chilliness, and feeling tense can interfere with introducing the catheter. The client's comfort will promote relaxation. The drape will protect bed linens from moisture.
5 Clean the genital and perineal area with warm soap and water. Rinse and dry. Wash your hands again.	Clean technique decreases the possibility of introducing organisms into the bladder.
6 Prepare urine drainage setup if indwelling catheter is to be inserted and separate urine collection system is used. Secure to bed frame according to manufacturer's directions.	This facilitates connection of the catheter to the drainage system and provides for easy access.
7 Open the sterile catheterization tray on overbed table using sterile technique.	Placement of equipment near the work site increases efficiency. Sterile technique protects the client and prevents the spread of microorganisms.
8 Put on sterile gloves. Grasp the upper corners of the drape and unfold the drape without touching unsterile areas. Fold back a cuff over gloved hands. Ask the client to lift her buttocks and slide the sterile drape under her with gloves protected by cuff.	The drape provides a sterile field close to the meatus. Covering the gloved hands will help keep the gloves sterile while placing the drape.
9 A fenestrated sterile drape may be placed over the perineal area exposing the labia.	The drape expands the sterile field and protects against contamination. Use of a fenestrated drape may limit visualization and is considered optional by some practitioners.
10 Place the sterile tray on the drape between the client's thighs.	This provides easy access to supplies.

(continued)

PROCEDURE 34-1 (continued)

Catheterizing the Female Urinary Bladder (Straight and Indwelling)

Action	Rationale
11 Open all supplies: **a** *If the catheter is to be indwelling,* test the catheter balloon. Remove the protective cap on the tip of the syringe and attach the syringe prefilled with sterile water to injection port. Inject appropriate amount of fluid. If the balloon inflates properly, withdraw fluid and leave the syringe attached to the port.	A balloon that does not inflate or that leaks needs to be replaced before insertion in the client.
b Pour antiseptic solution over cotton balls or gauze. Open the specimen container if specimen is to be obtained.	It is necessary to open all supplies and prepare for the procedure while both hands are sterile.
c Lubricate 1 to 2 inches of the catheter tip.	Lubrication facilitates the insertion of the catheter and reduces trauma to the tissues.

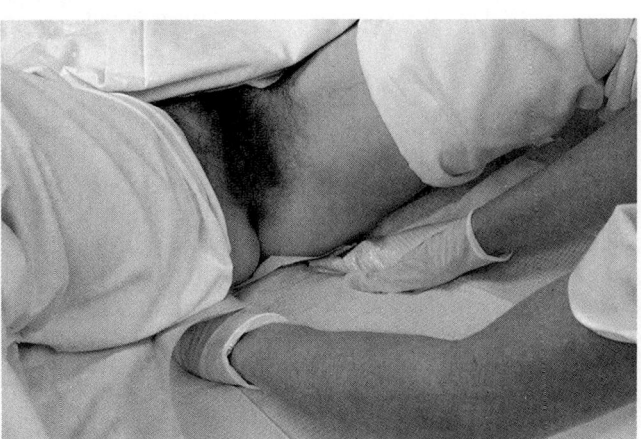

Action 8: Keeping sterile gloves protected while positioning drape under client.

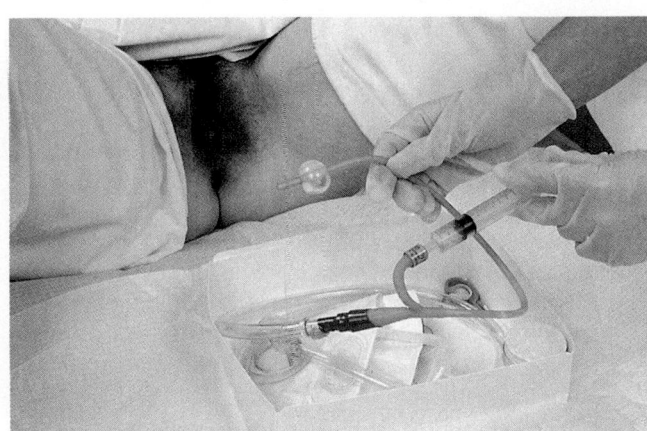

Action 11a: Testing the balloon.

Action	Rationale
12 With the thumb and one finger of your nondominant hand, spread the labia and identify the meatus, as shown in figure. Be prepared to maintain separation of the labia with one hand until urine is flowing well and continuously.	Smoothing the area immediately surrounding the meatus helps to make it visible. Allowing the labia to drop back into position may contaminate the area around the meatus, as well as the catheter. Your nondominant hand is now contaminated.
13 Using cotton balls held with forceps, clean both labial folds and then directly over the meatus. Move the cotton ball from above the meatus down toward the rectum. Discard each cotton ball after one downward stroke.	Moving from an area where there is likely to be less contamination to an area where there is more contamination helps prevent the spread of organisms. Cleaning the meatus last helps reduce the possibility of introducing organisms into the bladder.
14 With the uncontaminated gloved hand, place the drainage end of the catheter in the receptacle. *For insertion of an indwelling catheter* that is preattached to sterile tubing and drainage container (closed drainage system), position the catheter and setup within easy reach on the sterile field.	This facilitates drainage of urine and minimizes risk of contaminating sterile equipment.

(continued)

PROCEDURE 3 4 - 1 *(continued)*

Catheterizing the Female Urinary Bladder (Straight and Indwelling)

Action	Rationale

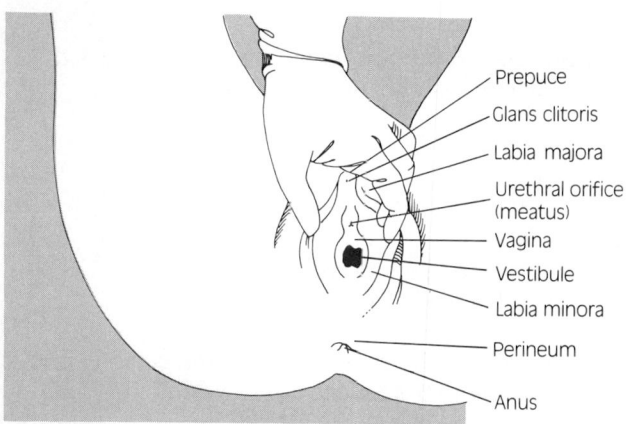

Action 12: Spreading the labia with nondominant hand to identify the meatus.

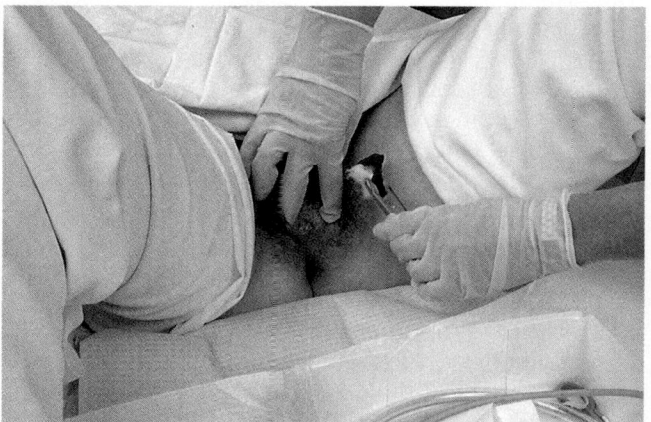

Action 13: Preparing to clean the labial folds.

15 Insert the catheter tip into the meatus 5 to 7.5 cm (2–3 inches) or until urine flows. Do not use force to push the catheter through the urethra into the bladder. Ask the client to breathe deeply, and rotate the catheter gently if slight resistance is met as the catheter reaches the external sphincter. *For an indwelling catheter,* once urine drains, advance the catheter another 1.3 to 2.5 cm (½ to 1 inch).

The female urethra is about 3.7 to 6.2 cm (1½ to 2½ inches) long. Applying force on the catheter is likely to injure mucous membranes. The sphincter relaxes and the catheter can enter the bladder easily when the client relaxes. Advancing an indwelling catheter an additional 1.3 to 2.5 cm (½ to 1 inch) ensures placement in the bladder and facilitates inflation of the balloon without damaging the urethra.

16 Hold the catheter securely with the nondominant hand while the bladder empties. Collect a specimen if required. Continue drainage according to agency policy.

Withdrawing and reinserting the catheter increase the chances of contaminating it. In general, no more than 750 mL of urine should be removed at one time. Pelvic floor blood vessels may become engorged from the sudden release of pressure leading to possible hypotensive episode.

17 Remove the catheter smoothly and slowly if a straight catheterization was ordered.

This causes less discomfort to the client.

18 *If the catheter is to be indwelling:*
   a Inflate the balloon according to the manufacturer's recommendations.

The balloon anchors the catheter in place in the bladder. Sterile water is used to inflate the balloon as a precaution in case the balloon ruptured.

   b Tug gently on the catheter after the balloon is inflated to feel resistance.

Improper inflation can cause client discomfort and malpositioning of catheter.

   c Attach the catheter to the drainage system if necessary.

Closed drainage system minimizes the risk of organisms being introduced into the bladder.

   d Secure to the upper thigh with a Velcro leg strap or tape. Leave some slack in the catheter to allow for leg movement.

Proper attachment prevents trauma to the urethra and meatus from tension on the tubing.

   e Check that the drainage tubing is not kinked and that movement of side rails does not interfere with catheter or drainage bag.

This facilitates drainage of urine and prevents the backflow of urine.

(continued)

PROCEDURE 34-1 *(continued)*

Catheterizing the Female Urinary Bladder (Straight and Indwelling)

Action

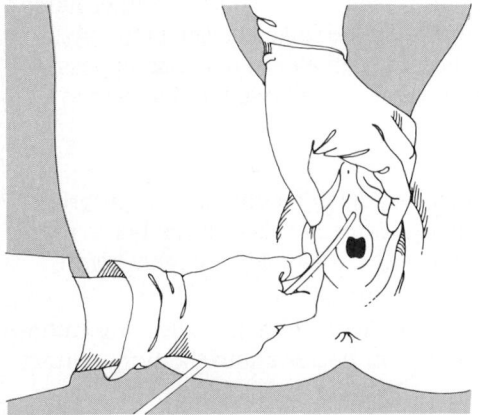

Action 15: Inserting the tip of the catheter into the meatus, using the uncontaminated gloved hand.

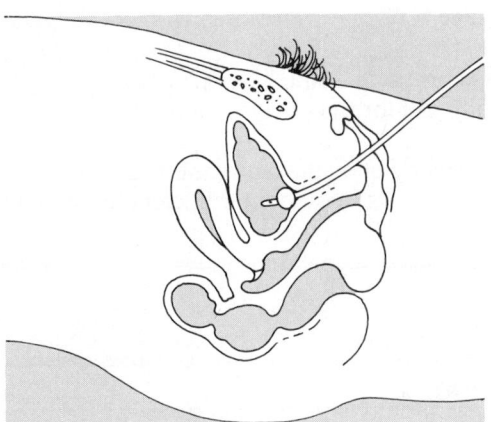

Action 18b: Tugging gently on catheter after balloon is in place to feel resistance.

Rationale

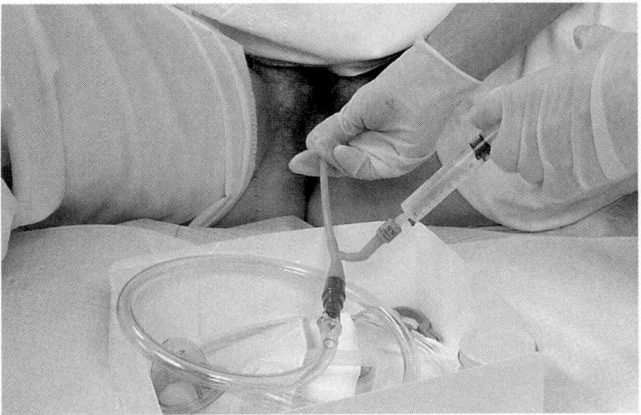

Action 18a: Injecting sterile water to inflate balloon.

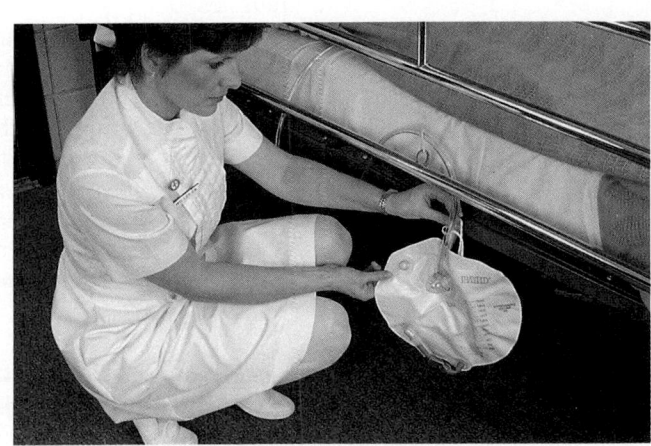

Action 18e: Checking position of drainage setup.

19 Remove the equipment and make the client comfortable in bed. Clean and dry the perineal area, if necessary. Care for the equipment according to agency policy. Send the urine specimen to the laboratory promptly or refrigerate it.

20 Wash your hands.

21 Record the time of the catheterization, the amount of urine removed, a description of the urine, the client's reaction to the procedure, and your name.

Urine kept at room temperature may cause organisms, if present, to grow and distort laboratory findings.

Handwashing deters the spread of microorganisms.

A careful record is important for planning the client's care.

(continued)

PROCEDURE 34-1 (continued)

Catheterizing the Female Urinary Bladder (Straight and Indwelling)

Age Considerations

If the client is a child, the size of the catheter must be adapted accordingly.

Elderly women may be uncomfortable in the lithotomy position, and require variable positions for catheterization. If the client is able to remain on her back, another nurse can assist her to flex her knees and hips, thus bringing the knees closer to the abdomen and allowing visualization of the urinary meatus. Catheterization also is possible with the client on her side in a modified Sims' position as discussed and shown in Figure 34-7.

Home Care Considerations

If self-catheterization must be performed in the home, clean technique is appropriate. The bladder's natural resistance to microorganisms normally found in the home makes sterile technique unnecessary. Rubber catheters must be washed thoroughly before boiling for 20 minutes. Dry and store properly for next usage.

A shower rather than a tub bath is recommended for clients with an indwelling catheter. Sitting in the bathtub may allow for easier access of bacteria into the urinary tract.

Special Considerations

If there is not an immediate flow of urine after the catheter has been inserted, several measures may prove helpful:

- Have the client take a deep breath, which helps to relax the perineal and abdominal muscles.
- Rotate the catheter slightly because a drainage hole may be resting against the bladder wall.
- Raise the head of the client's bed to increase pressure in the bladder area.
- Place a gloved finger in the vagina to digitally feel for the position of the catheter through the anterior vaginal wall.
- Temporarily leave a catheter that has inadvertently been placed in the vagina in place as a guide while the nurse regloves and inserts another sterile catheter directly above it into the urinary meatus.

PROCEDURE 34-2

Catheterizing the Male Urinary Bladder (Straight and Indwelling)

Equipment

Sterile catheterization kit that
contains:
  Sterile gloves
  Sterile drapes (one of which is
    fenestrated)
  Antiseptic solution
  Lubricant
  Cotton balls or gauze squares

Forceps
Straight or indwelling catheter
Prefilled syringe
Basin (base of kit usually serves
  as this)
Specimen container
Flashlight or lamp

Urine collection bag and drainage
  tubing (may be connected to sterile indwelling catheter if a closed
  drainage system is used)
Velcro leg strap or tape
Disposal bag
Waterproof pad or Chux

Action	Rationale
1 Assemble the equipment and follow actions 1 through 3 for female catheterization in Procedure 34-1.	

(continued)

PROCEDURE 34-2 *(continued)*

Catheterizing the Male Urinary Bladder (Straight and Indwelling)

Action

Rationale

2 Position the client on his back with the thighs slightly apart. Drape the client so that only the area around the penis is exposed.

This prevents unnecessary exposure.

3 Follow actions 5 to 7 for female catheterization in Procedure 34-1.

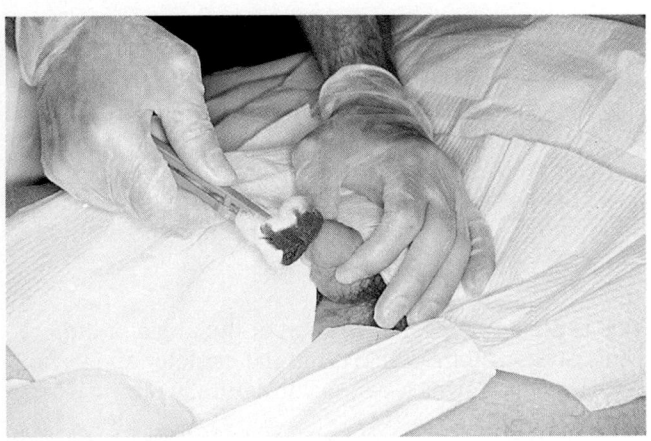

Action 3: Clean the area of the meatus.

4 Put on sterile gloves. Open the sterile drape and place on the client's thighs. Place the fenestrated drape with the opening over the penis.

This maintains a sterile working area.

5 Place the catheter set on or next to the client's legs on the sterile drape.

The sterile setup should be arranged so that the nurse's back is not turned to it, nor should it be out of the nurse's range of vision.

6 Open all supplies:
   a *If the catheter is to be indwelling,* test the catheter balloon. Remove the protective cap on the tip of the syringe and attach the syringe prefilled with sterile water to the injection port. Inject appropriate amount of fluid. If balloon inflates properly, withdraw fluid and leave syringe attached to port.

A balloon that does not inflate or that leaks must be replaced before insertion in the client.

   b Pour antiseptic solution over cotton balls or gauze. Open the specimen container if specimen is to be obtained.

It is necessary to open all supplies and prepare for the procedure while both hands are sterile.

7 *Generously* lubricate the catheter for about 15 to 18 cm (6 to 7 inches).

Generous lubrication is especially important because of the length and tortuousness of the male urethra. The lubricant decreases friction.

8 Lift the penis with your nondominant hand, which is then considered contaminated. Retract the foreskin in the uncircumcised male client. Clean the area at the meatus with a cotton ball held with a forceps. Use a circular motion, moving from the meatus toward the base of the penis for three cleansings.

The hand touching the penis becomes contaminated. Cleansing the area around the meatus and under the foreskin in the uncircumcised male client helps prevent infection. Moving from the meatus toward the base of the penis prevents bringing organisms to the meatus.

(continued)

P R O C E D U R E   3 4 - 2 *(continued)*

Catheterizing the Male Urinary Bladder (Straight and Indwelling)

Action	Rationale
9 Hold the penis with slight upward tension and perpendicular to the client's body. Ask the client to bear down as if voiding. With your dominant hand, place the drainage end of the catheter in the receptacle. *For insertion of an indwelling catheter* that is preattached to sterile tubing and drainage container (closed drainage system), position the catheter and setup within easy reach on the sterile field.	Holding the penis up with slight traction helps straighten the urethra.
10 Insert the tip into the meatus. Advance the catheter 15 to 20 cm (6 to 8 inches) or until urine flows. Do not use force to introduce the catheter. If the catheter resists entry, ask the client to breathe deeply and rotate the catheter slightly. *For an indwelling catheter,* once urine drains, advance the catheter another 1.3 to 2.5 cm (½ to 1 inch). Lower the penis.	The male urethra is about 20 cm long. Deep breaths or slight twisting of the catheter may ease the catheter past resistance at the sphincters. Advancing an indwelling catheter an additional 1.3 to 2.5 cm (½ to 1 inch) ensures its placement in the bladder and facilitates inflation of the balloon without damaging the urethra.
11 Follow Actions 16 through 21 for female catheterization in Procedure 34-1 except that the catheter may be secured to the upper thigh or lower abdomen with the penis directed toward the client's chest. Slack should be left in the catheter to prevent tension.	This is done to prevent irritation at the angle of the penis and scrotum. Slack left in the catheter allows for penile erection, which can occur naturally during sleep.

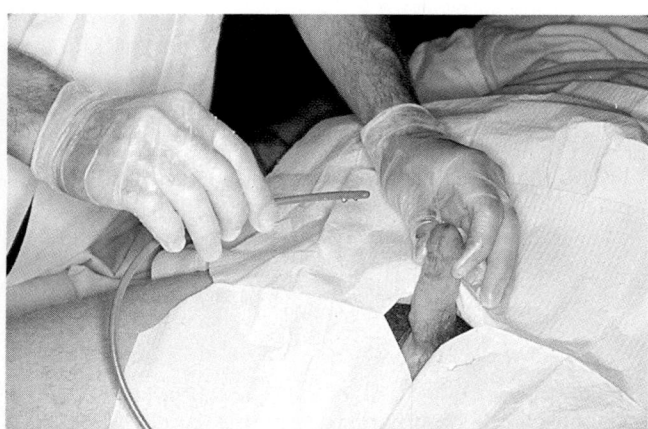

Action 9: Preparing to insert the catheter.

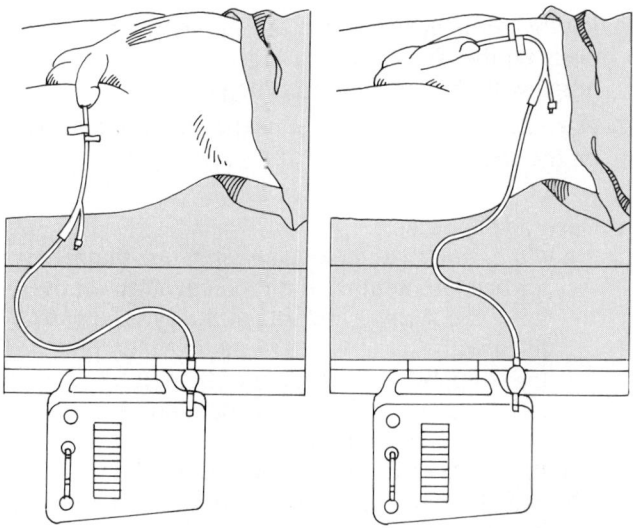

Action 11: Secure the catheter to the upper thigh or lower abdomen, allowing slack to prevent tension.

Age Considerations

If the client is a child, the size of the catheter must be adapted accordingly.

Home Care Considerations

If self-catheterization must be performed in the home, clean technique is appropriate. The bladder's natural resistance to microorganisms normally found in the home makes sterile technique unnecessary. Rubber catheters must be washed thoroughly before boiling for 20 minutes. Dry and store properly for next usage.

- Clip the drainage tubing to the bottom bed linen to help hold the drainage tube in the proper place while the client is in bed. This helps prevent pooling of urine in the drainage tubing.
- Keep the drainage bag off the floor at all times to reduce the risk of infection. The floor is grossly contaminated!

Irrigating the Indwelling Catheter The flushing of a tube, canal, or area with solution is called **irrigation**. The purpose of a catheter irrigation is to restore or maintain its patency. Procedures 34-3 and 34-4 describe how to irrigate an indwelling catheter.

Continuous or frequent irrigations may be ordered when blood clots or other debris threaten to block the catheter. In the past, the procedure was done routinely for almost all indwelling catheters, but because this is another means of introducing pathogens, it is now recommended that an irrigation should be done only when there is a demonstrated need. A sterile irrigation set is required each time the catheter is irrigated. Natural irrigation of the catheter through increased fluid intake by the client is the preferred technique.

Preferably, the client who needs frequent irrigation so that the catheter and tubing remain patent will have a triple-lumen catheter with continuous irrigation (Procedure 34-5).

(Text continues on p. 880)

P R O C E D U R E 3 4 - 3

Irrigating the Catheter Using the Closed System

Equipment

Sterile basin or container
Gauze squares or cotton balls with disinfectant or alcohol swabs
Waterproof drape
30- to 50-mL syringe with 18- or 19-gauge needle

Sterile irrigating solution (at room temperature or warmed to body temperature)
Bath blanket
Disposable gloves

Action	Rationale
1 Assemble equipment. Wash your hands. Explain the procedure and its purpose to the client.	Organization facilitates performance of task. Handwashing deters spread of microorganisms. An explanation encourages client cooperation and reduces apprehension.
2 Provide for privacy by closing the curtains or door and draping the client with the bath blanket.	The procedure may be embarrassing for the client.
3 Assist the client to a comfortable position and expose the aspiration port on the catheter setup. Place the waterproof drape under the catheter and aspiration port.	This provides for adequate visualization. The drape protects the client and the bed from leakage.
4 Open the sterile supplies. Pour sterile solution into the sterile basin. Aspirate irrigant (30 to 50 mL) into the sterile syringe and attach the capped sterile needle. Don gloves.	This prevents the spread of microorganisms and contact with blood or body substances.
5 Disinfect the aspiration port with alcohol swabs or gauze square with antiseptic solution.	This prevents the spread of microorganisms.
6 Clamp or fold the catheter tubing distal to the aspiration port.	This directs the irrigating solution into the bladder.
7 Remove the cap and insert the needle into the port. Gently instill solution into the catheter.	Gentle irrigation prevents damage to the lining of the bladder.
8 Remove the needle from the port. Unclamp the tubing and allow irrigant and urine to drain. Repeat the procedure as necessary.	Gravity aids drainage of urine and irrigant from the bladder.

(continued)

PROCEDURE 34-3 (continued)

Irrigating the Catheter Using the Closed System

Action	Rationale
9 Assess the client's response to the procedure and the quality and amount of drainage. Document on the client's chart.	This provides accurate documentation of the procedure.
10 Record the amount of irrigant used on the intake and output record. Subtract this from the urine output when totaled.	Subtracting irrigant total from drainage in urine collection bag provides accurate recording of urine output.
11 Remove equipment and discard uncapped needle and syringe in appropriate receptacle. Remove gloves and wash your hands. Make client comfortable.	Handwashing deters the spread of microorganisms. Proper disposal of needle prevents the nurse accidentally puncturing self.

PROCEDURE 34-4

Irrigating the Catheter Using the Open System

Equipment

Sterile irrigation tray with
   Sterile container and basin
   Sterile Asepto or Toomey syringe
Disposable gloves (optional)
Gauze squares or cotton balls with
   disinfectant or alcohol swabs

Sterile irrigating solution (at room
   temperature or warmed to body
   temperature)
Bath blanket
Sterile cover for tip of drainage
   tubing

Action	Rationale
1 Follow actions 1 and 2 in Procedure 34-3.	
2 Assist the client to a comfortable position and expose the connection between the catheter and the drainage tubing. Position a waterproof drape under the catheter.	This provides for adequate visualization. The drape protects the client and the bed from leakage.
3 Open the sterile supplies. Don gloves. Pour sterile solution into the sterile container. Remove the tip from the Asepto syringe and aspirate irrigant (30 mL) into the syringe.	This prevents the spread of microorganisms.
4 Clean the catheter junction with a gauze pad and disinfectant or alcohol swab.	This prevents the spread of microorganisms into bladder tissue.
5 Disconnect the catheter and drainage tube. Place the sterile cover over the drainage tip and secure drainage tubing on the bed. Hold catheter tubing 2.5 cm (1 inch) from its open end.	This avoids contaminating the sterile drainage system with microorganisms.
6 Position the sterile basin beneath the catheter. Insert the tip of the Asepto syringe into the catheter and gently irrigate with solution.	Gentle irrigation is less traumatic to the lining of the bladder.

(continued)

PROCEDURE 34-4 *(continued)*

Irrigating the Catheter Using the Open System

Action	Rationale
7 Remove the syringe, keeping the bulb compressed, and allow drainage to return by gravity flow into the basin. If there is no return, gently aspirate the solution from the catheter. Continue with irrigation as ordered by the physician.	Gravity aids the drainage of urine and irrigant from the bladder. Irrigation maintains patency of the urinary drainage system.

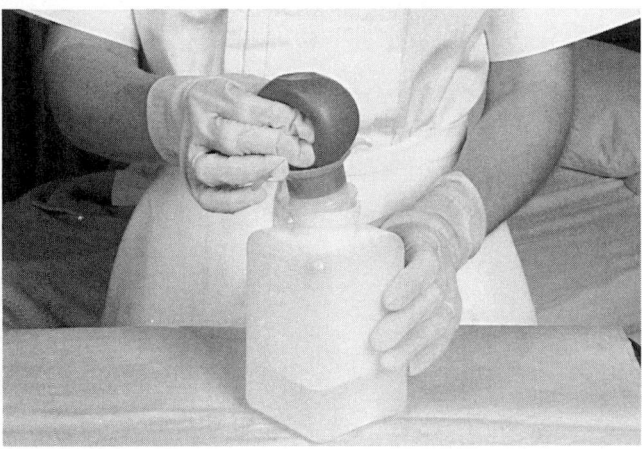

Action 3: Aspirating irrigant into syringe.

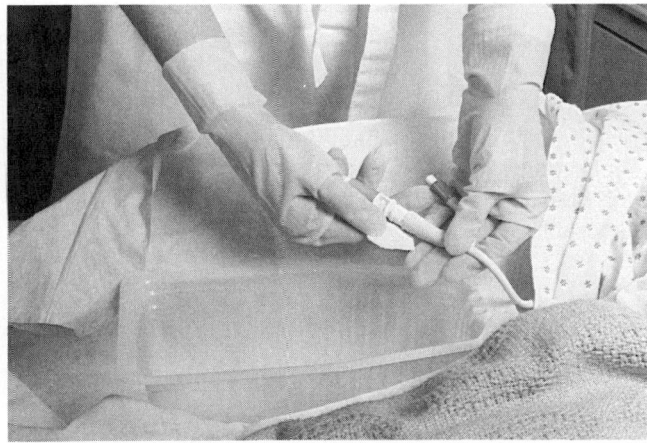

Action 4: Disinfecting the aspiration port.

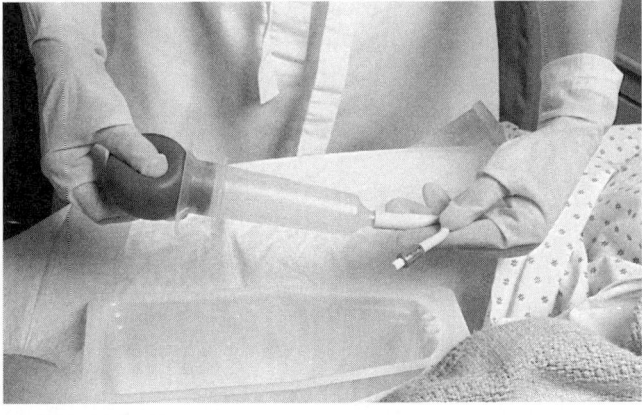

Action 6: Gently instilling solution.

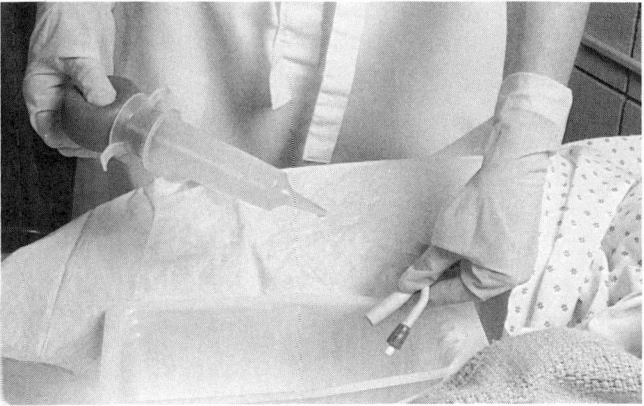

Action 7: Remove syringe, keeping bulb compressed, and allow drainage to return by way of gravity flow into basin.

Action	Rationale
8 Reattach the drainage tube to the catheter, being careful not to contaminate the system. Secure with tape or a Velcro leg strap. Remove gloves.	This prevents entry of microorganisms. The tape or the Velcro leg strap discourages separation of the catheter and the tubing.
9 Document the client's response to the procedure and the quality and amount of drainage on the client's chart.	This provides accurate documentation of the procedure.
10 Remove the equipment and make the client comfortable. Wash your hands.	Handwashing deters the spread of microorganisms.

P R O C E D U R E 3 4 - 5

Giving a Continuous Bladder Irrigation

Equipment

Sterile irrigating solution (at room temperature or warmed to body temperature), usually 2000-mL bags

Sterile tubing with drip chamber and clamp for connection to irrigating solution

IV pole

Three-way Foley catheter in place in client's bladder

Foley drainage setup (tubing and collection bag)

Bath blanket

Disposable gloves (optional)

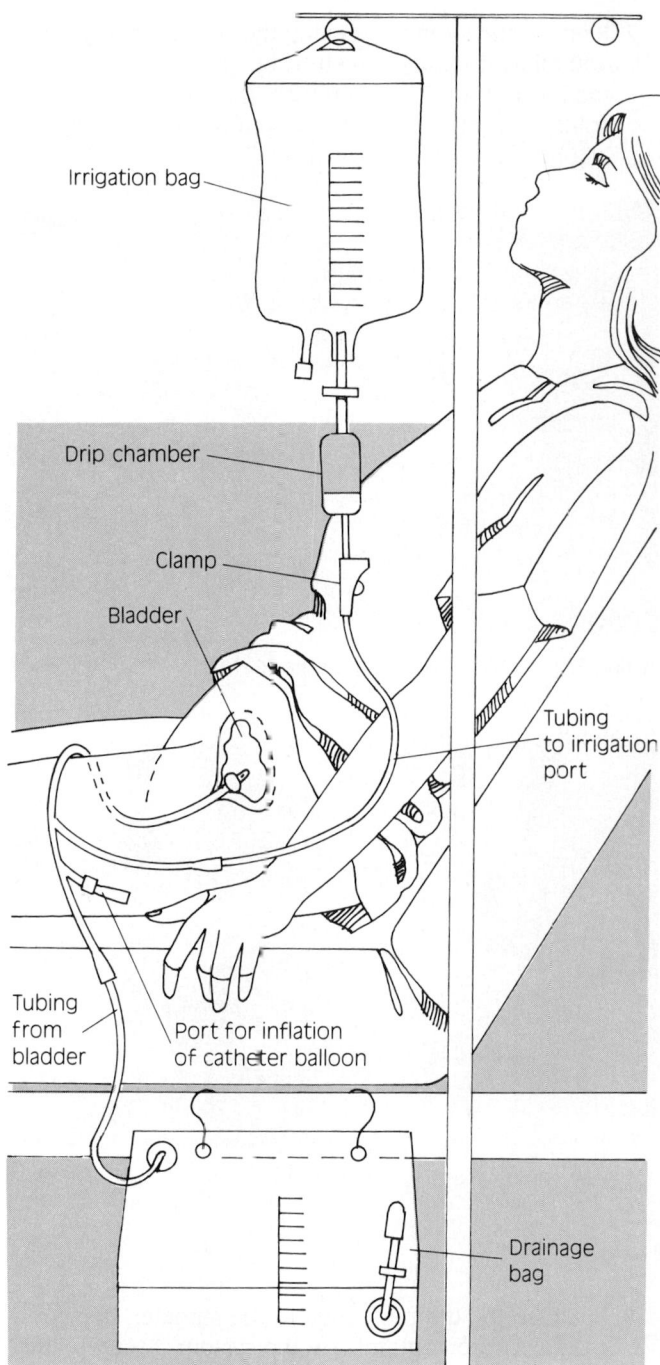

Irrigation bag

Drip chamber

Clamp

Bladder

Tubing to irrigation port

Tubing from bladder

Port for inflation of catheter balloon

Drainage bag

Continuous irrigation.

(continued)

Giving a Continuous Bladder Irrigation

Action	Rationale
1 Explain the procedure and its purpose to the client.	An explanation encourages client cooperation and reduces apprehension.
2 Assemble the equipment.	Organization facilitates performance of tasks.
3 Wash your hands	Handwashing deters the spread of microorganisms.
4 Provide for privacy by closing the curtains or door and draping the client with the bath blanket.	The procedure may be embarrassing for the client.
5 Prepare the sterile irrigation bag for use as directed by the manufacturer. Secure the clamp and attach the sterile tubing with drip chamber to the container. Hang the bag on IV pole 2½ to 3 feet above the level of the client's bladder. Release the clamp and remove the protective cover on the end of the tubing without contaminating it. Allow the solution to flush the tubing and remove air. Reclamp.	Irrigation solution continuously bathes the lining of the bladder and keeps the catheter patent. Flushing the tubing before irrigation clears air from the tubing that might cause bladder distention.
6 Using sterile technique, attach the irrigation tubing to the irrigation port of the three-way Foley catheter. If a closed system is used, tubing may already be connected to the irrigation port on the catheter.	Sterile technique prevents the spread of microorganisms into the bladder.

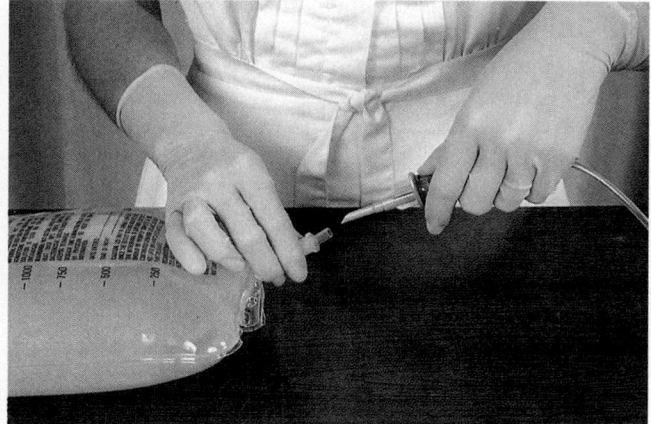

Action 5: Inserting spike into container of irrigating solution.

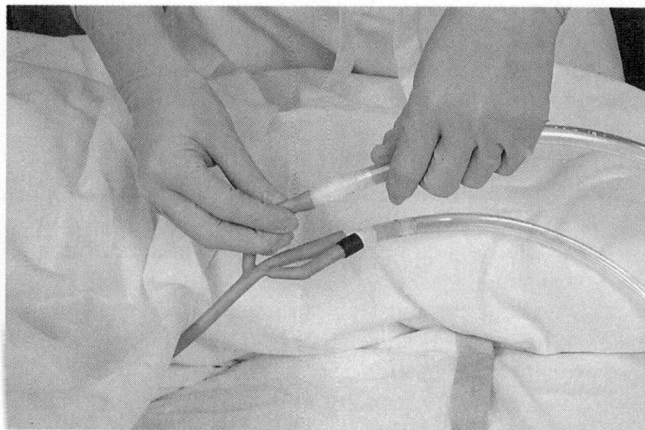

Action 6: Attaching irrigation tubing to irrigation port of three-way Foley catheter using sterile technique.

Action	Rationale
7 Release the clamp on the irrigation tubing and regulate the flow according to the physician's order.	This allows for continual gentle irrigation without causing discomfort to the client.
8 As irrigation is completed, clamp the tubing. Do not allow the drip chamber to empty. Disconnect the empty bag and attach a full irrigation bag. Continue as ordered by the physician.	This eliminates the need to separate tubing from the catheter and clear air from the tubing. Opening the drainage system provides access for introduction of microorganisms.
9 Assess the client's response to the procedure and the quality and amount of drainage. Document on the client's chart.	This provides accurate documentation of the procedure.
10 Record the amount of irrigant used on the intake and output record. Don gloves and empty the drainage collection bag as each new container is hung and record.	This ensures accurate recording of urine output. Gloves protect against exposure to blood, body substances, and microorganisms.
11 Wash your hands.	Handwashing deters the spread of microorganisms.

Caring for the Client The following are nursing measures used when caring for a client with an indwelling catheter:

- Be sure to wash hands before and after caring for a client with an indwelling catheter. Wear gloves to protect against possible exposure to blood and body substances.
- Clean the perineal area thoroughly, especially around the meatus, twice a day and after each bowel movement.
- Use soap or detergent and water to clean the perineal area, and rinse the area well. Do not use powders and lotions after cleaning. Some authorities recommend cleaning the area around the meatus with an antiseptic, for example, povidone-iodine (Betadine).
- Apply a topical antibiotic ointment at the meatus, as ordered.
- Make sure that the client maintains a generous fluid intake. This helps prevent infection and irrigates the catheter naturally by increasing urine output.
- Encourage the client to be up and about, as ordered.
- Note the volume and character of urine, and record observations carefully. The urine can be observed through the drainage tubing and in the collecting container. The usual procedure is to note and record the amount of urine on the client's intake-and-output record every 8 hours. The collecting container is calibrated, but the volume markings are only approximations. The urine should be emptied into a graduated container that is accurately calibrated for correct determination of output.
- Do not open the drainage system to obtain urine specimens or to measure urine. If the tubing becomes disconnected, wipe the ends of both tubes with antiseptic solution before reconnecting. When emptying the drainage bag, make sure the drainage spout does not touch a contaminated surface.
- Teach the client the importance of personal hygiene, especially the importance of careful cleaning after having a bowel movement and thorough washing of hands frequently.
- Promptly report any signs of infection. These include a burning sensation and irritation at the meatus, cloudy urine, a strong odor to the urine, an elevated temperature, and chills.
- Help keep the urine acid in character, since acidity retards bacterial growth. Plain water in increased amounts, cranberry juice, prune juice, and ascorbic acid are helpful in acidifying urine.
- Help the client take a tub or shower bath when permitted. The catheter should be clamped temporarily if the collecting container is higher than the bladder at any time. In a tub, with the catheter clamped, the container can be hung over the side of the tub. Care should be taken so that the catheter does not remain clamped after the bath. In a shower, the container can be attached to the client's leg, in which case clamping the tube usually is unnecessary.

- Plan to change indwelling catheters only as necessary. If rolling the drainage tubing between the hands frees the tubing of sandy particles, it is time to change the catheter. The usual interval between catheter changes varies from 5 days to 2 weeks. The less often a catheter is changed, the less the likelihood that an infection will develop.

Teaching Clients Clients who have indwelling catheters should be taught how the system functions and how they can assist with their care. Teaching points include keeping the tubing free of kinks, maintaining a constant downward flow of the urine, maintaining an adequate fluid intake, and promptly reporting any unusual symptoms.

Removing the Indwelling Catheter The removal of an indwelling catheter and the aftercare of the client should include the following nursing measures:

- Don disposable gloves.
- Be *sure the balloon is deflated before attempting to remove the catheter*. This is done by inserting a syringe into the balloon valve and aspirating the fluid initially used to inflate the balloon. Carefully check the size of the balloon so you know how much fluid to remove before proceeding. Do *not* cut the tubing with scissors.
- Have the client take several deep breaths to relax while gently removing the catheter. Wrap the catheter in a towel or disposable, waterproof drape.
- Clean the area at the meatus thoroughly with antiseptic swabs after the catheter is removed.
- See to it that the client's fluid intake is generous, and record the client's intake as well as time and amount of output for at least 24 hours or according to agency policy. Instruct the client to void into the bedpan or urinal.
- Inform the client that it may take a little while for the bladder to reestablish voluntary control and that an accident is not unusual.
- Tell the client that there may be a slight burning sensation the first time or two the client voids after the catheter is removed.
- Observe the urine carefully for any abnormalities.
- Record and report any unusual signs, such as discomfort, a burning sensation when voiding, bleeding, and changes in vital signs, especially the client's temperature. Be alert to any signs of infection, and report them *promptly*.

Teaching Self-Catheterization

Medical asepsis practices are used by clients who self-catheterize. There is less danger of nosocomial urinary tract infection when the procedure is done at home rather than in a hospital. Research has shown that the technique is safe. The procedure for self-catheterization is essentially the same as that used by the nurse to catheterize a client. The following are some differences, which should be emphasized when teaching self-catheterization:

Remembering my first hospital experiences, I would have to say that doing my first catheterization was the scariest. I was working with a nurse on the maternity floor. Our patient had not voided in more than 8 hours and seemed to be in great discomfort. We palpated her abdomen to see if her bladder was distended, and it was. Because she didn't have an urge to void, we decided to straight cath her to lessen her discomfort. The nurse I was working with turned and handed me the kit. She said, "You know what to do, right?" Automatically I replied, "Sure."

My heart began to race. Of course I knew the procedure, but I never actually did it on a real person. Not only was I nervous about doing the procedure, but I also didn't want to make her labor more painful. The nurse, out of courtesy, asked the patient if she minded if I did the procedure. Thank God the patient had a soft side for a beginner. Smiling she looked at me and said, "You know what you're doing right?" Again I said, "Sure." I began setting up to begin my mission. To my amazement, I really did remember how to prepare for a catheterization. I even was amazed that my sterile procedure wasn't bad for the first time. When it was time to insert the catheter, I took a deep breath. Thankfully, it went in nice and smooth, and I reached the bladder in seconds. The urine began flowing through rapidly. It seemed like it would never stop. Amazingly, it filled the container. I removed the catheter, cleaned up, and let out my breath.

In summary, I was glad that I had the experience to do a catheterization. The nurse told me that I did a good job, which made me feel good. Also, my patient thanked me for relieving some of her discomfort and gave me a reassuring smile. As I look back now, it wasn't as bad as I had myself believe it would be. Even though it's invasive to the patient, sometimes it's necessary. I want to do everything I can to help my patients. Now, I look at all my new adventures as helping my patients feel better.

—Alysia Paxson, Holy Family College,
   Philadelphia

- The client voids first and then inserts the catheter for residual urine.
- The male client uses a comfortable position in bed or a sitting or standing position. The female client may sit on a toilet or lay in bed in a comfortable position.
- A good light is important, especially for the female client.
- The female client can locate the meatus with the use of a mirror but should learn to insert the catheter using the touch technique. She more easily locates the urinary meatus by developing an awareness of the different sensations when the clitoris, urinary meatus, and vagina are touched. The fingers on the nondominant hand locate the meatus by placing the index finger on the clitoris and the third and fourth fingers at the vagina. A female self-catheterization aid has been developed to help in locating the urinary meatus (Webber-Jones, 1991).
- The client should press down with the abdominal muscles to remove as much urine from the bladder as possible before removing the catheter.
- The interval between catheterizations will vary. At first, catheterization may be necessary every 2 to 3 hours, but the interval can gradually be increased. According to Webber-Jones (1991), an oral intake greater than 2 qt (about 2000 mL) daily and catheterized amounts greater than 450 mL (about 1 pint) usually indicate the need to catheterize five times a day.
- The client must wash reusable plastic equipment well in soap or detergent and water, and rinse, dry, and store it in a clean, covered container.
- A minimum of 1500 mL (1.6 quart) of fluid a day is recommended for adults.

Applying a Condom Catheter

When voluntary control of urination is not possible for male clients, an alternative to an indwelling catheter is the **condom catheter**. This soft, pliable device made of plastic or rubberized material is applied externally to the penis. It is connected to tubing and a leg bag during the day and a drainage bag at night, and thus allows the client to be dressed and to participate in activities without problem. Instructions for applying a condom catheter are given in Procedure 34-6.

PROCEDURE 34-6

Applying a Condom Catheter

Equipment

Condom sheath in appropriate size
Basin of warm water and soap
Washcloth and towel
Bath blanket

Disposable gloves (optional)
Elastic strip or Velcro strap
Reusable leg bag with drainage
    tubing or urinary drainage setup

Action

1 Explain the procedure to the client.

2 Assemble the equipment. Prepare urinary drainage setup or reusable leg bag for attachment to the condom sheath.

3 Wash your hands.

4 Assist the client to the supine position. Close the curtain or door. Use the bath blanket and sheet to expose only the client's genital area.

5 Don disposable gloves. Wash the genital area with soap and water, rinse, and dry thoroughly.

6 Roll the condom sheath outward onto itself. Grasp the penis firmly with your nondominant hand. Apply the condom sheath by rolling it onto the penis with your dominant hand. Leave 2.5- to 5-cm (1 to 2-inch) space between the tip of the penis and the end of the condom sheath.

7 Apply the elastic or Velcro strap in a snug but not tight manner. Do not allow the elastic or Velcro to come in contact with the skin.

8 Connect the condom sheath to the drainage setup. Avoid kinking or twisting of the drainage tubing.

Rationale

This provides reassurance and promotes client co-operation.

This provides for an organized approach to the task.

Handwashing deters the spread of microorganisms.

This provides privacy for the client.

Washing removes urine, secretions, and microorganisms. The penis must be clean and dry to minimize skin irritation.

Rolling the condom sheath outward allows for easier application. The space prevents irritation to the tip of the penis and allows for free drainage of urine.

The elastic or Velcro strap should secure the condom sheath but not interfere with blood circulation to the penis.

The collection device keeps the client dry. Kinked tubing encourages backflow of urine.

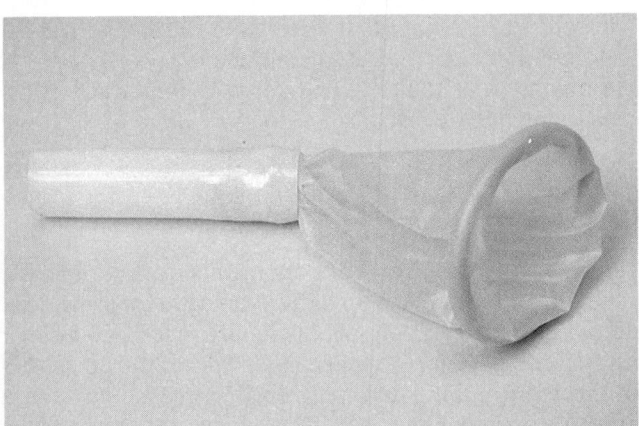

Condom sheath.

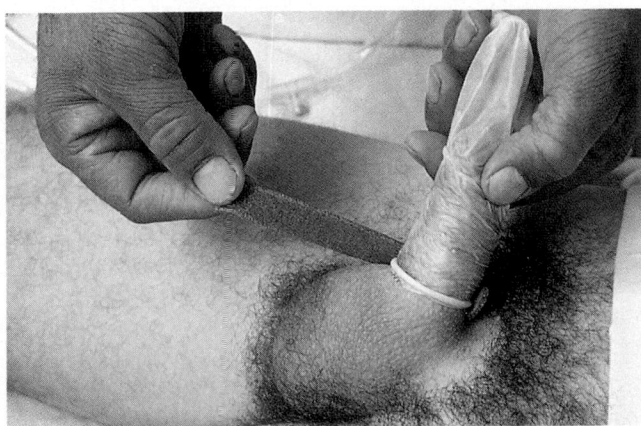

Action 7: Application of a Velcro strap at the base of the condom sheath.

(continued)

PROCEDURE 34-6 *(continued)*

Applying a Condom Catheter

Action	Rationale

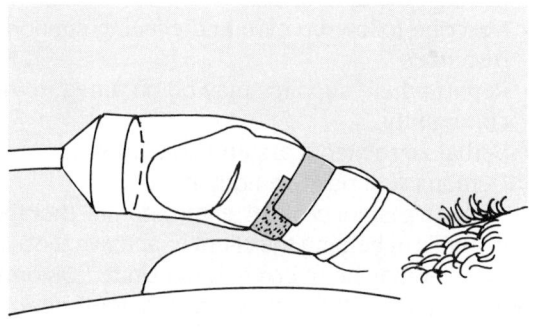

Action 8: Drawing of extra space at end of sheath and smoothing tubing to drainage unit.

9 Remove the equipment. Place the client in a comfortable, safe position. Wash your hands.

This provides a safe, comfortable setting for the client. Handwashing deters the spread of microorganisms.

10 Assess the client's response and record observations on the client's chart.

This provides accurate documentation and observation of urine output.

Nursing care includes vigilant skin care to prevent excoriation. The condom should be removed daily and the penis washed with soap and water, carefully dried, and inspected for irritation. The manufacturer's instructions for applying the condom should be followed because there are several variations. In all cases, care must be taken to fasten the condom securely enough to prevent leakage, yet not so tightly as to constrict the blood vessels in the area. The tip of the tubing should be kept 2.5 to 5 cm (1 to 2 inches) beyond the tip of the penis to prevent irritation to the sensitive glans. Maintaining free urinary drainage is another nursing priority because tubing may become kinked. To prevent urine from excoriating the glans, the tubing that collects urine from the condom should be positioned to draw urine away from the penis.

Assisting With Urinary Diversions

Obstructions or tumors in the urinary tract may require some clients to have the urinary flow diverted surgically. An **ileal conduit** is a surgical diversion of the ureters to the ileum rather than the bladder. This separated section of the small intestine is then brought to the abdominal wall, where urine is excreted through a stoma or artificial opening on the body surface created surgically. Figure 34-8 shows how the ureters are diverted in an ileal conduit. Other types of surgery for urinary diversion also are performed, and except for the location of the stoma, the nursing care is similar. Such diversions usually are permanent, and the client wears an external appliance to collect the urine, since voluntary control over elimination of the urine from the stoma is not possible.

The client who has an ileal conduit must adapt to an altered body image and usually needs assistance in coping. The time required for adaptation varies, and the adjustment often can be promoted by numerous sources of support, such as family, friends, nurses, physicians, and people with a similar health problem. Most of all, the client needs to

FIGURE 34-8

Location of an ileal conduit. The ureters are brought to the ileum of the small intestine and a stoma is made where the urine is excreted. (Redrawn after *Types of Ostomies.* Copyright 1979. Hollister Inc. All rights reserved.)

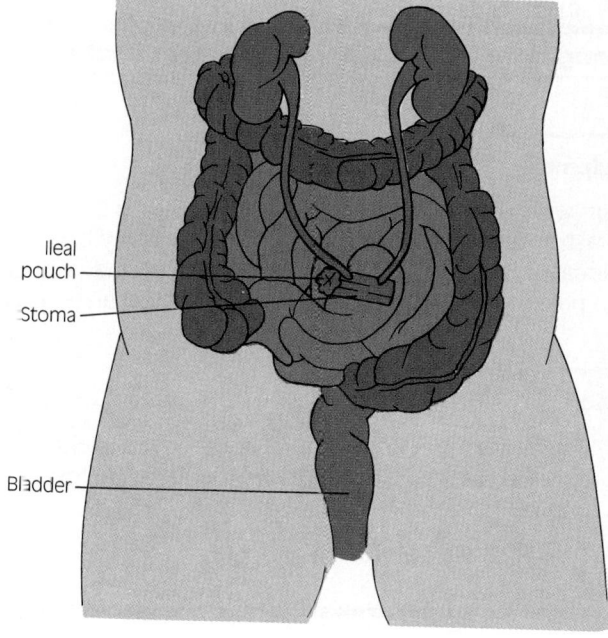

Ileal pouch

Stoma

Bladder

understand that an active, useful life is compatible with a urinary diversion.

Appliances to Collect Urine Typically, the external appliance is a soft rubber or plastic pouch that is either reusable or disposable. The upper part of the pouch has a firm faceplate several inches in diameter that has an opening the size of the stoma. Some faceplates are detachable from the pouch. The plate surface is firmly secured around the stoma opening with a moisture-proof adherent so that no urine leakage can occur. Many clients also use an elasticized belt worn around the waist for added support. The lower end of the pouch may have a drainage valve, which is used for emptying the pouch.

The pouch should be emptied before it becomes heavy with the weight of urine and causes the seal to loosen. For most people, this means emptying the appliance several times a day. Urine-collection receptacles designed to be placed under the bed are available for attachment to the appliance at night.

Changing the Urinary Appliance The frequency of changing the appliance varies with the type being used. The appliance should be changed after a time of low fluid intake, such as early morning. Urine production will be less at this time, which makes changing the appliance easier. Procedure 34-7 describes how to change an appliance worn over an ileal conduit.

Teaching the Client Nursing care is directed toward client education and the achievement of optimal self-care. As responsibility for self-care is assumed, the client should be taught to make the necessary observations, to be aware of indications of problems, and to recognize when to seek assistance. For these goals to be met, the client needs to be able to do the following:

- Explain the cause for the urinary diversion and the rationale for treatment
- Demonstrate self-care behaviors that effectively manage the diversion
- Describe follow-up care and existing support resources
- Report where supplies may be obtained in the community
- Verbalize related fears and concerns
- Demonstrate positive body image

The assistance of an enterostomal therapist can be invaluable in helping the client to achieve these outcomes. The client may be referred to the United Ostomy Association for further information and helpful periodicals. Detailed discussion of other aspects of caring for a client with a urinary diversion can be found in clinical texts.

Evaluating

The nurse evaluates the effectiveness of a plan of care to promote healthy urinary functioning by checking whether the client has met the individualized client goals specified in the plan. Nursing care is considered effective if the client expresses satisfaction with the regular voiding pattern and is able to:

- Produce a sufficient quantity of urine to maintain fluid, electrolyte, and acid–base balance
- Empty the bladder completely at regular intervals without discomfort

---

P R O C E D U R E 3 4 - 7

Changing a Stoma Appliance on an Ileal Conduit

Equipment

Basin with warm water, soap, towel, washcloth or cotton balls
Graduated container
Skin protectant or barrier

Sterile 2 × 2 gauze squares
Ostomy bag cut to the correct stomal size (with adhesive-backed faceplate, if available)

Ostomy belt (optional)
Adhesive cement (optional for reusable pouches)
Disposable gloves

Action	Rationale
1 Explain the procedure and encourage the client to observe or participate if possible. Provide for privacy.	Observing or assisting with procedure encourages self-acceptance.
2 Assemble the equipment.	Organization facilitates performance of task.

(continued)

Changing a Stoma Appliance on an Ileal Conduit

Action	Rationale
3 Wash your hands and don disposable gloves.	Handwashing deters the spread of microorganisms. Gloves protect the nurse from blood, body substances, and microorganisms.
4 Have the client sit or stand if able to assist with procedure or assume supine position in bed.	These positions result in less abdominal folds and facilitate removal and application of the device.
5 Empty the pouch being worn into the graduated container (before removing if it is reusable and not attached to straight drainage).	Having the pouch empty before handling it reduces the likelihood of spilling the excretions. The physician may have ordered recording of intake and output.
6 Gently remove the pouch faceplate from the skin.	The seal between the surface of the faceplate and the skin must be broken before the faceplate can be removed. Harsh handling of the appliance can damage the skin and impair the development of a secure seal in the future.
7 Discard the pouch appropriately if disposable, or wash reusable pouch in lukewarm soap and water and allow to air dry.	Thorough cleaning and airing of the appliance reduce odor and deterioration. For aesthetic and infection-control purposes, used appliances should be discarded appropriately.
8 Clean the skin around the stoma with soap and water or a commercial cleaner using washcloth or cotton balls. Make sure you remove all of old adhesive from the skin.	Cleaning the skin removes excretions and old adhesive and skin protectant. Excretions or a buildup of other substances can irritate and damage the skin.
9 Gently pat dry. Make sure the skin around the stoma is thoroughly dry. Assess the stoma and the condition of the surrounding skin.	Careful drying prevents trauma to the skin and stoma. An intact, properly applied urinary collection device protects skin integrity. Any change in the color and size of the stoma may indicate circulatory problems.
10 Place a gauze square or two over the stoma opening.	Continuous drainage must be absorbed to keep the skin dry during the appliance change.
11 Apply a skin protectant to a 5-cm (2-inch) radius around the stoma, and allow it to dry completely, which takes about 30 seconds.	The skin needs protection from the excoriating effect of the excretion and appliance adhesive. Allowing the protectant to dry completely enhances its effectiveness.
12 If necessary, enlarge the size of the faceplate opening to fit the stoma.	The appliance should fit snugly around the stoma, with only 1/16 to 1/8 inch of skin visible around the opening. A faceplate opening that is too small can cause trauma to the stoma. Exposed skin will be irritated by urine if the opening is too large.
13 Apply adhesive to the faceplate or remove the protective covering from the disposable faceplate, carefully position the appliance, and press it in place, moving from the center outward. Remove the gauze squares from the stoma before applying the pouch.	The appliance is effective only if it is properly positioned and securely adhered. Commercial deodorants may be used if odor is a problem.
14 Secure the optional belt to the appliance and around the client.	An elasticized belt helps support the appliance for some people.
15 Remove or discard the equipment and assess the client's response to the procedure. Wash your hands and remove gloves.	The client's response may indicate acceptance of the ostomy as well as the need for health teaching. Handwashing deters the spread of microorganisms.
16 Record the appearance of the stoma and the surrounding skin as well as the client's reaction to the procedure.	A careful record is important for planning the client's care.

- Develop a plan to modify any factors that contribute to current urinary problems or that might adversely affect urinary functioning in the future

- Correct unhealthy urinary habits, such as delaying voiding, drinking insufficient water, and abusing diuretics

 # NURSING PROCESS

in Clinical Practice

Once a urinary problem is detected, the nurse implements each phase of the nursing process to ensure correct identification and treatment of the problem. To identify and manage the urinary problem correctly, the nurse must possess the knowledge and clinical skills described earlier in this chapter. Following in outline format are the focused assessment priorities, client goals, nursing interventions, and evaluative criteria for common nursing diagnoses.

Altered Urinary Elimination related to dysuria
Altered Urinary Elimination related to maturational enuresis
Incontinence (five types with varying causes)
Urinary Retention related to varying causes
High Risk for Infection related to indwelling catheter

Altered Urinary Elimination Related to Dysuria

Dysuria, or difficult urination, is most often associated with a sensation of pain or burning. Clients report feeling the need to void but having great difficulty and pain in starting the stream. Common in women, dysuria is associated with lower urinary tract infections and irritation of the urethral meatus after sexual intercourse or caused by use of bath and feminine hygiene products.

Assessment

- Interview the client for report of painful or burning sensation while voiding and presence of fever, chills, nausea, or flank pain.
- Identify potential causative factors:
  - Infection
  - Sexual activity 1 to 2 days before symptoms
  - Liquid detergent or bubble bath in bath water
  - Examine urine for cloudiness, foul odor, hematuria, and proteinuria.

Planning: Client Goals

The client will:
- Report absence of pain and burning during urination
- Describe appropriate self-care measures to prevent recurrence

Interventions

- Instruct the client about the probable cause of the dysuria, and reassure the client that the distressing symptoms will be relieved with treatment.

- Teach perineal care to include wiping from front to back after voiding and the need to clean the perianal region with soap and water after defecation and intercourse. Female clients also should be instructed to void before and after intercourse to flush the lower urinary tract of bacteria. Because the urethra in the female is short and close to the vagina and anus, bacteria from these areas can easily migrate to the urethral meatus and ascend the urinary tract.
- Encourage a fluid intake of 2000 to 3000 mL to dilute infected urine and flush the system.
- If indicated, assist the client to alter urinary pH by dietary manipulation. Large quantities of water and cranberry juice may acidify the urine and be helpful in reducing bacterial growth. If urine alkalization is warranted to soothe an irritated bladder, eating more vegetables and fruits may be helpful.
- Sitz baths promote relaxation of tense muscles and facilitate healing of an irritated urethral meatus.
- Administer prescribed medications to treat the pathology underlying dysuria.

Evaluative Criteria

The client meets the previously stated goals.

Altered Urinary Elimination Related to Maturational Enuresis

Enuresis is involuntary urination after an age when continence should be present. *Nocturnal enuresis* is bed-wetting that occurs while a person is sleeping, and *diurnal enuresis* occurs when a person is awake. In *primary enuresis*, the child has never had a long period of dryness; in *secondary enuresis*, the pattern of bed-wetting follows a period of dryness of weeks or months. An identifiable stress, such as the birth of a sibling or parental divorce, often precedes the onset of secondary enuresis. It is helpful for parents to understand that enuresis is primarily a maturational problem that usually ceases between ages 6 and 8.

Assessment

- Interview the child and parents to determine
- Pattern of bed-wetting and precipitating factors (if present)
- Response of family members to the child
- History of toilet training
- Familial history of enuresis

- Assess bladder capacity by measuring voided specimen after the child has been instructed to delay voiding as long as possible. Use at least three recordings. Small bladder capacity is less than 300 mL.

Planning: Client Goals

- Child will develop day and nighttime control over urination
- Parents will respond constructively to child

Interventions

- Instruct the parents that enuresis usually is a maturational problem that the child will outgrow with assistance, and that punishing or shaming the child can have harmful effects.
- Share with the child that many other children bed-wet and that this problem will be outgrown.
- If both the parents and the child are motivated, use responsibility and reinforcement therapy. The child can keep a calendar of dry days and nights and contract for rewards.
- If the child has a small bladder capacity, encourage daytime bladder-stretching by helping the child to postpone voiding after drinking fluids.
- If the child is a sound sleeper, limit fluids at bedtime and have the child void immediately before retiring.
- If the child gets too absorbed in daytime play to respond to a full bladder, teach the child how to sense a full bladder and the importance of stopping to void. Reinforce dry days.
- Explore with the family various laundry aids.
- Assist the family to evaluate the pros and cons of a conditioning therapy that involves an alarm system, as well as other therapies.

Evaluative Criteria

The clients meet the previously stated goals.

Urinary Incontinence

Urinary incontinence is the inability to retain urine in the bladder after the age of toilet training. Conservatively, at least 10 million American adults are incontinent (Newman et al., 1991). Katherine Jetter, executive director of HIP (Help for Incontinent People), reports that 1 of every 25 Americans and Canadians is incontinent (HIP Media Packet, 1991). About 30% of elderly people living in the community and at least 50% of nursing home residents are affected (U.S. National Institutes of Health, 1989a). Incontinence is a special problem for elderly people, who often experience decreasing control over micturition and who may find it more difficult to reach a toilet in time to void because of mobility problems or dexterity problems in undressing. The statistics are alarming on two accounts. The discomfort, odor, and embarrassment of urine-soaked clothing can greatly diminish a person's self-concept and cause the person to feel like a social outcast. Urinary incontinence also can cause health care providers to be negatively disposed toward clients (Yu et al., 1991).

Many people believe that incontinence is a normal consequence of the aging process, and they are embarrassed to discuss it with their physicians or health care providers. Certainly there are age-related changes that affect urinary function, but urinary incontinence can be treated, and individualized interventions can help the client to lead a normal life. Advertisements for adult disposable undergarments have increased public awareness about urinary incontinence, but they fail to mention possible treatment alternatives.

In 1986, the North American Nursing Diagnosis Association defined five types of incontinence:

Functional incontinence: The state in which a person experiences an involuntary, unpredictable passage of urine

Reflex incontinence: The state in which a person experiences an involuntary loss of urine, occurring at somewhat predictable intervals when a specific bladder volume is reached

Stress incontinence: The state in which a person experiences a loss of urine of less than 50 mL, occurring with increased abdominal pressure

Total incontinence: The state in which a person experiences a continuous and unpredictable loss of urine

Urge incontinence: The state in which a person experiences involuntary passage of urine, occurring soon after a strong sense of urgency to void

Common causes for each type are listed in the Nursing Diagnoses display.

The Agency for Health Care Policy and Research recently issued clinical practice guidelines and recommendations when caring for adults with urinary incontinence. The focus of this guideline includes the following points:

- Identification and evaluation of incontinence and related problems
- Treatment with behavioral measures, drugs, and surgery
- Public and professional education (United States Department of Health and Human Services, 1992).

Based on the magnitude of this problem, the American Nurses Association and the Association of Rehabilitation Nurses also support this guideline.

Assessment

- Establish a data base to identify the type and severity of incontinence and the effect it is having on daily living. Newman et al. (1991) recommends assessment of the following:
  - Medical history, including history of a cerebrovascular accident, back problem, head injury, or neurovascular problem that affects the bladder; urologic surgery; number and routes of births
  - Drug therapy, particularly any medications possibly contributing to incontinence

R E S E A R C H   I N   N U R S I N G   **Making a Difference**

Urinary Elimination

Urinary incontinence is not a disease, but rather a symptom of other, underlying medical, psychological, or environmental problems. It is an embarrassing, potentially disabling, and costly health problem. Until the past decade, incontinence was seen as an inevitable outcome of the aging process. In recent years, nursing research has helped dispel this myth by examining urinary incontinence from three general perspectives—development of an assessment tool, management techniques for homebound elderly people, and the effectiveness of behavioral inverventions used by independent elderly people at home.

Related Research

Miller, J. (1990). Assessing urinary incontinence. *Journal of Gerontological Nursing, 16*(3), 15–19.

This study was conducted to determine the reliability of the Incontinence Monitoring Record to record patterns of incontinence in selected residents in an intermediate-care nursing home. An educational program and training session was provided for the nursing assistants responsible for the assessment of the incontinence episodes. Reliability testing further supported at least 80% agreement between all nursing assistants instructed in the use of this tool.

Thomas, A., & Morse, J. (1991). Managing urinary incontinence with self-care practices. *Journal of Gerontological Nursing, 17*(6), 9–14.

Thomas and Morse conducted interviews and summarized responses of active people living at home who reported problems with bladder control. Most of the participants had sought medical advice but depended on self-care practices such as restricting fluids, frequent toileting, and use of various absorbent products to manage their incontinence. Nurses were not viewed as being actively involved in the assessment or treatment of incontinence, although an incontinence clinic staffed by nurses was perceived as a solution to this problem.

Rose, M., Baigis-Smith, J., Smith, D., & Newman, D. (1990). Behavioral management of urinary incontinence in homebound older adults. *Home Healthcare Nurse, 8*(5), 10–14.

This study evaluated the effectiveness of behavioral interventions such as Kegel exercises, habit and relaxation training, and dietary modifications coupled with a bowel regimen on homebound elderly people who were periodically incontinent. The results supported the use of these nursing strategies to reduce urinary incontinence in both ambulatory and frail people in the home setting. Nursing involvement also had a beneficial impact on the caregivers of incontinent elderly people.

Summary

Incontinence research presents implications for changing current methods of nursing practice. The diverse causes of urinary incontinence and the various environmental settings must be considered as nurses strive to identify the most successful and clinically realistic methods of significantly improving urinary incontinence.

- Bowel profile, particularly normal schedule, consistency, and history of bowel incontinence
- Diet—how much does the client eat and drink daily, and alcohol intake
- Bladder profile—record of incontinent episodes and precipitating factors
- Environmental evaluation—distance to toilet, height of toilet seat, ability of client to manage own toileting, grab bars and lighting in the bathroom
- Identify high-risk populations. According to Heller and associates (1989), other causative factors that need to be assessed include:
  - Immobility
  - Slowed or unsteady gait
  - Fecal impaction or constipation
  - Confusion or lack of awareness
  - Urinary tract infection or vaginal infections
- Use of diuretics, sedatives, tranquilizers, and antipsychotics
- Depression
- Lack of privacy
- Communication problem
- Inconvenient toilet facilities

Planning: Client Goals

The client will:
- Eliminate or reduce incontinent episodes
- Explain the cause of incontinence and the rationale for treatment
- Participate in a bladder-training or reconditioning program
- Use appropriate incontinent aids (if indicated)
- Maintain skin integrity

- Demonstrate positive body image
- Participate in desired social activities

Interventions

As soon as medical evaluation of the client's problem has been made, nursing measures should be directed toward helping to restore normal functioning.

- Explain that efforts will be made to help the client. This is important to the client.
- Encourage a generous fluid intake—as much as 1800 to 2400 mL daily. Incontinent clients often voluntarily limit fluid intake in an effort to decrease urine output. These clients need to be helped to understand the relation between adequate fluid intake and total body functioning.
- Encourage the client routinely to make an effort to void shortly after taking fluids. Voluntary efforts to either control or start voiding may be sufficiently stimulating to help restore function for some clients.
- Take chronically ill and elderly incontinent clients to the bathroom or offer a bedpan or urinal every 2 to 3 hours. This practice, called *prompted voiding*, sometimes helps start at least some control over incontinence. Praise when they remain continent also appears effective.
- Teach perineal or Kegel exercises if possible. These exercises consist of contracting the muscles as though urination is to be halted. This is followed by relaxing muscles in the area, as though about to start to void. The exercises should be done 15 times each morning and afternoon and 20 times each night. They help strengthen muscles that control voiding.
- Use hygienic measures to keep the incontinent client dry, clean, and comfortable. Great skill often is required to prevent discomfort caused by wet clothing and linens. The ammonia in the urine and lying on wet linen can quickly irritate the skin and soon lead to the development of pressure ulcers.
- Try an external appliance for incontinent male clients, as indicated. Various types of appliances are available. These devices fit over the penis and are secured by straps. A collection bag usually is attached to the client's leg to permit the client to be up and about.
- Use absorbent pads and waterproof garments for female clients. Absorbent, waterproof briefs are available for incontinent clients and are especially effective for women. External appliances have not been found to be particularly comfortable or effective for incontinent women.
- Demonstrate tact and understanding while caring for an incontinent client. Offering emotional support and allowing the client to talk about the problem and to assist with decisions about personal care often are helpful.
- Refer the client to HIP, a nonprofit client advocacy group to educate the public about urinary incontinence (HIP, PO Box 544, Union, SC 29379, 803

579-7900), or The Simon Foundation, a support group for incontinence (The Simon Foundation, Box 835, Wilmette, Illinois 60091, 1 800 23-SIMON).

As a last resort, an indwelling catheter or intermittent clean catheterization may be necessary when other measures prove inadequate.

Under certain conditions, voluntary control of voiding is permanently impaired, but the reflex act of micturition remains intact. Clients with this condition may benefit from a formal *bladder training program*. This behavioral technique, also referred to as *bladder drill*, uses a bladder chart and teaches clients to void at short intervals and then gradually progress, over a period of time, to voiding at longer intervals. Studies indicate success rates of 10% to 15%, especially with stress and urge incontinence (U.S. National Institutes of Health, 1989a). It requires the motivation and cooperation of the client and health personnel.

The nurse should keep in mind that management of the emotional problems of clients with urinary incontinence often is as important for the nurse as management of the physical problems.

Evaluative Criteria

The client meets the previously stated goals.

Urinary Retention Related to Varying Etiologies

Retention occurs when urine is produced normally but not excreted from the bladder. The bladder continues to fill, and may distend to hold 3000 to 4000 mL of urine. In adults, the micturition reflex normally is triggered when the bladder holds 250 to 450 mL of urine. Retention is suspected when clients report

- Difficulty voiding despite urge to void
- Frequent small voidings (less than 50 mL)
- Discomfort in the pubic area
- Urine output that is much less than fluid intake

Palpation and percussion above the symphysis pubis are used to assess bladder distention. The abdomen swells as the bladder rises above the level of the symphysis pubis. The height of the bladder can be determined by palpating with light pressure on the abdomen. Physicians may order a client catheterized for **residual urine** to determine if urine is being retained in the bladder after voiding. All but 1 to 3 mL of urine normally is excreted from the bladder with each voiding. The client is catheterized after voiding, and both the amount of urine voided and that collected by catheterization are recorded.

Retention often is temporary, commonly after surgery that involves the lower abdomen, pelvis, bladder, or urethra, especially if ambulation is delayed or fluid intake is minimal. Any mechanical obstruction, such as swelling at the meatus, which often occurs after childbirth, or an enlarged prostate in men, may cause retention. The cause also may be psychic or due to certain disease conditions. Injuries to the spinal cord may cause permanent retention.

Urine that pools in the bladder predisposes the client to urinary tract infection.

Assessment

- Strict fluid intake and output; record time and amount of voidings.
- Note complaints of pain in the pubic area, swelling, urgency, frequency, dysuria.
- Palpate and percuss above the symphysis pubis.
- Catheterize for residual urine if indicated (ordered).

Planning: Client Goals

The client will:
- Verbalize the importance of emptying the bladder as soon as possible
- Empty the bladder completely as evidenced by:
  - Quantity of urine voided (24-hour output about equal to fluid intake)
  - Normal pattern of voiding reestablished (each voiding more than 50 mL)
  - Flattened pubic area
  - Absence of complaints
- Demonstrate no signs of urinary tract infection

Interventions

- Use nursing measures to stimulate micturition:
  - Provide privacy.
  - Help client to assume natural position.
  - Offer warm fluids to drink.
  - Warm the bedpan.
  - Run tap water within client's hearing.
  - Pour warm water over the perineal area.
  - Place client's hands in warm water.
  - Manually press on the client's abdomen.
- Administer prescribed analgesics, if appropriate, to promote comfort.
- If independent nursing measures fail to produce bladder emptying, contact a physician.
- If prescribed, administer bethanechol chloride (Urecholine), a parasympathomimetic agent that stimulates micturition.
- Catheterization may be ordered. Nursing measures should be exhausted before resorting to catheterizing clients with retention because of the danger of urinary tract infection.

Evaluative Criteria

The client meets the previously stated goals.

High Risk for Infection Related to Indwelling Catheter

Urinary tract infections are second only to respiratory tract infections in frequency of occurrence. Of special importance to nurses is that urinary tract infections are the most common type of hospital-acquired (nosocomial) infections in the United States and Canada. Urinary tract infections account for 53% of all nosocomial infections, and urinary catheters have been implicated in 85% of these (Sawyer, 1989).

Catheterization predisposes to urinary tract infection for the following reasons:
- The introduction of the catheter through the urethra provides a direct route for microorganisms to travel up the urinary tract to the bladder.
- Catheter-induced local irritation to the urethra or bladder predisposes to infection.
- The catheter interferes with the most important defense against bacterial urinary tract infection, the unobstructed flow of urine throughout the urinary tract and regular, complete evacuation of the bladder.
- Clients who require catheterization often have diseases or other conditions that interfere with the body's immune system, thereby decreasing the efficiency of the urinary tract's reaction to bacteriuria.

In summary, clients being catheterized are a highly vulnerable population and demand vigilant nursing care to prevent urinary tract infection. Breaks in aseptic technique may result in serious and even fatal consequences.

Assessment

- Note client complaints of frequency, urgency, dysuria, and nocturia.
- Palpate the suprapubic area for tenderness.
- Urinalysis: Urine may be dark yellow or pinkish red, and cloudy with or without sediment, bacteriuria, and hematuria.
- Urine culture and sensitivity: More than 100,000/mL bacterial colonies; sensitivity disks indicate bacterial sensitivity, intermediate sensitivity, or resistance to a given antibiotic agent.
- With worsening urinary tract infections, fever, chills, nausea, vomiting, and malaise may be present.
- Note that about half of clients with significant bacteriuria are asymptomatic. This is especially true for elderly clients.

Planning: Client Goals

The client will:
- Have a negative urine culture
- Demonstrate no signs of urinary tract infection

Interventions

Prevention
- Force fluids to 2500 to 3000 mL/day.
- Teach client appropriate hygiene (careful cleaning of perineal area after each voiding and bowel movement; wiping front to back).
- Observe urine for color, odor, amount, and frequency.
- Use strict asepsis with catheter insertion and maintenance unless clean technique is indicated. (Inter-

mittent clean catheterization is recommended for long-term maintenance at home when a catheter is required for bladder emptying. The reduced number and types of bacteria present in the home environment decrease the likelihood of nosocomial infection.)

Treatment

- Obtain urine for urinalysis and for urine culture and sensitivity.
- Administer antimicrobial medication as ordered. En-

courage client to continue medication for the entire period prescribed (usually 10 days).
- Ensure adequate hydration by oral or intravenous route.
- Monitor intake and output.
- Maintain thorough perineal hygiene.

Evaluative Criteria

The client meets the previously stated goals.

CASE STUDY

Mrs. Jaspers is an alert 83-year-old woman whose husband of 59 years died 6 months ago. Although Mrs. Jaspers was adamant about wanting to live independently in her own home, arthritis severely restricted her movement and ability to manage. After a hospitalization for pneumonia, she was transferred to a nursing home 1 month ago. Admitting medical diagnoses included hypertension, osteoarthritis, and depression.

Assessment Findings

A comprehensive nursing assessment of Mrs. Jaspers performed 1 month after her admission to the nursing home included the following notations:
- Continent of urine on admission
- At present, incontinent of urine one or two times a day; often found wet in the morning; states it is "too much bother to get into the bathroom"
- Sits in chair in room unless encouraged and assisted to walk, although capable of independent ambulation with care; progressive muscle atrophy and joint stiffness
- No identifiable pathology underlying incontinence
- Medications include a diuretic for hypertension and a tricyclic antidepressant
- Reddened skin in the perineal area

Nursing Diagnoses

Functional Incontinence related to difficult transition to nursing home and mobility deficit
Impaired Skin Integrity related to functional incontinence

Planning: Client Goals

Because Mrs. Jaspers is alert, the nurse works collaboratively with her to develop a plan designed to reestablish urinary continence. The nurse enters the planning phase understanding the relation between Mrs. Jaspers' urinary continence and her physical well-being and self-esteem. After discussion, Mrs. Jaspers indicates minimal acceptance of the following client goals.

Short-Term Goals

By the next monthly assessment, 5/1/93, the client will:
- Verbalize the importance of getting to bathroom toilet when she first feels the need to void
- Demonstrate the ability to walk independently to the bathroom (using cane) to toilet herself
- Demonstrate satisfactory perineal hygiene
- Decrease urinary incontinent episodes to less than three or four per week
- Demonstrate healing of the reddened perineal area

Long-Term Goal

The client will:
- Maintain urinary continence after eliminating incontinent episodes

See the care plan for details of the nursing strategies used to achieve these goals.

Implementation

In implementing the care plan, the nurse needs the following specialized abilities:
- Strong assessment skills (interviewing and physical assessment) to carefully identify the problem and its cause
- Knowledge of pathologic and nonpathologic basis for urinary incontinence and successful treatment strategies
- Interpersonal skills to communicate to Mrs. Jaspers empathy for her situation and the hope that with help, better outcomes are a real possibility
- Teaching, counseling, and caregiver skills to empower Mrs. Jaspers to value and reestablish urinary continence
- Interpersonal and leadership skills to motivate the nursing staff to help Mrs. Jaspers reestablish urinary continence
- Accountability and patience

Documentation

Sample documentation of nursing interventions follows.

Traditional Note Format

4/3/93, nursing

This AM, after an incontinent episode, Mrs. Jaspers began to talk about how hard it is to get adjusted to living here, and commented, "I feel like just giving up." We talked about the importance of being as independent as possible and the dangers of becoming passively dependent. Nursing teaching and counseling included values of independently adhering to usual toileting schedule and importance of perineal hygiene. Two hours later, after lunch, Mrs. Jaspers walked to bathroom and toileted herself. Progress with urinary continence will continue to be monitored. Ability definitely present but encouragement needed.

C. Taylor, RN

SOAP Format

4/24/93, 11 AM, nursing

#1 Functional Incontinence related to difficult transition to nursing home and mobility deficit

S: "I'm too weak today to walk to the bathroom. Why don't you put one of those pads on me that some of the other residents wear?"

O: Incontinent of urine after 2 days of complete dryness

A: Is capable of voluntary control of urination; temporary regression

P: Diagnostic: Continue to explore her desire to be independent and today's reason for regressive behavior.
Educative: Reinforce importance of urinary continence; communicate that this is the staff's expectation of her, and verbally reinforce next period of dryness.

Evaluation

Short-term goal achievement is evaluated at next monthly assessment. See the nursing care plan for related evaluative statements and revisions of the plan of care. Long-term goal achievement is an ongoing evaluation.

NURSING CARE PLAN

for Mrs. Jaspers

Nursing Diagnosis:	Functional Incontinence related to difficult transition to nursing home and mobility deficit as manifested by incontinence of urine one or two times a day; feeling toileting is too much bother; mobility deficits secondary to osteoarthritis; taking a diuretic and antidepressant.
Long-Term Goal:	Client maintains urinary continence after eliminating incontinent episodes.
Goal:	By the next monthly assessment, 5/1/93, the client will: • Verbalize the importance of getting to bathroom or toilet when she first feels the need to void

Nursing Actions	Rationale	Evaluative Statement
Assess the value the client attaches to voluntary control of urination and urinary continence; counsel appropriately.	Unless the client is committed to the plan of care, goal achievement is impossible.	5/1/93 Goal partially met. Client has commented on the importance of regular toileting but still finds this "too much trouble" some days.
Teach the importance of complete bladder emptying at regular intervals and the harmful effects of ignoring the urge to void.	Client understanding of the causes and harmful effects of urinary incontinence may motivate desire for reestablishment of voluntary control.	Revision: Reinforce value. <div align="right">D. Mora, RN</div>
Assess client's normal voiding habits at home and assist her to reestablish these. Initial reminders to toilet herself may be necessary.	Respect for the client's normal voiding schedule and patterns communicates nursing's sincere concern for the individual and encourages client achievement of goals.	

(continued)

NURSING CARE PLAN *(continued)*

for Mrs. Jaspers

Goal: By the next monthly assessment, 5/1/93, the client will:
- Demonstrate the ability to walk independently to the bathroom (using cane) to toilet herself

Nursing Actions	**Rationale**	**Evaluative Statement**
Assess the client's ability to toilet herself independently. Work consistently with her to increase activity tolerance: encourage short walks throughout the day to increase mobility.	One response to experiencing the multiple losses associated with aging is to surrender all control and become increasingly dependent. Non–pathology-based incontinence is less likely to occur if the daily living of the person keeps her more mobile, flexible, oriented, and motivated. An older person who seeks to take control and has a positive self-image is more continent.	5/1/93 Goal met. Client can safely walk to bathroom using cane and toilet herself when she wants to. *D. Mora, RN*
Refer client to occupational therapy for assistance with diagnosis and treatment if necessary.	The specialized skills of the occupational therapist may facilitate relearning toileting skills.	
Communicate clearly that the client is expected to use the toilet to urinate. Refrain from using incontinent briefs or pads. Talk with family about client's having sufficient undergarments to allow changes as needed until control is reestablished.	Understanding that the staff *expects* continence and is committed to working with the client to achieve it is a powerful client motivator.	

Goal: By the next monthly assessment, 5/1/93, the client will:
- Demonstrate satisfactory perineal hygiene

Nursing Actions	**Rationale**	**Evaluative Statement**
Assess client's motivation and ability to be clean, dry, and comfortable.	Client may not understand how easily skin irritation can occur and danger of pressure ulcers.	5/1/93 Goal not met. Client repeatedly neglects AM perineal care.
Teach perineal hygiene.	Keeping the perineal area clean and dry promotes intact skin around the urinary meatus and the perineal area. Proper hygiene measures also decrease the possibility of bacteria or organisms migrating into the bladder.	*Revision:* Reteach both the importance and procedure of perineal care. Assess each AM. *D. Mora, RN*

(continued)

NURSING CARE PLAN (continued)

for Mrs. Jaspers

Goal: By the next monthly assessment, 5/1/93, the client will:
- Decrease urinary incontinent episodes to less than three or four per week

Nursing Actions	Rationale	Evaluative Statement
Communicate to client that the nurses *care* about her reestablishing urinary continence and believe she can do this. Use verbal reinforcement to reward "dry" days.	A common feeling of recently institutionalized elderly people is *abandonment* and the sense that no one cares; response: "Why should I?" Communicating that the client's progress toward goal achievement is valued by the nurses is an excellent encouragement to continue progress.	5/1/93 Goal met. Client in last week was completely dry for 4 of 7 days. Recorded four incontinent episodes. *D. Mora, RN*
Chart incontinent episodes and monitor progress; discuss this with client.	This records progress with incontinent episodes and provides positive reinforcement.	

Nursing Diagnosis: Impaired Skin Integrity related to functional incontinence as manifested by reddened perineal area (skin still intact)

Long-Term Goal: Client will maintain intact skin in the perineal area

---

Goal: By next monthly assessment, 5/1/93, the client will:
- Demonstrate healing of reddened perineal area

Nursing Actions	Rationale	Evaluative Statement
Assess skin for breakdown each AM and PM and after each incontinent episode.	Perineal care is often neglected or assigned to the least trained personnel in care settings. Skin irritation not detected and treated early may progress to serious pressure ulcers.	5/1/93 Goal partially met. Perineal area is less inflamed. *Revision:* Continue to monitor perineal hygiene. No need for protective ointment. *D. Mora, RN*
Teach the client the importance of washing this area carefully with soap and water each AM and after incontinent episodes. Teach the importance of always cleaning and wiping the perineum from front to back to prevent autoinfection. Until incontinent episodes are eliminated, a protective waterproof ointment may be indicated.	The woman who is doing self-care may neglect it entirely or use incorrect technique.	
Cotton underwear should be worn. Nylon pantyhose, girdles, tight-fitting pants should be avoided.	Nylon products tend to hold moisture and may minimize airflow to the perineal area.	

KEY POINTS

- Urinary elimination, a natural process in which the body excretes waste products and material that exceed bodily needs, usually is taken for granted. When urinary problems arise, the nurse realizes that many clients consider urination a private act and may become embarrassed when they need to discuss urination or require assistance with elimination. The nurse implements nursing interventions accordingly.
- Healthy urinary elimination presupposes well-functioning kidneys, ureters, urinary bladder, and urethra. Problems in any of these areas can affect both the amount and the quality of the urine formed and the manner in which it is expelled from the body.
- Other factors that affect urination include growth and development, food and fluid intake, life-style variables, psychologic variables, activity and muscle tone, pathologic conditions, and medications.
- A comprehensive assessment of the urinary system includes the collection of data about voiding patterns and urinary problems and the physical assessment of the kidneys, bladder, urethral meatus, skin integrity, and urine. These findings may need to be correlated with the results of diagnostic tests and procedures for examining urine and the urinary tract.
- Identification of client health problems often is aided by the nurse's careful monitoring of fluid intake and output, collection of urine specimens, and testing of urine specimens for abnormalities.
- Nursing diagnoses may be written specifically addressing problems in urinary functioning (incon-

tinence, pattern alteration, and retention) and identifying the effect urinary problems have on other areas of human functioning (eg, anxiety, comfort, skin integrity).
- Nursing attention to the client's usual voiding schedule, need for privacy, natural position while voiding, and hygiene habits will help ensure the client's comfort and satisfactory urine output. Other measures facilitating normal urination include promoting an optimal fluid intake, strengthening tone in the perineal and abdominal muscles, and using specific measures (eg, running tap water) to initiate voiding.
- The client with cognitive, sensory, motor, neurologic, or endurance deficits may need nursing assistance with the toilet, bedpan, commode, or urinal. Family members also may need to be taught how to assist the client with elimination needs.
- Urinary catheterization may be indicated to relieve urinary retention, obtain select urine specimens, measure residual urine, or empty the bladder before and during surgery and before certain diagnostic procedures. Catheterization is considered the most prominent cause of nosocomial infections, and should be avoided whenever possible.
- Obstructions or tumors in the urinary tract may require some people to have the urinary flow diverted surgically. In the ileal conduit, the ureters are connected to the ileum, and a stoma is created on the abdominal wall. Nursing care is directed toward client education and the achievement of optimal self-care.

STUDY QUESTIONS

1. The nurse collects a urine specimen for routine urinalysis from a client. She is aware that
   a. a sterile specimen is required
   b. standing at room temperature for a prolonged period may alter the urine chemistry
   c. the external meatus should be cleaned with antiseptic soap and water before voiding
   d. a clean-catch midstream specimen is required
2. Which statement would be correct to teach the client in regard to healthy urinary functioning?
   a. drinking more than 2000 mL of fluid per day will cause fluid retention
   b. the healthy adult should drink four to six 8-oz glasses of water per day
   c. because of greater thirst sensitivity, children will drink required amounts of fluid without being reminded
   d. caffeine-containing beverages should be monitored to prevent excess intake
3. When a person has a fever or diaphoresis, the urine output will be which of the following?

a. decreased and highly concentrated
b. decreased and highly dilute
c. increased and concentrated
d. increased and dilute

4. The physician has ordered an indwelling catheter inserted in a hospitalized male client. The nurse is aware that
   a. the male urethra is more vulnerable to injury during insertion
   b. normally a clean technique is required
   c. the catheter is inserted 2 to 3 inches into the meatus
   d. usually smaller catheters are necessary because of the size of the urethra
5. Nursing care for a client with an indwelling catheter includes
   a. irrigation of the catheter with 30 mL of normal saline solution every 4 hours
   b. disconnecting and reconnecting the drainage system quickly to obtain a urine specimen
   c. encouraging a generous fluid intake if permitted

d. informing the client that burning and irritation at the meatus are normal and should subside within a few days

6. After surgery, Ms. Young is having difficulty voiding. Which nursing action will cause increased difficulty with voiding rather than stimulation of voiding?
    a. pour warm water over Ms. Young's fingers
    b. have Ms. Young ignore the urge to void until her bladder is full
    c. use a warm bedpan when Ms. Young feels the urge to void
    d. stroke Ms. Young's leg or thigh

7. Mrs. Chang has a neurologic condition that requires her to do self-catheterization at home. The visiting nurse teaches her that
    a. she should limit fluids to decrease the amount of times necessary to self-catheterize
    b. sterile technique is required to prevent a nosocomial infection
    c. dorsal recumbent position should be used consistently
    d. the plastic catheter should be washed thoroughly, dried, and stored for reuse

8. The inability to void although the kidneys are producing urine and it enters the bladder is known as
    a. urgency
    b. retention
    c. oliguria
    d. dysuria

9. Mrs. D'Ambrosia, an alert, ambulatory, elderly nursing home resident, voids frequently and has difficulty making it to the bathroom on time. As the nurse plans her care, she is aware that
    a. incontinence is to be expected in a woman Mrs. D'Ambrosia's age
    b. 1 of every 10 nursing home residents is incontinent
    c. Kegel exercises at regular intervals throughout the day may be helpful
    d. an indwelling catheter should be inserted as soon as possible

10. Mrs. D'Ambrosia's inability to retain urine in the bladder is probably defined as
    a. urge incontinence
    b. reflex incontinence
    c. functional incontinence
    d. total incontinence

11. A client taking Pyridium (a urinary tract analgesic) should be cautioned that her urine color may change to
    a. pale yellow
    b. green
    c. orange-red
    d. brown

12. Mr. Bales is 60 years old and alert. He is timid and reluctant to talk about his urinary retention problem. Which part of this plan could create stress for Mr. Bales and possibly increase his inability to urinate?
    a. assist client in assuming his normal voiding position
    b. pull curtains around client to provide privacy during voiding
    c. stay with client while voiding
    d. offer the urinal on a regular schedule

13. Which of the following is a nursing priority when caring for a male client with a condom catheter?
    a. preventing the tubing from kinking to maintain free urinary drainage
    b. not removing the catheter for any reason
    c. fastening the condom securely to prevent the possibility of leakage
    d. maintaining bed rest at all times to prevent the catheter from slipping off

14. If you read the nursing diagnosis, Altered Urinary Elimination related to maturational enuresis, you would recognize that your client is which of the following?
    a. an adult over age 65 who is incontinent
    b. a child over age 4 who has involuntary urination
    c. a 12-month-old child who has involuntary urination
    d. a client with neurologic damage resulting in bladder dysfunction

15. Data must be collected to evaluate the effectiveness of a plan to reduce urinary incontinence in the older adult client. Of the data below, which is least necessary for the evaluation process?
    a. the incontinence pattern
    b. state of physical mobility
    c. medications being taken
    d. age of the client

Answers With Rationale

1. The correct response is *b*. For a routine urinalysis, a clean specimen is adequate. The external meatus does not need to be cleaned with an antiseptic, as is required for a clean-catch midstream specimen.

2. The correct response is *d*. Caffeine intake should be limited because it is irritating to the bladder mucosa. It is recommended that a healthy adult drink 8 to 10 8-oz glasses of fluid daily. Unless a disease process is present, this will not cause fluid retention. Children frequently need to be reminded to drink fluids.

3. The correct response is *a*. Fever and diaphoresis cause the kidneys to conserve body fluids. Thus, the urine is concentrated and decreased in amount.

4. The correct response is *a*. Because of its length, the male urethra is more prone to injury and re-

quires that the catheter be inserted 6 to 8 inches or until urine flows. This procedure requires surgical asepsis to prevent introducing bacteria into the urinary tract. Larger catheters are used for male catheterization.

5. The correct response is *c*. A generous fluid intake promotes healthy urinary tract functioning. Irrigation may introduce bacteria into the urinary tract and is not routinely ordered. The drainage system should never be disconnected to obtain a specimen, since this may provide the opportunity for bacteria to enter the urinary tract. Burning and irritation may indicate that an infection is present and should never be disregarded.

6. The correct response is *b*. Ignoring the urge to void makes urination even more difficult and should be avoided. The other activities are all recommended nursing activities to promote voiding.

7. The correct response is *d*. For self-catheterization at home, the catheter may be reused as long as it is cleaned and dried properly. Fluids should be encouraged, not limited, and clean technique and varied positions to insert the catheter are appropriate when the client is at home.

8. The correct response is *b*. Urgency is a strong desire to void. Oliguria is scanty or greatly diminished amount of urine voided in a given time. Dysuria is difficulty urinating.

9. The correct response is *c*. Kegel exercises may help a client regain better control of the micturition process. Incontinence is not a normal consequence of aging, and at least half of nursing home residents may be incontinent. An indwelling catheter is the last choice of treatment.

10. The correct response is *a*. Reflex incontinence frequently occurs with neurologic impairment, and functional incontinence is more likely related to sensory, cognitive, or mobility deficits. Total incontinence is caused by trauma or neurologic impairment.

11. The correct response is *c*. Pyridium is noted for turning the urine orange-red, and the client needs to be aware of this.

12. The correct response is *c*. Mr. Bales will be embarrassed if the nurse remains with him as he attempts to void and is more likely to have difficulty voiding.

13. The correct response is *a*. The catheter should be removed daily to prevent skin excoriation, and should not be fastened too tightly or restriction of blood vessels in the area is likely. Confining a client to bed rest increases the risk of other hazards related to immobility.

14. The correct response is *b*. Maturational enuresis is involuntary urination after an age when continence should be present. The 12-month-old child is not expected to be continent, and incontinence and neurologic damage are not maturational problems.

15. The correct response is *d*. Incontinence is not a natural consequence of the aging process. All the other factors are necessary information for the plan of care.

BIBLIOGRAPHY

Andresen, G. (1989). A fresh look at assessing the elderly. *RN, 52*(6), 28–39.

Brady, S. (1988). Getting the kinks out of a bladder drainage system. *RN, 51*(2), 39–40.

Breitenbucher, R. (1990). Minimizing urinary incontinence in the nursing home. *Geriatrics, 45*(12), 32–40.

Brink, C., Sampselle, C., Wells, T., Diokno, A., & Gillis, G. (1989). A digital test for pelvic muscle strength in older women with urinary incontinence. *Nursing Research, 38*(4), 196–199.

Carpenito, L. (1992.) *Nursing diagnoses: Application to clinical practice* (4th ed.). Philadelphia: Lippincott.

Doughty, D. (ed.). (1991). *Urinary and fecal incontinence: Nursing management.* St. Louis: Mosby–Year Book.

Fuller, J., & Schaller-Ayers, J. (1990). *Health assessment: A nursing approach.* Philadelphia: Lippincott.

Hahn, K. (1988). Think twice about urinary incontinence. *Nursing, 18*(1), 65–67.

Heller, B., Whitehead, W., & Johnson, L. (1989). Incontinence. *Journal of Gerontological Nursing, 15*(5), 16–23.

HIP (Help for Incontinent People). Media Packet, 1991.

Hu, T., Kaltreider, D., & Igon, J. (1989). Incontinence products: Which is best? *Geriatric Nursing, 10*(4), 184–186.

Hu, T., Kaltreider, D., & Igon, J. (1990). The cost-effectiveness of disposable versus reusable diapers: A controlled experiment in a nursing home. *Journal of Gerontological Nursing, 16*(2), 19–24.

Kaltreider, D., Hu, T., Igou, J., Yu, L., & Craighead, W. (1990). Can reminders curb incontinence? *Geriatric Nursing, 11*(1), 17–19.

Lincoln, R., & Roberts, R. (1989). Continence issues in acute care. *Nursing Clinics of North America, 24*(3), 741–753.

McConnell, E. (1991). Clinical do's and don'ts: How to use a urinometer. *Nursing, 21*(10), 28.

McGuire, E. (1990). Identifying and managing stress incontinence in the elderly. *Geriatrics, 45*(6), 44–52.

Moore, K. (1991). Intermittent catheterization: Sterile or clean? *Rehabilitation Nursing, 16*(1), 15–18.

Morton, P. (1989). *Health assessment in nursing.* Springhouse, PA: Springhouse.

Newman, D. (1989). The treatment of urinary incontinence in adults. *Nurse Practitioner, 14*, 21–24, 26–28, 31–32.

Newman, D., & Jakovac-Smith, D. (1989). Incontinence in elderly homebound patients. *Holistic Nurse Practitioner,* 4(1), 52–60.

Newman, D., & Smith, D. (1989). Incontinence: The problem patients won't talk about. *RN, 52*(3), 42–45.

Newman, D., Lynch, K., Smith, O., & Cell, P. (1991). Restoring urinary continence. *American Journal of Nursing, 91*(1), 28–34.

Ouslander, J., Leach, G., Staskin, D., Abelson, S., Blaustein, J., Marishita, L., & Raz, S. (1989). Prospective evaluation of an assessment strategy for geriatric urinary incontinence. *Journal of the American Geriatric Society, 37*, 715–724.

Palmer, M. (1990). Urinary incontinence. *Nursing Clinics of North America, 25*(4), 919–931.

Palmer, M., et al. (1989). Do nurses consistently document incontinence? *Journal of Gerontological Nursing, 15*(12), 11–15.

Pritchard, V. (1988). Geriatric infections: The urinary tract. *RN, 51*(5), 36–38.

Sawyer, D. (1989). Potential for infection: A nursing diagnosis for the patient with an indwelling catheter. *Focus on Critical Care, 16*(1), 46–52.

Scheve, A., Engel, B., McCormick, K., & Leahy, E. (1991). Exercise in continence. *Geriatric Nursing, 12*(3), 124.

Staab, A., & Lyles M. (1990). *Manual of geriatric nursing.* Glenview, IL: Scott, Foresman/Little Brown Higher Education.

U.S. Department of Health and Human Services, Agency for Health Care Policy and Research. (March 1992). *Urinary incontinence in adults.* Rockville, MD: Author.

U.S. National Institutes of Health (1989a). Reaching a consensus on incontinence. *Geriatric Nursing, 10*(2), 78–80.

U.S. National Institutes of Health (1989b). Urinary incontinence in adults. *Jouraⁱ of the American Medical Association, 261*, 2685–2690

VanderMeer, J., & Weatherly, K. (1990). Nursing management of the undeflatable Foley catheter balloon. *Home Healthcare Nurse, 8*(6), 39–43.

Webber-Jones, J. (1991). Performing clean, intermittent self-catheterization. *Nursing, 21*(8), 56–59.

Wells, T. (1990). Conquering incontinence. *Geriatric Nursing, 11*(3), 133–135.

Yu, L., Johnson, K., Kaltreider, D., Hu, T., Brannon, D., & Ovy, M. (1991). Urinary incontinence: Nursing home staff reaction toward residents. *Journal of Gerontological Nursing, 17*(11), 34–41.

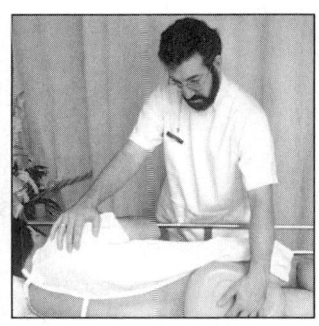
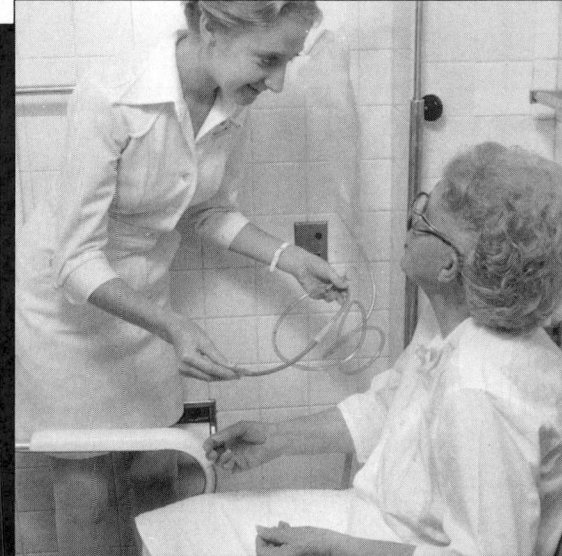

Bowel Elimination

OBJECTIVES

After studying this chapter, the learner should be able to:

Define key terms used in the chapter.

Describe the physiology of bowel elimination.

Identify 10 variables that influence bowel elimination.

Assess bowel elimination using appropriate interview questions and physical assessment skills.

Assist with the following diagnostic measures: stool collection for laboratory analysis and direct and indirect visualization studies of the gastrointestinal tract.

Develop nursing diagnoses that correctly identify bowel elimination problems amenable to nursing therapy.

Demonstrate how to (1) promote regular bowel habits (timing, positioning, privacy, nutrition, exercise); (2) use cathartics, laxatives, and antidiarrheals; (3) empty the colon of feces (enemas, rectal suppositories, rectal catheters, digital removal of stool); (4) design and implement bowel training programs; and (5) use comfort measures to ease defecation.

Plan, implement, and evaluate nursing care related to select nursing diagnoses that involve bowel problems.

KEY TERMS

bowel movement
bowel training program
cathartic
chyme
colon
colostomy
constipation
diarrhea
endoscopy
enema
fecal impaction
feces
flatulence
flatus
hemorrhoids
ileostomy
impaction (fecal)
incontinence (bowel)
laxative
occult blood
ostomy
peristalsis
stoma
stool
suppository
Valsalva maneuver

Bowel Elimination

35

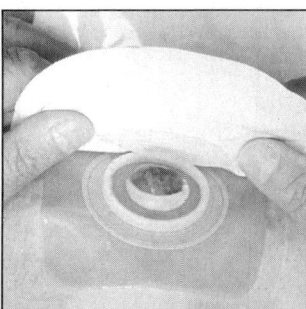

Elimination of the waste products of digestion is a natural process critical to human functioning. Clients differ widely in their expectations regarding bowel elimination, their usual pattern of defecation, and the ease with which they can and do speak of bowel problems. Although most people have experienced minor acute bouts of diarrhea or constipation, some clients experience severe or chronic bowel elimination alterations that affect fluid and electrolyte balance, hydration, nutritional status, skin integrity, comfort, and, particularly, self-concept. Because many of the clients that nurses encounter are experiencing illnesses that affect bowel elimination or undergoing diagnostic testing and pharmacologic or surgical treatment that affects functioning, nurses need to be knowledgeable in both preventing and treating bowel problems.

Study of this chapter will provide the student with knowledge of the physiology of bowel elimination and the multiple factors that influence this process. A practical guide to assess bowel elimination is presented that includes a description of nursing responsibilities related to diagnostic studies of the gastrointestinal tract. Numerous examples of nursing diagnoses are offered.

Goals are suggested for both the nurse and the client, and nursing strategies are described in detail. In the section titled Nursing Process in Clinical Practice, focused assessment, planning, implementation, and evaluation guides are offered for select nursing diagnoses of common bowel elimination problems—constipation, bowel incontinence, and diarrhea. These guides and the concluding case study illustrate how the nurse's knowledge of bowel elimination may be combined with specific nursing interventions and caring to successfully resolve bowel elimination problems.

FIGURE 35-1

Organs of the gastrointestinal system.

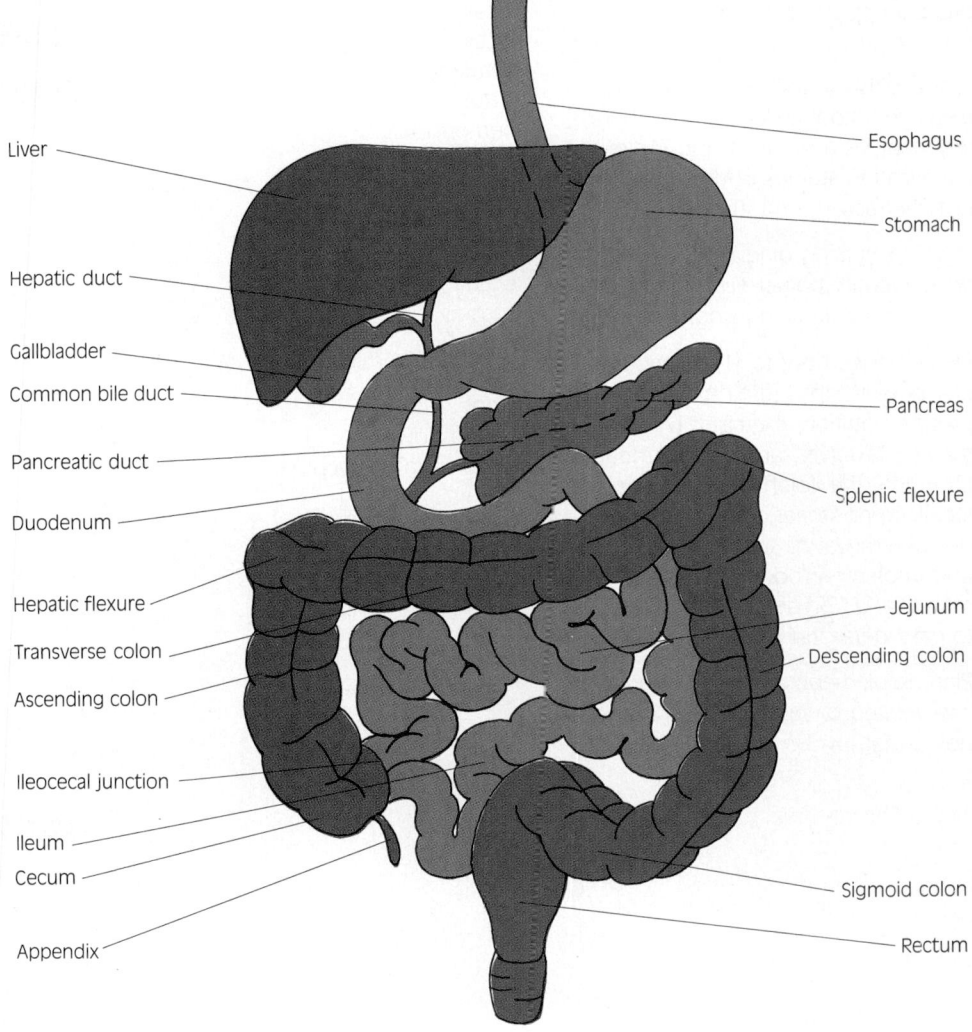

Liver

Hepatic duct

Gallbladder

Common bile duct

Pancreatic duct

Duodenum

Hepatic flexure

Transverse colon

Ascending colon

Ileocecal junction

Ileum

Cecum

Appendix

Esophagus

Stomach

Pancreas

Splenic flexure

Jejunum

Descending colon

Rectum

Sigmoid colon

Physiology

Large Intestine

The large intestine, the primary organ of bowel elimination, is the lower or distal part of the alimentary tract. It extends from the ileocecal valve to the anus. Waste products of digestion, termed **chyme**, are received by the large intestine from the small intestine. About 1500 mL of chyme is processed daily by the large intestine and most is absorbed in the proximal portion of the colon, except for about 100 mL of fluid that is eliminated in the feces. Functions of the large intestine include the completion of absorption, the manufacture of certain vitamins, the formation of feces, and the expulsion of feces from the body.

The length of the large intestine in adults is about 1.5 m (about 59 inches), but variations have been observed in normal people. The width of the colon varies. At its narrowest point, the colon is about 2.5 cm (1 inch) wide; at its widest point, it is about 7.5 cm (3 inches). Its diameter decreases from the cecum to the anus.

The barrier between the large intestine and the ileum of the small intestine is the ileocecal, or ileocolic, valve. This valve normally prevents contents from entering the large intestine prematurely and prevents waste products from returning to the small intestine.

The waste contents pass through the ileocecal valve and enter the cecum, which is the first part of the large intestine. It is situated on the right side of the body, and to it is attached the vermiform process or appendix. When waste products enter the large intestine, the contents are liquid or watery. While passing through the large intestine, they absorb water. About 800 to 1000 mL of liquid is absorbed daily by the intestinal tract. This absorption of water accounts for the formed, semisolid consistency of the normal stool. When absorption does not occur properly—as when the waste products pass through the large intestine at a rapid rate—the stool is soft and watery. If the stool remains in the colon too long, or if too much water is absorbed, the stool becomes dry and hardened.

From the cecum, the contents enter the colon, which is divided into several parts. The ascending colon extends from the cecum upward, toward the liver, where it turns to cross the abdomen. This turn is the hepatic flexure. The transverse colon crosses the abdomen from right to left. The turn from the transverse colon to form the descending colon is the splenic flexure. The descending colon passes down the left side of the body, from the splenic flexure to the sigmoid or pelvic colon. When the waste products reach the distal end of the colon, they are called **feces**, and when excreted, feces are called the **stool**.

The sigmoid colon contains feces ready for excretion, and empties into the rectum, which is the last part of the large intestine. The rectum is about 12 cm (about 5 inches) long, 2.5 cm (1 inch) of which is the anal canal. Three transverse folds of tissue normally are present in the rectum. These folds may help to hold the fecal material in the rectum temporarily. In addition, there are vertical folds, each of which contains an artery and a vein. Abnormally distended veins are called **hemorrhoids**.

The rectum is empty except during and immediately before defecation. Feces are excreted from the rectum through the anal canal and the anus, which is about 2.5 to 3.8 cm (1 to 1.5 inches) long.

The anatomy of the gastrointestinal tract is shown in Figure 35-1.

The muscles of the colon are innervated by the autonomic nervous system. The parasympathetic system stimulates movement, and the sympathetic system inhibits movement. Contractions of the circular and longitudinal muscles of the intestine (**peristalsis**) occur every 3 to 12 minutes and continually move waste products along the length of the intestine (Fig. 35-2). Mass peristaltic sweeps occur one to four times each 24-hour period in most people, propelling the fecal mass forward. This movement is unlike the frequent peristaltic rushes that occur in the small intestine. Mass peristalsis often occurs after food has been ingested. This accounts for the urge to defecate that frequently is observed after meals. Timing nursing interventions to evacuate bowel contents with this natural urge to defecate is helpful. One third to one half of ingested food waste products normally is excreted in the stool within 24 hours and the remainder, within the next 24 to 48 hours.

Anal Canal and Anus

The internal sphincter in the anal canal and the external sphincter at the anus control the discharge of feces and intestinal gas, or **flatus**. The internal sphincter consists of smooth-muscle tissue and is involuntary. The innervation

F I G U R E 3 5 - 2

Peristaltic movements in the intestine.

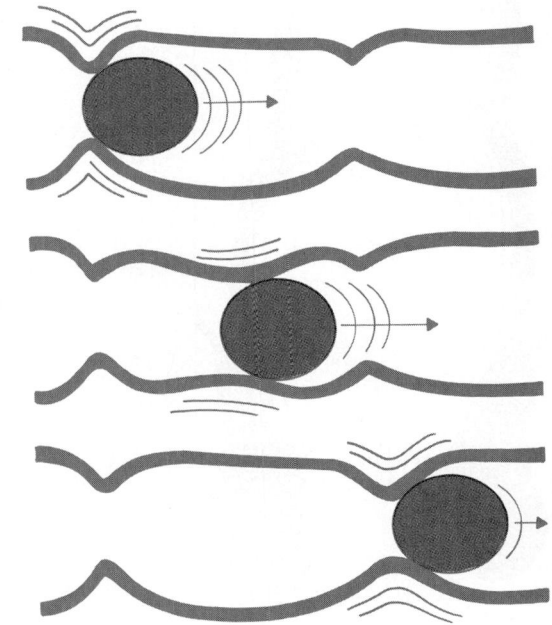

of the internal sphincter occurs through the autonomic nervous system. Motor impulses are carried by the sympathetic system (thoracolumbar), and inhibitory impulses by the parasympathetic system (craniosacral). These two divisions of the autonomic nervous system function antagonistically to each other in a dynamic equilibrium.

The external sphincter at the anus has striated muscle tissue and is, therefore, under voluntary control. The levator ani muscle reinforces the action of the external sphincter and is controlled voluntarily. Interference with the normal functioning of elimination from the intestines can occur in health as it can during illness. It can be affected by the amount and quality of fluid or food intake, the degree of activity, and emotional states.

Figure 35-3 shows these structures.

Act of Defecation

Defecation is the emptying of the intestines and often is called a **bowel movement**. Two centers govern the reflex to defecate. One is situated in the medulla, and a subsidiary one is in the spinal cord. When parasympathetic stimulation occurs, the internal anal sphincter relaxes and the colon contracts. The defecation reflex is stimulated chiefly by the fecal mass in the rectum. When the rectum is distended, the intrarectal pressure rises, the defecation reflex is stimulated by the muscle stretch, and the desire to eliminate results. The external anal sphincter is constricted or relaxed at will. If the desire to defecate is ignored, defecation often can be delayed voluntarily.

F I G U R E 3 5 - 3

Interior view of the rectum and the anal canal.

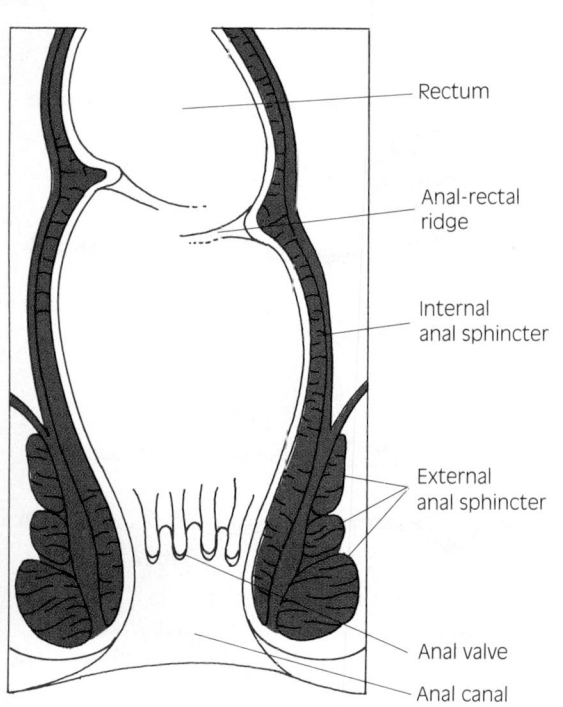

- Rectum
- Anal-rectal ridge
- Internal anal sphincter
- External anal sphincter
- Anal valve
- Anal canal

During the act of defecation, several additional muscles aid the process. Voluntary contraction of the muscles of the abdominal wall, fixing of the diaphragm, and closing of the glottis aid in increasing intraabdominal pressure up to four or five times the normal pressure that aids in expelling feces. This technique, termed the **Valsalva maneuver**, may be contraindicated in people with cardiovascular problems and other illnesses. Simultaneously, the muscles on the pelvic floor contract and aid in drawing the anus over the fecal mass.

Ease in defecation is aided by (1) flexing the thigh muscles, which increases abdominal pressure, and (2) assuming a sitting position, which increases downward pressure on the rectum.

Normal Defecation

The act of defecation usually is painless. Normally, it is associated with the regularity and type of stool. If the bowels move at regular intervals and the stools are formed and soft, functional problems of frequency of elimination seldom occur. Nurses find that many people show concern if they do not have a daily bowel movement. The normal frequency of bowel movements cannot be stated arbitrarily. Although many adults pass one stool each day, healthy people have been observed to have more frequent or less frequent bowel movements. Some people have a bowel movement two or three times a week; others, as often as two or three times a day.

Factors Affecting Bowel Elimination

Developmental Considerations

Age affects what a person eats and the body's ability to digest nutrients and eliminate wastes. There is a marked difference between the stools of an infant and those of an older person. Because clients often are reluctant to discuss bowel habits and stool characteristics, nurses need to be familiar with bowel concerns pertinent to each developmental group. These are highlighted in Table 35-1 with related nursing interventions.

Daily Patterns

Most people have regular patterns of bowel elimination that include frequency, timing considerations, position, and place. Changes in any of these may upset a person's routine and lead to constipation. For example, many people defecate after breakfast, when the gastrocolic and duodenocolic reflexes cause mass propulsive movements in the large intestine. If this urge to defecate is ignored because the person finds the time inconvenient, the feces remains in the rectum until the defecation reflex is again initiated. Meanwhile water continues to be absorbed from the unexpelled feces, which makes it dry, hard, and painful to pass.

TABLE 35-1

Developmental Variations in Bowel Elimination With Related Nursing Interventions

	Developmental Variations	Related Nursing Interventions
Infant	Stool characteristics depend on whether the infant is being fed breast milk or cow's milk. Breastfed babies have frequent yellow to golden stools of salvelike consistency. With cow's milk feedings, the stools vary from yellow to brown, are firmer, and have a stronger fecal odor because of the decomposition of protein. Both stools may have curds and mucus. Infants have no voluntary control over bowel elimination.	Parents should be advised that the number of stools an infant passes can vary greatly. In the first 4 months, breastfed infants average two to four stools daily and bottle-fed infants one or two stools daily. By the time the infant is 1 year old, he or she may only have one stool daily.

Parents may mistake the infant's liquid stool for diarrhea. Loose stools may be related to overfeeding or too much corn syrup in the formula. Real diarrhea requires evaluation.

The initial treatment for constipation is dietary manipulation; consistent use of suppositories and laxatives is to be discouraged. Infants with persistent constipation should be evaluated for structural defects. |
| Toddler | Between ages 18 and 24 months, the nerve fibers innervating the anal sphincter become fully developed and voluntary control of defecation becomes possible. Voluntary defecation requires intact muscular, sensory, and nervous structures. Successful bowel training includes:
1. Toddler demonstrates awareness of the need to defecate and communicates this (grunting, tugging at diaper, special word).
2. Toddler wants to avoid the discomfort of involuntary defecation and wishes to please the significant person managing bowel training.
3. Significant person has clearly and consistently communicated expectations, praises and reinforces successful behavior, does not punish accidents. Daytime bowel control is normally attained by 30 months. | The parents' approach to toilet training and understanding of the need for physiologic maturity should be assessed. Guidance may be offered to ensure that the process of toilet training strengthens the parent–child relationship. It is critical for parents to understand that a child should never be punished or shamed for elimination accidents or for a lack of readiness to become toilet-trained.

Toddlers who are toilet-trained may regress when hospitalized until they become comfortable in their new environment. Children who feel hostile to parents or staff may retaliate by soiling. Scolding or disgust only reinforces this behavior, and the only constructive approach is to seek out the underlying cause, which is most often some form of emotional turmoil. |
| Child or adolescent adult | Defecation patterns vary in quantity, frequency, and rhythmicity. | Each comprehensive nursing assessment should include questions about the client's bowel habits. Many people may not understand the significance of changes in bowel habits or may worry needlessly about normal stool characteristics or bowel habits. The use of over-the-counter laxatives and enemas should be evaluated. |
| Older adult | Decreased physical activity, decreased gastrointestinal motility, and changes in nutritional habits make constipation a chronic problem for many elderly people. Abuse of laxatives and enemas may cause rebound diarrhea and negatively affect other body systems. | Strenuous teaching of the importance of nonpharmacologic remedies for constipation is needed. These include regular exercise, increased fiber in the diet, decreased animal fat and refined sugar, and increased fluid intake. |

The position most people assume for defecation is squatting or sitting slightly forward with the thighs flexed. In this position, increased pressure is placed on the abdomen as well as downward pressure on the rectum; both facilitate defecation. It is difficult to obtain the same results when seated on a bedpan, and embarrassment may further inhibit defecation.

Lastly, for many people, defecation is a private affair that can be done easily only in the comfort of one's own bathroom. Defecation in a shared hospital room with only a curtain separating one from a roommate or other people may be difficult.

Food and Fluid

Both the type and the amount of foods eaten and the amount of fluids ingested affect elimination. Healthy elimination is facilitated by a high-fiber diet and a daily fluid intake of 2000 to 3000 mL. High-fiber foods increase the bulk in fecal material. As the bulk of feces expands, it places pressure on the intestinal wall, which serves as a stimulus for peristalsis. When fecal material moves quickly through the intestine, there is less time for water to be reabsorbed, and the resultant stool is soft and easily passed. There also is less time for toxins to be absorbed from feces by the colon. Many believe that these toxins play an important role in colon cancer.

People digest and tolerate food very differently. This variation is determined in part by one's culture. Traveling to a different country and eating the native foods may result in severe indigestion and elimination problems. Differences in water also may affect elimination when traveling. Lactose intolerance is common. People who lack the enzyme lactase, which helps to break down the simple sugar lactose found in milk and milk products, cannot digest milk. Food intolerances may result in diarrhea, gaseous distention, and cramping.

In addition to high-fiber, bulk-producing foods, other general food classifications that influence bowel elimination include the following:

Constipating foods—processed cheese, lean meat, eggs, and pasta

Foods with laxative effect—certain fruits and vegetables (eg, prunes), bran, chocolate, spicy foods, alcohol, and coffee

Gas-producing foods—onions, cabbage, beans, cauliflower

Activity and Muscle Tone

Regular exercise improves gastrointestinal motility and muscle tone, whereas inactivity decreases both. Adequate tone in the abdominal muscles, the diaphragm, and the perineal muscles is essential to ease in defecation. Clients who are on prolonged bed rest are prime candidates for constipation.

Life-Style

Many individual, family, and sociocultural variables influence a person's usual elimination habits. The long-term effects of bowel training may result in a person's (1) acceptance of bowel elimination as a normal life process, (2) preoccupation with bowel elimination, or (3) feeling that bowel elimination is a "dirty" process. Rituals associated with bowel elimination, cleanliness considerations, the language used to talk about bowel elimination or reluctance to discuss it, individual responses to involuntary passage of flatus (gas), and so forth vary widely among individuals. A person's daily schedule, occupation, and leisure activities may contribute to a habit of defecating at regular times or to an irregular pattern.

Psychological Variables

Emotional stress affects the body in many ways. In some people, anxiety seems to have a direct effect on gastrointestinal motility, and diarrhea can be expected to accompany periods of high anxiety. During the fight-or-flight response, when the body mobilizes itself for intense action, blood is shunted away from the stomach, and intestines and gastrointestinal motility slow. Chronic worriers and certain personality types who tend to hold on to problems and feelings may experience frequent constipation.

Pathologic Conditions

Numerous pathologic processes may result in changes in a person's usual bowel elimination. When a client reports that his or her stool is now narrower or ribbonlike, it is important for the nurse to consider the possibility of a tumor in the colon forming an obstruction to normal stool passage and to report this finding to the physician. Similarly, if a parent reports that a child's stools are frequent, bulky, greasy, and foul smelling, one possible explanation is cystic fibrosis; this would need to be ruled out if other clinical manifestations are present. Changes in stool characteristics or frequency may, therefore, be one of the first clinical manifestations of a disease, and their evaluation may lead to the diagnosis of the disease.

Pathologic conditions that may result in diarrhea include diverticulitis, infection, malabsorption syndromes, neoplastic diseases, diabetic neuropathy, hyperthyroidism, and uremia. Conditions that predispose to constipation include diseases within the colon or rectum, injury to or degeneration of the spinal cord, and megacolon. Conditions that traumatize the stomach or intestines or that interfere with normal digestion may change the color, contents, odor, and appearance of the stool, making stool assessment an important diagnostic task for nursing.

Medications

Medications are available to either promote peristalsis (cathartics and laxatives) or inhibit peristalsis (antidiarrheal medications). These are discussed later in the chapter.

Other types of medications may affect bowel elimination and stool characteristics. Narcotic analgesics (opioids), antacids containing aluminum, and anticholinergic medications all have the potential to cause constipation by decreasing gastrointestinal motility. Many medications have diarrhea as an adverse effect. Twenty percent of the time, antibiotic use is accompanied by diarrhea (Rowland, 1989). The use of antidiarrheal drugs in this situation is not recommended, since it further prolongs the exposure of the intestinal mucosa to the irritating effect of the antibiotics or toxins. The diarrhea may be severe enough to warrant cessation of the drug.

Medications may influence the appearance of the stool for a variety of reasons. Any drug with the potential to cause gastrointestinal bleeding (eg, anticoagulants, aspirin products) may result in the stool appearing pink to red to black; iron salts result in a black stool from the oxidation of iron; antacids may cause a white discoloration or speckling in the stool; and antibiotics may cause a green-gray color because of impaired digestion.

Diagnostic Tests

Clients may need to fast for diagnostic studies. Additionally, the stress of hospitalization and waiting for the results of the study combined with changes in food intake can severely alter usual elimination patterns. Bowel cleansing by use of cathartics or enemas is a prerequisite for certain diagnostic studies of the gastrointestinal tract.

Surgery and Anesthesia

Direct manipulation of the bowel during abdominal surgery inhibits peristalsis, causing a condition termed paralytic ileus. This temporary stoppage of peristalsis normally lasts 24 to 48 hours, and during this time, food and fluids are withheld. If this condition persists, it may cause distention and symptoms of acute obstruction and may require surgical intervention. General anesthetic agents that are inhaled also inhibit peristalsis by blocking the parasympathetic impulses to the intestinal musculature. Local and regional anesthetics have little effect on peristalsis.

Nurse as Role Model

Before intervening to help clients develop healthy bowel elimination patterns, it is important for nurses to assess the adequacy of their own bowel elimination habits and patterns. If you are unable to meet the following goals, you may want to take the time now to revise your own health practices, so that you will be an effective role model for clients. Use the assessment checklist to see how well you are meeting bowel elimination needs. The nurse:

- Has a normal bowel elimination pattern without discomfort
- Responds to the normal urge to defecate
- Includes in each day's nutritional intake sufficient high-fiber foods and fluid to promote peristalsis and reduce stool retention
- Identifies many ways to increase fiber and fluid in different types of diets
- Exercises vigorously for 15 to 30 minutes three or four times a week
- Responds to changes in stool characteristics (or frequency) by seeking their cause and getting medical assistance when necessary

Assessing

Nursing History

Because many clients are reluctant to initiate a discussion of their bowel status, nurses should include pertinent bowel elimination questions in each comprehensive nursing history (see display Focused Assessment Guide).

If the client is experiencing any disturbance in bowel elimination, a more detailed assessment is conducted with attention directed to each of the factors that may influence bowel elimination (described earlier).

Clients who are critically ill or who have impaired cognition may be incapable of reporting their bowel status accurately. In this instance, nurses need to record the client's daily bowel status to be alert to impending problems. While making daily rounds, the nurse asks the client who is a reliable historian, "Did you move your bowels yesterday

---

PROMOTING WELLNESS

Bowel Elimination

Use the assessment checklist to determine how well you are meeting your need for bowel elimination. Then develop a prescription for self-care by choosing appropriate behaviors from the list of suggestions.

Assessment Checklist

almost always / sometimes / almost never

1. I have a regular bowel elimination pattern, satisfactory to support comfort and activities of daily living.
2. I eat a diet high in fiber.
3. I exercise regularly.
4. I have an adequate intake of fluids.

Self-Care Behaviors

1. Accept individual patterns of defecation as normal.
2. Eat a balanced diet, including high-fiber foods, such as fruits, vegetables, and nuts.
3. Follow a regular exercise program with 30 to 45 minutes of activity three to four times a week.
4. Do not ignore the urge to defecate.
5. Establish a routine, if needed (1 hour after meals is usually best).
6. Avoid prolonged use of over-the-counter medications or enemas to treat constipation.

F O C U S E D   A S S E S S M E N T   G U I D E

Bowel Elimination

Factors to Assess	Questions and Approaches
Usual patterns of bowel elimination	How often do you move your bowels?
	Any special time of the day?
	What does your stool look like?
	• Frequency
	• Time of day
	• Description of usual stool characteristics (amount, consistency, shape, color, odor)
Recent changes in bowel elimination	Have you noticed any changes in your stool recently?
	Have you noticed any blood in your stool?
	Have you noted a difference in the appearance of your stool (narrowing, presence of mucus)?
Aids to elimination	Do you use anything to help move your bowels?
	• Natural aids (liquids, food)
	• Pharmacologic aids (laxatives)
	• Enemas
Problems with bowel elimination	Are your bowels causing you any problem now?
	• Nature of disturbance
	• Onset and frequency
	• Causes (*physical:* food and fluid intake, exercise status, history of surgery or illnesses influencing GI tract; *psychosocial*; *medicine related*
	• Severity
	• Symptoms
	• Interventions attempted and results
Presence of artificial orifices	What is your usual routine with your colostomy or ileostomy?
	Do you have any problems with it?

or today?'' and charts the response. If the client cannot offer this information, the nurse who is assisting with bowel elimination records daily stools.

Physical Assessment

Assessment of bowel elimination includes physical assessment of the abdomen, anus, and rectum. (This is discussed in Chapter 24.) Described below are examination techniques that may be helpful when assessing the functioning of the gastrointestinal tract.

Abdomen

The sequence for abdominal assessment proceeds from inspection–auscultation–percussion to palpation. Auscultation is done before palpation because palpation may disturb normal peristalsis. The client is comfortably positioned in the supine position with the abdomen exposed and the chest and pubic area draped. The bladder should be emptied.

Inspection   The nurse first observes the contour of the abdomen, noting any masses or areas of distention. Peristalsis is not visible except in very thin clients and when observed (visible waves) may indicate an intestinal obstruction.

Auscultation   The nurse uses a warmed stethoscope to listen for bowel sounds in a systematic, clockwise manner in all abdominal quadrants. The frequency and character of bowel sounds are noted. Bowel sounds are audible clicks and gurgles produced by the movement of air and flatus in the gastrointestinal tract. They usually are high-pitched, gurgling, and soft. Their frequency may range from 5 to 34 bowel sounds per minute, depending on the rate of peristalsis. Of significance are absent or infrequent bowel sounds, indicating hypoperistalsis or paralytic ileus (no decision should be made until the nurse has listened for 5 minutes), or abnormally intense and frequent bowel sounds (borborygmus), indicating hyperperistalsis. Bowel sounds usually are described as being audible, hyperactive, hypoactive, or inaudible.

Percussion The nurse next percusses all quadrants of the abdomen in a systematic, clockwise manner to identify any masses, fluid, or air in the abdomen. A resonate sound or tympany is expected over the abdomen and stomach because these are hollow organs. With practice, the nurse can distinguish normal resonance from the hyperresonance that occurs when excess flatus is trapped in the intestines. An intestinal obstruction sounds dull on percussion. Areas of increased dullness may be caused by fluid, a mass, or a tumor.

Palpation Both light and deep palpation in each quadrant are next performed by the skilled nurse, noting muscular resistance, tenderness, enlargement of organs, and masses. The beginning nurse quickly learns the feel of a distended abdomen.

Anus and Rectum

The skill of the nurse examiner determines the extent of the rectal examination. A superficial examination is performed each time a nurse washes a client's anal area or assists with bowel evacuation. The client is most often positioned in left Sims' position.

Inspection and Palpation The nurse first examines the anal area for cracks, nodules, distended veins (hemorrhoids), masses, or polyps. A fecal mass may be observed distending the anus. A gloved and lubricated finger is next inserted through the anus into the rectum to assess sphincter tone and smoothness of mucosal lining, and to note the presence of masses, polyps, hardened stool, bleeding, or abnormal discharge. The perineal area also is inspected for areas of skin irritation or breakdown secondary to diarrhea or fecal incontinence.

Stool Characteristics

Nurses are responsible for observing and recording information about the client's stool. Table 35-2 describes characteristics of a normal stool and presents special considerations to take into account when observing a stool. Anything unusual should be reported and recorded. Passing little or no gas or unusual amounts also should be recorded and reported.

The frequency with which the client has bowel movements is noted and recorded. Frequency is recorded as I, II, III, or i, ii, iii, and so on. Noting and recording the frequency of the client's bowel movements are important parts of nursing care. Figure 35-4 is an example of an agency form used to collect specific information about the amount and characteristics of stool. Any additional unusual observations are described in the nurses' notes on the client's permanent record. When auxiliary personnel or the client assumes this responsibility, the nurse should check at regular intervals to see that it is being done correctly.

Ideally, populations at high risk for bowel elimination problems will be identified, and such problems will be pre-

---

> **Warning Signs of Colon Cancer**
>
> - Change in the bowel elimination pattern
> - Blood in the stools
> - Rectal or abdominal pain
> - Change in the character of the stool
> - Sensation of incomplete emptying after bowel movement

---

vented or minimized through vigilant nursing care. The nurse also must be aware of clinical manifestations of colon cancer, since early detection significantly improves survival statistics (see display). To perform these assessments accurately, the nurse needs a thorough knowledge of the factors that contribute to these problems and of pertinent assessment priorities. These may be found later in the chapter, in the section titled Nursing Process in Clinical Practice.

Assisting With Diagnostic Studies

The nurse often is responsible for caring for clients with elimination problems who are undergoing diagnostic testing. General nursing responsibilities for diagnostic studies are discussed in Chapter 27. Following are specific guidelines for nursing's role with stool collection and direct and indirect visualization studies.

Stool Collection The nurse is responsible for obtaining the specimen according to agency procedure, labeling the specimen, and ensuring that the specimen is transported to the laboratory in a timely manner. The institution's policy and procedure manual or laboratory manual must be checked to determine specifics regarding the amount of stool needed, the time frame during which stool is to be collected, and the type of specimen container to use.

Medical aseptic techniques are imperative. Whether agency policy dictates the use of universal precautions, body isolation precautions, or other specific isolation procedures, disposable gloves should be worn when any contact or handling of a stool specimen is likely. Handwashing before and after glove use is essential. Care also must be taken not to contaminate the outside of the specimen container with stool. Specimens should be packaged, labeled, and transported to the laboratory according to the specific agency policy in a manner that guarantees that there is no leakage of the specimen.

Specific instructions the nurse needs to give the client when collecting a stool specimen may include the following:

- Void first because the laboratory study may be inaccurate if the stool contains urine.
- Use a clean or sterile bedpan or the bedside commode, depending on the specific specimen required.

TABLE 35-2

The Stool: Normal Characteristics and Special Considerations for Observation

Characteristic	Normal Finding	Special Considerations for Observation
Volume	Variable	The volume of the stool depends on the amount the person eats and the nature of the diet. For example, a diet high in roughage produces more feces than a soft, bland diet. Consistently large diarrheal stools suggest a disorder in the small bowel or proximal colon; small, frequent stools with urgency to pass them suggest a disorder of the left colon or rectum.
Color	Infant: Yellow Adult: Brown	The brown color of the stool is due to stercobilin, a bile pigment derivative. The rapid rate of peristalsis in the infant causes the stool to be yellow. The color of the stool is influenced by diet. For example, the stool will be almost black if the person eats red meat and dark green vegetables, such as spinach. The stool will be light brown if the diet is high in milk and milk products and low in meat. The absence of bile may cause the stool to appear white or clay-colored. Certain drugs influence the color of the stool. For example, iron salts cause the stool to be black. Antacids cause it to be whitish. Bleeding high in the intestinal tract causes a stool to be black owing to the digestion of the blood. Bleeding low in the intestinal tract will result in fresh blood in the stool. The stool darkens with standing.
Odor	Aromatic; may be affected by foods ingested	The characteristic odor of the stool is due to indole and skatole, caused by putrefaction and fermentation in the lower intestinal tract. The odor of the stool is influenced by its pH value, which normally is neutral or slightly alkaline. Excessive putrefaction causes a strong odor. The presence of blood in the stool causes a unique odor.
Consistency	Soft, semisolid, and formed	The consistency of the stool is influenced by fluid and food intake and gastric motility. The less time stool spends in the intestine (or the shorter the intestine), the more liquid the stool. Many pathologic conditions influence consistency.
Shape	Formed stool is usually about 1 inch (2.5 cm) in diameter and has the tubular shape of the colon, but may be larger or smaller, depending on the condition of the colon.	A gastrointestinal obstruction may result in a narrow, pencil-shaped stool. Rapid peristalsis thins the stool. Increased time spent in the large intestine may result in a hard, marblelike fecal mass.
Constituents	Waste residues of digestion: bile, intestinal secretions, shedded epithelial cells, bacteria, and inorganic material (chiefly calcium and phosphates); seeds, meat fibers, and fat may be present in small amounts.	Internal bleeding, infection, inflammation, and other pathologic conditions may result in abnormal constituents. These include blood, pus, excessive fat, parasites, ova, and mucus. Foreign bodies also may be found in the stool.

- Defecate into the required container rather than the toilet bowl because the laboratory study may be hindered by the water in the bowl.
- Do not place toilet tissue in the bedpan or specimen container because contents in the paper may influence laboratory results.

- Notify the nurse when the specimen is available, so that it may be collected and transported to the laboratory in the required manner.

  To place a specimen in a laboratory container, the nurse should use two clean tongue blades and gloved hands. Usually 1 inch (2.5 cm) of formed stool or 15 to 30 mL

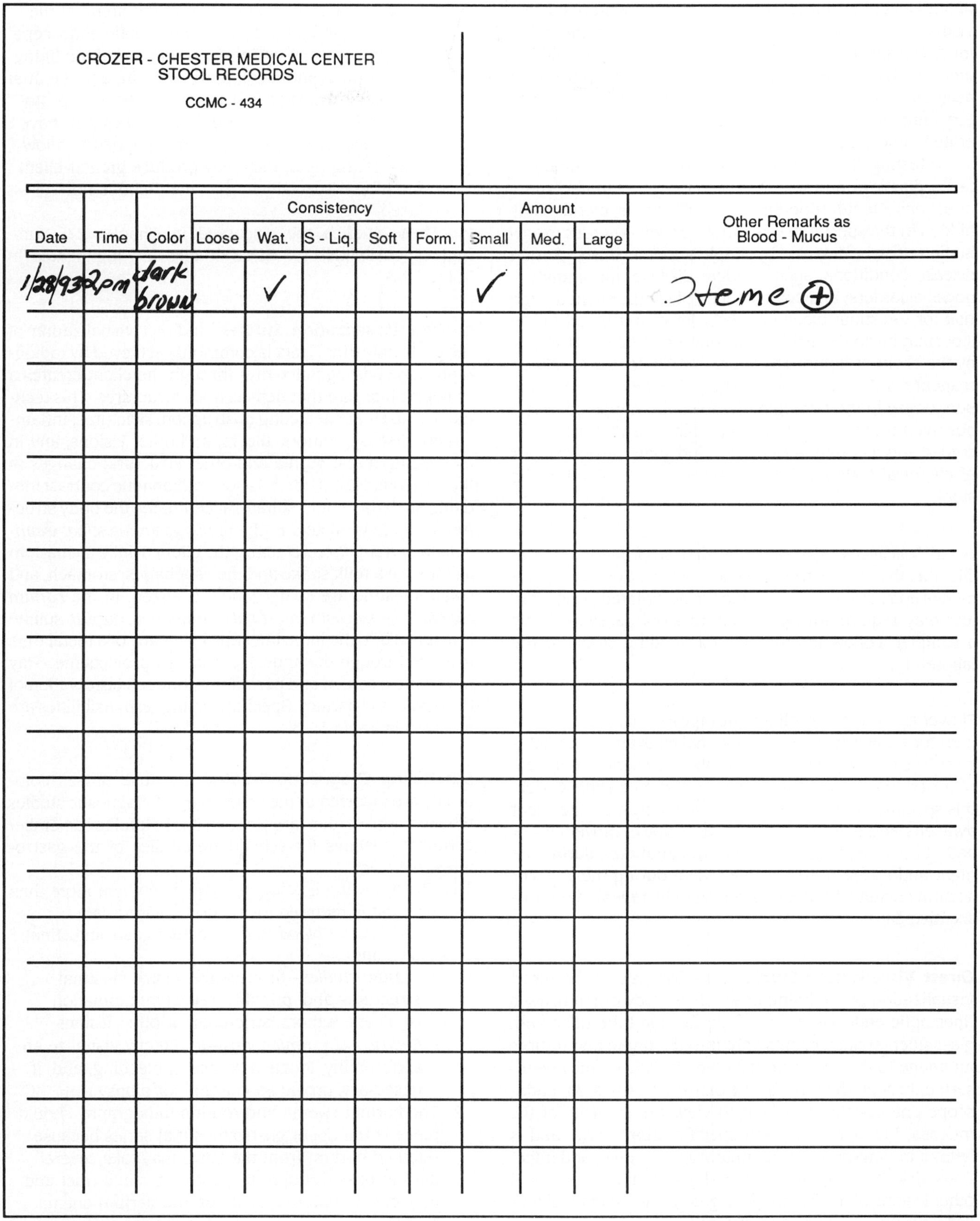

CROZER - CHESTER MEDICAL CENTER
STOOL RECORDS

CCMC - 434

| Date | Time | Color | Consistency | | | | | Amount | | | Other Remarks as Blood - Mucus |
			Loose	Wat.	S - Liq.	Soft	Form.	Small	Med.	Large	
1/28/93	2pm	dark brown		✓				✓			Heme ⊕

FIGURE 35-4

Example of a stool record.

of liquid stool is sufficient. If portions of the stool include visible blood, mucus, or pus, include these with the specimen. The specimen also should be free of barium and enema solution. Because a fresh specimen produces the most accurate results, the specimen should be sent to the laboratory immediately. If this is not possible, it should be refrigerated, unless contraindicated.

If testing the stool for pH or blood, use commercial tapes, dipsticks, and solutions according to manufacturer's directions. **Occult blood** in the stool—that is, blood that is hidden in the specimen or cannot be seen on gross examination—can be detected by simple screening tests. Certain disease conditions, such as ulcer disease, inflammatory bowel disorders, and colon cancer, place the client at high risk for intestinal bleeding. Tests for occult blood in the stool may be done quickly by the nurse in the clinical area or by the client at home. These are simply done and rely on reagent substances to detect the presence of the enzyme peroxidase in the hemoglobin molecule. A blue color is a positive finding, indicating occult blood, and must be recorded and reported. A Hematest and guaiac test are types of chemical tests used to determine occult blood in the stool.

Timed Specimens Consider the first stool passed by the client as the start of the collection period. Collect a specimen of *every* stool passed within the designated period (the test may require saving the entire stool passed or only a sample). Follow instructions for sending stools to the laboratory.

Pinworms Use clear cellophane tape for collecting a specimen for pinworms (frosted tape makes examination difficult). The tape is placed directly over the client's anal area, removed immediately, and then placed on a slide. Collect this specimen in the morning, immediately after the client awakens and before the client has a bowel movement or bath. Pinworms tend to come to the anal area during the night and retreat into the anal canal during the day. For accurate results, this test may need to be repeated on consecutive days.

Direct Visualization Studies **Endoscopy** is the direct visualization of the lining of a hollow body organ using a fiber-optic endoscope (ie, a long flexible tube filled with glass fibers that transmits light into the organ and returns an image to the scope's optical head). Pincers may be inserted through the tube for the biopsy of tissues. An endoscope enables the physician to view the integrity of the mucosa, blood vessels, and specific organ parts, and is helpful in diagnosing inflammatory, ulcerative, and infectious diseases; benign and malignant neoplasms; and other lesions of the esophageal, gastric, and intestinal mucosa. Studies include the following:

Esophagogastroduodenoscopy—visual examination of the lining of the esophagus, the stomach, and the upper duodenum with a flexible, fiber-optic endoscope

Colonoscopy—visual examination of the lining of the large intestine with a flexible, fiber-optic endoscope

Proctosigmoidoscopy—visual examination of the lining of the distal sigmoid colon, the rectum, and the anal canal using two rigid instruments (tubes)—a protoscope and a sigmoidoscope. These tubes also have an attached light source and are equipped to allow biopsy. Being rigid, they may produce greater client discomfort, especially in the client who is not relaxed.

These studies are discussed in Chapter 27. Nursing responsibilities for these studies are highlighted in Table 35-3.

Indirect Visualization Studies Indirect visualization of the gastrointestinal tract is commonly achieved by radiography. The passage of x-rays through the client creates a radiograph or film that depicts body structures. This technique is useful in detecting obstruction, strictures, inflammatory disease, tumors, ulcers, and other lesions, and in diagnosing hiatal hernia and other structural changes in the gastrointestinal tract. Use of a radiopaque contrast medium, such as barium sulfate, accentuates the body structures being visualized. In the *upper gastrointestinal examination* and *small-bowel series*, the client drinks the barium sulfate like a milk shake and the esophagus, stomach, and small intestine are coated and visualized. In the *barium enema* or *lower gastrointestinal examination*, barium sulfate is instilled into the large intestine by means of a rectal tube inserted through the anus. Fluoroscopy projects the x-ray films onto a screen and permits continuous observation of the flow of the barium. Specific nursing responsibilities are included in Table 35-3.

Scheduling Diagnostic Studies Because nurses commonly are involved in the scheduling of diagnostic studies when multiple orders are written, it is helpful to remember certain guidelines for scheduling studies of the gastrointestinal tract.

1. The following is a logical sequence when more than one test is required for accurate diagnosis:
   * *Fecal occult blood test*—to detect gastrointestinal bleeding
   * *Barium studies*—to visualize gastrointestinal structures and, possibly, reveal inflammation or ulcers, tumors, strictures, or other lesions
   * *Endoscopic examinations*—to directly visualize an abnormality, locate a source of bleeding, and, if necessary, provide a channel for biopsy
2. The barium enema and routine radiography should precede the upper gastrointestinal series because retained barium from the latter may take several days to pass through the gastrointestinal tract and may cloud anatomic detail on the barium enema studies.
3. Noninvasive procedures usually take precedence over invasive procedures, such as endoscopic studies, when sufficient diagnostic data can be

(Text continues on p. 915)

TABLE 35-3

Diagnostic Studies of the Gastrointestinal Tract

Test and Purpose	Client Preparation	Nursing Care During Test	Client Aftercare
Esophagogastroduodenoscopy			
• Allows visual examination of the esophagus, stomach, and upper duodenum • Indicated for clients with hematemesis, melena, or substernal or epigastric pain and in postoperative clients with recurrent or new symptoms • Assists in the diagnosis of inflammatory, ulcerative, and infectious diseases; tumors, and structural abnormalities • Allows biopsy, removal of foreign objects, and coagulation of bleeding	1. Explain to the client: • Nature and purpose of the test • Directions for fasting (6 to 12 hours before the test; check guidelines) • That the test requires about 30 minutes and involves the passage of a flexible tube through the mouth (client may experience gagging or sense of fullness; cannot speak during this time) • Dentures need to be removed; mouth guard often used to protect natural teeth • Client will be awake, although a sedative (and sometimes an anticholinergic drug to decrease GI secretions) is administered • A bitter-tasting local anesthetic is sprayed into the mouth and throat to decrease sensation (tongue will feel swollen temporarily—difficulty swallowing) 2. Ensure that informed consent is signed. 3. Assist client into hospital gown and complete agency protocol for testing (empty bladder, remove jewelry, and so forth). 4. Administer prescribed sedative, anticholinergic, and, if ordered, an analgesic.	• Position client in left lateral or left Sims' position. • Provide emotional support. • Obtain baseline vital signs. • Check that IV is in place; administer prescribed medications. • Place any tissue or cell specimens in properly labeled containers with preservatives and send to laboratory. • Observe for untoward responses; have emergency resuscitative equipment available.	• Check vital signs according to agency protocol. • Withhold food and fluids until the gag reflex returns. • Observe for signs of perforation: pain, persistent difficulty swallowing, vomiting blood, or black stools. • Explain to the client that it is normal to sense throat soreness and hoarseness for several days; warm, saline gargles and, lozenges may help.
Colonoscopy			
• Allows visual examination of the large intestine • Indicated for clients with histories of constipation and diarrhea, persistent rectal bleeding, or lower abdominal pain when results of proctosigmoidoscopy and the barium enema are negative or inconclusive • Assists in the diagnosis of inflammatory and ulcerative bowel disease, colonic stricture, and tumors	1. Explain to the client: • Nature and purpose of the test • Directions for dietary and bowel preparation (clear liquid diet for 48 hours before test; laxative evening before test; and tap water or sodium biphosphate enema 3 to 4 hours before test) • Test involves passage of a well-lubricated flexible tube through	• Position client on left side with knees flexed; drape to avoid embarrassment. • Provide emotional support. • Assist in positioning client (client may need to assume supine position to aid scope's advance). • Place any tissue or cell specimens in properly labeled containers with preservatives and send to laboratory. • Watch closely for untoward responses; have	• Check vital signs according to agency protocol. • Resume usual diet after client recovers from sedation. • Observe for signs of bowel perforation: rectal bleeding, abdominal pain and distention, fever, malaise. • If polyp was removed, inform client it is normal to see some blood in stool. • Inform client it is helpful and usual to expel large amounts of flatus—urge not to withhold.

(continued)

T A B L E   3 5 - 3 (continued)

Diagnostic Studies of the Gastrointestinal Tract

Test and Purpose	Client Preparation	Nursing Care During Test	Client Aftercare
Colonoscopy			
• Allows biopsy, removal of polyps by electrocautery	the anus; air is used to distend the intestine during the procedure; urge to defecate and to pass gas are to be expected • Relaxation is important; breathe deeply and exhale through mouth • Sedative may be administered 2. Ensure that informed consent is signed. 3. If client is unable to complete bowel preparation, administer the prescribed laxative and enema. 4. Assist client into hospital gown and complete agency protocol for testing (empty bladder, remove jewelry, and so forth). 5. Administer sedative if prescribed.	emergency resuscitative equipment available.	
Proctosigmoidoscopy			
• Allows visual examination of the lining of the distal sigmoid colon, the rectum, and the anal canal • Indicated for clients with recent changes in bowel habits, lower abdominal and perineal pain, prolapse on defecation, and passage of mucus, blood, or pus in stool • Assists in the diagnosis of inflammatory, infectious, and ulcerative bowel disease and tumors; and in detection of hemorrhoids, polyps, fissures, fistulas, and abscesses within the rectum and canal	1. Explain to the client: • Nature and purpose of the test • That the test involves three steps: *Digital examination* *Sigmoidoscopy:* a 10- to 12-inch (25 to 30 cm) rigid scope is inserted into the anus to visualize the distal sigmoid colon and rectum *Proctoscopy:* a 2¾-inch (7-cm) rigid scope is inserted into the anus to examine the lower rectum and anal canal • Directions for dietary and bowel preparation (these vary; check agency protocol; most involve clear liquid diet and, possibly, fasting and may include an enema before the test) • Both the examiner's finger and the scopes are well lubricated; they may feel cool and stimulate urge to defecate; air is used to distend the intestine and client may feel urge to pass gas	• Position client in knee–chest or left lateral position and drape to avoid embarrassment. • Provide emotional support. • Instruct client to bear down as scope is passed through the anal sphincter. • Place any tissue or all specimens in properly labeled container with preservatives and send to laboratory.	See client aftercare for colonoscopy.

(continued)

TABLE 35-3 (continued)

Diagnostic Studies of the Gastrointestinal Tract

Test and Purpose	Client Preparation	Nursing Care During Test	Client Aftercare
Proctosigmoidoscopy	• Relaxation is important and eases discomfort; breathe deeply and exhale through mouth 2. Ensure the informed consent is signed. 3. If the client is unable to complete the bowel preparation, administer any prescribed laxatives or enemas. 4. Administer local anesthetic if prescribed to minimize discomfort of rectal inflammation.		
Upper Gastrointestinal (UGI) and Small-Bowel Series			
• Fluoroscopic examination of the esophagus, stomach, and small intestine after ingestion of barium sulfate • Indicated for clients with upper GI symptoms (difficulty swallowing, regurgitation, burning, or epigastric pain), signs of small-bowel disease (diarrhea, weight loss), and signs of GI bleeding (hematemesis, melena) • Assists in the diagnosis of strictures, ulcers, tumors, regional enteritis, and malabsorption syndrome, and in the detection of hiatal hernia, diverticula, varices, and motility disorders	1. Explain to the client: • Nature and purpose of the test • Need to maintain a low-residue diet for 2 to 3 days before the test and to fast and avoid smoking after midnight the day of the test • That the UGI with the small-bowel series can take up to 6 hours to complete • That he or she will be on a rotating x-ray table and will need to assume different positions • That a chalky-tasting barium contrast mixture (16 to 20 oz) will be given to drink before the test 2. Ensure that an informed consent is signed. 3. Assist client to get into hospital gown and to remove jewelry or any objects that would interfere with the x-ray.	• A technician in the radiology department cares for the client during the test.	• Before allowing the client to resume food and fluids, check to be sure that additional x-rays have not been ordered. • Encourage fluids to prevent dehydration. • Administer the posttest cathartic prescribed by agency policy; if there is any question about its advisability for a particular client check with the physician. • Explain to the client the necessity of his or her eliminating the barium and that it will lighten the color of the stool the next few days. • If the cathartic and increased fluid intake do not result in the elimination of the barium within 2 to 3 days, notify the physician. • Encourage extra rest because this test is fatiguing.
Barium Enema			
• Radiographic examination of the large intestine after rectal instillation of barium sulfate (single-contrast technique) or barium sulfate and air (double-contrast technique) • Indicated for clients with altered bowel habits, lower abdominal pain, or the passage of blood, mucus, or pus in the stool	1. *Nursing alert:* Review the client's history for any evidence of ulcerative colitis or active GI bleeding, which would prohibit the use of the standard bowel preparation procedure of laxatives and enemas. Consult with the physician to determine a safe bowel preparation program.	A technician in the radiology department cares for the client during the test.	• Before allowing the client to resume food and fluids, check to be sure that additional x-rays have not been ordered. • Encourage fluids to prevent dehydration. • Encourage rest because this test and the preceding bowel preparation exhaust most clients.

(continued)

T A B L E   3 5 - 3 (continued)

Diagnostic Studies of the Gastrointestinal Tract

Test and Purpose	Client Preparation	Nursing Care During Test	Client Aftercare

Barium Enema
 	
 • Assists in the diagnosis of colorectal cancer and inflammatory disease and in the detection of polyps, diverticula, and structural changes in the larger intestine
	2. Explain to the client:
	 • Nature and purpose of the test (test takes 30 to 45 minutes)
	 • Importance of following the prescribed dietary and bowel preparation because residual fecal material interferes with accurate test results
	   a. Dietary modifications may include a low-residue diet for 1 to 3 days before the test, clear liquids the evening before the test, and increased water and clear liquid intake for 12 to 24 hours before the test.
	   b. A cathartic is usually administered the afternoon or evening before the test and cleansing enemas (tap water) until clear (not to exceed three) the evening before the test or that morning.
	 • That he or she will be on a tilting x-ray table and will need to assume different positions
	 • That he or she may experience cramping pains or the urge to defecate as the barium (500 to 1500 mL) is instilled in the rectum; relaxation and deep breathing may ease this discomfort
	 • That it is important to retain the entire barium enema to get good visualization (keeping the anal sphincter tightly contracted against the rectal tube helps)
	 3. Ensure that an informed consent is signed.
	 4. Assist the client into a hospital gown and prepare for transport to radiology following agency protocol.
			• Administer the prescribed cathartic or cleansing enema to promote elimination of the barium and to prevent fecal impaction and bowel obstruction; instruct the client that barium will lighten the color of the stool.
			 • If the barium is not eliminated within 2 to 3 days, notify the physician.

(Adapted from Fishback, F. [1992]. *A manual of laboratory diagnostic tests* (4th ed., pp. 647–653, 734–736, 745–751). Philadelphia: Lippincott.)

obtained. (In some instances, endoscopic studies may be done before barium studies to ensure visualization.)

Diagnosing

Bowel Elimination as the Problem When analysis of assessment data points to a bowel elimination problem that can be prevented or resolved by independent nursing intervention, a nursing diagnosis is developed. Common alterations in bowel elimination for which a nursing diagnosis may be identified include the following:

Constipation
Colonic Constipation
Perceived Constipation
Diarrhea
Bowel Incontinence

Whenever alterations in bowel elimination require new self-care behaviors (eg, colostomy management), Knowledge Deficit may be an appropriate nursing diagnosis. Examples of specific causes and defining characteristics for these problems are given in the display.

Bowel Elimination as the Etiology Problems of bowel elimination also may affect other areas of human functioning. In the nursing diagnoses that follow, problems of bowel elimination are the etiology for other problems:

Altered Growth and Development related to parents' misconceptions about bowel and bladder training
Altered Nutrition: Less Than Body Requirements, related to loss of appetite from flatulence or impaction
Anxiety related to lack of voluntary control of fecal elimination and significant others' response to ostomy
Body Image Disturbance related to ostomy, need to wear disposable adult briefs
Fluid Volume Deficit related to prolonged diarrhea
Impaired Skin Integrity related to prolonged diarrhea, fecal incontinence
Ineffective Individual Coping related to inability to accept permanent ostomy
Knowledge Deficit: Bowel Training, related to no previous experience
Pain related to intestinal distention, prolonged constipation or impaction, fecal incontinence, hemorrhoids
Self-Care Deficit: Toileting, related to mobility deficit, weakness, confusion
Self-Esteem Disturbance related to need for assistance with toileting, fecal incontinence
Sexual Dysfunction related to perceived change in body image, lack of interest, loss of self-esteem

Planning: Client Goals

Nursing measures for clients without specific bowel elimination problems are directed toward the client's achievement of the following goals. The client will:

- Have a soft, formed bowel movement every 1 to 3 days without discomfort
- Explain the relation between bowel elimination and dietary fiber, fluid intake, and exercise
- Relate the importance of seeking medical evaluation if changes in stool color or consistency persist

Specific client goals for common bowel elimination problems are presented later in the chapter.

Implementing

Promoting Regular Bowel Habits

Regular bowel habits can be promoted in both well and ill clients by attention to timing, positioning, privacy, nutrition, and exercise.

Timing Once the nurse knows when a client usually experiences the urge to defecate (this occurs most often about an hour after meals when mass colonic peristalsis occurs), the nurse offers whatever assistance is needed to help the client to the bathroom, commode, or bedpan at this time. It is important not to schedule nursing care or treatments during this time. Many clients feel uncomfortable about requesting time for elimination. It is helpful for the nurse to communicate to all clients the importance to heed this natural urge and that postponing it only results in constipation and other problems.

Positioning The squatting position best facilitates defecation, but most clients routinely use a sitting position while leaning a bit forward. Most clients who are able to use the bedside commode or bathroom toilet have little difficulty assuming this posture, although they may need support. An elevated toilet seat may be ordered for clients with orthopedic problems who cannot lower themselves to a toilet seat.

Clients who need to use the bedpan in bed benefit from having the head of the bed elevated 30 degrees, unless this is contraindicated. This eliminates the hyperextension of the back that occurs when a client who is lying flat attempts to lift the hips onto the pan. Once the head of the bed is elevated, the client raises the hips by bending the knees, digging in the heels, and lifting the hips upward. An overhead trapeze may be helpful to clients with weak lower extremities. The head of the bed should not be raised more than 45 degrees because this makes it harder to lift the hips straight up. Positioning a client with a bedpan is described in Procedure 35-1. Many clients on bed rest appreciate having moistened hand-wipes at the bedside to substitute for handwashing after toiletry. Bedpans should be emptied, cleaned, and returned to the client's bedside stand promptly.

Privacy Because elimination is considered a private act by most people, nurses must respect the client's need to be alone while defecating, unless the client's weakness makes this impossible. Bedside drapes should be pulled around

(Text continues on p. 918)

NURSING DIAGNOSES FOR COMMON PROBLEMS

Bowel Elimination

Problem	Related Factors	Sample Defining Characteristics
Constipation	• Decreased fiber in diet • Decreased fluid intake • Inactivity • Delaying defecation when urge is present • Abuse of laxatives • Use of constipating medications (antacids, narcotic analgesics [opioids], anticholinergics) • Change in routine • Pain associated with defecation	• "I feel bloated and know I have to move my bowels but I can't." • "Whenever I'm constipated I feel lethargic and lose my appetite." • Reports straining during defecation with little result • Passes small "marbles" of dry, hard stool • Decreased frequency • Decreased frequency of bowel sounds or changes in abdominal growling • Straining often results in small amount of bleeding from swollen external hemorrhoids • Reports feeling rectal fullness or pressure in rectum • Headache
Colonic Constipation	• Decreased fiber intake • Decreased fluid intake • Inactivity • Immobility • Lack of privacy • Abuse of laxatives • Stress • Change in routine • Metabolic alterations	• Decreased frequency • Passed small hard, dry stool • Reports straining at stool • "I have pain when I move my bowels." • Reports feeling bloated • Palpable mass • Reports feeling rectal pressure
Perceived Constipation	• Culture • Family health beliefs • Faulty appraisal • Impaired thought processes	• Expectation of daily bowel movement with resulting abuse of laxatives, enemas, suppositories • Expected passage of stool at the same time every day
Diarrhea	• Food intolerance (coarse, greasy, or spicy foods) • Food or drug allergies • Abuse of laxatives • Alteration in normal bacterial flora of the intestine (antibiotic therapy) • Emotional stress • Intestinal infection • Colon disease and other diseases • Surgical alterations	• Loose liquid stools, increased frequency • Urgency with soiling • Reports of abdominal pain and cramping • Increased frequency of bowel sounds
Bowel Incontinence	• Gross constipation with impaction and subsequent overflow • Organic changes in neural innervation of the rectum • Local causes (inflammation, cancer of rectum, prolapsed anus, semifluid stool) • Extreme debilitation • Cognitive impairment	• Involuntary passage of stool (stool characteristics vary) • "I'm sorry, I couldn't get into the bathroom (or onto the bedpan) quickly enough." • "It came so fast I couldn't hold it back." • History of constipation with sudden development of oozing diarrhea stool

PROCEDURE 35-1

Offering and Removing a Bedpan or Urinal

Equipment

Bedpan or urinal
Toilet tissue
Handwashing supplies
Disposable gloves

Cover for bedpan or urinal (use
  Chux or disposable cover if others
  not available)

Action

1 Bring the bedpan or urinal and equipment to bed-side. Don disposable gloves.

2 Warm the bedpan, if is is made of metal, by rinsing it with warm water.

3 Place an adjustable bed in the high position.

4 Place the bedpan or urinal on the chair next to the bed or on the foot of the bed. Fold the top linen back just enough to allow for placement of bedpan or urinal.

5 If the client needs assistance to move onto the bed-pan, have him or her bend the knees and rest some of his or her weight on the heels. Lift the client by placing one hand under the lower back, and slip the bedpan into place with the other hand.

Rationale

Having equipment on hand saves time by avoiding un-necessary trips to the storage area. Gloves protect against exposure to blood and body substances.

A cold bedpan feels uncomfortable and may make it dif-ficult for the client to void. Plastic bedpans do not re-quire warming.

Having the bed in the high position reduces strain on the nurse's back while assisting the client onto the bedpan.

Folding back the linen in this manner prevents unneces-sary exposure while still allowing the nurse to place the bedpan or urinal.

The client uses less energy as the nurse assists by lifting him or her onto the bedpan. The nurse uses less energy when the client can assist by placing some of his or her weight on the heels.

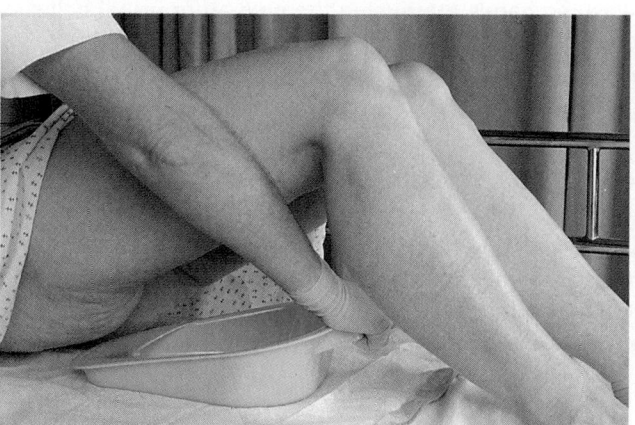

Action 5: Placing a fracture pan under buttocks.

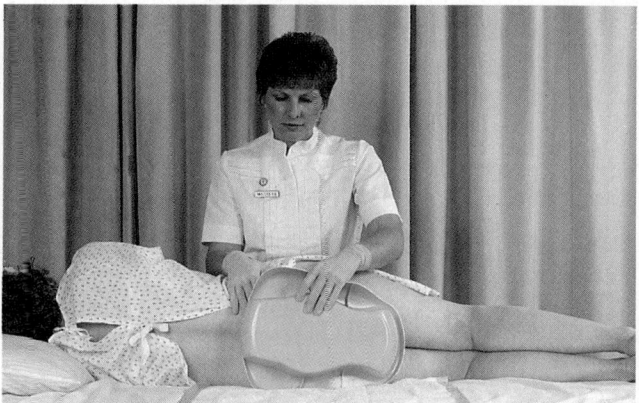

Action 6: Placing bedpan against buttocks while client is on his side. (Photos © B. Proud.)

6 If the client is helpless, two people may be required to lift him or her onto the bedpan. Or, the client may be placed on his or her side, the bedpan is placed against the buttocks, and the client is rolled back onto the bedpan, as shown.

Having two people lift a helpless client causes less strain on the nurse's back. Rolling the client takes less energy than lifting the client onto a bedpan.

(continued)

PROCEDURE 3 5 - 1 *(continued)*

Offering and Removing a Bedpan or Urinal

Action	Rationale
7 When the bedpan is in the proper place, the client's buttocks rest on the rounded shelf of the bedpan, as shown. For male clients, the urinal is properly placed between slightly spread legs with the penis positioned in it and with the urinal resting on the bed.	Having the bedpan or urinal in the proper place prevents spilling contents onto the bed and prevents injury to the skin from a misplaced bedpan.
8 If permitted, raise the head of the bed as near to the sitting position as tolerated.	This position makes it easier for the client to void or defecate, avoids strain on the client's back, and allows gravity to aid in elimination.
9 Place call device and toilet tissue within easy reach. Leave the client if it is safe to do so. Use side rails appropriately.	Falls can be prevented when the client does not have to reach for items he or she needs. Side rails are an additional safety precaution. Leaving client alone, if possible, promotes self-esteem and respects privacy.
10 Remove the bedpan in the same manner in which it was offered, being careful to hold it steady. If necessary to assist the client, don disposable gloves, wrap tissue around the hand several times, and wipe the client clean, using one stroke from the pubic area toward the anal area. Discard tissue, and use more until the client is clean. Place the client on his or her side, and spread the buttocks to clean the anal area. Cover bedpan.	Holding the pan steady prevents spilling its contents. Cleaning an area from front to back minimizes fecal contamination of the vagina and urinary meatus. Cleaning the client after he has used the bedpan prevents offensive odors and irritation to the skin.
11 Do not place toilet tissue in the bedpan if a specimen is required or if measurement of elimination is required. Have a receptacle handy for discarding the tissue.	Toilet tissue mixed with a specimen makes laboratory examination more difficult and interferes with accurate output measurement.
12 Offer the client supplies to wash and dry his or her hands, assisting as necessary.	Washing hands after using the bedpan or urinal helps prevent the spread of organisms.
13 Empty and clean the bedpan and urinal. Wash your hands. Record according to agency procedure.	Provides adequate documentation. Handwashing helps prevent the spread of organisms.

Modifications

A fracture bedpan may be substituted when it is difficult or uncomfortable to use a regular bedpan.

If it is difficult to slide client onto the bedpan, powder may be used on the resting surfaces of the pan to eliminate friction. Powder should not be used if a specimen is required because contamination could result.

---

the client using a bedside commode or bedpan. Well clients who cannot defecate in a public restroom or strange environment may need assistance in developing a workable schedule of defecation that makes use of private toilet facilities.

Nutrition Clients with elimination problems may need a dietary analysis to determine which foods and fluids are contributing to their problem and which may help in its treatment. General dietary recommendations to promote regular defecation include a fluid intake of 2000 to 3000 mL and a high-fiber intake. Water is recommended as the fluid of choice because other fluids (ie, coffee, tea, and juice) may have a diuretic effect instead (Ellickson, 1988). Increasing fiber intake without sufficient fluid intake can result in severe gastrointestinal problems, including fecal impaction. Specific recommendations are as follows:

Constipation Increase high-fiber foods (fruits, vegetables, whole-grain cereals and bread) and fluid intake (fruit

FOCUS ON THE OLDER ADULT

Nursing Strategies for Bowel Elimination Problems Affecting Older Adults

Constipation

- Determine normal bowel pattern.
- Encourage drinking of six to eight glasses of water per day if medical condition permits.
- Implement regular physical exercise routine, even if bedridden.
- Discourage laxative use (particularly mineral oil, cascara, and castor oil) and recommend use of bulk-forming agents (ie, Metamucil) instead.
- Increase fiber in diet moderately and gradually.
- Evaluate drug regimen for medications that constipate (ie, iron, calcium supplements, antacids, and antidepressants).
- Teach client to avoid straining and the Valsalva maneuver.
- Encourage client to eat regular meals and avoid highly processed foods.
- Encourage remaining on the toilet or commode for 20-minute periods.
- Emphasize that bowel pattern may change and lack of a daily bowel movement does not always indicate constipation.

Diarrhea

- Carefully document the occurrence of diarrhea episodes.
- Assess for fecal impaction.
- Monitor for dehydration and fluid and electrolyte imbalance.
- Evaluate diet for possible cause:
  Lactase deficiency
  Food poisoning
  Foods with high sorbitol content
  Foods high in sugar
  Raw seafood
  Improperly cooked or refrigerated food
- Encourage use of yogurt or buttermilk if diet permits to restore normal intestinal flora.

Flatulence

- Avoid foods known to produce gas.
- Encourage slower eating and thorough chewing of food.
- Increase physical activity.

---

juices, especially prune and hot liquids). Specific recommendations for bowel problems that affect older adults are included in the display.

Diarrhea   Prepare and store food properly. Avoid highly spiced foods or laxative-type foods such as raw fruits and vegetables. Encourage foods with low fiber content. Replace lost fluids and electrolytes with weak tea, water, bouillon, clear soup, gelatin; if diarrhea is severe, intravenous therapy may be needed.

Flatulence   Excessive formation of gases in the stomach or intestines is known as **flatulence**. When the gas is not expelled and accumulates in the intestinal tract, the condition is referred to as *intestinal distention* or *tympanites*. Gas-producing foods, such as beans, cabbage, onions, cauliflower, and beer, often predispose to flatulence and distention. Avoiding these foods may be helpful for people with ostomies who are concerned about odor.

Ostomies   Clients with ostomies need to experiment with their diets to see which foods result in the regular evacuation of a moderate amount of stool. A low-fiber diet usually is recommended. High-fiber foods, which could block the passage to the stoma, should be avoided; these include foods with skins, seeds, and shells (eg, raw fruits, popcorn, sunflower seeds, and nuts).

Exercise   Regular exercise improves gastrointestinal motility and aids in defecation. Well clients should be encouraged to incorporate three to five periods of regular exercise into each week's schedule. Ill clients should be ambulated as soon as possible and should be instructed about the relation between inactivity, and constipation, distention, and impaction. Bedside exercises may be helpful for the immobilized client.

Clients with weak abdominal and perineal muscles who are using a bedpan may be helped by the following exercises:

Abdominal Settings   Instruct the client who is lying in a supine position to tighten and hold the abdominal muscles for 6 seconds and then to relax them. This should be repeated several times each waking hour.

Thigh Strengthening   Flex and contract the thigh muscles by slowly bringing the knees up to the chest—one at a time—and then lowering them to the bed. This also should be performed several times for each knee each waking hour.

Teaching About Cathartics, Laxatives, and Antidiarrheals

Constipation and diarrhea are further discussed at the end of the chapter in Nursing Process in Clinical Practice.

Cathartics and Laxatives

Cathartics and **laxatives** are drugs that induce emptying of the intestinal tract. Sometimes used interchangeably, cathartics exert a stronger effect on the intestines than laxatives. Some of these drugs, such as castor oil, cascara, senna, phenolphthalein, and bisacodyl (Dulcolax), act chemically by stimulating peristalsis. Others, such as magnesium sulfate and psyllium hydrophilic mucilloid (Metamucil), act by increasing the intestinal bulk, which promotes additional mechanical stimulation on the intestine. Still others, such as mineral oil and dioctyl sodium sulfosuccinate (Colace), act on the fecal material itself by softening it. Another frequently used laxative is milk of magnesia. It has antacid properties in small dosages and laxative properties when taken in larger doses (refer to Table 35-4 for a summary of the types of laxatives).

Laxatives have their rightful place in health care. They are necessary at times for people whose activity is limited or whose food intake is poor. They also are used for emptying the intestinal tract in preparation for surgical or diagnostic exploration. Their occasional use is not harmful for most people, but all efforts should be taken to prevent a person from becoming dependent on this means of stimulating defecation. Because many laxatives are available as nonprescription drugs, and because modern advertising promotes their use, many people take them frequently on their own initiative, whether they need them or not.

Most people are aware that laxatives have a chemical action and, therefore, should not be taken when there is abdominal pain because of the danger of intestinal pathology and subsequent harm from increased peristalsis. Although many people take laxatives because they believe that they are constipated, most are unaware that habitual use of laxatives is the most common cause of chronic constipation.

Nurses often are in a position to help clients who abuse laxatives. Breaking the laxative habit, from both a physical and a psychological viewpoint, is not easy for a person who has come to depend on laxatives. It often requires a great deal of patience, support, and teaching by the nurse. The person also frequently needs to be helped with diet, fluid intake, activity, and regularity of habits.

T A B L E   3 5 - 4

Classification of Laxatives

Type	Action	Advantages	Caution
Bulk-forming (eg, Metamucil)	Psyllium, grain, or synthetic product that causes stool to absorb water and swell, thus stimulating peristalsis	Usually act within 24 hours	May interfere with absorption of calcium and iron and certain drugs Should not be given to bedridden clients or those with intestinal strictures May be expensive
Emollient/stool softener (eg, Colace)	Agents with detergent activity that allow water and fat to penetrate and lubricate the stool	Recommended for those who must avoid straining	Lubricant component of drug may interfere with absorption of fat-soluble vitamins
Lubricant (eg, mineral oil)	Lubricant absorbed from intestinal tract and softens stool, making it easier to pass	Usually effective within 8 hours	May interfere with absorption of fat-soluble vitamins Aspiration of drug may result in a lipid pneumonia
Stimulant (eg, Dulcolax)	Promotes peristalsis by irritating the intestinal mucosa or stimulating nerve endings in intestinal wall	Works more quickly than bulking agents	Most abused laxatives on the market Cause lazy bowel syndrome May affect absorption of vitamin D and calcium Not recommended for elderly clients due to prolonged action Alters electrolyte transport
Saline-osmotic (eg, Fleets)	Draws water into intestine and stimulates peristalsis	Use when rapid cleansing desired	Should not be used by elderly people Can produce dehydration Not recommended in clients with kidney disease or heart failure

Bowel Elimination

Normal bowel elimination in clients is an ongoing goal for nurses. Nursing assessment provides for early identification of bowel alterations and aids in the development of an individualized plan of care. Changes in bowel elimination patterns are distressing to clients. Nursing interventions help alleviate this stress and promote the emotional as well as the physical well-being of the client.

Related Research

Lara, L., Troop, P., Beadleson-Baird, M. (1990). The risk of urinary tract infection in bowel incontinent men. *Journal of Gerontological Nursing, 16*(5), 24–26.

This research conducted among male residents in a nursing home confirmed that bowel incontinence is significantly related to the incidence of urinary tract infections in men. Three times as many bowel-incontinent male residents developed urinary tract infections compared with those who were continent. These findings emphasize the need for a rapid nursing response to incontinence episodes to prevent transmission of gastrointestinal organisms to the urethra of vulnerable clients.

Brown, M., & Everett, I. (1990). Gentler bowel fitness with fiber. *Geriatric Nursing, 11*(1), 26–27.

Nurses in a long-term care setting developed a bowel-management protocol that included use of a fiber supplement recipe in conjunction with additional fluid intake, regularly scheduled abdominal and pelvic exercise sessions, and a specific toileting routine for each resident. Results in 3 months indicated that those residents in the experimental program required less laxatives while maintaining bowel regularity. Additionally, the fiber supplement proved less expensive than the previously required laxative doses.

Summary

Nursing research of bowel elimination is limited. Studies by other health care professionals do not provide enough information to help in making decisions. Problems in bowel elimination are commonly identified and treated by nurses, supporting the need for further research on normal and altered patterns of bowel elimination.

Antidiarrheals

Antidiarrheal medications usually are reserved for treatment of chronic diarrhea and not recommended initially for acute episodes of diarrhea. Acute diarrhea may occur as the result of a viral or bacterial infection, reactions to medications, or alterations in diet, and is characterized by its sudden onset and a duration of several hours to several days. The duration of chronic diarrhea (more than 3 to 4 weeks) and the many possible causative agents (secondary disease states, surgery, laxative and alcohol abuse, and radiation and chemotherapeutic agents) usually necessitate pharmacologic intervention in addition to fluid and electrolyte replacement. Whatever the type of diarrhea, every effort should be made to identify and eliminate its underlying cause. The most effective nonspecific antidiarrheal medications are the opiates (eg, opium tincture [Paregoric]) and related opiate derivatives (eg, loperamide [Imodium]), which act systemically to reduce intestinal hypermotility and slow peristalsis.

Clark, Queener, and Karb (1990) discuss some implications for use of the various antidiarrheal agents:

- Using opiates to treat diarrhea that is caused by poisons, toxins, or infections may actually prolong the diarrhea because it slows peristalsis and results in additional exposure of the intestinal mucosa to the causative agent.
- Dose requirements of opiates used for treatment of diarrhea usually are smaller than those for analgesia.

- The over-the-counter availability of loperamide (Imodium) requires client awareness of possible adverse effects and dependence with long-term use.
- Some antidiarrheal medications may cause drowsiness, and clients need to be cautioned about the hazards of driving or performing certain tasks when using these drugs.
- The commonly occurring "traveler's diarrhea" may be effectively treated with bismuth subsalicylate (Pepto-Bismol), which can produce black stools.

It is important for the nurse to focus on eliminating the cause of the diarrhea and replacing lost fluid as well as treating the symptoms. Some commercially available products, such as Gatorade, may prove helpful. Malseed and Harrigan (1989) suggest the BRAT routine (*b*ananas, *r*ice, *a*pplesauce, and *t*ea) as one protocol for providing a bland diet while replacing fluids and electrolytes during acute episodes of diarrhea.

Decreasing Flatulence

In addition to avoiding irritating foods, other nursing interventions are helpful in decreasing flatus. Having the client move about in bed and walk promotes peristalsis and the escape of flatus. Reclining after meals should be avoided.

A rectal tube also may be used to help gas escape. The introduction of the tube helps to stimulate peristalsis and provides a passageway for the escape of flatus. The procedure for inserting a rectal tube is as follows:

- Use a 22 to 34 French tube for adults; smaller sizes are used for children.
- Position the client on his or her side, and drape the client properly when preparing to insert a rectal tube.
- Lubricate the rectal tube to reduce irritation to mucous membranes when inserting it.
- Separate the buttocks well so that the anus is in plain view, and introduce the rectal tube beyond the anal canal into the rectum for about 10 cm (about 4 inches). It may be inserted a bit further if it is noted that no flatus is being removed.
- Attach the rectal tube to a piece of tubing of sufficient length to reach a small collection container, which can be attached to the bed frame. Or, place the end of the tube in a specimen container or urinal placed between the client's legs. These techniques allow any discharge that empties through the rectal tube to be caught.
- Leave the rectal tube in place for a short period—no longer than about 20 minutes; the tube no longer acts as a stimulant for peristalsis if left in place longer. If distention is not relieved, use the rectal tube intermittently every 2 to 3 hours, as necessary.
- Have the client assume various positions to help move flatus along the intestinal tract toward the anus. Gas is lighter than fluids and solids, and it will rise. Positions that help gas rise include lying on the abdomen, assuming the knee–chest position, and positioning the upper part of the body over the edge of the bed while the lower part rests across the bed. Do not use these positions if they are contraindicated or unsafe for the client.
- Confer with the physician if these measures bring no relief. An enema, a suppository, or a medication may be prescribed to help bring relief.

Emptying the Colon of Feces

Several methods are used to help promote elimination of feces—enemas, suppositories, rectal catheters, and digital removal of stool.

Enemas

An **enema** is the introduction of a solution into the large intestine, usually for the purpose of removing feces. The instilled solution distends the intestine, may irritate intestinal mucosa, and thus increases peristalsis.

Types of Enemas Enemas are classified as cleansing, retention, or return-flow enemas.

Cleansing Enemas Cleansing enemas are given to remove feces from the colon. They are used for four common purposes:
- To relieve constipation or fecal impaction
- To prevent involuntary escape of fecal material during surgical procedures
- To promote visualization of the intestinal tract by x-ray film or instrument examination

T H R O U G H

T H E   E Y E S

O F   A   S T U D E N T

"Administer soapsuds enema." Oh please, not *my* patient, not *me*. Oh what that word meant, what I would have to do . . . and could I really do it? Oh sure I could . . . I just kept telling myself that, like the little train that could. I kept saying, "I think I can, I think I can."

I went to read up on how to correctly administer an enema. I was to give a soapsuds enema that I needed to prepare myself in a bag with long tubing attached; it resembled an IV bag. It was obvious that I needed some assistance—oh no, that meant my instructor would be in the room also. I didn't know what was worse.

I went through the procedure first with my instructor. Later I ventured into the patient's room and explained to him what I was going to do, thus preparing him for the ordeal.

I rolled the tip of the tubing in KY jelly and inserted it into the rectum. The patient moaned and groaned while my instructor lent her support. Then suddenly something went haywire: the patient started to get up, the tubing started to come out, and my instructor was yelling, "Clamp the tubing." By that time, it was too late. The tubing was out and squirting like a fountain, wetting the patient and giving me a bath. I eventually dragged myself out of the room after cleaning up the mess, not knowing whether to laugh or cry.

I really thought that was the worst day of my life, but I got over it and I look back and laugh, and so does my instructor.

—Frances Faries, Holy Family College, Philadelphia

• To help establish regular bowel function during a bowel training program

The most frequent types of solutions used for cleansing enemas are tap water, normal saline solution, soap solution, and hypertonic solution. These are described in Table 35-5. Hypotonic (tap water) and isotonic (normal saline solution) enemas are large-volume enemas that result in rapid colonic emptying. The large volumes of solution (adults, 500 to 1000 mL; infants, 150 to 250 mL) may present a danger to clients with weakened intestinal walls. These solutions often require special preparation and equipment. Hypertonic solution preparations are available commercially and are administered in smaller volumes (adult, 70 to 130 mL). These solutions draw water into the colon, which stimulates the defecation reflex. They may be contraindicated in clients for whom sodium retention is a problem.

Retention Enemas Retention enemas are retained in the bowel for a prolonged period for different reasons.

Oil-retention enemas—lubricate the stool and intestinal mucosa, making defecation easier. About 150 to 200 mL of solution is administered to adults.

Carminative enemas—help to expel flatus from the rectum and provide relief from gaseous distention. Common solutions include the milk-and-molasses enema (equal parts) and the MGW enema (30 mL of magnesium sulfate, 60 mL of glycerine, and 90 mL of warm water).

Medicated enema—used to administer medications that are absorbed through the rectal mucosa

Anthelmintic enemas—administered to destroy intestinal parasites

Nutritive enemas—administer fluids and nutrition rectally

Return-Flow Enemas *Return-flow,* or *Harris flush, enemas* are used to expel flatus. For an adult, 100 to 200 mL of a solution is instilled into the rectum and sigmoid colon and then the solution container is lowered so that the solution flows back into the container. This process is repeated five or six times, and the alternating flow of solution stimulates peristalsis and aids in the expelling of flatus. The procedure is terminated when abdominal distention is relieved. If the return solution becomes thick with feces, it is replaced by fresh solution.

Equipment Commercially prepared enema kits include a flexible bottle containing hypertonic solution with an attached prelubricated firm tip about 5 to 7.5 cm (2 to 3 inches) in length. Its ease of use makes it particularly convenient in the home setting. Clients can readily administer their own enema in many instances.

For the tap water, saline solution, or soap solution enema, a container, rubber or plastic tubing with side openings near its distal end, a tubing clamp, lubricant, and the solution are necessary. Pitchers with a funnel attached to the tubing for introducing the solution may be used as solution containers. Although the commercially prepared equipment is sterile, and any reusable equipment is sterilized between clients in a health agency, the procedure for administering an enema requires clean or medical asepsis technique, not sterile technique. Disposable gloves protect the caregiver from exposure to blood, body substances, and microorganisms.

Client Preparation Because the enema is a common procedure, many clients understand its use and how it is administered. Other clients who have not experienced an enema before need an explanation of its purpose, what they can expect, and how they can participate. The procedure offers an excellent opportunity for health teaching because many people are not familiar with the functioning of the intestinal tract. Failure to observe one or more of these principles may be responsible for the clients' considering the procedure a disagreeable one.

TABLE 35-5

Commonly Used Enema Solutions

Solution	Amount	Action	Time to Take Effect	Adverse Effects
Tap water (hypotonic)	500–1000 mL	Distends intestine, increases peristalsis, softens stool	15 min	Fluid and electrolyte imbalance, water intoxication
Normal saline (isotonic)	500–1000 mL	Distends intestine, increases peristalsis, softens stool	15 min	Fluid and electrolyte imbalance, sodium retention
Soap	500–1000 mL (concentrate at 3–5 mL/1000 mL)	Distends intestine, irritates intestinal mucosa, softens stool	10–15 min	Rectal mucosa irritation or damage
Hypertonic	70–130 mL	Distends intestine, irritates intestinal mucosa	5–10 min	Sodium retention
Oil (mineral, olive, or cottonseed oil)	150–200 mL	Lubricates stool and intestinal mucosa	30 min	

Most clients think that solutions are to be expelled as soon as possible. When a solution is to be retained, care should be taken to have the client understand this.

Administering an Enema Using a Large Volume of Solution The procedure for administering a cleansing enema using either a large volume of solution or a commercially prepared solution is described in Procedure 35-2.

Administering an Enema Using a Hypertonic Solution Administering a cleansing enema using a hypertonic solution differs somewhat from the procedure described in Procedure 35-2.

- The equipment is included in the commercially prepared sets. The only additional equipment needed is the bedpan for the bedridden client and a disposable waterproof pad to protect bed linens.
- It is unnecessary to warm the hypertonic solution. Administer it at room temperature, and warm it only if it is very cold.
- The side-lying position usually is used. The knee–chest position helps to distribute the solution throughout the lower intestinal tract and is recommended if the client is able to assume it. Lubrication of the rectal tips is recommended, even though they are prelubricated.
- The solution is forced into the rectum by applying gentle pressure on the collapsible solution container. It should take 1 to 2 minutes to administer the enema.

Administering an Oil-Retention Enema The procedure for giving an oil enema differs from that of giving a cleansing enema in certain respects:

- A small rectal tube is used. The small size helps to reduce intestinal contractions so that the client can retain the oil more easily. Oil enemas are available in commercial kits similar to those for the hypertonic-solution enema. The kits contain a small rectal tube.
- Oil is given at body temperature to minimize muscle contractions caused by a warmer or cooler solution.

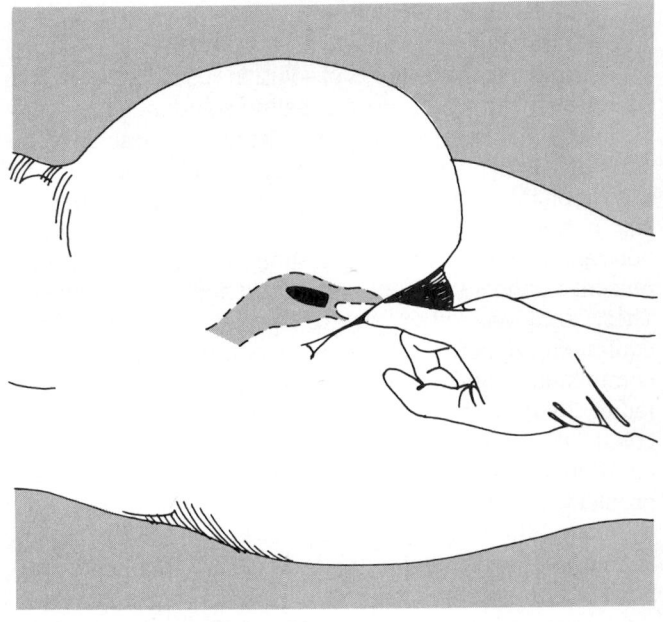

F I G U R E 3 5 - 5

Rectal suppositories should be introduced into the anus well beyond the internal sphincter.

- The client should be instructed to retain the oil for at least 30 minutes for best cleansing results.

Rectal Suppositories

A **suppository** is a conical or oval solid substance shaped for easy insertion into a body cavity and designed to melt at body temperature (Fig. 35-5). Various rectal suppositories are available. Some act as fecal softeners, others have direct action on the nerve endings in the rectal mucosa, and some liberate carbon dioxide when moistened. Fecal softeners are useful when the stool is very hard; substances

(Text continues on p. 928)

G U I D E L I N E S F O R N U R S I N G C A R E

Inserting a Rectal Suppository

- Use a glove for protection while inserting the suppository.
- Have the client lie on either side, and pie-fold top linens over him or her.
- Lubricate the suppository and fingertips to reduce irritation on intestinal mucosa while inserting the suppository.
- Separate the buttocks and then have the client relax by breathing through the mouth while the suppository is inserted.
- Introduce the suppository well beyond the internal sphincter (4 inches for adults and 2 inches for children and infants) so that the suppository is in the rectum, where its effect is desired.
- Avoid embedding the suppository in the fecal mass. Correct placement when there is stool in the rectum is between the stool and the rectal mucosa.
- Be sure the client understands that he or she is to retain the suppository, usually for 30 to 45 minutes after insertion.
- Encourage the client to walk about if ambulatory; this often helps promote peristalsis.

PROCEDURE 35-2

Administering a Cleansing Enema

Equipment

Disposable enema set
Water-soluble lubricant
Solution as ordered by physician:
  Temperature:
  For adult—105°–110°F (40°–43°C)
  For children—100°F (37.7°C)
  Amount: Will vary, depending on
  type of solution, age of the per-
  son, and the client's ability to
  retain the solution. Average
  cleansing enema for an adult
  may range from 750 to 1000 mL.

Necessary additves (soap, salt,
  and so forth)
Bath thermometer
Waterproof pad
Bath blanket
Bedpan and toilet tissue
IV pole
Disposable gloves
Paper towel
Washcloth, soap, towel or
  Handi-wipes

Action	Rationale
1 Assemble the necessary equipment. Warm solution in amount ordered, and check temperature with a bath thermometer if available. If tap water is used, adjust temperature as it flows from faucet.	Organization facilitates performance of task. If bath thermometer is not available, warm to room temperature or slightly higher, and test on inner wrist.
2 Explain the procedure to the client and plan where he or she will defecate. Have a bedpan, commode, or nearby bathroom ready for his use.	The client is better able to relax and cooperate if he or she is familiar with the procedure and knows everything is in readiness when he feels the urge to defecate. Defecation usually occurs within 5 to 15 minutes.
3 Wash your hands.	Handwashing deters the spread of microorganisms.
4 Add enema solution to container. Release the clamp and allow fluid to progress through tube before reclamping.	This causes any air to be expelled from the tubing. Although allowing air to enter the intestine is not harmful, it may further distend the intestine.
5 Position waterproof pad under the client.	This protects bed linen.
6 Provide for client's privacy. Position and drape the client on the left side (Sims' position) with anus exposed or on the back, as dictated by client comfort and condition.	The client's comfort and warmth help him relax. The exact position of the reclining person has not been found to alter results of an enema significantly.
7 Put on disposable gloves.	This protects the nurse from microorganisms in the feces.
8 Elevate the solution so that it is 45 cm (18 inches) above the level of the client's anus. Plan to give the solution slowly over a period of 5 to 10 minutes. The container may be hung on an IV pole or held in the nurse's hands at the proper height.	Gravity forces the solution to enter the intestine. The amount of pressure determines the rate of flow and pressure exerted on the intestinal wall. Giving the solution too quickly causes rapid distention and pressure in the intestine, resulting in too rapid expulsion of the solution, poor defecation, or damage to the mucous membrane.
9 Generously lubricate the end of the rectal tube for 5 to 7 cm (2 to 3 inches). A disposable enema set may have a prelubricated rectal tube.	This facilitates passage of the rectal tube through the anal sphincter and prevents injury to the mucosa.

(continued)

P R O C E D U R E 3 5 - 2 (continued)

Administering a Cleansing Enema

Action

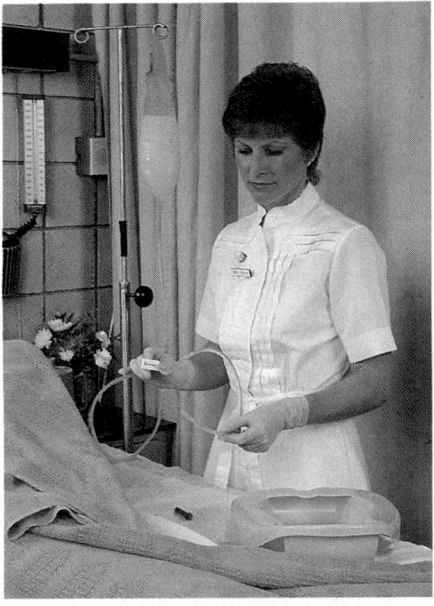

Rationale

Action 8: Preparing to administer the enema.

10 Lift the buttock to expose the anus. Slowly and gently insert the rectal tube 7 to 10 cm (3 to 4 inches). Direct it at an angle pointing toward the umbilicus.

Good visualization of the anus helps prevent injury to tissues. The anal canal is about 2.5 to 5 cm (1 to 2 inches) in length. The tube should be inserted past the internal sphincter. Further insertion may damage intestinal mucous membrane. The suggested angle follows the normal intestinal contour. Slow insertion of the tube minimizes spasms of the intestinal wall and sphincters.

11 If the tube meets resistance while inserting it, permit a small amount of solution to enter, withdraw the tube slightly and then continue to insert it. Do not force entry of the tube. Ask the client to take several deep breaths.

Resistance may be due to spasms of the intestine or failure of the internal sphincter to open. The solution may help to reduce spasms and relax the sphincter, thus making continued insertion of the tube safe. Forcing a tube may injure the intestinal wall. Taking deep breaths helps relax the anal sphincter.

12 Introduce the solution slowly over a period of 5 to 10 minutes. Hold tubing all the time that solution is being instilled. Commercial preparations may be administered by compressing container with hands, according to package directions.

Introducing the solution slowly helps prevent rapid distention of the intestine and a desire to defecate.

13 Clamp the tubing or lower the container if the client has the desire to defecate or cramping occurs. Client also may be instructed to take small, fast breaths or to pant.

These techniques help relax muscles and prevent the expulsion of the solution prematurely.

14 After solution has been given, clamp the tubing and remove the tube. Have paper towel ready to receive tube as it is withdrawn. Have the client retain the solution until the urge to defecate becomes strong, usually in about 5 to 15 minutes.

This amount of time usually allows muscle contractions to become sufficient to produce good results.

15 Remove disposable gloves from inside out and discard.

This protects the nurse from contact with any microorganism.

(continued)

PROCEDURE 35 - 2 *(continued)*

Administering a Cleansing Enema

Action

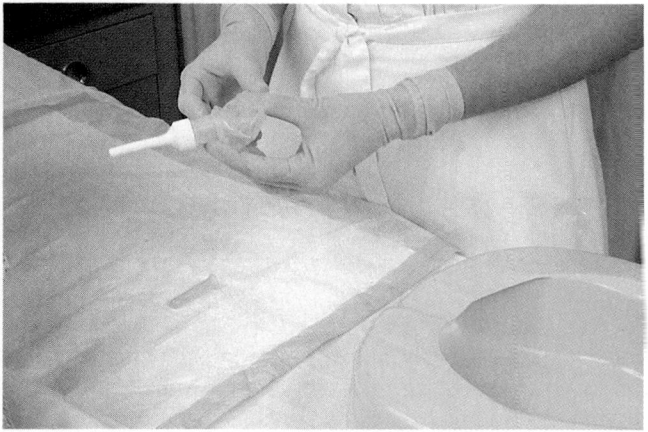

Technique for compressing Fleets enema container.

Rationale

16 When the client has a strong urge to defecate, place him or her in a sitting position on a bedpan or assist to a commode or to the bathroom.

The sitting position is most natural and facilitates the act of defecation.

17 Record the character of the stool and the client's reaction to the enema. Remind the client not to flush commode before nurse inspects results of enema.

The nurse needs to observe and record the results. Additional enemas may be necessary if physician has ordered enemas "until clear."

18 Assist client if necessary with cleaning of anal area. Offer washcloth, soap, and water to wash his hands.

Deters spread of microorganisms.

19 Leave the client clean and comfortable. Care for the equipment properly.

There is abundant growth of bacteria in the intestine, which can be spread to others when equipment is not properly cared for.

20 Wash your hands.

Handwashing deters the spread of microorganisms.

Age Considerations

Infirm or elderly clients who are unable to retain the enema solution should receive the enema while on the bedpan in the supine position. For comfort, the head of the bed can be elevated 30 degrees if necessary and pillows used appropriately. Disposable gloves protect the hands as the enema is being expelled.

Parents should be encouraged to assist in relieving anxiety and encouraging cooperation when young children require enemas.

Modify amount of solution according to client's ability to tolerate procedure and size of client.

Home-Care Considerations

Give enema in area that is as close to bathroom as possible. If using bedpan or commode, have it readily accessible.

Inform client about availability of commercially prepared solutions and equipment.

Special Considerations

The limit for "enemas until clear" usually is three. Check with the physician before continuing with additional enemas because fluid and electrolyte imbalance can occur.

that stimulate the rectal nerves are helpful for people with weak muscle tone or poor innervation. The carbon dioxide suppositories liberate about 200 mL of gas, which causes distention, thus producing stimulation and elimination impulses. See Nursing Guidelines for Inserting a Rectal Suppository.

Rectal Indwelling (Foley) Catheters

Indwelling catheters may be used in some institutions for clients with uncontrollable diarrhea after chemotherapy, antibiotic therapy, or tube feedings. Birdsall (1986) reported that the rectal catheters successfully maintained skin integrity and allowed liquid stool to be accurately measured.

The chief advantage of a rectal indwelling catheter over a straight rectal tube is that the balloon helps to seal the sphincter and prevents the continuous oozing of stool. The catheters also are used with comatose clients who need retention enemas like polystyrene sulfonate (Kayexalate) and neomycin but are unable to retain the enema solution. The procedure includes the following:

- Inserting a 28 or 30 French catheter (for an adult) about 5 to 7.6 cm (about 2 to 3 inches) into the rectum (the catheter should not be introduced into the sigmoid colon). This is a clean, not a sterile, procedure.
- Inflating the balloon with saline solution or air and gently pulling back on the catheter so that the balloon sits at the internal sphincter
- Attaching the indwelling catheter to a drainage bag
- Deflating the balloon for a few minutes *every hour* to relieve pressure (failure to do this may result in rectal necrosis)
- Changing the rectal catheter and drainage bag every day or more frequently if it becomes messy. (*Recommendation:* Have two catheters for each client. Clean each one after use and store in a sterile towel until needed to reduce the risk of nosocomial infections.) The catheter should not be flushed while in place because this may worsen the diarrhea.

Relatively little research supports the safety of this procedure. Some nurses claim that the rectal indwelling catheter stimulates sensory nerve fibers in the rectum and then increases peristalsis and worsens diarrhea. Others are concerned about the danger of rectal perforation and the development of mucosal necrosis. A physician's order is needed for this procedure, and the client needs to be carefully monitored.

Fecal Incontinence Pouch

An alternative measure to protect perianal skin from repeated episodes of fecal incontinence is the fecal incontinence pouch. Lincoln and Roberts (1989) state that this device can be secured around the anal opening and attached to gravity drainage, allowing liquid stool to accumulate in a collection bag. It is best applied before the perianal area becomes excoriated, but a skin barrier is effective if this has already occurred. Nursing responsibilities include careful assessment and documentation of the perianal skin condition and attentive management of the drainage system. The bag should be changed at least every 72 hours, or sooner if it is not intact or leakage has occurred. Families, particularly, may need explanation and support to understand the benefits of this system.

Digital Removal of Stool

A **fecal impaction** is prolonged retention or an accumulation of fecal material that forms a hardened mass in the rectum. It is common for a fecal impaction to prevent the passage of normal stools. Small amounts of fluid may go around the impacted mass. In fact, liquid fecal seepage and no passage of normal feces are symptomatic of the existence of an impaction.

If a client with a fecal impaction is unable to expel the fecal mass voluntarily, and oil and cleansing enemas fail to break up the mass, it is necessary to break up the impaction manually. This procedure may cause great discomfort to the client and cause irritation of the rectal mucosa, bleeding, and slowed heart rate by vagal stimulation. A physician's order is necessary for this procedure. The following techniques are recommended:

- Have a second person assist with the procedure. The second person can assure and comfort the client while the first person works to break up the mass.
- Place the client in a side-lying position for the convenience of the nurses.
- Place a bedpan in the bed so that pieces of removed feces can be deposited into it.
- Drape the client by pie-folding top linens back.
- Use clean gloves for the procedure; the intestinal tract is not sterile.
- Lubricate the forefinger generously to reduce irritating the rectum, and insert the finger *gently* into the anal canal. The presence of the finger added to the mass tends to cause discomfort for the client when work is not done slowly and gently. To minimize discomfort, a local anesthetic may be used. Weidner (1992) reports the following technique:
  - Place 1 to 2 mL of lidocaine on the gloved forefinger into the rectum as far as possible, remove immediately, and wait 5 minutes before proceeding with the digital removal. This should not be attempted without a physician's order.
- Work the finger around and into the hardened mass to break it up and then remove pieces of it.
- Remove the impaction at intervals if it is severe. This helps to avoid discomfort as well as irritation, which can injure intestinal mucosa.
- Use an oil-retention enema as necessary. The enema may be given before attempts are made to break up and remove an impaction digitally. Or, it may be ordered after digital attempts fail. A cleansing enema often is ordered after an oil-retention enema.

Figure 35-6 demonstrates this procedure. Many clients find that a sitz bath or tub bath after this procedure soothes the irritated perineal area.

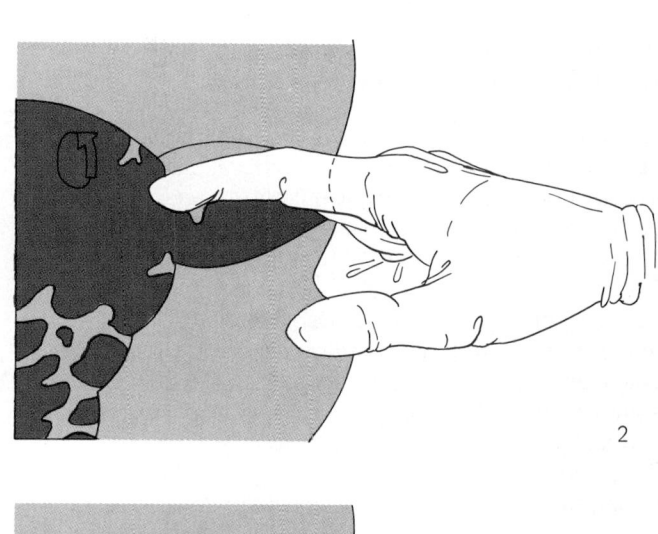

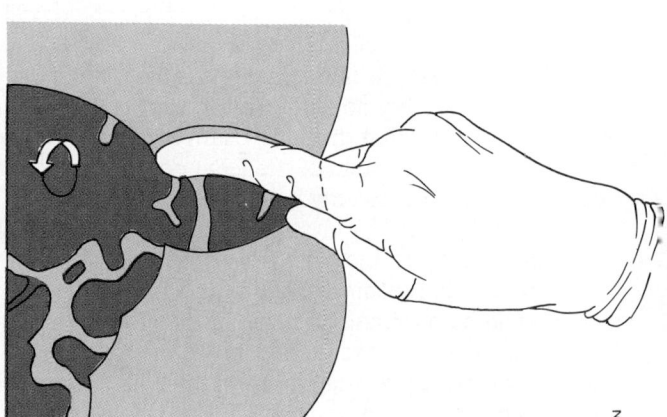

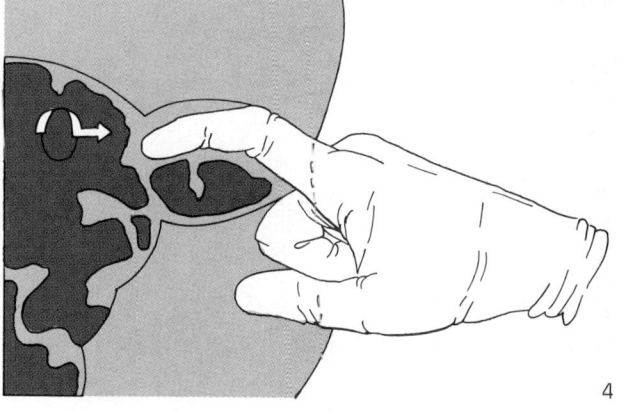

FIGURE 35-6

Digital removal of fecal impaction.

Designing and Implementing Bowel Training Programs

Clients with a history of chronic constipation and impaction and those who are incontinent of stool may benefit from a **bowel training program**. The purpose of this program is to manipulate factors within the person's control (food and fluid intake, exercise, time for defecation) to produce the elimination of a soft, formed stool at regular intervals without laxative support. This effort to regain bowel control may be initiated in the health care setting or implemented in the client's home. Steps in a bowel training program include the following:

- Explaining the program and its aim to the client in an effort to enlist the client's full participation
- Assessing the client's bowel elimination patterns and identifying factors that promote or hinder defecation
- Designing a plan to modify contributing life-style variables: (1) increase fluid intake to 2500 to 3000 mL—include hot drinks or fruit juices known to promote peristalsis for the client; (2) increase the fiber content of the diet; and (3) increase exercise if possible
- Starting the program with a clean bowel (rectal examination for impaction—remove if present)

- Maintaining a daily training routine for 14 to 21 days until a regular pattern of defecation without laxatives is established:
  - Thirty minutes before the client's usual defecation time (note this in plan) administer a cathartic suppository (eg, Dulcolax) to stimulate peristalsis.
  - Note the time it usually takes for the suppository to work and when the client has an urge to evacuate (usually 15 minutes to an hour). Assist the client to the bathroom or commode or onto a bedpan.
  - Allow the client privacy and ample time for evacuation (usually 20 to 30 minutes is adequate); avoid both rushing the client and abandoning the client on the bedpan or commode for prolonged periods.
  - Share the client's success and offer positive verbal reinforcement and encouragement; refrain from criticizing the client who is unsuccessful.
- Communicating that patience may be necessary before regular elimination patterns resume—project a "can do" mentality

When the client has established a pattern of regular defecation, continue to offer assistance with toileting at the successful time but discontinue use of the laxative.

Meeting Needs of Clients With Bowel Diversions

Sometimes surgical procedures are required to create an opening into the abdominal wall for fecal elimination. The intestinal mucosa is brought out to the abdominal wall, and a **stoma** is formed by suturing the mucosa to the skin. The word *ostomy* is a general term for an opening into the body; it usually is used to refer to an opening created for the excretion of body wastes. An **ileostomy** allows fecal content from the ileum to be eliminated through the stoma. A **colostomy** permits feces from the colon to exit through the stoma. Figure 35-7 shows the location of an ileostomy and variously placed colostomies.

An ileostomy or a colostomy may be either temporary or permanent. Temporary ostomies are done to allow the

FIGURE 35-7

Location of various colostomies and the location of an ileostomy.

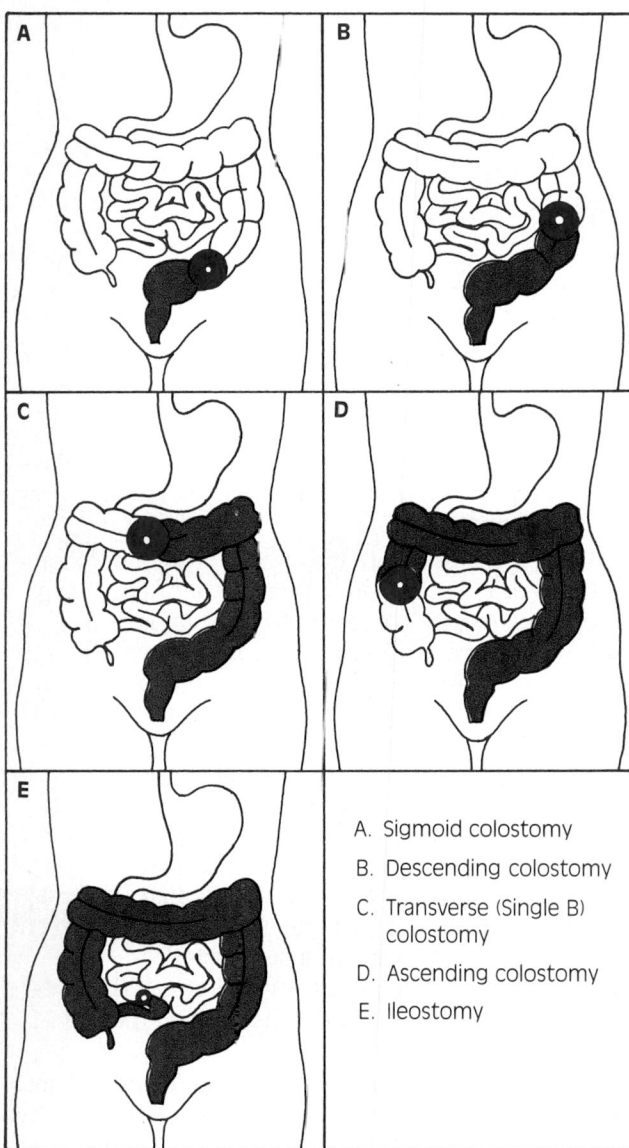

A. Sigmoid colostomy

B. Descending colostomy

C. Transverse (Single B) colostomy

D. Ascending colostomy

E. Ileostomy

intestine to repair itself after inflammatory disease, some types of intestinal surgery, or injury. Permanent ostomies are done as the result of debilitating intestinal diseases or cancer of the colon or rectum. Clinical texts further discuss pathophysiologic conditions for which ostomies are required.

Colostomy and Ileostomy Care   The client with an ostomy needs physical and psychological support both preoperatively and postoperatively. This support can come from people who are close to the client as well as from members of the health team and from people who have had similar experiences. The ostomy requires specific physical care for which the nurse is initially responsible. The following guidelines help to promote physical and psychological comfort for the ostomy client:

- Keep the client as free of odors as possible. The application of a temporary appliance after surgery or during the time of the first dressing change postoperatively can eliminate much of the fecal odor from a bulky dressing. The ostomy appliance should be emptied frequently.
- Check the client's stoma regularly. The color should be dark pink to red. Bleeding around the stoma and its stem should be minimal. The size of the stoma stabilizes within 4 to 6 weeks. Report any abnormal color, bleeding, or excessive edema promptly. If an abdominal dressing is in place, it also should be checked frequently for drainage and bleeding.
- Keep the skin around the stoma site (peristomal area) clean and dry. If care is not taken to protect the skin around the stoma, irritation or infection may occur. A leaking appliance frequently is responsible for skin erosion.
- Measure the client's fluid intake and output. Check the ostomy appliance for the quality and quantity of discharge. Intake and output should be recorded every 4 hours for the first 3 days after surgery. If the client's output decreases while intake remains stable, the condition should be reported promptly.
- Explain each aspect of care to the client, and explain what his or her role will be when he or she begins self-care. Client teaching is one of the most important aspects of colostomy care.
- Encourage the client to participate in care and to look at the ostomy. It is expected that the client will experience emotional depression during the early postoperative period. The nurse can help the client to cope by listening, explaining, and being available and supportive. A visit from a representative of the local ostomy support group may be helpful. The client usually begins to accept his or her altered body image when he or she is willing to look at the stoma, makes neutral or positive statements concerning the ostomy, and expresses interest in learning self-care.

Changing the Ostomy Appliance   The ostomy appliance should protect the skin, collect the fecal discharge, and

Changing an Ostomy Appliance

- Wear disposable gloves to protect against exposure to blood, body fluids and excretions, and microorganisms.
- Select a bag with the appropriately sized stomal opening, or cut a circle on the adhesive backing of the stomal appliance $1/16$ to $1/8$ inch larger than the stoma. Peel back the paper covering the adhesive backing of the stomal appliance. Figure 35-8 illustrates this.
- Position the hole of the appliance over the stoma, and place the appliance in position by pressing it gently but firmly on the area immediately around the stoma. Figure 35-9 shows the nurse placing the appliance over a colostomy stoma.
- If a belt is to be used, attach it to the stomal appliance. The belt provides extra support for keeping the appliance in place, especially when the client is ambulatory.
- Close the bottom of the appliance with the closure clip if an open-ended one is used. Empty the bag as often as required.

- Remove the bag every 2 to 3 days. Make sure the peristomal area is free of irritation or excoriation (a breakdown of the epidermis). Protect the skin appropriately.
- Remove the appliance carefully to avoid pulling off the outer layer of skin.
- Use warm water or a mild solvent to facilitate removal of the appliance. If a solvent is used, wash it from the skin with warm water.
- Cleanse the peristomal skin gently with warm water and a *mild* soap. Avoid hard rubbing and harsh cleansing agents. Some authorities recommend not using soap because of its irritating effects on the skin.
- Rinse the skin well, gently pat it dry, and apply a protective skin barrier. Use the skin-protecting agent required by agency policy. Karaya Gum Powder is a common agent. Allow the skin barrier to dry thoroughly.
- Measure the stomal size with a measuring guide if a new appliance is to be used.

control odor. For the first few days after surgery, most clients wear an open-ended appliance that allows for drainage of fecal material without removing the appliance. The drainage bag is cleansed by injecting warm water into the bag and allowing it to drain, as necessary. (See Guidelines for Nursing Care—Changing an Ostomy Appliance, and Figs. 35-8 and 35-9).

Colostomy Irrigation Ileostomies are not irrigated because the fecal content of the ileum is liquid, which cannot be controlled. Irrigations may be used to help regulate some colostomies. Various factors, such as the site of the colostomy in the colon and the client's and physician's preferences, determine whether or not a colostomy is irrigated.

FIGURE 35-8

The paper is peeled from the adhesive backing of the colostomy appliance before it is placed over the stoma. The Karaya ring around the opening fits over the stoma. For purposes of demonstration, gloves have not been worn but are recommended to prevent possible exposure to blood, body fluids and excretions, and microorganisms. (Courtesy of Convatec, a Squibb Company.)

FIGURE 35-9

The colostomy appliance is pressed into place. The stomal opening should be about $1/8$ inch larger than the diameter of the stoma. For purposes of demonstration, gloves have not been worn but are recommended to prevent possible exposure to blood, body fluids and excretions, and microorganisms. (Courtesy of Convatec, a Squibb Company.)

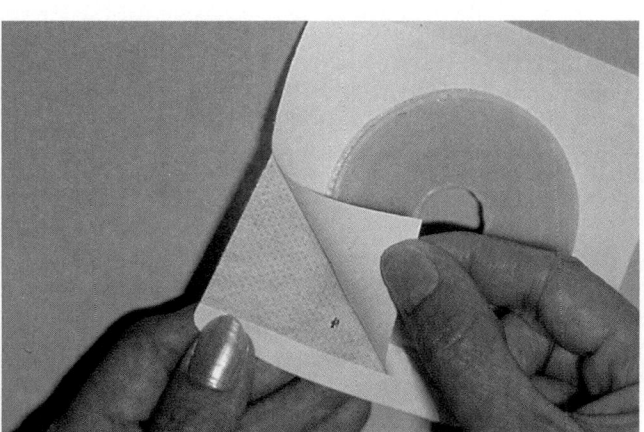

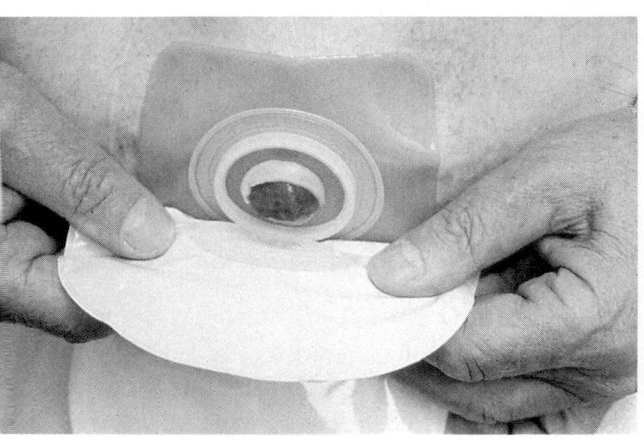

If an irrigation is to be done, the nurse should familiarize the client with the technique to be used. The nurse should explain the procedure, demonstrate the equipment, and explain how the return fluid can be directed into a bedpan, commode, or toilet bowl. It also may be helpful to have a family member learn the irrigation techniques in case there are times when the client cannot do the irrigation himself or herself. The procedure for irrigating a colostomy is similar to that for administering an enema, except that the irrigating catheter is inserted into an abdominal stoma instead of into the anus. A commercially obtained irrigation set usually has all the equipment needed and comes with explicit directions.

In many health agencies, ostomy care, colostomy irrigations, and client teaching are done by specially trained enterostomal therapists.

Long-Term Ostomy Care   The client can live an active and useful life with an ostomy. He or she should be aware of community resources to assist him, such as home health care nurses, special clinics, and ostomy support groups. The client should be encouraged to seek medical follow-up care on a regular basis.

Ostomy clients are encouraged to avoid foods high in fiber content initially, as well as any other foods that cause them to have diarrhea or excessive amounts of flatus. By gradually adding new foods, the ostomy client can build up to a normal diet. He or she may choose to avoid some foods that are bothersome.

Health teaching about medication use frequently is overlooked for the client with an ostomy. Madda (1991) offers the following helpful guidelines:

- Remind the client that some medications discolor the stool and cause unusual odors.
- Encourage the client to check the ostomy bag after starting on new medication to make sure the medication has been completely dissolved.
- Review the common drugs that cause constipation.
- Ileostomy clients need to be particularly alert about drug absorption problems, since the small bowel is where most absorption occurs. They should use liquid, chewable, or injectable forms rather than long-acting, enteric-coated, or sustained-release medications. Laxatives and enemas are dangerous because they may cause severe fluid and electrolyte imbalance.

Clients with ostomies should be taught various methods of odor control. The chlorophyll content in dark green vegetables helps to deodorize the feces when these vegetables are included in the diet. Bismuth subgallots, which can be purchased at drug stores and which can be taken with meals, help to lessen fecal odor. Benedict and Haddad (1989) recommend that 2 tbsp of a nonalcoholic mouthwash be placed in the ostomy bag for better odor control, and McKenzie and Gallacher (1989) suggest that enteric-coated peppermint oil capsules be ingested to mask fecal odor.

Some clients can achieve control over fecal elimination from a colostomy by regular irrigations and by habitual emptying of the colon at a certain time each day. Few clients with an ileostomy gain any degree of control of the excretion of wastes and seldom may dispense with the use of an appliance, except for short periods.

Normal activity, including work, can be resumed. Direct physical contact sports and heavy lifting should be avoided. The client can go swimming and needs to wear only gauze or a large adhesive bandage over the stoma.

Providing Comfort Measures

Comfort measures related to defecation include working with the client to develop a bowel elimination routine that results in the easy passage of a soft, formed stool, being attentive to perineal hygiene and the maintenance of skin integrity and using warm moist heat (sitz bath or tub bath) to soothe the perineal area. Clients with hemorrhoids may require special comfort measures, such as the application of topical medications to reduce inflammation and the administration of stool softeners.

Evaluating

The nurse evaluates the effectiveness of a plan of care to promote regular bowel elimination by checking to see if the client has met the individualized client goals specified in the plan. Nursing care is considered effective if the client expresses satisfaction with his or her regular pattern of defecation and the ability to comfortably pass a soft, formed stool without the use of medications or laxatives. The plan of care is most successful when the client is able to:

- Verbalize the relation between bowel elimination and nutrition, fluid intake, exercise, and stress management
- Develop a plan to modify any factors that contribute to current bowel problems or that might adversely affect bowel functioning in the future
- Correct unhealthy bowel habits, such as ignoring the urge to defecate and abusing laxatives and enemas

 ## NURSING PROCESS

in Clinical Practice

Once a bowel elimination problem is detected, the nurse implements each phase of the nursing process to ensure its correct identification and treatment. The nurse who wants to correctly identify and manage the bowel elimination problem must possess the knowledge and clinical skills described earlier in this chapter. What follows in outline format are focused assessment priorities, client goals, nursing interventions, and evaluative criteria for the nursing diagnoses:

Constipation
Bowel Incontinence
Diarrhea

In the case study that follows, a plan of care is developed to address the elimination needs of a pediatric client with severe diarrhea.

Constipation

Constipation is the passage of dry, hard stools. Decreased gastric motility slows the passage of feces through the large intestine, resulting in increased fluid absorption from the fecal mass and the dry, hard stool. Straining often accompanies defecation. Some people may be constipated and yet have a daily bowel movement, whereas others who regularly defecate no more than three times a week are not constipated. The habits of elimination vary greatly among healthy people.

Assessment

- Assess bowel elimination patterns noting (1) decrease in the usual number of bowel movements; (2) dry, hard stools; (3) straining and difficult evacuation; (4) abdominal distention; (5) swollen hemorrhoids; and (6) complaints of headache, lassitude, anorexia, low back pain, or irritability.
- Identify contributing factors: insufficient fluid intake, low-fiber diet, lack of exercise, environmental changes, delaying defecation when urge is present, abuse of enemas or laxatives, use of constipating drugs, mental stress or depression, neurologic degeneration.
- Identify high-risk populations: (1) clients on bed rest who take constipating medications (narcotic analgesics [opioids], anticholinergics), (2) clients who reduce fluids or bulk in their diet, (3) depressed people, and (4) clients with central nervous system disease or local lesions that cause pain.

Planning: Client Goals

The client will:
- Have a soft, formed bowel movement every 1 to 3 days without straining or discomfort
- Modify life-style variables that contribute to constipation (specify, eg, increase fluid intake to 2000 to 2800 mL, increase fiber in diet, incorporate three to five periods of regular exercise into week's routine)

Interventions

- Encourage the client to respond to the urge to defecate and to establish a routine for having a bowel movement when the urge is most likely to be present.

Ignoring the urge is a common cause of constipation. Most people experience an urge after a meal, especially breakfast.
- Provide privacy, and allow sufficient time to defecate when stress is at a minimum. Lack of privacy, being under stress, and rushing usually will quickly eliminate the urge to defecate. Emotions tend to cause spasticity, producing *hypertonic* or *spastic constipation*.
- See to it that the client's food and fluid intake are conducive to having a bowel movement. Balanced food content and varied bulk are important to produce fecal matter and promote its movement in the intestinal tract. Fresh fruits, vegetables, and bran cereals increase intestinal bulk, whereas such foods as lean meats, rice, and eggs leave little residue. Ingesting sufficient fluids is important to help prevent a dry, hard stool. Many people find that drinking such fluids as hot water or prune juice on awakening promotes elimination. Adequate hot meals rather than small cold meals stimulate peristalsis.
- Teach the client the importance of exercise and activity. Studies clearly have shown that lack of activity leads to poor muscle tone, a poor appetite, and sluggish intestinal activity.
- Position the client so that defecation is promoted. The squatting position, which allows maximum use of abdominal muscles, is best, but few people find this position comfortable. The sitting position, or semisitting position for bedridden clients, is most often used.
- Encourage the client to seek medical attention when minor rectal or anal problems, such as hemorrhoids or small linear ulcers called *anal fissures*, affect elimination. They cause discomfort, which causes the person to ignore the urge to defecate as long as possible.
- Teach the client to minimize the use of over-the-counter constipating drugs and to consult with the physician about limiting the use of constipating drugs when possible.
- Use laxatives, enemas, and suppositories as a last resort or temporary treatment. Various measures to stimulate defecation are presented earlier in the chapter.

Evaluative Criteria

The client meets the previously stated goals.

Bowel Incontinence

Bowel incontinence is the inability of the anal sphincter to control the discharge of fecal and gaseous material. The cause of incontinence usually is an organic disease, resulting either in a mechanical condition that hinders the proper functioning of the anal sphincter or in an impairment in the nerve supply to the anal sphincter. Mental illnesses also may be responsible for the client's indifference to the passage of stool. Although bowel incontinence seldom is a threat to life, incontinent clients suffer embarrassment and may become emotionally disturbed.

Assessment

- Assess bowel elimination pattern, noting onset of bowel incontinence and regularity and number of incontinent episodes. Note stool characteristics. Rule out impaction by rectal examination.
- Identify contributing factors: gross constipation with impaction and subsequent overflow, organic changes in neural innervation of the rectum, local causes (cancer of rectum, prolapsed anus, semifluid stool), mental illnesses resulting in indifference to passage of stool, extreme debilitation.
- Assess effects of incontinence on self-concept.
- Examine perineal area for skin breakdown.

Planning: Client Goals

The client will:
- Eliminate incontinent episodes (or reduce their number) if this is realistic
- Demonstrate appropriate self-care measures (or receive related nursing measures): perineal hygiene, use of absorbent pads or waterproof briefs, and so forth
- Demonstrate no signs of perineal excoriation
- Participate in bowel training program to time defecation and reduce the risk of accidents

Interventions

- Take into account that the client suffers embarrassment. The client requires emotional support and understanding.
- Note when incontinence is most likely to occur, and place the client on a bedpan at those times. If there is no pattern, offer a bedpan at regular intervals, such as every few hours.
- Keep the skin clean and dry by using proper hygienic measures. Pressure ulcers may develop when such measures are overlooked.
- Change bed linens and clothing as necessary to avoid odor, skin irritation, and embarrassment. Disposable bed pads and moisture-proof undergarments often are used. Form-fitting briefs and absorbent pads may be worn by the client.
- Confer with the physician about the use of a suppository or a daily cleansing enema. These measures empty the lower colon regularly and often help to decrease incontinence. Bowel training programs may be helpful.

The nurse should keep in mind that emotional problems of clients with diarrhea and bowel incontinence are as important for the nurse to manage as the physical problems.

Evaluative Criteria

The client meets the previously stated goals.

Diarrhea

Diarrhea is the passage of excessively liquid and unformed stools. Frequent bowel movements do not necessarily mean that diarrhea is present, although clients with diarrhea usually pass stools at frequent intervals. Diarrhea often is associated with intestinal cramps. Nausea and vomiting may be present as well as blood in the stools. Diarrhea is protective in nature when its cause is the presence of irritants in the intestinal tract.

Diarrhea may have a functional basis. The client may have allergies to ingested food or drugs. The abuse of cathartics as well as certain dietary indiscretions may cause diarrhea. Diseases in parts of the body other than the intestinal tract may be at the root of the trouble. Examples include uremia and certain cardiavascular and neurologic disorders.

Diarrhea may be caused by certain intrinsic conditions that exist in the intestine itself. These include viral, bacteriologic, fungal, protozoan, and metazoan invasions; alterations in the normal bacterial flora of the intestine; antimicrobial therapy; fistulas; inflammatory conditions, such as ulcerative colitis; and tumors in the intestinal tract.

If the cause of the diarrhea is psychological, the nurse may be able to play an important part in assisting the client to understand the cause. Situations in daily living may be disturbing to him. Diarrhea, however, may be associated with deep-seated emotional problems that require psychological counseling.

Large amounts of fluids and electrolytes may be lost relatively quickly in the presence of diarrhea. This is especially true with infants and young children; if neglected, such loss may easily place a youngster's life in jeopardy. Giving fluids other than by mouth may be necessary when diarrhea is present. If oral intake is possible, cold fluids and rich foods, especially sweets, should be avoided.

Assessment

- Assess bowel elimination patterns, noting (1) increased frequency or intensity of bowel movements; (2) increased fluid content in stool, greenish color, mucus, or blood; (3) increased bowel sounds; (4) whether diarrhea is acute, chronic, or recurrent; (5) fecal soiling; (6) being awakened at night to defecate; (7) complaints of abdominal pain and cramping, generalized weakness and fatigue, nausea and vomiting, fever.
- Assess anal and perineal area for excoriation.
- Identify contributing factors: recent travel, food intolerance, food or drug allergies (new medication), emotional stress, abuse of laxatives, alteration in the normal bacterial flora of the intestine (after antibiotic therapy), colon disease and other diseases, intestinal infection, surgical alterations.
- For clients with chronic diarrhea, assess effect on person's self-image and physiologic and social function-

ing. Note problems with hydration, nutritional status skin integrity, sleep, performance of usual self-care activities, and social interactions. Note abnormal laboratory values (electrolyte levels and hematocrit).

Planning: Client Goals

The client will:

- Reestablish usual defecation patterns (soft, formed stool) or experience less diarrhea
- Modify contributing factors when possible (specify, eg, eliminate certain foods from diet, practice stress management techniques, and so forth)
- Maintain skin integrity in anal and perineal areas
- Demonstrate signs of adequate hydration and nutritional status

Interventions

- Recognize that diarrhea is an embarrassing problem. The client is in need of emotional support and needs to know that the nurse is there to help.
- Answer the client's call signal promptly. The client with diarrhea often cannot control the urge to defecate. It may be necessary to place a bedpan within easy reach but out of sight to prevent embarrassment.
- Whenever possible, remove the cause of diarrhea. Discontinuation of medications that cause diarrhea usually results in a return to normal defecation within 1 to 3 days.
- If there is any indication of an impaction, a rectal

examination should be performed before using antidiarrheal medications.
- Maintain the client's fluid and electrolyte balance. A nonirritating diet is important until symptoms subside. Cold fluids and rich foods aggravate the problem.
- Give special care to the region around the anus, where skin irritation is common. Keep the area clean and dry. Use skin creams, ointments, or powders as necessary. Avoid toilet tissue when it irritates, and use something softer, such as cotton balls, to clean and dry the area.
- Rectal indwelling (Foley) catheters are now being used in some instances for clients with uncontrollable diarrhea after chemotherapy, antibiotic therapy, and tube feedings. The procedure is described earlier in the chapter.
- Once diarrhea stops, it is important to promote a return to normal bowel flora. Fermented dairy products, such as buttermilk or yogurt, aid this process.
- When diarrhea is a regular or intermittent phenomenon that interferes with daily living, clients need additional counseling regarding judicious use of medications, individualized dietary modifications, fluid balance, skin protection, special clothing, and strategies to permit social interactions (eg, preplanning seating on a plane or in a theater or restaurant to be near a bathroom).

Evaluative Criteria

The client meets the previously stated goals.

CASE STUDY

Jeremy Green, aged 4, height 45 inches (114.3 cm), weight 36 lb (16.3 kg), was placed in day care when his mother returned to work 6 months ago. He presents at the hospital with a diagnosis of viral gastroenteritis.

Assessment Findings

The admitting nurse questions Jeremy's mother about the duration, frequency, and amount of his diarrhea and the appearance and consistency of the stools. Treatment since the onset of diarrhea is noted, including any food or fluids the child has taken. Physical assessment is directed to signs of dehydration and the abdominal examination. The nurse records the following assessment note:

> 5/6/93
>
> Four-year-old white male child admitted with complaints of diarrhea beginning 3 days ago. Seen today by pediatrician, who recommended admission and work-up to rule out causes other than viral. Mother reports liquid stools (no observable pus,

blood, or mucus) six to seven times daily beginning 5/4/93 (amount "one to two cups"). Urgency results in soiling of pants. Child has sipped boiled skim milk and Coke and ate a small amount of broth and a few pretzels but has no appetite; complains of nausea; vomiting ×2 on 5/4. Child is pale, and eyes are sunken. Skin is warm and dry with decreased turgor; mucous membranes are dry. Hyperactive bowel sounds. Ht 45 in, wt 36 lb, T−99.8 Ⓣ P−88 R−18. Mother reported several other children in same day-care center are out sick with diarrhea.

> *D. Levitsky, RN*

Nursing Diagnosis

The admitting nurse develops a plan of care for Jeremy that includes several nursing diagnoses. The one that will be developed in this case study is as follows:

    Diarrhea related to unknown cause (possibly viral, rule out malabsorption of lactose and other causes)

Planning: Client Goals

The nurse works collaboratively with Jeremy and his parents, explaining that a plan of care is being developed to maintain Jeremy's well-being until the diarrhea is brought under control. The nurse recognizes Jeremy's distress both at losing control over defecation and at needing to be hospitalized. The family supports the following client goals. At the time of discharge, the client will:

- Voluntarily pass a formed stool of usual consistency (experience less or no diarrhea)
- Exhibit decreased bowel sounds
- Demonstrate signs of fluid and electrolyte balance:
  - Improved skin turgor
  - Moist mucous membranes
  - Normal eyeball
- Demonstrate signs of improved nutritional status:
  - Eat low-fiber diet without abdominal cramping, nausea, or vomiting
  - Maintain admission weight (or gain weight)
- Show no signs of skin breakdown in the perianal area
  See the nursing care plan, which details the nursing strategies used to achieve these goals.

Implementation

In implementing the plan of care, the nurse needs the following specialized abilities:

- Strong interpersonal skills to work effectively with children and their families
- Thorough knowledge of child development, normal bowel elimination, causes and manifestations of diarrhea and related problems, and successful treatment strategies
- Strong assessment skills (interviewing and physical assessment) to carefully identify and label the child's problems and their cause

- Ability to create a secure, comfortable, and developmentally stimulating environment for the child
- Ability to provide safe physical care to the child aimed at promoting optimal functioning of all body systems
- Teaching and counseling skills to meet the child's and parents' needs
- Interpersonal and leadership skills to work with the nursing staff and health care team to implement the plan of care
- Personal accountability

Documentation

Sample documentation of a nursing intervention follows.

SOAP Format

> 5/7/93, nursing
> #1 Diarrhea related to unknown cause (possibly viral, rule out malabsorption of lactose and other causes)

S: "My tummy doesn't hurt so much any more."
O: Liquid stools decreased to two in past 24 hours; negative report on stool culture
A: Diarrhea is resolving—cause may have been temporary lactose intolerance after acute viral diarrhea (mother had been giving child boiled skim milk)
P: Continue plan of care. Add rice cereal and bananas to diet. Reintroduce milk and milk products last—alert parents to monitor child for lactose intolerance.

D. Levitsky, RN

Evaluation

Short-term goal achievement is evaluated before discharge. See the care plan for related evaluative statements and revisions of the plan of care.

 N U R S I N G   C A R E   P L A N

for Jeremy Green

Nursing Diagnosis:	Diarrhea related to unknown cause (possibly viral, rule out malabsorption of lactose and other causes) as manifested by passage of liquid stools (1 to 2 cups) for 3 days; urgency with fecal soiling; anorexia, nausea, vomiting twice on day 1; signs of dehydration: decreased skin turgor, dry mucous membranes, sunken eyeballs
Long-Term Goal:	Client reestablishes usual pattern of bowel elimination.
Goal:	At the time of discharge, the client will: • Voluntarily pass a formed stool of usual consistency (experience less or no diarrhea)

Nursing Actions	Rationale	Evaluative Statement
Assess and chart frequency and amount of diarrhea, stool characteristics, precipitating factors, and	This assists in identifying the cause of the diarrhea.	5/8/93 Goal partially met. No recurrence of liquid stools for 24 hours.

(continued)

NURSING CARE PLAN (continued)

for Jeremy Green

accompanying manifestations (gastrointestinal symptoms, hyperactive bowel sounds).

Revision: Continue to monitor.

D. Lentsky, RN

Goal: At the time of discharge, the client will:
- Exhibit decreased bowel sounds

Nursing Actions	**Rationale**	**Evaluative Statement**
Work collaboratively with the physician to identify the cause of the diarrhea. Obtain stool specimens and send to laboratory.	Correct treatment depends on identification of the cause of the diarrhea. Viral diarrhea is usually self-limiting and lasts 24 to 72 hours. Prolonged diarrhea after acute viral illness may be from temporary malabsorption of lactose or other simple sugars.	5/8/93 Goal met. Bowel sounds are normal. *D. Lentsky, RN*
Instruct Jeremy and his parents (if they want to participate in care) on correct enteric precautions for handling stool.	To prevent transmissions of infectious diarrhea to others.	
Increase frequency and length of rest periods and discourage strenuous activity.	Exercise and activity stimulate peristalsis.	
Administer prescribed antidiarrheal medication and observe for adverse effects.	Antidiarrheal medications may cause drowsiness and dizziness.	

Goal: At the time of discharge, the client will:
- Demonstrate signs of fluid and electrolyte balance: (1) improved skin turgor, (2) moist mucous membranes, and (3) normal eyeballs

Nursing Actions	**Rationale**	**Evaluative Statement**
Continue to assess hydration status and be alert to signs of electrolyte imbalance.	Reestablishing normal fluid and electrolyte balance by replacing ongoing fluid losses and providing maintenance fluids is a priority for the child with severe and prolonged diarrhea. Diarrhea stools contain large amounts of water and often are relatively low in sodium and high in potassium.	5/8/93 Goal partially met. Skin turgor improved, eyeballs normal, mucous membranes still dry. *Revision:* Continue to encourage PO fluids. Enjoys clear chicken broth and half-strength gelatin products. *D. Lentsky, RN*
Administer prescribed intravenous therapy and clear liquids—note client response as new fluids and foods are added to the diet.	There is no ideal oral replacement fluid. Some may cause diarrhea or provide inappropriate amounts of electrolytes.	
Chart daily weight.	Daily weights are the most accurate indicator of fluid balance.	
Monitor intake and output. Note concentration of urine.	Urine becomes more concentrated when a person is dehydrated.	

(continued)

N U R S I N G   C A R E   P L A N *(continued)*

for Jeremy Green

Goal: At the time of discharge, the client will:
  • Demonstrate signs of improved nutritional status: (1) eats low-fiber diet without abdominal cramping, nausea, or vomiting; and (2) maintains or increases admission weight

Nursing Actions	Rationale	Evaluative Statement
Discontinue milk products and solid foods. Until the diarrhea resolves, offer a combination of clear liquids (half-strength apple juice or gelatin products; commercial products: Lytren, Pedialyte, 5% glucose water): 30 mL/hr for first 8 hours, then 60 to 90 mL every 1 to 2 hours if number of stools lessens.	If one fluid is used exclusively, inappropriate amounts of electrolytes may be provided. Commercial preparations tend to be expensive. Objective is to provide the necessary water, electrolytes, and minimal calories in a milk-free and solid-free diet—until the diarrhea resolves.	5/8/93 Goal met. Tolerating rice cereal and bananas. Gained 1 lb since admission. *D. Lentsky, RN*
As gastrointestinal symptoms subside, advance to other liquids and solids (bananas, apple sauce, and rice cereal solidify stool)—milk should be the last liquid added.	Adding new fluids and foods slowly enables intolerances to be quickly detected.	

Goal: At the time of discharge, the client will:
  • Show no signs of skin breakdown in the perianal area

Nursing Actions	Rationale	Evaluative Statement
Assess the perianal area after each passage of stool and note any irritation.	Perianal irritation is a common problem with severe diarrhea. The goal of treatment is prevention.	5/8/93 Goal partially met. Small area of excoriation remains around anus. Continue plan. *D. Lentsky, RN*
Wash and dry the area carefully after each episode of diarrhea and apply protective ointment (as ordered or per agency protocol).	Keeping the skin clean and dry and protected with a waterproof ointment or skin barrier may prevent breakdown.	

K E Y   P O I N T S

• Bowel elimination, a natural process in which the body excretes the waste products of digestion, is an essential component of healthy body functioning.
• Problems with bowel elimination may affect fluid and electrolyte balance, nutritional status, skin integrity, and self-concept.
• Healthy bowel elimination presupposes a well-functioning gastrointestinal tract. The large intestine is the primary organ of bowel elimination.

• *Defecation* and *bowel movement* are the terms used to describe the emptying of the intestines. People vary in the frequency of their bowel movements. The aim is to have the bowels move regularly and for the stools to be formed, soft, and passed without discomfort.
• Factors that affect bowel elimination include growth and development, daily patterns, food and fluid intake, activity and muscle tone, life-style variables, psychological variables, pathologic conditions, medications, diagnostic tests, surgery, and anesthesia.

- A comprehensive assessment of bowel elimination includes the collection of data about usual patterns of elimination; recent changes in these patterns; aids to elimination; elimination problems; physical assessment of the abdomen, anus, and rectum; and stool characteristics. These findings may need to be correlated with the results of diagnostic studies of the stool and gastrointestinal tract.
- When caring for a debilitated, confused, or unconscious client, the nurse needs to monitor bowel status daily to identify and treat bowel elimination problems early. Nursing care is directed to the prevention of bowel problems.
- Endoscopic examinations using a lighted tube allow the direct visualization of the gastrointestinal tract and are helpful in the diagnosis of inflammatory, ulcerative, and infectious diseases; neoplastic diseases; and lesions of the esophageal, gastric, and intestinal mucosa.
- Indirect visualization of the gastrointestinal tract is achieved through radiography. Important nursing responsibilities are assisting the client to complete a safe and effective dietary and bowel preparation program and ensuring that the client eliminates the contrast medium (barium sulfate) used in the study. Standard bowel preparation agents may be contraindicated for some clients.
- Nursing diagnoses may be written to specifically address problems in bowel elimination (constipation, diarrhea, bowel incontinence) and to identify the effect bowel elimination problems have on other areas of human functioning (anxiety, comfort, self-concept, skin integrity).
- Regular bowel elimination may be promoted in both well and ill clients by attention to timing, positioning, privacy, nutrition, and exercise. Clients need to understand the importance of heeding the urge to defecate and the relation between bowel elimination, and nutrition and exercise.
- Specific nursing strategies for bowel elimination include use of cathartics, laxatives, and antidiarrheals; techniques for emptying the colon of feces (enemas, rectal suppositories, rectal Foley catheters, the fecal incontinence pouch, and digital removal of stool); bowel training programs; and comfort measures.
- Although laxatives have valid uses, they frequently are abused. Many people who take laxatives for what they think is constipation do not realize that the habitual use of laxatives is the most common cause of chronic constipation.
- A physician's order may be needed before the nurse digitally removes a fecal impaction because this may result in irritation of the rectal mucosa and bleeding, and because vagal stimulation can decrease the heart rate.
- The purpose of a bowel training program is to manipulate factors within the person's control (food and fluid intake, exercise, time of defecation) and to achieve the elimination of a soft, formed stool at regular intervals without laxative support.
- The client with a bowel diversion needs physical and psychological support both preoperatively and postoperatively. The nurse works collaboratively with the physician and enterostomal therapist to ensure that the client and family can manage the care of the bowel diversion after discharge.
- Clients with acute or chronic constipation, impaction, diarrhea, incontinence, or flatulence require special nursing care. These problems, if uncorrected, may seriously affect the client's comfort, self-concept, and other areas of physical functioning.

STUDY QUESTIONS

1. The nurse encourages Mr. Brown to avoid foods that have a laxative effect. He is instructed to avoid
   a. cheese
   b. alcohol
   c. eggs
   d. pasta
2. Which of the following is a true statement about the effects of medication on bowel elimination?
   a. Diarrhea occurs with antibiotic use about 20% of the time.
   b. Anticoagulants cause a white discoloration of the stool.
   c. Narcotic analgesics increase gastrointestinal motility.
   d. Iron salts impair digestion and cause a green stool.
3. Mr. Jones has a fecal impaction. The nurse correctly administers an oil-retention enema by
   a. administering a large volume of solution (500 to 1000 mL)
   b. mixing milk and molasses in equal parts for an enema
   c. instructing the client to retain the enema for at least 30 minutes
   d. following the return-flow or Harris flush procedure
4. As the nurse prepares to assist Mrs. Perez with her newly created ileostomy, she is aware that
   a. an appliance will not be required on a continual basis
   b. the size of the stoma stabilizes within 2 weeks
   c. irrigation is necessary for regulation
   d. fecal drainage will be liquid

5. The class of laxative that acts by causing stool to absorb water and swell is
   a. bulk forming
   b. emollient
   c. lubricant
   d. stimulant

6. Mr. Toney is nervous about a colonoscopy scheduled for tomorrow. The nurse describes the test by explaining that
   a. it allows visual examination of the esophagus and stomach
   b. it allows visual examination of the large intestine
   c. it is a radiographic examination of the large intestine
   d. it is a fluoroscopic examination of the small intestine

7. A bowel training progran includes all the following steps *except*
   a. maintaining daily training routine for 2 to 3 weeks until a regular pattern is established
   b. increasing fluid intake to 2500 to 3000 mL
   c. administering an enema once a day to stimulate peristalsis
   d. allowing ample time for evacuation

8. Your client complains of excessive flatulence. Which food, if eaten regularly, may be responsible for this?
   a. meat
   b. cauliflower
   c. potatoes
   d. ice cream

9. The barium enema should be done before the upper gastrointestinal series because of which of the following?
   a. Retained barium may cloud the colon.
   b. Barium can cause lower gastrointestinal bleeding.
   c. The physician orders in that sequence.
   d. Barium is absorbed readily in the lower intestine.

10. Nurses should recommend to their clients the avoidance of habitual use of laxatives. Which of the following is the rationale for this?
    a. They will cause a fecal impaction.
    b. They will cause chronic constipation.
    c. They change the pH of the gastrointestinal tract.
    d. They inhibit the intestinal enzymes.

11. Which of the following is the physiology behind a hypertonic solution enema?
    a. bowel mucosa irritation
    b. diffusion of water out of colon
    c. osmosis of water into colon
    d. softening of fecal contents

12. Which of the following is the nursing rationale for deflating a rectal Foley catheter every hour?
    a. expels flatus
    b. reduces the risk of infection
    c. prevents rectal necrosis
    d. allows the diarrhea to drain adequately

13. During removal of a fecal impaction, which of the following could occur because of vagal stimulation?
    a. bradycardia
    b. atelectasis
    c. tachycardia
    d. cardiac tamponade

14. Which of the following would be a common nursing diagnosis for the client with an ileostomy?
    a. Body Image Disturbance
    b. Constipation
    c. Altered Growth and Development
    d. Fluid Volume Excess

15. Your client who is experiencing flatulence would be helped if he were placed in which of the following positions?
    a. Trendelenburg position
    b. knee–chest position
    c. semi-Fowler's position
    d. Fowler's position

Answers With Rationale

1. The correct response is *b*. All the foods listed except alcohol have a constipating effect.

2. The correct response is *a*. Anticoagulants may result in the stool having a pink to red to black appearance, whereas iron salts also cause a black stool. Narcotic analgesics decrease gastric motility.

3. The correct response is *c*. The usual amount of solution administered with a retention enema is 150 to 200 mL for an adult. The milk-and-molasses mixture is a carminative enema that helps to expel flatus, as does the Harris flush procedure.

4. The correct response is *d*. An appliance usually is required on a continual basis because the fecal drainage is liquid. Stoma size usually stabilizes

within 4 to 6 weeks, and irrigation is not necessary because fecal matter is liquid.

5. The correct response is *a*. Emollients lubricate the stool; lubricants soften the stool, making it easier to pass; and stimulants promote peristalsis by irritating the intestinal mucosa or stimulating nerve endings in the intestinal wall.

6. The correct response is *b*. An esophagogastroduodenoscopy allows visual examination of the esophagus and stomach. The radiographic examination of the large intestine is a barium enema, and a fluoroscopic examination of the small intestine is an upper gastrointestinal series.

7. The correct response is *c*. All are correct in a bowel

training program except for administration of a daily enema. A cathartic suppository is used 30 minutes before the client's usual defecation time to stimulate peristalsis.

8. The correct response is *b*. Cauliflower is a gas-producing food that results in flatulence.

9. The correct response is *a*. The barium enema should always precede the upper gastrointestinal series because retained barium from the latter may take several days to pass through the gastrointestinal tract and cloud anatomic detail on the barium enema studies.

10. The correct response is *b*. Habitual use of laxatives is the most common cause of chronic constipation.

11. The correct response is *c*. Hypertonic solutions draw water into the colon by osmosis, thus stimulating the defecation reflex. Oil solutions soften fecal contents, and soap solutions distend the intestine and irritate the bowel mucosa.

12. The correct response is *c*. Failure to deflate a rectal Foley catheter may result in rectal necrosis. Deflating the catheter balloon does not interfere with passage of flatus or liquid stool but makes it more likely that the catheter may become dislodged. This procedure has no effect on the development of an infection.

13. The correct response is *a*. Removing a fecal impaction manually may result in stimulation of the vagal nerve and a resulting bradycardia.

14. The correct response is *a*. Constipation will not occur with an ileostomy, since the drainage is liquid. Growth and development are not affected by the formation of an ileostomy. Fluid volume excess is unlikely to occur because the drainage is liquid and probably continual.

15. The correct response is *b*. Because gas rises, the knee–chest position facilitates the passage of flatus.

BIBLIOGRAPHY

Benedict, P., & Haddad, A. (1989). Postop teaching for the colostomy patient. *RN, 52*(3), 85–90.

Birdsall, C. (1986). Would you put a Foley in the rectum? *American Journal of Nursing, 86*(9), 1050.

Carpenito, L. (1992). *Nursing diagnosis: Application to chemical practice* (4th ed.). Philadelphia: Lippincott.

Cerrato, P. (1989). Is America really constipated? *RN, 52*(5), 81–86.

Cerrato, P. (1990). Diarrhea: The usual suspect may not be to blame. *RN, 53*(8), 73–75.

Clark, J., Queener, S., & Karb, V. (1990). *Pharmacological basis of nursing practice* (3rd ed.). St. Louis: Mosby.

Doughty, D. (Ed.). (1992). *Urinary and fecal incontinence: Nursing management*. St. Louis: Mosby–Year Book.

Ellickson, E. (1988). Bowel management plan for the homebound elderly. *Journal of Gerontological Nursing, 14*(1), 16–19.

Fischbach, F. (1992). *A manual of laboratory diagnostic tests* (4th ed.). Philadelphia: Lippincott.

Fuller, J., & Schaller-Ayers. (1990). *Health assessment: A nursing approach*. Philadelphia: Lippincott.

Kemp, M. (1990). Troubleshooting ostomy problems. *Geriatric Nursing, 11*(5), 233–236.

Kuhn, J., & Flaherty, J. (1990). Helping ostomy patients back to independence. *Journal of Gerontological Nursing, 16*(6), 27–30.

Lincoln, R., & Roberts, R. (1989). Continence issues in acute care. *Nursing Clinics of North America, 24*(3), 741–753.

Madda, M. (1991). Helping ostomy patients manage medications. *Nursing, 21*(3), 47–49.

Malseed, R., & Harrigan, G. (1989). *Textbook of pharmacology and nursing care*. Philadelphia: Lippincott.

McKenzie, J., & Gallacher, M. (1989). A sweet smelling success. *Nursing Times, 85*(27), 48–49.

Rousseau, P. (1988). Treatment of constipation in the elderly. *Postgraduate Medicine, 84*(4), 339–349.

Rousseau, P. (1990). Aging and chronic constipation. *Geriatric Medicine, 9*(3), 35–43.

Rowland, M. (1989). When drug therapy causes diarrhea. *RN, 52*(12), 32–35.

Shoaf, L. (1991). Fluid and fiber: Needs and drug implications. *Nursing Homes, 40*(2), 16–20.

Staab, A., & Lyles, M. (1990). *Manual of geriatric nursing*. Glenview, IL: Scott, Foresman/Little Brown Higher Education.

Wadle, K. (1990). Diarrhea. *Nursing Clinics of North America, 25*(4), 901–907.

Weidner, B. (1992). Constipation: Removing an impaction. *Nursing, 22*(4), 78.

Yakabowich, M. (1990). Prescribe with care: The role of laxatives in the treatment of constipation. *Journal of Gerontological Nursing, 16*(7), 4–11.

Yen, P. (1989). Tummy trouble. *Geriatric Nursing, 10*(6), 301.

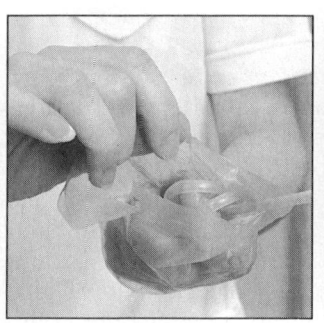
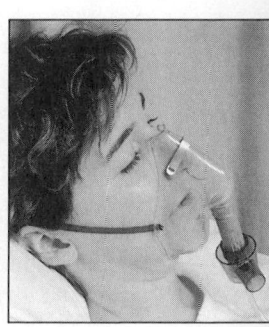

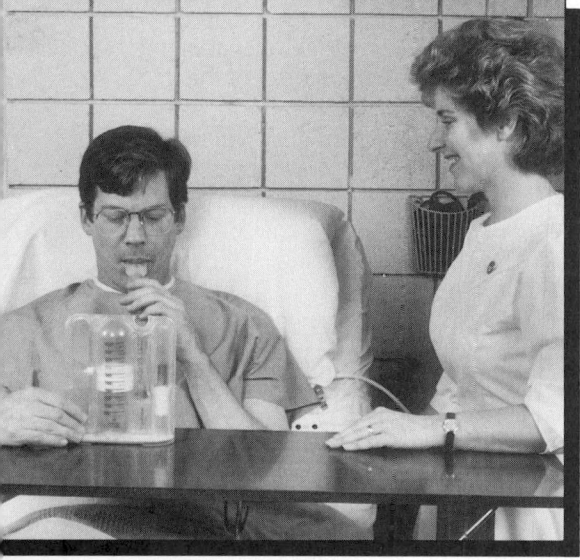

Oxygenation

36

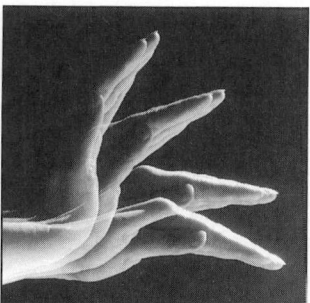

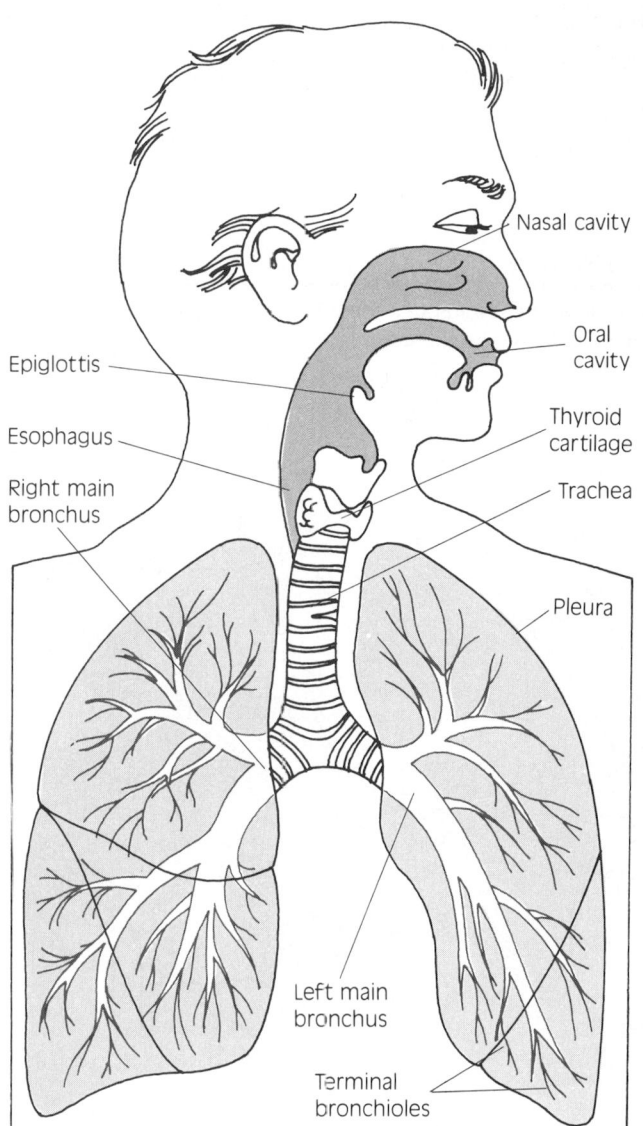

Most people take respiratory functioning for granted, but adequate respiratory functioning is necessary for life. Living cells require oxygen. The air passages must remain patent (ie, open) for oxygen to enter the system. Any condition that interferes with normal functioning must be reduced or eliminated to prevent pulmonary distress, which could lead to death.

Normal functioning depends on essentially three factors:

- The integrity of the airway system to transport air to and from the lungs
- A properly functioning alveolar system in the lungs to oxygenate venous blood and to remove carbon dioxide from the blood
- A properly functioning cardiovascular system to carry nutrients and wastes to and from body cells

Study of this chapter will provide the nurse with knowledge of the physiology, general purpose, and general factors affecting respiratory functioning. Practical suggestions for performing a comprehensive respiratory assessment are given. Sample interview questions for both a general and focused respiratory history are presented along with information and data collected from the nursing examination. The incorporation of results from laboratory and radiology studies is addressed in the assessment. After analyzing the data, it is important to decide whether the respiratory data lead to the problem statement, indicate another problem, or are the possible cause of a problem. Numerous examples of nursing diagnoses are given. Client goals and specific nursing strategies for implementation are described. In the section entitled Nursing Process in Clinical Practice, focused assessment planning, implementation, and evaluation guides are offered for selected nursing diagnoses related to alteration in respiratory functioning—Impaired Gas Exchange, Ineffective Breathing Pattern, and Ineffective Airway Clearance. These guides and the concluding case study illustrate how the nurse's knowledge of respiratory functioning is combined with skilled nursing interventions to successfully resolve respiratory problems.

Physiology of Respiration

A brief review of basic anatomy and physiology will aid the reader in understanding assessment findings and rationale for nursing interventions (Fig. 36-1). The main organs of respiration, the lungs, are located within the thoracic cavity. The right lung has three lobes, and the left has two lobes. Each lobe is further subdivided into segments or lobules. The right lung has 10 bronchopulmonary segments; the left has 8. The lungs extend from the base at the level of the diaphragm to the apex (top), which is above the first rib. The heart lies between the right and left lung. The lungs comprise elastic tissue that is capable of stretching or recoiling. Normally, the elastic fibers are partially stretched at all times, partially filling the thoracic cavity.

The *pleurae* is a two-layered membrane: the visceral pleura covers the lungs, and the parietal pleura lines the thoracic cavity. These two are continuous with one another and form a closed sac. There is normally a potential space between them, not an actual space. Pleural fluid between the membranes acts as a lubricant and as an adhesive

FIGURE 36-1

The organs of the respiratory tract.

Nasal cavity

Oral cavity

Thyroid cartilage

Trachea

Pleura

Epiglottis

Esophagus

Right main bronchus

Left main bronchus

Terminal bronchioles

943

agent to hold the lungs in an expanded position. Pressure within the pleural space is always subatmospheric (ie, negative). This constant intrapleural negative pressure is essential for normal ventilation.

The airway system provides a pathway for the transport and exchange of oxygen and carbon dioxide. The upper airway comprises the nose, pharynx, larynx, and epiglottis. Its main function is to warm, filter, and humidify inspired air. The lower airway, known as the tracheobronchial tree, includes the trachea, right and left main-stem bronchus, segmental bronchi, and terminal bronchioles. The major functions are conduction of air, mucociliary clearance, and production of pulmonary surfactant. Cilia, microscopic hairlike projections, propel sheets of mucus toward the upper airway so the mucus can be removed (by cough) after it has trapped cells, particles, and infectious debris. Surfactant, a detergent-like phospholipid, reduces surface tension of the fluid lining the alveoli. When surfactant production is reduced, the lung becomes stiff and the alveoli collapse.

The actual lung is composed of **alveoli**, small air sacs at the end of the terminal bronchioles (Fig. 36-2). These structures are the site of gas exchange. The average adult has more than 300 million alveoli.

The lungs and circulation act together to bring gases to body tissues for gas exchange. Movement of oxygen into the lungs by way of the airway system during inspiration

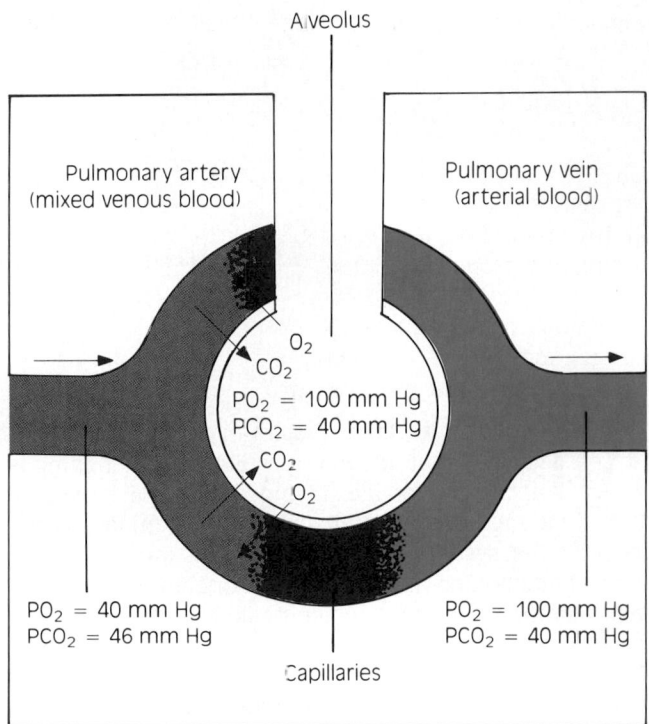

F I G U R E   3 6 - 3

Diagram of gas exchange in the alveolus.

F I G U R E   3 6 - 2

Alveoli and the intrapulmonary circulatory system where gas exchange takes place.

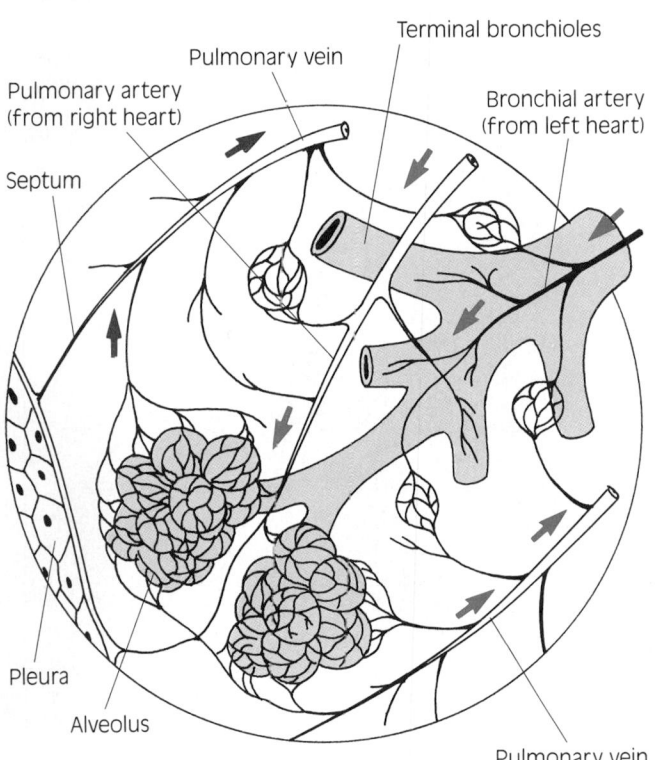

and removal of carbon dioxide by the airway system during exhalation is **ventilation**. Respiration occurs at the terminal alveolar capillary system, where there is an exchange of gases between the air and blood (Fig. 36-3). Diffusion refers to the movement of oxygen and carbon dioxide between the air (in the alveoli) and the blood (in the capillaries). The appropriate gas moves passively from an area of higher concentration to an area of lesser concentration.

The process of ventilation has two phases. **Inhalation**, the active phase, involves movement of muscles and thorax to bring air into the lungs. **Exhalation**, the passive phase, is the movement of air out of the lungs. The medulla in the brain stem immediately above the spinal cord is the respiratory center. It is stimulated by the increased concentration of carbon dioxide and hydrogen ions and, to a lesser degree, by the decreased amount of oxygen in the arterial blood. Chemoreceptors in the aortic arch and carotid bodies are also sensitive to the same arterial blood gas levels and can activate the medulla. Stimulation of the medulla increases the rate and depth of ventilation so carbon dioxide and hydrogen are blown off and oxygen levels are increased. The medulla sends an impulse down the spinal cord to the respiratory muscles to stimulate a contraction leading to inhalation. If the system is intact, the diaphragm, the major respiratory muscle, contracts and descends into the abdomen. The thoracic cavity enlarges. Lungs expand in response to pressure changes in the intrapleural space and the lung. Inhalation ceases when atmospheric air pressure and pulmonary air pressure are equal.

Exhalation occurs, and the lungs return to their resting position.

General Principles of Respiration

The following eight basic principles guide action in promoting respiratory functioning. First, *all living cells require oxygen, which the body cannot store*. The body must at all times maintain a properly functioning respiratory system. Environmental oxygen, usually readily available under normal conditions, must be accessible to the body. Environmental oxygen may be in short supply, such as at high altitudes where oxygen concentration in the air is low, and in the presence of toxic fumes, in which the air has reduced concentrations of oxygen.

Second, *the air passageways must remain patent for respiration to occur*. Respiratory gases are transported from the nose to the alveoli and are then returned. Obstruction in any part of the normal passageways impedes respiration. Obstruction can occur from a foreign substance, such as a piece of food, a coin, a toy, or liquids, as in the case of a drowning victim. Obstruction can also arise from tissues or secretions within the body (eg, excessive or thickened secretions, tumor growths, or edema in the respiratory tract). A decrease in the size of air passages due to constriction or to poor sitting, standing, and lying positions can impede respiration.

Third, *muscle movements provide the physical force essential for respiration*. The diaphragm and the intercostal muscles are responsible for normal inspiration and expiration (Fig. 36-4). Accessory muscles of the abdomen, neck, and back are used to maintain respiratory movements at times when breathing is difficult. The condition of the body's musculature can affect the process of respiration. For example, a depression of the respiratory center and pulmonary congestion with inadequate respiratory efforts are conditions that interfere with the normal movement of air into and out of the lungs.

Fourth, *the pressure changes resulting from expansion and contraction of the thoracic cavity produce pulmonary gas exchanges*. Incomplete lung expansion or lung collapse, known as **atelectasis**, prevents the pressure changes and the exchange of gas by diffusion in the lungs. Atelectatic areas of the lung cannot fulfill a function of respiration. Examples of conditions that predispose to atelectasis include obstructions of the airway by foreign bodies, mucus, constricted airways, external compression by tumors or enlarged blood vessels, and immobility.

Fifth, *adequate fluid intake is essential to respiratory functioning*. Fluid is necessary for the production of watery mucus normally present in the respiratory tract and for ciliary action. This covering of mucus also protects the underlying tissues from irritation and infection. A few milliliters of fluid between the pleural surfaces allow the lungs to move easily along the chest wall as they expand and contract. In its absence, filling and emptying of the lungs are difficult.

Sixth, *ventilation depends on the extent of perfusion in the area*. **Ventilation** is the movement of air in and out of the lungs. **Perfusion** is the passing of fluid, in this case, the blood, through tissue. The amount of blood flow through the lungs is a factor in the amount of oxygen and other gases that are exchanged. The amount of blood present in any given area of lung tissue depends partially on whether the person is sitting, standing, or lying down. The perfusion of lung tissue also depends on activity. Greater activity results in increased cellular oxygen need and cardiac output and, consequently, in increased blood return to the lungs. In addition, perfusion depends on an adequate blood supply and proper cardiovascular functioning to carry oxygen and carbon dioxide to and from the lung tissues.

Seventh, *oxygen and carbon dioxide must move through the alveoli and be carried to and from body cells by the blood*. Oxygen is carried two ways in the body. It is dissolved in plasma, but because oxygen is insoluble in liquids, little oxygen is carried in this way. The hemoglobin in red blood cells has a strong affinity for oxygen, and, therefore, most oxygen is carried in the body by red blood cells in the form of oxyhemoglobin. Hemoglobin carries carbon dioxide easily. Any abnormality in the alveoli or in the blood's constituents influences proper internal respirations.

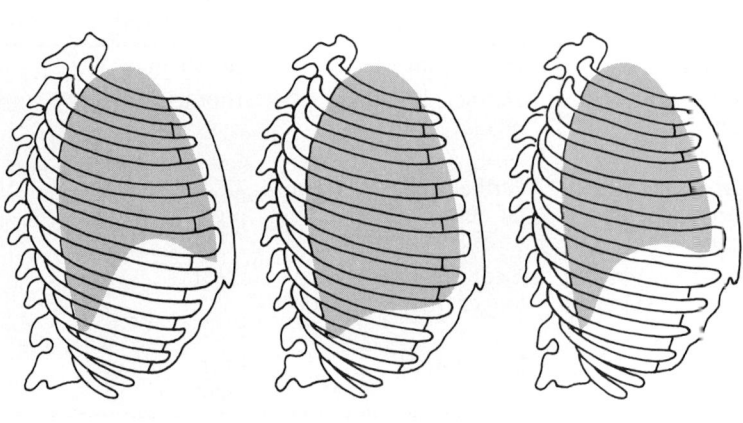

A   **B**   **C**

FIGURE 36-4

(A) With maximum expiration, the elevated diaphragm and depressed ribs shorten the length of the thoracic cavity and decrease the anteroposterior diameter. (B) At maximum inspiration, the diaphragm descends, lengthening the thoracic cavity and elevating the sternum and ribs to increase the anteroposterior diameter of the chest cavity. (C) End of normal expiration.

Eighth, *there must be an exchange of oxygen and carbon dioxide between the blood and body cells*. Conditions that influence the passage of oxygen and carbon dioxide through cell walls adversely affect internal respiration. Certain metabolic abnormalities can alter normal gas exchange at cell walls.

If a problem exists in any part of the respiratory process, **hypoxia**, an inadequate amount of oxygen available to cells, may occur. The most common symptoms of hypoxia are *dyspnea* (difficulty breathing), an elevated blood pressure with a small pulse pressure, increased respiratory and pulse rates, paleness, and cyanosis. Anxiety and restlessness are also common signs of hypoxia. Hypoxia is often caused by **hypoventilation**, a decreased rate or depth of air movement into the lungs. The effects of chronic hypoxia are detected in all body systems and include altered thought processes, headaches, chest pain, enlarged heart, anorexia, constipation, decreased urinary output, decreased libido, weakness of extremity muscles, and muscle pain. At the other extreme is **hyperventilation**, the increased rate and depth of ventilation above the body's normal metabolic requirements. This is discussed in more detail in the section entitled Diagnosing.

Developmental Variations

Birth necessitates many adaptations in the newborn. The most blatant of these changes occur with the lungs, because they change from fluid-filled organs to air-filled structures. The normal infant's chest is small, the airways are short, and aspiration is a potential problem. The respiratory rate is more rapid in the infant than in any other age group (Table 36-1). As alveoli increase in number and size, adequate oxygenation is accomplished at lower respiratory rates. Respiratory rates stabilize in young adulthood.

Respiratory activity is abdominal in the infant. The infant's chest wall is so thin that ribs, sternum, and xiphoid space process are easily noted because of little musculature. The infant has a rounded chest wall where anteroposterior diameter (ie, the measurement from the front to back of the thorax) equals transverse diameter. Occasional fine crackles at the end of deep inspiration noted on auscultation in the infant's thorax are normal.

In the preschool and school-age child, some subcutaneous fat is deposited on the chest wall so landmarks are less prominent than in the infant. Muscular development is also more noticeable. Transverse diameter and anteroposterior diameter ratio reaches adult configurations of 1:2 by age 6 years. The preschool child's eustachian tubes, bronchi, and bronchioles are elongated and less angular, so the number of routine colds and infections decreases until they enter school. Also, young children usually have not had the opportunity to develop antibodies for the variety of viruses and bacteria encountered. Good handwashing techniques and tissue etiquette are practices to be encouraged. Most children at this age experience colds or upper respiratory infections, but some have more serious problems of otitis media, bronchitis, and pneumonia. At the end of late childhood and during adulthood, the immune system is sufficiently seasoned to protect the person from most infections.

There are specific physical changes in elderly people that are unrelated to any pathology. Bony landmarks are more prominent because of the loss of subcutaneous fat. Kyphosis (curvature of the spine) contributes to the older person's appearance of leaning forward. Barrel chest deformity may result in a widening of the anterior–posterior diameter. In the absence of any abnormal findings with the physical examination, this is known as senile emphysema. The tissues and airways of the respiratory tract (including alveoli) become more rigid with age. Power of respiratory and abdominal muscles is reduced so the diaphragm moves less efficiently. These alterations increase the risk of disease, especially pneumonia.

T A B L E   3 6 - 1

Respiratory Variations in the Life Cycle				
	Infant [Birth–1 year]	**Early Childhood (1–5 years)**	**Late Childhood (6–12 years)**	**Aged Adult (65+ years)**
Respiratory rate	30–60/min	20–40/min	15–25/min	16–20/min
Respiratory pattern	Abdominal breathing, irregular in rate and depth	Abdominal breathing, irregular	Thoracic breathing, regular	Thoracic, regular
Chest wall	Thin, little muscle, ribs and sternum easily seen	Same as infant's but with more subcutaneous fat	Further subcutaneous fat deposited, structures less prominent	Thin, structures prominent
Breath sounds	Loud, harsh crackles at end of deep inspiration	Loud, harsh expiration longer than inspiration	Clear inspiration is longer than expiration	Clear
Shape of thorax	Round	Elliptical	Elliptical	Barrel shaped or elliptical

Factors Affecting Respiratory Functioning

A variety of factors affect adequate respiratory functioning. Six important factors are included here.

Levels of Health

People with renal or cardiac disorders often demonstrate a compromise in respiratory functioning due to fluid overload. People with chronic illnesses often have muscle wasting and poor muscle tone, including those of the respiratory system. (Developmental variations were discussed previously in this chapter.)

Development

Physical changes such as scoliosis (curvature of the spine) influence breathing patterns so that air trapping occurs. There is a statistically significant correlation between obesity and chronic bronchitis. Obese people are often short of breath with activity and thus participate in little exercise. The alveoli at the base of the lungs are rarely stimulated to expand fully.

Narcotic Analgesics (Opioids)

These chemical agents depress the medullary respiratory center so that the rate and depth of respirations are decreased. This is especially noted with the use of morphine and meperidine (Demerol). One must be alert to the potential of respiratory arrest when administering any narcotic or sedative.

Life-Style

Sedentary activity patterns do not encourage the expansion of alveoli and the development of pulmonary exercise patterns (deep breathing). People who exercise routinely three to six times per week (eg, aerobics, walking, swimming) are better able to respond to stressors to respiratory health. Cigarette smoking (active and passive) is a major contributor to lung disease and respiratory distress.

Environment

It is impossible to pinpoint all effects of air pollution, but researchers have demonstrated a statistically high correlation between air pollution and cancer and lung diseases. A person with adequate respiratory functioning who is exposed to air pollution experiences stinging of eyes, coughing, choking, headache, and dizziness. People who have experienced an alteration in respiratory functioning in the past are often unable to continue self-care activities in a polluted environment.

Psychological Health

Individuals responding to stress might demonstrate excessive sighing or hyperventilation breathing patterns. Generalized anxiety has been implicated by some scientists in establishing enough bronchospasm to produce an episode of bronchial asthma. Those experiencing an alteration in respiratory functioning develop some anxiety as a result of a physical disorder.

Nurse as Role Model

Nurses working with clients to initiate changes in health habits that affect respiration must also examine themselves as a factor in the success of the plan. Clients use nurses as role models in achieving healthy life-styles. Nurses dealing with stresses from professional and personal aspects of their own lives sometimes channel their energies into destructive behaviors. If the nurse wishes to encourage optimal respiratory functioning, he or she must demonstrate behaviors that support a healthy life-style. With this goal in mind, the nurse will do the following:

- Maintain adequate fluid intake and proper nutrition
- Use deep breathing exercises
- Evaluate his or her own use of nicotine
- Incorporate a plan to reduce smoking and then stop smoking on a specific target date
- Reduce activity patterns (ie, rest at home) in the presence of infection
- Create a pollution-reduced environment by avoiding use of strong perfumes, aftershaves, or other scents
- Arrange to have a tuberculin test (PPD) done annually
- Schedule three to four periods of exercise per week

Assessing Respiratory Functioning

The health history is an essential component of assessing respiratory functioning. Either the client or the accompanying person can provide information. The nursing examination combined with laboratory findings can provide information to identify client's strengths, the nature of the problem, its course, related signs and symptoms, onset, frequency, and effect on activities of daily living. The nurse decides, based on the findings, what problems can be treated independently by nursing. Other problems are referred to the physician for decisions on treatment.

Nursing History

The nursing history, an important clinical tool in the early steps of the nursing process, always includes a respiratory component. The information gained provides data on why

PROMOTING WELLNESS

Oxygenation

Use the assessment checklist to determine how well you are meeting oxygenation needs. Then develop a prescription for self-care by choosing appropriate behaviors from the list of suggestions.

Assessment Checklist

almost always / sometimes / almost never

1. I breathe easily, without discomfort and without feeling short of breath.
2. I exercise regularly.
3. I maintain normal weight for my height and body frame.
4. I live in an environment free of pollution.
5. I avoid substances (tobacco, chemicals) that cause respiratory problems.

Self-Care Behaviors

1. Follow a regular exercise program with 30 to 45 minutes of moderate activity three or four times a week.
2. Maintain normal body weight.
3. Obtain medical evaluation for chest pain, problems with breathing, chronic cough with sputum or blood.
4. Avoid smoking cigarettes, cigars, or pipes.
5. Avoid chemical substances that cause respiratory depression.
6. Maintain a pollution-free environment (as much as possible).
7. Support federal and community efforts to keep the air free of pollution.
8. Avoid exposure to second-hand smoke (from another's cigarette) when possible.

---

a client needs nursing care and what kind of care is required to maintain a sufficient intake of air. Interview questions are used to identify current or potential health deviations, client actions for meeting this need and their effects, contributing factors, use of aids to improve intake of air, and effect on current life-style and relationships with others.

Before starting the interview, ascertain that the client and accompanying people are comfortable. If the client is in any respiratory distress, appropriate actions should be initiated to relieve symptoms. The accompanying people can answer questions to provide a data base. The nurse can expand this when the client is able to provide information. If the clinical condition of the client indicates that no emergency interventions are necessary, a comprehensive history can be obtained.

When a health deviation is noted during the data collection, the nurse needs to collect as much descriptive information as possible, verifying whether the status of the problem changed suddenly or slowly. Sample questions are given in the accompanying display.

Physical Assessment

The basic examination of the lungs and respiratory status are discussed in Chapter 24. The nurse proceeds in a well-organized manner with a sequence of inspection, palpation, percussion, and auscultation.

Inspection Observation of the chest normally shows that the contour is slightly convex with no sternal depression.

The anteroposterior diameter should be less than the transverse diameter. Any abnormalities in thoracic structure should be described or sketched (see Fig. 24-32 for examples). The contour of the intercostal spaces should be flat or depressed. Movement of the chest should be symmetric. The skin at the thorax should be warm and dry and exhibit even distribution of color with no cyanosis or pallor. Note any scars; origin would have been recorded in the history under previous surgery or accidents. Observe the respiratory rate and rhythm for 1 full minute. Normally, respirations are quiet and nonlabored. Any flaring of nostrils, intercostal restriction, tachypnea, or bradypnea suggests a health deviation that necessitates further evaluation.

Palpation The trachea should be equidistant from each clavicle. Skin temperature should be the same as the rest of the body. Respiratory excursion is measured by placing one's hand on the client's posterior thorax at the tenth rib with both thumbs almost touching the vertebrae. While the client takes a few deep breaths, the nurse's thumbs should move 5 to 8 cm symmetrically at maximal inspiration (see Fig. 24-34). To assess vocal **fremitus** (the capacity to feel sound on the chest wall), the nurse should place his or her palm surface to the client's chest wall, avoiding bony areas (eg, scapulae); the nurse should detect equal vibrations as the client says some multisyllable word (eg, "ninety-nine"). Bilaterally equal mild fremitus should be detected with the greatest intensity noted at anterior and posterior base of neck and along trachea and large bronchi (see Fig. 24-34). Increased fremitus is noted in clients with pneumonia, because solid tissue conducts sound well. Conversely, clients

FOCUSED ASSESSMENT GUIDE

Respiration

Factors to Assess	Questions and Approaches
Usual patterns of respiration	How would you describe your breathing patterns? Do you have allergies? Do you smoke? Do you live with a smoker or are there smokers in your workplace?
Recent changes	Have you noticed any changes in your breathing pattern (out of breath, cough, pain)? Do you have chest pain?
Cough	How much and how often do you cough? Is the cough related to the time of day or any activity? What is it like (dry, bubbly, hoarse)? Do you have a history of allergies? Do you ever wheeze? Are you exposed to dust? Fumes? Where do you work? What kind of work? How are you treating the cough?
Sputum	Do you ever cough up and spit out mucus? How much do you spit out and do you associate it with anything (time of day, environment)? What color is it? Is it ever blood tinged? What is its odor?
Chest pain	On a scale of 0 to 5 (5 being very painful), how severe is the pain? Where is the pain? Is the pain worse with inspiration? Expiration? Cough? Does the pain radiate? What measures are you using to relieve the pain?
Dyspnea	Is it constant or remittent or related to any activity? How do different positions affect it? How does it affect your daily activities? Is any part of your body bluish during the breathing problem? What do you do during and after the breathing attack? Have you ever been told that you have asthma? Emphysema? Tuberculosis? Heart disease? Do you think the problem is getting worse or staying the same?
Fever	Have you had pneumonia recently? Do you have any contact with people who have tuberculosis? Do you have night sweats? Are others in your household well or ill? Have you traveled anywhere recently? What medications are you using? Have you been exposed to any pollutants?
Fatigue	Have you noticed you feel more tired lately? Are you getting your normal amount of sleep at night? Has your sleep at night been affected by any difficulty breathing? Do you become easily fatigued when you climb stairs? Has your pattern of daily activity changed lately?

with chronic obstructive pulmonary disease (COPD) have decreased fremitus, because air does not conduct sound well. The presence or absence of crepitation, masses, edema, or tenderness should be noted.

Percussion Percussion is performed posteriorly as the client pulls shoulders forward; examination proceeds down the client's back, comparing one side to the other. Anterior and lateral thorax can be examined with the client in a supine position. The nurse must listen to the intensity and quality of each sound as the chest wall and underlying structures are set in motion. Resonance, a loud hollow, low-pitched sound, is heard over the normal lung. Emphysematous lungs produce a loud, low, booming sound called hyperresonance. A flat sound is detected over bone or heavy muscle. A dull sound with medium pitch and intensity is percussed on the liver (fifth intercostal space at the right midclavicular line). Tympany is a high-pitched, loud, drumlike sound produced over the stomach. Dullness over the lung field occurs when fluid or solid tissue replaces normal lung tissue in the pleural space and requires further investigation.

Auscultation The nurse should move from apex to base with the stethoscope comparing one side with the other side. Normal breath sounds are of three types: *vesicular* (low pitch, soft expiration and heard over most of lung); *bronchial* (high pitch and loud expiration and heard over trachea and peripheral lung); and *bronchovesicular* (medium pitch and medium expiration and heard over upper anterior chest and intercostal area; see Fig. 24-38). The client should breathe through the opened mouth slowly. Nasal breathing produces false abnormal breath sounds. Hyperventilation is conducive to syncope and client distress. If any abnormal breath sound is detected, the nurse should instruct the client to cough and should auscultate again for at least two breaths. A recording of location, change in breath sounds after coughing, and phase of respiration (eg, expiration) in which abnormal sound was heard is imperative.

Adventitious sounds can be divided into four categories: (1) crackles (formerly called rales); (2) gurgles (formerly called rhonchi); (3) wheezes; and (4) rubs. **Crackles** are noncontinuous sounds that occur when air moves through airways that contain fluid. They are produced by a delayed reopening of deflated airways. Crackles can be further classified as fine, medium, or coarse. Fine crackles, high-pitched sounds heard toward the end of inspiration, indicate congestion. Rubbing strands of hair between your fingers creates a sound similar to fine crackles. Usually, they are first detected in the lung bases, usually cannot be cleared with coughing, and may be ausculated in a client who has pneumonia. Medium crackles are a lower-pitched moist sound heard halfway through inspiration and are produced as air moves through fluid in slightly larger airways. Clients with pulmonary edema exhibit these and cannot clear them by coughing. Coarse crackles are loud, bubbly noises heard during inspiration and expiration and not cleared by coughing. They result from fluid in the larger airways and indicate increasing pulmonary congestion (Stevens & Becker, 1988). **Gurgles** are continuous, musical sounds audible in expiration or inspiration, or both. Gurgles or rhonchi reflect obstruction in large upper airways due to secretions or edema. They can sometimes be cleared with coughing and sound like snoring. **Wheezes** are high-pitched squeaky sounds heard on expiration and sometimes on inspiration. They originate in smaller bronchi or

bronchioles and are often detected in asthmatics. A **pleural friction rub** is a dry grating sound caused by inflammation of pleural surfaces. It is usually heard on inspiration and expiration, is unaltered by coughing, and resembles the sound made by rubbing leather surfaces.

Common Methods to Assess Respiratory Functioning

In addition to the nursing history and physical examination, various laboratory and radiologic tests described in Table 36-2 provide further assessment data that can aid in the formation of nursing diagnoses. These tests are not distinctive of a particular disease but they do reflect how well the respiratory system is functioning. Figure 36-5 demonstrates a pulse oximetry unit used for measuring oxygen saturation (SaO_2) of arterial blood.

The nurse must always be alert for common clinical manifestations that may indicate an airway emergency (see the accompanying display). Specific disease processes and conditions leading to acute respiratory failure as well as specific clinical manifestations are discussed in a medical–surgical textbook.

(*Text continues on p. 955*)

F I G U R E   3 6 - 5

Pulse oximetry unit used to measure oxygen saturation (SaO_2) of arterial blood.

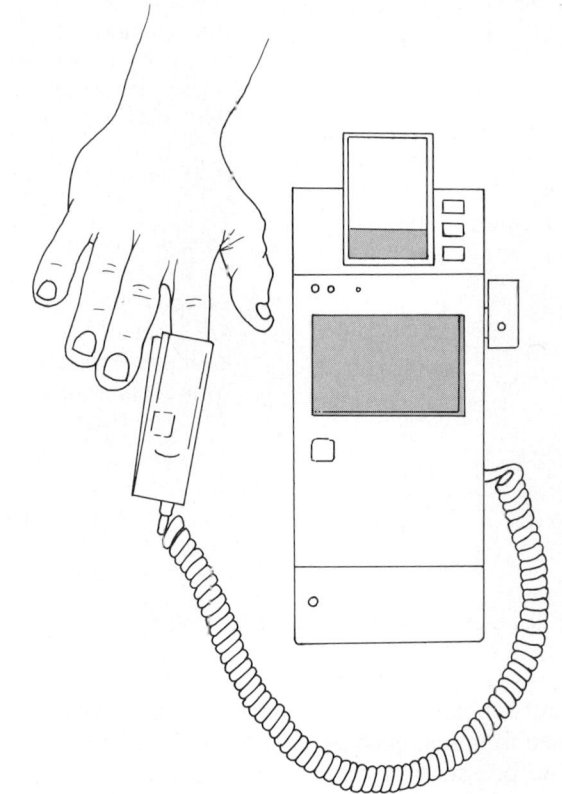

TABLE 36-2

Common Methods to Assess Respiratory Functioning

Definition and Purpose	Normal Values	Nursing Implications

Spirometry measures lung capacity, volumes, and flow rates with the use of an instrument called a **spirometer.**

Spirometry helps evaluate the pulmonary status and the efficacy of treatment. Corrections are made for age, sex, weight, and height.	*Tidal volume* (TV): The amount of air inspired and expired in a normal respiration. Normal is 500 mL. *Inspiratory reserve volume* (IRV): The amount of air that can be inspired beyond tidal volume. Normal is 3500 to 4300 mL. *Expiratory reserve volume* (ERV): The amount of air that can be exhaled beyond tidal volume. Normal is 1200 to 1500 mL. *Residual volume* (RV): The amount of air remaining in the lungs after a maximal expiration. Normal is 1200 to 1500 mL. *Vital capacity* (VC): The maximal amount of air that can be exhaled following a maximal inhalation. Normal is 4000 to 4800 mL. *Forced vital capacity* (FVC): The maximal amount of air that can be inhaled followed by a fast maximal forced exhalation with greatest effort. FVC differs from VC in that VC does not require a forced inhalation, and the person exhales normally. Normal is 4800 mL. *Functional residual capacity* (FRC): FRC is equal to the expiratory reserve volume plus the residual volume. Normal is 2400 to 3000 mL. A normal range is 75% to 125% of normal FRC. *Total lung capacity* (TLC): The tidal volume plus the residual volume. Normal is 5500 mL.	The client's understanding and cooperation are important to successful study. Explanations should include teaching the client to wear a nose clip and a mouthpiece for breathing. Suffocation will not occur. The examination is not painful but it is fatiguing. The client should wear comfortable clothing. Tight clothing, such as a girdle or belt, may restrict breathing. Drugs affecting the respiratory tract, such as bronchodilators, are withheld before the examination so that test results reflect the client's present status. There is no special aftercare, but the client may need extra rest.

Arterial blood gas and pH analysis examine arterial blood to determine the pressure exerted by oxygen and carbon dioxide in the blood and the blood pH.

A blood sample is used to measure gas components in arterial blood and the pH of blood. It reflects quality of ventilation and perfusion.	The pressure of carbon dioxide (pCO_2) is normally 35 to 45 mm Hg. The pressure of oxygen (pO_2) is normally 80 to 100 mm Hg The pH is normally between 7.35 and 7.45.	The procedure for obtaining arterial blood is uncomfortable, more so than an injection into a vein, muscle, or subcutaneous tissue, and the client should be prepared for this. The arm is usually used to obtain a blood sample. The radial artery or an artery in the inner aspect of the elbow is used. Occasionally, the femoral artery is entered. A pressure dressing is applied at the entry site for 3 minutes and watched for evidence of bleeding.

(continued)

T A B L E   3 6 - 2 *(continued)*

Common Methods to Assess Respiratory Functioning

Definition and Purpose	Normal Values	Nursing Implications

Pulse oximetry is a noninvasive technique that measures the oxygen saturation (SaO_2) of arterial blood.

Pulse oximetry is useful for monitoring people on oxygen, those at risk for hypoxia, and postoperative clients, and effectively records trends in oxygen saturation (SaO_2). It is not a replacement for arterial blood gas analysis but can be used selectively as adjunct therapy.	A range of 95% to 98% is considered normal oxygen saturation (SaO_2).	The appropriate type of sensor and location should be selected. Use an alcohol swab to cleanse the monitoring site and remove any artificial nails or nail polish if the finger is selected. Movement, low perfusion (eg, peripheral vascular disease), and cigarette smoking can affect the SaO_2 value. Always check that the alarms for high and low SaO_2 and high and low pulse rate are turned on before leaving the room. Prevent pressure necrosis by moving the sensor at prescribed intervals. It is important to be aware of the client's hemoglobin level before evaluating oxygen saturation because this test measures only the percentage of oxygen carried by the available hemoglobin. Even a client with a low hemoglobin could appear to have a normal SaO_2 because most of that hemoglobin is saturated yet not have enough oxygen to meet body needs.

Cytologic study of respiratory secretions involves a study of sputum and cells it contains.

A cytologic study is done primarily to study cells that may be malignant, determine organisms causing infection, and identify blood or pus in the sputum.	Sputum is free of abnormal cells and of pus, blood, and bacteria.	Sputum is best obtained in the morning, before breakfast, after secretions have accumulated in the respiratory tract during the night. Usually, specimens are collected on 3 successive days.
		It is best to have the client brush his or her teeth and rinse the mouth so that saliva and oral debris do not contaminate the specimen. The client should be taught that sputum is matter ejected from the lower respiratory tract through the mouth and that saliva is an unsatisfactory specimen.
		The client should be instructed to inhale deeply and cough deeply on exhalation. About 1 teaspoon of sputum is needed for a specimen.
		The sputum should be coughed directly into a sterile specimen container, which is then covered with a sterile lid, properly labeled, and sent to the laboratory
		A note should be made on the client's record about the character of the sputum, including amount, appearance, and odor.
		If a specimen cannot be obtained, an induced sputum specimen may be required.

(continued)

TABLE 36-2 *(continued)*

Common Methods to Assess Respiratory Functioning

Definition and Purpose	Normal Values	Nursing Implications

Endoscopy is the direct visualization of a body cavity. A *bronchoscope* is used to examine the bronchi and a *laryngoscope* is used to examine the larynx. These are lighted, tubular instruments.

Definition and Purpose	Normal Values	Nursing Implications
Respiratory endoscopy is used to view lesions, obtain a biopsy, improve drainage, remove foreign substances, and drain abscesses.	No obstructions are normally found in respiratory passageways, and tissues appear normal.	An informed consent is necessary for endoscopy. Endoscopic examinations are uncomfortable for most clients, especially the bronchoscopy, and the client should be prepared for this. The client should be without food or fluid for 4 to 6 hours before endoscopy to avoid the risk of aspirating stomach contents. An analgesic, sedative, or tranquilizer is generally given about 30 minutes before endoscopy. The client should be taught that there may be gagging when local anesthesia is applied to the throat and there is a feeling that one cannot swallow or breathe. However, the airway remains open. Aftercare includes withholding fluids and food, usually for 1 or 2 hours, until the client can swallow and cough. Vital signs should be checked for signs of atelectasis and pneumonitis. Warm gargles may be used to relieve irritation in the pharynx once the gag reflex has returned. The client should be observed for **hemoptysis,** which is sputum containing blood, and for excessive bleeding, especially if a biopsy has been obtained. If contrast media were used during the examination, the client should be helped and encouraged to cough to rid the bronchial tree of the material.

Skin tests determine antigen–antibody reactions.

Definition and Purpose	Normal Values	Nursing Implications
In intradermal tests, antigens, those to which the client may have been previously exposed, are injected into the superficial layer of skin with a needle and syringe or a sterile four-pronged lancet to evaluate immune response. Patch and scratch tests, applied to hairless portions of the client's body, are used to evaluate the immune system's ability to respond to known allergens.	Negative reactions indicate a lack of sensitivity. Positive reactions, which indicate a positive antigen–antibody reaction, are discussed in clinical texts.	Check the client's history for hypersensitivity to any of the test antigens. If positive, notify physician before performing tests. These skin tests are not usually performed with infants because of their immature immune system. If the client is an outpatient, instruct him or her to return at the appropriate time to have the test results read. Do not perform tests in areas with acne, dermatitis, or excessive hair. On the chart, record the test, time, date, method, and site of administration. After reading the results, document the reaction noting amount of erythema or induration.

(continued)

T A B L E 3 6 - 2 (continued)

Common Methods to Assess Respiratory Functioning

Definition and Purpose	Normal Values	Nursing Implications
Radiography is an x-ray examination of the lungs and thoracic cavity.		
X-ray examinations of the lungs are done to help diagnose pulmonary diseases and to determine the progress of development of disease.	The bony thoracic and soft tissues have normal positions, symmetry, and shape.	There is no special preparation for flat films of the chest, and the examinations are without discomfort. The client should be taught that clothing and jewelry from the waist up must be removed and that the client will be asked to hold his or her breath when the x-ray film is taken.
Lung scan is the recording on a photographic plate of the emissions of radioactive waves from a substance injected into a vein as it circulates through the lung.		
A *perfusion scan* (Q scan) is done to measure integrity of pulmonary blood vessels and evaluate blood flow abnormalities (eg, pulmonary emboli). A *ventilation scan* (V scan) is done to detect ventilation abnormalities (especially in clients with emphysema). Both scans used together provide greater and more accurate diagnostic information than either test used solely.	Q scan shows no increased uptake of radioactive drug. V scan shows no abnormalities	Explain procedure to client. In a Q scan, the radiologist injects radiopharmaceutical into a peripheral vein. Scan of chest is done in x-ray department. Client lies under the camera for 20 to 40 minutes. Ventilation scan is done after the perfusion scan. Scan is completed in x-ray department after client inhales radioactive gas by mask and then exhales it out of the lungs to room air. In 8 hours, the radioactive isotope disintegrates and is cleared from the circulation.
Thoracentesis is an aspiration of fluid or air from the pleural space (see Chapter 27).		
Thoracentesis provides a fluid sample for diagnostic purposes or a tissue sample for biopsy. It is also used to relieve pulmonary compression and respiratory distress in clients with a variety of disorders.	This sample should be negative for blood, bacteria, viruses, or abnormal cells.	Informed consent is necessary. Remind client that pressure, not pain, is felt after the local anesthetic is injected. Vital signs and breath sounds are checked before and after the procedure. Expose the entire chest for the procedure, and shave aspiration site. This sterile procedures necessitates the client to lie on the unaffected side or to sit with the overbed table supporting the head and arms. After the catheter is removed, the site is covered with a sterile dressing and observed for any drainage. Chest x-ray is usually done as part of the procedure to verify no complications. Documentation of amount of fluid, color, viscosity, and client response should appear in the nursing notes.

Recognizing Airway Emergencies

Common Clinical Manifestations

Universal distress signal (clutching throat with both hands)

and

Inability to speak or cough
Pain with respiration
Hemoptysis
Frothy white or pink sputum
Presence of adventitious breath sounds
Dyspnea

Diagnosing

Alterations in Respiratory Function as the Problem

After the assessment is completed and the data are examined, the nurse concludes either that there is no problem at this time or that there is an actual or potential respiratory problem that is amenable to independent or interdependent nursing action. Nursing diagnoses indicating alterations in respiratory functions are as follows:

Ineffective Airway Clearance
Ineffective Breathing Pattern
Impaired Gas Exchange

These three nursing diagnoses are discussed in detail at the end of this chapter in the section entitled Nursing Process in Clinical Practice.

Common etiologies for these diagnoses are inability to maintain proper position, pain or fear of pain, viscous secretions, fatigue, decreased level of consciousness, lack of knowledge, smoking, allergy, mechanical obstruction, medications, and decreased elasticity of lungs.

Examples of these diagnoses, etiologic factors, and defining characteristics are given in the accompanying display.

Alterations in Respiratory Function as the Etiology

Alteration in respiratory functioning may affect other areas of human functioning. Examples of other nursing diagnoses resulting from alterations in respiratory functioning are the following:

Activity Intolerance related to shortness of breath
Anxiety related to feeling of suffocation
Pain related to pleurisy
Impaired Verbal Communication related to endotrachial intubation
Ineffective Individual Coping related to frequent hospitalization due to acute symptoms of COPD
Diversional Activity Deficit related to loss of ability to perform specific activities due to shortness of breath
Fatigue related to impaired oxygen transport system
Fear related to disabling respiratory illness
Dysfunctional Grieving related to loss of normal respiratory functioning
Altered Health Maintenance related to smoking
Noncompliance With _____ [eg, Performance of Daily Respiratory Exercises] related to side effects of therapy
Altered Nutrition: Less Than Body Requirements, related to difficulty breathing

---

NURSING DIAGNOSES FOR COMMON PROBLEMS

Respiration

Problem	Related Factors	Sample Defining Characteristics
Ineffective Airway Clearance	Thick yellow secretions, fever, fatigue, dehydration, poor nutrition	"I never feel as though I am getting enough air." Seventy-year-old man with a 20-year history of COPD, recent development of pneumonia. He is pale with circumoral cyanosis. His respiratory rate is 40 per minute and shallow. Rhonchi are auscultated bilaterally. He does not sit quietly in chair or on bed. He cannot walk length of room without coughing episode, which produces little sputum.
Impaired Gas Exchange	Smokes one pack per day; works with asbestos in auto factory; has had a cold for 7 days	Cyanotic 50-year-old man. Using pursed-lip breathing while sitting on emergency room stretcher. Sitting hunched forward with overbed table supporting arms. Altered blood gases show respiratory acidosis. Admits to shortness of breath, nausea, and ankle edema for 1 week.
Ineffective Breathing Pattern	Anxious about results of cardiac catheterization and possible cardiac surgery	Hyperventilating, tachypneic (40 minutes). "I have a tingling feeling in my fingers."

Altered Oral Mucous Membrane related to presence of endotrachial tube

Powerlessness related to inability for self-care due to COPD

Self-Esteem Disturbance related to loss of normal respiratory functions

Sleep Pattern Disturbance related to orthopnea and bronchodilators

Social Isolation related to inability to walk to usual "people places"

High Risk for Suffocation related to child playing with a plastic bag

High Risk for Aspiration related to reduced level of consciousness

Important Distinctions   Each nursing statement identifies what is wrong with the client and suggests client goals. The etiology of the problem directs nursing interventions. The nurse, analyzing the assessment data must decide if the alteration in respiratory functioning:

- Is the problem
- Is contributing to a different problem
- Is a sign or symptom of a problem

Altered respiratory functioning can fit into all three categories. Let's examine how ineffective airway clearance in a 17-year-old asthmatic baseball player who is waiting to hear from the college of his choice plays a role in three different nursing diagnoses:

Ineffective Airway Clearance related to pollen exposure, exercise, and stress of questionable college admission. The airway clearance is the problem statement. Nursing interventions are directed to reducing exposure to pollens, specific stressors, and timing or degree of exercise. The outcome will be that the client achieves effective airway clearance.

Activity Intolerance related to ineffective airway clearance during and after baseball games, fatigue, and stress. Here, the activity intolerance is the problem statement and ineffective airway clearance is just one of the many factors contributing to the problem. All the nursing interventions are directed to improving the tolerance for activity.

Ineffective Individual Coping related to stress of career choices and stress of performance during baseball games as demonstrated by recent increase in episodes of asthmatic attacks. In this case, the ineffective airway clearance is a symptom of the client's real problem—ineffective coping. Nursing interventions are directed to reducing stressors. When the client is able to improve the use of his coping skills, the expected outcome is that the number of asthma attacks will decrease.

Each nursing diagnosis is unique to the situation, and the etiology varies with each client. The nurse, with the client, decides which problem is the priority. With creativity and patience, the nurse arrives at a nursing diagnosis that clearly directs nursing interventions and client goals. However, there might be interventions initiated by another member of the health care team for the nurse to follow (eg,

the prescription for administering medications). This would be the dependent aspect of nursing practice. The interdependent aspect refers to problems in which the nurse and other health care team members collaborate to treat (eg, nurses monitoring side effects of prescribed medications).

Planning: Client Goals

Whenever nurses care for clients with an alteration in respiratory functioning, nursing measures are supportive of the following general client goals. The client will:

- Demonstrate improved gas exchange in his or her lungs by an absence of cyanosis or chest pain
- Relate causative factors, if known, and relate adaptive method of coping with the factors
- Preserve pulmonary function by maintaining optimal level of activity
- Demonstrate self-care behaviors that provide relief from symptoms and prevent further pulmonary problems

When the client's physical, psychosocial, and spiritual conditions contribute to alterations in respiratory function, individualized client goals are developed with the client's input. For example: "By March 15, the client will be able to walk up one flight of steps at home without dyspnea."

Implementing

Establishing a Trusting Nurse–Client Relationship

Most people with a deviation in respiratory functioning experience anxiety as a result of symptoms and an actual or potential loss of independence. Oxygen deficits, particularly in elderly people, negatively affect all aspects of their daily living. The accompanying display focuses on oxygen problems and nursing education strategies for this particular group.

The nurse needs to create an environment that is likely to reduce anxiety. Immediate discomfort should be treated. Use of effective listening skills and accurate observation validates a caring attitude. Nurses must seek to understand clients' life experiences and habits without prejudging them. Clients often bring a fear of stigma into a professional relationship (especially with detrimental health habits), and this impedes the application of nursing interventions. The client who believes the nurse is genuinely concerned about him or her and the family is more willing to work toward achieving mutually desirable goals.

Promoting Proper Breathing

Deep Breathing

Habits of breathing that are not conducive to maximal respiratory functioning are common in well and ill people. Some people develop a pattern of shallow breathing or

FOCUS ON THE OLDER ADULT

Nursing Strategies for Oxygen Problems Affecting Older Adults

Decreased Gas Exchange and Increased Work of Breathing

- Encourage rest periods as necessary.
- Teach stair-climbing techniques.
- Encourage cessation or moderation of smoking.
- Teach breathing exercises.
- Remind about avoiding air pollutants.
- Caution about effect of extreme weather conditions.
- Instruct to avoid narcotics and sleeping pills.
- Discuss home management with client and family.
- Teach avoidance of infection and preventive measures (ie, flu vaccination).
- Use pillows as necessary to sleep.
- Encourage moderate exercise as tolerated.
- Encourage smaller, more frequent meals.

Decreased Ventilation and Effective Cough

- Encourage increased fluid intake, especially water, as allowed.
- Use cool-mist humidifier.
- Encourage attendance at pulmonary exercise rehabilitation program.
- Discourage use of over-the-counter medications.
- Teach how to splint thorax and cough effectively.
- Instruct in use of supplemental oxygen.
- Teach avoidance of milk products if they are troublesome.

walk with a caved-in–appearing chest wall. Ill people, for any number of reasons, may limit respiratory efforts. Hypoventilation occurs when there is a decreased amount of air entering and leaving the lungs. Deep-breathing exercises to produce hyperventilation, a condition in which there is more than the normal amount of air entering and leaving the lungs, are often used to overcome hypoventilation.

The nurse instructs the client to make each breath deep enough to move the bottom ribs. Unless there is a nasal condition that prohibits or prevents normal breathing, the client should start slow, deep ventilations nasally and expire slowly through the mouth. Breathing through the nose warms, filters, and humidifies the air. Respiratory status, motivation, and general clinical condition dictate the timing of this exercise, done hourly while awake or four times daily.

FIGURE 36-6

Teaching the client to use the incentive spirometer. (Photo © 1992 B. Proud.)

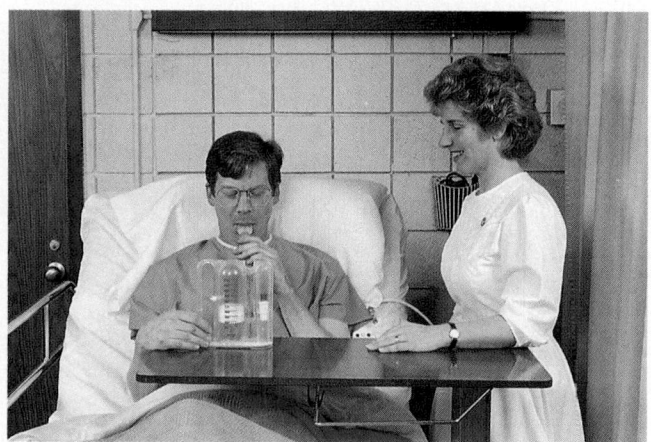

In incentive spirometry (Fig. 36-6), the client takes a deep breath and observes the results of his or her efforts registered on the spirometry equipment as the client sustains that maximal inspiration. Incentive spirometry keeps the alveoli from collapsing so that gas exchange can occur and secretions can be cleared and expectorated. Instructions are necessary before using incentive spirometry equipment. This intervention offers immediate positive reinforcement to the client for his or her breathing efforts.

Breathing Exercises

Breathing exercises are designed to aid the client to achieve more efficient and controlled ventilations, to decrease the work of breathing, and to correct respiratory defects.

Abdominal or Diaphragmatic Breathing

Many people with COPD have a tendency to breathe in a shallow, rapid, and exhausting pattern. This type of upper chest breathing can be changed to diaphragmatic breathing, reducing the rate, increasing the tidal volume, and reducing the functional residual capacity. The client is instructed to place one hand on the stomach and the other on the middle of the chest. The client then should breathe in slowly through the nose, letting the abdomen protrude as far as it will go. Next, he or she should breathe out through pursed lips while contracting the abdominal muscles. One hand should be pressing inward and upward on the abdomen. These steps should be repeated for 1 minute followed by rest for 2 minutes. The breathing pattern should be practiced several times during the day, and eventually it becomes automatic.

Pursed-Lip Breathing Clients who experience dyspnea and feelings of panic often obtain control of the respiration by using pursed-lip breathing. This exercise trains the muscles to prolong exhalation, increasing airway pressure during expiration and loosening the amount of airway trapping and resistance. To do this, the client inhales through the nose while counting to three and exhales slowly and evenly against pursed lips while tightening the abdominal muscles. During exhalation, the client counts to seven. To purse the lips, the client should position the lips as though he were sucking through a straw or whistling. While walking, the client should inhale while walking two steps and then exhale through pursed lips while taking the next four steps and then repeat the cycle. Before teaching these techniques, the nurse should practice them alone and then with a partner.

Managing Chest Tubes

Clients who develop fluid (pleural effusion), blood (hemothorax), or air (pneumothorax) in the pleural space require the assistance of a chest tube to drain these substances and allow the compressed lung to reexpand. A chest tube is a firm plastic tube with drainage holes in the proximal end that is placed in the pleural space, secured with a suture and tape, and attached to a drainage system that may or may not include suction. Other components of the system may include an air seal to prevent air from re-entering the chest once it has escaped and a suction control chamber that protects against excess suction pressure in the pleural cavity (Carroll, 1991). Most health care agencies currently use molded plastic, three-compartment disposable chest drainage units in place of the one-, two-, or three-bottle system. Placement of the chest tubes in the chest cavity is determined by the type of drainage. To drain air, the tube is placed higher in the chest, whereas gravity forces fluids to settle at the base of the lung, thus requiring a lower tube.

Nursing responsibilities include assisting with insertion and removal of a chest tube and, once the tube is in place, monitoring the client's respiratory status and vital signs, checking the dressing, and maintaining the patency and integrity of the drainage system. Figure 36-7 illustrates a chest drainage system.

Promoting and Controlling Coughing

The presence of excessive fluids or secretions in an organ or body tissue is called *congestion*, and a person with secretions or fluid in the lungs is said to have congested lungs. If the cough is dry, the client is said to be congested with a **nonproductive cough**. If the cough produces respiratory tract secretions, the client is referred to as being congested with a **productive cough**. Thick respiratory secretions are sometimes called **phlegm**. A client who is coughing with no congestion or secretions produced is described as being noncongested with a nonproductive cough.

Cough Mechanism   The cough mechanism (Fig. 36-8) consists of an initial irritation; a deep inspiration; a quick, tight closure of the glottis together with a forceful contrac-

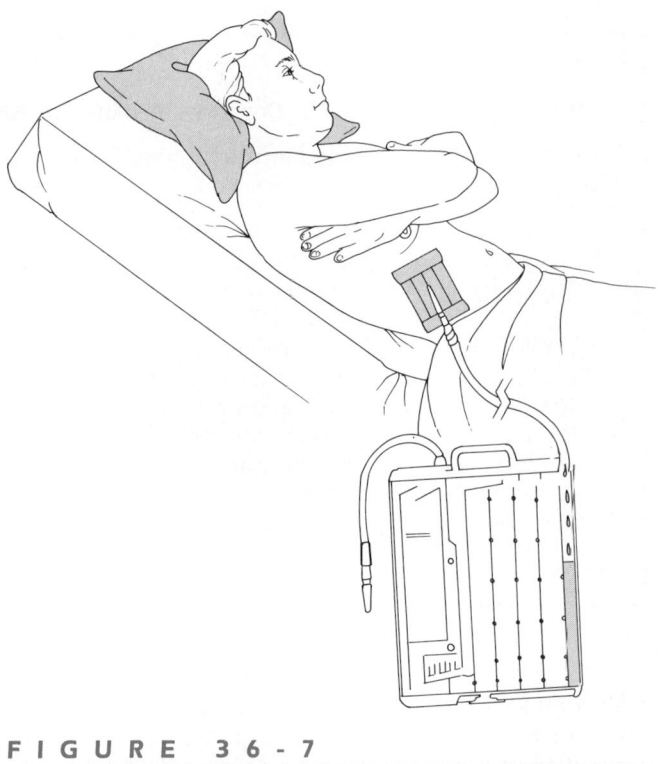

F I G U R E   3 6 - 7

A chest drainage system attached to a client.

tion of the expiratory intercostal muscles; and the upward push of the diaphragm. This causes an explosive movement of air from the lower to the upper respiratory tract. To be effective, a cough should have enough muscle contraction to force air to be expelled and to propel a liquid or a solid on its way out of the respiratory tract. This is most effective when the client is sitting upright with feet flat on the floor. A

F I G U R E   3 6 - 8

(A) A cough begins with a deep inspiration, distending the trachea and hyperinflating the lungs. (B) After inspiration, the glottis closes while intercostal and abdominal muscles contract forcibly. (C) When intrathoracic pressure reaches a high level, the glottis opens slightly, the diaphragm is pushed up, producing an explosive movement of air.

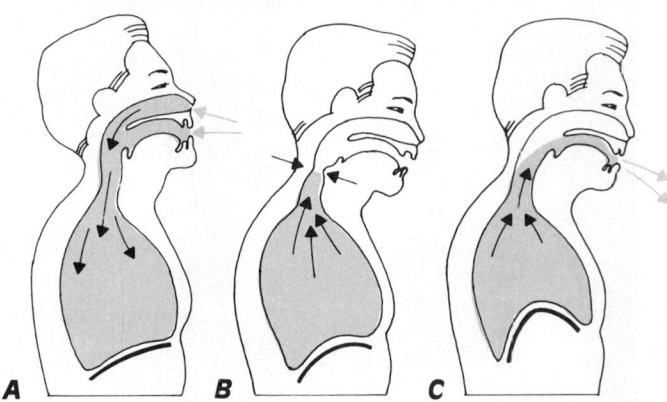

A   **B**   **C**

cough is a cleaning mechanism of the body. It is a means of helping to keep the airway clear of secretions and other debris.

Voluntary Coughing When a cough does not occur as a result of reflex stimulation of the cough-sensitive areas, it can be induced voluntarily. Teaching the client to cough voluntarily is an important aspect of preoperative and post-operative care. Although the teaching of deep breathing and coughing is relatively easy, experience has shown that it is difficult to have the client follow through and do them on his or her own. Frequent reminders throughout the day are necessary for many clients. Having a specific schedule on the nursing care plan is advised. Coughing early in the morning after rising removes phlegm that accumulated during the night. Coughing before meals improves the taste of food and oxygenation. At bedtime, coughing removes any buildup of phlegm and improves sleep patterns. For a client who is unable to cough voluntarily, manual stimulation over the trachea and prolonged exhalation can be helpful. If neither of these methods is successful, mechanical endotracheal suctioning with a catheter is used sometimes.

Involuntary Coughing Involuntary coughing often accompanies respiratory tract infections and irritations. It helps clear the airway if it is productive, but it is fatiguing and irritating when it is nonproductive. Medication may control involuntary coughing. Observations of the characteristics of breathing and coughing are necessary to determine the appropriate type of medication.

Cough Suppressants Suppressants are drugs that depress a body function, in this case, the cough reflex. Codeine, which is present in many cough preparations, is generally considered the preferred cough suppressant ingredient. However, codeine can be addictive. Because of possible abuse, many states require a physician's prescription for its use. Dextromethorphan hydrobromide is considered by some authorities to be as effective as codeine, and it is not addictive. Diphenhydramine hydrochloride, a potent antihistamine, is an effective cough suppressant. However, drowsiness (also common in other antihistamines) is a side effect of its use. Therefore, it may not be safe to use when the person must remain alert, as when driving a car.

An irritating nonproductive cough in people without congestion may be appropriately treated with suppressants. Inappropriate suppression of the cough in a person with respiratory congestion can result in harmful retention of the secretions.

Expectorants Expectorants are drugs that facilitate the removal of respiratory tract secretions by reducing the secretion viscosity. Clients with extremely tenacious secretions may need the secretions liquefied so the cough can be effective. In that way, the nonproductive cough of a person with lung congestion can become productive. An expec-torant used by a person who does not have congestion is inappropriate. Ammonium chloride, terpin hydrate, and ipecac have been widely used as expectorants in cough preparations. Adequate fluid intake and air humidification are considered effective expectorants by some authorities.

Lozenges Mild nonproductive coughs in people without congestion can often be relieved by lozenges. A *lozenge* is a small, solid medication intended to be held in the mouth until it dissolves. Lozenges generally control coughs by the local anesthetic effect of benzocaine. The local anesthetic can act on sensory and motor nerves by controlling the primary irritation and by inhibiting afferent and efferent impulses.

Teaching About Cough Preparations Because cough preparations are so readily available and people who purchase them are usually eager for relief, the consumer sometimes takes excessive amounts of more than one type. The nurse can offer health teaching about the appropriate choice of expectorants and suppressants. Also, the nurse should teach other misuses of cough mixtures. For example, cough syrups with a high sugar or alcohol content can disturb the metabolic balance of people with diabetes mellitus. Preparations containing antihistamines have an anticholinergic action, which can cause serious problems for people with glaucoma, or cause urinary retention in men with prostate enlargement. Other cough preparations can be detrimental to people with hypertension and with thyroid and cardiac diseases. In addition, prolonged use of self-prescribed cough preparations can conceal more serious health problems.

Promoting Comfort

Positioning Helping an incapacitated client assume a position that allows free movement of the diaphragm and expansion of the chest wall promotes ease of respiration. For example, sitting in a slumped position, which permits the abdominal contents to push upward on the diaphragm, results in less lung expansion during inspiration. People with dyspnea and orthopnea are most comfortable in a high Fowler's position because the accessory muscle can then be used easily to promote respiration. Recent research has demonstrated that turning bedridden clients from side to side every 2 hours may not always promote improved oxygenation. A client with most types of unilateral lung disease may have improved arterial oxygen levels when alternated between semi-Fowler's position and lying with the undiseased lung down for 60 to 90 minutes. This position provides for optimal gas exchange in the unimpaired lung, thus possibly hastening recovery and improving comfort (Yeaw, 1992).

Maintaining Adequate Fluid Intake Secretions can be kept thin by having the client drink 2 to 3 qt (1.9 to 2.9 L) of clear fluids daily. The client's fluid intake should be increased to the maximum that his or her health state can tolerate. The client who has an elevated temperature, who is breathing through the mouth, who is coughing, or who is losing excessive body fluids in other ways should have special attention focused on his or her intake. If there is incidence of right side heart failure, fluid intake should not exceed 1½ qt (1.4 L) daily. Milk products (milk, ice cream, yogurt, cheese, and so forth) work to thicken secretions and congestion. Clear fluids include water, tea, coffee, apple juice, broths, fruit ices, and plain flavored gelatin.

Providing Humidified Air When air humidity is low, artificial means for humidifying inspired air may be advisable. The inspiration of dry air removes the normal moisture in the respiratory passages, which is essential for protection from irritation and infection. Room humidifiers may be helpful for some clients. Electric vaporizers that produce steam or cool mist are available. Authorities believe the therapeutic value of one over the other has not been demonstrated. A cool-mist vaporizer does not present dangers with burns because it does not generate heat or hot water. However, it can provide the medium for pathogen growth if inadequately cleaned. The steam vaporizer does not present this problem.

Percussing Cupping (Fig. 36-9) is the manual percussion of lung areas to loosen pulmonary secretions so that they can be expectorated with greater ease. Percussion by cupping with the client supine or prone is carried out as follows:

1. Cup the hand by holding it in a rigid, dome-shaped position.
2. Strike rhythmically over the lobes of the lungs to be drained while keeping your wrists, elbows, and shoulders relaxed. Move the cupped hands from the client's lower ribs to the shoulders in back, and from the lower ribs to the top of the chest in front.
3. Listen for a hollow sound while percussing. The client should experience no pain. You are probably

not cupping the hand enough and are slapping the client's skin if the sound is not hollow and the client is uncomfortable.

4. Do not percuss on bare skin. The client may wear a gown or underclothing.
5. Do not percuss below the ribs or over the spine or breasts because of the danger of tissue damage.
6. Use percussion for 30 to 60 seconds over an area several times a day, but up to 3 to 5 minutes for clients with tenacious secretions.

The client may learn to percuss anterior surfaces of his or her chest wall. Family members are often taught to percuss posterior surfaces. Also, mechanical devices are available for percussion on the chest wall.

Vibrating Vibration involves the nurse's rhythmic contraction and relaxation of the arm and shoulder muscles while holding the hands flat on the client's chest wall. The purpose is to help loosen respiratory secretions so that they can be expectorated with ease. Vibration (Fig. 36-10) is carried out as follows:

1. Place your hands flat on the client's chest wall, where vibration is desired, and hold the hands side by side with the fingers extended and together. Some authorities prefer placing one hand on top of the other.
2. Ask the client to inhale deeply and then exhale slowly.
3. While the client exhales, vibrate the chest wall by contracting and relaxing your arm and shoulder muscles rhythmically and quickly.
4. Stop vibration on the client's inhalations.
5. Do not vibrate over the client's breasts, spine, sternum, and lower rib cage.
6. Use vibration for several minutes several times a day.
7. Plan to deliver a vibration frequency of about 200 per minute.

FIGURE 36-9

The cupping position and action of the hand in manual percussion of lung area.

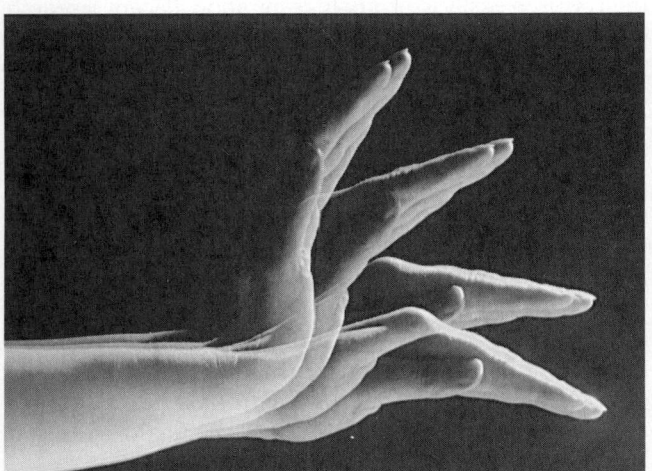

FIGURE 36-10

The position and action of the hands to use vibration to loosen respiratory secretions in the lungs.

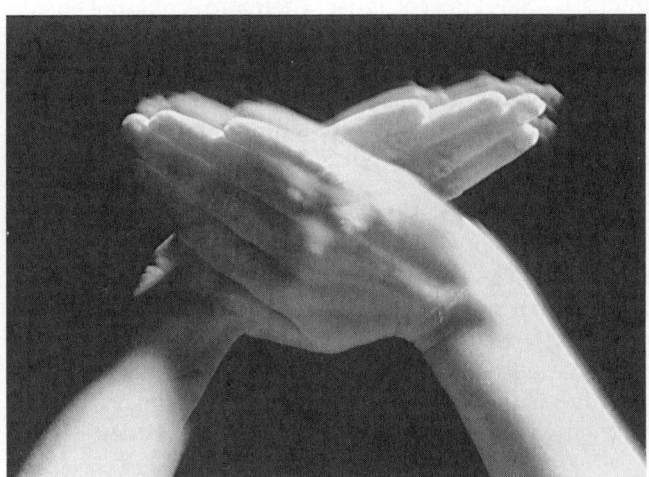

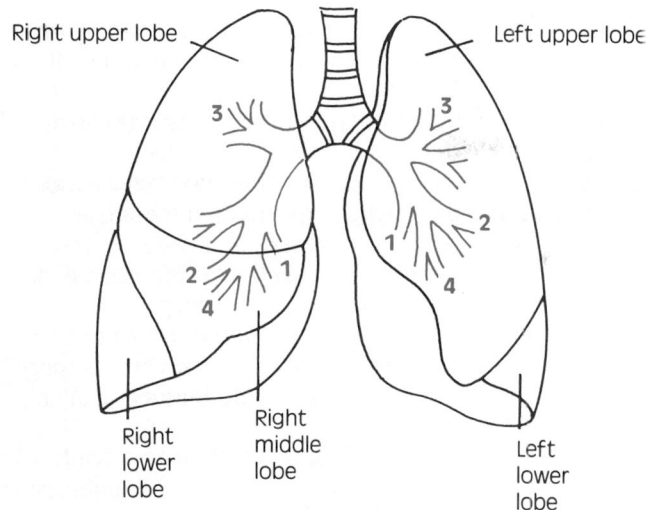

Family members can be taught to use vibration on the client's chest wall. Also, mechanical devices are available for vibrating the chest wall.

Providing Postural Drainage In **postural drainage**, gravity is used to drain secretions from the lungs. The person is positioned in a way that promotes the drainage of secretions from smaller pulmonary branches into larger ones, where they can be removed by drainage or coughing (Fig. 36-11). Postural drainage is often preceded by vibra-

F I G U R E   3 6 - 1 1

Postural drainage. Shown are four positions that use the force of gravity to assist the drainage of secretions from the smaller bronchial airways into the main bronchi and trachea so the client is able to cough them up.

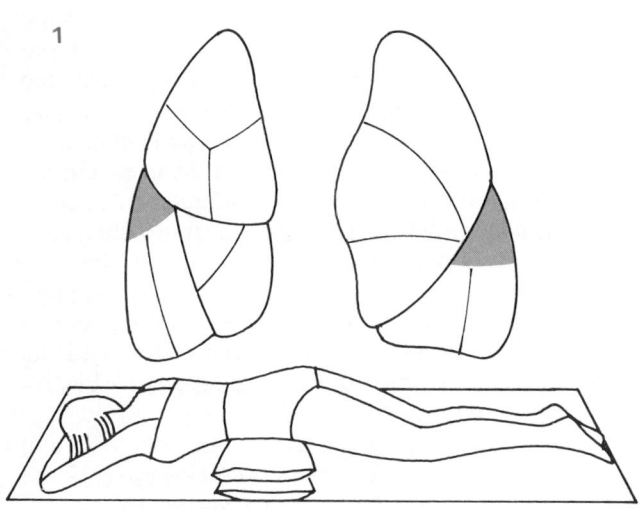

Lower lobes, superior segments

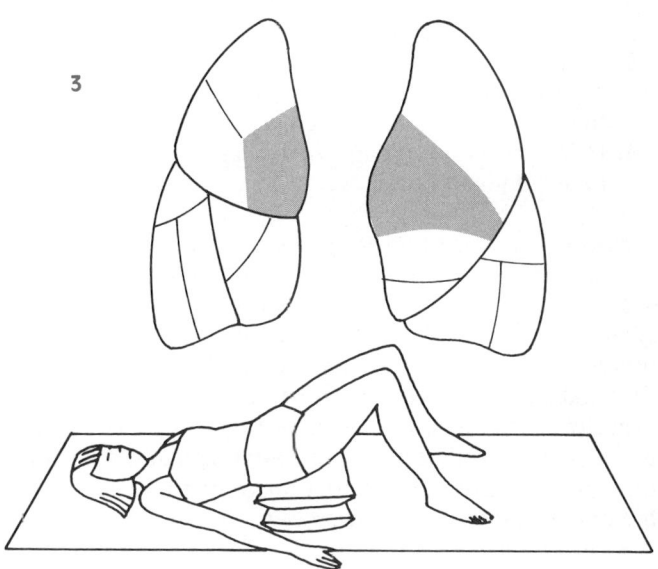

Upper lobes, anterior segment

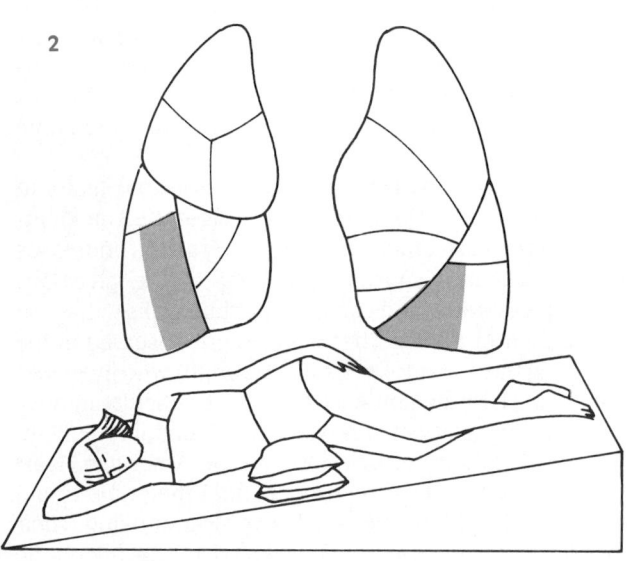

Lower lobes, anterior basal segment

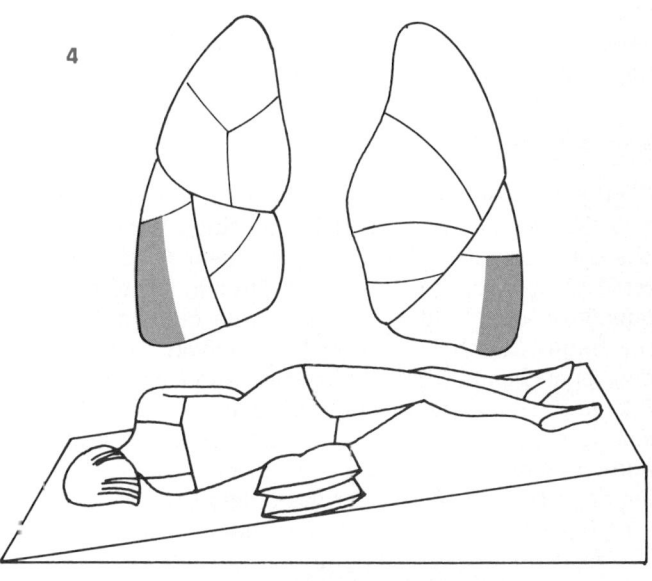

Lower lobes, lateral basal segment

tion, percussion, or both. Postural drainage is carried out as follows:

1. Have tissues and an emesis basin close at hand for the client to use when coughing and expectorating secretions.
2. Place the client in an appropriate position to promote drainage from the lobes of the lungs, as follows:
   - Use a high Fowler's position to drain the apical sections of the upper lobes of the lungs.
   - Place the client in a lying position, half on the abdomen and half on the side, right and left, to drain the posterior sections of the upper lobes of the lungs.
   - Place the client lying on the left side with a pillow under the chest wall to drain the right lobe of the lung.
   - Place the client in Trendelenburg's position to drain the lower lobes of the lungs.
3. Carry out postural drainage two to four times a day for 20 to 30 minutes. Discontinue the drainage if the client begins to feel weak or faint.
4. Delay postural drainage after meals for 1 to 2 hours to avoid vomiting.

Maintaining Good Nutrition People who are working hard at breathing often do not have energy for eating. Assessment of nutritional status is determined by measuring client's height, weight, upper arm circumference, serum protein levels, and nitrogen balance. Special attention and deliberate planning should be directed to adequate intake of proteins, vitamins, and minerals. Six small meals should be distributed over the course of the day instead of the usual three meals. Meals should be arranged 1 to 2 hours after breathing treatments and exercises.

Meeting Respiratory Needs With Medications Although treating clients with medications is a dependent nursing intervention, monitoring client response and side effects to medication is an independent nursing action. Table 36-3 shows some common medications for respiratory functioning, side effects, and nursing implications.

Using Inhalers

Clients use inhalers to disperse fine particles of medication into the deeper passages of the respiratory tract where absorption occurs. Inhaled medications may be administered to open narrowed airways (bronchodilators) or to liquefy or loosen thick secretions (mucolytic agents). A metered-dose inhaler or nebulizer delivers a controlled dose of medication with each compression of the canister. Clients need instruction to use inhalers effectively and safely. Overuse of inhalers may result in serious side effects and eventual ineffectiveness of the medication. The following are guidelines for proper use of inhalers:

1. Explain, demonstrate, and encourage client to manipulate inhaler apparatus.
2. Remove mouthpiece cover and shake inhaler well.
3. Fully exhale through the nose and place mouthpiece into mouth grasping securely with teeth and lips (see Fig. 42-24). Some recommend that the inhaler be held 1½ inches (4 cm) in front of the mouth rather than placed in the mouth. This facilitates movement of the medication into the trachea and lungs rather than being deposited on the tongue or pharynx.
4. Release one dose by pressing down on medication canister while inhaling slowly and deeply.
5. Hold breath for 5 to 10 seconds after inhalation before exhaling slowly through pursed lips.
6. Follow physician's order regarding frequency of inhaler use.

Package inserts accompanying medication also reinforce correct technique for using inhalers.

Teaching Clients to Maintain Pollution-Free Environments

In addition to applying the previously discussed interventions, the client also needs to assess the environment and make adjustments where possible to factors that impair respiratory functioning. The client must actively plan to prevent exposure to pollutants. This might involve a job change, use of protective equipment, enforcement of existing laws by government agencies, or subcontracting jobs. Dusting and vacuuming of office and home must be done minimally twice per week. If it is the client who must perform the tasks, a mask prevents some symptoms of respiratory distress. Exposure to industrial or occupational hazards (eg, paint, varnish, gaseous fumes, and asbestos) must be restricted.

In the United States and Canada, fine pollutants that pose a hazard to health are monitored closely. They are carbon monoxide, sulfur dioxide, total suspended particulates, ozone, and nitrogen dioxide. On days when pollutant levels are significantly elevated, morbidity and mortality rates among people with preexisting pulmonary disease are greatly increased. Thus, on those days when pollution alerts are announced, the client with an alteration in respiratory functions should decrease activity level, stay indoors, and use an air conditioner, electronic air cleaner, or air filter. If pollen alters respiratory functions, the same principles apply.

Cigarette smoking is the most important risk factor in pulmonary disease. The inhalation of cigarette smoke increases airway resistance, reduces ciliary action, increases mucus production, causes thickening of the alveolar-capillary membrane, and causes bronchial walls to thicken and lose their elasticity. These effects are observed in the smoker and the nonsmoker (child and adult) who lives with the smoker. Habitual smokers find great difficulty in quitting or reducing smoking and need much encouragement. The American Lung Association and the American Heart Association offer many free educational materials to aid and support the client who is trying to stop smoking. Their addresses and phone numbers are listed in local telephone directories. Nurses are in a prime position to present accu-

TABLE 36-3

Medications Used to Improve Respiratory Functioning

Medication	Activity	Route	Side Effects	Nursing Implications
Epinephrine	Relaxes muscles that line bronchi and bronchioles	IV, SQ	Tremors, anxiety, insomnia, headache, palpitations, elevated blood pressure, vomiting	Position client upright to prevent aspiration if vomiting occurs. Monitor heart rate, respirations, breath sounds, and blood pressure every 15 minutes. May repeat medication within 15 minutes with an order.
Isoproterenol (Isuprel)	Bronchodilator	Inhaler	Same as with epinephrine but milder	Monitor heart rate. Demonstrate proper use of inhaler. Warn client not to exceed prescribed frequency of doses.
Metaproterenol (Alupent)	Bronchodilator	PO, inhalation	Same as with epinephrine	Same as with epinephrine
Theophylline (aminophylline)	Bronchodilator	PO, IV, rectally	Nausea, vomiting, rapid heart rate, diuresis, irritability, vertigo, convulsions	Monitor vital signs closely. Force fluids as clinical status allows. Monitor serum theophylline levels, especially if client does not respond to drug or severe side effects develop.
Corticosteroids (ACTH, prednisone, dexamethasone)	Reduces inflammation	PO, IV	Fluid retention, hypertension, mood swings, weight gain, gastritis, hyperglycemia	Reduce sodium intake. Make client and family aware of potential for labile emotions. Weigh daily in morning. Monitor blood pressure and blood sugar. Warn client to follow administration directions accurately. Instruct client about correct use of inhaler.
Antihistamines	Blocks histamine and relieves congestion of an allergic origin	PO	Drowsiness, anorexia, constipation, dry mouth, blurred vision, urinary retention	Warn client to use only with physician's advice in presence of bronchial asthma. Do not mix with alcohol, tranquilizers, or sedatives. Client should avoid driving or using machinery. Observe clients for prolonged bleeding if they are using warfarin anticoagulants.
Cromolyn sodium (Intal)	Prevents the release of histamines, serotonin, prostaglandin by the mast cell in an antigen–antibody reaction in asthma.	Inhaler	Cough	Remind client this is used to prevent asthma attacks, not to treat acute episodes. This drug contains lactose and will cause diarrhea in lactose-deficient clients. Inform client that this is effective only if taken routinely (two to four times per day).

IV, intravenous; SQ, subcutaneous; PO, oral.

rate information regarding the deleterious effects of smoking and to encourage the decision to stop smoking or never to start smoking.

Providing Supplemental Oxygen

The amount of oxygen the client uses for inspiration can be increased by providing a supplemental supply. The provision of therapeutic oxygen is called oxygen therapy, and is usually prescribed by the physician. Oxygen therapy can frighten clients. Explanations from the nurse regarding procedures and purpose play a major role in reducing this fear. The client should be encouraged to discuss anxieties. If oxygen is given in an emergency, explanations concurrent with administration are appropriate.

Sources of Oxygen

Therapeutic oxygen is supplied from a wall outlet or a portable cylinder. The wall outlet source can be prepared for use quickly. The oxygen is supplied from a central source through a pipeline, usually at 50 to 60 pounds per square inch (psi) of pressure. A specially designed flowmeter (Fig. 36-12) is attached to the outlet and opens it. A valve makes regulation of oxygen flow possible.

Oxygen can also be dispersed under pressure in steel cylinders or tanks. The tank is delivered with a protective cap to prevent accidental force against the cylinder outlet. When a standard, large-sized cylinder is full, its contents are under more than 2000 psi of pressure. The force behind an accidentally partially opened outlet could cause the tank to take off like an uncontrolled, dangerous jet. Smaller

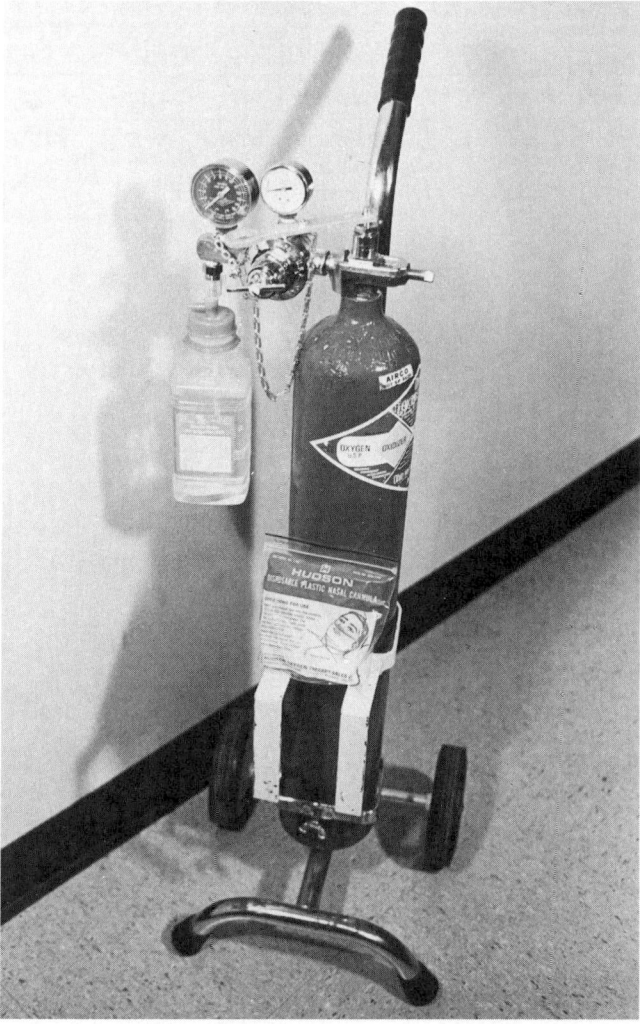

F I G U R E   3 6 - 1 3

A small cylinder of oxygen is in readiness for an emergency or transfer situations. The regulators and humidifier bottle are attached and ready to use.

cylinders are available for emergency, ambulatory, and home use. The principles and precautions are the same for all size cylinders.

To release oxygen safely and at a desirable rate, a regulator is used. The regulator has two gauges. The one nearest the tank shows the pressure or amount of oxygen in the tank. The other gauge indicates the number of liters per minute of oxygen being released. Figure 36-13 shows an oxygen tank with its regulator.

The oxygen cylinder and the regulator must be handled cautiously. The oxygen cylinder should be transported carefully, preferably strapped onto a wheeled carrier to avoid possible falling and breaking the outlet. The cylinder should be stabilized securely in a properly fitting stand.

Because of the possibility of dust and other particles becoming lodged in the outlet of the tank and being forced in the regulator, the tank is primed with two hands before a regulator is applied. The handle of the tank is turned slightly

F I G U R E   3 6 - 1 2

Flowmeter of a piped-in oxygen-delivery system.

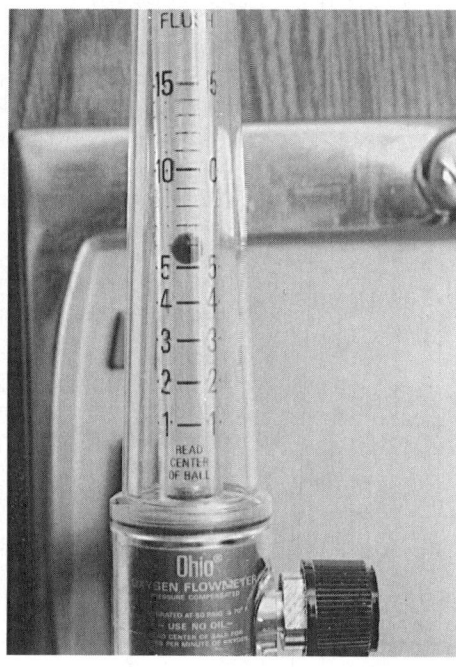

counterclockwise. This releases a small amount of oxygen and flushes out the outlet. The cylinder is closed again by turning the handle clockwise. The force with which the oxygen is released from this opening causes a loud, hissing sound that startles most people. Thus, clients and visitors need to be prepared for the noise with an appropriate explanation. It is recommended that tanks be primed away from the bedside.

Oxygen Flow Rate

The flow rate of oxygen, measured in liters per minute, is used to regulate the amount of oxygen available to the client. The rate varies depending on the condition of the client and the route of administration of the oxygen. The flow rate does not necessarily reflect the oxygen concentration actually inspired by the client, because there is leaking and mixing with atmospheric air. More precise doses are usually prescribed in terms of percent of inspired oxygen. To regulate oxygen concentration accurately, analysis of samples of the air mixture the client is actually inhaling is recommended every 4 hours. Several types of commercial oxygen analyzers are available.

A physician prescribes the rate of oxygen administration. The nurse must monitor closely the flow rate for clients with chronic lung conditions, such as emphysema. Normally, excessive levels of carbon dioxide in the blood stimulate respirations. However, the chemoreceptors of clients with chronic lung disease become insensitive to carbon dioxide and respond to hypoxia to stimulate breathing. If excessive oxygen is given, the stimulus to breathe is removed and the client may stop breathing completely. Most clients with chronic lung disease can tolerate oxygen with a nasal cannula at 2 L/min but arterial blood gas analysis should be monitored closely.

Humidifying Oxygen

Controversy exists about the benefits of humidifying oxygen before delivering it to the client by way of a nasal cannula. Previously it was believed that unless oxygen was humidified, there was excessive drying of the mucous membranes lining the respiratory tract. Research has indicated that in low-flow oxygen (less than 4 L/min) delivered by nasal cannula, humidification is unnecessary and elimination of this practice would result in significant reductions in time and dollars. Campbell and colleagues (1988) surveyed medium-sized American hospitals and reported that routine humidification of nasal cannula oxygen remains a common practice. Problems with a dry nose and dry throat were equally prevalent in those who received humidified oxygen versus nonhumidified oxygen. These authors concluded that routine humidification is not justified for this particular circumstance.

Distilled or sterile water is commonly used to humidify oxygen. Cahill and Heath (1990) suggest that tap water may be safely used instead to humidify low-flow oxygen therapy. They recommend that local tap water initially be cultured to determine the presence of bacterial contamination and approved by the hospital infection control committee before widespread use. Using tap water instead of sterile water is viewed as a reasonable method of reducing hospital costs.

Precautions for Oxygen Administration

Oxygen, which constitutes 20% of normal air, is a tasteless, odorless, colorless gas. It supports combustion. To prevent fires and injuries, the following precautions must be taken:
- Avoid open flames in the client's room.
- Place No Smoking signs in conspicuous places in the client's room. Instruct client and visitors on the hazard of smoking with oxygen in use.
- Check to see that electric equipment used in the room, such as electric bell cords, razors, radios, and suctioning equipment, is in good working order and emits no sparks.
- Avoid wearing and using synthetic fabrics that build up static electricity.
- Avoid using oils in the area. Oil can ignite spontaneously in the presence of oxygen.

Oxygen Administration

Oxygen can be administered by nasal cannula, nasal catheter, transtracheal catheter, simple mask, partial rebreather mask, nonrebreather mask, Venturi mask, and tent.

Nasal Cannula A **nasal cannula**, also called nasal prongs, is probably the most commonly used aid to breathing. The cannula is a disposable, plastic device with two protruding prongs for insertion into the nostrils; the cannula is connected to an oxygen source with a humidifier and flowmeter. The cannula does not impede eating or speaking. Procedure 36-1 explains oxygen administration by nasal cannula.

Nasal Catheter A nasal, or oropharyngeal, catheter (Fig. 36-14) is another efficient means for administering oxygen.

FIGURE 36-14

A nasal catheter for administering oxygen. (Photo © 1987 Ken Kasper.)

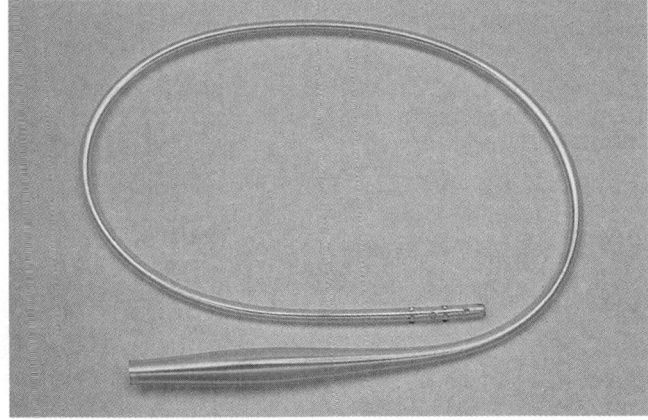

PROCEDURE 36-1

Administering Oxygen by Nasal Cannula

Equipment

Flowmeter connected to oxygen
supply
Humidifier with sterile distilled
water (optional with low-flow
system)

Nasal cannula and tubing
Gauze to pad tubing over ears
(optional)

Action

1 Explain procedure to client and review safety precautions necessary when oxygen is in use. Place No Smoking signs in appropriate areas.

2 Wash your hands.

3 Connect the nasal cannula to the oxygen setup with humidification, if one is in use. Adjust the flow rate as ordered by physician. Check that oxygen is flowing out of prongs.

Rationale

Oxygen supports combustion.

Handwashing deters the spread of microorganisms.

Oxygen forced through a water reservoir is humidified before it is delivered to the client, thus preventing dehydration of the mucous membranes. Recent research has questioned the necessity of humidification with low-flow oxygen delivery by way of cannula.

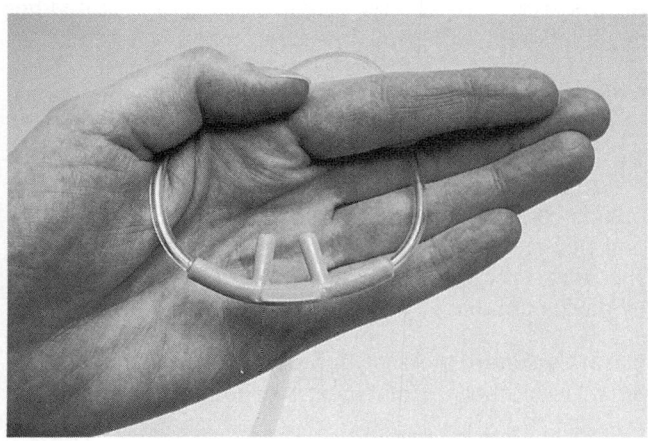

Nasal cannula.

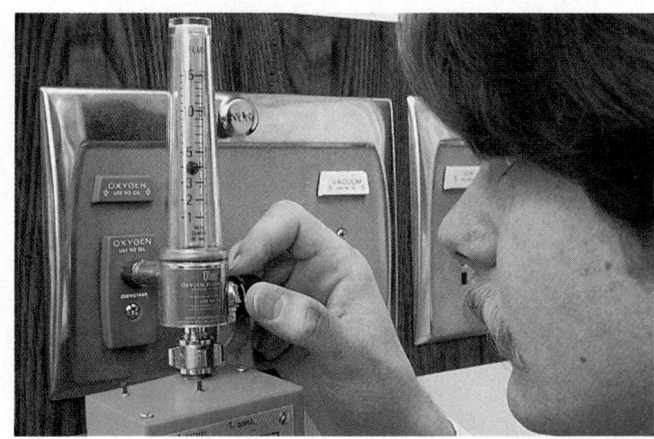

Action 3: Adjusting flow rate.

4 Place the prongs in the client's nostrils. Adjust according to type of equipment.
   a Over and behind each ear with adjuster comfortably under chin *or*
   b Around the client's head

5 Use gauze pads at ear beneath the tubing as necessary.

6 Encourage client to breathe through his or her nose with mouth closed.

7 Wash your hands.

8 Assess and chart client's response to therapy.

Correct placement of the prongs and fastener facilitates oxygen administration and comfort for the client.

Pads reduce irritation and pressure and protect the skin.

Provides for optimal delivery of oxygen to client.

Handwashing deters the spread of microorganisms.

Client's respirations, color, breathing pattern, and chest movements indicate effectiveness of oxygen therapy.

(continued)

PROCEDURE 36-1 (continued)

Administering Oxygen by Nasal Cannula

Action

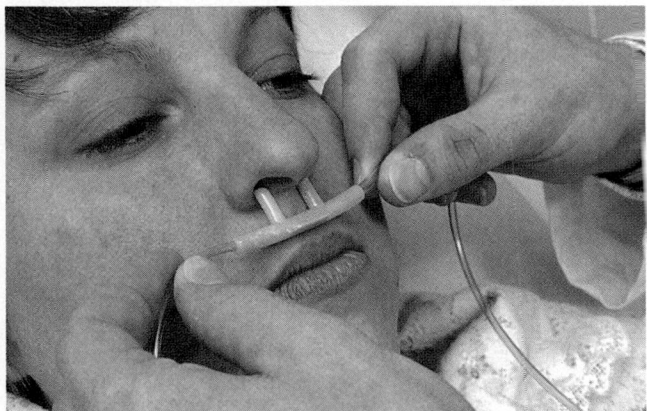

Action 4: Placing cannula prongs in nostrils.

Rationale

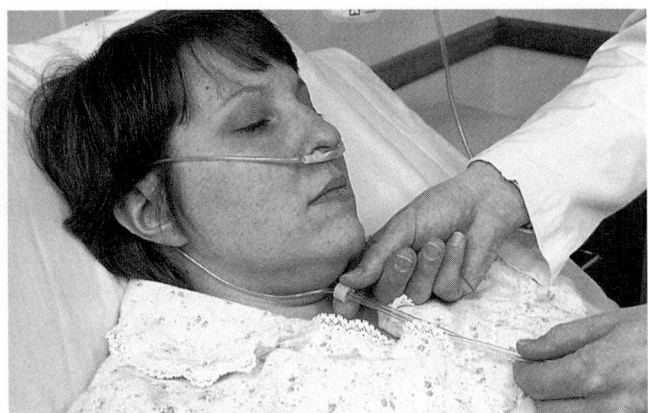

Action 4: Adjusting for comfort.

9 Remove and clean the cannula and assess nares at least every 8 hours or according to agency recommendations. Check nares for evidence of irritation or bleeding.

The continued presence of the cannula causes irritation and dryness of the mucous membranes. Lubricant counteracts the drying effects of oxygen.

Home Care Considerations   Clients may require oxygen administration to continue in the home setting. Portable oxygen cylinders are used most frequently and an indicator on the setup alerts the client or family member to call for a refill. Caregivers require instruction concerning safety precautions with oxygen use and an understanding of the rationale for the specific liter flow of oxygen.

It is inserted into the throat through one nostril and must be changed to the other nostril every 8 hours. Gastric distention often occurs because the gas flow can be misdirected into the stomach.

Transtracheal Oxygen Delivery Clients using continuous supplemental oxygen therapy have another alternative—transtracheal oxygen delivery. A small catheter is inserted into the trachea under local anesthesia. Clients usually report improved mobility, comfort, appearance, and lower cost with this delivery system. A transtracheal catheter does not interfere with talking, eating, or drinking and delivers oxygen throughout the respiratory cycle rather than just at inspiration. This system does require that the client or family assume responsibility for daily catheter care. A transtracheal oxygen setup is illustrated in Figure 36-15.

Face Masks Disposable and reusable face masks are available in plastic and rubber. The mask should be fitted carefully to the client's face to avoid leakage of oxygen. It

should be comfortably snug but not tight against the client's face. The most commonly used types of masks include the simple face mask, the partial rebreather mask, the nonrebreather mask, and the Venturi mask. Procedure 36-2 describes actions and rationale in using face masks.

The *simple oxygen mask* connects to oxygen tubing, a humidifier, and a flowmeter, just as the nasal cannula does. At a flow rate of 6 to 10 L/min, the mask delivers 35% to 60% oxygen. This mask has vents on its sides that allow room air to leak in at many places, thereby diluting the source oxygen. Often it is used when an increased delivery of oxygen is needed for short periods (ie, less than 12 hours). This mask should cover the nose and the mouth if the client breathes through the mouth.

The *partial rebreather mask* is equipped with a reservoir bag for the collection of the first parts of the client's exhaled air. The air is mixed with 100% oxygen for the next inhalation. The client rebreathes about one third of the expired air from the reservoir bag. The remaining exhaled air exits through vents. The use of this type of mask permits the conservation of oxygen. This bag should deflate slightly

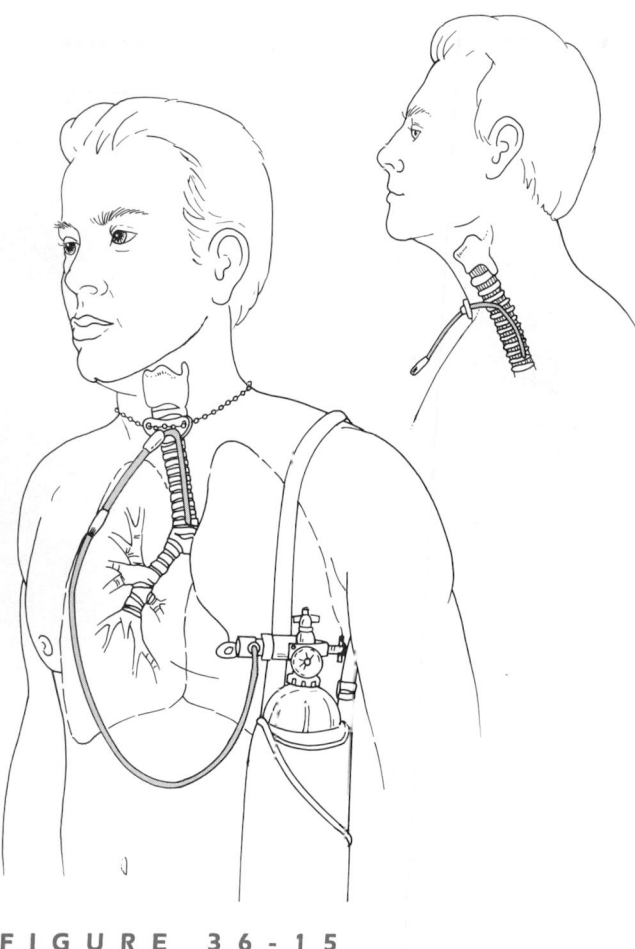

F I G U R E   3 6 - 1 5

A transtracheal oxygen setup.

with inspiration. If it deflates completely, the flow rate should be increased until only a slight deflation is noted.

The *nonrebreather mask* provides the highest concentration of oxygen with a mask to a spontaneously breathing client. It is similar to the partial rebreather mask except two one-way valves prevent conservation of exhaled air. The reservoir bag is filled with oxygen that enters the mask on inspiration. Exhaled air escapes through side vents. This mask can also be used to administer other gases.

The *Venturi mask* gets its name from the Venturi effect, which allows the mask to deliver the most precise concentrations of oxygen. This mask has a large tube with an oxygen inlet. As the tube narrows, the pressure drops, causing air to be sucked in through side ports. These ports are adjusted according to the prescription for oxygen concentration. It is a nursing responsibility to make sure the ports are always open. If these are occluded by linens, clothing, or a client rolling on it, the oxygen delivered might be at an unsafe concentration.

Oxygen Tent   Oxygen also can be administered by way of a tent, a light, portable structure made of clear plastic and attached to a motor-driven unit. The motor helps to circulate and cool the air in the tent. The cooling device func-

tions on the same principles as an electric refrigeration unit. A thermostat in the unit keeps the tent at the temperature considered most comfortable for the client. The tent fits over the top part of the bed so that the client's head and thorax are in the tent. It has side openings through which nursing care can be administered. It is commonly used with pediatric clients who need a cool and highly humidified air flow (eg, clients with pneumonia). The tent does not allow the maintenance of a satisfactory or precise oxygen concentration and thus, is usually not used outside of pediatrics. See Procedure 36-3.

Using Artificial Airways

Oropharyngeal and Nasopharyngeal Airways

An oropharyngeal (Fig. 36-16) or nasopharyngeal airway is a semicircular tube of plastic or rubber inserted into the back of the pharynx through the mouth or nose in the spontaneously breathing client. It is used to keep the tongue clear of the airway and to permit suctioning of secretions. It is often used for postoperative clients until they regain consciousness.

Endotracheal Tube

An **endotracheal tube** is a polyvinylchloride airway that is inserted through the nose or the mouth into the trachea using a laryngoscope as a guide. It is used to administer oxygen by mechanical ventilator, to suction secretions easily, or to bypass upper airway obstructions (eg, tongue or tracheal edema). Though uncomfortable and easier to manipulate with the tongue, orotracheal insertion is often the method of choice, especially in an emergency, because insertion is easier and a larger size tube can be used making breathing easier. Placement of the tube by way of the nasotracheal route, though tolerated better by clients, is more difficult and requires the use of a narrower tube. Most commonly, a cuffed endotracheal tube is used that prevents

F I G U R E   3 6 - 1 6

The plastic disposable airway is inserted through the mouth (oropharyngeal airway) and is shaped to follow the contour of the mouth and upper respiratory tract. When placed properly, the airway holds the tongue so that it cannot drop back and into the throat. It can be suctioned easily if secretions accumulate.

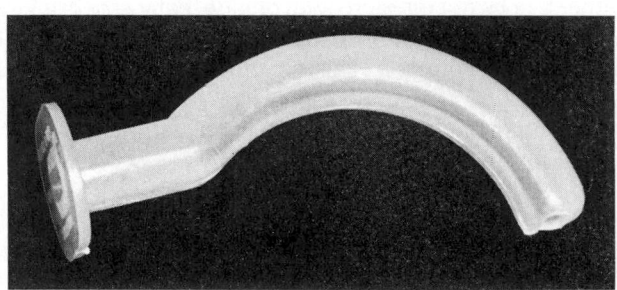

PROCEDURE 36-2

Administering Oxygen by Mask

Equipment

Flowmeter connected to oxygen supply
Humidifier with sterile distilled water

Face mask specified by physician
Gauze to pad elastic band (optional)

Action	Rationale
1 Explain procedure to client and review safety precautions necessary when oxygen is in use. Place No Smoking signs in appropriate areas.	Oxygen supports combustion. Explanation alleviates anxiety.
2 Wash your hands.	Handwashing deters the spread of microorganisms.
3 Attach the face mask to the oxygen setup with humidification. Start the flow of oxygen at the specified rate.	Oxygen forced through a water reservoir is humidified before it is delivered to the client, thus preventing dehydration of the mucous membranes.
4 Position the face mask over the client's nose and mouth. Adjust it with the elastic strap so that the mask fits snugly but comfortably on the face.	A loose or poorly fitting mask will result in oxygen loss and decreased therapeutic value. Masks may cause feeling of suffocation, and client needs frequent attention and reassurance.
5 Use gauze pads to reduce irritation on the client's ears and scalp.	Pads reduce irritation and pressure and protect the skin.
6 Wash your hands.	Handwashing deters the spread of microorganisms.
7 Remove the mask and dry the skin every 2 to 3 hours if the oxygen is running continuously. Do not powder around the mask.	The tight-fitting mask and moisture from condensation can irritate the skin on the face. There is danger of inhaling powder if it is placed on the mask.
8 Assess and chart client's response to therapy.	Client's respiratory rate and pattern, color, and so forth, indicate effectiveness of oxygen therapy.

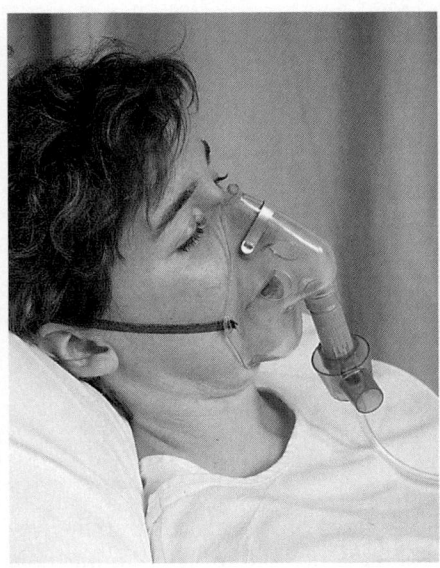

Venturi mask.
(Photos © 1987 Ken Kasper.)

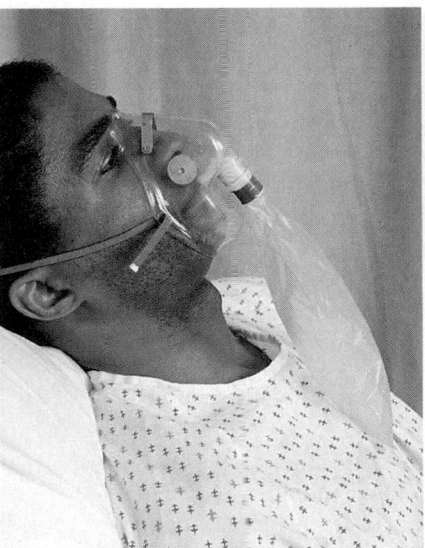

Nonrebreather mask.

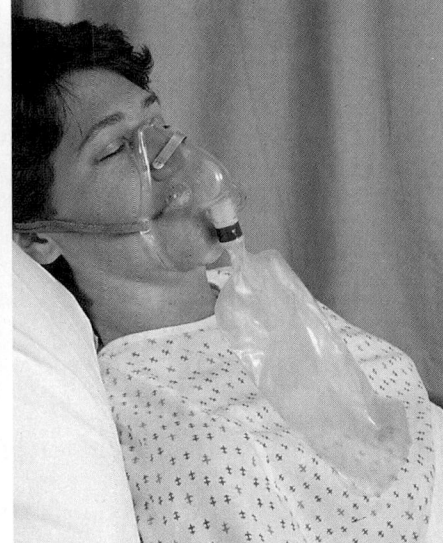

Partial rebreather mask.

P R O C E D U R E 3 6 - 3

Administering Oxygen by Tent

Equipment

Oxygen tent with tubing, flow
   regulator, and oxygen analyzer
Oxygen source
Humidifier

Sterile distilled water
Bath blankets
Ice

Action	Rationale
1 Explain procedure to client and family.	This reassures client and facilitates cooperation.
2 Gather equipment.	This provides for organized approach to task.
3 Wash your hands.	Handwashing deters the spread of microorganisms.
4 Use bath blanket to cover plastic mattress. Place second bath blanket over bottom sheet.	Bath blanket minimizes potential for static electricity from plastic mattress. Additional bath blanket is used to provide warmth and absorb moisture.
5 Prepare tent and position over bed. Attach to oxygen source.	Tent allows oxygen to be delivered in a confined environment.
6 Fill ice trough or start refrigeration component.	Ice or refrigeration unit cools the air in the tent.
7 Fill nebulizer or humidifier to recommended level with sterile distilled water. Turn on flowmeter and adjust oxygen flow to deliver required amount. Use oxygen analyzer now and recheck at least every 4 hours.	Humidification of oxygen prevents excessive drying of the respiratory tract. Oxygen analyzer measures oxygen concentration.
8 Place client in tent. Observe all safety precautions.	Oxygen supports combustion.
9 Secure tent between folded top sheet and under mattress.	Oxygen is heavier than air. If tent is not secure, oxygen content may be decreased.
10 Wash your hands.	Handwashing deters the spread of microorganisms.
11 Open tent as little as possible by organizing nursing care.	This maintains oxygen content in tent.
12 Assess client at frequent intervals (vital signs, color, response to therapy). Monitor equipment on a frequent basis.	Oxygen toxicity may develop in response to exposure to a high concentration of oxygen.
13 Change gown and linens as necessary. Edges of tent may be loosened, and tent may be secured with bath blanket under client's chin when performing hygienic care or other procedures.	This provides warmth and comfort.
14 Record type of therapy and client's response.	Keeping records provides accurate documentation of procedure.

air leakage and bronchial aspiration of foreign material, and allows more precise control of oxygen and mechanical ventilation (Fig. 36-17). Careful monitoring of endotracheal cuff pressure decreases the risk of tracheal necrosis. The smallest amount of air that results in an airtight seal between the trachea and the tube is desirable and less likely to result in complications.

Tracheostomy

A *tracheostomy* is an artificial opening made into the trachea. The curved **tracheostomy tube** inserted into this opening is made of flexible polyvinylchloride (Teflon), nylon, silicone, or metal and comes in multiple sizes with varied angles. An obturator that guides the placement of

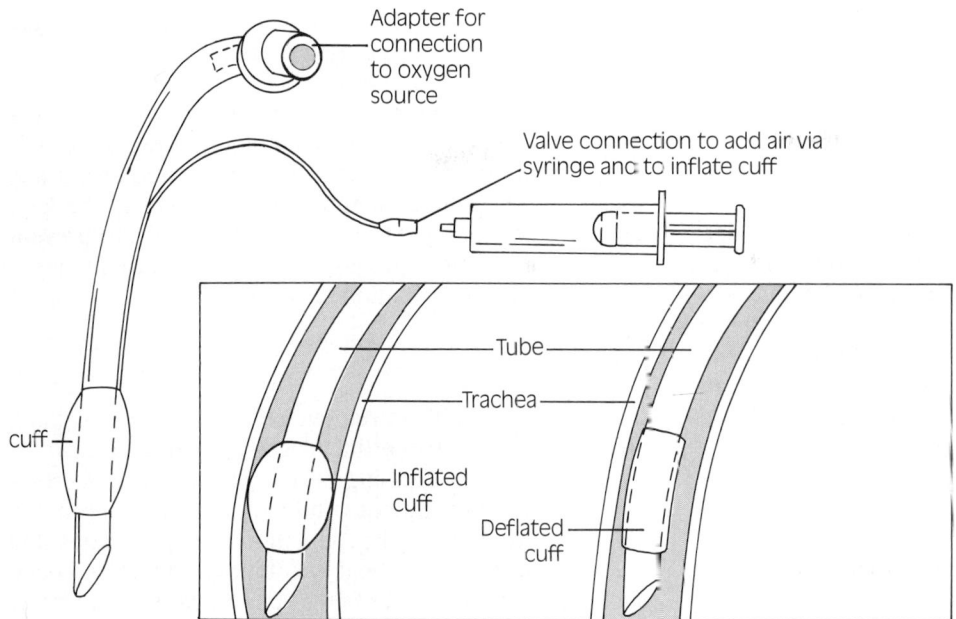

FIGURE 3 6 - 1 7

(*A*) Parts of a cuffed endotracheal tube. (*B*) Tube in place with the cuff inflated. (*C*) Tube in place with the cuff deflated.

the cannula is inserted into the tube during insertion and is removed once the outer cannula is in place (Fig. 36-18). Some tubes have two cannulas. The outer cannula remains in place in the trachea while the inner cannula is removed for cleaning. The newer plastic tubes have disposable inner cannulas. Single cannula tubes are more commonly used for children. Tracheostomy tubes may be either cuffed or uncuffed. The inflated cuff seals the opening around the tube against air leakage, prevents aspiration, and permits mechanical ventilation. (Figure 36-18 displays several types of tracheostomy tubes.) The practice of deflating cuffed tubes for a short interval every few hours is no longer

considered an effective method of preventing ischemic damage to the tracheal mucosa (Mapp, 1988). Newer tracheal cuffs are low pressure and can be maintained at lower than tracheal capillary pressure.

A tracheostomy tube is inserted for a variety of reasons (eg, to replace an endotracheal tube, to provide a method to mechanically ventilate, to bypass an upper airway obstruction, or to remove tracheobronchial secretions). It is inserted in the operating room or intensive care unit under sterile conditions using local anesthesia. The tracheostomy tube is held in place by tapes fastened around the client's neck. Usually, a sterile, square gauze pad that has been

FIGURE 3 6 - 1 8

Two types of tracheostomy sets—noncuffed (*A*) and cuffed (*B*).

Noncuffed

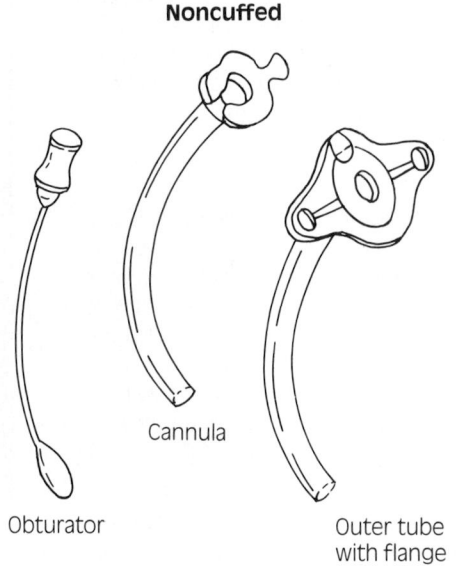

Cuffed

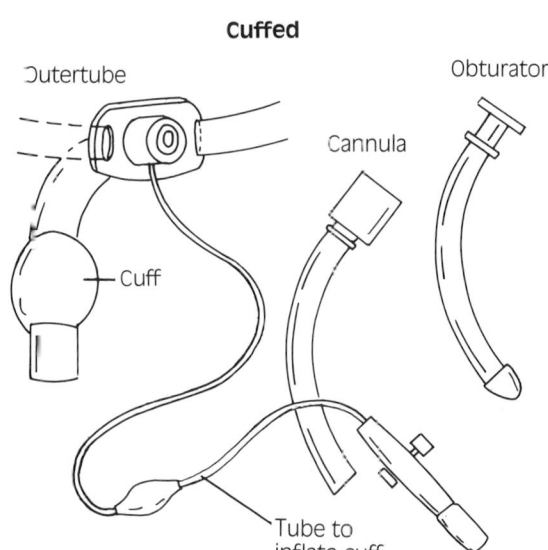

precut by the manufacturer is placed between the skin and outer wings of the tube before the tube is tied. This tracheostomy dressing must be kept dry to prevent infection and skin irritation. The tracheostomy can be temporary or permanent.

Nursing responsibilities may include regularly checking cuff pressure, although some tubes have a pressure-release valve that prevents pressure from increasing to damaging levels. Also, because the tracheostomy tube bypasses the natural humidifying and heating mechanisms in the nose and mouth, the oxygen must be heated and humidified to prevent secretions from becoming dry.

The tracheostomy tube must remain free from foreign objects and nonsterile materials. Cotton balls, loose threads from dressings, needles, and other small objects must be kept away from the opening. Suctioning to remove secretions is completed using the sterile technique described in Chapter 26. The frequency of suctioning varies with the amount of secretions present, but it should be done often enough to keep ventilation effective and as effortless as possible. The wound around the tube and the inner cannula, if one is present, should be cleaned at least every 8 hours. A newly inserted tracheostomy tube may require attention every 1 to 2 hours.

The tracheotomized client is unable to speak. The client's care should include consideration of his or her impaired ability to communicate. Communication tools (eg, writing board, letters, vocabulary cards) should be kept close at hand along with the call light or bell. To prevent anxiety, this client requires reassurance and frequent explanations and anticipation of needs.

Suctioning

If the client is unable to remove secretions with coughing after the application of artificial airways, secretions can be aspirated with a suctioning device (Procedure 36-4). Suctioning irritates the mucosa and removes oxygen from the respiratory tract. Thus, the client must be hyperoxygenated before suctioning. Tracheal suctioning, also called deep suctioning, may be performed by passing a sterile catheter through the mouth (orotracheal); through the nose (naso-

---

RESEARCH IN NURSING Making a Difference

Oxygenation

All body cells require oxygen to function, and supplying the body with oxygen is fundamental to life. Both of the following studies have important implications for tailoring client care to promote efficient gas exchange. Nursing is challenged with meeting the unique needs and enhancing the quality of life of clients who are experiencing the sense of helplessness that usually accompanies an oxygen deficit.

Related Research

Ashley, M. J. (1989). Concerns of sleep apnea patients with tracheostomies. *Western Journal of Nursing Research, 11*(5), 600–608.

In this study, clients, though ambulatory and active, with sleep apnea that necessitated a tracheostomy, indicated varying degrees of physical and emotional discomfort. Because the current health care system is characterized by decreased lengths of stay, minimal time before discharge was available for providing psychosocial support to these clients and their families. All expressed a need for follow-up care to help them deal with the fear, anxiety, and life-style changes following a tracheostomy. Nurses can alleviate concerns about daily functioning and altered self-image by providing a comfortable, open environment for clients to share their concerns. Additionally, this study group suggested a redesigned tracheostomy tube that is more flexible, comfortable, and less conspicuous.

Ogburn-Russell, L., & Johnson, J. (1990). Oxygen saturation levels in the well elderly: Altitude makes a difference. *Journal of Gerontological Nursing, 16*(10), 26–30.

The purpose of this study was to identify differences in oxygen saturation levels of well elderly at varying altitudes. Findings suggest that normal oxygen saturation levels of this group are lower than those of younger people regardless of place of residence. At moderate altitudes, test results for the elderly subjects were at the lower limits of normal. Nurses need to be aware of the effects of altitude on oxygen saturation in this age group because it affects physiologic functions such as tissue oxygenation, wound healing, and cardiopulmonary activity. Any changes in oxygen saturation should be evaluated and compared with the individual's normal level.

Summary

Interference with oxygen requirements necessitates a comprehensive approach by the nurse that involves monitoring respiratory status, recognizing deviations from normal, and meeting the unique needs of individual clients. Oxygen deficits, besides being life-threatening, also frequently result in alteration in life-style and body image. By recognizing physiologic and psychosocial concerns, the nurse facilitates the client's ability to cope with alterations in oxygen needs.

PROCEDURE 36-4

Suctioning the Nasopharyngeal and Oropharyngeal Areas

Equipment

Portable or wall suction unit with tubing
Sterile suction catheter with Y-port
Sterile water or saline

Sterile disposable container
Sterile gloves
Towel or waterproof pad

Action	Rationale
1 Determine the need for suctioning.	Suctioning should be done only when secretions have accumulated or adventitious breath sounds are audible. This minimizes trauma to airway mucosa.
2 Explain procedure to client.	This provides reassurance and promotes cooperation.
3 Assemble equipment.	This provides for organized approach.
4 Wash your hands.	Handwashing deters spread of microorganisms.
5 Adjust bed to comfortable working position. Lower side rail closer to you. Place the client in a semi-Fowler's position if conscious. An unconscious client should be placed in the lateral position facing you.	Having the client in a sitting position helps him or her to cough and makes breathing easier. Gravity also facilitates the insertion of the catheter. Lateral position prevents the airway from becoming obstructed and promotes drainage of secretions.
6 Place towel or waterproof pad across client's chest.	This protects bed linens.

7 Turn suction to appropriate pressure:
  a Wall unit
    Adult: 110 to 150 mm Hg
    Child: 95 to 110 mm Hg
    Infant: 50 to 95 mm Hg
  b Portable unit
    Adult: 10 to 15 mm Hg
    Child: 5 to 10 mm Hg
    Infant: 2 to 5 mm Hg
	Negative pressure must be at a safe level or pneumothorax may occur.

8 Open sterile suction package. Set up sterile container touching only the outside surface, and pour sterile saline or water into it.	Sterile normal saline or water is used to lubricate the outside of the catheter, thus minimizing irritation of mucosa as it is being introduced.
9 Don sterile gloves. The dominant hand that will handle the catheter must remain sterile while the nondominant hand is considered clean rather than sterile.	Handling the sterile catheter with a hand wearing a sterile glove helps prevent introducing organisms into the respiratory tract and the clean glove protects the nurse from microorganisms.
10 With sterile gloved hand, pick up sterile catheter and connect to suction tubing that is held with unsterile hand.	Sterilization can be maintained.
11 Moisten the catheter by dipping it into the container of sterile saline. Occlude Y-tube to check suction.	Lubricating the inside of the catheter with saline helps move secretions in the catheter.
12 Estimate the distance from the earlobe to the nostril, and place thumb and forefinger of gloved hand at that point on the catheter.	Ensures that catheter remains in pharynx rather than trachea.

(continued)

P R O C E D U R E 3 6 - 4 (continued)

Suctioning the Nasopharyngeal and Oropharyngeal Areas

Action

Rationale

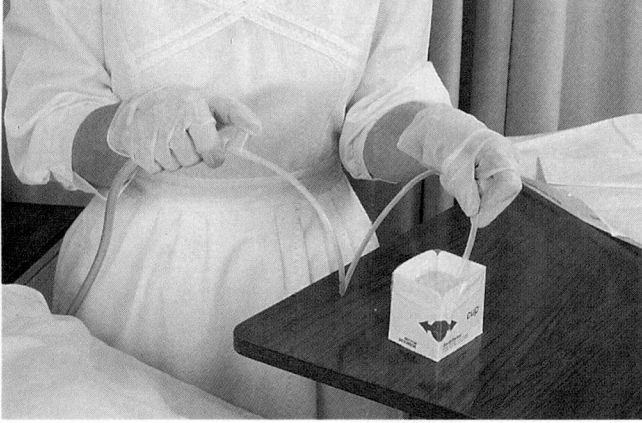

Action 11: Moisten the catheter by dipping it into the sterile saline container and occluding Y-tube to check suction.

13 Gently insert the catheter with the suction off by leaving the vent on the Y-connector open. Slip the catheter gently along the floor of an unobstructed nostril toward the trachea to suction the naso-pharynx. Or, insert the catheter along the side of the mouth toward the trachea to suction the oro-pharynx. Never apply suction as the catheter is introduced.

Using suction while inserting the catheter can cause trauma to the mucosa and removes oxygen from the respiratory tract. Coughing is induced when the trachea is touched. This helps the client raise secretions.

14 Apply suction by occluding the suctioning port with your thumb and gently rotate the catheter as it is being withdrawn. Do not allow the suctioning to continue for more than 10 to 15 seconds at a time.

Turning the catheter as it is withdrawn helps clean all surfaces of the respiratory passageways. Suctioning the client for longer than 10 to 15 seconds robs the respira-tory tract of oxygen, which may result in hypoxia.

15 Flush the catheter with saline and repeat suctioning as needed and according to client's toleration of procedure.

Flushing cleans and clears catheter and lubricates it for next insertion.

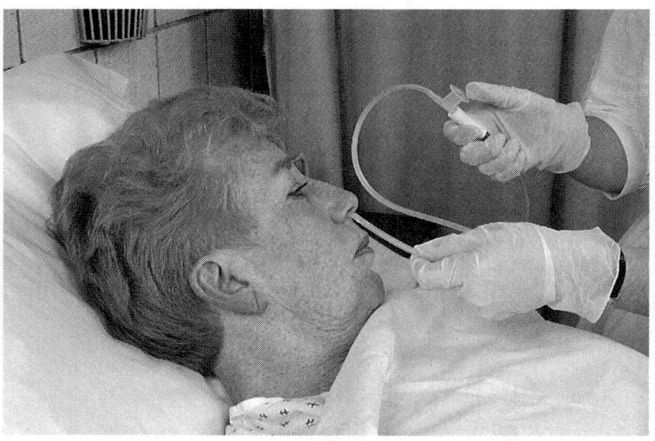

Action 13: Inserting the catheter.

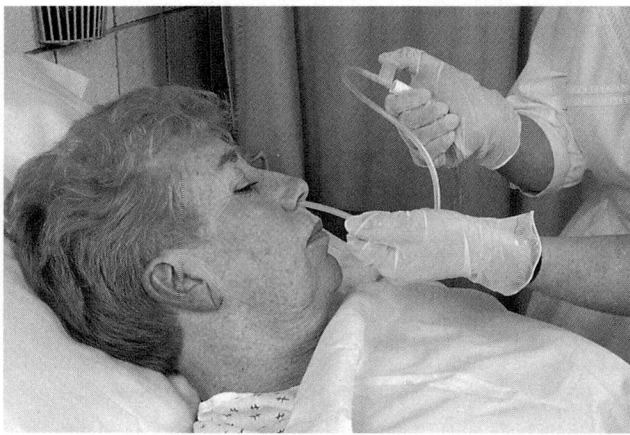

Action 14: Occluding port and rotating catheter while with-drawing.

(continued)

PROCEDURE 36-4 (continued)

Suctioning the Nasopharyngeal and Oropharyngeal Areas

Action	Rationale
16 Allow at least 20- to 30-second interval if additional suctioning is needed. The nares should be alternated when repeated suctioning is required. Do not force catheter through the nares. Encourage client to cough and deep breathe between suctionings.	Normal breathing between suctioning helps compensate for any hypoxia induced by the previous suctioning.
17 When suctioning is completed, remove gloves inside out and dispose of gloves, catheter, and container with solution in proper receptacle. Wash your hands.	Handwashing prevents transmission of microorganisms.
18 Use auscultation to listen to chest and breathing sounds to assess the effectiveness of suctioning.	Listening to chest and breathing sounds helps determine whether the respiratory passageways are clear of secretions.

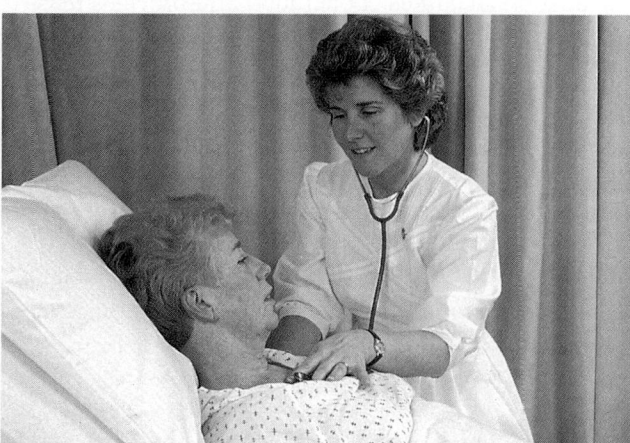

Action 18: Assessing effectiveness of suctioning. Photos © 1992 B. Proud.)

Action	Rationale
19 Record the time of suctioning and the nature and amount of secretions. Also note the character of the client's respirations before and after the suctioning.	Records of nursing measures used help assess, evaluate, and coordinate care.
20 Offer oral hygiene after suctionings.	Respiratory secretions that are allowed to accumulate in the mouth are irritating to mucous membranes and unpleasant for the client.

tracheal); through an endotracheal tube; or through a tracheostomy tube. Procedure 36-5 describes suctioning the tracheostomy. When performed correctly, suctioning provides comfort, relieves respiratory distress, and is painless. When performed incorrectly, it can increase anxiety and pain and cause respiratory arrest. Possible complications include infection, cardiac arrhythmias, hypoxia, mucosa trauma, and death. The suctioning catheter should be small enough not to occlude the airway being suctioned but large enough to remove secretions. Several sizes of soft, plastic, clear catheters are available. A newer silicone catheter does not require lubrication.

The nurse should wear gloves on both hands to prevent infection. The client's color; heart rate; and secretion color, amount, and consistency should be monitored continuously. If cyanosis, excessively slow or rapid heart rate, or suddenly bloody secretions are noted, the nurse should stop suctioning immediately. The client should be ventilated with oxygen, and the physician should be notified.

(Text continues on p. 978)

PROCEDURE 36-5

Suctioning the Tracheostomy

Equipment

Portable or wall suction device with connecting tubing
Sterile suction kit containing the following or gather separately:
Sterile suction catheter of appropriate size with Y-port
  Infants: 6–8 F
  Children: 8–10 F
  Adults: 12–16 F
Sterile container

Sterile glove
Sterile normal saline
Clean towel or sterile drape (optional)
Goggles (or glasses) and mask (optional)
Gown (optional)
Resuscitation bag connected to 100% oxygen

Action	Rationale
1 Explain procedure to client and reassure him or her that you will interrupt procedure if the client indicates respiratory difficulty.	Explanation facilitates cooperation and provides reassurance for client. Any procedure that compromises respiration is frightening for the client.
2 Gather equipment and provide privacy for client.	This provides for organized approach to task.
3 Wash your hands.	Handwashing deters spread of microorganisms.
4 Assist the client to a semi-Fowler's or Fowler's position if conscious. An unconscious client should be placed in the lateral position facing you.	Sitting position helps client to cough and breathe easier. This position also uses gravity to aid in the insertion of catheter. Lateral position prevents the airway from becoming obstructed and promotes drainage of secretions.

5 Turn suction to appropriate pressure:
  a Wall unit
    Adult: 110 to 150 mm Hg
    Child: 95 to 110 mm Hg
    Infant: 50 mm Hg
  b Portable unit
    Adult: 10 to 15 mm Hg
    Child: 5 to 10 mm Hg
    Infant: 2 to 5 mm Hg
	Negative pressure must be at safe level or damage to tracheal mucosa may occur.

6 Place clean towel, if being used, across client's chest. Don goggles, mask, and gown, if necessary.	Towel protects client and bed linens. Wearing protective equipment prevents contamination of the caregiver's mucous membranes.

7 Open sterile kit or set up equipment, and prepare to suction:
  a Place sterile drape, if available, across client's chest.
  b Open sterile container and place on bedside table or overbed table without contaminating inner surface. Pour sterile saline into it.
  c Prepare resuscitator bag and preoxygenate client for several breaths unless copious secretions are present.
  d Don sterile gloves or one sterile glove on dominant hand and clean glove on nondominant hand.
  e Connect sterile suction catheter to suction tubing that is held with unsterile gloved hand.
	Drape protects client and bed linens.
	
	This maintains sterile setup.
	
	This prevents hypoxia during suctioning. If secretions are copious, hyperventilating will move secretions farther into the respiratory tract.
	Gloves maintain sterility of procedure and protect the nurse from microorganisms.
	
	Sterile technique helps prevent introducing organisms into the respiratory tract.

(continued)

PROCEDURE 36-5 (continued)

Suctioning the Tracheostomy

Action	Rationale

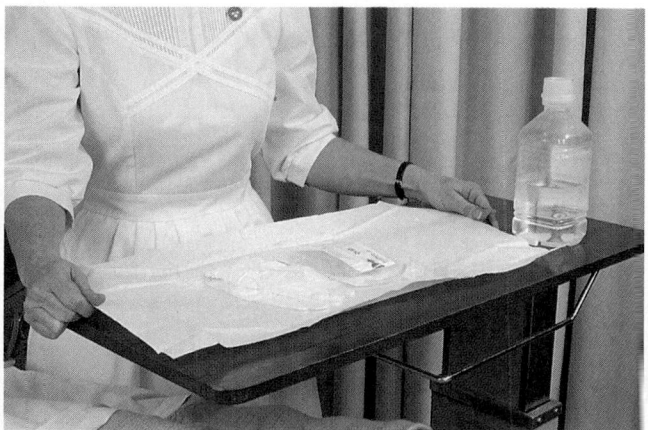

Action 7: Opening the sterile kit.

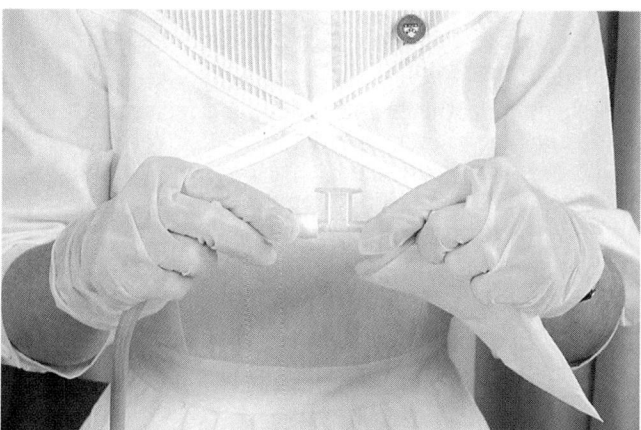

Action 7e: Connecting catheter to suction tube.

8 Moisten the catheter by dipping it into the container of sterile saline unless it is one of the newer silicone catheters that do not require lubrication.

Lubricating the inside of catheter with saline helps move secretions in the catheter. Silicone catheters do not require lubrication.

9 Remove oxygen delivery setup with unsterile gloved hand if it is still in place.

This exposes tracheostomy tube.

10 Using sterile gloved hand, gently and quickly insert catheter into the trachea. Advance about 10 to 12.5 cm (4 to 5 inches) or until client coughs. *Do not occlude Y-port when inserting catheter.*

Using suction when inserting catheter can cause trauma to mucosa and removes oxygen from the respiratory tract.

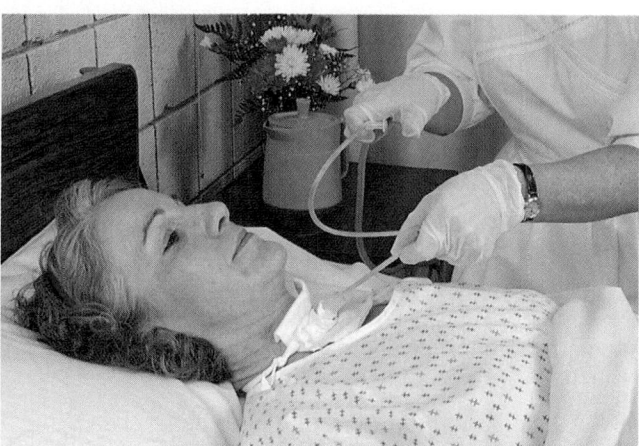

Action 10: Inserting catheter with Y-port open.

11 Apply intermittent suction by occluding Y-port with thumb of unsterile gloved hand. Gently rotate catheter with thumb and index finger of sterile gloved hand as catheter is being withdrawn. Do not allow suctioning to continue for more than 10 seconds.

Turning the catheter while withdrawing it helps clean surfaces of respiratory tract and prevents injury to tracheal mucosa. Suctioning for longer than 10 seconds may result in hypoxia.

(continued)

PROCEDURE 36-5 (continued)

Suctioning the Tracheostomy

Action

Rationale

Encourage client to cough and deep breathe between suctionings.

12 Flush the catheter with saline and repeat suctioning as needed and according to client's toleration of procedure. Allow client to rest at least 1 minute between suctionings, and replace oxygen delivery setup if necessary.

Flushing cleans and clears catheter and lubricates it for next insertion. Allowing time interval and replacing oxygen delivery setup helps compensate for hypoxia induced by the previous suctioning.

13 When procedure is completed, turn off suction and disconnect catheter from suction tubing. Remove gloves inside out and dispose of gloves, catheter, and container with solution in proper receptacle. Wash hands.

This prevents transmission of microorganisms.

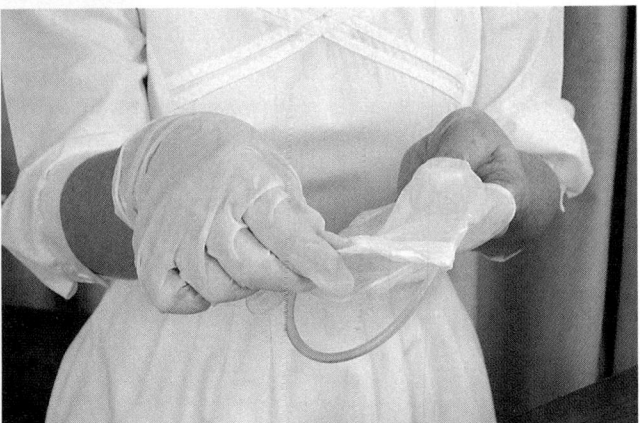

Action 13: Removing glove over catheter. (Photos © 1992 B. Proud.)

14 Adjust client's position. Auscultate chest to evaluate breath sounds.

Auscultation helps determine if respiratory passageways are cleared of secretions.

15 Record the time of suctioning and the nature and amount of secretions. Also note the character of client's respirations before and after suctioning.

This provides accurate documentation and provides for comprehensive care.

16 Offer oral hygiene.

Respiratory secretions that accumulate are irritating to mucous membranes and unpleasant for the client.

Special Considerations

If secretions are thick and tenacious, instill 3 to 5 mL of saline into the trachea using a syringe with the needle removed. Suction again for secretions.

Assisting Ventilation

Mechanical ventilators are used to assist or completely control ventilation. These machines are used with critically ill clients in conjunction with endotracheal or tracheos-tomy tubes. (The reader is referred to the general literature and other clinical texts that discuss the use of mechanical ventilators in great detail.)

Another mechanical device used to assist ventilation is *intermittent positive-pressure breathing* (IPPB). This is a method of providing a specific amount of air, oxygen, and aerosolized medication under increased pressure to the respiratory tract when other simpler approaches have proved ineffective. IPPB forces deeper inspiration by positive-pressure inhalation and then permits passive exhalation. The amount of pressure varies with each client.

The physician prescribes this therapy, and it is delivered by the respiratory therapist or the nurse. Treatments are provided with the client in an upright position upon first arising and at bedtime. Often, it is also done twice during the day depending on the needs of the client. IPPB usually induces coughing, and the nurse should encourage the client to expectorate as much of the secretions as is possible. The client receiving IPPB inhales the mist through a mouthpiece or a face mask. Before each treatment, the nurse should remind the client to inhale slowly and deeply to allow the lungs to be filled. The client should exhale as completely as is possible before the next inspiration. Avoid treatment immediately preceding or following meals to prevent vomiting or depressed appetite.

Ambu Bag and Mask

In emergency situations, the *ambu bag* (Fig. 36-19) is used to assist ventilation for clients whose respirations have ceased. With the client's head tilted back, jaw pulled forward, and airway cleared, the mask is held tightly over the client's nose and mouth. The operator's other hand compresses the bag at a rate that approximates normal respiratory rate (eg, 16 to 20 breaths per minute in the adult). The one-way valve in the mask allows exhaled air to escape. Artificial ventilation can be sustained until spontaneous breathing starts, until other mechanical assistance is available, or until death is confirmed. The bag is self-inflating.

Most bag and mask ventilators can accommodate an oxygen tube to increase the oxygen supply to the client. Many also have an adapter so they can be directly connected to a tracheostomy or endotracheal tube for manual ventilation of an intubated client.

FIGURE 36-19

The ambu bag and mask is used for assisting ventilation in emergency situations.

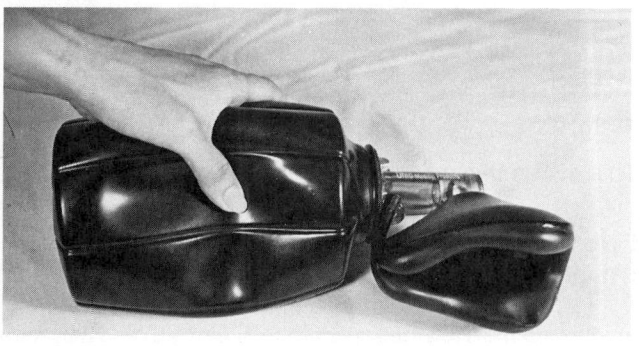

Clearing an Obstructed Airway

Foreign body obstruction of the airway usually occurs during eating. In adults, meat is the most common cause. In children, any variety of foods or objects have obstructed the upper airway. The National Safety Council reported 3100 deaths due to upper airway obstruction in 1987 (American Heart Association, 1987). The term *cafe coronary* has been used to describe foreign body upper airway obstruction that was mistaken for a heart attack (Kitay & Shafer, 1989). A semiconscious or unconscious client can develop airway obstruction because the tongue covers the pharynx as it falls back, obstructing the upper airway. The tongue is the most common cause of airway obstruction.

Foreign bodies can cause either partial airway obstruction or complete airway obstruction. In partial airway obstruction with good air exchange, the client can cough forcefully. This person should be allowed and encouraged to cough and breathe spontaneously. At this time, the nurse should not interfere with the client's efforts to expel the object.

Good air exchange can progress to poor air exchange, indicated by weak, ineffective cough, high-pitched noises while inhaling, increased breathing difficulties, and cyanosis. This should be managed the same way as complete airway obstruction.

With complete airway obstruction, the victim is unable to speak or cough. The client may demonstrate the universal distress signal (ie, clutching his or her throat with both hands). Immediate action is necessary or the client will become unconscious as the brain becomes hypoxic. Once complete airway obstruction has been established, the Heimlich maneuver (abdominal thrusts) should be provided. Application of this procedure for the conscious and unconscious adult is described in Procedure 34-6.

Administering Cardiopulmonary Resuscitation

CPR is the combination of mouth-to-mouth breathing, which supplies oxygen to the lungs, and chest compressions, which circulate blood. It is often described as the ABCs of basic life support:

*A*irway: Tip the head and check for breathing. The respiratory tract must be opened so air can enter.

*B*reathing: If the victim does not start to breathe spontaneously after the airway is opened, give two slow, full breaths.

*C*irculation: Check the pulse. If the victim has no pulse, artificial circulation must be started with breathing.

CPR should be started for any situation in which either breathing alone or breathing and heart beat are absent. The brain is sensitive to hypoxia and will sustain irreversible damage after 4 to 6 minutes of no oxygen. The faster CPR is initiated, the greater the chance of survival. Actions for CPR are described in Procedure 36-7.

(Text continues on p. 985)

P R O C E D U R E   3 6 - 6

Clearing an Obstructed Airway

Conscious Adult

Action

1 Assess victim. Ask, "Are you choking?" Determine if victim can speak or cough.

2 If victim is obstructed, initiate abdominal thrusts (Heimlich maneuver):

  a Stand behind victim.

  b Wrap arms around victim's waist.

  c Make a fist with one hand with thumb outside of fist. Place thumb side of fist against victim's abdomen above navel and well below xiphoid process.

  d Grasp fist with the other hand, and press upward with quick, firm thrusts.

  e Continue distinct thrusts until foreign body is expelled or victim becomes unconscious.

Rationale

Inability to speak or cough indicates that airway is obstructed.

Firm abdominal thrusts force exhalation of air through the victim's airway and aid in dislodging obstruction.

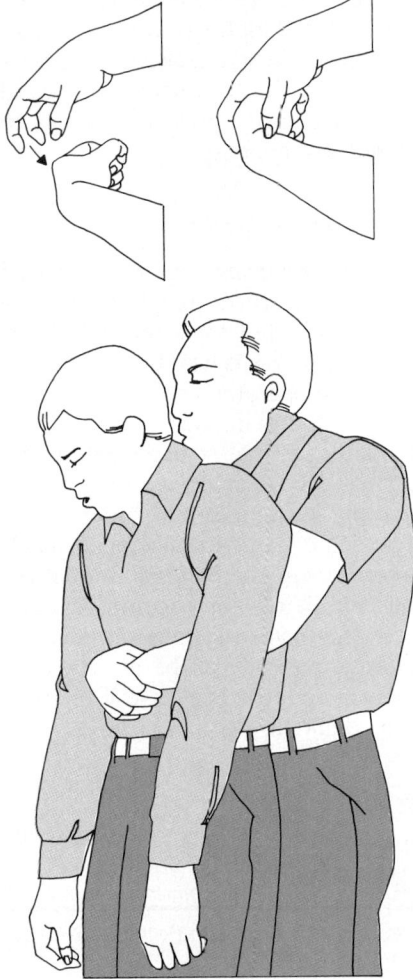

Action 2: Rescuer positioning to perform abdominal thrusts on conscious adult.

Unconscious Adult

Action

1 Assess victim's unresponsiveness. Gently shake shoulder and ask, "Are you ok?" Call for help.

2 Position victim on back on a flat, firm surface. Support head and neck and turn as a unit.

Rationale

This determines need for CPR.

Firm surface provides for maximum effect from abdominal thrusts.

(continued)

PROCEDURE 3 6 - 6 (continued)

Clearing an Obstructed Airway

Action

3 Tilt victim's head backward by placing hand on forehead. Place fingers of other hand underneath victim's jaw and lift upward and forward. If neck injury is suspected, use jaw-thrust maneuver. This is accomplished by using both hands to grasp the angle of the lower jaw and lift, thus bringing the mandible forward.

4 Determine breathlessness by placing ear over victim's mouth and observing chest.

5 Attempt ventilation if breathless. Seal victim's mouth and nose properly. If resistance is met, reposition victim's head and attempt to ventilate again. If anyone responds to call for help, send them to activate emergency medical service system.

6 Initiate abdominal thrusts (Heimlich maneuver):
   a Straddle victim's thighs.
   b Place heel of one hand against victim's abdomen above navel and well below xiphoid process.
   c Place second hand directly on top of first hand.
   d Press upward with quick, firm thrusts.
   e Perform 6 to 10 distinct abdominal thrusts.

Rationale

Either methods opens the airways. The jaw-thrust maneuver opens the airway without extending the neck.

If victim is breathing, expired air can be heard and felt on cheek as well as observed as chest rises and falls.

If airway is not positioned properly or is obstructed, resistance is felt when ventilating. Air will not enter lungs, and chest will not rise.

Firm abdominal thrusts force exhalation of air through the victim's airway and aid in dislodging obstruction.

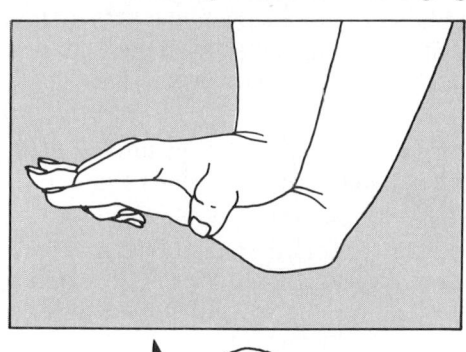

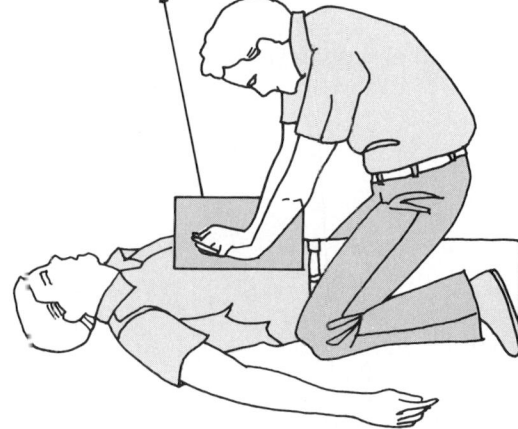

Action 6: Rescuer positioning for abdominal thrusts on unconscious adult.

7 Perform finger sweep using jaw lift to open mouth.

8 Attempt ventilation again using proper maneuver. If unable to ventilate, repeat sequence of thrusts, finger sweep, and ventilations until successful.

Finger sweep detects the expelled foreign body and removes it, thus preventing foreign body from being forced back into airway.

Forceful ventilation in unconscious victim may bypass obstruction and enable aeration of lungs.

(continued)

PROCEDURE 3 6 - 6 (continued)

Clearing an Obstructed Airway

Action	Rationale
9 If successful in ventilation, continue with normal resuscitation procedure; pulse check, chest compression, and breathing.	Once airway is open, the need for continued intervention must be established.

Special Considerations Use chest thrusts rather than abdominal thrusts on a pregnant woman or obese victim. Place fist on middle portion of sternum and thrust backward.

PROCEDURE 3 6 - 7

Administering Cardiopulmonary Resuscitation on an Adult (One Rescuer)

Action	Rationale
1 Assess victim's unresponsiveness. Gently shake shoulder and ask, "Are you ok?" If bystander is present, send him or her to activate the EMS system while you begin CPR. If alone, activate the EMS system immediately after unresponsiveness has been determined.	Assessment determines need for CPR. Immediate call to EMS system increases survival rates.
2 Position victim on back on a flat, firm surface. Support victim's head and neck and turn as a unit.	Firm surface provides for maximum compression and proper positioning.
3 Tilt victim's head backward by placing hand on forehead. Place fingers of other hand underneath victim's jaw and lift upward and forward. If a neck injury is suspected, use the jaw-thrust maneuver (see Procedure 36-6, Unconscious Adult, action 3).	Head tilt opens the airway.
4 Determine breathlessness by placing ear over victim's mouth and observing chest.	If victim is breathing, expired air can be heard and felt on cheek as well as observed as chest rises and falls.

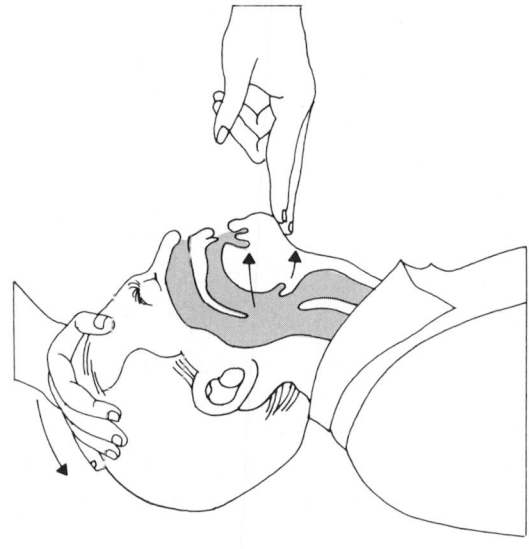

Action 3: Establishing open airway.

(continued)

PROCEDURE 3 6 - 7 *(continued)*

Administering Cardiopulmonary Resuscitation on an Adult (One Rescuer)

Action	Rationale
5 Remove dentures if they are loose; if snug, leave them in place.	Loose dentures may block the airway. If they are snug, they help seal the mouth.
6 Keeping head tilted backward, pinch the victim's nose shut with thumb and fingers of hand that is on forehead. Seal your lips tightly around victim's mouth or use a pocket face mask. Ventilate two times at 1.5 to 2 seconds per inspiration. Observe victim's chest rise and lift face away from victim between breaths.	Pinching the nose shut allows maximum ventilation with no escape of air through nostrils. Force of breathing needs to be sufficient so that chest visibly rises when air is forced into victim's mouth and falls with victim's passive exhalation.
7 Determine pulselessness by feeling for carotid pulse on near side of victim while maintaining head tilt with other hand (5 to 10 seconds). Send anyone who responds to call for help to activate EMS system.	Carotid artery is large, centrally located, and ordinarily readily accessible. A 5- to 10-second pause is needed to adequately assess for pulselessness.

8 Begin chest compressions if pulse is absent:
  a Kneel by victim's shoulders.
  b Locate the xiphoid process on sternum by following the lower rib to notch on sternum where rib meets. Measure 4 to 5 cm (1.5 to 2 inches) above the xiphoid process, about the width of two fingers.
  c Place heel of one hand on this point and position the heel of other hand on top of first hand. Preferably, the fingers should interlock. Bring your shoulders over your hands and keep your elbows locked and arms straight.
	Kneeling facilitates proper position.
	Proper hand position keeps pressure off the xiphoid process and prevents injury to underlying organs and ribs.
	
	Interlocking the fingers helps keep them off the victim's ribs, where pressure may cause fractures of the ribs. This position, with the elbows and arms straight, allows for best exertion of pressure on the sternum over the heart.

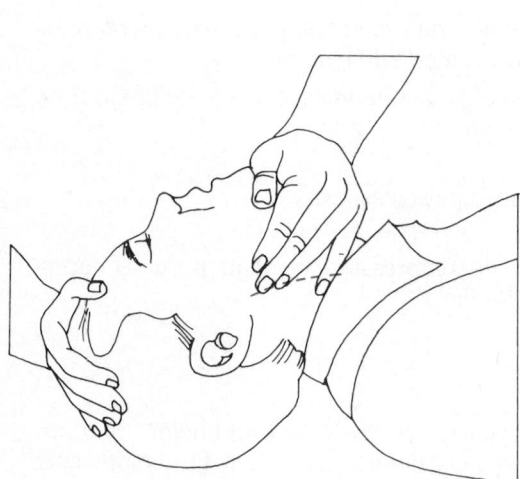

Action 7: Assessing carotid pulse.

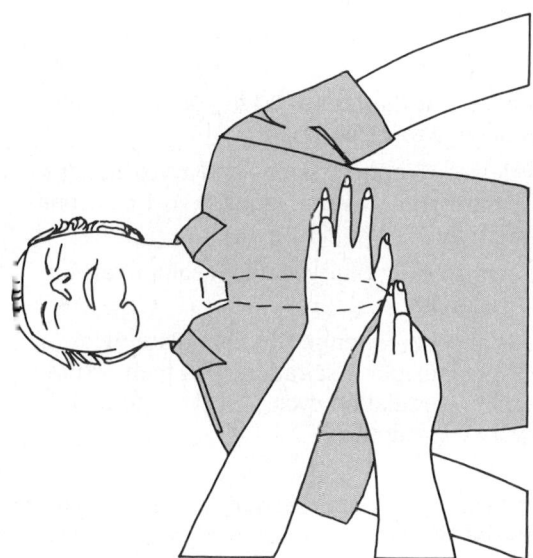

Actions 8b and 8c: Locating site for compression.

(continued)

P R O C E D U R E   3 6 - 7   (continued)

Administering Cardiopulmonary Resuscitation on an Adult (One Rescuer)

Action

Rationale

d Use body weight to depress victim's sternum about 4 to 5 cm (1.5 to 2 inches). Relax pressure immediately but keep hands on sternum during up stroke.

The depression of the sternum with pressure causes the heart to be compressed against the vertebral column, forcing blood into the aorta and pulmonary arteries. Relaxation of pressure allows the heart to expand and re-fill. Keeping the hands in place over the sternum helps administer regular and even compressions.

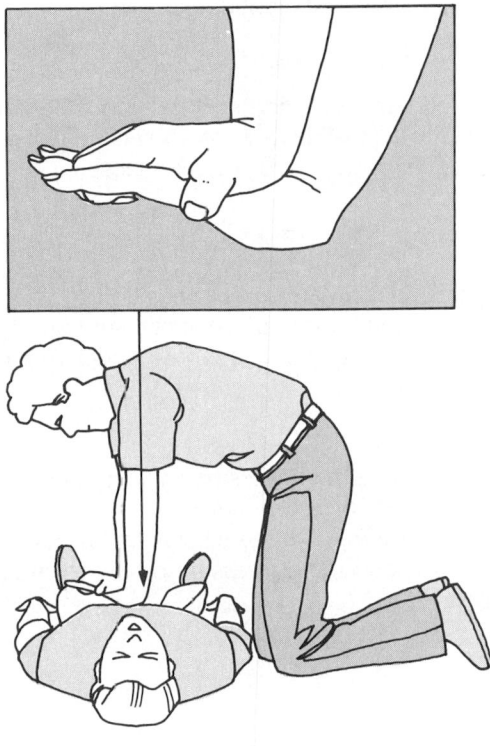

Actions 8c and 8d: Rescuer positioning and action of compression.

e Compress at the rate of 80 to 100 per minute (15 every 9 to 11 seconds).

This compression rate maintains adequate blood pressure and flow to maintain cell integrity.

9 Do 4 cycles of 15 compressions and 2 ventilations. Observe chest rise on ventilations (1 to 1.5 seconds per inspiration).

This provides for maintenance of adequate blood flow and oxygenation.

10 Reassess cardiopulmonary status. Feel for carotid pulse (5 seconds).

This determines pulselessness.

11 If pulse is absent, continue CPR. Ventilate twice (1 to 1.5 seconds per inspiration) and then resume compression/ventilation cycles. Feel for carotid pulse every few minutes.

Continuation of compression/ventilation rate is necessary to sustain life.

Special Considerations

Second rescuer should announce to first rescuer, "I know CPR. Can I help?" Second rescuer then does pulse check (action 10) and continues with action 11. First rescuer should assess adequacy of second rescuer's ventilations (observe chest rise) and compressions (check pulse).

In October 1992, the American Heart Association published revised CPR protocols. Several changes the AHA recommended include (1) early activation if a person is found unconscious and breathless rather than 1 minute of CPR and then telephoning for help and (2) the initial two breaths are slower and more deliberate (1.5 to 2 seconds each). Even though there may not be contact with a client's blood or body fluids during CPR, it is recommended that gloves be worn. The American Heart Association requires that all health care professionals learn mouth-to-mask breathing through a one-way valve during a one- or two-person rescue in addition to mouth-to-mouth breathing (Willens, 1991). Laypeople learn mouth-to-mouth breathing with a simple protective shield device but mouth-to-mouth breathing is still considered safe, particularly in the more common situation in which the rescue involves a family member or person known to the rescuer. No evidence links the human immunodeficiency virus to saliva, but the shield device does eliminate contact with the client's saliva during artificial breathing. (Figure 36-20 provides an example of a mouth-to-mask breathing device.)

Research aimed at reducing mortality in victims of cardiac arrest is focusing on the use of abdominal compressions, in conjunction with or alternating with chest compressions. Abdominal compressions are performed with open hands placed over the umbilicus area and appear to increase cardiac output. Results have been encouraging

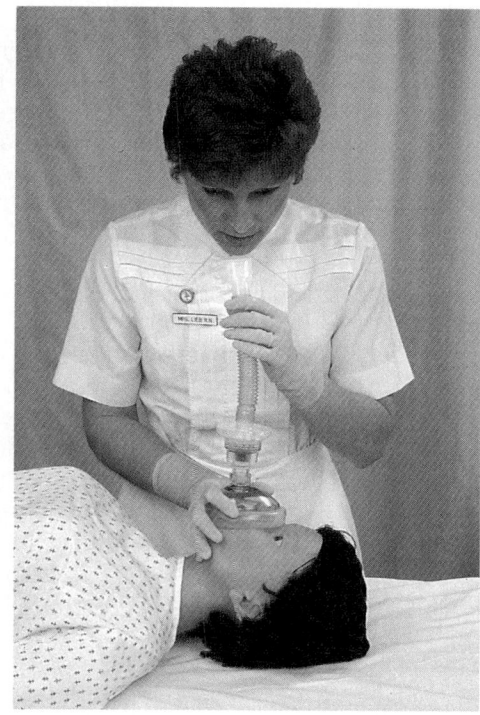

FIGURE 36-20

Using a face mask with a one-way valve for CPR. (Photo © 1992 B. Proud.)

PROCEDURE 36-8

Administering Cardiopulmonary Resuscitation on an Adult (Two Rescuers)

Action	Rationale
1 Rescuer who will ventilate initiates airway assessments. Sequence continues as for one rescuer (Procedure 36-7, actions 1 to 6).	Assessment determines need for CPR.
2 After pulselessness is determined, first rescuer states, "No pulse."	This indicates clearly to second rescuer to initiate compression sequence.
3 Compressor gets into position, locates anatomic landmarks and begins chest compressions. Correct ratio of compressions to ventilations is 5:1 with a compression rate of 80 to 100 per minute. Stop compressing for each ventilation. Continue for a minimum of 10 cycles.	The rate of 10 to 15 regularly spaced breaths per minute is considered necessary to supply the victim with sufficient oxygen to maintain cell integrity.
4 Compressor calls for switch when fatigued and gives clear signal. Compressor completes fifth compression, and ventilator completes ventilation after fifth compression. Rescuers switch simultaneously. Person who becomes ventilator does 5-second pulse check, states, "No pulse" (if pulse absent), and ventilates once. Person who becomes compressor then begins compressions at a 5:1 ratio.	It is important to carry out CPR without interruption to ensure adequate flow of oxygenated blood to maintain cell integrity.

in monitored settings where resuscitation began almost immediately, but their value outside the hospital in less-controlled situations is unknown (Coleman, 1992; Meyer, 1992).

The automated external defibrillator (AED) has also proved effective in reducing deaths attributed to cardiac arrest. This device is easy to use and quickly delivers a shock to the heart muscle that is intended to interrupt ventricular fibrillation, a frequent cause of cardiac arrest. Debate about the effectiveness of this intervention during CPR is ongoing (Coleman, 1992).

The procedure for CPR by two rescuers is given in Procedure 36-8. When there are two rescuers, they may switch positions during CPR to relieve fatigue. There should be no break in the rhythm and regularity of rescue breathing and cardiac compressions during this switch in positions. The technique for administering CPR to children and infants differs slightly from adult CPR. These techniques are discussed in depth in the basic life support course, which all health professionals should take before administering care in the health field.

Most professional organizations recommend and support widespread efforts to teach CPR to laypeople and all health professionals. Mannequins for practice can be obtained from the American Heart Association, the National Red Cross, and health agencies. It is a professional responsibility to maintain proficiency in CPR skills. This necessitates periodic practice with mannequins (adult and infant). CPR should be administered quickly and accurately, without hesitation, when an emergency arises.

Evaluating

Evaluation is an ongoing and deliberate part of the nursing process that involves the nurse, client, family, and other health care team members. It includes a comparison of the client's health status and the previously defined goals and an examination of the client's projected progress in meeting those goals. All involved in the evaluation process need to identify effective interventions and to identify reasons for any failures in achieving goals. Adjustments in the nursing care plan must be made accordingly.

NURSING PROCESS

in Clinical Practice

The nurse uses all phases of the nursing process when identifying and treating alterations in respiratory functioning. The nurse's knowledge and application of clinical skills described in this chapter play a major role in treating respiratory problems. This section addresses assessment priorities, client goals, nursing interventions, and evaluation criteria for those common types of respiratory problems treated by nurses:

Impaired Gas Exchange
Ineffective Breathing Pattern
Ineffective Airway Clearance

In the case study that follows, nursing care is described for a young child with an alteration in respiratory functioning.

Impaired Gas Exchange

Impaired gas exchange is the state in which the person experiences an actual or potential decreased passage of gas (oxygen or carbon dioxide) between the alveoli of the lungs and the vascular system (Carpenito, 1992).

Assessment

- Use interview questions directed to the client and significant others to determine exactly what is the problem.
- Determine if the client's perception of the impaired gas exchange corresponds to actual physiologic changes.

- Explore the client's life-style and physical and mental health for contributing factors.
- Examine the client for signs of impaired gas exchange (eg, tachypnea, abnormal breath sounds, cough, neck vein distention, or barrel chest).
- Check lab and radiology data for more information (chest x-ray, pulse oximetry readings, arterial blood gas results, hemoglobin, protein levels, and so forth).
- Observe client's technique when dealing with actual or perceived impaired gas exchange.
- Assess client's effectiveness in dealing with impaired gas exchange.

Planning: Client Goals

The client will:
- Identify causes of the impaired gas exchange
- Incorporate adequate pulmonary hygiene techniques into the daily routine
- Institute life-style changes to eliminate factors contributing to impaired gas exchange
- Seek treatment for early signs of infection
- Use breathing techniques with ease to decrease the work of breathing

Interventions

- Instruct client to cough properly and deep breathe four times a day (30 minutes before meals and at bedtime).

- Demonstrate and encourage client use of diaphragmatic breathing and pursed-lip breathing.
- Encourage good oral hygiene.
- Arrange (or encourage home manager to arrange) four or five small meals per day.
- Assist client to drink 2 to 3 qt of clear fluid each day. Keep a container of favorite juice at client's side.
- Incorporate a period of regular exercise into each day.
- Encourage client to socialize with others (friends, respiratory support group, church, and so forth).
- Use simple explanations (written and verbal) on medications, their actions, dose, timing, and side effects.
- Explore with client and others who live with him or her methods to reduce pollution in home or work environment.
- Use air conditioner on high pollution days.
- Avoid using respiratory irritants.
- If the client smokes, discuss the idea of reducing smoking with the goal of stopping the smoking habit.

Evaluative Criteria

The client meets the previously stated goals.

Ineffective Breathing Pattern

Ineffective breathing pattern is a state in which the person experiences an actual or potential loss of adequate ventilation related to an altered breathing pattern (Carpenito, 1992).

Assessment

- Use interview questions directed to the client and significant others to determine the nature of the problem, its probable cause, and its effect on life-style.
- Examine client and assess respiratory rate, rhythm, symptoms of anxiety or pain.

Planning: Client Goals

The client will:
- Demonstrate effective respiratory rate and rhythm
- Identify possible contributing factors
- Evaluate adaptive coping mechanisms when dealing with stress or anxiety

Interventions

- Demonstrate conscious controlled breathing and encourage client to use it during periods of anxiety or activity.
- Maintain a safe environment. Same nurses always work with this client. Maintain eye contact during conversation.
- If fear is the cause, encourage client to ventilate concerns. Reduce cause of fear, if feasible.

- If there is a strong emotional component, discuss with client the development of effective coping skills with professional counseling.
- If pain is present, use appropriate methods for comfort (eg, position, analgesics, blankets, and so forth).

Evaluative Criteria

The client meets the previously stated goals.

Ineffective Airway Clearance

Ineffective airway clearance is a state in which the person experiences a real or potential threat to the passage of air through the respiratory tract related to partial or complete airway obstruction (Carpenito, 1992).

Assessment

- Use interview questions directed to client or significant others to determine nature of the problem and its suspected cause.
- Examine the client and assess for signs of airway obstruction (eg, abnormal or absent breath sounds, inability to move secretions, cyanosis, restlessness, ineffective cough, nasal flaring).
- Evaluate laboratory studies (eg, arterial blood gases, pulse oximetry, tidal volume, vital capacity).
- Assess client's coughing techniques and other pulmonary hygiene practices.
- Verify client's ability to maintain a position that prevents aspiration and allows for complete opening of the airway.

Planning: Client Goals

The client will:
- Maintain good body alignment to ensure effective air exchange
- Maintain fluid intake so secretions are thin
- Demonstrate appropriate use of controlled coughing and diaphragmatic breathing techniques
- Follow medication regimen accurately and be able to state drug actions, dose, and side effects

Interventions

- Ausculate client's breath sounds every 4 hours.
- Encourage client to cough effectively or suction every 2 to 4 hours.
- Keep client's head elevated at least 45 degrees or maintain side-lying position to maintain an open airway.
- Splint incisions (if any) for support. Treat pain with analgesics as needed.
- Force favorite fluids (2 to 3 qt) unless cardiac or renal disturbances prevent this intake.

- Arrange periods of rest around activity (eg, 8 AM: After the walk down the hall, the client can sleep for 1 hour).
- Use praise liberally to encourage efforts and work.
- Review (orally and in writing) medications, their dose, actions, side effects, and possible interactions.
- Let the client and caregiver know about support groups in the area.

- Encourage family to contact the American Lung Association for free pamphlets.

Evaluative Criteria

The client meets the previously stated goals.

CASE STUDY

Freddie is a 1-year-old alert, well-developed child who has been a client on the pediatric unit for 3 days with status asthmaticus. He has had two other admissions for acute asthma during which he responded quickly to intravenous and inhalation bronchodilators. During this hospitalization, either his mother, a teacher, or his father, a psychologist, has stayed with him. Other relatives are caring for Freddie's 9-year-old sister and 5-year-old brother.

Freddie interacts happily with staff as long as a parent is within sight. Gross and fine motor coordination are appropriate for his age. His vocabulary consists of 25 words. History is from his mother, who is a reliable source. Child has had a clear nasal discharge with slight, intermittent, nonproductive cough for 3 days with no change in appetite or activity pattern.

On day of admission, he attended the day-care center as usual. After being there for 3 hours, his cough became more frequent and respirations became more labored. The caregivers were not alarmed because he continued to eat, drink, nap, and play in usual pattern. Mother states that when she arrived in the afternoon to pick up the boys, she discovered this child to be using his intercostal and neck muscles excessively with every breath. His respirations were 50 per minute, labored, and accompanied by a grunt. By the time she arrived home, he was pale and fitful and was crying weakly. Respirations were 60 per minute and circumoral, and peripheral cyanosis was noted. The pediatrician advised lung evaluation in the emergency department. While there, three subcutaneous injections of epinephrine were administered 5 minutes apart. The child did not respond satisfactorily, so he was admitted for intraveneous aminophylline and steroid administration.

In addition to the history of asthma, Freddie is allergic to eggs and peanuts and has eczema on his face, arms, legs, and upper back. His current medications include metaproterenol sulfate (Alupent) every 8 hours; a topical steroid (Lidex Cream); and a multivitamin and mineral supplement (Poly-Vi-Sol Chewable Tabs), 0.5 mL daily. No one in the family smokes. The caregivers at the day-care center smoke outside the building. The day-care center is clean and had the rugs shampooed the night before this child's illness. This child had no sputum production or fever. Immunizations are current.

Assessment Findings

Respiratory rate, 44 breaths/min
Irregular rhythm
Excessive use of accessory muscles
Nonproductive, frequent cough
Rhonchi and expiratory wheeze noted
Pale, no cyanosis
Blood pressure, 100/60; heart rate, 120 beats/min
Restless child who naps for only 20 to 30 minutes at intervals day and night
Arterial blood gases: normal values
Chest x-ray: normal
Poor appetite, vomiting one or two times daily
Up early in morning
Sweat test: negative for cystic fibrosis

Nursing Diagnosis

Ineffective Airway Clearance related to exposure to unknown allergens, bronchospasm, overproduction of thick mucus

Planning: Client Goals

Freddie's parents state that they are willing to do anything to improve his current respiratory state and to prevent further need for hospitalization.

Short-Term Goals

During the staff conference, the head nurse, two staff nurses, and Freddie's mother developed several short-term goals. Within the next 48 hours, the client will:

- Have less rhonchi throughout thorax
- Have no vomiting and no aspiration
- Eat six small meals and drink at least three 8-oz bottles per 24 hours
- Have optimal movement of air in and out of lungs

Long-Term Goal

The family will:

- Go home in 5 days and state that they feel comfortable in providing medications and inhalation to this child

Implementation

In activating this care plan, the professional nurse needs the following specialized abilities:

- Strong assessment skills
- Understanding of normal respiratory functioning and health deviations
- Knowledge of multiple factors that contribute to health deviations and their severity
- Knowledge of which deviations can be independently treated by nurse
- Interpersonal communication skills necessary to work with clients of all ages and their families
- Teaching and counseling skills to help the family understand the relationship between environment (dust, stuffed animals, pets, pollution, and so forth) and the development of the client's respiratory difficulties and to initiate the necessary changes
- Interpersonal and leadership skills to motivate the nursing staff to value the family's long- and short-term goals and to work with the entire health care team (physicians, dietary, respiratory therapy)
- Accountability

Documentation

Sample documentation of nursing interventions follows.

Traditional Note Format

12/1/93, nursing

Family and staff conference to discuss Freddie's respiratory disturbance initiated by primary nurse's concern. Present were Freddie's mother; MJ (primary nurse); TK (head nurse); TR (head of respiratory department); and MM and LQ (staff nurses). Primary nurse presented findings from assessment and nursing examination. Discussion centered on strategies to control airway edema and reduce wheezes, re-duce coughing episodes and control vomiting, and prevent further bronchospasms and edema resulting from exposure to allergens in environment. See care plan. Client progress will be evaluated in 4 days during nursing grand rounds, 12/5/93.

Mary Jones, RN

SOAP Format

12/1/93, 9 AM, nursing

#1 Ineffective Airway Clearance related to exposure to allergens, bronchospasm, and overproduction of mucus.

S: "My son's chest is still very congested, and he is still wheezing. When will he be well enough to go home? Will he be all right when we go home?"

O: Rhonchi and expiratory wheezes noted throughout anterior and posterior thorax, vomiting food and mucus after breakfast every morning, aminophylline infusing intravenously, steroids, acetaminophen, and antibiotic administered orally as ordered.

A: Ineffective airway clearance related to exposure to allergens, bronchospasm, and overproduction of mucus.

P: 1. Control airway edema and reduce wheezes and rhonchi.
 2. Reduce coughing episodes and control vomiting.
 3. Prevent further bronchospasm resulting from exposure to allergens in environment.

E: Reevaluate respiratory status at nursing grand rounds on 12/5/93.

Mary Jones, RN

Evaluation

Short-term goal achievement is evaluated at the next scheduled assessment. Long-term goal achievement is a lengthier process.

 NURSING CARE PLAN

for Freddie

Nursing Diagnosis:	Ineffective Airway Clearance related to exposure to allergens, viral infection, bronchospasm, overproduction of mucus
Long-Term Goal:	This family will return home in 5 days expressing confidence in administering oral and inhalation medications.

Goal: By 12/5/93, the client will:
- Have rare episodes of coughing and no vomiting

Nursing Actions	**Rationale**	**Evaluative Statement**
Hold meals until inhalation treatments are done.	Bronchodilators stimulate coughing and often cause vomiting if given after meals.	12/4/93 Goal met. Freddie has not vomited in 2 days and has 2-hour intervals between coughing episodes.

(continued)

N U R S I N G   C A R E   P L A N *(continued)*

for Freddie

Avoid milk products.	Milk accelerates the production of mucus.
Offer clear juices every 3 hours in a bottle or cup.	Clear liquids help to liquefy secretions and prevent dehydration.
Perform percussion during morning and evening bath.	Percussion loosens pulmonary secretions so they are more easily expectorated.

Goal: By 12/5/93, the client's parents will:
• Remove dust-collecting toys

Nursing Actions	Rationale	Evaluative Statement
Give parents allergy pamphlets from American Lung Association.	Adequate information reinforces instruction given by health care providers.	12/2/93 Goal met. Parents removed furry toys from hospital room.
Review with both parents methods to reduce exposure to possible allergens at home.	Constant exposure to allergens (dust, mold, mildew, and so forth) and irritants (perfume, smog, cleaners, and so forth) produces bronchospasm and stimulates copious mucus production. Medications are most effective when allergens are removed.	
Encourage parents to examine day-care environment. Explore options with them.	Environment in daycare may contain allergens. The least irritating setting is desirable.	

K E Y   P O I N T S

- The functioning units of the respiratory system are the alveoli, where the actual exchange of oxygen and carbon dioxide between the lung and circulation occurs. Airways conduct available gases during inhalation and exhalation phases of ventilation.
- There are normal variations in respiratory functioning unique to specific ages that allow appropriate oxygenation to meet cellular needs. These differences involve chest shape, breath sounds, and presence of landmarks. In addition to age, other factors affect adequate respiratory functioning—level of health, growth and development, environment, and psychological health. Persons with health deviations in respiratory functioning can initiate changes to improve the work of breathing.
- The health history is an essential component of respiratory function assessment. The client's physical examination and laboratory findings can provide information to identify the nature of the problem, its course, related signs and symptoms, onset and frequency, and effect on everyday living.

- Nursing diagnoses can be written to address inadequate breathing patterns, ineffective airway clearance, and impaired gas exchange. Nursing diagnoses also can be written to address how altered repiratory functioning has an effect on other areas of human functioning (eg, anxiety).
- Nursing interventions to promote adequate respiratory functioning include promoting effective breathing and coughing exercises, maintaining adequate fluid intake, maintaining good nutrition, promoting comfort by positioning, providing supplemental oxygen, using medications to promote adequate respiratory functioning, and educating clients to maintain a pollution-free environment.
- Evaluation is ongoing. The health-care team and the client examine progress toward achieving the established goals. The plan is modified based on client's response to nursing actions.

STUDY QUESTIONS

1. A client has a fractured rib and is breathing less often and with less depth because of the pain. This is best described as
   a. fremitus
   b. hyperventilation
   c. pleural friction rub
   d. hypoventilation

2. When auscultating Mr. Chang's breath sounds, the nurse detects a high-pitched squeaky sound heard on expiration. She assesses this as
   a. rales or crackles
   b. wheezes
   c. gurgles or rhonchi
   d. pleural friction rub

3. Air that develops in the pleural space is referred to as
   a. pneumothorax
   b. pleural effusion
   c. hemothorax
   d. atelectasis

4. When planning care for a client with chronic lung disease who is receiving oxygen by way of a nasal cannula, the nurse expects that
   a. the oxygen must always be humidified
   b. the rate will be 2 L/min or less
   c. arterial blood gases must be drawn every 4 hours to determine flow rate
   d. the rate will be 6 L/min or more

5. The highest concentration of oxygen is provided by the
   a. partial rebreather mask
   b. nonrebreather mask
   c. simple mask
   d. Venturi mask

6. Which of the following is a correct statement about pulse oximetry measurement?
   a. A range of 95% to 98% is considered normal oxygen saturation.
   b. Oximetry measurement measures oxygen saturation of venous blood.
   c. Cigarette smoking does not affect oxygen saturation values.
   d. Pulse oximetry is a replacement for arterial blood gas analysis.

7. The nurse correctly performs oropharyngeal suctioning on a client by
   a. using clean technique
   b. applying suction as the catheter is introduced
   c. flushing the catheter with saline between catheter insertions
   d. limiting suctioning to 25- to 30-second intervals at one time

8. Effective cardiopulmonary resuscitation by one rescuer on an adult requires that the rescuer

   a. remove the adult's dentures before beginning artificial breathing
   b. determine pulselessness by checking femoral pulse
   c. depress the sternum 1½ to 2 inches during chest compressions
   d. continue a ratio of five compressions to one ventilation for four cycles

9. Mr. Parks has chronic obstructive pulmonary disease. The nurse has taught him pursed-lip breathing that helps him by
   a. increasing carbon dioxide, which stimulates breathing
   b. teaching him to prolong inspiration and shorten expiration
   c. helping liquefy his secretions
   d. decreasing the amount of air trapping and resistance

10. A client has suddenly had a cardiac arrest. What is the critical time that the nurse must keep in mind before irreversible brain damage occurs?
    a. 1 to 3 minutes
    b. 2 to 4 minutes
    c. 4 to 6 minutes
    d. 8 to 10 minutes

11. David White is in the hospital with a medical diagnosis of viral pneumonia. He is getting oxygen by way of a simple face mask. Why must the mask fit snugly over the client's face?
    a. It prevents mask movement and consequent skin breakdown.
    b. It helps the client feel secure.
    c. It maintains carbon dioxide retention.
    d. It aids in maintaining expected oxygen delivery.

12. The nurse was suctioning her client through a tracheostomy tube and was careful to not occlude the Y-port when inserting the suction catheter because it would
    a. prevent suctioning from occurring
    b. cause trauma to the tracheal mucosa
    c. break the sterile technique
    d. suction out all the carbon dioxide

13. The Heimlich maneuver is described in which of the following statements?
    a. arms encircling person's waist from behind with firm abdominal thrusts
    b. quick, forceful blow with fist on client's sternum
    c. fingers sweeping out foreign objects from client's mouth
    d. sharp blow on center of client's back

14. Which of the following blood gas values are considered within the normal range?
    a. pH, 7.25 to 7.35; pCO_2, 25 to 35 mm Hg; pO_2, 50 to 100 mm Hg

b. pH, 7.35 to 7.45; pCO$_2$, 45 to 50 mm Hg; pO$_2$, 90 to 100 mm Hg

c. pH, 7.35 to 7.45; pCO$_2$, 35 to 45 mm Hg; pO$_2$, 80 to 100 mm Hg

d. pH, 7.30 to 7.40; pCO$_2$, 30 to 45 mm Hg; pO$_2$, 70 to 100 mm Hg

15. Abdominal breathing, 30 to 60 breaths/min with an irregular pattern of rate and depth, would closely describe the breathing patterns of what age group?
   a. aged adult
   b. infant
   c. early childhood
   d. late childhood

Answers With Rationale

1. The correct response is *d*. Hypoventilation is a decreased rate or depth of air movement into the lungs. Hyperventilation is an increased rate and depth of ventilation, whereas fremitus is the vibration of the chest wall that can be palpated. A pleural friction rub is a dry grating sound caused by inflammation of pleural surfaces.

2. The correct response is *b*. Crackles and gurgles are not described as squeaky and the pleural friction rub is a dry, grating sound.

3. The correct response is *a*. Fluid in the pleural space is referred to as a *pleural effusion* and blood in the pleural space is called *hemothorax*. *Atelectasis* is an incomplete expansion or collapse of the lungs.

4. The correct response is *b*. A rate higher than 2 L/min may destroy the hypoxic drive that stimulates respirations in the medulla in a client with chronic lung disease. Oxygen delivered at low rates does not necessarily have to be humidified, and arterial blood gases are not required at regular intervals to determine flow rate.

5. The correct response is *b*. The nonrebreather mask provides the highest concentration of oxygen to a spontaneously breathing client.

6. The correct response is *a*. Pulse oximetry measures oxygen saturation levels of arterial blood, is affected by cigarette smoking, and is an adjunct therapy, not a replacement for arterial blood gas analysis.

7. The correct response is *c*. The nurse should use sterile technique, should not apply suction as the catheter is being introduced, and suctioning should be limited to 10- to 15-second intervals to avoid causing hypoxia.

8. The correct response is *c*. Dentures are usually left in place to provide for a better seal for breathing and should be removed only if they are loose. The carotid pulse is most easily checked for lack of a pulse. Compression/ventilation ratio for one rescuer CPR is 15:2.

9. The correct response is *d*. Pursed-lip breathing prolongs expiration, increases airway pressure, and loosens the amount of airway trapping and resistance. Doing pursed-lip breathing correctly diminishes carbon dioxide retention.

10. The correct response is *c*. After 4 to 6 minutes without oxygen, irreversible brain damage can occur.

11. The correct response is *d*. A snug-fitting mask is necessary to deliver expected rates of oxygen. A simple face mask does not trap carbon dioxide and cause retention.

12. The correct response is *b*. Occluding the Y-port causes suction and may traumatize the tracheal mucosa if applied when the catheter is inserted.

13. The correct response is *a*. The Heimlich maneuver involves abdominal thrusts to clear an obstructed airway.

14. The correct response is *c*. These are the normal arterial blood gas ranges for pH, carbon dioxide, and oxygen.

15. The correct response is *b*. Respirations in the infant are more rapid and have not stabilized. As alveoli increase in number and size, the respiratory rate is lower.

BIBLIOGRAPHY

American Heart Association. (1987). *Instructor's manual for basic life support*. Dallas: Author.

Anderson, S. (1990). ABGs: Six easy steps to interpreting blood gases. *American Journal of Nursing, 90*(8), 42–45.

Beare, P., & Myers, J. (1990). *Adult health nursing*. St. Louis: Mosby.

Bolgiano, C. (1990). Administering oxygen therapy: What you need to know. *Nursing, 20*(6), 47–51.

Cahill, K., & Heath, J. (1990). Sterile water used for humidification in low-flow oxygen therapy: Is it necessary? *American Journal of Infection Control, 18*(1), 13–17.

Campbell, E., Baker, M. & Crites-Silver, P. (1988). Subjective effects of humidification of oxygen for delivery by nasal cannula. *Chest, 93*(2), 289–293.

Carabott, F., Kipling, D., Manger, G., & King-Pankratz, H. (1990). Teaching families tracheotomy care. *Canadian Nurse, 86*(3), 21–22.

Carnevali, D., & Patrick, M. (1986). *Nursing management for the elderly.* Philadelphia: Lippincott.

Carpenito, L. (1992). *Nursing diagnosis: Application to clinical practice* (4th ed.). Philadelphia: Lippincott.

Carroll, P. (1989). Safe suctioning. *Nursing, 18*(9), 48–51.

Carroll, P. (1991). What's new in chest tube management? *RN, 54*(5), 34–40.

Caruana, S. (1990). Myths and facts about tracheal tubes. *Nursing, 20*(6), 30.

Coleman, S. (1992). Cardiac issues in CPR: What the future might hold. *Nursing, 22*(4), 54–57.

Ellstrom, K. (1990). What's causing your patient's respiratory distress? *Nursing, 20*(11), 57–61.

Erickson, R. (1989a). Mastering the ins and outs of chest drainage. *Nursing, 18*(5), 36–43.

Erickson, R. (1989b). Mastering the ins and outs of chest drainage, part II. *Nursing, 18*(6), 46–49.

Finesilver, C. (1992). Perfecting the art: Respiratory assessment. *RN, 55*(2), 22–29.

Fischbach, F. (1992). *A manual of laboratory tests* (4th ed.). Philadelphia: Lippincott.

Fuller, J., & Schaller-Ayers, J. (1990). *Health assessment.* Philadelphia: Lippincott.

Gift, A. (1990). Dyspnea. *Nursing Clinics of North America, 25*(4), 955–963.

Grandstrom, D., & Wierzbicki, L. (1989). A better way to deliver long-term oxygen therapy. *RN, 52*(9), 58–67.

Juip, M., & Harned, J. (1988). Giving mouth-to-mouth ventilations. *Nursing, 18*(12), 48–49.

Kitay, G., & Shafer, N. (1989). Cafe coronary: Recognition, treatment, and prevention. *Nurse Practitioner, 14*(6), 35–46.

Macnee, C. (1991). Perceived well-being of persons quitting smoking. *Nursing Research, 40*(4), 200–203.

Mapp, C. (1988). Trach care: Are you aware of all the dangers? *Nursing, 17*(7), 34–42.

Mathews, P., Mathews, L. M., & Mitchell, R. (1992a). Airway monitoring: What the future holds. *Nursing, 21*(2), 49–51.

Mathews, P., Mathews, L. M., & Mitchell, R. (1992b). Artificial airways: Resuscitation guidelines you can follow. *Nursing, 21*(1), 53–59.

McConnell, E. (1991). Minimizing respiratory problems. *Nursing, 21*(11), 34–39.

Melini, L. (1989). A non-invasive way to measure oxygen saturation. *RN, 52*(1), 79.

Meyer, C. (1992). Doing the CPR two-step. *American Journal of Nursing, 92*(3), 15.

Miracle, V., & Allnutt, D. (1990). How to perform basic airway management. *Nursing, 19*(4), 55–60.

Nield, M., Kim, M., & Patel, M. (1989). Use of magnitude estimation for estimating the parameters of dyspnea. *Nursing Research, 38*(2), 77–80.

Shemansky, C. (1991). Choking: Clear and present danger for elders. *Geriatric Nursing, 12*(2), 68–70.

Sonnesso, G. (1991). Are you ready to use pulse oximetry? *Nursing, 20*(8), 60–64.

Spearing, C., & Cornell, D. (1987). Incentive spirometry: Inspiring your patient to breath deeply. *Nursing, 17*(9), 50–51.

Spyr, J., & Preach, M. (1990). Pulse oximetry. *RN, 53*(5), 38–45.

Staab, A., & Lyles, M. (1990). *Manual of geriatric nursing.* Glenview, IL: Scott, Foresman.

Stevens, S., & Becker, K. (1988). How to perform picture-perfect respiratory assessment. *Nursing, 18*(1), 57–63.

Webster, J., & Kadah, H. (1991). Unique aspects of respiratory disease in the elderly. *Geriatrics, 46*(7), 31–43.

Wesmiller, S., Hoffman, L., & Wiseman, M. (1989). Understanding transtracheal oxygen delivery. *Nursing, 18*(12), 43–47.

Whitney, J. (1990). The measurement of oxygen tension in tissue. *Nursing Research, 39*(4), 203–205.

Willens, J. (1991). B.C.L.S. forecast: Big changes in the wind. *Nursing, 21*(11), 53–56.

Willens, J., & Copel, L. (1989). Performing CPR on infants. *Nursing, 19*(3), 47–53.

Willens, J., & Copel, L. (1989). Performing CPR on adults. *Nursing, 19*(1), 34–43.

Yeaw, E. (1992). How position affects oxygenation: Good lung down? *American Journal of Nursing, 92*(3), 26–29.

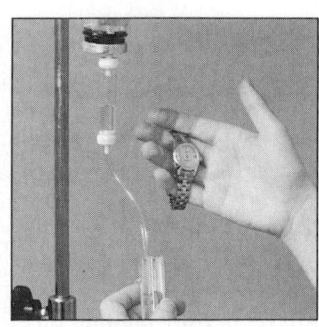
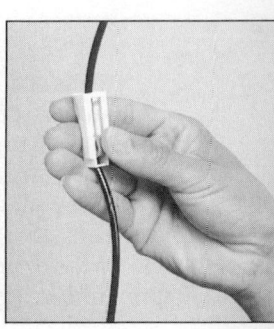

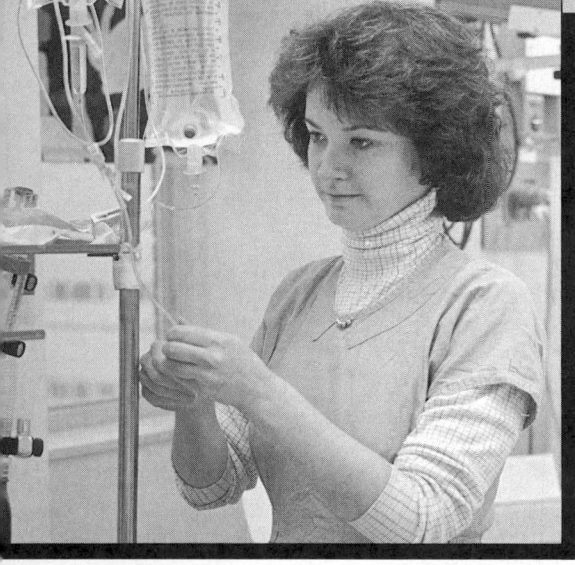

Fluid, Electrolyte, and Acid–Base Balance

37

OBJECTIVES

After studying this chapter, the learner should be able to:

Define key terms used in the chapter.

Describe the functions of body fluids, the two main compartments where fluids are located in the body, and factors that affect variations in fluid compartments.

Describe the functions, sources and losses, and regulation of main electrolytes of the body.

Explain the principles of osmosis, diffusion, active transport, and filtration.

Describe how thirst and the organs of homeostasis function to maintain fluid homeostasis.

Describe the role of buffer systems and respiratory and renal mechanisms in achieving acid–base balance.

Identify the etiologies, defining characteristics, and treatment modalities for common fluid, electrolyte, and acid–base disturbances.

Perform a fluid, electrolyte, and acid–base balance assessment.

Describe the role of dietary modification, modification of fluid intake, medication administration, intravenous therapy, blood replacement, and total parenteral nutrition in resolving fluid, electrolyte, and acid–base imbalances.

Plan, implement, and evaluate nursing care related to select nursing diagnoses involving fluid, electrolyte, and acid–base imbalances.

KEY TERMS

acid
acidosis
active transport
alkali
alkalosis
anion
base
blood transfusion
buffer
cation
cellular fluid
central venous catheter
colloid osmotic pressure
dehydration
diffusion
edema
electrolyte
embolus
extracellular fluid
filtration
filtration pressure
fluid volume deficit
fluid volume excess
hydrostatic pressure
interstitial fluid
intracellular fluid
intravascular fluid
intravenous fluid
ion
metabolic acidosis
metabolic alkalosis
milliliter
oncotic pressure
osmolality
osmosis
pH
respiratory acidosis
respiratory alkalosis
solute
solvent
speed shock
third-space fluid shift
total parenteral nutrition

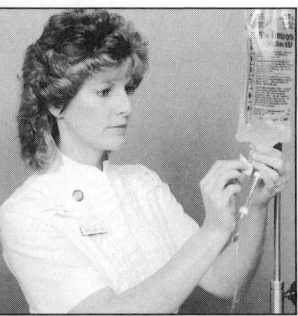

- It serves as a medium to transport such substances as hormones, enzymes, blood platelets, and red and white blood cells.
- It is important for cellular metabolism and proper cellular chemical functioning.
- It is the solvent for electrolytes and nonelectrolytes.
- It helps maintain normal body temperature.
- It helps digestion and promotes elimination.
- It is necessary for the manufacture of the body's secretions.

Body Fluid Compartments

The two main compartments, or spaces, in which fluids are located in the body are the **intracellular fluid** (ICF) and **extracellular fluid** (ECF). ICF is the fluid within the cell. It constitutes about 40% of an adult's body weight or 70% of the total body water. ECF is all the fluid outside of cell walls. It constitutes about 20% of an adult's body weight or 30% of total body water. ECF includes intravascular and interstitial fluids. **Intravascular fluid** or plasma is the liquid constituent of blood, (ie, fluid found within the vascular system). **Interstitial fluid** is the fluid in which tissue cells are bathed; it includes lymph. The term *total body water* or fluid (TBW or TBF) refers to the total amount of water in the body expressed as a percentage of body weight. Figure 37-1 illustrates a breakdown of total body fluid. Figure 37-2 is a microscopic visualization of body fluid distribution.

Water may constitute anywhere from 45% to 75% of a healthy person's body weight; the importance of fluid balance to health is readily apparent. Under usual conditions, virtually every organ and system in the body helps in some way to maintain fluid balance. Nurses routinely encounter in their practice clients with serious and even life-threatening fluid, electrolyte, and acid–base balance disturbances. One of nursing's most important roles is the prevention of these disturbances in high-risk populations by vigilant nursing care.

Study of this chapter will provide the student with basic knowledge of the principles of fluid, electrolyte, and acid–base balance and the etiologies, defining characteristics, and nursing interventions for common disturbances. Sample interview questions for performing a fluid balance nursing history are presented along with information on specific physical assessment measures and laboratory studies. Numerous examples of nursing diagnoses are offered. Client goals and specific nursing strategies for promoting fluid balance are described. These include dietary modification; modification of fluid intake; medication administration; and assisting with intravenous (IV) therapy, blood replacement, and total parenteral nutrition (TPN). In the section entitled Nursing Process in Clinical Practice, focused assessment, planning, implementation, and evaluation guides are offered for surgical and oncology clients with fluid balance nursing diagnoses. These guides and the concluding case study illustrate how the nurse's knowledge of fluid, electrolyte, and acid–base balance is combined with skilled nursing interventions and caring to successfully resolve fluid balance problems.

Physiology

Body Fluids

Water is the primary body fluid and is the most important nutrient of life. Whereas life can be sustained for many days without food, it can be sustained for only a few days without water.

The following are the primary functions of water in the body:
- It serves as a medium for transporting nutrients to cells and wastes from cells.

FIGURE 37-1

Total body fluid represents 50% to 60% of body weight of a normal adult.

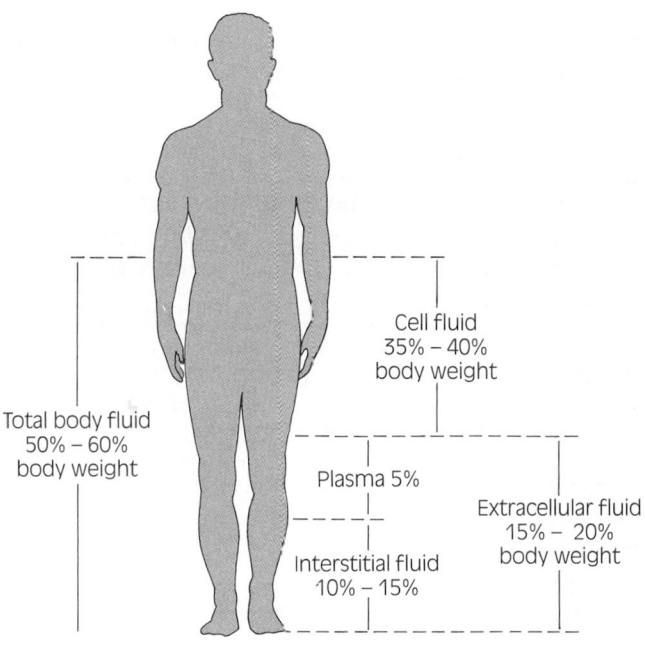

Cell fluid
35% – 40%
body weight

Total body fluid
50% – 60%
body weight

Plasma 5%

Extracellular fluid
15% – 20%
body weight

Interstitial fluid
10% – 15%

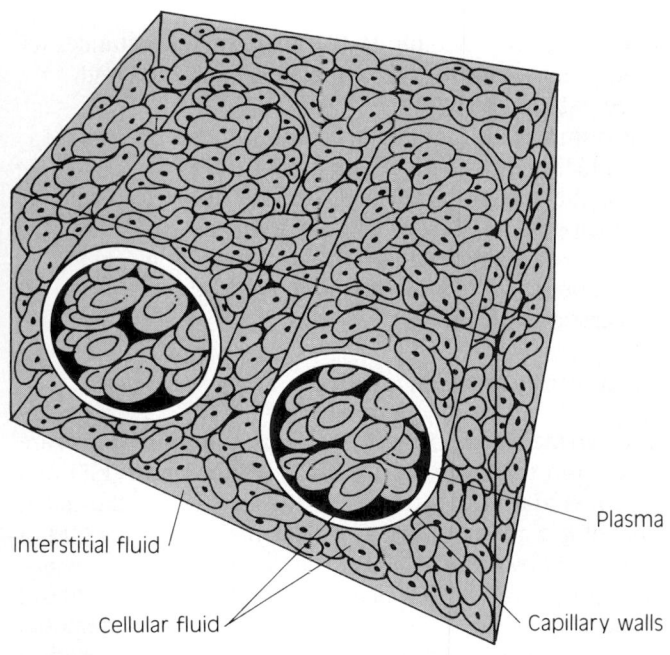

Plasma

Interstitial fluid

Cellular fluid

Capillary walls

F I G U R E 3 7 - 2

Microscopic visualization of body fluid distribution.

Variations in Fluid Content

In a healthy person, total body water constitutes about 45% to 75% of the body's weight. Variations depend on such factors as the person's age, lean body mass, and sex. Table 37-1 illustrates age-related changes in total body water and in the various water compartments of the body. An infant, especially one born prematurely, has considerably more body fluid than an elderly person. Infants also have relatively more ECF than adults. Because ECF is more easily lost from the body than ICF, infants are more prone to fluid volume deficits (FVDs).

Total body water also depends on the build of a person. Because fat tissues contain a small amount of water whereas lean tissue is rich in water, the more obese the

T A B L E 3 7 - 1

Average Percentages of Water in Relation to Body Weight in People of Different Ages in the Various Water Compartments of the Body

Water Compartment	Infant (%)	Adult (%)		Elderly Person (%)
		Man	Woman	
Extracellular				
Intravascular	4	4	5	5
Interstitial	25	11	10	15
Intracellular	48	45	35	25
Total body water	77	60	50	45

person, the smaller the percentage of total body water when compared with body weight. In an obese male, total body water can be as little as 50% of body weight; in an obese female, total body water can be as little as 42% of body weight. Because females tend to have proportionally more body fat than males, they also have less body fluid than males. Similarly, the decreasing percentage of body fluid in elderly people is related to the decrease in lean body mass in favor of fat.

Electrolytes

Certain compounds in solution dissociate to form ions by the process of ionization. An **ion** is an atom or molecule carrying an electric charge in solution. Substances capable of breaking into electrically charged ions when dissolved in a solution are called **electrolytes**. Some ions develop a positive charge and are called **cations**. Others develop a negative charge and are called **anions**.

If molecules in the body's chemical compounds remain intact, they are called nonelectrolytes. In the human body, urea and glucose are nonelectrolytes. **Solvents** are liquids that hold a substance in solution; **solutes** are substances that are dissolved in a solution. Water is the solvent in the body that makes up solutions with solutes. The solutes are electrolytes and nonelectrolytes.

Measurement of Electrolytes

The unit of measure used to describe electrolytes is expressed in terms of their chemical combining power, or chemical activity. Because the weight of an ion is not related to its combining power, a standard without regard for weight has been developed to compare the chemical activity of electrolytes.

The standard used to describe the chemical activity of electrolytes is the chemical activity of 1 milligram (mg) of hydrogen. The milliequivalent (mEq) is used in the United States as the unit of measure to describe the chemical activity of an electrolyte. One milliequivalent is chemically equivalent to the activity of 1 mg of hydrogen. Stated inversely, 1 mg of hydrogen exerts 1 mEq of chemical activity. This is true whether the comparison with hydrogen is made with a cation or an anion. Hence, 1 mEq of any cation is equivalent to 1 mEq of any anion.

Using the milliequivalent system, the total cations in the body are normally equal to the total anions. In healthy people, the milliequivalents per liter for electrolytes in the body vary within a relatively narrow range. When electrolytes are not in normal balance, the person is in a state of risk or jeopardy.

Regulation of Electrolytes

The chief functions of electrolytes include regulation of water distribution, regulation of acid–base balance, and maintenance of a balanced degree of neuromuscular excitability (Ulrich, 1989). There are many different kinds of electrolytes in the body. This section summarizes information about the most prevalent ones. Electrolyte disturbances are discussed later in the chapter.

Sodium (Na⁺) The cation sodium is the chief electrolyte of ECF. It moves easily between intravascular and interstitial spaces and moves across cell membranes by active transport. Many chemical reactions in the body are influenced by sodium, particularly in nervous-tissue cells and muscle-tissue cells.

Functions
- Maintains the isotonicity and volume of body fluids
  - Controls water distribution throughout the body
  - Is the primary regulator of ECF volume
  - Also influences intracellular fluid volume
- Participates in the generation and transmission of nerve impulses
- Is an essential electrolyte in the sodium–potassium pump

Sources and Losses
- Average daily requirements for sodium are not known precisely, but in North America, the average adult intake is estimated to be between 2 and 7 g, and the usual daily sodium requirement for adults is about 100 mEq.
- Sodium is found in many foods, particularly bacon, ham, sausage, catsup, mustard, relish, processed cheese, canned vegetables, bread, cereal, and salted snack food. It is found in table salt (sodium chloride), which is about 46% sodium.
- Sodium excesses are eliminated primarily by the kidneys; small amounts are lost in feces and perspiration.

Regulation
- Sodium normally is maintained in the body within a relatively narrow range, and deviations quickly result in a serious health problem. For this reason, health practitioners often speak of the "primacy of sodium."
- Salt intake regulates sodium concentrations.
- Sodium is conserved through reabsorption in the kidneys, a process stimulated by aldosterone.
- The normal extracellular concentration of sodium is 135 to 145 mEq/L (mmol/L).

Potassium (K⁺) Potassium is the major cation of ICF. Potassium and sodium work reciprocally. For example, an excessive intake of sodium results in an excretion of potassium, and vice versa.

Functions
- Is the chief regulator of cellular enzyme activity and cellular water content
- Plays a vital role in such processes as the transmission of electric impulses, particularly in nerve, heart, skeletal, intestinal, and lung tissue; protein and carbohydrate metabolism; and cellular building
- Assists in regulation of acid–base balance by cellular exchange with H⁺

Sources/Losses
- Average daily requirements for potassium are not known precisely, but about 40 to 60 mEq daily is ordinarily adequate.
- A well-balanced diet contains adequate quantities of potassium. Leading food sources include bananas, peaches, figs, dates, apricots, oranges, prunes, melons, raisins, broccoli, and potatoes. Meat and dairy products contain good amounts of potassium.
- Potassium is excreted primarily by the kidneys. The kidneys have no effective method of conserving potassium. Therefore, deficits develop readily if excreted in excess without being replaced simultaneously.
- Gastrointestinal (GI) secretions contain potassium in large quantities. Some is also found in perspiration and saliva.

Regulation
- Cellular K⁺ is conserved by the sodium pump when Na⁺ is excluded.
- The kidneys conserve K⁺ when cellular K⁺ is decreased.
- Aldosterone secretion triggers K⁺ excretion in urine.
- The normal range for serum potassium is 3.5 to 5 mEq/L.

Calcium (Ca²⁺) Calcium is the most abundant electrolyte in the body. Up to 99% of the total amount of calcium in the body is found in bones and teeth in ionized form. It works intimately with phosphorus.

Functions
- Is necessary for nerve-impulse transmission, blood clotting, and muscle contraction
- Is needed for vitamin B_{12} absorption and for its use by body cells
- Acts as a catalyst for many cell chemical activities
- Is necessary for strong bones and teeth
- Establishes thickness and strength of cell membranes

Sources/Losses
- The average daily requirement for calcium is about 1 g for adults. Higher amounts are required, according to body weight, for children, for pregnant and lactating women, and postmenopausal women.
- It is found in milk, cheese, and dried beans. Some calcium is present in meats and vegetables.
- Use of calcium is stimulated by vitamin D.
- It leaves bones and teeth to maintain normal blood-calcium levels, if necessary.
- It is excreted in urine, feces, bile, digestive secretions, and perspiration.

Regulation
- When ECF calcium levels decrease, the parathyroid glands increase the secretion of parathyroid hormone (PTH), which acts on bones to increase the release of calcium into the blood, and acts on the kidney tubules and the intestinal mucosa to increase the reabsorption of calcium from the kidneys and the intestine.

- A high serum phosphate concentration causes a secondary depression of serum calcium; a low serum phosphate concentration may cause a secondary elevation of serum calcium.
- Calcitonin, a hormone secreted by the thyroid gland, has an opposite effect on calcium than PTH. Increases in calcitonin reduce serum calcium concentration.

Magnesium (Mg^{2+}) Most of the cation magnesium is found within body cells. It is present in heart, bone, nerve, and muscle tissues. Magnesium is the second most important cation of ICF.

Functions
- Is important for the metabolism of carbohydrates and proteins
- Is important for many vital reactions related to the body's enzymes
- Serves to help maintain electric activity in nervous membranes and muscle membranes

Sources and Losses
- The average daily adult requirement for magnesium is about 18 to 30 mEq; children require larger amounts.
- Magnesium is found in most foods but especially in vegetables, nuts, fish, whole grains, peas, and beans.

Regulation
- Magnesium levels in the body are largely controlled by the kidneys.
- Plasma concentrations of magnesium range from 1.3 to 2.1 mEq/L.

Chloride (Cl^-) Chloride, the chief extracellular anion, is found in blood, interstitial fluid, and lymph, and in minute amounts in ICF.

Functions
- Acts with sodium to maintain the osmotic pressure of the blood
- Plays a role in the body's acid–base balance
- Is important in buffering action when oxygen and carbon dioxide exchange in red blood cells (RBCs)
- Is essential for the production of hydrochloric acid in gastric juices

Sources/Losses
- Average daily requirements of chloride are unknown, but its intake is usually the same as sodium.
- It is found in foods high in sodium, in dairy products, and meat.

Regulation
- It is normally paired with sodium, and excreted and conserved with sodium by the kidneys.
- Chloride deficits lead to potassium deficits, and vice versa.
- Normal serum chloride levels range from 95 to 105 mEq/L (mmol/L).

Bicarbonate (HCO_3^-) The bicarbonate molecule is an anion. It is the major chemical base buffer within the body and is found in both ECF and ICF.

Function
- Is essential for acid–base balance; bicarbonate and carbonic acid constitute the body's primary buffer system

Regulation
- Bicarbonate levels are regulated primarily by the kidneys.
- Bicarbonate is ordinarily readily available as a result of carbon dioxide formation in the process of metabolism.
- In plasma, bicarbonate varies indirectly with intracellular potassium.
- Normal bicarbonate levels range between 25 and 29 mEq/L (mmol/L).

Phosphate (PO_4^-) The phosphate ion is the major anion in body cells. It is a buffer anion in both ICF and ECF.

Functions
- Helps maintain acid–base balance
- Has important chemical reactions in the body; for example, phosphorus is necessary for many B vitamins to be effective, helps promote nerve and muscle action, and plays a role in carbohydrate metabolism
- Is important for cell division and for the transmission of hereditary traits

Sources/Losses
- Average daily requirements for phosphorus are similar to those of calcium.
- It is found in most foods but especially in beef, pork, and dried peas and beans.
- It is metabolized in the same manner as calcium.

Regulation
- Phosphate is regulated by PTH and by activated vitamin D.
- Calcium and phosphate are inversely proportional; an increase in one results in a decrease in the other.
- The normal range of phosphate is 2.5 to 4.5 mEq/L (mmol/L).

Additional Electrolytes The anion sulfate is found primarily within cells and is associated with cellular protein. Excesses are excreted by the kidneys. The organic-acid anions are normally intermediary in cell metabolism. The major one in the body is lactic acid. The protein anion functions in the process of diffusion to move substances to and from the capillaries. Plasma proteins include albumin, globulin, and fibrinogen.

Other electrolytes are required for proper cell functioning, but they are found only in traces in the body. One example is chromium. A well-balanced diet ordinarily ensures an adequate supply of trace substances in the body.

Fluids in various compartments of the body differ from one another in terms of their constituents. For example, ICF has higher concentrations of certain electrolytes than ECF. Figure 37-3 illustrates differences in the electrolyte composition of body fluids according to the compartments in which the fluids are found.

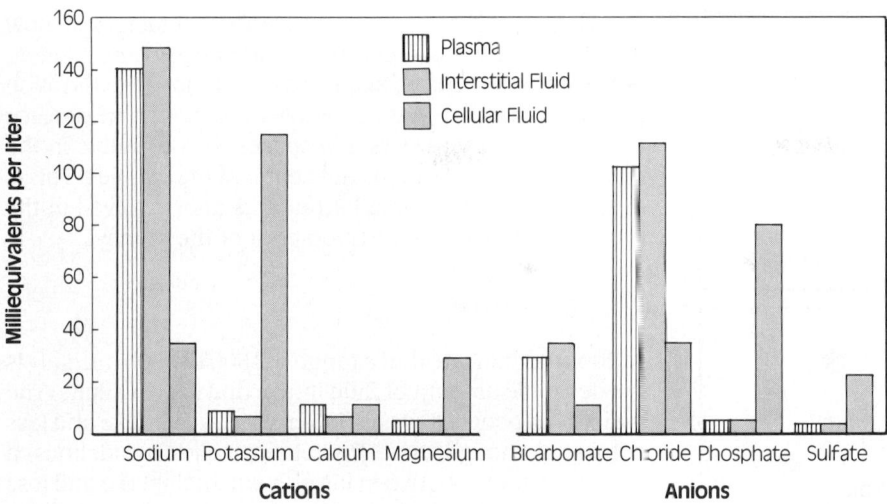

Electrolyte composition of normal body fluids.

Fluid and Electrolyte Movement

ECF takes nourishment to each body cell and receives each cell's waste products. These exchanges, which normally result in fluid balance and homeostasis, are essential to life. The most common routes for transporting materials to and from intracellular compartments are osmosis, diffusion, active transport, and filtration.

Osmosis   The membranes of the body's cells are semipermeable. This makes it possible for water, a pure solvent, to be transported through cell walls. **Osmosis** is the most important method of transporting body fluids. Water shifts and, hence, fluid balance, depend heavily on this mode of transport.

Through the process of osmosis, the solvent water passes from an area of lesser solute concentration to an area of greater solute concentration until equilibrium is established. As a result, the volume of more concentrated solution increases, and the volume of the weaker solution decreases. The greater the difference in the concentration of the two solutions on each side of a semipermeable membrane, the greater the osmotic pressure. Figure 37-4 illustrates the process of osmosis.

Diffusion   **Diffusion** is the tendency of solutes to move freely throughout a solvent. The solute moves from an area of higher concentration to an area of lower concentration (ie, "downhill") until equilibrium is established. Gases move about by diffusion. For example, if an open pan of water is left in a room, evaporation occurs as the water molecules disperse themselves evenly about the room. Oxygen and carbon dioxide exchange in the lung's alveoli and capillaries occurs by diffusion.

Active Transport   **Active transport** is a process that requires energy for the movement of substances through a cell wall, from an area of lesser concentration to an area of higher concentration. Adenosine triphosphate, released from a cell, makes it possible for certain substances to acquire energy needed to pass through a cell wall. Although the process is not entirely understood, the energy requirements are affected by characteristics of the cell membrane, specific enzymes, and concentrations of ions. This process explains the so-called pump mechanism and is illustrated in Figure 37-5 using sodium and potassium as examples. If diffusion can be called "coasting downhill," active transport can be called "pumping uphill." Substances believed to use active transport are amino acids; glucose, but in certain places only, such as in the kidneys

Through the process of osmosis, body fluids are transported through cell walls. The solvent water moves from an area of lesser solute concentration to one of greater solute concentration until equilibrium is established.

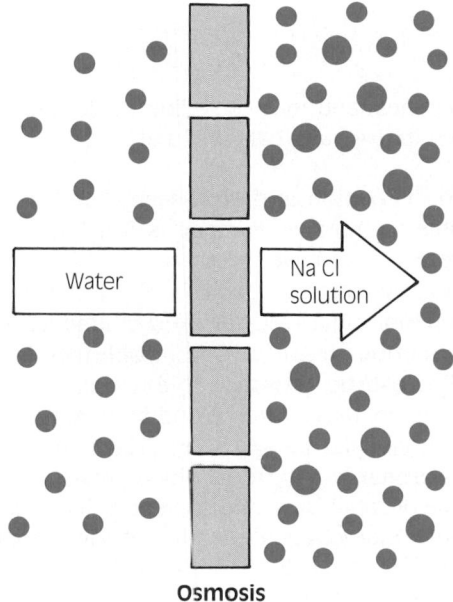

Osmosis

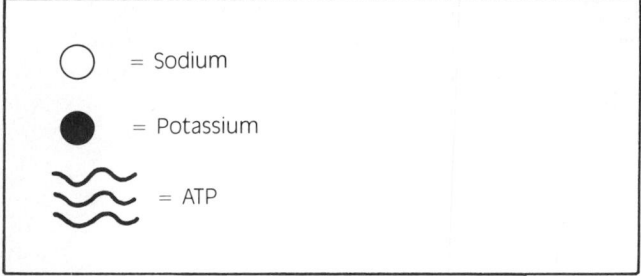

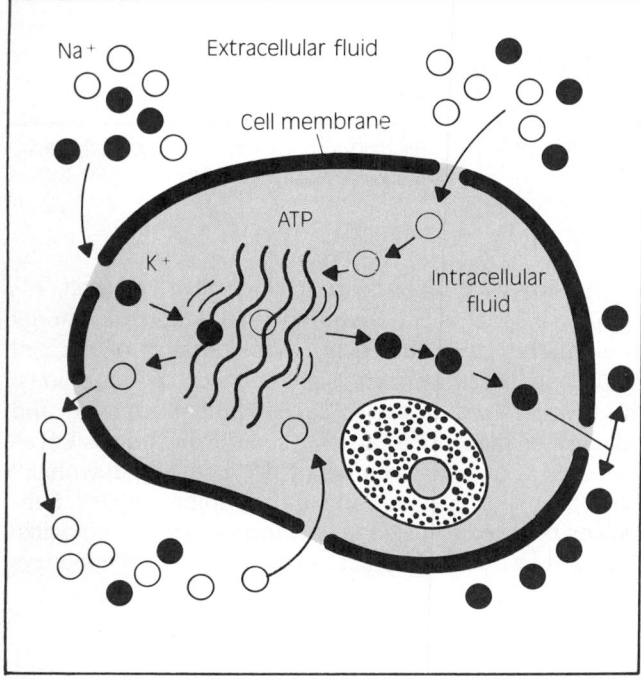

Active transport. Sodium that diffuses into the cell through a pore in the cell membrane is actively pumped out of the cell by a carrier system (*wavy lines*). Similarly, potassium that diffuses out of the cell is actively replaced by the carrier system.

and intestines; and ions of sodium, chloride, potassium, hydrogen, phosphate, calcium, and magnesium.

Filtration   **Filtration** is the passage of a fluid through a permeable membrane. Passage is from an area of high pressure to one of lower pressure.

Certain substances, such as plasma proteins, which have high molecular weights, exert **colloid osmotic pressure**, or **oncotic pressure** on permeable membranes in the body. **Hydrostatic pressure** is force exerted by a fluid against the container wall. Blood hydrostatic pressure is the pressure of plasma and blood cells in the capillaries; it depends primarily on arterial blood pressure on the arteriolar side of capillaries, and on venous blood pressure on the venular side of capillaries. **Filtration pressure** is the difference between colloid osmotic pressure and blood hydrostatic pressure.

These pressures are significant to understand how fluid leaves arterioles, enters the interstitial compartment, and eventually returns again to the venules. The filtration pressure is positive in the arterioles and, hence, helps force or filter fluids into interstitial spaces; it is negative in the venules and, hence, helps fluid enter at the venules. This is illustrated in Figure 37-6 Filtration is also involved in the proper functioning of the glomeruli of the kidneys.

Fluid Balance

Authorities indicate that a range of 1500 to 3500 mL daily is the desirable amount of fluid intake and loss in adults. The majority of people have a 2500-mL average intake and loss per day. Although these figures are helpful guidelines, a person's balance between his or her actual intake and loss must be considered when assessing nursing needs. A person's intake should normally be approximately balanced by his or her output or fluid loss. A general rule is that in the healthy adult, the output of urine normally approximates the ingestion of liquids; and the water from food and oxidation is balanced by the water loss through the feces, the skin, and the respiratory process. The intake should be within the desirable average range. The intake–output balance may not always exist in a single 24-hour period but should normally be achieved within 2 to 3 days.

Fluid Sources   Water is derived from several sources for the body.

Ingested Liquids   This source makes up the largest amount of water normally taken into the body. Fluid intake is primarily regulated by the thirst mechanism. Located within the hypothalamus, the thirst control center is stimulated by intracellular dehydration and decreased blood volume.

Water in Food   This is the second largest source of water for the body. The amount ingested depends on dietary items. For example, melons and citrus fruit are high in water content, whereas cereal and dried fruits have a relatively low water content.

Water from Metabolic Oxidation   Water is an end product of the oxidation that occurs during the metabolism of food substances. This source also varies with different types of nutrients. For example metabolism of 100 g of fat produces 107 g of water, whereas 100 g of carbohydrate yields 55 g of water, and 100 g of protein produces 40 g of water. Therefore, a person whose diet is high in fat has a proportionately greater amount of water resulting from metabolic processes than a person whose diet is high in protein.

Fluid Losses   Water is lost from the body through the kidneys and intestinal tract, and through the skin as perspiration. Water is also lost in insensible ways. *Insensible water loss* is unperceptible. For example, in addition to perspiration, which is perceptible, an invisible amount of water is lost from the skin constantly through evaporation. Insensible loss from the lungs is moisture exhaled through the

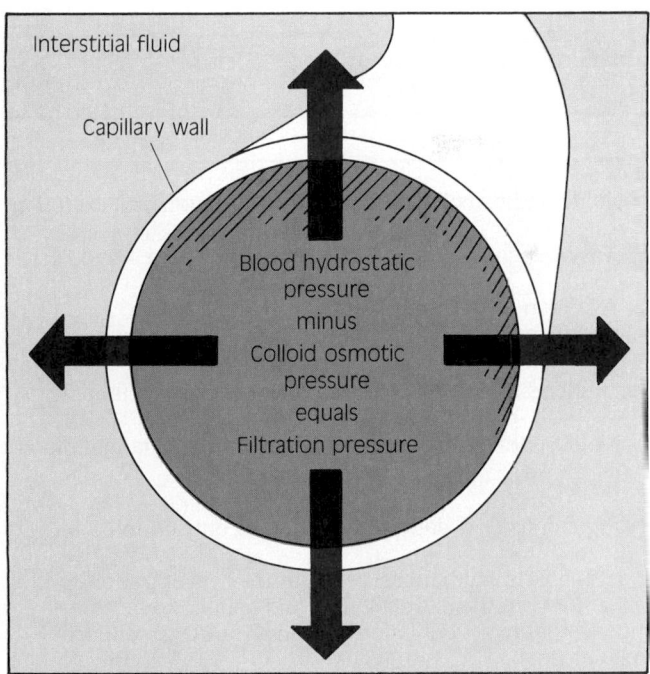

Arteriole: The pressure within the arteriole is **positive** and hence, fluid is forced into interstitial fluid.

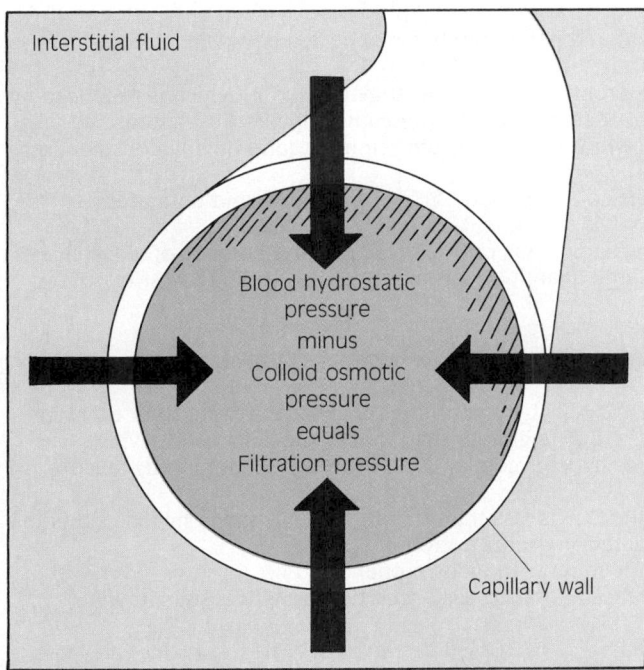

Venule: The pressure within the venule is **negative** and hence, fluid is forced into the venule.

FIGURE 37-6

Filtration, which is the tendency of solutes to move from an area of higher pressure to an area of lower pressure. (*Top*) *Arteriole:* The pressure within the arteriole is positive and, hence, fluid is forced into interstitial fluid. (*Bottom*) *Venule:* The pressure within the venules is negative and, hence, fluid is forced into the venule.

breath. Water losses vary according to the person and the circumstances.

Figure 37-7 illustrates fluid intake and output balance in healthy adults. Deviations from normal ranges for balance of water intake and output should alert the nurse to impending problems and possibly preventable imbalances.

Homeostatic Mechanisms Fluid homeostasis normally functions automatically and effectively. Almost every organ and system in the body helps in some way to maintain fluid homeostasis. The following are the primary organs of homeostasis. Functions are highlighted in Table 37-2. Fluid balance is threatened when any organ fails to function properly.

Kidneys The kidneys are frequently referred to as the master chemists of the body. They normally filter 170 L of plasma daily in the adult while excreting only 1.5 L of urine.

FIGURE 37-7

In health, fluid intake and fluid losses are about equal. The amounts indicated are average adult daily fluid sources and losses.

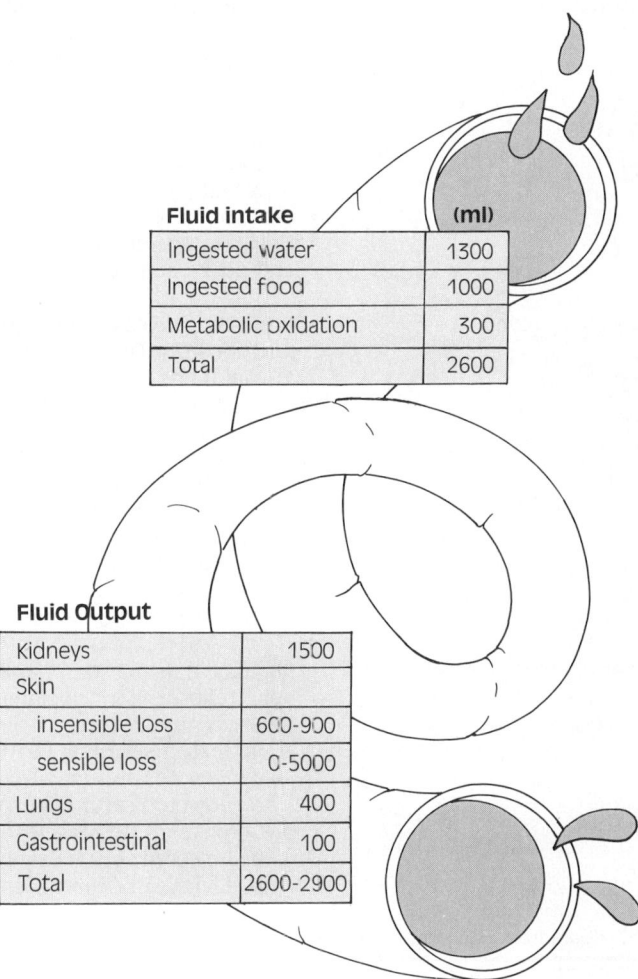

Fluid intake	(ml)
Ingested water	1300
Ingested food	1000
Metabolic oxidation	300
Total	2600

Fluid Output	
Kidneys	1500
Skin	
insensible loss	600-900
sensible loss	0-5000
Lungs	400
Gastrointestinal	100
Total	2600-2900

TABLE 37-2

Homeostatic Mechanisms That Maintain the Composition and Volume of Body Fluid Within Narrow Limits of Normal

Organs of Homeostasis	Functions
Kidneys	• Regulate extracellular fluid (ECF) volume and osmolality by selective retention and excretion of body fluids. • Regulate electrolyte levels in the ECF by selective retention of needed substances and excretion of unneeded substances • Regulate pH of ECF by excretion or retention of hydrogen ions • Excrete metabolic wastes (primarily acids) and toxic substances
Heart and blood vessels	• Circulate blood through the kidneys under sufficient pressure for urine to form (pumping action of the heart) • React to hypovolemia by stimulating fluid retention (stretch receptors in the atria and blood vessels)

Lungs	• Eliminate about 13,000 mEq of hydrogen ions (H^+) daily, as opposed to only 40 to 80 mEq excreted daily by the kidneys
	• Act promptly to correct metabolic acid–base disturbances; regulate H^+ concentration (pH) by controlling the level of carbon dioxide (CO_2) in the extracellular fluid as follows:
	  1. Metabolic alkalosis causes compensatory hypoventilation, resulting in CO_2 retention (increases acidity of the extracellular fluid).
	  2. Metabolic acidosis causes compensatory hyperventilation, resulting in CO_2 excretion (decreases acidity of the extracellular fluid).
	• Remove approximately 300 mL of water daily through exhalation (insensible water loss) in the normal adult

Adrenal glands	• Regulate blood volume and sodium and potassium balance by secreting aldosterone, a mineral corticoid secreted by the adrenal cortex
	  1. The primary regulator of aldosterone appears to be angiotension II, which is produced by the renin–angiotensin system. A decrease in blood volume triggers this system and increases aldosterone secretion, which causes sodium retention (and thus water retention) and potassium loss.
	  2. Decreased secretion of aldosterone causes sodium and water loss and potassium retention.
	• Cortisol, another adrenocortical hormone, has only a fraction of the potency of aldosterone.
	• However, secretion of cortisol in large quantities can produce sodium and water retention and potassium deficit.

Pituitary gland	• Stores and releases the antidiuretic hormone (ADH), which makes the body retain water; functions of ADH include:
	  1. Maintains osmotic pressure of the cells by controlling renal water retention or excretion
	    a. When osmotic pressure of the ECF is greater than that of the cells (as in hypernatremia—excess sodium—or hyperglycemia), ADH secretion is increased, causing renal retention of water.
	    b. When osmotic pressure of the ECF is less than that of the cells (as in hyponatremia), ADH secretion is decreased, causing renal excretion of water.
	  2. Controls blood volume (less influential than aldosterone)
	    a. When blood volume is decreased, an increased secretion of ADH results in water conservation.
	    b. When blood volume is increased, a decreased secretion of ADH results in water loss.

Parathyroid glands	• Regulate calcium (Ca^{2+}) and phosphate (HPO_4^{2-}) balance by means of PTH; PTH influences bone reabsorption, calcium absorption from the intestines, and calcium reabsorption from the renal tubules.
	  1. Increased secretion of PTH causes
	    a. Elevated serum calcium concentration
	    b. Lowered serum phosphate concentration
	  2. Conversely, decreased secretion of PTH causes
	    a. Lowered serum calcium concentration
	    b. Elevated serum phosphate concentration

(Data from Metheny, N. M. [1992]. *Fluid and electrolyte balance* [2nd ed.]. Philadelphia: Lippincott.)

They selectively retain electrolytes and water and excrete wastes and excesses. Renal failure results in serious fluid and electrolyte problems.

Cardiovascular System The cardiovascular system is responsible for pumping and carrying nutrients and water throughout the body.

Lungs The lungs regulate oxygen and carbon dioxide levels of the blood. The regulation of the carbon dioxide level is especially crucial in maintaining acid–base balance, and is explained later in this chapter.

Adrenal Glands The adrenal glands secrete aldosterone, which is known as the great sodium conserver of the body. The hormone also helps save chloride and water, and causes potassium to be excreted as indicated.

Pituitary Gland The posterior lobe of the pituitary gland stores ADH, which is manufactured in the hypothalamus. Neurons called *osmoreceptors* are sensitive to changes in the concentration of ECF and send appropriate impulses accordingly to release ADH.

Thyroid Gland Thyroxine, released by the thyroid gland, increases blood flow in the body. This in turn increases renal circulation, which results in increased glomerular filtration and urinary output.

Parathyroid Glands The parathyroid glands secrete parathyroid hormone, which regulates the level of calcium in ECF.

Gastrointestinal Tract The GI tract absorbs water and nutrients that enter the body through this route.

Nervous System The nervous system acts as a switchboard and inhibits and stimulates mechanisms that influence fluid balance. It functions chiefly as the regulator of sodium and water intake and excretion. The thirst center is located in the hypothalamus.

Acid–Base Balance

Body fluids must maintain a normal acid–base balance to sustain health and life. Acidity or alkalinity of a solution is determined by its concentration of hydrogen ions (H^+) and hydroxyl ions (OH^-). An **acid** is a substance containing hydrogen ions that can be liberated or released. An **alkali** is a **base**, which is a substance that can accept or trap a hydrogen ion. The following equations illustrate:

Equation: An acid releases hydrogen, as follows:

$$H_2CO_3 \rightarrow H^+ + HCO_3^-$$

Carbonic releases hydrogen to form bicarbonate
acid   ion   base

Equation: A base traps hydrogen, as follows:

$$HCO_3^- + H^+ \rightarrow H_2CO_3$$

Bicarbonate traps hydrogen to form carbonic
base   ion   acid

Equation: A base traps hydrogen, as follows:

$$OH^- + H^+ \rightarrow H_2O$$

Hydroxyl traps hydrogen to form water
ion from   ion
a base

The unit of measure used to describe acid–base balance is pH, which is an expression of hydrogen-ion concentration and the resulting acidity of a substance. The pH scale ranges from 1 to 14. Neutrality of a solution is 7; an example is pure water. Because pH is based on a negative logarithm, as the hydrogen ions increase and a solution becomes more acid, the pH becomes less than 7. When the concentration of the hydroxyl ions exceeds the concentration of hydrogen ions, the solution is alkaline and the pH is greater than 7. Gastric secretions that are strongly acidic have an approximate pH of 1 to 1.3, whereas strongly alkaline pancreatic secretions have an approximate pH of 10.

Normal blood plasma is slightly alkaline and has a normal pH range of 7.35 to 7.45. When the normal pH range is exceeded in either direction, the person develops signs and symptoms of illness, and if the condition goes on unabated, death results. **Acidosis** is the condition characterized by a proportionate excess of hydrogen ions in ECF in which the pH falls below 7.35. **Alkalosis** occurs when there is a proportionate lack of hydrogen ions and the pH exceeds 7.45. Figure 37-8 illustrates normal pH, acidosis, and alkalosis, and also the points at which death can be expected to occur.

The narrow range of normal pH is achieved by three major homeostatic regulators of hydrogen ions: (1) buffer systems, (2) respiratory mechanisms, and (3) renal mechanisms. A **buffer** is a substance that prevents body fluids from becoming overly acidic or alkaline. The body has three buffer systems: (1) the carbonic acid–sodium bicarbonate buffer system, (2) the phosphate buffer system, and (3) the protein buffer system.

Buffer Systems

Carbonic Acid–Sodium Bicarbonate Buffer System The most important buffer system of the body is the carbonic acid–sodium bicarbonate system. This system buffers up to 90% of the H^+ of ECF. The following two equations illustrate the system:

Equation: A strong acid plus sodium bicarbonate yields a weak acid, as follows:

$$HCl + NaHCO_3 \rightarrow NACl + H_2CO_3$$

Strong   added   sodium   yields salt and weak
hydrochloric to   bicarbonate   carbonic
acid   base   acid

Equation: A strong base plus a weak acid yields a weak base, as follows:

$$NaOH + H_2CO_3 \rightarrow NaHCO_3 + H_2O$$

Strong   added carbonic yields weak   and water
sodium   to   acid   sodium
hydroxide   buffer   bicarbonate
base   base

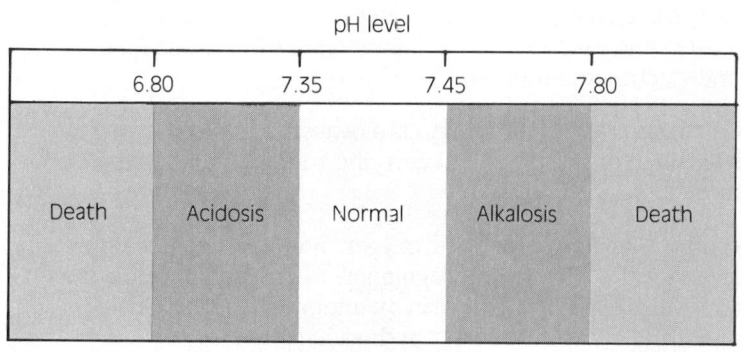

pH level				
6.80	7.35	7.45	7.80	
Death	Acidosis	Normal	Alkalosis	Death

Bicarbonate 20 parts

Carbonic acid 1 part

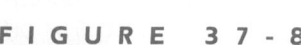

FIGURE   37-8

Acid–base balance. Note that acidosis is used to describe the condition when pH is between 6.80 and 7.35. When the fluid acidity falls below 7, the person is gravely ill or dying.

The ratio of carbonic acid to the base bicarbonate is important for acid–base balance. Normal ECF has a ratio of 20 parts bicarbonate to 1 part carbonic acid. The exact quantities are unimportant for acid–base balance as long as they remain in a 20 : 1 ratio.

Phosphate Buffer System   Phosphate salts are formed in the kidneys by exchanging a sodium ion for a hydrogen ion in the conversion of alkaline sodium phosphate (Na_2HPO_4) to acid sodium phosphate (NaH_2PO_4). The acid sodium phosphate is then excreted. This occurs in the following way:

Equation: The conversion of sodium phosphate to acid sodium phosphate occurs as follows:

$$Na_2HPO_4 + H^+ \rightarrow NaH_2PO_4 + Na^+$$

Alkaline   and   hydrogen   yields   acid sodium   and   sodium
sodium   phosphate
phosphate

Protein Buffer System   The third buffer system is a mixture of plasma proteins and the globin portion of hemoglobin in RBCs. Because plasma proteins and hemoglobin possess groups that can combine with or liberate hydrogen ions, they tend to minimize changes in pH and serve as excellent buffering agents over a wide range of pH values. The following equations illustrate the oxygenation of hemoglobin as it proceeds in conjunction with the bicarbonate buffer system:

Equation: The high oxygen pressure in the lungs forces oxygen into hemoglobin converting it to oxyhemoglobin:

$$HHb + O_2 \rightarrow HbO_2 + H^+$$

Hemoglobin   and   oxygen   yields   oxyhemoglobin   and   hydrogen
in red cell   from   goes in red cell   ion in
air   to tissues   red cell

Equation: The hydrogen ions are promptly neutralized by bicarbonate ions producing carbonic acid:

$$H^+ + HCO_3^- \rightarrow H_2CO_3$$

Hydrogen ion   and   bicarbonate ion   yields   carbonic acid
just made   in red cell and   in red cell
from tissues

Equation: Carbonic acid decomposes to water and carbon dioxide, which departs by exhaling:

$$H_2CO_3 \rightarrow H_2O + CO_2$$

carbonic acid   yields   water   and   carbon dioxide
just made in   leaves lungs in
red cell   exhaled air

Respiratory Control of H^+ Balance

The lungs are the primary controller of the body's carbonic-acid supply. They have a huge surface area from which CO_2 can readily diffuse and they can bring about rapid changes in H^+ when needed. Carbon dioxide is constantly produced by cellular metabolism and enters ECF. As it does, the carbon dioxide and water are acted upon by the enzyme carbonic anhydrase to produce carbonic acid. The following equations illustrate how carbonic acid is produced and broken down:

Equation: The production of carbonic acid occurs as follows:

$$CO_2 + H_2O \xrightarrow[\text{yields}]{\text{(carbonic anhydrase)}} H_2CO_3$$

Carbon   and   water   carbonic
dioxide   acid

Equation: The breakdown of carbonic acid occurs as follows:

$$H_2CO_3 \xrightarrow[\text{yields}]{\text{(carbonic anhydrase)}} H_2O + CO_2$$

Carbonic   water   and   carbon
acid   dioxide

Carbon dioxide is excreted by exhalation. As the amount of carbon dioxide in the blood increases, the sensitive respiratory center in the medulla is stimulated and increases the rate and depth of respirations to eliminate more carbon dioxide. When the blood level of carbon dioxide is below normal, the center decreases the rate and depth of respirations to retain the carbon dioxide so that carbonic acid can be formed and the delicate balance maintained. This total respiratory process also occurs frequently and nearly as rapidly as the buffering action in the carbonic acid–sodium bicarbonate system.

Renal Control of H⁺ Balance

The concentration of bicarbonate in the plasma is regulated by the kidneys through the production of ammonia (NH_3), the excretion of hydrogen ions, and by forming additional bicarbonate as needed. The kidneys regulate hydrogen and bicarbonate ions in the following ways:

Equation: The reabsorption of bicarbonate becomes possible when a sodium ion combines with bicarbonate to form sodium bicarbonate, which is taken up in the kidney tubules, as follows:

$$Na^+ \quad + \quad HCO_3^- \quad \rightarrow \quad NaHCO_3$$

Sodium and bicarbonate yields sodium bicarbonate

Equation: As a result of amino acid metabolism, ammonia (NH_3) is formed in the kidney tubules, where it unites with hydrogen to form an ammonium ion (NH_4^+), which, in turn, unites with chloride (Cl^-) to form ammonium chloride (NH_4Cl) for excretion, as follows:

$$NH_3 \quad + \quad H^+ \quad \rightarrow \quad NH_4^+$$

Ammonia and hydrogen yields ammonium

$$NH_4^+ \quad + \quad Cl^- \quad \rightarrow \quad NH_4Cl$$

Ammonium and chloride yields ammonium chloride

Acid–base regulation by the kidneys occurs more slowly than by the carbonic acid–sodium bicarbonate system or by respiratory regulation. It may take up to 3 days for fluid pH to be restored by the kidneys. The pH of urine varies, depending on the ions that are being excreted, but generally it is in the 4.5 to 8.2 range.

Disturbances in Fluid, Electrolyte, and Acid–Base Balance

Nurses commonly encounter disturbances in fluid, electrolyte, and acid–base balance while caring for acutely or chronically ill clients. Although many of these disturbances are interrelated and may occur together, they are presented singly for the purpose of study.

Fluid Imbalances

Fluid imbalances occur when the body's compensatory mechanisms are unable to maintain a homeostatic state. Fluid imbalances may relate to either volume or distribution of water or electrolytes.

Fluid Volume Deficit   Fluid volume deficit (FVD) is a deficiency in the amount of both water and electrolytes in ECF, but the water and electrolyte proportions remain near normal. The state is commonly known as *hypovolemia*. Both osmotic- and hydrostatic-pressure changes force the interstitial fluid into the intravascular space. As the interstitial space is depleted, its fluid becomes hypertonic, and cellular fluid is then drawn into the interstitial space, leaving cells without adequate fluid to function properly.

Dehydration is sometimes used as a synonym for hypovolemia, but this is technically inaccurate. **Dehydration** refers only to a decreased volume of water, but water is not decreased without electrolyte changes also. *Hydration* is the union of a substance with water and is often used to indicate that there is normal water volume in the body.

FVDs result from the loss of body fluids, especially if fluid intake is simultaneously decreased. Table 37-3 summarizes FVD, common problems, and general nursing interventions. Specific interventions are presented later in this chapter.

The very young and elderly people and those individuals fatigued or weakened by illness are particularly susceptible to hypovolemia. A weight loss of 5% for adults and 10% for infants can occur rapidly. A 5% weight loss is considered to be pronounced fluid deficit, and an 8% loss or more is considered severe. A 15% weight loss owing to fluid deficiency usually threatens life.

Third-space fluid shift refers to a distributional shift of body fluids into body spaces such as the pleural, peritoneal, pericardial, or joint cavities, the bowel, or into the interstitial space (plasma-to-interstitial shift). Once trapped in these spaces, the fluid is not easily exchanged with ECF and a deficit in ECF volume is created. Treatment is directed toward correction of the cause of the third-space shift.

Fluid Volume Excess   Excessive retention of water and sodium in ECF in near-normal proportions results in a condition termed **fluid volume excess**. It is also called *hypervolemia*. Overhydration is commonly used as a synonym for hypervolemia, but strictly speaking, this is inaccurate. *Overhydration* refers only to above-normal amounts of water in extracellular spaces. Malfunction of the kidneys, causing an inability to excrete the excesses, is the most common cause. When water is retained in excessive amounts, so is sodium.

Because of the increased extracellular osmotic pressure from the retained sodium, fluid is pulled from the cells to equalize the tonicity. By the time the intracellular and extracellular spaces are isotonic to each other, an excess of both water and sodium are in ECF, while the cells are nearly depleted. The excessive ECF may accumulate in tissue spaces; this is known as **edema**. Edema is most frequently seen around the eyes, fingers, ankles, and sacral space (Fig. 37-9). It may result in a weight gain in excess of 5%. When the excess fluid remains in the intravascular space, the concentration of solids in the blood is decreased.

Interstitial-to-plasma shift is the movement of fluid from the space surrounding the cells to the blood. This shift, also called hypervolemia, is a compensatory response to volume or osmotic-pressure changes of the intravascular fluid. While the body attempts to maintain normal balance in all fluid spaces, if circumstances demand, the intravascular fluid is usually protected at the expense of interstitial fluid and ICF.

(Text continues on p. 1008)

Fluid Volume Disturbances: Related Factors, Defining Characteristics, and Nursing Interventions

Related Factors	Defining Characteristics	Nursing Interventions
Summary of Fluid Volume Deficit		

Loss of water and electrolytes, as in
• Vomiting
• Diarrhea
• Excessive laxative use
• Fistulas
• GI suction
• Polyuria
• Fever
• Excessive sweating
• Third-space fluid shifts
 	
Decreased intake, as in:
• Anorexia
• Nausea
• Inability to gain access to fluids
• Inability to swallow fluids
• Depression
	Weight loss over short period (except in third-space losses)
	• 2% (mild deficit, such as 2.4 lb in 120-lb person or 1 kg in a 54.5-kg person)
	• 5% (moderate deficit, such as 6 lb in 120-lb person or 2.1 kg in a 54.5-kg person)
	• 8% or more (severe deficit, such as 10 lb or more in 120-lb person or 4.5 kg or more in a 54.5-kg person)
	
	Decreased skin and tongue turgor
	
	Dry mucous membranes
	
	Urine output less than 30 mL/hr in adult
	
	Postural hypotension (systolic pressure drops by more than 15 mm Hg when client moves from lying to standing or sitting position
	
	Weak, rapid pulse
	
	Slow-filling peripheral veins
	
	Decreased body temperature, such as 95° to 98°F (35° to 36.7°C) unless infection is present
	
	CVP less than 4 cm H_2O in vena cava
	
	BUN elevated out of proportion to serum creatinine
	
	Specific gravity (SG) high (urine)
	
	Hematocrit elevated
	
	Flat neck veins in supine position
	
	Marked oliguria, late
	
	Altered sensorium
	
	Cold extremities, late
		1. Assess for presence, or worsening of FVD (see defining characteristics).
		2. Administer oral fluids if indicated.
		  • Consider the client's likes and dislikes when offering fluids.
		  • Consider the type of fluid the client has lost and replace appropriately.
		  • If the client is reluctant to drink because of oral discomfort, select fluids that are nonirritating to the mucosa, and provide frequent mouth care (offer saline gargles and apply lubricant to lips).
		  • Offer fluids at frequent intervals.
		  • Explain the need for fluid replacement to the client and attempt to gain his or her cooperation.
		  • Administer prn medications if nausea is present to provide relief before fluids are offered.
		3. Consider the following interventions for clients with impaired swallowing:
		  • Assess gag reflex and ability to swallow water before offering solid foods; have a suction apparatus on hand.
		  • Position the client in an upright position with head and neck flexed slightly forward during feeding (tilting the head backward during swallowing predisposes to aspiration because this position opens the airway).
		  • Provide thick fluids or semisolid foods (such as puddings or gelatin). These are more easily swallowed because of their consistency and weight than are thin liquids.
		4. If the client is unable to eat and drink, discuss possibility of tube feedings with the physician.
		5. Consult with the physician for parenteral fluid directives if the client is unable to consume fluids by the enteral route.
		6. Monitor response to fluid intake, either orally or parenterally. If therapy is adequate, one should observe
		  • Increased urinary volume, toward 40 to 60 mL/hr in adult
		  • If previously hypotensive, increased blood pressure toward normal
		  • Return of pulse rate to baseline
		  • Improved sensorium and sense of vitality
		  • Improved skin and tongue turgor
		(continued)

Fluid Volume Disturbances: Related Factors, Defining Characteristics, and Nursing Interventions

Related Factors	Defining Characteristics	Nursing Interventions
		• Decreased dryness of oral mucosa • Increased CVP, toward normal • Normal, or no worse, breath sounds • Decreased urinary SG as urinary volume increases • Increased body weight, toward preillness level 7. Monitor clients with tendency for abnormal fluid retention (such as renal or cardiac problems) for signs of overload during aggressive fluid replacement. 8. Turn client frequently; apply moisturizing agents to skin and massage bony prominences to avoid skin breakdown. 9. Give frequent oral care.

Summary of Fluid Volume Excess

Compromised regulatory mechanisms: • Renal failure • Congestive heart failure • Cirrhosis of liver • Cushing's syndrome Overzealous administration of sodium-containing IV fluids Excessive ingestion of sodium-containing substances in diet or sodium-containing medications	Weight gain over short period • 2% (mild excess, such as 2.4-lb gain in 120-lb person or 1 kg in a 54.5-kg person) • 5% (moderate excess, such as 6-lb gain in 120-lb person or 2.7 kg in a 54.5-kg person) • 8% or more (severe excess, such as 10-lb or more gain in 120-lb person or 4.5 kg or more in a 54.5-kg person) Peripheral edema (excess of fluid in interstitial space) Distended neck veins Distended peripheral veins Slow-emptying peripheral veins CVP over 11 cm H_2O in vena cava Moist rales in lungs Polyuria (if renal function is normal) Ascites, pleural effusion (when FVE is severe, fluid transudates into body cavities) Decreased BUN (due to plasma dilution) Decreased hematocrit (also due to plasma dilution) Bounding, full pulse Pulmonary edema, if severe	1. Assess for the presence, or worsening of fluid volume excess (FVE). 2. Encourage adherence to sodium-restricted diet, if prescribed. Assist dietitian in diet instruction. 3. Instruct clients requiring sodium restriction to avoid over-the-counter drugs without first checking with the health care adviser. 4. When fluid retention persists despite adherence to dietary sodium intake, consider hidden sources of sodium, such as water supply or use of water softeners. 5. When indicated, encourage rest periods. Lying down favors diuresis of edema fluid. 6. Monitor the client's response to diuretics. Discuss significant findings with physician. 7. Monitor rate of parenteral fluids and the client's response. Discuss significant findings with physician. 8. Teach self-monitoring of weight and intake and output measurements to clients with chronic fluid retention (such as those with congestive heart failure, renal disease, or cirrhosis of liver). 9. Monitor for worsening of underlying cause of FVE. 10. If dyspnea and orthopnea are present, position the client in semi-Fowler's position to favor lung expansion. 11. Turn and position the client frequently; be aware that edematous tissue is more prone to skin breakdown than is normal tissue.

(Data from Metheny, N. M. [1992]. *Fluid and electrolyte balance* [2nd ed.]. Philadelphia: Lippincott.)

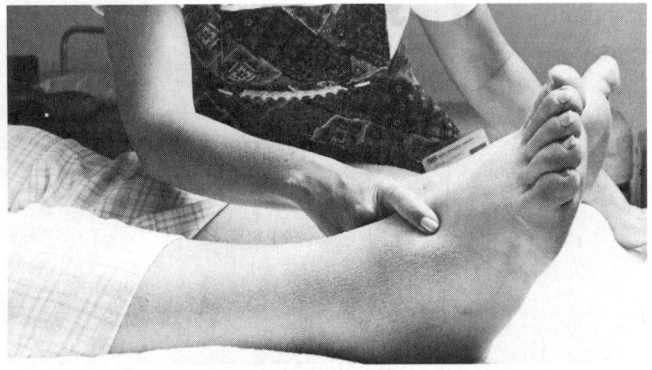

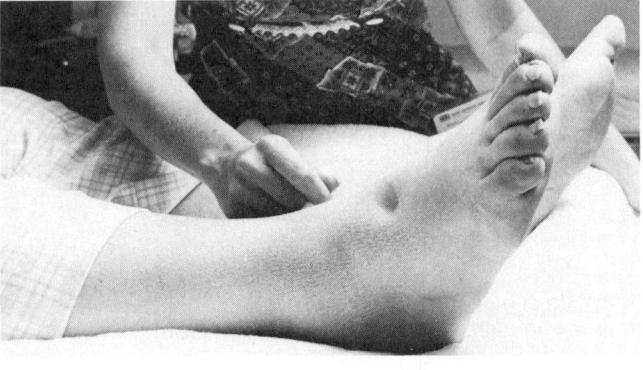

F I G U R E 3 7 - 9

(Top) The nurse depresses an area near the ankle of the client where edema is present. *(Bottom)* An indentation of edematous tissues remains after the nurse releases pressure.

Table 37-3 summarizes FVEs, examples of common problems likely to produce them, and common nursing interventions. Specific nursing interventions for these problems are presented later in this chapter.

Electrolyte Imbalances

When clients present with deficits or excesses of sodium, potassium, calcium, magnesium, or phosphate, special nursing care is required. Table 37-4 highlights etiologic factors, defining characteristics, nursing interventions for common electrolyte imbalances, and specific nursing strategies to prevent these problems.

Hyponatremia and Hypernatremia *Hyponatremia* refers to a sodium deficit in ECF. Osmotic pressure changes result in ECF moving into the cells. When this occurs, a typical sign is fingerprints over the sternum, that is, an examiner's fingerprints tend to remain on the client's skin over the sternum when pressure is applied with the fingers. The phenomenon results from tissue plasticity as fluid moves into cells in excess amounts. *Hypernatremia* refers to a surplus of sodium in ECF. Because of the increased extracellular osmotic pressure, fluids move from the cells, leaving them without sufficient fluid.

Hypokalemia and Hyperkalemia *Hypokalemia* refers to a potassium deficit in ECF. When the extracellular potassium level falls, potassium moves from the cell, creating an intracellular potassium deficiency. Sodium and hydrogen ions are then retained by the cells to maintain isotonic fluids. These electrolyte shifts not only influence normal cellular functioning but also influence the pH of ECF. Muscle tissues are generally the first to demonstrate a potassium deficiency. *Hyperkalemia* refers to an excess of potassium in ECF. Although this condition occurs less frequently than hypokalemia, it can be hazardous. The transmission of stimuli through heart muscle is slowed or prevented, and cardiac arrest eventually occurs if hyperkalemia is not corrected.

Hypocalcemia and Hypercalcemia *Hypocalcemia* refers to a calcium deficit in ECF. If the condition is prolonged, calcium is taken from the bones. This results in **osteomalacia**, which is characterized by soft and pliable bones. *Hypercalcemia* refers to an excess of calcium in ECF. Hypercalcemia presents an emergency situation because the condition often leads to cardiac arrest.

Hypomagnesemia and Hypermagnesemia *Hypomagnesemia* refers to a magnesium deficit. The body's potassium level also drops because the kidneys tend to excrete more potassium when magnesium supplies are poor. As a result, hypomagnesemia and hypokalemia often occur together. A magnesium deficit is ordinarily treated with the administration of magnesium sulfate. *Hypermagnesemia* refers to a magnesium excess. It is a rare condition, but it does occur when the kidneys fail to excrete magnesium and when excessive amounts are used therapeutically.

Hypophosphatemia and Hyperphosphatemia *Hypophosphatemia* refers to a below-normal serum concentration of inorganic phosphorus. Although this may indicate phosphorus deficiency, multiple factors may lower serum phosphate levels while total body phosphorus stores are normal. *Hyperphosphatemia* refers to above-normal serum concentrations of inorganic phosphorus.

Acid–Base Imbalances

Acid–base imbalances can be assessed by using laboratory plasma findings. The pH of plasma indicates balance or impending acidosis or alkalosis. In addition, however, a study of the blood's oxygen and carbon dioxide gases is important. The partial pressures of these gases, or their tensions, are determined by the use of a nomogram, which reflects the chemical and physical activities of the two gases. The partial pressure of carbon dioxide is abbreviated pCO_2; for oxygen, it is pO_2. When the pO_2 is low, hemoglobin carries less than normal amounts of oxygen; when the pO_2 is high, the hemoglobin carries more oxygen. The pCO_2 is influenced almost entirely by respiratory activity. When

(Text continues on p. 1016)

Electrolyte Disturbances: Related Factors, Defining Characteristics, and Nursing Interventions

Related Factors	Defining Characteristics	Nursing Interventions

Hyponatremia

Related Factors	Defining Characteristics	Nursing Interventions
Loss of sodium, as in: • Loss of GI fluids • Use of diuretics • Adrenal insufficiency • Salt-losing nephritis • Osmotic diuresis Gains of water, as in: • Excessive administration of D_5W • Psychogenic polydipsia • Excessive water administration with hypotonic tube feedings Disease states associated with SIADH (a form of hyponatremia): • Oat-cell carcinoma of lung • Carcinoma of duodenum or pancreas • Head trauma • Stroke • Pulmonary disorders (abscesses, pneumonia, tuberculosis) Pharmacologic agents that may impair renal water excretion, such as: • Nicotine • Morphine • Barbiturates • Acetaminophen	Anorexia Nausea Vomiting Lethargy Confusion Muscle cramps Fingerprinting over sternum Muscular twitching Seizures Coma Papilledema Hemiparesis Serum Na below 135 mEq/L Serum osmolality less than 285 mOsm Urinary Na level varies with cause of hyponatremia	1. Identify clients at risk for hyponatremia. 2. Monitor fluid losses and gains. Look for loss of sodium-containing fluids, particularly in conjunction with low-sodium intake. 3. Monitor for presence of gastrointestinal symptoms, such as anorexia, nausea, vomiting, and abdominal cramping. 4. Monitor for central nervous system changes, such as lethargy, confusion, muscular twitching, and convulsions. Be aware that more severe neurologic signs are associated with very low sodium levels that have fallen rapidly due to water overloading. 5. Monitor laboratory data for serum sodium levels less than normal. 6. Check specific gravity of urine. 7. With clients able to consume a general diet, encourage foods and fluids with a high sodium content. For example, broth made with one beef cube contains about 900 mg of sodium; 8 oz (250 mL) of canned tomato juice contain about 700 mg of sodium. 8. Be familiar with the sodium content of commonly used parenteral fluids. Monitor clients with cardiovascular disease receiving sodium-containing fluids closely for signs of circulatory overload, such as moist rales in the lungs. 9. Use extreme caution when administering hypertonic saline solutions (3% or 5% NaCl). Be aware that these fluids can be *lethal* if infused carelessly. 10. Avoid giving large water supplements to clients receiving isotonic tube feedings, particularly if routes of abnormal sodium loss are present or water is being retained abnormally. 11. Monitor clients with decreased adrenal function for signs of acute adrenocortical insufficiency (adrenal crisis) when they are exposed to severe stress (such as surgery, trauma, emotional upset, excessive heat, or prolonged medical illness). Look for extreme weakness, acute onset of nausea and vomiting, hypotension, confusion, and even shock.

Hypernatremia

Related Factors	Defining Characteristics	Nursing Interventions
Deprivation of water, most common in those unable to perceive or respond to thirst Hypertonic tube feedings with inadequate water supplements Increased insensible water loss (as in hyperventilation) Water diarrhea Ingestion of salt in unusual amounts Excessive parenteral administration of sodium-containing solutions: • Hypertonic saline (3% or 5% NaCl)	Thirst Elevated body temperature Tongue dry and swollen, sticky mucous membranes Severe hypernatremia • Disorientation • Hallucinations • Lethargy when undisturbed • Irritable and hyperreactive when stimulated • Focal or grand mal seizures, coma Serum Na above 145 mEq/L Serum osmolality above 295 mOsm Urinary SG greater than	1. Identify clients at risk of hypernatremia. 2. Monitor fluid losses and gains. Look for abnormal losses of water or low water intake, and for large gains of sodium as might occur with ingestion of proprietary drugs with a high sodium content (such as Alka-Seltzer, an effervescent antacid). Also, consider that prescription drugs may have a high sodium content. Of course, one should look for excessive intake of high sodium foods. 3. Monitor for changes in behavior, such as restlessness, disorientation, and lethargy. 4. Look for excessive thirst and elevated body temperature. If present, evaluate in relation to other signs. 5. Monitor serum sodium levels as indicated. 6. Prevent hypernatremia in debilitated clients unable to perceive or respond to thirst by offering them fluids at regular intervals. If fluid intake remains inadequate, consult with the physician to plan an alternate route

(continued)

T A B L E 3 7 - 4 (continued)

Electrolyte Disturbances: Related Factors, Defining Characteristics, and Nursing Interventions

Related Factors	Defining Characteristics	Nursing Interventions
Hypernatremia • 7.5% sodium bicarbonate • Isotonic saline Profuse sweating Diabetes insipidus Heatstroke Drowning in sea water Hypertonic saline accidentally introduced into maternal circulation during therapeutic abortion	1.015, provided water loss is from nonrenal route	for intake, either by tube feedings or by the parenteral route. 7. If tube feedings are used, give sufficient water to keep the serum sodium and the BUN level within normal limits. Be aware that the higher the osmolality of the feeding, the greater the need for water supplements. 8. Monitor the client's response to corrective parenteral fluids by reviewing serial sodium levels and by observing for changes in neurologic signs. With gradual decrease in the serum sodium level, the neurological signs should improve, not worsen. Be aware that the serum sodium should be dropped gradually.
Hypokalemia Diarrhea Vomiting or gastric suction Potassium-losing diuretics (such as furosemide and thiazides) Steroid administration Carbenicillin, sodium penicillin, amphotericin B Hyperaldosteronism Hyperalimentation Poor intake, as in anorexia nervosa, alcoholism, potassium-free parenteral fluids Osmotic diuresis (as occurs in uncontrolled diabetes mellitus or mannitol administration) Renal tubular acidosis Cushing's syndrome	Fatigue Anorexia, nausea, and vomiting Muscle weakness Decreased bowel motility (intestinal ileus) Cardiac arrhythmias Increased sensitivity to digitalis toxicity Polyuria, nocturia, dilute urine (if hypokalemia is prolonged) Mild hyperglycemia Postural hypotension Serum K below 3.5 mEq/L Paresthesias or tender muscles ECG changes: Flattened T waves ST segment depression	1. Be aware of clients at risk for hypokalemia and monitor for its occurrence. Hypokalemia can be life-threatening; it is important to detect it early. 2. Assess digitalized clients at-risk for hypokalemia especially closely for symptoms of digitalis toxicity because hypokalemia potentiates the action of digitalis. Be aware that the physician usually prefers to keep the serum potassium level above 3.5 mEq/L in digitalized clients. 3. Take measures to prevent hypokalemia when possible. a. Prevention may take the form of encouraging extra potassium intake for at-risk client (when the diet allows). b. When hypokalemia is due to abuse of laxatives or diuretics, education of the client may help alleviate the problem. 4. Administer oral potassium supplements when prescribed. 5. Be aware that clients may not need potassium supplements if they are using salt substitutes because these substances usually contain sizable amounts of potassium. Educate clients regarding the use of salt substitutes. 6. Be thoroughly familiar with the critical facts related to administering potassium intravenously. 7. Be aware that any client experiencing life-threatening symptoms, such as arrhythmias or paralysis, requires urgent replacement of potassium.
Hyperkalemia Pseudohyperkalemia: • Tight tourniquet • Hemolysis of sample • Leukocytosis • Thrombocytosis Decreased potassium excretion: • Oliguric renal failure • Potassium-conserving diuretics • Hypoaldosteronism High potassium intake, especially in presence of renal insufficiency:	Vague muscular weakness is usually first sign Cardiac arrhythmias, bradycardia, and heart block can occur Paresthesias of face, tongue, feet, and hands Flaccid muscle paralysis (spreads from legs to trunk and arms; respiratory muscles may be affected) GI symptoms such as nausea, intermittent intestinal colic, or diarrhea may occur	1. Be aware of clients at risk for hyperkalemia and monitor for its occurrence. Hyperkalemia is life threatening; it is imperative to detect it early. 2. Take measures to prevent hyperkalemia when possible by following guidelines for administering potassium safely, both intravenously and orally. a. Follow rules for safe administration of potassium. b. Avoid administration of potassium-conserving diuretics, potassium supplements, or salt substitutes to clients with renal insufficiency. c. Caution clients to use salt substitutes sparingly if they are taking other supplementary forms of potassium or are taking potassium-conserving diuretics (eg, spironolactone, triamterene, and amiloride).

(continued)

T A B L E 3 7 - 4 (continued)

Electrolyte Disturbances: Related Factors, Defining Characteristics, and Nursing Interventions

Related Factors	Defining Characteristics	Nursing Interventions

• Improper use of oral potassium supplements
• Rapid or excessive administration of IV potassium
• Rapid transfusion of aged blood
• High-dose potassium penicillin
• Foods high in potassium (such as dried apricots)
 	
Shift of potassium out of cells:
• Acidosis
• Tissue trauma
• Malignant cell lysis
	ECG changes: tall, peaked T waves, absent P waves, widened QRS complex.
	
	Serum K above 5.0 mEq/L (mmol/L)
		d. Caution hyperkalemic clients to avoid foods high in potassium content. Some of these are coffee, cocoa, tea, dried fruits, dried beans, whole-grain breads, and milk desserts. Meat and eggs also contain substantial amounts of potassium. (Foods with minimal potassium content include butter, margarine, cranberry juice or sauce, ginger ale, gumdrops or jellybeans, lollypops, root beer, sugar or honey.)
		3. To avoid false reports of hyperkalemia, take the following precautions:
		  a. Avoid prolonged use of tourniquet while drawing blood sample
		  b. Do not allow client to exercise extremity immediately before drawing blood sample
		  c. Take blood sample to laboratory as soon as possible (serum must be separated from cells within 1 hour after collection)
		  d. Avoid drawing blood specimen from a site above an infusion of potassium solution (or any solution for that matter).
		4. Be familiar with usual treatment regimens for hyperkalemia and factors related to their safe implementation.

Hypocalcemia
 	
Surgical hypoparathyroidism (may follow thyroid surgery or radical neck surgery for cancer)
 	
Malabsorption
 	
Vitamin D deficiency
 	
Acute pancreatitis
 	
Excessive administration of citrated blood
 	
Primary hypoparathyroidism
 	
Alkalotic states (decreased ionized calcium)
 	
Hyperphosphatemia
 	
Medullary carcinoma of thyroid
 	
Hypoalbuminemia (as in cirrhosis, nephrotic syndrome, and starvation)
 	
Hypomagnesemia
 	
Decreased ultraviolet exposure
	Numbness, tingling of fingers, circumoral region, and toes
	
	Cramps in muscles of extremities
	
	Hyperactive deep-tendon reflexes (such as patellar and triceps)
	
	Trousseau's sign
	
	Chvostek's sign
	
	Mental changes, such as confusion and alterations in mood and memory
	
	Convulsions (usually generalized but may be focal)
	
	Spasm of laryngeal muscles
	
	Cardiac manifestations; ECG shows prolonged QT interval
	
	Spasms of muscles in abdomen (can simulate acute abdominal emergency)
	
	Total serum calcium level below 8.5 mg/dL or ionized level below normal (below 50%)
	
	Sulkowitch's test shows light precipitation
		1. Be aware of clients at risk for hypocalcemia and monitor for its occurrence.
		2. Be prepared to take seizure precautions when hypocalcemia is severe.
		3. Monitor condition of airway closely because laryngeal stridor can occur.
		4. Take safety precautions if confusion is present.
		5. Be aware of factors related to the safe administration of calcium replacement salts.
		6. Educate people in high-risk groups for osteoporosis (especially postmenopausal women not on estrogen therapy) as to the need for dietary calcium intake. If adequate amounts are not consumed in the diet (as is often the case), calcium supplements should be considered.
		  a. Most sources recommend that the calcium intake for these individuals be 1000 to 1500 mg each day. Of course, the best way for healthy people to ensure an adequate calcium intake is to eat a wide variety of foods from the four food groups daily.
		  b. As stated in *a*, calcium supplements may be necessary for people unable to consume enough calcium in the diet, such as those who do not tolerate milk or dairy products well. Numerous preparations can be obtained over the counter and consumers need advice in selecting suitable products. It appears that calcium is best absorbed when taken in divided doses, rather than all at once. Also, it is suggested that some of the calcium be taken at bedtime because calcium loss accelerates during sleep. (Antacids containing aluminum may increase bone loss, and their use is discouraged in people having bone health problems; among these products are Rolaids, Tempo, Di-Gel, Gaviscon, Gelusil, and Mylanta.)

(continued)

T A B L E 3 7 - 4 *(continued)*

Electrolyte Disturbances: Related Factors, Defining Characteristics, and Nursing Interventions

Related Factors	Defining Characteristics	Nursing Interventions
Hypocalcemia		

c. Some postmenopausal women are advised by their physicians to take estrogen. For those who cannot take estrogen, synthetically produced calcitonin is now available by prescription.

d. Encourage people with a tendency to form renal stones to consult their physicians before greatly increasing their calcium intake. Also, it is important to encourage these people to drink no less than 2 to 3 qt of fluid a day to protect against stone formation.

7. Educate people at risk for osteoporosis about the value of regular physical exercise in decreasing bone loss.

8. To prevent osteoporosis in later years, educate young women about the need for a normal diet to ensure adequate calcium intake. Also, discuss the calcium-losing aspects of alcohol and nicotine use.

Hypercalcemia

Related Factors	Defining Characteristics	Nursing Interventions
Hyperparathyroidism	Muscular weakness	
Malignant neoplastic disease:	Tiredness, listlessness, lethargy	
• Solid tumors with metastases (breast, prostate, and malignant melanomas)	Constipation	
• Solid tumors without bony metastases (lung, head and neck, and renal tumors)	Anorexia, nausea, and vomiting	
• Hematologic tumors (lymphoma, acute leukemia, and myeloma)	Decreased memory span, decreased attention span, and confusion	
Prolonged immobilization	Polyuria and polydipsia	
Large doses of vitamin D	Renal stones	
Overuse of calcium-containing antacids or calcium supplements	Neurotic behavior progressing to frank psychoses may occur (reversible with correction of hypercalcemia)	
Thiazide diuretics	Cardiac arrest may occur in hypercalcemic crisis	
Milk–alkali syndrome	ECG shows shortened QT interval	

Defining Characteristics (continued):

Bone changes seen on film in chronic hypercalcemia

Itching and ocular changes (band keratopathy)

Serum calcium over 10.5 mg/dL

Sulkowitch's test shows dense precipitation

Nursing Interventions:

1. Be aware of clients at risk for hypercalcemia and monitor for its presence.

2. Increase client mobilization when feasible; recall that immobilization favors hypercalcemia.

3. Encourage the oral intake of sufficient fluids to keep the client well hydrated. Sodium-containing fluids should be given, unless contraindicated by other conditions, because sodium favors calcium excretion.

4. Discourage excessive consumption of milk products and other high-calcium foods.

5. Encourage adequate bulk in the diet to offset the tendency for constipation.

6. Take safety precautions if confusion or other mental symptoms of hypercalcemia are present. Explain to the client and family that the mental changes associated with hypercalcemia are reversible with treatment.

7. Be aware that cardiac arrest can occur in clients with severe hypercalcemia; be prepared to deal with this emergency.

8. Be aware that bones may fracture more easily in clients with chronic hypercalcemia because bone resorption has been excessive, weakening the bony structure. Transfer clients cautiously.

9. Educate home-bound oncology clients with a predisposition for hypercalcemia, and their families, to be alert for symptoms that occur with this condition and to report them to the health care providers before they become severe.

10. Be alert for signs of digitalis toxicity when hypercalcemia occurs in digitalized clients.

11. Help prevent formation of calcium renal stones in clients with long-standing hypercalcemia or immobilization by
   a. Forcing fluids to maintain a dilute urine, thus avoiding supersaturation of precipitates.
   b. Encouraging fluids that yield an acid-ash (such as prune or cranberry juice) because a urinary pH less than 6.5 favors calcium deposits.

(continued)

T A B L E 3 7 - 4 (continued)

Electrolyte Disturbances: Related Factors, Defining Characteristics, and Nursing Interventions

Related Factors	Defining Characteristics	Nursing Interventions
		c. Preventing urinary stasis by turning the immobilized client frequently, elevating the head of the bed, and having the client sit up if this can be tolerated. d. Encouraging weight-bearing and ambulation as soon as possible.
Hypomagnesemia		
Chronic alcoholism, particularly during withdrawal Intestinal malabsorption syndromes Diarrhea Nasogastric suction Aggressive refeeding after starvation (as in TPN) without adequate magnesium replacement Prolonged administration of magnesium-free maintenance IV fluids Diabetic ketoacidosis Hyperaldosteronism (either primary, or secondary, as in congestive heart failure or cirrhosis) Drugs: • Diuretics • Aminoglycoside antibiotics (such as gentamicin) • Cisplatin • Excessive doses of vitamin D or calcium supplements • Citrate preservative in blood products Pancreatitis Thyrotoxicosis Hyperparathyroidism Others: • Burns • Sepsis • Hypothermia	Neuromuscular irritability • Increased reflexes • Coarse tremors • Positive Chvostek's and Trousseau's signs • Convulsions Cardiac manifestations • Tachyarrhythmias • Increased susceptibility to digitalis toxicity • ECG changes in severe cases: PR and QT interval prolongation, widened QRS complex, ST segment depression, and T-wave inversion Mental changes • Disorientation in memory • Mood changes • Intense confusion • Hallucinations Serum magnesium level below 1.3 mEq/L or 1.8 mg/dL (0.8 mmol/L). Usually symptoms don't appear until serum magnesium is over 1 mEq/L (0.8 mmol/L). Hypocalcemia and hypokalemia frequently occur with severe hypomagnesemia.	1. Be aware of clients at risk for hypomagnesemia and monitor for its presence. 2. Assess digitalized clients at risk for hypomagnesemia especially closely for symptoms of digitalis toxicity because a deficit of magnesium predisposes to toxicity. 3. Be prepared to take seizure precautions when hypomagnesemia is severe. 4. Monitor condition of airway, because laryngeal stridor can occur. 5. Take safety precautions if confusion is present. 6. Be familiar with magnesium replacement salts and factors related to their safe administration. 7. Be aware that magnesium-depleted clients may experience difficulty in swallowing. 8. When magnesium deficit is due to abuse of diuretics or laxatives, educating the client may help alleviate the problem. 9. Be aware that most commonly used IV fluids have either no magnesium or a relatively small amount. When indicated, discuss need for magnesium replacement with physician. 10. For clients experiencing abnormal magnesium losses, but able to consume a general diet, encourage the intake of magnesium-rich foods (such as green vegetables, nuts and legumes, and fruits such as bananas, oranges, and grapefruits).
Hypermagnesemia		
Renal failure (particularly when magnesium-containing medications are administered) Adrenal insufficiency Excessive magnesium administration during treatment of eclampsia	Early signs (serum magnesium level of 3 to 5 mEq/L) • Flushing and a sense of skin warmth (due to peripheral vasodilation) • Hypotension (due to blockage of sympathetic ganglia as well as to a direct effect on smooth muscle)	1. Be aware of clients at risk for hypermagnesemia and assess for its presence. When hypermagnesemia is suspected, assess the following parameters: • Vital signs: Look for low blood pressure and shallow respirations with periods of apnea • Patellar reflexes: If absent, notify physician because this usually implies a serum magnesium level greater than 7 mEq/L. If allowed to progress, cardiac or respiratory arrest could occur.

(continued)

T A B L E   3 7 - 4 (continued)

Electrolyte Disturbances: Related Factors, Defining Characteristics, and Nursing Interventions

Related Factors	Defining Characteristics	Nursing Interventions
Hypermagnesemia		
Hemodialysis with excessively hard water or with a dialysate inadvertently high in magnesium content Untreated ketoacidosis	• Nausea and vomiting Drowsiness, hypoactive reflexes, and muscular weakness (can occur at a serum magnesium level of 4 to 7 mEq/L) Depresses respirations (can occur at a serum magnesium level of 10 mEq/L) Coma (can occur at a serum magnesium level of 10 to 15 mEq/L) Cardiac abnormalities • Sinus bradycardia, prolonged PR, QRS, and QT intervals (at serum magnesium levels of 7.1 to 10 mEq/L) • Heart block and cardiac arrest in diastole (can occur at a serum magnesium level of 15 to 20 mEq/L) Weak or absent cry in newborn	• Level of consciousness: Look for drowsiness, lethargy, and coma. 2. Do not give magnesium-containing medications to client with renal failure or compromised renal function. (Be particularly careful in following "standing orders" for bowel preparation for x-ray because some of these include the use of magnesium citrate.) 3. Caution clients with renal disease to check with their health care providers before taking over-the-counter medications. 4. Be aware of factors related to safe parenteral administration of magnesium salts.
Hypophosphatemia		
Glucose administration Refeeding after starvation Hyperalimentation Alcohol withdrawal Diabetic ketoacidosis Respiratory alkalosis Phosphate-binding antacids Recovery phase after severe burns	Paresthesias Muscle weakness (perhaps manifested as decreased strength of hand grasp and difficulty speaking) Muscle pain and tenderness Mental changes, such as apprehension, confusion, delirium, and coma Cardiomyopathy Acute respiratory failure (perhaps related to chest muscle weakness) Seizures Decreased tissue oxygenation Joint stiffness Serum phosphate below 2.5 mg/dL	1. Identify clients at risk for hypophosphatemia. • Particularly at risk are extremely malnourished clients being started on TPN or large caloric intake by tube feeding (refeeding syndrome in starving clients). • Also at great risk are alcoholic clients undergoing withdrawal therapy and initial treatment with intravenous fluids. • Similarly at great risk are clients with diabetic ketoacidosis during the early treatment period with insulin and intravenous fluids. 2. Monitor clients at risk for the presence of hypophosphatemia. See *Defining Characteristics*. 3. Be aware that severely hypophosphatemic clients are thought to be at greater risk for infection because of changes in white blood cells. 4. Administer IV phosphate products cautiously. Be aware that they should be administered slowly in dilute infusion solutions to avoid phosphate intoxication. Frequent monitoring of serum phosphorus levels is required to guide therapy. 5. Be aware that in adults the usual maintenance dose of phosphorus is 10 to 15 mmol/L of TPN solution. However, maintenance doses may not be sufficient if the client is in a high anabolic state. Allowances must also be made for existing phosphorus deficit. 6. Be aware of the need to introduce hyperalimentation *gradually* in clients who are malnourished. Gradual introduction of the feeding solution is less apt to be associated with rapid shifts of phosphate into the cells. Monitor rates of TPN flow frequently.

(continued)

TABLE 37-4 (continued)

Electrolyte Disturbances: Related Factors, Defining Characteristics, and Nursing Interventions

Related Factors	Defining Characteristics	Nursing Interventions
		7. Be aware that sudden increase in the serum phosphorus level can cause hypocalcemia. For this reason, serum calcium levels should be monitored. Watch for twitching around the mouth, laryngospasm, positive Chvostek's sign, paresthesias, arrhythmias, and hypotension.
		8. Because it is possible to give too much phosphorus when administering phosphate solutions, monitor for signs of hyperphosphatemia and of the salt in which it is administered.
		9. Monitor for diarrhea in clients taking oral phosphorus supplements; consult with physician if it persists or becomes severe.
		10. Mix powdered oral phosphorus supplements with chilled or iced water to make them more palatable. Also, palatability may be increased by refrigerating the solution made from the powder.
Hyperphosphatemia Renal failure Chemotherapy, particularly for acute lymphoblastic leukemia and lymphoma Large intake of milk, as in treatment of peptic ulcer Use of cow's milk in infants Excessive intake of phosphate-containing laxatives Overzealous administration of phosphorus supplements, orally or intravenously Excessive use of Fleet's phosphosoda as enema solution, particularly in children and people with slow bowel elimination Large vitamin D intake (increased phosphorus absorption) Hypoparathyroidism Hyperthyroidism	Short-term consequences: symptoms of tetany, such as tingling of fingertips and around mouth, numbness, and muscle spasms Long-term consequences: precipitation of calcium phosphate in nonosseous sites, such as the kidney, joints, arteries, skin, or cornea. Serum phosphate above 4.5 mg/dL	1. Identify clients at risk for hyperphosphatemia. 2. Monitor for signs of tetany, such as tingling sensations in the fingertips and around the mouth, and presence of muscle cramps or positive Chvostek's and Trousseau's signs in at-risk clients. Be aware that these symptoms are probably due to hypocalcemia induced by the high phosphate level and are most likely to occur in clients who have taken in a high phosphate load. 3. Be aware that soft-tissue calcification can be a long-term complication of a chronically elevated serum phosphate level. Calcification may occur in sites such as the kidney, arteries, joints, and cornea. Monitor for signs of these complications. 4. Administer prescribed oral and IV phosphate supplements cautiously and monitor serum phosphorus levels periodically during their use. 5. When appropriate, instruct clients that use of phosphate-containing laxatives may result in acute phosphate poisoning. 6. Be aware that phosphate-containing enemas can result in hyperphosphatemia if used injudiciously, particularly in children and those with slow bowel emptying. Instruct clients accordingly. 7. When a low-phosphorus diet is prescribed, instruct clients to avoid foods high in phosphorus content. Such foods include hard cheese or cream, nuts and nut products; while grain cereals (eg, bran and oatmeal); dried fruits, dried vegetables; special meats such as kidneys and sardines and sweetbreads; and desserts made with milk.

(Data from Metheny, N. M. [1992]. *Fluid and electrolyte balance* [2nd ec.]. Philadelphia: Lippincott.)

pCO_2 is low, carbonic acid leaves the body in excessive amounts; when the pCO_2 is high, there are excessive amounts of carbonic acid in the body. The following equations illustrate:

Equation: When the pCO_2 exceeds normal, carbonic acid has increased, as follows:

$$CO_2 + H_2O \rightarrow H_2CO_3$$

Equation: When the pCO_2 is below normal, carbon dioxide leaves the body in excessive amounts, as follows:

$$H_2CO_3 \rightarrow CO_2 + H_2O$$

The measure of pH, pCO_2, and pO_2 is almost universally carried out in clinical laboratories at 37°C (98.6°F) using arterial whole blood. Many blood gas instruments have microprocessors that can calculate bicarbonate, CO_2 content, base excess, and oxygen saturation. Alternatively, these values can be determined from nomograms or figures. Laboratory levels for ABGs are given later in the chapter.

Acid–base imbalances occur when the carbonic acid or bicarbonate levels become disproportionate. When there is a single primary cause, these disturbances are known as respiratory acidosis or alkalosis and metabolic acidosis or alkalosis, which are defined and described in the sections that follow. These disturbances are a result of an upset in acid–base balance, as follows:

- A respiratory disturbance alters the carbonic-acid portion:
  - Respiratory acidosis and alkalosis are the results of respiratory phenomena.
  - Compensation occurs to restore balance in the kidneys by either trying to conserve or excrete more bicarbonate.
- A metabolic disturbance alters the bicarbonate portion:
  - Metabolic acidosis and alkalosis are almost entirely the result of metabolic processes.
  - The primary organs for compensation to restore balance are the lungs, which either try to conserve or excrete more carbon dioxide, which is available in weakly ionized carbonic acid.

Table 37-5 summarizes acid–base imbalances. Complicated clinical situations may occur when respiratory and metabolic imbalances coexist.

Respiratory Acidosis Respiratory acidosis is a primary excess of carbonic acid in ECF. Any decrease in alveolar ventilation that results in retention of carbon dioxide can cause respiratory acidosis. Because the lungs are the source of the problem, they are unable to participate in compensation. As the carbonic acid content increases, the kidneys attempt to retain more bicarbonate and increase their hydrogen excretion. Thus,

respiratory acidosis = high pCO_2 because of alveolar hypoventilation

Respiratory Alkalosis Respiratory alkalosis is a primary deficit of carbonic acid in ECF. It is the result of increased alveolar ventilation and, therefore, a decrease in carbon dioxide. An increase in respiratory rate and depth causes the carbon dioxide loss because the carbon dioxide is excreted faster than normal.

Because of the deficit of carbon dioxide, which is a respiratory stimulant, depression or cessation of respirations eventually occurs. Because the lungs are the source of the problem, they are unable to participate in compensation. Therefore, the kidneys attempt to alleviate the imbalance by increasing the bicarbonate excretion and by retaining more hydrogen. Thus,

respiratory alkalosis = low pCO_2 because of alveolar hyperventilation

Metabolic Acidosis Metabolic acidosis is a proportionate deficit of bicarbonate in ECF. The deficit can occur as the result of an increase in acid components or an excessive loss of bicarbonate. The lungs attempt to increase the carbon dioxide excretion by increasing the rate and depth of respirations. The kidneys attempt to compensate by retaining bicarbonate and by excreting more hydrogen. If the body is unable to achieve normal balance, the person may lose consciousness as metabolic acidosis increases, and death eventually results. Thus,

metabolic acidosis = low bicarbonate. Nonvolatile acid is present to use up HCO_3^- in disproportionate amounts, or HCO_3^- is lost in disproportionate amounts

Metabolic Alkalosis Metabolic alkalosis is a primary excess of bicarbonate in ECF. This may be the result of excessive acid losses or increased base ingestion or retention. The body attempts to compensate by retaining carbon dioxide. The respirations become slow and shallow, and periods of no breathing may occur. The kidneys attempt to excrete potassium and sodium with the excessive bicarbonate, and retain hydrogen in carbonic acid. Thus,

metabolic alkalosis = high bicarbonate. Nonvolatile acid is lost and is not using up HCO_3^-, or HCO_3^- is gained in disproportionate amounts

Nurse as Role Model

Nurses wishing to be a role model of self-care behaviors that promote fluid, electrolyte, and acid–base balance should meet the following goals. The nurse will:

- Daily ingest the quantity and type of fluids (to include six to eight glasses of water) that promote healthy hydration and urinary functioning

TABLE 37-5

Acid–Base Disturbances: Related Factors, Defining Characteristics, and Nursing Interventions

Related Factors	Defining Characteristics	Nursing Interventions
Respiratory Acidosis (Carbonic Acid Excess)		

Acute respiratory acidosis:
- Acute pulmonary edema
- Aspiration of a foreign body
- Atelectasis
- Pneumothorax, hemothorax
- Overdosage of sedatives or anesthetic
- Position on operating room table that interferes with respirations
- Cardiac arrest
- Severe pneumonia
- Laryngospasm
- Mechanical ventilation improperly regulated

Chronic respiratory acidosis:
- Emphysema
- Cystic fibrosis
- Advanced multiple sclerosis
- Bronchiectasis
- Bronchial asthma

Factors favoring hypoventilation:
- Obesity
- Tight abdominal binders or dressings
- Postoperative pain (as in high abdominal or chest incisions)
- Abdominal distention from cirrhosis or bowel obstruction

Acute respiratory acidosis
- Feeling of fullness in the head ($PaCO_2$ causes cerebrovascular vasodilation and increased cerebral blood flow, particularly when over 60 mm Hg)
- Mental cloudiness
- Dizziness
- Palpitations
- Muscular twitching
- Convulsions
- Warm, flushed skin
- Unconsciousness
- Ventricular fibrillation may be first sign in anesthetized patient (related to hyperkalemia)
- Arterial blood gases (ABGs)
  - pH below 7.35
  - $PaCO_2$ over 45 mm Hg (primary)
  - HCO_3^- normal or only slightly elevated

Chronic respiratory acidosis
- Weakness
- Dull headache
- Symptoms of underlying disease process
- ABGs
  - pH below 7.35 or within lower limits of normal
  - $PaCO_2$ over 45 mm Hg (primary)
  - HCO_3^- over 26 mEq/L (mmol/L) (compensatory)

Treatment is directed at improving ventilation; exact measures vary with the cause of inadequate ventilation. Pharmacologic agents are used as indicated. For example, bronchodilators help reduce bronchial spasm; antibiotics are used for respiratory infections. Pulmonary hygiene measures are used, when necessary, to rid the respiratory tract of mucus and purulent drainage. Adequate hydration (2 to 3 L/day) is indicated to keep the mucous membranes moist and thereby facilitate removal of secretions. Supplemental oxygen is used as necessary.

A mechanical respirator, used cautiously, may improve pulmonary ventilation. One must remember that overzealous use of a mechanical respirator may cause such rapid excretion of carbon dioxide that the kidneys will be unable to eliminate excess bicarbonate with sufficient rapidity to prevent alkalosis and convulsions. For this reason, the elevated $PaCO_2$ must be decreased slowly.

Respiratory Alkalosis (Carbonic Acid Deficit)

Extreme anxiety (most common cause)

Hypoxemia

High Fever

Early salicylate intoxication (stimulates respiratory center)

Gram-negative bacteremia

Central nervous system lesions involving respiratory center

Pulmonary emboli

Thyrotoxicosis

Excessive ventilation by mechanical ventilators

Pregnancy (high progesterone level sensitizes the respiratory center to CO_2: physiologic)

Lightheadedness (a low $PaCO_2$ causes cerebral vasoconstriction and thus decreased cerebral blood flow)

Inability to concentrate

Those of decreased calcium ionization (numbness and tingling of extremities and circumoral paresthesia; more likely to occur if respiratory alkalosis develops rapidly)

Hyperventilation syndrome
- Tinnitus
- Palpitations
- Sweating
- Dry mouth
- Tremulousness
- Precordial pain (tightness)
- Nausea and vomiting
- Epigastric pain
- Blurred vision
- Convulsions and loss of consciousness (may be partly due to cerebral ischemia, caused by cerebral vasoconstriction)

If the cause of respiratory alkalosis is anxiety, the client should be made aware that the abnormal breathing practice is responsible for the symptoms accompanying this condition. Instruct the client to breathe more slowly (to cause accumulation of carbon dioxide) or to breathe in a closed system (such as a paper bag) is helpful. Usually a sedative is required to relieve ventilation in very anxious patients. (If alkalosis is severe enough to cause fainting, the increased ventilation ceases and respirations revert to normal.)

Treatment for other causes of respiratory alkalosis is directed at correcting the underlying problem.

(continued)

T A B L E 3 7 - 5 (continued)

Acid–Base Disturbances: Related Factors, Defining Characteristics, and Nursing Interventions

Related Factors	Defining Characteristics	Nursing Interventions
Respiratory Alkalosis (Carbonic Acid Deficit)		
	ABGs • pH over 7.45 • $PaCO_2$ below 35 mm Hg (primary) • HCO_3^- under 22 mEq/L (mmol/L) (compensatory)	

Metabolic Acidosis (Base Bicarbonate Deficit)

Related Factors	Defining Characteristics	Nursing Interventions
Normal anion gap: • Diarrhea • Intestinal fistulas • Ureterosigmoidostomy • Hyperalimentation • Acidifying drugs (such as ammonium chloride) • Renal tubular acidosis (RTA) High anion gap: • Diabetic ketoacidosis • Starvational ketoacidosis • Lactic acidosis • Renal failure • Ingestion of toxins (such as salicylates, ethylene glycol, and methanol)	Headache Confusion Drowsiness Increased respiratory rate and depth (may not become clinically evident until HCO_3^- is quite low) Nausea and vomiting Peripheral vasodilation (may be present, causing warm, flushed skin) Decreased cardiac output when pH falls below 7; bradycardia may develop ABGs • Fall in pH to below 7.35 • HCO_3^- under 22 mEq/L (mmol/L) (primary) • $PaCO_2$ under 35 mm Hg (compensation by lungs) • Base excess always negative Hyperkalemia is frequently present (except in RTA, diarrhea, and use of acetazolamide)	Treatment is directed toward correcting the metabolic defect. If the cause of the problem is excessive intake of chloride, treatment obviously focuses on eliminating the source. When necessary, bicarbonate is administered.

Metabolic Alkalosis (Base Bicarbonate Excess)

Related Factors	Defining Characteristics	Nursing Interventions
Vomiting or gastric suction Hypokalemia Hyperaldosteronism Cushing's syndrome Potassium-losing diuretics (eg, thiazides, furosemide, ethacrynic acid) Alkali ingestion (bicarbonate-containing antacids) Parenteral $NaHCO_3$ administration for cardiopulmonary resuscitation Abrupt relief of chronic respiratory acidosis	Those related to decreased calcium ionization, such as: • Dizziness • Tingling of fingers and toes • Circumoral paresthesia • Carpopedal spasm • Hypertonic muscles Depressed respiration (compensatory action by lungs) ABGs • pH above 7.45 • Bicarbonate over 26 mEq/L (mmol/L) (primary) • $PaCO_2$ over 45 mm Hg (compensatory) • Base excess always positive Hypokalemia often present Serum Cl relatively lower than Na	Treatment is aimed at reversal of the underlying disorder. Sufficient chloride must be supplied for the kidney to absorb sodium with chloride (allowing the excretion of excess bicarbonate). Treatment also includes restoration of normal fluid volume by administration of sodium chloride fluids (because continued volume depletion serves to maintain the alkalosis).

(Data from Metheny, N. M. [1992]. *Fluid and electrolyte balance* [2nd ed.]. Philadelphia: Lippincott.)

Fluid and Electrolyte Balance

Use the assessment checklist to determine how well you are meeting fluid and electrolyte needs. Then develop a prescription for self-care by choosing appropriate behaviors from the list of suggestions.

Assessment Checklist

almost always	sometimes	almost never	
☐	☐	☐	1. I drink six to eight glasses of water every day.
☐	☐	☐	2. I am aware of early signs of dehydration or fluid retention.
☐	☐	☐	3. I limit sugar, alcohol, and caffeine in my diet.
☐	☐	☐	4. I am alert for any sudden variations in my weight.
☐	☐	☐	5. I am aware of fluid and electrolyte imbalances that may be associated with intake of certain medications.
☐	☐	☐	6. I diet sensibly when I need to lose weight.

Self-Care Behaviors

1. Consume approximately 1½ quarts of water daily.
2. Maintain normal body weight.
3. Avoid consuming excess amounts of products high in salt, sugar, and caffeine.
4. Limit alcohol intake because of its diuretic effect.
5. Obtain medical evaluation for any ongoing indications of fluid imbalance.
6. Monitor side effects of medications, especially diuresis and diarrhea.

- Evaluate use of fad diets, diuretics, laxatives, and alcohol, identifying potential risks to health
- Identify situations of high risk for fluid and electrolyte imbalance and intervene appropriately

Assessing

The pathophysiology underlying both acute and chronic illness, trauma, and select therapeutic interventions may all place a client at high risk for fluid, electrolyte, and acid–base imbalances. Once present, these imbalances can seriously compromise the client's health status and may prove life-threatening. Nursing assessment is directed toward the following:

- Identification of clients at high risk for fluid, electrolyte, and acid–base imbalance
- Determination that a specific imbalance is present, identification of the nature of imbalance, severity, etiology, and defining characteristics
- Determination of the effectiveness of the care plan

Important assessment parameters include the nursing history and nursing examination, record of fluid intake and output, daily weight, and laboratory studies.

Nursing History

Each comprehensive nursing history should include questions that allow the nurse to assess the client's fluid, electrolyte, and acid–base balance. The accompanying Fo-

cused Assessment Guide includes interview questions helpful in identifying the client's usual pattern of fluid intake and elimination and the client's evaluation of his or her hydration status and awareness of particular problems. Interview questions should also assist in the identification of clients at high risk for imbalances. Risk factors include the following:

- The pathophysiology underlying both acute and chronic illness (eg, diabetes mellitus, congestive heart failure, renal failure)
- Abnormal losses of body fluids (eg, prolonged or severe vomiting and diarrhea, draining wounds, fistulas). Table 37-6 lists imbalances that result from fluid loss of specific body fluids.
- Burns and trauma
- Therapies with the potential to disrupt fluid and electrolyte balance (eg, medications such as diuretics and steroids, treatments such as IV therapy and TPN)

Physical Assessment

Metheny (1992) recommends that the nurse pay attention to certain parameters when assessing a client's fluid and electrolyte status:

- Comparison of total intake and output of fluids
- Urine volume and concentration
- Skin and tongue turgor
- Degree of moisture in oral cavity
- Body weight
- Thirst

F O C U S E D   A S S E S S M E N T   G U I D E

Fluid, Electrolyte, and Acid–Base Balance

Factors to Assess	Questions and Approaches
Usual pattern of fluid intake	Describe the amount and types of fluids you usually drink in a 24-hour period. Have there been any recent changes?
Usual pattern of fluid elimination	Describe your usual voiding/urination habits.
	Any recent changes in frequency or amount?
	Is your body losing fluids in any other major way? • Vomiting • Diarrhea • Excessive perspiration • Fistula
Client's evaluation of hydration status	Do you think there is an approximate balance between your fluid intake and output?
	Have you noticed any signs that your body is experiencing too much or too little hydration (difficulty breathing, edema, dry skin and mucous membranes, thirst)?
History of disease process	Is there any history of disease process or injury that might disrupt fluid and electrolyte balance (eg, diabetes mellitus, cancer, burns)?
Medication history	Do you take any medications or treatments that might disrupt fluid and electrolyte balance (eg, steroids, diuretics, total parenteral nutrition, dialysis)?
Fluid, electrolyte, and acid–base imbalances, and contributing factors	Are you aware of any specific fluid, electrolyte, or acid–base problems you may be experiencing? • Nature • Onset of problem and frequency • Causes • Severity • Symptoms • Intervention attempted and results

T A B L E   3 7 - 6

Imbalances Resulting From Fluid Loss of Specific Body Fluid

Fluid Lost	Imbalances Likely to Occur	Fluid Lost	Imbalances Likely to Occur
Gastric juice	Extracellular fluid volume deficit Metabolic alkalosis Sodium deficit Potassium deficit Tetany (if metabolic alkalosis is present) Ketosis of starvation Magnesium deficit	Pancreatic juice	Metabolic acidosis Sodium deficit Calcium deficit Extracellular fluid volume deficit
		Sensible perspiration	Extracellular fluid volume deficit Sodium deficit
Intestinal juice	Extracellular fluid volume deficit Metabolic acidosis Sodium deficit Potassium deficit	Insensible water loss	Water deficit (dehydration) Sodium excess
		Wound exudate	Protein deficit Sodium deficit Extracellular fluid volume deficit
Bile	Sodium deficit Metabolic acidosis	Ascites	Protein deficit Sodium deficit Plasma-to-interstitial fluid shift Extracellular fluid volume deficit

- Tearing and salivation
- Appearance and temperature of skin
- Facial appearance
- Edema
- Vital signs
- Neck and hand vein filling
- CVP
- Neuromuscular irritability

When suspecting imbalance of particular electrolytes, knowledge of their defining characteristics should guide the assessment (see Table 37-4). Table 37-7 presents select nursing considerations for each of these parameters, findings in a healthy adult, and significant findings.

Measuring Fluid Intake and Output

When either the physician or nurse orders that a client's fluid intake and output be continuously measured, the client, his or her family, and all caregivers should be alert to the need to measure all fluids entering and leaving the body—to the extent that this is possible. The client's condition dictates the strictness of the intake and output mea-surement. Adherence to the guidelines in the accompanying display helps eliminate common errors in measuring fluid intake and output.

Daily Weights

Because of the numerous sources of inaccuracies in fluid intake and output measurement, the recording of a client's daily weight may offer a more accurate depiction of fluid balance status. Guidelines for accurate weight measurement include weighing the client at the same time each day, preferably in the morning before breakfast and after the first morning void; with the same or similar clothing; and on the same scale.

Laboratory Studies

Laboratory tests are helpful in determining whether fluid, electrolyte, and acid–base balance exists. Standard tests include the following (tables of normal values are given in Appendix B).

(Text continues on p. 1027)

GUIDELINES FOR NURSING CARE

Measuring Fluid Intake and Output

As soon as measured intake and output is ordered for the client, the client and family are instructed that the nurse needs a record of all fluids entering the body and all fluid output. A simple explanation of why this is being done is offered as well as specific instructions as to how the client can help to keep his or her record accurate. Some clients may need to be reminded during nursing rounds each morning that this measurement will continue.

The client's plan of care and nursing Kardex are used to communicate to nursing personnel the need to measure fluid intake and output. A sign posted in the client's room and bedside form for recording intake and output are helpful reminders for both the client and nurses.

The client's fluid intake includes the following:

- All fluids and foods that are liquid at room temperature (ice cream, gelatin dessert [Jell-O], and so forth)

   Use the agency's designation of specific volumes for common food containers (eg, juice glass = 90 mL; milk carton = 240 mL).

   Remind the client that sips of water or other fluids in between meals need to be recorded; small disposable calibrated cups at the bedside facilitate accurate measurement.

   Remember that liquid medications or water taken with pills may significantly increase the fluid intake of some clients.
- All parenteral fluids

- Other fluids taken into the body: subcutaneous fluids, fluids instilled into drainage tubes, enema solutions

The client's fluid output includes the following:

- Urine; vomitus; diarrhea; drainage from fistulas, wounds, and ulcers; and drainage from suctioning devices. Calibrated measuring devices should be readily available for accurate measurement. Disposable, calibrated urine collection containers that fit under the toilet seat are available for ambulatory clients. Urine or liquid feces in diapers or bed clothes, vomitus on clothing or bed linens, wound drainage saturating dressings, and so forth, need to be estimated.
- Heavy perspiration should be noted on the output record especially when the client's clothing or bed linens are soaked.
- Hyperventilation (water vapor loss) should also be noted on the output record. Record rate and depth of respirations.

   Both intake and output should be measured whenever possible, rather than estimated. Output measurement is described in Chapter 34. Failure to record intake or output when it is measured may result in being forgotten.

   Intake and output totals are generally recorded for each 8-hour shift and totaled each 24 hours. At the conclusion of each shift, the alert client should be questioned about his or her intake and output.

T A B L E 3 7 - 7

Parameters to Be Considered in Clinical Assessment for Fluid, Electrolyte, and Acid—Base Balance

Assessment Parameters	Nursing Considerations	Findings In Healthy Adult	Significant Findings
Comparison of total intake and output of fluids	• Records may be initiated by the nurse for any client with a real or potential water or electrolyte problem. • Intake should include all fluids taken into the body (oral fluids, foods that are liquid at room temperature, IV fluids, subcutaneous fluids, fluids instilled into drainage tubes as irrigants, tube feeding solutions and water, even enema solutions in clients requiring strict fluid intake recording) • Output should include urine, vomitus, diarrhea, drainage from fistulas, and drainage from suction apparatus. Perspiration and drainage from lesions should be noted and estimated. Prolonged hyperventilation should also be noted because it is an important route of water vapor loss.	• Fluid intake about equals fluid output—when averaged over 2 or 3 days. • Range of 1500 to 3500 mL fluid intake and loss; 2000 mL is average adult intake and loss per day. • Output of urine normally approximates the ingestion of liquids; water from food and oxidation is balanced by the water loss through feces, the skin, and the respiratory process.	• when the total intake is substantially less than the total output, the client is in danger of fluid volume deficit. • When the total intake is substantially more than the total output, the client is in danger of fluid volume excess.
Urine volume and concentration	• Measure all fluid losses according to routes. • Use a device calibrated for small volumes of urine when hourly urine volumes need to be measured. • Account for factors that can alter urinary output: 1. Amount of fluid intake 2. Losses from skin, lungs, and GI tract 3. Amount of waste products for excretions 4. Renal concentrating ability 5. Blood volume 6. Hormonal influences (primarily aldosterone and ADH)	• Normal urinary output is about 1 mL/kg of body weight per hour (for the average adult: 1500 mL/24 hr, which is equivalent to about 40 to 80 mL/hr). • Stress may diminish the 24-hour urine volume in the adult to 750 to 1000 mL (or 30 to 50 mL/hr) because of increased aldosterone and ADH secretion. • The range of specific gravity if from 1.003 to 1.035. Urine osmolality ranges between 500 mOsm and 800 mOsm/kg (mmol/kg).	• A low urine volume with a high specific gravity indicates fluid volume deficit. • A low urine volume with a low specific gravity indicates renal disease. • A high urine volume suggests fluid volume excess. • Urine volume is increased in conditions with high solute loads, such as diabetes mellitus, high protein tube feedings, and fever. • Hypovolemia causes decreased renal perfusion and thus oliguria; hypervolemia causes increased urinary volume if the kidneys are functioning normally.
Body weight	• Because of the common inaccuracies in recording intake and output, body weight is believed to be a more accurate indicator of fluid gained and lost. • Guidelines for weighing clients: 1. Use the same scale each time. 2. Measure weight at the same time each day: in the morning before breakfast and after voiding.	• A client's dry weight should remain relatively stable.	• Rapid variations in weight closely reflect changes in body fluid volume. • A rapid loss of body weight occurs when the total fluid intake is less than the total fluid output. 1. Rapid loss of 2% total body weight (TBW) indicates mild fluid volume deficit. 2. Rapid loss of 5% TBW indicates moderate fluid volume deficit.

(continued)

T A B L E   3 7 - 7 (continued)

Parameters to Be Considered in Clinical Assessment for Fluid, Electrolyte, and Acid–Base Balance			
Assessment Parameters	**Nursing Considerations**	**Findings in Healthy Adult**	**Significant Findings**
	3. Be sure the client is wearing the same, or similar clothing (clothing should be dry). 4. If the client is unable to stand on a small, portable scale, use a bed scale. • A client may have a severe fluid volume deficit even though body weight is essentially unchanged when there is a third-space loss of body fluid.		3. Rapid loss of 8% or more of TBW indicates severe fluid volume deficit. • A rapid gain of body weight occurs when the total fluid intake is greater than the total fluid output. 1. Rapid gain of 2% TBW indicates mild fluid volume excess. 2. Rapid gain of 5% TBW indicates moderate fluid volume excess. 3. Rapid gain of 8% or more of TBW indicates severe fluid volume excess. • A rapid gain or loss of 1 kg (2.2 lb) of body weight is about equal to the gain or loss of 1 L of fluid.
Skin turgor (elasticity)	• Pinch the client's skin over the sternum, inner aspect of the thighs, or forehead. • Some prefer to test skin turgor in children over the abdominal area and on the medial aspect of the thighs. • Skin turgor can vary with age, nutritional state, and even race and complexion. Observations are most meaningful if done sequentially before the development of a fluid balance abnormality.	• Pinched skin immediately falls back to its normal position when released. • Reduced skin turgor is common in older clients (those more than 55 to 60 years of age) because of a primary decrease in skin elasticity.	• In a person with a fluid volume deficit, the skin flattens more slowly after the pinch is released; the skin may remain elevated for many seconds. • Severe malnutrition, particularly in infants, can cause depressed skin turgor even in the absence of fluid depletion.
Tongue turgor	• Unlike skin turgor, tongue turgor is not affected appreciably by age and thus is a useful assessment for all age groups.	• Tongue has one longitudinal furrow.	• In the person with fluid volume deficit there are additional longitudinal furrows and the tongue is smaller. • Sodium excess causes the tongue to look red and swollen.
Moisture and oral cavity	• A dry mouth may be the result of fluid volume deficit or of mouth breathing. When in doubt, the nurse should run a finger along the oral cavity and feel the membrane where the cheek and gum meet; dryness in this area indicates a true fluid volume deficit.	• Mucous membranes in oral cavity are moist.	• Dryness of the membrane where the cheek and gum meet indicates fluid volume deficit. • Dry sticky mucous membranes are noted in sodium excess. (The oral cavity feels like flypaper.)
Tearing and salivation		• Tearing and salivation decrease normally with age.	• The absence of tearing and salivation in a child is a sign of fluid volume deficit; it becomes obvious with a fluid loss of 5% of TBW.
Appearance of skin and skin temperature			• Metabolic acidosis can cause warm, flushed skin (due to peripheral vasodilation).

(continued)

T A B L E 3 7 - 7 *(continued)*

Parameters to Be Considered in Clinical Assessment for Fluid, Electrolyte, and Acid–Base Balance

Assessment Parameters	Nursing Considerations	Findings in Healthy Adult	Significant Findings
Facial appearance			• Severe fluid volume deficit causes the skin to be pale and cool as a result of vaso-constriction, which occurs to compensate for hypovolemia. • A person with a severe fluid volume deficit has a pinched and drawn facial expression. • A fluid volume deficit of 10% of body weight causes decreased intraocular pressure causing the eyes to appear sunken and to feel soft to the touch
Edema (excessive accumulation of interstitial fluid)	• Pitting edema (phenomenon manifested by a small depression that remains after one's finger is pressed over an edematous area and then removed) may be indicated by using plus signs to indicate the amount, ranging from +1 (barely perceptible edema) to +4 (severe edema). See Figure 37-9. • Measurement of an extremity or body part with a millimeter tape, in the same area each day, is a more exact method of measurement. • An excess of interstitial fluid may accumulate predominantly in the lower extremities of ambulatory clients and in the presacral region of bed-ridden clients. • The presence of periorbital (around the eyes) edema or pedal edema should prompt one to look for edema in other parts of the body.	• No edema	• Clinically edema is not usually apparent in the adult until the retention of 5 to 10 lb of excess fluid occurs. • Pitting edema is not evident until at least a 10% increase in weight has occurred. • Formation of edema may be localized (as in thrombophlebitis) or generalized (as in heart failure, cirrhosis of liver, or nephrotic syndrome). Edema of congestive heart failure, liver cirrhosis, or nephrotic syndrome is the result of sodium retention. • There is no peripheral edema with only water retention (as occurs with excessive secretion of ADH). Instead, there is a cellular swelling that can be detected by pressing one's finger over the sternum and producing a visible fingerprint.
Body temperature	• Because fever increases the loss of body fluids it is important that temperature elevations be detected early and appropriate interventions be taken. • Body temperature and other vital signs should be assessed at the nurse's discretion.	• Baseline temperature: diurnal variations	• There is an elevation of body temperature in hypernatremia (dehydration) probably related to lack of available fluid for sweating. Also, dehydration has a direct effect on the hypothalamus. • There is a decrease in body temperature in fluid volume deficit, when uncomplicated by infection (probably as a result of decreased metabolism). • Fever increases the loss of body fluids

(continued)

Parameters to Be Considered in Clinical Assessment for Fluid, Electrolyte, and Acid–Base Balance

Assessment Parameters	Nursing Considerations	Findings in Healthy Adult	Significant Findings
			1. Increased metabolism produces more metabolic wastes and increased urinary output.
			2. Fever also causes hyperpnea, an increase in breathing that results in extra vapor loss through the lungs.
			• A temperature elevation between 101°F (38.3°C) and 103°F (39.4°C) increases the 24-hour fluid requirement by at least 500 mL, and a temperature above 103°F increases it by at least 1000 mL.
Pulse		• Baseline pulse rate, rhythm, and volume	• Tachycardia is usually the earliest sign of the decreased vascular volume associated with fluid volume deficit. It may also be associated with deficits of magnesium or potassium.
			• Excesses of magnesium or potassium can cause decreased heart rate.
			• Irregular pulse rates also occur with potassium imbalances and magnesium deficit.
			• Pulse volume is decreased in fluid volume deficit and increased in fluid volume excess.
Respirations		• Baseline respiratory rate, rhythm, and qualities	• Deep, rapid respirations may be a compensatory mechanism for metabolic acidosis or a primary disorder causing respiratory alkalosis.
			• Slow, shallow respirations may be a compensatory mechanism for metabolic alkalosis or a primary disorder causing respiratory acidosis.
			• Weakness or paralysis of respiratory muscles is likely in severe hypokalemia or hyperkalemia and in severe magnesium excess.
			• Moist crackles, in the absence of cardiopulmonary disease, indicate fluid volume excess.
Blood pressure	• Whenever a fluid imbalance is suspected, check the client's blood pressure while he or she is lying down, sitting, and standing.	• Baseline blood pressure	• A fall in systolic pressure greater than 15 mm Hg from the lying to the sitting or standing position (postural hypotension) usually indicates fluid volume deficit.

(continued)

TABLE 37 - 7 (continued)

Parameters to Be Considered in Clinical Assessment for Fluid, Electrolyte, and Acid–Base Balance			
Assessment Parameters	**Nursing Considerations**	**Findings in Healthy Adult**	**Significant Findings**
			• Hypotension may occur with magnesium excess (first occurring at a level of 3 to 5 mEq/L). • Hypertension can occur with magnesium deficit and with fluid volume excess.

Neck veins and central venous pressure (CVP)	• The jugular veins provide a built-in manometer for following changes in CVP.
	 • To estimate CVP, the nurse:
	   1. Positions the client in a semi-Fowler's position (head of bed elevated to a 30- to 45-degree angle), keeping the neck straight
	   2. Removes any of the client's clothing that could constrict the neck or upper chest
	   3. Provides adequate lighting to visualize effectively the external jugular veins on each side of the neck
	   4. Measures the levels to which the veins are distended on the neck or above the level of the manubrium
	 • More accurate assessments of blood volume are obtained by measuring CVP with a manometer or by hemodynamic monitoring with a device that measures pressures in both sides of the heart.
		• Normally, when the client is supine, the external jugular veins fill to the anterior border of the sternocleidomastoid muscle. With the client positioned sitting at a 45-degree angle, the venous distentions normally should not extend higher than 2 cm above the sternal angle.
		 • Pressure in the right atrium is usually 0 to 4 cm H_2O; pressure in the vena cava is about 4 to 11 cm H_2O.
			• A low CVP may indicate:
			   1. Decreased blood volume
			   2. Drug-induced vasodilation (causing pooling of blood in peripheral veins).
			 • A high CVP may indicate:
			   1. Increased blood volume
			   2. Heart failure
			   3. Vasoconstriction

Neuromuscular irritability	• When imbalances in calcium, magnesium, and sodium are suspected it is important to assess clients for increased or decreased neuromuscular irritability • To test for *Chvostek's sign*, the facial nerve should be percussed about 2 cm anterior to the earlobe.	• Negative response	• Clients with hypocalcemia or hypomagnesemia respond positively with a unilateral twitching of the facial muscles, including the eyelid and lips.
	• To test for *Trousseau's sign*, place a blood pressure cuff on the arm and inflate above systolic pressure for 3 minutes.	• Negative response	• A positive response is the development of carpal spasm.

(continued)

TABLE 37-7 *(continued)*

Parameters to Be Considered in Clinical Assessment for Fluid, Electrolyte, and Acid–Base Balance

Assessment Parameters	Nursing Considerations	Findings in Healthy Adult	Significant Findings
	• A deep tendon reflex is elicited by briskly tapping a partially stretched tendon with a rubber percussion hammer, preferably over the tendon insertion of the muscle. The broad head of the hammer is used to stroke easily accessible tendons and the pointed end for less accessible tendons.	• The response in the prospective muscle is a sudden contraction (2+).	• Deep tendon reflexes may be hyperactive in the presence of hypocalcemia, hypomagnesemia, hypernatremia, and alkalosis.
	• The muscle being tested should be slightly stretched and the client should be relaxed.		• Deep tendon reflexes may be hypoactive in the presence of hypercalcemia, hypermagnesemia, hyponatremia, hypokalemia, and acidosis.
	• Reflexes usually graded on a 0 to 4+ scale 0 = no response 1+ = somewhat diminished, but present 2+ = normal 3+ = brisker than average and possibly but not necessarily indicative of disease 4+ = hyperactive		
• Behavior • Sensation • Fatigue level	• Because these changes are often vague, they are best evaluated in context with specific imbalances.		

(Data from Metheny, N. M. [1992]. *Fluid and electrolyte balance* [2nd ed.]. Philadelphia: Lippincott.)

Complete Blood Count This basic screening test provides a determination of the total number of RBCs and values for hemoglobin and hematocrit. Significant values include the following:
- Increased hematocrit values: Found in severe dehydration and shock (when hemoconcentration rises considerably)
- Decreased hematocrit: Found with acute, massive blood loss, and with hemolytic reaction following transfusion of incompatible blood
- Increased levels of hemoglobin: Found in hemoconcentration of the blood
- Decreased levels of hemoglobin: Found with severe hemorrhage and following a hemolytic reaction

Serum Electrolytes This screening test performed routinely upon hospital admission provides information on plasma levels of select electrolytes. Commonly determined are plasma levels of sodium, potassium, chloride, and bicarbonate ions.

Urine pH and Specific Gravity Both the urine pH and SG may be obtained by dipstick measurement on a fresh voided specimen or through laboratory analysis. The urine pH expresses the strength of the urine as a dilute acid or a base solution and measures the free hydrogen ion concentration of the urine. SG is a means by which the kidney's ability to concentrate urine is measured. The range of SG depends on the state of hydration and varies with urine volume and the load of solutes to be excreted. Normal values range from 1.003 to 1.035 (concentrated urine—1.025 to 1.030 or more; dilute urine—1.001 to 1.010).

Arterial Blood Gases ABGs are obtained to determine the adequacy of oxygenation and ventilation and to assess acid–base status. Blood gas analysis provides values for pH, pCO_2, HCO_3^-, pO_2, and oxygen saturation. When interpreting blood gases:

1. Determine whether the pH is alkalotic (>7.45) or acidotic (<7.35).
2. Next, check the pCO_2 (respiratory parameter) and HCO_3^- (metabolic parameter) to identify the cause of the pH change. Acidosis is caused by high carbon dioxide levels (hypoventilation) or low bicarbonate levels. Alkalosis is caused by low carbon dioxide levels (hyperventilation) or high bicarbonate levels.
   a. In respiratory acid–base imbalances, the pH and pCO_2 values are inversely abnormal.
   b. In metabolic acid–base imbalances, the pH and HCO_3^- values are both high or both low:

Respiratory acidosis	↓ pH <7.35	↑ PCO_2	Normal HCO_3^-
Metabolic acidosis	↓ pH <7.35	Normal PCO_2	↓ HCO_3^-
Respiratory alkalosis	↑ pH >7.45	↓ PCO_2	Normal HCO_3^-
Metabolic alkalosis	↑ pH >7.45	Normal PCO_2	↑ HCO_3^-

3. Determine whether the body is compensating for the pH change.

   Examples:

pH	7.25	Decreased	Metabolic acidosis (both the pH and HCO_3^- are decreased); decreased pCO_2 indicates respiratory compensatory attempt—hyperventilation
PCO_2	31	Decreased	
HCO_3^-	12	Decreased	

pH	7.16	Decreased	Respiratory acidosis pH is decreased whereas
pCO_2	70	Increased	
HCO_3^-	31	Increased	pCO_2 is increased (ie, inversely abnormal); increased HCO_3^- indicates renal compensatory attempt

Lindell and Wesmiller (1989) suggest an alternate method of interpreting ABGs:

1. Determine the primary state by circling the appropriate pH analysis.

   pH < 7.35—acidosis
   pH > 7.35—alkalosis

2. Determine the primary cause by circling the appropriate pCO_2 and HCO_3 analysis.

   pCO_2 > 45—acidosis
   pCO_2 < 35—alkalosis
   HCO_3^- < 22—acidosis
   HCO_3^- > 26—alkalosis

3. Determine the acid–base disorder by matching terms.

   Example:

   pH = 7.25—(acidosis) ⎫
   pCO_2 = 31—alkalosis ⎬ metabolic acidosis
   HCO_3^- = 12—(acidosis) ⎭

a. When the pH indicates acidosis, call the disorder:
   Respiratory acidosis if the pCO_2 also indicates acidosis
   Metabolic acidosis if the HCO_3 indicates acidosis

   Example:

   pH = 7.49—(alkalosis) ⎫
   pCO_2 = 30—(alkalosis) ⎬ respiratory alkalosis
   HCO_3^- = 24—normal ⎭

b. When the pH indicates alkalosis, call the disorder:
   Respiratory alkalosis if the pCO_2 also indicates alkalosis
   Metabolic alkalosis if the HCO_3 indicates alkalosis

4. Look at the total picture and determine if compensation has occurred. Compensation is classified as follows:
   Absent if:
      pH abnormal
      One component abnormal
      Second component within normal range
   Partial if:
      pH abnormal
      One component abnormal
      Second component beginning to change
   Complete if:
      pH within normal range
      One component abnormal
      Second changed to move pH within normal range

Diagnosing

Fluid and Electrolyte Disturbances as the Problem

When assessment data point to fluid and electrolyte problems amenable to nursing therapy, they receive one of three diagnostic labels:

   Fluid Volume Excess
   Fluid Volume Deficit
   High Risk for Fluid Volume Deficit

Excess fluid volume may result from greatly increased fluid intake, or more frequently from decreased excretion such as occurs in progressive renal disease and with certain cancers. FVDs may result from decreased intake, increased excretion of fluids, fluid shifts, and from the special need for fluids and electrolytes created by strenuous exercise, extreme heat or dryness, and conditions (eg, fever) that increase the metabolic rate. The accompanying display presents contributing factors and defining characteristics for these diagnoses.

The nurse's analysis of assessment data may also lead to the diagnosis of specific electrolyte or acid–base disturbances that are termed collaborative problems because they require joint intervention by nursing and medicine (see Tables 37-4 and 37-5).

NURSING DIAGNOSES FOR COMMON PROBLEMS

Fluid and Electrolyte Balance

Problem	Related Factors	Sample Defining Characteristics
Fluid Volume Excess	Pathophysiologic factors: renal failure, decreased cardiac output, liver disease, abnormal fluid accumulations, hormonal problems	• "I've noticed that my wedding ring is tight . . . also my clothes don't fit as well as they used to. I guess I've gained some weight." • Reports dyspnea with exertion, feeling weak and fatigued • Pitting edema in feet, ankles, lower legs • Taut, shiny skin • Jugular venous distention
	Situational factors: excessive IV infusion	• Bounding pulse, increased from baseline • Shallow, rapid respirations, rales • Increased blood pressure
	Nutritional factors: excessive sodium intake, low protein intake	• 10-lb (4.5-kg) weight gain over past month • Fluid intake greater than output • "Sometimes I can't catch my breath and I feel like my heart is pounding away." • "I feel bloated."
Fluid Volume Deficit High Risk for Fluid Volume Deficit	Decreased fluid intake: imposed fluid restrictions, inability to obtain or swallow fluids (debilitation, oral pain), depression	• "After I got the flu I got so weak I couldn't get out of bed. . . . I think I was out of it for a couple of days." • Increased pulse and respirations • Dry oral mucosa, cracked lips, furrowed tongue • Scanty urine output
	Abnormal fluid loss: vomiting; diarrhea; abnormal drainage; excessive use of laxative, enemas, diuretics; blood loss; diaphoresis; burns	• "I'm thirsty all the time." • "I've been vomiting and I have diarrhea—several times a day." • Weight loss: 5 lb (2–3 kg) • Urine is concentrated (specific gravity, 1.035). • Fluid output greater than fluid intake • Neck veins collapsed when lying flat • Decreased skin turgor
	Increased need for fluids: strenuous exercise, extreme heat or dryness, fever (increased metabolic rate)	• Skin is warm to touch, moist, and flushed • Increased temperature, pulse, respirations • Decreased blood pressure

Fluid and Electrolyte Disturbances as the Etiology Disturbances in fluid, electrolyte, and acid–base balance may affect many other areas of human functioning. Sample diagnoses follow:

Activity Intolerance related to dyspnea on exertion

Anxiety related to pulmonary edema

Ineffective Breathing Pattern related to compensatory mechanism by lungs (hypoventilation or hyperventilation)

Decreased Cardiac Output related to decreased blood volume, shock

High Risk for Injury related to neuromuscular irritability, cardiac arrhythmia

Knowledge Deficit: Harmful Effects of Abuses of Dieting, Alcohol, Diuretics, Laxatives, and Enemas, related to no previous experience

Altered Oral Mucous Membrane related to dehydration

Impaired Skin Integrity related to dehydration, edema

Altered Thought Processes related to cerebral edema, mental confusion or disorientation, convulsions

Altered Tissue Perfusion: [specify type] related to decreased cardiac output

Altered Urinary Elimination related to decreased kidney perfusion secondary to decreased plasma volume

Planning: Client Goals

Nursing care for any client supports the following client goals. The healthy adult client will:

- Maintain an approximate balance between fluid intake and fluid output (average about 2500 mL fluid intake and output over 3 days)
- Maintain a urine SG within normal range (1.010 to 1.025)
- Practice self-care behaviors to promote fluid, electrolyte, and acid–base balance—maintain adequate intake of fluid and electrolytes; respond appropriately to body's signals of impending fluid, electrolyte, or acid–base imbalance

When an imbalance exists, the client will:

- Relate relief of symptoms (specify) after implementation of treatment regimen (eg, 1 month after decreasing sodium intake client reports 4 lb [1.8 kg] weight loss)

Implementing

Nursing interventions to prevent or correct fluid, electrolyte, and acid–base imbalances include dietary modification, modification of fluid intake, medication administration, IV therapy, blood and blood products replacement, and TPN.

Preventing Fluid Imbalances

An adequate fluid intake and a well-balanced, nutritious diet with appropriate adjustments throughout the life cycle are basic essentials to promote fluid balance. The following are some of the basic items the nurse needs to consider to help prevent fluid imbalances:

- Be familiar with common events in life that lead to fluid imbalances, and observe the client carefully.
- Note the client's present fluid and food intake, and learn what his or her previous eating and drinking patterns have been. Learn whether the client has used fad diets, which may lead to imbalances.
- Note whether thirst is excessive or whether the client experiences little or no thirst. Thirst is a subjective sensation and an important factor in determining water intake and, eventually, output through the kidneys.

Thirst is poorly understood, although both psychologic and physiologic factors appear to be involved.

- Be aware of excessive losses of fluids from the body, and attempt to prevent losses when possible. Vomiting, pronounced perspiration, diarrhea, draining wounds, and excessive urinary output, for example, may cause excessive losses.
- Consider ways in which the client's medical regimen may lead to imbalances. For example, many drugs to stimulate urine formation increase the elimination of potassium. If food supplements high in potassium are not included in the diet or if drug therapy is not started, hypokalemia often follows. Adrenocorticosteroids may lead to sodium and water retention and to excessive potassium excretion.
- Learn whether the client has been "treating" himself or herself and, as a result, threatening fluid balance. Common practices that threaten fluid balance include the indiscriminate use of enemas, laxatives, antacids, and over-the-counter drugs to promote urination.
- Consider conditions that induce destructive effects on the body as threats to fluid balance. Examples include immobilization, trauma, burns, surgical procedures, and exposure to toxic agents.
- Teach clients to observe for fluid imbalances and to report them promptly. Examples include rapid weight gains and losses; swollen fingers, feet, and ankles; puffy eyelids; muscle weakness; change in skin sensations; and scanty or profuse urine production.
- Help clients and their families understand the significance of maintaining fluid balance and preventing imbalances.
- Be aware that normal physiologic changes associated with aging impact on the elder client's ability to maintain fluid balance. Dehydration is a common fluid and electrolyte disorder in this population and the accompanying display suggests specific nursing strategies to prevent and correct fluid and electrolyte imbalance.

Developing a Dietary Plan

Simple dietary changes may help to resolve fluid and electrolyte disturbances. After doing a nutritional assessment to identify actual or potential imbalances and food preferences, the nurse can initiate teaching. It is important to involve both the client and the person who prepares the meals in the development of the nutritional plan. The plan should include foods that both help to resolve the fluid or electrolyte imbalance and are acceptable to the client. For example, for FVD, increase foods with high water content (eg, citrus fruit, melons, celery); for hypokalemia, increase foods with high potassium content (eg, bananas, citrus fruits, apricots, melons, broccoli, potatoes); for hypernatremia, avoid foods high in sodium (eg, processed cheese, lunch meats, canned soups and vegetables, salted snack foods); eliminate use of table salt.

When given a list of foods, the client should be able to identify those that can be eaten freely or moderately as well

FOCUS ON THE OLDER ADULT

Nursing Strategies for Ensuring Fluid Balance in Older Adults

Decrease in Total Body Weight

- Ensure that oral intake is at least 1500 mL for 24 hours.
- Assess for signs of dehydration or fluid retention.
- Assess 24-hour intake and output for consistency and balance.
- Teach family to notify physician when persistent diarrhea or vomiting occur.
- Assess skin turgor and mucous membranes.
- Be aware of schedule for diagnostic tests (and associated dietary and fluid restrictions).
- Assess medication history for drugs that have a diuretic action or require additional fluid intake.

Altered Sense of Thirst

- Offer fluids at regular intervals.
- Replace fluids as necessary either orally or IV.
- Investigate individual fluid preferences.
- Provide assistance or assistive devices for encouraging fluid intake.

Loss of Nephrons and Decreased Renal Blood Flow

- Record output accurately.
- Note appearance and specific gravity of urine.
- Check laboratory values for abnormal levels.

---

as those that should be avoided. Both the client and person responsible for food preparation should be able to describe a 24-hour diet plan compatible with the recommended modifications.

Modifying Fluid Intake

Depending on the nature of the fluid or electrolyte imbalance, a client's fluids may need to be increased, decreased, or modified in terms of types of fluids ingested. The nurse is responsible for

- Identifying the appropriate fluid modification (with certain illnesses, the physician may order fluid directives [eg, "Restrict fluids to 1000 mL/d"])
- Determining if the client understands the rationale for the fluid modification, is motivated to comply with the modification, and is capable of compliance (eg, a bedridden client who needs to increase fluid intake cannot do this independently)
- Developing and implementing a care plan based on the preceding information. For example, three clients with the same tendency to retain fluids may need different nursing care. One has never learned that the high-sodium beverages she frequently drinks are contributing to her problem. One teaching session may be sufficient to resolve her fluid imbalance. A second client has a history of poor self-care behaviors. Intelligent and the recipient of much health education in the past, this client has no need for further teaching. Nursing time is best invested in counseling and exploring why the client fails to value his health sufficiently to comply with the treatment regimen. Until the client values the proposed fluid modification, compliance will probably be poor. The third client is a frail elderly woman with pneumonia and a history of congestive heart failure who depends on the nursing staff

for care. Her fluid intake will be determined by the fluids offered her by the nursing staff.

Increasing Fluids

An above-average intake of fluids is prescribed for certain clients. The usual order reads, "Force fluids," and indicates the amount of fluid the client is to have in each 24-hour period. The care plan should specify the amount of fluid to be ingested in 24 hours (for hospitalized clients shift totals are helpful [eg, 7 to 3, 1200 mL; 3 to 11, 900 mL; 11 to 7, 300 mL]) and the client's food preferences. Fluids should be chosen that best provide the calories and electrolytes needed by the client.

A variety of techniques is recommended to help the client take more than average amounts of fluids:

- Explain to the client in language he or she can understand, the specific goal of taking the daily amount of fluid prescribed for the client. This helps promote motivation and is more meaningful than simply telling the client to increase fluid intake.
- Set short-term or interim goals with the client. Examples include a glass of water every hour, a particular beverage by the time a television program is finished, or a pitcher of water by lunch. Most clients try to reach goals that they help to set, even when they do not feel thirsty.
- Plan to offer a proportionately larger amount of fluid during the early hours of the client's waking day. The client is usually able to take fluids relatively easily after having few or no fluids during sleeping hours.
- Try to avoid making it necessary to offer large amounts of fluid before sleep. This helps prevent disturbing rest because the client needs to urinate.
- Encourage as wide a variety of liquids as possible to make larger intake more interesting and palatable. If

clients dislike taking fluids (a common problem with children) or have swallowing difficulties, offering a gelatin dessert (Jell-O), flavored frozen water (Popsicles), water ice, and so forth may meet with more success.

- Keep fluids readily available for the client. It is distressing to see people who are unable to secure their own fluids left with an unfilled water pitcher, an empty glass, a full pitcher out of reach, or a pitcher too heavy to lift.
- Serve fluids at the appropriate temperature. For example, the client is likely to drink more when iced liquids are iced and cold, and coffee and tea when they are hot but not so hot that the client is likely to burn himself or herself.
- Use attractive, clean, and easily handled cups and glasses, a practice that helps to encourage the client's desire to take fluids.
- Have the client assist in keeping a record of his or her intake when this is possible. This often serves as a motivating factor to increase fluid intake.
- Provide support, understanding, and encouragement because forcing fluid intake for the person experiencing no thirst can be uncomfortable.

Increasing the fluid intake of clients is among the most common nursing care objectives. Often, creativity and con-siderable patience by the nurse are necessary to reach desired goals. The display indicates nursing interventions that focus on maintaining fluid balance. Fluids may also be replaced through nasogastric, gastrostomy, or jejunostomy tubes (see Chapter 33).

Restricting Fluids

Restricting the client's fluid intake is sometimes necessary. The usual order reads, "Restrict fluids," and indicates the amount of fluid the client is to have in each 24-hour period.

A variety of techniques is recommended to help the client who is to have a restricted fluid intake:

- Explain to the client, in language he or she can understand, the specific goal of taking the daily amount of fluid prescribed. This often helps promote motivation and is more meaningful to the client than simply telling him or her to restrict fluid intake.
- Discuss with the client the time intervals at which fluids will be served. Usually, it is best to offer fluids between meals because food often helps to relieve some feelings of thirst.
- Set short-term or interim goals for offering fluids at 1- or 2-hour intervals when this seems helpful and when the client can cooperate.
- Serve ice chips instead of water from time to time.

RESEARCH IN NURSING Making a Difference

Fluid and Electrolyte Balance

Monitoring and maintaining fluid and electrolyte balance in clients is a major component of nursing care. The elderly population is particularly at risk for imbalances, which can be life-threatening. Unfortunately, little research has been carried out by nurses with respect to fluid and electrolyte status.

Related Research

Adams, F. (1988). How much do elders drink? *Geriatric Nursing 8*(4), 218–221.

This study compared fluid intake between institutionalized and noninstitutionalized elderly people with a focus on amount, time pattern, and type of fluids. Most participants in this research, regardless of setting, reported limited intake after 6 PM, with the highest intake in the afternoon. The amount of fluid intake (40% of which was water) was significantly higher for those clients living at home. Institutionalized clients drank less water and fluids in general, with most of the fluid intake occurring with meals or medications. Because the nursing home residents appeared to depend more on a caregiver for assistance with fluid intake, nurses can have a significant impact on increasing fluid intake while considering individual preferences.

Gaspar, P. (1988). What determines how much patients drink? *Geriatric Nursing 8*(4), 221–224.

The results of this research indicated that water intake among nursing home residents is inadequate and identified seven variables that were associated with maintaining an adequate water intake in this population. Age, sex, length of institutionalization, number of visitors, medications, sensory ability, and functional ability appeared to significantly affect water intake in these clients. Diligent nursing assessment can identify residents at risk for inadequate intake and suggest opportunities for increasing fluid intake in dependent elderly people. This study also implied the need for ongoing education efforts with all nursing home personnel about maintaining adequate fluid intake in residents.

Summary

Routine nursing interventions that focus on fluid and electrolyte status include daily maintenance of intake and output records, monitoring client's weight, and monitoring laboratory values. Additional research is needed to determine more effective ways nurses can help clients of all ages maintain fluid and electrolyte balance.

When they melt, the water is about one half of its volume when frozen.

- Use small glasses or cups so that the container appears to contain more fluid than it actually does. Large containers partially full make the amount of fluid seem smaller than it actually is.
- Provide oral hygiene at regular intervals so that the client's mouth remains clean. Lubricate the lips and mucous membranes as indicated.
- Allow the client to rinse the mouth with water when he or she can cooperate without swallowing this fluid and exceeding the intake limit.
- Avoid offering the client dry, salty, or sweet foods and fluids, because they tend to increase thirst.
- Avoid offering the client hard candy or gum. They were often thought to relieve thirst by stimulating salivation. The sugar content increases oral tonicity and temporarily draws fluids to the mouth membranes. After about 15 to 30 minutes, the membranes are even more dry than before. Sugarless gum may be offered to some clients.
- Divert the client's attention from thirst by involving him or her in various activities to the degree that he or she is able to participate.
- Keep fluids not intended for the client out of sight.
- Have the client assist in keeping an intake record when possible. This may serve as a motivating factor to limit fluid intake.
- Provide understanding, support, and encouragement because limiting fluid intake for the person experiencing thirst is uncomfortable.

Administering Medications

Clients with fluid, electrolyte, and acid–base imbalances are often prescribed medications as part of the therapeutic regimen. Nurses need to be knowledgeable about the therapeutic effects of mineral–electrolyte preparations and diuretics as well as alert for adverse effects of other medications such as steroids and hormone replacements.

Mineral–Electrolyte Preparations Mineral–electrolyte preparations are frequently prescribed to correct electrolyte imbalances. Nursing responsibilities include

- Accurate administration consistent with manufacturer's guidelines (eg, dilute oral potassium supplements to disguise the unpleasant taste and decrease gastric irritation; monitor ABGs for increased pH after each 50 to 100 mEq of sodium bicarbonate to avoid overtreatment and metabolic alkalosis)
- Knowledge of the intended therapeutic effect and evaluation (eg, with magnesium sulfate, look for decreased restlessness and irritability, decreased muscle tremors, and control of convulsions)
- Observation for adverse effects (eg, with sodium chloride injection, observe for hypernatremia and circulatory overload)
- Observation for drug interactions (eg, drugs that increase the effects of minerals and electrolytes include acidifying agents, alkalinizing agents, cation exchange resin, iron salts, and potassium salts)
- Teaching the clients appropriate self-care behaviors

Diuretics Diuretics are drugs that increase renal excretion of water, sodium, and other electrolytes. Although helpful in treating clients with FVE, they have the potential to cause dehydration and serious electrolyte deficiencies. Clients need careful monitoring and education while on diuretic therapy.

Administering Intravenous Therapy

A relatively common form of therapy for handling fluid disturbances is the use of various solutions infused IV. The physician is responsible for prescribing the kind and amount of solution to be used. The nurse is responsible for initiating, monitoring, and discontinuing the therapy. As is true with other therapeutic agents, the nurse should understand the client's need for IV therapy, the type of solution being used, its desired effect, and untoward reactions that may occur. Contents of selected water and electrolyte solutions with comments about their use are presented in Table 37-8.

Equipment Sterile technique is observed when a vein is entered. Disposable infusion tubing and needles are used to help eliminate many possible sources of contamination and to reduce the cost of equipment aftercare.

Equipment varies according to the manufacturer. The nurse is responsible for being familiar with the equipment used in the agency where he or she cares for clients. Typically, solutions for infusions are dispensed in either 1-L or 500-mL glass or plastic bottles or in plastic bags. The plastic bags collapse under atmospheric pressure as the solution enters the client's vein. Rigid containers, such as glass bottles, cannot collapse. Therefore, they have an air vent that allows air to replace fluid as it enters the client's vein. Small 50- and 100-mL solution bags are available to administer medications IV.

Tubing is attached to the solution container. The rate of flow is manually controlled by a clamp or constricting device on the tubing. A device called a dripmeter or dripchamber connects the solution bottle and tubing and permits the number of drops per minute of solution to be determined.

There are a variety of needles and catheters commonly used for the IV infusion. IV catheters, increasingly being used for IV therapy, are plastic tubes that have been mounted on a needle or are threaded through a needle for insertion. Single- or double-winged infusion needles (butterflies) are short-beveled, thin-walled needles with plastic flaps. They are used because of the ease in handling and stabilizing them. The flaps, or wings, are brought together tightly in the nurse's fingers and are used to hold the needle securely as it is being inserted. Other equipment necessary to start an IV infusion is listed in Procedure 37-1.

(*Text continues on p. 1039*)

TABLE 37-8

Contents of Selected Water and Electrolyte Solutions With Comments About Their Use	
Solution	**Comments**

5% dextrose in water (D_5W)
  No electrolytes
  50 g of dextrose
	Supplies about 170 cal/L and free water to aid in renal excretion of solutes
	Should not be used in excessive volumes in clients with increased ADH activity or to replace fluids in hypovolemic patients

0.9 % NaCl (isotonic saline)
  Na^+ 154 mEq/L
  Cl^- 154 mEq/L
	Not desirable as a routine maintenance solution because it provides only Na^+ and Cl^-, which are provided in excessive amounts

0.45% NaCl (1/2-strength saline)
  Na^+ 77 mEq/L
  Cl^- 154 mEq/L
	A hypotonic solution that provides Na^+, Cl^-, and free water Na^+ and Cl^- provided in fluid allows kidneys to select and retain needed amounts
	Free water desirable as aid to kidneys in elimination of solutes

0.33% NaCl (1/3-strength saline)
  Na^+ 56 mEq/L
  Cl^- 56 mEq/L
	A hypotonic solution that provides Na^+, Cl^- and free water
	Often used to treat hypernatremia (because this solution contains a small amount of Na^+, it dilutes the plasma sodium while not allowing it to drop too rapidly)

3% NaCl
  Na^+ 513 mEq/L
  Cl^- 513 mEq/L
	Grossly hypertonic solutions used only to treat severe hyponatremia

5% NaCl
  Na^+ 855 mEq/L
  Cl^- 855 mEq/L
	Dangerous solutions

Lactated Ringer's solution
  Na^+ 130 mEq/L
  K^+ 4 mEq/L
  Ca^{++} 3 mEq/L
  Cl^- 109 mEq/L
  Lactate (metabolized to bicarbonate) 28 mEq/L
	A roughly isotonic solution that contains multiple electrolytes in approximately the same concentrations as found in plasma (note that this solution is lacking in Mg and PO_4)
	Used in the treatment of hypovolemia, burns, and fluid lost as bile or diarrhea
	Useful in treating mild metabolic acidosis

Other isotonic multiple electrolyte solutions
  Plasma-Lyte 148 (Travenol)
  Isolyte S (McGaw)
  Normosol R (Abbott Hospital Prods)
  Na^+ 140 mEq/L
  K^+ 5 mEq/L
  Mg^{++} 3 mEq/L
  Cl^- 98 mEq/L
  HCO_3^- 50 mEq/L (or equivalent)
	Isotonic solution that can be used to replace extracellular fluid loss
	Because of relatively high bicarbonate content, can be used to correct mild acidosis

Hypotonic multiple electrolyte solutions
  Plasma-Lyte 56 (Travenol)
  Normosol-M (Abbott Hospital Prods)
  Na^+ 40 mEq/L
  K^+ 13 mEq/L
  Mg^{++} 3 mEq/L
  Cl^- 40 mEq/L
  HCO_3^- 16 mEq/L (or equivalent)
	Hypotonic solution that supplies free water as well as electrolytes

Sodium lactate solution, 1/6 M
  Na^+ 167 mEq/L
  Cl^- 167 mEq/L
	A roughly isotonic solution used to correct severe metabolic adidosis (lactate is metabolized to bicarbonate in 1 to 2 hours by the liver)
	Not used in clients with liver disease (lactate cannot be converted to bicarbonate in such individuals); also, not used in clients with oxygen lack (unable to adequately convert lactate to bicarbonate)

Sodium bicarbonate, 5%
  Na^+ 595 mEq/L
  Cl^- 595 mEq/L
	A hypertonic solution used to correct severe metabolic acidosis
	Should be cautiously administered at a slow rate, under careful volume control
	Should be administered only with extreme caution to salt-retaining clients (eg, those with cardiac, renal, or liver damage)

Ammonium chloride, 2.14%	Acidifying solution used to correct severe metabolic alkalosis Due to high ammonium content, must be administered cautiously to clients with compromised hepatic function

(Data from Metheny, N. M. [1992]. *Fluid and electrolyte balance* [2nd ed.]. Philadelphia: Lippincott.)

PROCEDURE 37-1

Starting an Intravenous Infusion

Equipment

IV solution
IV infusion set
IV tubing
Needle (angiocatheter, intracath, standard needle, butterfly)
Tourniquet
Antiseptic swabs
IV pole

Tape
Electronic infusion device (if ordered)
Dressings with Betadine or other antiseptic ointment
Armboard, if needed
Clean disposable gloves

Action	Rationale
1 Gather all equipment and bring to bedside. Check IV solution and medication additives with physician's order.	Having equipment available saves time and facilitates accomplishment of task. Ensures that client receives the correct IV solution and medication as ordered by physician.
2 Explain procedure to client.	Explanation allays client's anxiety.
3 Wash your hands.	Handwashing deters the spread of microorganisms.
4 Prepare IV solution and tubing: a Maintain aseptic technique when opening sterile packages and IV solution	This prevents spread of microorganisms.
b Clamp tubing, uncap spike, and insert into entry site on bag or bottle as manufacturer directs.	This punctures the seal in the IV bag or bottle.
c Squeeze drip chamber and allow it to fill at least half way.	Suction effect causes fluid to move into drip chamber. Also prevents air from moving down the tubing.

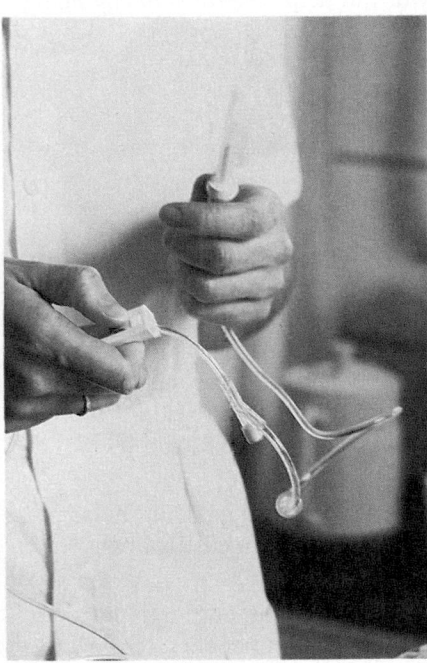

Action 4b: Clamping tubing.

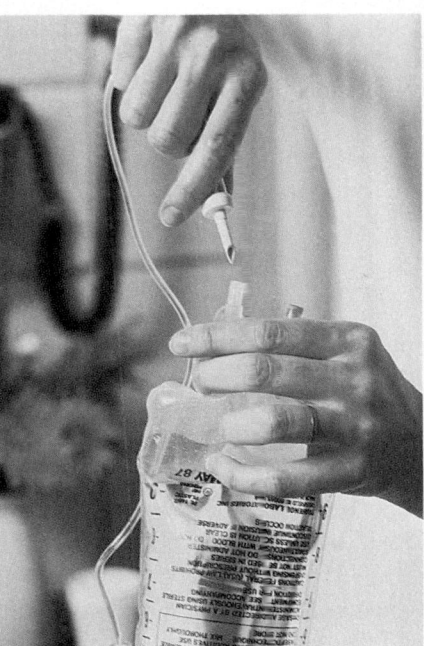

Action 4b: Inserting spike.

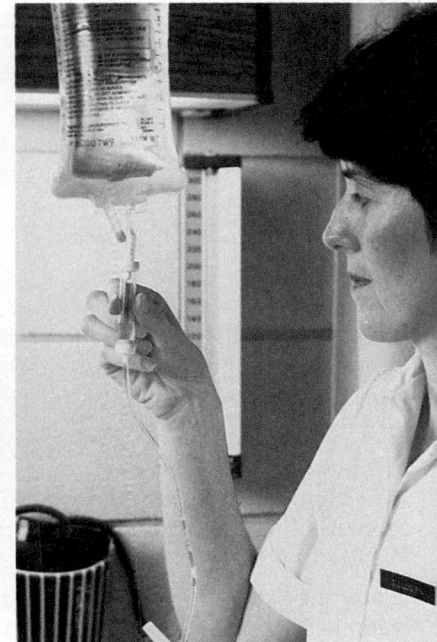

Action 4c: Squeezing drip chamber.

(continued)

Starting an Intravenous Infusion

Action	Rationale
d Remove cap at end of tubing, release clamp, and allow fluid to move through tubing. Allow fluid to flow until all air bubbles have disappeared. Close clamp and recap end of tubing maintaining sterility of setup.	This removes air from tubing that can, in larger amounts, act as an air embolus.
e If an electronic device is to be used, follow manufacturer's instructions for inserting tubing and setting infusion rate.	This ensures correct flow rate and proper use of equipment.
5 Have the client in a low Fowler's position in bed.	The supine position permits either arm to be used and allows for good body alignment. The low Fowler's position is usually most comfortable for the client.
6 Select an appropriate site and palpate accessible veins.	The selection of an appropriate site decreases discomfort for the client and possible damage to body tissues.
7 If the site is hairy and agency policy permits, shave a 2-inch area around the intended site of entry.	It is difficult to clean the site of entry in the presence of hair because hair can harbor microorganisms. Adhesive tape will adhere better and may be removed more easily if hair is removed from site.
8 Apply a tourniquet 5 to 6 inches above the venipuncture site to obstruct venous blood flow and distend the vein. Direct the ends of the tourniquet away from the site of entry. Check to be sure that the radial pulse is still present.	Interrupting the blood flow to the heart causes the vein to distend. Interruption of the arterial flow impedes venous filling. Distended veins are easy to see, palpate, and enter. The end of the tourniquet could contaminate the area of injection if directed toward the site of entry.
9 Ask the client to open and close his or her fist. Observe and palpate for a suitable vein. Try the following techniques if a vein cannot be felt:	Contraction of the muscles of the forearm forces blood into the veins, thereby distending them further. Lowering the arm below the level of the heart, tapping the vein, and applying warmth help distend veins by filling them with blood.
a Release the tourniquet and have the client lower his or her arm below the level of the heart to fill the veins. Reapply tourniquet and gently tap over the intended vein to help distend it.	
b Remove tourniquet and place warm compresses over the intended vein for 10 to 15 minutes.	
10 Don clean, disposable gloves.	Care must be used when handling any blood or body fluids to prevent transmission of HIV and other bloodborne infections.
11 Cleanse the entry site with an antiseptic solution. Use a circular motion to move from the center outward for several inches.	Cleansing that begins at the site of entry and moves outward in a circular motion carries organisms away from the site of entry. Organisms on the skin can be introduced into the tissues or the bloodstream with the needle.
12 Use the nondominant hand, placed about 1 inch or 2 inches below entry site, to hold the skin taut against the vein.	Pressure on the vein and surrounding tissues helps prevent movement of the vein as the needle is being inserted.
13 Enter the skin gently with the needle held in dominant hand, bevel side up, at a 30- to 45-degree angle, and when the needle is through the skin, lower the needle until it is nearly parallel to the skin.	This allows needle to enter the vein with minimal trauma and deters passage of the needle through the vein.

(continued)

Starting an Intravenous Infusion

Action	Rationale

While following the course of the vein, advance the needle or catheter into the vein. A sensation of "give" can be felt when the needle enters the vein.

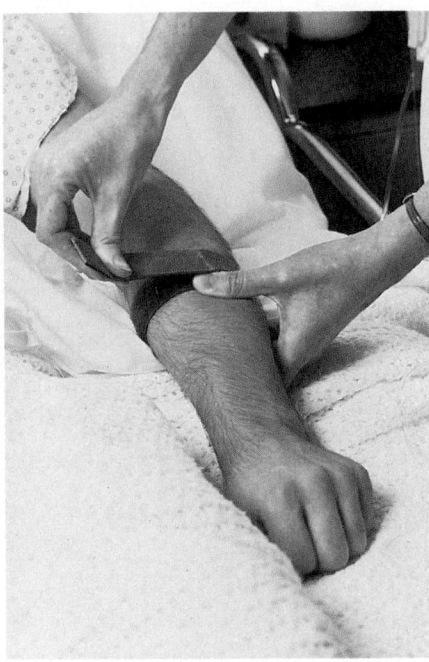

Action 8: Applying tourniquet.

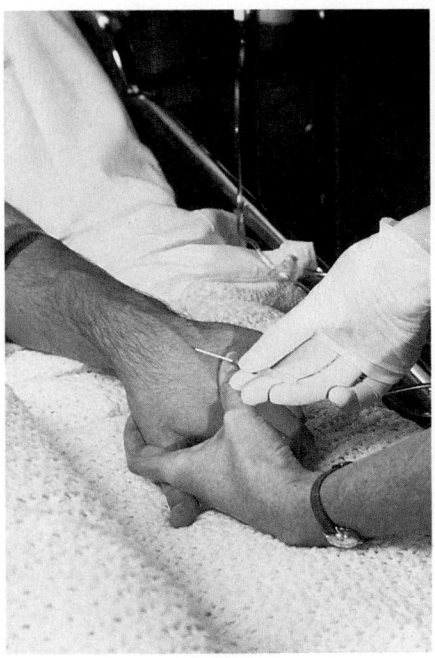

Action 13: Entering vein.

14 When blood returns through the lumen of the needle, advance the need farther into the vein. The exact technique depends on the type of needle used. With an angiocatheter, the needle is removed, leaving the catheter in place.

The tourniquet causes increased venous pressure resulting in automatic backflow. Having the needle placed well into the vein helps to prevent dislodgement of the needle.

15 Quickly remove protective cap from the IV tubing and attach the tubing to the catheter or needle. Stabilize the catheter or needle with nondominant hand and release the tourniquet with your other hand.

Bleeding is minimized and patency of the vein is maintained if the connection is made smoothly between the catheter and tubing.

16 Start the flow of solution promptly by releasing the clamp on the tubing. Examine the tissue around the entry site for signs of infiltration.

Blood clots readily if intravenous flow is not maintained. If needle accidentally slips out of vein, solution will accumulate and infiltrate into surrounding tissue.

17 Support the needle with small piece of gauze under the hub, if necessary, to keep the needle properly positioned in the vein.

The pressure of the wall of the vein against the bevel of the needle interrupts the rate of flow of the solution. The wall of the vein can be easily punctured by the needle.

18 An antiseptic ointment may be applied to the needle's site of entry with a sterile dressing according to agency policy. Remove soiled gloves and discard appropriately.

Dressing and antiseptic ointment reduce skin contamination and protect against infection.

(continued)

P R O C E D U R E   3 7 - 1   *(continued)*

Starting an Intravenous Infusion

Action	Rationale
19 Loop the tubing near the site of entry, and anchor with tape to prevent pull on the needle, as illustrated in figure.	The smooth structure of the vein does not offer resistance to the movement of the needle. The weight of the tubing is sufficient to pull the needle out of the vein if it is not well anchored.
20 Mark the date, time, and type and size of the needle used for the infusion on the tape anchoring the tubing.	Personnel working with the infusion will know what type of needle is being used and when it was inserted. Protects client and IV site from infection.

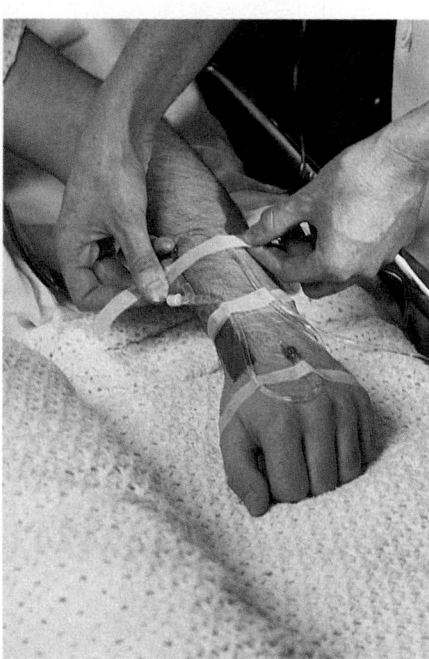

Action 19: Looping and anchoring tubing.

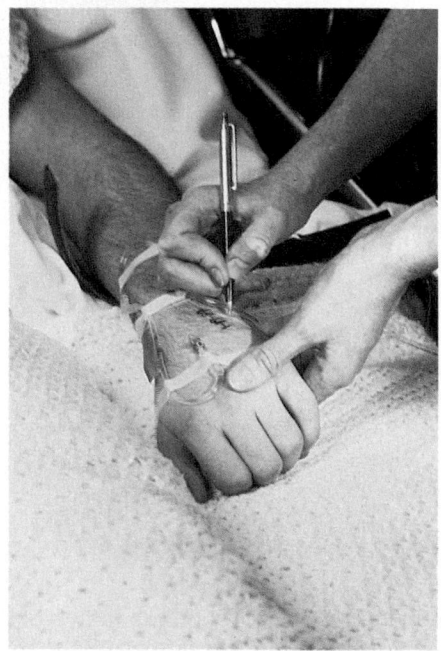

Action 20: Marking pertinent information on tape.

21 Anchor arm to an armboard for support, if necessary.	An armboard protects against change in the position of the vein and acts as a reminder to the client to minimize movements of his or her arm.
22 Adjust the rate of solution flow according to the amount prescribed or follow manufacturer's directions for adjusting flow rate on infusion pump.	The physician prescribes the rate of flow.
23 Remove all equipment and dispose in proper manner. Wash hands.	Handwashing deters the spread of microorganisms.
24 Document the procedure and client's response. Chart time, site, device used, and solution.	This provides accurate documentation and ensures continuity of care.
25 Return to check flow rate and observe for infiltration 30 minutes after starting infusion.	This documents client's response to infusion.

Age Considerations	Tape is more likely to tear the thinner, more fragile skin of an elderly client. Special skin preparations (eg, Skin Prep) can be applied to the skin before taping.
	In elderly clients, it may be necessary to delay rotating peripheral IV sites after a certain amount of days due to limited availability of locations.

(continued)

PROCEDURE 37-1 *(continued)*

Starting an Intravenous Infusion

Special Considerations

The Landry Vein Light Venoscope is a new device developed to locate veins that are not easily seen or palpated. It consists of two fiber-optic probes that are placed on the skin several inches apart and shine an intense light into the client's subcutaneous tissue. The veins appear as dark lines under the skin. The venoscope can be used on any age or size client but requires a dimly lit or dark environment (Gonsoulin & Broussard, 1991).

Recent studies have questioned the value of transparent dressings used with the insertion of central and venous catheters. A major drawback may be an increased risk of developing an infection. The gauze dressing is being reevaluated for use with IV insertion sites at some institutions (Meyer, 1992).

A 1% lidocaine solution injected intradermally into the IV start-up site significantly reduces the pain associated with inserting an IV needle or catheter. Research continues on the safety of this technique (Dick, Maree, & Gray, 1992).

Other Venous Access Devices The **central venous catheter (CVC)** is usually introduced into the subclavian or internal jugular veins and passed to the superior vena cava just above the right atrium. In the United States, its use is becoming more common; some 3 million CVCs are inserted annually (Viall, 1990). Traditionally only used in critical care situations, CVCs are now common on medical–surgical units and in home care. They provide access for a variety of IV fluids and medications as well as a means for hemodynamic monitoring. CVCs may be used for short (up to 4 weeks) or long-term periods and have a single, double, or triple lumen or entry port (see Fig. 37-10 for an example of CVC placement). Long-term CVCs are made of flexible silicone rubber rather than the polyurethane used for short-term access and are less likely to result in thrombus formation. The Groshong long-term CVC is unique because pressure-sensitive valves seal off each lumen, further reducing the risk of complications and simplifying routine catheter maintenance. A short-term CVC may be inserted at the bedside under sterile conditions, whereas a long-term catheter is surgically inserted in the operating room and the proximal portion of the catheter is tunneled through subcutaneous fascia to an exit point on the chest wall below the nipple line. Both types of catheter require a chest x-ray to confirm proper placement before infusion of IV solutions begins. An occlusive dressing protects the insertion site. (See Special Considerations for Procedure 37-1 for recent information about occlusive dressings.)

Nursing responsibilities with CVCs include changing the dressing according to agency policy at least every 72 hours, carefully assessing for any sign of infection, changing injection caps on the lumens, and flushing with a heparin solution to prevent clotting and blockage of the lumen.

Peripherally inserted central catheters (PICs) are a type of venous access that can be introduced into the basilic or cephalic veins by way of the antecubital space and ad-

FIGURE 37-10

Placement of triple-lumen central venous catheter.

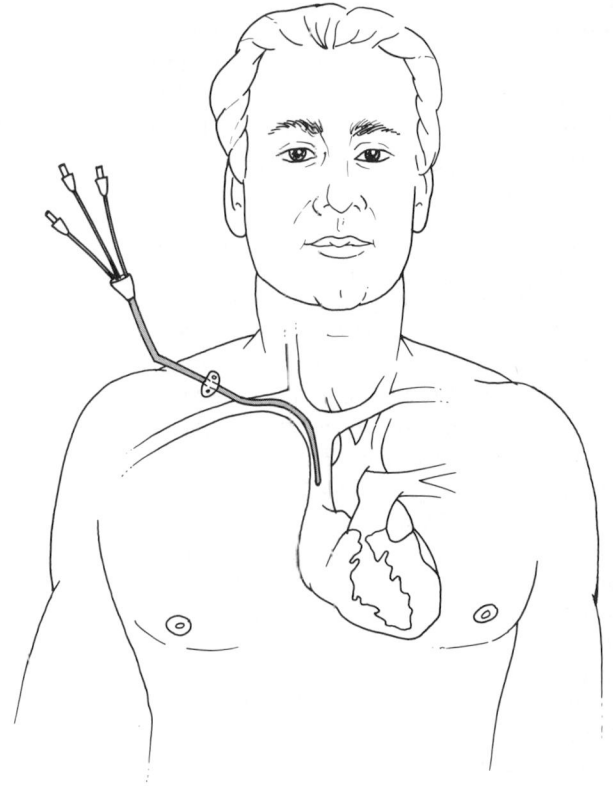

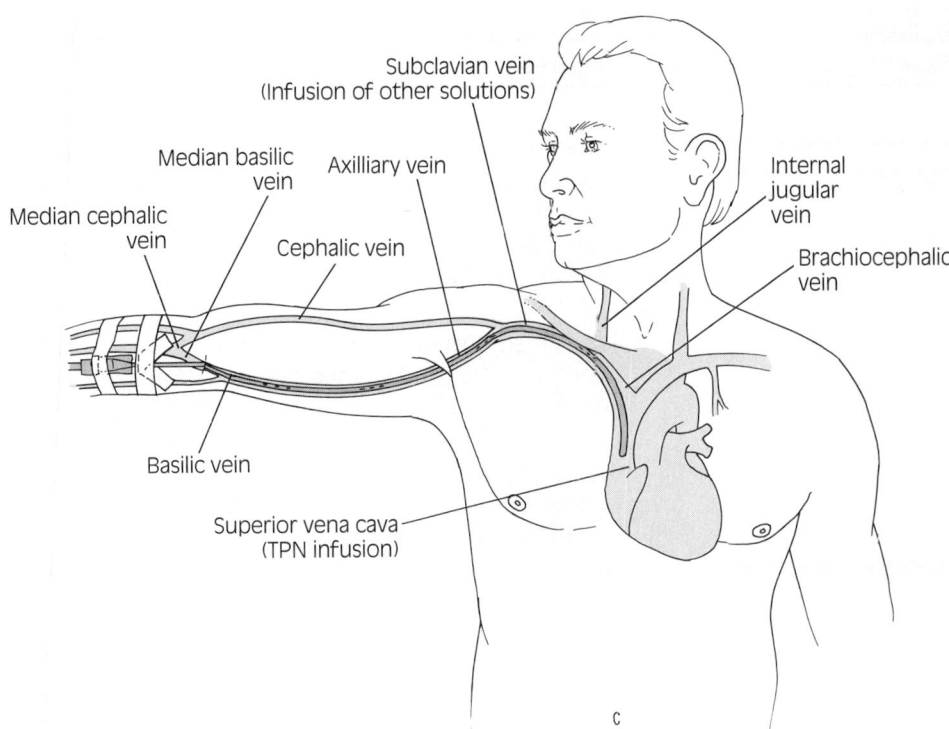

FIGURE 37-11

Placement of peripherally inserted central catheter.

vanced as far as the superior vena cava (Fig. 37-11). X-ray verification is always required if the tip of the catheter is advanced beyond the axillary vein. They may be single- or double-lumen catheters. In some areas of the country, registered nurses are permitted by their state boards of nursing to insert these catheters (Hadaway, 1991). Indications for use of PICs include administration of IV antibiotics for an extended period (2 to 6 weeks); infusion of parenteral nutrition; chemotherapy; continuous narcotic infusions; and long-term rehydration (Rountree, 1991). According to several studies, the average dwell time for PICs in hospitalized and home care clients is around 20 days (Kyle & Myers, 1990; Markel & Reynen, 1990).

Nursing responsibilities include sterile dressing changes per agency schedule and protocol, routine heparin or saline flushes to maintain patency, and careful observation for any complications of PIC therapy such as phlebitis, cellulitis, infiltration, and infection or sepsis. The decreased risk of complications as well as the other benefits of comfort, simplicity of insertion, and length of dwell time make PICs an excellent alternative for some clients.

Another type of long-term CVC is an *implanted port*. The catheter tip is again placed in the subclavian or internal jugular vein but the proximal end or port is implanted in a subcutaneous pocket of the chest wall so that no external parts of the system are visible. Newer implanted ports are currently available for placement in the antecubital area of the arm and are referred to as peripheral access system ports or PAS ports. Initially, implanted ports were intended for chemotherapy but recently have also been used in home care clients as a route for TPN or IV antibiotics. A special angled needle is inserted through the skin and rubber sep-

tum and into the port reservoir (Fig. 37-12). Nurses have many opportunities for health teaching about medical and surgical asepsis and meticulous skin care as they care for clients with implanted ports.

Site Selection   Suitability of veins for IV infusions varies with individual circumstances. Selection should be determined after considering several factors.

Accessibility of a Vein

- Determine the most desirable accessible vein. The lower cephalic vein, accessory cephalic vein, and the basilic vein are good sites for infusion. The superficial veins on the dorsal aspect of the hand can also be used successfully for some people. Figure 37-13 illustrates common infusion sites on the arm and hand. Either arm may be used for IV therapy. If the client is right-handed and both arms appear to be equally usable, usually the left arm is selected to free the right arm for the client's use.
- Determine accessibility based on the client's condition. For example, a person with severe burns on both forearms does not have vessels available in these areas.
- Avoid the antecubital veins for long-term infusions. They are not a good choice for infusion because of the need to limit flexion of the client's arm for an extended period. These vessels are quite satisfactory for blood withdrawal or for small amounts of IV medication administration.
- Avoid veins in the leg, unless other sites are inaccessible, because of the danger of stagnation of peripheral circulation and possible serious complications.

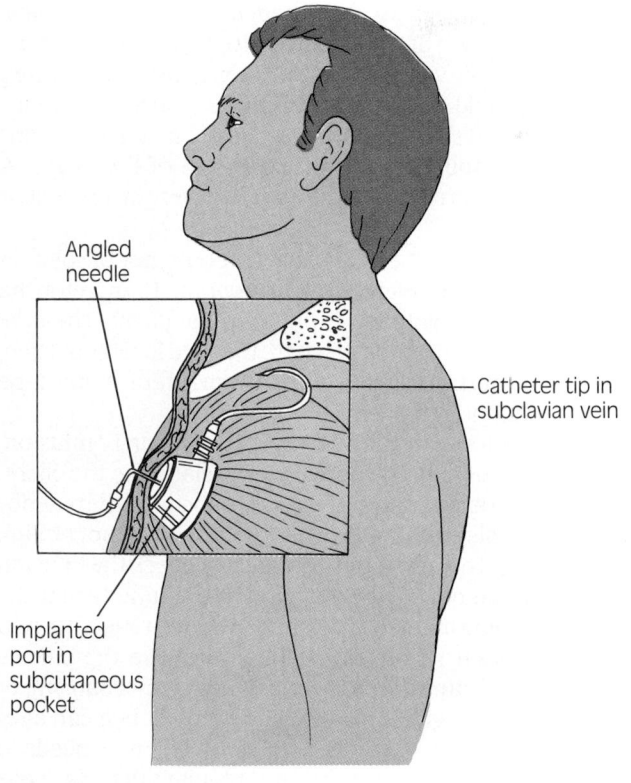

FIGURE 37-12

Placement of an implanted port with the tip in the subclavian vein. Angled needle is inserted through skin and rubber septum into port.

- Avoid veins in surgical areas. For example, infusions in the arm should not be given on the same side as recent extensive breast surgery because of vascular disturbances in the area.
- Select scalp veins for infants because of their accessibility and because of relative ease of preventing dislocation of the needle.

Condition of the Vein
- Determine the condition of the vein. Thin-walled and scarred veins, especially in some elderly clients, make continued infusion a problem. Experience helps the nurse acquire skill in palpating veins to determine their general condition.

Type of Fluid To Be Infused
- Select a vein appropriate for the solution. Hypertonic solutions, those containing irritating medications, those administered at a rapid rate, and those with a high viscosity should be given in a large vein to minimize vessel trauma and to facilitate the rate of flow.

Anticipated Duration of Infusion
- Select a site where restriction in movement is kept to a minimum.
- Change sites every 48 to 72 hours, if possible, starting with sites as distal as possible and moving in a proximal direction on the alternate arms.

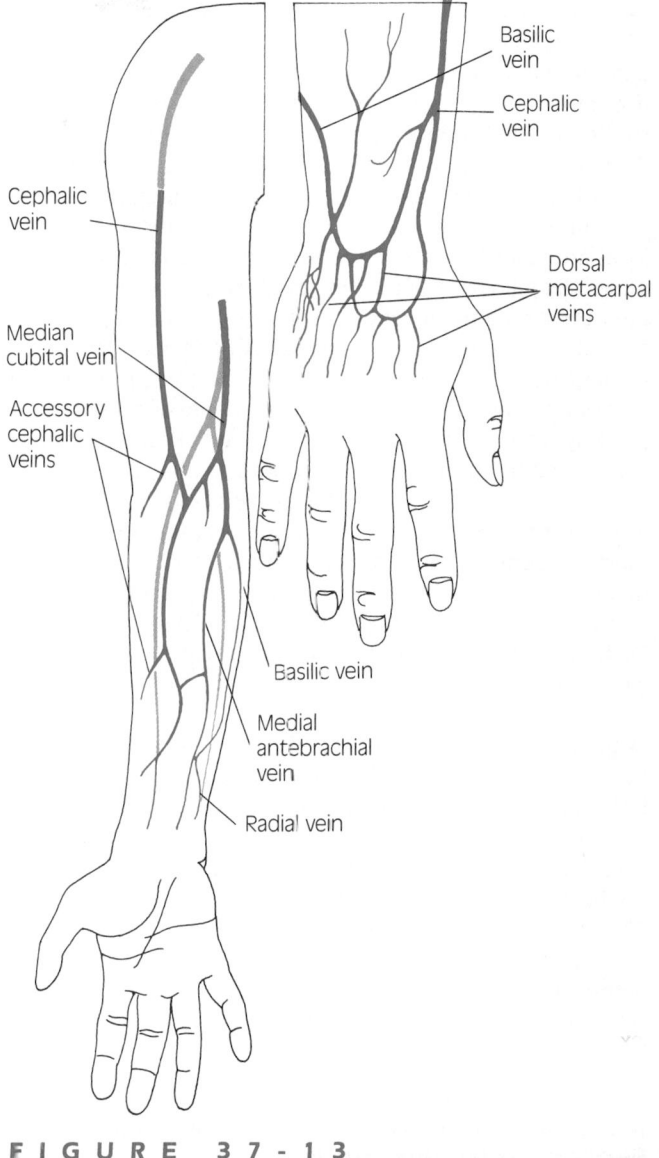

FIGURE 37-13

Infusion sites on the ventral and dorsal aspects of the lower arm and hand.

Other
- Select a vein large enough to accommodate the needle to be used.
- Select a site that is naturally splinted by bone, such as the back of the hand or the forearm.
- Select a site distal to the heart, and move proximally, as necessary, to find an appropriate injection site.
- Select a site while moving toward the heart, and away from a damaged vein.

Starting an Intravenous Infusion Before the infusion is started, a final check should be made of the solution to ensure that it is clear and contains no particles or precipitates. This check is especially important when substances have been added to the solution, because some additives create precipitates. Inline filters to help reduce the risk of contamination are commercially available to filter the solution immediately before it enters the client's vein. Filters are routinely recommended for any client receiving long-term IV therapy, total parenteral nutrition, or IV chemotherapy.

It has been suggested by Dick and colleagues (1992) that an intradermal injection of 1% lidocaine solution (a local anesthetic) at the venipuncture site considerably reduced the pain associated with an IV start. Fifteen seconds after the lidocaine injection has formed a small wheal, the needle or catheter can be inserted with minimal discomfort through the wheal. Reluctance to use lidocaine is related to fear of an allergic reaction and complaints of burning and stinging from the lidocaine injection itself. Researchers are continuing to study the effectiveness of this technique.

The nurse should wash hands well before starting the infusion because of the threat of infections posed by IV therapy. Centers for Disease Control guidelines recommend that gloves be worn as a preventive measure against human immunodeficiency virus (HIV) and hepatitis B virus. Techniques for starting an IV infusion are described in Procedure 37-1.

Regulating and Monitoring   The nurse is responsible for maintaining the proper flow rate while assuring the comfort and safety of the client. The physician prescribes the flow rate. The amount of solution to be infused within a specified period is indicated. The rate is then determined on the basis of drops of solution to be infused every minute. This is called the drip rate.

The drop factor, or drops per milliliter of solution, is determined by the size of the opening in the infusion apparatus. It varies with the company producing the product.

Most health agencies use the products of a single company. The most common drop factors are 10, 15, 20, and 60 drops per milliliter. Sixty drops per milliliter is used most often when small fluid volumes are important, such as with infants and small children. Adapters may be added to common infusion tubings to reduce the size of the drops. A method for determining flow rate is given in Procedure 37-2.

A time tape can be placed on the container of solution to provide a quick reference for the nurse to monitor the rate at which the solution is entering the client. The tape gives an hourly indication of where the fluid level should be, based on the nurse's calculation of the drip rate. A time tape is illustrated in Figure 37-14.

Many factors can alter the rate of flow of an IV infusion, such as the height of the container in relation to the client, the client's blood pressure, the client's position, the patency of the IV needle or catheter, infiltration, and a knot or kink in the tubing. The nurse can periodically check the infusion and determine quickly by glancing at the time tape if the solution is being infused at the proper hourly rate. If it is not, the nurse again regulates the flow. Because the client's movements, disturbances of the regulation mechanism, or change in the height of the infusion bottle or bed can alter the flow rate, even after it is regulated, the nurse needs to continue to check on the infusion at regular intervals. It has been reported that standard IV administration sets lose up to one half of their initial flow rate during the first hour of infusion because of tubing flexibility, and therefore the rate needs adjustment.

Maintenance of the flow rate is important because of the implications relative to the client's fluid balance. Too slow a flow may result in either the occurrence of deficits because the input is not balancing the loss, or in delaying

---

P R O C E D U R E   3 7 - 2

Regulating IV Flow Rate

Action	Rationale
1 Check physician's order for IV solution.	This ensures that correct solution is being given with the correct medications and determines the exact time period for administration of IV.
2 Check patency of IV line and needle.	Any interference with patency influences IV flow rate.
3 Verify drop factor (number of drops in 1 mL) of the equipment in use.	Drop factor of the equipment varies according to manufacturer and will be displayed on outer package. Equipment labeled *microdrop* or *minidrip* is standard and delivers 60 gtt/mL, but macrodrip delivery systems vary. Some of the more common types of equipment according to manufacturer are:

Travenol Macrodrip	10 gtt/mL
Abbott Macrodrip	15 gtt/mL
McGaw Macrodrip	15 gtt/mL

(continued)

Regulating IV Flow Rate

Action	**Rationale**
4 Calculate the flow rate: **a** *Standard formula* $$\text{gtt/min} = \frac{\text{volume (mL)} \times \text{drop factor (gtt/mL)}}{\text{time (in minutes)}}$$ EXAMPLE—Administer 1000 mL 5% D/W over 10 hours (set delivers 60 gtt/1 mL). $$\text{gtt/min} = \frac{1000 \text{ mL} \times 60}{600 \text{ (60 min} \times 10 \text{ h)}}$$ $$= \frac{60,000}{600}$$ $$= 100 \text{ gtt/min}$$	Standard formula for calculating IV flow rate produces the correct number of gtt/min.
b *Short formula using milliliters per hour* $$\text{gtt/min} = \frac{\text{milliliters per hour}}{\text{time (60 min)}} \times \text{drop factor (gtt/mL)}$$ EXAMPLE—Administer 1000 mL 5% D/W over 10 hours (set delivers 60 gtt/1 mL). Find milliliters per hour by dividing 1000 mL by 10 hours: $$\frac{1000}{10} = 100 \text{ mL/hr}$$ $$\text{gtt/min} = \frac{100 \text{ mL} \times 60}{60 \text{ min}}$$ $$= \frac{6000}{60}$$ $$= 100 \text{ gtt/min}$$	Short formula results in calculations using smaller numbers by using milliliters per hour. This is particularly useful for calculating drip rates when infusing piggyback IV medication.
5 Count drops per minute in drip chamber (number of gtt/15-sec interval × 4 = gtt/min). Hold watch beside drip chamber.	Holding watch next to drip chamber allows eyes to focus on drops and second hand on watch to provide accurate count.
6 Adjust IV clamp as needed and recount drops per minute.	Clamp regulates flow rate into drip chamber.
7 Mark IV container according to agency policy and manufacturer's recommendations. Use a time tape or label to measure amount to be infused at timed intervals.	This allows for comparison of volume actually infused with scheduled infusion rate.
8 Monitor IV flow rate at frequent intervals. Document client's response to infusion at prescribed rate.	This provides for observation of IV infusion and ensures accurate documentation of client's response to IV infusion.

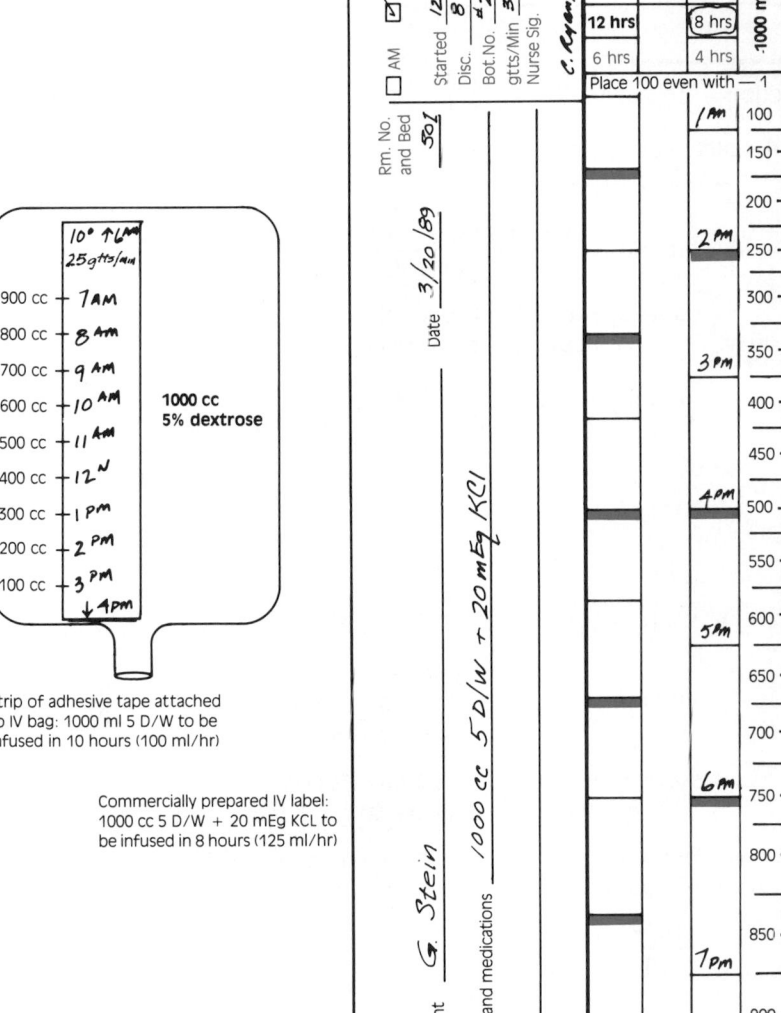

Strip of adhesive tape attached
to IV bag: 1000 ml 5 D/W to be
infused in 10 hours (100 ml/hr)

Commercially prepared IV label:
1000 cc 5 D/W + 20 mEg KCL to
be infused in 8 hours (125 ml/hr)

F I G U R E   3 7 - 1 4

Time tapes. Use of time tapes enables the nurse
to quickly evaluate if the IV solution is infusing
according to schedule and to regulate the drip
rate if needed.

the restoration of the balance. Infusing IV fluid too rapidly can overtax the body's capacities to adjust to the increase in the water volume or the electrolytes it contains. Nurses who allow infusions to get behind schedule and increase the rate to catch up may be seriously insulting the client's compensatory mechanisms and jeopardizing the client's well-being.

Electronic infusion devices (EIDs) limit the amount of fluid to be infused at any one time and in some hospitals are used to regulate all IV infusions. They can automatically regulate the flow rate at preset limits and notify the nurse by an alarm system when air is in the tubing, the flow is obstructed, or the solution level of the bottle or bag is getting low. Either a pump or controller may be used, but many health care facilities select pumps because their accuracy is greater, alarms are triggered less easily, and there are fewer

IV-related problems (Millam, 1988). Pumps totally control the delivery rate by exerting positive pressure based on preset limits when resistance develops. Controllers do not rely on pressure to control solution flow but rely on the height of the IV container in relation to the IV site to affect flow rate over time. An infiltrated IV with a pump EID may not recognize an infusion problem if pressure build-up from the leaking solution in subcutaneous tissues is not significant enough to trigger the alarm.

A newly marketed pump monitoring device is expected to more quickly detect an infiltrated IV solution. Syringe pumps are also available. They deliver small amounts of fluid, 100 mL or less, and are particularly useful with children. There are portable models on the market also, which are handy for the ambulatory client. An infusion pump is shown in Figure 37-15.

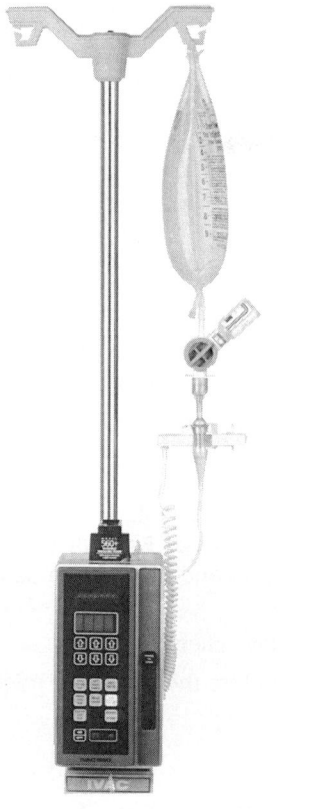

FIGURE 37-15

This is an example of an infusion pump. It is a positive-pressure pump that automatically regulates the flow rate. The alarm on this model is activated by an empty fluid container, an occluded tubing, or an unobtainable drop rate. (Courtesy of Ivac Corporation, San Diego, CA.)

Changing Solution and Tubing If more than one bottle of solution is ordered for the client, the nurse attaches the additional bottles. The method by which this is done depends on the procedure of the agency. Some IV equipment is designed to simplify the procedure by making it possible to attach additional bottles with a tandemlike arrangement. Because infusions often are continued after the responsibility for a client's care changes from one nurse to another, it is a good practice to agree on one common method for managing infusions. Without such uniformity, serious errors can occur, or valuable time is lost in checking and rechecking. One method for changing the solution and tubing is presented in Procedure 37-3.

Caring for the Infusion Site Scrupulous care of the infusion site should be observed to help control contamination and to help prevent the introduction of microorganisms into the bloodstream. Regular dressing changes and tubing replacements are important means of preventing infection. Hospital policy should be followed in relation to changing dressings and tubing.

It is best to change the needle or catheter and the site of entry to a vein every 48 to 72 hours. The longer the needle remains in place, the greater the chances of complications, such as infection and phlebitis. Under certain circumstances, the nurse must use discretion in deciding how often to change the infusion site. For example, the client who is receiving long-term chemotherapy quickly runs out of suitable veins. Procedures 37-4 and 37-5 explain how to monitor an IV site and how to change an IV dressing.

A controversial aspect of the care of the insertion site concerns irrigation of the needle. An irrigation is sometimes used when the needle begins to clog with blood and the client does not have other good sites for starting another infusion. *The procedure should not be used unless agency policy recommends it.*

Complications The client can be an important source of information regarding the possibility of complications associated with IV therapy. If the client is uncomfortable, the nurse should check to see that the infusion is entering the vein as intended, that the flow rate is not too rapid, and that the client's position is satisfactory. Anxiety over the implications of an infusion can also cause discomfort for the client.

Local complications such as infiltration, phlebitis, and thrombophlebitis occur more frequently than systemic complications. Systemic complications (eg, fluid overload, embolus, infection), however, are more serious and may be life-threatening. Table 37-9 defines these complications, noting common causes, signs and symptoms, and pertinent nursing considerations.

Converting a Primary Line to a Heparin Lock When a continuous IV is no longer necessary, the primary IV line can be converted to a heparin lock, which provides venous access for intermittent or emergency medications. A heparin lock consists of a plastic tube with a sealed injection port on the end that is connected to an indwelling needle or catheter. Periodic injection with heparin or saline according to agency policy is required to keep the catheter patent. Procedure 37-6 describes this technique.

Discontinuing the Infusion When the amount of solution the physician has ordered has been infused, the nurse assumes responsibility for discontinuing the infusion. If the needle or catheter are to be removed, the adhesive strips and sterile dressing are removed, the needle or catheter is removed in line with the vein, and pressure is immediately applied to the site. A dry sterile gauze pad is preferable to an alcohol preparation to apply pressure to the site because alcohol tends to burn and does not stop blood flow from the puncture wound. If the client is able to do so, he or she may be asked to hold the pressure for a minute or more.

If the client's arm or leg has been immobilized for several hours or longer, the nurse should manipulate it carefully in an attempt to put the joint through range of motion and passively move the muscles of the area.

(*Text continues on p. 1054*)

PROCEDURE 37-3

Changing IV Solution and Tubing

Equipment

For solution change:
  IV solution as ordered by physician
For tubing change:
  Administration set
  Sterile gauze
  Tape or label

Sterile dressings and antiseptic
  solutions/ointments (according to
  agency recommendations)
Clean disposable gloves

Action	Rationale
1 Gather all equipment and bring to bedside. Check IV solution and medication additives with physician's order.	Having equipment available saves time and facilitates accomplishment of task. Ensures that client receives the correct IV solution and medication as ordered by physician.
2 Explain procedure to client.	Explanation allays client's anxiety.
3 Wash your hands.	Handwashing deters the spread of microorganisms.

To Change IV Solution

Action	Rationale
4 Carefully remove protective cover from new solution container and expose entry site.	This maintains sterility of IV solution.
5 Close clamp on tubing.	Clamping stops the flow of IV fluid during change of solution.
6 Lift container off IV pole and invert it. Quickly remove the spike from the old IV container being careful not to contaminate it.	This maintains sterility of IV setup.
7 Steady new container and insert spike. Hang on IV pole.	This allows for uninterrupted flow of new solution.
8 Reopen clamp on tubing and adjust flow.	Opening clamp regulates flow rate into drip chamber.
9 Label container according to agency policy. Record on intake and output record and document on chart according to agency policy. Discard used equipment in proper manner. Wash your hands.	This ensures accurate continuation and administration of correct IV solution. Handwashing deters the spread of microorganisms.

To Change IV Tubing and Solution

Action	Rationale
10 Follow actions 1 through 4.	
11 Open the administration set and remove protective covering from infusion spike. Using sterile technique, insert into new container.	This maintains sterility of IV setup.
12 Close clamp on new tubing. Hang IV container on pole and squeeze drip chamber to fill at least halfway.	Gravity and suction effect cause fluid to move into drip chamber. This action also prevents air from moving down the tubing.
13 Remove cap at end of tubing, release clamp, and allow fluid to move through tubing until all air bubbles have disappeared. Close clamp and recap end of tubing maintaining sterility of setup.	This removes air from tubing that can, in larger amounts, act as an air embolus.

(continued)

PROCEDURE 37 - 3 (continued)

Changing IV Solution and Tubing

Action

Rationale

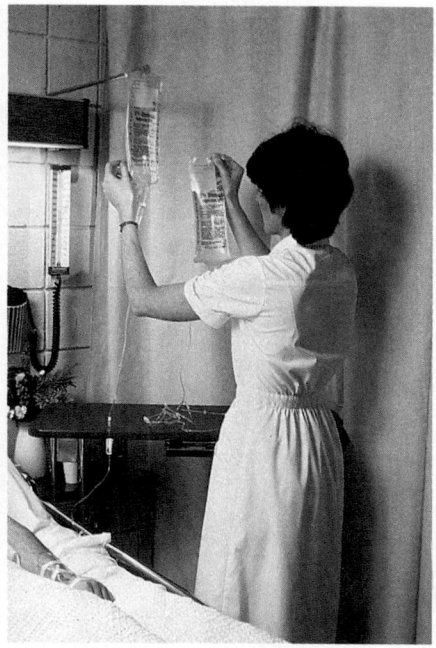

Action 12: Hanging new bag and tubing.

14 Loosen tape at IV insertion site. Don clean, disposable gloves. Carefully remove dressing and tape.

Care must be used when blood contact is possible. This prevents transmission of HIV and other blood-borne infections. Removing dressing provides access to needle hub necessary for tubing change.

15 Place sterile gauze square under needle hub.

Gauze absorbs any leakage when tubing is disconnected from needle.

16 Place new IV tubing close to client's IV site and slightly loosen protective cap.

This facilitates removal of cap and attachment to needle hub.

17 Clamp the old IV tubing. Steady the needle hub with nondominant hand until change is completed. Remove tubing with dominant hand using a twisting motion.

This stabilizes needle and prevents inadvertently dislodging it.

18 Set old tubing aside. While maintaining sterility, carefully remove cap and insert sterile end of tubing into the needle hub. Twist to secure it. Remove soiled gloves.

This maintains sterility of IV setup.

19 Open the clamp.

Opening clamp allows solution to flow to client.

20 Reapply sterile dressing to site according to agency protocol (see Procedure 37-5).

This deters entry of microorganisms at site.

21 Regulate the IV flow according to physician's order (see Procedure 37-2).

This ensures that client receives IV solution at the prescribed rate.

(continued)

P R O C E D U R E   3 7 - 3   (continued)

Changing IV Solution and Tubing

Action

22 Attach to IV tubing tape or label that states date, time, and your initials. Label container and record procedure according to agency policy. Discard used equipment in proper manner and wash hands.

23 Record client's response to IV infusion.

Rationale

This documents IV tubing change. Handwashing deters the spread of microorganisms.

This ensures accurate documentation of client's response.

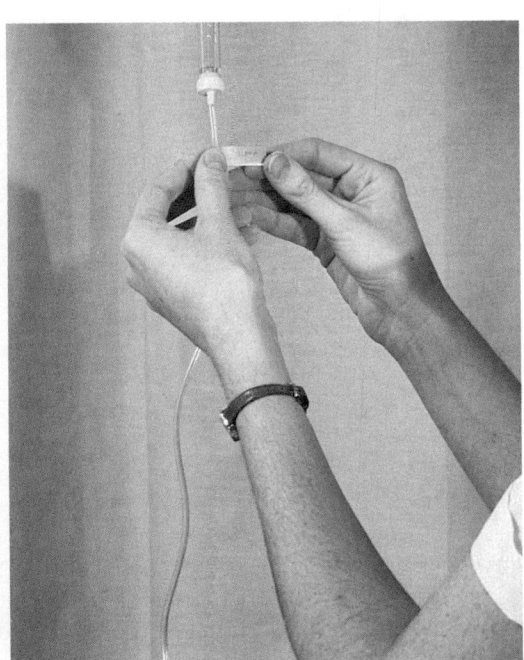

Action 22: Labeling IV tubing.

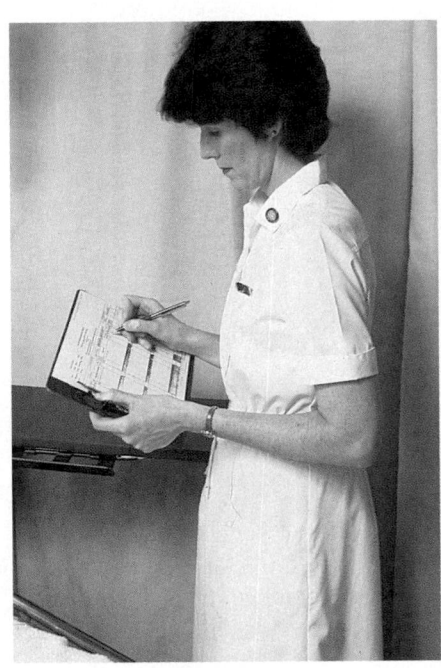

Action 23: Recording client's response to infusion.

P R O C E D U R E   3 7 - 4

Monitoring an IV Site and Infusion

Action

1 Monitor IV infusion at least once every hour. More frequent checks may be necessary if medication is being infused:

   a Check physician's order for IV solution.

   b Check drip chamber and time drops if IV is not regulated by an infusion control device.

   c Check tubing for anything that might interfere with flow. Be sure that clamp is in the open position. Observe dressing for leakage of IV solution.

Rationale

Promotes safe administration of IV fluids and medication. Too rapid administration of medications can result in the development of speed shock.

This ensures that correct solution is being given at the correct rate and in the proper sequence with the correct medications.

This ensures that flow rate is correct.

Any kink or pressure on tubing may interfere with flow. Leakage may occur at connection of tubing with hub of needle or catheter and allow for loss of IV solution.

(continued)

P R O C E D U R E   3 7 - 4   (continued)

Monitoring an IV Site and Infusion

Action

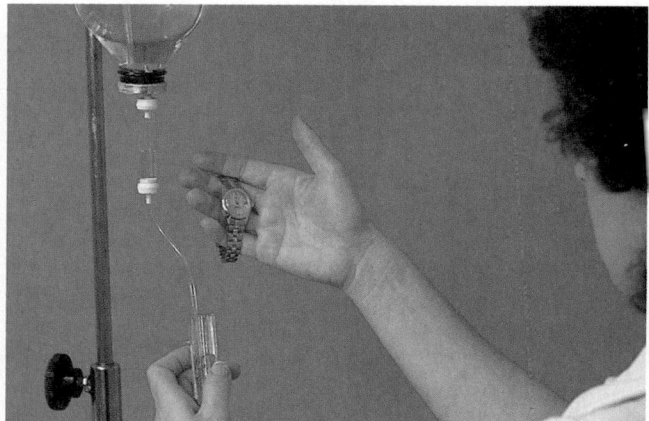

Action 1b: Timing drops.

Rationale

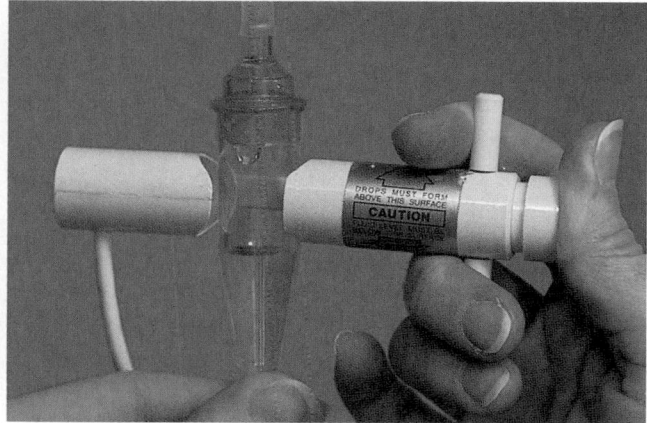

Action 1b: Placing electronic eye for infusion control device.

d Observe settings, alarm, and indicator lights on infusion control device if one is being used.

2 Inspect site for swelling, pain, coolness, or pallor at site of insertion, which may indicate infiltration of IV. This necessitates removing IV and restarting at another site. Another method of validating whether IV is infiltrated involves applying a tourniquet above the insertion site. If IV needle is in the vein the solution will stop flowing.

3 Inspect site for redness, swelling, heat, and pain at the IV site, which may indicate phlebitis is present. IV will need to be discontinued and restarted at another site. Notify physician if you suspect that phlebitis may have occurred.

Observation ensures that infusion control device is functioning and that alarm is in ON position.

Needle may become dislodged from vein, and IV solution may flow into subcutaneous tissue.

Chemical irritation or mechanical trauma cause injury to the vein and can lead to the development of phlebitis.

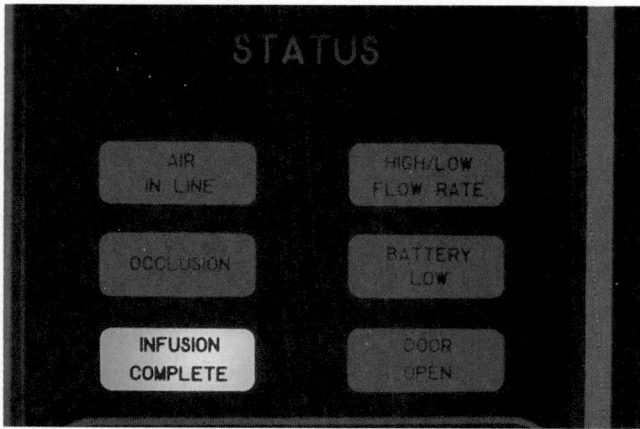

Action 1d: Checking indicator lights on infusion control device.

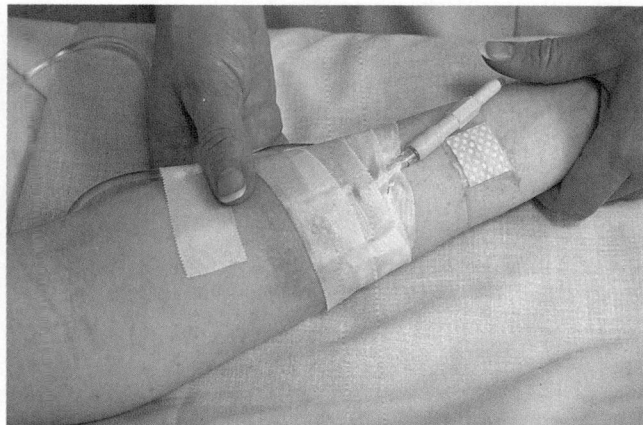

Action 3: Example of inflammation surrounding infusion site.

(continued)

P R O C E D U R E 3 7 - 4 (continued)

Monitoring an IV Site and Infusion

Action	Rationale
4 Check for local or systemic manifestations that indicate an infection is present at the site. IV will be discontinued and physician notified. Never disconnect IV tubing when putting on client's hospital gown.	Poor aseptic technique may allow bacteria to enter the needle or catheter insertion site or tubing connection.
5 Be alert for additional complications of IV therapy. a Circulatory overload can result in signs of cardiac failure and pulmonary edema. Monitor intake and output during IV therapy.	Infusing too much IV solution results in an increased volume of circulating fluid.
b Bleeding at the site is most likely to occur when the IV is discontinued.	Bleeding may be caused by anticoagulant medication.
6 If possible, instruct client to call for assistance if any discomfort is noted at site, solution container is nearly empty, or flow has changed in any way.	This facilitates cooperation of client and safe administration of IV solution.
7 Document IV infusion, any complications of therapy, and client's reaction to therapy.	This provides accurate documentation and ensures continuity of care.

P R O C E D U R E 3 7 - 5

Changing an IV Dressing

Equipment

Sterile gauze (2 × 2 or 4 × 4) or
  transparent polyurethane dressing
Povidone-iodine (Betadine) solution
  or swabs
Adhesive remover
Povidone-iodine ointment (or other
  antiseptic ointment recommended
  by agency)

Alcohol swabs
Tape
Clean disposable gloves

Action	Rationale
1 Assess client's need for dressing change.	Agency policy determines interval for dressing change (every 24 to 72 hours). The presence of moisture or a nonadhering dressing increases risk of bacterial contamination at the site.
2 Gather equipment and bring to bedside.	Having equipment available saves time and facilitates the performance of the task.
3 Explain procedure to client.	Explanation allays client's anxiety.
4 Wash your hands. Don clean disposable gloves.	Handwashing deters the spread of microorganisms. Gloves prevent transmission of HIV and other bloodborne infections.

(continued)

PROCEDURE 37 - 5 (continued)

Changing an IV Dressing

Action	Rationale
5 Carefully remove old dressing but leave tape that anchors IV needle or catheter in place. Discard in proper manner.	This prevents dislodging of IV needle or catheter.
6 Assess IV site for presence of inflammation or infiltration. Discontinue and relocate the IV if noted.	Inflammation or infiltration causes trauma to tissues and necessitates removal of the IV needle or catheter.
7 Loosen tape and gently remove, being careful to steady catheter or needle hub with one hand.	Tape stabilizes needle and prevents inadvertently dislodging it.
8 Use adhesive remover to initiate cleansing procedure at site.	Process removes adhesive residue and facilitates attachment of new dressing.
9 Cleanse the entry site with povidone-iodine solution. Use a circular motion to move from the center outward. Follow with alcohol cleansing.	Cleansing in a circular motion while moving outward carries organisms away from the entry site. Use of antiseptic solutions reduces the number of microorganisms on the skin surface.
10 Reapply tape strip to needle or catheter at entry site.	Tape anchors needle or catheter to prevent dislodgement.
11 Apply povidone-iodine ointment to the entry site if agency policy recommends this.	Antiseptic ointment reduces skin contamination and protects against infection.
12 Apply sterile gauze or transparent polyurethane dressing over entry site. Remove gloves and dispose properly.	Dressing protects site and deters contamination with microorganisms.
13 Secure IV tubing with additional tape if necessary. Label dressing with date, time of change, and initials. Check that IV flow is accurate and system is patent.	Label documents IV dressing change.
14 Discard equipment properly and wash hands.	Handwashing protects against spread of microorganisms.
15 Record client's response to dressing change and observation of site.	This provides accurate documentation and ensures continuity of care.

PROCEDURE 37 - 6

Converting a Primary Intravenous Access to a Heparin Lock

Equipment

Heparin lock (also called male adaptor or leur lock)	Saline, Nonpreservative saline, or Heparin Flush (1 mL) prepared in a	Alcohol wipe Tape
Clean disposable gloves	syringe with a 25-gauge needle or	Plastic clamp or hemostat
4 × 4 gauze pad	according to agency policy	

Action	Rationale
1 Gather equipment and verify physician's order.	Having equipment available saves time and facilitates the task; ensures that the procedure has been ordered by the physician.

(continued)

PROCEDURE 37 - 6 *(continued)*

Converting a Primary Intravenous Access to a Heparin Lock

Action	Rationale
2 Explain the procedure to the client.	Explanation allays the client's anxiety.
3 Wash your hands.	Handwashing deters the spread of microorganisms.
4 Assess the IV site.	Complications such as infiltration or phlebitis necessitate discontinuation of the IV infusion at that site.
5 Use a plastic clamp or hemostat to close off primary line.	Protects client and nurse from inadvertent blood loss when IV and tubing are disconnected.
6 Don clean gloves.	Gloves protect the nurse from contact with the client's blood.
7 Place gauze 4 × 4 sponge underneath IV connection hub between IV catheter and tubing.	Gauze absorbs any blood leakage when IV and tubing are disconnected.
8 Stabilize hub of IV catheter with nondominant hand. Use dominant hand to quickly twist and disconnect IV tubing from the catheter, discard it, and attach heparin device to hub without contaminating the tips of the catheter and the lock.	This maintains sterility of IV setup.
9 Cleanse lock entry with an alcohol wipe.	Cleansing removes surface bacteria at the heparin lock entry site.
10 Insert the syringe needle into the heparin lock port and gently flush catheter with saline, nonpreservative saline, or heparin flush as per agency policy. Remove syringe carefully.	This maintains patency of the IV access line.

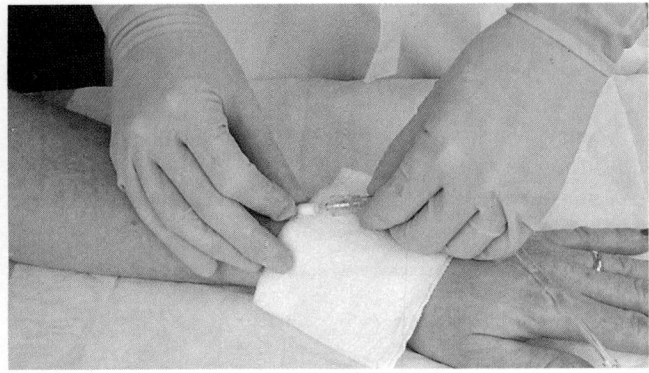

Action 8: Disconnecting tubing from IV catheter.

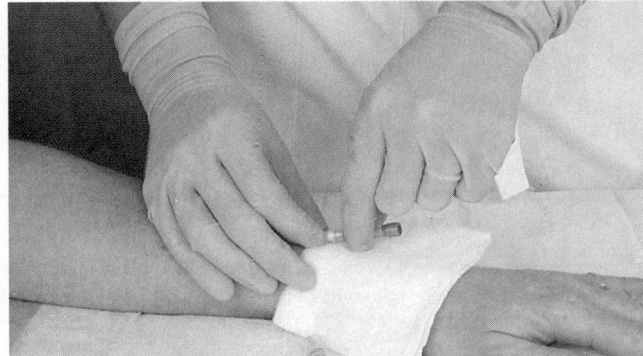

Action 8: Attaching heparin lock to IV catheter hub.

Action	Rationale
11 Tape heparin lock securely in place.	Tape secures the heparin lock and IV in place.
12 Chart on IV administration record or medication Kardex per institutional policy.	Accurate documentation is necessary to prevent error.

TABLE 37-9

Complications Associated With Intravenous Infusions

Name and Definition	Causes	Signs and Symptoms	Nursing Considerations
Infiltration: The escape of fluid into the subcutaneous tissue	• Dislodged needle • Penetrated vessel wall	Swelling; pallor; coldness; or pain around the infusion site; significant decrease in the flow rate	• Check the infusion site often for symptoms. • Discontinue the infusion if symptoms occur. • Restart the infusion at a different site. • Limit the movement of the extremity with the IV.
Phlebitis: An inflammation of a vein	• Mechanical trauma from needle or catheter • Chemical trauma from solution • Septic (due to contamination)	Local, acute tenderness; redness; warmth; and slight edema of the vein above the insertion site	• Discontinue the infusion immediately. • Apply warm, moist compresses to the affected site. • Avoid further use of the vein. • Restart the infusion in another vein.
Thrombus: A blood clot	• Tissue trauma from needle or catheter	Symptoms similar to phlebitis IV fluid flow may cease if clot obstructs needle	• Stop the infusion immediately. • Apply warm compresses as ordered by the physician. • Restart the IV at another site. • *Do not rub or massage the affected area.*
Speed shock: The body's reaction to a substance that is injected into the circulatory system too rapidly	• Too rapid a rate of fluid infusion into circulation	Pounding headache; fainting; rapid pulse rate; apprehension; chills; back pains; and dyspnea	• If symptoms develop, discontinue the infusion immediately. • Report symptoms of speed shock to the physician immediately. • Monitor vital signs if symptoms develop. • Use the proper IV tubing. A microdrip (60 gtt/mL) should be used on all pediatric clients. • Carefully monitor the rate of fluid flow. • Check the rate frequently for accuracy. A time tape is useful for this purpose.
Fluid overload: The condition caused when too large a volume of fluid infuses into the circulatory system	• Too large a volume of fluid infused into circulation	Engorged neck veins; increased blood pressure; and difficulty in breathing (dyspnea)	• If symptoms develop, slow the rate of infusion. • Notify the physician immediately. • Monitor vital signs. • Carefully monitor the rate of fluid flow. • Check the rate frequently for accuracy.
Embolus: A foreign body or air in the circulatory system	• Thrombus dislodges and circulates in the blood • Air enters the vein through the infusion line	Dependent on whether the embolism causes an obstruction or infarction in the circulatory system	• Check the site regularly to identify signs of phlebitis. • Do not allow air to enter the infusion line. • Treat phlebitis with the utmost caution.

(continued)

Complications Associated With Intravenous Infusions

Name and Definition	Causes	Signs and Symptoms	Nursing Considerations
Infection: An invasion of pathogenic organisms into the body	• Nonsterile technique used in starting infusion • Improper care of infusion site • Contaminated IV solution	Fever; malaise; and pain, swelling, inflammation, or discharge at IV insertion site	• Report any sudden pain or breathing difficulty immediately. • Use scrupulous aseptic technique when starting an infusion. • Change the dressing over the site regularly. • Change IV tubing every 24 hours if agency policy permits. • Always wash hands before working with the IV.

The following information is recorded when the infusion has been completed:

• The date and time the infusion was completed
• The kind and amount of solution infused
• The name of the person discontinuing the infusion
• Symptoms of any adverse reactions
• Signs of the desired effects of the infusion

Replacing Blood and Blood Products

A **blood transfusion** is the infusion of whole blood or a blood component such as plasma, RBCs, or platelets into the venous circulation. Whole blood is infrequently used because the various components can be easily separated and used for replacement therapy. The person receiving the blood is the *recipient*. The person giving the blood is the *donor*.

Typing and Crossmatching   Before blood can be given to a person, it must be determined that the blood of the donor and that of the recipient are compatible. If incompatible, clumping and hemolysis of the recipient's blood cells results. The laboratory examination to determine a person's blood type is called *typing*. The process of determining compatibility between blood specimens is *crossmatching*.

Blood Types   The four main blood groups in the ABO system of blood typing are A, B, AB, and O. Some of these groups are broken down into still more subgroups.

Blood type is an inherited trait and is determined by the type of antigens and antibodies present in the blood. An *antigen* is a substance that causes the formation of antibodies. An *antibody* is a protein substance developed in the body in response to the presence of an antigen that has in some way gained access to the body. An *agglutinin* is an antibody that causes a clumping of specific antigens. People who have type-A blood have an A antigen in their RBCs; those with type-B blood have B antigens in their cells; those in the AB group have A and B antigens; and people with

type-O blood have neither A nor B antigens in their RBCs. People in each blood group have the agglutinins to the red cell antigens that they lack. Group-A people have the agglutinin for B; group-AB people have no agglutinins for A and B, whereas group-O people have both A and B agglutinins in their blood serum. Assume a person with type-O blood is transfused with blood from either a person with group-A or group-B blood. There would be destruction of the recipient's red cells because his or her anti-A or anti-B agglutinins would react with the A or B antigens in the donor's red cells. From this example, it can be seen why group-AB people are often called universal recipients, because people in this blood group have no agglutinins for either A or B antigens, and group O people are often called universal donors because they have neither A nor B antigens.

Rh Factor   The Rh factor is an inherited antigen in human blood. There are five antigens in the Rh system, but the one designated D is of first concern. A person whose blood contains a D antigen is called Rh positive; an Rh-negative person lacks D. It is important that an Rh-negative person receive blood from another Rh-negative person. If Rh-positive blood is injected into an Rh-negative person, the recipient develops anti-Rh agglutinins. Subsequent transfusion with Rh-positive blood may cause serious reactions with clumping and hemolysis of RBCs.

The Rh factor is of special importance during pregnancy because Rh incompatability between mother and fetus is often the problem when an infant has hemolytic disease. An Rh-negative mother who gives birth to an Rh-positive child is given RhoGam (an anti-Rh gamma globulin) within 72 hours after birth to prevent the development of permanent active immunity to the Rh antigen.

Selection of Blood Donors   The selection of blood donors must be done with care. Not only must the donor's blood be accurately typed, but it is also important to determine whether the donor is free from diseases, such as acquired immunodeficiency syndrome (AIDS) and hepatitis. The virus causing these diseases can be transmitted to the recipient. People who have allergies usually are not used, nor are those with a history of a chronic disease, such as tuberculosis, certain types of cancer, and hemophilia. As a further precaution, some blood banks do not accept blood from a donor who has been immunized recently because of a possible allergic reaction to the blood.

The donor is examined carefully at the time of donation and receives specific information about eligibility as well as a confidential method to allow or disallow the distribution of their donated blood. Prospective donors are questioned about high risk behaviors such as unsafe sex, IV drug abuse, and the presence of any of the signs and symptoms of AIDS. Individuals may give blood only if blood count, temperature, pulse, respiration, and blood pressure are within normal range.

In the early 1980s, a number of people contracted AIDS after receiving contaminated blood. Although careful screening of both donors and donated blood has greatly decreased the likelihood of this happening, both blood donors and recipients continue to have many questions regarding safety. *There is no way that donors may contract AIDS or any other disease by giving blood* because single-use sterile setups are used for each donor. Some clients who know in advance that they will need blood request to be allowed to have family members or themselves (autologous transfusion) donate the blood. Autotransfusion eliminates the danger of transmitting cross-infection from donor to recipient. This practice is growing in popularity.

Blood Extracts   Some people do not need all of the constituents of whole blood. For example, one may need RBCs but not the blood plasma and its constituents. RBCs in concentrated form are called packed RBCs and may be used in the following situations:
- Client with anemia suffering with a low RBC count
- Client with cardiovascular failure, to increase his or her blood volume and RBCs while avoiding cardiovascular overload
- Client with GI bleeding, to maintain adequate hemoglobin levels without increasing blood pressure, which would likely lead to more bleeding.

In other situations, only plasma is required, such as when plasma protein or the blood's clotting factor is in low supply. Fresh frozen plasma is particularly useful in emergencies for immediate restoration of fluid because serum presents no compatibility problems and time need not be lost seeking donors and matching blood. It is also an excellent blood-volume expander when time is of essence, an example being for the person who is severely burned and losing plasma rapidly from burn areas. Components of plasma that are used therapeutically include human albumin (hypovolemic shock, albuminemia, liver failure); cryoprecipitates (bleeding due to hemophilia or disseminated intravascular coagulation); and gamma globulins—the antibody-containing part of plasma (gamma globulin deficiencies).

Platelet infusion is indicated for treatment or prevention of bleeding associated with deficiencies in the number or function of a client's platelets. The demand for platelets has noticeably risen over the past several decades and specialized products and preparation methods have been developed to reduce the risk of complications and improve the client's response to platelet therapy.

Initiating the Transfusion   The procedure for starting a blood transfusion (Procedure 37-7) is basically the same as for an IV solution. If possible, larger veins should be selected because no smaller needle or catheter than a No. 19 gauge should be used. This size is necessary because of the viscosity of blood.

Transfusion Reactions   When preparing and administering the transfusion, the nurse should take every precaution to prevent the occurrence of transfusion reactions through scrupulous technique. Table 37-10 describes some potential transfusion reactions. A nurse should stay with the client for at least 5 to 10 minutes after starting a blood transfusion and then check the client every 15 minutes while the client receives blood. A transfusion reaction can be serious.

Giving Total Parenteral Nutrition

Hypertonic solutions consisting of dextrose, amino acids, and select electrolytes and minerals may be infused using a central vein by a procedure known as **total parenteral nutrition**. Used in cases of severe malnutrition, TPN is directed to
- Reestablish and maintain positive nitrogen balance
- Increase or maintain weight
- Correct metabolic complications

This procedure and the related nursing responsibilities are described in Chapter 33.

Evaluating

When evaluating the effectiveness of the care plan aimed at promoting healthy fluid, electrolyte, and acid–base balance, the nurse pays attention to the following parameters:
- Are the client's drinking and eating patterns supplying the fluid and electrolytes he or she needs? Are food and fluid likes and dislikes interfering with the implementation of the care plan? Is the client having any difficulties with oral fluids, tube feedings, IV therapy, or TPN?
- Is the client's urine output approximately equal to the fluid intake? Does the client void at least once each shift (except when sleeping)? Do urine characteristics (color, odor, SG) indicate healthy functioning of the kidneys and excretion of fluids?

(Text continues on p. 1059)

PROCEDURE 37-7

Administering a Blood Transfusion

Equipment

Blood product

Blood administration set (tubing with inline filter and Y for saline administration

0.9% Normal saline

IV pole

Intravenous line with a #18 or #19 needle or catheter

Disposable gloves

Action

1 Determine if client knows reason for transfusion. Ask if the client has had a transfusion or transfusion reaction in the past.

2 Explain procedure to client. Check for signed consent for transfusion if required by agency. Advise client to report any chills, itching, rash, or unusual symptoms.

3 Wash your hands and put on clean gloves.

4 Hang container of 0.9% normal saline with blood administration set to initiate IV infusion and follow administration of blood.

Rationale

This directs teaching before beginning transfusion.

Explanation provides reassurance and facilitates cooperation. Prompt reporting of any reaction to transfusion necessitates stopping immediately.

Handwashing deters the spread of microorganisms. Gloves protect against accidental exposure to the client's blood.

Dextrose may lead to clumping of red blood cells and hemolysis. Filter in blood administration set removes particulate material formed during storage of blood.

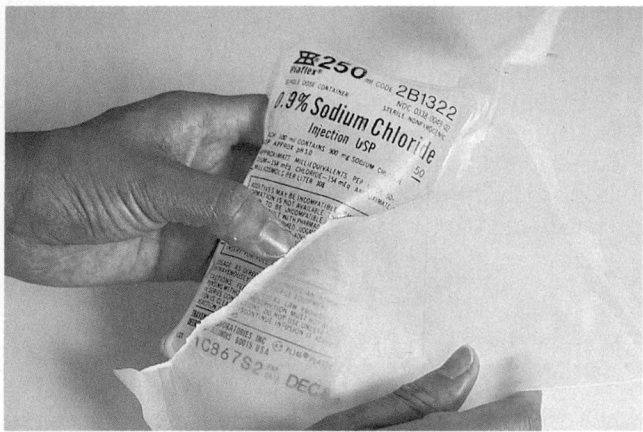

Normal saline container.

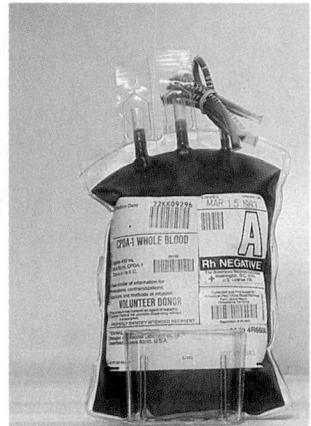

Unit of packed red blood cells.

5 Start intravenous with #18 or #19 catheter if not already present (see Procedure 37-1). Keep IV open by starting flow of normal saline.

6 Obtain blood product from blood bank according to agency policy.

7 Complete identification and checks as required by agency:
  a Identification number
  b Blood group and type

Large-bore needle or catheter is necessary for infusion of blood products. The lumen must be large enough not to cause damage to red blood cells.

Blood must be stored in refrigerated unit at carefully controlled temperature (4°C).

Some agencies require two registered nurses to verify information:
  Verifies that unit numbers match
  Verifies that ABO group and Rh type are the same

(continued)

Administering a Blood Transfusion

Action	Rationale
c Expiration date	Safe storage of blood is limited to 35 days before red blood cells begin to deteriorate.
d Client's name	Never administer blood to a client without a name band.
e Inspect blood for clots	If clots are present, blood should be returned to blood bank.
8 Take baseline set of vital signs prior to beginning transfusion.	Any change in vital signs during the transfusion may indicate a reaction.
9 Start infusion of the blood product:	
a Prime in-line filter with blood.	Priming is necessary if blood is to flow properly.
b Start administration slowly (no more than 2 mL/min for the first 15 minutes).	Transfusion reactions typically occur during this period, and a slow rate will minimize the volume of red blood cells infused. If there have been no adverse effects during this time, the infusion rate is increased.
c Check vital signs every 5 minutes for first 15 minutes.	If complications occur, they can be observed, and the blood can be stopped immediately.
d Observe client for flushing, dyspnea, itching, hives, or rash.	These symptoms may be early indication of a transfusion reaction.

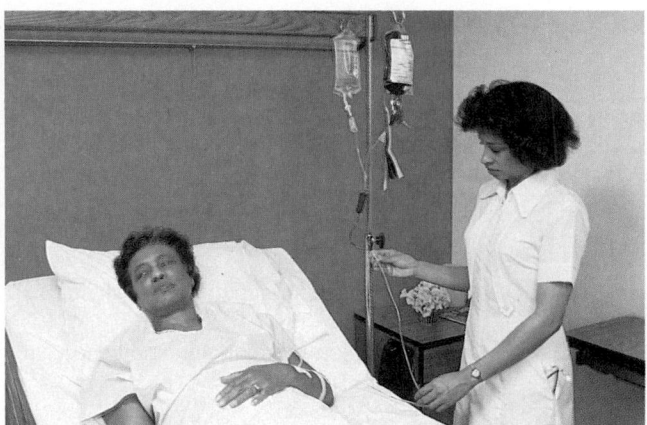

Action 9a: Priming the in-line filter.

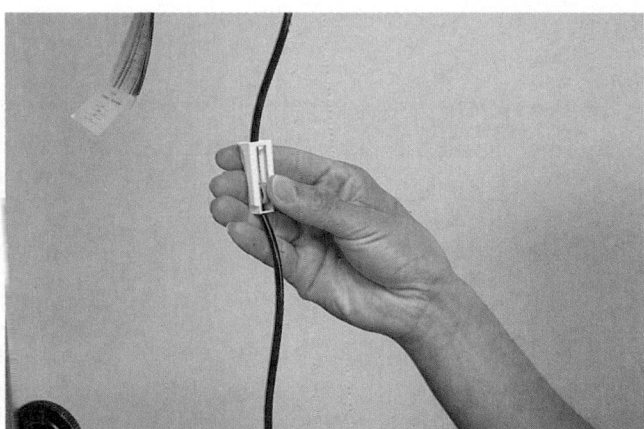

Action 9b: Starting infusion of blood slowly.

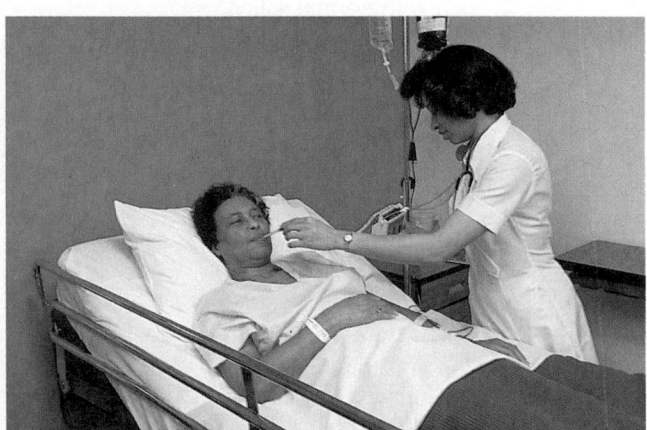

Action 9c: Checking vital signs.

(continued)

P R O C E D U R E 3 7 - 7 (continued)

Administering a Blood Transfusion

Action	Rationale
e Use a blood warming device, if indicated, especially with rapid transfusions through a CVP catheter.	Rapid administration of cold blood can result in cardiac arrhythmias.
10 Maintain the prescribed flow rate as ordered and assess frequently for transfusion reaction. Stop blood transfusion and allow saline to flow if you suspect a reaction. Notify physician and blood bank.	Rate must be carefully controlled, and client's reaction must be monitored on a frequent basis.
11 When transfusion is complete, infuse 0.9% normal saline.	Saline prevents hemolysis of red blood cells and clears remainder of blood in IV line.
12 Record administration of blood and client's reaction as ordered by agency. Return blood transfusion bag to blood bank according to agency policy.	This provides for accurate documentation of client's response to blood transfusion.

Special Considerations   Electronic infusion devices may be used to maintain prescribed rate but must be specifically designed for use with blood transfusions.

T A B L E 3 7 - 1 0

Transfusion Reactions

Reaction	Signs and Symptoms	Nursing Activity
Allergic reaction: Allergy to transfused blood	Hives, itching Anaphylaxis	• Stop transfusion immediately and keep vein open with normal saline. • Notify physician stat. • Administer antihistamine parenterally as necessary.
Febrile reaction: Fever develops during infusion	Fever and chills Headache Malaise	• Stop transfusion immediately and keep vein open with normal saline. • Notify physician. • Treat symptoms.
Hemolytic transfusion reaction: Incompatibility of blood product	Immediate onset Facial flushing Fever, chills Headache Low back pain Shock	• Stop infusion immediately and keep vein open with normal saline. • Notify physician stat. • Obtain blood samples from site. • Obtain first voided urine. • Treat shock if present. • Send unit, tubing, and filter to lab. • Draw blood sample for serologic testing and send urine specimen to the lab.
Circulatory overload: Too much blood administered	Dyspnea Dry cough Pulmonary edema	• Slow or stop infusion. • Monitor vital signs. • Notify physician. • Place in upright position with feet dependent.
Bacterial reaction: Bacteria present in blood	Fever Hypertension Dry, flushed skin Abdominal pain	• Stop infusion immediately. • Obtain culture of client's blood and return blood bag to lab. • Monitor vital signs. • Notify physician. • Administer antibiotics stat.

- Are abnormal sources of fluid loss (vomiting, diarrhea, draining wounds, fistula, and so forth) responding to treatment? Are these losses effectively being replaced by the designated therapy? Are the signs of FVD improving?
- Do the client's weight and record of fluid intake and output indicate fluid balance?
- Are the signs and symptoms that initially manifested fluid, electrolyte, or acid–base imbalances absent or improved? Has therapy created any troublesome new signs or symptoms?

- Is the client now able to manage his or her own care (ie, practice self-care behaviors to maintain fluid, electrolyte, and acid–base balance)? Can the client describe appropriate responses to potential future problems?

This evaluation should be ongoing as the care plan is implemented. As the client achieves short-term goals, these should be noted and reinforced. Before nursing care is terminated, the client (and family) should be able to independently promote fluid, electrolyte, and acid–base balance.

NURSING PROCESS

in Clinical Practice

When identifying and treating fluid, electrolyte, and acid–base balance problems categorized as nursing diagnoses, the nurse uses each phase of the nursing process. Quality care depends on the nurse's possession of the knowledge and clinical skills described earlier in this chapter. In this section, the special fluid, electrolyte, and acid–base balance needs of two target populations are explored—surgical clients and oncology clients. Both groups of clients are at increased risk for fluid, electrolyte, and acid–base balance problems.

In the case study that follows, nursing care is described for a client with an FVD related to prolonged diarrhea.

The Surgical Client

Clients undergoing surgery are at high risk for fluid, electrolyte, and acid–base balance problems preoperatively, intraoperatively, and postoperatively for many reasons:
- The pathology that underlies the need for surgery
- Aggressive diagnostic testing
- The stress of anesthesia and surgery
- Postoperative treatment
- Effects of surgery
  Potential nursing diagnoses include the following:

Preoperative
Fluid Volume Deficit related to fluid restrictions for diagnostic tests or pathology that results in decreased fluid intake (anorexia, intestinal obstruction) or abnormal fluid losses (vomiting, draining fistula)

Intraoperative
Fluid Volume Deficit related to bleeding, which, if severe, may cause shock and acute renal failure or actual fluid loss and third-space fluid shift during surgical procedure

Postoperative
Fluid Volume Deficit related to vomiting, gastric suction, or oral fluid restriction secondary to ileus following abdominal surgery
Fluid Volume Excess related to increased antidiuretic hormone secondary to surgery and anesthesia, al-
dosterone secretion, or overadministration of isotonic electrolyte solutions

Assessment

Preoperative
- Obtain baseline vital signs, body weight.
- Review laboratory data to ensure normal electrolytes and a hematocrit at 33% or higher (because transport of oxygen to cells depends on an adequate hemoglobin level). Notify physicians of any abnormalities so these can be corrected before surgery.
- Use intake and output records (and daily weights if fluid balance problems are suspected) and assessment of urine characteristics to assess fluid balance.
- Check for malnutrition (muscles with a wasted appearance—decreased strength, pale skin that breaks down easily, listlessness and apathy, dull, dry hair that falls out easily).

Postoperative
- Monitor vital signs according to agency policy and client's condition. Tachycardia and hypotension may indicate severe FVD. Changes in respirations and abnormal breath sounds are key indicators of acid–base and fluid volume disturbances.
- Maintain accurate intake and output record that includes intraoperative fluid intake and output. Ensure in adults an hourly urine output of 30 to 50 mL. Factors that contribute to decreased urinary volume in the postoperative period include the following:
  - Stress reaction (healthy physiologic response to surgery)
  - Hypovolemia resulting from fluid loss incurred in surgery
  - Preoperative dehydration
  - Subtle accumulation of fluid at the surgical site
  - Disturbance in myocardial function causing decreased blood flow to the kidneys
  - Renal failure, a serious cause of postoperative oliguria (Metheny, 1992)
- Assess for signs of electrolyte imbalance (see Table 37-4).

Planning: Client Goals

Preoperative

The client will:

- Enter surgery in fluid balance as evidenced by the following:
  - Stable body weight
  - Urine output of 30 to 50 mL/hr
  - Urine SG of 1.010 to 1.025
- Enter surgery in electrolyte balance as evidenced by normal laboratory values for sodium, chloride, potassium, and bicarbonate

Postoperative

The client will:

- Maintain approximately equal fluid intake and output
- Maintain urine output of 30 to 50 mL/hr
- Maintain stable body weight
- Maintain stable vital signs
- Be free of signs indicating fluid, electrolyte, or acid–base disturbance

Interventions

The best intervention for fluid, electrolyte, and acid–base disturbances is *prevention*.

- Before client's surgery, offer oral foods and fluids that the client likes and that are most likely to result in fluid, electrolyte, and nutritional balance.
- Bring any suspected abnormality to the physician's attention and execute orders for fluid or electrolyte replacement, strategies to reduce excesses, and so forth.
- Assist in identifying contributive factors and reduce or eliminate these factors, if possible.
- Administer IV fluids as prescribed and maintain accurate drip rates to prevent underinfusion or overinfusion.
- As soon as the client is able to tolerate oral fluids (check for swallowing reflex and bowel sounds), begin oral fluid replacement with fluids the client prefers.
- In clients with severe fluid imbalances, an indwelling Foley catheter may need to be inserted so that hourly urine outputs can be monitored.

Evaluative Criteria

The client meets the previously stated goals.

The Oncology Client

Most clients with cancer experience problems with fluid and electrolyte regulation during their illness. These problems are related to the following:

- Faulty regulation or availability of calcium, uric acid, sodium, potassium, phosphate
- Altered hormonal regulation (malignant tumors may produce hormones that interfere with water and electrolyte balance: ADH, PTH, osteoclastic activating factor, adrenocorticotropic hormone)

- Third-space fluid accumulation related to malignant effusions into the peritoneal, pericardial, or pleural compartments, or to edema resulting from blocked lymphatic drainage or venous return
- Treatment-related imbalances (Metheny, 1992)

Sample nursing diagnoses for the client with cancer include the following:

Fluid Volume Deficit or High Risk for Fluid Volume Deficit related to anorexia and vomiting (may be secondary to chemotherapy or radiation therapy), prolonged gastric suction, or third-space fluid shifts into the peritoneal, pericardial, or pleural compartments

Fluid Volume Excess: Edema related to obstruction of lymphatic drainage or venous return secondary to tumor pressure

Assessment

- Assess for the signs and symptoms that accompany electrolyte disturbances associated with specific tumors and treatment modalities.
- Weigh clients daily or weekly for signs of fluid deficit or excess. FVD is characterized by decreased skin turgor, decreased urinary output, concentrated urine, and postural hypotension. Clients with third-space fluid shifts have an *increase* in total body fluid, thus no decrease in weight, although clinically their condition is described as FVD.
- Be alert for signs of third-space fluid shifts:
  - Peritoneal—increased abdominal girth
  - Pleural—difficulty breathing
- Assess for signs of dependent edema; check the feet and ankles of people who sit or stand for long periods and the back and sacral area of the bedridden client.
- Assess for the development of weeping edema (leakage of fluid through the pores).

Planning: Client Goals

The client will:

- Take in sufficient fluids (oral if possible) to maintain fluid balance as evidenced by the following:
  - Normal skin turgor
  - Moist mucous membranes
  - Stable body weight
  - Baseline blood pressure
- Report (demonstrate) relief of symptoms of dehydration, third-space fluid shifts, edema, or other electrolyte disturbances
- Exhibit decreased dependent edema
- Describe self-care behaviors to prevent future fluid and electrolyte disturbances

Interventions

Interventions vary according to the nature of the fluid, electrolyte, or acid–base disturbance. To prevent problems, the client should be encouraged to drink sufficient fluids (about 2500 mL for the adult) and to eat nutritious meals.

- Clients with anorexia may need to be taught how to choose times when their systems will best tolerate food and fluids to ingest high-calorie liquids with key electrolytes.
- Clients with abnormal fluid losses may need to be taught the importance of fluid replacement.
- Clients with FVDs resulting from third-space fluid shifts may require IV fluid replacement; however, this also increases the volume of fluids trapped in the third space (eg, pleural cavity) and increase the client's discomfort. The client needs to be carefully monitored for signs of fluid overload during the administration of IV fluids.
- Clients with dependent edema require frequent position changes and a skin care program to prevent skin breakdown. Special mattresses are helpful.
- See Tables 37-3 through 37-5 for nursing interventions to treat specific fluid, electrolyte, and acid–base balance disturbances.

Evaluative Criteria

The client meets the previously stated goals.

 ## CASE STUDY

Gerry Stein is a 22-year-old Jewish man who is a senior in the pre-med program at a large state university. Although his grades were poor his first year in college, he currently is an honors student and plans to take the MCATs in 2 weeks. His overwhelming ambition is to be accepted into a prestigious medical school and to become a psychiatrist. He presents at the campus health clinic.

Assessment Findings

A comprehensive nursing assessment of Mr. Stein yields the following data:

- History of problems with diarrhea since his junior year in high school; treatment—kaolin and pectin (Kaopectate) and limiting his food and fluid intake; believes diarrhea is stress related; no medical evaluation to date
- Has had two or three loose bowel movements per day for the past week with urgency and occasional incontinence; believes this is related to anxiety about performance on MCATs and need for good grades; always thirsty but afraid to drink much; urine output is decreased and he noted it is darker in color and has a stronger odor
- Nursing examination: Temperature, 99.8°F (37.6°C); pulse, 92 beats per minute; respirations, 18; blood pressure, 100/60; skin and mucous membranes are pale and dry; weight is 4 lb less than usual (current weight 170 lb)

Nursing Diagnosis

Mr. Stein will receive a thorough medical work-up to rule out irritable bowel syndrome and inflammatory disorders of the bowel. Meanwhile, several nursing diagnoses are identified and a care plan is developed. Among the diagnoses is:

Fluid Volume Deficit related to prolonged diarrhea and decreased fluid intake

Planning: Client Goals

Mr. Stein expresses serious concern about his ability to continue to cope with the diarrhea, "Up until now, my problem has been manageable." He understands the importance of fluid and electrolyte balance and is highly motivated to practice any new self-care behaviors that will help to decrease the diarrhea so he can get on with his studies. He is supportive of the following goals.

Short-Term Goals
By the next week's visit on 3/24/93, the client will:

- Describe two effective means he has used to cope with stress
- Report that his diarrhea is eliminated or decreased to one or two episodes per day
- Demonstrate improved fluid and electrolyte balance as evidenced by:
  - Maintenance of current weight (170 lb)
  - Moist mucous membranes
  - Report of increased urinary output

Long-Term Goal
The client will:

- Demonstrate signs of fluid and electrolyte balance

Implementation

In implementing the care plan, the nurse needs the following specialized abilities:

- Strong assessment skills and knowledge of causative factors of diarrhea and means to eliminate them—and knowledge of the etiologies, defining characteristics, and treatment of fluid and electrolyte imbalances
- Interpersonal skills to facilitate the nurse's ability to empathize with Mr. Stein regarding his stressors and to communicate realistic hope that his situation can be improved as well as competence and caring as the nursing plan is implemented

- Knowledge of effective stress management techniques
- Teaching and counseling skills to assist Mr. Stein to develop the self-care behaviors that will enable him to live with his chronic condition with minimal discomfort and complications
- Accountability

Documentation

Sample documentation of the client's first return visit follows.

Traditional Note Format

3/24/93, nursing

    Mr. Stein returned to the clinic reporting that his diarrhea is decreased to one to two episodes per day and that he has an appointment with a gastroenterologist. He believes that modifying his diet, increasing rest periods, and medications (loperamide hydrochloride to control diarrhea and methylcellulose to increase the consistency of stool) were of great help. He still does not know how he can reduce his stress level. Nursing examination revealed temperature, 98.9°F (37.1°C); pulse, 88 beats/min; respirations, 18; blood pressure, 110/60; weight, 169 lb; skin and mucous membranes less dry than on

previous visit. States he has not noted much change in urine output but possibly less concentrated.

C. Ryan, RN

SOAP Format

3/24/93, 6 PM, nursing
#2 Fluid Volume Deficit related to prolonged diarrhea and decreased fluid intake

S: "I certainly feel better. I still have one or two loose bowel movements a day but I'm drinking more and seem less dry." Reports no noticeable change in urine output but urine "may be" less concentrated.
O: 98.8°F (37.1°C), 88, 18, 110/60, 1-lb weight loss (170 to 169 lb), skin and mucous membranes less dry
A: FVD responding to treatment
P: Continue care plan; reinforce follow-up with gastroenterologist

C. Ryan, RN

Evaluation

Short-term goal achievement is evaluated weekly. See Nursing Care Plan for evaluative statements and revisions of the care plan. Long-term goal achievement is an ongoing evaluation by client.

NURSING CARE PLAN

for Mr. Stein

Nursing Diagnosis:	Fluid Volume Deficit related to prolonged diarrhea and decreased fluid intake as evidenced by 4-lb weight loss, dry skin and mucous membranes, and report of decreased urine output and concentrated urine
Long-Term Goal:	Client will continue to demonstrate signs of fluid and electrolyte balance.

Goal: By next week's visit, 3/24/93, the client will:
- Describe two effective means he has used to cope with stress

Nursing Actions	Rationale	Evaluative Statement
Explore with the client (1) what he finds most stressing at present, (2) the control he believes he has over these stressors, and (3) the adequacy of his past and present stress management strategies.	Assisting the client to eliminate and reduce stress where possible and learn to cope better with unavoidable stress (identify and eliminate causative factors) is critical in controlling stress-related diarrhea.	3/24/93 Goal not met. Client reports little progress in coping with stress. With MCATs 1 week away, he feels more tense than ever before. Reports no time to explore stress management techniques.
Assess for other factors contributing to diarrhea and fluid volume deficit.	Diarrhea may have a functional basis.	*Revision:* Goal is appropriate. Encourage visit to counseling center if not before MCATs then as soon as possible afterward.
Teach relation between stress and bouts of diarrhea.	Stress may result in increased intestinal mobility.	
Refer to counseling center on campus for assistance with stress management.	Professional assistance may facilitate identification and management of stressful situation.	*C. Ryan, RN*

(continued)

NURSING CARE PLAN *(continued)*

for Mr. Stein

Goal: By the next week's visit, 3/24/93, the client will:
- Report that his diarrhea is eliminated or decreased to one or two episodes per day

Nursing Actions	**Rationale**	**Evaluative Statement**
Teach client to link causative factors with diarrhea and to note anything that brings relief or assists in establishment of usual pattern of defecation.	Being able to make these connections helps client to assume charge of own condition and to reinforce preventive strategies and successful relief measures.	3/24/93 Goal met. Client reports diarrhea decreased to one or two episodes per day. *Recommendation*: Advise client that it is important to keep appointment with gastroenterologist because relief may only be temporary. *C. Ryan, RN*
Make sure client understands diet: chemically and mechanically non-irritating diet high in calories, protein, and minerals; exclude foods such as cocoa, chocolate, alcohol, cold or carbonated beverages, citrus juices; try frequent, small meals.	Some clients fear eating because it stimulates the gastrocolic reflex and may result in a stool. Eating the proper diet actually reduces bowel irritation and decreases peristalsis.	
Teach client proper use of prescribed medications.	Loperamide hydrochloride controls diarrhea, and methylcellulose increases consistency of stool.	

Goal: By next week's visit, 3/24/93, the client will:
- Demonstrate improved fluid and electrolyte balance as evidenced by (1) maintenance of present weight (170 lb), (2) moist mucous membranes, and (3) report of increased urinary output

Nursing Actions	**Rationale**	**Evaluative Statement**
Explore with client workable plan for oral replacement of fluids.	Collaboration with client to determine acceptable sources of fluid intake may allay his fear that fluid intake causes diarrheal episodes.	3/24/93 Goal partially met. Client reports diarrhea decreased to once or twice a day. Two days there was no diarrhea. Weight, 169 lb. Mucous membranes are moist. Urine output is increased. *C. Ryan, RN*
Have client note which calorie- and electrolyte- (sodium and potassium) rich fluids he can tolerate. Increase fluid intake to maintain a normal urine specific gravity.	Increased fluid intake is necessary to compensate for excessive loss in diarrhea and to reestablish fluid balance.	
Instruct client to weigh himself every other day and to note changes in the volume or appearance of his urine.	All other things being equal, weight loss is a good indicator of continued fluid volume deficit. Other signs include decreased urinary output and high specific gravity.	
Teach client defining characteristics of electrolyte imbalances associated with prolonged diarrhea—hyponatremia and hypokalemia.	Excreted stool pulls electrolytes with it, especially sodium and potassium.	

KEY POINTS

- Whereas life can be sustained for many days without food, it can be sustained for only a few days without water.
- There are two major compartments for body fluids: (1) intracellular fluid, which is the fluid within cells, and (2) extracellular fluid, located outside of body cells, which includes intravascular fluid (plasma) and interstitial fluid (fluid in which tissue cells are bathed).
- A person's age, lean body mass, and sex can all influence the distribution of body fluids in the different compartments. Because lean tissue has higher water content than fat, thin people, females, and younger people tend to have higher percentages of total body water in relation to body weight than obese, male, and older people because of their increased lean body mass.
- Sodium and chloride are the principal ions of ECF; potassium and phosphate are principal ions of ICF.
- The most common routes for transporting fluid and electrolytes among the body compartments are osmosis, diffusion, active transport, and filtration.
- In a healthy adult, fluid intake and loss should average about 2500 mL over 2 to 3 days. The output of urine generally approximates the ingestion of liquids; water from food and oxidation is balanced by the water loss through the feces, the skin, and the respiratory process.
- Deficiencies in the amount of both water and electrolytes in ECF in near-normal proportions are termed *fluid volume deficits*. Excessive retention of water and electrolytes in ECF is termed *fluid volume excess*.
- To prevent the serious complications that can result from untreated electrolyte imbalances, nurses must be familiar with the etiologies, defining characteristics, and treatment of imbalances of sodium, potassium, calcium, magnesium, and phosphate.
- Normal blood plasma is slightly alkaline and has a normal pH range from 7.35 to 7.45. Slight deviations in either direction (acid–base imbalances) if untreated may result in death.
- The narrow range of normal pH is achieved by complex buffer systems (bicarbonate, phosphate, protein) and specific respiratory and renal mechanisms.
- Failure of acid–base regulating mechanisms may result in respiratory or metabolic disturbances, which can be acidosis or alkalosis.

- Risk factors for fluid, electrolyte, and acid–base imbalances include pathologies involving homeostatic regulators of fluid balance (eg, diabetes mellitus, congestive heart failure, renal failure); abnormal losses of body fluids; burns and trauma; and therapies with the potential to disrupt fluid and electrolyte balance (eg, medications such as diuretics and steroids, IV therapy, TPN).
- Pertinent assessment measures include maintaining accurate intake and output records, recording daily weights, observing for the signs and symptoms that characterize specific imbalances, and monitoring results of laboratory studies.
- Nursing diagnoses may be developed in which the fluid imbalance is the problem statement: Fluid Volume Deficit or Fluid Volume Excess, or the etiology: Pain related to edema, impaired oral mucous membrane related to dehydration.
- Nursing interventions are directed to maintaining a client's fluid, electrolyte, and acid–base balance; to preventing disturbances; and to correcting imbalances.
- When fluids are being encouraged or restricted, it is important that both the nursing staff and client understand the target amount of fluid to be taken each shift and that the client's fluid preferences be respected.
- Nurses administering IV fluids should accurately prepare the prescribed solution; understand the desired effect of treatment and possible adverse responses; and assume responsibility for initiating, monitoring, and, when ordered, discontinuing the therapy.
- Complications associated with IV infusions include infiltration, phlebitis, thrombus, speed shock, fluid overload, embolus, and infection.
- Administering blood transfusions requires a careful pretransfusion assessment of the client, accurate identification and matching of the blood to be transfused with its intended recipient, and ongoing monitoring of the client throughout the transfusion for transfusion reactions. These include hemolytic, febrile, allergic, and hypervolemic reactions.
- In TPN, hypertonic solutions of dextrose, amino acids, and select electrolytes and minerals—capable of reestablishing positive nitrogen balance and weight gain—are infused using a central vein.

STUDY QUESTIONS

1. Plasma, the liquid constituent of blood, is correctly identified as
   a. interstitial fluid
   b. intravascular fluid
   c. intracellular fluid
   d. 40% of total body fluid
2. Potassium functions as
   a. the chief electrolyte of extracellular fluid

b. the most abundant electrolyte in the body
c. the major cation of intracellular fluid
d. the chief extracellular anion

3. The movement of the solvent water from an area of lesser solute concentration to an area of greater solute concentration until equilibrium is established is known as
    a. osmosis
    b. diffusion
    c. active transport
    d. filtration

4. The most accurate indication of fluid balance status is
    a. intake and output
    b. skin turgor
    c. complete blood count
    d. daily weight

5. After assessing the following arterial blood gas values (pH, 7.30; pCO$_2$, 32; HCO$_3^-$, 14), the nurse correctly identifies
    a. respiratory acidosis
    b. respiratory alkalosis
    c. metabolic acidosis
    d. metabolic alkalosis

6. Mrs. Podralski, a client in the hospital, has been encouraged to increase her fluid intake. The nurse can best facilitate this by
    a. explaining the mechanisms involved in transporting fluids to and from intracellular compartments
    b. keeping fluids readily available for the client
    c. emphasizing the long-term goal of increasing fluids when she returns home
    d. planning to offer the larger amount of fluids in the evening

7. As the nurse prepares to assist the physician with insertion of a short-term CVC, she is aware that
    a. this catheter usually remains in place for 2 to 3 months
    b. the catheter is introduced by way of the basilic or cephalic veins in the antecubital space
    c. nursing responsibility includes changing the CVC dressing at least once weekly
    d. a chest x-ray is required to confirm placement

8. The nurse alertly assesses the acid–base balance of a client because she is aware that the client will be unable to effectively control his carbonic acid supply. This is most likely a client with badly damaged
    a. kidneys
    b. lungs
    c. adrenal glands
    d. blood vessels

9. Having the client breathe more slowly or breathe in a paper bag would be the most helpful intervention for the problem of
    a. respiratory acidosis (carbonic acid excess)
    b. respiratory alkalosis (carbonic acid deficit)
    c. metabolic acidosis (base bicarbonate deficit)
    d. metabolic alkalosis (base bicarbonate excess)

10. Which of the following is the most common etiologic factor related to the nursing diagnosis of fluid volume excess?
    a. increased need for fluids secondary to fever
    b. abnormal fluid loss from vomiting
    c. excessive IV infusion
    d. decreased fluid intake secondary to depression

11. In evaluating for complications of IV therapy, which of the following is evidence that the IV has infiltrated?
    a. In the past hour, only 50 mL of fluid has infused.
    b. The insertion site is red, hot, and swollen.
    c. The client's temperature has risen to 101°F (38.3°C).
    d. The site is pale, cool, swollen and painful.

12. For a client at risk for hyperkalemia, it is important to teach the client to avoid certain foods. Included in the foods to avoid would be
    a. Carrots and squash
    b. Canned soups and potato chips
    c. bananas, apricots, broccoli
    d. whole grain cereals

13. Your client has multiple injuries after an automobile accident and you are to start IV therapy. His right arm is in a cast. Which site would you choose for venipuncture?
    a. left antecubital
    b. dorsal aspect of either foot
    c. right hand
    d. left forearm

14. For clients who are receiving IV therapy, the nurse should
    a. change the IV catheter and entry site daily
    b. change the tubing every 8 hours
    c. increase the rate to catch up if the correct amount has not been infused at the end of the shift
    d. monitor the flow rate at least every hour

15. While a client is receiving blood, the nurse should evaluate for transfusion reaction
    a. 15 minutes after the infusion is started
    b. after the blood is all infused
    c. every hour
    d. every 15 minutes

Answers With Rationale

1. The correct response is *b*. Intravascular fluid or plasma is extracellular fluid and composes 5% of total body fluid.

2. The correct response is *c*. Sodium is the chief electrolyte of extracellular fluid, calcium is the most abundant electrolyte in the body, and chloride is the chief extracellular anion.

3. The correct response is *a*. Gases move about by diffusion. Active transport is a process that requires energy for the movement of substances through a cell wall from an area of lesser to higher concentration. Filtration is the passage of fluids through a permeable membrane from an area of high pressure to one of low pressure.

4. The correct response is *d*. Intake and output are not always as accurate and may involve a subjective component. Measurement of skin turgor is subjective and the complete blood count does not necessarily reflect fluid balance.

5. The correct response is *c*. Metabolic acidosis equals low bicarbonate. Acidosis equals low pH. Decreased pCO$_2$ represents a respiratory compensatory attempt.

6. The correct response is *b*. Explanation of the fluid transportation mechanisms is inappropriate and it does not focus on the immediate problem of increasing fluid intake. Meeting short-term goals provides further reinforcement and additional fluids should be taken earlier in the day.

7. The correct response is *d*. Short-term CVCs remain in place up to 4 weeks, are introduced into the subclavian or internal jugular vein, and dressings should be changed according to agency policy but at least every 72 hours.

8. The correct response is *b*. The lungs are the primary controller of the body's carbonic acid supply.

9. The correct response is *b*. Breathing more slowly or breathing into a closed system causes accumulation of carbon dioxide to reverse carbonic acid deficit.

10. The correct response is *c*. The other alternatives are related to fluid volume deficit.

11. The correct response is *d*. A decrease in flow rate may indicate an infiltration but is not as significant as the other signs of a pale, cool, swollen and painful site. Phlebitis is an inflammatory process and results in redness, warmth, and possibly a temperature elevation.

12. The correct response is *c*. Hyperkalemia is an elevated serum potassium level and bananas, apricots, and broccoli are foods high in potassium content and should be avoided in this situation.

13. The correct response is *d*. Based on the condition of the right arm, this is not a choice. The left forearm is preferable to the antecubital space of the left arm or the lower extremities.

14. The correct response is *d*. IV catheter and entry site should be changed every 48 to 72 hours in most circumstances. Tubing is changed according to agency policy but not at the frequency of every 8 hours. Increasing the rate may lead to fluid overload.

15. The correct response is *d*. The nurse should closely observe a client for the first 5 to 10 minutes and then check the client every 15 minutes while he or she is receiving the blood transfusion.

BIBLIOGRAPHY

Bowman, M., Eisenberg, P., Katz, B., & Metheny, N. (1989). Effect of tube-feeding osmolarity on serum sodium levels. *Critical Care Nurse, 9*(1), 22–28.

Boykoff, S., Boykoff, S., Boxwell, A., & Boxwell, J. (1988). 6 Ways to clear the air from an IV line. *Nursing, 18*(2), 46–48.

Brenner, M., & Welliver, J. (1990). Pulmonary and acid–base assessment. *Nursing Clinics of North America, 25*(4), 761–770.

Butler, S. (1989). Current trends in autologous transfusion. *RN, 52*(11), 44–54.

Carpenito, L. (1992). *Nursing diagnosis: Application to clinical practice* (4th ed.). Philadelphia: Lippincott.

Dick, M., Maree, S., & Gray, J. (1992). How to boost the odds of a painless IV start. *American Journal of Nursing, 92*(6), 49–50.

Drago, S. (1992). Banking on your own blood. *American Journal of Nursing, 92*(3), 64.

Fischbach, F. (1992). *A manual of laboratory tests* (4th ed.). Philadelphia: Lippincott.

Gasparis, L., et al. (1989). IV solutions: Which one's right for your patient? *Nursing, 19*(4), 62–64.

Gahart, B. (1992). *Intravenous medications: A handbook for nurses and allied health professionals* (8th ed.). St. Louis: Mosby–Year Book.

Gonsoulin, S., & Broussard, P. (1991). Shedding light on IV therapy. *Nursing, 21*(12), 62–64.

Gullatte, M. (1989). Managing an implanted infusion device. *RN, 52*(1), 44–49.

Hadaway, L. (1991). IV tips. *Geriatric Nursing, 12*(2), 78–81.

Hahn, K. (1989). Monitoring a blood transfusion. *Nursing, 18*(10), 20–21.

Handerhan, B. (1991). Computing the anion gap. *RN, 54*(7), 30–31.

Janusek, L. (1989). Metabolic acidosis: Pathophysiology, signs, and symptoms. *Nursing, 19*(7), 52–53.

Janusek, L. (1990). Metabolic alkalosis: Pathophysiology—the resulting signs and symptoms. *Nursing, 19*(6), 52–53.

Kyle, K., & Myers, J. (1990). Peripherally inserted central catheters: Development of a hospital-based program. *Journal of Intravenous Nursing, 13*(5), 287–290.

Lenox, A. (1990). IV therapy: Reducing the risk of infection. *Nursing, 20*(3), 60–61.

Lindell, K., & Wesmiller, S. (1989). Using arterial blood gases to interpret acid–base balance. *Orthopaedic Nursing, 8*(3), 31–34.

Markel, S., & Reynen, K. (1990). Impact on patient care: 2652 PIC catheter days in the alternative setting. *Journal of Intravenous Nursing, 13*(6), 347–351.

Mathewson, M. (1989). Intravenous therapy. *Critical Care Nursing, 9*(2), 21–36.

Metheny, N. (1990). Why worry about IV fluids? *American Journal of Nursing, 90*(6), 50–55.

Metheny, N. (1992). *Fluid and electrolyte balance: Nursing considerations* (2nd ed.). Philadelphia: Lippincott.

Meyer, C. (1992). Transparent dressings' clear disadvantage. *American Journal of Nursing, 92*(6), 14.

Millam, D. (1988). Managing complications of IV therapy. *Nursing, 18*(3), 34–42,

Miller, J. (1989). Intravenous therapy in fluid and electrolyte imbalance. *Professional Nurse, 4*(5), 237–241.

Mims, B. (1991). Interpreting ABGs. *RN, 54*(3), 42–46.

Mueller, K., & Boisen, A. (1989). Keeping your patient's water level up. *RN, 52*(7), 65–68.

National Blood Resource Education Program's Nursing Education Working Group. (1991). Transfusion nursing: Trends and practices for the '90s. *American Journal of Nursing, 91*(6), 42–52.

Newton, G. (1988). A better way to chart IV therapy. *RN, 51*(7), 26–28.

Querin, J., & Stahl, L. (1990). 12 simple sensible steps for successful blood transfusions. *Nursing, 19*(10), 68–81.

Rinard, G. (1989). Water intoxication. *American Journal of Nursing, 89*(12), 1635–1638.

Rosen, G. (1990). Home parenteral nutrition. *Caring, 9*(5), 34–36.

Rountree, D. (1991). The PIC catheter: A different approach. *American Journal of Nursing, 91*(8), 22–26.

Sherman, J., & Sherman, R. (1989). I.V. therapy that clicks. *Nursing, 19*(5), 50–51.

Sommers, M. (1990). Rapid fluid resuscitation: How to correct dangerous deficits. *Nursing, 20*(1), 52–53.

Sumner, J. (1988). Preserving IV power if fluids are restricted. *RN, 51*(8), 26–28.

Sympson, G. (1991). CATR: A new generation of autologous blood transfusion. *Critical Care Nurse, 11*(4), 60–64.

Taylor, D. (1990a). Respiratory acidosis: Pathophysiology, signs, and symptoms. *Nursing, 19*(9), 52–53.

Taylor, D. (1990b). Respiratory alkalosis: Pathophysiology, signs, and symptoms. *Nursing, 20*(8), 60–61.

Thomason, S. (1991). Using a Groshong central venous catheter. *Nursing, 21*(10), 58–60.

Ulrich, B. (1989). *Nephrology nursing: Concepts and strategies*. Norwalk, CT: Appleton & Lange.

Viall, C. (1990). Your complete guide to central venous catheters. *Nursing, 20*(2), 34–41.

Walpert, N. (1990). An orderly look at calcium disorders. *Nursing, 19*(7), 60–64.

Whitney, R. (1991). Comparing long-term central venous catheters. *Nursing, 21*(4), 70–71.

Woodtli, A. (1990). Thirst: A critical care nursing challenge. *Dimensions of Critical Care Nursing, 9*(1), 6–15.

Yarnell, R., & Craig, M. (1991). Detecting hypomagnesemia: The most overlooked electrolyte imbalance. *Nursing, 21*(7), 55–57.

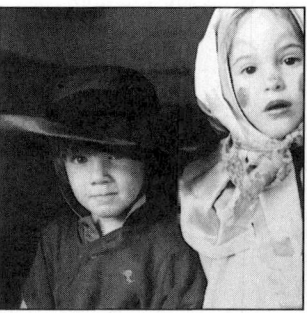

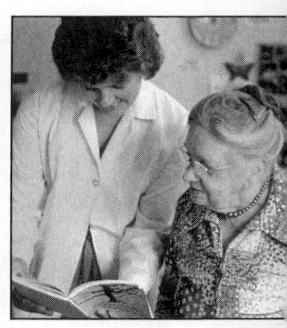

Promoting Healthy Psychosocial Responses

Each individual person is a composite of interrelated physiologic and psychosocial dimensions; alterations in one dimension affect all of the others. Unit VIII discusses psychosocial considerations in holistic client care, focusing on self-concept, sensory stimulation, sexuality, and spirituality.

One's self-concept can serve as a positive strength; if altered, it can interfere with meeting other needs. Nursing interventions to maintain, strengthen, or change self-concept are basic to all aspects of client care.

Intact and functioning senses are necessary for life, normal growth and development, and pleasurable experiences. Alterations in any of the senses require caring, knowledgeable, and individualized nursing interventions to meet needs and prevent further overload or deprivation.

Sexuality and spirituality are important components of human functioning. These dimensions are an integral part of each person's identity and are critical elements in holistic client care. To facilitate sexual and spiritual wellness, nurses must develop self-awareness in these areas and become comfortable with values and practices different from their own. Nursing interventions and therapeutic interpersonal skills are used to elicit concerns, identify needs, implement teaching, make referrals, and demonstrate empathic acceptance and caring.

Unit VIII provides the knowledge base for promoting healthy psychosocial responses in clients. Using the nursing process, interventions can be planned and implemented to meet needs and support strengths in both health and illness.

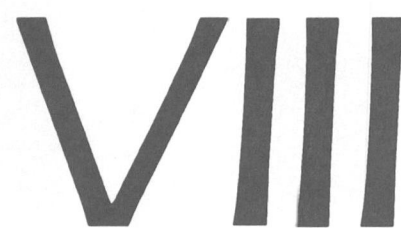

VIII

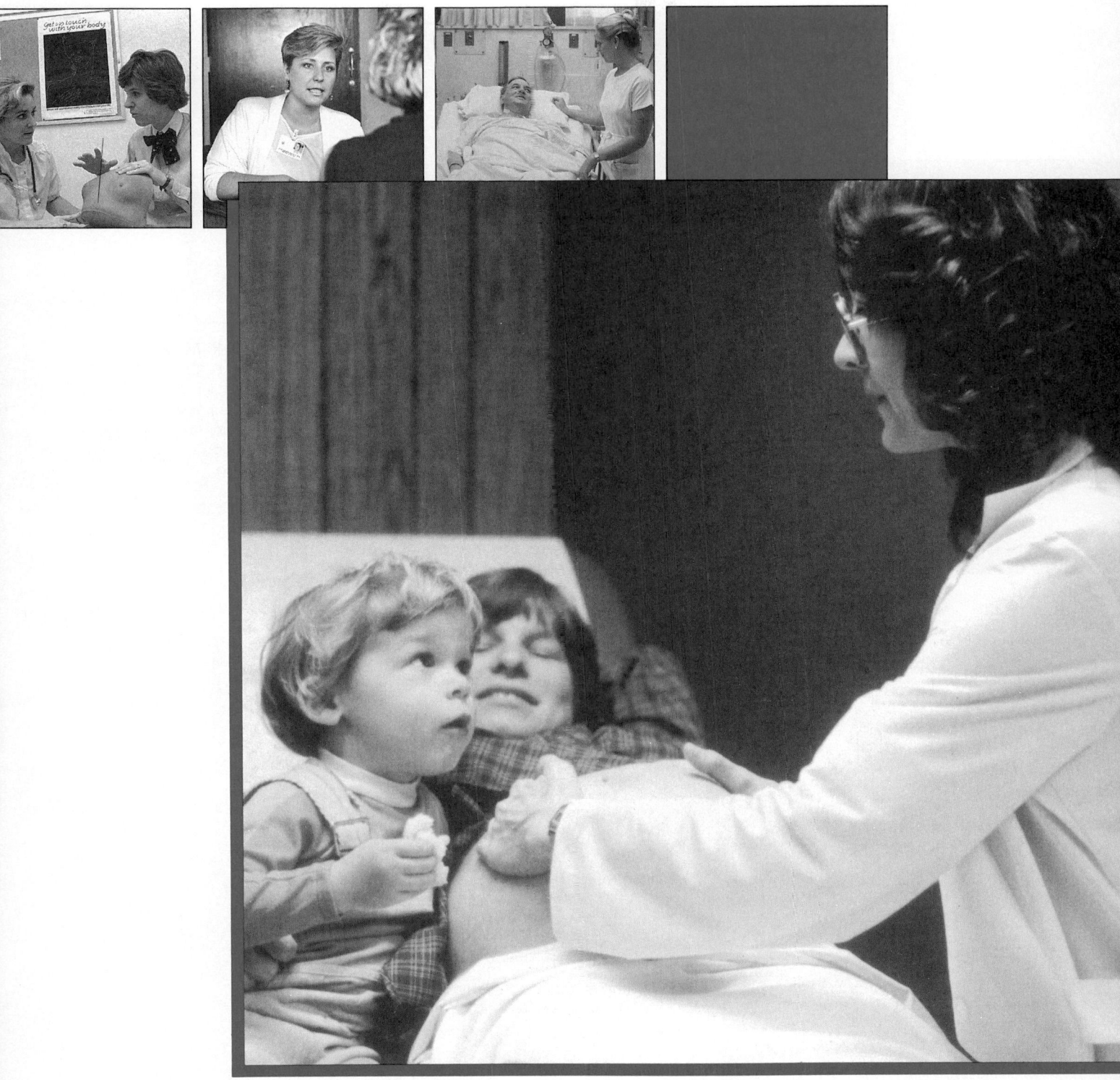

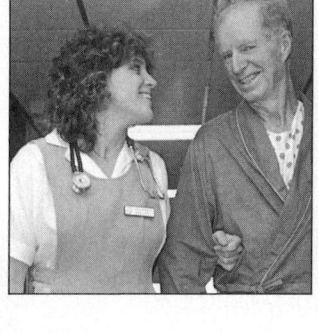

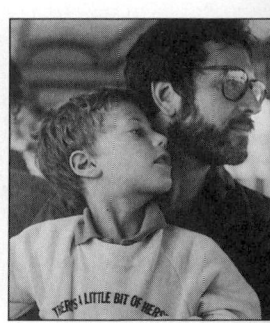

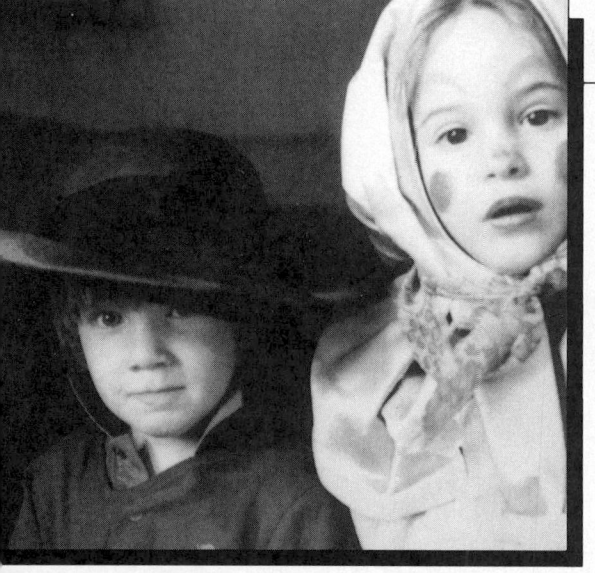

Self-Concept

OBJECTIVES

After studying this chapter, the learner should be able to:

Define key terms used in the chapter.

Identify three dimensions of self-concept—self-knowledge, self-expectation, self-evaluation (self-esteem)

Describe major steps in the development of self-concept.

Differentiate positive and negative self-concept and high and low self-esteem.

Identify six variables that influence self-concept.

Use appropriate interview questions and observations to assess a client's self-concept.

Develop nursing diagnoses to correctly identify disturbances in self-concept (body image, self-esteem, role performance, personal identity).

Describe nursing strategies that are effective in resolving self-concept problems.

Plan, implement, and evaluate nursing care related to select nursing diagnoses for disturbances in self-concept.

KEY TERMS

body image
ideal self
personal identity
role performance
self-actualization
self-concept
self-esteem
social self
subjective self

38

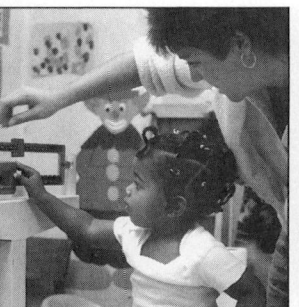

Overview of Self-Concept

Dimensions of Self-Concept

Self-concept is the mental image or picture of self. All the feelings, beliefs, and values associated with "I" or "me" compose self-concept. Included in the notion of self-concept are the following:

Body image: How I experience my body
Subjective self: How I see myself, who I think I am
Ideal self: Self I would like to be or feel I should be
Social self: Way I feel others see me (Atwater, 1990)

The dimensions of self-knowledge, self-expectations, and self-evaluation describe self-concept (Calhoun & Acocella, 1989; Fig. 38-1). People with a positive self-concept have broad and diversified knowledge of the self, realistic expectations, and high self-esteem.

Self-Knowledge: "Who Am I?" A person's self-knowledge includes basic facts (age, race, occupation), which place that person in social groups, and a listing of qualities or traits, which describe typical behaviors, feelings, moods, and other characteristics (generous, hot-headed, ambitious, intelligent, sexy). Although some labels cannot be changed, (eg, sex, age, and race), most are unstable and subjective.

Self-Expectations: "Who or What Do I Want to Be?" Expectations for the self flow from the ideal self, the self I want to be or think I should be. These expectations often develop early in childhood and are based on the image of a role model. These expectations may be healthy or unhealthy. Many contemporary thinkers are expressing concern that many children currently identify as their heroes rock stars or pimps, prostitutes, and drug dealers rather than parents, government leaders, or other professional people.

Self-Evaluation: "How Well Do I Like Me?" Self-esteem is the evaluative component of the self-concept, sometimes termed self-respect, self-approval, or self-worth. According to Maslow (1954), all people "have a need or desire for a stable, firmly based, usually high evaluation of themselves, for self-respect or self-esteem, and for the esteem of others" (p. 90). Accordingly, he identified two subsets of esteem needs: (1) self-esteem needs (strength, achievement, mastery and competence, confidence in the face of the world, independence, and freedom) and (2) respect needs or the need for esteem from others (status, dominance, recognition, attention, importance, and appreciation).

Coopersmith (1967) identified the four bases of self-esteem as (1) significance—the way a person feels he or she is loved and approved of by the people important to that person; (2) competence—the way tasks that are considered important are performed; (3) virtue—the attainment of moral-ethical standards; and (4) power—the extent to

As people move through the hierarchy of human needs to a higher level, needs for self-esteem and self-actualization occur as discussed in Chapter 7. **Self-esteem** is the need to feel good about oneself and to believe that others also hold one in high regard. **Self-actualization** is the need to reach one's potential through full development of one's unique capability. A critical component of both of these needs is self-concept. One's self-image or self-concept has the power to either encourage or thwart personal growth.

People who think of themselves as born losers most likely will not be motivated to learn self-care behaviors in response to illness or trauma. Nursing efforts aimed at teaching such people are doomed to failure until the client values himself or herself enough to want to invest energy in self-care. On the other hand, clients may desperately want to modify their self-concept and self-care behaviors and have no idea how to do it. Nursing assistance can help them explore factors in self-esteem. The experience of illness, diagnostic testing, and treatment can severely threaten the self-concept of a client. Nurses sensitive to the self-concept needs of clients can use each nurse–client interaction to enhance the client's sense of self and to assist the client in resolving self-concept disturbances.

Study of this chapter provides the student with knowledge of the dimensions of self-concept, formation of self-concept, and key factors affecting self-concept. Practical interview guides are offered for assessing self-concept. Strategies for enhancing the self-esteem of the nurse are provided. Numerous examples of nursing diagnoses are given, and specific nursing strategies for assisting clients to meet the self-concept goals are described. In the section Nursing Process in Clinical Practice, focused assessment, planning, implementation, and evaluation guides are offered for the nursing diagnoses Body Image Disturbance and Self-Concept Disturbance. Self-Concept Disturbance is not a North American Nursing Diagnosis Association diagnostic label but is often used initially as a broad diagnostic category until a client's problem can be further specified.

These guides and the concluding case study illustrate how the nurse's knowledge of self-concept may be combined with skilled nursing interventions and caring to successfully resolve disturbances in self-concept.

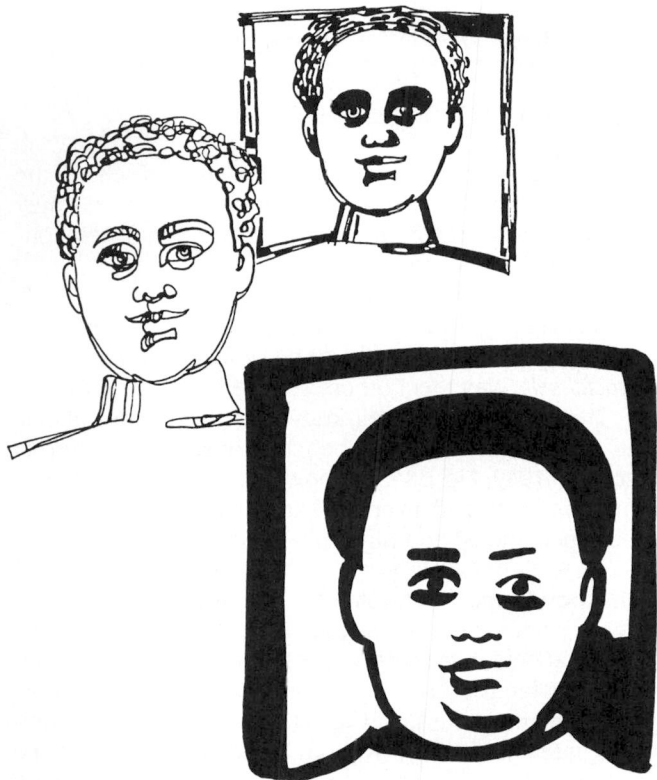

FIGURE   38-1

The dimensions of self-knowledge, self-expectation, and self-evaluation describe our self-concept. Here, the artist characterizes himself visually in a self-portrait. We all describe and present our concept of self in our actions and associations, as well as in our self-descriptions.

which a person influences his or her own and others' lives. According to Coopersmith, people with high, medium, and low self-esteem differ in their expectations of the future, in their affective reactions, and in their basic styles of adapting to environmental demands. People with high self-esteem are accustomed to being well received and successful. They are able to approach people, tasks, and new situations freely, with confidence in their ability to interact and to get along with people and to respond successfully to life's challenges.

Formation of Self-Concept

A person is not born with a self-concept. Rather, it is a social creation that develops as a result of interactions with others. Steps in the formation of self-concept include the following:

1. An infant learns that the physical self is different from the environment. If basic needs are met and warmth and affection are experienced, the child begins life with positive feelings about self.
2. The child next internalizes (incorporates into self) other people's attitudes toward self (Fig. 38-2). Par-

ents play the most influential role here; peers play the second most influential role.
3. The child or adult internalizes the standards of society.

Coleman, Morris, and Glaros (1987) identified the following psychological conditions that foster healthy development of the self in children (Fig. 38-3):

- Emotional warmth and acceptance
- Effective structure and discipline
  - Clearly defined standards and limits, so that children understand what goals, procedures, and conduct are approved
  - Adequately defined roles for both older and younger members of the family
  - Established methods of handling children that produce the desired behavior, discourage misbehavior, and deal with infractions when they occur

FIGURE   38-2

The child internalizes other persons' attitudes toward him or her. His or her self-esteem is based on his feeling of being loved and approved of. Parents play the most influential role in the formation of the child's self-concept.

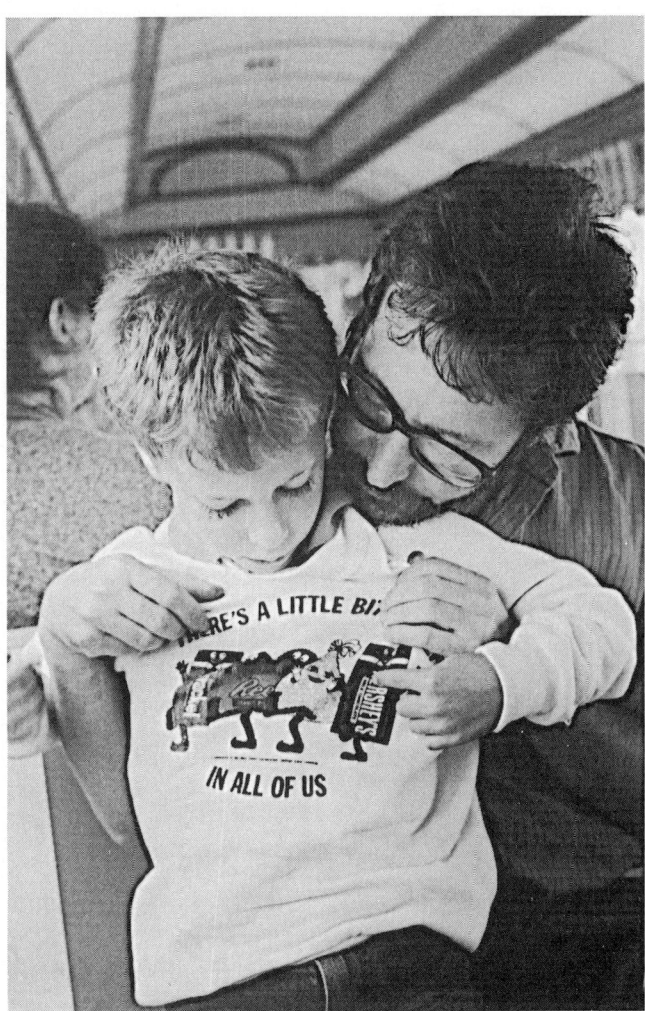

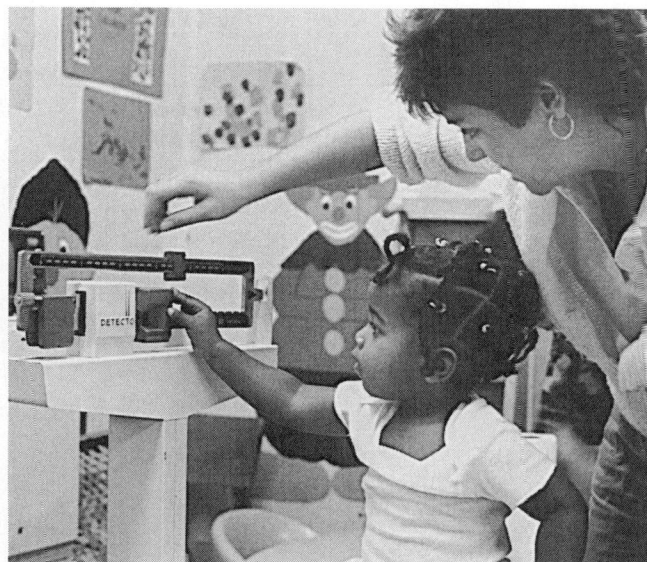

FIGURE 38-3

Conditions fostering healthy development of the self in children include emotional warmth and acceptance; effective structure and discipline; encouragement of competence, self-confidence, and ability to meet challenges; appropriate role models; and a stimulating and responsive environment. (Photo by Gates Rhodes, courtesy of School of Nursing, University of Pennsylvania.)

- Encouragement of competence and self-confidence
- Helping children meet challenges
- Appropriate role models
- A stimulating and responsive environment

Formation of self-concept is further understood in the developmental theories, especially in Erikson's stages of development, Piaget's cognitive developmental stages, and Havighurst's developmental tasks (see Chapters 10 and 11).

Threats to Self-Concept

Anxiety is a threat to self-concept. According to psychoanalysts, the ego uses many different methods to protect itself from anxiety. Among these methods are coping and defense mechanisms. (Anxiety and coping and defense mechanisms are discussed briefly in Chapter 9.)

Factors Affecting Self-Concept

Almost any life experience can influence a person's self-concept. Key factors include developmental considerations, culture, internal and external resources, history of success and failure, stressors, and illness or trauma.

Developmental Considerations

As a person matures, the criteria that mark the experiences necessary for a positive self-concept change. (See the preceding discussion of formation of self-concept.) Although the infant needs a supportive environment in which all human needs are met, the growing child needs the freedom to explore and develop the ability to meet increasing personal needs. Table 38-1 highlights developmental changes affecting self-concept, related nursing implications, and potential self-concept disturbances.

Culture

As a child internalizes the values of parents and peers, culture begins to influence a sense of self. If the culture is relatively stable, little tension may be experienced between what culture expects of the child and what the child expects of self. When parents, peers, and the adult world confront the child with different cultural expectations, the sense of self may be confused. For example, an adolescent may realize his or her parents live by the work ethic and believe it is necessary to rise early every day and put in a full day's work. The adolescent's peer group has few demands placed on it and encourages the adolescent to hang out with the group. The adolescent's vocational aptitudes, meanwhile, are leading him or her to consider a music career in a rock group, which will keep the adolescent out late many nights doing something the parents do not classify as work.

Internal and External Resources

The personal strengths an individual recognizes, develops, and uses are powerful but subjective determinants of self-concept. One person may use humor as both an effective coping mechanism and as a successful interpersonal tool. Another person may use humor to avoid facing conflict and may feel bad about being known as a joker or clown. External resources such as a network of support people, adequate finances, and organizational supports are also subjective determinants of self-concept. Generally, the more resources a person has and uses wisely, the better the feelings about self.

History of Success and Failure

People with a history of repeated failure (in school, friendships, work, or marriage) may perceive themselves as failures and actually perpetuate this image by unconsciously instructing others to treat them this way. They may come to fear success and actually find it easier to fail even though they do not like themselves that way. Thus, failure influences an individual's self-concept negatively, and his or her self-concept instructs the person to continue to fail. On the other hand, one successful experience conditions a person to strive for the next success and a positive self-concept is forged that expects success and makes it happen.

T A B L E 3 8 - 1

Developmental Changes Affecting Self-Concept

Developmental Period	Changes Affecting Self-Concept	Implications for Nursing	Potential Causes of Disturbances in Self-Concept
Infancy	• No self-concept at birth • Beginning differentiation of self and nonself	• Teach parents the critical importance of providing consistent and affectionate parenting • Assess if the parents have reasonable expectations of the infant: sleeping, eating, other awake behaviors	• Unmet basic human needs • Lack of adequate body and sensory stimulation • Parents' lack of acceptance of the infant's appearance or behavior
Childhood	• An intact body is important to the young child, who fears bodily mutilation • During middle childhood, a sense of being trusted and loved, of being competent and trustworthy develops • Differences between self and others are strong	• If invasive procedures are indicated, explain simply to the child what is being done and offer the child support • Assess the parents' ability to provide the type of developmental environment in which the child's self-concept can evolve positively	• Dysfunctional family • Too much or too little structure • Sensory perceptual impairments
Adolescence	• Development of secondary sex characteristics; rapid body changes • Emphasis on sexual identity • Parental influences on self-concept are often rejected; peers become more important; movement is toward development of own identity	• Assess adolescent's self-knowledge and understanding of body changes • Counsel adolescent regarding mature and healthy use of independence he or she craves • Provide anticipatory guidelines regarding hazards to life, health, human functioning	• Inability to accept body • Inability to resolve competing pulls to be both a child and an adult • Unhealthy peer pressure
Adulthood	• Society places emphasis on intactness of body, fitness, energy, sexuality, style, sophistication, beauty • Important to meet role expectations well	• Assess how realistic the adult's expectations are and the incentive they provide for growth and development • Assist client to deal constructively with negative influences in self-image • Preretirement counseling	• Inability to fulfill conflicting role expectations • Failure to accept role responsibility (eg, parenting responsibilities) • Unreasonable expectations • Irreversible body change related to trauma, illness • Unsatisfying job • Failure to develop new goals to give meaning and purpose to life
Later years	• Declining physical and possibly mental abilities	• Assess how the older person is adjusting to effects of aging • Counsel regarding meaningful use of time • Explore resources	• Loss of significant work (retirement); feelings of uselessness • Death of spouse, significant others • Diminished physical attractiveness, strength, overall health • Multiple stressors • Fear of dependency

Stressors

Life stressors (marriage, divorce, an exam, a new job, a gray hair, a fire) may call forth a personal response and mobilize an individual's talents that results in good feelings about oneself. Stressors may also evoke maladaptive responses that diminish the self-concept. Examples of these include withdrawal, depression, extreme anxiety, and substance abuse. How the person perceives the stressor (threat, challenge, defeat) and his or her ability to mobilize personal strengths and other resources are determined largely by that person's self-concept, which then is influenced by the response the person chooses.

Aging, Illness, or Trauma

Because most people take a healthy body for granted, the diminishment of physical attractiveness or functioning, the

Self-Concept

Use the assessment checklist to determine how well you are meeting your need for positive self-concept. Then develop a prescription for self-care by choosing appropriate behaviors from the list of suggestions.

Assessment Checklist

almost always	sometimes	almost never	
☐	☐	☐	1. I have established appropriate expectations and goals for myself.
☐	☐	☐	2. I have effective and satisfying relationships with others.
☐	☐	☐	3. I cope effectively with change and loss.
☐	☐	☐	4. I accept and feel good about myself.

Self-Care Behaviors

1. Accept normal variations in physical appearance and capabilities.
2. Use problem-solving and decision-making strategies to define expectations and set goals.
3. Set priorities and accept that no one person can be all things to all people.
4. Forget past mistakes; carrying around "excess baggage" is unhealthy.
5. Emphasize strengths and abilities in self.
6. Take an active part in group activities in school, work, church, or the community.
7. Volunteer time, talents, or services.
8. Avoid alcohol or drugs.
9. Live life one day at a time.

---

suggestion of disease, or sudden impact of trauma may pose serious threats to the self. People vary greatly in their response to aging, illness, and trauma.

Nurse as Role Model

Before nurses can successfully identify and resolve self-esteem disturbances in clients, they must be comfortable with themselves and possess a certain measure of self-esteem. Important goals for the nurse's personal esteem are the following:

- Identify basic unmet human needs, exploring positive means to meet these needs
- Schedule time every day to meet personal needs
- Assess the effect of feedback from significant others on self-esteem
- Describe personal strengths accurately
- Develop a realistic plan to achieve goals for personal growth and development

Specific strategies for developing self-esteem in relation to one's professional practice follow (Fig. 38-4):

Dispel the myth that it is necessary to know all there is to know about nursing to be a good nurse. At no one point in time does any nurse ever have it all together. Acceptance of the need to learn new theories or new procedures frees you from having to practice defensively (ie, pretend to be on top of every new development) and is a great stimulus for professional growth and development.

Realistically evaluate strengths and weaknesses. Build a periodic review into your practice and be fair in your self-evaluation. "I think I'm giving better care than

ever before and I know my clients are appreciative, but I'm sensing a lot of tension between myself and a couple of the other nurses. . . . "

Accentuate the positive. Many of us have a knack for forgetting the 99 things we did well and focusing on our one error. Errors need to be taken seriously and

FIGURE 38-4

Two strategies for developing one's own professional self-esteem as a nurse are to recognize that it is okay to ask questions about things you do not know or about which you are uncertain and, in doing so, to develop team self-esteem. (Photo by Gates Rhodes, courtesy of School of Nursing, University of Pennsylvania.)

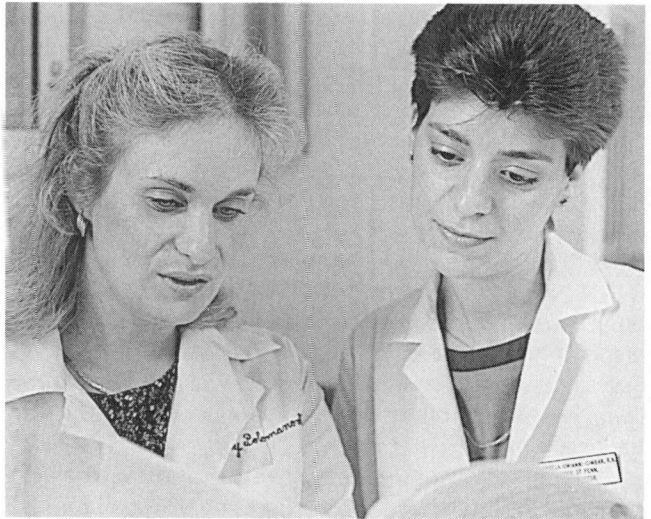

evaluated but not to the exclusion of overlooking positive accomplishments

Develop a conscious plan for changing weaknesses into strengths. Professional growth and development depend on strong motivation to become better at what you do. "Realizing that I never know what to say when a client receives bad news, I can try to avoid these clients or consciously plan to develop better interpersonal skills." Nurses are tremendous resources for each other. Tapping into each other's strengths is a great way to mutually build self-esteem. "You always seem to know the right thing to say or do with clients. Do you mind if I observe for a while and then 'try on' some of your behaviors?"

Work to develop team self-esteem. A basic interpersonal principle that seems to work well in practice is to offer to others what you want yourself. Because our sense of self is strongly influenced by the feedback we receive from others, positive reinforcement of our strengths and sincere offers to help correct deficiencies are needed by everyone.

Actively demonstrate your commitment to nursing and concern about nursing's public image. To feel good about yourself, you need to be able to experience pride in your profession. Active participation in professional organizations can offer many personal rewards—not the least of which is enthusiasm and pride in being a nurse. Monitoring the media's portrayal of nursing and providing appropriate feedback contributes to individual and corporate nursing self-esteem.

High-Risk Factors for Self-Concept Disturbances

Personal Identity Disturbance

- Developmental changes
- Trauma
- Gender dissonance
- Cultural dissonance

Body Image Disturbance

- Loss of body part or function
- Disfigurement
- Developmental changes

Self-Esteem Disturbance

- Unhealthy interpersonal relationships
- Failure to achieve developmental milestones
- Failure to achieve life goals
- Failure to live up to personal moral code
- Sense of powerlessness

Altered Role Performance

- Loss of valued role
- Ambiguous role expectations
- Conflicting role expectations
- Inability to meet role expectations

Assessing Self-Concept

The nurse assessing self-concept focuses on the client's personal identity, body image, self-esteem, and role performance. A general assessment of self-concept should be included in every comprehensive nursing assessment. It is as important to identify and label a client's positive self-concept as it is to note problems. Positive self-concept can be used as a key strength when working with clients to achieve other health goals. Clients experiencing illness or trauma that results in body disfigurement or altered functioning or life crises that arrest development and thwart the achievement of life goals are at high risk for problems related to self-concept and should be assessed more carefully. If problems surface during the interview, a more thorough assessment should be carried out. The accompanying displays highlight elements common to any self-concept assessment and high-risk factors. The discussion that follows offers specific interviewing guides for each element in the assessment.

It is important for the nurse conducting this assessment to realize the limitations of self-reporting. A client may give what he or she believes are the desired or socially acceptable responses to interview questions. "Why, of course I like myself. I'm a pretty good person. Yes, I have friends." For this reason the nurse must evaluate the client's responses in relation to observations made about the client and what is known about the client from other sources. The accompanying display outlines behaviors often associated with low self-concept. When the nursing assessment reveals a clustering of these behaviors, it is important to discuss this finding with the client. This is especially true when there is a discrepancy between the client's words and behavior. "You've told me that you feel in control of your situation right now and are committed to the treatment plan, but I notice you've broken three therapy appointments this month and you did mention that you are drinking more heavily. . . . "

Personal Identity

When assessing self-concept, the information needed first is the client's description of self. **Personal identity** describes an individual's conscious sense of who he or she is. "How would you describe yourself to others?" The nurse pays special attention to the labels used by the client and the order in which they appear. Calhoun and Acocella (1989) have recommended the following exercise:

FOCUSED ASSESSMENT GUIDE

Self-Concept

Factors to Assess	Questions and Approaches
Personal identity	How would you describe yourself to others? • Personal characteristics and traits • Strengths
Body image	Describe your body to me. What do you like most/least about your body? Is there anything about your body that you would like to change?
Self-esteem	Do you like who you are? Who would you like to be? Who or what has influenced your self-expectations? Are these expectations realistic? • Significance: Does it bother you when you feel unloved or unappreciated by those who are important to you? • Competence: How do you feel about your ability to do the things in life that are important to you? • Virtue: Are you satisfied with the way you are able to live up to your moral standards? • Power: To what extent do you feel able to control what happens to you in life? How does this make you feel?
Role performance	How do you feel about your ability to do all the things your roles demand of you? Are these roles satisfying for you?

Defining Characteristics of Low Self-Concept

Refusal to touch or look at a body part

Refusal to look into a mirror

Unwillingness to discuss a limitation, deformity, or disfigurement

Refusal to accept rehabilitation efforts

Inappropriate attempts to direct own treatment

Denial of the existence of a deformity or disfigurement

Increasing dependence on others

Signs of grieving—weeping, despair, anger

Refusal to participate in own care or take responsibility for self-care (self-neglect)

Self-destructive behavior (alcohol, drug abuse)

Displaying hostility toward healthy people

Withdrawal from social contacts

Changing usual patterns of responsibility

Showing change in ability to estimate relation of body to environment

(Carpenito, L. J. [1992]. *Nursing diagnosis: Application to clinical practice* [4th ed.]. Philadelphia: Lippincott, 711–712.)

As an exercise in understanding how people organize knowledge about themselves, make a list of ten labels that you feel identify you (for example, "student," "Italian American," "opera fan," "premed major"). Put the most important label first and then list the others in order of decreasing importance. (What if the order were reversed?) To what extent do you think your way of organizing information about yourself affects your behavior? (p. 63)

It is important to discover if individuals are comfortable with their perceived identity. Developmental changes, trauma, and cultural and gender dissonance may all place a client at risk for personal identity disturbances.

Client Strengths Many clients focus naturally on their deficiencies; asking pointed questions about personal strengths can help a client identify positive factors:

"What are some of your personal strengths . . . qualities you are proud of . . . things you do well?"

"What special talents or abilities do you have?"

"What has helped you cope in the past when things were tough?"

Body Image

When body image disturbances are suspected, the nurse can specifically ask the client how he or she would describe his or her body to another person. When illness or trauma has resulted in a temporary or permanent alteration in body image, the nurse should assess the nature of the threat, the meaning the client attaches to the threat, the adequacy of the client's coping strategies, and the resources and supports available to the client.

Self-Esteem

Once a client has shared perceptions of self, the nurse questions if the client likes himself or herself, if the client is pleased with his or her expectations and the progress the client is making to realize them.

"Tell me what you like about yourself."

"What would you change about yourself if you could?"

Using Makay and Gaw's (1975) graphic description of self-esteem as the discrepancy between the "real self" (what we think we really are) and the "ideal self" (what we think we would like to be or think we should be), the nurse can obtain a quick indication of a client's self-esteem by having the client plot two points on a line—real self and ideal self (Fig. 38-5). The greater the discrepancy, the lower the self-esteem; the smaller the discrepancy, the higher the self-esteem.

A person's ideal self may differ dramatically from the current sense of self and positively or negatively influence behavior and personal development. If indicated, the nurse questions the client about self-expectations:

"You've told me something about who you are, how you view yourself now. Tell me who you would like to be in the future."

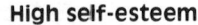

High self-esteem

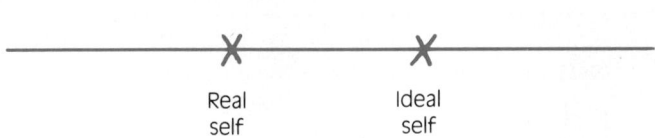

Real   Ideal
self   self

Low self-esteem

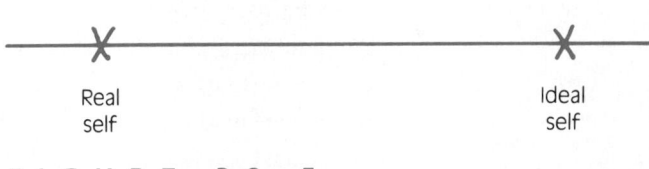

Real   Ideal
self   self

F I G U R E   3 8 - 5

The client who perceives his or her real self as relatively close to the ideal self has high self-esteem. The client who perceives his or her real self as far from the ideal self has low self-esteem.

"What life goals are important to you?"

"Where do you see yourself 5 years from now? In 10 years?"

"Are these expectations realistic?"

"Are your expectations stemming from who you would *like* to be or from who you think you *should* be?"

"Who or what has influenced your self-expectations?"

The nurse is assessing if the client possesses life goals that are positively motivating personal development. Unrealistic expectations need to be identified, and their source needs to be explored with the client. For example,

"You seem to feel that it is necessary to be all things to all people—no matter what this costs you. How might this belief have developed? Is it helpful to you?"

"What I'm hearing is that your performance must always be perfect, that although you allow others to make mistakes, you cannot allow yourself this luxury. . . . Tell me more about this."

"Then, unless you graduate at the top of your class you will not be satisfied? Why is this so important? Is this type of achievement realistic with your abilities? What will this success both benefit and cost you?"

"You state you have no goals for the future . . . when you wake up each morning what gets you out of bed? What keeps you moving?"

If this exercise indicates the need for a more detailed assessment, the nurse next explores the concepts of significance, competence, virtue, and power.

Significance

"Are there people in your life with whom you share a close relationship?"

Sample Recording

The following self-concept assessment was recorded on the nursing history of a 17-year-old, single, new mother of a healthy newborn:

Describes herself as a strong, healthy, fun-loving person who is "going to make it." Is unafraid of new parenting responsibilities. Identifies the following as strengths: experience with younger brothers and sisters; program for single parents in her high school; strong motivation to make something of herself (plans on getting associate degree in x-ray technology); support of family and friends; and belief that "God will help me." Expresses concern about always being able to make the right decisions about going out with friends, dating, and so forth. Views motherhood as an achievement about which she is proud. Basically has positive self-concept with high self-esteem.

M. LeBon, RN

"Many people have 'people' problems. Are your relationships causing you any problems right now?"

"To what extent do you feel loved and approved of by the key people in your life?"

"Does it bother you when you feel unloved or when others fail to appreciate you?"

"In what ways do you let family members and friends know that you like them or are proud of their accomplishments?"

Competence

"What are the things you need to do to feel important?"

"Is anything interfering with your ability to execute these tasks?" ("How does this make you feel?")

"How important to you is it to feel that others value your work?"

Virtue

"Tell me something about the moral–ethical principles that govern your life."

"How must you live to describe yourself as a 'good' person?"

"How do you feel about your ability to live this way?"

"Describe any difficulties you experience in living up to your moral principles that you would like to discuss."

"In what ways can the nurses help you to better live according to your moral standards?"

Power

"How important is it to you to 'be in control' of your life (health)?"

"To what extent did you feel 'in control' of your life (health) before this illness (trauma, crisis, and so forth)?"

"To what extent do you feel 'in control' of your life (health) currently?"

"What is it that makes you feel not in control?"

"How might you change this? How can nurses help you to develop and gain more control?"

Role Performance

We all play many roles. Our ability to successfully execute societal expectations regarding role-specific behaviors, **role performance**, is easily compromised by illness and injury. If a nurse suspects this might be contributing to a self-concept disturbance, the following questions are indicated:

"What major roles describe you—son, daughter, spouse, parent, employer or employee, student, club member, and so on?"

"How important is it to you to be good in each of these roles?"

"Tell me how successful you think you are in each of these roles."

"What roles or expectations would you change if you could?"

"If you feel 'incompetent' or less than successful in some of these roles, why? What is preventing you from being more successful? What can you do about this? How might I help you?"

Diagnosing

Disturbances in Self-Concept as the Problem Specific disturbances in self-concept that can be treated by independent nursing interventions receive one of four nursing diagnostic labels:

Body Image Disturbance

Self-Esteem Disturbance (Chronic Low Self-Esteem or Situational Low Self-Esteem)

Altered Role Performance

Personal Identity Disturbance

Common etiologies and defining characteristics for these diagnoses are found in the accompanying display.

Disturbance in Self-Concept as the Etiology Because disturbances in self-concept have the potential to affect so many other areas of human functioning, they may serve as etiologies for numerous problem statements. Examples of these follow:

Impaired Adjustment related to change in health status (increasing dependency, need for ongoing medical evaluation and treatment, and so forth)

Anxiety related to irreversible change in body image (eg, amputation, mastectomy, burn); delayed development of secondary sex characteristics (body image); discrepancy between real and ideal self (self-esteem); perceived incompetence in important roles; loss of key roles (child or spouse dies, separation, retirement, graduation)

Ineffective Individual Coping related to inability to identify personal strengths, low self-esteem, "I know I can't manage this"; role conflict

Anticipatory or Dysfunctional Grieving related to change in body image, loss of key roles

Altered Health Maintenance related to low self-esteem—"why bother?"

Hopelessness related to low self-esteem, overwhelming role demands, belief that nothing will change (destiny is controlled externally)

Knowledge Deficit: How to Help Children Develop High Self-Esteem, related to lack of experience with parenting

Noncompliance: (specify) related to low self-esteem

Altered Parenting related to disturbance in role performance (rejection of parent role)

Post-Trauma Response related to disturbance in personal identity

Self-Care Deficit related to learned helplessness, low self-esteem, "I can't"

NURSING DIAGNOSES FOR COMMON PROBLEMS

Disturbances in Self-Concept

Problem	Related Factors	Sample Defining Characteristics
Body Image Disturbance	Irreversible changes in body image—amputation, mastectomy, hysterectomy, colostomy, scars, burns, disfiguring skin disorder	"Look at me. Nothing can ever be the same again. I feel less whole. When I look in the mirror all I see is my (stump, missing breast, scar). I know when others look at me they feel repulsed or at the very least pity me."
	Effects of treatment (eg, braces, casts)	Thirteen-year-old female adolescent with scoliosis wearing a Milwaukee brace (covers pelvic area and has rods in the front and back which extend up to the chin): "I feel dumb in this thing . . . it's bad enough that my back is crooked but this makes me look like a freak. Besides, it's hot. Must I wear it to school?"
	Difficulty accepting development of secondary sex characteristics or delayed development of same	Fifteen-year-old male adolescent, sophomore in high school, height 5'1", weight 88 lb; "When am I going to grow up and start looking like the other guys in my class?" No pubic hair, penis, testes, and scrotum are the same size and proportion as in childhood.
	Extreme thinness or obesity	Twenty-year-old woman, height 5'7"; weight 98 lb; works out for 30 min three times a day in addition to 100 sit-ups a day: "When I look in the mirror I see fat!"
		Twenty-year-old woman, height 5'7"; weight 200 lb: "I hate my body . . . I've been fat all my life and I'm always on a diet. Why can't I be like everyone else?"
Self-Esteem Disturbance	Feeling unloved or unapproved of by significant others	Twelve-year-old son of parents in the process of getting a divorce: "No matter what I do to make my dad like me he acts like I don't exist. When he's home he fights with mom, but mostly he's away. I wouldn't even care if he yelled at me so long as he noticed me. I wonder why he doesn't like me?"
	Feelings of incompetence	Forty-two-year-old car salesperson, with company for 18 years: "What's wrong with me? I do my job, I'm also never absent, I have a good sales record, but I keep getting passed over for promotions. I think I'm too old to move to a different company, but I don't want to just sell cars for someone else for the rest of my life!"
	Failure to live according to personal moral ethical code	Thirty-three-year-old single female computer programmer: "I should have known I'd get pregnant—I deserve it. I knew I was wrong to go to bed with this guy. Basically I've tried to live the way I think I should all my life up until now. What if something's wrong with the baby because of my sin?"
	Powerlessness	Sixty-seven-year-old alert widow with degenerative joint disease: "It may be hard for me to move around now, but darn it—there's nothing wrong with my mind. The kids think they are helping me by making all my decisions but they aren't. I'm not a doddering old lady in a nursing home."
Altered Role Performance	Rejection of role	Twenty-two-year-old mother 2 days after birth of her second son (first son is 15 months old): "I don't know who my husband got to watch our son. I never wanted to be a mother anyway. My husband and I have never had any time for ourselves—and things aren't going to get any better."

(continued)

NURSING DIAGNOSES FOR COMMON PROBLEMS

Disturbances in Self-Concept (continued)

Problem	Related Factors	Sample Defining Characteristics
	Role conflict Role fatigue Multiple life stressors	Twenty-one-year-old, full-time junior nursing student who failed a major exam, is married and the mother of an 18-month-old daughter; works every other weekend in a hospital as an electrocardiogram technician: "I'm trying so hard to get my grades up, but I don't know what else I can do. My husband seems to be losing patience with me more and more and I sometimes feel awful about neglecting my daughter. I'd stop working but we need the money. I want nursing so bad but I'm getting awfully tired."
	Changing personal resources (physical health, mental abilities, motivation)	Fifty-year-old college chemistry teacher begins exhibiting signs of early Alzheimer's disease; forgets where she is and what she is doing; began rambling in class and saying things that made no sense—much to the class's amusement. Later cried and called herself "stupid."
Personal Identity Disturbance	Unresolved crisis	Eighty-eight-year-old man who lost his wife 6 months ago; wife took care of all his needs; sits alone in the house all day: "We always did everything together. I wish I had died first. What shall I do?"
	Declining physical, mental, or sensory abilities	Same 88-year-old man 3 months after admission to long-term care institution, medical diagnosis "rule out depression/dementia"; has become increasingly withdrawn, never initiates conversation; responses to questions are sometimes inappropriate: "What do you mean, what's my name? Who cares? I want to go home to my wife."
	Rejection of membership in minority group	Fifteen-year-old Cambodian girl recently emigrated to the United States with family; in constant conflict with parents as she rejects her family's culture in hopes of fitting in with peer group: "Sometimes I feel like I no longer know who I am or how I should act. I feel lonely inside and afraid."

Sensory/Perceptual Alterations related to disturbance in personal identity (ability to distinguish between self and nonself)

Altered Sexuality Patterns related to changed body image, disturbance in self-concept

Impaired Social Interaction or Social Isolation related to low self-esteem, disturbance in personal identity

Altered Thought Processes related to disturbance in personal identity

High Risk for Self-Directed Violence related to disturbance in self-concept, overwhelmed by failure to live according to moral–ethical standards

Important Distinctions When assessment data point to an alteration in self-concept, the nurse's first task is to determine if the altered self-concept is the problem, the cause of the problem (etiology), or merely a sign that a problem exists (defining characteristics). Self-concept data seem to fit well in all three categories. It is important that an accurate determination be made because this directs the goals developed for the client and related nursing interventions.

For example, the following three different diagnoses might be written for a 25-year-old woman who is recently divorced:

1. Self-Esteem Disturbance related to perceived failure in role of wife (recent divorce) as manifested by neglect of personal appearance and inability to accept positive reinforcement

Assessment data point to a disturbance in self-esteem as the priority problem. Nursing energies will be directed to helping the client evaluate herself positively despite the stress of the divorce.

2. Altered Health Maintenance related to decreased self-esteem as manifested by failure to follow through on referrals (support group, stress-management class, and so forth); "Why bother? Nothing ever works for me anyway."

Here, low self-esteem is contributing to the client's problem of failing to follow through with health-seeking behaviors. Nursing energies will be best directed to improving the client's use of health resources; one of the means used will be to help her to value herself enough to choose healthy behaviors.

3. Ineffective Individual Coping related to inability to accept recent divorce as manifested by low self-esteem statements: "I never should have gotten married—my mother said I'd be a rotten wife." "I know I can't make it on my own." "Why did he do this to me?"

Here, low self-esteem statements are the cues that led to the identification of the problem statement. One of the criteria used to evaluate nursing intervention to increase the client's coping skills will be a reduction in or elimination of low self-esteem statements.

Planning: Client Goals

Whenever nurses care for clients, nursing measures need to be supportive of the following client goals. The client will:

- Describe self realistically, identifying both strengths and deficiencies
- Verbalize realistic expectations for self based on who he or she would like to be
- Verbalize that self is liked or at least okay
- Communicate his or her feelings and needs in a way that is comfortable and effective in meeting needs
- Nurture relationships in which needs for love and worth are mutually met (significance)
- Assume role-related responsibilities with confidence (competence)
- Express satisfaction with ability to live according to one's moral–ethical standards (virtue)
- Demonstrate confidence in ability to accomplish what is desired (power)

Client goals for specific disturbances in self-concept are presented later in this chapter.

Implementing

Nursing interventions to assist clients to develop and maintain a positive self-concept may vary tremendously from one client to another. Nurses must be comfortable with their own self-image before they can address image problems in clients. Specific nursing strategies addressed in this section include helping clients identify and use personal strengths, helping high-risk clients maintain a sense of self, changing the self-concept, and working with parents and educators to develop self-esteem in children and adolescents.

Helping Clients Identify and Use Personal Strengths

When confronted with a major stressor, many people forget that they have histories of successful coping and numerous personal strengths. Clients at high risk for giving up are those with low self-esteem or multiple stressors perceived as being overwhelming.

Although attributing strength to a client sounds like something nurses would do naturally, nurses frequently fall into the trap of doing for clients (ie, solving their problems, rather than helping them to identify and tap their personal power and strengths). Moreover, clients continually instruct nurses about how they should be perceived, and some clients successfully communicate a manipulative helplessness that encourages the nurse's taking charge. An appropriate nursing response in this case is, "I wonder why you want me to speak with your physician about treatment alternatives. I am sure you would feel much better hearing this information firsthand. If you'd like I will stay here while you talk with the physician."

Clients experiencing powerlessness may need help to recognize their strengths. Examples of personal strengths include healthy functioning body, cognitive abilities, emotional strengths, communication strengths, other interpersonal skills, sense of life meaning and purpose, belief system that is a strength, social support network, meaningful work, hobbies, other interests, education, life experience, and past history of effective coping. A good sense of humor, belief in a loving God, healthy nutritional state, ability to make decisions, and sense of self-worth are all personal strengths that may better equip a person to respond to life's challenges.

Specific strategies nurses can use to help clients identify and use personal strengths include the following:
- Encouraging clients to identify their strengths
- Replacing self-negation with positive thinking
- Noticing and reinforcing client strengths
- Encouraging clients to will for themselves the strengths they desire and to try them on

Helping High-Risk Clients Maintain a Sense of Self

People who are acutely ill are often separated not only from their strengths but also from any real sense of self. One client, a college president who was recovering from serious complications after surgery for ovarian cancer, shared the following:

When I was very sick, I felt utterly weak and devoid of any personal strength. During this time, how I felt about myself was totally dependent on how the doctors and nurses approached me. My esteem was at their mercy. If they came into my room and did something to me without talking to me or talked as if I were not present, then I felt like a nonperson, unworthy of their care. But if they approached me gently and caringly and spoke with me, then I felt like a human again, worthy of human respect and care. Once I started feeling stronger, then I could fight feelings of depersonalization. But when I was really sick, my feelings of worth were totally determined by the behaviors of others.

Nurses can help clients maintain a sense of self and worth by doing the following:

- Speaking respectfully to the client and addressing the client by name whenever entering the client's room
- Offering the client a simple explanation before initiating any procedure
- Moving the client's body respectfully if the client is unable to do this
- Respecting the client's privacy and sensitivities

This type of caring does not require additional nursing time or energy. It does require from the nurse continual reaffirmation that nursing is a person-centered profession and that nothing is more important at any moment of a nurse's workday than the person being served.

Changing a Negative Self-Concept

The time is ripe for change when a client realizes that a negative self-concept is hindering personal development. A nurse working in a setting that allows long-term nurse–client relationships may intervene to assist the client in modifying self-concept. At the outset, it must be remembered that the self-concept is firmly entrenched and that by nature it resists change. See the interventions for the self-concept disturbance diagnosis at the end of this chapter.

Working With Parents and Educators to Develop Self-Esteem in Children and Adolescents

Nurses who work in practice settings where they have access to groups of parents or teachers can offer specific guidelines for creating developmental environments that build high self-esteem.

Children are most likely to develop high self-esteem when parents do the following:
- Frequently communicate unconditional regard for the child (use body language and words to let the child know he or she is *liked*)
- Communicate a range of acceptable behaviors
- Challenge the child to explore strengths and limitations
- Celebrate the child's competencies and accomplishments
- Assist the child to respond to mistakes responsibly and to learn from them

Because some parents and educators may not have experienced these helps to personal growth themselves, it is beneficial for the nurse to role model these behaviors when interacting with children.

Dinkmeyer (1970) called on educators to arrange learning experiences in ways that strengthen a child's self-esteem and enable the child to meet social, emotional, and academic needs. Dinkmeyer recommended that the learning atmosphere be characterized by the following:
- A mutual respect and trust by teacher and child
- A focus on mutual alignment of purposes by teacher and child
- A feeling on the part of students that they belong to the group
- An environment where it is safe for the child to look at inner needs, hopes, and wishes

- An opportunity to express needs that, if not articulated and clarified, hamper the learning process
- An emphasis on the importance of self-evaluation in contrast to evaluation by others
- A climate marked by identification, recognition, acceptance, and appreciation of individual differences
- An emphasis on growth from dependence to independence
- Situations in which limits are most often a result of natural and logical consequences and not merely reflection of the personal needs of the teacher*

Important learning tasks for children include understanding and accepting oneself and understanding feelings; others; independence; goals and purposeful behavior; mastery, competence, and resourcefulness; emotional maturity; and choices and consequences.

Developing Self-Esteem in Older Adults

The many losses associated with aging, for example, diminished strength and physical health, interpersonal losses, retirement, and shrinking income, make older adults especially vulnerable to disturbances in self-concept, particularly chronic low self-esteem. Society's generally negative view of aging compounds the problem. Nurses interacting with older people need to understand that simple measures such as addressing older clients respectfully, communicating that you take their concerns seriously, noticing and affirming their personal strengths, and interacting with them as individuals as opposed to members of a homogeneous group, can greatly enhance the older person's self-esteem. In the accompanying display, nursing interventions are highlighted for specific self-concept disturbances.

Evaluating

Nurses who are sensitive to the relation between self-concept and general well-being consistently evaluate the effect the nursing care plan has on the client's self-concept. For example, while educating a client with hypertension for whom life-style counseling was recommended, the nurse may detect that the client is feeling extremely guilty about his or her smoking, dietary habits, and lack of exercise. "Why should I even try to change any of these things now. I made myself sick so I may as well live with the punishment." If the care plan is to be effective, the nurse must first help this client value himself or herself and the client's health sufficiently to want to make the necessary changes.

When the care plan includes specific interventions to assist clients with disturbances in body image, self-esteem, role performance, and personal identity, then the nurse listens carefully to the client's self-report and observes cli-

---

* List reprinted by permission of American Guidance Service, Circle Pines, MN 55014. *Developing understanding of self and others* (Manual DUSO-D1) by Don Dinkmeyer, Sr. Copyright 1970. Rights reserved.

F O C U S O N T H E O L D E R A D U L T

Nursing Strategies to Promote Self-Esteem in Elderly People

Personal Identity

- When an older person's sense of self is threatened, assist him or her to find meaning in the experience, to regain mastery to the extent that this is possible, and to realistically evaluate the adequacy of his or her coping strategy.
- Teach older people to identify and develop a game plan for confronting anxiety-producing situations.
- Help to identify and secure intervention for treatable depressions.
- Remedy treatable causes of self-identity disturbances such as pain, abusive living arrangements, and substance abuse.

Body Image

- Notice and affirm positive physiologic characteristics of elderly people.
- Teach preventive self-care measures that reduce discomforting signs of aging (eg, exercise, which maintains muscle mass and joint flexibility; proper nutrition; and basic hygiene and skin care measures).
- Explore new activities (including hobbies) that are within the changing physical capabilities of the older person.

Self-Esteem

- Assist older people to identify and use personal strengths.

- Communicate that you value older people simply for who they are (unconditional affirmation)—know and use the name they prefer, ask them questions about their life, interests, or values.
- When appropriate, use the expertise of older people and ask their advice; let them know you value their life experience.
- Engage older people in activities in which they can be successful.
- Allow older people to make tough decisions and to confront challenging situations when appropriate; teach protective family members the value of older adults confronting situations that invite their continued growth.
- Empower older people to meet their own needs: provide necessary knowledge, teach new behaviors, instill the belief that they "can manage."

Role Performance

- Explore with older people the many roles they have fulfilled throughout their lifetime; invite reminiscences.
- Facilitate grieving over valued roles that are no longer able to be performed.
- Remedy, whenever possible, factors that prevent older people from engaging in valued roles.
- Explore new roles.

---

ent behaviors to see if the disturbances are being resolved. Basically, the client should be:
- Comfortable with body image and able to use it effectively to meet human needs
- Able to describe self positively

- Able to meet realistic role expectations without undue anxiety and fatigue
- Capable of interacting appropriately with environment while recognizing self to be a separate and distinct entity

 NURSING PROCESS

in Clinical Practice

When identifying and treating disturbances in self-concept categorized as nursing diagnoses, the nurse uses each phase of the nursing process. Quality care depends on the nurse's possession of the knowledge and skills described earlier in this chapter. What follows in outline format are the assessment priorities, client goals, nursing interventions, and evaluative criteria for two common types of self-concept disturbances treated by nurses:

Body Image Disturbance
Self-Concept Disturbance *related to faulty thinking (distortions and denials, faulty categorizing, and inappropriate standards)*

In the case study that follows the development of these diagnoses, nursing care is described for a woman with low self-esteem.

Body Image Disturbance

Disturbances in body image are common given the current emphasis on physical appearance. In a 2000-person survey conducted in 1985, 34% of the men and 38% of the women disagreed with the statement, "I like my looks just the way they are" (Cash, Winstead, & Janda, 1986). In general, people who like their appearance, fitness, health, and sexual attractiveness tend to feel happier and more adjusted.

Disturbances in body image result from multiple causes. As a child gains control over body parts and functioning, this control is integrated into the self. Anything that threatens this control is perceived as a threat to the self. A child being prepared for surgery may become hysterical when asked to put on a hospital gown and remove all personal clothing including underpants. This action may leave the body too vulnerable in the child's eye. Similarly, an injection or any other penetrating device may threaten the child's sense of self. For adults, loss of control of body parts and functioning is especially traumatic. Normal aging, loss of breast or uterus, loss of memory, mobility, or sexual functioning are all significant stressors. McCloskey (1976) described the concept of "spread" that occurs when a person's attitude about a part of his or her body spreads to his or her entire concept of self. McCloskey noted two major types of boundary disturbances:

1. Body wall changes but the client "keeps" the old body boundary (may explain the phantom pain some clients feel in amputated limbs). *Example:* Woman with a history of obesity (210 lb) who currently is a size 14 continues to buy clothes that would look good on an obese person and to think herself overweight.

2. Client changes a body boundary even though his or her body wall remains intact. *Example:* A man whose left side is paralyzed after a stroke may refuse to believe that this side is still a part of his body—despite efforts to make him conscious of it—because he cannot feel it or move it.

Assessment

- Once a body image disturbance is suspected, carefully interview and observe the client to identify the nature of the threat to the person's body image (functional significance of the part involved, importance of physical appearance, and visibility of the part involved); the meaning the client attaches to the threat; the adequacy of the client's coping abilities; response of family members and significant others; and help available to the client and his or her family (McCloskey, 1976).
- Assess the client's response to the deformity or limitation, including changes in independence–dependence patterns and in socialization and communication (Carpenito, 1987).
  - Response to deformity or limitation
    - *Adaptive responses:* Exhibits signs of grief and mourning (shock, disbelief, denial, anger, guilt, acceptance)
    - *Maladaptive responses:* Continues to deny and to deal with the deformity or limitation, engages in self-destructive behavior, talks about feelings of worthlessness or insecurity, equates deformity or limitation with whole person, shows a change in ability to estimate relationship of body to environment

- Independence–dependence patterns
  - *Adaptive responses:* Assumes responsibility for care (makes decisions); develops new self-care behaviors; uses available resources; interacts in a mutually supportive way with family
  - *Maladaptive responses:* Assigns responsibility for his or her care to others; becomes increasingly dependent or stubbornly refuses necessary help
- Socialization and communication
  - *Adaptive responses:* Maintains usual social patterns; communicates needs and accepts offers of help; serves as support for others
  - *Maladaptive responses:* Isolates himself or herself; exhibits superficial self-confidence; unable to express needs (becomes hostile, ashamed, frustrated, depressed)

Planning: Client Goals

The client will:
- Describe his or her body positively, integrating the change in body part or functioning into his or her self-concept
- Verbalize or demonstrate acceptance of irreversible body changes
- Develop new abilities to compensate for irreversible losses
- Use his or her body effectively to meet basic human needs
- Demonstrate by appearance and self-care behaviors (hygiene, exercise, nutrition) a respect for his or her body
- Maintain maximal independence while accepting necessary help
- Continue preexisting social patterns

Interventions

Interventions for body image disturbances vary according to the nature of the disturbance. Interventions may include any combination of the following:
- Establish a trusting relationship with the client. Allow the client to openly share his or her feelings. Sitting quietly by the client for a few minutes with a few words such as, "How are things?" or "Gee, it must be hard to lie there after all you've been through . . ." communicates to the client your willingness and readiness to share his or her experience.
- Support the client through the various stages of loss, grief, and mourning (shock, disbelief, denial, anger, guilt, acceptance), remembering that there is no one right way to proceed through these stages. Rather, clients may move fluidly in and out of various stages, sometimes returning to earlier stages. Some clients may need to learn that it is okay to cry, to be angry, to feel depressed.
- Use play therapy with children so they can describe their feelings and work through their grief using the nonthreatening medium of dolls or animals.

- Role model for the client a healthy acceptance of the client's body. Be careful that facial expressions, words, or body positioning do not communicate to the client disgust, fear, or rejection.
- While communicating support to the client who is slow to develop and use appropriate self-care behaviors, firmly insist that the client participate in his or her care to the extent that the client is able. Whenever possible, provide the client with honest answers to his or her questions or put the client in touch with the appropriate person to give the answers.
- Strengthen the decision-making ability of the client by honestly exploring alternatives; help the client to imagine living with the consequences of different courses of action.
- Reinforce the client's personal strengths and help the client and family to identify all possible resources.
- Assess the response of the client's significant others and intervene if they negatively influence the client.

Evaluative Criteria

The client meets the previously stated goals.

Self-Concept Disturbance

Many of the clients with whom nurses interact, especially on a long-term basis, may be interested in modifying some aspect of a negative self-concept that is related to faulty thinking. Common analogies of negative self-concepts include distortions and denials, faulty categorizing, and inappropriate standards—perfectionism, conventionality, "What the other guy thinks" (Calhoun & Acocella, 1983).

Distortions and Denials

A woman who was taught early in life that a woman's place is in the home may systematically have distorted or denied any talents or feelings that she thought were inconsistent with being a full-time wife and mother. For example, if she enjoyed math and did well in her math courses in high school, rather than feel good about this she might think it abnormal and consciously limit her study of math. If a guidance counselor recommended college to her, she might laugh off the suggestion.

Nursing diagnosis: Negative (Limited) Self-Concept related to a long history of distorting and denying her abilities and desires

Faulty Categorizing

A positive self-concept is characterized by a broad image of the self. The more labels we can attach to ourselves, the more self-information we are able to assimilate and make part of us. An adolescent who repeatedly hears from his or her father that he or she is no good and who consistently characterizes himself or herself this way may reject genuine affirmations of the adolescent's positive qualities and strengths from other family member, peers, teachers, and so forth. Moreover, the adolescent may choose to act in ways that reinforce his or her image of being no good.

Nursing diagnosis: Negative Self-Concept related to inability to recognize and "own" positive qualities, strengths ("I'm no good")

Inappropriate Standards

At the root of the negative self-concepts of some clients may be an unrealistic ideal self. With all the emphasis in society on being number one, many people hold *perfectionistic standards* that they will never be able to meet. In describing their self-expectations, these clients may reveal that they must always get an *A* to feel good about themselves, or always be the center of everyone's attention and love. Anything less is viewed as failure.

Conventionality offers another set of problems for the person who uncritically accepts all his or her culture dictates. When the person's feelings or preferred actions conflict with society's standards, then that person concludes that something must be wrong with him or her. Because sick-role behaviors are dictated by many cultures, the person who finds he or she cannot suffer in silence or, conversely, cannot express his or her pain or grief vocally, may feel alienated from his or her culture. An older person whose family is considering nursing home placement may find this more difficult to accept if the culture is one in which family members traditionally respect and care for aged members at home.

Changing the Self-Concept

Analyzing the Problem

- Isolate the basic problem label.
- Describe your problem in situational terms.
- Search for correlations, watching out especially for negative self-talk.
- Review the background of your problem to check for causes:
    Distortions and denials
    Faulty categorizing
    Perfectionism
    Conventionality
    Other people's judgments

Changing the Self-Concept

- Set a goal.
- Gather new information about this aspect of yourself.
- Engage in cognitive restructuring:
    Listen to your old self-talk.
    Talk back to this old self-talk, cross-examining it to get at the reality.
    Act on your back-talk, substituting new behavior to accompany your new, more rational self-talk.

(Adapted from Calhoun, J. F., & Acocella, J. R. [1989]. Psychology of adjustment and human relationships [3rd ed.]. New York: Random House.)

Exploring and Developing the Positive

Example: Twenty-year-old new mother who perceives herself as "a failure in everything I try"; states husband feels childrearing is the woman's responsibility and she is terrified.

Immediate goal: Develop confidence in parenting skills, see herself as a good mother
- Explore and reinforce the client's personal qualities and strengths that will help her to reach her goal.

> "You look like a natural mother when you hold your baby; some women are afraid at the beginning to even hold their infants."

> "That's good that you are talking with your baby. Babies quickly sense how a parent feels about them."

- Teach the client how to substitute positive self-talk for negative self-talk.

> *Negative self-talk* (mother during feeding): "She's awfully fussy tonight I mustn't be doing this right. . . . It was probably dumb luck that she took to breast so well this morning. . . ."

> *New positive self-talk:* " . . . but she fed so well this morning and the nurse said her weight is good. I wonder what else might be making her fussy . . . maybe she's wet. . . . "

"What the other guy thinks" is the third faulty standard. Allowing others to define ideal behavior sets up a person for constant failure because it is impossible to please everyone. The young executive who tries to live up to the expectations of his or her boss, peer group at work, spouse and children, and college friends, is bound to lose himself or herself in the process.

> *Nursing diagnosis:* Negative Self-Concept related to unrealistic self-expectations (perfectionism, conventionality, "What the other guy thinks")

Assessment

- Assess how accurately the client is able to describe himself or herself; note in particular the use of negative labels and their significance for the client.

- Determine whether the client is motivated to modify the self-concept. Does the client see a relationship between a negative self-concept and self-defeating thoughts, feelings, and behaviors?
- Teach the client to choose a day on which he or she will write down every self-critical thought that enters his or her mind. At the end of the day, the client should review the list and ask three questions:
  - What is the standard (perfectionism, conventionality, other people's judgments) on which this self-criticism is based?
  - From whom do you think you picked up this standard?
  - Do you really subscribe to the standard wholeheartedly? (Calhoun & Acocella, 1989)

Planning: Client Goals

The client will:
- Describe the relation between self-concept and behavior
- Identify faulty thinking that reinforces a negative self-concept (distortions and denials, faulty categorizing, inappropriate standards)
- Integrate positive self-knowledge into self-concept
- Report feeling better about himself or herself

Interventions

- See the display titled Changing the Self-Concept.
- Once the client has identified faulty thinking patterns (negative self-talk) that reinforce the negative self-concept, teach the client to "red flag" this behavior as soon as he or she is aware of it happening. The goal is to replace the negative self-talk with talk that will develop a more positive self-image.
- Help the client explore the positive dimension of himself or herself that he or she wishes to develop and incorporate this new knowledge into the self-concept. For an example, see the display titled Exploring and Developing the Positive.

Evaluative Criteria

The client meets the previously stated goals.

CASE STUDY

Melissa Motsky is a 31-year-old married woman, mother of three children (aged 12, 10, and 8), and junior-level nursing student. She works every other weekend as a nurse's aide. She has just received a letter from the nursing division head informing her that she is in academic jeopardy and will fail out of the program unless her grades improve. She presents this to her adviser.

Assessment Findings

After talking with Ms. Motsky, who calls herself a failure and who cries as she describes her situation at home, her faculty adviser suspects a serious self-esteem problem and helps her to list factors contributing to her current sense of failure and low self-esteem. The following list is generated:

Significance
- Receives little understanding, affection, approval from husband. "I stay with him because of the kids. I started back to school because I had to get out of the house and want to make something of myself. He doesn't understand this."
+ "Children are very supportive but get impatient when I have to study and can't spend time with them."

Competence
- Feels a failure in all the roles that are important to her—wife, mother, and, now, student. "I jeopardized everything to go back to school—if I fail, it's all over for me. There just isn't enough time or energy to do anything well."
+ "They do love me at work, though, which makes me feel like nursing is what I should be doing."

Virtue
- "I've always believed that hard work pays off and that if you were faithful to your duty you'd be rewarded by the 'good life'—I'm beginning to doubt that. Maybe I'm a fool for trying so hard."
+ "I do still try and live according to my beliefs and feel okay about this. I treat others as I'd like to be treated."

Power
- "I always believed I could do anything I put my heart and soul into. But I can't seem to change my marriage and if I fail out of school that will be the end of all my dreams."

Key indicators of low self-esteem that also surfaced in the interview included overeating (10-lb weight gain during the past year); difficulty sleeping; fatigue; new sensitivity to criticism; and expressions of feeling unloved, alone, and no longer able to manage. Personal strengths included history of "can do" mentality, high motivation to succeed, and past history of success as mother and nurse's aide.

Nursing Diagnosis

Situational Low Self-Esteem related to decreased sense of significance, competence, virtue, and power.

Many nursing diagnoses could be developed for Ms. Motsky. This was given high priority because her nursing adviser felt it to be a key to other problems.

Planning: Client Goals

Ms. Motsky is eager to try anything that will help her to feel better about herself and enable her to perform better academically. "I'd like to start feeling like myself again." She cautions her adviser that she does not have much time to devote to this because she obviously needs to spend every spare minute studying. In response to her adviser's question, "What personal goals would you like to achieve in the next month," she suggests the following goals.

Short-Term Goals
By this time next month, I will demonstrate increased self-esteem as evidenced by:
- Expression of positive statements about myself
- Report of ability to receive negative feedback from family, school, and so forth, without falling apart
- Passing grade on next quarterly exam
- Ability to verbalize that the way I am living my life is okay
- Report of two recent instances when my power was effective in accomplishing what I desired

Long-Term Goal
I will:
- Consistently maintain sufficient self-esteem to successfully develop and achieve new life goals.

See the Nursing Care Plan developed to aid Ms. Motsky in accomplishing her goals.

Implementation

To assist Ms. Motsky in meeting her goals, the nurse needs the following specialized abilities:
- Belief that a person's self-esteem influences all aspects of his or her functioning and a commitment to addressing this human need (ie, holistic orientation)
- Empathy for the multiple role expectations the client is experiencing and ability to identify and mobilize the client's inner strengths so that a *realistic* plan can be developed to assist the client to *satisfactorily* meet necessary role expectations
- Knowledge of etiologies and defining characteristics for disturbances in self-esteem and specific nursing strategies to enhance self-esteem
- Interpersonal skills to communicate to client that he or she is important, cared about, competent, good, and that the client possesses within self the power and strength to turn the situation around
- Ability to correctly decide that it is wise to encourage this student to continue in the nursing program, whereas another student of lesser ability would be assisted to reevaluate his or her career goals
- Teaching, counseling, and advocacy skills
- Accountability (ability and willingness to encourage student and follow-up on the student's progress; celebrate goal achievement or make realistic plans if student should fail out of program)

Documentation

Sample documentation of Ms. Motsky's initial visit to her adviser follows:

Traditional Note Format

10/2/93, nursing
    Melissa Motsky presented today after receiving academic jeopardy letter. She is strongly motivated to complete nursing program successfully and seems to have the ability to do this. Current multiple

life stressors—lack of support from husband; need to mother three children (12, 10, 8); part-time nurse's aide job (necessary for financial reasons); and current academic jeopardy (test grades 68, 74) are all contributing to her low self-esteem and overwhelming sense of being a failure. We together developed a care plan that it is hoped will help her to do better academically as well as begin to feel better about herself. See attached. She will return 11/2/93 at 10 AM for follow-up.

C. Taylor, RN

SOAP Format

10/2/93, 12:30 PM, nursing
  #1 Academic jeopardy—Melissa Motsky

S: "I jeopardized everything to go back to school—if I fail, it's all over for me."

Reports lack of support from husband; grief that she does not have enough time for children; failure of personal work ethic ("hard work pays off"); and sense of powerlessness.
O: Nursing II quarterly exam grades: 68, 74; weight gain of 10 lb during past year; facial and body expressions of fatigue, profuse tears
A: Disturbance in Self-Esteem related to decreased sense of significance, competence, virtue, and power
P: See attached care plan.

C. Taylor, RN

Evaluation

Short-term goal achievement will be evaluated informally as student is met at school and formally at the next month's conference. Long-term goal achievement is an ongoing personal evaluation.

NURSING CARE PLAN

for Mrs. Motsky

Nursing Diagnosis:	Situational Low Self-Esteem related to decreased sense of significance, competence, virtue, and power as manifested by expressions of being a failure, powerlessness, fatigue, tears, weight gain, low academic performance (test grades 68, 74)
Long-Term Goal:	Client will consistently maintain sufficient self-esteem to successfully develop and achieve new life goals.

Goal:	By this time next month, 11/2/93, the client will demonstrate increased self-esteem by: • Expressing positive statements about herself

Nursing Actions	**Rationale**	**Evaluative Statement**
Assist client to rediscover and "own" personal strengths: identify personal qualities and strengths that have pleased her in the past and explore why this has changed; recommend that she make at least one positive statement about herself each morning and evening.	Clients can lose touch with their strengths, especially when multiple stressors seem to create impossible demands.	11/3/93 Goal partially met. Client's statements are of the "This is good, *but . . .*" variety. "I think I'm doing better in school but I don't know if it will continue." *Recommendation:* Continue to identify and reinforce personal strengths. <div align="right">*C. Taylor, RN*</div>
Consistently interact with the client as if she had the power to weather the crisis successfully (ie, "will" strength to her). Role-model positive self-concept behaviors.	Once the client senses that an authority believes in her power and expects her to use it, she may internalize this knowledge and act on it.	

Goal:	By this time next month, 11/2/93, the client will demonstrate increased self-esteem by: • Reporting ability to receive negative feedback without falling apart

(continued)

NURSING CARE PLAN *(continued)*

for Mrs. Motsky

Nursing Actions
Explore with client to what degree she allows the opinions of others to influence her self-concept.

Teach how the self-concept filters life experiences; thus, if I feel that I am a failure, I may interpret the words and behaviors of others as confirming this, even though that was not their intention.

Explore with the client ways she can enhance her self-concept independently of others (eg, take time each day for herself). Encourage client to draw on personal strengths.

Teach the client how to analyze feedback constructively and respond appropriately; *cancel negative thinking.* For example, client receives care plan back with many corrections and the notation, "sloppy work."

Maladaptive response: "She hates me. See, this proves I'll never be a good nurse. I wasted my time even doing this."

Adaptive response: "I spent as much time as I had on this . . . now let me see what I did wrong. Maybe I should make an appointment with my instructor so she can show me how to improve."

Rationale
Significance—sense of being loved and approved of by significant others—is a critical component of self-esteem.

Principle of self-consistency: once I am down I may reinforce this by distorting what I feel, hear, and experience.

This facilitates internal locus of control versus external. Spending time on self communicates that self is valuable.

It is important to break the cycle of negative thinking, which reinforces negative self-concept.

Evaluative Statement
11/3/93 Goal partially met. Client reports being able to handle everything except put-downs from her husband.

Recommendation: Explore origin of power she has given to her husband to influence her sense of self and what she wants to do about this.

C. Taylor, RN

Goal: By this time next month, 11/2/93, the client will demonstrate increased self-esteem by:
• Getting a passing grade on her next quarterly examination

Nursing Actions
Explore study skills with client; recommend study group.

Discuss importance of how she *perceives* present situation. If present failures are equated with *defeat,* she may be unable to mobilize her resources to succeed; if present failures represent *challenge,* it may call forth her best efforts and result in success.

Rationale
Poor study skills may also be contributing to her low academic performance. A study group will meet both her social and academic needs.

The meaning given to present stressor can dramatically affect the client's response to it and condition her for success or failure.

Evaluative Statement
11/3/93 Goal met. Grade: 82

C. Taylor, RN

(continued)

✒ NURSING CARE PLAN (continued)

for Mrs. Motsky

Discuss importance of breaking cycle of failure leading to another failure.	If this short-term goal is met, it will set the stage for future successes and contribute to the client's positive self-concept.

Goal: By this time next month, 1/2/93, the client will demonstrate increased self-esteem by:
- Verbalizing that the way she is living her life is okay

Nursing Actions	**Rationale**	**Evaluative Statement**
Assist client to examine her moral–ethical standards; explore sources of these standards and if the client feels comfortable with them.	Moral–ethical standards may be uncritically internalized and place the client in conflict.	11/3/93 Goal met. Client stated: "I guess I'm living the best way I know how right now. If things are meant to be different someone is going to have to show me how."
Identify unrealistic standards; client may need "permission" to be human.	Unrealistic standards (perfectionism, conventionality) may constantly undermine the client's self-esteem.	*Recommendation:* Reinforce self-acceptance.
Refer if appropriate for counseling.	Support groups on campus (counseling centers, ministries) may be able to meet client's needs.	*C. Taylor, RN*

Goal: By this time next month, 11/2/93, the client will demonstrate increased self-esteem by:
- Reporting two recent instances when personal power was effective in accomplishing desired goals

Nursing Actions	**Rationale**	**Evaluative Statement**
Identify and affirm client's use of personal power to accomplish goals.	A negative self-concept may deny or distort personal successes; outside intervention may be necessary to bring these to consciousness.	11/3/93 Goal met . . . with difficulty. Needed considerable prompting to identify successful use of her personal power. Was ready to attribute passing grade to luck rather than her own efforts.
		Recommendation: Have client make daily record of her use of personal power and results.
		C. Taylor, RN

KEY POINTS

- Self-concept is the mental image or picture of self. It has the power to encourage or thwart personal growth and development.
- Included in the notion self-concept are body image, how I experience my body; subjective self, how I see myself; ideal self, the self I want to be; and social self, way I feel others see me.

- It is helpful to explore the self-concept by assessing self-knowledge, self-expectations, and self-evaluation or self-esteem. Self-esteem is a measure of a person's satisfaction with his or her significance, competence, virtue, and power.

- Self-concept is a social creation. An infant, born without a self-concept, develops positive feelings about self if basic needs are met and warmth and affection are experienced.
- A positive self-concept is characterized by stable and diversified self-knowledge, realistic self-expectations, and positive self-evaluation and acceptance of self.
- High self-esteem is characterized by positive expectations of the future, ability to approach others freely because of a history of being well received and successful, and ability to approach new tasks and situations freely—confident of own ability to get along.
- Life experiences both affect and are affected by a person's self-concept. Key factors influencing self-concept are developmental state, culture, internal and external resources, history of success and failure, stressors and illness or trauma.

- The nurse who wishes to effectively meet the self-concept needs of clients needs to be comfortable with self, his or her abilities, and his or her needs before the nurse can interact therapeutically with clients. It is important for the nurse to role-model positive self-concept behaviors.
- Because a client may offer the responses the interviewer wants rather than what is really felt, client responses should be evaluated in relation to observations the nurse makes of the client's behaviors.
- Nursing diagnoses may be written specifically addressing disturbances in self-concept: negative self-concept, disturbances in body-image, self-esteem, role competence, and personal identity, or identifying the effect these disturbances have on other areas of human functioning (eg, coping, health maintenance, powerlessness).

STUDY QUESTIONS

1. Robert, aged 19, has Down's syndrome and is mildly mentally retarded with an intelligence quotient of 82. He told his nurse, "I'm a good helper. You see I can carry these trays because I am so strong. But I'm not very smart so I have just learned to help with the things I know how to do." Robert most likely has
   a. a negative self-concept and low self-esteem
   b. a negative self-concept and high self-esteem
   c. a positive self-concept and fairly high self-esteem
   d. a positive self-concept and low self-esteem

2. Jerry was having academic difficulty in all his college courses, and during a counseling session he was asked to make a list of 20 words that describe him. After 15 minutes, Jerry listed the following: 19 years old, male, named Jerry, and declared he couldn't think of anything else. Jerry has demonstrated
   a. lack of self-esteem
   b. deficient self-knowledge
   c. unrealistic self-expectation
   d. inability to evaluate himself

3. Jerry, who is in counseling because he is having academic difficulty, was able to list only three facts, traits, or qualities that describe himself. His counselor then asked him to list facts, traits, or qualities that he would like to be descriptive of himself or which he thinks he should have. Jerry quickly listed 25, all of which were characteristic of a successful man. When asked if he knew anyone like this, he replied, "My father." This discrepancy between Jerry's description of himself as he is and as he would like to be indicates
   a. positive self-concept
   b. Jerry's modesty (lack of conceit)

   c. body image disturbance
   d. low self-esteem

4. David and his wife have decided that she will get a job so that David can go to pharmacy school as he has wanted to do for some time. Their three teenagers, who were involved in the decision, are also getting jobs to buy their own clothes. David plans to work 12 to 16 hours weekly. He states, "I was always an A student, but I may have to settle for Bs now because I don't want to neglect my family and I need to work a few hours so my wife won't have to work overtime." David's self-expectations are
   a. realistic and positively motivating his development
   b. unrealistic and negatively motivating his development
   c. unrealistic but positively motivating his development
   d. realistic but negatively motivating his development

5. Which of the following statements made by a parent of a child you are seeing in clinic needs to be followed up with teaching about how to foster healthy development of the self in children?
   a. "I love my child so much I 'hug him to death' every day."
   b. "I think children need challenges, don't you?"
   c. "My husband and I both grew up in very restrictive families. We want our children to be free to do whatever they want."
   d. "My husband and I have different ideas about discipline but we're talking this out because we know it's important for Johnny that we be consistent."

6. Which intervention would you take first to assist a mother who states that she feels incompetent as a mother of a teenage daughter?

a. recommend that she discipline her daughter more strictly and consistently

b. make a list of things her husband can do to help her improve

c. assist the mother to identify both what she believes is preventing her success and what she can do to improve

d. explore with the mother what the daughter can do to improve her behavior

7. Which of the following clients is *least* likely to develop problems related to self-concept?

   a. 55-year-old female television news reporter undergoing a hysterectomy (removal of uterus)

   b. young clergyperson whose vocal cords are paralyzed following a motorbike accident

   c. 32-year-old accountant who survives a massive heart attack

   d. 23-year-old model who has just learned that she has breast cancer

For questions 8 to 11, read the client data below and use the following letters to indicate the diagnosis the data suggest (each response may be used only once):

   a. Personal Identity Disturbance

   b. Body Image Disturbance

   c. Self-Esteem Disturbance

   d. Altered Role Performance

8. _____ Juanita Sanchez has only been in the United States 3 months and has recently suffered the loss of her husband and job. She states that nothing feels familiar, "I don't know who I am supposed to be here," and she misses home (Nicaragua) terribly.

9. _____ Jim Boa, a sophomore in high school, has missed a great amount of school this year because of leukemia. He said he feels like he is falling behind in everything and misses "hanging out at the mall" with his friends most of all.

10. _____ "Why did I have to be born into a family of big bottoms and short fat legs! No one will ever ask me out for a date . . . oh why can't I have long thin legs like everyone else in my class? What a frump I am."

11. _____ Marissa Yule, a 33-year-old businessperson, is now in counseling attempting to deal with a long-repressed history of sexual abuse by her father. "I guess I should feel satisfied with what I've achieved in life but I'm never content and nothing I achieve makes me feel good about myself." "I hate my father for making me feel like I'm no good. This is an awful way to live."

12. Nancy, aged 36, who was divorced 5 years earlier, entered the emergency department with severe burns and cuts on her face after an auto accident in a car driven by her fiancé of 3 months. Three

weeks later, her fiancé has not yet contacted her. Nancy states that he is so busy and she is too tired to visit anyway. Nancy frequently lies with her eyes closed and head turned away. These data suggest that

   a. there is no disturbance in self-concept

   b. this client has ego strength and high self-esteem but may have a disturbance of body image

   c. the area of self-esteem has very low priority at this time and should be ignored until much later

   d. it is probable that there are disturbances in self-esteem and body image

13. Which of the nursing interventions below is *least* likely to assist a severely ill client with cancer to maintain a positive sense of self?

   a. making it a point to address the client by name each time you enter the room

   b. fatiguing the client as little as possible by performing all procedures in silence

   c. continuing to respect the client's privacy and sensitivities

   d. offering the client a simple explanation before moving her in any way

14. Doris, aged 16, has a nursing diagnosis of Body Image Disturbance related to severe acne. In planning nursing care, an appropriate goal for this nursing diagnosis is, "The client will

   a. make above *B* grades in all tests at school"

   b. demonstrate by diet control and skin care increased interest in control of acne"

   c. report that she feels more self-confidence in her music and art, which she enjoys"

   d. express that she is very smart in school"

15. A 4½-year-old boy required stitches for a laceration on the eyebrow. After the doctor held him, visited with him, explained what was going to be done and that his eye would get better and look just like it did before, the boy placed his hands under his hips as instructed and quietly permitted the procedure. He then expressed pride in himself. Evaluation of the effect of this health care experience is best expressed in which of the following?

   a. The doctor did an excellent job.

   b. The child's self-esteem was enhanced, fear of bodily mutilation decreased, and the parents were given an excellent role model.

   c. The child was made the center of attention and the situation exaggerated, thus encouraging the child to become self-centered.

   d. These interventions consumed too much physician time to be evaluated positively.

Answers With Rationale

1. The correct response is *c*. The data point to Robert's having a positive self-concept, "I'm a good

helper," and fairly high self-esteem (realizes his strengths and limitations). The statement "But I'm not very smart" is accurate and is not an indication of a negative self-concept.

2. The correct response is *b*. Jerry's inability to list more than three items about himself indicates deficient self-knowledge. There are not enough data provided to determine if he lacks self-esteem, has unrealistic self-expectations, or is unable to evaluate himself.

3. The correct response is *d*. Low self-esteem is characterized by great discrepancy between the ideal and real selves. There are no data in this item to suggest that Jerry has either a positive self-concept or a body image disturbance. The data do indicate something more serious than modesty.

4. The correct response is *a*. David's self-expectations are realistic, given his multiple commitments, and seem to be positively motivating his development.

5. The correct response is *c*. Each option with the exception of *c* correctly addresses some aspect of fostering healthy development in children. Because children need effective structure and development, giving them total freedom to do as they please may actually hinder their development.

6. The correct response is *c*. The first intervention priority with a mother who feels incompetent to parent a teenage daughter is to assist the mother to identify what is preventing her from being an effective parent and then to explore solutions aimed at improving her parenting skills. The other interventions may prove helpful but they do not directly address the mother's problem with her feelings of incompetence.

7. The correct response is *a*. Based simply on the facts given, the 55-year-old news reporter would be least likely to experience a body image or role performance disturbance because she is beyond her child-bearing years and the hysterectomy should not impair her ability to report the news. The young clergyperson's inability to preach, the 32-year-old's massive myocardial infarction, and the model's breast resection have much greater potential to result in self-concept problems.

8. The correct response is *a*. An unfamiliar culture coupled with traumatic life events and loss of husband and job has resulted in this client's total loss of her sense of self: "I don't know who I am supposed to be here." Her very sense of identity is at stake, not merely her body image, self-esteem, or role performance.

9. The correct response is *d*. Important roles for Jim are being a student and a friend. His illness is preventing him from doing either of these well. This self-concept disturbance is basically one that concerns role performance.

10. The correct response is *b*. Clearly, this client's concern is with his or her body image.

11. The correct response is *c*. Marissa's self-concept disturbance is mainly one of devaluing herself, and thinking that she is no good. This is a self-esteem disturbance.

12. The correct response is *d*. The traumatic nature of Nancy's injuries, her fiancé's failure to contact her, and Nancy's response, that is, her withdrawal, all point to potential problems with both body image and self-esteem. It is not true that self-esteem needs are of low priority.

13. The correct response is *b*. Each option with the exception of *b* should assist the client to maintain a positive sense of self. Working in silence with the client may be preferable to idle chatter but the ideal is to address the client by name, give simple explanations of procedures, and communicate that he or she is a person of worth by simple words of caring.

14. The correct response is *b*. All of these client goals may be appropriate for Doris, but the only goal that directly addresses her body image disturbance is *b*.

15. The correct response is *b*. The physician enhanced the child's self-esteem by teaching him how to participate effectively, decreased his fear of bodily mutilation by telling him that his eyebrow would heal and look normal, and gave the parents an excellent role model.

BIBLIOGRAPHY

Abood, D. A., & Conway, T. L. (1992). Health value and self-esteem as predictors of wellness behavior. *Health Values, 16*(3), 20–26.

Atwater, W. E. (1990). *Psychology of adjustment* (4th ed.). Englewood Cliffs, NJ: Prentice-Hall.

Baird, S. E. (1985). Development of a nursing assessment tool to diagnose altered body image in immobilized patients. *Orthopedic Patients, 4*(1), 47–54.

Bensink, G. W., Godbey, K. L., Marshall, M. J., & Yarandi, H. N. (1992). Institutionalized elderly: Relaxation, locus of control, self-esteem. *Journal of Gerontological Nursing, 18*(4), 30–36.

Calhoun, J. F., & Acocella, J. R. (1989). *Psychology of adjustment and human relationships* (3rd ed.). New York: Random House.

Carpenito, L. J. (1992). *Nursing diagnosis: Application to clinical practice* (4th ed.). Philadelphia: Lippincott.

Cash, T. F., Winstead, B. A., & Janda, L. H. (1986). The great American shape-up. *Psychology Today, 20*(4), 30–37.

Coleman, J. C., Morris, C. G., & Glaros, A. G. (1990). *Contemporary psychology and effective behavior* (7th ed.). Glenview, IL: Scott, Foresman.

Coopersmith, S. (1967). *The antecedents of self-esteem.* San Francisco: Freeman.

Crouch, M. A., & Straub, V. (1983). Enhancement of self-esteem in adults. *Family and Community Health, 6*(2), 65–78.

Darling-Fisher, C. S. (1985). Impairment of body image. In M. M. Jacobs & W. Geels (Eds.), *Signs and symptoms in nursing*. Philadelphia: Lippincott.

Davidhizar, R. (1991). Ten strategies for increasing your self-confidence. *Imprint, 38*(3), 105–108.

Dinkmeyer, D., Sr. (1970). Developing understanding of self and others (Manual DUSO-D1). Circle Pines, MN: American Guidance Service.

Gilbert, R. (1983). The evaluation of self-esteem. *Family and Community Health, 6*(2), 29–49.

Granger, R. (1990). How to feel good about being you. *American Journal of Nursing, 90*(4), 14.

Harris, M. (1986). Helping the person with an altered self-image. *Geriatric Nursing, 72*(2), 90–92.

Janelli, L. M. (1986). The realities of body image. *Journal of Gerontological Nursing, 12*(10), 23–27.

Jenny, J. (1990). Self-esteem: A problem for nurses. *Canadian Nurse, 86*(11), 19–21.

LeMone, P. (1991). Analysis of a human phenomenon: Self-concept. *Nursing Diagnosis, 2*(3), 126–130.

Long, K. A., & Hamlin, C. M. (1988). Use of the Piers-Haris self-concept scale with Indian children: Cultural considerations. *Nursing Research, 37*(1), 42–46.

Maslow, A. (1954). *Motivation and personality*. New York: Harper & Row.

McCloskey, J. C. (1976). How to make the most of body image theory in nursing practice. *Nursing, 6*(5), 68–72.

Meisenhelder, J. B. (1986). Self-esteem in women: The influence of employment and perception of husband's appraisals. *Image: Journal of Nursing Scholarship, 18*(1), 8–14.

Muhlenkamp, A. F., & Sayles, J. A. (1986). Self-esteem, social support, and positive health practices. *Nursing Research, 35*(6), 334–338.

Norris, J., & Kunes-Connell, M. (1985). Self-esteem disturbance. *Nursing Clinics of North America, 20*(4), 745–761.

Otto, H. (1965). The human potentialities of nurses and patients. *Nursing Outlook, 13*(8), 32–35.

Pensiero, M., & Adams, M. (1987). Dress and self-esteem. *Journal of Gerontological Nursing, 13*(10), 11–17.

Reasoner, R. W. (1983). Enhancement of self-esteem in children and adolescents. *Family and Community Health, 6*(2), 51–64.

Rutkowski, B. L. (1985). 6 steps to building your confidence. *Nursing Life, 6*(1), 26–29.

Schmitt, D. (1989). Linda had lost her looks—and her will to live. *Nursing, 29*(7), 43–45.

Stanwyck, D. J. (1983). Self-esteem through the life span. *Family and Community Health, 6*(8), 11–28.

Taft, L. B. (1985). Self-esteem in later life: A nurse's perspective. *Advances in Nursing Science, 8*(1), 77–84.

Taylor, C. (1982). The need for self-esteem. In H. Yura & M. B. Walsh (Eds.), *Human needs 2 and the nursing process*. Norwalk, CT: Appleton-Century-Crofts.

Whall, A. L. (1987). Self-esteem and the mental health of older adults. *Journal of Gerontological Nursing, 13*(4), 41–42.

Williamson, M. L. (1987). The nursing diagnosis of body image disturbance in adolescents dissatisfied with their physical characteristics. *Holistic Nursing Practice, 1*(4), 52–59.

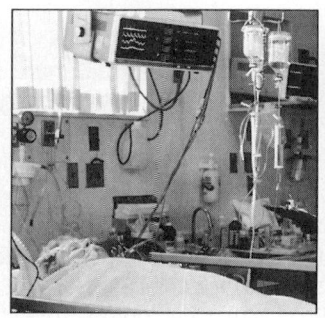
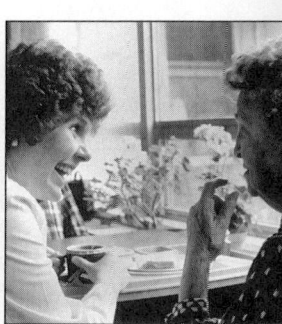

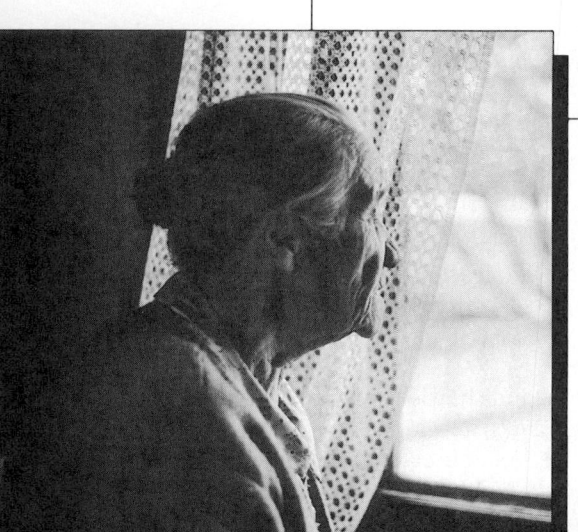

Sensory Stimulation

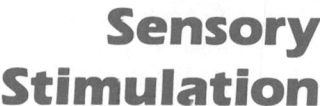

OBJECTIVES

After studying this chapter, the learner should be able to:

Define key terms used in the chapter.

Describe the four conditions that must be met in each sensory experience.

Explain the role of the reticular activating system in sensory experience.

Identify etiologies and perceptual, cognitive, and emotional responses to sensory deprivation and sensory overload.

Perform a comprehensive assessment of sensory functioning using appropriate interview questions and physical assessment skills.

Develop nursing diagnoses that correctly identify sensory/perceptual alterations that may be treated by independent nursing intervention.

Describe specific nursing strategies to prevent sensory alterations, to stimulate the senses, and to assist clients with sensory difficulties.

Develop a nursing care plan to assist clients meet individualized sensory/perceptual goals.

Implement individualized nursing strategies that successfully resolve the client's individualized sensory/perceptual alterations.

Evaluate the nursing care plan using specified criteria.

KEY TERMS

arousal
auditory
cultural care
deprivation
gustatory
kinesthesia
olfactory
perception
presbycusis
presbyopia
reception
reticular activating system
sensoristasis
sensory deprivation
sensory overload
sensory/perceptual alterations
stimulus
tactile
visceral
visual

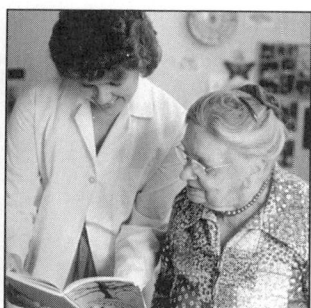

A person's senses are vital to survival, growth and development, and the experience of bodily pleasure. Intrinsic to each of the following experiences is intact sensory functioning:

- Being able to smell smoke and interpret this as potentially life threatening, I can protect myself from fire.
- Seeing a client smile when I walk into his or her room and hearing the client say, "I couldn't have gone through this week without you," bolsters my professional confidence and self-esteem and encourages me to offer quality nursing to others.
- Feeling someone's gentle hands stroke my body, I luxuriate in feelings of care, pleasure, and sensual delight.

Many of the clients nurses encounter have impaired sensory functioning, which places them at high risk of injury and altered growth and development and decreases their well-being. Moreover, the stress of illness or trauma and the need for diagnosis and treatment may quickly result in sensory deprivation or overload with serious disturbances in visual, perceptual, cognitive, or emotional functioning.

Study of this chapter provides the student with knowledge of the process of sensation, the role of the arousal mechanism, sensory alterations, and factors affecting sensory stimulation. Practical suggestions are given for performing an assessment of sensory functioning. Examples are given of nursing diagnoses identifying specific sensory/perceptual alterations, as are many diagnoses describing the effects of altered sensory functioning on other areas of human functioning. Client goals for preventing and managing sensory alterations are described. Specialized nursing interventions for vision- or hearing-impaired, confused, or unconscious clients are presented. In the section Nursing Process in Clinical Practice, focused assessment, planning, implementation, and evaluation guides are offered for select nursing diagnoses of sensory deprivation related to inadequate parenting, to the effects of aging, and to unfamiliar culture.

The Sensory Experience

Components and Conditions

The two components of any sensory experience are reception and perception. **Sensory reception** is the process of receiving data about the internal or external environment through the senses. The senses by which individuals maintain contact with the external environment are vision (**visual**); hearing (**auditory**); smell (**olfactory**); taste (**gustatory**); and touch (**tactile**). The kinesthetic and visceral senses arise internally from muscles and hollow organs, respectively, and are the basic orienting systems. (**Kinesthesia** refers to awareness of positioning of body parts and body movement; **visceral** pertains to inner organs.) **Sensory perception** is the conscious process of selecting, organizing, and interpreting data from the senses into meaningful information. Perception is influenced by the intensity, size, change, or representation of stimuli, as well as by past experiences, knowledge, and attitudes.

For a person to receive data necessary to experience the world, four conditions must be met:

- A stimulus, an agent, act, or other influence capable of initiating a response by the nervous system, must be present.
- A receptor or sense organ must receive the stimulus and convert it to a nerve impulse.
- The nerve impulse must be **conducted** along a nervous pathway from the receptor or sense organ to the brain.
- A particular area in the brain must receive and translate the impulse into a sensation.

Arousal Mechanism

To receive stimuli and respond appropriately, the brain must be alert or aroused. The **reticular activating system** (RAS), located in the core of the brain stem, mediates arousal. According to Schultz (1965), the arousal state of the RAS is a general drive state, which he called **sensoristasis**. Nerve impulses from all the sensory tracts reach the RAS, which then selectively allows certain impulses to reach the cerebral cortex and be perceived. With its many ascending and descending connections to other areas of the brain, the RAS serves to monitor and regulate incoming sensory stimuli and thereby maintain, enhance, or inhibit cortical arousal.

A stimulus must be variable or irregular to evoke a response. The body quickly adapts to constant stimuli; thus the repeated stimulus of a continuing noise such as city traffic or a noxious odor eventually goes unnoticed. This phenomenon is termed *adaptation*. Impulses that are not acted on when received may be used at a later date. The memory process involves the storage of that material. For example, thought and memory are used when a new sensory experience occurs and the organism uses a response based on previous knowledge and experience.

Sensory Alterations

When admitted to a health agency, the client is confronted with stimuli that are different in quality and quantity to the accustomed stimuli. For example, the client confined to bed rest may receive many fewer stimuli, whereas the client undergoing multiple diagnostic tests may receive a greater than normal level of sensory input. These and other typical experiences are likely to result in the client's having sensory alterations. Behavioral changes in hospitalized clients have been reduced because more attention is being paid to the use of color and sound and increased privacy and social interaction. Factors contributing to severe sensory alteration (intensive care unit psychosis) include sensory overload, sensory deprivation, sleep deprivation, and cultural care deprivation. Table 39-1 provides an overview of sensory deprivation and sensory overload with related nursing interventions.

Sensory Deprivation

Sensory deprivation results when a person experiences decreased sensory input or input that is monotonous, unpatterned, or meaningless. With decreased sensory input, the RAS is no longer able to project a normal level of activation to the brain and the individual may hallucinate simply to maintain an optimal level of arousal (MacKinnon-Kesler, 1983). Factors placing a client at high risk for sensory deprivation include the following:

- An environment with decreased or monotonous stimuli (institutionalized clients, clients confined to a small living area at home, clients on bed rest or in isolation, and so on)
- Impaired ability to receive environmental stimuli (clients with sensory alterations: impaired vision or hearing; clients with bandages or casts that interfere with vision, hearing, or tactile stimulation; clients with affective disorders who "close out" the environment, and so on)
- Inability to process environmental stimuli (clients with spinal cord injuries or brain damage, clients who are confused or disoriented, clients taking prescribed or recreational drugs that affect the central nervous system)

Effects of sensory deprivation include perceptual, cognitive, and emotional disturbances:

Perceptual responses—inaccurate perception of sights, sounds, tastes, smells, and body position, coordination, and equilibrium; mild to gross distortions ranging from daydreams to hallucinations

Cognitive responses—inability to control the direction of thought content; decreased attention span and ability to concentrate; difficulty with memory, problem solving, and task performance

Emotional responses—inappropriate emotional responses: apathy, anxiety, fear, anger, belligerence, panic, depression; rapid mood changes (see Table 39-1 for additional information)

Sensory Overload

Sensory overload is the condition that results when a person experiences so much sensory stimuli that the brain is unable meaningfully to respond to or ignore the stimuli.

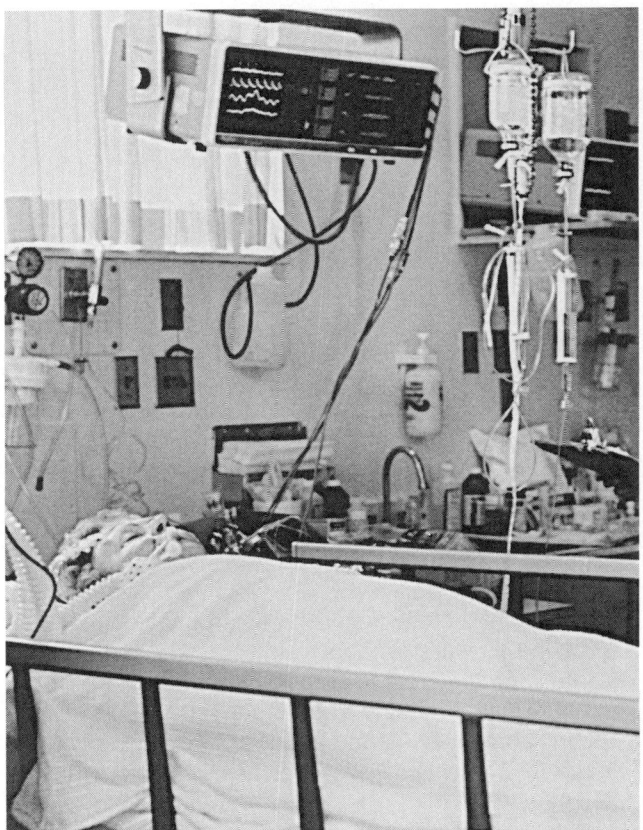

F I G U R E   3 9 - 1

Illness, pain and medication stress the individual's capacity to process normal sensory stimuli. In addition, the hospital environment of strange sights, sounds, odors, and people can cause symptoms of sensory overload in some clients. (Photo by Gates Rhodes, courtesy of School of Nursing, University of Pennsylvania.)

The person feels out of control and may exhibit all of the manifestations observed in sensory deprivation. The amount and quality of stimuli necessary to produce overload may differ greatly from one individual to another and are influenced by factors such as age, culture, personality, and life-style.

In some clients, especially those coming from a quiet environment with unvarying stimuli, the experience of being hospitalized quickly results in sensory overload. In such clients, the brain is assaulted by the constant presence of strangers who not only demand to be spoken to but who also touch and poke at the body; by the strange sights, odors, sounds, and feels of the unfamiliar environment; by the constant presence of pain or discomfort from dressings, IVs, drainage tubes, or endotracheal tubes; and by the ever-present worries about the meaning and course of the illness. Nursing assistance is directed to reducing distressing stimuli and helping the client to gain control over the environment (see Table 39-1).

T A B L E 3 9 - 1

Overview of Sensory Deprivation and Sensory Overload

Sensory Deprivation   Insufficient quantity or quality of stimuli; may result from decreased sensory input or monotonous, unpatterned, and unmeaningful input

Defining Characteristics	Contributing Factors	Clients at Risk
Physical behaviors: drowsiness, excessive yawning *Escape behaviors*: eating, exercising, sleeping, running away to escape the deprived environment *Changes in perception*: unusual body sensations; preoccupation with somatic complaints (dry mouth, palpitations, difficulty breathing, nausea); change in body image; illusions and hallucinations *Changes in cognitive behavior*: decreased attention span, inability to concentrate, decreased problem solving and task performance *Changes in affective behavior*: crying, increased irritability and annoyance over small matters, confusion, panic, depression	Decreased environmental stimuli: institutionalized environment; separation from significant others and usual sources of stimuli; treatments that decrease access to stimuli, such as bed rest or isolation *Impaired ability to receive environmental stimuli*: impaired vision, hearing, taste, smell, touch resulting from treatments such as bandages or body casts that interfere with reception of stimuli, or as a result of depression and other affective disorders *Inability to process environmental stimuli*: spinal cord injuries, brain damage, confusion, dementia, medications that depress the central nervous system	Institutionalized clients, especially those in long-term care settings Clients with communicable disease (eg, AIDS) Clients confined to bed Clients with sensory alterations (eg, impaired vision or hearing, or clients with eye patches or body casts) Clients who are depressed Clients from a different culture Clients with a disturbance of the nervous system

Nursing Interventions

Maintain sufficient level of arousal by increasing sensory stimuli from all sensory modalities:

- Instruct the client in self-stimulation methods: counting, singing, reading, reciting poetry.
- Structure meaningful tangible stimuli into client's external environment; include a variety of people, ideas, sensations; a pet may provide excellent stimulation.
  - *Visual stimulation*
    - Colorful sheets, pajamas, robes
    - Colorful uniform tops for the nurse
    - Face-to-face human contact
    - Clocks, calendars, wrist watches
    - Pictures, flowers, greeting card
  - *Auditory stimulation*
    - Call person by name
    - Conversation that communicates caring as well as orients client
    - Reading to the client
    - Television, radio
  - *Gustatory and olfactory stimulation*
    - Attention to oral hygiene and properly fitting dentures
    - Food of different textures, colors, temperatures served attractively
    - Smelling food before eating it and recalling pleasurable aromas from the past
    - Seasoning foods or having favorite foods brought from home
  - *Tactile stimulation*
    - Back rubs
    - Turning and repositioning   Foot soaks
    - Passive range-of-motion exercises   Hugs
    - Hair brushing, combing, washing   Touching of arms or shoulders

(continued)

T A B L E   3 9 - 1 (continued)

Overview of Sensory Deprivation and Sensory Overload

Defining Characteristics	Contributing Factors	Clients at Risk

• *Cognitive input*
   Orient client to environment
   Encourage client participation in self-care
   Discuss current events or client's occupation, hobbies, or interests
   Reinforce reality without arguing with a client who is hallucinating.
     "No, I don't see a man standing there but the linen hamper may be confusing you."
• *Emotional input*
   Encourage client to share fears, concerns, and perceptions; reassure client that illusions and misperceptions do occur with sensory deprivation.
• Incorporate culturally assistive, supportive, facilitative acts into nursing care.
• *Caution:* Because it can be difficult to distinguish the behavioral manifestations of sensory deprivation from sensory overload, introduce more stimulation cautiously. If the added stimulation only increases the client's maladaptive behaviors, consider reducing sensory input because the client may be experiencing sensory overload.		

Sensory Overload	Excessive stimuli over which an individual feels little control; brain is unable meaningfully to respond to or ignore stimuli	
Similar to those observed in sensory deprivation Elderly clients and clients who have suffered a stroke are more likely to experience confusion or agitation. Young clients are more likely to seek the comfort of their parents' embrace to block out sensory overload.	*Increased internal stimuli:* pain, pressure and discomfort of intrusive tubes (eg, intravenous lines [IVs], catheters; endotracheal tubes, nasogastric tubes), worry about state of health or need to make treatment decisions *Increased external stimuli:* unfamiliar healthcare environment, such as lights, noises, sounds, odors, movement, and constant presence of strangers, many of whom touch the body; intrusive procedures such as diagnostic tests and treatments; scratchy linens *Inability perceptually to disregard or selectively ignore some stimuli:* nervous system disturbances, medications such as caffeine that stimulate the central nervous system arousal mechanism	Any acutely or chronically ill client Clients in pain Client with intrusive monitoring or treatment equipment Hospitalized clients, especially those in critical care settings Clients with disturbances of the nervous system

Nursing Interventions
• Provide a consistent, predictable pattern of stimulation to help the client develop a sense of control over the environment.
• Offer simple explanations before procedures, tests, and examinations.
• Establish a schedule with the client for routine care such as eating, bathing, turning, positioning, coughing, and exercise.
• Speak calmly with the client and move slowly; communicate confidence.
• Explore with the client what stimuli are most distressing and develop a plan to reduce or eliminate these (eg, incoming phone calls, visitors); ear plugs or pain medication may be indicated.
• Be careful not to cause sensory deprivation.
• Identify and, wherever possible, eliminate culturally inappropriate stimuli.

(Adapted from Lee, K. A. [1991]. Sensory overload, sensory deprivation, and sleep deprivation. In M. L. Patrick, S. L. Woods, R. F. Craven, J. S. Rokosky, & P. M. Bruno [Eds.], *Medical–surgical nursing* [2nd ed.]. Philadelphia: Lippincott.)

Cultural Care Deprivation

Sensory deprivation, sensory overload, and sleep deprivation are all related to or affected by an individual's cultural practices, values, and beliefs. Kloosterman (1991) suggests that the concept missing in current practices concerning severe sensory alteration is "culturally congruent care." **Cultural care deprivation** is described as "a lack of culturally assistive, supportive, or facilitative acts" (p. 121). The nurse who is sensitive to the client's culture attempts to determine what constitutes acceptable levels of stimuli from the client's viewpoint. For example, touching in certain cultures is viewed as a natural and welcome custom whereas other cultures may view touching as insulting or offensive. Kloosterman noted that different cultures have rules on how, where, and for what purpose the human body may be touched. Similarly, clients may find comfort in cultural and religious symbols of care and healing that are absent in a hospital environment.

Factors Affecting Sensory Stimulation

There appears to be considerable variation in the amount of stimuli different individuals consider optimal. Factors influencing the amount and quality of stimuli needed to maintain cortical arousal include developmental considerations, culture, personality and life-style, stress, and illness and medication.

Developmental Considerations

Different types of sensory stimulation are needed for growth as sensory receptors and organs and the nervous system mature. Although the newborn is capable of rudimentary perceptual discriminations at birth, many neural pathways are immature and must be stimulated to develop, become refined, and function adequately. Appropriate stimulation includes soothing; holding; rocking and changes of position (tactile and kinesthetic sensations); singing and being talked to (auditory sensations); and changing patterns of light and shade, such as through the use of mobiles and bright objects (visual sensations). Developmentally appropriate play develops the child's muscles and coordination, provides an outlet for surplus physical energy, develops communication skills, furnishes sources of learning, acts as a stimulant to creativity, develops social skills, teaches sex roles, provides an outlet for the release of emotional energy, and develops self-insights.

Sensory functioning tends to progressively decline throughout adulthood as the result of aging or chronic illness. The adult may experience the need to compensate for the loss of one type of stimulation by increasing other sources of sensory stimuli.

Culture

An individual's culture may dictate the amount of sensory stimulation considered normal. For example, the amount of touching a child experiences in a Puerto Rican family may be different from that experienced by a child in a German family. Similarly, male and female roles may be culturally defined; for example, although the male is expected to respond to the challenge of out-of-the-home sensory stimuli, the female who attempts to do so may be scorned if her place is considered to be in the home. Ethnic norms, religious norms, income group norms, and the norms of subgroups within a culture all influence the amount of sensory stimulation sought by an individual and perceived as meaningful.

Personality and Life-Style

Apart from a person's culture, different personality types demand different levels of stimulation. One person may thrive on a steady stream of fast-paced changes and excitement, whereas another may feel best when daily routines are rigidly structured and life sends no challenges necessitating changes. Life-style choices can dramatically influence the quantity and quality of stimuli received by an individual. The nurse who elects to work in the emergency room of a large city hospital is exposed to vastly different stimuli than the nurse working on a small unit in a residential long-term care setting.

Stress

Increased sensory stimulation may be sought during periods of low stress simply to maintain cortical arousal. During high-stress periods, multiple stressors may already be overloading the sensory system, and decreased sensory stimulation is desired. The stress of physical illness, pain, hospitalization, testing, surgery, and treatment may provide more stimulation than an individual can process and respond to without assistance.

Illness and Medication

Illness can affect the reception of sensory stimuli (eg, diminution of the sense of touch associated with diabetes and cerebrovascular disease) and their transmission and perception (eg, neurologic disorders, dementias). Medications that alert or depress the central nervous system may interfere with the perception of sensory stimuli. Certain medications also may contribute to impaired sensory functioning by decreasing reception (eg, captopril, an antihypertensive agent, can cause taste alteration; aspirin can cause tinnitus—ringing in the ears).

Nurse as Role Model

Sensitivity to the important role sensory functioning plays in a person's well-being guides the nurse to promote personal well-being. Awareness of one's own sensory functioning and the stimulation in one's own life is a stepping stone to providing proper stimulation to clients. The nurse works to achieve the following goals. The nurse will:

- Evaluate the quantity and quality of sensory stimuli present in both the home and at work
- Identify stimuli important to self-development as a person (mental, physical, and spiritual health) and as a professional nurse
- Manipulate the environment to decrease distressing stimuli and increase positive stimuli
- Practice nursing, conscious of the need to promote optimal sensory functioning in clients

Assessing Sensory Functioning

When assessing a client for sensory disturbances, the nurse interviews the client and examines the client for sensory deficits and manifestations of sensory deprivation or overload. Examination of the client's environment is included in the assessment to determine whether it is providing adequate sensory stimulation for healthy development. The assessment may be structured using the components of the sensory experience—stimulation, reception, and transmission—perception—reaction, the components of the sensory experience. Because clients may adapt to sensory impairments, it may be helpful to include someone the client knows well (eg, spouse or parent) in the assessment to see if that person has noticed behavioral characteristics in the client that suggest a sensory disturbance (eg, "I've noticed he turns the television volume much louder than ever before").

Stimulation

Assess if there have been any recent changes in sensory stimulation, for example, reduction of stimulation from one or more sensory modalities ("Since my husband died no one touches me anymore. It sounds crazy but I'm hungry to be touched!") or new or unusual stimulation ("Ever since my granddaughter moved in with me, my house is always noisy. I can't stand the constant noise and her smoking."). Assess if the type of stimulation present is developmentally appropriate. High-risk clients for problems related to stimulation include children in nonstimulating environments, elderly clients, terminally ill clients, clients on bed rest, clients in isolation, and clients requiring intensive nursing in a critical care setting.

Reception

Assess for anything that may interfere with sensory reception and describe any corrective devices you use for sensory impairments (eyeglasses, contacts, hearing aids). The accompanying display highlights assessment strategies for each sense. High-risk clients for reception problems include people with visual, auditory, or other sensory impairments.

Transmission–Perception–Reaction

High-risk clients for transmission–perception–reaction problems include confused clients and clients with nervous system impairments. Everyday interactions afford the nurse multiple opportunities to assess clients' abilities to transmit, perceive, and react to stimuli.

Defining Characteristics of Sensory Deprivation and Overload

Complete the assessment of the client's sensory functioning by assessing for specific indicators of sensory deprivation or overload (see Table 39-1), including boredom, inactivity, slowness of thought, daydreaming, increased sleeping, thought disorganization, anxiety, panic, illusions, or hallucinations (Schiefer, 1982). It is important to know the client's usual state to be able to identify changes stemming from sensory deprivation or overload.

Physical Assessment

Physical examinations related to the senses are discussed in Chapter 24. Ear and eye tests, whether performed by a physician or nurse, should be considered when planning care. Problems with the neurologic system indicate the necessity of further assessment of the sensory experience.

Diagnosing

Sensory/Perceptual Alterations as the Problem When assessment data point to sensory disturbances that can be treated independently by nursing interventions, nursing diagnoses are developed and labeled **sensory/perceptual alterations**. These alterations may be further specified as visual, auditory, gustatory, olfactory, tactile, or kinesthetic. *Sensory deprivation* and *sensory overload* may also be used to further specify the sensory/perceptual alteration and in some cases may be the etiology.

Common etiologies for sensory/perceptual alterations include the following:

- Altered environmental stimuli, excessive or insufficient
- Altered sensory reception, transmission or integration
- Chemical alterations, endogenous (eg, electrolytes) or exogenous (eg, drugs)
- Psychological stress

Sample nursing diagnoses in which the sensory/perceptual alteration is the problem are listed in the accompanying display.

Sensory/Perceptual Alterations as the Etiology Because sensory/perceptual alterations affect many other

Sensory Stimulation

Factors to Assess	Questions and Approaches
Stimulation	"Does your current environment overly, insufficiently, or appropriately stimulate you?"
	"Are you bored? Why?"
	"Are you able to read? Watch television? Knit? Why not?"
	"Are there other people in your home during the day? Do you spend much time together? How do you spend the time?"
	"Who visits you while you are in the hospital?"
	Note reduction in the patterns or meaningfulness of stimulation in each sensory modality; changes in stimulation other than decreases (eg, new or unusual stimulation); or developmental appropriateness of stimulation.
Reception	"Does anything interfere with the functioning of your senses?"
	"Describe any corrective devices you use for sensory impairments."
Assess for visual disturbances.	"Please read my name tag (or this page of print)."
	Note if the client can correctly identify objects directly in front of the eyes as well as those requiring peripheral vision.
	Note eye rubbing; squinting; movements indicating faulty vision (bumping into furniture, overreaching or underreaching for objects); changes in the appearance of the eye (cataracts, swelling); and complaints of eye pain, spots, halos, or other visual disturbances.
Assess for auditory disturbances.	"Repeat the words that I will speak softly close to each ear."
	Note if the client is able to hear equally well from both ears, distinguish voices, locate the direction of a sound, if the client needs to face the person speaking and relies on lip reading, if the client's responses to questions include blank looks, many nods, smiling, or inappropriate responses indicating faulty hearing.
	Note complaints of ringing or buzzing in ears.
Assess for gustatory (taste) disturbances.	"Close your eyes, stick out your tongue, and tell me if what I place on your tongue is sweet, sour, bitter, or salty."
	"Have you been experiencing any strange tastes (bitter, metallic) or aftertastes lately?"
	Note if the client is able to differentiate sweet, sour, bitter, or salty tastes or reports unusual, persistent taste sensations.
	Note deficient oral hygiene, ill-fitting dentures, braces, or anything else that might contribute to gustatory disturbances.
Assess for olfactory (smell) disturbances.	"Close your eyes and tell me what you smell."
	"Have you smelled odors lately that others cannot smell or have you been especially sensitive to odors?" Note if the client can correctly identify common odors (coffee, vanilla) or has noticed increased sensitivity to odors.
Assess for tactile (touch) disturbances.	"Close your eyes and tell me when you feel something (brush skin with cotton ball), if what you feel is dull or sharp (use both ends of safety pin), hot or cold (use items from food tray). Now, keep your eyes closed and tell me what I am placing in your hand (coin, cotton ball, paper clip)."
	Note if the client can correctly sense touch and distinguish sharp and dull, hot and cold, and different shapes.

(continued)

FOCUSED ASSESSMENT GUIDE

Sensory Stimulation *(continued)*

Factors to Assess	Questions and Approaches
	Note if the client reports decreased sensation in any part of the body; numbness, pins and needles, tingling; or abnormal sensitivity to pain or touch.
	Note if the client withdraws from being touched.
Assess for kinesthetic and visceral disturbances.	"Have you noticed any changes in the way you perceive your body?"
	"Do you feel any unusual pressure or pain inside your body?"
	Note if the client seems unsure of his or her body parts or body position and if he or she experiences new internal sensations (fullness, pressure, pain).
Transmission– perception–reaction	"Are you aware of any problems with your nervous system?"
	"Have you found it difficult to communicate verbally?"
	Note consciousness, orientation, appropriateness of responses, ability to perform usual self-care activities, ability to follow simple commands, decision-making abilities, pathology affecting central nervous system, or prescribed or recreational drug use that affects the central nervous system.
Behavioral manifestations of sensory deprivation or overload	
Perceptual responses	Mild to gross sensory distortions (illusions, hallucinations)
Cognitive responses	Thought disorganization, slowness of thought, decreased attention/concentration, difficulty with problem solving and task performance
Emotional responses	Rapid mood changes, anxiety, panic

areas of human functioning, they serve as etiologies for multiple problem statements. Examples of these follow:

Activity Intolerance related to impaired balance and coordination (kinesthetic alteration)

Anxiety related to paranoia stemming from hearing impairment, sensory deprivation (specify setting), sensory overload

Impaired Verbal Communication related to difficulty receiving, transmitting, and perceiving sensory stimuli

Ineffective Individual Coping related to sensory overload (multiple stressors)

Diversional Activity Deficit related to impaired vision or hearing

Altered Growth and Development related to non-stimulating home environment

High Risk for Injury related to decreased or impaired sensation (specify visual, auditory, tactile, kinesthetic)

Knowledge Deficit: Means to Compensate for Sensory Impairment (Blindness, Deafness, and so forth), related to lack of previous experience with this problem, unavailability of resources

Knowledge Deficit: Providing a Developmentally Stimulating Environment, related to lack of experience with children's growth and development

Impaired Physical Mobility related to impaired balance and coordination (kinesthetic alteration)

Altered Parenting: Failure to Provide Stimuli for Growth related to lack of knowledge, decreased motivation to provide for child's growth and development

Powerlessness related to inability to interact meaningfully with environment

Self-Care Deficit: (specify) related to visual impairment, auditory impairment, tactile impairment

Body Image Disturbance related to kinesthetic impairment (distorted sense of body parts), sensory deprivation

Self-Esteem Disturbance related to sensory/perceptual alterations (specify visual, auditory, and so forth)

Altered Role Performance related to sensory/perceptual alteration (blindness, deafness, and so forth)

Personal Identity Disturbance related to sensory deprivation or overload

Sexual Dysfunction related to decreased sensation

Impaired Skin Integrity related to absent tactile sensation (injury)

Sleep Pattern Disturbance related to sensory deprivation or overload

Impaired Social Interaction related to inability to receive and process interactional stimuli

NURSING DIAGNOSES FOR COMMON PROBLEMS

Sensory/Perceptual Alterations

Problem	Related Factors	Sample Defining Characteristics
Sensory/Perceptual Alteration: Sensory Deficit or Excess		
Visual	Eye patches following surgery	"I never realized before how sight-dependent I am. I don't know what time of day it is now unless I have the radio on or smell food coming in."
		"It's frightening not to know who is in my room and what they are doing."
		Client observed sitting in room with blank facial expression; frequently comments on how bored he or she is and how slowly time is passing; hesitant to move about room without assistance although he or she has been oriented repeatedly
Auditory	Effects of aging	"You're right. I don't always hear what people are saying anymore so I try not to get involved in conversations. If people insist on talking, I just nod and hope I'm giving the right response."
		Able to hear moderately spoken word close to right ear; cannot hear same from left ear; often startled when someone approaches from left side
		Sits close to television and radio; loud volume, no history of hearing testing
Gustatory or olfactory	Chemotherapy	"I always seem to have a bitter taste in my mouth now and can't stomach certain foods at all that I used to enjoy, like beef, tomatoes, coffee. . . . I also can't take sweets and I used to be a real sweets junkie."
		"Sometimes the very smell of certain foods or even the thought of eating nauseates me."
		Client has been receiving vincristine (cancer chemotherapeutic agent) for past 3 months; some nausea and vomiting; history of poor oral hygiene
Tactile	Psychological stress	"I don't know why I feel this way, but I'm hypersensitive to any touch. If anyone even brushes against me I feel burning pain. Even the weight of my clothes against my skin bothers me. I'm trying to move my body as little as possible and keep it protected—but that's obviously impossible when even a breeze assaults me."
		Client observed holding the body stiffly looking like he or she does not know what to do with the arms and legs; dressed only in a loose-fitting outfit; reports that he or she sits at home all day afraid to go out
Kinesthetic	Clinitron bed therapy	"I've been in this bed for 2 weeks now and I've lost all sense of my body . . . it's a curious weightless feeling that I have . . . sort of like floating in Jell-O. I'm no longer sure where my body begins and ends, and when I try to lift an arm or leg I feel like I'm in slow motion. I hope I'll be able to walk when I get out of here."
Sensory/Perceptual Alteration: Sensory Deprivation	Isolation	"One of the worst things that has happened to me since I found out I had AIDS is that everyone is afraid of me—and no one touches me. I'm so lonely. I've always needed a lot of people around."

(continued)

NURSING DIAGNOSES FOR COMMON PROBLEMS

Sensory/Perceptual Alterations (*continued*)

Problem	Related Factors	Sample Defining Characteristics
		"Here in the hospital I think I'm going crazy. I can't leave this room. Everyone who comes in looks the same dressed in those yellow gowns. Lately I've seen some bizarre things that I know can't be real. I look at the clock and it turns into a swirling sun with a sad face that keeps coming closer and closer to me and I'm terrified I'll burn up if it gets too close. That's crazy isn't it? I'm really losing it now."
		Disturbed sleep for past 2 weeks; during the day yawns excessively and catnaps; limited attention span; states he or she is unable to concentrate on anything.
Sensory/Perceptual Alteration: Sensory Overload	Trauma of rape and aftercare	"When is everyone going to stop touching me? First he wouldn't stop. Now everyone here is poking at me, looking at me, asking me hundreds of questions. . . . Why did I have to report this and come to the hospital? Oh please leave me alone. Get out of here everyone."

Social Isolation related to visual or auditory impairment

Altered Thought Processes (specify: illusions, hallucinations, decreased attention or concentration, and so forth) related to sensory deprivation or overload

iors for visual impairment, hearing impairment, or other sensory impairment
• Verbalize acceptance of the sensory deficit

Planning: Client Goals

In whatever setting nurses encounter and care for clients, optimal sensory stimulation is a priority and nursing care is supportive of the following client goals. The client will:
• Live in a developmentally stimulating and safe environment
• Exhibit a level of arousal that enables the brain to receive and meaningfully organize patterns of stimulation
• Demonstrate intact functioning of the senses: vision, hearing, taste, smell, touch, kinesthetic and visceral awareness
• Maintain orientation to time, place, and person
• Respond appropriately (verbally and nonverbally) to sensory stimuli while executing self-care activities
Clients with impaired sensory functioning require individualized goals similar to the following. The client will:
• Report feeling safe and in control of the environment
• Describe different types of meaningful stimuli present in the environment
• Demonstrate (describe) appropriate self-care behav-

Implementing

The nurse can assist clients to improve sensory functioning by teaching clients and significant others means to stimulate the senses, teaching clients with intact and impaired senses appropriate self-care behaviors, and interacting therapeutically with impaired clients. Safety is always a special concern for clients with sensory alterations. Nurses are responsible for ensuring that the client's environment is as free of danger as possible and for assisting the client to develop new self-care behaviors to compensate for sensory impairments. Safety considerations are discussed in Chapter 25. In this section, the nursing interventions described are preventing sensory alteration, stimulating the senses, meeting the needs of visually impaired as well as hearing impaired people, communicating with a confused person, and communicating with an unconscious person.

Preventing Sensory Alteration and Stimulating the Senses

The most effective means by which sensory alteration can be managed is prevention. The key to prevention is, with the client's help, to create a functional and meaningful

RESEARCH IN NURSING Making a Difference

Appropriate Level of Stimuli

Identifying which patterns of stimuli are most promotive of human well-being for different clients is an ongoing challenge for nurses. In the studies that follow, nursing research targeted two specific client populations—preterm infants and cognitively impaired institutionalized elderly people—and explored which patterns of interaction facilitated well-being.

Related Research

Harrison, L. L., & Woods, S. (1991). Early parental touch and preterm infants. *Journal of Obstetric, Gynecologic, and Neonatal Nursing, 20*(4), 299–306.

Thirty-six parents were videotaped during visits with their preterm infants in a neonatal intensive care unit (NICU) to describe characteristics of parental touch. Ideally, this descriptive study will serve as a basis for designing controlled experiments to evaluate the effects of parental touch on premature infants. If a data base can be developed that identifies early interaction patterns predictive of subsequent maladaptive parent–infant relationships, parents in need of extra support and guidance can be identified and assisted early.

Burgener, S. C., & Barton, D. (1991). Nursing care of cognitively impaired institutionalized elderly. *Journal of Gerontological Nursing, 17*(4), 37–43.

In this study, nonverbal as well as verbal nursing staff behaviors were related to behaviors of demented elderly people, especially smiling, eye contact, and manipulating the environment to avoid difficult encounters. Use of verbal distraction or redirection, praise, and light-hearted, playful approaches were often found to be helpful when the demented elder became upset or paranoid.

Summary

It is important for nurses to continue to identify those patterns of interacting with clients that provide meaningful stimuli that facilitate the client's growth and development and sense of well-being. Clients with sensory impairments may have special needs.

---

environment while keeping limitations in mind. The creation of such an environment requires careful observation, analysis, and creative planning.

Numerous nursing measures can be considered in planning care. Appropriate measures for implementing depend on the circumstances. Well-being is promoted by offering care that provides rest and comfort (see Chapters 31 and 32). Client discomfort should be controlled whenever possible. The nurse should be aware of the need for sensory aids and prostheses, such as eyeglasses, contact lenses, hearing aids, dentures, canes, and artificial limbs, and these should be made available as needed. Physical activity and exercise, which help maintain normal sensory perceptions and decrease the likelihood of sensory alteration, should be encouraged (exercises are discussed in Chapter 30).

Stimulate as many senses as possible. Varied sights, sounds, smells, body positions, and textures can be helpful in providing a variety of sensations. Be aware of cultural factors and take them into consideration when offering nursing care. This is especially important when caring for clients from cultures other than your own.

Explain procedures to the client because a more informed client is better able to handle fears, frustration, and confusion. Explanations also help prevent the client from feeling that space and body are invaded. Individuals experiencing perceptual and thought distortions should have the opportunity to acknowledge that fact. The opportunity to discuss such experiences and be reassured that they are normal and usually temporary generally eases anxiety.

Teaching is a significant nursing responsibility. The nurse can aid clients in sensory self-stimulation and guide parents in stimulation of their infants and children. Table 39-2 gives helpful suggestions for teaching clients about sensory stimulation.

Meeting the Needs of Visually Impaired Clients

When caring for a client with a sensory deficit, it is important for the nurse to check with the physician if the problem is temporary, permanent, partial, or complete and the degree to which the problem is likely to affect the client's everyday functioning. The nurse cannot develop a realistic teaching plan without this information.

The nurse's first priority is to teach clients self-care behaviors to maintain vision and prevent blindness. Lindberg and Kruszewski (1983) offered the following suggestions:

• Avoid rubbing eyes.
• Avoid eyestrain.
• Avoid damage from ultraviolet rays.
• Protect eyes from foreign bodies.
• Keep eyeglasses clean, protected, adjusted.
• Avoid nonprescription eyedrops and seek attention for symptoms.

T A B L E 3 9 - 2

Suggestions for Stimulating the Senses

Sense	Client	Nurse
Vision	Surround yourself with different colors and with an environment that changes (walk through a mall, sit by a window where you see people come and go). Develop a sensitivity to changes in nature (weather patterns, dawn to night cycle, changing seasons, changes in a plant or animal). Use visual devices to keep oriented (watches, calendars, newspaper, television). Use crossword puzzles and games to stimulate mental activities. Create favorite scenes in your mind, paying attention to tiny details.	Wear visually stimulating and comforting colors. Keep meaningful visual stimuli such as photos, greeting cards, toys, or flowers near client. Position clients with impaired mobility where they can see out a window or watch local traffic on the unit.
Hearing	Decrease or eliminate distressing auditory stimuli (change bedroom, talk with family members about noise of stereos and other such equipment, use earplugs, use headphones to listen to soft music). Develop sensitivity to different sounds (music, chirping birds, night sounds, different voices). Use the telephone to maintain contact with family and friends. Use television, radio, cassettes to keep current and to stimulate mental activities. Recall favorite sounds of the past with the situations in which they were heard.	Speak in a warm and pleasant tone and communicate caring to the client. Use your voice to orient client to environment and current situation (eg, procedure, treatment). Avoid speaking about the client to others within the client's hearing. Remember that clients overhearing snatches of conversation outside their room often presume it is about *them!* Decrease extraneous noise (intercom, movement of carts, loud conversations of staff); use carpets and sound-absorbing material whenever possible.
Taste	Experiment with foods of different tastes (seasonings), colors, temperature, and textures; realize that as taste buds age, things will no longer taste the same. Practice thorough oral hygiene and have regular dental examinations. Recall foods that tasted especially good in the past and the events surrounding these tastes (eg, grandparent baking cookies or homemade bread).	Consult with the dietitian about preparing meals with varied taste sensations; serve meals attractively. Perform routine oral hygiene for clients who are unable to do this for themselves.
Smell	Consciously savor smells that are pleasant; decrease or eliminate noxious odors. Recall pleasant aromas or smells from the past and the events surrounding them (eg, smell of the ocean as the vacation house was neared, smell of fresh pine in the house at Christmas, the body scent of a loved person or animal).	Keep the client's room well ventilated, using opportunities when the client is out of the room to air it out. Remove dressings, drainage, and any equipment with odors from the client's room as quickly as possible. Encourage clients to focus on pleasant or familiar smells, such as coffee, newspaper, or flowers. Avoid wearing heavy perfumes.
Touch	Consciously surround yourself with different textures and let yourself feel and enjoy them (scratchy afghan; a puppy's moist, wet tongue; soft petal of a flower; smooth silk scarf; mug of hot chocolate). Allow these textures to evoke memories of past tactile experiences (grandchild's hug may bring back memories of hugs from own children, scrap of fabric may recall a prom dress or wedding gown or baby blanket). Recognize need to be touched and tell someone, "I need a hug today!" Receive tactile stimulation from a pet.	Include different textures in the client's environment (silky pillow sham from home, soft sheepskin, wooley blanket). Respect the client's need and desire to be touched or not touched (touch the client's forearm or shoulder, hug the client). Use physical care (bath time, foot soaks, hair care, back massages, turning and positioning, passive range of motion) to provide tactile stimulation. Limit intrusive procedures and times when the client needs to be uncomfortably manipulated.

(continued)

T A B L E   3 9 - 2 (*continued*)

Suggestions for Stimulating the Senses		
Sense	**Client**	**Nurse**
General Nursing Strategies in the Hospital or Other Residential Care Setting		Encourage the client to participate in activities that require exploration of the environment (exercise, feeling, tasting, touching, moving, listening).
		Use conversation to explore areas of interest to the client.
		Encourage the client to share feelings.
		Familiarize the environment by encouraging the client to wear own clothes and keep personal items nearby.
		Suggest the use of self-stimulation techniques—humming, singing, whistling, reciting, memory review, and problem solving.

- Avoid cleaning eyes or contact lenses with soiled articles.
- Use caution with aerosol sprays.
- Use caution with ammonia, lye, and so on.
- Visit your physician frequently if you are prone to eye problems.
- Know the danger signals that indicate serious eye problems: persistent eye redness; pain or discomfort, especially after injury; visual disturbances; crossing eyes; growth on or near the eyes; discharge or increased tearing; or pupil irregularities.

The following guidelines are recommended for communicating with people who are visually impaired:
- Acknowledge your presence in the client's room. Identify yourself by name.
- Speak in a normal tone of voice. Remember that the blind person is unable to pick up most nonverbal cues during communication.
- Explain the reason for touching the person before doing so.
- Keep the call light or bell within easy reach of the person and place the bed in the lowest position.
- Orient the person to sounds in the environment.
- Orient the person to the arrangement of the room and its furnishings. Clear pathways for the person and do not rearrange furnishings. Clarify this fact with housekeeping personnel also.
- Assist with ambulation by walking slightly ahead of the person, allowing the person to grasp your arm.
- Stay in the person's field of vision if the person has partial or reduced peripheral vision.
- Provide diversions using other senses.
- Indicate to the person when the conversation has ended and when you are leaving the room.

Meeting the Needs of Hearing Impaired Clients

Temporary hearing losses are most often *conductive* in nature, that is, they are due to a problem with the external or middle ear (wax buildup, foreign body obstruction, infection). *Sensorineural hearing losses* are caused by inner ear or central nervous system problems and may not be totally correctable. Health teaching to prevent hearing problems includes the following recommendations from Lindberg and Kruszewski (1983):
- Avoid excessive noise.
- Avoid inserting sharp objects into ears.
- Avoid excessive cleaning of ears.
- Avoid practices that can cause infection; treat infection early.
- Know the symptoms of hearing loss: asking frequently that statements be repeated, inability to hear at a distance, need to see the person who is talking, leaning forward or turning an ear toward the speaker, answering inappropriately, talking too loudly, inability to carry on a phone conversation, strained facial expression (pp. 307, 312).

The following are recommended guidelines for communicating with people with hearing deficits:
- Orient the person to your presence before initiating conversation. This may be done by moving so you can be seen or by *gently* touching the person.
- Decrease background noises (television, radio) if possible before you speak.
- Position yourself so the light is on your face and the person can see your lips and expressions.
- Talk directly to the person while facing the person or angle the chair so that your voice reaches the ear that hears best. If the person is able to lip-read, use simple sentences and speak in a quiet, natural manner and pace. Be aware of nonverbal communication.
- Do not chew gum, cover your mouth, or turn away when talking with the person.
- Demonstrate or pantomime ideas you wish to express, as appropriate.
- Use sign language or finger spelling, as appropriate.
- Write any ideas that you cannot convey to the person in another manner.

Communicating With a Confused Person

The client who lacks the mental ability to process environmental stimuli may be aware of this inability and find it frustrating. This client needs the nurse's support to make adjustments to this limitation. Other clients may be oblivious to the deficiency. In both instances, the nurse must protect the safety of the client while providing optimal sensory stimulation. Nursing interventions include the following:

- Using frequent face-to-face contact to communicate the social process (use touch when appropriate, walk arm in arm, hug, give a back rub)
- Speaking calmly, simply, and directly to the client and allowing sufficient time for the client to think before responding
- Orienting and reorienting the client to the environment and filling the client's personal space with as many personal objects as possible
- Using conversation, watches, clocks, calendar, newspaper, television, radio, and other such devices to orient the client to time, place, and person
- Clearly communicating that the client is expected to perform all self-care activities of which the client is capable
- Keeping the emphasis on client strengths rather than on deficiencies and verbally reinforcing strengths
- Offering the client simple explanations for care, new activities, and so on
- Varying environmental stimuli gradually while keeping the environment structured enough that the client feels comfortable and at home
- Using objects from the client's past (baseball, picture of a train, photograph) to spark reminiscences and discussions
- Reinforcing reality if the client is delusional

Communicating With an Unconscious Person

The following are recommended guidelines for communicating with an unconscious client:
- Be careful of what is said in the person's presence. Hearing is believed to be the last sense lost in the unconscious person, and therefore the person is often likely to hear what is being said, even though there does not appear to be a response.
- Assume the person can hear you. Talk with the person in a normal tone of voice about things you would ordinarily discuss.
- Speak to the person before touching. Remember that touch can be an effective means of communicating with the unconscious person.
- Keep environmental noises at as low a level as possible. This helps the person focus on the communication.

Evaluating

While implementing a nursing care plan designed to decrease excessive sensory stimuli or increase meaningful stimuli, the nurse evaluates the effectiveness of the plan by observing for a decrease in the behavioral manifestations of sensory deprivation or overload. It may be concluded that the care plan is working if a client who had begun to withdraw and spend most of the day lying in bed with a blank facial expression appears more alert and begins to initiate conversations and to take an interest in personal care. The nurse also evaluates the client's ability to interact appropriately with the environment while practicing necessary self-care behaviors. The client's achievement of the individualized goals specified in the care plan is evaluated at set times.

The nurse also evaluates the client's need for nursing versus ability to manage the care plan independently. Ideally, the client and family learn to manipulate the environment to promote optimal sensory stimulation for growth and development. Clients with specific sensory impairments are evaluated for their knowledge of the impairment, acceptance and management of the treatment regimen, and ability to perform necessary self-care activities.

 N U R S I N G   P R O C E S S

in Clinical Practice

The nurse uses each phase of the nursing process when identifying and treating sensory/perceptual alterations categorized as nursing diagnoses. Quality care depends on the nurse's knowledge and clinical skills as described earlier in this chapter. Following in outline format are the assessment priorities, client goals, nursing interventions, and evaluation criteria for two common types of age-related sensory deprivation problems:

Sensory/Perceptual Alterations: Sensory Deprivation related to parent's inability to provide a developmentally stimulating environment

Sensory/Perceptual Alterations: Chronic Sensory Deprivation related to effects of aging and institutionalization

In the case study that follows the development of these diagnoses, nursing care is described for a non–English-speaking client who is experiencing mixed sensory deprivation and overload on admission to the maternity unit in a large teaching hospital.

Sensory Deprivation Related to Inadequate Parenting

Sensory organs and nerve fibers need early sensory stimulation to develop normally both structurally and functionally. Parents may fail to provide a developmentally stimulating environment for their child for many reasons:

- Lack of knowledge of the child's growth and development needs
- Lack of motivation to promote the child's development
- Inadequate resources—parenting skills, finances, and so on

Assessment

- Use well-baby/child visits to monitor the child's development (gross motor behavior, fine motor, adaptive, language, personal–social).
- Assess if the child is receiving the stimulation and interactional experiences with the environment necessary to develop optimally. For example, if an infant is slow to crawl, see if parents and caretakers are providing supervised time to explore the environment on the floor versus leaving the infant in a baby chair, swing, or some other device all day. Similarly, if a child's expressions are dull and the child's language development is slow, assess the quality of human interaction and communication the child is receiving.
- Assess if the child's sensory/perceptual abilities are intact; identify sensory impairments and make appropriate referrals.
- If a lack of environmental stimulation is suspected, assess for possible etiologies: parents' lack of knowledge, motivation, skill, or resources; inadequate child care outside the home; other such factors.

Planning: Client Goals

The child will:
- Appear alert and interested in the environment
- Demonstrate improved sensory stimulation by achieving targeted developmental milestones (specify)
  The parents will:
- Identify the relation between sensory stimulation and the child's development
- Suggest reasons for the child's limited sensory experiences to date
- Describe a realistic and developmentally appropriate plan to increase visual, auditory, olfactory, gustatory, and tactile stimulation for the child
- Verbalize commitment to the plan

Interventions

Interventions should be tailored to the etiology of the problem. If the parents are eager to participate in the care plan and simply lack knowledge:
- Offer suggestions for increasing environmental stimulation and role model appropriate interactional behaviors.
  - *Visual:* Vary colors in the child's environment, increase access to out-of-the-home stimulation (parks, stores, fire engines, and other such stimuli), offer the child books with interesting pictures, and limit television.

- *Auditory:* Talk with and sing or hum to the child, read stories to the child, have the child join a storytelling group at the library, teach the child to become sensitive to nature's sounds or other sounds in the environment.
  - *Olfactory:* Allow the child to identify and distinguish different odors; role model for the child savoring special aromas (pizza coming out of the oven).
  - *Gustatory:* Encourage the child to experiment with foods of different tastes, shapes, colors, textures, and temperatures; recognize that children enjoy finger foods, foods that are crispy, chewy, or bubbly.
  - *Tactile:* Increase body contact with the child by means of games and sports as well as through demonstrative affection (hugs, holding child in lap, stroking face, and so on); if possible, allow the child to select a pet.
- Discuss with the parents developmentally appropriate play activities for children that will enable the child to learn social behavior, develop cognitive abilities, develop gross and fine motor skills, and work through emotional conflicts.
- Refer parents to parenting education group. If the parents lack the motivation to provide a developmentally stimulating environment for the child, intensive counseling is indicated with follow-up to ensure that the child is receiving adequate care. Counseling should explore the parents' experiences as children, the meaning the child holds for the parents, and the probability that the parents will learn and be motivated to use adequate parenting skills. If parents are resistant to counseling and child neglect is suspected, the nurse is legally responsible to report the family for evaluation.
- If lack of resources is contributing to the parents' difficulty in stimulating the child's development, available resources are explored. A referral to social services may be indicated.

Evaluative Criteria

The child and parents meet the previously stated goals.

Chronic Sensory Deprivation Related to Effects of Aging

Although the phenomenon of acute sensory deprivation has been carefully studied by nurses and other researchers, less attention has been paid to chronic sensory deprivation, a condition experienced by many elderly people. The elderly person who has multiple sensory deficits or who lives in a deprived environment is a prime candidate for chronic sensory deprivation. Symptoms of this disorder are most likely gradual in onset and are all too often mistaken for senility (Gioiella & Bevil, 1985).

Assessment

To define the extent of the problem and its etiologies, Gioiella and Bevil recommend careful data collection in the following seven areas: (1) sensory status; (2) level of mobility; (3) preferred stimulation level; (4) sensory, perceptual, and social environment; (5) mental status; (6) behavioral changes; and (7) personal resources. Using assessment guidelines presented earlier in this chapter, the nurse assesses the elderly person's vision, hearing, taste, smell, touch, and kinesthetic and visceral awareness. It is critical to understand that some older people have a need to deny sensory impairment and may evolve remarkable compensatory abilities. Behavioral changes (eg, withdrawal or the paranoia that many hearing-impaired elderly clients demonstrate) may be the best indicator of an underlying sensory problem.

Sensory Status

The senses of vision, hearing, and touch (and to a lesser degree, taste and smell) all decline with age. Moreover, many of the chronic illnesses experienced by elderly people impair sensory functioning. Common sensory problems include vision problems such as cataracts; **presbyopia** (condition of aging in which decreased elasticity of the lens hinders accommodation to close vision); glaucoma and macular degeneration; hearing problems such as **presbycusis** (age-related hearing loss in which there is decreased ability to distinguish higher frequencies); diminution of touch with diabetes and cerebrovascular disease; and altered body sense or awareness associated with restricted mobility and arthritis, cardiovascular and respiratory diseases, and neurologic disorders involving some degree of paralysis.

Level of Mobility

The less mobile an elderly client is, the more the client depends on the immediate environment and the more likely he or she is to experience sensory deprivation in an impoverished environment. The nurse needs to determine the client's physical ability to ambulate; the need for supportive devices (braces, canes, walkers, wheelchairs, railings, ramps); the client's motivation to be mobile; the presence of external factors hindering mobility ("I'm afraid if I go out of the house I'll be mugged"); and the need for support services (physical therapy, walking partner, transportation assistance, planned reinforcement).

Preferred Stimulation

Individuals vary greatly in the amount of stimulation they need. One older client sitting quietly may be enjoying reminiscences that effectively stimulate the brain whereas another client may be utterly bored and becoming disoriented.

Sensory, Perceptual, and Social Environment

The client's environment is assessed to determine if it presents a sufficient *variety* of meaningful sensory, cognitive, and emotional stimulation. Determine if each sense is being stimulated, if the client's mental abilities are being challenged, and if different emotions are being evoked. In caring families there often is a tendency to "do for" the older person, which may be counterproductive. The older person who has no need to meet everyday demands may feel useless and lose abilities not being used.

Mental Status

Changes in mental status or behavior may be the first indication of sensory deprivation. Assess for disorientation to time, place, or person; altered ability to concentrate or problem solve; and perceptual changes such as illusions or hallucinations.

Behavioral Changes

Significant behavioral changes include personality changes such as boredom and apathy, restlessness, withdrawal, and paranoia; alterations in sleep–wake patterns; decreased attention to personal hygiene and appearance; change in responses to others and communication patterns; and rapid mood swings.

Personal Resources

It is important to assess how well the client has coped with stresses in the past and the adequacy of supports available to the client currently.

Planning: Client Goals

The client will:
- Demonstrate orientation to time, place, and person
- Demonstrate interest in everyday self-care activities
- Demonstrate a decrease in the perceptual, cognitive, and emotional responses indicating sensory deprivation (specify)
- Actively participate in a plan to increase sensory stimulation

The client's caretakers (family, nursing staff) will:
- Identify factors contributing to sensory deprivation
- Develop a realistic plan to increase sensory, cognitive, and emotional stimulation

Interventions

- Make every effort to correct client's sensory impairments (eg, medical evaluation and treatment of sensory deficits; correct use and care of eyeglasses, contact lenses, hearing aids, ambulation aids).
- Ensure that the client has adequate periods of rest and that daytime activities prevent boredom and catnapping. Discourage the use of sedatives. Assess the central nervous system effect of any other medications the client is taking.
- Implement the plan to increase sensory stimulation (see Table 39-2). Homebound or institutionalized elderly people may benefit greatly from visits by chil-

dren. Pet therapy is an excellent source of stimulation. Simple activities like rolling a colorful, large, soft ball among four people seated at a table can effectively stimulate multiple senses (vision, hearing, touch, kinesthetic) for confused clients. Exercise classes for elderly clients also provide excellent stimulation.

- Make a concerted effort to increase the client's mobility and encourage changes in the environment. Use family and community resources to get the homebound client out of the house. Implement a plan to assist institutionalized clients to visit other parts of the institution, to get outside, and to participate in scheduled social events. Volunteers may be extremely helpful once committed to a plan of action.

- When interacting with the elderly client, communicate that the client is important and valued and make your expectations known.

- Avoid endorsing confusion. Gently reorient the client to reality whenever delusional statements are made.

- Keep the environment safe for the client.

Evaluative Criteria

The client and caretakers meet the previously stated goals.

CASE STUDY

Two days ago, Mrs. Philomela Palikias delivered by cesarean section a 32-week-old, small-for-gestational-age infant girl weighing 3 lb, 8 oz. Because of her size and respiratory distress, the infant was placed in NICU. Postpartal assessments indicate that Ms. Palikias's physical progress is satisfactory. However, the nurses are concerned about her mental status. Ms. Palikias arrived in the United States 3 months ago with her husband. Both speak only Greek and neither has family in the United States.

Assessment Findings

Recorded in the client's progress notes the evening of her second postpartal day is the following nursing assessment:

> 12/4/93, 9 PM, nursing
>
> Client refused to get out of bed again this evening—demonstrates no interest in seeing baby; to date has not ambulated to NICU. Refusing to learn and participate in self-care activities—expressing breast milk or performing perineal care. Nurses throughout the day reported sudden mood changes—apathy, frustration, panic, and hostility. Unable to find someone who speaks Greek to serve as translator. Husband does not speak English but appears concerned about his wife.
>
> *N. Gable, RN*

Nursing Diagnosis

Sensory/Perceptual Alterations: Mixed Sensory Deprivation and Overload related to unfamiliar hospital environment (different culture) and stress of cesarean birth and infant's prematurity

Planning: Client Goals

The nurse recognizes that the client's behaviors are most likely related to her:

- Being in a strange environment in which she cannot communicate
- Lacking familiar supports
- Being bombarded by new stimuli: cesarean birth; discomfort and pain; fear about the baby; fear about her parenting skills; strangers handling her body for reasons she does not understand; unfamiliar sights, sounds, smells, tastes, and touches of the hospital environment; unfamiliar feel of her own body (postsurgery and postdelivery)

The nurse's first move is to search the hospital (and outside community, if necessary) to find an interpreter to explain to Ms. Palikias what is happening. With the assistance of the interpreter, the nurse and client agree on the following goals.

Short-Term Goals

Before discharge, the client will:

- Demonstrate increased comfort in the hospital environment (absence of mood swings, apathy, frustration—panic, hostility)
- Resume usual self-care activities
- Demonstrate interest in her baby by visiting NICU, holding the baby, expressing her milk, and so on

Long-Term Goal

The client will:

- Develop communication strategies that will enable her to control the amount and quality of sensory stimulation she receives from her environment

Implementation

The nurse needs the following specialized abilities in implementing the care plan:

- Knowledge of and respect for different cultures and their influence on health and human functioning
- Ability to empathize with a young woman experiencing multiple stressors (sensory overload) with few customary supports

- Strong interpersonal skills and creative ability to communicate well to non–English-speaking client using body language, services of interpreter, and so on
- Strong assessment skills and knowledge of factors contributing to sensory alterations and of nursing interventions to prevent and treat sensory alterations
- Knowledge and clinical skills of maternity nursing
- Ability to communicate to client that what she is experiencing is understandable and that help is available
- Teaching and counseling skills to prepare the client to assume new mothering role with confidence
- Ability and willingness to go the extra mile with this client to ensure she is not lost in the system and discharged without receiving the assistance she needs
- Interpersonal and leadership skills to help the nursing staff view this client as a challenge and together to be committed to her care plan
- Human caring, compassion, strong sense of accountability for delivering quality care

Documentation

Sample documentation of the first session with the interpreter follows.

Traditional Note Format

12/5/93, 10 AM, nursing
   First session with interpreter and client at 9 AM. Client's face brightened as soon as she heard someone speak to her in Greek. Basically, client shared she did not care too much about what was happening to her but she was terrified about the baby and afraid of what everyone was doing to the baby. Di-

rected interpreter to orient client to her environment, daily routine, and NICU. Client appeared anxious when she first saw baby but looked content when able to hold her. Scheduled teaching session for tomorrow AM when interpreter will come for 1 hour. Client currently resting comfortably.

R. Traner, RN

SOAP Format

12/5/93, 9 PM, nursing
   #4 Sensory/Perceptual Alterations: Mixed Sensory Deprivation and Overload related to unfamiliar hospital environment and stress of cesarean birth and infant's prematurity

S: —
O: Cried after husband left this evening; refused postpartal check; turned away from nurses
A: Still feels overwhelmed by newness of all that is happening to her and tries to shut out what she cannot handle
P: Continue to intervene with help of interpreter; focus on helping client develop more control over her situation; proceed at slow pace; referral to social services for follow-up care

N. Gable, RN

Evaluation

Short-term goal achievement is evaluated each shift. See the care plan for related evaluative statements. Long-term goal achievement is ongoing.

NURSING CARE PLAN

for Mrs. Palikias

Nursing Diagnosis:	Sensory/Perceptual Alteration: Mixed Sensory Deprivation and Overload related to unfamiliar hospital environment (different culture) and stress of cesarean birth and infant's prematurity
Signs and Symptoms:	Demonstrating no interest in baby or self-care activities; limited ability to concentrate on new tasks (pericare, expressing breast milk); sudden mood changes—apathy, frustration, panic, hostility
Long-Term Goal:	Client will develop communication strategies that will enable her to control the amount and quality of sensory stimulation she receives from the environment.
Goal:	Before discharge, the client will: • Demonstrate increased comfort in the hospital environment (decreased or absent mood swings—apathy, frustration, panic, hostility)

(continued)

NURSING CARE PLAN (continued)

for Mrs. Palikias

Nursing Actions	Rationale	Evaluative Statement
Secure assistance of an interpreter and work with the interpreter to do the following:		12/6/93 Goal met. Client is quiet but no longer apathetic, fearful, or hostile. Moving about in hospital with more confidence.
• Orient the client to her surroundings (explaining reasons for equipment, procedures, treatment)	Sensory deprivation results from *meaningless*, unpatterned stimuli; once the client understands her environment she can respond to it appropriately.	*N. Gable, RN*
• Reassure the client that what she is experiencing is normal given her recent stresses (moving to new country, cesarean birth of first child, infant's prematurity)	Clients experiencing strange perceptual, cognitive, and affective responses to sensory deprivation and overload often fear they are going crazy and hesitate to share their feelings.	
• Determine the client's needs	The client herself is best able to voice her needs.	
Have the interpreter teach the nurse several Greek words and make recommendations about how the client can personalize her environment, such as having her husband provide her with usual food, music, and other familiar items.	Contributing to sensory deprivation is the absence of familiar sounds (native languages, sights, tastes, or scents. Having access to familiar food and the like may reduce sensory deprivation.	
See if the interpreter can explain usual customs regarding childbirth and aftercare in Greece.	Including culturally familiar childbirth and aftercare customs in the plan of care enhances client wellbeing and cooperation in the plan of care.	
Limit the number of nurses and other persons interacting with the client; attempt to have the same nurse caring for her each shift.	A trusting nurse–client relationship can develop	
Schedule care to allow for uninterrupted periods of sleep and rest.	Sleep deprivation contributes to other sensory alterations.	

Goal:	Before discharge, the client will:
	• Resume independent self-care activities

Nursing Actions	Rationale	Evaluative Statement
Use services of interpreter to teach client importance of ambulating and becoming independent again in self-care measures.	Regaining independence enhances client's sense of wellbeing.	12/6/93 Goal partially met. Client is ambulating, but she resists pericare and is fearful when expressing breast milk.
Have interpreter write simple directions for follow-up care, times when baby may be visited after	Cognitive responses to sensory deprivation and overload include decreased attention span and	*Recommendation:* Continue teaching with assistance of interpreter.
		N. Gable, RN

(continued)

N U R S I N G   C A R E   P L A N (continued)

for Mrs. Palikias

Nursing Actions	Rationale	Evaluative Statement
client is discharged, and so on. Share these instructions with the client's husband.	concentration and problem-solving ability. Written instructions and husband's knowledge reinforce the client's learning.	
See if husband has bilingual friends or work acquaintances who might be willing to help the client when she gets home until she has established a comfortable routine of care for the baby and is knowledgeable about community resources.	Careful discharge planning is necessary to ensure that the client can manage new parenting responsibilities in an unfamiliar country.	

Goal: Before discharge, the client will:
• Demonstrate interest in her baby by visiting the neonatal intensive care unit, holding the baby, expressing her milk, and other such activities.

Nursing Actions	Rationale	Evaluative Statement
Learn and respect cultural norms for new mothering behaviors.	Nursing care that is not culturally sensitive is deficient.	12/6/93 Goal met. Client is now visiting baby in the unit on her own.
Assist the client to ambulate to unit to see the baby; if interpreter is available, have the person explain equipment surrounding the baby and answer the client's questions about the baby.	The client may be refusing to visit the unit to protect herself from barrage of frightening stimuli (sensory overload); the goal is for her to become familiar with the unit so she is able to focus on bonding with her daughter.	*N. Gable, RN*

KEY POINTS

• The senses of vision, hearing, smell, taste, and touch keep an individual in contact with the external environment. The kinesthetic and visceral senses arise from muscles and hollow organs, respectively, and orient the individual to the internal environment.

• The brain must be alert or aroused to receive stimuli and respond appropriately. The reticular activating system, with its many ascending and descending connections to other areas of the brain, monitors and regulates incoming sensory stimuli and thus maintains, enhances, or inhibits cortical arousal.

• Sensory alterations occur when a person experiences decreased sensory input or input that is monotonous, unpatterned, or meaningless (sensory deprivation); or excessive sensory input such that the brain is unable to respond meaningfully (sensory overload).

• Responses to both sensory deprivation and overload include perceptual changes (mild to gross distortions or hallucinations); cognitive changes (decreased attention and concentration, decreased problem-solving ability); and affective changes (apathy, anxiety, fear, panic, anger, depression, or rapid mood swings).

• Clients at high risk for sensory deprivation include those experiencing decreased environmental stimuli (homebound or institutionalized clients, clients on bed rest or in isolation) and those with impaired ability to receive or process environmental stimuli (clients with sensory deficits, clients from a different culture, clients with certain affective disorders and disturbances of the nervous system, clients with bandages or casts that interfere with sense reception, clients taking medications that affect the central nervous system).

- Clients at high risk for sensory overload include acutely ill clients, clients in critical care settings, clients in pain, clients with intrusive and discomforting monitoring or treatment equipment, and clients with disturbances of the nervous system.
- Factors affecting sensory stimulation include age, culture, personality and life-style, stress, illness, and medication.
- A comprehensive nursing assessment of sensory functioning includes an examination of the client for sensory deficits and manifestations of sensory deprivation or overload and an examination of the client's environment to see if it is providing adequate sensory stimulation for healthy development.
- Nursing diagnoses may be written specifically addressing sensory/perceptual alterations (visual, auditory, olfactory, gustatory, tactile, sensory deprivation, sensory overload) or identifying the effect sensory/perceptual alterations have in other areas of human functioning (eg, verbal communication, self-care, social interaction, thought processes).

- Small modifications in a client's environment and in the nurse's pattern of interacting may be all that is needed to prevent sensory alterations.
- Sensory deprivation during a child's formative years may yield permanent results because sensory organs and nerve fibers need early sensory stimulation to develop normally both structurally and functionally. Parents may fail to provide a developmentally stimulating environment for their child because of lack of knowledge, decreased motivation, or inadequate resources.
- The elderly person who has multiple sensory deficits or who lives in a nonstimulating environment is at high risk for chronic sensory deprivation. Symptoms of this disorder are frequently mistaken for senility.

STUDY QUESTIONS

1. The major components of any sensory experience are
   a. the kinesthetic and visceral senses
   b. reception and perception
   c. the intensity, size, change, or representation of stimuli
   d. vision, hearing, smell, taste, and touch
2. Four conditions necessary for a person to receive data and experience the world are
   a. a stimulus, a receptor, an intact nerve pathway, and a functioning brain
   b. the visual, auditory, olfactory–gustatory, and tactile senses
   c. the basic orienting systems arising from muscles, joints, hollow organs, and movement
   d. the reticular activating system, variable stimuli, memory, and motivation
3. By monitoring and regulating incoming sensory stimuli, this system maintains, enhances, or inhibits cortical arousal
   a. general adaptation system
   b. kinesthetic/visceral system
   c. reticular activating system
   d. sensory/perceptual system
4. You notice that Mr. Wong, who has cataracts, is sitting closer to the television than usual. The etiology of his sensory problem is
   a. altered environmental stimuli
   b. altered sensory reception
   c. altered nerve impulse conduction
   d. altered impulse translation

5. Should you learn that Mr. Wong, who is 85 years old, also has presbycusis, you would want to
   a. obtain large print written material
   b. speak distinctly using lower frequencies
   c. decrease tactile stimulation
   d. initiate a safety program to prevent falls
6. Peter Almone is in the last stages of AIDS, which is now affecting his brain as well other major organ systems. He confides to you that he feels terribly alone because most of his friends are afraid to visit. The etiology of his sensory alterations is most likely related to
   a. stimulation
   b. reception
   c. transmission–perception–reaction
   d. all of the above
7. Which of the following factors is least likely to place a client at high risk for sensory deprivation?
   a. an environment with decreased or monotonous stimuli
   b. impaired ability to receive environmental stimuli
   c. impaired ability to process environmental stimuli
   d. impaired ability to respond to environmental stimuli
8. Which of the following clients is at greatest risk for sensory deprivation?
   a. elderly man confined to bed at home after a stroke

b. adolescent in an oncology unit working on homework supplied by friends

c. woman in labor

d. toddler in a play room awaiting same-day surgery

9. A client in an intensive care burn unit for 1 week is in pain much of the time, and has his face and both arms heavily bandaged. His wife visits every evening for 15 minutes at 6, 7, and 8 PM. A heart monitor beeps for a client on one side and another client moans frequently. These data suggest that the client probably

a. has sufficient sensory stimulation

b. has deficient sensory stimulation

c. has excessive sensory stimulation

d. has both sensory deprivation and overload

10. Richard's spinal cord was severed and he is paralyzed from the waist down. In making an assessment of this client, it is most important to assess which component of the sensory experience?

a. transmission of tactile stimuli

b. adequate stimulation in the environment

c. reception of visual and auditory stimuli

d. general orientation and ability to follow commands

11. An 11-year-old 6th grader whose grades have dropped has difficulty completing her work on time, frequently rubs her eyes, and squints. Her visual acuity on a Snellen's eye chart was 160/20. Based on these data, the most appropriate nursing diagnosis is

a. Knowledge Deficit related to visual impairment

b. Altered Role Performance (Student) related to visual impairment

c. Body Image Disturbance related to visual impairment

d. Altered Growth and Development related to visual impairment

12. Of the four items listed below, the best nursing intervention to prevent sensory alterations for a man with a severe hearing deficit who reads lips well is

a. turn the radio or television volume up very loud and close the door to his room

b. prevent embarrassment and emotional discomfort as much as possible

c. provide daily opportunity for him to participate

in a social hour with six or eight people

d. encourage daily participation in exercise and physical activity

13. In a boarding home where most clients have slight-to-moderate visual or hearing impairment, and some are periodically confused, the nurse's first priority in caring for sensory concerns is to

a. maintain safety and prevent sensory deterioration

b. insist that every client participate in as many self-care activities as possible

c. emphasize and reinforce individual client strengths

d. encourage reminiscence and life review in groups

14. The nursing diagnosis for 8-month-old Sally was Sensory/Perceptual Alterations: Sensory Deprivation related to inadequate parenting. Since that time, both parents have attended parenting classes. However, both parents work while Sally stays with her 86-year-old grandmother who is visually impaired. The parents provide appropriate stimulation in the evening. At an evaluation conference at age 11 months, Sally lay on the floor sucking her thumb and rocking her body. Her facial expression was dull and she vocalized only in a low monotone uh-h-h. Your best evaluation concerning Sally's sensory deprivation is that

a. her parents lack motivation to provide necessary stimulation

b. her grandmother is unable to improve Sally's care

c. sally's sensory deprivation is still severe

d. this is normal behavior for a child of Sally's age

15. Which of the following nursing interventions should NOT have been implemented for an elderly woman in a nursing home who walked out the door unobserved and was was hit by a car? The nursing diagnosis was Sensory/Perceptual Alterations: Chronic Sensory Deprivation related to the effects of aging:

a. Ignore when the client is confused or go along to prevent embarrassment.

b. Encourage self-care and independent decisions.

c. Take walks around the grounds and to the garden daily.

d. Provide daily contact with children, community people, and pets.

Answers With Rationale

1. The correct response is *b*. Reception and perception are the major components of any sensory experience. All other choices are merely part of the sensory experience.

2. The correct response is *a*. A stimulus, a receptor, an intact nerve pathway, and a functioning brain are the four conditions necessary for a person to receive data and experience the world.

3. The correct response is *c*. The reticular activating system maintains, enhances, or inhibits cortical arousal by monitoring and regulating incoming sensory stimuli.

4. The correct response is *b*. Cataracts are interfering with the client's ability to receive visual stimuli—altered sensory reception. The nature of incoming stimuli, the conduction of nerve impulses, and the translation of incoming impulses in the brain are not a problem here.

5. The correct response is *b*. Presbycusis is a normal loss of hearing as a result of the aging process. Speaking distinctly in lower frequencies is indicated. The other choices refer to interventions for other sensory problems.

6. The correct response is *d*. This client is receiving decreased environmental stimuli (eg, from his friends); is more than likely experiencing problems with reception because of major organ involvement; and his impaired brain function will impair impulse transmission–perception–reaction.

7. The correct response is *d*. The other options all pertain to components of the sensory experience that, if impaired, may place a client at high risk for sensory deprivation. An impaired ability to respond to environmental stimuli places a client at risk for problems other than sensory deprivation.

8. The correct response is *a*. The client confined to bed rest at home is at risk of having his environmental stimuli greatly reduced. The other clients are all in environments where environmental stimuli are at least adequate.

9. The correct response is *d*. This client's bandages may result in deficient sensory stimulation (sensory deprivation) and the monitors and other sounds in the intensive care burn unit may cause a sensory overload. All other options are incomplete responses.

10. The correct response is *a*. Below-the-waist paralysis makes the transmission of tactile stimuli a problem. Although the other options may be assessed, they are indirectly related to his paralysis.

11. The correct response is *b*. An important role for an 11-year-old is that of student. Her impaired vision is clearly disturbing her role performance as a student as evidenced by her lower grades. Although the other options may also represent accurate diagnoses for this client, they do not flow from the data that were presented.

12. The correct answer is *c*. Providing daily opportunities for this client to participate in a social hour builds on his strength of being able to lip-read and provides sufficient sensory stimulation to prevent sensory deprivation resulting from his hearing loss.

13. The correct answer is *a*. Safety is a basic physiologic need that must be met before higher-level needs such as love and belonging, self-esteem, and self-actualization can be met.

14. The correct response is *c*. Although the data show that the parents have been motivated to improve their parenting skills, it is clear from the data presented that Sally's sensory deprivation is still severe. The data suggest that the grandmother was not improving Sally's care, but there is nothing to suggest that she is *unable* to do so if shown how.

15. The correct response is *a*. Even if well-motivated, ignoring a client's confusion to prevent embarrassment may be dangerous, as it was in this case where the appropriate safety precautions were never implemented. The other options are all appropriate for this client.

BIBLIOGRAPHY

Alleyne, B. C. (1989). Hearing loss: Can knowing what it costs society help reduce its occurrence? *Canadian Journal of Public Health, 80*(6), 463–464.

Andrews, J. F., & Wilson, H. F. (1991). The deaf adult in the nursing home. *Geriatric Nursing, 12*(6), 279–283.

Blank, D. M., & Mattes, R. D. (1990). Sugar and spice: Similarities and sensory attributes. *Nursing Research, 39*(5), 290–293.

Bolin, R. H. (1974). Sensory deprivation: An overview. *Nursing Forum, 13*(3), 240–258.

Broussard, A. B. (1990). Incorporating infant stimulation concepts into prenatal classes. *Journal of Obstetric, Gynecologic, and Neonatal Nursing, 19*(5), 381–387.

Brown, I. A. (1985). Sensory deprivation: An overview. *Journal of Neurosurgery Nursing, 17*(5), 273–279.

Burgener, S. C., & Barton, D. (1991). Nursing care of the cognitively impaired institutionalized elderly. *Journal of Gerontological Nursing, 17*(4), 37–43.

Burnside, I. M. (1973). Touching is talking. *American Journal of Nursing, 73*(12), 2060–2063.

Christian, E. (1989). Sounds of silence: Coping with hearing loss and loneliness. *Journal of Gerontological Nursing, 15*(11), 4–9, 33–34.

Cole, J. (1991). Cuddles for kids. *Canadian Nurse, 87*(3), 30–31.

Gioiella, E., & Bevil, C. (1985). Nursing care of the aging client. Norwalk, CT: Appleton-Century-Crofts.

Glynn, N. J. (1992). The music therapy assessment tool in Alzheimer's patients. *Journal of Gerontological Nursing, 18*(1), 3–9.

Harrison, L. L. (1990). Minimizing barriers when teaching hearing-impaired clients. *MCN, 15*(2), 113.

Harrison, L. L., & Woods, S. (1991). Early parental touch and preterm infants. *Journal of Obstetric, Gynecologic, and Neonatal Nursing, 20*(4), 299–306.

Janken, J. K. (1990). Auditory sensory/perceptual alteration: Suggested revision of defining characteristics. *Nursing Diagnosis, 1*(4), 147–154.

Johnson, S. M., Omery, A., & Nikas, D. (1989). Effects of conversation on intracranial pressure in comatose patients. *Heart and Lung, 18*(1), 56–63.

Kee, C. C. (1990). Sensory impairment: Factor X in providing nursing care to the older adult. *Journal of Community Health Nursing, 7*(1), 45–52.

Kloosterman, N. D. (1991). Cultural care: The missing link in severe sensory alteration. *Nursing Science Quarterly, 4*(3), 119–122.

Kolanowski, A. M. (1992). The clinical importance of environmental lighting to the elderly. *Journal of Gerontological Nursing, 18*(1), 10–14.

Koniak-Griffin D., & Ludington-Hol S. M. (1988). Developmental and temperament outcomes of sensory stimulation in healthy infants. *Nursing Research, 37*(2), 70–76.

Lindberg, J. B., & Kruszewski A. Z. (1983). Special senses and the environment. In J. Lindberg, M. Hunter, & A. Kruszewski (Eds.), *Introduction to person-centered nursing* (pp. 297–315). Philadelphia: Lippincott.

MacKinnon-Kesler, S. (1983). Maximizing your ICU patient's sensory and perceptual environment. *Canadian Nurse, 79*(5), 41–45.

Mayers, K., & Griffin, M. (1990). The play project: Use of stimulus objects with demented patients. *Journal of Gerontological Nursing, 16*(1), 32–35.

Newman, D. (1990). Assessment of hearing loss in elderly people: The feasibility of a nurse administered screening test. *Journal of Advanced Nursing, 15*(4), 400–409.

Norris, C. M. (1985). Primitive pleasure as the basic human state. *Advances in Nursing Science, 8*(1), 25–43.

Oehler, J. M. (1991). Beyond technology: Meeting developmental needs of infants in NICUs. *Maternal–Child Nursing, 16*(3), 148–151.

Palumbo, M. V. (1990). Hearing access 2000: Increasing awareness of hearing impaired. *Journal of Gerontological Nursing, 16*(9), 26–31, 37–38.

Ross, V., Echevarria, K. H., & Robinson, B. (1991). Geriatric tinnitus: Causes, clinical treatment, and prevention. *Journal of Gerontological Nursing, 17*(10), 6–11.

Schiefer, C. C., Sr. (1982). The need for effective perception. In H. Yura & M. Walsh (Eds.), *Human needs 2 and the nursing process* (pp. 155–203). Norwalk, CT: Appleton-Century-Crofts.

Schultz, D. (1965). *Sensory restriction: Effects on behavior.* New York: Academic Press.

Suedfeld, P. (1985). Stressful levels of environmental stimulation. *Issues in Mental Health Nursing, 7*(1/4), 83–104.

Sullivan, J. (1990). Neurologic assessment. *Nursing Clinics of North America, 25*(4), 795–809.

Yazdanfar, D. J. (1990). Assessing the mental status of the cognitively impaired elderly. *Journal of Gerontological Nursing, 16*(9), 32.

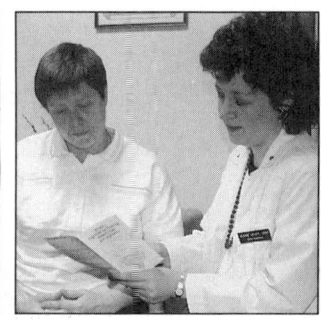
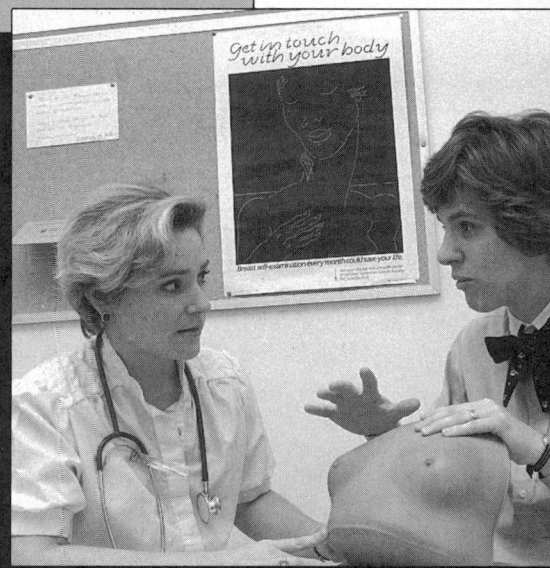

Sexuality

40

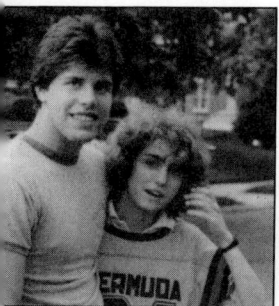
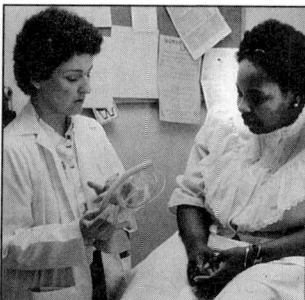

When people visit a health care facility, they bring all aspects of their individuality with them. This includes sexuality, which permeates a person's life both in illness and in wellness. **Sexuality** is the degree to which a person exhibits and experiences maleness or femaleness physically, emotionally, and mentally. Sexuality is defined not only by a person's genitalia but also by attitudes and feelings. It can also be defined as learned behaviors in how a person reacts to his or her own sexuality and by how one behaves in relationships with others. Sexuality is an integral part of a person's identity and is present in one's demeanor through actions, communications, and physical appearances. A person's sexuality is therefore a concern in professional nursing care.

This chapter discusses reproductive anatomy and physiology, the sexual response cycle, and factors that affect sexuality. Obtaining a sexual history as part of a comprehensive client history is presented as well as interview questions that specifically address a client with a sexual dysfunction. Nursing priorities with regard to assessment of the reproductive system are presented along with the progressive steps of the examination. Analysis of assessment data is discussed with examples of corresponding nursing diagnoses. The section Nursing Process in Clinical Practice provides the nurse with a format that uses assessment data, planning, interventions, and evaluations for nursing diagnoses that pertain to concerns with sexuality (Sexual Dysfunction: Inhibited Sexual Desire; Altered Sexuality Patterns: Change in Sexual Expression; Knowledge Deficit: Contraceptive Methods; and Body Image Disturbance: Surgical Removal of a Breast). The case study and care plan provide the nurse with examples of how the information presented in the chapter can be used in a clinical setting to nurture and promote aspects of sexuality in clients.

Physiology

Female

The female genitalia are represented by both internal and external structures. The external genitalia are illustrated in Figure 24-51. The appearance of these structures varies slightly among individuals.

External Genitalia

The *mons pubis* is actually a pad of fatty tissue that lies over the part of the bony pelvis called the *symphysis pubis*. In the physically mature female, the mons pubis is covered with coarse *pubic hair*. It contains many nerve endings that make the mons pubis sensitive to touch and pressure. The *labia majora* consist of two rounded folds of fatty tissue. The outer lips separate downward from the mons pubis and meet again below the vaginal introitus. The labia majora contain a multitude of sebaceous and sweat glands. They respond to touch during sexual activity. The *labia minora* are the smaller lips located within the labia majora. They are thin and sensitive structures and are pale pink in color. When stimulated by touch, the labia minora may turn a darker pink or even red due to the presence of many blood vessels. The labia minora have no hair and are smooth in texture.

The *clitoris* is found above the urinary meatus at the joining of the labia minora, called the *clitoral hood*. The clitoris is a small button-like structure similar to the male penis in its reaction to stimuli. The clitoris contains erectile tissue, blood vessels, and nerves. It is extremely sensitive. The opening of the vagina lies between the urinary meatus and the anus. It may contain a structure called the *hymen*, which is a thick membrane with no apparent function. At one time, the hymen was thought to represent *virginity* (not having experienced sexual intercourse); however, this is erroneous. Remnants, or "tags," of the hymen may be noted at the vaginal introitus in both sexually active and inactive women.

Internal Genitalia

The internal genitalia—the ovaries, fallopian tubes, uterus, and vagina (Fig. 40-1)—are located deep within the pelvis of the female. The female body normally contains two ovaries, one on each side of the body. The ovaries closely resemble an almond in size and shape. At the time of a female child's birth, each ovary contains some 200,000 to 400,000 follicles. This number steadily decreases until puberty, when 100,000 to 200,000 follicles remain, and the number continues to decline over the reproductive years. The process of ovulation is discussed later in this chapter. The ovaries also secrete the hormones estrogen and progesterone.

The *fallopian tubes* are slender structures that extend from either side of the uterus and end in a fringed fashion near each ovary. Their function is to transport a mature *ovum* (female reproductive cell) from an ovary to the uterus. Fertilization of the ovum by a sperm usually occurs in the tube. The fertilized ovum then travels the rest of the way to the uterus, where it implants. An unfertilized ovum travels the same path but does not implant. It is eventually expelled from the body during the menses. Because the lumen of each tube is so narrow, it can easily be damaged by the effects of infection and surgery.

The *uterus* is a pear-shaped organ about 3 inches long located between the urinary bladder and the rectum. Its

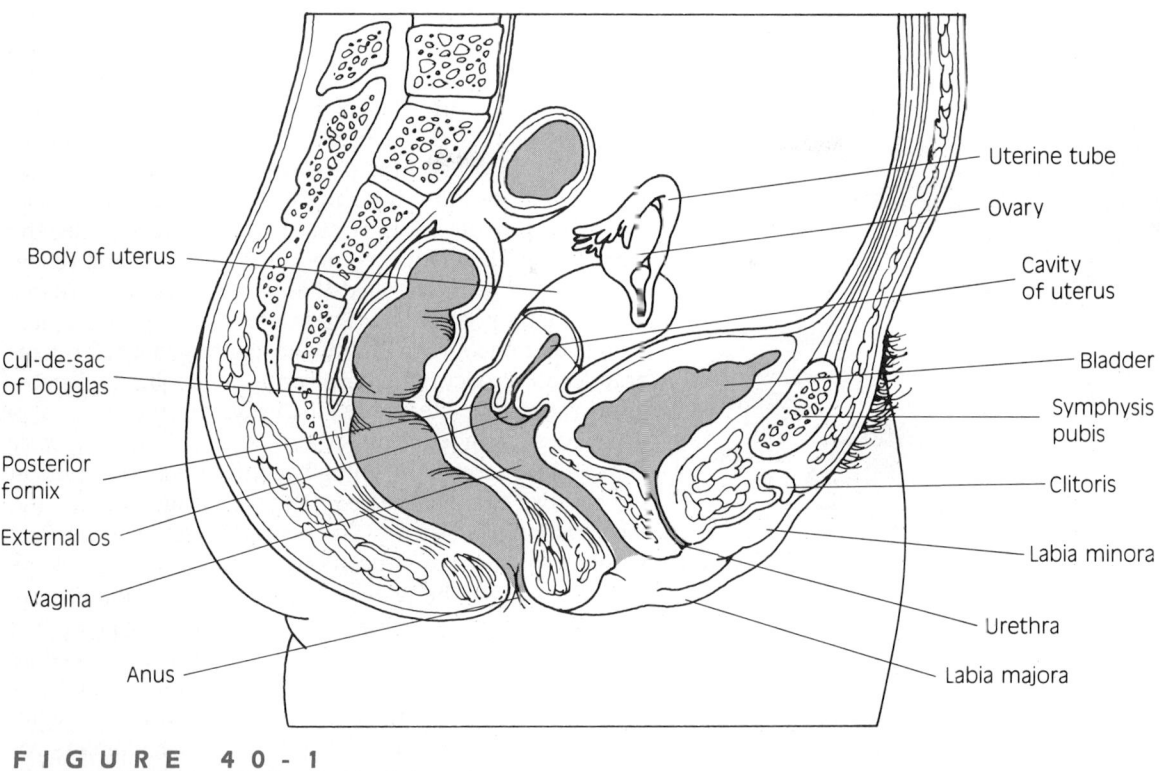

FIGURE 40-1

Sagittal section of the female reproductive organs.

Labels: Body of uterus, Cul-de-sac of Douglas, Posterior fornix, External os, Vagina, Anus, Uterine tube, Ovary, Cavity of uterus, Bladder, Symphysis pubis, Clitoris, Labia minora, Urethra, Labia majora

primary purpose is to house and nurture a *pregnancy* (the condition of carrying a developing embryo in the uterus). The uterus comprises three layers: the outermost layer, the *perimetrium*, consists of elastic tissue; the middle layer, the *myometrium*, is muscular; and the innermost layer, the *endometrium*, comprises tissue that thickens and sloughs off with the menses. The *cervix* is the structure at the lower portion of the uterus that connects the uterus and the vagina. The cervix is usually closed. However, during the birth process, it dilates and thins out extensively to permit the birth of a baby. The cervix is a smooth, pink-colored structure that possesses few nerve endings. When touched, the sensation resembles that of touching the end of one's nose.

The *vagina* is a tubular, hollow organ that lies between the urinary urethra and the rectum. Its size and shape are individual among women. The walls of the vagina are composed of ruga or ribbed tissue. The vagina serves three purposes: it is (1) a receptacle for the penis during sexual intercourse, (2) a birth canal for the passage of a baby, and (3) an exit for menstrual flow from the uterus. During sexual activity, the walls of the vagina secrete, or "sweat," a thin watery material, sometimes in copious amounts. This lubrication is necessary for the comfortable placement and movement of the penis in the vagina.

Breasts

Although the breasts are not considered part of the internal or external genitalia, they are an important aspect of the female's physical sexuality. The breasts consist of fatty and glandular tissues and the nipples. Their size and shape vary widely among women. The nipples are pale to deep pink in color. Caressing of the breasts can be pleasurable during sexual activity, and many women can be brought to orgasm by this action alone.

Menstrual Cycle

Menstruation is a cycle during which the body prepares for the presence of a fertilized ovum. Each cycle is about 28 days long but may vary from as short as 21 days to as long as 40 days. The first menstrual period, called **menarche**, is experienced around age 12 years. Again, the age of menarche is individual and may occur at age 8 years to age 17 years. **Menopause**, the cessation of a woman's menstrual activity, occurs between the ages of 45 and 55 years. The woman may experience irregular menses over time before menstruation ends.

The menstrual cycle is controlled by a series of reactions that rely on feedback from the ovaries to the pituitary gland. Actually two cycles occur simultaneously, one in the ovaries and one in the uterus (Fig. 40-2).

In the ovaries, in a typical 28-day cycle, the phase from day 4 to 14 is called the *follicular phase*. During this phase, a number of follicles mature but only one produces a mature ovum. At the same time, in the uterus, the endometrium is becoming thick and velvety in preparation for receiving a fertilized egg. This phase in the uterus is called the *prolifera-*

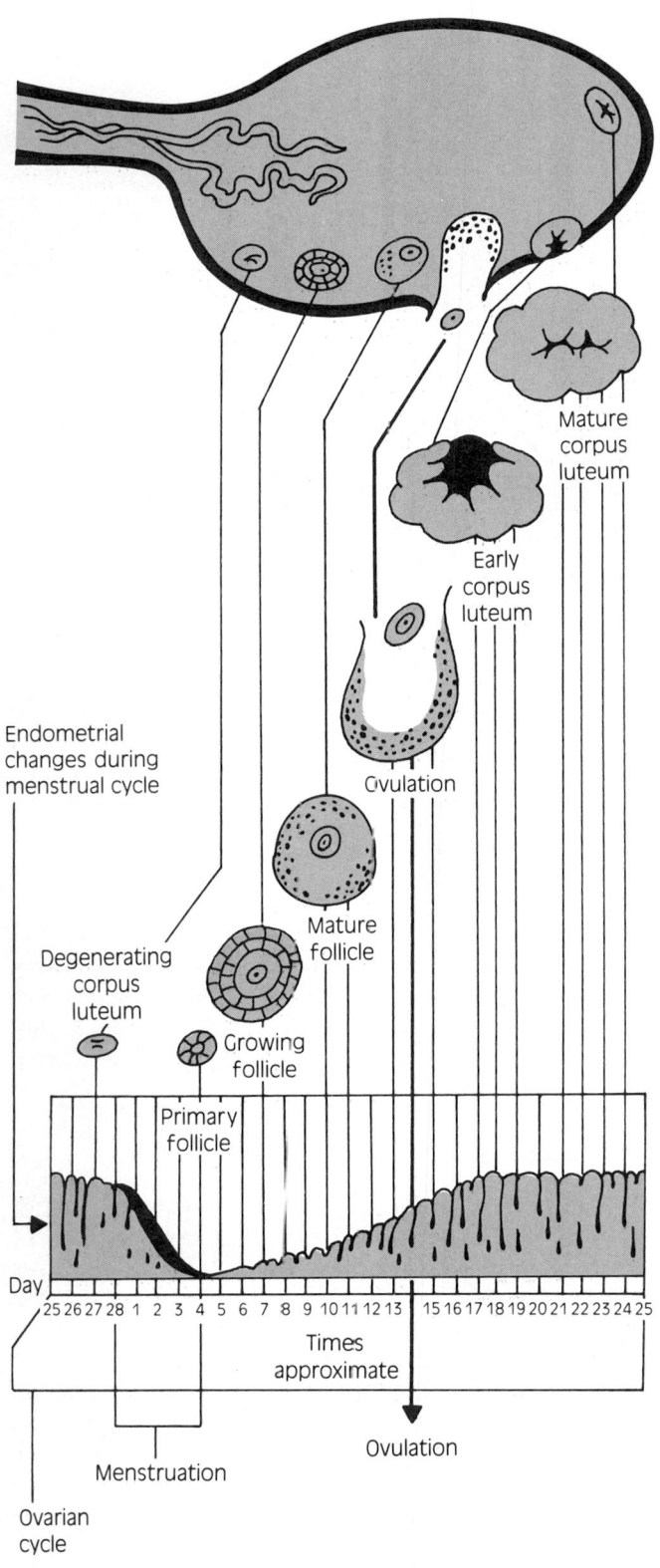

Endometrial changes during menstrual cycle

Degenerating corpus luteum

Mature corpus luteum

Early corpus luteum

Ovulation

Mature follicle

Growing follicle

Primary follicle

Day

25 26 27 28 1 2 3 4 5 6 7 8 9 10 11 12 13 15 16 17 18 19 20 21 22 23 24 25

Times approximate

Ovulation

Menstruation

Ovarian cycle

F I G U R E   4 0 - 2

Schematic representation of one ovarian cycle and the corresponding changes in the endometrium.

tion phase. **Ovulation** occurs on day 14. The mature ovum ruptures from the follicle and the surface of the ovary and is swept into the fallopian tube. If sperm are present, the ovum is fertilized at this time. Some women can detect ovulation by the presence of a sharp, cramping pain over the ovulating ovary. This pain is called *mittelschmerz*, or middle pain, because it occurs in the middle of the cycle. From day 15 to day 28, the phase in the ovaries is called the *luteal phase.* The leftover empty follicle fills up with a yellow pigment and is then called the *corpus luteum*, or yellow body. The purpose of the corpus luteum is to produce hormones that encourage a fertilized egg to grow. If fertilization does not occur, the corpus luteum begins to disintegrate. During the luteal phase in the ovaries, the uterus also undergoes changes. This phase is called the *secretory phase.* The endometrial lining becomes thick. However, in the absence of a fertilized egg, the corpus luteum dies and the endometrial lining disintegrates. At day 28, the **menses**, or the menstrual flow, begin as a result of the uterus shedding the useless portion of its endometrium.

The menses lasts for 3 to 7 days, the average length of flow being 5 days. The menstrual discharge is a bloody fluid that also contains endometrial debris, mucus, and enzymes. It is odorless until exposed to the air, when a light, fleshy, pungent odor may be noticed by the woman. Deodorized pads and tampons do little to minimize odor and can cause a chemical irritation to the vulva and vagina. Good hygiene and regular bathing are much more effective during the menses to prevent odor. Normal blood loss averages between 30 and 80 mL. Pads and tampons should be changed frequently to prevent odor and irritation from wetness. Women using tampons should be advised to read and follow the manufacturer's suggestions to reduce the risk of toxic shock syndrome. Usually the flow is the heaviest and is bright red in color on the first day or two of the menses, gradually tapering off in amount to light brown staining. Many women experience some degree of discomfort either premenstrually or at the time of the menses.

There is no scientific rationale supporting abstinence from sexual activity during the menses. Many women enjoy sex during the menses due to the increase in vascularity in the pelvic region, which heightens enjoyment. Men may also enjoy the warm wetness the menstrual flow provides to the vagina. If the flow is heavy, a diaphragm can be used to hold back the flow until sexual activity ceases or a towel can be placed under the woman's buttocks to protect bedding. Women who experience abdominal cramping during the menses, or dysmenorrhea, find that sexual activity and orgasm relieve their discomfort.

Premenstrual (Tension) Syndrome Menstrual cycle-related distress, commonly called PMS, reportedly occurs in 50% to 90% of the female population. PMS is characterized by the appearance of one or more of the following several days before the onset of menstruation: irritability, emotional tension, anxiety, mood changes, headache, breast tenderness, and water retention. Although it is often used to explain unusual behavior (and has been used as a legal defense) its etiology is still uncertain (both physiologic and psychogenic theories have been postulated) as are its effects on women's roles and relationships. Most of the current PMS literature perpetuates a twofold myth: (1) biology and physiology are destiny (many females do and should experience premenstrual distress) and (2) female biology and physiology result in psychiatric disorder, destruction, and violence (Winter, Ashton, & Moore, 1991). Nurses have a great role to play in researching PMS and ensuring that women and the public correctly understand its effects.

Male

Unlike female genitalia, the male genitalia are found primarily outside the body. These structures are illustrated in Figure 24-53. The *testes*, which are about the size of walnuts, feel smooth and are freely movable within the scrotum. The *scrotum* is the loose baglike structure that houses the testes. Normally two testes are present. The testes produce **sperm** and the hormones necessary for the maintenance of male sex characteristics. The primary hormone secreted by the testes is *testosterone*, which is responsible for a man's deep voice, beard growth, and body hair.

The scrotum hangs between a man's upper thighs. The area around the base of the penis and the scrotum is covered with pubic hair. The looseness of the scrotum is intentional to provide expansion and contraction. When exposed to cool temperatures, the scrotum contracts and draws the testes closer to the body for warmth. In warm temperatures, the scrotum become loose and allows the testes to hang farther away from the heat of the body. The testes are sensitive organs and can suffer discomfort, sometimes extreme, if handled roughly or jostled about. It is important that a man wear a properly fitted athletic support, or jockstrap, when engaged in strenuous physical activity. However, the continuous use of a support can cause the temperature within the scrotum to rise and the delicate sperm to die because of constant exposure to high temperatures. Snug-fitting garments such as tight blue jeans can have the same effect on a man's fertility. The scrotum can be a source of sexual pleasure when lightly stroked, fondled, or caressed during sexual activity.

Tubules from the testes drain into the *epididymis*, which in turn drains into the *vas deferens* and *ejaculatory ducts*. These ducts then drain directly into the urethra. It is believed that the vas deferens acts as a reservoir for sperm between ejaculations.

The seminal vesicles, prostate gland, and Cowper's glands produce a liquid called *seminal plasma*. The seminal plasma and the sperm collectively make up the *semen*. The plasma aids in the transport of sperm and also provides energizing nutrients for the sperm. It contains a form of sugar (fructose), mucus, salts, water, base buffers, and coagulators to aid the sperm in their journey. Semen is a thick, creamy white fluid with the consistency of mucus or egg whites. The normal amount of semen per ejaculate is 2 to 6 mL. A fertile man dispels 120 to 160 million sperm per ejaculate. Cowper's glands produce small droplets of fluid during sexual activity that neutralize the acidity of the male urethra and aid in the transport of sperm. This fluid may contain sperm. Therefore, contraceptive measures, if used, must be taken before this fluid can be introduced into the woman's vagina.

The *penis* is a tubular structure located above the scrotum. It functions to eliminate urine from the bladder, to ejaculate semen and impregnate a woman, and as a sex organ for sexual pleasure. It consists of the shaft and the *glans* (head of the penis). In the uncircumcised male, the glans is covered by loose skin (*foreskin*) that can be retracted. In the circumcised male, the foreskin has been surgically removed and the glans is exposed. Penis size and shape vary among individuals. Normally the penis is soft and flaccid and 2½ to 4 inches long. The dimensions of the penis in no way dictate the man's ability to perform effectively during sexual activity. When an **erection** occurs, the blood vessels in the shaft of the penis become congested and the penis becomes hard and erect. The size of the penis during an erection may increase to 5½ to 7 inches in total length. The penis, particularly the glans, is extremely sensitive to stimulation. Stroking and handling of the shaft of the penis are also pleasurable during sexual activity. Stimulation to prompt the penis to an erection is varied. A full bladder on awakening in the morning can cause an erection. Fantasy, memories of a past sexual encounter, and accidental brushing by an attractive stranger can all lead to an erection. An erection in the male does not always signify desire for sexual activity. Exposure of the male client by the nurse during a bed bath may cause an erection. An erection is a normal physiologic response and not something the man can voluntarily control. The erection ceases if no further stimulation is added.

Ejaculation is the expulsion of semen by the rhythmic contractions of the penis. The penis engages in short, jerky movements that produce a spurt of semen with each motion. The period of ejaculation is short and the penis becomes flaccid after ejaculation. Many males, particularly adolescent boys, may experience a phenomenon known as **nocturnal emission**, or "wet dream." These ejaculatory episodes occur during sleep without physical stimulation. They are perfectly normal and do not represent any sort of deviation.

Male breasts contain little real breast tissue, but they still may be stimulated during sexual activity. Although the area of sensitivity is usually limited to the nipple and areola, its stimulation can be as pleasurable an experience for the male as it is for a female.

Sexual Response Cycle

The physiologic responses to sexual activity of female and male are more similar than different (Fig. 40-3). Also, body response is essentially the same regardless of the source of stimulation; that is, fantasy, masturbation, and sexual intercourse between two individuals can all bring about the same body reactions. The sexual response cycle is not lim-

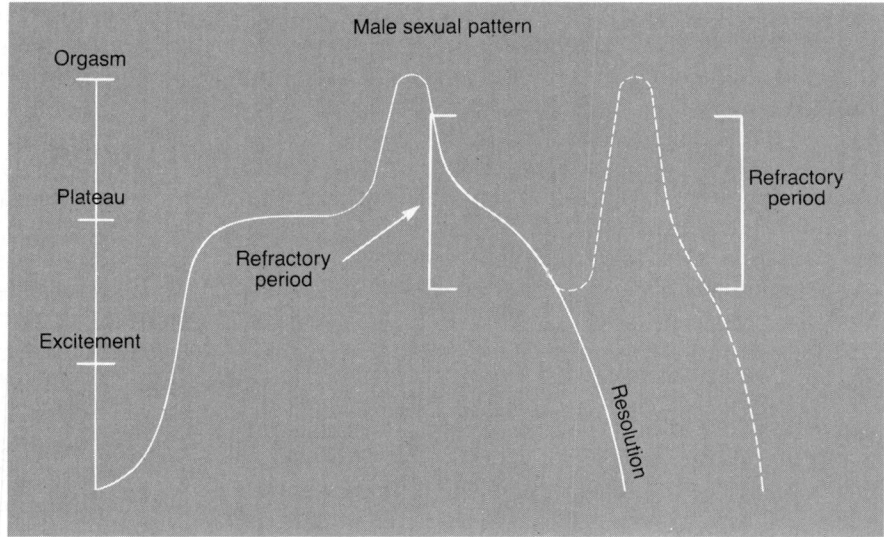

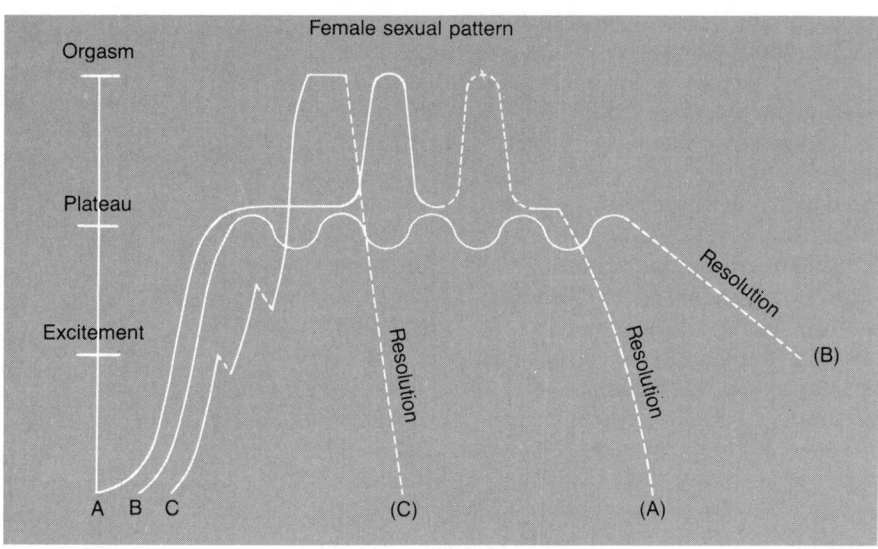

F I G U R E 4 0 - 3

Male and female sexual response patterns. There are three female patterns shown. (A) Steady progression to plateau stage is followed by intense orgasm; subsequent orgasms may occur; resolution is slower. (B) Slower progression to plateau stage is followed by minor surges toward orgasm, causing prolonged pleasurable feelings without definitive orgasm; resolution is slowest. (C) Rapid progression to plateau stage with some peaks and dips; one intense orgasm follows with rapid resolution. This most closely resembles the male pattern. (Reeder, S. J., & Martin, L. L. L. [1992]. *Maternity nursing* [17th ed.]. Philadelphia: Lippincott.)

ited to the genital organs but is a total body response that causes many physiologic changes throughout the body. Masters and Johnson, two researchers best known for their work on sexual response (Woods, 1984), divided the response cycle into the four phases of (1) excitement, (2) plateau, (3) orgasm, and (4) resolution, with a smooth progression from one phase to the next. Although only physiologic response is discussed here, the reader should keep in mind that the emotional and mental involvement of sexual response contributes a great deal to the pleasure and satisfaction of sexual activity.

The human body contains many **erogenous zones**, which are areas that, when stimulated, cause sexual arousal and desire. The genitals are an obvious source of sexual pleasure for both men and women, but other areas of the body are also considered erogenous zones. The skin of the body is the largest erogenous zone. Other areas include the ears, lips, thighs, and breasts. Some people can reach orgasm simply by stimulation of erogenous zones other than the genitals. The most important body organ for sexual arousal and stimulation is the brain. It allows individuals freedom to enjoy a sexual experience but also may prevent satisfaction by inhibitions, doubts, and guilt.

Excitement

The *excitement phase* is initiated by erotic stimulation and arousal. Some of the physiologic changes common in both men and women include increase in heart rate and blood pressure and the appearance of a pink flush to the skin. This sex flush, which is more evident in women than in men, spreads over the face, neck, back, and upper torso of the body. Congestion of the genitals with increased blood flow begins in the excitement phase and causes even more arousal. The length of the excitement phase varies greatly among individuals and even from one experience to another. Women usually enjoy a more prolonged period of stimulation than do men.

During the excitement phase, the breasts of the woman swell and the nipples become erect and hard to the touch. Lubrication of the vagina seeps to the outside of the body along the vulvar creases and makes stimulation of the genitals more pleasurable by decreasing friction. The upper two thirds or so of the vagina enlarge and expand. The clitoris enlarges and emerges slightly from the clitoral hood. The labia also enlarge and separate and turn a deep rosy red in color with arousal.

The first obvious sign of arousal in the man is an erection of the penis caused by increased pelvic congestion of blood. The scrotum noticeably elevates, thickens, and enlarges. The skin of the penis and scrotum turns a deep reddish-purple in response to congestion and arousal. Male nipples may also harden and become erect.

Plateau

The intensity of the **plateau phase** is greater than that of excitement but not enough to begin orgasm. Desire and arousal continue to build and intensify. The length of time of this phase varies from a few minutes to 15 to 20 minutes. In the female, the clitoris retracts and disappears under the clitoral hood. It is thought that the clitoris performs in this mysterious way as the body's protection against overstimulation. In the male, secretions from Cowper's glands may appear at the glans of the penis during the plateau phase.

Orgasm

The term **orgasm** defines the climax and sexual explosion of the tension built over the preceding phases. Orgasm lasts a matter of seconds, but it is an extremely intense reaction. Characteristic of the orgasm phase are the involuntary spasmodic contractions of the genital organs. The number of contractions felt by the individual depends on the intensity of the orgasm.

The orgasm phase in the female begins with a heightened feeling of physical pleasure followed by overwhelming release and involuntary contractions of the genitals. Loss of muscular control can also be seen in spastic contractions and twitching of the arms and legs. The number of contractions can be as few as 4 or as many as 20. Areas of the body that contract spasmodically are the uterus, anal sphincter, rectum, and urethral sphincter. It currently is believed that women achieve orgasm in a variety of ways. Although some women can achieve orgasm by penile thrusting in the vagina alone, most women need clitoral stimulation to reach orgasm.

Involuntary spasmodic contractions of the genitals occur in the male during orgasm. These occur in the penis, epididymis, vas deferens, and rectum. The male orgasm is most often accompanied by ejaculation of semen from the urinary meatus of the penis. It is not necessary for ejaculation and orgasm to occur simultaneously. Rather, it is a coincidence that the two events usually happen at the same time.

Resolution

The *resolution phase* is characterized by a return to normal body functioning present before the excitement phase. Feelings of relaxation, fatigue, and fulfillment are common. Some people may also have a need to be held, fondled, and caressed. Physical demonstrations of affection may initiate the sexual response cycle once again. The woman is physiologically capable of immediate response to sexual stimulation. Because of this, many women can achieve multiple orgasms. The man experiences a period during which he is incapable of sexual response, called the *refractory period*. The length of the refractory period is individual. It may be a few minutes or even days before the man's body responds readily to continued sexual stimulation.

Sexual Expression

The methods by which a person or people gain satisfaction through sexual stimulation are varied. Also, a number of factors are involved in the degree to which a sexual experience is enjoyable. Touch, smell, sight, sounds, feelings, thoughts, and fantasy can all contribute to sexual fulfillment in any form of expression chosen by individuals. Feelings of love for another person are also closely associated with desire. Fantasies can greatly aid sexual stimulation and are quite normal.

Masturbation

Masturbation is a technique of sexual expression in which an individual practices self-stimulation. Many myths and misinformation surround the issue of masturbation. Masturbation is a means of learning what is preferred by a person during stimulation and what feels good. Men masturbate by holding and stroking the shaft of the penis. Women find manual stimulation of the clitoris enjoyable, although variations of technique are numerous. People masturbate regardless of sex, age, or marital status. People who do not masturbate usually abstain because of a sense of guilt or wrongness associated with self-stimulation. Masturbation is not dirty and will not lead to blindness, nor will it cause insanity.

Sexual Intercourse

Sexual intercourse between a man and a woman is the most common image that comes to mind when sexuality is mentioned. Unlike other animals, humans must learn how to engage in sexual intercourse. The act of intercourse, or **coitus**, usually begins by stimulation of the senses in some way, followed by a period of activity known as **foreplay**. Petting is part of foreplay and can be simple stroking of the breasts, arms, back, and neck without genital involvement or may lead to mutual masturbation and orgasm. Many adolescents engage in petting without further sexual involvement. However, the progressive steps of intercourse are merely shades of gray. An adolescent couple may find themselves involved in the sexual act without any preparation or forewarning.

Penetration The act of placing the penis in the vagina, or **penetration**, can be accomplished by various positions. The most common position in Western cultures is the missionary position, which places the woman horizontally under the man. (This position was named *missionary* by the Polynesians because it was the preferred position used for intercourse by religious missionaries.) Other positions may be more stimulating and comfortable. Clitoral stimulation is difficult to achieve in the missionary position. Lying side by side, female on top, and rear entry are some examples of coital positions that make clitoral stimulation more successful. Some people are so inhibited they need permission to engage in alternate sexual positions.

When the penis is pushed into the vagina, the man begins rhythmic thrusting movements of his hips to stroke the penis back and forth along the vaginal walls. The woman may match her partner's hip movements with movements of her own body. These movements continue until orgasm is attained by one person or both people. Simultaneous orgasms, or both people attaining orgasm at the same moment, are difficult to achieve. Preoccupation with attaining simultaneous orgasms may disrupt the ultimate intimacy and satisfaction possible during the coital experience.

The period after coitus is just as significant as the events leading up to it. Caressing, hugging, and kissing actually deepen the intimacy shared by the couple and should be nurtured and not rushed.

Variant Forms

Stimulation by using the mouth and tongue on the genitals may be used during foreplay or as a method to reach orgasm. *Cunnilingus* is stimulation of the female genitals by licking and sucking the clitoris and surrounding structures. *Fellatio* is stimulation of the male genitals by licking and sucking the penis and surrounding structures. These techniques may be used singularly or simultaneously.

Sodomy, the act of introducing the penis into the rectum, is still considered illegal in some areas. Once a finger or the penis is placed in the rectum, it should not be introduced into the vagina without thorough cleansing, because many organisms present in the rectum can cause subsequent vaginal infections. Care should be exercised to avoid injury to the delicate rectal mucosa, and lubrication is essential for comfort.

Sadism refers to the practice of gaining sexual pleasure while inflicting abuse on another person. *Masochism* refers to gaining sexual pleasure from the humiliation of being abused. When practiced together, the act is called *sadomasochism*. *Fetishism*, usually practiced by a male, is sexual arousal with the aid of an inanimate object not generally associated with sexual activity. Items such as shoes, leather, rubber, and women's undergarments may be used.

Transvestism is sexual arousal of a man when he wears clothing normally worn by a woman. Most transvestites are heterosexual and many are married and have children. Transvestites usually have a great need to keep their habit a secret from others and indulge in cross dressing in private or choose to wear women's undergarments that are not easily detectable.

The extent to which people practice variants of sexual expression may range from totally harmless to compulsive in nature. Nurses must be able to provide care to these individuals as they do to any other consumers of health care.

Factors Affecting Sexuality

Many factors influence and affect a person's sexuality and thus differentiate personal feelings regarding sexuality. That is, the brain rather than the genitals plays the most significant role in how people perceive themselves as sexual beings.

Developmental Considerations

The process of human development affects the psychosocial, emotional, and biologic aspects of life, and these in turn affect an individual's sexuality. Sexuality is the only distinguishing trait present at conception. From birth onward, gender, or sex, influences behavior throughout life. See Table 40-1 for a summary of sexuality throughout the life span and nursing implications for each stage.

Culture

The manner in which sexuality is perceived by a society of people in turn influences the individual. Every culture has its own norms regarding sexual identity and behavior. To some degree, culture dictates the duration of sexual intercourse, methods of sexual stimulation, and sexual positions. In some cultures, women may be expected merely to tolerate sex, whereas in others, the woman's participation is encouraged.

Religion

Some view organized religion as having a generally negative effect on the expression of sexuality. Many forms of sexual expression other than male–female coitus are considered unnatural by some religions. Also, over time, the concept of virginity came to be synonymous with purity and sex became synonymous with sin. Double standards and rigid regulations have inflicted a considerable amount of guilt and anxiety on many individuals. A number of sexual dysfunctions can be related to the individual's anguish over the negative connotation of sex as dictated by some

Sexuality

Use the assessment checklist to determine how well you are meeting your sexuality needs. Then develop a prescription for self-care by choosing appropriate behaviors from the list of suggestions.

Assessment Checklist

almost always | sometimes | almost never

1. I feel good about my sexual identity.
2. I have satisfying relationships with others.
3. I accept sexual needs as a normal part of life.
4. I am comfortable with physical actions that indicate love and belonging (such as touching and hugging).

Self-Care Behaviors

1. Avoid stereotyping typical gender roles.
2. Learn the biologic aspects of sexual functioning.
3. Ask questions about sexual needs and sexual activity when necessary.
4. Enjoy close relationships with others who love you.
5. Give a hug to someone you love.
6. Accept touch from others as a sign of caring and affection.
7. Practice safer sex (eg, use contraceptives or condoms, and choose partner carefully).
8. Recognize how age, illness, or disability influences sexual needs and expression.

religious groups. Most major religions are currently re-examining their teachings on sexuality in response to challenges posed by their members. Many have recognized the importance of solid sex education within the realm of the church.

Ethics

Healthy sexuality depends on freedom from guilt and anxiety. What one person believes is wrong may be perfectly natural and correct to another. Some individuals, however, may feel that certain forms of sexual expression are bizarre and the people that participate in them are perverted. If the sexual expression is performed by consenting adults, is not harmful to them, and is practiced in privacy, it is not considered a deviant behavior. Individuals should personally decide with which aspects of sexual expression they are comfortable. Frequently, all an individual needs to alleviate guilt and consequently enhance sexual satisfaction is permission from a health care provider to engage in a different form of expression.

Life-Style

Modern life-styles greatly affect sexuality and its expression. Both men and women are exposed to stress, and many are under considerable strain to perform and function in the workplace as well as at home. Stressors may be external, such as job and financial demands, or internal, such as a competitive nature. These varied responsibilities

place a time restraint on communication between a couple, as well as on the energy level and motivation for sexual satisfaction. Although some couples view sexual activity as a release from the stressors of everyday life, most place sex far from the top of the list of things to do. It is crucial to a relationship's survival that a couple set aside priority time if not for lovemaking, then for intimate quiet contact.

Sexual Orientation

Most adults develop a sexual orientation resulting from childhood experiences (Table 40-1). Sexual orientation refers to the preferred sex of the partner of an individual. Homosexual people prefer sexual activity with a person of the same sex. Heterosexual people prefer sexual activity with a person of the opposite sex. Heterosexuality and homosexuality can be placed at opposite ends of a continuum with many variations in between. **Bisexuality** refers to a person who finds pleasure with both an opposite-sex or same-sex partner. Homosexual or heterosexual people may have bisexual relationships at times.

Heterosexuality Heterosexuality is the most common form of sexual orientation among humans, and coitus between a man and woman is their most common form of sexual expression. Although some people feel coitus should only occur in a marital relationship, it also occurs premaritally, extramaritally, and postmaritally.

Premarital sex is the practice of coitus before marriage. The standard for sexual **abstinence** before marriage has

T A B L E 4 0 - 1

Developmental Aspects of Sexuality Through the Life Span

Stage	Characteristics	Nursing Implications and Teaching Guidelines
Infancy: Birth to 18 mo	• Needs affection and tactile stimulation • Boys have penile erections and girls have orgasmic potential • Gradually can differentiate self from others • Obtain pleasure from touching genitals • Dressed according to gender • Toys are gender related	• Avoid early weaning to prevent oral deprivation. • Encourage parents to provide ample physical touch, deprivation of which may cause physical and mental underdevelopment. • Self-manipulation of genitals is normal behavior; avoid denoting this as "bad." • Avoid confusion of sex by consistent use of male or female role reinforcement.
Toddler: Age 1–3 yr	• Establishes control over bowels and bladder • Both sexes enjoy fondling genitals • Able to identify own gender • Develops vocabulary related to anatomy	• Allow toddler to designate his or her readiness to toilet-training. Strict measures may lead to compulsive behaviors later. • Punishment of genital fondling may lead to guilt and shame regarding sexual behavior later in life. • Use proper terms for body parts.
Preschool: Age 4–6 yr	• By age 6, sexuality has been internalized and preference for sexual partners determined • Methods of play and dress are in accordance with gender • Enjoys exploring body parts of self and playmates • Engages in masturbation	• Parents may cause anxiety in the child by intolerance of inconsistency of sex-role behavior. • Negative overreaction by parents of child's masturbating behavior can lead to a belief that the genitals and sex are bad and dirty.
School-age: Age 6–10 yr	• There is attachment to the parent of the opposite sex • Tendency toward having same-sex friends • Curiosity about sex and sharing of fears • Increasing self-awareness	• Same-sex preference for relationships is not related to heterosexual or homosexual tendencies. • Give child the information desired in a clear, factual form. May look to peers for information that may be incorrect.
Preadolescence: Age 10–13 yr	• Puberty begins for most boys and girls with development of secondary sex characteristics • Menarche takes place • May test behavioral limits	• Information is necessary regarding body changes to alleviate fears. This information should be given to the young person before pubertal changes begin. • Parents need to find a satisfactory middle ground for role setting. Rules that are either too rigid or too lenient can interfere with the development of self-confidence and internal value system. • Treat body image changes with a positive attitude to prevent poor self-image.
Adolescence: Age 13–19 yr	• Begins to develop opposite-sex relationships • Sexual fantasies are common • Masturbation is common • May begin to partake in sexual activity ranging from light to heavy petting to full genital intercourse • Girls concerned with reputations and self-image • Boys preoccupied with competitiveness of sexual activity • Incidence of adolescent pregnancies is increasing	• Parents share their beliefs and moral value systems with their children. • Teenagers may share their feelings with parents. If not taken seriously, may lead to lack of trust and communication gap. • Teens need information regarding contraceptive measures and the potential for contracting sexually transmitted diseases.

(continued)

T A B L E   4 0 - 1 (*continued*)

Developmental Aspects of Sexuality Through the Life Span

Stage	Characteristics	Nursing Implications and Teaching Guidelines
Young adulthood: Age 20–35 yr	• Premarital sex is common • Although many young adults choose co-habitation instead of marriage, most marry and begin families before age 30 • Knowledge regarding sexual response and activity increases pleasure of relationship • May experiment with various sexual expressions • Develops own value system and respects values of other people • Many couples share financial responsibilities as well as household tasks	• Encourage communication between partners regarding sexual needs and differences. • Teach use of abstinence and contraceptive measures to prevent unwanted pregnancies. • Counsel against promiscuous behavior to guard against sexually transmitted diseases and loss of trust of partner. • Daily communication is necessary to vent stresses and work out difficulties.
Adulthood: Age 35–55 yr	• Bodily changes as a result of menopause • Couples focus on quality rather than quantity of sexual experiences • Divorce is common • Grown children begin their own lives and sexual experiences • Sexual satisfaction may actually increase due to loss of fear of pregnancy	• Both men and women need positive reinforcement of what is good about themselves and their relationships. • Teach parents that *empty nest syndrome* (feelings of loss caused by children leaving) is common. Accentuate positive aspects of this situation. • Encourage couple to use this period as one of renewal for themselves.
Late adulthood and elderly: Age 55 yr and older	• Orgasms may become shorter and less intense in both men and women • Vaginal secretions decrease and period of resolution in men lengthens • May feel need to conform to stereotypes regarding the aging process and cease sexual activity • Fear of loss of sexual abilities	• Sexual activity need not be hindered by age. • Teach couples that adaptation to bodily changes is possible with use of comfortable positions for intercourse and increased time for stimulation. • Teach alternatives to coitus, such as caressing, hugging, and stroking, when coitus is impossible because of illness or disability. • Couples who have been consistently sexually active throughout their lives may continue their intimate relationship for as long as they desire.

been a cultural and religious norm in many societies for centuries. Abstinence and virginity have been perceived as more important for women to maintain than for men. This double standard appears to be changing as increasing numbers of women report having premarital sexual relationships, especially in western societies. Extramarital sexual relationships are usually a symptom of a troubled marriage and rarely the cause of the failure of a strong one. Extramarital relationships are often the product of stress-filled lives and sexual dissatisfaction at home and are destructive to a marriage relationship.

Homosexuality Homosexuality occurs in both males and females. The term **gay** is synonymous with male homosexual. A **lesbian** is a female homosexual. The sexual behaviors of the heterosexual and the homosexual are the same except for penile–vaginal penetration. The primary difference between a heterosexual and a homosexual is in the gender of the preferred sex partner and not in a particular type of behavior.

Homosexuality has been considered an illness or deviant behavior, but in 1974 the American Psychiatric Association removed homosexuality from the category of mental illness. Although this move and certain research findings eliminated some of the stigma attached to homosexuality, society as a whole has made slow progress in accepting the gay movement.

Transsexuality A transsexual is a person of a certain biologic sex with the feelings of the opposite sex. The person feels trapped within the body of the wrong sex. The reason, or etiology, behind this is unknown, although many factors are believed to be involved. For many transsexuals, the solution for this agonizing problem is to change their bodies to match their inner feelings through surgery and hormone therapy.

Health State

A healthy body, mind, and emotions are necessary for sexual wellness. Any trauma or stress that interferes with an individual's ability to perform daily functions certainly also affects the expression of sexuality. Illness is no exception.

Chronic Pain   Many chronic illnesses are accompanied by constant pain, and an individual with persistent pain may not desire any sexual contact. However, the desire for human warmth and contact does not cease because of pain. Altered or modified positions for coitus are sometimes necessary; these are discussed in more detail later in this section.

Diabetes Mellitus   Diabetes mellitus is a hormonal disease in which the body is deficient in the amount of insulin secreted by the pancreas. Although almost all hormonal disorders affect sexuality in some way, diabetes is the most prevalent and well known. *Erectile dysfunction*, or **impotence**, is a great concern among diabetic men. Treatment to date depends largely on the degree of erectile ability lost. Some men may be candidates for a penile prosthesis, which was developed in 1973. The prosthesis is surgically implanted below the base of the penis and inflation of the device produces an erection when sexual activity is desired.

It is not uncommon for diabetic women to experience loss of ability for orgasm (**orgasmic dysfunction**). Difficulty experiencing arousal and loss of vaginal lubrication have also been reported. Frequent *Monilia* infections of the vagina are also common and cause discomfort during coitus.

Cardiovascular Disease   Cardiovascular disease is prevalent in North America. It is known that the sexual response cycle can greatly increase the demands of the heart and other structures. A person with a cardiovascular disease may experience much anxiety over the effect the illness will have on sexuality and sexual functioning.

Hypertension   The most significant difficulty a hypertensive person faces regarding sexuality is that the medication used to control the disease frequently causes a change in sexual functioning. These sexual dysfunctions may be relieved by modifying the dose of the medication or switching to a different medication.

Myocardial Infarction (Heart Attack)   The primary goal after a myocardial infarction (MI) is to allow the heart ample time to heal. Activities of daily living, including sexual activity, should be resumed gradually and stressors such as overexertion, alcohol consumption, and emotional upheavals should be avoided. In an uncomplicated MI, sexual activity may begin around week 3 of recovery, beginning with masturbation to partial erection in the male. Generally, this activity is gradually increased until 3 months after the MI when sexual intercourse may be resumed (Woods,

1984). A comfortable position should be assumed that places the least stress on the affected partner.

Diseases of the Joints and Mobility   Joint diseases and disorders affect young and old people. Pain, fatigue, stiffness, and loss of range of motion can accompany any of the dozens of known diseases of the joints. The disease itself does not affect sexual functioning, although the manifestation of it can cause discomfort and anxiety.

Surgery and Body Image   Surgery is performed to remove diseased tissue and repair body organs. It usually requires an incision with resulting scars. The most devastating kinds of surgery are those used to remove cancerous tissue and surrounding structures. The client is almost always distressed over a diagnosis of cancer and possible death. After surgery, people need to cope and adjust to major alterations to their bodies. Changes in body image also affect a person's self-perception as a sexual being.

Mastectomy is a surgical procedure to remove a breast and its surrounding tissue. After such surgery, a woman's return to sexual functioning depends on many factors, such as support of her partner, the value placed on the breast by the man or woman, and fear of discomfort during sexual activity.

An *ostomy* is a surgical opening placed on the outside of the body to allow for the passage of secretions and elimination into a closed drainage bag. The grief over the loss of the natural means to eliminate waste, such as urine or feces, accompanies learning to live with an obvious artificial device. Many people are anxious as to how this apparatus will affect their sexual lives and how accepting sexual partners will be of it.

Spinal Cord Injuries   Thousands of people are victims of spinal cord injuries each year as a result of various types of accidents. This type of injury almost always results in some degree of permanent disability. These people face multiple adaptations in normal living styles, including those related to mobility, bowel and bladder control, sexual functioning, and role expectations. The extent of remaining sexual response after a spinal cord injury depends primarily on the level and extent of the injury. Ejaculation and orgasm are most likely to remain with low spinal injuries. Women are more likely to experience orgasm than men but complain more about the lack of physical sensations during the excitement phase than do men. Many people find that other erogenous zones become more easily stimulated after the injury.

Mental Illness   Various psychological and physical disorders can cause mental illness. The mind plays a powerful role in sexuality and any disruption of its functioning will no doubt cause a disturbance in some way to sexual functioning. Even a disorder such as mild depression can affect desire and sexual functioning. Sometimes it is difficult for the partner of a client who has developed a mental illness to continue the sexual relationship. People afflicted with Alzheimer's disease can lose the memory of any contact with a partner or spouse. At times, clients with mental illness act out in a sexual manner, such as touching themselves or discarding their clothing at inappropriate times and places.

Sexually Transmitted Diseases   The term *sexually transmitted disease* (STD) is used to describe diseases that are almost always transmitted through direct sexual contact. The number of cases and varieties of STDs has increased over the years and many currently are at epidemic proportions. STDs are hard to control because the partner or partners also need treatment. This is usually difficult if the partner is promiscuous or a one-time contact. It is believed that to have sexual contact with one person is also to have sexual contact with everyone else that person has had contact with in the past. The only clear way to avoid exposure to an STD is for a virginal person to have sexual contact with another virgin. Some STDs can be treated easily and effectively, whereas others have longstanding implications. For instance, women may suffer severe consequences from an STD by developing pelvic inflammatory disease (PID). The resulting adhesions from PID cause much damage to delicate reproductive structures and may lead to infertility. Furthermore, other STDs are deadly because there is no cure and no effective treatment. Acquired immunodeficiency syndrome (AIDS) is an example of a deadly STD. Table 40-2 lists the more common types of STDs and their signs and symptoms and corresponding treatment.

Medications

Medications are used to halt a disease, cure an illness, and promote and stabilize body functions. Some medications are necessary to prevent severe illness and even death. Some medications have side effects that may affect sexual functioning. Illegal drugs are used by some people because of their ability presumably to heighten the sexual experience. These drugs can have serious and even deadly side effects of their own. Table 40-3 lists some of the categories of medications and their possible effects on sexual functioning.

Nurse as Role Model

A nurse's attitudes, biases, and prejudice regarding sexuality are readily transmitted to clients through the nurse's actions, manner of speech, avoidance of certain circumstances, and types of discussion. The level of knowledge a nurse has about sexual issues can inhibit or promote discussion of sexual health. The nurse who does not have a sound knowledge base of reproductive anatomy and physiology, sexual response, sexual expression, and other issues surrounding sexuality will be unable effectively to assess, teach, or counsel the client with sexual concerns. The nurse must also feel comfortable with self as a sexual being.

Nursing goals to enhance interactions with clients and to promote individual sexual wellness are as follows. The nurse will be able to:
- Define individual sexuality
- Assess degree of comfort with sexual issues
- Feel comfortable as a sexual being
- Develop self-awareness regarding sexual topics
- Develop communication skills that promote discussion of sexual concerns with clients
- Practice responsible sexual expression

Sexual Harassment

Nurses in different types of health care settings have experienced work-related sexual harassment. Sexual harassment may be defined as "any unwelcome verbal or physical advance or sexually explicit statement—such as leers, pats, grabs, jokes, requests for dates, and even rape—that interferes with your ability to do your job by making you feel humiliated, intimidated or uncomfortable" (Horsley, 1990, p. 69). It is important for nurses to recognize that harassment can often be effectively stopped when confronted early. Specific measures to stop harassment are highlighted in the accompanying display.

Assessing

Sexual History

The comprehensive health history should include information regarding a client's reproductive and sexual health, depending on the circumstances in which the client is receiving care. As a rule, three general categories of clients should have a sexual history recorded by the nurse:
- Any inpatient or outpatient client who is receiving care for pregnancy, STD, infertility, or contraception
- Any client who is currently experiencing a sexual dysfunction or problem
- Any client whose illness will affect sexual functioning and behavior in any way

Information is best obtained from the client by beginning with nonthreatening questions and progressing to more sensitive concerns (see the accompanying display). Clients usually have no difficulty answering questions regarding their bodies and general reproductive issues such as, "When did your menstrual periods first begin?"

Clients should understand why the nurse needs information about their intimate sexual functioning. Nurses should explain to clients that this information may be helpful in assisting them in the care plan. The sexual history is a vital portion of the reproductive history. It also assists the nurse in identifying any sexual problems or concerns. It is an excellent opportunity for the nurse to teach by helping the client confront fears and allay myths. There are four general levels of sexual history suggested by Watts (1979):

TABLE 40-2

Sexually Transmitted Diseases

Disease	Characteristics	Treatment
Acquired immunodeficiency syndrome (AIDS)	• Human immunodeficiency virus (HIV) • Positive ELISA and Western Blot tests • Incidence high in IV drug users and homosexual and bisexual men; increased heterosexual transmission • Fatigue, diarrhea, weight loss, enlarged lymph nodes, fever, anorexia, and night sweats	• No cure, but treatment is directed toward delayed disease progression, opportunistic diseases, and relief of symptoms
Cervical intraepithelial neoplasia (CIN) Cervical cancer	• Abnormal Pap smears • Women with multiple sex partners, women who began sexual activity before age 18, and women whose partners have multiple female partners • Asymptomatic • Possible vaginal bleeding or spotting	• Depends on extent and stage of dysplasia • Surgical removal of cervix and other surrounding structures if severe; cryosurgery and laser treatment also used
Chlamydia trachomatis Nongonococcal urethritis (NGU) *Chlamydia*	• The most prevalent STD to date • Intracellular bacteria • Vaginal discharge, burning on urination, urinary frequency, dysuria, and urethral soreness • Many women are asymptomatic.	• Tetracycline, 500 mg PO qid for 7 days, or erythromycin, 500 mg PO qid for 7 days, for both partners; single dose azithromycin 1 g
Cytomegalovirus (CMV)	• A virus in the same family as herpes and Epstein-Barr • May be asymptomatic or may be confused with another disease such as pneumonia, mononucleosis, or hepatitis • Not exclusively sexually transmitted	• No specific treatment; aimed at relief of symptoms; may be passed in utero and affect newborn
Nonspecific vaginitis *Gardnerella vaginalis*	• Mixed anaerobic bacteria • Foul-smelling, thin, grayish white vaginal discharge • Male partners are asymptomatic.	• Metronidazole (Flagyl), 500 mg PO bid for 7 days, for both partners; alcohol must not be consumed while taking medication.
Neisseria gonorrhoeae "The clap" or "the drip" Gonorrhea	• Gram-negative bacteria • Both men and women may be asymptomatic. • Symptoms in men: purulent penile discharge, dysuria, frequency of urination • Symptoms in women: dysuria, abnormal menses, vaginal discharge, pelvic inflammatory disease • Symptoms of pharyngitis if oral sex practiced • May be accompanied by chlamydial infection • Detected by gonorrhea culture of cervix or penile discharge from men • Newborns exposed at birth are at risk for blindness and pneumonia. • Untreated gonorrhea can result in infertility, skin rash with lesions, and acute arthritis.	• Ceftriaxone, 250 mg IM (single dose) effective against PPNG, pharyngeal, and anorectal • Alternatively, tetracycline, 500 mg by mouth qid for 7 days, *plus* aqueous procaine penicillin G, 4.8 million units IM, *plus* probenecid, 1 g by mouth. • Cultures should be repeated 1 week after treatment.
Herpes simplex virus type 1 and 2 "Cold sores" Herpes	• A DNA virus • Lesions develop mostly in oral and genital areas. • Appear as single or multiple painful vesicles, which rupture and form ulcer-like lesions; these form scabs as they heal. • First infections last about 10 to 14 days, whereas subsequent infections are shorter in duration. • Recurrences are usually preceded by prodromal symptoms of tingling and fullness.	• No cure. • The antiviral drug acyclovir is used in treatment: acyclovir, 200 mg PO five times per day. • Areas of lesions should be kept clean and dry. • Use analgesics to reduce pain as well as topical anesthetics. • Avoid sexual contact while lesions are present. • May be transmitted to newborn at birth.

(continued)

TABLE 40-2 (continued)

Sexually Transmitted Diseases

Disease	Characteristics	Treatment
Human papilloma virus (HPV) Condylomata acuminata Genital warts Venereal warts	• A DNA virus • Pale, soft, papillary lesions found around the internal and external genitalia, and perianal and rectal areas of the body; vary in size • Profuse watery vaginal discharge, dyspareunia, intense pruritus, and vulvar irritation • Women with HPV are at risk for developing cervical cancer. • Male partner may or may not have lesions.	• Treat male partner if he has lesions. • Podophyllum 10% to 25% in tincture of benzoin may be applied to external lesions. Wash off in 1 to 4 hours. Repeat treatment until lesions are gone. • Cryosurgery and carbon dioxide laser surgery may also be used. • Use condoms or abstain from sex.
Treponema pallidum Syphilis	• A spirochete detected through serologic blood test (VDRL, RPR, STS) • Three stages to disease if left untreated *Primary:* Single painless genital lesion 10 days to 3 months after exposure *Secondary:* Generalized skin rash, enlarged lymph nodes, fever that may appear 2 to 4 weeks after appearance of primary lesion; may last for several years *Latent:* Usually no clinical symptoms present for as long as 20 years; may continue to involve and damage neurologic and cardiovascular organs; dementia, confusion, paralysis, and paresis may occur	• Treat both partners. • Benzathine penicillin G, 2.4 million units IM if of less than 1 year's duration; increase dosage and length of treatment if unknown duration of disease or longer than 1 year. • Repeat serology studies. • Avoid sexual contact or use condoms.
Trichomoniasis "Trich" *Trichomonas vaginalis*	• Protozoan with flagella • Identified on wet-mount microscopic examination of vaginal discharge • May be identified on Pap smear • Males usually asymptomatic • Foul-smelling vaginal discharge, thin, foamy, and green in color, causes itching of vulva and vagina, burning on urination and dyspareunia; "strawberry" cervix may be seen on speculum examination	• Treat both partners. • Metronidazole (Flagyl), 2 g PO at one time; avoid alcohol consumption. • Avoid sex or use condoms.

(Data from Baldwin, K., & Goodwin, K. [1985]. The Papanicolaou smear. *Journal of Nurse–Midwifery 30*[6]: 327–331; Bourcier, K., & Seidler, A. [1987]. *Chlamydia* and condylomata acuminata: An update for the nurse practitioner. *Journal of Obstetric, Gynecologic, and Neonatal Nursing 16*[1], 17–21; Fromer, M. [1983]. *Ethical issues in sexuality and reproduction.* St. Louis: Mosby; Hatcher, R. et al. [1986]. *Contraceptive technology.* New York: Irvington; Hill L., & Smith, M. [1990]. *Self-care nursing* [2nd ed.]. Englewood Cliffs, NJ: Prentice-Hall.)

Level 1: Sexual history as part of a comprehensive health history—obtained by a nurse

Level 2: Sexual history—obtained by a nurse with education and training in sexuality

Level 3: Sexual problem history—obtained by a sex therapist

Level 4: Psychiatric/psychosocial history—obtained by a psychiatric nurse clinician

Each level acquires more specific information from the client regarding sexual health and also requires the interviewer to have more sophisticated preparation and skills. The professional nurse usually performs a sexual history on level 1.

The nurse sets the tone or atmosphere for the interview. The nurse's attitudes will greatly affect the client's response to the sexual history, and clients will be more cooperative if they sense the nurse's security and ease during the interview. Privacy is essential for the sexual history; doors should be closed and no interruptions allowed. Sit close to the client and speak in a quiet, relaxed, objective tone of voice. Use eye contact and open body posture. The client needs to know what will happen to this information and who will have access to it. The nurse needs to explain to the client that no one will have access to this information unless it is significant to the client's care. Reproductive health information should be obtained from the client first, followed by the client's sexual health history. The best approach is to begin with general open-ended questions and progress to more specific ones. The nurse should use the language used by the client. If not, clients may be reluctant to tell the caregiver that they do not understand certain terms for fear of appearing ignorant or fool-

TABLE 40-3

Medications and Their Effects on Sexual Functioning

Drug	Effect on Sexual Functioning
Amyl nitrite	Peripheral vasodilator used in the past for treating angina; has become popular as sex enhancer among male homosexuals in particular; when inhaled at time of orgasm, the resulting vasodilation is felt to cause an intensified orgasmic release. Loss of erection, hypotension, and faintness may occur.
Anticonvulsants	Dilantin (phenytoin) has sedative effects, which may decrease desire and reduce sexual response.
Antidepressants	
Tricyclic compounds	Similar to antihypertensive drugs. Male impotence is significant.
Monoamine oxidase inhibitors	Male impotence and ejaculatory dysfunction in 25% to 30% of men.
Lithium carbonate	Decreases serum testosterone in men. Some antidepressants have been found to cause prolonged painful erections known as *priapism*; one such drug is trazodone.
Antihistamines	May have sedative effect that decreases desire; may also cause decreased vaginal lubrication.
Antihypertensives	
Methyldopa	May decrease desire in both male and female clients.
Clonidine	Erectile failure in 24% of men; no adverse effect on female clients.
Reserpine	Decreased desire in women; erectile and ejaculation dysfunctions in men.
Antipsychotics	Causes decreased desire in 10% to 20% of clients; may also cause erection and ejaculatory dysfunctions. Small amount of the antipsychotic drug may be found in the semen. The partner may experience resulting genital rash. Wear condoms while on therapy.
Antispasmodics	These drugs relax smooth muscle; male impotence may occur.
Barbiturates	In low initial doses, sexual pleasure may be increased due to loss of inhibitions. However, long-term use commonly causes decreased desire and orgasmic dysfunction. Male impotence is not uncommon.
Cocaine	Reported to increase quality of sexual experience. Chronic use, however, results in sexual dysfunction and loss of desire in both men and women.
Ethyl alcohol	In moderate amounts, decreases inhibitions and consequently improves sexual functioning. Continued consumption decreases sexual functioning. Chronic alcoholics are impotent and often sterile. Testicular damage and permanent dysfunction are common. Female alcoholics experience decreased desire and orgasmic dysfunction.
Marijuana	Release of inhibitions may cause feeling of increased sexual functioning. Marijuana users have increased incidence of decreased desire and male impotence.
Narcotics	Serious impairment of sexual functioning with increased dependence. Erectile and ejaculatory dysfunctions common in men. Testosterone levels and amount of semen decreased. High incidence of decreased desire occurs in both men and women.

(Data from Fuentes, R. [1983]. Sexual side effects. What to tell your patients, what not to say. *RN, 46*[2], 34–41; Woods, N. F. [1984]. *Human sexuality in health and illness* St. Louis, MO: Mosby.)

Specific Measures to Stop Sexual Harassment

Confrontation: Look the harasser in the eye and tell him or her you do not like this behavior and want it to stop.

Documentation: Document specific instances of harassment (words and acts, your response, date, time, and place and the names of any witnesses). Put the details of these incidents in a letter and send it to the harasser again, indicating that you do not like this behavior and want it to stop. Send the letter by way of registered mail.

Written complaint: If the behavior does not stop, submit a written complaint to administration (use appropriate channels).

Government complaint: If all else fails, file a complaint with the Equal Employment Opportunity Commission.

(Horsley, J. E. [1990]. Don't tolerate sexual harassment at work. *RN, 53*[1], 69, 72, 75.)

FOCUSED ASSESSMENT GUIDE

Sexuality

Factors to Assess	Questions and Approaches
Reproductive history	Ask women their date of menarche, date of last menstrual period, duration and length of flow in days, number of pregnancies, living children, miscarriages, abortions, method of birth control. Ask men the number of children they have fathered and method of birth control used. Ask both men and women of childbearing age if they have any concerns about their fertility and determine if there is any interest in the new reproductive technologies and genetic testing options.
History of sexually transmitted diseases	"Do you or a sexual partner have a history of sexually transmitted diseases? Many people today have questions about sexually transmitted diseases that they are reluctant to express. Do you have any questions? Have you noticed any signs that might indicate a problem?"
Sexual self-care behaviors	"Do you perform the breast-self exam [testicular-self exam] on a monthly basis? When was your last gynecologic [urologic] examination (Pap smear, mammogram)? Is there a family history of breast disease, ovarian cancer, testicular cancer, colon cancer? With all the attention on safer sex today and responsible parenting, many people have questions about their sexual self-care behaviors. Do you have any such concerns?" [It is important for nurses to ascertain if clients possess the knowledge, attitudes, and skills necessary to promote their own sexual health and that of others.]
Sexual self-concept	
Sexual identity	"How do you feel about yourself as a man or woman? Is anything changing the way you feel about yourself?"
Sexual body image	"Many people have concerns about their sexual body image. Are you comfortable with your physical maleness or femaleness? Have you experienced any physical changes (eg, baldness, weight loss or gain, impotence, menopause, mastectomy, hysterectomy, sterilization) that are troubling to you?"
Sexual self-esteem	"We all have certain expectations of ourselves. Are you comfortable with the way you are currently expressing yourself sexually and meeting your sexual needs?"
Sexual role performance	"Has anything interferred with your ability to be a spouse, sexual partner, parent (any other valued sex-related roles)?"
Sexual functioning	"It's not unusual for people with health concerns [name specific medical problem, if appropriate] to have questions related to sexuality and sexual functioning. Do you have any questions or concerns that I can help you with? Has anything [if appropriate substitute the name of a specific disease, surgery, or medication] changed your ability to function sexually?" [Asking clients if they have questions about resuming their usual sexual activity is an appropriate part of discharge planning for many clients.]

ish. For example, the client may choose the term *come* to mean climax or orgasm.

It is useful to begin questions with "many people like" or "many people feel." This gives clients security in knowing they are not alone in how they feel and are encouraged to talk about their problems or concerns. An example of this type of questioning is the following: "Many people feel that it's helpful to discuss your concerns about sex with your partner. What do you think about this?"

Annon (cited in Reamy, 1984) has described one method of obtaining information from a client with a sexual problem. This method elicits information in a short time:

- Description of the problem: "How would you describe the problem?"
- Onset and cause of the problem: "What do you think caused the problem or what was happening when you first noticed it?"
- Past attempts at resolution: "What have you tried in the past to correct the problem?"
- Goals of the client: "What do you wish to accomplish?"

A narrative form of recording a sexual history is generally used because it allows the interviewer to document the data in many of the client's own words. If a client is seeking help for a sexual problem, a more specific format will be used in recording information obtained by a skilled therapist.

Sexual Dysfunction

Sexual dysfunction is a problem that prevents an individual or couple from engaging in or enjoying satisfactory sexual intercourse and orgasm. Dysfunctions may occur as a result of physiologic malfunctions, conflicts with cultural norms, interpersonal problems, or any combination of these. Anxieties and fears concerning the sexual act are most always present. Clients with severe sexual dysfunctions require intensive professional therapy from a qualified sex therapist. It is hypothesized that sexual dysfunctioning is a problem of considerable magnitude. A few of

the major dysfunctions are briefly discussed here and in Table 40-4.

Male Sexual Dysfunctions **Erectile failure**, also called **impotence**, is the inability of a man to attain or maintain an erection to such an extent that he cannot have satisfactory intercourse. Common causes of impotence include various illnesses, treatments for these illnesses, and personal anxieties.

Premature ejaculation is the condition when a man consistently reaches ejaculation or orgasm before or soon after entering the vagina. The result is that his partner usually does not have time to reach sexual satisfaction. Causes of the problem are rarely physical in nature.

Retarded ejaculation, also called *ejaculatory incompetence*, refers to a man's inability to ejaculate into the vagina

T A B L E   4 0 - 4

Sexual Dysfunction and Nursing Assessment	
Sexual Dysfunction	**Assessment Priorities**
Male	
Erectile failure (impotence)	• History of diabetes, spinal cord trauma, cardiovascular disease, surgical procedure, alcoholism • Use of certain medications such as antihypertensives, antidepressants, or illicit drugs • Determine degree of mental depression that may be present • Obtain specific information regarding the degree of impotence, length of time of disorder, continuing life factors
Premature ejaculation	• Assess what client defines as his dysfunction and ability to control ejaculation • Assess any causative relationship factors, such as anxiety, guilt, lack of time, new partner, and so on
Retarded ejaculation	• History of neurologic disorders, Parkinson's disease, or use of certain medications • Same assessment priorities as for premature ejaculation
Female	
Inhibited sexual desire	• Use of oral contraceptives or other hormonal therapy, use of alcohol or certain medications • History of sexual abuse, rape or incest, depression, or other sexual dysfunctions • Assess any other contributing or relationship factors.
Orgasmic dysfunction	• Assess knowledge level regarding sexual response cycle and anatomy • Assess communication pattern between the client and her partner • Assess usual sexual pattern and behavior between client and her partner • Assess any other contributing factors
Dyspareunia	• History of diabetes, hormonal imbalance, vaginal infection, endometriosis, urethritis, cervicitis, or rectal lesions • Use of antihistamines, alcohol, tranquilizers, or illicit drugs • Assess client's ability for vaginal lubrication during sexual act • Assess client's use of coital positions • Assess use of cosmetic or chemical irritants to genitals such as deodorant tampons, contraceptive creams, or jellies or condoms • Physical assessment of internal and external genitalia • Assess any other contributing factors
Vaginismus	• Assess knowledge regarding anatomy and sexual response • Assess pattern of sexual activity: how often, level of arousal, orgasm • Assess presence of other sexual dysfunctions • History of sexual abuse, trauma, or rape • Assess client's feelings regarding her partner • Assess any other causative factors, such as fear of pregnancy, anxiety, guilt • Physical assessment of internal and external genitalia

or to suffer with delayed intravaginal ejaculation. The causes of this problem are similar to those of impotence. When it occurs after having experienced normal ejaculations, the cause is most probably due to interpersonal problems.

Female Sexual Dysfunctions   Inhibited sexual desire consists of an inhibition in sexual arousal so that congestion and vaginal lubrication are absent or minimal. Causative factors may be anxiety, negative emotions, fear, interpersonal problems, or physical factors.

Orgasmic dysfunction is defined as the inability of a woman to reach orgasm. The causes are similar to those of inhibited sexual desire.

Dyspareunia is painful intercourse. Although it is most often described by women, some men may also suffer from this disorder. The cause is usually physical in nature, although psychological problems such as fear and anxiety can cause pain in some women.

Vaginismus is a rare condition in which the vaginal opening closes tightly and prevents penile penetration. Vaginismus is due to involuntary spastic contractions of muscles at and around the vaginal opening and the levator ani muscles. The cause of vaginismus may be physical, psychologic, or both.

Physical Assessment

Physical examination of the reproductive or genitourinary system for either male or female clients is necessary under the following circumstances:

- As part of a routine physical examination
- Annual women's health care, including Pap smear
- Suspicion of an STD
- Suspicion of pregnancy
- Work-up for infertility
- Unusual lump, discharge, or unusual appearance of the genital organs noticed by the client
- Request for birth control
- Change in urinary function

The examiner may routinely perform a complete physical examination along with assessment of the reproductive system if the client has not had contact with the health care system within 1 year or if assessment findings of a complete examination would be useful in diagnosing an ailment or complaint of the client.

The nurse should initially ask whether the client has experienced this type of examination in the past if this information is not evident by the client's records. Depending on the client's knowledge base, the nurse should explain the progressive steps of the examination and what the client may feel during the examination. This will give the client some feeling of control and security during the examination. The nurse's responsibilities during an examination of the reproductive system are as follows:

- To provide information to the client regarding the examination

- To teach the client
- To provide support for the client during the examination
- To assist the examiner, if appropriate, with any procedures or laboratory studies

Female

Examination of body parts that are considered private and not usually viewed by others is embarrassing for some women. Many physical examinations are performed by nurse practitioners in women's health facilities. However, many examiners are male physicians. It is the responsibility of the nurse present at such an examination to anticipate anxiety and discomfort on the part of the client. In some cultures, the spouse must be present if his wife is to be examined. Preparation for and discussion of the examination are covered in Chapter 24, as is breast examination. The breast examination provides an excellent opportunity to assess the woman's knowledge of breast self-examination and to teach her how to examine her breasts properly. Breast self-examination is discussed later in this chapter.

The woman should be informed before the examiner touches her. This information greatly diminishes a woman's reflex to jump when her external genitalia are initially palpated and consequently prevents tightening of the pelvic muscles. Her relaxation eliminates much of the discomfort of the examination.

The vaginal speculum, as illustrated in Figure 24-1, is a two-bladed instrument used to open the vagina and to inspect the cervix and vaginal walls. Its use can cause discomfort if the client is not assisted to relax or if the wrong size speculum is used. It is helpful to show the speculum to the woman and explain its function beforehand. A Papanicolaou's stain test (Pap smear) is performed of the cervix, and cultures may be taken while the speculum is in place. The speculum is slowly withdrawn from the vagina while the examiner notes the condition of the vaginal walls.

A bimanual examination is performed to assess internal structures. The examiner introduces the gloved index and middle fingers of one hand into the client's vagina while the other hand lies on the client's lower abdomen. The cervix is palpated for movement, tenderness, and consistency. The areas around the cervix are also palpated. The uterus is examined by palpation between the internal and external hands for size, shape, contour, and consistency and for the presence of lumps or lesions.

The client is assisted to a sitting position by instructing her first to push back on the examining table from the stirrups to avoid straining the back. A running commentary about assessment findings by the examiner is necessary throughout the examination to teach the woman about her body as well as to assist her to relax and remove the mystery of a pelvic examination. Mirrors may be used to educate women about body parts they have never examined.

Male

The examination of the male genitalia is described in Chapter 24. Examination of the man's breast should always be included in the nursing examination. Although cancer of the male breast is rare, it can occur. The breast tissue and underlying muscle mass are palpated for lesions and the nipples are assessed for presence of discharge.

The external male genitalia should be examined with gloved hands. The perineum and anal sphincter are best inspected with the client lying on his side with the knees bent. The prostate gland is palpated through the rectum. The client can be assisted in this portion of the examination if he is asked to bear down against the examiner's finger as it is placed within the rectum.

The male client should be given the same consideration during the genitourinary examination as the female client. All procedures should be explained and the client's involvement in the examination encouraged.

Diagnosing

Sexual Dysfunction as the Problem Before a nursing diagnosis can be made regarding a sexual problem, the assessment data collected by the nurse must be carefully reviewed to determine if the situation can be corrected by independent nursing interventions. Although many problems of sexuality experienced by a client in a health care situation are amenable to nursing action, some require the expertise of other specialties. For example, an impotent diabetic client who would benefit from a penile implant needs medical consultation. A client with a serious sexual dysfunction or who practices a destructive sexual expression needs intensive therapy by a clinical psychologist, sex therapist, or counselor. Appropriate referrals by the nurse should follow the identification of such problems. Either of two diagnoses, Sexual Dysfunction or Altered Sexuality Patterns, is used to describe problems of sexuality amenable to nursing intervention. A related diagnosis is Rape-Trauma Syndrome.

Sexual dysfunction may be specified as erectile failure (impotence); premature ejaculation; retarded ejaculation; inhibited sexual desire; orgasmic dysfunction; vaginismus; or dyspareunia. Common etiologies for sexual dysfunction include effects of medication (specify); effects of alcohol consumption; effects of disease process (specify); history of abuse (specify rape, incest); feelings of depression; guilt; anxiety; fear of rejection; miscommunication with partner; fear of pain; effects of birth control method (specify); lack of knowledge; or effects of surgical procedure (specify). The nursing diagnosis Altered Sexuality Patterns can be further specified by loss of desire (to abstinence); increased desire

---

F O C U S   O N   T H E   O L D E R   A D U L T

Talking With Elderly People About Sexuality

The many losses associated with aging leave elderly people with special needs for love and affection. Unfortunately many health care professionals simply assume that older people have no health concerns related to sexuality. Factors that can inhibit sexual activity in elderly adults include the following:

- Societal expectations that sexual activity somehow belongs to the young and beautiful
- Rigid moral principles
- Decreased self-esteem
- Physical factors: age-related body changes, the effects of fatigue, illness, medications
- The attitudes of health care professionals who ignore or demean expressions of sexual needs by elderly people
- Institutional factors such as policies preventing sexual activity between competent, consenting older adults

Nurses who are sensitive to these factors can initiate a discussion about sexuality with elderly clients by asking the following questions. If questioning results in the older person's discomfort, do not press for information not needed for medical reasons.

"Many older people talk about feeling lonely. Are there people with whom you feel close who meet your needs for love and affection?"

"Are you sexually active currently?" [or] "Are you comfortable with your current level of sexual activity?"

"Is there anything interfering with your ability to be as sexually active as you would like? Physical limitations? Attitudes, beliefs, values? No partner?" [In a long-term care setting, institutional factors may inhibit sexual activity.]

"In what physical ways do you express and receive affection?" [kissing, hugging, hand-holding, coitus, oral or manual genital stimulation]

"Do you have any concerns about sexually transmitted diseases?"

"Is there any information you would like from me that would help you to better meet your needs for love and affection?" "Are there any questions or concerns you have that we haven't addressed?"

(to promiscuity); or change in sexual expression. Common etiologies for Altered Sexuality Patterns include stress (lifestyle, job, family, finances, marital conflict); isolation from partner; effects of pregnancy (specify); feelings of depression; loss of privacy; loss of communication with partner relationship change (new partner); effects of disease process (sexual position, frequency, mode of expression); change in body image; change in self-concept; or loss of partner. A representative sample of some nursing diagnoses concerning sexuality is given in the accompanying display.

Sexual Dysfunction as the Etiology   Changes in sexuality can affect other areas of human functioning. In the following nursing diagnoses, problems of sexuality are the etiology of another problem:

Impaired Adjustment related to loss of sexual partner, loss of sexual body part

Anxiety related to fear of pregnancy, loss of sexual functioning or desire, effects of disease process on sexual functioning

Pain related to sexual position, penile penetration, effects of genital surgery, lack of vaginal lubrication

Ineffective Individual Coping related to effects of body image on sexual expression, change in sexual partner

Fear related to pain during sexual intercourse, history of sexual abuse

NURSING DIAGNOSES FOR COMMON PROBLEMS

Sexuality

Problem	Related Factors	Sample Defining Characteristics
Sexual Dysfunction: Erectile Failure	Use of antihypertensive medication	• 45-year-old man with 3-year history of hypertension • Maintained normotensive on reserpine, 0.25 mg daily • "I have had trouble keeping an erection. My wife and I haven't made love in months. We don't talk about it anymore. I guess that part of my life is over." • Client appears resigned and saddened.
Sexual Dysfunction: Dyspareunia	Effects of menopausal process	• 54-year-old female whose last menses was 1 year ago • "Whenever my husband and I make love, my vagina burns and stings." • States decrease in vaginal lubrication during past several months
Altered Sexuality Patterns: Change in Sexual Expression	Loss of privacy due to hospitalization	• 23-year-old man hospitalized for past 6 weeks with injuries resulting from car crash; has been in traction for fractured right femur • "I can't take this place anymore! Everyone barges in here whenever they want to—nobody cares about my feelings—a guy can't even act like a guy around here. I wish I could be alone with my wife for a while with no interruptions."
Altered Sexuality Patterns: Loss of Desire	Change in body image due to body-altering surgery	• Surgery for bowel cancer with construction of permanent colostomy 1 month ago • "I know the colostomy was necessary to save my life, but it is so disgusting. I'll never be able to have a relationship with my husband again. It's a real turn-off to me—just imagine what he'll think—how can I expect him to want to make love to a freak?"
Alteration in Comfort: Pain	Abduction of hips in sexual positioning	• 60-year-old woman with history of osteoarthritis for 6 years • "The act of intercourse hurts my hips so bad that I'm in pain the whole next day. I don't want to stop having intercourse with my husband, but I'm going to have to if this pain gets worse." • Client states that the missionary position is the only position used during sex with her husband throughout their 40-year marriage.

Anticipatory Grieving related to loss of sexual functioning, effects of surgical excision of genital body part

Altered Growth and Development related to sexual exploitation or abuse, sexual guilt, effects of hormonal imbalance, lack of information about sexuality

Knowledge Deficit (specify: Contraceptive Methods, Spread of STDs, Sexual Response, Genital Anatomy, Modes of Sexual Expression, Self-Examination, Effects of Disease or Medications) related to misinformation, sexual myths, lack of interest in learning, cognitive limitation

Body Image Disturbance (specify: Surgical Excision of Genital Body Part, Loss of or Gain in Body Weight) related to fear of rejection

Impaired Social Interaction related to effects of marital separation or divorce

Social Isolation related to fear of contraction of STD, fear of sexual encounter

Planning: Client Goals

It is important for nurses to value sexuality as an important aspect of who the client is and how the client is identified as a unique human. Specific client goals to promote sexual wellness will be determined.

The client will:

- Define individual sexuality
- Establish open patterns of communication with significant others
- Develop self-awareness and body awareness
- Practice responsible sexual expression (eg, by 5/1/93, the client will use rubber condoms with all sexual encounters)

Specific client goals will depend on the nature of the client's problem or concern. Client goals should be client oriented, that is, something the client desires to do or has the ability to accomplish. For example, it is not enough to advise a method of birth control; rather, the nurse needs to know which method the client is motivated and able to use.

Implementing

Establishing a Trusting Nurse–Client Relationship

It is impossible to address or help a client's sexuality if trust has not developed between the nurse and the client. The

T H R O U G H

T H E   E Y E S

O F   A   S T U D E N T

I knew it was going to happen sooner or later. Male nurses are not unheard of in this day and age, but some people just aren't yet ready for us. Especially Ethel, a 68-year-old black woman with a deep religious conviction. I concluded this because she called on Jesus for help when I told her that I was her student nurse for the day, and that I would be giving her a bath.

"You're my nurse?" she said. "Help me, Jesus . . . No, no, you just go on and help somebody else, honey. I've already had my bath," she insisted.

Accordingly, I told her she was mistaken and that I understood her anxiety. Then I proceeded to exaggerate the truth by saying that I had done this before, when really I had given baths before, but not to members of the opposite sex. She thought *she* was having anxiety!

Next I asked my instructor, Lynn, for help. She quickly assessed the situation and tried to comfort Ethel by vouching for my professional character and abilities, but still no go. Then I tried appealing to her logic.

"This is a hospital where male doctors examine you all the time. Why is this any different?" I asked. "Because you are *not* a doctor" was her logical reply.

I felt inadequate. I could not give this women the care she needed because of my gender. Luckily, in the next bed, Michele was about to give her client a bath. She offered to give Ethel her bath if I would help her with her clients.

Consequently, Ethel got her bath, and I learned that a nurse has to be flexible as well as willing to ask for and accept help when the client's quality of care is at stake. This is something I hope to remember throughout my nursing career.

—Daniel E. Zirolli, Delaware County Community College, Media, Pennsylvania

nurse needs to project an objective, nonthreatening, and nonjudgmental attitude and an aura of confidentiality. The nurse's anticipating client concerns and needs through awareness of the client's behavior and verbal and nonverbal cues also helps the client trust the nurse later on with information of an intimate nature. It is important to establish respect for the individual and empathy before sexual topics are discussed. An empathic nurse considers all of an individual's circumstances and life experiences and views them from a therapeutic, not a pitying, approach. Only when the nurse is accepted as a trusted caring person will the client relay details of private life, including concerns of a sexual nature.

Teaching the Client

Most nursing interventions pertaining to a client's sexuality encompass teaching to promote wellness. Major goals of client teaching are a change in knowledge, a change in client attitude, or a change in behaviors. In some situations, clients need assistance in defining or redefining their sexuality and its importance to their lives. Offering information, dispelling fears, and providing positive reinforcement are some ways nurses can assist clients to increase their knowledge about their bodies and sexual functioning. Clients may need assistance in modifying behaviors or learning new skills to increase the quality of sexual health and functioning.

Sexual Myths and Body Awareness

Many people believe things about sex that they have heard from family, friends, or as part of their culture that are simply not true or not based on scientific data. The nurse may refute sexual myths (Table 40-5) and teach factual information during the assessment or while providing care.

Clients may need assistance in becoming familiar with what they believe and feel about their sexual selves. The nurse can be helpful in a situation in which a client has difficulty accepting or developing his or her sexuality by promoting self-confidence and a good self-concept in the client. When clients feel comfortable about themselves and their sensual feelings, they can begin to focus on how they feel about their sexual functioning and specific sexual expressions.

Getting to know one's physical body is important to healthy sexual development. Every man and woman, sexually active or not, needs to be aware of the appearance of his or her individual genitalia. Some people, because of their background, feel ashamed and repulsed by their bodies. Others feel that touching the body is dirty and may feel guilt and anxiety in stimulating themselves. Clients need assistance in improving body awareness if any of these issues are present. Clients become accustomed to looking at their bodies by looking at nonthreatening anatomy first and then proceeding to the genitals. This can be done in the shower or with the use of a mirror. Knowing what looks normal can be of great importance in reporting the development of an

unusual appearance later on. After clients have developed some degree of comfort in looking at their bodies, they can progress to experiencing touch. Again, clients should progress from nonthreatening parts of the body until the genitals can be touched without stress.

A good exercise for women in developing body awareness is the use of *Kegel exercises*. These exercises promote good vaginal tone by localizing and strengthening the *pubococcygeal* muscle. A woman can locate this muscle by stopping a stream of urine midway through urination. Contracting this muscle can be repeated at any time of the day in any circumstance because its performance is undetectable. Women who practice Kegel exercises have found that sexual satisfaction is greatly improved.

Self-Examination

It is important for both men and women to learn to examine themselves through inspection and palpation of sexual body parts. Many conditions, some life threatening, can be detected when self-examination is performed. Early detection of cancer is crucial to its control and cure. The presence of some STDs may also be detected by self-examination.

Breast Self-Examination   The importance of breast self-examination (BSE) lies in its routine monthly performance, which helps the person to become familiar with what is normal. BSE should be performed after each menses or once a month for a postmenopausal woman. Any contact with a female client in the health care delivery system should include assessment of her knowledge and practice of BSE.

The steps in performing BSE are shown in Figure 40-4 and are as follows:

1. Stand before a mirror with hands on hips to inspect the breasts. Look for the presence of indentations, dimpling, or odd position of a nipple. Any discharge from a nipple is abnormal unless the woman is nursing. Changes in size or shape of breasts should be reported.

2. Lie on the bed with a small pillow under the shoulder on the side of the breast to be examined, and the arm over the head. Using the opposite hand, palpate the breast starting at the outer edge of the breast, using small circular motions of the flat portions of the fingers. Work inward in a clockwise manner toward the nipple. The nipple should be gently squeezed to detect the presence of any discharge. This procedure should be repeated for the opposite breast. Any unusual lump or tenderness should be reported to a health care professional.

Testicular Self-Examination   Male clients need to be taught to perform monthly assessment of the testicles. Although testicular cancer is not widespread, it can be easily detected and prognosis is good if found early. A good time to examine the testes is during a shower, when the scrotum

T A B L E 4 0 - 5

Sexual Myths and Facts to Refute Them

Myths	Facts
Each person is born with a certain amount of sexual drive, which if over-drawn in youth leaves little reserve for later years.	Actually, the correlation between sexual activity and length of time it persists throughout life is just the opposite. The more consistently sexually active a person is, the longer the activity continues into the later years of life.
The need for expressing one's sexuality becomes less important in the latter half of one's life.	Physiologically, sexual desire and ability do not decrease markedly after middle age. The expression of one's sexuality, as an integral part of development, follows the overall pattern of health and physical performance.
Sexual abstinence is necessary in training for sports.	Physiologically, the achievement of orgasm is rarely more demanding than most activities encountered in daily life. The desire for sleep that often follows is most commonly due to factors other than physical exhaustion from sexual activities. There is no scientific evidence that sex "weakens" a person.
Excessive sexual activity can lead to mental illness.	The biologic significance of human sexuality has no greater effect on total development than any other necessary biologic function. There is no scientific basis for believing that one will develop a mental or physical illness with excessive or no sexual activity.
Wet dreams are indicators of sexual disorders.	Erotic dreams that culminate in orgasms are normal common physiologic phenomena in at least 85% of men. They can occur at any age after puberty. Some women also report in clinical studies that their sexual dreams culminate in orgasm. In women, this phenomenon is believed to increase with advancing age.
Because of the anatomic nature of the sex organs, women are passive and men are aggressive.	Physiologic studies disprove this myth by showing the woman to be far from passive. Maximum gratification requires each partner to be both passive and aggressive in participating mutually and cooperatively.
It is unnatural for a woman to have as strong a desire for sex as a man—women should not enjoy sex as much as men.	These myths have been reinforced by a society that has traditionally taught women that they are to suppress sexual desires to gain love, security, and society's respect, based on the assumption that it is the basic nature of women to be submissive, dependent, and subordinate. Physiologic studies indicate that, in some respects, the woman's sex drive is not only as strong but may be even stronger than that of the man.
Women who have multiple orgasms or who readily come to climax are nymphomaniacs or promiscuous.	Physiologic studies at this time suggest that we do not know women's sexual potential; these studies indicate that there is a wide range of intensity and duration of orgasmic experience, and the potential for multiple or frequent orgasms within a brief period is not at all uncommon. Therefore, women normally may have greater orgasmic capacity than men with regard to duration and frequency of orgasm.
There is a difference between vaginal orgasm and clitoral orgasm.	Physiologic misunderstanding has produced the myth of separate clitoral and vaginal orgasms rather than their interrelations. Female orgasm is normally initiated by clitoral stimulation, but because it is a total body response, there are marked variations in intensity and timing. There is no reason to believe that the female response to the sex act is due to a vaginal rather than a clitoral orgasm.
A mature sexual relationship requires the man and woman to achieve simultaneous orgasm.	Although simultaneous orgasm may be desirable, it is unrealistic. Often it is possible only under the most ideal circumstances, and is not a determinant of sexual achievement or of satisfaction (except to someone who accepts this as dogma).
It is dangerous to have intercourse during menstruation.	Because the source of the menstrual flow is from the uterus rather than the vagina, there is no basis for concern about tissue damage to the vagina. Actually, the desire for sex increases during the menses as a result of increased pelvic vasocongestion. There is no physiologic basis for abstinence during the menses.
The larger penis has greater possibilities for producing orgasm in the woman.	Physiologically, there is practically no relation between the size of a man's penis and his ability to satisfy a woman sexually. Furthermore, there is little correlation between penile size and body size and their relation to sexual potency.
The face-to-face coital position is the proper, moral, and healthy one.	Recent knowledge of human sexual practices dispels this myth with the recognition that there is no normal or single most acceptable sexual position. Whatever position offers the most pleasure and is acceptable to both partners is correct for them. Any variation is normal, healthy, and proper if it satisfies both partners.
The ability to achieve orgasm is an indicator of a person's sexual responsiveness.	Achievement of a satisfactory sexual response is the result of numerous physical, psychological, and cultural influences. Too often the physical fact of orgasm (or lack of orgasm) is taken to be symbolic of sexual responsiveness and seen out of context of the entire relationship between man and woman.

becomes warm and loose. Men should also be taught the importance of examining their breasts.

The steps in TSE, shown in Figure 40-5, are as follows:

1. The thumb and the fingers of each hand are used to palpate each testicle simultaneously. The client should systematically palpate the testes for the presence of lumps or differences in texture. The testes should feel smooth.

2. The epididymis is palpated above each testicle. The epididymis feels soft and not as smooth as a testicle.

3. The spermatic cord, or vas deferens, extends upward from the scrotum toward the base of the penis and should be palpated for firmness and smoothness in texture.

Contraception

Clients choose **contraception** for many reasons and may contact health care providers for information on birth control or contraceptive methods. Some people use contraception for the orderly spacing of pregnancies in a family. Others use a contraceptive method to prevent pregnancy from occurring until a family is desired. Some people choose a permanent method to prevent the possibility of pregnancy from ever occurring.

The best method available to prevent a pregnancy is sexual abstinence. For many people, however, this is not an acceptable method. All contraceptive methods have distinct advantages and disadvantages. It is the responsibility of the nurse to understand and explain thoroughly the available methods so the client can choose one that will best meet his or her unique situation and needs.

Natural Family Planning Natural family planning methods are available to everyone but using them effectively requires motivation and understanding of male and female reproductive anatomy and physiology. There are four basic natural family planning methods: calendar (rhythm method), basal body temperature (BBT), ovulation (Billing's method), and symptothermal.

The *rhythm* or *calendar* method is based on a woman's monthly menstrual cycle in determining safe and unsafe

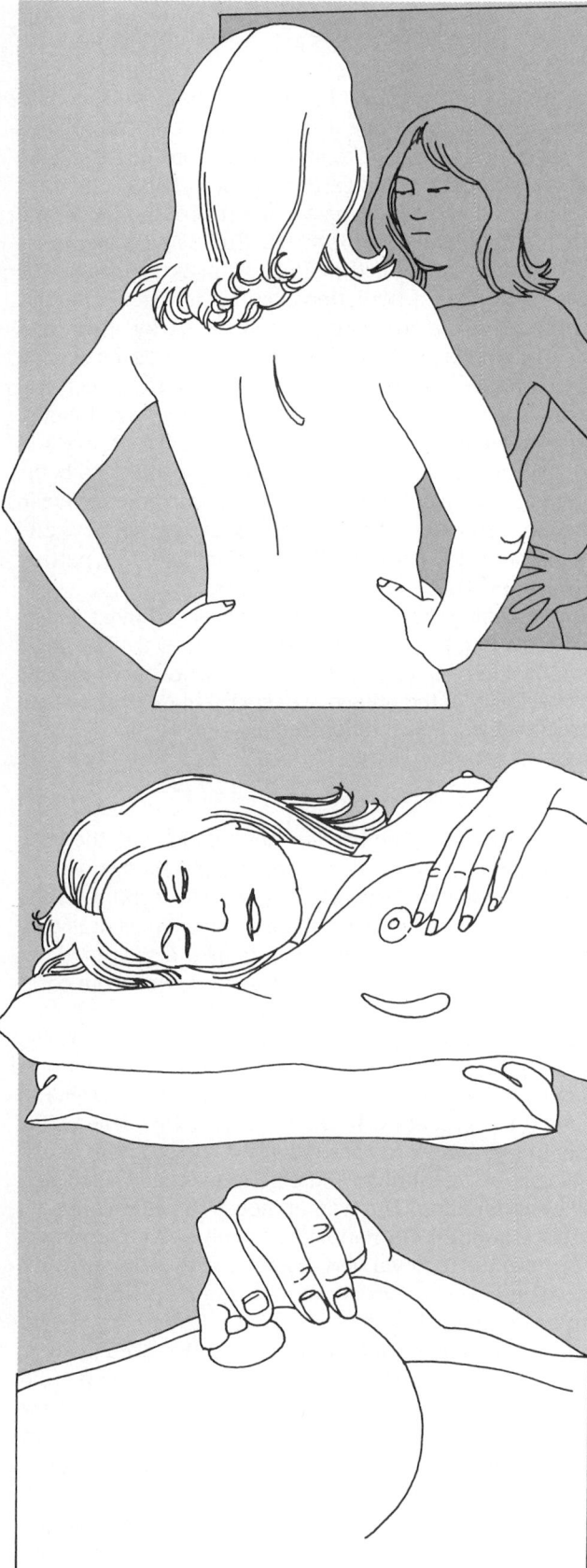

F I G U R E 4 0 - 4

Breast self-examination is to be performed once a month. It is begun with inspection using a mirror. Attention is given to contours of the breast and to the skin. Pressing down on the hips serves to tense pectoralis major muscles to inspect for any retraction of the skin. Palpatory examination is performed in a supine position with the side to be examined elevated on a pillow or blanket. Self-examination is completed with a squeeze of the nipple to detect abnormal discharge.

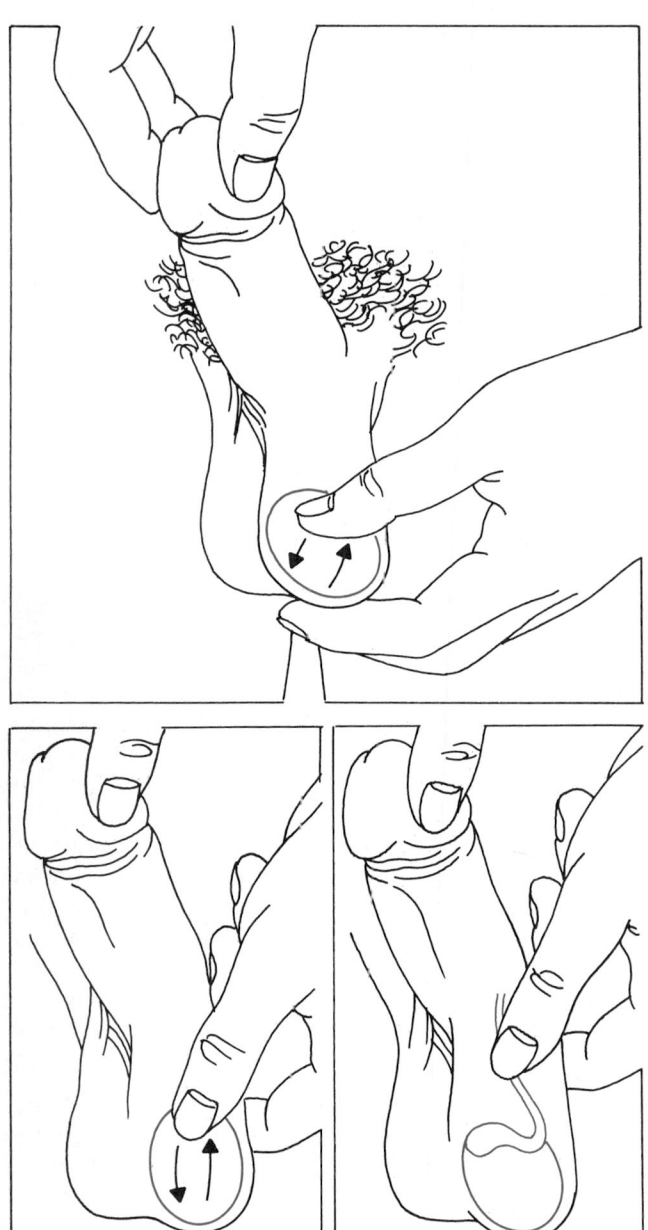

FIGURE 40-5

Testicular self-examination is to be performed once a month. A convenient time is after a warm bath or shower when the scrotum is relaxed. Both hands are used to palpate the testis; the normal testicle is smooth and uniform in consistency. (A) With the index and middle finger under the testis and the thumb on top, roll the testis gently in a horizontal plane between the thumb and fingers, feeling for any evidence of a small lump or abnormality. (B) Follow the same procedure for palpation in the vertical plane. (C) Locate the epididymis (cordlike structure on the top and back of the testicle that stores and transports sperm). Repeat the examination for the other testis; it is normal to find one testis larger than the other. Any evidence of a small, pea-size lump should be checked by a physician. It may be due to an infection or a tumor growth.

days. It is an inappropriate method for a woman with irregular cycles. The unsafe days are regarded as periods for sexual abstinence because these days are optimal for conception. The *BBT* method is based on the body's response to hormones and ovulation. The woman takes and records her temperature on awakening every morning. A sudden drop in temperature indicates ovulation. This method restricts sexual activity to the second half of the menstrual cycle after ovulation has occurred. The *Billing's* method is based on the changes in the cervical mucus throughout the menstrual cycle. As ovulation occurs, the mucus changes considerably in consistency, becoming sticky, clear, and slippery like an egg white. This method requires the woman to be aware of and have the ability to assess her cervical mucus. The *symptothermal* method combines a number of signs of ovulation, including the rise in BBT, changes in cervical mucous, and variations of the cervix. Both the ovulation and symptothermal methods can be effective in avoiding pregnancy if mutual understanding, support, and motivation exist between the woman and her partner (Fehring, 1991).

Coitus interruptus, one of the oldest and most widely used contraceptive methods, is the withdrawal of the penis from the vagina before ejaculation. Its drawbacks include the possibility of the presence of sperm in Cowper's gland secretions before ejaculation and the stress it places on the man's sexual experience.

Barrier Methods The barrier methods include the condom, diaphragm, cervical cap, and vaginal sponge used in combination with a spermicidal agent. The *diaphragm* has been used in various forms since ancient times. It is currently marketed as a large dome-shaped device made of latex rubber that mechanically prevents semen from coming into contact with the cervix. It is also used to hold a quantity of spermicidal jelly in place against the cervix. The diaphragm is placed in the vagina before sexual activity. It fits between the pelvic notch at the front of the vagina to behind the cervix at the back. It should not be detected by either the woman or her partner when correctly situated in the vagina. A diaphragm must be individually fitted at a pelvic examination. The woman needs to be familiar with her body and able to handle her genitals for diaphragm placement and removal. The diaphragm must be worn during each episode of sexual activity and consistently used with a spermicidal agent.

The traditional *condom,* or "rubber," is used by men, although it is appropriate for a woman to have them available for her partner's use. The condom is rolled over the erect penis and collects the semen after ejaculation occurs. If the condom does not have a nipple receptacle end, leave a small space at the end of the condom to collect sperm (this prevents breakage). The condom is readily and conveniently available over the counter. The condom has had a surge of popularity with the recent increased incidence of AIDS and other STDs among single people. A new female condom known as the *vaginal pouch* may offer women greater protection from STDs than male condoms and equal protection from unwanted pregnancy.

The *cervical cap* currently is not universally available. Its mechanism of action is similar to that of the diaphragm. The cervical cap is a thimble-shaped rubber device that is placed over the cervix and may be left there for up to 3 days at a time. Not all women can wear a cervical cap because of individual anatomic differences. There is some evidence to suggest that the cervical cap can cause cervical inflammation and increase risk of pelvic infection.

Spermicides are used with barrier methods but can also be used alone. Spermicides come in creams, jellies, foams, and suppositories. Although readily available, spermicides are not as effective alone as when combined with another method, such as a diaphragm or a condom.

The *vaginal sponge* is a barrier method that contains a spermicide. It has been available over the counter for several years. The sponge not only acts as a barrier between the semen and the cervix but also serves as a reservoir to hold semen. The vaginal sponge does carry some risk of toxic shock syndrome (TSS) and is contraindicated for use in women who have a past history of TSS. It is important for women who use the vaginal sponge to follow package directions carefully and to remove the sponge within 24 hours. The vaginal sponge is about as effective as the diaphragm.

Intrauterine Device The intrauterine device (IUD) is an object that is placed by a physician or nurse practitioner within the uterus to prevent implantation of fertilized ovum. The precise mechanism by which it works is unknown. Although it has a high effectiveness rate and requires little care or motivation on the part of the client, the IUD has many serious side effects and resulting complications. It is an excellent method for women who have completed their families but are not ready or willing to take the final step toward sterilization. Owing to the litigation resulting from complications caused by the IUD, it has been taken off the market by most IUD-producing pharmaceutical companies. Although the IUD may reappear in the future, all women who currently have an IUD in place should seek assistance from a health care provider to have it removed. Women wearing a Progestasert IUD should check for the presence of the string in the vagina after every menses and should have the IUD replaced every year.

Hormonal Methods Hormonal methods are based on the feedback mechanism of hormones of the menstrual cycle. Synthetic estrogens and progestin chemical compounds are used in the form of a pill, shot, or implant to prevent ovulation.

The *oral contraceptive* ("the pill") is the most common contraceptive method and the most popular method for

---

RESEARCH IN NURSING Making a Difference

Women and HIV Infection

Nurses are in a unique position to provide holistic care, education, and counseling, to coordinate services, and to conduct and disseminate research about HIV and AIDS; they can also provide leadership as advocates for women through professional and political action.

Related Research

Williams, A. B. (1991). Women at risk: An AIDS educational needs assessment. *Image: Journal of Nursing Scholarship, 23*(4), 208–213.

To acquire the information nurses need to develop education and support programs for women at risk for AIDS, a qualitative needs assessment of 21 women at risk through their own injection drug use or as the heterosexual partners of injection drug users, was conducted. Citing the great need for professional advocacy and support her interviews documented, the author urged nurses to become advocates for the inclusion of women's concerns in the development of public health policy and education. "It is difficult to encourage women to seek treatment for drug dependence, HIV-1 counseling and testing, or abortion counseling when access to these services is limited" (p. 213).

Smeltzer, S. C., & Whipple B. (1991). Women and HIV infection. *Image: Journal of Nursing Scholarship, 23*(4), 249–256.

In this article, the authors reviewed what is known about HIV infection and AIDS in women and alerted nurses to the special issues concerning women and HIV infection so that they can use this information in their research, education, and practice. "HIV transmission to women will continue as long as they remain unequal partners in society. Prevention programs must be aimed at empowering women to initiate behavior change and to maintain healthy sexual behaviors. These programs must be considered in terms of political and economic empowerment" (p. 255).

Summary

Smeltzer and Whipple noted that public policy, research, and education and treatment programs have basically ignored the special needs of women infected with HIV. Awareness of and increased attention to the issues of sexism and lack of empowerment and their effect on all women must continue to be addressed.

women in their twenties. Most of the harmful side effects and dangers associated with taking the pill are related to the estrogen component. However, most pills currently available contain a small dose of 35 μg of estrogen. The pill has many beneficial noncontraceptive effects. It has been shown to protect women against the development of breast, ovarian, and endometrial cancer (Dickerson, 1983). Taken consistently and as prescribed, the pill is almost 100% effective in guarding against pregnancy. However, the cost may be prohibitive to some women. The woman must also be motivated to take a pill every day at the same time. A health history and physical examination by a health care provider are necessary to obtain a prescription for oral contraceptives. Some women should not take the pill in the presence of certain physiologic disorders or diseases. Smoking increases the risks associated with oral contraceptives.

Sterilization Although male and female sterilization methods can be surgically reversed, the results are not always satisfactory and the methods should therefore be regarded as permanent and irreversible. Sexual desire and ability are unaffected by sterilization.

Sterilization in the woman is accomplished by surgically severing the fallopian tubes. This procedure is known as a *tubal ligation* and prevents travel of the ovum down the tube. Currently, tubal ligation is usually performed on an outpatient basis. Some physicians can also perform the tubal ligation under local anesthesia. Postoperative care and recovery time are required after a tubal ligation.

Sterilization in the man is accomplished by surgically severing the vas deferens, which prevents sperm from entering the semen. The *vasectomy* is usually performed in a physician's office under local anesthesia. It is important that the man know that he and his partner must use an alternate form of contraception until he has produced two semen analyses with zero sperm. It usually takes about 4 to 6 weeks for all stored sperm to be eliminated from the ductal system of the male.

Coerced Contraception Implantable long-lasting contraceptives that gradually release progestin for up to 5 years, such as Norplant, are currently available. Because effectiveness does not depend on client compliance and use can be monitored easily by checking for the implants in the woman's arm, Norplant immediately initiated controversy in the press, legislative arena, and courts for fear it might be used for coerced contraception. Some suggested the use of financial incentives for welfare recipients who agreed to use Norplant and others recommended its use as part of a sentence or plea agreement for offenses such as child abuse, child endangerment, and murder. At issue is whether an individual's right to privacy outweighs the state's interest in limiting unwanted pregnancies (Rhodes, 1991).

Coping With Special Sexual Needs

The nurse can do much for clients to facilitate their coping with sexual concerns generated by diseases and their treatments. Anticipatory guidance and information should be offered to the client. The importance of open communication with the partner should be stressed. The nurse should include the partner in teaching. Discussion about possible sexual positions is useful and can aid in eliminating pain during coitus. The client can use drawings in selecting possible sexual positions. The client will also find that intercourse may be more comfortable if pain medication is taken before beginning any sexual activity.

When teaching clients about medications, it is important to include known possible sexual alterations to prevent future anxiety and also depression. Clients should alert their physicians if these side effects are experienced. Often a drug dosage can be modified or the drug changed if sexual functioning is affected. Otherwise, clients may opt to discontinue the medication on their own rather than sacrifice optimal sexual functioning, if this is an important aspect of life.

Nurses also need to be aware of the special concerns and issues surrounding the care of a homosexual client. Homosexuals have the same right to health care as do heterosexuals. The homosexual has the right to information and the right to confidentiality just like anyone else.

Responsible Sexual Expression

Clients need to know how best to gain satisfactory sexual experiences and yet behave responsibly in their activities. Responsible sexuality encompasses these major areas: the form of sexual expression, the prevention of unwanted pregnancy, the prevention of spread of STDs, and sex education.

The form of sexual expression used by clients should not inflict unwanted harm on themselves or others. When the sexual expression encroaches on the rights of others, it is neither healthy nor desirable. Sexual acts that violate another's rights are usually considered to be acts of aggression or hostility rather than stemming from sexual need or desire. Acts of rape in particular are motivated by the need to dominate and humiliate the victim.

The prevention of an unwanted pregnancy must be a conscious decision. Anyone considering the possibility of a sexual encounter who is unprepared for pregnancy should refrain from intercourse or seek out a contraceptive method either from a health care provider or from the pharmacy; it is too late to think about contraception during sexual intercourse. To practice responsible sexuality, the contraceptive method must be used consistently and according to instructions.

The incidence of the various STDs is widespread. The only absolute method to avoid an STD is to remain a virgin until marriage, to marry a person who is a virgin, and henceforth never to have sex with anyone else. When this is

RESEARCH IN NURSING Making a Difference

Gender Gap in Research

Nurses have been in the forefront of the movement calling for increased research in women's health issues and the inclusion of more women in clinical trials. The studies that follow both address key women's health issues in vulnerable populations.

Related Research

Jemmott, L. S., & Jemmott, J. B., (1991). Applying the theory of reasoned action to AIDS risk behavior: Condom use among black women. *Nursing Research, 40*(4), 228–234.

This study tested hypotheses regarding attitudinal and normative influences on intentions to use condoms, a practice that would reduce women's risk of sexually transmitted HIV infections. Participants were 103 sexually active, unmarried black female undergraduates in an area with a high rate of reported AIDS cases among women. The results suggest that the theory of reasoned action that has been successfully applied to a wide range of preventive health behaviors in diverse populations may apply to an important HIV-associated behavior among black women, resulting in a reduction of the devastating effect of AIDS.

Hall, L. A., Gurley, D. N., Sachs, B., & Kryscio, R. J. (1991). Psychosocial predictors of maternal depressive symptoms, parenting attitudes, and child behavior in single-parent families. *Nursing Research, 40*(4), 214–220.

This study identified psychosocial predictors of depressive symptoms among low-income, single mothers and investigated the effects of maternal psychosocial factors, depressive symptoms, and parenting attitudes on children's behavior. High depressive symptoms were present in 134 (59%) of the 225 mothers in the sample and were associated with greater everyday stressors, fewer social resources, and greater use of avoidance coping. This study identified areas for intervention to enhance the well-being of low-income, single-mother families.

Summary

Nursing is providing leadership in researching women's health issues, which until recently have been greatly underinvestigated. Women and children are already benefiting from nursing's commitment to these research priorities.

---

impractical, other practices that can decrease a person's exposure to STDs are the following:

- The client should limit the number of sexual partners. The risk of an STD rises with the addition of each new partner.
- If a partner has symptoms of an STD, the client should abstain from any sexual activity.
- If the client is in doubt about possible exposure, he or she should report to a health care facility for examination.
- If the client does contract an STD, all partners should be notified and advised to seek treatment.
- The use of condoms is advocated for protection against STDs as well as against pregnancy. The client should keep a box of condoms on hand if monogamy is not practiced within the relationship.

Sex education is critical to healthy sexual development and safe sexual behaviors. Information received from peers and friends is almost always inadequate and erroneous. Parents should be taught to answer children's questions immediately and accurately.

Meeting Sexuality Needs of the Hospitalized Client

A hospital experience puts a strain on a person's individuality and sexual self. Illness may diminish feelings of sexual desire. Therefore, it can be a good sign of a client's improving health if sexual interaction is desired with the partner. This necessitates anticipatory guidance on the part of the nurse, because many clients may hesitate to make such a request for fear of being ridiculed. Often a client merely desires the privacy to hold and caress the partner. The intimacy of this act often fulfills feelings of longing to be needed and loved.

There are many ways nurses can advocate for a client's sexual needs. Some may seem obvious and commonplace, whereas others may necessitate nurses' coming to terms with their own sexuality (see the display titled Advocating Clients' Sexual Needs).

Counseling the Client Regarding Sexuality

Not all clients with sexual concerns need intensive therapy. Some clients benefit greatly by the presence of another to listen to verbally expressed concerns. Voicing their concerns allows clients the opportunity to put information into perspective and gain a clearer focus on what the problem really is and how to solve it. Nurses counseling clients need to refrain from offering their own advice because what is right for one person may be wrong for another. Also, offering false reassurances such as, "It will be all right" is unproductive. Rather, the nurse needs to adopt an objec-

---

Advocating Clients' Sexual Needs

- All clients should be accepted as sexual beings with the right to be treated with dignity and with sensitivity to their feelings.
- All clients have the right to some degree of privacy regardless of the circumstances surrounding their hospitalization.
    Anticipate the client's desire for privacy by the simple act of drawing a curtain or closing a door.
    Clients should be given the option of wearing their own sleepwear to promote sexual identity.
- Potentially shaming situations for the client should be anticipated.
    Give information regarding what the procedure is and why it needs to be done, and acknowledge that the client's embarassment is normal and understandable.
- Health care providers should not simply take for granted that clients do not mind intrusive or embarassing procedures performed on their bodies and private parts.
- Clients have a right to question the physician regarding sexual needs or future sexual functioning.
    Anticipate these questions for the client.

Ask clients if they have any concerns regarding sexuality that can be answered by the nurse.
Nurses can interface with the physician to obtain information required by the client.
- The atmosphere within the hospital unit needs to allow for sexual expression between clients and their partners.
- Confidentiality is a right of every hospitalized client.
    Do not promise confidentiality if that promise cannot be kept.
    Allow no one access to the client's personal records who is not directly involved in the client's care.
    Allow no information regarding clients to escape into idle conversation.
- All clients should be referred to formally as Mr., Mrs., Miss, Ms., according to the client's preference.
- Visitors, including a visiting spouse, should be referred to as people with genders, rather than as "the visitor."
- Clients should be allowed to keep some personal possessions, if it is practical to do so.

---

tive, empathic, and receptive attitude to facilitate an open communication between nurse and client.

Annon (cited in Hatcher et al., 1986) developed a model, termed PLISSIT, for counseling to be used by therapists and nontherapists for clients with sexual problems. The four stages to this model, each increasing in intensity with the seriousness of the client's problem, are listed in the display entitled Model for Counseling Clients With Sexual Problems (PLISSIT).

Evaluating

To evaluate the care plan for the client's sexuality needs, the nurse needs to use information from the client for most client goals. It is unrealistic and inappropriate for the nurse to evaluate the client by observing expression of client sexuality. However, the nurse can evaluate how the client is progressing toward sexuality-oriented goals by appear-

---

Model for Counseling Clients With Sexual Problems (PLISSIT)

P—*Permission giving:* The nurse may make a suggestion that the client can use. Permission giving is not the same as advice. Permission giving implies giving the client freedom to choose to do something that the authority figure (such as a nurse) deems to be a positive alternative. It may be something the client wanted to do all along. For example,
    Client: "Aren't some sexual positions perverted?"
    Nurse: "Many people enjoy using different positions for sex. Some positions are more pleasurable to some couples than others. You and your partner have the right to use any position for sex that you desire."

LI—*Limited information:* Specific factual information is required by the client. It often involves some aspect of anatomy and physiology or the specifics of certain sexual expressions.
SS—*Specific suggestions:* Clients need very specific instructions regarding a useful technique. Many clients have a sexual dysfunction for which they are seeking intervention and correction.
IT—*Intensive therapy:* Used primarily by therapists, it involves issues such as marriage, self-concept, and sexual desire, to name a few. If the first three levels of counseling presented were unsuccessful, intensive therapy is indicated.

---

ance, level of self-confidence, and manner. For example a client who has expressed feelings of anxiety in the past over a sexual concern should be observably more confident and free of anxiety if client goals are being met. The nurse also needs to question the client about progress toward goals. Some goals need to be stepping goals, because not all client problems are easily resolved with one-time intervention and direction.

One line of questioning when evaluating a client's progress is as follows: "In what ways have you been able to achieve [orgasm, increased desire, comfortable intercourse, erection]?" "What methods seemed most effective?" "Which were not?" "What do you think should be the next step?" The nurse should determine from this interaction with the client if something more needs to be accomplished. It is not enough to assume that because a set of goals has been met the client is satisfied with the results.

 NURSING PROCESS

in Clinical Practice

The nurse uses each phase of the nursing process when identifying and treating problems of sexuality categorized as nursing diagnoses. Quality care depends on the nurse's possession of the knowledge and clinical skills described earlier in this chapter. Numerous nursing diagnoses can be written to address problems of sexuality depending on specific client assessment data. The four nursing diagnoses chosen for review here are examples of the types of diagnoses that can be developed. The following outlines the assessment priorities, client goals, nursing interventions, and evaluative criteria for sexual concerns treated by nurses.

Sexual Dysfunction: Inhibited Sexual Desire
Altered Sexuality Patterns: Change in Sexual Expression
Knowledge Deficit: Contraceptive Methods
Body Image Disturbance related to breast removal

The case study in Chapter 29 addresses feminine hygiene concerns. In the case study in this chapter, nursing care is described for an adolescent client with a knowledge deficit.

Sexual Dysfunction: Inhibited Sexual Desire

For information on inhibited sexual desire, the reader is referred to the section of this chapter on sexual dysfunctions. It is important to identify the causative factors of inhibited desire. This is difficult due to the often complex nature of the problem. Therefore, an accurate and thorough assessment is crucial.

Assessment

- Assess the client's past ability for sexual arousal to determine if this is a new problem or a chronic one.
- Assess the client's interest for sexual activity.
- Assess for other contributing factors such as change in relationship or stressors (life-style, finances, job, children).
- Assess medications the client is currently taking (prescription and nonprescription) alcohol consumption.
- Assess the client's physical and mental status for presence of guilt, fear, anxiety, depression, fatigue.

- Assess the client's relationship with the current partner and also the quality of communication patterns.
- Use Annon's set of questions during interviewing to determine specific data related to the problem (see the previous section Sexual History).

Planning: Client Goals

The client will:
- Report an increase in sexual desire
- Identify factors in life-style that may be affecting desire
- Promote changes in life-style to relieve factors contributing to decreased desire
- Initiate open communication pattern with partner

Nursing Interventions

The nursing interventions used for assisting the client to develop an increase in sexual desire actually stem from the causative factors involved in creating the problem initially. A thorough assessment is critical to identify these causative factors. The following interventions specifically address inhibited sexual desire caused by stressful life-style:
- Assist the client to identify the specific stressor.
- Assist the client to determine if the stressor can be modified or controlled.
- Plan sexual activity for the time of day when stressors are minimized. (It may be helpful to block out on a calendar a 1- or 2-hour period on specific days.)
- Advise the client to initiate honest dialogue with the partner regarding the plan.
- Use the blocked-out period for stroking and relaxing to focus in on partner.
- Stress that sexual intercourse need not always be the goal of this exercise and not to feel stressed if it does not occur, because this would defeat the purpose of the exercise.

Evaluative Criteria

The client meets the previously stated goals. Refer the couple to the appropriate resource for more intensive therapy if inhibited desire persists.

Altered Sexuality Patterns: Change in Sexual Expression

Altered Sexuality Patterns is a broad diagnosis with many interpretations for use in nursing practice. Loss of desire, increased desire, and change in sexual expression are three dimensions of the problem that are defined more specifically as follows:

1. Loss of desire may also be interpreted as loss of opportunity or involuntary abstinence. The problem can be further specified by any number of causative factors.
2. Increased desire may also be interpreted as preoccupation with sexual activity. An example would be the beginning of a new sexual relationship. Although this in itself is rarely a problem for the individual, it could be if the desire leads to promiscuous or nondiscriminating behaviors.
3. A change in sexual expression may be a problem if it is involuntarily imposed on the client and the partner. Any disease process, the aging process, isolation from the partner, or life stressors can change the mode of sexual expression for the couple. Change in sexual expression is discussed in more detail in this section.

A disruption in a client's usual mode of sexual expression can cause stress and anxiety in the client's relationship. Although nursing actions cannot change medical conditions or reverse pathophysiology, nurses can assist clients to adapt to the changes in their lives.

Assessment

Assessment is important because it helps the nurse identify the specific etiologic factors that are amenable to nursing action. The reader is referred to the preceding section Diagnosing for a list of possible etiologic factors. As an example of the nursing process in clinical practice, the effects of disease process on sexual expression are used.

- Use the three interview questions regarding relationships, feelings of sexuality, and sexual functioning to determine the significance of the problem (see the section Sexual History earlier in this chapter).
- Assess past sexual behaviors such as frequency, sexual positions, favored methods of foreplay, use of oral–genital sex, or sexual intercourse.
- Assess importance of each activity and what will remain the same or constant.
- Assess what has changed or will change for the client and partner as a result of the disease or surgery.
- Assess communication patterns between the client and partner.

Planning: Client Goals

The client will:
- Identify positive aspects of the current sexual relationship
- Identify at least three viable alternatives to altered sexuality pattern
- Express satisfaction with change in sexual expression

Nursing Interventions

Nursing measures are needed to assist the client to discover possible alternatives to the change in sexual expression that will prove satisfying to the client and the partner.

If the preferred sexual position has been altered:
- Allow the client to voice any preferences regarding alternative sexual positions
- Give the client permission to use alternative sexual positions
- Teach the client regarding the use of alternative positions: use charts or diagrams, and give specific instructions

If frequency of sexual activity has been altered:
- Review past frequency of sexual activity
- Identify options for increasing frequency (ie, increase desire, increase opportunity, increase privacy)
- Take pain medication, if indicated, before any sexual activity

If method of sexual activity has been altered:
- Review with the client and partner their feelings regarding the use of oral–genital stimulation and mutual masturbation
- Give the client permission to use alternative modes of sexual expression
- Give the client specific information about the use of alternative activities
- Encourage open communication between the client and partner to express their satisfaction or dissatisfaction with the activated care plan

Evaluative Criteria

The client meets the previously stated goals. Any client who does not meet the stated client goals or whose problem is severe should be referred to an appropriate resource for further intensive therapy.

Knowledge Deficit: Contraceptive Methods

Many areas of knowledge deficit can be identified and treated by nurses. Some examples as they pertain to sexuality are reproductive anatomy and physiology, sexual response cycle, modes of sexual expression, self-examination, spread of STDs, contraceptive methods, and effect of disease and medications on sexual functioning.

To illustrate how the nursing process in clinical practice can be used for a knowledge deficit of a sexual concern, knowledge deficit about contraceptive methods is used as an example here. For a discussion of the various contraceptive methods currently available, the reader is referred to the pertinent section of this chapter.

Assessment

- Determine past use of contraceptive methods.
- Assess effectiveness and satisfaction with past methods.
- Assess the client's current knowledge of contraceptive methods.
- Assess frequency of the client's sexual activity.
- Identify any methods that are unacceptable to the client.
- Assess motivation of the client to use certain methods.
- Assess the client's level of comfort with manipulation of genital body parts.
- Obtain complete client history and perform a physical examination if indicated.

Planning: Client Goals

The client will:
- Choose a contraceptive method that the client is motivated to use
- List the adverse effects or danger signs associated with the contraceptive method
- List the steps needed to use the contraceptive method effectively
- Use the contraceptive with every act of sexual intercourse
- Choose a back-up method
- Report back to the health care setting for follow-up as directed

Nursing Interventions

- Describe in terms at the client's level of understanding each contraceptive method for which the client needs information (give objective information in matter-of-fact manner to avoid bias by nurse).
- Describe the effectiveness of each method and side effects or possible complications.
- Instruct the client in the use of a chosen method, giving step-by-step instructions.
- Advise the client of the importance of having a back-up method on hand.
- Instruct the client in the use of the back-up method.
- Have the client obtain a physical examination if indicated by the chosen contraceptive method (eg, the pill).
- Instruct the client to report back in a specified period for follow-up of use of method if indicated (follow-up visits to a health care facility are important, particularly if a client elects to use the pill).

Evaluative Criteria

The client meets the previously stated goals.

Body Image Disturbance Related to Breast Removal

Any change in one's physical body needs to be integrated into one's mental image of that body. Because the body plays such a large part in the expression of sexuality, any disturbance in body image will no doubt have some effect on the expression of sexuality for the client.

In this section, a disturbance in body image as the result of the loss of a breast is illustrated. The effect of mastectomy on a woman's sexuality depends largely on how much significance she places on her breasts. Also, some women find stimulation of their breasts during foreplay a satisfying component of sexual activity. Some men place a great deal of sexual emphasis on women's breasts as well.

The fears experienced by some women after surgery include the fear of rejection by society and fear of rejection by the sexual partner. A woman may feel she has been mutilated and is defective as a woman and sex partner. Some women may choose to hide the surgical site from their partners by undressing in the dark or by wearing a bra to bed. Although a stable marriage should not be threatened by illness and surgery, many marriages cannot bear the stress of the trauma of a mastectomy because of other contributing factors. The fear of causing revulsion in her partner and the possibility of the partner ending the relationship also cause much anxiety to the postoperative mastectomy client.

Assessment

Assessment should include review of preoperative relationship factors between the woman and her partner because these will be helpful in determining the causative factors of disturbed body image and provide clues for effective nursing intervention.
- Assess the client's feelings regarding herself as a woman, wife, and sexual partner (use the interview questions listed in the section Sexual History earlier in this chapter).
- Assess the client's fears regarding change in her femininity, sexual relationship, and images of herself as a person.
- Assess the client's concerns regarding the illness, treatment, and prognosis.
- Assess the value placed on the lost breast by the client (and by her sexual partner if appropriate).
- Assess the client's support system, including family and close friends.

Planning: Client Goals

The client will:
- List positive aspects of her body
- List positive aspects of sexual relationship
- Maintain open communication patterns with her partner

- Enhance physical appearance and positive features with use of feminine clothing, make-up, and breast prosthesis if desired
- Report satisfactory sexual activity
- Verbalize integration of mastectomy into body image

Nursing Interventions

- Support the client as she examines her thoughts and feelings about her lost breast.
- Encourage the client to talk openly with her partner regarding her feelings and fears.
- Provide positive reinforcement by identifying the client's positive aspects.
- Instruct the client that as she recovers from surgery, desire for sexual closeness will return.

- Advise the client to strive to continue previous behaviors with partner.
- Inform the client that much attractive clothing is currently available to minimize the effects of mastectomy.
- Give the client information as desired regarding breast prosthesis and reconstructive surgery.
- Contact Reach for Recovery or other support people to assist client in adaptation to mastectomy.

Evaluative Criteria

The client meets the previously stated goals. Refer the client to the appropriate resource for intensive therapy if goals are not achieved.

CASE STUDY

Pete is a 13-year-old adolescent boy attending the area health clinic. He is nervous as he explains to the nurse his need for health care. He has noticed "sticky white stuff" around his penis and bed clothes on arising some mornings and fears he may be ill. Pete has also expressed concern over his lack of knowledge regarding sexuality. He has heard a lot of stories from his friends but does not feel he can talk to his parents because the subject has never been broached at home. Also, although Pete is a virgin, he is beginning to feel pressured by his friends, who boast of many sexual experiences.

Assessment Findings

After spending time in conversation with Pete, the nurse gathered the following data:
- Pete is experiencing nocturnal emissions and has little scientific knowledge about their source.
- Pete is anxious over the stories regarding sex he has heard from his friends.
- There is no communication or dialogue at home with parents about issues of sexuality.
- Pete is having feelings of insecurity and anxiety over his present virginal status, which he feels he should change.
- Peer pressure from friends is also a concern.

Nursing Diagnosis

Knowledge Deficit: Adolescent Sexuality Concerns related to misinformation and absent family-based sex education

Planning: Client Goals

The nurse will work together with Pete to develop a care plan to correct misinformation and relieve his anxiety.

Planning will be directed toward correcting myths and supplying Pete with accurate information. Because Pete has a negligible knowledge base on sexuality, the care plan should allow for ongoing sessions to augment the initial information (see the Nursing Care Plan). The nurse should outline this plan with Pete to be certain it is acceptable to him.

Short-Term Goals

By the end of the teaching session on 8/1/93, the client will:
- Describe the nature of nocturnal emissions
- Differentiate sexual myths from sound knowledge
- List the positive aspects of abstinence
- Relate unprotected intercourse to pregnancy
- Describe the use of rubber condoms (if appropriate)
- Express a decrease in anxiety

Although Pete did not express an interest in contraception at this initial interview, he should have some knowledge regarding condoms before he leaves. It is possible that he may not return to the clinic for future teaching and may not receive this information before he becomes sexually active.

Long-Term Goal

The client will:
- Develop a knowledge base of sexuality (according to his stage of growth and development and level of understanding) that promotes his sexual health

Implementation

In implementing the care plan, the nurse needs the following specialized abilities:
- Strong assessment skills of interviewing a client with concerns of sexuality

- Interpersonal communication skills to build rapport with an adolescent client
- Nonjudgmental attitude to avoid bias, which would impede trusting nurse–client relationship
- Strong knowledge base of human sexuality, including anatomy and physiology, growth and development, sexual myths, and current issues of sexuality
- Teaching skills to provide client with necessary information and skills
- Counseling skills to diffuse client anxiety over sexual growth and development
- Sense of own sexuality and comfort with sexual issues

Documentation

Sample documentation of the client's first visit follows.

Traditional Note Format

8/1/93, 11 AM, nursing

Nursing consultation with 13-year-old client regarding anxiety over cause and source of nocturnal emissions. Client also expressed concern about sexual myths he has heard from friends. Stated that much peer pressure exists to become sexually active. Client admits to possessing little knowledge regarding sexual issues. Feels he cannot discuss sexuality with parents, because it is not a topic that has been brought up in the past at home. Will conduct initial teaching session with client to provide information and decrease anxiety about priority concerns. Client is agreeable to return to clinic for at least three more teaching sessions to further expand knowledge base of sexuality.

R. Gordon, RN

SOAP Format

8/1/93, nursing

#1 Knowledge Deficit: Adolescent Sexuality Concerns related to misinformation and absent family-based sex education

S: "I'm afraid I might have a disease because of the sticky white stuff I find on my penis in the morning. . . . All I know about sex is what I hear from the guys."

O: Concern over source and cause of nocturnal emission. No information about sexuality discussed at home. Client's information received from friends. Feels pressure from peers to become sexually active.

A: Healthy 13-year-old male desiring information on sexuality

P: Begin initial teaching session today on:
1. Nocturnal emissions
2. Sexual myths
3. Sexual abstinence and use of rubber condoms; will plan three more teaching sessions of sexuality issues

R. Gordon, RN

Evaluation

Short-term goals are evaluated after the initial session. Long-term goal will be evaluated as an ongoing process after each future teaching session.

 NURSING CARE PLAN

for Pete

Nursing Diagnosis:	Knowledge Deficit: Adolescent Sexuality Concerns related to misinformation and absent family-based sex education
Long-Term Goal:	Client will develop sound knowledge base of sexuality according to his stage of growth and development and level of understanding to decrease anxiety.
Goal:	By the end of the teaching session, the client will: • Describe the nature of nocturnal emissions

Nursing Actions	Rationale	Evaluative Statement
Assess client's present knowledge base on nocturnal emission and the source of his information.	It is necessary to discover what the client does know and to build on that knowledge.	8/1/93 Goal met. Client able to describe the source of nocturnal emissions.
Use terms that the client has used and language at the level of the client's understanding.	This facilitates comprehension.	*R. Gordon, RN*

(continued)

NURSING CARE PLAN *(continued)*

for Pete

Nursing Actions	Rationale	Evaluative Statement
Teach the client about nocturnal emissions: • Nocturnal emissions, or "wet dreams," are normal in men of all ages and that they are particularly common in the teen years. They are not the result of disease. • They occur during sleep as the result of erotic dreams. The "white sticky stuff" is the result of ejaculation of semen from the penis. • This is an involuntary action over which the male has no control.	Knowledge decreases anxiety.	

Goal: By the end of the teaching session, the client will:
• Differentiate sexual myths from sound knowledge

Nursing Actions	Rationale	Evaluative Statement
Assess what client has heard from peers regarding sexual information:	The nurse can then specifically address the myths to which the client has been exposed.	8/1/93 Goal met. Client was able to differentiate between truth and sexual issues and what is myth.
Myth 1: "A large penis is better for sex than a small one."	This enables the client to develop a positive sexual body image based on fact.	*R. Gordon, RN*
Truth: No relation exists between the size of a penis and the man's ability to perform sexually. When a penis becomes erect, it reaches sufficient size to engage in sexual intercourse.		
Myth 2: "Jerking off causes blindness. It is a dirty habit."	The client is given permission to engage in a sexual activity of a masturbatory nature.	
Truth: Masturbation or self-stimulation is a natural and healthy outlet for sexual urges. Men and women of all ages masturbate. Masturbation can also teach the person what feels good and what does not. Every person has the right to masturbate if he or she wishes to do so.		
Myth 3: "It looks bad for a guy to be a virgin—everybody's doing it."	The client is given permission to abstain from sexual activity and not to feel pressured by friends. Almost 39% of teens have had sex by age 16 years.	
Truth: No one, whether male or female, should feel pressured into sexual activity at any age. Engaging in sexual activity carries with		

(continued)

NURSING CARE PLAN (continued)

for Pete

Nursing Actions	Rationale	Evaluative Statement
it a great deal of responsibility and concerns of pregnancy and spread of STDs. No one needs to know of another person's status if the person chooses not to discuss it.		

Goal: By the end of the teaching session, the client will:
- List the positive aspects of abstinence in a sexual relationship

Nursing Actions	Rationale	Evaluative Statement
Assess the client including previous discussion of sexual myths and knowledge.	Giving the client all the information necessary allows him to make an informed decision.	8/1/93 Goal partially met. Client able to verbally list all positive aspects of abstinence but is still undecided.
Instruct the client on the positive aspects of abstinence, including the following:		*Revision:* Reinforce to client that this is a personal decision that he can make for himself with a good knowledge base. Also, he does not have to make a firm decision for or against abstinence immediately. He should take time to think about this information.
• Engagement in any sexual activity should be a personal decision and not the result of pressure from friends.		
• Abstinence will guarantee protection from pregnancy and from most sexually transmitted diseases.	Many young people think they are immune to the consequences of their actions. Therefore, it is important to stress that pregnancy and STDs are very probable results of sexual intercourse.	*R. Gordon, RN*
• People can show affection for each other without sexual involvement.	It is difficult to understand and undertake all the implications of a sexual relationship during the teen years. The client learns that a successful sexual relationship requires intimacy, love, and sharing; it should not be merely an outlet for sexual feelings.	
• Every person has the right to say no.	The client has permission to refuse an activity in which he is not sure he wishes to engage.	

Goal: By the end of the teaching session, the client will:
- Describe the correct use of rubber condoms

Nursing Actions	Rationale	Evaluative Statement
Assess what the client knows about rubber condoms and their use.	Since client is undecided over whether to initiate a sexual relationship in the future, it is prudent to give him information to protect against pregnancy and STDs.	8/1/93 Goal met. Client successfully listed the steps in using a condom.
		R. Gordon, RN

(continued)

NURSING CARE PLAN (continued)

for Pete

Nursing Actions	Rationale	Evaluative Statement
Inform the client that rubber condoms are available over the counter in drug stores. Prices will vary according to type and style.	Client should know where to purchase condoms and the variety available.	
Teach client the steps in using rubber condoms:	Client should know how to use condoms safely.	
• Roll condom onto the penis as soon as it becomes erect.	Protects against sperm from secretions from Cowper's glands	
• If condom does not have a nipple receptacle end, leave a small space at end of condom to collect semen.	Provides a pocket to collect semen and prevents breakage	
• Immediately after ejaculation, remove penis and condom from vagina by holding onto base of condom.	Prevents spillage of semen into the vagina	
• Discard condom.	Condoms are not meant to be used over. A new condom is used for each act of intercourse.	
Advise the client to use a condom with every act of intercourse. Spermicides used with condom increase effectiveness.	To be as effective as possible, the condom should be used with every act of intercourse. The rubber condom used with spermicide is effective against pregnancy and the spread of STDs. The woman's use of a spermicide foam in the vagina increases effectiveness.	

Goal: By the end of the teaching session, the client will:
• Express a decrease in anxiety

Nursing Actions	Rationale	Evaluative Statement
Assess client's anxiety level by verbal and nonverbal behavior.	Client was anxious when he came into clinic. It is important to evaluate level of anxiety before he leaves. If he is still anxious, reassessment should occur because plan of care may have been unsuccessful.	8/1/93 Goal met. Client expressed relief that he is normal. Would like to bring a friend to next session.
		Future teaching sessions to include these topics identified by client:
		• STDs, particularly AIDS
		• Pregnancy—occurrence and prevention
		• Sexual expression
		• Further discussion of sexual myths
		R. Gordon, RN

KEY POINTS

- Sexuality is a human component that is inadequately understood.
- Sexuality defines maleness and femaleness and is evident in behaviors, physical appearances, and relationships with others.
- Nurses are concerned with clients' sexuality because individuals bring with them to a health care setting all aspects of what makes them human.
- A sound knowledge base of female and male reproductive anatomy and physiology, the sexual response cycle, and factors that affect sexuality is important for the nurse to be an effective teacher, counselor, and advocate in dealing with clients with sexual concerns.
- Factors that affect sexuality include developmental stage, culture, religion, ethics, life-style, sexual orientation, health state, and medications.
- Obtaining a comprehensive history and performing a physical assessment are paramount before nursing care can be planned for a client with a sexual concern. However, the collection of a sexual history is not appropriate in all health care situations. Clients who should have at least a brief sexual history recorded are clients with concerns of a reproductive nature, clients experiencing a sexual dysfunction, and clients whose illness or treatment will affect their sexual functioning.
- The physical assessment of reproductive anatomy can be stressful and uncomfortable for both male and female clients. Because the major portion of female genitalia is internal, the examination is invasive and may be frightening. The nurse should provide support and information before and during the pelvic examination to create a positive experience for the woman.
- Problems associated with sexuality are rarely simple and clear-cut due to the integral nature of sexuality. Clients may need assistance to talk through their concerns before definitive nursing diagnoses can be formulated.
- Nursing diagnoses can be written specifically to address Altered Sexuality Patterns and Sexual Dysfunction. The effect of sexual concerns on other areas of human functioning can also be identified (eg, Body Image Disturbance, Anxiety, Impaired Adjustment).
- Nurses who are good role models in promoting healthy sexuality have developed a definition of their own sexuality, have developed a self-awareness of their beliefs, and possess a knowledge base of sexual topics and issues.
- Nursing interventions that promote healthy sexuality include establishing a trusting nurse–client relationship, advocating for hospitalized clients' sexual needs, counseling clients regarding sexual concerns, and teaching clients about sexuality-related subjects.
- Client education, which includes topics of self-examination, contraceptive methods, and responsible sexual expression, can be implemented in many health care situations.

STUDY QUESTIONS

1. The female counterpart to a male penis is the
   a. clitoris
   b. vagina
   c. hymen
   d. labia majora
2. Fertilization of the ovum by the sperm usually occurs in the
   a. uterus
   b. fallopian tube
   c. ovary
   d. vagina
3. The primary hormone secreted by the testes is
   a. estrogen
   b. progesterone
   c. semen
   d. testosterone

4. The sexual response cycle is
   a. limited to the genitalia
   b. a total body response
   c. limited to the erogenous zone
   d. divided into two phases, excitement and resolution
5. Male orgasm always consists of
   a. ejaculation of semen
   b. 15 to 20 contractions
   c. involuntary spasmodic contractions of the genitals
   d. 4 to 10 contractions
6. A 16-year-old girl confides to the school nurse, "Something must be wrong with me. I'm the only one in my class who doesn't have her period yet." The nurse's best **initial** response is

a. recommend a thorough medical examination to rule out medical disease

b. explain that menarche can be experienced as early as 8 years and as late as 17 years

c. question her about life stresses that might be retarding the start of her period

d. question her about the age at which her mother and maternal grandmother and aunts experienced menarche

7. You are asked, "Is it okay to enjoy intercourse during menses?" Your answer is best based on the knowledge that

a. there is no scientific rationale to support abstinence from sexual activity during menses

b. intercourse during menses is more likely to damage sensitive tissues in the vagina

c. women should not have intercourse during the time of the month when they are "unclean"

d. women have been oppressed for too long and need to regain control of their bodies

8. When exposure of a male client during the bed bath results in an erection, the best nursing response is to

a. explain that this is a natural physiologic response and offer to leave the room if the client wishes

b. leave the room quickly to allow the client to regain control

c. state firmly that this behavior makes you uncomfortable and that you expect it to stop

d. ask that client if he is experiencing anxiety about his ability to be sexually active after his illness

9. When a young mother confides to you that she is concerned about her toddler who frequently fondles his genitals, you should

a. explain that it is not too early to begin teaching the youngster what is "bad" or unacceptable behavior

b. stress the importance of the parent's "setting limits" by using negative reinforcement

c. explain that it is perfectly natural for toddlers to enjoy fondling their genitals

d. stress that this may signal a medical/psychiatric problem that requires evaluation

10. An 87-year-old client asks you if you think it's wrong for her to masturbate. Your best response is,

a. "I thought you were too old for that!"

b. "Do you really do that?"

c. "How do you feel about it?"

d. "Why don't you ask your physician?"

11. The statement below that reveals a correct knowledge of sexuality is

a. "My small penis makes it hard for me to satisfy a woman sexually."

b. "Because sex 'weakens a person,' the coach insists we abstain before big games."

c. "Something must be wrong with me. I know women aren't supposed to enjoy sex as much as men."

d. "I think all the attention being paid to achieving simultaneous orgasms is misplaced."

12. Which of the following statements indicates a need for contraceptive teaching?

a. "Because breastfeeding isn't a foolproof contraceptive, we plan to use a condom as soon as we are sexually active again."

b. "My partner always withdraws before ejaculation, so we are not worried about pregnancy."

c. "My husband and I are highly motivated to make natural family planning work so that we can have our children when we are ready."

d. "I understand that I should always use a spermicidal agent with my diaphragm."

13. When teaching young clients about sexually transmitted diseases, it is important to communicate

a. abstinence is an unrealistic, old-fashioned idea

b. having sexual contact with one person is to have contact with everyone else with whom that person has had sexual contact

c. adolescents are less likely to contract a sexually transmitted disease because they are generally healthier than adults

d. with prompt medical treatment all sexually transmitted diseases can be cured without long-standing complications

14. In 1974, the American Psychiatric Association removed which of the following from the category of mental illness?

a. transsexuality

b. bisexuality

c. homosexuality

d. heterosexuality

15. During the admission history, Mrs. Victor tells you that she experiences extreme pain during intercourse. An appropriate nursing diagnosis would be

a. Fear related to pain during sexual intercourse

b. Body Image Disturbance related to painful intercourse

c. Ineffective Individual Coping related to pain

d. Pain related to dyspareunia

Answers With Rationale

1. The correct response is *a*. The clitoris is the female counterpart to the male penis because they are similar in their reaction to stimuli. The vagina, hymen, and labia majora are not similarly responsive to stimuli.

2. The correct response is *b*. Fertilization of the ovum by the sperm usually occurs in the fallopian tube, not the uterus, ovary, or vagina.

3. The correct response is *d*. The primary hormone secreted by the testes is testosterone, not estrogen or progesterone (female sex hormones). Semen, seminal plasma, and sperm are not hormones.

4. The correct response is *b*. The sexual response cycle is clearly a total body response and is not limited to the genitalia nor to the erogenous zones. There are more than two phases in the sexual response cycle.

5. The correct response is *c*. By definition, the male orgasm always consists of involuntary spasmodic contractions of the genitals. The other options are all possible but unnecessary.

6. The correct response is *b*. The nurse's first priority is to inform the client that, at 16 years, she is still within the normal age span for experiencing menarche (8 to 17 years). Once this is done, a more detailed history may be taken.

7. The correct response is *a*. If a client asks about enjoying intercourse during the menses, it is important to base your response on fact (there is no scientific rationale to support abstinence from sexual activity during menses) rather than on a religious, cultural, or personal belief. Option *b* is simply false.

8. The correct response is *a*. Explaining to the client that this is a natural physiologic response and giving him time to regain control will decrease any embarrassment he is experiencing. Option *b* (leaving the room without comment) might be interpreted as signifying disapproval. Option *c* clearly communicates disapproval and option *d* is premature.

9. The correct response is *c*. The appropriate response to this mother's concern is the factual information that this is developmentally appropriate behavior. Options *a* and *b* communicate incorrectly that this is abnormal behavior that ought to be curbed. Option *d* is false.

10. The correct response is *c*. Option *a* is based on the myth that elderly people do not have any sexual needs. Option *b* implies disapproval. Option *d* refers to the physician a question the nurse should be able to answer. Asking the client how she feels (option *c*) opens the door for a frank discussion of the client's concerns and will surface any false information or negative beliefs the client holds.

11. The correct response is *d*. Placing too much attention on achieving simultaneous orgasm can detract from the overall sexual experience. The other options are all common sexual myths.

12. The correct response is *b*. Withdrawing before ejaculation is no guarantee that no sperm have been released because, during sexual activity, Cowper's glands produce small droplets of fluid that may contain sperm. The other options are all statements that reveal a correct understanding of contraceptive measures.

13. The correct response is *b*. Having sexual contact with one person is to have contact with everyone else that person has had contact with is the only factually correct response. Option *a* may be held by some nurses but is a personal belief that many would challenge. Options *c* and *d* are false.

14. The correct response is *c*. Homosexuality was removed from the category of mental illness in 1974 by the American Psychiatric Association.

15. The correct response is *d*. The data point to a nursing diagnosis of Pain related to dyspareunia (painful intercourse). The client has not mentioned fear and no data point to a disturbance in body image or to ineffective coping.

BIBLIOGRAPHY

Abrums, M. (1986). Health care for women. *Journal of Obstetric, Gynecologic, and Neonatal Nursing, 15*(3), 250–255.

Baldwin, K., & Goodwin K. (1985). The Papanicolaou smear. *Journal of Nurse–Midwifery, 30*(6), 327–331.

Bernharrd, L., & Dan, A. (1986). Redefining sexuality from women's own experiences. *Nursing Clinics of North America, 21*(1), 125–135.

Bourcier K., & Seidler, A. (1987). *Chlamydia* and condylomata acuminata: An update for the nurse practitioner. *Journal of Obstetric, Gynecologic, and Neonatal Nursing, 16*(1), 17–21.

Buczny, B. (1992). Impotence in older men: A newly recognized problem. *Journal of Gerontological Nursing, 18*(5), 25–30.

Cholewinski, J. T., & Burge, J. M. (1990). Sexual harassment of nursing students. *Image: Journal of Nursing Scholarship, 22*(2), 106–110.

Dickerson, J. (1983). The pill: A closer look. *American Journal of Nursing, 83*(10), 1393–1398.

Fehring, R. J. (1991). New technology in natural family planning. *Journal of Obstetric, Gynecologic, and Neonatal Nursing, 20*(3), 199–205.

Fromer, M. (1983). Ethical issues in sexuality and reproduction (2nd ed.). St. Louis: Mosby.

Fuentes, R. J., Rosenberg, J. M., & Marks, R. G. (1983). Sexual side effects. What to tell your patients, what not to say. *Registered Nurse, 46*(2), 34–41.

Googe, M., & Mook, T. M. (1983). The inflatable penile prosthesis: New developments. *American Journal of Nursing, 83*(7), 1044–1047.

Gruen, S. M., Hayes, E., & Fritsch-deBruyn, R. (1991). Setting up a school-based sexual education program to help prevent AIDS and other STDs. *Nurse Practitioner, 16*(8), 47–51.

Hammond, D. (1984). Screening for sexual dysfunction. *Clinical Obstetrics and Gynecology, 27*(3), 732–737.

Hatcher, R., Guest, S., Stewart, F., Stewart, G. K., Trussell, J., Cerel, S., & Kates, W. (1990). *Contraceptive technology* (15th ed.). New York: Irvington.

Herold, E. S., Fisher, W. A., Smith, E. A., & Yarher, W. A. (1990). Sex education and the prevention of STD/AIDS and pregnancy among youths. *Canadian Journal of Public Health, 81*(2), 141–145.

Hill, L., & Smith, N. (1990). *Self-care nursing* (2nd ed.). Englewood Cliffs, NJ: Prentice-Hall.

Horsley, J. E. (1990). Don't tolerate sexual harassment at work. *RN, 53*(1), 69, 72, 75.

Katzin, L. (1990). Chronic illness and sexuality. *American Journal of Nursing, 90*(1), 54–59.

King, J. (1992). Helping patients choose an appropriate method of birth control. *MCN, 17*(2), 91–95.

Kisker, E. (1985). Teenagers talk about sex, pregnancy, hand contraception. *Family Planning Perspective, 17*(2), 83–90.

LaBrie, P. M., & Lafond, J. S. (1991). Sexualite et cardiopathies. *Canadian Nurse, 87*(6), 34–35.

Leppert, P. (1985). Adolescent anxiety at first pelvic examination. *Medical Aspects of Human Sexuality, 19*(7), 24–32.

Morrison-Beedy, D. (1989). Sexual assessment and the aging female. *Nurse Practitioner, 14*(12), 38–39, 42ff.

Penninger, J. (1985). After the ostomy: Helping the patient reclaim his sexuality. *RN, 48*(4), 46–50.

Pollard, M., & Baker, E. (1985). Straight talk on sex for the older patient. *RN, 48*(2), 17–18.

Reamy, K. (1984). Sexual counseling for the nontherapist. *Clinical Obstetrics and Gynecology, 27*(3), 781–788.

Relf, M. V. (1991). Sexuality and the older bypass patient. *Geriatric Nursing, 12*(6), 294–296.

Renshaw, D. (1985). Sex, age, and values. *Journal of American Geriatric Society, 33*(9), 635–643.

Reznichek, C. G., & Reznichek, R. (1990). The problem most men won't talk about. *RN, 55*(3), 28–32.

Rhodes, A. M. (1991). Norplant and the 'coerced contraception' controversy. *MCN, 16*(5), 277.

Sarazin, S. K., & Seymour, S. F. (1991). Causes and treatment options for women with dyspareunia. *Nurse Practitioner, 16*(10), 30–41.

Semmens, J., & Semmens, E. (1984). Sexual function and the menopause. *Clinical Obstetrics and Gynecology, 27*(3), 717–723.

Stockard, S. (1991). Caring for the sexually aggressive patient: You don't have to blush and bear it. *Nursing, 21*(11), 72–73.

Talashek, M. L., Tichy, A. M., & Eping, H. (1990). Sexually transmitted diseases in the elderly: Issues and recommendations. *Journal of Gerontological Nursing, 16*(4), 33–42.

Tillmann, J. (1992). Syphilis: An old disease, a contemporary perinatal problem *Journal of Obstetric, Gynecologic, and Neonatal Nursing. 21*(3), 209–213.

Touchstone, D. M., & Davis, D. D. (1992). Consider chlamydia. *RN, 55*(2), 32–35.

Varnhagen, C. K. (1991). Sexually transmitted diseases and condoms: High school students' knowledge, attitudes, and behaviors. *Canadian Journal of Public Health, 82*(2), 129–132.

Watts, R. (1979). Dimensions of sexual health. *American Journal of Nursing, 79*(9), 1568–1572.

Weisberg, M. (1984). Physiology of female sexual function. *Clinical Obstetrics and Gynecology, 27*(3), 697–706.

Willard, M., Heaberg, G., & Pack, J. (1986). The educational pelvic examination. Women's responses to a new approach. *Journal of Obstetric, Gynecologic, and Neonatal Nursing, 15*(2), 135–139.

Williams, A. B. (1992). The epidemiology, clinical manifestations and health maintenance needs of women infected with HIV. *Nurse Practitioner, 17*(5), 27–44.

Winter, E.J.S., Ashton, D. J. & Moore, D. L. (1991). Dispelling myths: A study of PMS and relationship satisfaction. *Nurse Practitioner, 16*(5), 34–45.

Woods, N. F. (1984). *Human sexuality in health and illness.* St. Louis: Mosby.

Yost, M. (1986). When your patient's problem is sexual dysfunction. *Contemporary OB/GYN, 28*(2), 171–185.

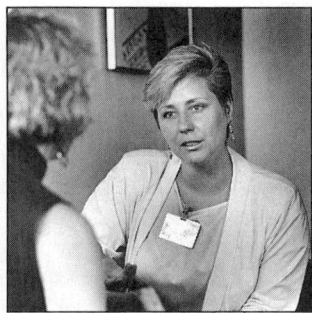
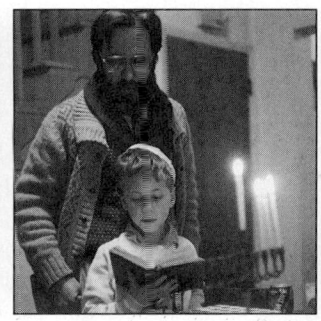
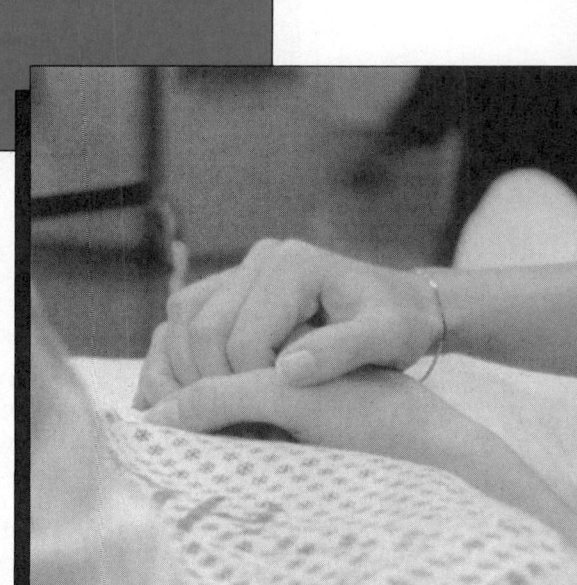

OBJECTIVES

After studying this chapter, the learner should be able to:

Define key terms used in the chapter.

Identify three spiritual needs believed to be common to all people.

Describe the influences of spirituality on everyday living, health, and illness.

Differentiate life-affirming influences of religious beliefs from life-denying influences.

Distinguish the spiritual beliefs and practices of the major religions practiced in the United States and Canada.

Identify five factors that influence spirituality.

Perform a nursing assessment of spiritual health, using appropriate interview questions and observation skills.

Develop nursing diagnoses that correctly identify spiritual problems.

Describe nursing strategies to promote spiritual health and state their rationale.

Plan, implement, and evaluate nursing care related to select nursing diagnoses involving spiritual problems.

KEY TERMS

agnostic
atheist
faith
religion
spiritual beliefs
spiritual distress
spirituality
spiritual needs

Spirituality

41

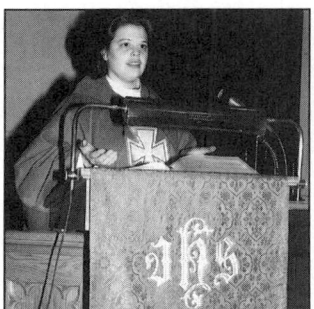

The "spirit" dimension of the person was recognized in ancient cultures. "The dual roles of priest and physician were generally held by one individual, and thus the functions and dictates of religion (pertaining to the spirit) and medicine (pertaining to the body) were closely interwoven" (O'Brien, 1982, p. 85). Over the years, however, medicine and religion evolved separately. Not until the holistic health movement took root was the person once again viewed as an integrated whole of body, mind, and spirit. Health care practitioners began again to probe the relationships among physical, psychologic, and spiritual health.

Nursing has always been a strongly holistic tradition and nurses have practiced nursing sensitive to the physical, psychosocial, and spiritual needs of people. According to Fish and Shelly (1978), there are three **spiritual needs** underlying all religious traditions and common to all people: (1) need for meaning and purpose, (2) need for love and relatedness, and (3) need for forgiveness. Although nurses may differ in their beliefs about how involved they should become in meeting clients' spiritual needs, it is impossible to nurse individuals well while ignoring the spiritual dimensions of health. Nurses can assist clients to meet spiritual needs by offering a compassionate presence; assisting in the struggle to find meaning and purpose in the face of suffering, illness, and death; fostering relationships (with God/humans) that nurture the spirit; and facilitating the client's expression of religious or spiritual beliefs and practices.

Study of this chapter provides the student with a knowledge base of spirituality. Practical suggestions for performing a spiritual assessment are given, along with specific interview questions. Sample nursing diagnoses are developed for common problems of spiritual distress (spiritual pain, alienation, anxiety, guilt, anger, loss, and despair). Related client and nurse goals and specific nursing strategies for promoting spiritual health are described. In the section Nursing Process in Clinical Practice, focused assessment, planning, implementation, and evaluation guides are offered for clients experiencing spiritual distress related to challenged beliefs and value systems. These guides and the concluding case study illustrate how the nurse's knowledge of spirituality may be combined with skilled nursing interventions and caring to resolve spiritual distress successfully.

Spirituality and Faith

Although the terms *spirituality, religion,* and *faith* are used interchangeably by some, there are distinctions. **Spirituality** is anything that pertains to a person's relationship with a nonmaterial life force or higher power. Whereas one person describes spirituality in terms of coming to know, love, and serve God, another speaks of transcending the limits of body and experiencing a universal energy. Spirituality may include **religion**, which refers to an organized system of beliefs about a higher power. Religions are often characterized by set forms of worship, spiritual practices, and codes of conduct. Thus a person may be deeply spiritual yet not profess a religion. The fact that people do not belong to an organized religion should not be interpreted by the nurse to mean that they have no spiritual needs. **Faith** generally refers to a confident belief in something for which there is no proof or material evidence. It can involve a person, idea, or thing, and it is usually followed by action related to the ideals or values of that belief.

An **atheist** is a person who denies the existence of a God, and an **agnostic** is one who holds that nothing can be known about the existence of a God. The agnostic and the atheist are guided by philosophies of living that do not include a religious faith. They deserve respect for what they choose to believe, just as do those who accept a particular religious creed.

Spirituality and Everyday Living

Spiritual beliefs and practices are associated with all aspects of a person's life, including health and illness. Aspects of a person's life commonly influenced by spirituality and religion include relationships with others, daily living habits, required and prohibited behaviors, and the general frame of reference for thinking about oneself and the world.

Religious influences may be life affirming or life denying.

> Life-affirming influences enhance life, give meaning and purpose to existence, strengthen one's feelings of self-worth, encourage self-actualization, and are health-giving and life-sustaining. Life-denying influences restrict or enclose life patterns, limit experiences and associations, place burdens of guilt on individuals, encourage feelings of unworthiness, and are generally health-denying and life-inhibiting. (Larue, 1981)

Spirituality, Health, and Illness

Spiritual beliefs are of special importance to nurses because of the many ways they can influence a client's level of health and self-care behaviors.

Guide to Daily Living Habits   Certain practices generally associated with health care may have religious significance for a client. For example, many religions prescribe dietary

Six Basic Spiritual Needs of Americans

George Gallup, who is chair of the George H. Gallup International Institute, recently identified six basic spiritual needs of contemporary Americans. His conclusions are based on a variety of religious research and were presented in a speech given at a meeting of the Theological Students Fellowship, Princeton Theological Seminary, on December 10, 1990.

The need to believe that life is meaningful and has a purpose. During a time when sociologists observe an obsession with self in America, 70% of Americans nevertheless believe it is important that life is meaningful and has a purpose. Yet as many as two thirds of people interviewed believe that "most churches and synagogues today are not effective in helping people find meaning in life." Here is a basic need apparently being only partially met. The fact is, significant numbers of people find churches irrelevant, unfulfilling, and boring.

The need for a sense of community and deeper relationships. "Radical individualism" continues to have a hold on the religious lives of Americans. Most Americans, for example, believe that one can be a good Christian or Jew if one does not attend church or synagogue. One of the poignant consequences of this separateness is loneliness. As we have discovered from surveys, as many as 3 people in 10 say they have been lonely "for a long period of time" in their lives, with half of these people saying this experience has affected their thoughts "a great deal."

The need to be appreciated and respected. This is certainly a basic and fundamental need, yet as many as one third of the American people have a low sense of self-worth or self-esteem, as a direct consequence of not being loved or appreciated. Low self-esteem brings with it a host of social problems, including alcohol and drug abuse, child and spouse abuse, lawlessness, and crime. Significantly, surveys suggest that the closer people feel to God, the better they feel about themselves. They are also more satisfied with their lives than are others, more altruistic, enjoy better health, and have a happier outlook. Furthermore, it has been found that experiencing the closeness of God is a key factor in the ability of people to forgive themselves and others.

The need to be listened to—to be heard. Americans overwhelmingly think the future of the church will be shaped to a greater extent by the laity than by the clergy. In specific terms, this means that the laity should play a greater role in the church, freeing up clergy to perform what the laity expects of them: to listen to people's religious needs and to provide spiritual counseling and inspiration. When the "unchurched" in one survey were asked what would most likely draw them back into the community of active worshippers, the lead reason given was "if I could find a pastor or rabbi with whom I could share my religious needs and doubts."

The need to feel that one is growing in faith. People like to feel that they are maturing spiritually; we go through passages in our faith lives, just as we do in our secular lives. It would appear that, basically, people aspire to lead good lives. Significant numbers of people have given thought to living a worthwhile life, to their relationship to God, to the basic meaning and value of their lives, and to developing their faith. People need help in understanding the significance of these experiences and in building on them.

The need for practical help in developing a mature faith. There is an urgent need to work closing the gap between belief and practice—to turn professed faith into lived-out faith.

(Used with permission.)

---

requirements and restrictions. Acceptable birth-control practices are determined by some religious faiths, as are some types of medical treatments.

Source of Support   It is common for many people to seek support from their religious faith during times of stress. This support is often vital to the acceptance of an illness, especially if the illness brings with it a prolonged period of convalescence or indicates a questionable outcome. Prayer, devotional reading, and other religious practices often do for the person spiritually what protective exercises do for the body physically (Fig. 41-1).

Source of Strength and Healing   The values derived from religious faith cannot be enumerated or evaluated easily. However, the effects attributable to faith are constantly in evidence to health care workers. People have been known to endure extreme physical distress because of strong faith. Clients' families have taken on almost unbelievable rehabilitative tasks because they had faith in the eventual positive results of their effort (Fig. 41-2).

Source of Conflict   There are times when religious beliefs conflict with prevalent health care practices. For example, the doctrine of the Jehovah's Witnesses prohibits blood

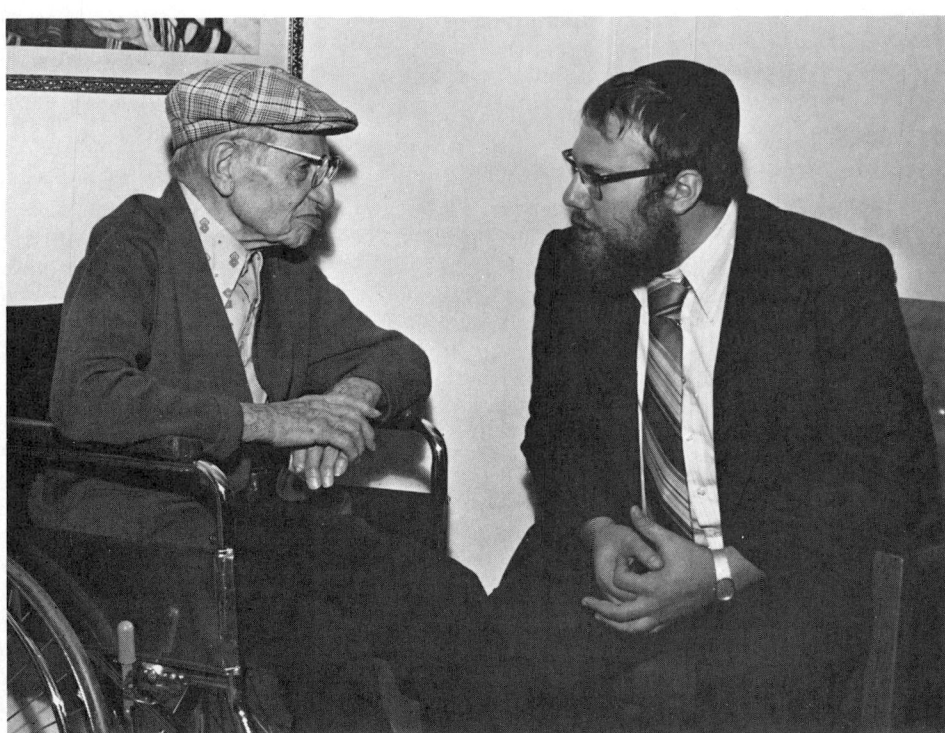

F I G U R E   4 1 - 1

The rabbi's visit is important for
this resident of a geriatric center.

transfusions. In the Islamic religion, humans are regarded
as largely helpless in controlling their environment, and
illness is accepted as their fate rather than something
against which action might be taken. Some Navajo Indians
use a lengthy religious ceremony to cure certain diseases,
such as tuberculosis. For some people, illness is viewed as
punishment for sin and therefore inevitable.

Such beliefs may require the health care worker to
modify a treatment plan to accommodate the person's religion. In some instances, acknowledgment of the client's

religious convictions and efforts by health practitioners to
accommodate the client's beliefs can result in quality
health care without violating the person's religious practices. In other situations, an objective explanation of alternative treatments and the predicted consequences of each
may help the client determine acceptable therapy. Whatever the person's decision about health care, the nurse
should remember that each person is unique and has a
right to pursue his or her own convictions, even though they
may differ from those of the health care provider.

F I G U R E   4 1 - 2

A group of retired people gather
for their weekly Bible study.

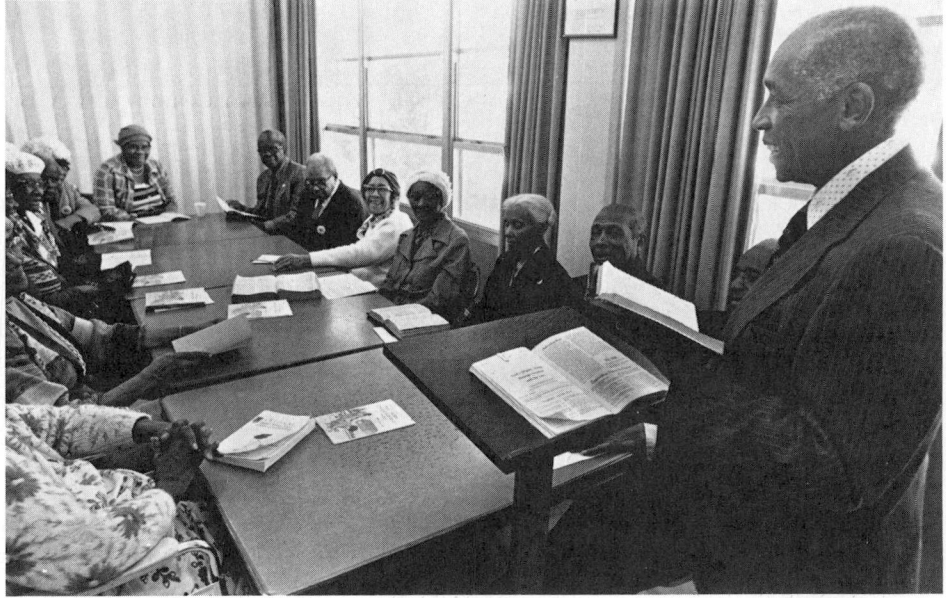

Cultural Care

After a year of legal struggles that took the case all the way to the U.S. Supreme Court, the parents of a Vietnamese refugee defeated an attempt by social workers to force their son to have corrective surgery on his two clubfeet. The surgery would have shattered the Hmong family's religious beliefs. They believe their son Kou was born with clubfeet so that a warrior ancestor whose own feet were wounded in battle could be released from a sort of spiritual entrapment. They do not regard Kou's clubfeet as a deformity but as a sign of good luck and they think their son is special because of it.

(Kurtzman, L. [1990, December 22]. Surgery for boy, 7, blocked. *Philadelphia Inquirer*, p. 3A.)

Major Religions

Nurses care for people from many different religious traditions. Although it is impossible for nurses to be knowledgeable about all religions, nurses are better able to meet the spiritual needs of clients when they understand the client's religious beliefs and practices. These can directly influence the client's response to illness and suffering, self-care practices such as diet and hygiene, birth and death rituals, gender roles, spiritual practices, and moral codes. Nurses who are unfamiliar with a client's religion can gain valuable knowledge by reading (Carson's [1989] *Spiritual Dimensions of Nursing Practice* is an invaluable resource) and through discussion with the client and the client's family and spiritual adviser. A brief discussion of major religious traditions follows.

Religions With a Western Philosophy

The three major religions with a Western philosophy are Judaism, Christianity, and Islam. Each is monotheistic; central to their sacred scripture is one God who personally created the world and who reveals himself through events in human history. The moral codes of these religions stress the honor of parents, honesty, kindness, and generosity as important social concerns and reject lying, stealing, slander, covetousness, and adultery (Carson, 1989).

Judaism

Judaism, the oldest continuous religion still practiced in Western civilization, is the foundation on which both Christianity and Islam were built. The formation of the Jewish people is closely bound with a divine revelation and with the commitment of the people to obedience to God's will.

The Jewish people have been called "the people of the Book," meaning that the Hebrew Bible has been the authority, guide, and inspiration of all the many forms that the religion of the Jews has taken in different periods and in different lands (Parrinder, 1983). There are currently three forms of Judaism: (1) Reform, (2) Conservative, and (3) Orthodox. Reform Judaism is more liberal that the other two in its beliefs, whereas Orthodox Judaism is the most traditional of the three.

Nurses caring for Orthodox Jews as well as some Conservative Jews need to be sensitive to their special needs in the areas of diet, birth rituals, male and female contact, and death. For observant Jewish clients, treatments and procedures should not be scheduled on the Sabbath (sundown Friday to sundown Saturday) and important holy days, provided this will not harm the client.

Christianity

Christianity, the largest religion in the world, embraces adherents to Roman Catholic, Eastern Orthodox, and Protestant faiths. The Christian way of life is centered on worship of the one God revealed to the world through Jesus Christ of Nazareth (lived AD 1st century), who is believed to be risen from the dead. Love of neighbor is a central tenet. Other beliefs include sin, redemption, salvation, and retribution or a final accounting with God at the end of life. The Christian tradition has always encouraged care for the sick. God, recognized as the author and giver and life, is also the healer. Most Christian clients accept medical science and many use prayer, faith healing, laying on of hands, and the sacraments in times of illness.

Roman Catholicism Dating its beginning from the time when the apostles first began to preach about Jesus of Nazareth, the Roman Catholic Church governed both the temporal world as well as the Church in the West until the 11th century. In AD 1054, theological differences resulted in the Western and Eastern Orthodox traditions. However, in both the Roman Catholic and Eastern Orthodox Churches, there is a high regard and concern for human life as a gift of God. There is a prolife stance that honors and respects the life of each person as a divine gift that requires development and enhancement.

Nurses caring for Roman Catholic clients should be aware of the importance of the sacraments of baptism, Eucharist, penance, and the anointing of the sick; dietary habits; sexual ethical norms; and the potential importance of private devotions.

Eastern Orthodox Factors contributing to the split between the Eastern and Western Churches include theological differences over the wording of the Nicene Creed regarding the Holy Spirit, the use of pictures and statues in the Churches, the sacraments, the marriage of priests, and the use of Greek or Latin in worship services. Patriarchs who rule the Eastern Orthodox Church are located in Istanbul, Alexandria, Antioch, and Jerusalem, as well as in Russia,

Serbia, Romania, Bulgaria, and Georgia. Important concerns for the sick include the administration of sacraments, dietary practices, rituals regarding death, and calendar differences.

Protestant Faiths Martin Luther, generally credited with starting the Protestant Reformation in 1517, concluded through his study of the Bible that a person's sins are forgiven by having a personal relationship with Jesus Christ and that God alone forgives through faith and not good works. The Protestant faith embraces a large number of denominations, most of which hold to Luther's beliefs in the final authority of the Bible, justification by faith, and the priesthood of all believers. Issues dividing diverse Protestant sects include ways of interpreting the message of the Bible, involvement of the Church with secular issues, and sacramental and worship differences. Nurses caring for Protestant clients need to assess how the client's beliefs and religious practices contribute to spiritual needs (Fig. 41-3).

F I G U R E   4 1 - 3

The Protestant faith embraces a large number of denominations. Some doctrines are common to most of these denominations, but individual practices and interpretations give each a distinct pattern. This group has chosen a female spiritual leader. (Photo by Isadore Faven.)

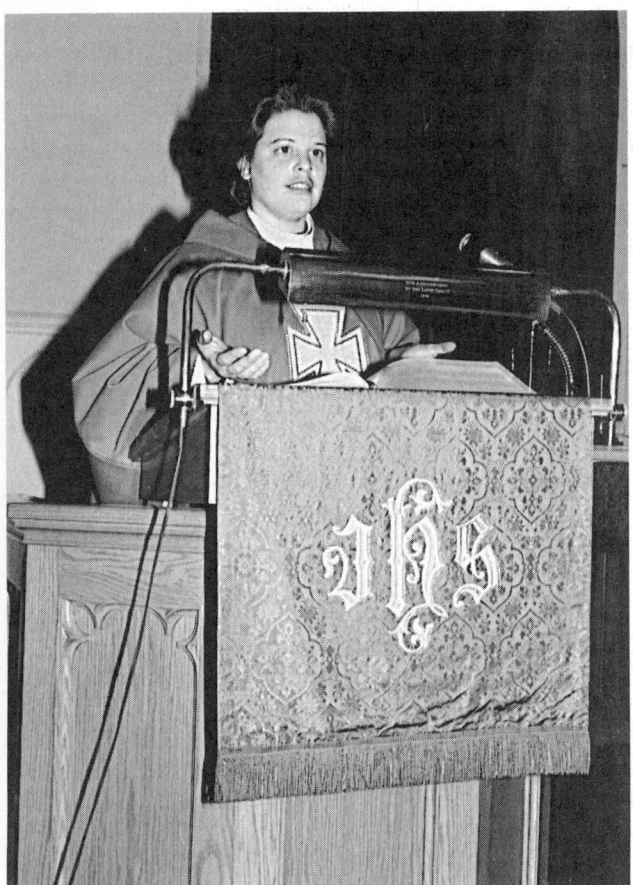

Islam

Islam, started by the prophet Muhammad in AD 580, is one of the largest and fastest-growing religions in the world. Major sects include the Sunni, the Shiites, and the Sufis. Followers of Islam believe in Allah, one God who is only one, all seeing, all hearing, all speaking, all knowing, all willing, and all powerful. Their religious duties include repetition of a creed; prayer five times each day facing Mecca preceded by washing, almsgiving, fasting during the sacred 9th month of Ramadan; and a pilgrimage to Mecca once during a lifetime. When caring for Muslim clients, it is helpful to understand the Koranic law and customs that influence birth, diet, care of women, death, and prayer rituals. Women are not allowed to make independent decisions and husbands need to be present when informed consent is sought.

American Muslim Mission (Black Muslim)

Adherents of the American Muslim Mission trace their religious beginnings to Muslim slaves who came to the United States from Islamic West Africa but who were prevented from practicing Islam and consequently lost knowledge of the practices of their faith. Accepting the Koran as their sacred scripture, current members of "the Nation of Islam" stress the importance of cooperation among blacks in business and education to build self-esteem. Members are encouraged to obtain health care provided by the black community. Malcolm X was one of this sect's most charismatic leaders and with others preached an end to white denomination and the establishment of an independent nation. Major tenets involve prayer rituals; dietary restrictions (prohibitions against pork and alcohol); hygiene (extreme cleanliness); life-style modifications;, and marital faithfulness.

Other Western faiths with which health care professionals should be familiar include Christian Science, Jehovah's Witnesses, Church of Jesus Christ of Latter-Day Saints (Mormons), Unification Church, and Unitarian Universalist Association of Churches and Fellowships (Table 41-1).

Religions With an Eastern Philosophy

Some areas of North America have citizens of Chinese, Korean, Japanese, and Indian descent, and there has been a recent influx of people from Southeast Asia. It is thus helpful for nurses to have some understanding of religions with an eastern philosophy. Buddhism, Confucianism, Daoism (Taoism), and Hinduism are highlighted in Table 41-2.

There is a growing acceptance of therapies rooted in Eastern approaches to medicine such as acupuncture, biofeedback, yoga, and rolfing. In Eastern medicine, health is closely related to personal attitudes and actions.

The healer's role is to impart deeper understanding of the ways of nature so that while promoting healing, he or she also educates clients in self-care. The

TABLE 41-1

Other Western Religions, Beliefs and Health Care Practices

Religion	Beliefs	Health Care Practices
Adventist	Believe in the individual's choice and God's sovereignty. The body is believed to be the temple of the Holy Spirit.	• The taking of all narcotics and stimulants is prohibited because the body is the temple of the Holy Spirit and should be protected. Many groups prohibit meat. • Many regard Saturday as the Sabbath. • Approach to health care is holistic.
Christian Scientist	They deny the existence of health crises; sickness and sin are errors of the human mind and can be overcome by altering thoughts, not by using drugs or medicines.	• They will use orthopedic services to set a bone but decline drugs and, in general, other medical or surgical procedures. • They do not allow hypnotism or any form of psychotherapy, which alters the "Divine Mind." • A Christian Science Practitioner may be called to administer spiritual support. • Alcohol and tobacco are not used.
Church of Jesus Christ of Latter Day Saints (Mormons)	Devout adherents believe in divine healing through the "laying on of hands," though many do not prohibit medical therapy. The Church maintains an extensive and well-funded welfare system, including financial support for the sick.	• Disapprove of alcohol, tobacco, and caffeinated beverages. • A special undergarment worn by some members should be removed only in an emergency.
Jehovah's Witnesses	They oppose the "false teachings" of other sects; opposition often extends to modern science, including medicine.	• Blood transfusions violate God's laws and therefore are not allowed. Alternative treatments include use of nonblood plasma expanders, surgical techniques to decrease blood loss, and autotransfusions through use of a heart–lung machine. • The courts have not supported the right of Jehovah Witness parents to refuse life-saving treatment for their children. • Use of alcohol and tobacco are discouraged.
Unification Church	God is the living, eternal person who represents universal love and care. God created the world and humans to reflect his nature. The goal of the Unification Church is to unite Christians everywhere as one family under God.	• Most members are still healthy young adults. There is little information available on their interactions with the health care team.
Unitarian Universal Association of Churches and Fellowships	Encourage creativity, reason, and living an ethical life. No member is required to adhere to a given creed or set of religious beliefs. The inherent worth and dignity of every person is affirmed.	• Free to accept what they take to be best for their health.

client, in turn, needs to recognize that body and mind are intimately related to each other. To be in command of this crucial interaction requires a practiced sensitivity and response to the needs of body and mind. (Carson, 1989. p. 129)

The health care community continues to struggle to combine the ancient wisdom of Eastern health practices with the sophisticated scientific and technological expertise of the West.

Native American Religions

The multitude of tribes in North America makes it difficult to generalize about Native American cultures and religions. There are however, two basic and contrasting orientations—the old hunting religions (as seen among the Shoshoni) and the new horticultural religions (as among the Zuni). Although all Native Americans look to natural spirits, or the spirits of nature, for revelation and power, the Shoshoni look more to animals and the sky, whereas the Zuni

T A B L E   4 1 - 2

Eastern Religions and Related Beliefs About Health, Illness, and Health Care Practices

Religion	Beliefs	Health Care Practices
Buddhism	Buddha or "the Great Physician" taught the Four Noble Truths to indicate the range of "suffering," its "origin," its "cessation," and the "way" that leads to its cessation. The real cause of human suffering is ignorant craving. The Noble Eightfold Path, which consists of right views, aspirations, speech, conduct, mode of livelihood, effort, mindfulness, and concentration, leads to the cessation of suffering.	• Buddhist hospitals for sick humans and sick animals antedated anything similar found in the West. • Buddhists do not outwardly proclaim healing through faith. However, spiritual peace and liberation from anxiety attained through the awakening to Buddha's wisdom may be an important factor in expediting healing and the recovery process. • Accepts modern science. The doctrine of avoidance of extremes is applied to the use of drugs, blood, vaccines. • Buddhism does not condone taking lives of any form. • Check with the client about any special diet restrictions and the observance of holy days.
Confucianism	Inherent in Confucianism is the appreciation of life and the desire to keep the body from untimely or unnecessary death.	• Appreciate life and desire to keep the body from untimely or unnecessary death. • Historically emphasized public health solutions to impending health problems.
Daoism (Taoism)	Health is a manifestation of the harmony of the universe, obtained through the proper balancing of internal and external forces. Implicit throughout the Daoist tradition is the tendency to understand salvation in the biomedical sense of health and qualitative improvement and prolongation of human life. The universal principle of the Tao is the mysterious biologic and spiritual life rhythm or order of nature.	• There is a "medicinal" concern for maintaining and prolonging human health and life (*sheng*). Knowing and living a natural life—following the Tao—is the secret of both health and sagehood. • Long tradition of seeking pragmatic medical techniques, along with its religious techniques of meditation and ritual for establishing a harmony of body and spirit, humanity, and nature (holistic approach).
Hinduism	Doctrine of Transmigration. Moral factors, linked with the all-embracing doctrine of "karma" were believed to be significant in promoting health or causing disease.	• Hindu medicine shows a surprising openness to new ideas, at least in respect to practical treatment. • Many Hindu dietary restrictions conform to individual sect doctrine. • The nurse administering medications should avoid touching the client's lips. • Certain prescribed rites are followed after death; disposal of the body is by cremation.

(Data in part from Reich, W. T. [Ed.]. [1978]. *Encyclopedia of bioethics*. New York: Free Press.)

look to plants and the underground. Features of the hunting religions include animal ceremonialism, quest for spiritual power, Male Supreme Being, annual ceremony of cosmic rejuvenation, few stationary cult places, shamanism, and life after death beyond the horizon or in the sky. Features of the horticultural religions include rain and fertility ceremonies, priestly ritual, goddesses and gods, yearly round of fertility rites, permanent shrines and temples, medicine society ritualism, and life after death in the underworld or among the clouds.

Unlike Western religions, Native American religions were handed down by tribes as oral traditions and have not been so dogmatically bound by what was handed down

from the past. Most share a similar worldview, a notion of cosmic harmony, emphasis on directly experiencing powers and visions, and a common view of the cycle of life and death. Understanding time cyclically, Native North Americans view each individual's life as a cycle of time from birth to death, with rituals marking the important changes of life—birth ceremonies, puberty rituals, initiation rites, and death rituals. Death is not an end but the beginning of new life either on this earth (reincarnation as another human or transmigration into some animal) or in a transcendent hereafter. Medicine men and women have specialized spirits from whom they receive the mission to cure and who help to cure the diseases of clients. Instructions in the ways of doctoring are received in visions. Common therapeutic measures are sucking, blowing, and drawing out with a feather fan; all are designed to remove the agent of the disease. Medicine men and women who fall recurringly into deep trances to save a person's life are called *shamans* (Hultkrantz, 1987).

Religion and Law, Ethics, and Medicine

Christian Scientists, Jehovah's Witnesses, and members of faith-healing groups are among those challenging the intricate web of rights and responsibilities among individual, society, church, and state. These religious bodies are asking for protection, under the veil of religious freedom, of their right to exercise individual decisions in accordance with scriptural interpretations, even though those decisions may result in the individual's own death or that of a family member, including a child. The most troubling cases are those in which treatable problems such as bacterial meningitis, diabetes, and bowel obstruction resulted in the death of minors whose parents chose religious means of healing over traditional medicine. The American Pediatrics Academy is currently urging that all child abuse, neglect, and medical neglect statutes be applied without potential or actual exemption for religious beliefs.

Perhaps even more troubling for nurses are situations in which family members insist on care deemed medically futile (ie, the likelihood of medical benefit is virtually nonexistent) because they believe that God is going to work a miracle. In these cases, simple nursing measures such as turning or bathing clients become occasions of pain and torment to both the client and nurse. Nurses are forced to administer care that they take to be cruel and abusive to conscious clients whose agonized dying is being needlessly prolonged. Unfortunately, there are no clear guidelines for drawing the line between promoting life and prolonging the dying process. Although nurses always have the moral right to withdraw from administering care that violates their personal moral code, this does not resolve the problem for the client. More dialogue is needed on the interaction between religion and law, ethics, and medicine. Ideally, the religious freedom of clients and their families is respected as is the moral autonomy of caregivers and the integrity of the healing professions.

Factors Affecting Spirituality

Among the many factors that can influence a person's spirituality, the most important are developmental considerations, family, ethnic background, formal religion, and life events.

RESEARCH IN NURSING Making a Difference

Spiritual Well-Being and Spiritual Care

The importance of spirituality to client well-being has been widely accepted within the nursing community. Developmental theorists include spirituality in describing concepts of personal integrity and self-actualization. Investigators have researched spirituality from such varying perspectives as religiousness, folk beliefs, and crisis.

Related Research

Piles, C. L. (1990). Providing spiritual care. *Nurse Educator, 15*(10), 36–41.

This study was designed to discover whether, or to what extent, spiritual care was being provided to clients manifesting evidence of spiritual needs. Responses to mailed questionnaires from 300 nurses randomly selected from throughout the United States demonstrated a need for spiritual care content in basic nursing programs. The author presents strategies for teaching students and practicing nurses how to provide spiritual care.

Nelson, P. B. (1990). Intrinsic/extrinsic religious orientation of the elderly: Relationship to depression and self-

esteem. *Journal of Gerontological Nursing, 16*(2), 29–37.

This study was designed to determine if there is a relationship between intrinsic and extrinsic religious orientation, depression, and self-esteem in noninstitutionalized elderly people (convenience sample of 68 elderly people). Results indicated that elderly people who are more intrinsically oriented to religion (ie, religion is a part of their daily activities) experience less depression and higher self-esteem.

Summary

Spirituality is an area that deserves further research by nurses. Ideally, research data will continue to direct effects to identify the spiritual needs of target populations as well as the specific nursing strategies that best meet those needs. Additional studies that focus on the preparation and needs of the nurse who administers spiritual care are also indicated.

Developmental Considerations

Because spirituality has to do with the nonmaterial realm of being, a child must have some capacity for abstract thought before beginning to understand the spiritual self and explore a relationship with a higher power. This is not to say that spirituality is meaningless for children.

David Heller (1985) interviewed 40 children, ages 4 to 12 years, affiliated with one of four major religions—Judaism, Roman Catholicism, Protestantism, or Hinduism—and discovered that the children had definite perceptions of God and preferred forms of prayer or spiritual exercises, which differed according to the age, sex, religion, and personality of the child. Central themes in all the children's descriptions of God included

- Notion of a God who works through human intimacy and the interconnectedness of lives
- Belief that God is involved in self-change and growth and transformations that make the world fresh, alive, and meaningful
- Attributing to God tremendous and expansive power and then showing considerable anxiety in the face of this power
- Image of light

As the child matures, life experiences usually influence and mature spiritual beliefs. With advancing years, the tendency to think about life after death prompts some individuals to reexamine and reaffirm their spiritual beliefs.

Family

A child's parents play a key role in the development of the child's spirituality. What is important is not so much what parents teach a child about God and religion, but rather what the child learns about God, life, and self from parents' behavior. Because the family is the first world the child experiences, his or her worldview is colored by experiences with parents and siblings.

Ethnic Background

Religious traditions differ among ethnic groups. There are clear distinctions between Eastern and Western spiritual traditions as well as among those of individual ethnic groups such as Native Americans. A person's culture and formal religion has much to do with whether the basic approach to religion is doing something, being someone, or continually striving for harmony.

Formal Religion

Each of the major religions discussed earlier in this chapter has several characteristics in common:
- Basis of authority or source of power
- A portion of scripture or sacred word
- An ethical code that defines right and wrong

- A psychology and identity so that its adherents fit into a group and the world is defined by the religion
- Aspirations or expectations
- Some ideas about what follows death (Murray & Zentner, 1989)

Life Events

Both positive and negative life experiences can influence spirituality and, in turn, are influenced by the meaning a person's spiritual beliefs attribute to them. For example, if two women who believe in a loving God both lose a child in a car accident, one may bitterly deny God's existence and stop going to church, whereas the other may spend more time in prayer asking God to help her understand and accept her loss. Similarly, a chain of successful life experiences (marriage, degree, promotion) may cause one person to assume success and experience no need for God, whereas for another it occasions deep gratitude and rejoicing.

Nurse as Role Model

Three spiritual needs are common to all people—the need for meaning and purpose, the need for love and relatedness, and the need for forgiveness (Fish & Shelly, 1978). These needs are common to nurses, whether they observe an established religion, believe in a spiritual essence, or recognize a field of power. As the nurse develops plans to be a spiritual role model to clients, the nurse develops goals for self. The nurse will:
- Hold spiritual beliefs that meet his or her need for meaning and purpose, love and relatedness, forgiveness
- Derive from these beliefs strength for everyday living, especially when confronting pain, suffering, and death in his or her professional practice
- Set aside regular periods to nurture his or her spiritual self
- Demonstrate in his or her interactions with others peace, inner strength, warmth, joy, caring, and creativity
- Respect the spiritual beliefs and practices of others even when they are different from the nurse's own
- Increase his or her knowledge of how the spiritual beliefs of clients influence their life-styles, responses to illness, health care choices, and treatment options
- Demonstrate sensitivity to the spiritual needs of clients
- Develop successful nursing strategies to assist clients in spiritual distress

Use the assessment checklist in the accompanying display to see how well you are meeting your own spirituality needs.

♥ PROMOTING WELLNESS

Spirituality

Use the assessment checklist to determine how well you are meeting spirituality needs. Then develop a prescription for self-care by choosing appropriate behaviors from the list of suggestions.

Assessment Checklist

(almost always / sometimes / almost never)

1. I am comfortable with my spiritual beliefs and values.
2. My beliefs meet my needs for love, belonging, forgiveness, meaning, and purpose.
3. I respect the belief systems of others.
4. I derive sufficient strength from my religious beliefs to meet each day's challenges.

Self-Care Behaviors

1. Explore personal values and beliefs of self and others.
2. Explore practices that are spiritually supportive.
3. Respect the belief systems of others.
4. Practice loving relationships with self and others.
5. Seek spiritual assistance to help cope with stress, crisis, or loss.

Assessing Spirituality

Nursing History

Because a person's spirituality and religious beliefs have the potential to influence every aspect of being, an assessment of the client's spirituality should be included in each comprehensive nursing history. Helpful assessment guides are offered by Fish and Shelly (1978), Stoll (1979), and O'Brien (1982). Data are gathered about the client's spiritual beliefs and practices, the effect of these beliefs on everyday living, spiritual distress, and spiritual needs. Sample questions are listed in the Focused Assessment Guide in the accompanying display.

The following questions are from O'Brien's (1982) Spiritual Assessment Guide:

Spiritual pain: Do you ever feel hurt or pain associated with the spiritual or religious beliefs that you hold? Do you feel pain related to uncertainty or nonbelief?

Spiritual alienation: Do you frequently feel far away from God? Does it seem that he is remote and far removed from your everyday life?

Spiritual anxiety: Are you afraid that God might not take care of your needs? That he might not be there when you need him?

Spiritual guilt: Have you ever done things that God would be angry at you for? Are you feeling badly about things that you have done or failed to do in your life?

Spiritual anger: Are you angry at God for allowing you to be ill? Do you ever feel like blaming God for your illness? Do you think God is unfair to you?

Spiritual loss: Do you ever feel that you have lost God's love? That you have broken or weakened your relationship with God? Has God turned his back on you?

Spiritual despair: Do you ever feel that there is no hope of having God's love? Of pleasing him? That God does not love you anymore? (p. 102)

If the client shares a spiritual problem, remember to use interview questions to determine the specific nature of the problem, its probable causes, related signs and symptoms, when it first began and how often it occurs, how it affects everyday living, the severity of the problem and whether it can be treated independently by nursing or needs to be referred, and how well the client is coping with the problem.

Nursing Observation

Because many clients may find it difficult to talk about their spiritual beliefs and problems, the nurse also observes the client's behavior for signs of spiritual distress. A family member or close friend may share significant observations.

"He's been awfully moody since his heart attack . . . I can't believe the change in him."

"I've never seen my father so depressed. He's never in his life been away from the Synagogue at Passover. I don't know how to help him."

FOCUSED ASSESSMENT GUIDE

Spirituality

Factors to Assess	Questions and Approaches
Spiritual beliefs	"Are there particular spiritual or religious beliefs that are important to you? Have these beliefs changed recently? Is your illness challenging these beliefs? Do your religious beliefs in any way dictate a course of action that puts you in conflict with what your physicians are recommending?"
Spiritual practices	"Describe your usual spiritual practices and anything interfering with your ability to perform them. Can I help in any way to secure the aids necessary for these practices (prayer shawl, Bible, crystals, beads, icon)?"
Relation between spiritual beliefs and everyday living	"Describe ways your spiritual beliefs affect everyday living (daily schedule, diet, hygiene, sense of self and the world, relationships). Do you find this influence to be healthy (life affirming) or destructive (life denying)?"
Spiritual deficit or distress	"Are your spiritual beliefs currently causing you any distress?"
Spiritual needs	"In what ways can I and the other nurses help you to meet your spiritual needs?" "Would you like me to contact your spiritual adviser or the hospital's pastoral care minister?"
Need for meaning and purpose	"In what ways do your religious beliefs help or hinder you to understand your current situation and face it with peace and courage?"
Need for love and relatedness	"In what ways do your religious beliefs help or hinder you to meet your need to love and be loved?"
Need for forgiveness	"In what ways do your religious beliefs help or hinder you to feel at peace?"
Significant behavioral observations	Be alert to sudden changes in spiritual practices, mood changes, sudden interest in spiritual matters, and sleep disturbances—all of which may point to unresolved spiritual needs.

Significant behavioral observations include sudden changes in spiritual practices (rejection, neglect, fanatical devotion); mood changes (frequent crying, depression, apathy, anger); sudden interest in spiritual matters (reading religious books or watching religious programs on television, visits to clergy); and disturbed sleep. A nurse who observes these behaviors should follow up with appropriate interview questions. Often problems with spiritual distress do not surface until well after a client's admission history and examination. Effective questions include

"You've been lying there so quietly . . . what are you thinking about?"

"After all you've been through you must have done a good bit of soul searching. . . . Experiences like these are enough to shake anyone's faith—how is yours holding up?"

Diagnosing

When assessment data point to a spiritual problem that can be treated by independent nursing intervention, it receives the label *Spiritual Distress*. This may be further specified as spiritual pain, alienation, anxiety, guilt, anger, loss, or despair (O'Brien, 1982). Common etiologies for spiritual distress include inability to reconcile current life situation (eg, illness, death of loved person, divorce) with spiritual beliefs ("God is all-powerful, all-loving, all-wise and he cares about me") or separation from the religious community or supports. Sample nursing diagnoses of spiritual distress are presented in the accompanying display.

Spiritual distress may affect other areas of human functioning. In the following nursing diagnoses, spiritual distress is the etiology of another problem.

Impaired Adjustment to Illness related to inability to reconcile illness with spiritual beliefs

Ineffective Individual Coping related to loss of religion as primary support (feels abandoned by God)

Fear related to feeling unprepared for death and afterlife experience

Dysfunctional Grieving: Despair related to belief that religion is meaningless

Hopelessness related to belief that no one cares—including God

Powerlessness related to feeling victimized by a tyrannical and arbitrary God

NURSING DIAGNOSES FOR COMMON PROBLEMS

Spiritual Distress*

Problem	Related Factors	Sample Defining Characteristics
Spiritual pain	Inability to accept death of son	A 46-year-old woman, agnostic, only son died 6 months ago (lung cancer)
		"I've often wondered throughout my life if there is a God—thought maybe if I had tried harder I'd have recognized him. Now I don't care if God exists or not because if he allows this I don't want to know him."
		"My son was my whole life; there's nothing left for me to live for."
		Lost 10 lb in 6 months since son died; leaves home only when necessary to purchase food, go to bank, and engage in other routine activities.
Spiritual alienation	Separated from "faith community"	A 72-year-old Orthodox Jewish man, recently admitted to Protestant nursing home following 3-week hospitalization for stroke
		"I guess Yahweh has written me off; first the stroke that killed half my body and then I'm abandoned here where I can't even observe the Sabbath."
		"I want to go home."
Spiritual anxiety	Challenged belief and value system	A 37-year-old previously healthy male executive recovering from massive myocardial infarction
		"My parents were strict Methodists, but when I left home for college I stopped going to church . . . never gave it much thought . . . there was always something else to do. I started going again but it never meant much."
		"I haven't exactly done anything awful but I've also not been a saint and I find myself wondering if there is a God what does he think of me."
		"Funny, I guess I thought I'd live forever. I sure never thought about dying and what happens after that."
		Often observed lying quietly in bed awake; asked to see minister.
Spiritual guilt	Failure to live according to religious rules	A 23-year-old, single, Baptist woman being treated for premenstrual syndrome
		"I was raised in a strict Baptist home but had to leave . . . I needed more room to be me. I like life here at the university but there's a restlessness in me I can't describe. I've dated several men, one or two I really liked, but I always do something to mess up the relationship. It would kill my mother if she knew I lived with Gary for 3 months."
		"What it really comes down to is my own sense of betraying myself, my family, and my religion. Who am I anyway?"
Spiritual anger	Inability to accept illness	A 38-year-old homosexual man recently diagnosed with AIDS
		"My parents are fundamentalists . . . all I ever heard at home was how much Jesus loves me . . . all the while my mom was beating the daylights out of me. . . . Does he love me? Does he love me so much that he had my parents throw me out when I finally told them I was gay? Does he love me so much that I got AIDS and now no one comes near me?"
		Facial features are tight; body held rigidly; speech is sharp, appears angry with God, the world, himself.

(continued)

NURSING DIAGNOSES FOR COMMON PROBLEMS

Spiritual Distress* (Continued)

Problem	Related Factors	Sample Defining Characteristics
Spiritual loss	Terminal illness; anticipatory grieving; inability to find comfort in religion	A 40-year-old mother of three sons who was diagnosed with ovarian cancer 18 months ago; currently in advanced stage of disease
		I've tried hard to do it all right . . . I read my Bible, prayed every day, went to church each Sunday, loved my husband and kids . . . why is this all happening to me? Why must I lose it all? Where is God now that I need him? Some mornings I wish I could shoot myself and end it all—instead another day drags on. Who can help me?''
		Cries frequently, no longer interested in everyday activities of family, no interest in praying, told family not to have pastor call anymore. "No one can help now.''
Spiritual despair	Feeling that no one (not even God) cares	A 92-year-old frail widow who lives alone in a two-room apartment; crippled with arthritis; has two married sons she has not seen for years.
		Says to community nurse who visits every week, "No one should have to live like this. If it weren't for the neighbor who comes on Saturday with a few groceries and you I'd be dead. I guess that would be for the best. It's been a long time since I felt like my living or dying would matter to anyone. Because I'm 92 now I guess even God doesn't want me. Couldn't you do something to put me out of my misery?''

*NANDA-approved nursing diagnosis label.

Self-Esteem Disturbance related to failure to live according to dictates of religion

Sexual Dysfunction related to values conflict

Sleep Pattern Disturbance related to spiritual distress

High Risk for Self-Directed Violence: related to feeling that life is meaningless

Planning: Client Goals

Nurses who are sensitive to the role spiritual beliefs play in influencing both a person's thoughts about self and the world and interactions with the world value spiritual health. Their interactions with any client who values spirituality are supportive of the following client goals. The client will:

- Identify spiritual beliefs that meet needs for meaning and purpose, love and relatedness, and forgiveness
- Derive from these beliefs strength, hope, and comfort when facing the challenge of illness, injury, or other life crisis
- Develop spiritual practices that nurture communion with inner self, with God, and with the world
- Express satisfaction with the compatibility of spiritual beliefs and everyday living.

Goals for clients in spiritual distress need to be individualized and may include some of the following. The client will:

- Explore the origin of spiritual beliefs and practices
- Identify factors in life that challenge spiritual beliefs
- Explore alternatives given these challenges: deny, modify, or reaffirm beliefs; develop new beliefs
- Identify spiritual supports (eg, spiritual reading, faith, community)
- Report or demonstrate a decrease in spiritual distress following successful intervention.

Implementing

There are a variety of interventions available to the nurse who wishes to help clients meet spiritual needs. Like other nursing skills, these interventions need to be practiced before the nurse is able to use them confidently, competently, and at the right moment. In this section, the following nursing interventions are presented: offering supportive presence, facilitating the client's practice of religion, nurturing spirituality, praying with a client, spiritual counseling, referring a client to a religious counselor, and resolving conflicts between spiritual beliefs and treatment.

Offering Supportive Presence

A nurse's gift of supportive presence must underlie all other types of intervention to meet spiritual needs. Supportive presence communicates value and respect. Chapter 20 presents basic communication skills helpful in establishing this type of presence.

The client who senses that the nurse is sincerely concerned and committed to helping meet human needs is better able to participate in the care plan. Clients who experience respect and affirmation from other humans find it easier to hold spiritual beliefs that meet their needs for meaning and purpose, love and relatedness, and forgiveness.

Facilitating the Client's Practice of Religion

The nurse can assist the hospitalized client in meeting spiritual needs. The following are means of helping the client continue normal spiritual practices in the unfamiliar environment of the hospital or care center:

- Familiarize the client with religious services and materials available within the institution.
- Respect the client's need for privacy or quiet during periods of prayer.
- Assist the client to obtain devotional objects and protect them from loss or damage.
- Arrange for the client wishing to receive the sacraments to do so.
- Attempt to meet the client's religious dietary restrictions.
- Arrange for the client's minister, priest, or rabbi to visit if the client so wishes.

If the client has a conflict between spiritual beliefs and the proposed medical therapy, the nurse can assist the client in discussing this with the physician.

Nurturing Spirituality

Some clients experiencing a need to get in touch with their spiritual self and to nurture their spiritual development may look to the nurse for direction. The person who lives life enmeshed in the action and noises of society may feel strangely uncomfortable when illness forces self-introspection. The nurse can be helpful in recommending means to develop a relationship with one's inner world and manifest spiritual energy in one's outer world (Hill & Smith, 1990). (See the accompanying display titled Nurturing Spirituality.)

Praying With a Client

Clients accustomed to regular periods of prayer but who feel too ill to pray as they would like or who enjoy praying with others may ask the nurse to pray with them or hope that the nurse will suggest this. Because there are many forms of prayer—quiet reflection, silent communion with God or higher power, reading or recitation of formal prayers, silent or loud calling on God or conversation with

---

Nurturing Spirituality

Ways to Develop a Relationship With One's Inner World

- Prayer
- Reflection or "quiet listening to one's essence"
- Communion with nature through walks in the park, woods, beach
- Enjoyment of music, drama, art, dance
- Inner dialogues with oneself or with a higher being
- Dream analysis

Ways to Manifest Spiritual Energy in One's Outer World

- Loving relationships with others
- Service to others in need
- Forgiveness of others
- Empathy, compassion, and hope
- Laughter, joyous expressions
- Participation in church services and activities and social gatherings

(Hill, L., & Smith, N. [1990]. *Self-care nursing* [2nd. ed.]. New York: Appleton & Lange.)

God, or reading the Bible—the nurse can take the lead from the client by asking, "How would you like us to pray?" The religious background of the client is considered along with the type of prayers that have been meaningful in the past. It is also helpful to ask the client if there is a particular prayer request.

The nurse unaccustomed to praying aloud or in public may find it helpful to have a Bible passage or formal prayer readily available. The prayer may also be a simple expression aloud of the client's needs and hopes. A sample follows:

> Lord God, our Creator and Healer, I entrust Mrs. Smith and her family to your loving care . . . bring peace to her mind and health and strength to her body. . . . Be with her [as her treatment begins today, as she goes for surgery, and so on]. . . . We remember all your blessings to us in the past and thank you. . . . We are confident of your help now as we claim your promises."

It is important not to use prayer to block communication with the client. Praying before a client feels ready to pray may communicate to the client a lack of interest in the client's feelings. Because prayer often evokes deep feelings, the nurse should be prepared to spend time with the client after sharing prayer to respond to these feelings (Fish & Shelly, 1978).

Spiritual Counseling

The client who feels that the nurse is sensitive to spiritual needs and comfortable in his or her own spirituality may choose to share spiritual concerns with the nurse rather than with a religious counselor. The nurse who feels able to counsel the client may assist the client to:

- Articulate spiritual beliefs
- Explore the origin of the client's spiritual beliefs and practices
- Identify life factors that challenge the client's spiritual beliefs (cause spiritual distress)
- Explore alternatives given these challenges: modify life-style; deny, modify, or reaffirm beliefs; develop new beliefs
- Develop spiritual beliefs that meet needs for meaning and purpose, care and relatedness, forgiveness

To be an effective spiritual counselor, the nurse must be open to different spiritual beliefs and forms of spiritual expression and supportive of the client's efforts to nurture spiritual growth.

Referring a Client to a Religious Counselor

Although not every nurse feels comfortable serving as a spiritual counselor, each nurse's responsibility is to identify when clients wish to see a religious counselor and to make the appropriate referral. Options include contacting the client's own spiritual adviser; contacting the institution's pastoral ministry department (if one exists); and using the institution's referral list of clergy in the local community. At times, a representative of the client's own religion may be unable to visit but a clergyperson from another faith may both be able to help and be welcomed by the client.

The nurse can assist the religious counselor by making the counselor feel welcome, answering questions about the client, directing the counselor to the client, and ensuring that the client is ready to receive the counselor. Preparations of the client's room for the visit may vary, but the following are generally recommended practices:

- The room should be orderly and free of unnecessary equipment and items.
- There should be a seat for the religious counselor at the bedside or near the client so that both can be comfortable during the visit.
- The top of the bedside table should be free of items and covered with a clean, white cover if a sacrament is to be administered.

- The bed curtains should be drawn to provide privacy if the client is in a unit with other clients and is unable to be moved to a more private setting.

Some clients and spiritual advisers may value the nurse's participation in prayers, rituals, or the administration of sacraments. When a nursing diagnosis of spiritual distress is made, the nurse and the religious counselor can often collaborate on the care plan and reinforce each other's efforts to assist the client to meet goals.

Resolving Conflicts Between Spiritual Beliefs and Treatments

Both the client and members of the client's family may experience conflict between a particular spiritual belief or religious law and proposed medical treatment or health option. The client may want the nurse's assistance when conferring with the spiritual adviser about a particular procedure. The nurse's role is to assist the client in obtaining the information needed to make an informed decision and to support the *client's* decision making. Because what the nurse says and the way it is said may powerfully influence the client's decision, it is important for the nurse to maintain objectivity.

Evaluating

The nurse working with a client and family to achieve specified goals to meet spiritual needs can use each client interaction to evaluate the care plan. Necessary to the evaluation are sensitivity to what the client is saying and not saying and observation of the client when alone as well as when interacting with the family and nurses.

In general, the nurse evaluates the client's ability to:

- Find meaning and purpose in the client's current condition
- Interact honestly with family, friends, and others who meet the client's need for love and relatedness
- Derive strength and peace from the client's spiritual beliefs
- Reconcile any interpersonal differences causing the client anguish (religious belief or law in conflict with medical therapy)

The nurse helps the client to determine if spiritual beliefs are generally life affirming or life denying and if there is harmony between these beliefs and the client's everyday life experiences.

 # N U R S I N G P R O C E S S

in Clinical Practice

The nurse uses each phase of the nursing process when identifying and treating spiritual problems categorized as nursing diagnoses. Quality care depends on the nurse's possession of the knowledge and skills described earlier in this chapter. Following in outline format are the assess-

ment priorities, client goals, nursing interventions, and evaluative criteria for a common spiritual problem encountered by nurses—spiritual distress. In the case study, nursing care is described for a middle-aged male client who has not practiced any formal religion recently and who, following a heart attack, is concerned about his relationship with God.

Spiritual Distress

Spiritual distress may result when an individual is unable to meet one or more of the basic spiritual needs for meaning and purpose, for love and relatedness, or for forgiveness (Fish & Shelly, 1978). Possible etiologies for these spiritual deficits include the following:

Deficit: Meaning and purpose

Inability to reconcile spiritual beliefs with illness, pain, suffering, impending death

No prior need to explore life or its meaning and purpose

Deficit: Love and relatedness

Human relationships to date have been painful.

Belief that people are bad and best dealt with as little as possible

Belief that God is a distant and uncaring superpower

Deficit: Forgiveness

Inability to forgive oneself or others for human failings

Belief that God is a harsh taskmaster who desires nothing less than perfection

When identifying spiritual deficits, it is important to remember that individuals have different spiritual needs and meet them differently. The meaning one person attributes to life may be different from that of another. It must be sufficient that it enables the individual to face each day with renewed energy for living in pursuit of some good.

Assessment

- Use interview questions and observations of the client's behavior to identify defining characteristics of each spiritual deficit.
  - Meaning and purpose: Statements reflecting sense of despair, hopelessness, powerlessness ("What's the use?" "Nothing matters any more . . . " "Why should I bother?"); apathy, indifference, listlessness, lethargy; decreased energy for daily living and for healing
  - Love and relatedness: Statements indicating loneliness, desire for meaningful relationships with God and people; statements describing God and humans as overwhelmingly negative (evil, hurtful, distant, indifferent, uncaring); decreased ability to interact with others (withdrawal, behaviors that alienate others); absence of visitors for hospitalized client
  - Forgiveness: Statements reflecting dissatisfaction with self, shame, guilt, desire for forgiveness, belief that one's failings are unforgivable; belief that God is punishing; anger, depression, cynicism; confessions of failings to others
- Identify attempts client has made or is making to resolve these deficits and their effectiveness.

- Assess the need for referral to a spiritual adviser.

Planning: Client Goals

The client will:
- Identify some spiritual belief that gives meaning and purpose to everyday life
- Move toward a healthy acceptance of the current situation: illness, pain, suffering, impending death
- Develop mutually caring relationships
- Verbalize satisfaction with relationship with God (if this is important)
- Express peaceful acceptance of limitations and failings
- Express ability to forgive others and to live in the present
- Demonstrate an "interior state of peace and joy; freedom from abnormal anxiety, guilt, or a feeling of sinfulness; and a sense of security and direction in the pursuit of one's life goals and activities" (O'Brien, 1982, p. 98)

Interventions

Deficit: Meaning and Purpose
- Explore with the client what has given the client's life meaning and purpose up to the present, sources of meaning for other people, and possible meanings for the client's current experience of illness, pain, suffering, or impending death.
- Refer the client to a spiritual adviser if the client wishes this.
- Explore with the client spiritual practices from which strength and hope might be derived (eg, prayer or reading scripture or other spiritual books).
- Recommend that the client read spiritual biographies or Harold Kuschner's (1983) book *Why Bad Things Happen to Good People* (available in paperback in most bookstores).
- Refer the client to the appropriate support groups (eg, self-help groups for people with stroke, cancer, and so on).

Deficit: Love and Relatedness
- Treat the client at all times with respect, empathy, and genuine caring.
- Encourage the client to talk about relationships with others and to identify the origin of negative beliefs about people.
- Encourage conversation about God as the client knows and experiences God (if God is part of the client's spiritual beliefs). If appropriate, introduce or reinforce the belief that God is a loving and personal God who is concerned about the client.
- Whenever possible, encourage and facilitate visits from the client's family, friends, and spiritual adviser.

Deficit: Forgiveness
- Offer a supportive presence to the client that demonstrates your acceptance of the client.

- Explore with the client the importance of *learning* to accept oneself and others, including both strengths and limitations.
- Explore negative images of God and others that make it difficult for the client to seek forgiveness and to believe that the client is forgiven.
- Explore the client's self-expectations and assist the client to determine how realistic these are.
- Allow the client to verbalize shame, guilt, and anger and counsel about the importance of expressing negative emotions in healthy ways. Refer the client to a spiritual adviser, if appropriate.
- Offer the client examples of how feelings of unforgiving toward others can end up hurting only the one who cannot forgive.

Evaluative Criteria

The client meets the previously stated goals.

CASE STUDY

Mr. Gargan is a 38-year-old divorced man on a step-down unit following treatment for a myocardial infarction. He owns a small car dealership. His religion is listed as Protestant. Frequently unable to sleep at night, Mr. Gargan often talks with the night nurse and once asked, "Did you ever give much thought to whether or not there is a God?" Sensing much concern behind this question, the nurse asks specific questions to determine if the client has spiritual needs that are not being met.

Assessment Findings

12/26/93, 2 AM
Client again unable to sleep and initiated discussion about God. States was raised in a Lutheran home where everyone went to church on Sunday and tried to live according to God's commandments. Upon leaving home, he stopped going to church (was never a value for his wife) and simply has not given much thought to religion—too busy running his business. Until now has not experienced any need for God. "But when I think how close I was to dying and that I've no idea what to expect after death—I'm actually scared. Do others feel this way?" Wants to explore religious beliefs—feels lack in his life. Said he would like to talk with hospital minister—will arrange for tomorrow.

E. Nolan, RN

Nursing Diagnosis

Spiritual Distress: Anxiety related to concerns about relationship with God

Planning: Client Goals

Mr. Gargan expresses his concerns about religion hesitantly and admits it is not easy for him to talk about religious matters. He also states that he has not been able to think about much else ever since his heart attack. The following short-term goals are suggested to him and he quickly endorses them: "I need to make some peace with God and really don't know how much time I have, so the sooner we start the better."

Short-Term Goals
Before discharge, the client will:
- Identify his religious beliefs
- Reconcile his life up until the present with God
- Verbalize that his spiritual beliefs have become a source of strength and peace rather than a source of anxiety
- Increase night sleep to at least 6 hours

Long-Term Goal
The client will:
- Develop spiritual beliefs that effectively meet his needs for meaning and purpose, love and belonging, and forgiveness

See the care plan designed to accomplish the preceding goals.

Implementation

Successful implementation of the care plan requires the following specialized nursing abilities:
- Holistic orientation to nursing, which values physical, psychologic, and spiritual health
- Sensitivity to the spiritual needs of clients and the ability and willingness to address these needs
- Respect for and knowledge of different spiritual beliefs (traditions) and the means people use to meet spiritual needs
- Ability to offer the client a supportive nursing presence, including listening skills, empathy, vulnerability, humility, and commitment, as he struggles with his spiritual anxiety
- Willingness to refer the client to a spiritual adviser and to work collaboratively with this person
- Interpersonal and leadership skills to motivate the entire nursing staff to value spiritual health and to better understand its role in facilitating cardiac rehabilitation

Documentation

A sample documentation written when the problem was first detected follows.

SOAP Format

> 12/26/93, 2 AM, nursing
> #9 Spiritual Distress

S: "I need to make some peace with God and really don't know how much time I have. . . . " Reports was raised in Lutheran home but has not practiced any formal religion for most of his adult life—up until now no need for God

O: Frequently unable to fall asleep at night—often observed lying quietly in bed with face tense

A: Spiritual Distress: Anxiety related to concerns about his relationship with God

P: 1. Add preceding diagnosis to problem list.
2. Refer to hospital minister in AM.
3. See care plan.

E. Nolan, RN

Sample documentation of nursing interaction with the client following the first visit of the hospital minister follows.

Traditional Note Format

> 12/27/93, 3 PM, nursing

B. Hanks, Protestant minister, here to see client at 1 PM. Afterward, client said he felt "a whole lot better." Reported minister had assured him that many people in the hospital with a serious illness go through exactly what he is experiencing now—and this thought seemed to decrease much of his anxiety. Minister had reinforced nurse's suggestion that he explore his religious beliefs and he has already jotted down some thoughts. "I knew you fixed bodies in hospitals but didn't know you fix souls, too." Client looking forward to minister's visit tomorrow.

G. Paris, RN

Evaluation

Short-term goal achievement is continuously evaluated before client's discharge. See the nursing care plan for evaluative statements. The client is taught how to evaluate the long-term goal because this will require ongoing evaluation.

 NURSING CARE PLAN

for Mr. Gargan

Nursing Diagnosis:	Spiritual Distress: Anxiety related to concerns about relationship with God
Long-Term Goal:	The client's spiritual beliefs will effectively meet his needs for meaning and purpose, love and belonging, forgiveness.

Goal:	Before discharge, the client will: • Identify his religious beliefs

Nursing Actions	Rationale	Evaluative Statement
Assist the client to (1) identify the spiritual beliefs he had as a child and the origin of these beliefs; (2) evaluate these beliefs in terms of his life experiences; and (3) reaffirm, modify, or reject these beliefs or develop new spiritual beliefs.	Life experiences may challenge religious beliefs that were uncritically held as a child.	12/30/93 Goal partially met. Client states he has a much clearer concept of God and no longer fears that God will reject him for ignoring him for so long . . . but believes he also has a lot to learn. *E. Nolan, RN*
Assist the client to assess whether his newly articulated spiritual beliefs are life-affirming or life-denying and the degree to which they meet his needs for meaning and purpose, love and relatedness, and forgiveness.	Because spiritual beliefs can exert positive (life-affirming) and negative (life-denying) influences on a person's life, individuals should have some criteria to use when evaluating their beliefs.	
Refer the client to the hospital minister for assistance with the above.	Client may value speaking with a minister.	

(continued)

N U R S I N G   C A R E   P L A N *(continued)*

for Mr. Gargan

Goal: Before discharge, the client will:
- Reconcile his life up until the present with God

Nursing Actions	**Rationale**	**Evaluative Statement**
Reassure the client that many persons get involved in day-to-day living to the extent that they forget about God and that in some religions persons believe that God uses illness and other stressors to invite people to rethink their spiritual beliefs. In these traditions, God is often pictured with open arms waiting to welcome a child home.	Images of a stern and unyielding God ready to strike down transgressors may contribute to a client's spiritual distress.	12/30/93 Goal met. "This minister has really helped. I wish I had talked to him a long time ago. I've carried so much guilt about my divorce and some other things—thought God would never forgive me. I feel so much more at peace now."
Refer the client to a spiritual advisor for help in experiencing forgiveness if he mentions guilt feelings.	Guilt often inhibits persons from seeking and experiencing the forgiveness they desire.	*E. Nolan, RN*
Communicate to the client the importance of people accepting themselves—with all their strengths and weaknesses.	Many persons have unrealistic self-expectations.	

Goal: Before discharge, the client will:
- Verbalize that his spiritual beliefs have become a source of strength and peace rather than anxiety

Nursing Actions	**Rationale**	**Evaluative Statement**
Encourage the client to compare the role of spiritual beliefs in his life before, during, and after hospitalization.	This highlights the positive and negative roles spiritual beliefs can play. It may motivate the client to continue searching if he values his present experience.	12/30/93 Goal met. "It's good to be able to feel more peaceful about whatever the future brings. I'm anxious to get out of here because there's a lot I want to do with God's help."
		E. Nolan, RN

Goal: Before discharge, the client will:
- Increase night sleep to at least 6 undisturbed hours

Nursing Actions	**Rationale**	**Evaluative Statement**
Nurse on the 11 to 7 shift checks on client at beginning of shift to make sure he is comfortable and ready for sleep.	Nursing supervision of the client at bedtime rules out other factors that may interfere with sleep.	12/30/93 Goal met. Client slept last night from midnight to 6 AM. Will continue to monitor.
Use power of suggestion to enhance sleep. "I'm sure when I check back you'll be sound asleep."	Suggestion has been shown to enhance the therapeutic effect of other interventions.	*E. Nolan, RN*
If sleep remains disturbed, try relaxation exercises or guided imagery (see Chapter 9).	As spiritual anxiety decreases, sleep should improve. If sleep does not improve, other contributing factors and interventions will need to be explored.	

KEY POINTS

- The tradition of nursing has always been strongly holistic and nurses have practiced nursing sensitive to the physical, psychosocial, and spiritual needs of clients.
- Spiritual needs underlying all religious traditions and common to all people include need for meaning and purpose, need for love and relatedness, and need for forgiveness.
- Spiritual beliefs and practices are associated with all aspects of a person's life—health and illness, relationships with others, daily living habits, required and prohibited behaviors, the general frame of reference for thinking about oneself and the world.
- Spiritual beliefs during illness may be an important source of support, strength, and healing but may also be a source of anxiety when they conflict with proposed medical therapy.
- It is important for the nurse to be knowledgeable about and respect the spiritual beliefs of clients.
- The nurse who demonstrates peace, inner strength, warmth, joy, caring, and creativity in interactions with others will be most effective when assisting clients to meet spiritual needs.
- A comprehensive nursing assessment of spirituality addresses spiritual beliefs and practices, relationship between spiritual beliefs and everyday living, indicators of spiritual distress, and unmet spiritual needs.
- Nursing diagnoses may be written that specifically address spiritual distress (spiritual pain, alienation, anxiety, guilt, anger, loss, or despair) or that identify the effect of spiritual distress on other areas of human functioning (Ineffective Individual Coping, Dysfunctional Grieving, Hopelessness, Powerlessness, Self-Esteem Disturbance).
- Nursing interventions that promote spiritual health include offering a supportive presence, facilitating the client's practice of religion, nurturing spirituality, praying with a client, spiritual counseling, referring a client to a religious counselor, and assisting clients to resolve conflicts between spiritual beliefs and treatment.

STUDY QUESTIONS

1. Which of the following statements most correctly differentiates between an agnostic and an atheist?
   a. The terms are used interchangeably, both believing there is no God.
   b. An agnostic denies that humans can know anything about God's existence, whereas an atheist denies God's existence.
   c. They both deny the need for a philosophy of living to guide their life.
   d. No aspect of an atheist's life is influenced by spirituality, whereas an agnostic has spiritual values.

2. A nurse who was raised a strict Roman Catholic stated she couldn't assist clients with their spiritual distress because she recognizes only a field power in each individual. She said, "My parents and I hardly talk because I've deserted my faith. Sometimes I feel real isolated from them and also God—if there is a God." Analysis of these data reveals which unmet spiritual need?
   a. need for meaning and purpose
   b. need for forgiveness
   c. need for love and relatedness
   d. need for strength for everyday living

3. Which statement is true concerning the influence of spirituality and religion on the various aspects of a person's life?
   a. All aspects of life may be influenced by spirituality.
   b. Activities of daily living (eating, bathing, sleeping, dressing) are rarely influenced by religion.
   c. Work and recreation are not influenced by religion.
   d. Whereas physical illness is seldom influenced by religion, mental illness frequently is.

4. A client whose last name was Goldstein was served on a paper plate a kosher meal ordered from a restaurant because the hospital made no provision for kosher food or dishes. Mr. Goldstein became angry and accused the nurse of insulting him. "I want to eat what everyone else does—and give me decent dishes." Analysis of these data reveals that
   a. the nurse should have ordered kosher dishes also
   b. the staff must have behaved condescendingly or critically
   c. Mr. Goldstein is a problem client and difficult to satisfy
   d. Mr. Goldstein was stereotyped and not consulted about his dietary preferences

5. You are *least* likely to encounter resistance to emergency life-saving surgery for a client from which of the following families?
   a. Christian Scientist family
   b. Faith Assembly Healer family
   c. Jehovah's Witness family
   d. Orthodox Jewish family

6. When the family desires baptism for an infant, it is imperative that the nurse provide for baptism to be done because
   a. baptism frequently postpones or prevents death or suffering

b. it is legally required that nurses provide for this care when the family makes this request

c. it is a nursing function to assure the salvation of the baby

d. lack of baptism when desired may increase the family's sorrow and suffering

7. Because the capacity for abstract thought develops as a child grows older, spirituality is understood differently by children of different ages. Which of the following statements is *false?*

a. Spirituality and perception of God is meaningless for the 4- to 5-year-old.

b. Even young children, 4 to 5 years, have definite perceptions of God and forms of worship.

c. Children's perceptions of their "spiritual self" mature as they mature.

d. Children, 5 to 11 years, may show anxiety concerning the power they believe God has.

8. The most important source of learning about his or her own spirituality for a child is

a. his or her church or religious organization

b. what parents say about God and religion

c. how parents behave in relationship to one another and their children, to others, and to God

d. the spiritual adviser for the family

9. Even though a detailed nursing history in which spirituality is assessed is taken on admission, problems with spiritual distress may not surface until days after admission. The probable explanation is that

a. clients usually want to conceal information about spiritual needs

b. clients are not concerned about spiritual needs until after their spiritual adviser visits

c. family members and close friends often initiate spiritual concerns

d. illness increases spiritual concerns, which may be difficult for clients to express in words

10. When a client needs spiritual counseling, the nurse who is comfortable with his or her own spirituality should

a. always call the client's own spiritual adviser

b. consult with the client about the spiritual adviser with whom he or she wishes to counsel

c. attempt to counsel the client and, if unsuccessful, make a referral

d. advise the client and spiritual adviser concerning health options and the correct decision

11. When assessment data point to a spiritual problem that can be treated by independent nursing intervention, it receives the NANDA-approved diagnostic label

a. Spiritual Alienation

b. Spiritual Despair

c. Spiritual Distress

d. Spiritual Pain

12. A client states she feels so isolated from her family

and church and even God "in this huge medical center so far from home." An appropriate goal for the client to relieve her spiritual distress is as follows. The client will

a. express satisfaction with the compatibility of her spiritual beliefs and everyday living

b. identify spiritual beliefs that meet her need for meaning and purpose

c. express peaceful acceptance of limitations and failings

d. identify spiritual supports available to her in this medical center

13. A man who is a declared agnostic is extremely depressed after losing his home, his wife, and his children in a fire. His nursing diagnosis is Spiritual Distress: Spiritual Pain related to inability to find meaning and purpose in his current condition. The most important nursing intervention to plan is

a. ask the client which spiritual adviser he would like you to call

b. recommend that the client read spiritual biographies or religious books

c. explore with the client what, in addition to his family, has given his life meaning and purpose in the past

d. introduce the belief that God is a loving and personal God

14. After having an abortion, the client told the visiting nurse, "I shouldn't have had that abortion because I'm Catholic, but what else could I do? I'm afraid I'll never get close to my mother or back in the Church again." She then talked with her priest about this feeling of guilt. Which evaluation statement shows a solution to the problem?

a. Client states, "I wish I had talked with the priest sooner. I now know God has forgiven me and even my mother understands."

b. Client has slept from 10 PM to 6 AM for three consecutive nights without medication.

c. Client has developed mutually caring relationships with two women and one man.

d. Client has identified several spiritual beliefs that give purpose to her life.

15. Mr. Brown's teenage daughter had been involved in shoplifting. He expressed much anger toward her and stated he could not face her, let alone discuss this with her. "I just will not tolerate a thief." Which of the following nursing interventions would you take to assist Mr. Brown with his deficit in forgiveness?

a. Assure him that many parents feel the same way.

b. Reassure him that many teenagers go through this kind of rebellion and that it will pass.

c. Assist the client to identify how unforgiving feelings toward others only hurt the one who cannot forgive.

d. Ask him if he is sure he has spent sufficient time with his daughter.

Answers With Rationale

1. The correct response is *b*. It is factually correct that an agnostic denies that humans can know anything about God's existence, whereas an atheist denies God's existence. The other options are factually incorrect.

2. The correct response is *c*. The data point to an unmet spiritual need to experience love and belonging given her estrangement from her family and God following her leaving the church. The other options may represent other needs this client has, but the data provided do not support them.

3. The correct response is *a*. It is true that spirituality can influence all aspects of a person's life, including activities of daily living, work and recreation, and all types of illnesses. The other options are incomplete or false.

4. The correct response is *d*. The nurse jumped to the premature and false conclusion with this client on the basis of his name alone that he would want a kosher diet.

5. The correct response is *d*. There is no teaching in the Hebrew scriptures that prohibits emergency lifesaving surgery. On the contrary, most Orthodox Jews would be highly motivated to have the surgery because of the high value attached to preserving life. All of the other groups mentioned might have religious grounds for refusing surgery.

6. The correct response is *d*. Failure to ensure that an infant baptism is performed when parents desire it may greatly increase the family's sorrow and suffering, and this is an appropriate nursing concern. Whether baptism postpones or prevents death and suffering (option *a*) is a religious belief that is insufficient to bind all nurses. There is no legal requirement regarding baptism; option *b* is false. Although some nurses may believe part of their role is to assure the salvation (option *c*) of the baby, this function would understandably be rejected by many.

7. The correct response is *a*. It is false that spirituality and perception of God is meaningless for the 4- to 5-year-old. All the other options are factually correct.

8. The correct response is *c*. Children learn most about their own spirituality from how their parents behave in relationship to one another, their children, others, and God. Less important sources of learning are each of the other options.

9. The correct response is *d*. It is factually correct that illness surfaces and may increase spiritual concerns, which many clients find difficult to express. The other options do not correspond to actual experience.

10. The correct response is *b*. Even when a nurse feels comfortable discussing spiritual concerns, he or she should always check first with clients to determine the spiritual adviser with whom they wish to counsel. Calling the client's own spiritual adviser (option *a*) may be premature if it is a matter the nurse can handle. Options *c* and *d* deny clients the right to speak privately with their spiritual adviser from the outset, if this is what they prefer.

11. The correct response is *c*. The only NANDA-approved nursing diagnosis among the options is *c*—Spiritual Distress. The other options may be further specifications of the broader diagnosis Spiritual Distress.

12. The correct response is *d*. Each of the four options represents appropriate spiritual goals. Identifying spiritual supports available to her in the medical center demonstrates a decreased sense of isolation.

13. The correct response is *c*. The nursing intervention, exploring with the client what, in addition to his family, has given his life meaning and purpose in the past, is more likely to correct the etiology of his problem, Spiritual Pain, than any of the other nursing interventions listed.

14. The correct response is *a*. Because this client's nursing diagnosis is Spiritual Distress: Guilt, an evaluative statement that demonstrates a diminishment of guilt is necessary. Only option *a*, "Client states, 'I wish I had talked with the priest sooner. I now know God has forgiven me and even my mother understands'" directly deals with guilt.

15. The correct response is *c*. The only nursing intervention that directly addresses the client's unmet spiritual need concerning forgiveness is option *c*. Options *a* and *b* may make him feel better initially, but neither option addresses his need to forgive. Option *d* is likely to make him feel guilty.

BIBLIOGRAPHY

Brittain, J. N., & Boozer, J. (1987). Spiritual care: Integration into a collegiate nursing curriculum. *Journal of Nursing Education, 26*(4), 155–159.

Burnhard, P. (1987). Spiritual distress and the nursing response: Theoretical considerations and counseling skills. *Journal of Advanced Nursing, 12*(3), 377–382.

Callahan, D., & Campbell, C. S. (Eds.). (1990). Theology, religious traditions, and bioethics: A special supplement. *Hastings Center Report, 20*(6), 18–19.

Carson, V. B. (1989). *Spiritual dimensions of nursing practice.* Philadelphia: Saunders.

Charnes, L. S. (1992). Meeting patients' spiritual needs: The Jewish perspective. *Holistic Nursing Practice, 6*(3), 64–72.

Clark, C. C., Cross, J. R., Deane, D. M., & Lowry, L. W. (1991). Spirituality: Integral to quality care. *Holistic Nursing Practice, 5*(3), 67–76.

Coles, R. (1990). *The spiritual life of children.* Boston: Houghton Mifflin.

Corinne, L., Baily, V., Valentin, M., Morantus, E., & Shirley, L. (1992). The unheard voices of women: Spiritual interventions in maternal–child health care. *MCN, 17*(3), 141–145.

Donley, R. (1991). Spiritual dimensions of health care. *Nursing and Health Care, 12*(4), 178–183.

Dossey, B. (Ed.). (1989). Spirituality and healing [entire issue]. *Holistic Nursing Practice, 3*(3).

Earhart, H. B. (Ed.). *Religious traditions of the world series.* San Francisco: HarperCollins.

Ellerhorst-Ryan, J. (1985). Selecting an instrument to measure spiritual distress. *Oncology Nursing Forum, 12*(2), 93–94, 99.

Ellis, D. (1980). Whatever happened to the spiritual dimension? *Canadian Nurse, 76*(9), 42–43.

Emblen, J. D. (1992). Religion and spirituality defined according to current use in nursing literature. *Journal of Professional Nursing, 8*(1), 41–47.

Fish, S., & Shelly, J. (1978). *Spiritual care: The nurse's role.* Downer's Grove, IL: InterVarsity Press.

Fowler, J. W. (1981). *Stages of faith: The psychology of human development and the quest for meaning.* San Francisco: HarperCollins.

Hauerwas, S. (1990). *Naming the silences: God, medicine, and the problem of suffering.* Grand Rapids: Erdmans.

Heller, D. (1985). The children's God. *Psychology Today, 19*(12), 22–27.

Henderson, K. J. (1989). Dying, God, and anger: Confronting through spiritual care. *Journal of Psychosocial Nursing and Mental Health Services, 27*(5), 17–21.

Highfield, M. F. (1992). Spiritual health of oncology patients. *Cancer Nursing, 15*(1), 1–8.

Hill, L. & Smith, N. (1990). *Self-care nursing* (2nd ed.). New York: Appleton & Lange.

Hultkrantz, A. (1987). *Native religions of North America.* San Francisco: HarperCollins.

Hungelmann, J., et al. (1989). Development of the JAREL spiritual well-being scale. In *Classifications of nursing diagnoses, proceedings of the eighth conference* (pp. 393–398).

Hutchings, D. (1991). Spirituality in the face of death. *Canadian Nurse, 87*(5), 30–31.

Krishnamoni, D. (1992). Pregnant teens. *Canadian Nurse, 88*(3), 20–21.

Krohn, B. (1989). Spiritual care: The forgotten need. *Imprint, 36*(1), 95–96.

Kuschner, H. S. (1983). *Why bad things happen to good people.* New York: Avon.

Larue, G. A. (1988). Religion and the aged. In I. M. Burnside (Ed.), *Nursing and the aged* (3rd ed.). St. Louis: Mosby.

Marty, M. E. (1990). The tradition of the Church in health and healing. *Second Opinion, 13*, 48–72.

Marty, M. E., & Vaux, K. L. (Eds.). *Health/medicine and the faith traditions.* New York: Crossroad.

Mayer, J. (1992). Wholly responsible for a part, or partly responsible for a whole? The concept of spiritual care in nursing. *Second Opinion, 17*(3), 26–55.

McHolm, F. A. (1992). A nursing diagnosis validation study: Defining characteristics of spiritual distress. In R. M. Carroll-Johnson (Ed.), *Classification of nursing diagnoses: Proceedings of the Ninth Conference* (pp. 112–119). Philadelphia: Lippincott.

Miller, J. F., & Powers, M. J. (1988). Development of an instrument to measure hope. *Nursing Research, 37*(1), 6–10.

Montgomery, C. P. (1992). The spiritual connection: Nurses' perceptions of the experience of caring. In D. A. Gaut (Ed.), *The presence of caring* (pp. 39–52). New York: National League for Nursing Press.

Murray, R. B., & Zentner, J. P. (1989). *Nursing assessment and health promotion strategies throughout the lifespan* (4th ed.). New York: Appleton-Lange.

Nelson, P. B. (1990). Intrinsic/extrinsic religious orientation of the elderly: Relationship to depression and self-esteem. *Journal of Gerontological Nursing, 16*(2), 29–37.

O'Brien, M. E. (1982). The need for spiritual integrity. In H. Yura & M. Walsh (Eds.), *Human needs 2 and the nursing process* (pp. 81–115). Norwalk, CT: Appleton-Century-Crofts.

Parrinder, G. (Ed.). (1983). *World religions.* New York: Facts on File Publications.

Peck, M. S. (1978). *The road less traveled.* New York: Simon & Schuster.

Piles, C. L. (1990). Providing spiritual care. *Nurse Educator, 15*(1), 36–41.

Pumphrey, J. B. (1977). Recognizing your patients spiritual needs. *Nursing, 8*(12), 64–69.

Reed, P. G. (1991). Spirituality and mental health in older adults: Extant knowledge for nursing. *Family and Community Health, 14*(2), 14–25.

Rew, L. (1986). Exercises for spiritual growth. *Journal of Holistic Nursing, 4*(1), 20–22.

Salladay, S. A. (1987). Spiritual care of clients. *Nursing and Humanities Newsletter, 5*(3), 8–9.

Salladay, S. A., & McDonnell, M. M. (1989). Spiritual care, ethical choices, and patient advocacy. *Nursing Clinics of North America, 24*(2), 543–549.

Shaffer, J. L. (Ed.) (1989). Spirituality and healing [entire issue]. *Holistic Nursing Practice, 3*(3).

Shaffer, J. L. (Ed.) (1991). Spiritual distress and critical illness. *Critical Care Nurse, 11*(1), 42–45.

Sommer, D. R. (1989). The spiritual needs of dying children. *Issues in Comprehensive Pediatric Nursing, 12*(2/3), 225–233.

Starck, P. L., & McGovern, J. P. (Eds.) (1992). *The hidden dimension of illness: Human suffering.* New York: National League for Nursing Press.

Stepnick, A., & Perry, T. (1992). Preventing spiritual distress in the dying client. *Journal of Psychosocial Nursing, 30*(1), 17–24.

Stoll, R. I. (1979). Guidelines for spiritual assessment. *American Journal of Nursing, 79*(9), 1574–1577.

Warren-Robbins, C. G., & Christiana, N. M. (1989). The spiritual needs of persons with AIDS. *Family and Community Health, 12*(2), 43–51.

Widerquist, J. G. (1992). The spirituality of Florence Nightingale. *Nursing Research, 41*(1), 49–55.

Wilson, D. R. (1989). The chaplain as a resource to families of patients in ICU. *Canadian Critical Care Nursing Journal, 6*(1), 10–12.

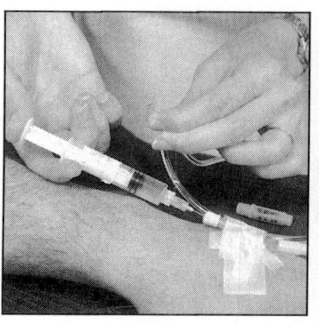
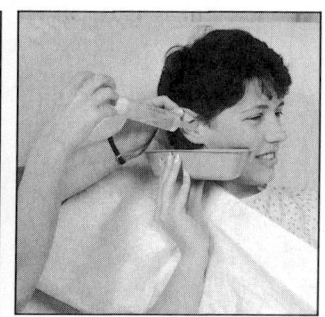
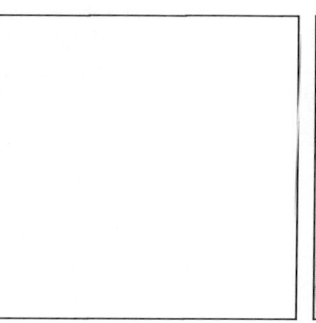
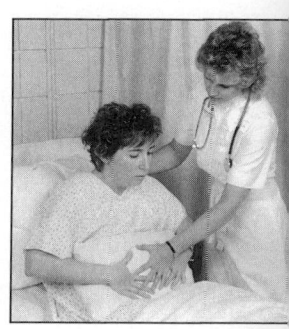

Promoting Optimal Health in Special Situations

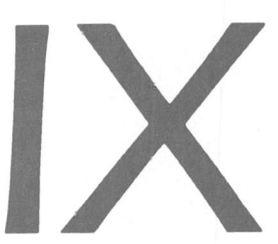

Through use of the nursing process, nurses give holistic care to promote wellness, prevent illness, restore health, and facilitate coping. These broad aims of holistic nursing are integrated when nursing care is focused on promoting optimal health in special situations. Unit IX discusses the nurse's role in situations that occur commonly in health care settings: medication administration, wound care, and care of the client having surgery. In each situation, the nurse uses knowledge and skill to carry out client care in a variety of roles. As caregiver, the nurse assesses, plans, implements, and evaluates nursing interventions to meet holistic physical and psychosocial needs and to provide safety and comfort. As communicator, teacher, and counselor, the nurse provides psychological support and meets knowledge deficits to facilitate coping, maximize strengths, and ensure client and family understanding and continuity of care. As researcher, the nurse uses research findings to ensure ongoing excellence in care and serves as a leader and advocate in working to keep the entire team focused on the individualized needs of the client and family.

The situations discussed in this unit are typical of the interdependent (or collaborative) aspects of nursing and medicine. The physician orders the medications, wound care, or surgical care; the nurse orders and implements nursing measures to promote client safety and knowledge and to facilitate optimal function or recovery. Although procedures and protocols are often used in these situations, nursing interventions are individualized to the unique needs of each person requiring care.

Unit IX provides the content and special skills necessary for knowledgeable, safe, and individualized nursing care when administering medications, caring for wounds, and caring for the client having surgery.

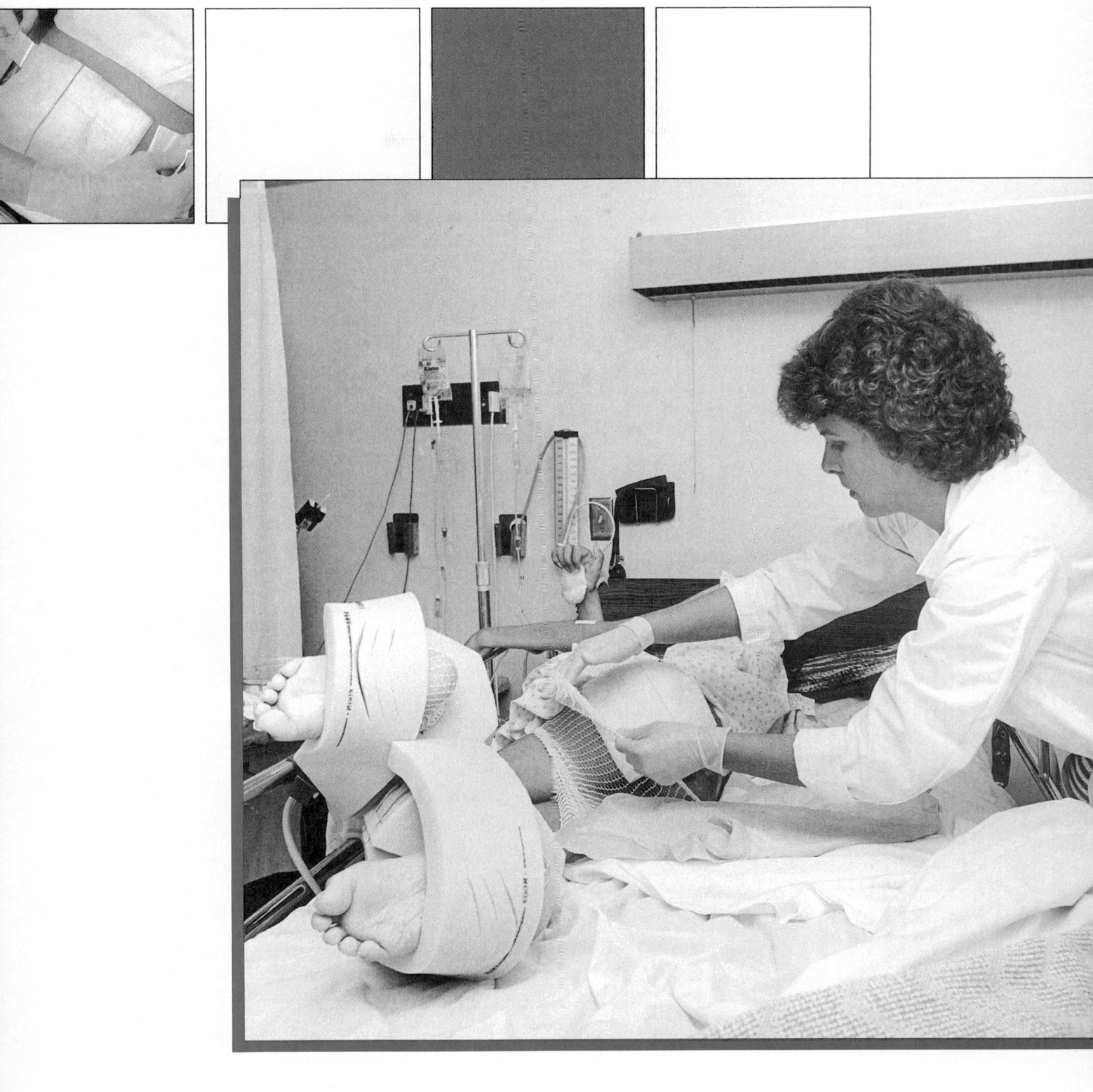

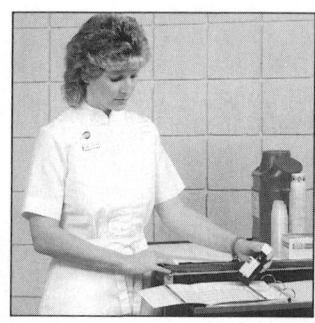

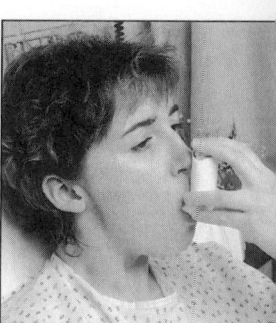

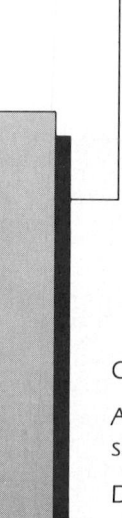

Medications

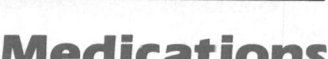

OBJECTIVES

After studying this chapter, the learner should be able to:

Define key terms used in the chapter.

Discuss drug legislation in the United States and Canada.

Describe drug names, types of preparation, and types of drug orders.

Identify drug classifications and actions.

Discuss adverse effects of drugs, including allergy, tolerance, cumulative effect, idiosyncratic effect, and interactions.

Obtain client information necessary to establish a medication history.

Calculate drug dosages, using the various systems of equivalents.

Describe principles used to safely prepare and administer medications orally, parenterally, topically, and by inhalation.

Develop teaching plans to meet client needs specific to medication administration.

KEY TERMS

absorption
ampule
anaphylactic reaction
antagonist effect
body surface area
bolus
chemical name
cumulative effect
distribution
drug
excretion
generic name
heparin lock
iatrogenic disease
idiosyncratic effect
inhalation
injections
instillation
intradermal injection
intramuscular injection
intravenous route
irrigation
medication
medication order
metabolism
official name
parenteral
pharmacodynamics
pharmacokinetics
pharmacology
piggyback infusion
prefilled cartridge
prescription
receptor
subcutaneous injection
synergistic effect
tandem infusion
topical application
trade name
vial
Z-track

42

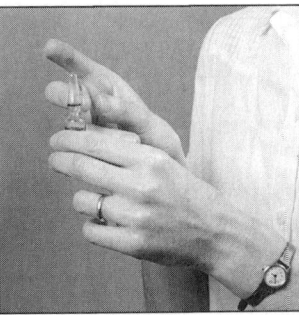

M edication administration is a basic nursing function that involves skillful technique and consideration of the client's development. Medications are prepared and administered with safety in mind. The nurse administering medications is expected to have a knowledge base concerning drugs, including drug names, preparations, classifications, adverse effects, and physiologic factors that affect drug action.

The nursing process can be applied to the fundamental nursing skill of medication administration. Assessment entails a comprehensive medication history as well as ongoing assessments of the client's response during and after drug therapy. Nursing diagnoses are developed from the assessment data. Client-centered outcomes are evaluated after implementation of the plan of care, tailored to the client's needs.

A **drug** or **medication** is any substance that modifies body functions when taken into the living organism. The study that deals with chemicals that affect the body's functioning is called **pharmacology**. A *pharmacist* is a person licensed to prepare and dispense drugs. The physician is legally responsible for prescribing medications. Legislation in some states grants nurse practitioners this privilege also. The physician or nurse practitioner conveys the medication plans to others by an order called a **prescription**. After the medication is prepared by the pharmacist, the nurse administers the medication to the client.

Some medications are given frequently, and the nurse becomes familiar with the facts concerning these drugs. Other medications may not be given by the nurse often, and the nurse needs to seek information before administering the drugs. Information about specific drugs is more appropriately discussed in pharmacology texts. Many references are available to nurses to help them develop a personal medication data base.

Drug Legislation

United States

In 1906 the Pure Food and Drug Act designated the United States Pharmacopeia (USP) and the National Formulary (NF) as official standards of drugs and empowered the federal government to enforce these standards. This legislation was updated in 1938 by the Federal Food, Drug and Cosmetic Act. The Food and Drug Administration is responsible for enforcing this law. Extensive testing of new drugs is required before they may be marketed for use. An amendment to the Federal Food, Drug and Cosmetic Act in 1952 distinguished prescription (legend) drugs from nonprescription (over-the-counter) drugs and provided directions for dispensing prescription drugs.

The Comprehensive Drug Abuse Prevention and Control Act, also known as the Controlled Substances Act, was passed in 1970. This law regulates the distribution of narcotics and other drugs of abuse. Such drugs have been categorized according to their therapeutic usefulness and potential for abuse. Government programs for the prevention and treatment of drug abuse were established.

Canada

Drug legislation in Canada includes the Canadian Food and Drug Act, passed in 1953, which addresses regulations for the manufacture and sale of drug substances. This law has been amended often. According to the act, drugs must comply with standards outlined in specific pharmacopeias and formularies (British Pharmacopeia, Canadian Formulary). The regulations of the Canadian Narcotic Control Act, enacted in 1961, restrict the sale, possession, and use of opiates, coca, and marijuana. Amendments made since 1961 include restrictions on methadone. Only authorized people can possess narcotics. Enforcement of this law has been the charge of the Royal Canadian Mounted Police.

Introduction to Pharmacology

Drug Preparations

Nomenclature

One drug can have several names. The **chemical name** is a precise description of the drug's chemical composition; it identifies the drug's atomic and molecular structure. This name is of significance to the pharmacist. The **generic name** is the name assigned by the manufacturer that first develops the drug. Often the generic name is derived from the chemical name. The **official name** is the name by which the drug is identified in the official publication, *United States Pharmacopeia and National Formulary* (USP and NF). The **trade name**, also referred to as the *brand name* or *proprietary name*, is selected by the drug company that sells the drug and is copyrighted. A drug can have several trade names when produced by different manufacturers.

Nurses should be familiar with a drug's generic and trade names. For example, acetaminophen (generic name) is known by such trade names as Tylenol, Tempra, and Liquiprin.

Types of Preparations

Drugs are available in many forms, or preparations. The form in which the drug is prepared may determine the route of administration. Some drugs may be prepared in only one form to be administered by a certain route. Others may be supplied in several preparations, which allow them to be given through various routes. One type of preparation may be desirable in a given situation. For example, a liquid preparation of a medication would be indicated for young children who are not able to swallow solid preparations such as tablets. Drug preparations are available for oral, topical, and injectable administration. Table 42-1 describes drug preparations commonly used by the nurse.

Classifications

How does the nurse organize the vast amount of information about medications? Where does the nurse begin the study of medications? It is recommended that the nurse focus on drug classifications.

Drugs can be classified from different perspectives. For example, drugs may be classified by body systems (eg, drugs that affect the respiratory system, drugs that affect the cardiovascular system), by the symptom relieved by the drug, or by the clinical indication for the drug (eg, analgesic, antibiotic).

Mechanism of Drug Action

Pharmacodynamics

Drugs act at the cellular level to achieve their desired effects. The process by which drugs alter cell physiology is called **pharmacodynamics** (Malseed & Girton, 1990). One mechanism of drug action is a drug–receptor interaction in which the drug interacts with one or more cellular structures to alter cell function. These specialized structures are called **receptor** sites. The drug fits the receptor as a key fits a lock. Drugs may also combine with enzymes to achieve the desired effect, which is referred to as a *drug–enzyme interaction*. Some drugs act on the cell membrane or alter the cellular environment.

Pharmacokinetics

Pharmacokinetics is the study of the movement of drug molecules in the body in relation to the drug's absorption, distribution, metabolism, and excretion.

Absorption Absorption is the process by which a drug is transferred from its site of entry into the body to the bloodstream. Absorption of a drug is influenced by several factors:

TABLE 42-1

Common Types of Drug Preparations

Preparation	Description
Capsule	Powder or gel form of an active drug enclosed in a gelatinous container
Elixir	Medication in a clear liquid containing water, alcohol, sweeteners, and flavor
Extended release	Preparation of a medication that allows for slow and continuous release over a predetermined period; may also be referred to as CR or CRT (controlled release), SR (sustained or slow release), SA (sustained action), LA (long acting), or TR (timed release)
Liniment	Medication mixed with alcohol, oil, or soap, which is rubbed on the skin
Lotion	Drug particles in a solution for topical use
Lozenge	Small oval, round, or oblong preparation containing a drug in a flavored or sweetened base, which dissolves in the mouth and releases the medication; also called *troche*
Ointment	Semisolid preparation containing a drug to be applied externally; also called an *unction*
Patch	Unit dose of medication applied directly to skin for diffusion through skin and absorption into the bloodstream
Pill	Mixture of a powdered drug with a cohesive material; may be round or oval
Powder	Single or mixture of finely ground drugs
Solution	A drug dissolved in another substance (eg, in an aqueous solution the drug has been dissolved in water)
Suppository	An easily melted medication preparation in a firm base such as gelatin that is inserted into the body (rectum, vagina, urethra)
Suspension	Finely divided, undissolved particles in a liquid medium; should be shaken before use
Syrup	Medication combined in a water and sugar solution
Tablet	Small, solid dose of medication, compressed or molded; may be any color, size, or shape; enteric-coated tablets coated with a substance that is insoluble in gastric acids to reduce gastric irritation by the drug

Route of administration: Injected medications usually are absorbed more rapidly than oral medications.

Drug solubility: Liquid medications are absorbed more rapidly than solid preparations. Liquid preparations do not have to be dissolved in the gastrointestinal fluids. Most drugs are weak acids and bases. When in solution, drugs are a mixture of ionized and un-ionized forms. The un-ionized form is more readily absorbed.

pH: The form in which the drug is found depends on the pH of the environment. Acidic drugs are well absorbed in the stomach. Drugs that are basic remain ionized or insoluble in an acid environment. These drugs are not absorbed before reaching the small intestine.

Local conditions at the site of administration: The more extensive the absorbing surface, the greater the absorption of the drug and the more rapid the effect. A client with burns would have poor absorption from an intramuscular injection. Food in the stomach can delay the absorption of some medications or enhance the rate of absorption of other drugs. Drug absorption can be manipulated with sustained-release preparations or enteric-coated preparations. Enteric-coated preparations are resistant to the digestive action of the stomach.

Drug dosage: A loading dose is higher than body capacity. A maintenance dose is a lower dosage that becomes the usual or daily dosage. Clients who receive digoxin or phenobarbital may receive loading does when therapy is initiated.

Distribution After a drug has been absorbed into the bloodstream, it is distributed throughout the body. The drug accumulates in specific tissues for its action. **Distribution** depends on the rate of perfusion and capillary permeability to the drug. Certain other factors may also influence distribution. The drug may bind to plasma proteins, which causes unequal distribution and may prevent the drug from reaching its intended site of action. The blood–brain barrier is poorly permeable to water-soluble drugs. Some drugs fail to penetrate the tissues of the central nervous system as readily as others. The placenta, on the other hand, is not a selective barrier to the distribution of drugs. Drugs move across the placenta readily, and many produce harmful effects in the fetus.

Metabolism Metabolism, or biotransformation, is the breakdown of the drug to an inactive form. The liver is the primary site for drug metabolism. Various processes and enzymes are involved in metabolism. Physiologic changes associated with aging or the presence of liver disease may complicate the process. The reader is referred to a pharmacology text for a further explanation of metabolism.

Excretion After the drug is broken down to an inactive form, **excretion** of the drug from the body occurs. Most drugs are excreted by the kidneys. The lungs are the primary route for the excretion of gaseous substances, such as inhalation anesthetics. Many drugs are excreted through the intestines. The sweat, salivary, and mammary glands also are routes of drug excretion.

Some medications may be contraindicated or dosages may need to be adjusted downward if renal excretion is affected by age or disease.

Factors Affecting Drug Action

Certain variables influence the action or effect of a medication.

Developmental Considerations

During pregnancy, most drugs are contraindicated because of their possible adverse effects on the fetus. A child's dose for medication is smaller than an adult's dose. Infants especially are responsive to medications because of the immaturity of their organs. Elderly people are responsive to medications because their bodies have experienced physiologic changes associated with the aging process, including decreased gastric motility, acid production, and blood flow, which affect drug absorption. Small body size, reduced weight, and reduced body water also alter distribution, as do decreases in cardiac output and organ perfusion. Decreased plasma binding increases the possibility of drug toxicity. Liver function declines with advancing age and changes in hepatic enzymes involved in drug metabolism. Blood flow to the liver decreases secondary to a decrease in cardiac output. Drugs are excreted more slowly from the body as a result of changes in kidney function. Receptor sensitivity is altered in elderly people and their sensitivity to certain drugs increases. The physiologic changes in elderly people that increase drug susceptibility are summarized in Focus on the Older Adult.

Weight

Expected responses to drugs are based largely on those reactions that occur when the drugs are given to healthy adults (ages 18 to 65, 150 lb [68 kg]). The nurse should be aware of the usual dose for a particular medication. Drug doses for children are calculated by weight or body surface area.

Sex

This variable refers to the difference in the distribution of body fat and fluids in men and women.

Genetic Factors

Differences in the responses of clients receiving the same medication may be attributed to genetic differences. Enzyme deficiencies or metabolic disturbances can alter the way the body handles the medication.

Altered Drug Response in Elderly People

Physiologic Basis	Adverse Reaction	Nursing Action
• Decreased gastric emptying time and increased pH of gastric juices	Stomach irritation and ulceration	Assess for symptoms of stomach discomfort. Test stools for blood.
• Increased adipose tissue and decreased total body fluid in proportion to the total body mass Decreased number of protein-binding sites Decline in liver function and enzyme production needed for drug metabolism Decreased kidney function, resulting in diminished filtration and excretion	Increased possibility of drug toxicity	Assess for early signs of drug interactions or toxicity. Monitor blood levels of drugs. Monitor laboratory values.
• Altered peripheral venous tone	More pronounced hypotensive effects from medications (particularly antihypertensives and diuretics)	Monitor vital signs. Caution client to change position slowly.
• Changes in blood–brain barrier allowing for easier penetration of fat-soluble drugs	Increased risk of dizziness and confusion, particularly with beta blockers	Assess for dizziness and light-headedness. Be aware of safety precautions.

Psychological Factors

The client's expectations of the medication affect the response to the medication, as, for instance, in studies of drug effects where some clients receive a placebo. A placebo is a pharmacologically inactive substance. In clinical drug trials, one group of clients receives the active drug, while another group receives a placebo to study the drug's effects. Some clients have the same response with the placebo as with the active drug.

Pathology

The presence of disease can affect drug action. The liver is the primary organ for drug breakdown. Pathologic conditions that involve the liver may slow down metabolism.

Environment

The client's environment may influence the response to medications. Sensory deprivation and overload may affect drug responses. The relative oxygen deprivation at high altitudes may increase sensitivity to some drugs (Shlafer & Marieb, 1989). The client who receives pain medication or a sedative in an active environment may not be able to benefit fully from the medication's effects.

Time of Administration

The presence of food in the stomach delays the absorption of orally administered medications. Some medications should be given with food to prevent gastric irritation, and the nurse should consider this when establishing a client's medication schedule. Human rhythms and cycles may also influence drug action.

Adverse Drug Effects

Therapeutic effect is the desired effect of the medication; it is the reason the drug was administered. Sometimes drug reactions are unpredictable and harmful. Adverse effects are effects that are not intended or desired.

An **iatrogenic disease** is caused unintentionally by drug therapy. *Drug allergy* occurs in a person who has been previously exposed to the drug and has developed antibodies. Drug allergies can be manifested in a variety of symptoms ranging from minor to serious. The reaction can occur immediately after the client receives the medication or be delayed for hours to days. Some of the signs and symptoms of a drug allergy are rash, urticaria, fever, diarrhea, nausea, and vomiting. A life-threatening immediate reaction is called an **anaphylactic reaction** and results in respiratory distress, sudden severe bronchospasm, and cardiovascular collapse. This reaction is treated with epinephrine, bronchodilators, and antihistamines.

Drug tolerance exists when the body becomes accustomed to a particular drug over a period of time. Larger doses of the drug must be given to the client to produce the same effects. A **cumulative effect** occurs when the body cannot metabolize one dose of a drug before another dose is administered. The drug is taken in more frequently than it is excreted, and each new dose increases the total quantity in the body than is excreted in the same period. An **idiosyncratic effect** is any abnormal or peculiar response to a drug that may manifest itself by overresponse, underresponse, or response different from the expected outcome. Elderly clients often have unpredictable or erratic responses to medications. Idiosyncratic effects are thought to be the result of genetic enzyme deficiencies that lead to an abnormal mechanism for drug breakdown.

In a *drug interaction*, the combined effect of two or more drugs acting simultaneously produces either an effect less than that of each drug alone (**antagonist effect**) or greater than that of each drug alone (**synergistic effect**). Alcohol and barbiturates, when taken together, create a synergistic effect. Nurses must be knowledgeable and alert for drug interactions and effects of drug therapy.

Assessing: The Medication History

Assessment of the client receiving medications begins during a nursing history, one component of which is the medication history. During the interview, the nurse's questions can be adapted or elaborated to meet the client's needs and level of understanding. The nurse should avoid using medical jargon that the client may not understand. Familiar terms the client or family recognize should be chosen. For instance, the client may refer to a diuretic as the "water pill" or to an anticoagulant as a "blood thinner."

Areas to be included in the medication history are listed in the Focused Assessment Guide.

Assessment is an ongoing process. The nurse not only assesses the client with regard to medications during the nursing history but also continues the assessment of the client during and after medication administration. A discussion of how the nurse would measure the client's response to medications is included in the evaluation section later in this chapter.

Diagnosing

Data that the nurse collects may lead to the development of several nursing diagnoses related to the medication administration experience. The following are examples of appropriate nursing diagnoses:

Altered Health Maintenance related to lack of knowledge about anticoagulant medication regimen
Altered Sexuality Patterns related to adverse effects of antihypertensive drug
Anxiety related to daily self-injection of insulin
Body Image Disturbance related to effects of chemotherapy
High Risk for Aspiration related to impaired swallowing of oral medications
High Risk for Poisoning related to confusion about medication dosages
Knowledge Deficit related to lack of interest in learning about medication regimen
Noncompliance With Medication Regimen related to adverse drug effects, cost of medications, confusion, lack of motivation, visual impairment, complexity of regimen
Sleep Pattern Disturbance related to consistent use of sedative-hypnotics

Planning for Medication Administration

Medication Orders

No medication may be given to a client without a **medication order** from a physician. Each health agency has a policy specifying the manner in which a physician writes an order. In most instances, orders are written on a form specifically designed for a physician's order. This becomes part of a client's permanent record.

Safe practice dictates that a nurse follow only a written order. A written order by a physician is least likely to result in error or misunderstanding. Under certain circumstances, such as in an emergency, a verbal order from the physician may be given to a registered nurse or a pharmacist. The legal implications for dispensing and administering an agent without a written order vary, and the nurse is cautioned to be familiar with the exact agency policy whenever called on to administer therapeutic agents. The legal implications of verbal orders are discussed in Chapter 6.

Usual hospital policy dictates that when a client is admitted, unless specific orders to the contrary are written, all drugs that the physician may have ordered while the client was at home are discontinued. This may prove to be a problem when a client brings medications from home to the hospital. To avoid the possibility of having the client continue taking the home medications while receiving the same ones or others under new orders, all medications should be sent home with the family or removed from the client's unit and placed in safekeeping. This requires an explanation to the client and the family of how the client's drug plan is to be implemented. In some inpatient facilities, clients keep their medications at their bedside and learn or continue to administer them as they would at home. It is believed that this approach helps to promote the clients'

FOCUSED ASSESSMENT GUIDE

Medications

Factors to Assess	Questions and Approaches
Previous and current drug use	What medications are you taking that the doctor prescribed for you?
	What over-the-counter medications are you taking on a regular basis?
	Do you use nonmedicinal drugs on a regular basis (eg, alcohol, caffeine, home remedies)?
	What is the reason for taking the medication?
	What medications have you taken during the past year and for what reasons?
Medication schedule	At what times do you take your medications?
	Is there any special way your medication has to be prepared (eg, crushing and mixing with applesauce)?
	Do you have any special method for remembering to take your medications?
Response to medications	Have the medications had the expected effects?
	Have you ever experienced any adverse or unexpected reactions to the medications?
	Is there a family history of this type of reaction to medication?
	Do you have any allergies to medications?
	What happens when you take this medication?
Attitude toward drugs and use of drugs	How do you feel about taking medications?
	Why do you take the medications?
Compliance with regimen	Do you understand the reason for taking the medications?
	Do you adhere to the medication schedule?
	Are there any problems that prevent you from adhering to the medication regimen?
Storage	Where are your medications stored at home?
	How long do you keep medications in the home?
	Can you show me any medications you have on hand?

independence. The nurse should be aware when clients are allowed to take their own medications while hospitalized and should know each agent's purpose and possible adverse effects. Also, a notation should be made on the client's plan of care, so that everyone knows the client has medications at the bedside.

When a client has had surgery or is transferred to another clinical service or another health agency, it is general practice that all orders related to drugs are discontinued, and new orders are written. To keep physicians aware of orders in effect, some hospitals specify a day of the week when orders are to be rewritten or they automatically are discontinued.

Types of Orders

There are several types of orders that a physician may write.

A *standing order* is carried out as specified until it is canceled by another order. Many physicians whose practices are limited to a particular clinical area have a specified set of written orders for all their hospitalized clients. These are also referred to as standing orders. Occasionally, a physician writes a standing order and its cancellation simultaneously; that is, the physician specifies that a certain order is to be carried out for a stated number of days or times. After the stated period has passed, the order is canceled automatically.

The physician may write an *"as needed"* (prn) *order* for medication. The client receives medication when it is requested or needed. A prn order commonly is written for postoperative pain medication.

Another type of order is called a *single order;* that is, the directive is carried out only once, at a time specified by the physician. Medication to be administered immediately before surgery is an example of a single order.

A *stat order* also is a single order but one that is carried out at once. A stat order for epinephrine or an anti-histamine would be carried out immediately for a client who is experiencing an anaphylactic drug reaction.

Parts of the Medication Order

The medication order consists of seven parts:
- Client's name
- Date and time the order is written
- Name of drug to be administered
- Dosage of the drug
- Route by which the drug is to be administered
- Frequency of administration of the drug
- Signature of person writing the order

Client's Name The client's full name is used. The middle name or initial should be included to avoid confusion with other clients. In most agencies, the client's full name and hospital number and the physician's name are mechanically imprinted on all sheets on the client's chart, including the physician's order sheet.

Date and Time the Order Is Written The date the order is written is given. In some situations, the time the order is written is included. Because the nursing staffs in inpatient agencies change several times during each 24-hour period, the date and time help to prevent errors of oversight as different nurses take charge of a unit. When an order is to be followed for a specified number of days, the date and time are important, so that the discontinuation date and time can be determined accurately. The length of time an order for a narcotic remains valid is determined by law. Therefore, the date and time the order is written are essential for determining when the order for a narcotic becomes invalid.

Name of Drug to Be Administered The name of the drug is stated in the order, either by the brand name or by the generic name. Certain brand names are well known, but the practice of using the generic name is considered safest and is required by some health care agencies.

If the nurse is unfamiliar with a drug, there are several sources for obtaining information. The USP and NF is the official source in the United States. In Canada, the *Compendium of Pharmaceutical Specialties* (CPS) is published with information written by the pharmaceutical companies. Most other countries have similar references that describe official therapeutic agents. Many agencies also provide their own book listing the official drugs commonly used by the agency. The *Physician's Desk Reference* (PDR) is another source of information. It is published by Medical Economics, Inc., from information supplied by pharmaceutical companies. In addition, the nurse may obtain information about drugs from the hospital pharmacist, the physician, and any of several texts written specifically for the nursing role in the management of drug therapy.

Dosage of the Drug The dosage of a drug can be stated in either the apothecary or the metric system. The metric system has been adopted internationally. A similar system (le Système international d'unités), abbreviated as SI, is used in Canada. It includes familiar metric units with some differences (eg, the base unit of weight is the kilogram, not the gram, and temperature is measured in Celsius). In SI, the spelling of liter is litre.

Apothecary measurements are being used less frequently. Self-administered drugs commonly are labeled in household measurements to facilitate administration. Most agencies post a table of common equivalent dosages for people who have learned to use one system and find that the agency for which they work uses the other system. Although these tables are convenient and useful, the nurse should be prepared to convert from one system to the other, since such tables are not available in every situation. The nurse should also be familiar with common equivalent measurements when using household equipment, such as teaspoons and tablespoons, since usually the home is not equipped with special measuring devices. The most common equivalents can be found in Appendix A.

Certain standard abbreviations are used to indicate drug amounts, and the nurse should know the common abbreviations before administering drugs. Table 42-2 lists some of the most commonly used abbreviations.

Route by Which the Drug Is to Be Administered The route to be used when administering a medication is stated clearly because some drugs can be given in more than one way and some may be used safely only through one route. Table 42-3 describes common routes by which medications are administered.

Frequency of Administration of the Drug The time and frequency with which a drug is to be administered usually are stated in standard abbreviations in the medication or-

TABLE 42-2

Common Abbreviations for Measures

Abbreviation	Unabbreviated Form
ʒ	Dram
gt	Drop
gtt	Drops
gr	Grain
g	Gram
μg or mcg	Microgram
mg or mgm	Milligram
mL or ml	Milliliter
m or min	Minim
ʒ or oz	Ounce
tbsp	Tablespoon
tsp	Teaspoon

T A B L E   4 2 - 3

Routes for Administering Drugs

Route	How Drug Is Administered	Term Used to Describe Route
Given by mouth	Having patient swallow drug	Oral administration
Given by way of respiratory tract	Having patient inhale drug	Inhalation
Given by injection	Injecting drug into	Administration by injection
	Subcutaneous tissue	Subcutaneous injection
	Muscle tissue	Intramuscular injection
	Corium (under epidermis)	Intradermal injection
	Vein	Intravenous injection
	Artery	Intraarterial injection
	Heart tissue	Intracardial injection
	Peritoneal cavity	Intraperitoneal injection
	Spinal canal	Intraspinal injection
	Bone	Intraosseous injection
Given by placing on skin or mucous membrane	Inserting drug into	
	Vagina	Vaginal administration
	Rectum	Rectal administration
	Placing drug under tongue	Sublingual administration
	Placing drug between cheek and gum	Buccal administration
	Rubbing drug into skin	Inunction
	Placing drug into direct contact with mucous membrane	Instillation
	Flushing mucous membrane with drug in solution	Irrigation
	Applying medicated patch to skin	Topical application

der. Common abbreviations used in writing prescriptions, including time and frequency, are listed in Table 42-4.

The nursing service department of inpatient facilities usually determines the hours at which routine drugs are given. For example, if certain drugs are to be given every 4 hours, the nursing service policy indicates the times. Every 4-hour administration may be at the times of 12 noon, 4 PM, 8 PM, 12 midnight, 4 AM, and 8 AM. Another agency may use the hours 1 PM, 5 PM, 9 PM, 1 AM, 5 AM, and 9 AM. If a drug is ordered to be given before or after meals, time of administration depends on the hours at which meals are served.

If a drug is to be given only once or twice a day, the decision as to which hours to use depends on the nature of the drug and the client's plan of care. Whenever possible, the client's choice of time should be considered.

Drugs should be administered punctually as ordered. A nurse administering drugs to several clients, however, cannot give all of the drugs exactly on the hour indicated. Agency policies vary, but a common one is that drugs should be administered within a half hour before or after the indicated hour. Thus a drug to be administered at 9 AM can be administered any time between 8:30 AM and 9:30 AM, using this policy. This policy does not apply to all drugs. A preoperative medication ordered to be given at 7:30 AM should be administered at that hour, since the time was planned in relation to the time surgery is to begin. This also holds true when clients are given drugs before certain diagnostic procedures and stat orders.

Signature of Person Writing the Order   The signature of the person writing the order follows the order. The signature is of importance for legal reasons because the authority to prescribe drugs is defined by state laws. Also, if there is a question about the order, the signature indicates who should be contacted.

Questioning the Medication Order

The nurse is legally responsible for drugs administered. Any drug order suspected to be in error should be questioned. The suspected error may be in any part of the order. The legal implications are serious in a situation in which there is an error in a drug order and in which the nurse could be expected, based on knowledge and experience, to have noted and reported the error.

On occasion, the nurse may not think that there is an error in the order but may not understand why the medication has been prescribed. In such instances, the nurse should ask how the order relates to the client's plan of care.

A drug to which the client is allergic may be inadvertently prescribed. The client may describe past adverse reactions with the drug. It is general practice to clearly indicate any drug allergies on the client's chart. The drug should not be given, and the order should be questioned when, in the nurse's judgment, the client is allergic to a drug. An allergic reaction can be life-threatening to the client.

A nurse may have difficulty reading an order. Guessing is gross carelessness. Rechecking with the person who wrote the order is the only safe procedure.

The nurse has the right to refuse to administer any medication that, based on knowledge and experience, may be harmful to the client. Although this situation seldom occurs, the nurse needs to understand that the client's safety is a primary objective in the administration of medications.

Checking the Medication Order

Agency policy specifies the manner in which the medication order is checked. Various systems are used. Nurses should be familiar with the system used in the agency where they care for clients and should implement it correctly to minimize errors in administering therapeutic agents.

Some agencies use a card system. In many institutions, the order is copied onto the client's medication record, often called a *Kardex*. Increasing numbers of health care facilities are computerizing client records, including medication records. The nurse is responsible for checking that the transcription of the medication order is correct by comparing it with the original order.

Medication Supply Systems

Medications are supplied in a number of ways. With a *stock supply* system, large quantities of medications are kept on the nursing unit. With an *individual supply* system, each client is supplied with the medication needed for a period of time. The nurse is responsible for accurately measuring the dosage from the medication containers. In the *unit dose* system, the pharmacist simplifies medication preparation by packaging and labeling each dosage for a 24-hour period. In some inpatient facilities, clients self-administer medications.

Most nursing units use a medication cart for the administration of medications. The cart contains individual drawers into which the medications for each client are placed. The drawer is labeled with the client's name. The nurse moves the cart from room to room when dispensing medications. A medication cart is shown in Figure 42-1.

Dosage Calculations

Systems of Measurement

Nurses need to be proficient in the use of weights and measures as well as systems of measurement to calculate drug dosages and prepare medications for administration. There are three systems of measurement in use for administering medications—the metric system, the apothecary system, and the household system.

Metric System The metric system is the most widely accepted and convenient system. The official system used in Canada is the SI, which is similar to the metric system. The basic units of measurement are the meter (linear), the liter (volume), and the gram (weight). The metric system is a decimal system, in which each unit can be divided into multiples of 10 (10, 100, 1000). To do calculations in the metric system, the decimal point is moved to the right or left. In the preparation of medications, the nurse usually uses the following metric units:

Weight
    1 kilogram = 1000 grams
    1 gram = 1000 milligrams
    1 milligram = 1000 micrograms

Volume
    1 liter = 1000 milliliters or cubic centimeters

TABLE 42-4

Common Abbreviations Used in Prescribing Medications

Abbreviation	Meaning
aa	Of each
ac	Before meals
ad lib	As desired
aq	Water
bid	Twice a day
c̄	With
cap	Capsule
DC	Discontinue
elix	Elixir
hs	At bedtime; hour of sleep
IM	Intramuscular
IV	Intravenous
IVPB	IV piggyback
KVO	Keep vein open
OD	Right eye
od	Every day
OS	Left eye
OU	Each eye
pc	After meals
PO	By mouth
per	By
prn	As needed; when necessary
q	Every
qd	Every day
qh	Every hour
q2h	Every 2 hours
qid	Four times a day
qod	Every other day
qs	Quantity sufficient
Rx	Take
s̄	Without
SC	Subcutaneous
stat	Immediately
supp	Suppository
susp	Suspension
tid	Three times a day
tinct	Tincture
ung	Ointment

RESEARCH IN NURSING Making a Difference

Strategies to Prevent Nurses From Making Medication Errors

Much has been documented about the incidence of medication errors, but little is known about the effectiveness of strategies to prevent their occurrence. An initial step is the identification of situations that place the nurse at risk to commit an error. Dosage calculation of deficiencies frequently are mentioned whenever data are reviewed. Various authors have focused on the ability of student nurses and registered nurses to correctly calculate medication doses as well as on the effect of annual medication tests for registered nurses on reducing medication errors.

Related Research

Worrel, P., and Hodson, K. (1989). Posology: The battle against dosage calculation errors. *Nurse Educator, 14*(2): 27–31.

Completed questionnaires returned from baccalaureate, associate, and diploma programs indicated that most nurse educators rely on faculty-developed tests to measure students' competency with drug dosage calculations. Variability in the specific format for setting up dosage calculation problems was the most startling inconsistency reported. Most schools continue to integrate drug calculation problems into nursing tests and quizzes but few view successful completion of a drug dose calculation test as a program outcome or criteria for graduation. Recommended measures to resolve these inconsistencies include review of admission criteria, with particular attention to SAT or ACT math score criteria; continual measurement of dosage calculation skills throughout the program and at graduation; consistent labeling and formula application for all students; evaluation of the use of math faculty rather than nursing faculty as a remediation resource; and consideration of computer-assisted instruction as an effective alternate to faculty teaching and testing.

Conklin, D., MacFarland, V., Kinnie-Sleeves, A., & Chenger, T. (1990). Medication errors by nurses: Contributing factors. *AARN Newsletter, 46*(1): 8–9.

Registered nurses working in two acute-care facilities in Calgary, Canada, identified factors that contributed to medication errors in their health care settings. In this research study, careless nursing actions, including calculation errors, were implicated most frequently as the cause of medication errors. Remedial responses that stressed accountability were recognized as important in minimizing errors and preserving professional self-esteem. Encouragement to report errors as well as regular medication updates by pharmacists or other nurses provided for improved standards of care on the units.

Ludwig-Beymer, P., Czurylo, K. Gattuso, M., Hennessey, K., & Ryan, C. (1990). The effect of testing on the reported incidence of medication errors in a medical center. *Journal of Continuing Education in Nursing, 21*(1): 11–17.

Results of this research study indicated that the registered nurses who are required annually to take a medication test did not experience a decreased medication error rate. A questionnaire that the nurses returned also indicated that more medication errors occurred than were accounted for on hospital incident reports. Nurses identified the factors they considered significant in reducing medication errors. These included checking the medication three times, length of time assigned to the patient, previous experience with medication errors, and familiarity with the medications. As a result of the nurses' recommendations, a videotape and an inservice program on medication errors are being evaluated as possible replacements for the annual medication test.

Summary

The potential for error always exists when nurses are administering medications. Concern about medication errors prompted these nurse researchers to recommend strategies that deal effectively with reducing their incidence. Closer monitoring of students' dosage calculation skills, consistent testing measures—including use of computer-assisted instruction to supplement instruction—and completion of a dose calculation test as an outcome measure at graduation are recommended to lessen the number of errors made by students. The medication error rate did not decline for a group of registered nurses in the practice setting required to take an annual medication calculation test. Inservice programs featuring reviews and updates by pharmacists are being evaluated as a replacement.

Converting Dosages It may be necessary to convert drug dosages to a different unit in the metric system. To convert a larger unit into a smaller unit, move the decimal point to the right (the new number is larger than the original). To convert a smaller unit into a larger unit, move the decimal point to the left (the new number is smaller than the original).

Example
0.5 g = ? mg
    Move decimal point three places to right.
    Answer = 500 mg
900 mg = ? g
    Move decimal point three places to the left.
    Answer = 0.9 g

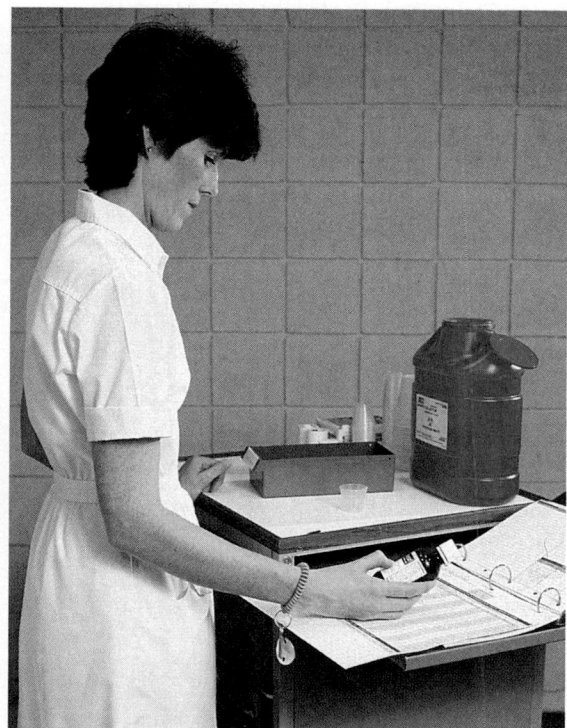

F I G U R E   4 2 - 1

The mobile medication cart and the Kardex are taken to the client's room when medications are given. Each client's medications are stored in a separate drawer. The nurse carefully checks the medication he or she will give with the Kardex to avoid errors. The cart is stored between uses in a locked room near the nurses' station.

Apothecary System The apothecary system is less convenient and precise than the metric system. It is used for only a few drugs. The basic unit of weight is the grain. The minim, dram, ounce, pint, and quart are used for volume. In the apothecary system, Roman numerals are used to express numbers (grains X) and quantities less than 1 are written in fraction form (grains ¼).

Household System The household system is the least accurate system of measurement. It is not widely used except in home settings. Teaspoon, tablespoon, teacup, and glass are commonly used household measures.

Equivalents of Measurement All three systems of measurement are in use in the United States. The nurse may be called on to convert dosages from one system to another. It is then extremely important that the nurse know and be able to calculate commonly used equivalents as listed in Appendix A.

Formulas for Computing Drug Dosages

Sometimes drugs are prepared and supplied in the amount ordered by the physician and the nurse can see that no calculation is necessary when checking the medication la-

bel. At other times, drugs are not prepared and supplied in the exact quantities called for in the medication order, and the nurse must do a dosage calculation to determine what quantity of medication the client is to receive.

Several formulas can be used to calculate drug dosages. One such formula consists of ratios to set up a proportion and can be used to calculate dosages for both solid and liquid preparations. A ratio shows the relation between numbers. A proportion contains two ratios. The nurse usually is seeking the quantity of on-hand medication that is equal to the desired dosage (the dosage ordered). The formula is as follows:

$$\frac{\text{dose on hand}}{\text{quantity on hand}} = \frac{\text{dose desired}}{\text{X (quantity desired)}}$$

The dosage must be in the same unit of measurement. This applies to the quantity as well. Dosages are on the top line of the proportion and quantities on the bottom line. After the numbers are placed in the proportion, the nurse cross-multiplies to find the desired quantity.

Example Amoxicillin 625 mg PO is ordered. It is supplied as a liquid preparation containing 250 mg in 5 mL. How much would the nurse administer?

$$\frac{250 \text{ mg}}{5 \text{ mL}} = \frac{625 \text{ mg}}{\text{X mL}}$$

cross-multiply:

$$3125 = 250X$$

$$X = 12.5 \text{ mL}$$

Example Phenobarbital gr i PO is ordered. It is available in 30-mg tablets. How many tablets would the nurse administer?

There are two systems of measurement in this problem. The nurse checks the list of equivalents to learn that 60 mg is equivalent to grains i.

$$\frac{30 \text{ mg}}{1 \text{ tablet}} = \frac{60 \text{ mg}}{\text{X tablets}}$$

$$60 = 30X$$

$$X = 2 \text{ tablets}$$

Another formula that can be used to calculate drug dosages is

$$\frac{\text{dose desired}}{\text{dose on hand}} \times \text{quantity on hand} = \text{desired quantity}$$

This formula can be used for both liquid dosages and fractions of tablets.

Pediatric Calculations

Pediatric dosages are calculated according to the child's weight or **body surface area** (BSA).

The *BSA formula* provides the most accuracy in calculating pediatric dosages because it considers weight and height. To find a child's BSA, the West nomogram is used (Fig. 42-2). The child's height is located by a point in the left-

Nomogram for Estimating Surface Area of Infants and Young Children

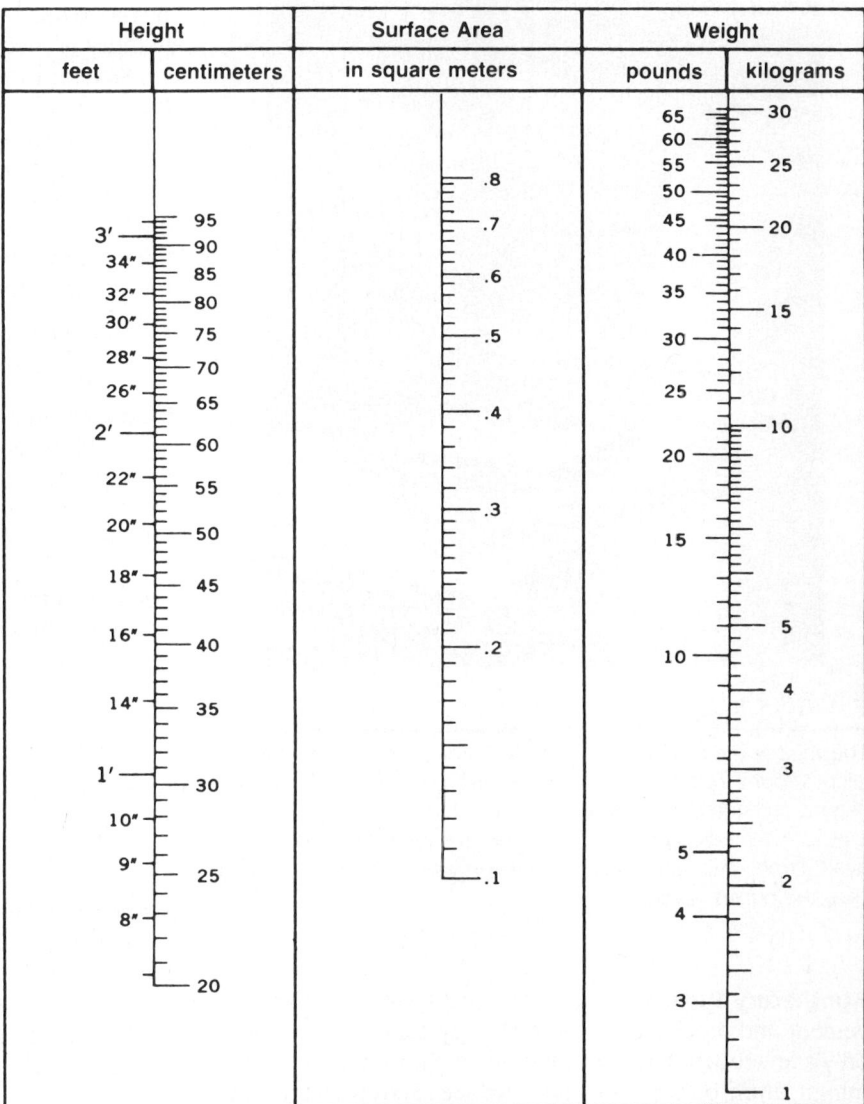

F I G U R E 4 2 - 2

West nomogram for calculating body surface area. (Behman, R. E., & Vaughn, V. C. [1987]. *Nelson textbook of pediatrics* [13th ed.]. Philadelphia: Saunders.)

hand column and the weight is located by a point in the right-hand column. The two points are connected with a line. The point at which the line crosses the surface area column is the child's BSA. The formula for calculating the child's dosage is

$$\frac{\text{BSA (child)}}{\text{BSA (adult)}} \times \text{adult dose} = \text{child's dose}$$

The average adult BSA is 1.7 square meters.

A less commonly used formula is *Clark's rule* for children age 2 years or younger. This formula assumes that the average adult weighs 150 lb (68 kg) and is calculated as follows:

$$\frac{\text{usual}}{\text{adult dose}} \times \frac{\text{weight of child in pounds}}{150} = \text{child's dose}$$

Accepted pediatric dosages according to milligram per kilogram per 24 hours for many drugs are listed in medication references.

Using Safety Measures While Preparing Drugs

Safety is of the utmost importance in preparing and implementing drug administration. The nurse observes the *three checks* and the *five rights* when administering medications.

Three Checks The label on the medication container should be checked three times during medication preparation. The label is read (1) when the nurse reaches for the container, (2) immediately before pouring the medication, and (3) when replacing the container to the drawer or shelf.

Five Rights The *five rights* help to ensure accuracy when administering medications. The nurse gives the (1) *right medication* to the (2) *right client* in the (3) *right dosage* through the (4) *right route* at the (5) *right time*. In some literature, seven rights are listed.

The importance of the three checks and the five rights cannot be overemphasized. The safe nurse does not allow automatic habits of preparing medications to replace constant thinking, purposeful action, and repeated checking for accuracy.

Maintaining a Safe Environment

An environment that promotes safety and good working habits contributes to accuracy in the preparation of drugs for administration. It is important that good lighting be available when preparing drugs. Also, the nurse who is preparing drugs should work alone. This practice helps to avoid distractions and interruptions, which may lead to errors.

After the nurse begins to prepare drugs for administration, they should not be left unattended. If it is imperative to leave for a short time, the drugs that have been prepared should be placed in a locked area. The nurse who prepares the medication also administers the drug and records the drug administration. When the nurse is not working at the medication cart, it should be locked.

Caring for Controlled Substances Safely

Controlled substances are kept in a double-locked drawer, box, or room. This precaution is observed as a safety measure. Narcotics or controlled substances may be ordered only by physicians who are registered with the Department of Justice, Bureau of Narcotics and Dangerous Drugs, or as specified by the Narcotic Control Act and Regulations (Canada). According to federal law, a record must be kept for each narcotic that is administered. Health care agencies provide forms for keeping such records, and these forms are kept with the narcotics. Although the forms differ, the following information usually is required—the name of the client receiving the narcotic, the amount of the narcotic used, the hour the narcotic was given, the name of the physician who prescribed the narcotic, and the name of the nurse who administered the narcotic. It is common practice to check narcotics daily at specified intervals. In hospitals, checking usually is performed at each shift change. The amount of narcotics on hand is counted, and each used narcotic must be accounted for on the narcotic record. A narcotic count that does not check must be reported immediately. The law requires these special precautions in the use of narcotics, to aid in the control of drug abuse. The nurse administering narcotics has an important responsibility to see that the federal law is observed. If for any reason a narcotic prepared for administration has to be discarded, it is best to have a second person act as a witness and have that person sign the narcotic sheet also.

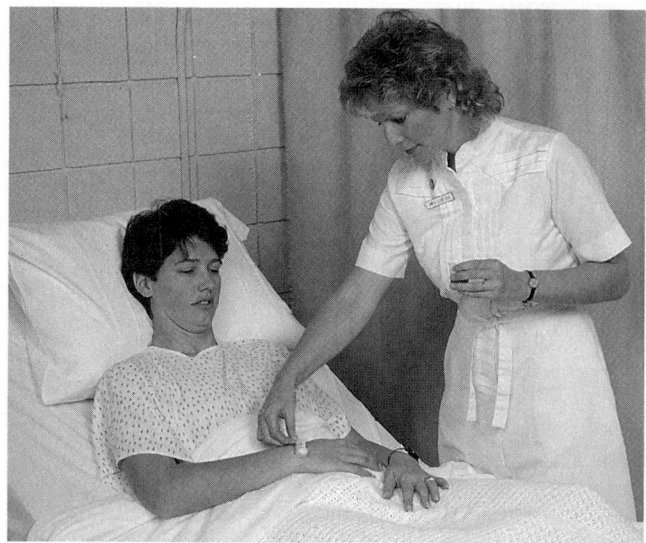

FIGURE 42-3

An essential step is to check the client's identification bracelet carefully before administering medications to ensure that the right medication is given to the right person.

Identifying the Client

The nurse prepares medications, considering safety at all times, as discussed in the previous sections. Positive identification of the client is essential to safe drug administration. Before administering the drug, the nurse must check carefully to see that the right drug is given to the right client. Clients in inpatient health care agencies usually wear identification bracelets. In Figure 42-3, the nurse is identifying the client by checking the identification bracelet. Also, the client should be asked to state his or her name if possible. It is considered unsafe to call the client by name because the client may respond even when the nurse has used an improper name.

Implementing: Administering a Medication

The nurse should remain with the client and see that the medication is taken. If the client receives several drugs, offer them separately so that if one is refused or dropped, positive identification can be made and the drug recorded or replaced. Never leave medications at the bedside for the client to take later. This is unsafe practice because the client may forget to take the medication or someone else may take the medication. The nurse records medication administration as soon as possible after the client takes the medication. Some agencies allow clients to self-administer certain drugs to promote the client's independence. The nurse should be familiar with agency policy on this matter. Nursing responsibilities for administering drugs are listed in the adjoining display.

Nursing Responsibilities for Administering Drugs

- Assessment of the client and clear understanding of why the client is receiving a particular medication
- Preparing the medication to be administered (ie, checking labels, preparing injections, observing proper asepsis techniques with needles and syringes)
- Accurate dosage calculations
- Administration of the medication (proper injection techniques, aids to help swallowing, topical methods)
- Documentation of medications given
- Monitoring the client's reaction and evaluating the client's response
- Educating the client regarding his or her medications and medication regimen

---

Administering Oral Medications

Drugs given orally are intended for absorption in the stomach and small intestine. The oral route is the most commonly used route of administration. It usually is the most convenient and comfortable and the safest for the client. After oral administration, drug action has a slower onset and a more prolonged but less potent effect.

There are certain situations in which oral medications would not be administered, such as when the client has difficulty swallowing, is unconscious, is to receive nothing by mouth, or is vomiting.

Oral medications are available in two forms—solid and liquid. Solid preparations include tablets, capsules, and pills. Some tablets are scored for easy breaking if a partial quantity is needed. Enteric-coated tablets are covered with a hard surface that impedes absorption until the tablet has left the stomach. Absorption takes place in the small intestine because the active ingredient of the drug is irritating to the stomach mucosa. Enteric-coated tablets should not be chewed or crushed.

Liquid preparations include elixirs, spirits, suspensions, and syrups. Some are water-based solutions and others are alcohol-based solutions. Liquid preparations should be prepared with an appropriate measuring device. Disposable, calibrated cups are available for the preparation of liquid medications. When liquids are being poured from a bottle, they should be poured from the side of the bottle opposite the label. This prevents drops from running onto the label, making it difficult to read. Hold the container and the bottle at eye level, and place the thumbnail on the line on the container that indicates the proper dosage. Because of surface tension, a meniscus (a curved convex surface) forms on the liquid in the measuring container. The liquid should be measured at the *bottom* of this meniscus.

Extractors to remove liquids from a bottle are commercially available. The extractor resembles a syringe and fits tightly into the bottle neck. The medication is withdrawn and then placed in a medication cup. The extractor has markings on it so that the proper dosage can be determined as the liquid is withdrawn. For clients who find it difficult to take liquids from a cup, the medication can be placed in the mouth directly from the extractor or from a syringe. The extractor or syringe should be placed between the gum and cheek, and the liquid given to the client slowly. These techniques help to prevent the client from choking and aspirating the medication.

If a label becomes difficult to read or accidentally comes off the container, the container should be returned to the pharmacy. A medication should never be given from a bottle without a label or with a label that cannot be read with accuracy. Because of the danger of error, unused medications should not be returned to their bottles. Care should be exercised in pouring, to prevent unnecessary loss. Medications should not be transferred from one pharmacy container to another. Many medication bottles now have an identification code number on them. If similar medications were mixed and a client had a reaction, it would be difficult to identify which drug was responsible. A medication with an unexpected precipitate should not be used, nor should one that has changed color.

Procedure 42-1 describes the techniques for preparing and administering oral medications.

Special Techniques

Certain drugs that are given orally discolor the teeth or damage the enamel. Such medications are mixed well with water or some other liquid vehicle; the client takes it through a drinking straw, and water is taken after administration. This practice reduces the strength of the drug that comes in contact with the teeth. Dilute hydrochloric acid is an example of a drug that damages tooth enamel and should be given well diluted and with a drinking straw.

Some clients object to the taste of certain medications. The following techniques are suggested to disguise or mask the objectionable taste.

- Sometimes it is necessary to crush a medication or add it to food so the client can swallow it. Some drugs cannot be crushed (eg, enteric-coated and sustained-release capsules). Table 42-5 lists commonly used medications that should not be crushed.
- Allow the client to suck on a small piece of ice for a few minutes before taking the medication. The ice numbs the taste buds, and the objectionable taste is less discernible.
- Store oily medications in the refrigerator. Cold oil is less aromatic than oil at room temperature.
- Place the medication in a syringe, and place the syringe well back on the tongue, being careful not to trigger the client's gag reflex. This places the medication on the part of the tongue where there are few taste buds.

(*Text continues on p. 1208*)

PROCEDURE 42-1

Administering Oral Medications

Equipment

Medication Kardex, cards, or record form
Medication cart or tray

Medication cups (disposable)
Straws
Water or juice

Action	Rationale
1 Gather equipment. Check each medication order against the original physician's order according to agency policy. Clarify any inconsistencies. Check the client's chart for allergies.	This comparison helps to identify errors that may have occurred when orders were transcribed. The physician's order is the legal record of medication orders for each agency.
2 Know the actions, special nursing considerations, safe-dose ranges, purpose of administration, and adverse effects of medications to be administered.	This knowledge aids the nurse in evaluating the therapeutic effect of the medication in relation to the client's diagnosis.
3 Wash your hands.	Handwashing prevents the spread of microorganisms.
4 Move the medication cart to the outside of the client's room or prepare for administration in the medication area.	Organization facilitates error-free administration and saves times.
5 Unlock the medication cart or drawer.	Locking of the cart or drawer safeguards each client's medication supply.
6 Prepare medications for one client at a time.	This prevents errors in medication administration.
7 Select the proper medication from the drawer or stock and compare with the Kardex or order. Check expiration dates and perform calculations if necessary:	Comparison of medication to physician's order reduces errors in medication administration. Verify calculations with another nurse if necessary. This is the *first* safety check.
a Place unit dose–packaged medications in a disposable cup. *Do not open wrapper* until at bedside. Keep narcotics and medications that require special nursing assessments in a separate container.	The label is needed for an additional safety check. Prerequisites to giving certain medications may include monitoring of certain vital signs.
b When removing tablets or capsules from a bottle, pour the necessary number into the bottle cap and then place the tablets in a medication cup. Break only scored tablets, if necessary, to obtain the proper dose.	Pouring medication into the cap allows for easy return of excess medication to bottle. Pouring tablets or capsules into the nurse's hand is unsanitary.
c Hold liquid medication bottles with the label against the palm. Use the appropriate measuring device when pouring liquids, and read the amount of medication at the bottom of the meniscus at eye level. Wipe the lip of the bottle with a paper towel.	Accuracy is possible when the appropriate measuring device is used and then read accurately. Liquid that may drip onto the label makes the label difficult to read.
8 Recheck each medication package, card, or preparation with the order as it is poured.	This is a *second* check to guard against a medication error.
9 When all medications for one client have been prepared, recheck once again with the medication order before taking them to the client.	This is a *third* check to ensure accuracy and to prevent errors.
10 Transport medications to the client's bedside carefully, and keep the medications in sight at all times.	Careful handling and close observation prevent accidental or deliberate disarrangement of medications.

(continued)

P R O C E D U R E 4 2 - 1 (continued)

Administering Oral Medications

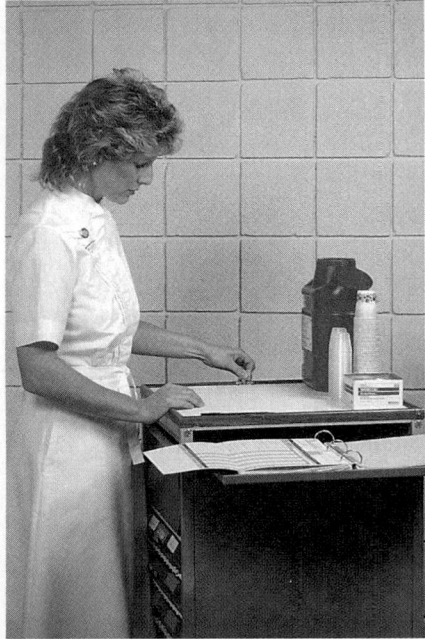

Action 5: Unlocking medication cart.

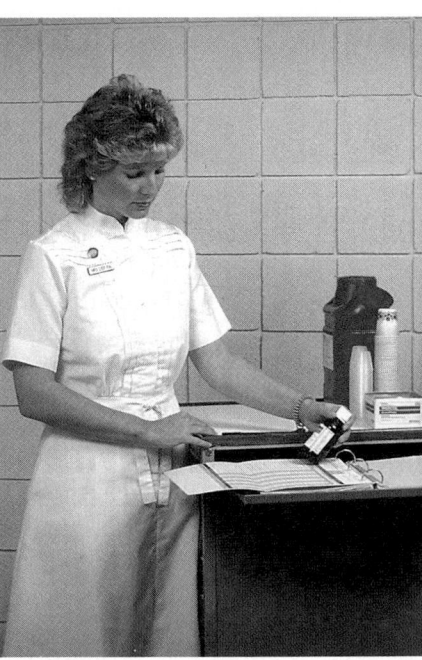

Action 7: Comparing medication with Kardex or order.

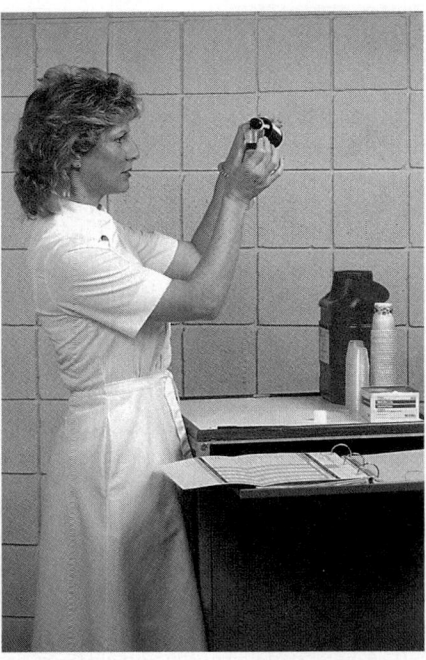

Action 7c: Measuring at eye level.

Action	Rationale
11 See that the client receives medications at the correct time.	Check agency policy, which may allow for administration within a period of 30 minutes before or 30 minutes after designated time.
12 Identify the client carefully. There are three correct ways to do this:	Identifying the client is the nurse's responsibility to guard against error.
a Check the name of the client's identification band.	This is the most reliable method. Replace the identification band if it is missing or inaccurate in any way.
b Ask the client his or her name.	This requires a response from the client, but illness and strange surroundings often cause clients to be confused.
c Verify the client's identification with a staff member who knows the client.	This is another way to double-check identity. Do not use the name on the door or over the bed because these may be inaccurate.
13 Complete necessary assessments before administration of medications. Check allergy bracelet or ask client about allergies. Explain the purpose and action of each medication to the client.	Assessment is a prerequisite to administration of medications.
14 Assist the client to an upright or lateral position.	Swallowing is facilitated by proper positioning.
15 Administer medications:	
a Offer water or other permitted fluids with pills, capsules, tablets, and some liquid medications.	Liquids facilitate swallowing of solid drugs. Some liquid drugs are intended to adhere to the pharyngeal area, in which case liquid is not offered with the medication.
b Ask the client's preference regarding medications to be taken by hand or in a cup and one at a time or all at once.	This encourages the client's participation in taking the medications.

(continued)

PROCEDURE 42-1 *(continued)*

Administering Oral Medications

Action	Rationale
c If the capsule or tablet falls to the floor, it must be discarded and a new one administered.	This prevents contamination.
d Record any fluid intake if intake and output measurement is ordered.	This provides for accurate documentation.
16 Remain with the client until each medication is swallowed. Unless the nurse has seen the client swallow the drug, it cannot be recorded that the drug was administered.	The client's chart is a legal record. Only with a physician's order can medications be left at the bedside.

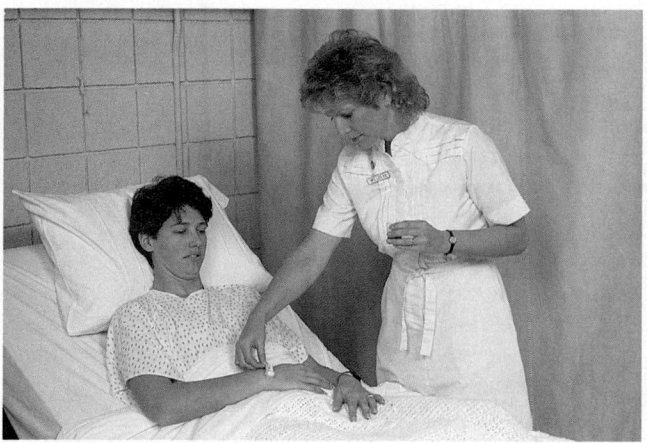

Action 12a: Checking client identity.

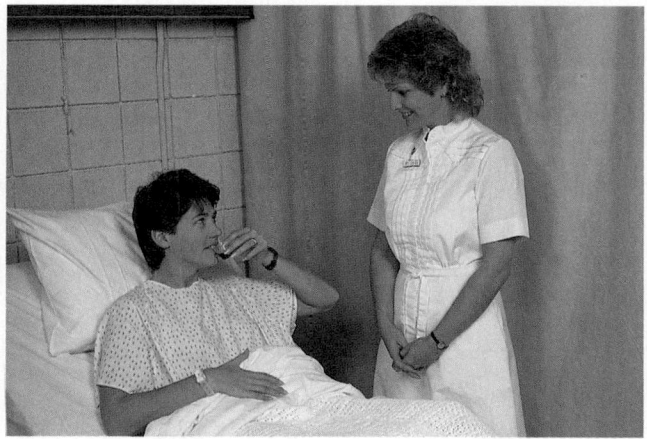

Action 16: Observing client swallowing medication. (Photos © Ken Kasper.)

Action	Rationale
17 Wash your hands.	Handwashing prevents the spread of microorganisms.
18 Record each medication given on the medication chart or record using the required format.	Prompt recording avoids the possibility of accidentally repeating the administration of the drug.
a If the drug was refused or omitted, record this in the appropriate area on the medication record.	This verifies the reason medication was omitted.
b Recording of administration of a narcotic requires additional documentation on a narcotic record stating drug count and other specific information.	Controlled substance laws necessitate careful recording of narcotic use.
19 Check on the client within 30 minutes to verify response to medication.	This provides opportunity for further documentation and additional assessment.

Age Considerations

Special devices are available in a pharmacy to ensure accurate dose calculations for young children and infants.

Elderly clients with arthritis may have difficulty opening child-proof caps. On request, the pharmacist can substitute a cap that is easier to open. A rubber band twisted around the cap may provide a more secure grip for older clients.

(continued)

P R O C E D U R E 4 2 - 1 *(continued)*

Administering Oral Medications

Home Care Considerations

Encourage the client to discard outdated prescription medications.

Discuss safe storage of medications when there are children and pets in the environment.

Devices are available to help the client remember to take medications as scheduled. These may be simple charts or appliances that can be made in the home, or more elaborate devices that can be purchased in a pharmacy or from the manufacturer.

Special Considerations

If the client questions a medication order or states that the medication is different from the usual dose, *always* recheck and clarify with the original order before giving medication.

If the client's level of consciousness is altered or his or her swallowing is impaired, check with the physician to clarify the route of administration or alternative forms of medication.

Provide a straw for the client who has to swallow a liquid medication that may have a harmful effect on the teeth or mucous membranes.

Clients with poor vision can request labels printed with larger type on medication containers. A magnifying lens also may prove helpful.

- Offer oral hygiene immediately after giving the medication.
- Give the medication with generous amounts of water or other liquids, if permitted, to dilute the taste.

Children Nurses find administration of medications to infants and children challenging as well as frustrating at times. Children under age 5 years have difficulty swallowing tablets and capsules. Most medications are available in liquid form. The following are helpful techniques in administering medications to children:

- Use a dropper to give infants or very young children liquid medications while holding them in a sitting or semisitting position. Place the medication between the gum and cheek to prevent possible aspiration.
- Crush uncoated tablets or empty a soft capsule and mix the medication with soft foods, such as potatoes or cereal, for clients who are likely to aspirate liquids. Proper absorption may not occur if coated tablets or hard capsules are added to food.
- Explain to the child when a medication has an objectionable taste if the child is old enough to understand. Failing to warn the child is likely to decrease the child's trust in the nurse.
- Care should be taken when selecting the food to be mixed with the medication. The item should not be an essential part of the child's diet such as formula or the child's favorite food. The child may refuse a food associated with medications.
- Praise the child for a job well done after he or she swallows the medication.

Elderly Clients Techniques for administering medications include the following:

- Allow extra time to administer medications to elderly clients because their reflexes may be slowed and their understanding of the treatment decreased.
- Elderly clients may experience some difficulty swallowing medications and may find it easier to take their medications when crushed or given in liquid form. Swallowing can be initiated by massaging the laryngeal prominence or the area just below the chin prominence. The pressure from the gentle massage creates the desire to swallow.
- Reevaluation of the drug dosage is necessary with the elderly client. Weight and age should be used as criteria for determining the dosage.
- The nurse would assist the elderly client to set up a home medication schedule. Some form of a weekly medication dispenser tray may be helpful.
- Monitor carefully for adverse effects associated with the drug regimen. These may be magnified in elderly clients.
- Teach clients the names of drugs rather than distinguishing them by color. Manufacturers may vary the colors of generic drugs, and the visual changes associated with aging may make it more difficult to identify medications by their color.

Administering Medications Through a Nasogastric Tube

Occasionally, a client with a nasogastric tube receives a medication through the tube. The insertion of the tube is

TABLE 42-5

Common Medications That Should Not Be Crushed*

Enteric Coated	Sustained-Release Tablets and Capsules
ASA Enseals	Actifed 12-hour
Asulfidine Entabs	Artane Sequels
Bisacodyl	Calan SR
Dulcolax	Cardizem
Easprin	Cardizem SR
Erythromycin base Filmtab	Chlor-Trimeton Repetab
Feosol	Compazine Spansule
Ferrous sulfate Enseals	Contac
Pancrease	Diamox Sequels
Triaminic	Dimetapp Extentabs
Tussagesic	Drixoral
	Elixophyllin SR
Sublingual, Buccal, and Miscellaneous	Feosol Spansule
	Inderal-LA
Feldene	Indocin SR
Isordil sublingual	Isordil Tembid
Isuprel Glossets	K-Tab
Nitrostat	Micro-K
	MS Contin
	Nitro-Bid
	Nitrospan
	Pavabid
	Procan SR
	Procardia XL
	Ritalin SR
	Slo-Bid Gyrocaps
	Slow-K
	Theo-Dur
	Thorazine Spansule

*For a complete list, refer to Mitchell, J., & Pawlickl, K. (1990). Oral dosage forms that should not be crushed: 1990 revision. *Hospital Pharmacy, 25*(4), 329–335.

described in Chapter 33. The following are suggestions for giving medications through the tube:
- Use liquid medications or crushed medications combined with liquid. If permitted, crushed medication may be mixed with 1 tbsp of applesauce and a small amount of warm water before being administered through the tube by way of a syringe. Solid medications are not given because they may obstruct the tube.
- Bring the liquid medication to room temperature. Cold liquids may cause client discomfort.
- Remove the clamp from the tube and use the recommended procedure for checking tube placement in the stomach *before* administering the drug.
- Pour the medication into a syringe barrel or funnel attached to the tube *after* determining tube placement and patency.
- Flush the tube with 30 mL of warm water before giving the medication and immediately after giving the medication. Flushing before may warn you if the tube is clogged and helps to maintain tube patency.

- Position the client in a semisitting position on the right side after removing the syringe barrel or funnel and after reclamping the nasogastric tube. This positioning helps the stomach to empty and helps to prevent regurgitation. If the medication is to remain in the stomach for a period of time, position the client on the left side.

Administering Medications Sublingually

Certain drugs, sublingual nitroglycerin being typical, are administered *sublingually*; that is, a tablet is placed under the client's tongue. This area is rich in superficial blood vessels, which allows the drug to be absorbed relatively rapidly into the bloodstream for quick systemic effects. This type of medication should not be swallowed but held under the tongue so that complete absorption can occur.

Administering Parenteral Medications

The term *enteral* means within the intestines; *parenteral* means outside the intestines or alimentary canal. Many people use the term parenteral to refer to injection routes only, although technically the term includes routes for administering agents given by inhalation, those placed on the skin, and most of those placed on the mucous membrane.

Table 42-3 defines terms used to describe various types of **injections**. Medications may be injected into an artery, the peritoneum, heart tissues, the spinal canal, and bones. Techniques for injecting medications into these areas are discussed in clinical texts. In most instances, physicians are responsible for these procedures, and the nurse acts as an assistant.

Absorption occurs more rapidly with injection than when other routes are used. It is also more nearly complete; therefore, the results are more predictable, and the desired dosage can be determined with greater accuracy. Giving drugs by injection is necessary if the drug is available in no other form. Injections are particularly desirable for clients who are irrational, unconscious, or having gastrointestinal disturbances. The injection of drugs is also used in emergencies because absorption and desired results occur rapidly.

Needles and Syringes

Needles are available in various lengths and gauges with different size bevels. Figure 42-4 shows the parts of a needle. Needle lengths vary from 1/2 to 2 inches (1.3 to 5.1 cm). The length of the needle is determined by the route of administration. The gauge is determined by the width of the needle. Needle gauges are numbered 18 through 27. As the diameter of the needle increases, the gauge number decreases. An 18-gauge needle is larger than a 27-gauge needle. The bevel of the needle is its sloped edge, designed to make a narrow, slit-like opening that closes quickly.

Syringes are supplied in various sizes. Most syringes are plastic and disposable. Some syringes are supplied with

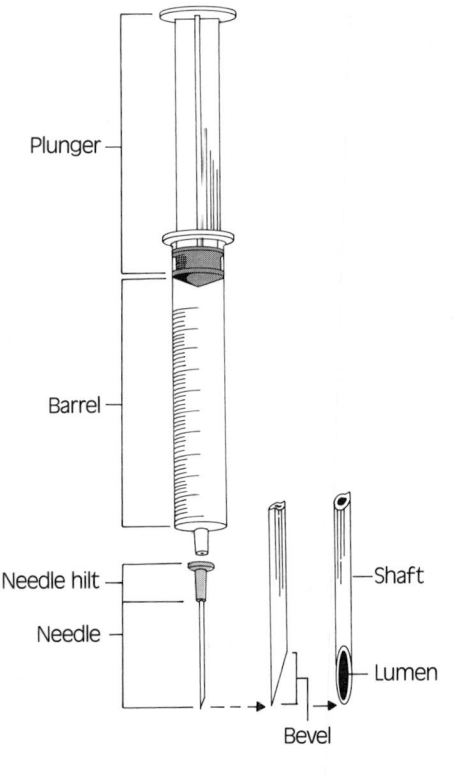

Plunger

Barrel

Needle hilt

Needle

Shaft

Lumen

Bevel

F I G U R E 4 2 - 4

Parts of a needle and syringe.

the needle attached, whereas others are not, in which case the nurse selects an appropriate needle. The parts of a syringe are shown in Figure 42-4.

The nurse chooses the equipment needed for an injection based on the following criteria:

Route of administration: A longer needle is required for an intramuscular injection than for an intradermal or a subcutaneous injection.

Viscosity of the solution: Some medications are more viscous than others and require a large-lumen needle to inject the drug.

Quantity to be administered: The larger the amount of medication to be injected, the greater the capacity of the syringe.

Body size: An obese person requires a longer needle to reach muscle tissue than a thin person.

Type of medication: There are special syringes for certain uses. An example is the insulin syringe used to inject insulin. Some medications, such as iron dextran injection (Imferon), are irritating to subcutaneous tissue. Therefore, a longer needle should be used to ensure proper placement of the medication in the muscle tissue.

After use, the needles and syringes are placed in puncture-resistant containers without being recapped. Most needlestick injuries occur during recapping. Additional measures to protect health care workers from accidental transmission of infectious diseases are discussed in Chapter 26.

Techniques of surgical asepsis must be strictly followed for parenteral injections to help avoid introducing organisms into the body. The parts of the syringe and needle that must be kept sterile during the procedure of preparing and administering an injection are the inside of the barrel, the part of the plunger that enters the barrel, the tip of the barrel, and the needle, except for the needle's hub.

Surgical asepsis applies to cleaning the skin for an injection. The skin is cleaned with alcohol or povidone–iodine (Betadine) in a circular motion, working from the center of the designated site outward. The skin is then considered clean enough to pierce with a sterile needle.

Preparing Medications for Administration by Injection

Drugs for administration by injection are packaged in several ways. Those that deteriorate in solution usually are dispensed as powders and are reconstituted immediately before injection. If drugs remain stable in solution, they usually are dispensed in ampules, bottles, or vials in an aqueous or oily solution or suspension.

Drugs may be dispensed in single-dose glass ampules, single-dose rubber-capped vials, multidose rubber-capped vials, and prefilled cartridges. Figure 42-5 shows several types of ampules and vials as well as a prefilled cartridge.

Ampules An **ampule** is a glass flask that contains a single dose of medication for parenteral administration. There is no way to prevent airborne contamination of any unused portion of medication once the ampule is opened. If all the medication is not used, the remainder must be discarded. Medication can be removed from an ampule by breaking its thin neck. The ampule can be inverted or placed on a flat surface to draw the solution into the syringe. Care must be taken not to contaminate the needle by touching the rim of the ampule. Procedure 42-2 shows how to remove medication from an ampule.

F I G U R E 4 2 - 5

Ampules, vials, prefilled cartridges, and holders.

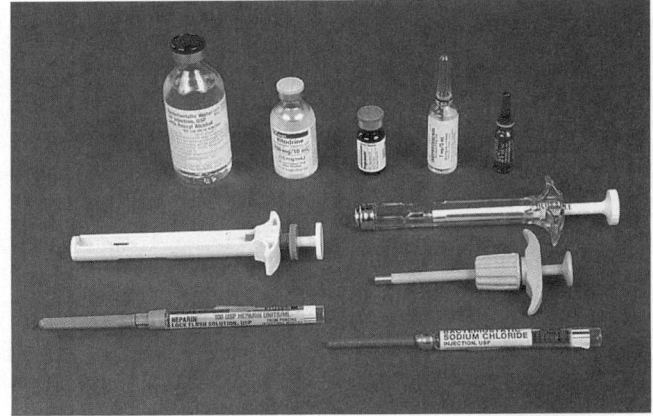

PROCEDURE 42-2

Removing Medication From an Ampule

Equipment

Sterile syringe and needle (size depends on medication being administered and client)

Ampule of medication
Medication card or Kardex

Alcohol swab or gauze pad
Filter needle (optional)

Action

1 Gather equipment. Check the medication order against the original physician's order according to agency policy.

2 Wash your hands.

3 Tap the stem of the ampule or twist your wrist quickly while holding the ampule vertically.

4 Wrap a small gauze pad or dry alcohol swab around the neck of the ampule.

5 Use a snapping motion to break off the top of the ampule along the prescored line at its neck. Always break away from your body.

Rationale

This comparison helps to identify errors that may have occurred when orders were transcribed.

Handwashing deters the spread of microorganisms.

This facilitates movement of medication in the stem to the body of the ampule.

This protects the nurse's fingers from the glass as the ampule is broken.

This protects the nurse's face and fingers from any shattered glass fragments.

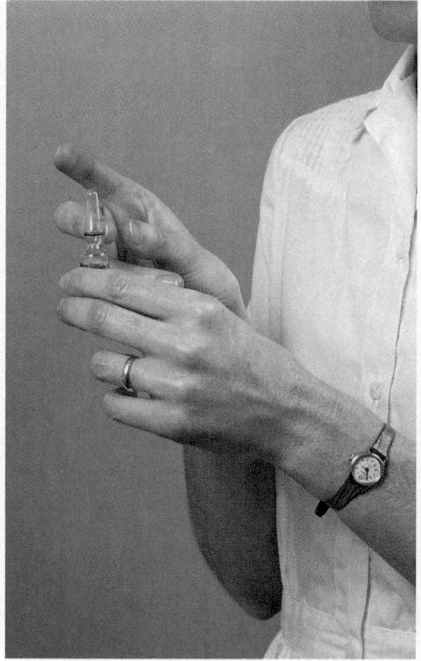

Action 3: Tapping stem of ampule.

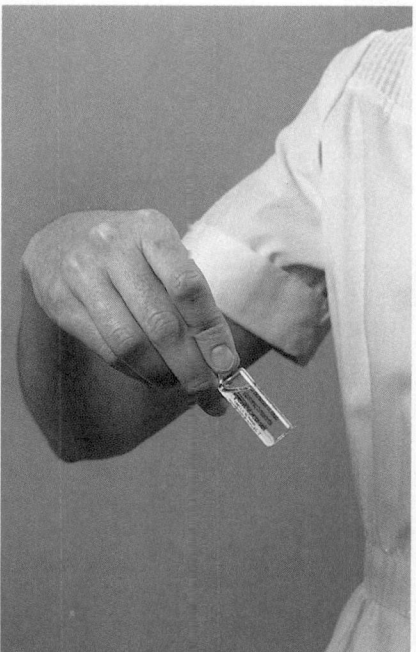

Action 3: Twisting motion of wrist while holding ampule.

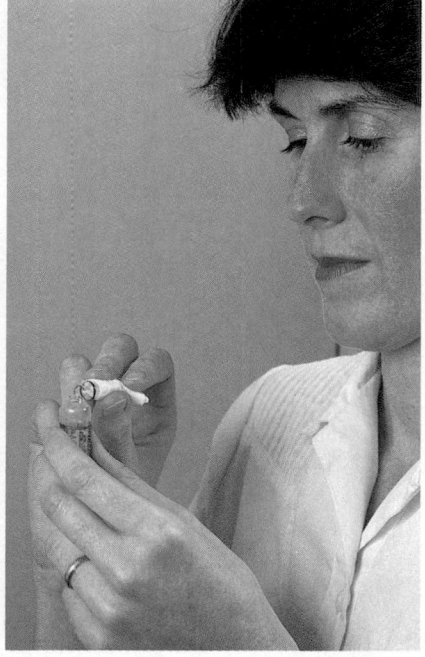

Action 5: Snapping off top of ampule.

6 Remove the cap from the needle by pulling it straight off. Insert the needle into the ampule, being careful not to touch the rim. (Some agencies recommend use of a filter needle when withdrawing solution from an ampule.)

The rim of the ampule is considered contaminated. (Use of a filter needle prevents the accidental withdrawing of small glass particles with the medication.)

(continued)

PROCEDURE 42-2 (continued)

Removing Medication From an Ampule

Action

Rationale

7 Withdraw medication in the amount ordered. Do not inject air into solutions. Use either of the following methods:

a Insert the tip of the needle into the ampule, which is *upright* on a flat surface, and withdraw fluid into the syringe.

b Insert the tip of the needle into the ampule and *invert* the ampule. Keep the needle centered and not touching the sides of the ampule. Remove the prescribed amount of medication.

The contents of the ampule are not under pressure; therefore, air is unnecessary and will cause the contents to overflow.

Surface tension holds the fluid in the ampule when inverted. If the needle touches the sides or is removed and then reinserted into the ampule, surface tension is broken and fluid runs out.

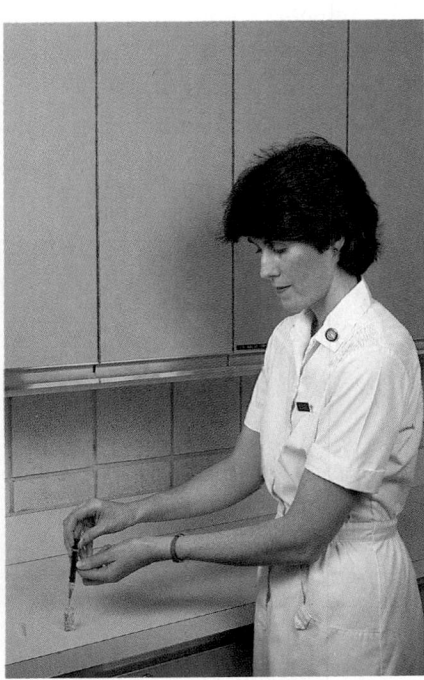

Action 7a: Withdrawing medication from upright ampule.

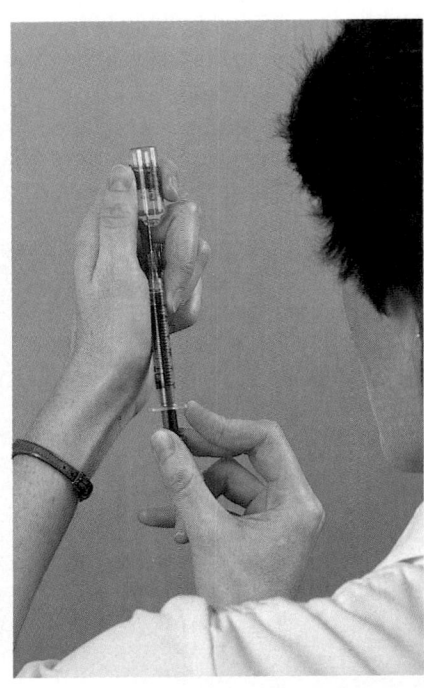

Action 7b: Withdrawing medication from inverted ampule. (Photos © Ken Kasper.)

8 Do not expel any air bubbles that may form in the solution. Wait until the needle has been withdrawn to tap the syringe and expel the air carefully. Check the amount of medication in the syringe and discard any surplus.

Ejecting air into the solution increases pressure in the ampule and can force the medication to spill out over the ampule.

9 Discard the ampule in a suitable container after comparing with the medication card or Kardex.

If all of the medication has been removed from the ampule, it must be discarded because there is no way to maintain sterility of contents in an opened ampule.

10 Cap the needle on the syringe.

This prevents contamination of the needle and protects the nurse against inadvertent needlesticks.

11 Wash your hands.

Handwashing deters the spread of microorganisms.

Vials As Figure 42-5 shows, a **vial** is a glass bottle with a self-sealing stopper through which medication is removed. For safety in transporting and storing, the single-dose rubber-capped vial usually is covered with a soft metal cap that can be easily removed. The rubber stopper that is then exposed is the means of entrance into the vial.

Some drugs are dispensed in vials that contain several doses. This means that the nurse can remove several doses from the same container. To facilitate removal of medication, the nurse injects air into the vial. The amount of air is the same as the desired quantity of solution. Procedure 42-3 shows how to remove medication from a vial.

Prefilled Cartridges Prefilled cartridges provide a single dose of medication. The nurse inserts the cartridge into a reusable holder. Before giving the injection, the nurse checks the dosage in the cartridge and clears the cartridge of excess air. Most prefilled cartridges are overfilled, and the nurse should eject any excess medication to give an exact dose and avoid a medication error. Tubex and Carpuject are two types of prefilled cartridges.

Mixing Medications in One Syringe

Preparation of medications in one syringe depends on how the medication is supplied. When using a single-dose vial and a multidose vial, air is injected into both vials and the medication in the multidose vial is drawn into the syringe first. This prevents the contents of the multidose vial from being contaminated with the medication in the single-dose vial. The nurse must ensure that the two drugs are compatible.

The steps to follow when preparing medications from two multidose vials in one syringe are as follow:

1. Inject air into vial A, keeping the needle from touching the medication.
2. Inject air into vial B and withdraw the quantity of medication needed.
3. Change the needle if possible. This prevents the contents of vial A from being contaminated with the contents of vial B.
4. Carefully withdraw the needed quantity of medication from vial A. The two medications are now combined in the syringe. Excess medication must not be reinjected into vial A because this may cause an imbalance in the two dosages.

This procedure is shown in Figure 42-6.

When preparing medications from an ampule and a vial, the medication in the vial is prepared first. The medication in the ampule is drawn up after the medication in the vial.

It is important for the nurse to be aware of drug incompatibilities when preparing medications in one syringe. Certain medications, such as diazepam (Valium), are incompatible with other drugs when combined in the same syringe. Other drugs have limited compatibility and should be administered within 15 minutes of preparation. Incompatible drugs may become cloudy or form a precipitate in the syringe. Such medications are discarded and re-prepared in separate syringes. A drug compatibility table should be available to nurses who are preparing medications.

Mixing Insulins in One Syringe

Insulin, a naturally occurring hormone produced by the islets of Langerhans in the pancreas, enables cells to use carbohydrates. Clients with diabetes mellitus produce no insulin or produce insulin in insufficient amounts. Several types of insulin are available for use by clients with diabetes mellitus. Insulins vary in their onset and duration of action and are classified as short-acting, intermediate-acting, and long-acting. Some insulins have a modifying protein that slows absorption. The modifying proteins are globin and protamine (NPH, globin zinc, protamine zinc).

Insulin dosages are calculated in units. The scale commonly used is U-100, which is based on 100 units of insulin contained in 1 mL of solution. An insulin syringe is calibrated in units also. Before administering insulin, the nurse should check the dosage with the physician's orders. Many clients with diabetes mellitus are regulated with a combination of two insulins (eg, regular and NPH insulins).

Procedure 42-4 gives the steps for mixing two types of insulins in the same syringe.

The importance of rotating injection sites for insulin administration cannot be overemphasized. A discussion of injection sites is included under Administering Medications Subcutaneously. Insulin should be stored in a cool place. It can be warmed before administration by rolling the vial between the palms. Some insulins are stable at room temperature.

Reconstitution of Powdered Medications

Several drugs, including many antibiotics, are supplied as powders in vials. A liquid, or *diluent*, must be added to the powder before it is administered as a solution. The technique of adding a diluent to a powdered drug is called *reconstitution*. Information needed for reconstitution and dosage calculation usually is located on the vial label. The nurse must know the amount and type of diluent to be added to the powder. Common diluents are sterile water for injection and 0.9% sodium chloride injection. After the diluent is added to the solution, the nurse reads the label further to determine the concentration of drug per milliliter of solution. This is essential to the dosage computation. If all the medication is not used at the time of reconstitution, the nurse refers to the vial label for storage instructions. Additional sources of information about reconstitution of medications are package inserts and the pharmacist. Figure 42-7 shows a package insert and the label of a vial that contains a powdered drug.

Administering Medications Intradermally

The intradermal route has the longest absorption time of all parenteral routes. For this reason, intradermal injections

P R O C E D U R E   4 2 - 3

Removing Medication From a Vial

Equipment

Sterile syringe and needle (size depends on medication being administered and client)

Vial of medication
Medication card or Kardex

Alcohol swab
Filter needle (optional)

Action

1 Gather equipment. Check medication order against the original physician's order according to agency policy.

2 Wash your hands.

3 Remove the metal or plastic cap on the vial that protects the rubber stopper.

4 Swab the rubber top with the alcohol swab.

5 Remove the cap from the needle by pulling it straight off. (Some agencies recommend use of a filter needle when withdrawing premixed medication from multidose vials.)

6 Pierce the rubber stopper in the center with the needle tip and inject the measured air into the space above the solution. (Do not inject air into the solution.) The vial may be positioned upright on a flat surface or inverted.

Rationale

This comparison helps to identify errors that may have occurred when orders were transcribed.

Handwashing deters the spread of microorganisms.

The metal cap prevents contamination of the rubber top.

Alcohol removes surface bacteria contamination. This is not necessary the first time the rubber stopper is entered but subsequent reentries into the vial require the use of alcohol cleansing.

Before fluid is removed, injection of an equal amount of air is required to prevent the formation of a partial vacuum because a vial is a sealed container. If not enough air is injected, the negative pressure makes it difficult to withdraw the medication. (Use of a filter needle prevents any solid material from being withdrawn through the needle.)

Air bubbled through the solution could result in withdrawal of an inaccurate amount of medication.

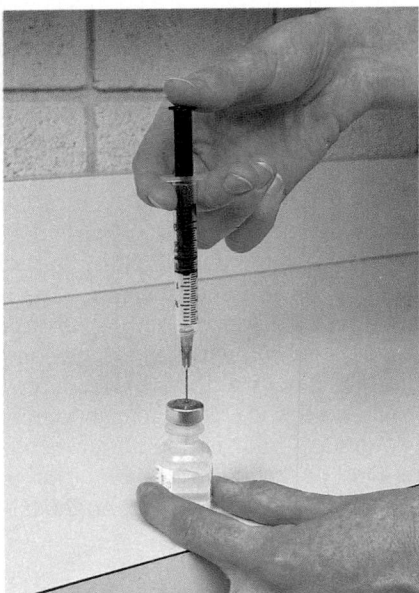

Action 6: Injecting air with vial upright.

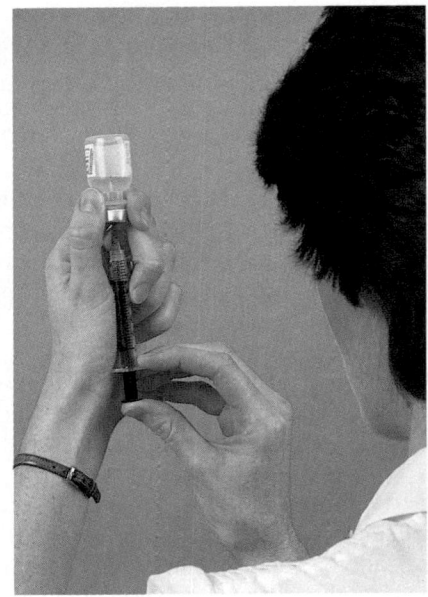

Action 6: Injecting air with vial inverted and needle above solution.

(continued)

PROCEDURE 43-3 (continued)

Removing Medication From a Vial

Action	Rationale
7 Invert the vial and withdraw the needle tip slightly so that it is below the fluid level.	This prevents air from being aspirated into the syringe.
8 Draw up the prescribed amount of medication while holding the syringe at eye level and vertically.	Holding the syringe at eye level facilitates accurate reading, and the vertical position makes removal of air bubbles from the syringe easy.
9 If any air bubbles accumulate in the syringe, tap the barrel of the syringe sharply and move the needle past the fluid into the air space to reinject the air bubble into the vial. Return the needle tip to the solution and continue withdrawal of the medication.	Removal of air bubbles is necessary to ensure accurate dose of medication.

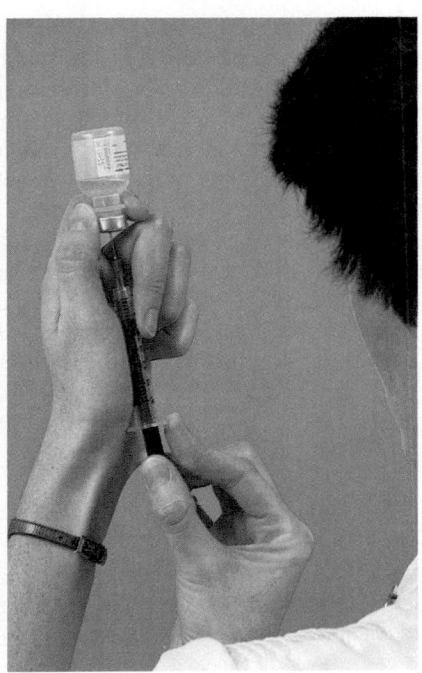

Action 8: Withdrawing medication at eye level.

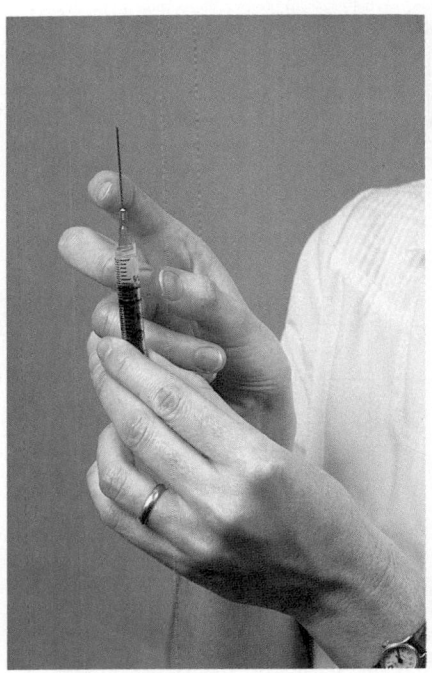

Action 9: Tapping to remove air bubbles. (Photos © Ken Kasper.)

10 Once the correct dose is withdrawn, remove the needle from the vial and cap it.	This prevents contamination of the needle and protects the nurse against accidental needlesticks.
11 If a multidose vial is being used, store the vial containing the remaining medication according to agency policy.	Because the vial is sealed, the medication inside remains sterile and can be used for future injections.
12 Wash your hands.	Handwashing deters the spread of microorganisms.

are used for diagnostic purposes, such as the tuberculin test and tests to determine sensitivity to various substances. The advantage of the intradermal route for these tests is that the body's reaction to substances is easily visible, and degrees of reaction are discernible by comparative study.

Intradermal injections are placed just below the epidermis. Sites commonly used are the inner surface of the forearm, the dorsal aspect of the upper arm, and the upper back. Equipment used for an intradermal injection includes a tuberculin syringe calibrated in tenths and hundredths of a milliliter. The dosage given intradermally is small, usually

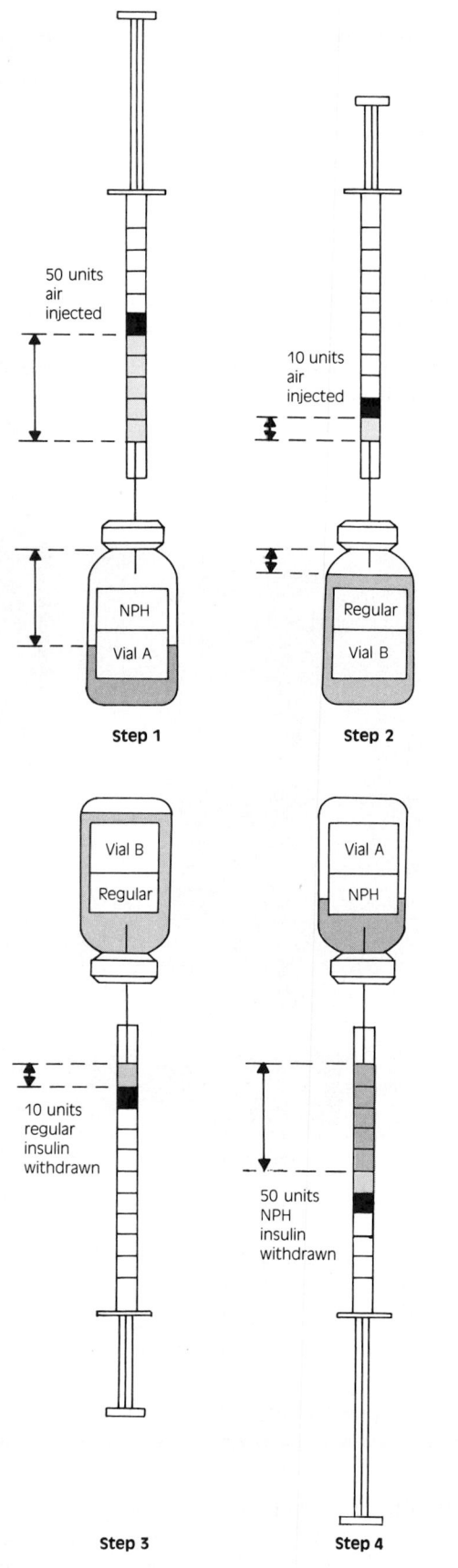

50 units
air
injected

NPH

Vial A

Step 1

10 units
air
injected

Regular

Vial B

Step 2

Vial B

Regular

10 units
regular
insulin
withdrawn

Step 3

Vial A

NPH

50 units
NPH
insulin
withdrawn

Step 4

F I G U R E 4 2 - 6

Mixing medications in one syringe.

less than 0.5 mL. A ¼- to ½-inch (0.6 to 1.3 cm) 26- or 27-gauge needle is used.

To administer an intradermal injection, the site is cleaned with alcohol in a circular motion, working from the center of the site outward. The nurse holds the client's skin taut with the nondominant hand and the syringe in the dominant hand with palm down to enable the needle to be inserted bevel upward at a 5- to 15-degree angle. The needle is inserted until the bevel is no longer visible and the medication is injected. A small raised area, or wheal, should be present at the injection site. To prevent hastened absorption, the site is not massaged after injection. The site of injection is recorded. The client should receive instructions about care and observation of the site and follow-up. Procedure 42-5 outlines and shows the procedure for administering an intradermal injection.

Administering Medications Subcutaneously

Subcutaneous tissue lies between the epidermis and the muscle. Because there is subcutaneous tissue all over the body, various sites are used for **subcutaneous injections**. These sites are the outer aspect of the upper arm, anterior aspects of the thigh, lower abdominal wall, and upper back. Figure 42-8 shows the sites on the body where subcutaneous injections can be given. This route is used to administer insulin, heparin, and certain immunizations.

Equipment used for a subcutaneous injection depends on the medication to be given. For instance, insulin is prepared with an insulin syringe. Heparin is prepared with a tuberculin syringe or supplied in a prefilled cartridge. A ½- to 1-inch 25-gauge needle is used for this route. Ordinarily, no more than 1 mL of solution is given subcutaneously.

(*Text continues on p. 1220*)

F I G U R E 4 2 - 7

Package insert and label for instructions on reconstituting powdered medications. (Photo © Ken Kasper.)

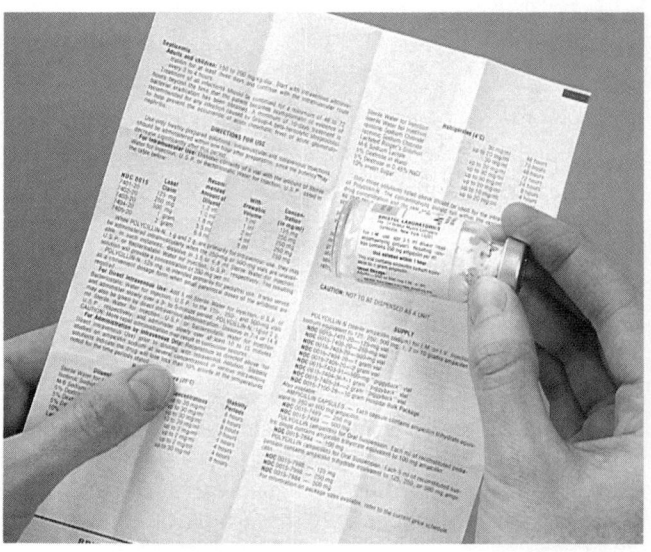

PROCEDURE 42-4

Mixing Insulins in One Syringe

Equipment

Two vials of insulin
Medication card or
  Kardex

Sterile insulin syringe with 25-gauge
  or 27-gauge needle
Alcohol swabs

Action	Rationale
1 Gather equipment. Check medication order against the original physician's order according to agency policy.	This comparison helps to identify errors that may have occurred when orders were transcribed.
2 Wash your hands.	Handwashing deters the spread of microorganisms.
3 If necessary, remove the metal cap that protects the rubber stopper on each vial.	The metal cap prevents contamination of the rubber top.
4 If insulin is a suspension, rotate the vial between your palms to mix before withdrawal.	Shaking vials creates froth that may interfere with withdrawal of accurate dose. Regular insulin is clear because it does not contain any modifying agents to slow its absorption.
5 Cleanse the rubber tops with alcohol swabs.	Alcohol removes surface bacteria contamination. This is not necessary the first time a metal cap is removed, but subsequent reentries into the vial require use of alcohol cleansing.
6 Remove cap from needle. Inject air into the modified insulin preparation (eg, NPH insulin). Use an amount of air equal to the amount of medication to be withdrawn. Do not allow the needle to touch the medication in the vial. Remove the needle.	Regular, or short-acting, insulin should never be contaminated with NPH or any insulin modified with added protein. Placing air in the NPH insulin first without allowing the needle to contact the insulin ensures that regular insulin is not contaminated with the additional protein in the NPH.
7 Inject air into the clear insulin without additional protein (eg, regular insulin). Use an amount of air equal to the amount of medication to be withdrawn. Do not bubble the air through the medication.	An equal amount of air must be injected into the vacuum to allow easy withdrawal of medication.

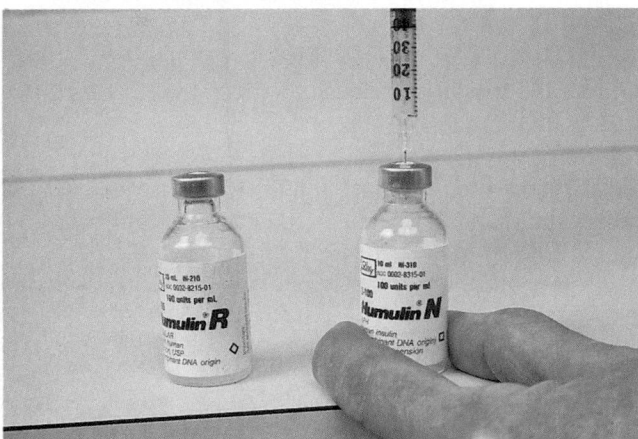

Action 6: Injecting air into modified insulin preparation.

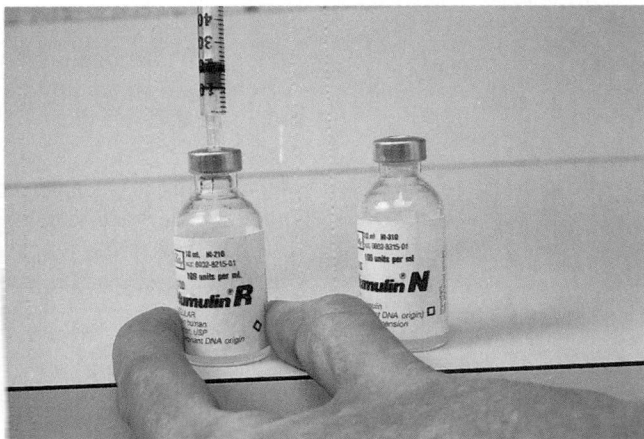

Action 7: Injecting air into clear insulin.

(continued)

P R O C E D U R E 4 2 - 4 *(continued)*

Mixing Insulins in One Syringe

Action

8 Invert the vial of clear insulin and aspirate the amount prescribed. Remove the needle from the vial.

9 Cleanse the rubber top of the modified insulin vial. Insert the needle into this vial, invert it, and withdraw the medication. Cap the needle.

Rationale

Regular insulin that contains no additional protein is not contaminated by insulin that contains globulin or protamine.

Previous addition of air eliminates need to create positive pressure. Capping the needle prevents contamination and protects the nurse against accidental needlesticks.

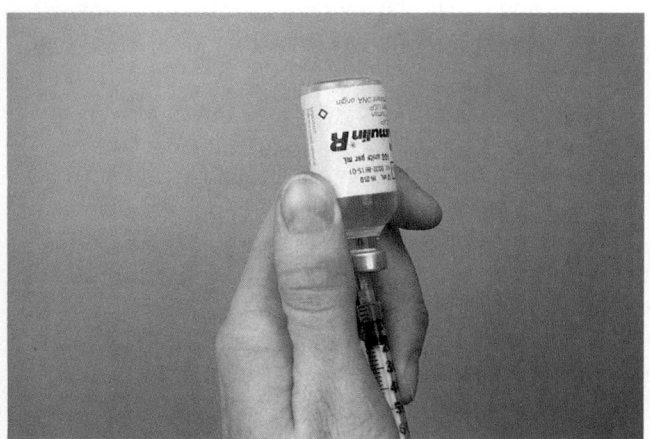

Action 8: Withdrawing clear insulin.

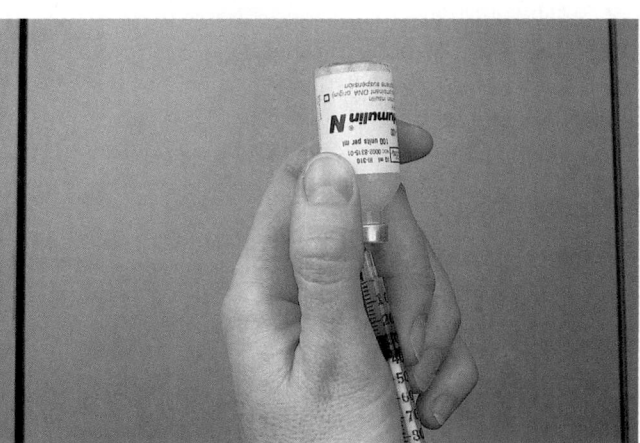

Action 9: Withdrawing modified insulin. (Photos © Ken Kasper.)

10 Store the vials according to agency recommendations.

11 Wash your hands.

Insulin need not be refrigerated but must be protected from temperature extremes.

Handwashing deters the spread of microorganisms.

Special Considerations

An insulin-dependent diabetic who is visually impaired may find it helpful to use a magnifying apparatus that fits around the syringe.

An insulin-cartridge pen (the Novalin Pen) is available that allows the client to dial the correct dose of insulin and press a button to quickly release the dose through a short, fine, 27-gauge needle.

Before attempting to explain or demonstrate devices that aid low-vision diabetics to prepare their medication, the nurse should attempt to use the device under similar circumstances. Practice using the aid with a blindfold in place, to detect any difficulties the client may experience.

PROCEDURE 42-5

Administering an Intradermal Injection

Equipment

Medication
Medication card or Kardex
Sterile syringe and needle (size
   depends on medication being
   administered and client)

Alcohol swab
Acetone and 2 × 2 sterile gauze
   square (optional)
Disposable gloves (optional)

Action	Rationale
1 Assemble equipment and check the physician's order.	This ensures that the client receives the right medication at the right time by the proper route. Many intradermal drugs are potent allergens and may cause a significant reaction if given in an incorrect dose.
2 Explain the procedure to the client.	Explanation encourages cooperation and reduces apprehension.
3 Wash your hands. Don disposable gloves (optional).	Handwashing deters the spread of microorganisms. Gloves protect from accidental exposure to blood but are not required by the CDC as long as some type of barrier (alcohol prep or gauze pad) is available to prevent the nurse's hands from contacting blood.
4 If necessary, withdraw medication from an ampule or vial as described in Procedures 42-2 and 42-3.	
5 Select an area on the inner aspect of the forearm that is not heavily pigmented or covered with hair. The upper chest or upper back beneath the scapulae also are sites for intradermal injections.	The forearm is a convenient and easy location for introducing an agent intradermally. Hair or lesions at the injection site may interfere with assessments of skin changes at the site.
6 Cleanse the area with an alcohol swab while wiping with a firm, circular motion and moving outward from the injection site. Allow the skin to dry. If the skin is oily, clean the area with a pledget moistened with acetone.	Pathogens on the skin can be forced into the tissues by the needle. Introducing alcohol into tissues irritates the tissues and is uncomfortable for the client. Acetone is effective for removing oily substances from the skin.
7 Use the nondominant hand to spread the skin taut over the injection site.	Taut skin provides an easy entrance into intradermal tissue.
8 Remove the needle cap with the nondominant hand by pulling it straight off.	The cap protects the needle from contact with microorganisms. This technique lessens the risk of an accidental needle stick.
9 Place the needle almost flat against the client's skin, bevel side up, and insert the needle into the skin so that the point of the needle can be seen through the skin. Insert the needle only about 1/8 inch.	Intradermal tissue is entered when the needle is held as nearly parallel to the skin as possible and is inserted about 1/8 inch.
10 Slowly inject the agent while watching for a small wheal or blister to appear. If none appears, withdraw the needle slightly.	If a small wheal or blister appears, the agent is in intradermal tissue.
11 Withdraw the needle quickly at the same angle that it was inserted.	Withdrawing the needle quickly and at the angle at which it entered the skin minimizes tissue damage and discomfort for the client.

(continued)

P R O C E D U R E 4 2 - 5 *(continued)*

Administering an Intradermal Injection

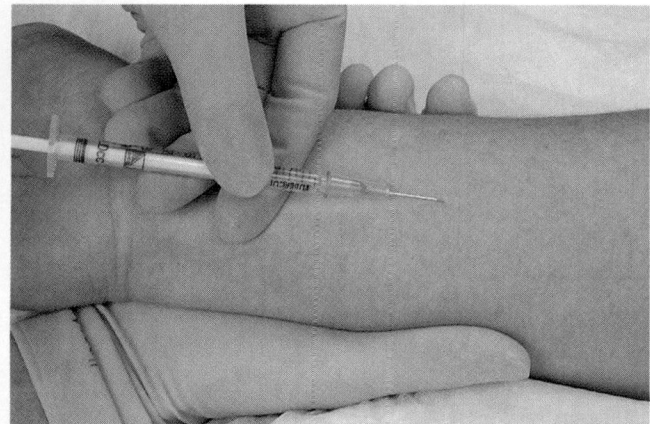

Action 9: Inserting the needle almost level with the skin.

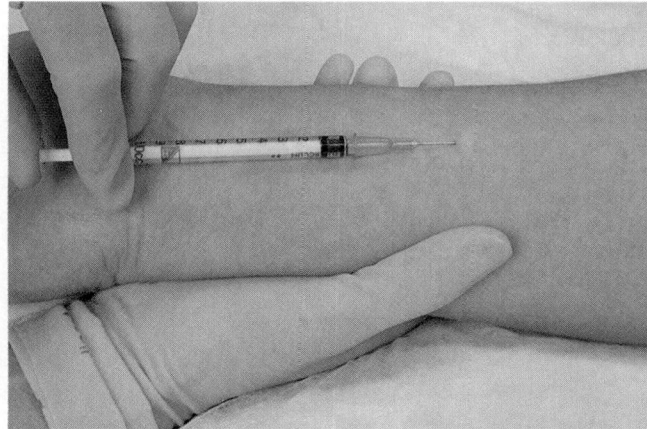

Action 10: Observing for wheal while injecting medication.

Action	Rationale
12 Do not massage the area after removing the needle.	Massaging the area where an intradermal injection is given may interfere with test results by spreading medication to underlying subcutaneous tissue.
13 Do not recap the used needle. Discard the needle and syringe in the appropriate receptacle.	Proper disposal of the needle protects the nurse from accidental injection. Most accidental puncture wounds occur when recapping needles.
14 Assist the client to a position of comfort.	This provides for the well-being of the client.
15 Remove gloves if worn, and dispose of them properly. Wash your hands.	Handwashing deters the spread of microorganisms.
16 Chart the administration of the medication.	Accurate documentation is necessary to prevent medication error.
17 Observe the area for signs of a reaction at ordered intervals, usually at 24- to 72-hour periods. Inform the client of this inspection. In some agencies, a circle may be drawn on the skin around the injection site.	This easily identifies the site of the intradermal injection and allows for careful observation of the exact area.

Giving larger amounts adds to the client's discomfort and may predispose to poor absorption.

The skin is cleaned for a subcutaneous injection in the same manner as for an intradermal injection. The nurse chooses the angle of needle insertion based on the amount of subcutaneous tissue present and the length of the needle. In most cases, a ⁵/₈-inch (1.6 cm) needle is inserted at a 45-degree angle and a ¹/₂-inch needle is inserted at a 90-degree angle. The client's size also may determine the angle of needle insertion. The amount of tissue that can be bunched or grasped is an indication. A 90-degree angle is used if 2 inches (5.1 cm) of tissue can be grasped at the site, and a 45-degree angle is recommended when 1 inch of

tissue is grasped. Stretching or spreading the skin taut allows for easier insertion of the needle.

After the needle is in place, the nurse gently pulls back on the plunger to determine that the needle has not entered a blood vessel. If blood enters the barrel of the syringe, the needle is removed and the medication, syringe, and needle should be discarded appropriately and a new dose prepared for administration at another site.

If no blood enters the barrel of the syringe, the medication is injected into the client. Aspiration of the plunger is not recommended with administration of subcutaneous heparin because this action can result in hematoma formation. The site is gently massaged, except in the case of

cle tissue. If a sore or inflamed muscle is entered, the muscle may act as a trigger area, and severe referred pain often results. It is best to palpate a muscle before injection. A site should be selected that does not feel tender to the client and where the tissue does not contract and become firm and tense.

Absorption occurs as in subcutaneous administration but more rapidly because of the greater vascularity of muscle tissue. The amount of 3 mL is considered the maximum to be given in one site.

Intramuscular Injection Sites An important point in the administration of an **intramuscular injection** is the selection of a safe site, one that is away from large nerves, bones, and blood vessels. When care is not taken, common complications include abscesses, necrosis and skin slough, nerve injuries, lingering pain, and periostitis (inflammation of the membrane covering a bone).

The sites for injecting intramuscular medications should be rotated when therapy requires repeated injections. The sites described in this chapter may all be used on a rotating basis. Whatever pattern of rotating sites is used, a description of it should appear in the client's nursing care plan.

Dorsogluteal Site The dorsogluteal site, located in the buttock, is a common site for administering intramuscular injections and can be located using anatomic landmarks. The posterior superior iliac spine and the greater trochanter are palpated. An imaginary line is drawn between the posterior superior iliac spine and the greater trochanter. The injection site is lateral and slightly superior to the midpoint of the line, as shown in Figure 42-9.

If the site is identified correctly, damage to the sciatic nerve is avoided. Palpation of anatomic landmarks ensures that the nurse has identified the injection site. The gluteal muscles are developed by walking; therefore, the dorsogluteal site is not to be used for children under age 3 years because their gluteal muscles are too small.

The site is so important that no injection into the buttock should be given without good visualization of the entire area and careful mapping to locate the proper site. This necessitates adequate exposure by lowering the undergarments. Merely raising one side of underclothing permits only a partial visualization of the area. It is recommended that the client be in a prone position with the toes pointed inward, or in the side-lying position with the upper knee flexed and the upper leg in front of the lower leg. These positions help to promote maximum muscle relaxation and, therefore, minimum discomfort. When the client is in a standing position, the gluteus muscle usually is tense.

Ventrogluteal Site The ventrogluteal site involves the gluteus medius and gluteus minimus muscles in the hip area. The ventrogluteal site is recommended for both adults and children. There are no large nerves or blood vessels in the injection area, it is removed from bone tissue, the area is

(*Text continues on p. 1225*)

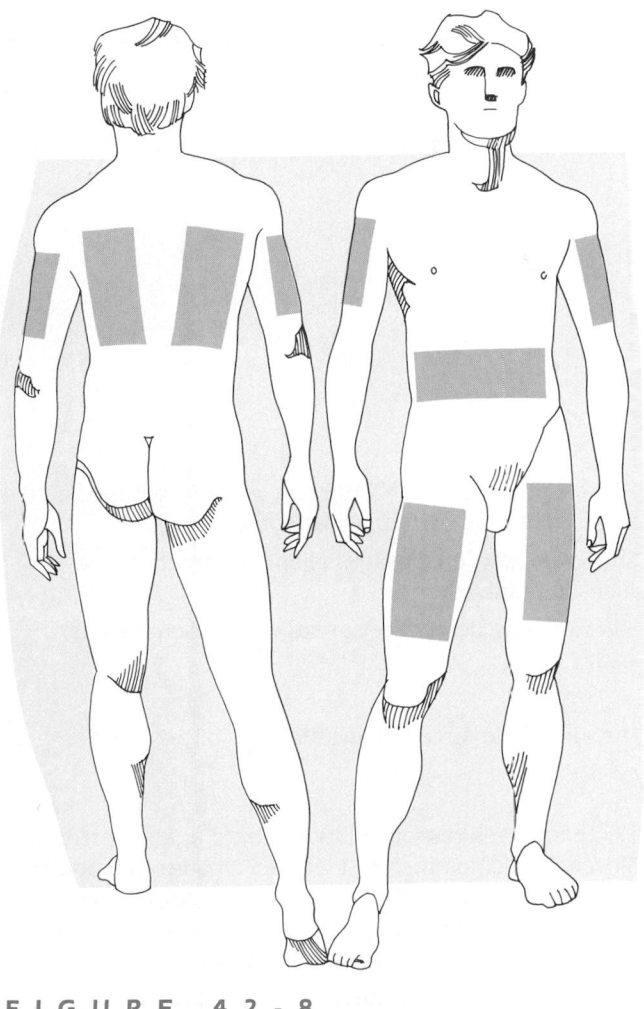

FIGURE 42-8

Sites on the body where subcutaneous injections can be given.

heparin and insulin because massaging the site can increase the rate of absorption of these agents. The site of administration is recorded in the client's record. Procedure 42-6 shows the procedure for administering medications subcutaneously.

It is necessary to rotate sites if the client is to receive frequent injections. This helps to prevent irritation and permits complete absorption of the medication. Clients who receive injections repeatedly in one site are likely to develop an area of hardened and tender tissue. A marked diagram incorporated into the client's plan of care is helpful for noting alternative sites. It is futile to rely on memory. Not even the client can always recall the site of the previous injection. Techniques for reducing discomfort in subcutaneous administrations are listed after the discussion Administering Medications Intramuscularly.

Administering Medications Intramuscularly

The intramuscular route often is used for drugs that are irritating because there are few nerve endings in deep mus-

P R O C E D U R E   4 2 - 6

Administering a Subcutaneous Injection

Equipment

Medication
Medication card or Kardex
A sterile syringe and needle (size
  depends on medication being
  administered and client)

Alcohol swabs
Disposable gloves (optional)

Action	Rationale
1 Assemble equipment and check the physician's order.	This ensures that the client receives the right medication at the right time by the proper route.
2 Explain the procedure to the client.	An explanation encourages client cooperation and reduces apprehension.
3 Wash your hands.	Handwashing deters the spread of microorganisms.
4 If necessary, withdraw medication from an ampule or vial as described in Procedures 42-2 and 42-3.	
5 Add air to the syringe according to agency policy (0.1 mL of air usually is added to a heparin injection).	The air bubble forces medication out of the needle.
6 Identify the client carefully. See Procedure 42-1, action 12. Close the curtain to provide privacy. Don disposable gloves (optional).	It is the nurse's responsibility to guard against error. Gloves protect against accidental exposure to blood but are not required by the CDC as long as some type of barrier (alcohol prep or gauze pad) is available to prevent the nurse's hands from contacting blood.
7 Have the client assume a position appropriate for the site selected:	Injection into a tense muscle causes discomfort.
a Outer aspect of upper arm—the client's arm should be relaxed and at the side of the body.	
b Anterior thighs—the client may sit or lie with the leg relaxed.	
c Abdomen—the client may lie in a semirecumbent position.	
d Scapular area—the client may be prone, on side, or in a sitting position.	
8 Locate the site of choice according to directions given in this chapter. Ensure that the area is not tender and is free of lumps or nodules.	Good visualization is necessary to establish the correct location of the site and avoid damage to tissues. Nodules or lumps may indicate a previous injection site where absorption was inadequate.
9 Clean the area around the injection site with an alcohol swab. Use a firm, circular motion while moving outward from the injection site. Allow the antiseptic to dry. Leave the alcohol swab in a clean area for reuse when withdrawing the needle.	Friction helps to clean the skin. A clean area is contaminated when a soiled object is rubbed over its surface.
10 Remove the needle cap with the nondominant hand, pulling it straight off.	The cap protects the needle from contact with microorganisms. This technique lessens the risk of an accidental needlestick.

(continued)

Administering a Subcutaneous Injection

Action	Rationale
11 Grasp and bunch the area surrounding the injection site or spread the skin at the site.	This provides for easy, less painful entry into the subcutaneous tissue. The decision to pinch or spread tissue at the injection site depends on the size of the client. If the client is obese, skin needs to be bunched to allow the needle to penetrate below the fatty layer in the subcutaneous tissue.
12 Hold the syringe in the dominant hand between the thumb and forefinger. Inject the needle quickly at an angle at 45 to 90 degrees, depending on the amount and turgor of the tissue and the length of the needle, as shown.	Subcutaneous tissue is abundant in well-nourished, well-hydrated persons and spare in emaciated, dehydrated, or very thin persons.

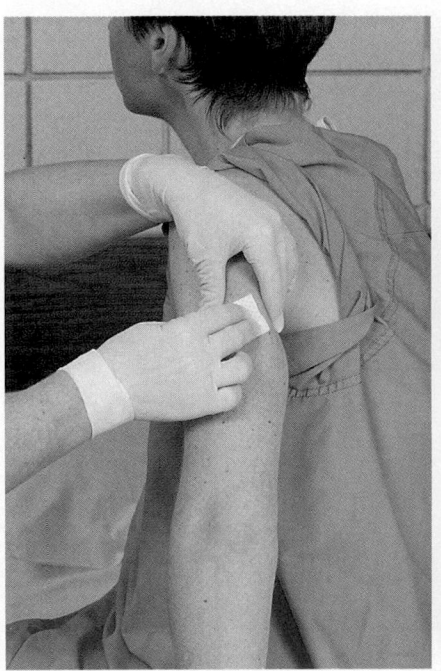

Action 9: Cleaning injection site.

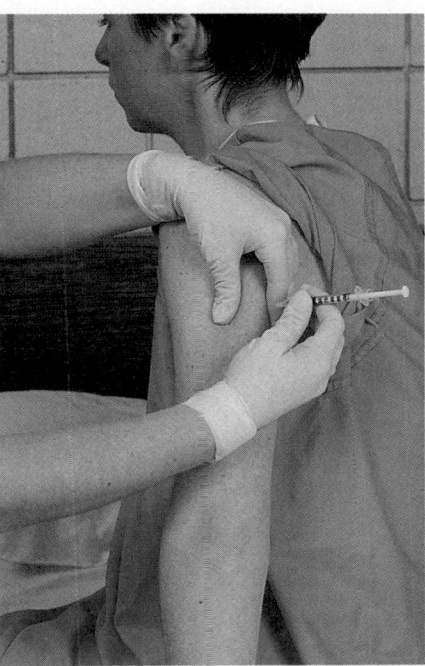

Action 11: Bunching tissue around injection site.

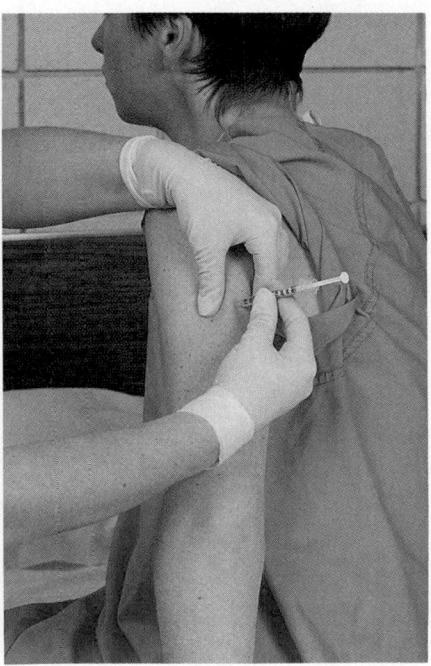

Action 12: Inserting needle.

13 After the needle is in place, release the tissue and immediately move your nondominant hand to steady the lower end of the syringe. Slide your dominant hand to the tip of the barrel.	Injecting the solution into compressed tissues results in pressure against nerve fibers and creates discomfort. The nondominant hand secures the syringe and allows for smooth aspiration.
14 Aspirate by pulling back gently on the plunger of the syringe to determine whether the needle is in a blood vessel. If blood appears, the needle should be withdrawn and the medication, syringe, and needle are discarded, and a new syringe with new medication prepared. (Most agencies recommend that a subcutaneous heparin injection should not be aspirated.)	Discomfort and possibly a serious reaction may occur if a drug intended for subcutaneous use is injected into a vein. Heparin, an anticoagulant, may cause bruising if aspirated.

(continued)

P R O C E D U R E   4 2 - 6 (continued)

Administering a Subcutaneous Injection

Action	Rationale
15 If no blood appears, inject the solution slowly.	Rapid injection of the solution creates pressure in the tissues, resulting in discomfort.
16 Withdraw the needle quickly at the same angle at which it was inserted, as shown.	Slow withdrawal of the needle pulls the tissues and causes discomfort. Applying countertraction around the injection site helps to prevent pulling on the tissue as the needle is withdrawn. Removing the needle at the same angle at which it was inserted minimizes tissue damage and discomfort for the client.

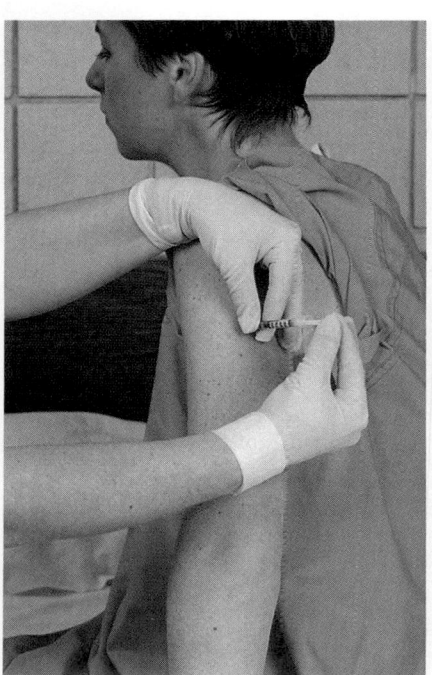 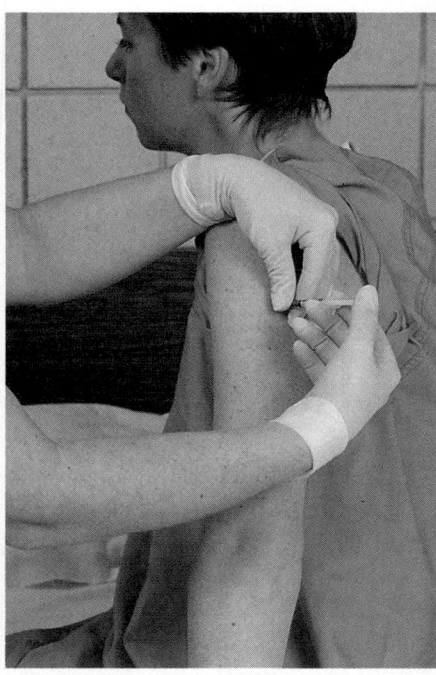 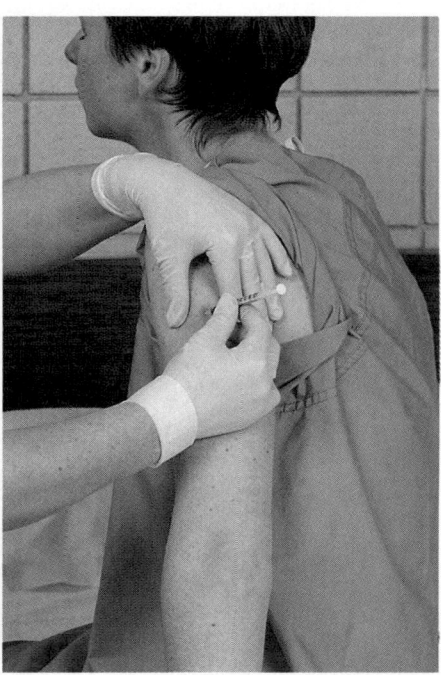

Action 14: Aspirating.　　　Action 15: Injecting medication.　　　Action 16: Withdrawing needle.
(Photos © B. Proud.)

Action	Rationale
17 Massage the area gently with the alcohol swab. (Do not massage a subcutaneous heparin or insulin injection site. Some institutions also recommend no massage after an insulin injection.)	Massaging helps to distribute the solution and hastens its absorption. Massaging the site of a heparin injection causes additional bruising. Massaging after an insulin injection may contribute to unpredictable absorption of the medication.
18 Do not recap the used needle. Discard the needle and syringe in the appropriate receptacle.	Proper disposal of the needle protects the nurse from accidental injection. Most accidental puncture wounds occur when recapping needles.
19 Assist the client to a position of comfort.	This provides for the well-being of the client.
20 Remove gloves if worn, and dispose of them properly. Wash your hands.	Handwashing deters the spread of microorganisms.

(continued)

PROCEDURE 42-6 *(continued)*

Administering a Subcutaneous Injection

Action	Rationale
21 Chart the administration of the medication.	Accurate documentation is necessary to prevent medication error.
22 Evaluate the response of the client to medication within an appropriate time frame.	Reaction to medication given by the parenteral route may occur within 15 to 30 minutes after injection.

Special Considerations

If a diabetic client is visually impaired, several insulin syringes may be preloaded and stored in the refrigerator for future use.

A poster or body log may be used to indicate sites for systematic rotation of insulin injections as well as to record the location of injections.

Refer the diabetic client to the American Diabetic Association for additional information and assistance.

---

clean because fecal contamination is rare at this site, and the client can be on the back, abdomen, or side for the injection. To relax the gluteal muscle, the client may flex the knees while lying on the back, point the toes inward while lying in the prone position, and flex the top leg in front of the lower leg in the side-lying position. Although any of the three positions just described may be used when injecting the ventrogluteal site, nurses increasingly prefer the side-lying position.

To locate the ventrogluteal site, the nurse places the palm over the greater trochanter, with the fingers facing the client's head. The right hand is used for the client's left hip and the left hand is used for the right hip to identify landmarks. The index finger is placed on the anterior superior iliac spine and the middle finger extends dorsally, palpating the crest of the ileum. A triangle is formed. The injection is made in the center of the triangle. Figure 42-10 shows injection of the ventrogluteal site.

Vastus Lateralis Site The vastus lateralis muscle is being recommended more frequently for the injection of medications. It is a thick muscle, and there is little or no danger of serious injury. There are no large nerves or vessels in proximity, and it does not cover a joint. The muscle covers the anterolateral aspect of the thigh. It is bounded by the midanterior thigh on the front of the leg and the midlateral thigh on the side. The thigh is divided into thirds horizontally and vertically. The injection is given in the *outer middle* third. This space provides a large number of injection sites. The syringe is held parallel to the surface of the bed. Figure 42-11 shows the location of this site. The vastus lateralis site is particularly desirable for infants and children, whose gluteal muscles are poorly developed.

Rectus Femoris Site The rectus femoris muscle is on the anterior part of the thigh. The site is used only when others

are contraindicated, since many clients find it uncomfortable. Some clients who must inject themselves at home use this site because of its convenience. The muscle is included in the sketch of the thigh in Figure 42-12.

Deltoid Muscle Site The deltoid muscle is located in the lateral aspect of the upper arm. It is not often used because it is a small muscle. The deltoid muscle is not capable of absorbing large amounts of solution. Damage to the radial nerve and artery is a risk of the deltoid site. Intramuscular injections into the deltoid muscle should be limited to 1 mL of solution and used only for adults. The deltoid muscle is not developed enough in infants and children to absorb medication adequately.

The deltoid muscle can be located by palpating the lower edge of the acromion process. A triangle is formed at the midpoint in line with the axilla on the lateral aspect of the upper arm. Hepatitis B virus vaccine is one medication that should be given in the deltoid muscle in adults to induce adequate levels of the antibody. Figure 42-13 shows the deltoid site.

Injection Procedure No more than 3 mL should be injected into a single injection site. Equipment commonly used for an intramuscular injection includes a 1- to $1\frac{1}{2}$-inch (2.5 to 3.8 cm) 20- to 22-gauge needle. The length of the needle should be selected with care before administering any intramuscular injection. The prepackaged loaded syringes usually have a needle that is 1 inch long. If there is any question about whether the belly of the target muscle can be reached, the needle should be exchanged for a longer one. A 2- to $2\frac{1}{2}$-inch (5.1 to 6.4 cm) needle may be necessary for an obese client. Evidence does not suggest that a short needle minimizes discomfort or that a longer one adds to discomfort. The characteristic of the client's anatomy should dictate needle length. The most important

THROUGH

THE EYES

OF A STUDENT

This day was like any other clinical day—up before dawn and in the hospital before most people even dream of being awake. I entered my client's room, knowing that she had had surgery less than 12 hours before my arrival, and introduced myself. I asked how she was feeling, to which she immediately responded, "I need pain medication—*now!*" I told her that I would check the medication orders and be back as soon as possible. I walked quickly to the medication Kardex, and there it was glaring at me in neatly printed black and white: "Demerol 100 mg IM q 3–4 hr prn." My mind raced as I thought, "I have never given an IM injection. There has to be something else ordered for pain." I knew that there wasn't. I found my clinical instructor and announced, "My client needs an IM injection," not "I have to give pain medication" or "I have to give some medication," just simply "I have to give an IM injection." Everything went surprisingly well as we prepared the medication, given the anxiety I was feeling. I went over the procedure one last time before entering the client's room.

We approached the client just in time for her to look at us in sheer terror and cry, "I hope that shot isn't for me; I hate them," which did nothing for my already shaking hands. I explained that she couldn't take a pill because she could not have anything by mouth because of the nature of her surgery. My instructor and I positioned the client on her side—a feat in itself—so that I could give her the shot in the dorsogluteal area. I marked the landmarks at least half a dozen times, wiped the area with alcohol, and asked her if she was ready for the injection. *Big mistake!* She swiftly replied, "No, but get it over with."

A little voice in my head repeated the words my technologies professor had said a million times, "Darting action is the key to a successful injection." So I aimed at the bull's-eye that appeared in front of my eyes. My hand, which seemed to be moving in slow motion, propelled downward at a 90-degree angle. Secretly I prayed that I would not hit my own hand. I must have closed my eyes because the next thing I remember was the loudest scream I had ever heard! I looked down and it was a bull's-eye, thank God, but the needle had not penetrated the muscle! The client successfully tensed her muscle tight enough to intercept the needle midflight. At that moment she relaxed, probably because she thought the worst was over, and I pushed the needle into place. I slowly drew back the plunger to make sure no blood appeared in the syringe. I began injecting the Demerol slowly, watching my hands shake as if I had just drunk a pot of coffee, and then I withdrew the needle and gently applied pressure over the site. It was over, I wanted to scream, "I did it!" but I kept my composure to feign the experience I lacked. Giving my first IM injection was not as bad as I thought it would be!

—Alison L. Moriarty, Georgetown University,
   Washington, DC

consideration is to use a needle with a tip that will reach deep into the muscle.

Just before injecting a medication intramuscularly, a small air bubble, about 0.2 to 0.3 mL, may be added to the syringe after the solution to be administered has been accurately measured. Figure 42-14 shows the air bubble in the syringe. This air bubble helps expel solution that is trapped in the shaft of the needle. Solution that remains in the needle shaft after the medication is injected is in danger of being pulled up through the tissues as the needle is withdrawn. If the drug is an irritating one, this causes discomfort to the client and may result in tissue damage. The air bubble also helps to trap the injected solution in intramuscular tissue. There is no danger of air embolism with this procedure.

To administer an intramuscular injection, the nurse cleans the site, spreads the skin taut with the nondominant hand, and inserts the needle in a dartlike manner at a 90-degree angle into the skin. The nurse aspirates the plunger and injects the medication if the needle is not in a blood

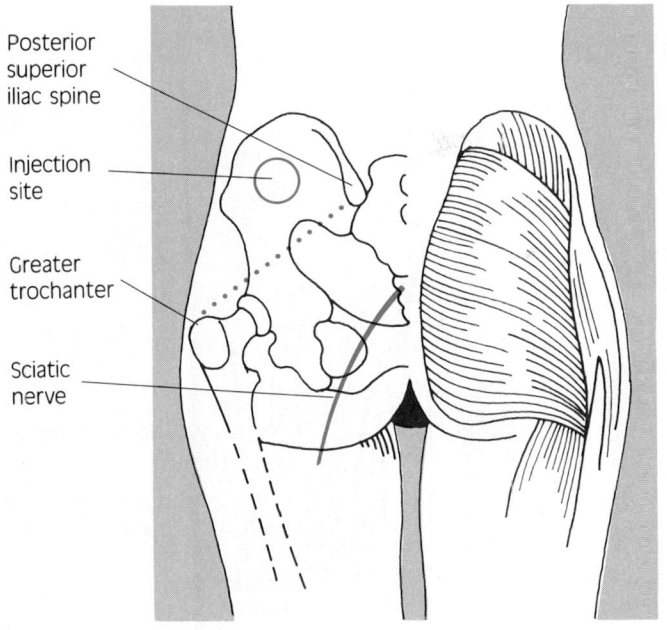

Posterior
superior
iliac spine

Injection
site

Greater
trochanter

Sciatic
nerve

FIGURE 42-9

The dorsogluteal site for administering an intramuscular injection is lateral and slightly superior to the midpoint of a line drawn from the trocanter to the posterior superior iliac spine. Correct identification of this site minimizes the possibility of accidentally damaging the sciatic nerve.

vessel. The site is gently massaged after the injection and recorded in the client's record. The procedure for administering an intramuscular injection is outlined in Procedure 42-7. Figure 42-15 compares the angles for needle insertion for all the injections.

Z-Track Technique The Z-track, or zig-zag, technique is used to administer medications that are highly irritating to subcutaneous tissues—for example, iron dextran injection (Imferon). Any intramuscular injection may be given using the Z-track technique. Taylor (1992) states that Z-track is the safest and most comfortable technique for giving any IM injection. This prevents seepage of the medication into the needle track and reduces the pain and discomfort, particularly for clients receiving injections over an extended period. An air lock of 0.2 to 0.3 mL is created after the medication is prepared in the syringe. A clean needle is attached to the syringe to prevent the injection of medication on the needle into superficial tissues. The needle should be a minimum of 1½ inches (3.8 cm) long; for obese people, a 3-inch (7.6-cm) needle may be required, so that there is no danger of injecting the medication into subcutaneous tissue. The dorsogluteal, ventrogluteal, or vastus lateralis sites can be used for this procedure. The skin is pulled to one side, about 1 inch (2.5 cm) laterally, and held in this position with the left hand for a right-handed person. The needle is inserted and aspirated for blood. The solution

is injected. For a dextran injection, the needle is allowed to remain in place for 10 seconds after injecting the medication. For other medications, the needle is withdrawn immediately and the displaced tissue is allowed to return to its normal position.

Light, steady pressure is applied over the site. The area may be massaged unless the manufacturer's directions on the drug label state that massage is contraindicated. The procedure for administering a Z-track injection is outlined in Figure 42-16.

Reducing Discomfort in Subcutaneous and Intramuscular Administrations

The following are recommended techniques to help reduce discomfort when injecting medications subcutaneously or intramuscularly:

- Select a needle of the smallest gauge that is appropriate for the site and solution to be injected.
- Be sure the needle is free of medication that may irri-

FIGURE 42-10

The ventrogluteal site is located by placing the palm on the greater trochanter and the index finger toward the anterior superior iliac spine. The middle finger is then spread posteriorly away from the index finger as far as possible. A V or triangle is formed by this maneuver. The injection is made in the middle of the triangle.

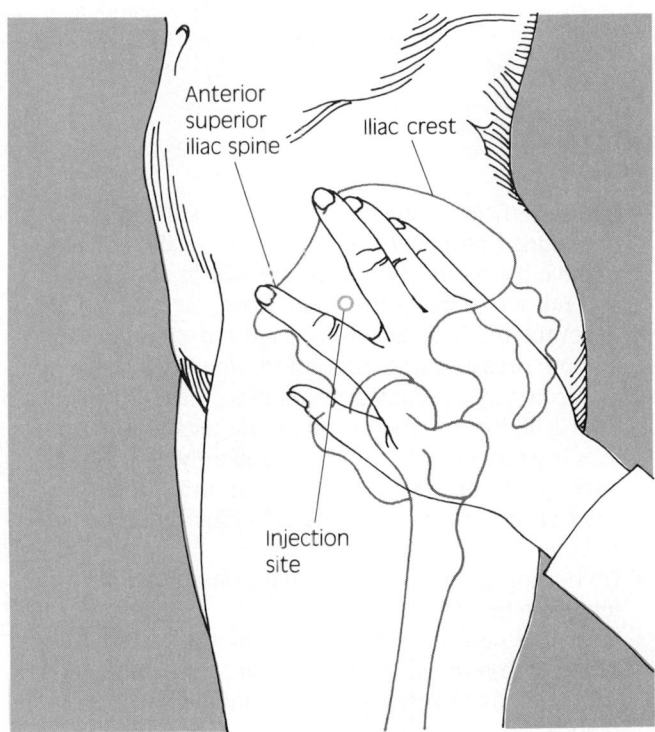

Anterior
superior
iliac spine

Iliac crest

Injection
site

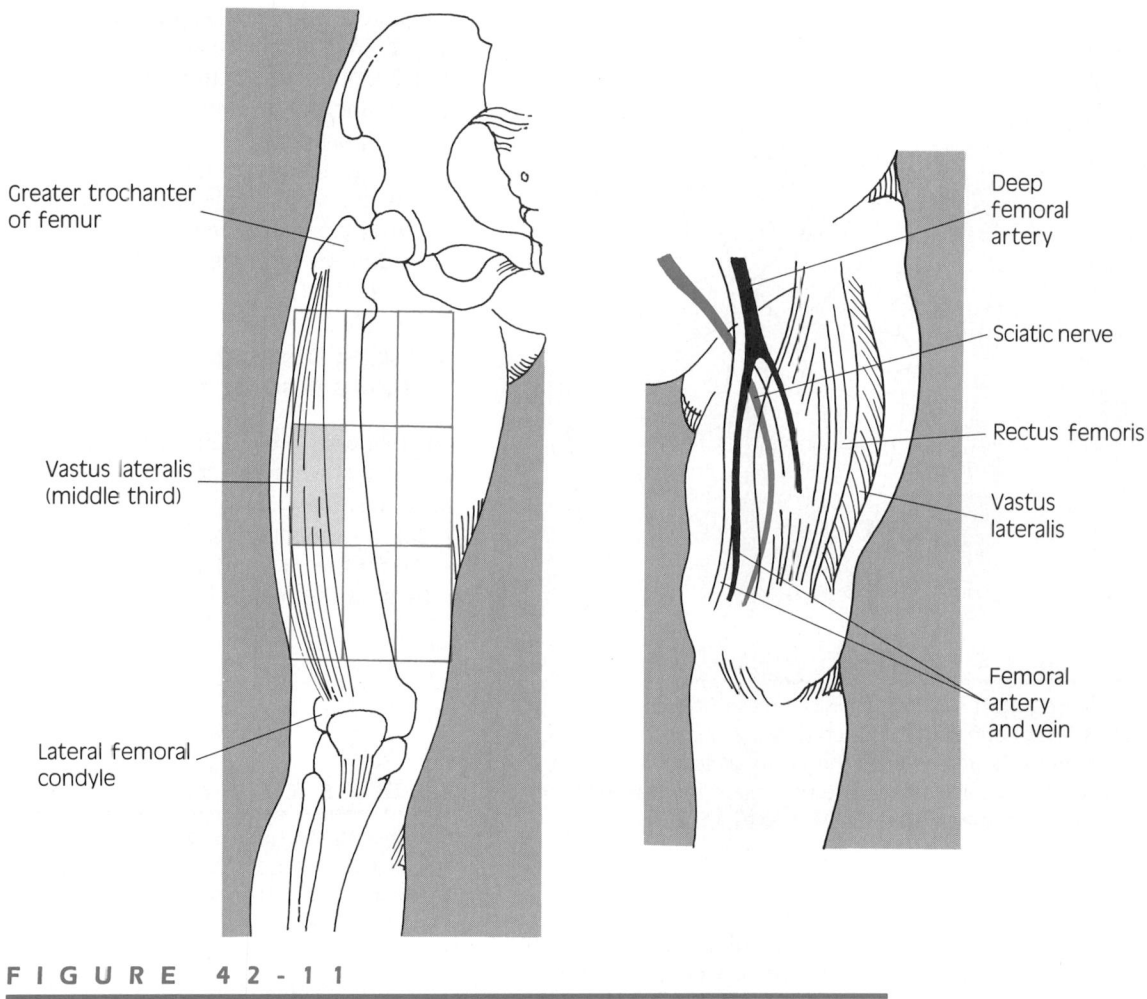

F I G U R E   4 2 - 1 1

The vastus lateralis site for intramuscular injections is identified by dividing the thigh into thirds horizontally and vertically. The injection is given in the outer middle third.

tate superficial tissues as the needle is inserted. Recommended procedure is to use two needles—one to remove the medication from the vial or ampule and a second one to inject the medication.

- Inject the medication into relaxed musculature. There is more pressure and discomfort when the medication is injected into a contracted muscle. Have the client lie on the abdomen while rotating the legs to point the toes inward. Or, when using the side-lying position, have the client flex the upper knee and place it in front of the lower leg. These positions relax the gluteal muscle.
- Do not inject areas that feel hard on palpation or tender to the client.
- Insert the needle with a dartlike motion without hesitation, and remove it quickly at the same angle at which it was inserted. These techniques help to reduce discomfort and tissue irritation.
- Do not administer more solution in one injection than is recommended for the site. Injecting more solution

creates excess pressure in the area and increases discomfort.
- Inject the solution slowly so that it may be dispersed more easily into the surrounding tissue.
- Massage the area after injection, unless this technique is contraindicated. Massage helps to spread the solution into surrounding tissues and hastens absorption by increasing circulation to the area.
- Allow the client who is fearful of injections to talk about the fears. Answer the client's questions truthfully, and explain the nature and purpose of the injection. Taking the time to offer support often allays fears that ordinarily add to the discomfort of the procedure for the client.
- Rotate the sites when the client is to receive repeated injections. Injections in the same site may cause undue discomfort, irritation, or abscesses in tissues.
- Use the Z-track technique for intramuscular injections to prevent leakage of medication into the needle track, thus minimizing the client's discomfort.

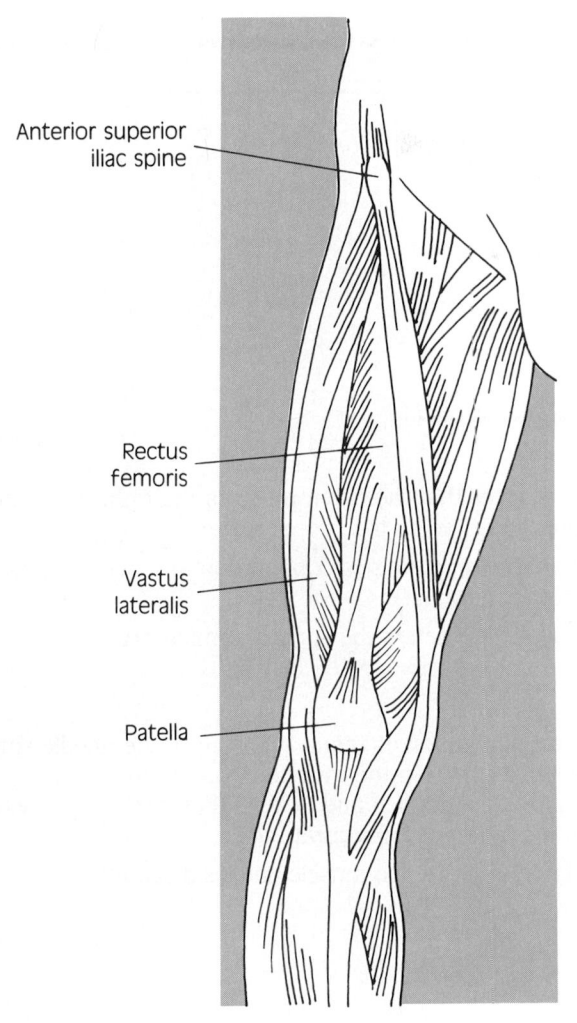

FIGURE 42-12

The rectus femoris site for intramuscular injections is used only when other sites are contraindicated.

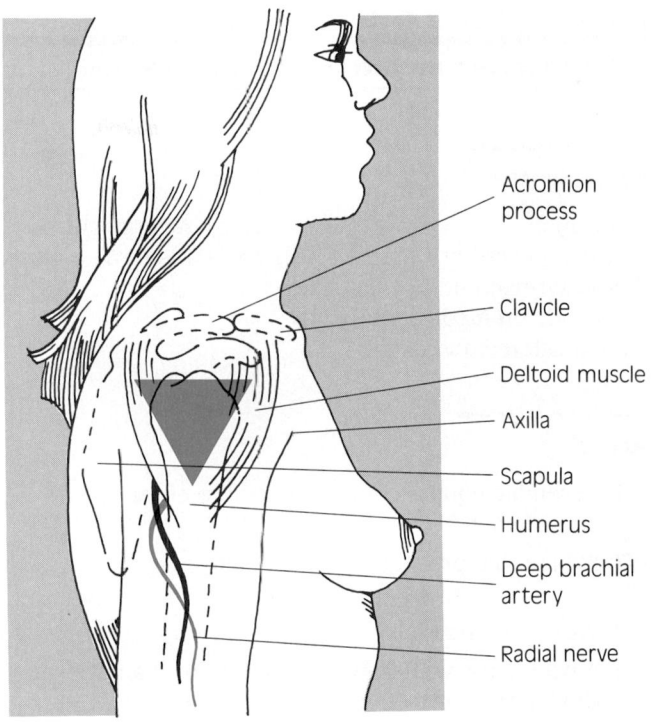

FIGURE 42-13

The deltoid muscle site for intramuscular injections is located by palpating the lower edge of the acromion process. At the midpoint, in line with the axilla on the lateral aspect of the upper arm, a triangle is formed.

FIGURE 42-14

An air bubble added to the syringe after the medication has been accurately measured helps to expel solution that is trapped in the shaft of the needle when the injection is given. It also helps to trap the injected solution in the intramuscular tissue.

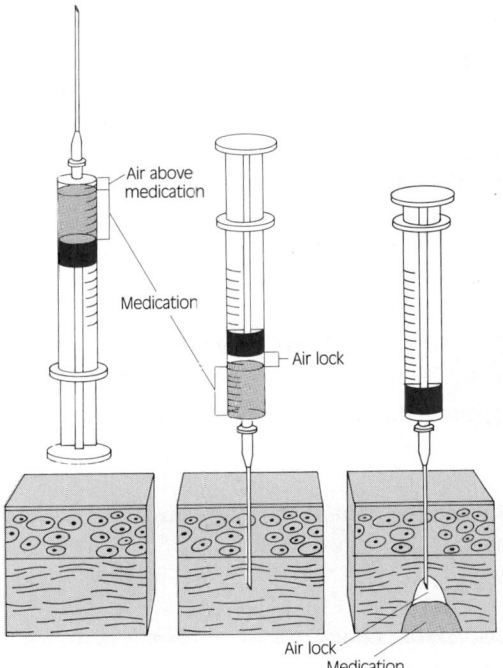

Administering Medications Intravenously

Medications administered intravenously have an immediate effect. The **intravenous route** is the most dangerous route of administration. Because the drug is placed directly into the bloodstream, it cannot be recalled nor can its actions be slowed. Intravenous administration would be the route chosen in an emergency situation when immediate absorption is required. There also are many clinical situations in which drugs are administered intravenously when an emergency does not exist. Patient-controlled analgesia allows the client to control administration of an intravenous analgesic for pain management and is discussed in Chapter 32. Procedure 37-1 describes the basic technique for administering an intravenous infusion.

There are several ways to administer medications intravenously. Medications may be added to the client's infusion solution. The recommended procedure is for the pharmacist to add the prescribed drug to a large volume of

(Text continues on p. 1232)

P R O C E D U R E   4 2 - 7

Administering an Intramuscular Injection

Equipment

Medication
Medication card or Kardex
Sterile syringe and needle (size depends on medication being administered and client)

Alcohol swab
Disposable gloves (optional)

Action	Rationale
1 Assemble equipment and check the physician's order.	This ensures that the client receives the right medication at the right time by the proper route.
2 Explain the procedure to the client.	Explanation encourages cooperation and alleviates apprehension.
3 Wash your hands.	Handwashing deters the spread of microorganisms.
4 If necessary, withdraw medication from an ampule or vial as described in Procedures 42-2 and 42-3.	
5 Add 0.2 mL of air to the syringe.	The air bubble forces medication out of the needle shaft and helps trap it in the muscle tissue. Some experts question this practice and believe that it interferes with administration of an accurate dose.

6 Provide for privacy. Have the client assume a position appropriate for the site selected.
  a Dorsogluteal—the client may lie prone with toes pointing inward or on the side with the upper leg flexed and placed in front of the lower leg.
  b Ventrogluteal—the client may lie on the back or side with the hip and knee flexed.
  c Vastus lateralis—the client may lie on the back or may assume a sitting position.
  d Deltoid—the client may sit or lie with arm relaxed.
	Injection into a tense muscle causes discomfort.

7 Locate the site of choice according to directions given in this chapter and ensure that the area is nontender and free of lumps or nodules. Don disposable gloves (optional).	Good visualization is necessary to establish the correct location of the site and avoid damage to tissues. Nodules or lumps may indicate a previous injection site where absorption was inadequate. Gloves protect against accidental exposure to blood but are not required by the CDC as long as some type of barrier (alcohol prep or gauze pad) is available to prevent the nurse's hands from contacting blood.
8 Clean the area thoroughly with an alcohol swab, using friction.	Pathogens present on the skin can be forced into the tissues by the needle.
9 Remove the needle cap by pulling it straight off.	The cap protects the needle from contact with microorganisms. This technique lessens the risk of an accidental needlestick.
10 Spread the skin at the site using your nondominant hand.	This makes the tissue taut and minimizes discomfort.

(continued)

PROCEDURE 42-7 *(continued)*

Administering an Intramuscular Injection

Action	Rationale
11 Hold the syringe in your dominant hand between the thumb and forefinger. Quickly dart the needle into the tissue at a 90-degree angle.	A quick injection is less painful. Inserting the needle at a 90-degree angle facilitates entry into muscle tissue.

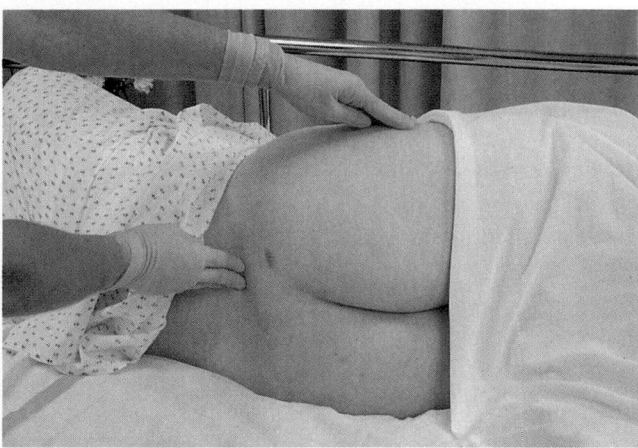

Action 7: Identifying landmarks for dorsogluteal injection site.

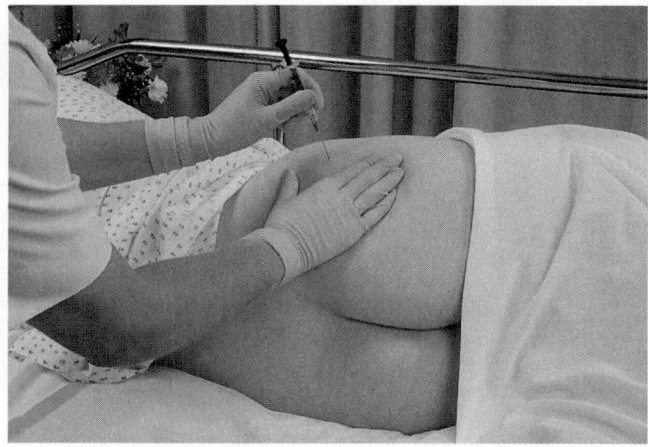

Actions 10 and 11: Spreading the skin at site and darting in at 90-degree angle.

Action	Rationale
12 As soon as the needle is in place, move your non-dominant hand to hold the lower end of the syringe. Slide your dominant hand to the tip of the barrel.	This acts to steady the syringe and allows for smooth aspiration.
13 Aspirate by slowly pulling back on the plunger to determine whether the needle is in a blood vessel. If blood is aspirated, discard the needle, syringe, and medication, prepare a new sterile setup, and inject another site.	Discomfort and possibly a serious reaction may occur if a drug intended for intramuscular use is injected into a vein.
14 If no blood is aspirated, inject the solution slowly, followed by the air bubble.	Injecting slowly helps to reduce discomfort by allowing time for the solution to disperse in the tissues.

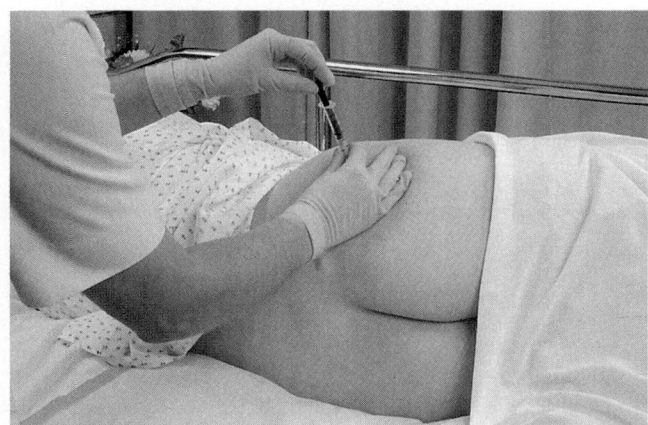

Action 13: Aspirating.

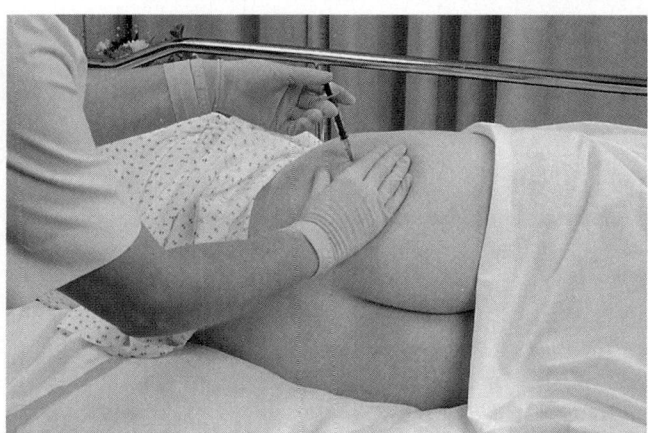

Action 14: Injecting.

(continued)

P R O C E D U R E 4 2 - 7 *(continued)*

Administering an Intramuscular Injection

Action	Rationale
15 Remove the needle quickly.	Slow removal of the needle pulls tissues and may cause discomfort.
16 Massage the injection site with the alcohol swab using gentle pressure.	Massaging helps to distribute the solution and hastens its absorption by increasing blood flow to the area.
17 Do not recap the used needle. Discard the needle and syringe in the appropriate receptacle.	Proper disposal of the needle protects the nurse from accidental injection. Most accidental puncture wounds occur when recapping needles.
18 Assist the client to a position of comfort.	This provides for the well-being of the client.
19 Remove gloves if worn, and dispose of them properly. Wash your hands.	Handwashing deters the spread of microorganisms.
20 Chart the administration of the medication.	Accurate documentation is necessary to prevent medication error.
21 Evaluate the response of the client to the medication within an appropriate time frame.	Reaction to medication given by the parenteral route may occur within 15 to 30 minutes after injection.

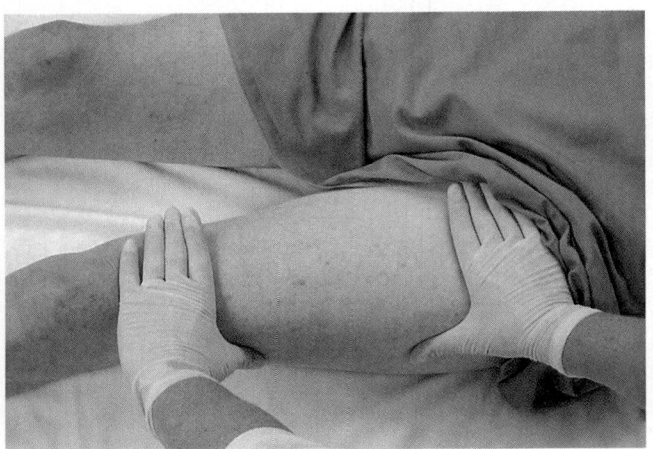

Action 7: Identifying vastus lateralis injection site.

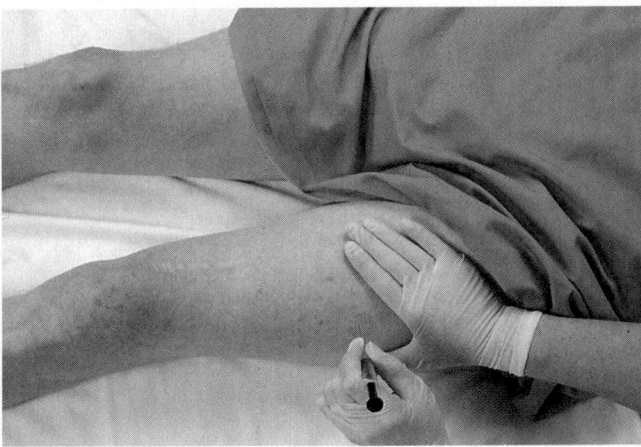

Action 11: Darting needle into the tissue. (Photos © B. Proud.)

Age Considerations

Safe administration of an intramuscular injection into an infant's vastus lateralis muscle may require use of a 1-inch needle rather than the commonly used ⅝-inch needle. A 1-inch needle consistently allows penetration into the muscle and safe administration of the medication.

intravenous solution, but sometimes the drug is added in the nursing unit, in which case sterile technique must be maintained. Steps for adding medications to intravenous solutions are given in Procedure 42-8.

When medication is administered by continuous infusion, the client receives it slowly and over a long period. Although sometimes this can be an advantage when it is desirable to give the medication slowly, it is a disadvantage when it is necessary for the client to receive the drug more quickly. Also, if for some reason all of the solution cannot be infused, the client will not receive the prescribed amount of the medication. The client receiving medication by a continuous intravenous infusion should be checked for possible adverse effects at least every hour.

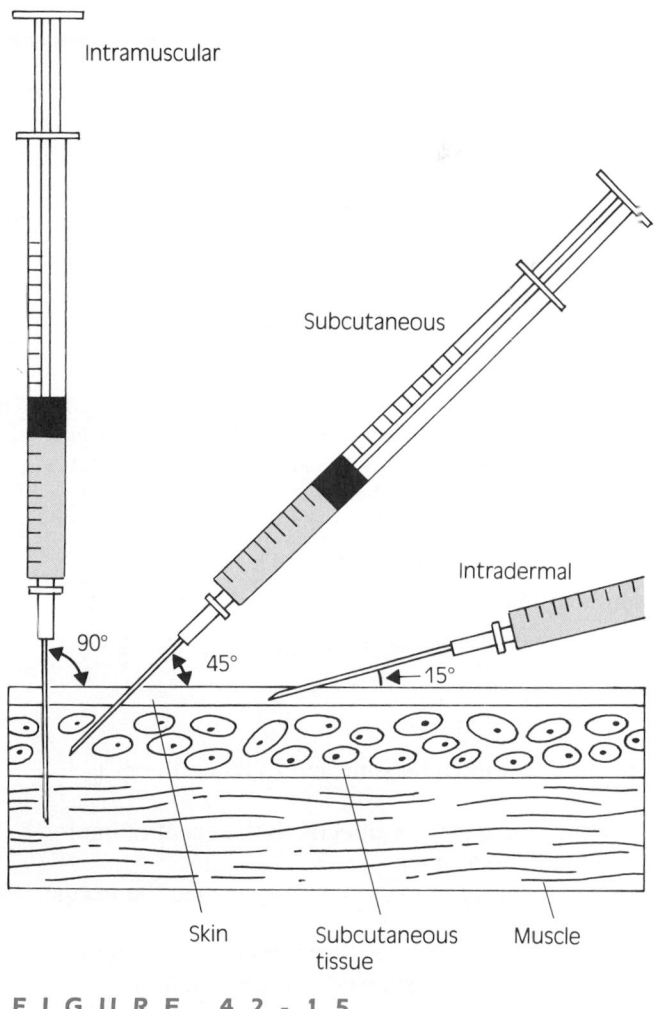

F I G U R E   4 2 - 1 5

Comparison of the angles of insertion for intramuscular, sub-cutaneous, and intradermal injections.

A medication can be administered as an intravenous **bolus**. A bolus dose of medication is a single injection of a concentrated solution administered directly into an intravenous line (see Procedure 42-9).

Medications can be administered by intermittent intravenous infusion. The drug is mixed with a small amount of the intravenous solution, such as 50 to 100 mL, and administered over a short period at the prescribed interval—for example, every 4 hours. The client with an intravenous line in place receives the solution containing the medication by way of a piggyback setup or a tandem setup (see Fig. 42-17). The intravenous **piggyback** delivery system requires the intermittent or additive solution to be placed higher than the primary solution container. An extension hook provided by the manufacturer provides for easy lowering of the main intravenous container. The port on the primary intravenous line has a backcheck valve that automatically stops the flow of the primary solution, allowing the secondary or piggyback solution to flow when connected. A **tandem** delivery setup is similar, except that both

solutions remain at the same height and there is no back-check valve at the secondary port on the primary line. If the two solutions are incompatible, the primary infusion may be temporarily clamped and the nurse must flush the primary intravenous tubing below the secondary port with a sterile solution (usually 0.9% sodium chloride solution) before and after the tandem intravenous administration. The nurse is responsible for calculating and manually adjusting the flow rate of the intravenous intermittent infusion or regulating the infusion with an infusion pump or controller. The intravenous piggyback setup is explained in Procedure 42-10.

Medications also can be placed in a controlled-volume administration set (Soluset, Buretrol) for intermittent intra-

(*Text continues on p. 1239*)

F I G U R E   4 2 - 1 6

The Z-track or zigzag technique is used to administer medications that are irritating to subcutaneous tissue. The skin is pulled to one side, blood is aspirated, and the solution is injected. When the needle is withdrawn and the displaced tissue is allowed to return to its normal position, the solution is prevented from escaping from the muscle tissue.

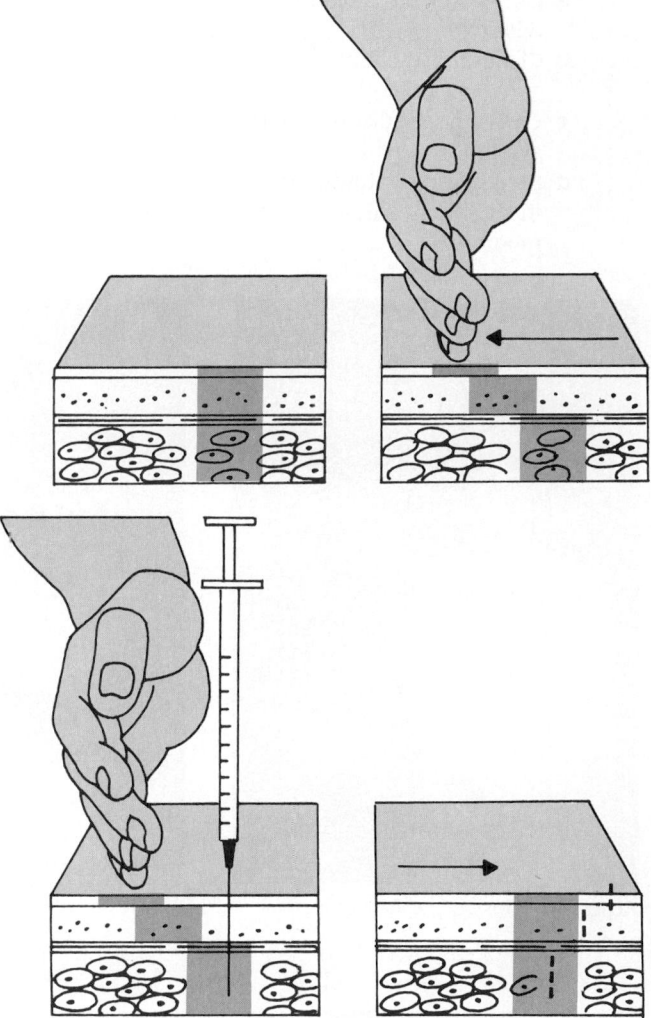

P R O C E D U R E   4 2 - 8

Adding Medications to an IV Solution Container

Equipment

Medication prepared in a syringe
  with a 19- to 21-gauge needle
Alcohol swab

IV fluid container (bag or bottle)
Label to be attached to the IV
  container

Action	Rationale
1 Gather all equipment and bring to the client's bedside. Check the medication order with the physician's order.	Having equipment available saves time and facilitates performance of the task. Checking the orders ensures that the client receives the correct medication at the correct time and in the right manner.
2 Explain the procedure to the client.	Explanation allays the client's anxiety.
3 Wash your hands.	Handwashing deters the spread of microorganisms.
4 Identify the client by checking the band on the client's wrist and asking the client his or her name.	This ensures that medication is given to the right person.
5 Add the medication to the IV solution that is infusing:	
a Check that the volume in the bag or bottle is adequate.	The volume should be sufficient to dilute the drug.
b Close the IV clamp.	This prevents backflow directly to the client of improperly diluted medication.
c Clean the medication port with an alcohol swab.	This deters entry of microorganisms when the needle punctures the port.
d Steady the container, uncap the needle, and insert the needle into the port. Inject the medication.	This ensures that the needle enters the container and medication can be dispersed into the solution.

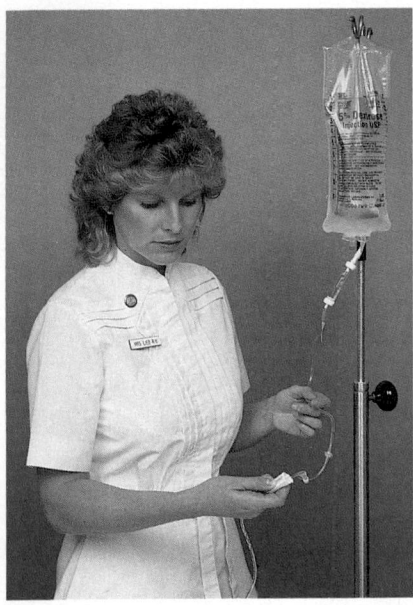

Action 5b: Closing the IV clamp.

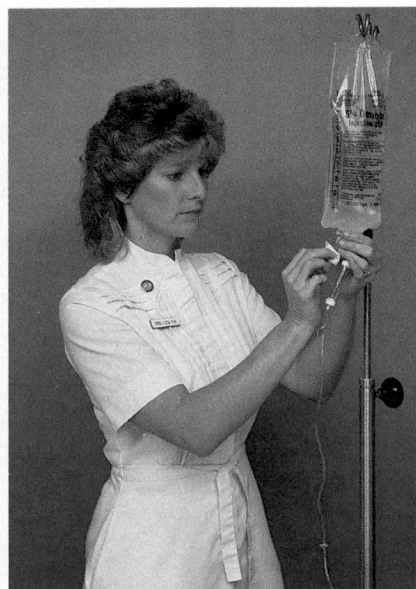

Action 5c: Cleaning the medication port.

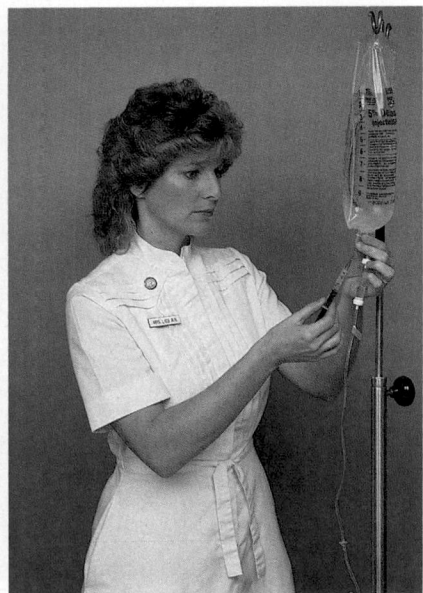

Action 5d: Inserting the needle into the port.

(continued)

PROCEDURE 42-8 (continued)

Adding Medications to an IV Solution Container

Action	Rationale

Action

e Remove the container from the IV pole and gently rotate the solution.

f Rehang the container, open the clamp, and readjust the flow rate.

g Attach the label to the container so that the dose of medication that has been added is apparent.

Rationale

This mixes the medication with the solution.

This ensures the infusion of the IV with medication at the prescribed rate.

This confirms that the prescribed dose of medication has been added to the IV solution.

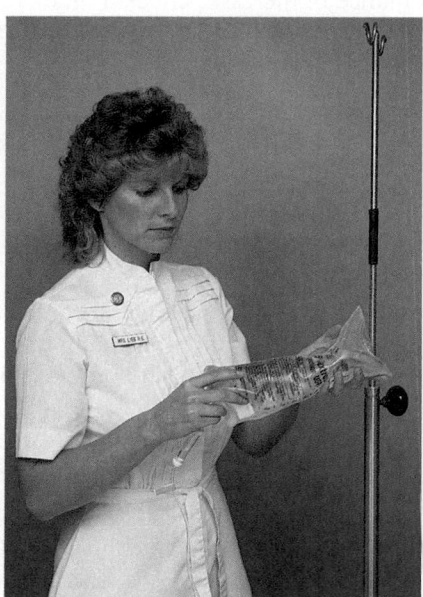

Action 5e: Rotating solution to distribute medication.

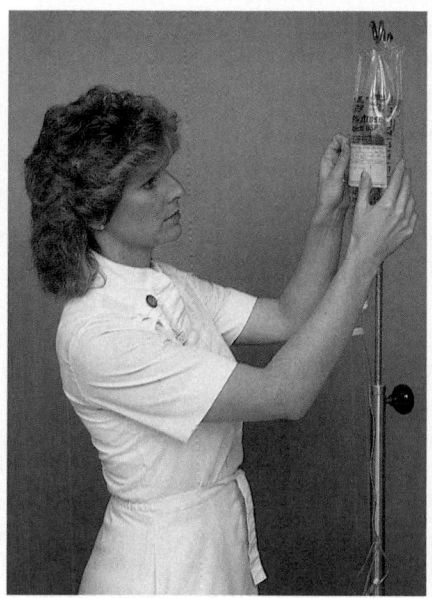

Action 5g: Labeling container to show medication. (Photos © Ken Kasper.)

6 Add the medication to the IV solution before infusion:

  a Carefully remove any protective cover and locate the injection port. Clean with an alcohol swab.

  This deters entry of microorganisms when the needle punctures the port.

  b Uncap the needle and insert into the port. Inject the medication.

  This ensures that the needle enters the container and that medication can be dispersed into the solution.

  c Withdraw the needle and insert the spike into the proper entry site on the bag or bottle.

  This punctures the seal in the IV bag or bottle.

  d With tubing clamped, gently rotate the IV solution in the bag or bottle. Hang the IV.

  This mixes medication with the solution.

  e Attach the label to the container so that the dose of medication that has been added is apparent.

  This confirms that the prescribed dose of medication has been added to the IV solution.

7 Dispose of equipment according to agency policy.

  This prevents inadvertent injury from the equipment.

8 Wash your hands.

  Handwashing deters the spread of microorganisms.

9 Chart the addition of medication to the IV solution.

  Accurate documentation is necessary to prevent medication errors.

10 Evaluate the client's response to medication within the appropriate time frame.

  Clients require careful observation because medications given by the IV route may have a rapid effect.

PROCEDURE 42-9

Adding a Bolus IV Medication to an Existing IV

Equipment

Medication prepared in a syringe with 23- to 25-gauge, 1-inch needle

Alcohol swab
Watch with second hand
Disposable gloves (optional)

Action	Rationale
1 Gather the equipment and bring to the client's bedside. Check the medication order with the physician's order.	Having the equipment available saves time and facilitates performance of the task. Checking the orders ensures that the client receives the correct medication at the correct time and in the right manner.
2 Explain the procedure to the client.	Explanation allays the client's anxiety.
3 Wash your hands.	Handwashing deters the spread of microorganisms.
4 Identify the client by checking the band on the client's wrist and asking the client his or her name.	This ensures that the medication is given to the right person.
5 Assess the IV site for the presence of inflammation or infiltration.	IV medication must be given directly into a vein for safe administration.
6 Select the injection port on the tubing that is closest to the venipuncture site. Clean the port with an alcohol swab.	Using the port closest to the needle insertion site minimizes dilution of the medication. Cleaning with alcohol deters entry of microorganisms when the needle punctures the port.
7 Uncap the syringe. Steady the port with your nondominant hand while inserting the needle into the center of the port.	This supports the injection port and lessens the risk of accidentally dislodging the IV or entering the port incorrectly.
8 Move your nondominant hand to the section of IV tubing just beyond the injection port. Fold the tubing between your fingers to temporarily stop the flow of the IV solution.	This minimizes the dilution of the IV medication with IV solution.
9 Pull back slightly on the plunger just until blood appears in the tubing.	This ensures injection of medication into a vein.
10 Inject the medication at the prescribed rate.	This delivers the correct amount of medication at the proper interval.

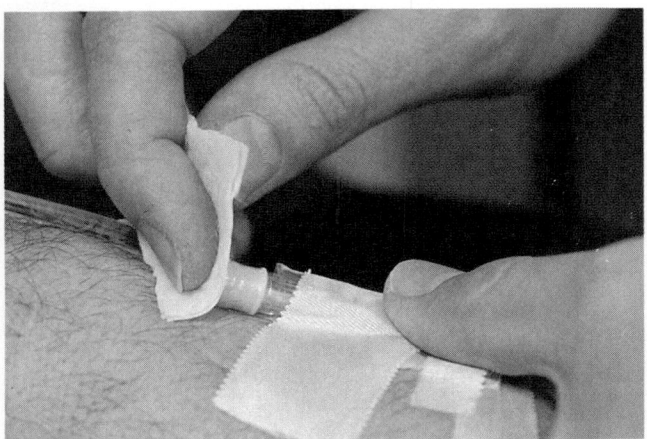

Action 6: Cleaning injection port.

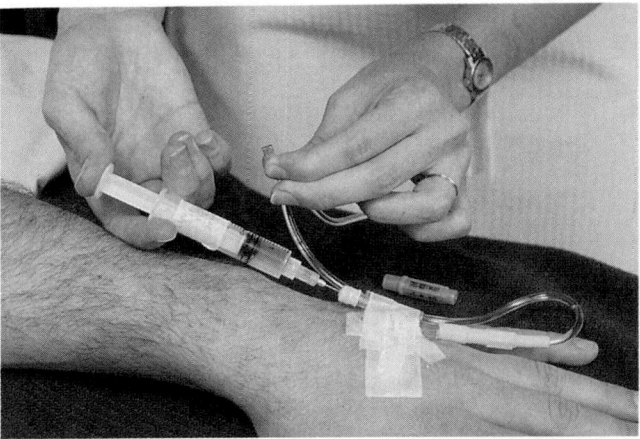

Action 10: Injecting medication while interrupting IV flow.

(continued)

PROCEDURE 4 2 - 9 (continued)

Adding a Bolus IV Medication to an Existing IV

Action	Rationale
11 Remove the needle. Do not cap it. Release the tubing and allow the IV to flow at the proper rate.	This prevent accidental needlestick.
12 Dispose of the needle and syringe in the proper receptacle.	Proper disposal of the needle prevents accidental injury and spread of microorganisms.
13 Wash your hands.	Handwashing deters the spread of microorganisms.
14 Chart the administration of the medication.	Accurate documentation is necessary to prevent medication errors.
15 Evaluate the client's response to the medication within the appropriate time frame.	The client requires careful observation because medications given by an IV bolus injection may have a rapid effect.

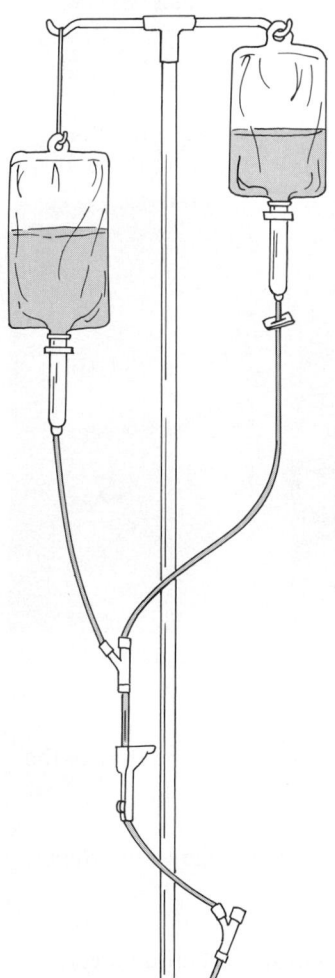

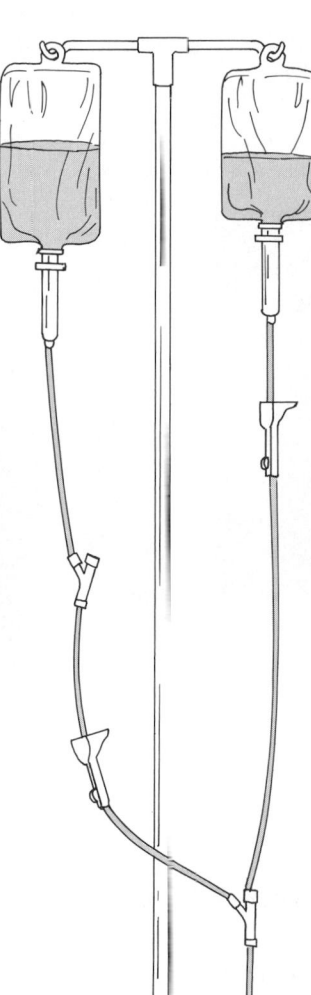

IV Piggyback delivery system   **IV Tandem delivery setup**

FIGURE 4 2 - 1 7

Piggyback and tandem setup for intermittent delivery of IV medications.

PROCEDURE 4 2 - 1 0

Administering Medications by IV Piggyback

Equipment

Medication preparation in labeled
  piggyback set (50 to 100 mL)
Secondary infusion tubing
  (microdrip or macrodrip)

Sterile needle (21 to 23 gauge)
Alcohol swab
Tape

Action	Rationale
1 Gather all equipment and bring to the client's bedside. Check the medication order against the original physician's order according to agency policy.	Having equipment available saves time and facilitates performance of the task. Checking the orders ensures that the client receives the correct medication at the correct time and in the right manner.
2 Explain the procedure to the client.	Explanation allays the client's anxiety.
3 Wash your hands.	Handwashing deters the spread of microorganisms.
4 Assess the IV site for the presence of inflammation or infiltration.	IV medications must be given directly into a vein for safe administration.
5 Attach the infusion tubing to the piggyback set containing diluted medication. Open the clamp and prime the tubing (see action 5, Procedure 42-8). Close the clamp. Connect the capped sterile needle to the sterile end of the tubing.	This removes air from the tubing and preserves the sterility of the setup.

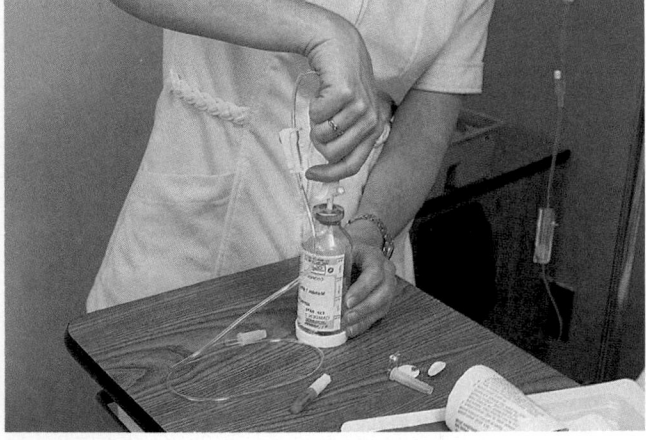

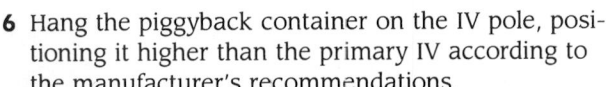

Action 5: Attaching infusion tubing to piggyback set containing medication.

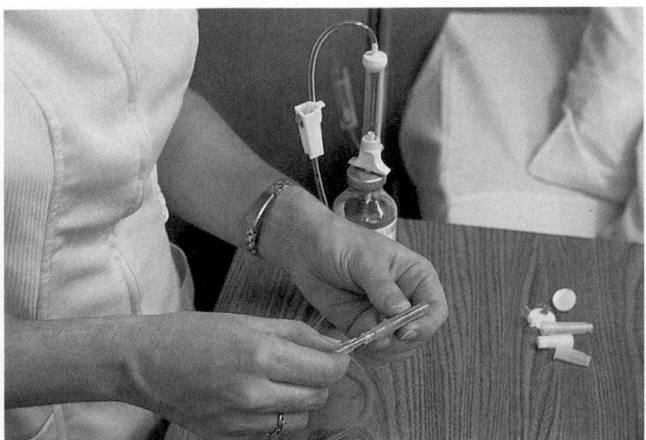

Action 5: Connecting capped sterile needle to tubing.

6 Hang the piggyback container on the IV pole, positioning it higher than the primary IV according to the manufacturer's recommendations.	The position of the container influences the flow of the IV fluid into the primary setup.
7 Identify the client by checking the identification band on the client's wrist and asking the client his or her name.	This ensures that the medication is given to the right person.
8 Use an alcohol swab to clean the secondary IV port.	This deters entry of microorganisms when the needle punctures the port.

(continued)

PROCEDURE 42-10 (continued)

Administering Medications by IV Piggyback

Action	Rationale
9 Remove the cap and insert the needle into the secondary port. Use a strip of tape to secure the secondary set tubing to the primary infusion tubing.	The tape stabilizes the needle in the infusion port and prevents it from slipping out.

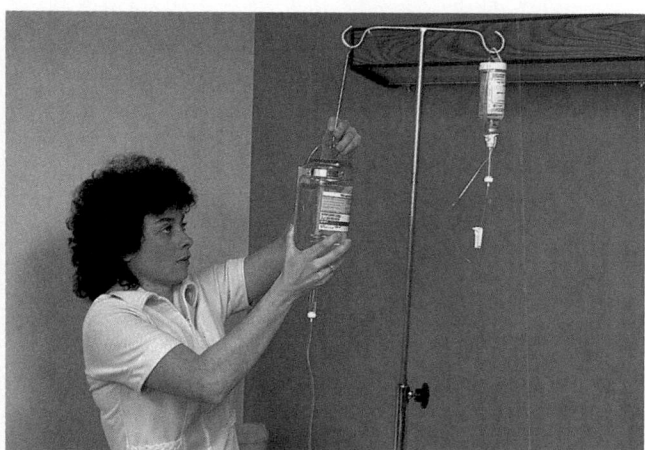

Action 6: Hanging on IV pole.

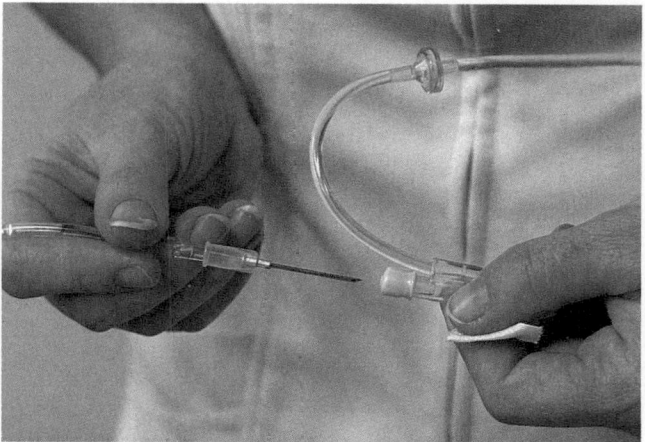

Action 9: Inserting needle into secondary port.

Action	Rationale
10 Open the clamp on the piggyback set and regulate the flow at the prescribed delivery rate. Monitor the medication infusion at periodic intervals.	Delivery over a 30- to 60-minute interval is a safe method of administering IV medication.
11 Clamp the tubing on the piggyback set when the solution is infused. Follow agency policy regarding disposal of equipment.	This reduces the risk of contaminating the primary IV setup.
12 Readjust the flow rate of the primary IV.	Piggyback medication administration may interrupt the normal flow rate of the primary IV. Readjustment of the rate may be necessary.
13 Wash your hands.	Handwashing deters the spread of microorganisms.
14 Chart the administration of medication after it has been infused.	Accurate documentation is necessary to prevent medication errors.
15 Evaluate the client's response to medication within the appropriate time frame.	The client requires careful observation because medications given by the IV route may have a rapid effect.

venous infusion. The medication is diluted with a small amount of solution and administered through the client's intravenous line (Procedure 42-11). This type of equipment is also used for infusing solutions into children and elderly clients when the volume of fluid infused must be carefully monitored.

A **heparin lock** is used for a client who requires intermittent intravenous medication but not a continuous intravenous infusion. This device consists of a needle or catheter connected to a short length of tubing capped with a sealed injection port. A heparin lock is shown in Figure 42-18. After the needle is in place in the client's vein, the needle and tubing are anchored to the client's arm so that the needle remains in place until the client no longer requires the repeated medication intravenously.

A heparin lock allows the client more freedom than a continuous intravenous infusion. The client is connected to the intravenous line when it is time to receive the medication and disconnected when the medication is completed. A saline flush rather than a heparin flush is used by many

P R O C E D U R E   4 2 - 1 1

Administering IV Medications by Volume-Control Administration Set

Equipment

Volume-control administration set
(50 to 100 mL)
Medication (in vial or
ampule)

Syringe with 20- or 21-gauge
needle attached
Alcohol swab
Medication label

Action

1 Gather all equipment and bring to the client's bedside. Check the medication order against the original physician's order according to agency policy.

2 Explain the procedure to the client.

3 Wash your hands.

4 Assess the IV site for the presence of inflammation or infiltration.

5 Withdraw medication from the vial or ampule into the prepared syringe. See Procedure 42-2 or 42-3.

6 Identify the client by checking the identification band on the client's wrist and asking the client his or her name.

7 Open the clamp between the IV solution and the volume-control administration set or secondary setup. Follow the manufacturer's instructions and fill with the desired amount of IV solution. Close the clamp.

8 Use an alcohol swab to clean the injection port on the secondary setup.

9 Remove the cap and insert the needle into the port while holding the syringe steady. Inject the medication. Mix gently with IV solution.

Rationale

Having equipment available saves time and facilitates performance of the task. Checking of the orders ensures that the client receives the correct medication at the correct time and in the right manner.

Explanation allays the client's anxiety.

Handwashing deters the spread of microorganisms.

IV medications must be given directly into a vein for safe administration.

The correct dose is prepared for dilution in the IV solution.

This ensures that medication is given to the right person.

This dilutes the medication in the minimal amount of solution. Reclamping prevents the continued addition of fluid to the volume to be mixed with the medication.

This deters entry of microorganisms when the needle punctures the port.

This ensures that the medication is evenly mixed with solution.

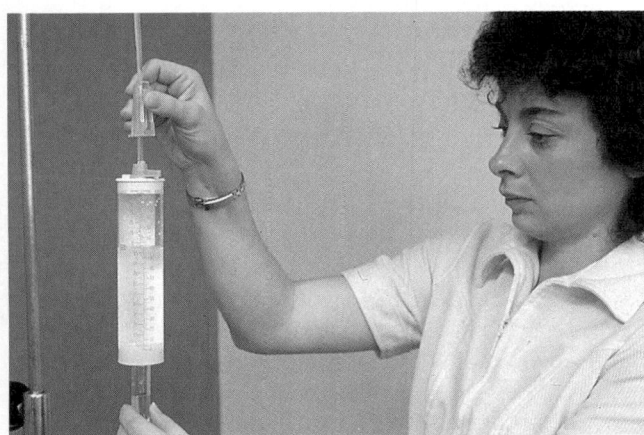

Action 7: Filling volume-control set.

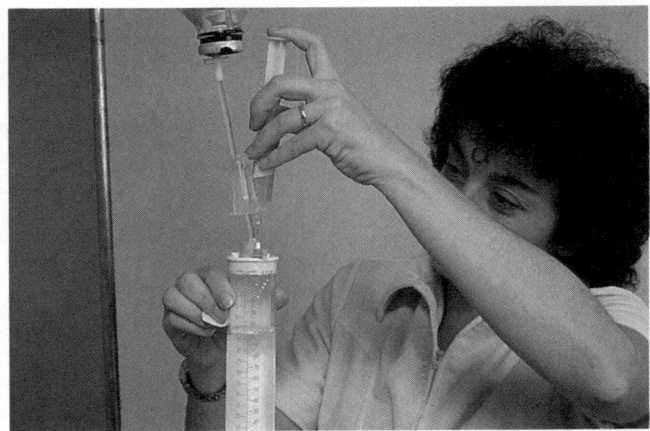

Action 9: Injecting medication.

(continued)

PROCEDURE 42-11 (continued)

Administering IV Medications by Volume-Control Administration Set

Action	Rationale
10 Open the clamp below the secondary setup and regulate at the prescribed delivery rate. Monitor the medication infusion at periodic intervals.	Delivery over a 30- to 60-minute interval is a safe method of administering IV medication.
11 Attach the label to the volume-control device.	This prevents medication error.
12 Place the syringe with the uncapped needle in the designated container.	Proper disposal of the needle prevents inadvertent needlestick.
13 Wash your hands.	Handwashing deters the spread of microorganisms.
14 Chart the administration of the medication after it has been infused.	Accurate documentation is necessary to prevent medication errors.
15 Evaluate the client's response to the medication within the appropriate time frame.	The client requires careful observation because medications given by the IV route may have a rapid effect.

institutions to maintain patency of the heparin lock. Using saline eliminates any possible systemic effects on coagulation or drug incompatibility that may occur when a heparin solution is used. The intermittent infusion is not started until the nurse confirms intravenous placement. The heparin lock is flushed after the infusion is completed to clear the vein of any medication and to prevent clot formation in the needle. The procedure for flushing an intravenous or heparin lock with saline is discussed in Procedure 42-12. The intravenous site is assessed for complications discussed in Chapter 37. If infiltration or phlebitis occurs, the heparin lock is removed and replaced in a new site.

Intermittent intravenous medication may be administered through a catheter placed in the subclavian vein. Medications are prepared under laminar flow in a sterile environment if they are to be administered through a central intravenous line, such as a Hickman catheter. Aseptic technique is observed when the nurse administers medications through a central intravenous line. All connections are cleaned with povidone–iodine for its antiseptic properties.

FIGURE 42-18

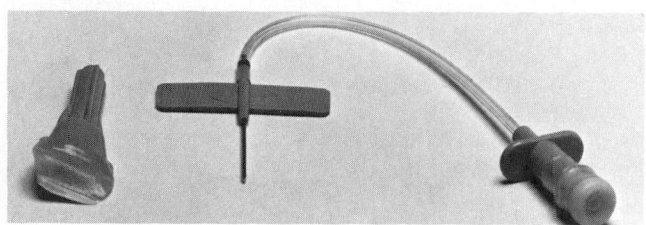

The heparin lock is a small IV tube with a self-sealing plug at the end into which medications can be injected.

Administering Topical Medications

When a drug is applied directly to a body site, it is called a **topical application**. Other terms used include the *dermal* and *mucosal route*.

Topical applications usually are intended for direct action on a particular site, although some systemic effect may also occur. The action depends on the type of tissue and the nature of the agent.

If the site of application is readily accessible, such as the skin, an agent can easily be placed on it. If it is a cavity, such as the nose, or is enclosed, such as the eye, it is necessary to use a mechanical applicator for introducing the drug.

Skin Applications

The skin is a mechanical and chemical barrier that protects the underlying tissues. It is a sense organ, having receptors that respond to touch, pain, pressure, and temperature. The skin helps in excretion, in regulating body temperature, and in storing essentials to the body, such as water, salts, and glucose.

When a drug is incorporated in an agent, such as an ointment, and rubbed into the skin for absorption, the procedure is referred to as an *inunction*. On normal skin, drugs are absorbed into the lining of the sebaceous glands. Absorption is hindered because of the protective outer layer of the skin, which makes penetration difficult, and because of the fatty substances that protect the lining of the glands. Absorption can be enhanced by cleaning the skin well with soap or detergent and water before administration and then rubbing the medicated preparation into the skin. Absorption can also be improved by using a drug mixed in an

(Text continues on p. 1244)

PROCEDURE 42-12

Introducing Drugs Through a Heparin or Intravenous Lock Using the Saline Flush

Equipment

Medication
Medication card, Kardex, or printout
Saline vial
Sterile syringe with 25-gauge
  needle
Alcohol swabs

Watch with second hand or digital
  readout
Disposable gloves
For bolus injection
  Sterile syringe with medication
  and 25-gauge needle

For intermittent IV delivery
  IV setup with 25-gauge needle
  attached to tubing
  Additional sterile 25-gauge needle
  Adhesive tape
  IV pump or controller (optional)

Action

1 Assemble the equipment and check the physician's order.

2 Explain the procedure to the client.

3 Wash your hands.

4 Withdraw 1 to 2 mL of sterile saline from the vial into the syringe as described in Procedure 42-3.

5 Don the clean gloves.

6 Administer the medication.
  For bolus IV injection·
  a Check the drug package for the correct injection rate for the IV push route.
  b Clean the port of the lock with an alcohol swab.
  c Stabilize the port with your nondominant hand and insert the needle on the syringe into the port.
  d Gently inject the medication, using a watch to verify correct injection rate. Do not force the injection if resistance is felt. If the lock is clogged, it has to be changed. Remove the medication syringe and needle when administration is completed.

Rationale

This ensures that the client receives the right medication at the right time by the proper route.

Explanation alleviates the client's apprehension about IV drug administration.

Handwashing deters the spread of microorganisms.

Using saline eliminates concern about drug incompatibilities and effect on systemic circulation that exists with heparin flush.

Gloves protect the nurse's hands from contact with the client's blood.

Using the correct injection rate prevents speed shock from occurring.
Cleaning removes surface bacteria at the heparin lock entry site.
This allows for careful insertion of the needle into the center circle of the lock.

Easy instillation of the medication usually indicates that the lock is still patent and in the vein.

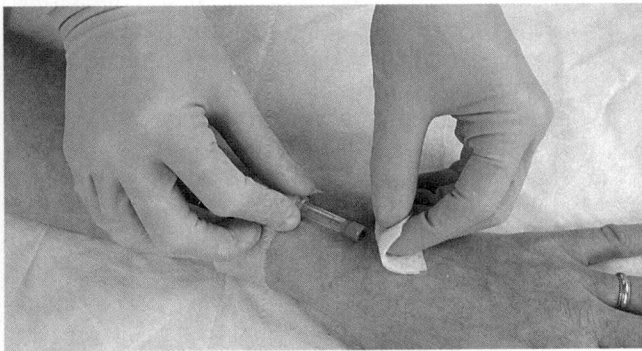

Action 6b: Cleaning the port (bolus injection).

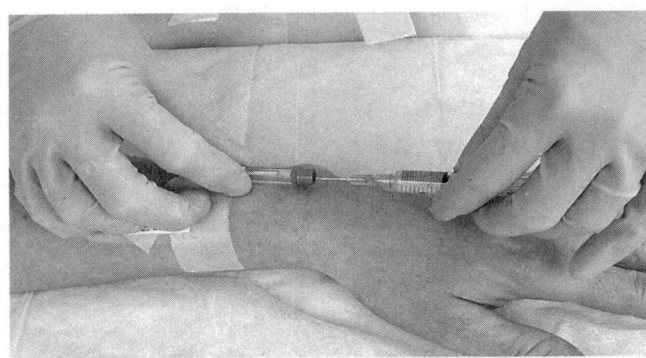

Action 6c: Stabilizing the port while inserting the needle (bolus injection).

(continued)

Introducing Drugs Through a Heparin or Intravenous Lock Using the Saline Flush

Action	Rationale
For administration of a drug by way of an intermittent delivery system:	
a Use a drug resource book to check for the correct flow rate of the medication. (The usual rate is 30 to 60 minutes.)	Using the correct injection rate prevents speed shock from occurring.
b Connect the infusion tubing to the medication setup according to the manufacturer's directions. Hang the IV setup on a pole. Open clamp and allow solution to clear IV tubing of air. Reclamp tubing.	This removes air from the tubing and preserves the sterility of the setup.
c Attach sterile 25-gauge needle to the end of the infusion tubing.	A small-gauge needle prevents damage to the lock.
d Clean the port of the lock with an alcohol swab. Stabilize the port with your nondominant hand and insert the needle on the tubing into the port. Secure with tape.	Cleaning removes surface bacteria at the lock entry site. Tape secures the needle in the lock port.
e Open the clamp and regulate the flow rate or attach to IV pump or controller according to manufacturer's directions. Close clamp when infusion is complete.	This ensures that the client receives the medication at the correct rate.
f Remove the needle from lock. Carefully replace the uncapped used needle on the tubing with a sterile covered needle. Allow the medication setup to hang on the pole for future use according to agency policy.	This prevents possible needlestick with contaminated needle. Agency policy specifies length of time for safe use of IV infusion tubing.
g Dispose of uncapped used needle appropriately.	This prevents possible needlestick injury.

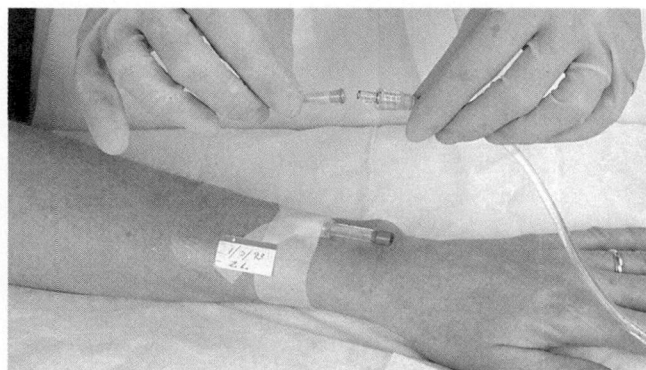

Action 6c: Attaching the sterile needle to the end of the infusion tubing (intermittent delivery).

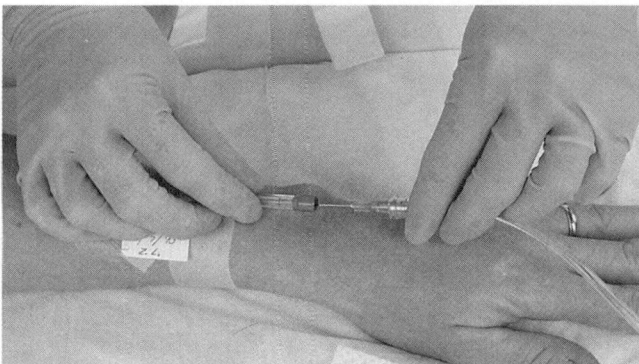

Action 6d: Stabilizing the port while inserting the needle into the port (intermittent delivery). [Photos © B. Proud.]

7 Insert the needle of the syringe containing saline and flush the reservoir with 1 to 2 mL of sterile saline. Remove the syringe and needle and discard in the appropriate receptacle. Remove gloves and discard appropriately.	Saline clears the line of medication with less of the systemic effects of the heparin flush.

(continued)

PROCEDURE 42-12 *(continued)*

Introducing Drugs Through a Heparin or Intravenous Lock Using the Saline Flush

Action	Rationale
8 Wash your hands.	Handwashing deters the spread of microorganisms.
9 The injection site and IV lock should be checked at least every 8 hours and a small amount of saline administered if medication is not given at least that often.	This ensures the patency of the system for continuing injections.
10 The heparin lock should be changed at least every 48 hours or according to agency policy. A clogged lock should be changed immediately.	Changing a heparin lock regularly and having it free of clotted blood reduces dangers of infection and emboli in the circulating blood.
11 Chart the administration of the medication or saline flush.	Accurate documentation is necessary to prevent medication error.

Safety Considerations   Some agencies recommend the use of single-dose saline vials without preservatives in the solution. Preservatives may be linked to an increased incidence of phlebitis with heparin locks.

---

ointment or added to a liniment that will mix with the fat in the gland lining. The following are typical preparations applied to skin areas and their primary purposes:

Powders—to promote drying of the skin and prevent friction on the skin

Ointments—to provide prolonged contact of a medication on the skin and soften the skin

Creams and oils—to lubricate and soften the skin and prevent drying of the skin

Lotions—to protect and soothe the skin

GUIDELINES FOR NURSING CARE

Applying Topical Medications

- Be sure the skin is dry and clean before applying anything on it. Previous preparations usually are removed before applying additional medication, except in the case of lotions used for soothing the skin.
- Clean the skin with detergent or soap and water before administering a preparation to the skin. This technique removes substances from the skin that will delay absorption of the drug and prevents debris from interfering with the desired actions.
- Apply local heat to the area, when indicated. This measure promotes absorption by improving blood circulation to the area.
- Shake lotions, which are suspensions of powder, before using so that the active ingredient reaches the skin in desired amounts. Apply lotions with cotton balls or gauze.
- Thoroughly massage creams and ointments into intact skin, or, if this is contraindicated, pat them onto the skin with the fingers.
- Warm the preparation in the hands or fingers if a large part of the body is to be covered, such as the back. This technique helps prevent the client from feeling chilly.
- Keep powders away from the nose and mouth to prevent the client from inhaling them. If they are applied on or near the face, apply then while the client exhales.
- Follow the manufacturer's directions regarding use of gloves for skin applications.
- Apply nitroglycerin ointment as prescribed in centimeters or inches, measuring the ordered amount on a special paper or plastic applicator.
- Always wear gloves when applying nitroglycerin ointment to the skin because some of the medication can be absorbed through the skin of your fingers.
- For a nitroglycerin transdermal patch, apply firm pressure, especially around edges, to ensure contact with the skin. Apply to a hairless site and remove the previous patch before applying the new one.
- Wear gloves, as indicated, especially when the client has a disease condition that is infectious.

Counterirritants—to relieve discomfort

Astringents and alcohol—to cool and dry the skin

See Nursing Guidelines for Applying Topical Medications.

Eye Instillations and Irrigations

The receptors for the sense of sight are located in the eye. The outer layer of the eyeball is called the *sclera*. The cornea is the transparent part of the sclera in front of the eyeball. The sclera is fibrous and tough, but the cornea is easily injured by trauma. For this reason, applications to the eye seldom are placed directly onto the eyeball.

Because direct application cannot be made onto the sensitive cornea, applications intended to act on the eye or the lids are placed onto, or instilled or irrigated into, the lower conjunctival sac.

The eye is a delicate organ, highly susceptible to infection and injury. Although the eye is never free of microorganisms, the secretions of the conjunctiva have a protective action against many pathogens. For maximum safety for the client, equipment, solutions, and ointments introduced into the conjunctival sac should be sterile. If this is not possible, the most careful measures of medical asepsis should be followed.

Eyedrops Instillation of eyedrops is performed for their local effects, such as for pupil dilatation or constriction when examining the eye or for treating an infection. The type and amount of solution depend on the purpose of the instillation.

Exposing the lower conjunctival sac is necessary for eye instillations. It is important to work carefully and gently to avoid injuring the conjunctiva and the eyeball when exposing the sac. This is particularly important when the lids are swollen, inflamed, or tender. See Nursing Guidelines for Instilling Eyedrops and Figure 42-19 for techniques used to expose the lower conjunctival sac and instill eyedrops.

Ointments Various types of medication in an ointment form may be prescribed for the eye. These ointments usually are used in the presence of a local infection or irritation. Eye ointments are dispensed in a tube. A small amount of ointment is distributed along the exposed lower conjunctival sac after the eyelids and eyelashes have been cleansed. About ½ inch of ointment is squeezed from the tube along the exposed sac. After the application, the eyes should be closed. The warmth helps to liquefy the ointment. Also, the client should be instructed to move the eye because this helps to spread ointment under the lids and over the surface of the eyeball.

Eye Irrigation An eye **irrigation** is performed to remove secretions from the eye. In an emergency, eye irrigation can

---

GUIDELINES FOR NURSING CARE

Instilling Eyedrops

- Offer the client paper tissues to remove solution and tears that may spill from the eye during the procedure.
- Clean the eyelids and eyelashes of any drainage with cotton balls or gauze pledgets moistened with normal saline solution because debris can be carried into the eye when the conjunctival sac is exposed. Use each cotton ball for only one stroke, moving from the inner toward the outer canthus to prevent carrying debris to the lacrimal ducts. (Disposable gloves should be worn if drainage is present.)
- Tilt the client's head back slightly if sitting, or place the client's head over a pillow if lying down. The head may be turned slightly to the affected side to prevent solution or tears from flowing toward the opposite eye.
- Draw up only sufficient solution required for the eyedrops. Hold the dropper with the bulb higher than the dropper. Allowing solution to enter the bulb by holding the bulb lower than the dropper may result in contaminating the solution with particles in the bulb. Unused solution should not be returned to a stock bottle. A monodrip plastic container also may be used to instill eyedrops.

- Have the client look up while focusing on something on the ceiling.
- Place the thumb or two fingers near the margin of the lower eyelid immediately below the eyelashes, and exert pressure downward over the bony prominence of the cheek. The lower conjunctival sac is exposed as the lower lid is pulled down.
- Hold the dropper close to the eye, but avoid touching the eyelids or lashes, which may startle the client and cause blinking. Also, avoid touching the eyeball with the dropper because this could easily injure the eye.
- Allow the prescribed number of drops to fall in the lower conjunctival sac. Do not allow drops to fall onto the cornea because of the danger of injuring it and the unpleasant sensation it causes the client.
- Release the lower lid after the eyedrops are instilled. Ask the client to gently close the eyes.
- Apply gentle pressure over the inner canthus to prevent the eyedrops from flowing into the tear duct. This minimizes the risk of systemic effects from the medication.

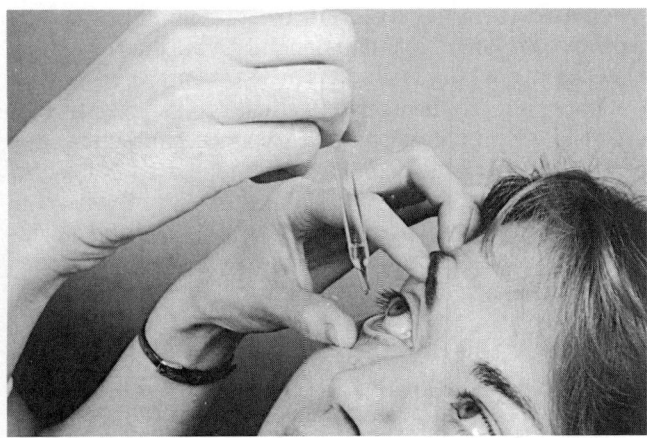

F I G U R E   4 2 - 1 9

The nurse exposes the lower conjunctiva of the eye, where he or she places eyedrops by having the patient look up and by applying pressure downward over the bony prominence of the cheek. If drainage is present, the nurse should wear disposable gloves. (Photo © Ken Kasper.)

be used to remove chemicals that may burn the eye. Copious amounts of tap water should be used to remove chemicals such as acid. The irrigation should continue for at least 15 minutes, and then professional help should be sought.

The techniques for administering a conjunctival irrigation are described in Procedure 42-13.

Ear Instillations and Irrigations

The ear contains the receptors for hearing and for equilibrium. It consists of the external ear, the middle ear, and the inner ear. The external ear consists of the auricle or pinna and the exterior auditory canal. The auditory canal serves as a passageway for sound waves. Drugs or irrigations are instilled into the auditory canal.

Drugs in solution are placed in the auditory canal for their local effect. They are used to soften wax, relieve pain, apply local anesthesia, destroy organisms, or destroy an insect lodged in the canal, which can cause almost intolerable discomfort.

The tympanic membrane separates the external ear from the middle ear. Normally, it is intact and closes the entrance to the middle ear completely. If it is ruptured or has been opened by surgical intervention, the middle ear and the inner ear have a direct passage to the external ear. When this occurs, instillations and irrigations should be performed with the greatest of care to prevent forcing materials from the outer ear into the middle ear and the inner ear. Sterile technique is used to prevent infection.

Ear Drops   The techniques listed in the Guidelines for Nursing Care are recommended to place drops in the external auditory canal.

G U I D E L I N E S   F O R   N U R S I N G   C A R E

Instilling Ear Drops

- Warm the solution to be instilled to body temperature to minimize discomfort for the client.
- Clean the external ear of drainage with cotton balls moistened with normal saline solution, as necessary. (Disposable gloves should be worn if drainage is present.)
- Place the client on the unaffected side in bed, or if ambulatory, have the client sit with the head well tilted to the side so that the affected ear is uppermost. This positioning prevents the drops from escaping from the ear.
- Draw up the amount of solution needed in the dropper. Excess medication should not be returned to a stock bottle.
- Straighten the auditory canal by pulling the cartilaginous portion of the pinna up and back in an adult and down and back in an infant or a child under age 3 years. In an adult, the auditory canal is directed inward, forward, and down. In a child, it is chiefly cartilaginous and almost straight, with the floor of the auditory canal resting on the tympanic membrane. Pulling on the pinna as described helps to straighten the canal properly for ear instillation.

- Hold the dropper in the ear with its tip above the auditory canal. For an infant or an irrational or restless client, protect the dropper with a piece of soft tubing to help prevent injury to the ear.
- Allow the drops to fall on the side of the canal. It is uncomfortable for the client if drops fall directly onto the tympanic membrane.
- Release the pinna after instilling the drops, and have the client maintain the position to prevent the escape of the medication.
- Gently press on the tragus a few times to help move the medication from the canal toward the tympanic membrane.
- Insert a loose, cotton wick when continuous application of the medication in the canal is desired. The wick should be removed 30 minutes after insertion. A tightly packed wick is contraindicated because it interferes with outward movement of secretions and may cause excessive pressure.
- Wait 5 minutes before instilling drops in the second ear, if ordered.

PROCEDURE 42-13

Administering an Eye Irrigation

Equipment

Sterile irrigating solution (warmed to 37°C [98.6°F])

Sterile irrigation set (sterile container and irrigating or bulb syringe)

Cotton balls

Emesis basin or irrigation basin

Disposable gloves (optional)

Waterproof pad

Towel

Action	Rationale
1 Explain procedure to client.	Explanation facilitates cooperation and reassures the client.
2 Assemble equipment.	This provides for an organized approach to the task.
3 Wash your hands.	Handwashing deters the spread of microorganisms.
4 Have the client sit or lie with the head tilted toward the side of the affected eye. Protect the client and the bed with a waterproof pad.	Gravity aids the flow of solution away from the unaffected eye and from the inner canthus of the affected eye toward the outer canthus.
5 Don disposable gloves if infection is present. Clean the lids and the lashes with a cotton ball moistened with normal saline or the solution ordered for the irrigation. Wipe from the inner to the outer canthus. Discard the cotton ball after each wipe.	Materials lodged on the lids or in the lashes may be washed into the eye. This cleaning motion protects the nasolacrimal duct and the other eye.
6 Place the curved basin at the cheek on the side of the affected eye to receive the irrigating solution. If the client is sitting up, ask him or her to support the basin.	Gravity aids the flow of solution.
7 Expose the lower conjunctival sac and hold the upper lid open with your nondominant hand.	The solution is directed onto the lower conjunctival sac because the cornea is sensitive and easily injured. This also prevents reflex blinking.

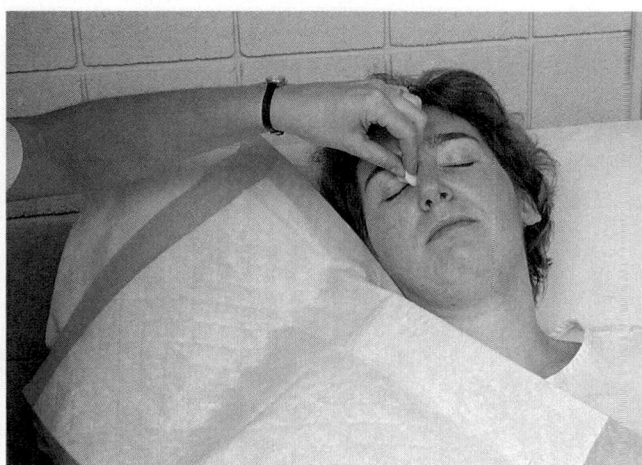

Action 5: Cleaning lids and lashes from inside of eye to outside.

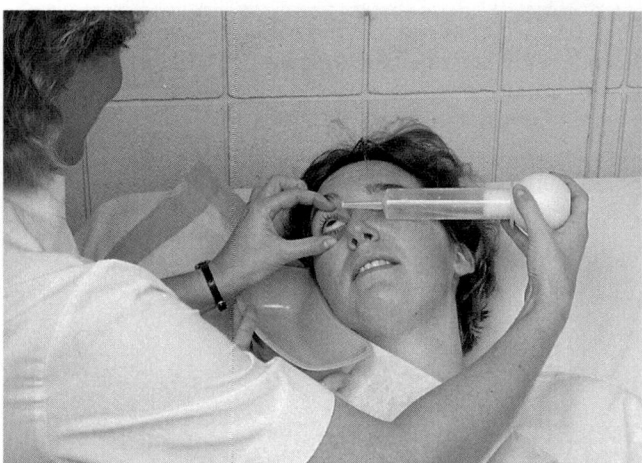

Action 7: Preparing to irrigate the eye. (Photos © Ken Kasper.)

(continued)

PROCEDURE 42-13 (continued)

Administering an Eye Irrigation

Action	Rationale
8 Hold the irrigator about 2.5 cm (1 inch) from the eye. Direct the flow of the solution from the inner to the outer canthus along the conjunctival sac.	This minimizes the risk of injury to the cornea. Solution directed toward the outer canthus helps to prevent the spread of contamination from the eye to the lacrimal sac, the lacrimal duct, and the nose.
9 Irrigate until the solution is clear or all of the solution has been used. Use only sufficient force gently to remove secretions from the conjunctiva. Avoid touching any part of the eye with the irrigating tip.	Directing solutions with force may cause injury to the tissues of the eye, as well as to the conjunctiva. Touching the eye is uncomfortable for the client.
10 Have the client close the eye periodically during the procedure.	Movement of the eye when the lids are closed helps to move secretions from the upper to the lower conjunctival sac.
11 Dry the area after the irrigation with cotton balls or a gauze sponge. Offer a towel to the client if the face and neck are wet.	Leaving the skin moist after an irrigation is uncomfortable for the client.
12 Wash your hands.	Handwashing deters the spread of microorganisms.
13 Chart the irrigation, appearance of the eye, drainage, and the client's response.	This provides accurate documentation.

Figure 42-20 shows a nurse about to instill drops into an adult's ear. Figure 42-21 shows the instillation of ear drops for a child.

Ear Irrigations Irrigations of the external auditory canal are ordinarily performed for cleaning purposes or for applying heat to the area. Typically, NSS, is used, although an antiseptic solution may be indicated for local action. An irrigation syringe is used in most instances. An irrigating container with tubing and an ear tip also may be used, especially if the purpose of the irrigation is to apply heat to the area. The techniques for administering an irrigation of the external auditory canal are described in Procedure 42-14.

FIGURE 42-20

The nurse pulls the pinna of the ear up and back to straighten the ear canal in adult patients. He or she then places eardrops on the side of the canal. Disposable gloves should be worn if drainage is present.

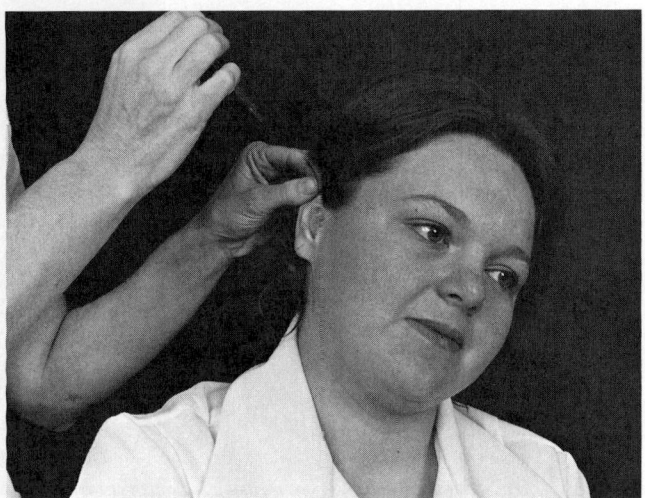

FIGURE 42-21

The nurse pulls the pinna of the ear down and back to straighten the auditory canal in children. He or she then places the eardrops on the side of the canal. Disposable gloves should be worn if drainage is present.

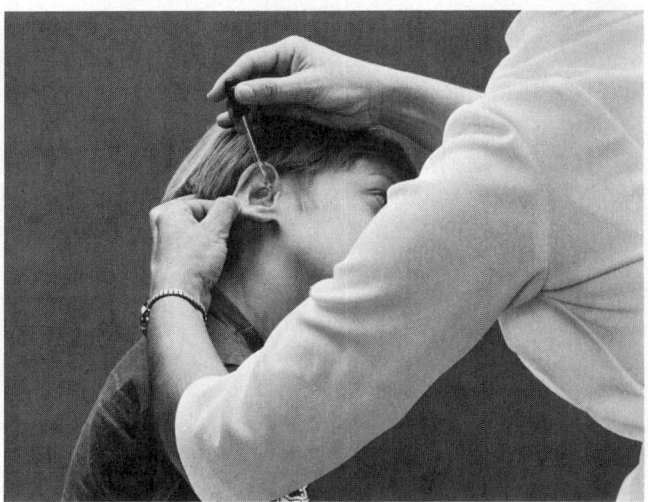

PROCEDURE 42-14

Administering an Ear Irrigation

Equipment

Prescribed irrigating solution
(warmed to 37°C [98.6°F])
Irrigation set (container and
irrigating or bulb syringe)

Emesis basin
Cotton-tipped applicators
Disposable gloves (optional)

Cotton balls
Waterproof pad

Action	Rationale
1 Explain the procedure to the client.	Explanation facilitates cooperation and provides reassurance for the client.
2 Assemble the equipment. Protect the client and bed linens with a moisture-proof pad.	This provides for an organized approach to the task.
3 Wash your hands.	Handwashing deters the spread of microorganisms.
4 Have the client sit up or lie with the head tilted toward the side of the affected ear. Have the client support a basin under the ear to receive the irrigating solution.	Gravity causes the irrigating solution to flow from the ear to the basin.
5 Clean the pinna and the meatus at the auditory canal as necessary with the applicators dipped in normal saline or the irrigating solution.	Materials lodged on the pinna and at the meatus may be washed into the ear.
6 Fill the bulb syringe with solution. If an irrigating container is used, allow air to escape from the tubing.	Air forced into the ear canal is noisy and therefore unpleasant for the client.
7 Straighten the auditory canal by pulling the pinna down and back for an infant and up and back for an adult.	Straightening the ear canal aids in allowing solution to reach all areas of the canal easily.
8 Direct a steady, slow stream of solution against the roof of the auditory canal, using only sufficient force to remove secretions. Do not occlude the auditory canal with the irrigating nozzle. Allow solution to flow out unimpeded.	Solution directed at the roof of the canal aids in preventing injury to the tympanic membrane. Continuous in-and-out flow of the irrigating solution helps to prevent pressure in the canal.

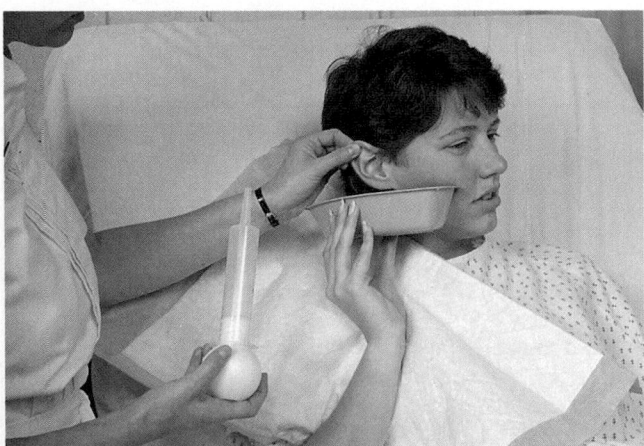

Action 7: Straightening the auditory canal.

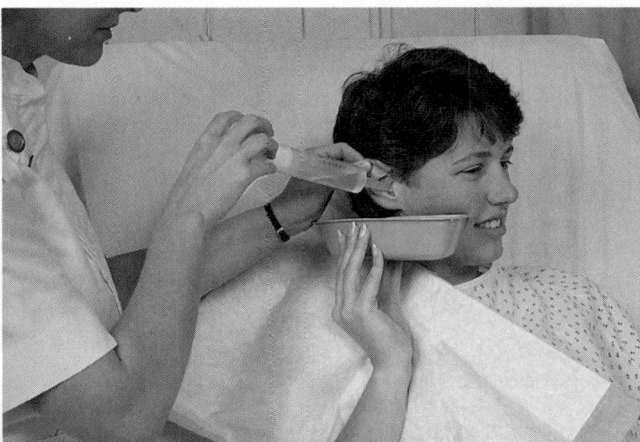

Action 8: Instilling irrigation fluid. (Photos © Ken Kasper.)

(continued)

PROCEDURE 4 2 - 1 4 *(continued)*

Administering an Ear Irrigation

Action	Rationale
9 When the irrigation is completed, place a cotton ball loosely in the auditory meatus and have the client lie on the side of the affected ear on a towel or an absorbent pad.	The cotton ball absorbs excess fluid and gravity allows the remaining solution in the canal to escape from the ear.
10 Wash your hands.	Handwashing deters the spread of microorganisms.
11 Chart the irrigation, the appearance of the drainage, and the client's response.	This provides accurate documentation.
12 Return in 10 to 15 minutes and remove the cotton ball and assess drainage.	Drainage or pain may indicate injury to the tympanic membrane.

Nasal Instillations

Besides serving as the olfactory organ, the nose functions as an airway to the lower respiratory tract and protects the tract by cleaning and warming the air taken in by inspiration. Cilia project on most of the surfaces of the nasal mucous membrane and are important in helping to remove particles of dirt and dust from the inspired air. The nose also serves as a resonator when speaking and singing.

Nasal instillations are used to treat sinus infections and nasal congestion. Medications that have a systemic effect, such as vasopressin, may also be prepared as a nasal instillation. The nose normally is not a sterile cavity, but because of its connection with the sinuses, medical asepsis should be carefully observed when using nasal instillations. See Nursing Guidelines for Instilling Nose Drops and Figure 42-22 for recommended techniques to instill nose drops.

Solutions that are instilled by drops may also be applied to the nasal mucous membrane by using a spray. A small atomizer is used. The end of the nose is held up, and the tip of the nozzle is placed just inside the nares and directed backward. Only sufficient force to bring the spray into contact with the membrane is used. Too much force may drive the solution and contamination into the sinuses and eustachian tubes.

Vaginal Applications

A healthy vagina contains few pathogens but many nonpathogenic organisms. The nonpathogens are important because they protect the vagina from the invasion of pathogens. The normal secretions in the vagina are acidic in reaction and further serve to protect the vagina from microbial invasion. Therefore, the normal mucous membrane is its own best protection.

GUIDELINES FOR NURSING CARE

Instilling Nose Drops

- Provide the client with paper tissues for the expectoration of secretions.
- Have the client sit up with head tilted well back. Or, if the client is lying down, tilt the head back over a pillow. These positions allow the solution to flow well back into the nares.
- Draw sufficient solution into the dropper for both nares. Excess solution should not be returned to a stock bottle.
- Hold up the tip of the nose and place the dropper just inside the nares, about one third of an inch. Instill

the prescribed number of drops in one naris and then into the other. Protect the dropper with a piece of soft tubing when the client is an infant or young child.
- Avoid touching the nares with the dropper because it may cause the client to sneeze.
- Have the client remain in position with the head tilted back for a few minutes to prevent the escape of the solution.

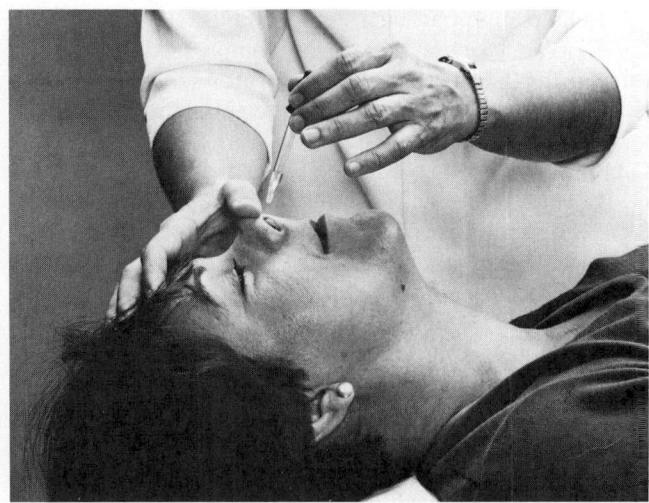

FIGURE 42-22

The nurse is preparing to instill nose drops. The patient's head is tilted back to facilitate proper placement of the medication.

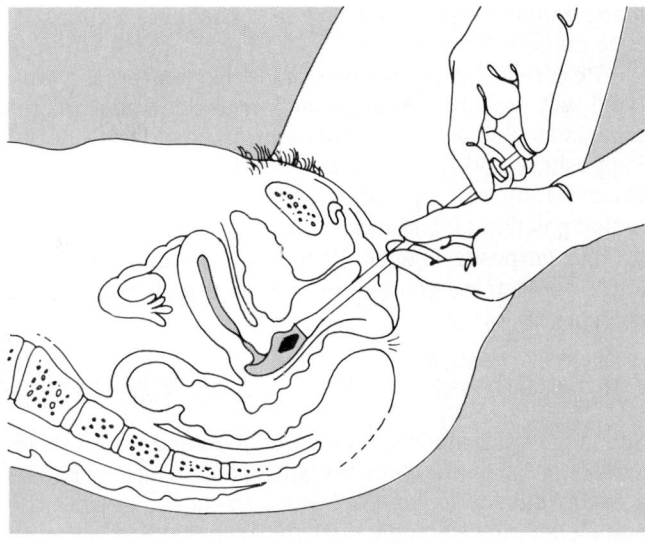

FIGURE 42-23

Cream or suppository vaginal preparations should be inserted well into the vagina using an applicator or a gloved hand.

Creams can be applied intravaginally, using a narrow, tubular applicator with an attached plunger. Suppositories that melt when exposed to body heat are also prepared for vaginal insertion. Suppositories should be refrigerated for storage.

The client should be asked to void before inserting the medication. The client is positioned lying on her back with the knees flexed. Privacy should be maintained with draping. Adequate light should be available to visualize the vaginal opening. See Nursing Guidelines for Vaginal Insertion of Suppository or Cream and Figure 42-23.

Rectal Instillations

Rectal suppositories are used primarily for their local action, such as a laxative and a fecal softener. Systemic effects are also achieved with rectal suppositories. Acetaminophen suppositories are used for an antipyretic effect, and

GUIDELINES FOR NURSING CARE

Vaginal Insertion of Suppository or Cream

- Fill a vaginal applicator with the prescribed amount of cream, or have a suppository ready.
- Lubricate the applicator with water, as necessary. A suppository may be lubricated with a water-soluble gel. Ordinarily, lubrication is unnecessary but may be used to reduce friction while inserting the applicator or suppository.
- Wear disposable gloves.
- Use clean aseptic technique to administer the medication.
- Spread the labia well with the fingers, and clean the area at the vaginal orifice with cotton balls and warm water to remove discharge, as necessary. With each cotton ball, use a single stroke moving from above the orifice downward toward the sacrum. These techniques prevent contamination of the vaginal orifice with debris surrounding the anus.

- Introduce the applicator gently in a rolling manner while directing it downward and backward to follow the normal contour of the vagina for its full length. Push the plunger to its full length, and then gently remove the applicator with the plunger depressed. After the applicator is properly positioned, the labia may be allowed to fall in place to free the nurse's hand for manipulating the plunger. Insert a suppository with gloved fingers well into the vagina.
- Ask the client to remain in the supine position for 5 to 10 minutes after insertion.
- Offer the client a perineal pad to collect excess drainage.
- Instruct proper techniques to the client who wants to administer vaginal suppositories and creams herself.

many antiemetics are available in suppository form to relieve nausea and vomiting.

Be sure to use a clean disposable glove to protect your hand and prevent contamination with feces and micro-organisms. See Nursing Guidelines for Inserting a Rectal Suppository and the accompanying figure in Chapter 35. Once the suppository is inserted, the client should remain in that position for 5 minutes, unless the suppository is for laxative purposes, in which case it must remain in position for 35 to 45 minutes or until the client feels the urge to defecate.

Administering Medications by Inhalation

The lungs are richly supplied with blood and have a large surface area. These characteristics allow drugs to be absorbed from the lower respiratory tract. The smaller the particles of inhaled medication, the lower in the respiratory tract the medication tends to travel. A disadvantage of using this route is that the drug dosage is difficult to establish.

Drugs classified as bronchodilators and decongestants commonly are administered by **inhalation**. They act to decrease resistance to air flow by enlarging the passageway. Decongestants are local vasoconstrictors. Bronchodilators promote relaxation of musculature in the tracheobronchial tree. The relaxed passages produce less resistance to air flow and provide an opened respiratory passageway. Bronchodilators are further discussed in Chapter 36.

Drugs for inhalation may be administered by a hand atomizer or a nebulizer. These devices work to cause increased pressure in the unit, which forces solution into a specially constructed strictured chamber. The force with which the solution is made to move through the stricture and to leave the container is sufficient to break the large droplets of medication into a mist.

F I G U R E 4 2 - 2 4

Inhaler. A bottle of medication is attached to a mouthpiece. After the client exhales, the mouthpiece is gripped with the lips, and while the client takes a deep inhalation slowly, the bottle is firmly pushed down on the mouthpiece to release one dose of medication. (Photo © Ken Kasper.)

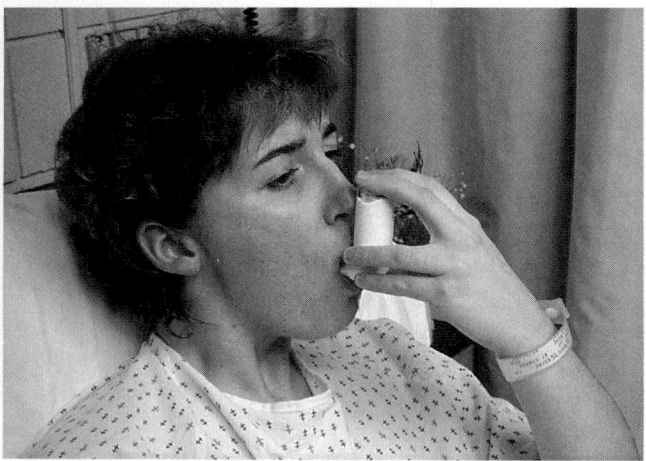

Nebulization can also be accomplished by using the force of an oxygen stream or compressed air passed through the fluid in a nebulizer or an atomizer. This method is valuable for clients who require inhalation of a drug several times a day when the hand atomizer or nebulizer is fatiguing. The oxygen stream is also useful in the production of vapors when high humidity is needed continuously for long periods. One of the most common means of administering a nebulized drug using air pressure is the intermittent positive-pressure breathing machine, discussed in Chapter 36.

A popular nebulizer now on the market supplies premeasured amounts of medication each time the nebulizer releases the drug in solution. This equipment helps to control the amount of medication the client receives and minimizes the dangers of overdosing when ordinary hand nebulizers are used. Figure 42-24 shows this nebulizer.

Documenting Medication Administration

The medication record is a legal document. Recording each dose of medication as soon as possible after it is given provides a documented record that can be consulted if there is any question as to whether the client received the medication. The nurse should not record medications before they are given. If the medications are not given, the medication record would show that the client received the medication when in fact that was not true.

Different forms are used for recording medications. The name of the medication, dosage, route of administration, time given, and nurse's initials are noted on the form. The site used for an injection should be recorded. The nurse's full signature must appear on the form for initial identification. Other specific client information may be required. For instance, the pulse rate may be recorded when administering some cardiac drugs or a description of the effects on the client's pain when administering analgesics.

Omitted Drugs Drugs may be omitted intentionally or inadvertently. The omission and the reason for it are documented on the client's record. Drugs may be omitted intentionally for the following reasons:

- The client is to have a diagnostic test and is to fast before the test. Oral drugs usually are omitted or their administration is delayed, depending on the physician's orders.
- The problem for which the medication is intended no longer exists. For example, a laxative has been ordered for a client. The client has had a bowel movement and no longer needs the laxative. The laxative is then omitted.
- The client is suspected of having an allergy to the medication. Any suspected allergy should be reported to the physician.

In an effort to reduce the incidence of medication errors, some hospitals are evaluating a bar code system similar to that used in grocery stores. One hospital is using a portable hand-held computer with a bar code scanner and keypad that scans the nurse's identification badge, the client's identification, and the medication's bar code. Not only is the current dosage to the right client at the right time confirmed, this information can also be integrated with a charting system as well as the hospital billing system (Carr, 1989).

Teaching Clients About Medications

In many cases, clients continue a prescribed medication regimen at home after discharge from the hospital. A factor that affects the client's compliance to the medication regimen at home is education about the prescribed medications. Teaching should be tailored to the client's level of understanding. Written instructions can be used as a reference for the client. The client should know the name of the drug, dosage, route of administration, and frequency. A common cause of errors in self-administration of medications is a lack of understanding about the dose and the frequency for taking the medication. The nurse should help the client establish a medication schedule that best fits the prescribed frequency of medications and the client's lifestyle. Clients can be taught to establish a medication routine by taking medications at the same time each day

Inadvertent omission of a drug should be reported as soon as it is detected to determine whether a dose should be administered at that time. For example, a certain medication given daily might be administered in the afternoon when it is discovered that it had been inadvertently omitted in the morning.

Refused Drugs If the client refuses a drug that is considered essential to the therapeutic regimen, the nurse should report this promptly. The nurse often can play an important role in determining the reason for the refusal and can help the client accept needed drugs. If reasonable efforts fail to accomplish this, it is unwise to continue urging the client who adamantly refuses a medication. Clients have the right to refuse therapy, and the nurse should recognize and respect that right. Refusals to take prescribed drugs and the manner in which the situation was managed should be described on the client's record and reported according to agency policy. Figure 42-25 shows a health agency medication record.

Medication Errors The conscientious nurse takes every precaution to avoid errors when administering therapeutic agents. Humans are subject to occasional poor judgment, however, and errors may occur.

Nursing actions that may result in medication errors are highlighted in the accompanying display.

Prompt acknowledgment of errors may minimize their possible detrimental effects. The following steps are recommended when a medication error occurs.
- Check the client's condition immediately when the error is noted.
- Notify the physician to discuss possible courses of action, which depend on the client's condition.

- Write a description of the error on the client's permanent record, including remedial steps that were taken.
- Complete a special form for reporting errors, as dictated by agency policy. These forms, called *accident, incident,* or *unusual occurrence reports,* require a full explanation of the situation and the steps that were taken after its commission. For legal reasons, it is essential that errors be described fully and accurately.

According to Long (1992), a peer review committee has effectively reduced medication errors in one hospital. After an error has occurred, the nurse completes a Medication Error Tool and receives varying types of counseling based on a score tallied from the form. Recommendations and suggestions for improvements from the committee concerning medication delivery protocols have also proved helpful.

Techniques of medication administration should be explained to the client and family. Before discharge from a health care facility, the client should practice the necessary techniques under the supervision of a nurse to acquire sufficient skill for safe administration. Many clients have learned to give themselves injections, as well as many other medications when the teaching has been well planned and the client is able and willing to learn.

The client should understand the desired effects of medications and possible adverse effects. The client should also be taught the symptoms of toxic drug effects and the exact course of action to take if symptoms occur.

The nurse must stress the importance of taking medications as prescribed and for as long as prescribed. A common error made by clients is simply omitting a drug, either through carelessness or because they believe that missing a dose is not important. Various aids are available to help nurses identify clients who are noncompliant and remind the client to take his or her medication on schedule. Medication containers that beep when a dose is due to be taken, scratch-off dots on a medication label, and an electronic cap that signals dosage time and records each time the cap is removed are compliance aids that are now available.

The client should be instructed not to alter the dosage without consulting the physician. Medications should not be discontinued when symptoms disappear. Drugs used to maintain health, such as those to control high blood pressure, need to be continued as ordered to avoid recurrence of symptoms.

Clients should be taught the importance of safe storage of medications. Keeping medications out of the reach of children can prevent accidental poisoning.

Caution the client not to share prescribed medications with other family members or with friends and neighbors. Inappropriate use of another person's drugs can have serious consequences.

Nurses have a teaching responsibility to society in relation to the abuse of any drug. Teaching may take place on an individual basis or on a family or community level. Drug abuse is a major public health concern worldwide, according to authorities on the subject, especially among teenagers and young adults. Not only is continued public and individual education indicated, nurses are also expected to
(*Text continues on p. 1256*)

CROZER-CHESTER MEDICAL CENTER
MEDICATION ADMINISTRATION + PARENTERAL THERAPY RECORD

FORM NS-MAR-1

Legend for Injection Sites

RA- Right Arm   RT- Right Thigh
LA- Left Arm   LT- Left Thigh
RB- Right Buttock   R.Abd.- Right Abdomen
LB- Left Buttock   L.Abd.- Left Abdomen

Allergies:

Penicillin

Operative Date:
Procedure:

STANDING ORDERS (MEDICATION ORDERED PER ROUTINE SCHEDULE OR WITH SPECIFIC NUMBER OF DOSES)

ORDER DATE & RN INIT.	EXP. DATE & TIME	MEDICATION, DOSAGE, FREQUENCY, ROUTE	HOURS	11/29 INJ. SITE	11/29 INIT.	11/30 INJ. SITE	11/30 INIT.	12/1 INJ. SITE	12/1 INIT.	12/2 INJ. SITE	12/2 INIT.	12/3 INJ. SITE	12/3 INIT.	12/4 INJ. SITE	12/4 INIT.	12/5 INJ. SITE	12/5 INIT.	12/6 INJ. SITE	12/6 INIT.	12/7 INJ. SITE	12/7 INIT.	12/8 INJ. SITE	12/8 INIT.
11/29/93 SM		Digoxin 0.25 mg po QD	10A	AC AR =88	AC	AC AR =92	AC	CL AR =86	CL														
11/29/93 SM		Lasix 20 mg QD po	10A	AC	AC	AC	AC	CL	CL														
11/29/93 SM		Trental 400 mg TID Po	10A	AC	AC	AC	AC	CL	CL														
			2P	AC	AC	AC	AC	CL	CL														
			6P	PR	PR	PR	PR	PR	PR														
11/29/93 SM		Slow K++ po QD	10A	AC	AC	AC	AC	(CL)	(CL)														
11/29/93 SM		Serax 15 mg Po q. 8°	6A	SP	SP	SP	SP	MS	MS														
			2P	AC	AC	AC	AC	CL	CL														
			10P	PR	PR	PR	PR	PR	PR														
11/29/93 SM		Procardia 20 mg po TID	10A	AC	AC	AC	AC	CL	CL														
			2P	AC	AC	AC	AC	CL	CL														
			6P	PR	PR	PR	PR	PR	PR														

SINGLE ORDERS (STAT, PRE-OP, ONE TIME DOSE, ON CALL, DIAGNOSTIC PREP)

ORDER DATE & RN INIT.	MEDICATION, DOSAGE, ROUTE	TO BE GIVEN DATE	TO BE GIVEN TIME	INJ. SITE	RN INIT.	ORDER DATE & RN INIT.	MEDICATION, DOSAGE, ROUTE	TO BE GIVEN DATE	TO BE GIVEN TIME	INJ. SITE	RN INIT.
11/29 PR	Dalmane 15 mg po now	11/29	11P	–	PR						
11/30	Dulcolax Tab. ĭĭĭ po at 6 pm	11/30	6P		PR						

F I G U R E 4 2 - 2 5

Example of a medication record.

PRN MEDICATIONS (ENTER DATE, TIME GIVEN, INJECTION SITE AND RN INITIALS)

ORDER DATE & RN INIT.	EXP. DATE & TIME	MEDICATION, DOSES, FREQUENCY, ROUTE		DOSES GIVEN											
11/29/93 SM		Tylox tab ii po q 3° prn	DATE	11/29	11/30										
			TIME	1q	3A										
			INJ. SITE												
			RN INIT.	AC	SP										
11/29/93 SM		Maalox 30 cc po q 6° prn	DATE												
			TIME												
			INJ. SITE												
			RN INIT.												
			DATE												
			TIME												
			INJ. SITE												
			RN INIT.												
			DATE												
			TIME												
			INJ. SITE												
			RN INIT.												
			DATE												
			TIME												
			INJ. SITE												
			RN INIT.												
			DATE												
			TIME												
			INJ. SITE												
			RN INIT.												
			DATE												
			TIME												
			INJ. SITE												
			RN INIT.												

PATIENT NAME:

PARENTERAL THERAPY			DOCUMENTATION FOR MEDICATION WITHHELD				
ORDER DATE & RN INIT.	I.V. SOLUTIONS	SCHEDULE	DATE	TIME	MEDICATION	REASON FOR WITHHOLDING	
11/29/93 SM	1000 cc D5W	q 8°	12/1	10A	Slow K tab ii	patient refused	

RN IDENTIFICATION						
INIT.	SIGNATURE	INIT.	SIGNATURE	INIT.	SIGNATURE
AC	a. Christopher RN				
PR	P Rogers RN				
SP	S. Pointer RN				
CL	C. Lewis RN				

Common Errors Made in Administering Medication

- Failure to understand why a medication is given or unfamiliarity with the drug
- Failure to check client's identification bracelet and failure to ask client his or her name
- Failure to check with the prescribing physician when orders are unclear
- Being careless and laying medication down before administering it
- Incorrect calculation of drug dosage

Medication Dos and Don'ts to Teach Clients

DOs

- Do read and follow directions for use.
- Do be cautious when using a drug for the first time.
- Do dispose of old prescription drugs and outdated over-the-counter medications.
- Do seek professional advice before combining drugs.
- Do seek professional advice when symptoms persist or return.
- Do get medical check-ups regularly.

DON'Ts

- Don't be casual about taking drugs.
- Don't take drugs you don't need.
- Don't overbuy and keep drugs for long periods.
- Don't combine drugs carelessly.
- Don't continue taking over-the-counter drugs if symptoms persist.
- Don't take prescription drugs not prescribed specifically for you.

---

teach by setting high standards for their own behavior and the use of drugs. The increasing incidence of impaired providers makes it imperative that nurses observe, document, and intervene, for the client's safety, if drug abuse by a professional caregiver is suspected.

Important dos and don'ts that should be noted when teaching clients about medications are listed in the accompanying display.

Evaluating the Client's Response to Medications

Drug effectiveness can be assessed in several ways. Clinical observation is the first method. Subjective data from the client (eg, "My pain has disappeared") can be collected. Objective data (eg, the client's vital signs) help the nurse evaluate medication effectiveness. The alert nurse assesses the client for adverse drug effects.

Measurement of drug levels in body fluids provides data about the client's response to a particular medication. For many drugs, including digoxin, theophylline, anti-convulsants, and aminoglycoside antibiotics, monitoring blood levels is an important component of therapy. The client is tested to determine if the drug level in the blood is within the therapeutic range. Drug dosages may be adjusted as a result of the serum drug level.

Monitoring systems can also assist the nurse in evaluating drug effectiveness. For the client with an arrhythmia, a cardiac monitor would show a change in heart rhythm.

KEY POINTS

- Medications have several names. The nurse should be aware of a drug's generic and trade names. Drugs can be classified by body system and by the symptom they relieve (clinical indication).
- Drugs are available in many forms. Some drugs are supplied in a number of preparations; others are available in only one form.
- Factors that influence drug absorption include route of administration, local conditions at the site of administration, drug solubility, pH, and drug dosage.
- Variables that influence the action of medications are age, weight, sex, genetic factors, psychological factors, illness, environment, and time of administration.

- Known adverse drug effects include iatrogenic disease, drug allergy, drug tolerance, cumulative effect, idiosyncratic reaction, and drug interactions.
- Assessment of clients receiving medications includes obtaining a comprehensive medication history.
- Components of a medication order are client's name, date and time order is written, name of the drug, dosage, route, frequency, and signature of the prescriber. The nurse questions any unclear medication order before the order is implemented.
- Pediatric dosages are calculated by the child's weight or body surface area.

- The nurse observes the *five rights* and *three checks* in medication preparation and administration. The nurse who prepares a medication administers the medication. The medication area is locked when not in use.
- The nurse identifies the client correctly before administering a medication and remains with the client until the medication is taken. The nurse records the medication on the client's record as soon as possible after administration.
- Selection of equipment for a parenteral injection is based on the route of administration, viscosity of the drug, quantity to be administered, type of medication, and client's body size.
- After use, needles should never be recapped and are placed in a puncture-resistant container. Most needlestick injuries occur during recapping.
- Sterile equipment is used to prepare a drug for injection.

- Modified insulin should never be subjected to a vial of unmodified insulin when preparing two insulins to be mixed in the same syringe.
- Proper site selection for an intramuscular injection should include palpation of anatomic landmarks. The Z-track method for an intramuscular injection is safer and less painful for most adults.
- Intravenous medications can be administered as a continuous infusion, as a bolus, or intermittently. A bolus dose and an intermittent infusion may be administered through the primary intravenous line or through a heparin lock. The nurse checks the placement of a heparin lock before administering any medication.
- Topical medications are applied to the skin and mucous membranes primarily for their local effects, although some systemic effects may occur.

STUDY QUESTIONS

1. The official name of a drug that is selected by the pharmaceutical company selling the drug and copyrighted by it is the drug's
   a. chemical name
   b. generic name
   c. official name
   d. trade name
2. The process by which a drug is transferred from its site of entry into the body to the bloodstream is known as
   a. absorption
   b. distribution
   c. metabolism
   d. excretion
3. A client has an abnormal unexpected response to a drug. This is defined as
   a. drug tolerance
   b. a cumulative effect
   c. an idiosyncratic effect
   d. an anaphylactic reaction
4. A medication order reads: "Digoxin, 0.125 mg PO qod." The nurse correctly gives this drug
   a. daily before bedtime
   b. by mouth every other day
   c. twice a day by way of the oral route
   d. once a week after recording an apical rate
5. In addition to checking a client's identification bracelet, the nurse can correctly verify his identity by
   a. asking Mr. Brown his name
   b. reading his name on the sign over the bed
   c. asking his roommate to verify his name
   d. asking, "Are you Mr. Brown?"

6. Medication needs to be administered by way of a nasogastric tube. Before giving the medication, it is important for the nurse to
   a. crush the enteric-coated pill for mixing in a liquid
   b. flush open the tube with 60 mL of very warm water
   c. check for proper placement of the nasogastric tube
   d. take the client's vital signs
7. The medication order reads: "Meperidine, 50 mg IM stat." A prefilled cartridge is available with a label reading 50 mg/1 mL. The cartridge contains 1.2 mL of meperidine. The nurse should
   a. give all the medication in the cartridge because it expanded when it was mixed
   b. call the pharmacy and request the proper dose
   c. refuse to give the medication
   d. dispose of 0.2 mL correctly before administering the drug
8. A client requires 40 units of NPH insulin and 10 units of regular insulin daily subcutaneously. The correct sequence when mixing insulins is
   a. inject air into the regular insulin vial and withdraw 10 units; then, using the same syringe, inject air into the NPH vial and withdraw 40 units of NPH insulin
   b. inject air into the NPH insulin vial, being careful not to allow the solution to touch the needle; next, inject air into the regular insulin vial and withdraw 10 units; then, withdraw 40 units of NPH insulin

c. inject air into the regular insulin vial, being careful not to allow the solution to touch the needle; next, inject air into the NPH insulin vial and withdraw 40 units; then, withdraw 10 units of regular insulin

d. inject air into the NPH insulin vial and withdraw 40 units; then, using the same syringe, inject air into the regular insulin vial and withdraw 10 units of regular insulin

9. Ms. Hall has an order for meperidine, 100 mg q 4 h prn. The nurse notes that according to Ms. Hall's chart, Ms. Hall is allergic to Demerol. The order for medication was signed by Dr. Long. Which of the following would be the correct procedure for this situation?

a. Administer the medication; the doctor knows best.

b. Call Dr. Long and ask that she change the medication.

c. Ask the supervisor to administer the medication.

d. Ask the pharmacist to provide a medication to take the place of Demerol.

10. The nurse manager on your unit prepared medications for Mr. Giles. She is called to the phone and asks you to give the client his medications. Which is the best response to this request?

a. Give Mr. Giles the medication and record it on his chart.

b. Tell the nurse manager that you do not have time and ask her to get someone else.

c. Tell the nurse manager that because you did not pour the medication, you cannot administer it.

d. Give the medication to Mr. Giles but have the nurse manager chart it.

11. Which of the following is the reason the intravenous method of medication administration is called the most dangerous route of administration?

a. The vein can take only a small amount of fluid at a time.

b. The vein may harden and become non-functional.

c. Blood clots may become a serious problem.

d. The drug is placed directly into the bloodstream and its action is immediate.

Answers With Rationale

1. The correct response is *d*. The chemical name identifies the drug's chemical composition and molecular structure. The generic name is assigned by the manufacturer who develops the drug, and the official name is the name that identifies the drug in the official publication.

2. The correct response is *a*. Distribution, metabolism, and excretion occur after the drug has been absorbed.

3. The correct response is *c*. Drug tolerance results when the body becomes accustomed to the drug

12. Mr. King is receiving heparin subcutaneously. Which of the following demonstrates correct technique for this procedure?

a. Aspirate before giving and gently massage after the injection.

b. Do not aspirate; massage the site for 1 minute.

c. Do not aspirate before or massage after the injection.

d. Massage the site of the injection; aspiration is not necessary but will do no harm.

13. A client refuses to take her noon medication, saying that she does not need it. Which of the following would be the best response?

a. Tell her that she must take the medication because the doctor ordered it.

b. Tell her that you went through a lot of preparation to get her medications ready and it's the least she can do.

c. Tell her that you don't care whether she takes the medications or not.

d. Tell her that you will return the medications to the cart but would like to discuss her reasons for refusing the medications.

14. The nurse discovers that she has made a medication error. Which of the following would be the first response?

a. Record the error on the medication sheet.

b. Notify the physician regarding course of action.

c. Check the client's condition to note any possible effect of the error.

d. Complete an incident report, explaining how the mistake was made.

15. The nurse takes an 8 AM medication to the client and properly identifies her. The client asks the nurse to leave the medication on the bedside table and states that she will take it with breakfast when it comes. What is the best response to this request?

a. Leave the medication and return later to make sure that it was taken.

b. Tell her that it is against the rules and take the medication with you.

c. Tell her that you cannot leave the medication but will return with it when breakfast arrives.

d. Take the drug from the room and record it as refused.

over time. A cumulative effect occurs when the body cannot metabolize one dose of a drug before another one is given. An anaphylactic reaction is a life-threatening immediate response to a drug that can result in respiratory distress and cardiovascular collapse.

4. The correct response is *b*. The abbreviation *qod* refers to every-other-day administration.

5. The correct response is *a*. A sign over the client's bed may not always be current and updated. The roommate is an unsafe source of information, and the client may not even hear his name and reply in the affirmative (eg. a person with a hearing deficit).

6. The correct response is *c*. Tube placement should always be checked before administering any medication to prevent the possibility of aspiration if the tube is not in the stomach. Enteric-coated pills should never be crushed, and very warm water may injure stomach mucosa. Taking the vital signs is not necessary unless a particular medication requires it before administration.

7. The correct response is *d*. Many of the cartridges are overfilled, and some of the medication needs to be discarded. Giving the excess medication in the cartridge may result in adverse effects for the client. For this dose, it is not necessary to call the pharmacy or refuse to give the medication, provided the order is written correctly.

8. The correct response is *b*. Regular or short-acting insulin should never be contaminated with NPH or any insulin modified with added protein. Placing air in the NPH vial first without allowing the needle to contact the solution ensures that the regular insulin will not be contaminated.

9. The correct response is *b*. The nurse is responsible for any medications he or she gives and must contact the doctor to inform her of the client's allergy to the drug. The nurse should not give the medication and might speak with the supervisor only if he or she is uncomfortable with the physician's response once she is notified. The nurse is legally un-

able to order a replacement medication, as is the pharmacist.

10. The correct response is *c*. The nurse should never give medications prepared by someone else, since she is responsible for what she administers.

11. The correct response is *d*. The intravenous route is a direct access to the bloodstream, and medications act quickly when given intravenously. The condition of the veins is not as important as the rapid effect of the medication administered by way of the intravenous route.

12. The correct response is *c*. Heparin that is given subcutaneously should not be aspirated or massaged, so as not to cause trauma or bleeding in the tissues.

13. The correct response is *d*. The client has the right to refuse medications, but the nurse should assess the client's reasons for refusal, document them, and report them to the physician.

14. The correct response is *c*. The nurse's first responsibility is the client, and careful observation is necessary to assess for any effect of the medication error. The other nursing actions are pertinent but only after checking the client's welfare.

15. The correct response is *c*. Safe nursing practice requires that a medication never be left at the client's bedside. It is not correct to say that the client has refused medication in this situation.

MEDICATION CALCULATION PROBLEMS

1. Metoprolol (Lopressor), 25 mg PO, is ordered. Metoprolol is available as 50-mg tablets. How many tablets would the nurse administer?

2. Phenytoin (Dilantin), 100 mg PO, is ordered to be given through a nasogastric tube. Phenytoin is available as 30 mg/5 mL. How much would the nurse administer?

3. Captopril (Capoten), 12.5 mg PO, is ordered. Captopril is available as 25-mg tablets. How many tablets would the nurse administer?

4. Potassium chloride (Micro-K), 20 mEq, is ordered. Potassium chloride is available as 10 mEq per tablet. How many tablets would the nurse administer?

5. Digoxin (Lanoxin), 0.0625 mg PO, is ordered. Digoxin is available as 0.125-mg tablets. How many tablets would the nurse administer?

6. Propantheline bromide (Pro-Banthine), 15 mg, is ordered. Propantheline bromide is available as 7.5-mg tablets. How many tablets would the nurse administer?

7. Ciprofloxacin (Cipro), 500 mg PO, is ordered. Ciprofloxacin is available as 250-mg tablets. How many tablets would the nurse administer?

8. Furosemide (Lasix), 20 mg PO, is ordered. Furosemide is available as 40-mg tablets. How many tablets would the nurse administer?

9. Theophylline elixir, 100 mg PO, is ordered by way of a percutaneous endoscopic gastrostomy tube. Theophylline elixir is available as 80 mg/15 mL. How much would the nurse administer?

10. Clonidine (Catapres), 0.1 mg PO, is ordered. Clonidine is available as 0.2-mg tablets. How many tablets would the nurse administer?

11. Vitamin K, 10 mg IM, is ordered. Vitamin K is available as 5 mg/mL. How much would the nurse administer?

12. Meperidine (Demerol), 35 mg IM, is ordered. Meperidine is available as 50 mg/mL. How much would the nurse administer?

13. Midazolam (Versed), 3 mg IM, is ordered. Midazolam is available as 5 mg/mL. How much would the nurse administer?

14. Hydroxyzine (Vistaril), 50 mg IM, is ordered. Hydroxyzine is available as 25 mg/mL. How much would the nurse administer?

15. Epoetin alfa (Epogen), 2000 units SC, is ordered. Epoetin alfa is available as 4000 units/mL. How much would the nurse administer?
16. Nalbuphine (Nubain), 1.5 mg IM, is ordered. Nalbuphine is available as 1 mg/mL. How much would the nurse administer?
17. Ocreotide acetate (Sandostatin), 50 μg SC, is ordered. Ocreotide is available as 100 μg/mL. How much would the nurse administer?
18. Morphine sulfate, 4 mg SC, is ordered. Morphine sulfate is available as 8 mg/mL. How much would the nurse administer?
19. Procholorperazine (Compazine), 7.5 mg IM, is ordered. Prochlorperazine is available as 5 mg/mL. How much would the nurse administer?
20. Glycopyrrolate (Robinul), 0.4 mg IM, is ordered. Glycopyrrolate is available as 0.2 mg/mL. How much would the nurse administer?

Answers to Medication Calculation Problems

1. $\dfrac{\text{dose on hand}}{\text{quantity on hand}} = \dfrac{\text{dose required}}{\text{X (quantity desired)}}$

    $\dfrac{50 \text{ mg}}{1 \text{ tablet}} = \dfrac{25 \text{ mg}}{\text{X}}$

    cross-multiply:

    $50\text{X} = 25$
    $\text{X} = 0.5 \text{ or } \frac{1}{2} \text{ tablet}$

2. $\dfrac{\text{dose on hand}}{\text{quantity on hand}} = \dfrac{\text{dose desired}}{\text{X (quantity desired)}}$

    $\dfrac{30 \text{ mg}}{5 \text{ ml}} = \dfrac{100 \text{ mg}}{\text{X}}$

    cross-multiply:

    $30\text{X} = 500$
    $\text{X} = 16.66 \text{ or } 17 \text{ ml}$

3. $\dfrac{\text{dose on hand}}{\text{quantity on hand}} = \dfrac{\text{dose desired}}{\text{X (quantity desired)}}$

    $\dfrac{25 \text{ mg}}{1 \text{ tablet}} = \dfrac{12.5 \text{ mg}}{\text{X}}$

    cross-multiply:

    $25\text{X} = 12.5$
    $\text{X} = 0.5 \text{ or } \frac{1}{2} \text{ tablet}$

4. $\dfrac{\text{dose on hand}}{\text{quantity on hand}} = \dfrac{\text{dose desired}}{\text{X (quantity desired)}}$

    $\dfrac{10 \text{ mEq}}{1 \text{ tablet}} = \dfrac{20 \text{ mEq}}{\text{X}}$

    cross-multiply:

    $10\text{X} = 20$
    $\text{X} = 2 \text{ tablets}$

5. $\dfrac{\text{dose on hand}}{\text{quantity on hand}} = \dfrac{\text{dose desired}}{\text{X (quantity desired)}}$

    $\dfrac{0.125 \text{ mg}}{1 \text{ tablet}} = \dfrac{0.0625 \text{ mg}}{\text{X}}$

    cross-multiply:

    $0.125\text{X} = 0.0625$
    $\text{X} = 0.5 \text{ or } \frac{1}{2} \text{ tablet}$

6. $\dfrac{\text{dose desired}}{\text{dose on hand}} \times \dfrac{\text{quantity}}{\text{on hand}} = \text{X (desired quantity)}$

    $\dfrac{15 \text{ mg}}{7.5 \text{ mg}} \times 1 \text{ tablet} = \text{X}$

    $2 \times 1 = 2 \text{ tablets}$

7. $\dfrac{\text{dose desired}}{\text{dose on hand}} \times \dfrac{\text{quantity}}{\text{on hand}} = \text{X (desired quantity)}$

    $\dfrac{500 \text{ mg}}{250 \text{ mg}} \times 1 \text{ tablet} = \text{X}$

    $2 \times 1 = 2 \text{ tablets}$

8. $\dfrac{\text{dose desired}}{\text{dose on hand}} \times \dfrac{\text{quantity}}{\text{on hand}} = \text{X (desired quantity)}$

    $\dfrac{20 \text{ mg}}{40 \text{ mg}} \times 1 \text{ tablet} = \text{X}$

    $\frac{1}{2} \times 1 = \text{X}$
    $\text{X} = \frac{1}{2} \text{ tablet}$

9. $\dfrac{\text{dose desired}}{\text{dose on hand}} \times \dfrac{\text{quantity}}{\text{on hand}} = \text{X (desired quantity)}$

    $\dfrac{100 \text{ mg}}{80 \text{ mg}} \times 15 \text{ ml} = \text{X}$

    $\dfrac{1500}{80} = \text{X}$

    $\text{X} = 18.75 = 19 \text{ mL}$

10. $\dfrac{\text{dose desired}}{\text{dose on hand}} \times \dfrac{\text{quantity}}{\text{on hand}} = \text{X (desired quantity)}$

    $\dfrac{0.1 \text{ mg}}{0.2 \text{ mg}} \times 1 \text{ tablet} = \text{X}$

    $\frac{1}{2} \times 1 = \text{X}$
    $\text{X} = \frac{1}{2} \text{ tablet}$

11. $\dfrac{\text{dose on hand}}{\text{quantity on hand}} = \dfrac{\text{dose desired}}{\text{X (quantity desired)}}$

    $\dfrac{5 \text{ mg}}{1 \text{ mL}} = \dfrac{10 \text{ mg}}{\text{X}}$

    cross-multiply:

    $5\text{X} = 10$
    $\text{X} = 2 \text{ mL}$

12. $\dfrac{\text{dose on hand}}{\text{quantity on hand}} = \dfrac{\text{dose desired}}{\text{X (quantity desired)}}$

$$\frac{50 \text{ mg}}{1 \text{ mL}} = \frac{35 \text{ mg}}{\text{X}}$$

cross-multiply:
$$50\text{X} = 35$$
$$\text{X} = 0.7 \text{ mL}$$

13. $\dfrac{\text{dose on hand}}{\text{quantity on hand}} = \dfrac{\text{dose desired}}{\text{X (quantity desired)}}$

$$\frac{5 \text{ mg}}{1 \text{ mL}} = \frac{3 \text{ mg}}{\text{X}}$$

cross-multiply:
$$5\text{X} = 3$$
$$\text{X} = 0.6 \text{ mL}$$

14. $\dfrac{\text{dose on hand}}{\text{quantity on hand}} = \dfrac{\text{dose desired}}{\text{X (quantity desired)}}$

$$\frac{25 \text{ mg}}{1 \text{ mL}} = \frac{50 \text{ mg}}{\text{X}}$$

cross-multiply:
$$25\text{X} = 50$$
$$\text{X} = 2 \text{ mL}$$

15. $\dfrac{\text{dose on hand}}{\text{quantity on hand}} = \dfrac{\text{dose desired}}{\text{X (quantity desired)}}$

$$\frac{4000 \text{ U}}{1 \text{ mL}} = \frac{2000 \text{ U}}{\text{X}}$$

cross-multiply:
$$4000\text{X} = 2000$$
$$\text{X} = 1/2 \text{ mL}$$

16. $\dfrac{\text{dose desired}}{\text{dose on hand}} \times \dfrac{\text{quantity}}{\text{on hand}} = \text{X (desired quantity)}$

$$\frac{1.5 \text{ mg}}{1 \text{ mg}} \times 1 \text{ mL} = \text{X}$$

$$1.5 \times 1 = \text{X}$$

$$\text{X} = 1.5 \text{ mL}$$

17. $\dfrac{\text{dose desired}}{\text{dose on hand}} = \dfrac{\text{quantity}}{\text{on hand}} = \text{X (desired quantity)}$

$$\frac{50 \text{ μg}}{100 \text{ μg}} \times 1 \text{ mL} = \text{X}$$

$$1/2 \times 1 = \text{X}$$

$$\text{X} = 1/2 \text{ mL}$$

18. $\dfrac{\text{dose desired}}{\text{dose on hand}} \times \dfrac{\text{quantity}}{\text{on hand}} = \text{X (desired quantity)}$

$$\frac{4 \text{ mg}}{8 \text{ mg}} \times 1 \text{ mL} = \text{X}$$

$$1/2 \times 1 = \text{X}$$

$$\text{X} = 1/2 \text{ mL}$$

19. $\dfrac{\text{dose desired}}{\text{dose on hand}} \times \dfrac{\text{quantity}}{\text{on hand}} = \text{X (desired quantity)}$

$$\frac{7.5 \text{ mg}}{5 \text{ mg}} \times 1 \text{ mL} = \text{X}$$

$$1.5 \times 1 = \text{X}$$

$$\text{X} = 1.5 \text{ mL}$$

20. $\dfrac{\text{dose desired}}{\text{dose on hand}} \times \dfrac{\text{quantity}}{\text{on hand}} = \text{X (desired quantity)}$

$$\frac{0.4 \text{ mg}}{0.2 \text{ mg}} \times 1 \text{ mL} = \text{X}$$

$$2 \times 1 = \text{X}$$

$$\text{X} = 2 \text{ mL}$$

BIBLIOGRAPHY

Abrams, A. (1991). *Clinical drug therapy* (3rd ed.). Philadelphia: Lippincott.

Adams, C. (1989). New strategies for avoiding medication errors. *Nursing, 19*(8), 39–45.

Alexander, D., & O'Quinn-Larson, J. (1990). When nurses are addicted to drugs: Confronting an impaired co-worker. *Nursing, 20*(8), 55–58.

Bayne, T., & Bindler, R. (1988). Medication calculation skills of registered nurses. *Journal of Continuing Education in Nursing, 19*(6), 258–262.

Bindler, R., & Bayne, T. (1991). Medication calculation ability of registered nurses. *Image: Journal of Nursing Scholarship, 23*(4), 221–224.

Boyer, M. (1991). *Math for nurses: A pocket guide to dosage calculation and drug preparation* (2nd ed.). Philadelphia: Lippincott.

Byington, K. (1991). Your guide to pediatric drug administration. *Nursing, 21*(8), 82–92.

Carpenito, L. (1991). *Nursing care plans and documentation: Nursing diagnoses and collaborative problems.* Philadelphia: Lippincott.

Carr, D. (1989). New strategies for avoiding medication errors. *Nursing, 19*(8), 39–45.

Clark, J., Queener, S., & Karb, V. (1990). *Pharmacological basis of nursing practice* (3rd ed.). St. Louis: Mosby.

Cobb, M. (1990). Dealing fairly with medication errors. *Nursing, 20*(3), 42–43.

Cole, M. (1989). Flushing heparin locks: Is saline flushing really cost-effective? *Journal of Intravenous Nursing, 12*(Suppl. 1), S23–S29.

Conklin, D., MacFarland, V., Kinnie-Sleeves, A., & Chenger, T. (1990). Medication errors by nurses: Contributing factors. *Alberta Association of Registered Nurses' Newsletter, 46*(1), 8–9.

Craft, K. (1990). Do you really know how to handle sharps? *RN, 53*(8), 33–35.

Cyganski, J., Donahue, J., & Heaton, J. (1987). The case for the heparin flush. *American Journal of Nursing, 87*(6), 796–797.

Deglin, J., Vallerand, A., & Russin, M. (1990). *Davis's drug guide for nurses* (2nd ed.). Philadelphia: Davis.

Dick, L. (1989). Warning: Take only as directed. *RN, 52*(10), 83–84,86,88.

Dunn, D., & Lenihan, S. (1987). The case for the saline flush. *American Journal of Nursing, 87*(6), 798–799.

Fuqua, R., & Stevens, K. (1988). What we know about medication errors: A literature review. *Journal of Nursing Quality Assurance, 3*(1), 1–17.

Graham, K., & McMahon, M. (1989). Medication incidents: A microgram of prevention. *Dimensions of Health Service, 66*(8), 21–24.

Hahn, K. (1989). Administering eye medications. *Nursing, 19*(9), 80.

Hahn, K. (1990). Brush up on your injection technique. *Nursing, 20*(9), 54–58.

Herget, M., & Williams, A. (1989). New aids for low-vision diabetics. *American Journal of Nursing, 89*(10), 1319–1322.

Keen, M. (1990). Get on the right track with Z-track injections. *Nursing, 20*(8), 59.

Lacombe, D. (1990). Avoiding a malpractice nightmare. *Nursing, 20*(6), 42–43.

Lenox, A. (1990). IV therapy: Reducing the risk of infection. *Nursing, 20*(3), 60–61.

Long, T. (1992). Pointing out medication errors. *American Journal of Nursing, 92*(2), 76–78.

Lorenz, B. (1990). Are you using the right IV pump? *RN, 53*(5), 31–36.

MacIsaac, A., Rivers, R., & Adamson, C. (1989). Multiple medications: Is your elderly patient caught in the storm? *Nursing, 19*(7), 60–64.

Malseed R., & Girton, S. (1990). *Pharmacology: Drug therapy and nursing considerations* (3rd ed.). Philadelphia: Lippincott.

McConnell, E. (1990). Giving intradermal injections. *Nursing, 20*(3), 70.

McGovern, K. (1988). 10 Golden rules for administering drugs safely. *Nursing, 22*(3), 49–56.

Mitchell, J., & Pawlickl, K. (1990). Oral dosage forms that should not be crushed: 1990 Revision. *Hospital Pharmacy, 25*(4), 329–335.

Palmieri, D. (1991). Clearing up the confusion: Adverse effects of medications in the elderly. *Journal of Gerontological Nursing, 17*(10), 32–35.

Purkiss, R., & Chung, S. (1990). Facing the fax. *Nursing Times, 86*(11), 57–59.

Rasic, E., et al. (1989). A new system for managing medication errors. *Nursing Management, 20*(5), 102–106.

Robers, P., Moore, T., & Svarstad, B. (1988). Nurse administration of sleep medication: A comparison of registered nurses and licensed practical nurses. *American Journal of Public Health, 78*(12), 1581–1582.

Santo-Novak, D., & Edwards, R. (1989). RX: Take caution with drugs for elders. *Geriatric Nursing, 10*(2), 72–75.

Scholz, D. (1990). Establishing and monitoring an endemic medication error rate. *Journal of Nursing Quality Assurance, 4*(2), 71–74.

Schwartz, L., & Lowe, D. (1989). Applying a theoretical framework for reducing medication errors in intensive care units. *Focus on Critical Care, 16*(6), 438–444.

Sherman, J., & Clinefelter, K. (1989). Medication variances: A multi-hospital comparison. *Nursing Management, 20*(5), 56–58.

Sherman J., & Sherman, R. (1989). IV therapy that clicks. *Nursing, 19*(5), 50–51.

Shlafer, M., & Marieb, E. (1989). *The nurse, pharmacology, and drug therapy.* Redwood City, CA: Addison-Wesley.

Taylor, H. (1992). Patients deserve painless injections. *RN, 55*(3), 25–26.

Todd, B. (1990). Prescription for the '90s. *Geriatric Nursing, 11*(3), 114–115.

Trainor, P. (1988). Over-the-counter drugs: Count them in. *Geriatric Nursing, 9*(5), 298–299.

Ward, L. (1990). Patient teaching for home IV therapy. *RN, 53*(4), 86–88.

Whaley, L., & Wong, D. (1989). *Essentials of pediatric nursing* (3rd ed.). St. Louis: Mosby.

Williams, P. (1989). How do you keep medicines from clogging feeding tubes? *American Journal of Nursing, 89*(2), 181–182.

Wordell, D. (1988). Should you crush that tablet? *Nursing, 18*(1), 48–49.

Worrell, P., & Hodson, K. (1989). Posology: The battle against dosage calculation errors. *Nurse Educator, 14*(2), 27–31.

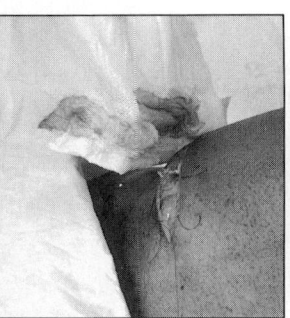
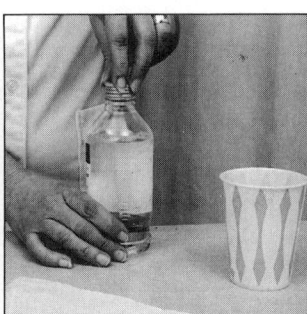

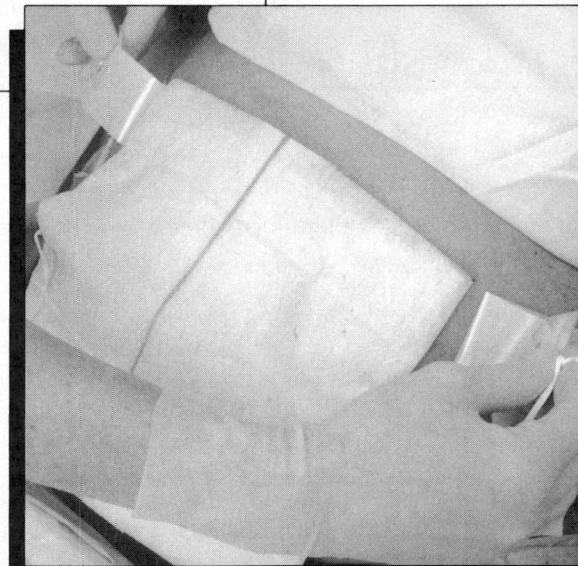

Care of Wounds

OBJECTIVES

After completing this chapter, the learner should be able to:

Define key terms used in the chapter.

Describe the physical and psychological effects of trauma to the body, with resultant wounds.

Discuss the processes involved in wound healing.

Describe wound complications, integrating factors that affect wound healing.

Summarize emergency wound assessment and care.

Describe the effects of the application of heat or cold.

Use the nursing process to knowledgably derive an individualized plan of care for the client with a wound, including the application of dressings and heat or cold.

KEY TERMS

abrasion
abscess
bandage
binder
capillarity
closed wound
compress
contusion
dehiscence
dressing
evisceration
exudate
granulation tissue
incision
laceration
open wound
pack
puncture
purulent
retention sutures
sanguineous
scar
serous
skin sutures
stab wound
wound

43

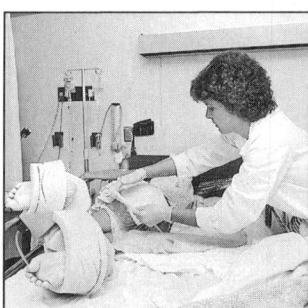

A ny alteration in the integrity of the skin is a **wound**. A wound may be accidental or intentional (as in the case of surgery) and may result in an increased risk for a person in terms of meeting basic needs and maintaining health. The care of the client with a wound requires nursing knowledge and skill, using the nursing process to plan and implement care that promotes healing; prevents further injury or illness; and facilitates coping with changes in self-concept and body image.

This chapter provides information about wounds, including the wound-healing process and factors that affect wound healing. Guidelines, rationale, and procedures for wound care (sterile dressing changes, dressings, and applications of heat and cold) are provided. The use of the nursing process is illustrated through selected nursing diagnoses for both the client with a wound and the client receiving applications of heat and cold. A sample care plan for one nursing diagnosis is included at the end of the chapter to illustrate the application of the nursing process in the clinical setting.

Functions of the Skin

The skin (or integument). the largest organ of the body, serves various functions in response to both the internal and the external environment. (A description of the anatomy and physiology of the skin, with related assessments in found in Chapter 24.) The functions of the skin are as follows:

- Provide protection for underlying tissues from the external environment. The potential for injury or infection is increased when the skin is undernourished, aged, traumatized, overly dry, or wet for long periods or when a physical illness is present.
- Control body temperature by the processes of radiation, conduction, convection, or evaporation (as described in Chapter 23)
- Provide sensory perception of pain, touch, heat, or cold
- Assist in the maintenance of the fluid and electrolyte balance of the body. Excessive sweating or drainage from the body results in the loss of water and salt (see Chapter 37).
- Use sunlight to synthesize vitamin D, necessary to calcium and phosphorus metabolism

- Communicate feelings and serve as a major component in self-concept and body image

This chapter, focusing on the care of wounds, is most concerned with the protective, sensory, and psychosocial functions of the skin.

Body's Reaction to Trauma

Wounds

The nurse cares for wounds, but only as one aspect of the nursing care given to the *client* with the wound. Using the nursing process, an individualized plan of care is developed to assess, to identify and prevent complications, to implement and evaluate skills essential to wound care, and to provide the necessary physical and emotional support so that healing, adaptation, and self-care are facilitated.

Types of Wounds

Wounds may be intentional or unintentional, open or closed. These broad classifications are discussed here; more specific descriptors are found in Table 43-1.

An *intentional wound* is the result of planned therapy or treatment that requires invasive measures. Examples of intentional wounds are those that result from surgical incisions, intravenous therapy, lumbar puncture, thoracentesis, and paracentesis. The wound edges are clean, and bleeding usually is controlled. Because the wound is made under sterile aseptic conditions with sterile supplies and skin preparation, the risk of infection is decreased and healing is facilitated.

Unintentional wounds occur from unexpected trauma, such as from accidents, forcible injury (such as stabbing, gun shots), and burns. Because the wounds occur in an unsterile environment, contamination is likely. Wound edges usually are jagged. multiple trauma is common, and bleeding is uncontrolled. These factors create a high risk for infection and a longer healing time.

An **open wound** occurs from intentional or unintentional trauma. The skin surface is broken, providing a portal of entry for microorganisms. Open wounds may be accompanied by bleeding, tissue damage, and increased risk for infection. A **closed wound** is the result of a blow, force, or strain sustained in traumatic situations such as a fall, an assault, or a motor vehicle accident. The skin surface is not broken, but soft tissue is damaged and internal injury and hemorrhage may occur.

Wounds may also be open or closed, clean or contaminated, superficial or deep. Table 43-1 lists the types, causes, descriptions, and implications of different types of wounds. Many wounds combine several descriptors; for example, an intentional wound to remove the appendix usually is a clean, open wound. In comparison, after an automobile accident, a person may have an unintentional, open laceration considered to be contaminated. Understanding the

TABLE 43-1

Types of Wounds and Risk of Infection

Type	Cause	Description and Implications
Contusion (bruise)	Blow from a hard object	A closed wound, results in soft-tissue damage and ruptured blood vessels; causes swelling and pain. If internal organs are contused, serious effects may result.
Incision	Made with a sharp instrument or needle	See intentional (open) wound.
Abrasion	An accidental injury or fall that scrapes or rubs off the skin surface; or an intentional dermatologic procedure	A painful open wound; involves only the skin
Laceration	Accidental trauma	Tissues are torn, and wound edges are ragged. Depth of wound varies, and affects risk of complications. Often caused by an unclean object, increasing risk of infection.
Puncture	Made by a sharp instrument or object that penetrates the skin and underlying tissue	May be intentional, or unintentional (see above)
Possibility and Degree of Contamination		
Clean	Surgical incision or closed wound	Contains no pathogenic organisms. Surgery did not enter the respiratory, gastrointestinal, or genitourinary systems.
Clean–contaminated	A specific surgery	Surgery enters the respiratory, gastrointestinal, or genitourinary system; risk of infection is increased.
Contaminated	Open accidental wounds, surgery with a major break in asepsis, or surgery with major contamination from the gastrointestinal system	Tissue becomes inflamed; risk of infection is high.
Infected	A wound with demonstrated pathogens; an old, traumatic wound; or a surgical incision into an infected area	Wound demonstrates inflammation, heat, purulent drainage, skin separation.

definitions and types of wounds prepares the nurse for wound care through assessing risk factors, implementing wound care, and evaluating wound healing.

General Principles of Tissue Healing

The following principles are used to guide action in promoting tissue healing. The healthy body has an innate capacity to protect and restore itself. Increasing the blood supply to the damaged area, walling off and removing cellular and foreign debris, and initiating cellular development are parts of the body's healing process. The healing process occurs normally, without assistance, although some care measures can help to support the process. For example, keeping the injured area free of debris by proper cleaning helps to promote tissue healing, as does positioning the wounded area to promote circulation to the part.

The body's ability to handle tissue trauma is influenced by the extent of the damage and by the person's general state of health. The capacity to deal adequately with an injury is limited when a healthy person sustains a massive injury, when the person has a chronic disease, or when the client is very young or very old. The promotion of wellness to im-

prove resistance to an insult to the body is partially directed toward maintaining adequate body reserves to deal with traumatic experiences.

The body's response to injury is more effective if proper nutrition has been maintained. Undernourished clients have difficulty mounting their cell-mediated defense system associated with T-lymphocyte activity. These clients may demonstrate diminished immune response to an antigen. Some leukocytic functions are diminished in the presence of protein deficiency. Undernourished clients, then, are at higher risk for developing a wound infection. Although the role of fatty acids in wound healing is not understood, it is known that certain quantities of glucose are necessary to meet the energy requirements of wound healing.

Various vitamins, minerals, and trace elements are needed for efficient wound healing. Vitamin A is necessary for collagen synthesis and epithelialization. Vitamin B complex serves as a cofactor of enzyme reactions needed for wound healing. Vitamin C is needed for collagen synthesis, capillary formation, and resistance to infection. Vitamin K is needed for the synthesis of prothrombin. Zinc, copper, and iron assist in collagen synthesis. Manganese serves as an enzyme activator.

The body responds systematically to trauma in any of its parts. Local physical responses to an injury cannot be separated from an overall body reaction. For example, an injured foot or hand or an abdominal incision can cause a variety of systematic reactions, which include increased body temperature, increased heart and respiratory rates, anorexia or nausea and vomiting, musculoskeletal tension throughout the body, and harmful hormonal changes. Adequate rest, relief of emotional stress, and sufficient nutrients and fluids are particularly important for the person undergoing a response to trauma.

The blood transports substances to and from injured tissue. An adequate blood supply is essential for the body's normal response to any injury. The blood brings increased amounts of leukocytes, erythrocytes, and platelets to the site of injury. Antibodies also are carried by the plasma. Increased circulation to the injured part provides for the removal of toxins and debris and allows for nutrients, oxygen, and other cell-building materials to be supplied. Areas of the body that have a good blood supply, such as the head and the neck, heal faster than areas in which the blood supply is not as great, such as the distal part of an extremity.

Intact skin and mucous membranes serve as first lines of defense against microorganisms. A break in the continuity of the skin or mucous membranes increases the likelihood of a wound infection. Surgical asepsis is used in caring for an open wound to minimize the possibility of pathogens entering the site. Precautions also are taken for people with closed wounds because the resistance of the damaged tissue is lowered and pathogenic organisms may be present. Careful handwashing before caring for a wound is probably the single most effective method for preventing wound infections.

Normal healing is promoted when the wound is free of foreign bodies, including bacteria. Healing does not start until foreign bodies are removed from the wound. Excessive exudate, dead or damaged tissue cells, pathogenic organisms, or embedded fragments of bone, metal, glass, or other substances can all act as foreign bodies. The body's rejection mechanisms are sufficient to remove many foreign substances. Sometimes mechanical means may be used to assist the process. In some situations, the body walls off a collection of pus or another foreign body, and healing occurs around it. This localized collection of pus is called an **abscess**. The person can be expected to develop symptoms at the unhealed site, although they may be delayed in their appearance.

Wound Healing

An injury to tissues results in two major responses—the stress response and the inflammatory response. All wounds follow the same phases in healing, although differences occur in the length of time required for each phase of the healing process and in the extent of granulation tissue formed.

Phases of Wound Healing

The phases of wound healing are described as they occur in the surgical wound (Cooper, 1990b) because this is the one that most commonly requires nursing care.

Inflammatory Phase The inflammatory phase begins with the incision for surgery and lasts through the third or fourth post-operative day. The two major physiologic activities are hemostasis and phagocytosis. The inflammatory response is immediate and prepares the tissues for healing.

As a major stressor, injury initiates the local adaptation syndrome (described in Chapter 9). As a result, there is first an immediate and brief constriction of blood vessels, allowing clotting of blood to seal the wound. This is followed by vasodilatation, allowing increased blood flow to the area, which permits white blood cells (leukocytes) to invade the area of injury and engulf bacteria and debris. About 24 hours after injury, a large phagocytic cell (a microphage) enters the area and secretes an angiogenesis factor that stimulates the formation of epithelial buds at the end of injured vessels so that reanastamosis can occur.

During the inflammatory phase, the client has a generalized body response, including a mildly elevated temperature, leukocytosis, and generalized malaise.

Proliferation Phase The proliferation phase begins about day 3 or 4 and lasts to about day 21. Fibroblasts rapidly synthesize collagens and ground substance. These two substances form the scaffold for the final repair of the wound. A thin layer of epithelial cells were formed across the wound during the inflammatory phase; now capillaries grow across the wound. This revascularization brings oxygen and nutrients required for continued healing. Fibroblasts also migrate from the bloodstream into the wound, depositing fibrin that stretches through the clot. A thin layer of epithelial cells forms across the wound, and blood flow across the wound is reinstituted. The new tissue, called **granulation tissue**, is highly vascular and reddish and bleeds easily.

The systemic symptoms should disappear, and the client looks and feels better. During this phase, adequate nutrition and oxygenation as well as prevention of strain on the suture line are important client care considerations.

Maturation Phase This final stage of healing begins about day 21 and can continue for as long as 1 to 2 years after injury. Collagen that has been haphazardly deposited in the wound is remodeled, making the healed wound stronger and more like adjacent tissue. New collagen continues to be deposited, which compresses the blood vessels in the healing wound, so that the scar eventually becomes a flat, thin, white, line. The **scar** is avascular collagen tissue that does not sweat, grow hair, or tan in sunlight.

Processes of Wound Healing

Wounds heal by one of three processes—primary, secondary, or tertiary intention (Fig. 43-1). Most surgical incisions

Primary Intention

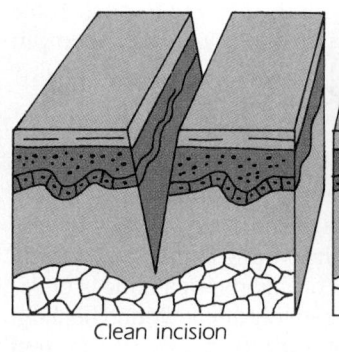
Clean incision

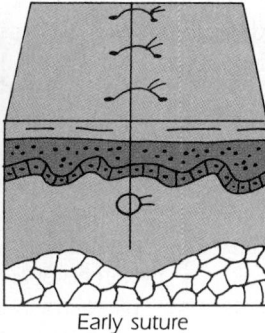
Early suture

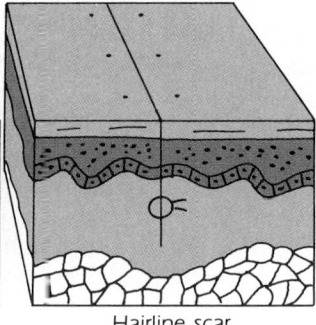
Hairline scar

- Wound is clean, in a straight line, with little loss of tissue
- All wound-edges are well approximated with sutures
- Usually rapid healing with minimal scarring

Secondary Intention

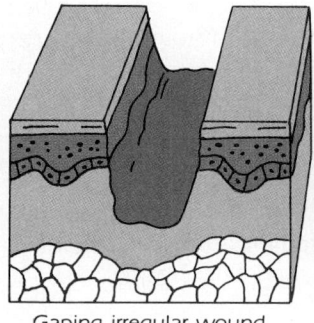
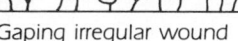
Gaping irregular wound

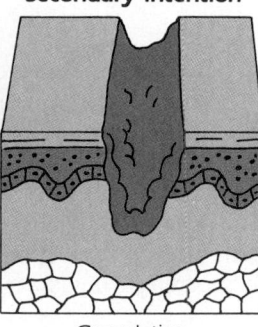
Granulation

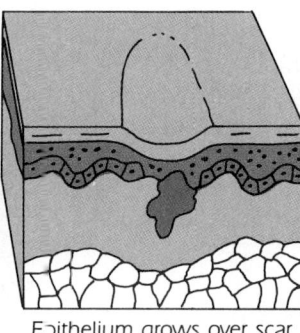
Epithelium grows over scar

- Large wound with considerable tissue loss
- Natural healing by formation of granulation tissue
- Healing takes longer and results in more scarring

Tertiary Intention

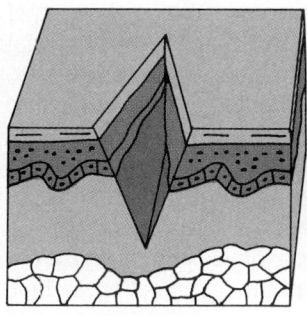
Wound

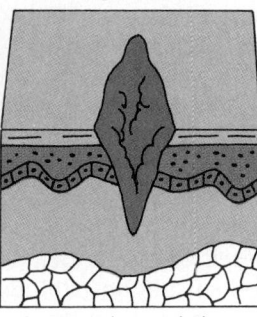
Increased granulation

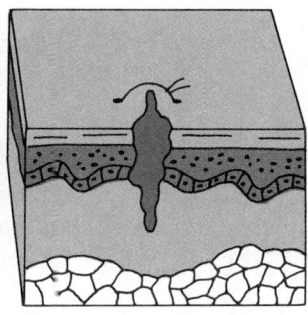
Late suturing with wide scar

- Time delay before wound is sutured
- Greater granulation, greater risk of infection, greater inflammatory reaction than primary intention
- Late suturing and more scarring

FIGURE 43-1

Types of wound healing.

and small sutured lacerations heal by *primary intention*. The wound is a clean, straight line with little loss of tissue. All wound edges are well approximated with sutures. These wounds normally heal rapidly with minimal scarring. *Secondary intention* healing takes place in large wounds that have considerable tissue loss, so that the edges cannot be approximated. Healing occurs by formation of granulation tissue. Because the wounds are more open, there is a greater chance of infection, healing time is longer, and scars are larger. *Tertiary intention* healing occurs when the interval between the wound's occurrence and its suturing is extended. This delay allows access for pathogens, so that there is an increased risk for infection. There also is a greater inflammatory reaction and more granulation tissue in comparison to healing by primary intention, so scars are large and less likely to shrink to a flat line.

Wound Drainage

During the first two phases of wound healing, the inflammatory response results in exudate that escapes from the wound. **Exudate** is composed of fluid and cells that escape from blood vessels and are deposited in or on tissue surfaces. This exudate is called *wound drainage* and is described as *serous* or *sanguineous* or, if infected, as *purulent*. These types of exudate can be further described as follows:

Serous—composed primarily of the clear serous portion of the blood and from serous membranes. Serous drainage is clear and watery.

Sanguineous—consists of large numbers of red blood cells and looks like blood. Bright red sanguineous drainage is indicative of fresh bleeding, whereas darker drainage indicates older bleeding.

Purulent—made up of white blood cells, liquefied dead tissue debris, and both dead and live bacteria. Purulent drainage is thick, often has a musty or foul odor, and varies in color, depending on the causative organism.

Drainage may be a mixture of these three types; surgical wounds most commonly have a mixture of serum and red blood cells, called *serosanguineous* drainage.

Factors Affecting Wound Healing

Developmental Considerations

Children and healthy adults heal more rapidly than do elderly people, in whom physiologic changes caused by aging have resulted in diminished fibroblastic activity and circulation. The older adult is more likely to have one or more chronic illnesses, with pathologic changes that impede the healing process (Jones & Millman, 1990). See the display Focus on the Older Adult.

Impaired Circulation and Oxygenation

A number of physical conditions can affect wound healing. The presence of large amounts of subcutaneous and tissue fat (which has fewer blood vessels) in obese people may slow wound healing because fatty tissue is more difficult to suture and more prone to infection, and takes longer to heal. Circulation may be impaired in elderly people and in people with peripheral vascular disorders, cardiovascular disorders, hypertension, or diabetes mellitus. Oxygenation of tissues is decreased in people with anemia or chronic respiratory disorders and in those who smoke.

Wound Condition

The specific condition of the wound affects how quickly and effectively the wound heals. For example, large, con-taminated, infected wounds or wounds that retain foreign bodies heal slowly. Some wounds may fail to heal. Table 43-1 describes types of wounds that are prone to complications.

Overall Client Wellness

Clients who have inadequate nutrition, are taking steroid drugs, or require postoperative radiation therapy have a high risk of delayed healing and wound complications. Additionally, the presence of a chronic physical illness or severe emotional stress can negatively affect wound healing. In some instances, it is necessary to improve nutritional status or treat underlying conditions before surgery is done.

Wound Complications

Wound complications increase the risk of generalized illness and death, lengthen the client's hospital stay, and add to health care costs. Wound complications include infection, hemorrhage, dehiscence, and evisceration.

Infection

Invasion of the wound by bacteria can occur at the time of trauma, during surgery, or at any time after the initial wound. A contaminated wound is more likely to become infected, as is a surgical wound resulting from a procedure that involves the intestines, in which the risk of contamination with fecal material is high. Symptoms of wound infection usually become apparent within 2 to 7 days after the injury or surgery. This means that with the trend toward decreased hospital stay, infection may appear after the client has left the hospital. Symptoms of infection include purulent drainage, increased drainage, pain, redness and swelling in and around the wound, increased body temperature, and increased white blood cell count. Nursing care of infected wounds is discussed later in this chapter.

F O C U S   O N   T H E   O L D E R   A D U L T

Factors That Affect Wound Healing in Older Adults

Changes in Skin

- Skin loses turgor and is more fragile.
- There is increased risk of further injury from cleaning agents and tape.

Nutrition

- Decreased secretion of enzymes and absorption of nutrients and minerals may have potential risk for altered nutrition, which would delay wound healing.

Potential for Infection

- Age reduces antibody production and functioning of the endocrine system, both of which increase susceptibility to infection.
- The incidence of chronic illnesses that compromise circulation and oxygenation of tissues (such as diabetes mellitus and cardiovascular problems) further decreases resistance to infection.

Hemorrhage

Hemorrhage may indicate a slipped suture, a dislodged clot from stress at the suture line or operative site, infection, or the erosion of a blood vessel by a foreign body (such as a drain). Postoperative wounds require careful nursing assessment so that hemorrhage is detected early. Hypovolemia may not be immediately evident. Therefore, dressing (and the wound under the dressing if possible) should be checked frequently during the first 48 hours after surgery and no less than every 8 hours thereafter. Early assessment findings of hemorrhage can include excessive thirst, increased pulse and respiratory rate, and generalized weakness. If excessive bleeding does occur, additional sterile pressure dressings or packing may be necessary, fluid replacement will probably be necessary, and surgical intervention may be required.

Dehiscence and Evisceration

Dehiscence and evisceration are the most serious postoperative wound complications. **Dehiscence** is the partial or total disruption of wound layers. **Evisceration** is the protrusion of viscera through the incisional area (see Fig. 43-2). These are frightening occurrences for both the client and the nurse. Careful nursing assessment can help to identify the predisposing signs of these events. An appreciable increase in the flow of serosanguineous fluid into the wound dressings between the 5th and 12th postoperative days is a clue to impending dehiscence (Flynn and Rovee, 1982). Wound disruption often is preceded by a sudden straining, such as coughing, sneezing, or vomiting. It is not

uncommon for the client to comment that "something has suddenly given way." If dehiscence or evisceration occurs, the wound area should be covered with sterile towels soaked in saline solution, and the physician should be notified immediately. Both these situations are emergencies that require prompt preparation for surgical repair.

Psychological Effects of Wounds

Trauma, with resultant wounds, causes psychological stress as well as physical injury. Because the skin functions as a sensory organ and plays a major role in the way we communicate with others and feel about ourselves, wounds require adaptation in the emotional as well as the physical dimensions of the traumatized person. Although stress and adaptation are highly individualized, there are actual and potential emotional stressors common to all clients with wounds. These stressors include pain, anxiety, fear, and alterations in self-concept.

Pain

Pain is part of almost any trauma, from a small cut on the finger to a large abdominal incision made during bowel surgery. Although pain can be considered to be a physical complication, there is a large psychological component as well. Pain from wounds often is increased by activities such as ambulating, coughing, moving in bed, and dressing changes. The actual pain may be worsened for the client by anticipatory apprehension of such activities. Nursing interventions to reduce pain through skill and explanations can greatly reduce emotional stress.

Anxiety and Fear

Anxiety and fear are common responses to a wound. Clients are apprehensive about the wound strength, how much privacy will be lost as the wound is cared for, and how they and others will react to the sights and smells of the wound. They may actually fear the sight of blood or the sight of what they consider mutilation of their bodies. As nurses care for clients with wounds, it is important that they be accepting and empathic, encourage ventilation of feelings, answer questions accurately and honestly, and avoid excessive exposure of body parts when giving wound care.

Alterations in Self-Concept

The self-concept of each person is that of a whole entity. When the skin and tissues are traumatized, that concept is changed, and the person must adapt and reformulate the concept of self. Wounds and scars that are visible to others, especially on the face, can leave the client with feelings of being conspicuous and ugly and of less worth. Large scars, such as those remaining from removal of a breast or from

FIGURE 43-2

Wound complications.

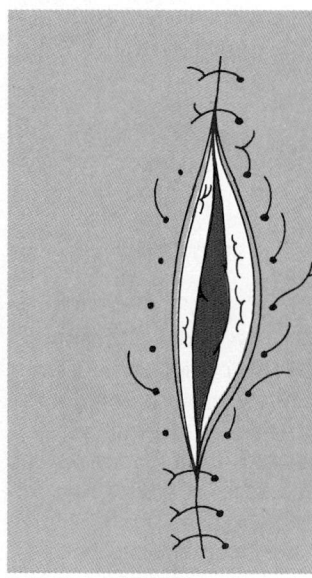
Dehiscence

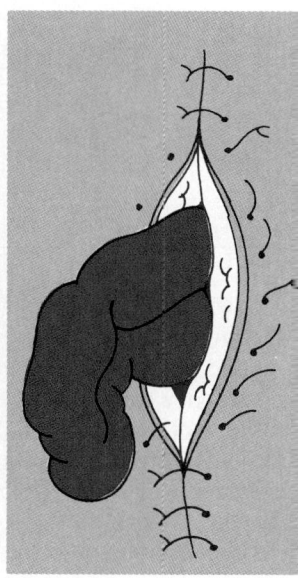
Evisceration

colostomy openings, can seriously impact sexuality, social relationships, and body image. When developing a plan of care, nurses must include interventions to resolve these concerns; referral to support groups or counselors may be necessary to facilitate coping and acceptance—by both the client and the family—of changes in body structure or function.

Nurse's Role in Wound Care

This section of the chapter discusses the nurse's role in the care of wounds, including the use of all phases of the nursing process in the clinical setting. A case study and sample care plan for one common nursing diagnosis is included at the end of the chapter to illustrate the application of knowledge and skills presented.

Assessing the Wound

Trauma to tissues can occur unexpectedly through a wide variety of accidental injuries, or it can be planned, as in surgical intervention. Nurses need to know how to assess clients and their wounds in both emergency and structured settings and to make appropriate interventions to meet client needs specific to the setting (see the accompanying display). This section focuses on the assessment and first aid for wounds from unplanned trauma as well as the assessment of surgical wounds.

Emergency Wound Assessment and Care

The following are general guidelines for emergency wound assessment and client care.

- The priority is assessment of the general condition of the wounded person. If the injury is serious, assess for an open and intact airway, spontaneous respirations, and a strong pulse. A helpful way to remember these important areas of assessment are by using the mnemonic ABC:

  A = airway
  B = breathing
  C = circulation

  (This pattern of assessments should be the priority in any emergency situation.)

- Assess the severity of the wound. In the case of major trauma or serious bleeding, either call 911 for emergency care or have someone else call while you remain with the injured person.
- Control bleeding from blunt trauma by applying ice during the first 24 to 48 hours.
- Control bleeding that is severe by applying direct pressure over the wound. If possible, cover the wound with a clean dressing.
- Assess for any other traumatic injuries—fractures, internal bleeding, spinal cord injuries, head injuries.

Emergency Assessments and Care of Specific Wounds

Type	Assessments and Interventions
Abrasion	• Assess extent and depth of wound. • Flush with running water and wash with soap and water. • If small, leave open; if large, cover with light dressing.
Laceration	• Assess length, depth, and location of wound. • Clean with soap and water. • Hold wound edges together with tape or a dressing. • Refer for further treatment, if necessary.
Puncture	• Assess cause (animal bite, out doors) and last tetanus shot. • Allow bleeding to flush out saliva or dirt. • Clean with soap and water. • Refer for further treatment, as necessary.
Impaled object	• Assess cardiopulmonary status. • *Do not* remove the object. • Control the bleeding by putting pressure around the object. • Secure immediate emergency care.
Amputations	• Assess blood loss and cardiopulmonary status. • Control bleeding by direct pressure to wound or over pressure points. • Elevate the affected extremity. • Place amputated digits or extremity in a sealed plastic bag and immerse bag in ice-filled container. • Secure immediate emergency care; transport amputated part with client.

- For anything other than a minor wound, be sure the injured person goes to an emergency department or emergency care facility. Immediate treatment reduces the risk of infection and decreases scar formation. If the person has not had a tetanus immunization within the past 5 years, it may be necessary for him or her to receive such an immunization.
- Instruct the person or his or her family members to immediately report redness, swelling, continued pain, or purulent or increased drainage.

Assessing the Surgical Wound

Surgical wounds are defined here as wounds that result from intentional surgical therapy or wounds that were unintentional but have been treated (cleaned and sutured). Wounds are assessed by inspection (sight and smell) and palpation and for appearance, drainage, and pain. Included in the assessment are drains or tubes, sutures, and signs of possible complications, as previously described.

Appearance   Included in assessing the appearance of a wound are the approximation of wound edges, color of the wound and surrounding area, drains or tubes, sutures, and signs of dehiscence or evisceration. The wound edges should be clean and well approximated, with a crust along the wound edges. The wound's edges initially are reddened and slightly swollen, but by the end of about a week, the skin should be closer to normal in appearance and the wound edges should be healed together. Skin surrounding the wound may at first be bruised, but this, too, returns to normal as blood is reabsorbed. If an infection is present, the wound is swollen, has increased redness, and feels hot. If dehiscence is impending or present, the wound edges are separated.

Skin sutures, which may be black silk, synthetic material, metal staples, fine wire, or metal skin clips, are used to hold tissue and skin together. **Retention sutures** are used to provide extra support for obese clients and for wounds with increased risk of dehiscence (Fig. 43-3). Most skin sutures are removed in 7 to 10 days. Silk and synthetic sutures are removed with a suture removal set (Fig. 43-4); staples are removed with a special staple remover. The steps in removing sutures and staples are summarized in the accompanying display. After the removal of skin sutures, Steri-Strips are sometimes applied across the healed wound to give additional support as the wound continues

Types of sutures

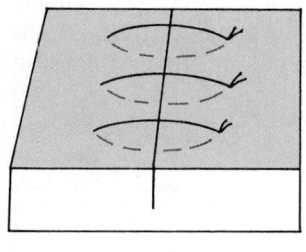

Plain interrupted

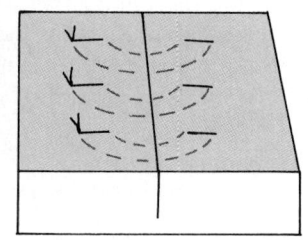

Mattress interrupted

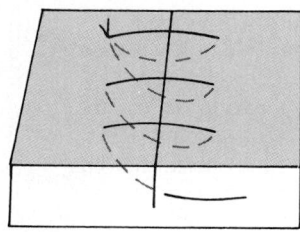

Plain continuous

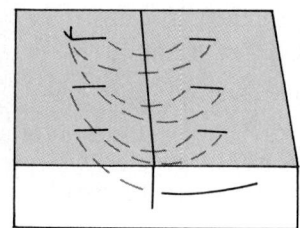

Mattress continuous

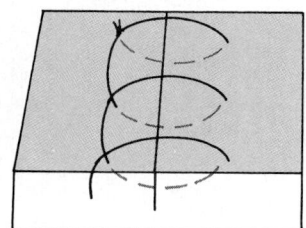

Blanket continuous

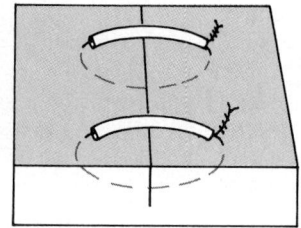

Retention

FIGURE   43-3

Types of sutures and techniques for removal.

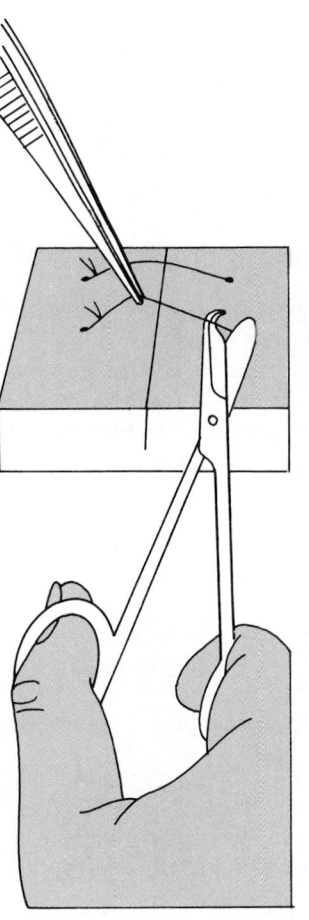

Removing interrupted sutures

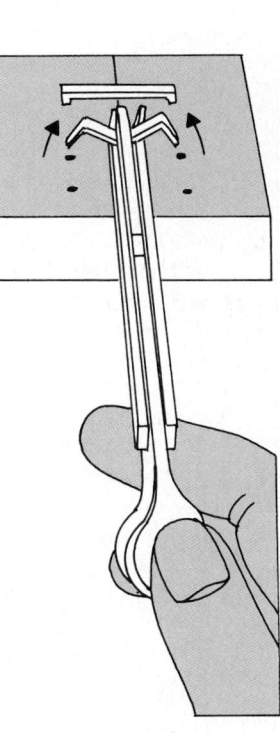

Removing staples

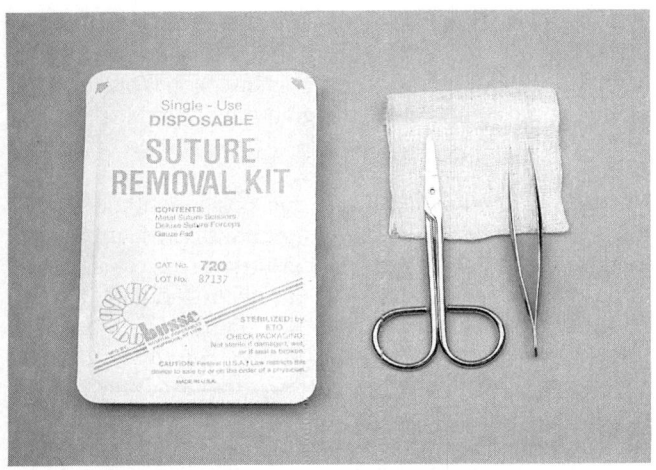

FIGURE 4 3 - 4

Suture removal kit. (Photo © Ken Kasper.)

to heal. The status of skin sutures is included in wound assessment.

Drains and tubes are inserted into or near a wound when it is anticipated that a collection of fluid in a closed area will delay healing. After a surgical procedure, the physician places one end of the tube or drain in or near the area

to be drained and passes the other end through the skin, either directly through the incision or through a separate opening called a **stab wound**. Drains and tubes may or may not be sutured in place; drains placed directly through the wound (for example, a Penrose drain) usually have a large safety pin in the part outside the wound to prevent them from slipping back into the incised area and are not sutured (Fig. 43-5). Tubes that are connected to suction or that have a built-in reservoir to maintain constant low suction usually are sutured to the skin (for example, a Jackson-Pratt drainage tube or a Hemovac). It is important to know which type of drain or tube was inserted during surgery, so that accurate assessment can be made. The patency and placement of tubes or drains are included in wound assessment. Table 43-2 describes the purpose and common use of selected drains and tubes.

Drainage The amount, color, odor, and consistency of wound drainage is assessed. The amount and color depend on the wound location and size, with larger wounds having more drainage. Wound drainage, as previously described, may be serous, serosanguineous, sanguineous, or, if infected, purulent. Purulent drainage usually has a musty or foul odor; it is thick and either yellow, green, or brown. Frankly sanguineous drainage is indicative of hemorrhage. Drainage can be assessed on the wound, on the dressings, in

GUIDELINES FOR NURSING CARE

Removal of Staples and Sutures

The removal of staples or sutures may be done by the physician or by the nurse with a physician's order. Agency protocol should be followed, but general guidelines are as follows:

- Use sterile techniques, following recommended CDC guidelines for care of wounds.
- Wash hands before and after the procedure.
- Explain the procedure to the client. Describe the sensation that will be experienced as a pulling or slightly uncomfortable experience.
- Use proper technique to remove and dispose of old dressings.
- Clean the incision from the center of the wound outward, using hospital policy and procedure for type of agent.
- Remove every other suture or staple to be sure wound edges are healed; if they are, remove remaining sutures or staples as ordered.
- Remove or reapply dressing, depending on physician preference and agency policy.
- Some physicians order Steri-Strip application to the healed wound after removal of staples or sutures to give additional support to the wound as it continues to heal. Follow agency protocol and physician preference for placement of these tapes.

Specifics for Suture Removal

- Use a sterile suture removal kit.
- Using the sterile forceps, grasp the knot of the first suture and gently lift the knot.
- Using the sterile scissors, cut one side of the suture below the knot close to the skin.
- Grasp the knot with the forceps and pull the cut suture through the skin (be sure to pull through the healed wound only the portion of the suture that has been inside the tissue).

Specifics for Staple Removal

- As directed on the package, gently position the sterile staple remover under the staple to be removed.
- Firmly close the staple remover to straighten the staple ends (do not lift upward while disengaging staple ends).
- Carefully lift upward with the closed staple remover to remove the staple from the incision line. It may be necessary to remove one end of the staple and then the other if it does not easily lift out.

and laboratory test results. *Infection* may cause generalized malaise, increased pain, anorexia, and an elevated body temperature and pulse rate; laboratory data include an elevated white blood cell count and, if a wound culture is done, a causative organism. *Hemorrhage* is further identified by restlessness, anxiety, a drop in systolic blood pressure, increased pulse and respiratory rates, decreased urinary output, and decreased hemoglobin levels and hematocrit.

Diagnosing

Nursing diagnoses made to identify human responses to alterations in health status as a result of a wound are written to guide nursing interventions that support wound healing and prevent complications. Additionally, holistic assessments and nursing care focus on the *client* with the wound, and identify problems in other functions or dimensions affected by the wound's presence.

In formulating nursing diagnoses for the client with a wound, the nurse must consider the assessment and nursing history information that support the specific diagnosis. Data used would include the following:
- Client's physical status, including age, presence or absence of other illnesses, health habits, and obesity
- Cause of the wound
- Location, size, and severity of the wound
- Support systems available
- Client's social and work history

Included below are examples of nursing diagnoses developed to describe actual or potential problems experienced by the client with a wound.

Altered Sexuality Patterns related to altered self-concept from change in appearance after colostomy

Anticipatory Grieving related to loss of left breast from surgical procedure to remove malignant tumor (scheduled for next day)

Anxiety related to lack of knowledge about postoperative care of left anterior thigh incision

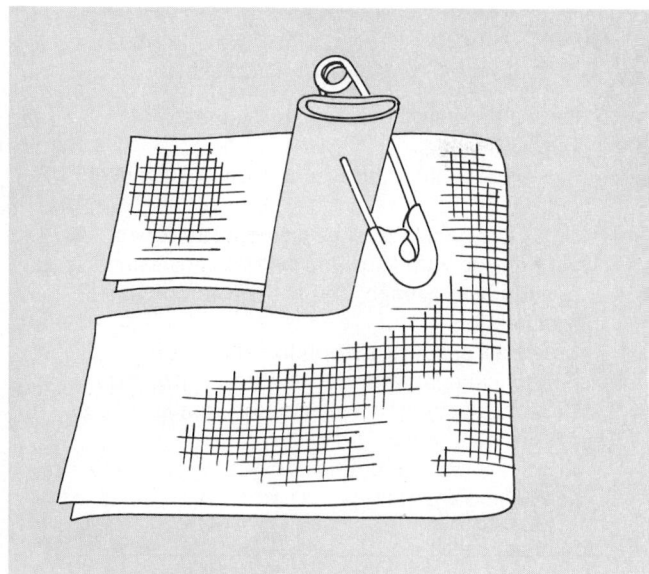

FIGURE 43-5

Penrose drain.

drainage bottles or reservoirs, or, depending on the location of the wound and the amount of drainage, under the client.

Pain If the client complains of increased or constant pain from the wound, or if wound edges are swollen with purulent or increased drainage, further assessments should be made and symptoms should be documented and reported. Pain, especially when accompanied by an increased or purulent flow of drainage, indicates delayed healing or the presence of an infection. Incisional pain usually is severest for the first 2 to 3 days and then progressively diminishes.

Related Assessments In addition to assessments of the wound, the nurse evaluates the client's general condition

TABLE 43-2

Common Types of Drains		
Type	Purpose	Example
Penrose	Provides sinus tract	After incision and drainage of abscess, in abdominal surgery
T-tube	For bile drainage	After gallbladder surgery
Jackson-Pratt	Decrease dead space by collecting drainage	After breast removal, abdominal surgery
Hemovac	Decrease dead space by collecting drainage	After abdominal, orthopedic surgery
Gauze, iodoform gauze, NuGauze	Allow healing from base of wound	Infected wounds, after removal of hemorrhoids

Self-Care Deficit: Bathing/Hygiene related to presence of infected midline abdominal wound

Body Image Disturbance related to multiple lacerations of face.

High Risk for Infection related to presence of chronic illness (diabetes mellitus) and lack of knowledge about care of foot ulcer

Pain related to large incision in right flank

Planning: Client Goals

Although many nursing diagnoses can be identified as appropriate for the client with a wound, there are so many different types of wounds that planning is highly individualized and specific. With the major goals of promoting health, preventing further injury or illness, and facilitating coping, nursing care for any client with a wound is focused on the following client goals. The client will:

- Demonstrate progressive healing of the wound, as evidenced by the following:
  - Wound edges closing together
  - Reduced swelling and redness of wound edges
  - Reduction in amount and color of drainage
  - Decreased wound pain
- Remain free of infection, with normal temperature and white blood cell count; absence of wound swelling, odor, and purulent drainage; and no increase in pain
- Practice self-care behaviors to promote healing by the following:
  - Washing hands appropriately
  - Keeping hands away from wound, wound drainage, and dressing
  - Maintaining fluid intake at appropriate levels
  - Selecting and eating a balanced diet, as ordered
- Verbalize and demonstrate wound and dressing care

In caring for the client with a wound, the nurse carries out interventions to promote wound healing, prevent further injury or alteration in skin integrity, prevent infection, promote physical and emotional comfort, and facilitate coping.

Implementing

The basic objective of wound care is to promote tissue repair and regeneration (Cuzzell & Stotts, 1990), so that skin integrity is restored. There are two methods of caring for wounds—the open method, in which no dressing is used to cover the wound, and the closed method, in which a **dressing** is used as a protective cover over the wound.

Most dressings, especially for the surgical wound, consist of three layers. The dressing applied directly over the wound, called the contact layer, allows drainage to pass into the middle layer. This layer should be able to be removed without causing further tissue damage. The middle

---

> **Advantages of Wound Dressings**
>
> - Dressings absorb drainage to help promote wound healing.
> - Dressings protect the wound from mechanical injury.
> - Dressings, when used as a pressure dressing or with elastic bandages, promote hemostasis, help prevent hemorrhage, and aid in wound edge approximation.
> - Dressings splint or immobilize the wound, facilitating healing and preventing further trauma.
> - Dressings prevent contamination from the external environment.
> - Dressings provide physical, psychological, and aesthetic comfort.

---

layer dressings absorbs the drainage, and the outer layer keeps the two inner layers in place (Flynn & Hackel, 1990).

Dressings have advantages and disadvantages. The advantages are listed in the display; the disadvantages are that dressings can rub or stick to the wound, causing further superficial injury. Dressings also can create a warm, damp, and dark environment—all components conducive to the growth of organisms, with resultant infection. Most wounds are covered with a dressing, and nurses are responsible for most dressing changes. This section deals with the supplies needed for dressing changes, guidelines for prevention of infection, and procedures for changing selected types of dressings.

Gathering Supplies for Dressings

Before changing a dressing, the nurse should gather needed supplies. The items may be gathered individually or they may be packaged in a sterile dressing tray. Some hospital units have special dressing carts, with all dressing supplies located in one area. The supplies needed vary with the type, location, and amount of wound drainage; the nursing care plan should include specifics about each client's dressing procedure and supplies. Materials and supplies include cleaning agents, materials to cover the wound (the dressing), and materials used to secure the dressing and support the wound.

Cleaning Agents Many possible antiseptic cleaning agents can be used to clean the wound. Some commonly used agents are Betadine, 70% alcohol, 3% hydrogen peroxide, and sterile normal saline solution. Some authorities question the use of any agent other than saline solution because of the caustic effect on skin, tissues, and granulating tissue of the other agents (Rodeheaver et al., 1982). The choice of cleaning agent largely depends on agency protocol and physician preference.

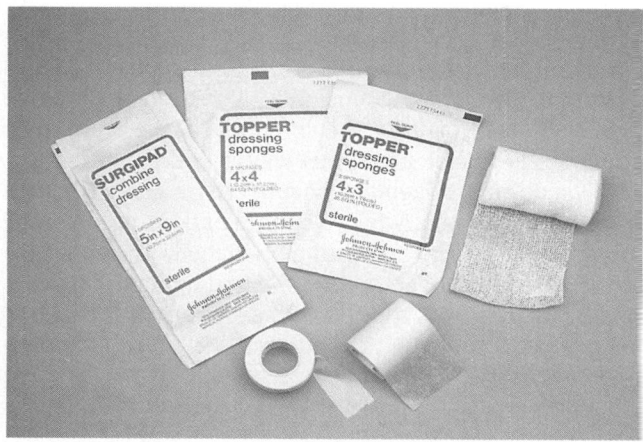

Various types of gauze dressings and tape. (Photo © Ken Kasper.)

Dressing Supplies The number and types of dressings used depend on the location and size of the wound as well as on the amount and type of drainage. In discussing dressings, supplies are defined as they are used from the incision outward. An incision line often is covered with sterile petrolatum gauze or a special gauze called Telfa. Telfa's shiny outer surface is applied to the wound and allows drainage to pass through and be absorbed by the center (or outer) absorbent layer. Both these protective dressings prevent outer dressings from adhering to the wound and causing further injury when removed.

Gauze dressings commonly are used to cover wounds (Fig. 43-6). These dressings come in various sizes (2 × 2 inches, 4 × 4 inches, 4 × 8 inches) and are commercially packaged as single units or in packs. Special gauze dressings (eg, Soft-Wick) are precut halfway to fit around drains or tubes. Larger dressings (8 × 10s, ABDs, Surgipads) are placed over the smaller gauzes and serve to absorb drainage and protect the wound from contamination or injury.

Transparent dressings (eg, Op-Site) are applied directly over a small wound or tube; these dressings are occlusive, decreasing the possibility of contamination while allowing visualization of the wound. This type of dressing often is used over intravenous sites, subclavian catheter insertion sites, and healing wounds.

Tape There are many kinds of tape, ranging in width from ½ to 4 inches (1-inch wide tape is the most commonly used). Table 43-3 summarizes the types and purposes of different tapes.

Bandages and Binders Bandages are strips of cloth, gauze (eg, roller gauze, Kerlix, Kling), or elasticized material (eg, Ace bandages) used to wrap a body part. They come packaged in rolls and vary in width from 1 to 6 inches. Bandages are used to secure dressings, apply pressure, and support the wound; they are especially useful in injuries of the extremities.

Binders are designed for a specific body part, and include slings, abdominal binders, chest binders, and T-binders. Binders may be made of cloth (flannel, muslin) or of an elasticized material that fastens together with Velcro.

Applying Bandages and Binders

General Principles

A bandage or binder promotes healing by preventing damage to wounds and skin by holding dressings on a wound and by offering the client comfort and security. The following principles guide action for applying bandages and binders.

Unclean bandages and binders may cause infection if applied over a wound or skin abrasion. This fact guides what may be a rather obvious action: bandages and binders should be kept clean and free of contamination. Medical asepsis is observed when applying bandages and binders. Skin abrasions and wounds are first covered with sterile

Types of Tape	
Type	**Purpose**
Adhesive (can cause occlusion, allergy, skin maceration, shearing)	Used for strength, support, and economy • To secure dressings and splints • To strap joints to prevent athletic injuries • To immobilize or stabilize body parts • To provide pressure • To approximate wound edges
Paper, plastic, acetate	Increased comfort, decreased allergic and skin problems • To close small wounds • To secure dressings
Microfoam	Used for compression or pressure dressings

T A B L E   4 3 - 3

dressings before clean bandages and binders are applied to protect the wound from trauma and contamination. Certain bandages and binders may be reused, but they should be changed if they become soiled or wet.

Prolonged heat and moisture on the skin may cause epithelial cells to deteriorate. This principle indicates that the area to be covered should be cleaned and dried thoroughly before applying a bandage or binder. An unnecessarily thick or extensive bandage should be avoided, so that the part being covered does not become excessively warm. Porous materials are preferable to nonporous materials because they allow air to circulate and perspiration to evaporate.

Placing and supporting the body part to be bandaged in the normal functioning position prevents deformities and discomfort and enhances circulation to the body part. Bandages and binders usually restrict some motion and often are intended to immobilize a part of the body. Therefore, it is important that the body part involved first be placed comfortably in the position of normal functioning.

Blood flow through tissues is decreased by applying excessive pressure on blood vessels. The healing process is impaired and tissue cells may die if the blood supply is inadequate to remove wastes and bring nourishment to the body part involved. The bandage or binder is applied with sufficient pressure to provide the amount of immobilization or support desired, to remain in place, and to secure a dressing if one is present. Pressure should not be so great, however, that circulation in the body part involved is impeded. Leaving a small portion of an extremity exposed, such as the fingers or toes, allows the nurse to assess for proper circulation in the bandaged area. Leaving a considerable portion of the end of an extremity exposed is likely to impede circulation if swelling in the exposed area occurs. For example, the heel should not be exposed when bandaging the foot and leg.

The tension of each bandage turn should be equal, and unnecessary and uneven overlapping of turns should be avoided. These techniques help to prevent undue and uneven pressure on tissues. Bony prominences over which bandages and binders must be placed are padded. Hollows in the body contour may be filled with padding to provide comfort and help maintain equal pressure from the bandage or binder. An extremity should be bandaged toward the trunk to promote venous return and impaired circulation in the distal part. After a bandage or binder has been applied, the body part is assessed frequently for signs of impaired circulation. In addition to being dangerous, a bandage applied too tightly is uncomfortable for the client.

Pins and knots, often used to secure a bandage or binder, are placed well away from the wound, a pressure point, or a tender and inflamed area. Pins and knots as well as seams in a bandage or binder cause undue and uneven pressure. They also cause discomfort for the client if located incorrectly.

A well-applied bandage or binder is comfortable, durable, neat, and clean. This is important for the client's emotional security as well as for promoting the best possible physiologic functioning of the body.

Applying Bandages (Fig. 43-7)

Applying Roller Bandages
A roller bandage is a continuous strip of material wound on itself to form a cylinder or roll. Plain gauze, elastic webbing, and stretchable roller bandages are made in various widths and lengths.

When the bandaging is begun, the free end is held in place with one hand while the other hand passes the roll around the body part. After the bandage is anchored, the roll is passed or rolled around the body part, taking care that equal tension is exerted with each turn. It is easier to keep tension equal by unwinding the bandage gradually and only as it is required.

Basic Turns for Applying Roller Bandages
Circular Turn When using the circular turn, the bandage is wrapped around the body part with complete overlapping of the previous bandage turn. It is used primarily for anchoring a bandage where it is begun and where it is terminated.

Spiral Turn When using the spiral turn, the bandage ascends in a spiral manner so that each turn overlaps the preceding one by one half or two thirds the width of the bandage. The spiral turn is useful when the body part being bandaged is cylindrical, such as the area around the wrist, the fingers, and the trunk.

Spiral-Reverse Turn A spiral-reverse turn is a spiral turn in which reverses are made halfway through each turn. Spiral-reverse turns are particularly effective for bandaging a cone-shaped body part, such as the thigh, the leg, or the forearm.

Figure-of-Eight Turn The figure-of-eight turn consists of making oblique overlapping turns that ascend and descend alternately. Each turn crosses the one preceding it so that it appears like the figure eight. It is effective for use around joints, such as the knee, the elbow, the ankle, and the wrist. Because it provides a snug bandage, it often is used for immobilization.

Spica The spica consists of ascending and descending turns that overlap and cross one another to form an angle. It is particularly useful for bandaging the thumb, the breast, the shoulder, the groin, and the hip.

Recurrent Bandage Sometimes this type of bandage is called a *stump bandage.* It is used for fingers and for the stump of an amputated limb. After a few circular turns to anchor the bandage, the initial end of the bandage is placed in the center of the body part being bandaged, well back from the tip to be covered. The bandage is passed back and forth over the tip, first on the one side and then on the other side of the center piece of bandage. Figure 43-7 shows how to apply a recurrent bandage to a stump, using the figure-of-eight turn to finish the bandage. Recurrent bandages also are used effectively for head bandages.

Roller Bandages

Circular Turn

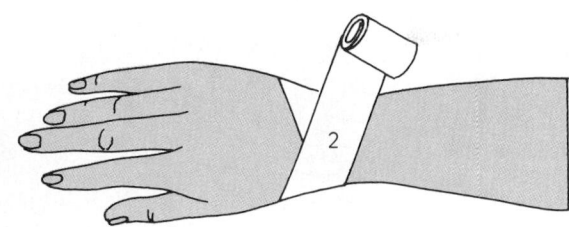

How the circular turn is started to anchor a roller bandage.

Spiral Turn

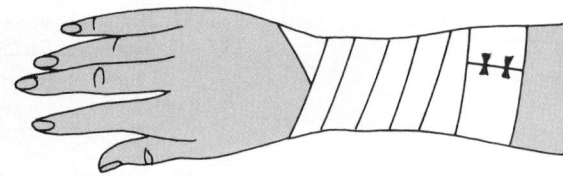

A spiral turn, which was performed after the bandage was anchored.

Spiral-Reverse Turn

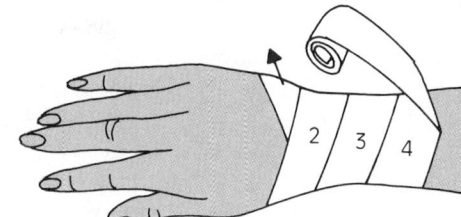

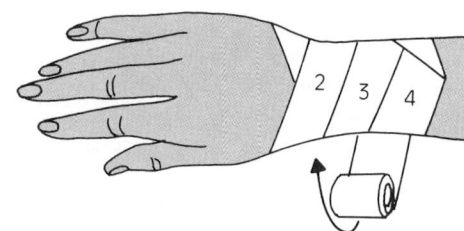

Figure-Eight

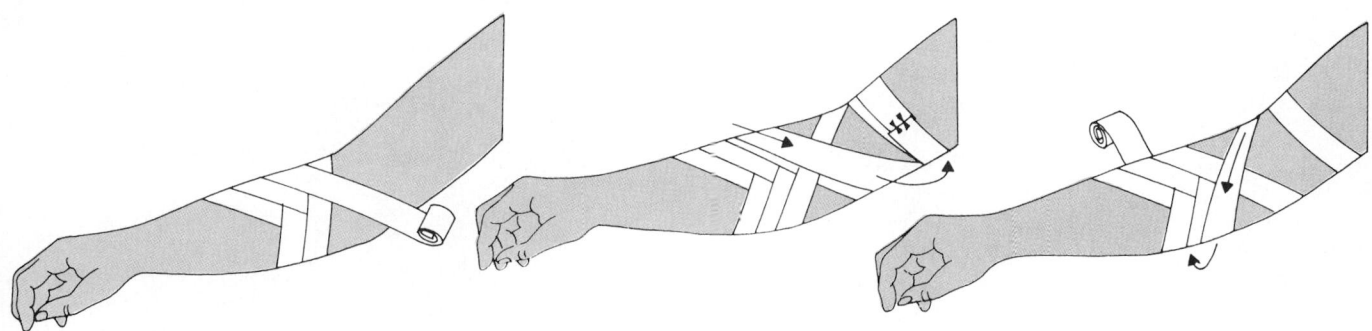

Spica

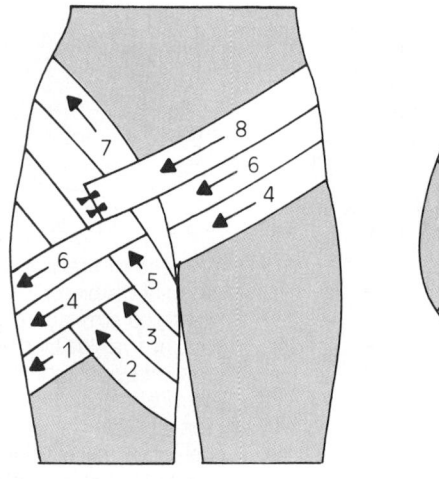

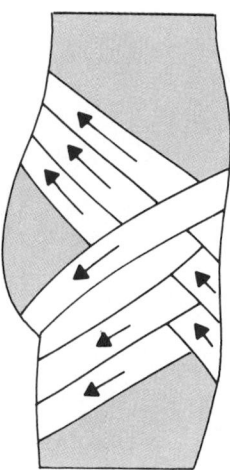

FIGURE 43-7

Techniques for applying various types of bandages.

Recurrent—Stump Bandage

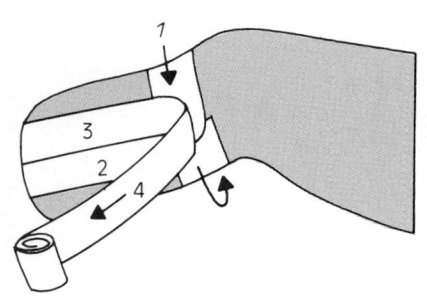
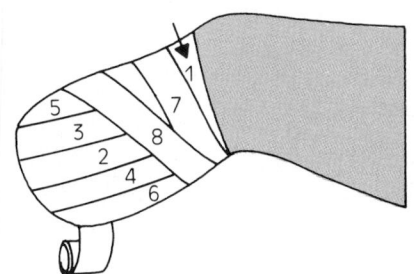
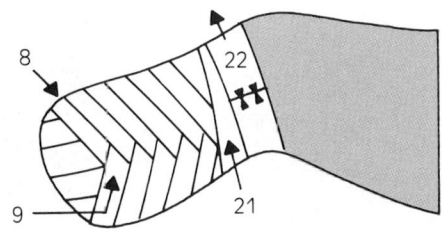

Binders

T-binders

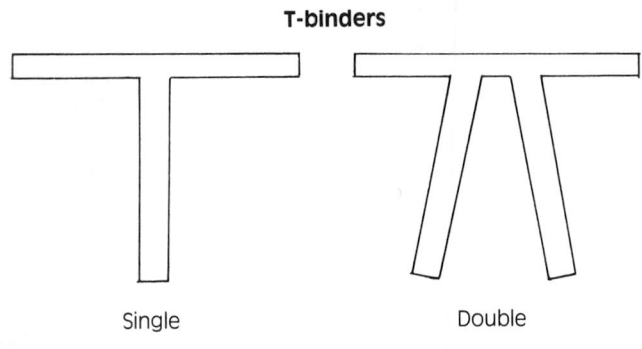

Single   Double

Many-Tailed Binders

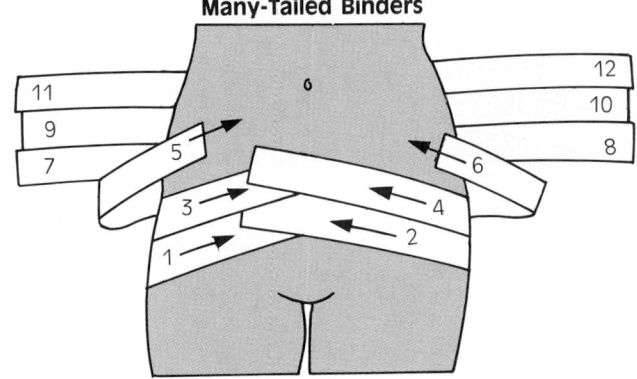

Slings

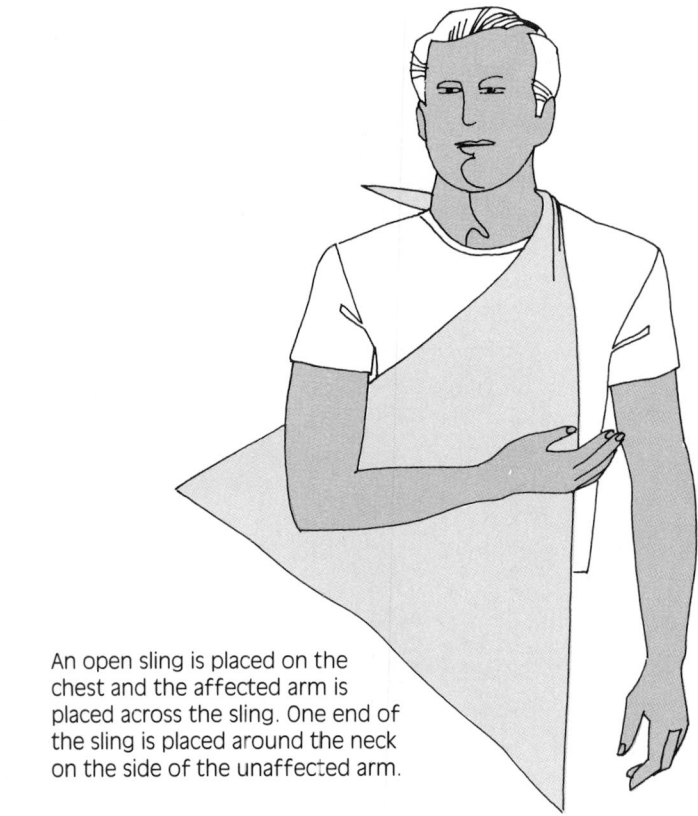

An open sling is placed on the chest and the affected arm is placed across the sling. One end of the sling is placed around the neck on the side of the unaffected arm.

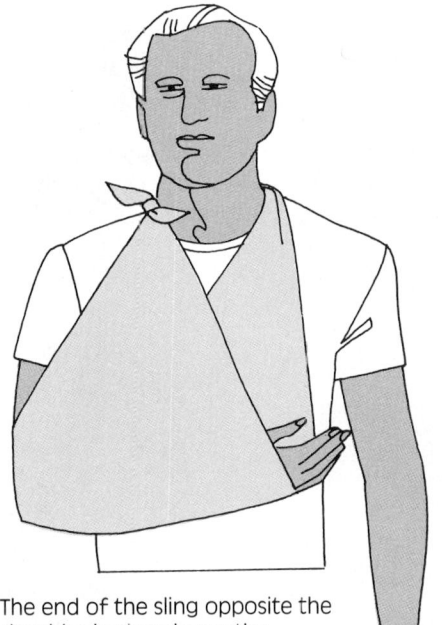

The end of the sling opposite the shoulder is placed over the affected arm, and the ends are tied at the side of the neck so that the knot does not rub over the cervical vertebra. The material at the elbow is folded neatly and may be secured with a pin placed behind the sling so that it is out of sight.

F I G U R E 4 3 - 7

(continued)

Whichever turn is being used, care should be taken to provide even overlapping of one half to two thirds the width of each bandage, except for the circular turn. All skin surfaces should be covered by the finished bandage to prevent pinching the skin between turns of the bandage. The bandage is completed well away from the wound or inflamed and tender areas. The terminal end of the bandage may be secured with adhesive, special clamps, or a safety pin, being careful to avoid undue pressure.

Removing Roller Bandages   It is best to cut a roller bandage with a bandage scissors to prevent excessive manipulation of the part. Cutting should be done on the side opposite the injury or the wound, from one end to the other, so that the bandage can be folded open for its entire length. If the bandage is to be reused, it may be unwound by keeping the loose end together and passing it as a ball from one hand to the other while unwinding it.

Applying Binders

T-Binders   A T-binder is so named because it looks like the letter T. T-binders are particularly effective for securing dressings on the rectum and perineum and in the groin. The single T-binder is used for female clients, and the double T-binder is used for male clients. The belt is passed around the waist and secured with safety pins. The single or double tails are passed between the legs and pinned to the belt.

Many-Tailed Binders   A many-tailed binder, or scultetus binder, consists of a rectangular piece of fabric, with tails that are each about 5 cm (2 inches) wide attached to its sides. The binder supports the abdomen or holds dressings on it or on the chest. When a scultetus binder is applied to the abdomen, the client lies on his or her back on the center of the binder. The lower end of the binder is placed well down on the hips, but not so low that it interferes with the use of a bedpan or with walking. The tails are brought out to the sides of the client's body, with the bottom tail in position to wrap around the lower part of the abdomen first. A tail from each side is brought up and placed obliquely over the abdomen until all tails are in place. The last tails are fastened with safety pins.

Sling   A sling is used to support an arm. Most health care agencies use commercial strap slings or sleeve slings. In the home setting, a large piece of cloth folded into a triangle can be used as a sling.

Straight Binders   A straight binder is a straight piece of material, usually about 15 to 20 cm (6 to 8 inches) wide and long enough to more than circle the torso. It is used for the chest and the abdomen. Straight binders may be pinned, or fastened with Velcro. A straight binder for the chest often is provided with shoulder straps so that it does not slip down on the trunk and may require tucks to fit the body's contours.

A binder around the chest wall should not be applied so tightly that it interferes with the client's breathing.

Changing the Dressing

The nurse prepares the client for the dressing change by explaining what will be done before starting the procedure. Proper screening is used to provide privacy. The client is assisted to a position that is comfortable and also convenient for the person changing the dressing (eg, raising the bed to a higher position during the procedure). The area is exposed while maintaining proper draping.

It is important to use appropriate aseptic techniques when changing the dressing. It is especially important to wash hands thoroughly before and after changing dressings and to follow Centers for Disease Control (CDC) guidelines, described in the accompanying display. Among the most common causes of nosocomial infections is carelessness in observing medical and surgical asepsis when changing dressings.

CDC Guidelines for Preventing Infection and Transmission of Human Immunodeficiency Virus in Wound Care

General Guidelines for Wounds

- Always wash hands before and after caring for a wound.
- Use sterile gloves or sterile forceps to touch a wound until the wound is sealed.
- Change dressings on both open and closed wounds when wet.
- Take a culture of any suspect drainage.

Precautions for Contact With Blood and Body Fluids

Blood and body fluid precautions should be consistently used for all clients.

- Wear gloves when touching blood, body fluids containing visible blood, an open wound, or nonintact skin of all clients and when handling items or surfaces soiled with blood or body fluids.
- Wash hands thoroughly after removing gloves and if contaminated with blood or with body fluids that contain visible blood.
- Take precautions to prevent injuries by needles, sharp instruments, or sharp devices.
- Do not give direct client care if you have open or weeping lesions or dermatitis.
- If procedures commonly cause droplets or splashing of blood or body fluids to which universal precautions apply, wear gloves, a surgical mask, and protective eyewear, as appropriate.

Cleaning a Wound and Applying a Clean Dressing

The wound is cleaned and the dressing changed as described in Procedure 43-1.

The nurse often is afforded an excellent opportunity for teaching while changing the client's dressing. Teaching becomes especially important when the client will be changing his or her own dressings after discharge from a health care agency. He or she can be encouraged to help to as much as possible, beginning with such assistance as preparing adhesive strips.

A client may be disturbed by the sight of his or her wound. The nurse should listen carefully to what the client is saying and observe for nonverbal communication as well. In some instances, the client may not want to look at the wound. This is apt to occur when a client has a wound that involves a change in normal body functions or appearance, such as a wound resulting from the removal of a breast, the amputation of an extremity, or the placement of a tube in a draining wound. Patience and emotional support help the client become accustomed to the sight of the wound in time.

Frequency of Changing Dressings

The frequency with which dressings should be changed cannot be stated categorically. It depends on the amount of drainage, the physician's preference, and the nature of the wound. It is customary for the physician to perform the first dressing change after surgery. The first dressing change usually is performed within 24 to 48 hours after surgery (Neuberger & Reckling, 1985). Thereafter, nurses change the dressings on an as-needed basis or daily. Frequency for dressing changes should be noted on the client's nursing care plan.

Documenting Wound Care

The nurse is responsible for caring for a wound and for noting factors that may be interfering with healing.

The nurse documents assessments and interventions each time wound care is given and describes the wound's appearance. If drainage is present, the kind and amount are described. If the client has a complicated dressing, details for caring for the wound should be described in the care plan. Many clients have preferences for when dressings are changed and how the dressings can be best arranged. They may become distressed if one nurse uses one method and another nurse uses a different one, even if both nurses use proper technique. An example of documentation follows:

1/12/93, 1 PM, nursing
Four-inch midline abdominal incision cleaned with 0.9% sterile NS. Wound edges well approximated, skin sutures intact. Crust along suture line, edges of incision slightly edematous and dark pink. Penrose drain present in lower ¼ of incision. Old dressing moderately saturated with serosanguine-

ous drainage. New dressing applied with sterile technique, using Telfa, four 4 × 4s, and two ABDs applied with nonallergic tape.

A. Sprengel, RN, CS

Removing Staples and Sutures

Sutures are removed when enough tensile strength has developed to hold the wound edges together during healing. This stage varies from client to client, depending on age, nutritional status, and wound location. Silk sutures should be removed within 6 to 8 days to prevent suture marks, even though collagen formation and remodeling takes at least 21 days altogether. That means the scar may still stretch and widen after the silk sutures have been removed. Special subcutaneous techniques have now been developed to minimize this problem. Small wound closure strips of adhesive (Steri-Strips) may now be applied directly to the wound to help hold it together. Unless otherwise directed, the nurse should not remove these Steri-Strips during wound care (Neuberger & Reckling, 1985). The guidelines for removing sutures and staples are included in the section on assessing the surgical wound.

Changing a Dressing for a Draining Wound

The basic care of a draining wound is similar to that of a wound with little or no drainage. The following techniques are important in caring for a draining wound.

Promoting Comfort If wound care is an uncomfortable procedure for the client, it is best to administer a prescribed analgesic or sedative 30 to 45 minutes before changing the dressing. It also is preferable to change the dressing midway between meals so that the client's appetite and mealtimes are not disturbed.

Maintaining Skin Integrity A protective ointment or paste may be applied to cleaned skin surrounding the draining wound. The ointment or paste acts as a protective barrier to prevent skin irritation and excoriation from wound drainage. Protecting the skin is particularly important when it is anticipated that the drainage period may be prolonged or when the person's skin is especially susceptible to irritation. The protective ointment or paste should be removed regularly, at least daily, and the skin should be cleaned thoroughly. It is best to remove the protective material with a minimal amount of rubbing to prevent epithelial cells from being injured by friction. It is recommended that the first layer of dressing material applied directly to a draining wound be nonabsorbent but hydrophilic (ie, capable of carrying moisture). This type of material allows drainage from the wound to pass from the first dressing without absorption to overlying absorbent layers of dressing. The advantage of such a dressing is that it does not hold the drainage in direct contact with the wound to cause maceration and reinfection. Also, the material tends not to

PROCEDURE 43-1

Cleaning a Wound and Applying Clean Dressing

Equipment

Sterile gloves
Gauze dressings or squares
Sterile dressing set or suture set
  (contains scissors and forceps)
Cleaning solution
Clean disposable gloves
Sterile basin (optional)

Sterile drape (optional)
Plastic bag for soiled dressings
Waterproof pad
Bath blanket
Tape or ties
Surgi-pads or A3Ds

Additional dressing supplies as
  needed or ordered (antiseptic ointments, extra dressings)
Acetone or adhesive remover (optional)
Sterile normal saline (optional)

Action	Rationale
1 Explain procedure to client.	An explanation encourages client cooperation and reduces apprehension.
2 Gather equipment.	This provides for organized approach to task.
3 Wash your hands.	Handwashing deters spread of microorganisms.
4 Check physician's order for dressing change. Note if drain is present.	This clarifies type of dressing.
5 Close door or curtain. Use bath blanket as needed when exposing area to be redressed. Position waterproof pad under client if desired.	This provides for privacy and warmth.
6 Assist client to comfortable position that provides easy access to wound area.	This provides for comfort.
7 Place opened, cuffed plastic bag near working area.	Soiled dressings may be placed in disposal bag without contaminating outside surfaces of bag.
8 Loosen tape on dressing. Use adhesive remover if necessary.	It is easier to loosen tape before putting on gloves.
9 Don clean disposable gloves, and remove soiled dressings carefully. Check position of drains before removing dressing. If dressing is not wet-to-dry application and is adhering to skin surface, it may be moistened by pouring a small amount of sterile saline onto it. Keep soiled side of dressing away from client's view.	This protects the nurse from handling contaminated dressings. Cautious removal of dressing is more comfortable for client and ensures that drain is not removed if one is present. Sterile saline provides for easier removal of dressing.
10 Assess amount, type, and odor of drainage.	Wound healing process or presence of infection should be documented.
11 Discard dressings in plastic disposal bag. Pull off glove inside out and drop it in bag.	This prevents spread of microorganisms by contaminated dressings
12 Using aseptic technique, open sterile dressings and supplies on work area.	Supplies are within easy reach, and sterility is maintained.
13 Open sterile cleaning solution, and pour over gauze sponges in plastic container or over sponges placed in sterile basin.	Sterility of dressings and solution is maintained.
14 Don sterile gloves (see Procedure 26-2).	Maintains surgical asepsis

(continued)

P R O C E D U R E   4 3 - 1 *(continued)*

Cleaning a Wound and Applying Clean Dressing

Action	Rationale
15 Clean wound or surgical incision. Use sterile forceps if desired.	
a Clean from top to bottom or from center outward.	Clean from least to most contaminated area.
b Use one gauze square for each wipe, discarding each square by dropping into plastic bag. Do not touch bag with forceps.	Previously cleaned area is not recontaminated.
c Clean around drain, if present, moving from center outward in a circular motion. Use one gauze square for each circular motion.	Move from least to most contaminated area.
d Dry wound using gauze sponge and same motion.	Moisture provides medium for growth of microorganisms.
e Apply antiseptic ointment if ordered.	Growth of microorganisms may be retarded and healing process improved.
16 Apply a layer of dry, sterile dressings over wound. Use sterile forceps if desired.	Primary dressing serves as a wick for drainage.
17 Cut sterile 4 × 4 gauze square to place under and around drain if one is present (see Fig. 43-5).	Drainage is absorbed and surrounding skin area is protected.
18 Apply second gauze layer to wound site.	This provides for increased absorption of drainage.

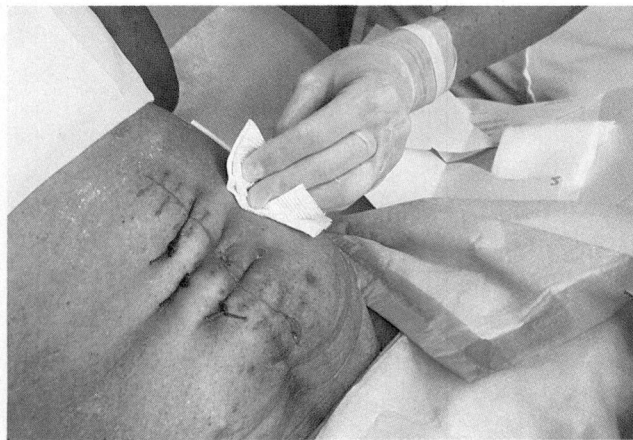

Action 15: Cleaning a surgical incision.

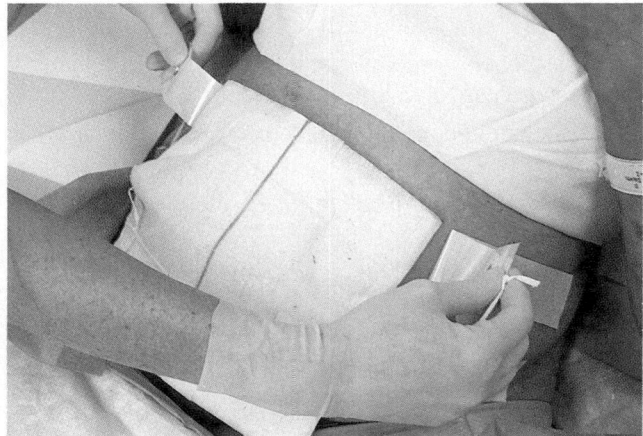

Action 19: Applying Montgomery straps over outer layer of dressing.

Action	Rationale
19 Place Surgi-pad or ABD dressing over wound as outermost layer.	Wound is protected from microorganisms in environment.
20 Remove gloves from inside out, and discard them in plastic waste bag. Apply tape or tie existing tapes to secure dressings.	Tape is easier to apply after gloves have been removed.
21 Wash hands. Remove all equipment, and make client comfortable.	This prevents spread of microorganisms.
22 Check dressing and wound site every shift. Record dressing change, appearance of wound, and describe any drainage in chart.	This provides accurate documentation of procedure.

(continued)

Cleaning a Wound and Applying Clean Dressing

Age Considerations	To keep a dressing intact or to prevent contamination of wound and supplies on an infant or young child, it may be necessary to restrain the child's hand. An old stocking or piece of stockinette may be used to encircle child's hand and then may be secured to the bed or crib with a tie or safety pin. Care must be taken not to compromise circulation to that extremity
Home Care Considerations	Reinforce need for thorough handwashing before and after dressing change. Have plastic bag available for safe disposal of soiled dressings and equipment. Boil any nondisposable equipment (eg, forceps) for 10 minutes to ensure sterility after washing carefully in warm soapy water. Inform client about availability of disposable wound care supplies.
Special Considerations	Client must be instructed that any break or interruption in the suture line may require immediate intervention and the surgeon should be notified immediately. Instruct client and family about significant changes that need to be reported to the nurse or physician. Encourage splinting of wound during activity (coughing, sneezing, sudden movement, or change in position).

stick to the wound, a characteristic that makes changing a dressing less uncomfortable for the client. Material to absorb and collect drainage is then placed on the first layer of nonabsorbent material.

The property of surface tension exhibited by liquids and the forces of cohesion and adhesion cause a column of liquid to rise in a fine tube or on a hair. This is called capillary action or **capillarity**. For example, absorbent cotton allows for greater capillarity than untreated cotton. Therefore, cotton-lined gauze sponges soak up more liquid than unlined sponges. Loosely packed gauze, the threads of which act as numerous wicks, enhances capillarity and allows for drainage to be directed upward and away from its source. Fluffed and loosely packed dressings, then, are more absorbent than tightly packed dressings and carry drainage up and away from the wound. The number of gauze sponges used in the dressing depends on the amount of drainage. The top of the dressing may be further protected by surgical or abdominal pads, which are thick, absorbent pads that help to absorb profuse drainage.

Because a draining wound requires more frequent changes of dressing than a wound without drainage, it is recommended that Montgomery straps be used to secure the dressing (Fig. 43-8). These straps do not require changing with each dressing, as tape strips do. Montgomery straps can be made or are available commercially. The adhesive end of the strap is placed on the skin well away from the wound. The end of the strap near the wound remains free because the adhesive side is turned back on itself. Gauze or woven strips passed through eyelets are tied over the wound to secure the dressing. When the dressing is changed, the strips are untied and turned back to allow

for wound care. After the fresh dressing is applied, the straps are retied to hold the dressing in place.

Preventing Infection and Promoting Healing In caring for wounds, the nurse uses principles of both medical and

FIGURE 43 - 8

Montgomery straps make it possible to care for a wound without removing adhesive strips with each dressing change.

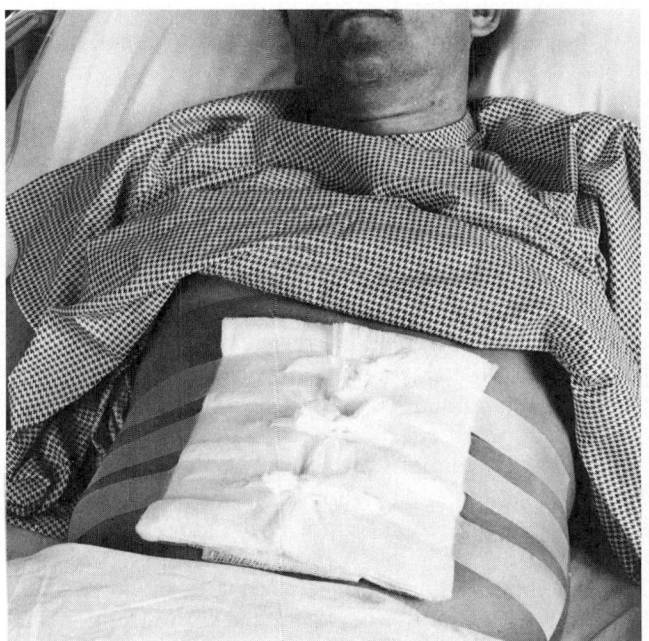

surgical asepsis. Nurses should make certain that precautions are taken to prevent infection of the wound by following CDC guidelines (described earlier).

Contamination occurs through a moist medium. Microorganisms can move from the external surface through the dressing to the wound if a dressing remains in place until it is saturated. In like manner, microorganisms can move from the wound to the outer surface of a saturated dressing. For this reason, dressings should not be allowed to become saturated. They should either be replaced with fresh dressings or be reinforced before drainage causes saturation.

A rubber tubular drain (Penrose), a sump tube, or a catheter may be placed in a wound to promote exudate drainage. Care must be used so that these devices are not dislodged when dressings are changed. A Penrose drain may be ordered to be shortened each day. This can be done by grasping the end of the drain with sterile forceps, pulling it out a short distance while using a twisting motion, and cutting off the end of the drain with sterile scissors. A sterile safety pin (or Klip) often is placed at the end of the drain so that it cannot slip down into the wound.

Closed drainage systems are now being used more often in place of incisional drains like the Penrose drain. Some studies show that the infection rate is cut nearly in half when drains are placed only when necessary and through a separate stab wound rather than in the incision itself.

Closed drainage systems consist of a drain connected to an electric suction machine or a portable closed drainage suction system (Fig. 43-9).

Portable closed drainage systems have directions for their use printed on the container itself. The nurse should avoid touching the open port when emptying the drainage. Reflux of drainage from a contaminated port could contaminate the wound itself. The use of a closed drainage system eliminates a potential source of microorganisms. The frequent dressing changes needed with the open Penrose drain (which empties directly onto a dressing) are no longer necessary (Neuberger and Reckling, 1985). Closed drainage systems also allow accurate measurement of drainage.

Collecting a Wound Culture If assessment of the wound and the drainage indicates a possible infection, a specimen of the drainage is obtained and sent to the laboratory for culture and sensitivity, as outlined in Procedure 42-2.

Irrigating and Packing a Wound An irrigation consists of directing a flow of solution over traumatized tissues. The purposes of an irrigation include cleaning the area of pathogens and other debris and applying local heat or an antiseptic to the area.

Nonsterile solutions are used if the wound is closed. Sterile equipment and solutions are required for irrigating an open wound, even in the presence of an existing infection.

The type and amount of solution vary with the condition of the wound. Sterile normal saline, an antiseptic, or an

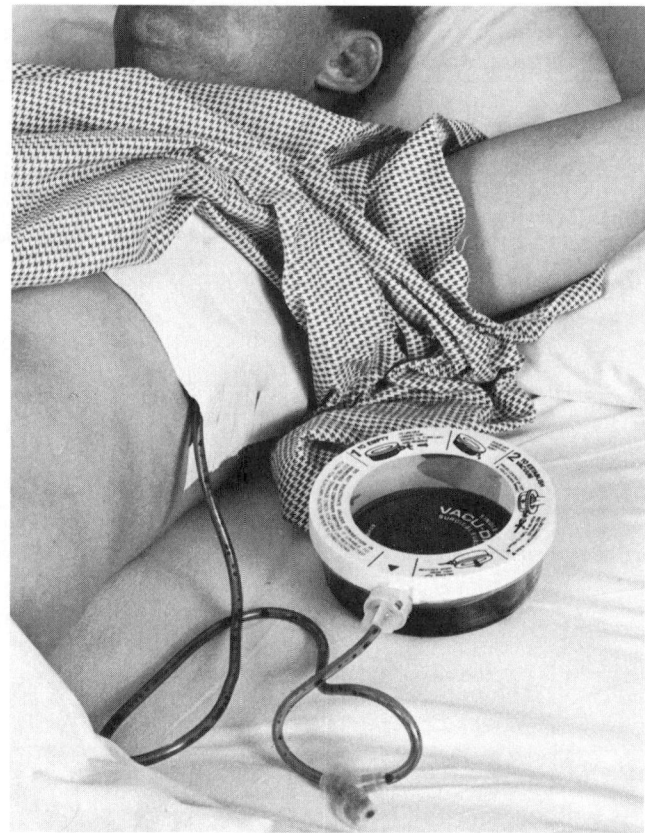

FIGURE 43-9

The portable suction apparatus shown here helps to remove drainage from the wound site.

antibiotic solution is used. Hydrogen peroxide may be the solution of choice because its oxygen-releasing ability cleans effectively. A sterile, large-volume syringe is used to hold the solution. Packing is placed in wounds to allow granulation tissue and healing by secondary intention to take place.

The techniques for irrigating a wound and inserting packing are described in Procedure 42-3.

Changing Dressings in Special Situations

Infected Wounds

CDC guidelines for minor abscesses, infected pressure ulcers, and minor skin or wound infections (which are *not* infections caused by *Staphylococcus aureus*, beta-hemolytic streptococcus, and *Clostridium perfringens*) include the following:

- Masks are not indicated.
- Use gowns if soiling is likely.
- Use gloves to touch infected materials.
- Wash hands after touching the client or potentially contaminated articles. Wash hands before taking care of another client.

(*Text continues on p. 1288*)

PROCEDURE 43-2

Collecting a Wound Culture

Equipment

Sterile Culturette tube with enclosed
  swab (or culture tube with
  individual swabs)
Sterile gloves
Clean disposable gloves

Plastic bag for soiled dressing
Label for Culturette tube
Laboratory requisition with rubber
  band or plastic bag

Action	Rationale
1 Explain procedure to client.	An explanation encourages client cooperation and reduces apprehension.
2 Gather equipment.	This provides for organized approach to task.
3 Wash your hands.	Handwashing deters the spread of microorganisms.
4 Don clean disposable gloves. Remove dressing and assess wound and drainage (see Procedure 43-1, actions 5 to 11).	This protects nurse from handling contaminated dressings.
5 Using aseptic technique, don sterile gloves and clean wound (see Procedure 43-1, action 15). Remove sterile gloves.	Previous drainage and skin flora are removed.
6 Twist cap to loosen swab in Culturette tube, or open separate swab and remove cap from culture tube, keeping inside uncontaminated.	Supplies are within easy reach, and sterility is maintained.
7 Don clean glove or new sterile glove, if necessary.	Use of Culturette does not require immediate contact with skin or wound. If contact with wound is necessary to collect specimen, wear sterile glove on that hand.
8 Carefully insert swab into drainage and roll gently. Use another swab if collecting specimen from another site.	Cotton tip absorbs wound drainage. This prevents cross-contamination of wound.
9 Place swab in Culturette tube, being careful not to touch outside of container. Twist cap to secure.	Outside of container is protected from contamination with microorganisms.
10 If using Culturette tube, crush ampule of medium at bottom of tube.	Swab with drainage can be surrounded by culture medium.

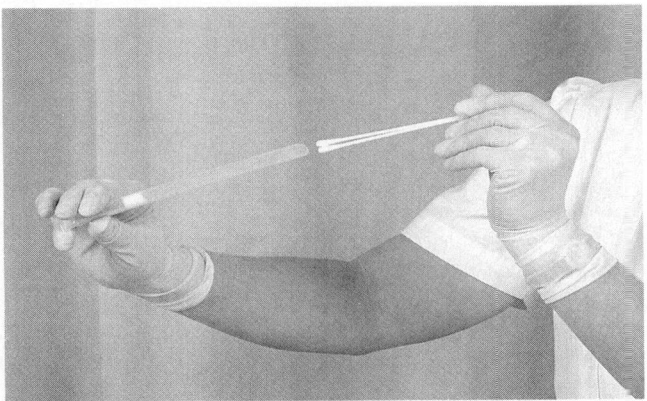

Action 9: Placing swab in a Culturette tube.

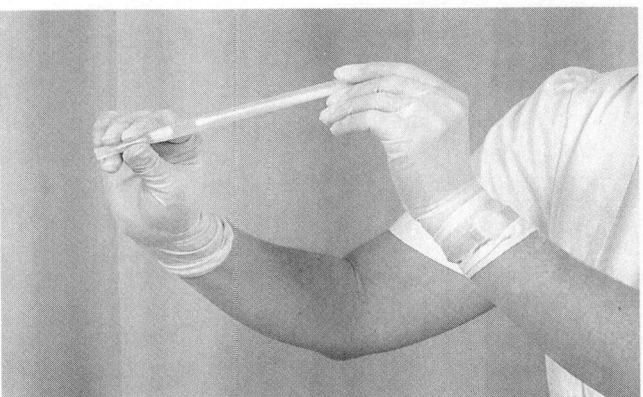

Action 10: Crushing ampule of medium at bottom of tube.
(Photos © B. Proud.)

(continued)

PROCEDURE 4 3 - 2 *(continued)*

Collecting a Wound Culture

Action	Rationale
11 Remove gloves from inside out, and discard them in plastic waste bag.	This prevents spread of microorganisms.
12 Wash your hands.	Handwashing deters the spread of microorganisms.
13 Apply clean dressing to wound (see Procedure 43-1, actions 16 to 20).	Drainage from wound is absorbed.
14 Wash your hands. Remove all equipment, and make client comfortable.	Handwashing deters the spread of microorganisms.
15 Label specimen container appropriately (client's name, date, time, nature of specimen). Attach laboratory requisition to tube with rubber band or place tube in plastic bag with requisition attached. Send to laboratory within 20 minutes.	This ensures proper identification of specimen. Overgrowth of other organisms can interfere with test results if specimen remains at room temperature for extended period.
16 Record collection of specimen, appearance of wound, and description of drainage in chart.	This provides for accurate documentation of procedure.

PROCEDURE 4 3 - 3

Irrigating a Sterile Wound and Inserting Packing

Equipment

Sterile irrigation set (basin, container for irrigant, irrigating syringe)
Prescribed irrigating solution (warmed to body temperature or 34°–37°C [93.2°–98.6°F])
Sterile soft catheter (optional)

Sterile gloves
Clean disposable gloves
Sterile dressing set or suture set (contains scissors and forceps)
Waterproof pad
Sterile gauze and surgipads or ABDs (for dressing change)

Plastic bag for soiled dressings
Packing gauze (as specified by physician)
Gown (optional)
Bath blanket
Tape

Action	Rationale
1 Explain procedure to client. Check physician's order for irrigation and packing of wound.	Explanation facilitates client cooperation. Clarified procedure and type of supplies required.
2 Gather equipment.	This provides for organized approach to task.
3 Wash your hands.	Handwashing deters the spread of microorganisms.
4 Close door or curtain. Use bath blanket as needed when exposing wound site.	This provides for privacy and warmth.
5 Position client so irrigating solution will flow from upper end of wound toward lower end. Place waterproof pad under client.	Gravity directs flow of liquid from least contaminated to most contaminated area. Waterproof pad protects client and bed linens.
6 Warm sterile irrigating solution to body temperature.	Warmed solution is more comfortable for client and promotes vasodilation.

(continued)

PROCEDURE 43-3 (continued)

Irrigating a Sterile Wound and Inserting Packing

Action	Rationale
7 Place opened, cuffed plastic bag near working area. Don gown if recommended.	Soiled dressings and packing may be placed in disposal bag without contaminating outside surfaces of bag. Gown protects uniform from contamination if splashing should occur.
8 Loosen tape on dressing, and put on clean glove to remove soiled dressings and packing.	Nurse is protected from handling contaminated dressings.
9 Assess amount, type, and odor of drainage. Observe condition of wound.	This provides information about wound healing process or presence of infection.
10 Discard dressings in plastic disposal bag. Remove glove inside out, and drop it in bag.	Spread of microorganisms by way of contaminated dressings is prevented.
11 Using aseptic technique, open sterile dressings and supplies on work area.	Supplies are within easy reach and sterility is maintained.

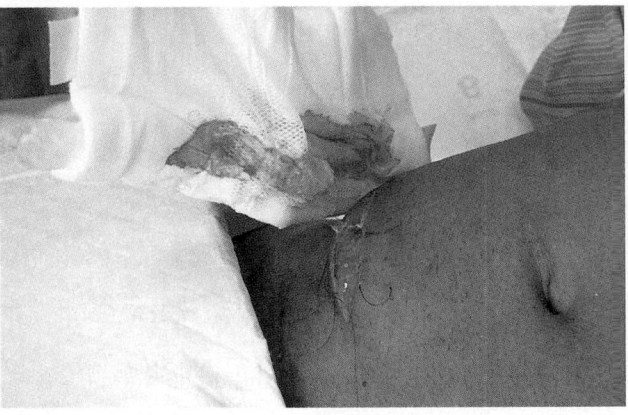

Action 9: Assessing wound drainage.

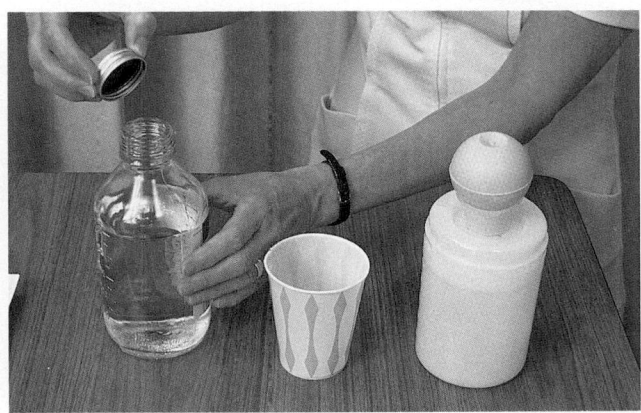

Action 11: Preparing sterile irrigating solution.

Action	Rationale
12 Pour warmed sterile irrigating solution into sterile container. Amount may vary from 200 to 500 mL depending on size of wound.	This facilitates wound irrigation.
13 Put sterile glove on dominant hand (see Procedure 26-2).	This maintains surgical asepsis.
14 Position the sterile basin below the wound to collect irrigation fluid with nondominant clean hand.	Irrigation is facilitated and client and bed linens are protected from contaminated fluid.
15 Use dominant gloved hand to fill syringe with irrigant. Gently direct a stream of solution into wound, keeping tip of syringe 1 inch (2.5 cm) above upper tip of wound. If using a catheter tip on syringe, insert it gently into wound to point of resistance.	Debris and contaminated solution flow from least contaminated to most contaminated area. Catheter allows introduction of irrigant into wound with small opening or one that is deep.
16 Continue irrigation until solution returns clear. Try to maintain a steady flow of solution.	Irrigation removes exudate and debris.

(continued)

P R O C E D U R E   4 3 - 3 *(continued)*

Irrigating a Sterile Wound and Inserting Packing

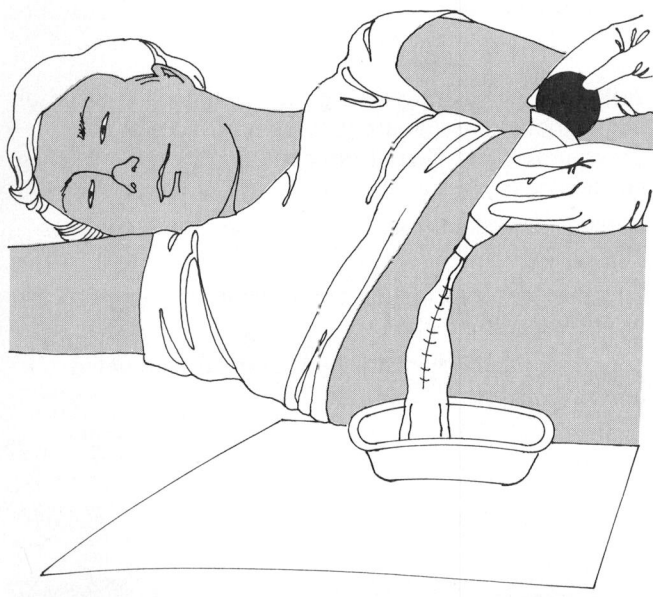

Action 15: Irrigating wound.

Action	**Rationale**
17 Use sterile forceps to gently insert sterile packing into wound. Be careful not to pack wound excessively. Cut packing with sterile scissors if necessary. Allow small strip of packing to protrude from small and deep wound for easier removal.	Packing may be used to absorb drainage and promote healing. Excessive packing of wound may impede blood flow and delay healing process.
18 Dry area around wound with a sterile gauze sponge.	Moisture provides medium for growth of microorganisms.
19 Apply layers of sterile dressing.	Drainage is absorbed and surrounding skin area is protected.
20 Remove gloves, and discard them in plastic waste bag. Apply tape to secure dressings.	Tape is easier to apply after gloves have been removed.
21 Wash hands. Remove all equipment, and make client comfortable.	This prevents spread of microorganisms.
22 Check dressing and wound site every shift. Record dressing change, insertion of packing, appearance of wound, and describe any drainage in chart.	This provides for accurate documentation of procedure.

- Discard and bag contaminated materials separately and label them before sending them for decontamination (Neuberger and Reckling, 1985).

  The CDC also recommends special techniques for the care of extensive wounds with purulent drainage. In particular, wounds infected with *S. aureus*, beta-hemolytic streptococcus, and *C. perfringens* (gas gangrene) require the use of these special techniques. When information about the causative organism is unknown, the CDC advises the use of these techniques for all infected and extensive wounds.

  The following special precautions should be taken when caring for extensive wounds with purulent drainage:

- Wash hands before wound care.
- Wear a gown while caring for the client's wound. This gown need not be sterile, unless there is danger of carrying organisms on a clean gown to an already debilitated client.
- Wear a mask while caring for the wound.
- Be prepared to use two pairs of sterile gloves, and change gloves between the removal of the old dressing and the application of the new dressing.
- Wash hands thoroughly between glove changes. An antimicrobial soap is recommended by many health care agencies.

- Use a no-touch technique when handling soiled dressings. Lift soiled dressings with a clamp or forceps. This prevents contamination of the hands.
- Place soiled dressings in a moisture-proof bag, which is then closed securely, double-bagged, and incinerated without being opened.
- Be sure to wash the hands again thoroughly after completing wound care. If organisms accumulate on the hands because proper technique was broken, the organisms not only are likely to be carried to others, but eventually may also become resident flora on the nurse's hands.

Open Wounds

Recommendations for the treatment of open wounds focus on facilitating healing. Research supports the harmful effects of such treatments as the use of full-strength Betadine and of wet-to-dry dressings (Cooper, 1990a). In caring for wounds, each wound is individually evaluated, and one (or more) of a variety of choices for dressing might be made.

New trends are for a wet-to-damp packing for open wounds. Cellular migration needed for tissue repair and healing is enhanced by a moist surface. Packing material is soaked in a solution (with normal saline solution being the solution of choice) and then wrung out so it is only slightly moist. A wet packing slows wound closure, increases the risk of bacterial growth, and can macerate surrounding tissue. Packing is applied loosely and only to the edges of the wound; it is then covered with a secondary dressing to absorb drainage. If the packing dries, it should be soaked with saline solution before it is removed (Wound-Care Update 91, 1991).

Chronic Wounds

Many types of special dressings are used to facilitate healing in chronic wounds. A brief discussion of each of these follows.

Transparent Adhesive Dressings   These semipermeable dressings allow an exchange of oxygen between the wound and the environment, protect against contamination, and maintain a moist wound environment. They are used for wounds with only minimal drainage.

Absorptive Dressings   Included as absorptive dressings are karaya powder, dextranomer beads, and copolymer starches. These dressings absorb drainage and maintain a moist surface by forming a gelatinous mass. Dextranomer and copolymer starch dressings are used for deep wounds with heavy drainage.

Hydrocolloid Dressings   Hydrocolloid dressings absorb drainage, maintain a moist wound surface, and decrease the risk of infection. They are used for shallow wounds that have minimal drainage. Polyurethane dressings are nonadhesive hydrocolloid dressings that must be taped down

to prevent wound contamination because they do not adhere to the wound surface. They may be used in conjunction with packing for deep, open wounds.

Hydrogel Dressings   Hydrogel dressings are oxygen-permeable and nonadhesive and maintain moisture. They are used for wounds that are not deep.

Synthetic Barrier Dressings   These are pastes that dry to form transparent, semipermeable dressings. Pores in the dried paste allow drainage to move from the wound to an absorbent dressing.

Preparing for Home Care of a Wound

With the trend toward earlier dismissal of the client from an inpatient setting to home care, teaching the client and his or her family about wound care is increasingly important. Although a nurse from a home health care or community health care agency may be needed to change dressings and provide wound care for complex situations, it is often family members who will do the procedure. To provide the continuity of care that is necessary to prevent infection and promote healing, the nurse must include teaching about wound care as part of discharge planning.

Each of the following components should be included in the teaching plan, and the client or family member who will be changing the dressing should demonstrate proper techniques in wound care and dressing change before the client is discharged.

- Dressing materials can be purchased from pharmacies, drug stores, discount stores, and medical supply stores. Consideration of the cost and ease of use is important.
- Signs and symptoms of infection (increased body temperature; malaise; reddened wound edges; drainage that is thick, green, odorous, or increased in amount; increased pain) should be reported immediately.
- Good nutrition and hydration are important. The diet should be high in proteins, zinc, iron, and vitamins.
- Modifications of activities of daily living and exercise patterns may be necessary until healing is completed.

Evaluating

Evaluating the effectiveness of the nursing care plan is based on the client goals. The plan of care for the client with a wound is effective if the client has a healed wound, has remained free of infection, and can carry out wound and dressing care by himself, if needed.

Heat and Cold Applications

Hot and cold agents are applied to an area of a client's body to bring about a local or systemic change in body temperature for various therapeutic purposes. Physiologic responses to heat and cold are modified by the method and duration of application, the degree of heat and cold applied, the client's age and physical condition, and the amount of body surface covered by the application. This section discusses the effects of heat and cold and uses the phases of the nursing process to define the nurse's responsibilities in caring for the client receiving applications of heat or cold.

Physiologic Responses to Heat and Cold

Heat and cold cause both local and systemic effects. Body temperature is regulated by cells in the hypothalamus in response to signals from thermal (heat and cold) receptors located close to the skin's surface. Stimulation of these receptors sends sensory messages to cells of the anterior hypothalamus to dissipate heat (by such mechanisms as vasodilation and sweating) or to the cells of the posterior hypothalamus to conserve heat (by vasoconstriction and shivering). Pain receptors, also located near the skin's surface, are activated if external temperatures are too hot or too cold.

Local Effects of Heat

The many benefits of heat are summarized in Table 43-4. Heat causes vasodilation of peripheral blood vessels, a mechanism that helps to dissipate heat from the body to the environment. Vasodilation also increases blood flow to a body part that is injured or has altered function. In turn, the supply of oxygen and nutrients to the area is increased and

venous congestion is decreased. Reduced viscosity of blood and increased capillary permeability improve the delivery of leukocytes and nutrients while also facilitating the removal of wastes and prolonging clotting time. These actions, combined with increased tissue metabolism, accelerate the inflammatory response to promote healing. Heat reduces muscle tension to promote relaxation and helps to relieve muscle spasms and joint stiffness. It decreases the viscosity of the synovial fluid in joint spaces. Heat also reduces pain through vasodilation and the relaxation effect.

Because of these local physiologic effects, heat in various forms is used to treat infections, surgical wounds, inflamed tissue, arthritis, joint and muscle pain, dysmenorrhea, and ischemia of peripheral tissue.

Local Effects of Cold

The effects of cold are opposite those of heat. The benefits of cold are listed in Table 43-4. Cold causes vasoconstriction of peripheral blood vessels, reducing blood flow to tissue. Decreased metabolic needs and capillary permeability combined with increased coagulation of blood at the wound site facilitate the control of bleeding and reduce edema formation. Cold also reduces muscle spasm, alters tissue sensitivity (producing numbness), and promotes comfort by relieving pain.

Cold, for these effects, is used after direct trauma (especially in closed wounds, trauma to muscles and bones, and burns) and in the treatment of arthritis.

Other Effects of Heat and Cold

The *systemic effects* of extensive heat are increased cardiac output, sweating, increased pulse rate, and decreased blood pressure. Application of heat to a large body area increases the blood flow to that area while decreasing it to another part of the body. Extensive cold produces systemic effects of increased blood pressure, shivering, and goose bumps. Another generalized response is found when the effects of heat or cold in one body part also are found in another area of the body; for example, the application of heat to the right leg results in vasodilatation in both legs.

The *rebound phenomenon* is important to the therapeutic value of heat and cold and to the safety of clients receiving such therapy. Heat produces maximum vasodilatation in 20 to 30 minutes; if heat is continued beyond that time, tissue congestion and vasoconstriction occur (for unknown reasons). With cold, maximum vasoconstriction occurs when the skin reaches 60°F (15°C); then vasodilation begins.

The ability of the body to *adapt* to heat and cold is an important consideration in this type of therapy. Heat and cold skin receptors are initially strongly stimulated by sudden changes in temperature. For the first few seconds after being stimulated, the response decreases rapidly, and then more slowly for the next 30 minutes, as the receptors adapt

T A B L E   4 3 - 4

Benefits of Heat and Cold	
Heat	**Cold**
Relaxes muscles	Relaxes muscle
Decreases pain	Decreases pain
Increases circulation	Decreases circulation
Relieves congestion	Reduces swelling
Raises body temperature, prevents infection	Prevents edema
Promotes healing	Reduces temperature
Has sedative effect	Retards bacterial growth
Reduces need for medication	Acts as local anesthetic; decreases need for analgesics
Reduces joint stress, reduces need for anti-inflammatory agents	Decreases oxygen supply to area
Promotes resolution of superficial infections, reduces need for antibiotics	Decreases metabolism
Relieves dysmenorrhea	

(Spencer, R. T., et al. [1989]. *Clinical pharmacology and nursing management* [3rd ed.]. Philadelphia: Lippincott.)

to the temperature. A hot application, even if the temperature remains constant, does not feel as warm after adaptation has taken place. Clients must be informed that increasing the temperature or lengthening the time of application can seriously damage tissues.

Assessing

Before initiating heat or cold applications, the nurse must assess the client's physical and mental status, the condition of the body area to be treated with heat or cold, and the condition of the equipment to be used. Those factors that influence the tolerance of heat and cold need to be carefully considered, and are the bases for the following questions:

- How long will the heat or cold be applied? As previously discussed, prolonged exposure increases tolerance, and rebound effects are undesirable.
- What body part is involved? Some body areas, such as the neck, perineum, and inner aspect of the forearm and wrist, are more sensitive to thermal changes.
- Is the skin intact? Open tissue or abraded skin is more sensitive to thermal changes.
- How large is the area? Applications of heat or cold to large areas of the body cause systemic responses and lower tolerance of temperature change.
- What is the client's age? Infants, children, and elderly people tolerate temperature changes less well than adults.
- What is the client's physical condition? Clients with certain alterations in health have reduced response to or tolerance of thermal changes, increasing the risk of injury.

Assessing Physical and Mental Status Assessing the client's physical status includes a health history and physical examination. A history of cardiovascular or peripheral vascular impairment, sensory impairment, and alterations in mental status (such as confusion or decreased level of consciousness) indicate caution with the use of heat or cold because of the danger of tissue damage. Heat should not be applied to an open wound immediately after the trauma; during hemorrhage; over noninflammatory edema; to an acutely inflamed area, a localized malignant tumor, the testes, or the abdomen of a pregnant female; or over metallic implants. Cold should not be used for open wounds or for clients with impaired peripheral circulation or allergy to cold.

Assessments would include response to stimuli (sharp and dull), color and appearance of body tissues, circulation (pulses, blanching sign, temperature, and color), level of consciousness, and orientation.

Assessing the Area of Application Although application of heat or cold to a specific body part is ordered by the physician, it is the nurse's responsibility to assess the area and evaluate the client's response to the applications. Baseline assessment data are used to ensure safety and to evaluate outcomes of therapy. The risk of damage to tissues is increased if the area is traumatized, has altered skin integrity (assess for open lesions, blisters, wounds, edema, bleeding, or drainage), or has altered circulation (assess color, temperature, pulses, and sensation). As with any assessment, bilateral body parts are compared for changes. Tissue that has decreased or absent pulses, is pale or cyanotic, and feels cold has decreased circulation. This increases the risk of injury from heat and cold.

Assessment findings of undesired responses to heat include localized redness, blistering, and pain (symptoms of burning). Systemic responses that may occur when large areas of the body are exposed to heat are primarily the result of peripheral vasodilatation, resulting in a drop in blood pressure and risk for loss of consciousness. In contrast, applications of cold to a large body surface area can cause vasoconstriction, with an increase in blood pressure. Localized responses to cold include pallor, cyanosis, numbness, and pain. Shivering is a normal body response to cold.

Assessing the Condition of Equipment The nurse is responsible for checking the equipment used and for maintaining client safety. Included is the condition of cords and plugs, heating or cooling elements, fluid leaks, and distribution and constancy of temperature.

Diagnosing

Heat and cold applications are initiated only with a physician's order; the nurse's role is interdependent, specific to the ordered therapy. The client's response to the heat or cold indicates possible nursing diagnoses. Collaborative problems include potential complications—hypothermia (specify body part), hyperthermia (specify body part), impaired circulation, tissue injury, and neurovascular deficits.

The following nursing diagnoses may be indicated:

High Risk for Altered Peripheral Tissue Perfusion related to use of ice packs to reduce edema after fractured left tibia and known decreased peripheral circulation

Anxiety related to lack of knowledge about treatment of infected wound on right upper arm with hot soaks

High Risk for Infection related to daily débridement of lacerations of left hand followed by hot soaks

High Risk for Injury related to decreased thermal perception and the application of a heat lamp to legs every 4 hours

Pain related to thrombophlebitis of left lower leg requiring use of aquathermia heating pad

Planning: Client Goals

Heat and cold are used for a wide variety of therapeutic purposes that are an essential part of planning individualized client care and form the basis for client outcomes.

Indications for Heat Applications

Promote Wound Healing Heat promotes wound healing in various ways. The increased blood supply resulting from vasodilatation increases cell metabolism by bringing additional nutrients to the injured tissue and by increasing waste and toxin removal. These phenomena promote wound healing. The blood also brings increased numbers of leukocytes to defend against infection. Heat hastens the physical and chemical processes of suppuration, which is the formation of pus. The pus becomes localized in the infected area, where it is then carried away by the circulatory and lymph systems or drains from the wound rather than spreading to surrounding tissues. Drainage is thereby also increased with heat applications.

Relieve Pain One of the most common uses of the local application of heat is to relieve pain. The exact mechanism is not clearly understood, although some investigators believe that heat decreases the perception of pain. Others theorize that in the presence of both heat and pain stimulation, the perception of either decreases.

Relieve Muscle Tension and Joint Stiffness Although the effects of the local application of heat do not occur deeply in the body, heat has a muscle-relaxing effect and, therefore, promotes rest and relaxation. The exact mechanism is not clearly understood. Heat also decreases the viscosity of synovial fluid and allows improved joint range of motion.

Warm Part of the Body Heat may be applied locally to warm the body. For example, by placing warmth on cold feet, heat is transmitted to the body by conduction.

Reduce Edema Heat facilitates the removal of excess fluid from the interstitial fluid spaces as blood supplies to the area are increased. As a result, increased absorption of fluid takes place in the capillaries. Excess fluid in the tissues is absorbed into the general circulation.

Indications for Cold Application

Relieve Pain Cold applications are used to limit the accumulation of fluid in the body's tissues. This occurs by the phenomenon of vasoconstriction and decreased circulation to the area, so that excess fluid cannot gather in an injured area to increase pressure and pain. Pain and muscle spasms also are relieved by the anesthetic effects of cold. Cold is especially useful in traumatic injuries and burns.

Limit Inflammation and Suppuration Cold causes vasoconstriction, decreases cell metabolism, and inhibits microbial activity. These mechanisms act to control the inflammatory process and suppuration.

Control Bleeding Cold application helps to control bleeding by means of vasoconstriction. Also, the decreased flow rate of blood and its increased viscosity promote blood clotting.

Planning: Client Goals

When applications of heat or cold are part of a care plan, the following outcomes are appropriate; specific outcomes should be chosen based on the purpose of the application. The client will:

- Verbalize increased comfort, as evidenced by decreased muscle spasms, increased ability to rest, decreased local inflammation, and decreased edema
- Demonstrate signs of wound healing
- Verbalize and demonstrate safe hot or cold application

The nurse's aims in applying heat and cold are (1) to promote wound healing, (2) to facilitate comfort, (3) to use knowledge and skill in carrying out the application, and (4) to follow safety measures when providing heat or cold therapy.

Implementing

Heat and cold are applied to the body as both moist and dry applications, using many forms and methods. Types of application and their definitions are described in the display. Temperatures for heat and cold applications are given in Table 43-5.

Client Teaching As with any other procedure, the nurse explains the purpose and steps of the application and the sensations that will be experienced. To promote safety, it is important to ask the client to report immediately any changes in sensation or discomfort; to provide a timer or clock; and to have the call light in reach. The client should be instructed not to move the application or adjust any controls.

Physician's Order An order is necessary for any type of heat or cold application. The order should include the type of application, body area to be treated, frequency of application, and length of time for each application. Guidelines are given in this chapter for various applications; specific details may vary according to agency protocol.

Applying Heat

Heat is applied by both dry and moist methods. Hot water bottles, electric heating pads, aquathermia pads, or chemical heat packs provide local heat by conduction (see Procedure 43-4). Dry heat by radiation is provided by heat lamps or heat cradles. Moist heat by conduction is provided by hot compresses or packs, sitz baths, or soaks.

Dry Heat

Hot Water Bags or Bottles Hot water bags have disadvantages: they may leak, their weight often makes them uncomfortable for the client, and there is a danger of burns from improper use. They are, however, relatively easy and inexpensive to use (see Procedure 43-4).

Electric Heating Pads The electric heating pad can be used to apply dry heat locally. It is easy to apply and relatively

Heat and Cold Applications

Dry Applications

Aquathermia (Aqua K) pad: A rubber pad of tubular construction that can be filled with distilled water. An electrical control unit heats the water and keeps it at an even temperature. This pad permits the maintenance of a constant temperature at the level prescribed by the physician; therefore, it is both safer and more effective than a hot water bottle or an electric heating pad.

Cold chemical packs: A rubberized or plasticized flat bag containing a chemical substance that is frozen and used as a cold, dry application to the body surface. It must be covered with a protected covering before application.

Heat cradle: A metal cradle in which several electric sockets are installed for luminous bulbs; a means of providing radiant heat.

Heat lamp: A gooseneck lamp containing a 60-watt bulb, applied 18 to 24 inches from the body site. The heat lamp provides dry-heat radiation.

Ice bag or collar: A rubber or plastic device filled with ice chips and covered with a protective fabric before application to the client's body site. Vasoconstriction of peripheral vessels is caused by cold application.

Ice glove: A rubber glove filled with ice chips, placed in a light covering, and applied to a body surface. It is usually used in a postoperative oral surgery client and for relief of discomfort of the perineum after childbirth.

Moist Applications

Alcohol or cold sponge baths: A means by which reduction of body temperature occurs from evaporation. Cool water or a combination of cool water and alcohol is applied to the skin.

Compresses: Compresses may be either moist (gauze) dressings or washcloths. A compress usually is applied to smaller body areas and must be changed frequently. Compresses may be either hot or cold, sterile or unsterile, as designated by the physician.

- Hot compresses use the principle of heat conduction and can be sterile or unsterile moist applications. Gauze is soaked in the solution designated by the physician. The excess fluid is wrung out of the gauze to be applied. Sterile precautions are indicated when the compress is to be applied to an open wound or to an organ, such as the eye, to prevent the entrance of microorganisms. An insulating, waterproof cloth is placed over the compress to aid in heat retention. Hot compresses hasten the suppurative process and improve circulation.
- Cold or ice compresses are usually made of gauze or washcloths. The application of cold to open wounds or to lesions that may rupture requires sterile technique. Cold diminishes the formation

and absorption of bacterial toxins. It also causes vasoconstriction, decreased tissue metabolism, and sensory anesthesia. It is used for contusions, sprains, and strains and for controlling hemorrhages. Cold compresses also may be used for an injured eye, headache, tooth extraction, or hemorrhoids. The material used for application is immersed in a basin (clean or sterile, as ordered) that contains pieces of ice and water or ordered solution. If sterile technique is used, the sterile solution bottle is set in the bowl of ice. Compresses should be changed frequently.

Packs: Packs are usually applied to an extensive area of body surface. They may be either cold or hot, sterile or unsterile, as designated in the order. Examples are as follows:

- Hot pack (fomentation) is a piece of heated, moist towel that is applied to a client's skin to provide superficial heat. The effect of moderate heat is vasodilation, lessened viscosity of the blood, increased tissue metabolism, as well as relief of pain, congestion, inflammation, swelling, and muscle spasms. Application to open wounds or lesions that may rupture should be done using sterile technique. A heating device may be used to keep the pack warm. If the sterile procedure is ordered, the solution, towels, and dry covering must be sterile as well as the gloves or forceps used for wringing them dry.
- A cool wet pack is composed of bath towels moistened in water cooled with a small amount of ice chips. After wringing, the towels are applied full length to cover the anterior and posterior trunk of the body and each extremity. The temperature of the water is maintained at 75°F (23.9°C). Ice bags may be placed at the axillae, groin, and head. The cool wet pack is used to reduce body temperature by evaporation. This procedure may be done under sterile conditions.
- Ice packs are used occasionally to lower the temperature of a client's limb before surgery or to decrease swelling. It is a method of hypothermia that should be used with caution. Plastic bags of ice, which are covered with a pillowcase or towel, are placed on the specified area. Lower body temperatures are used for checking inflammation and suppuration by decreasing blood supply, slowing cellular metabolism, and inhibiting microbial activity. Extreme cold can destroy tissue if the length of application is excessive, however.

Soaks: A soak usually refers to the immersion of a part of the body, such as a foot or a hand, or may refer to wrapping the part with gauze and saturating it with fluid. The soak may be done under sterile conditions.

(Wieck, L., King, E. E., & Dyer, M. [1986]. *Illustrated manual of nursing techniques* [3rd ed., pp. 419–420]. Philadelphia: Lippincott.)

TABLE 43-5

Temperatures for Heat and Cold Applications		
Description	**Temperature Range**	**Example**
Very cold	Below 59°F (15°C)	Ice bags
Cold	59°–65°F (15°–18°C)	Cold pack
Cool	65°–80°F (18°–27°C)	Cold compress
Tepid	80°–98°F (27°–37°C)	Alcohol sponge bath
Warm	98°–105°F (37°–41°C)	Aqua-K pad
Hot	105°–115°F (41°–46°C)	Hot soak
Very hot	Above 115°F (46°C)	Hot water bottle

safe to use and provides constant and even heat. Improper use can, however, result in injury. The following are recommended techniques for using an electric heating pad:

- Avoid pins to secure a heating pad. There is danger of electric shock if a pin touches a wire.
- Place a covering over the pad, preferably one that is moisture-proof. Prevent wet and moist conditions around the pad. Short-circuiting the heating element may cause an electric shock to occur. The pad should not be covered too heavily. Heat may accumulate and burn the client when it cannot dissipate normally from the pad.
- Place a heating pad anteriorly or laterally to a body part, not under a portion of the body. If the heating pad is between the client and the mattress, there may be inadequate heat dissipation. This could cause the client or bed linens to be burned.
- Use a heating pad with a selector switch that cannot be turned up beyond a safe temperature. After heat has been applied and a certain amount of adaptation of heat receptors takes place, the client often increases the heat when the switch is not permanently preset because the pad does not seem sufficiently warm. Many people have been burned by turning up the heat in an electric pad because they thought that the pad was too cool.
- Assess the client's skin at regular intervals for the effects of excessive exposure to heat.
- Be sure to check agency protocol for use of heating pads; a release form may need to be signed.

Aquathermia Pads   Aquathermia (Aqua-K) pads are commonly used in health care agencies for various health problems, including back pain, muscle spasms, thrombophlebitis, and mild inflammation (Fig. 43-10). These devices are safer than a heating pad but still must be checked carefully. Guidelines for using aquathermia pads are as follows (see also Procedure 43-4):

- The temperature setting usually is set and locked before application.
- If the distilled water in the reservoir runs low, more is added at the top of the control unit. Tap water is not used.

- An application should last only 20 to 30 minutes.
- Assess the client's skin frequently for signs of burning.

Heat Lamps   Heat lamps provide dry heat to increase circulation to a small area, such as a pressure ulcer. They are available with either infrared or regular 40- to 60-watt bulbs. The lamps (often gooseneck type) are placed 18 to 30 inches (46 to 76 cm) from the area to be treated and applied for 15 to 20 minutes. Precautions for use are as follows:

- Clean and dry the area before the treatment to prevent burning.
- Do not cover the lamp or place it under bedclothes.
- Assess skin exposed to the heat every 5 minutes.

Heat Cradles   A heat cradle is a metal half-circle frame that encloses the body part to be treated with heat. A series of 25-watt bulbs, 16 to 18 inches (41 to 46 cm) from the client, provides heat over a larger area. The cradle may be covered with a sheet. Treatments usually take 15 minutes. Precautions should be taken to prevent burning, as for a heat lamp.

Hot Packs   Commercial hot packs provide a specified amount of dry heat for a specific period. Instructions on the package describe how to activate the pack.

Moist Heat

Warm Moist Compresses   Sterile warm moist compresses are used to treat open wounds to promote circulation and wound healing (especially if infected) and to reduce edema. To maintain heat—because moist heat evaporates and cools rapidly—the compresses must be changed frequently and be covered with a heating agent (hot water bottle, heating pad, Aqua K pad) or plastic wrap. Procedure 43-5 describes the application of warm sterile compresses to an open wound.

Sitz Baths   As a means of applying tepid or hot water to the pelvic or rectal area, clients are placed in a tub filled with sufficient water to reach the umbilicus. These baths are called *sitz baths*. Special tubs and chairs or basins that fit onto the toilet seat are available. They are designed so that the client's buttocks fit into a rather deep seat that is filled

Applying an External Heating Device

Equipment

Hot water bag
  Cover for bag
  Water at the appropriate
    temperature:
    46.1° to 51.6°C (115° to 125°F) for
      older children and adults
    40.5° to 43.3°C (105° to 110°F) for
      infants, young children, elderly
      people, diabetics, unconscious
      clients

Bath thermometer
Aquathermia pad
  Electrically controlled unit
  Distilled water
  Cover for pad
  Gauze bandage or tape
    (to secure pad)

Action	Rationale
1 Explain the procedure to the client.	This facilitates cooperation and provides reassurance for client.
2 Assess condition of skin where heat is to be applied.	Impaired circulation may affect sensitivity to heat. Elderly people and very young children have the least tolerance to applications of heat.
3 Assemble necessary equipment, and close door or curtain if privacy is desired.	Organization facilitates performance of task.
4 Wash your hands.	Handwashing deters the spread of microorganisms.

Hot Water Bag

Action	Rationale
5 Check temperature of water with bath thermometer or test on inner wrist. Rinse bag with water, empty, and then fill.	This provides for application of heat within the acceptable range for individual. Rinsing bag with warm water warms the rubber.
6 Fill hot water bag one-half to two-thirds full.	Hot water bottle molds more easily to area and puts less pressure on site.
7 Expel remaining air from bag in one of two ways: Place the bag on a flat surface, permit the water to come to the opening, and then close the bag; or, hold the bag up, twist the unfilled portion to remove the air, and then close the bag. Fasten top securely. Check for leaks.	Air reduces pliability of bag. Securing the top prevents leakage of water and discomfort for client.
8 Cover bag with towel or other protector, and apply hot water bottle to prescribed area.	This protects skin from direct contact with rubber. Heat travels by conduction from one object to another.
9 Assess condition of skin and client's response to heat at frequent intervals. Do not exceed prescribed length of time for application of heat. Remove hot water bag if excessive swelling, redness, or pain occurs, and report to physician.	Maximum therapeutic effects from application of heat occur within 20 to 30 minutes. Extended use of heat (beyond 45 minutes) results in tissue congestion and vasoconstriction. This *rebound phenomenon* results in increased risk to client of burns from application of heat.
10 After removal, record client's response and dispose of equipment appropriately.	This provides for accurate documentation of procedure.
11 Wash your hands.	Handwashing deters the spread of microorganisms.

(continued)

PROCEDURE 43-4 *(continued)*

Applying an External Heating Device

Action	Rationale

Aquathermia Pad

12 Check that distilled water is at appropriate level. Use key to adjust temperature at 40.5°C (105°F) if it has not already been preset. Plug in unit, and warm pad before use if manufacturer recommends.

Water temperature is regulated by key. Presetting the temperature eliminates risk of client adjusting the temperature.

13 Cover pad with pillowcase or other protector, and apply to prescribed area. Do not allow client to lie on pad if applying to back. Client should assume prone position and place aquathermia pad on back.

This protects skin from direct contact with rubber or source of heat. Pressure reduces dissipation of heat.

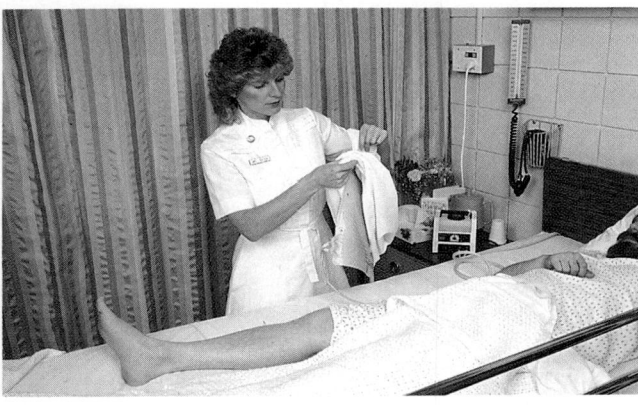

Action 13: Covering pad with pillowcase. (Photo © Ken Kasper.)

14 Secure with gauze bandage or tape. Never use safety pins to hold pad in place.

Hold pad in position on client. Pins may puncture and damage the pad.

15 Same as actions 9 to 11.

Same as actions 9 to 11.

---

with water of the desired temperature; the legs and the feet remain out of the water. The basins are disposable and economical for home or health care agency use. A regular bathtub is not as satisfactory for a sitz bath because the heat causes generalized vasodilation, altering the effect desired.

The following are recommended techniques for administering a sitz bath:

- Test the water in a sitz bath with a thermometer before the client enters the tub. If the purpose of the sitz bath is to apply heat, water at a temperature of 43° to 46°C (109° to 115°F) for 15 minutes produces relaxation of the parts involved after a short initial period of contraction. Warm water should not be used if considerable congestion is already present.
- If the purpose of the sitz bath is to produce relaxation or to help to promote healing in a wound by cleaning it of discharge and debris, then water at a temperature

of 34° to 37°C (93° to 99°F) is used. Check agency protocols for correct temperature.

- Assist the client into the tub and position him or her properly. The client should be able to sit in the basin or tub with his or her feet flat on the floor. There should be no pressure on the sacrum or thighs.
- Wrap a bath blanket around the client's shoulders to protect the client from feeling chilly and from exposure.
- Observe the client closely for signs of weakness and fatigue. Discontinue the bath if the client exhibits faintness, pallor, a rapid pulse rate, or nausea.
- Test the water in the tub several times, and keep it at the desired temperature. Additional hot water may be added by pouring it slowly from a pitcher or by opening the hot water faucet a little bit. The water should be agitated by stirring it as hot water is added to prevent burning the client.

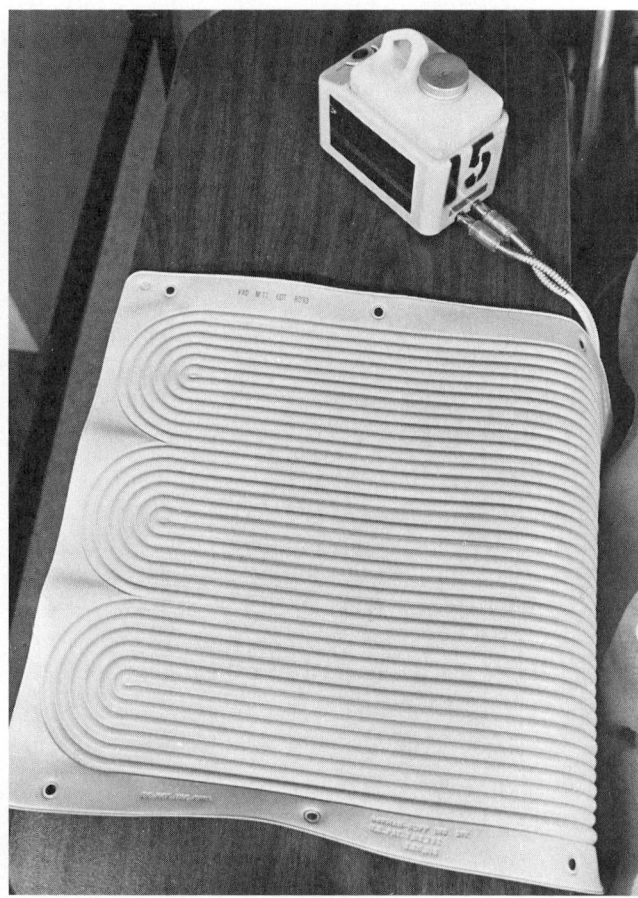

F I G U R E 4 3 - 1 0

The Aquathermia (Aqua-K) pad is an electrical device that can be set to maintain water at a constant temperature and circulate it through the coils of the plastic pad. The pad can be used to provide dry heat, or it can be placed over a moist dressing to provide moist heat.

- Do not leave the client alone unless it is safe to do so.
- Help the client out of the tub when the bath is completed. A sitz bath should take 15 to 30 minutes. Help the client dry, and cover the client adequately.

Warm Soaks The immersion of a body area into warm water or a medicated solution is called a soak. The purposes of soaks vary: to increase blood supply to a locally infected area; to aid suppuration; to aid in cleaning large, sloughing wounds, such as burns; to improve circulation; and to apply medication to a locally infected area. A soak has the added advantage of making manipulation of a painful area much easier because the body part is buoyed up by the weight of water it displaces. General guidelines for administering a warm soak include the following:

- If a soak is prescribed for a large wound, such as might cover an entire arm or lower leg or even an area of the torso, a compromise with sterile technique

usually is made. The container into which the body area is placed is sterilized before use if possible; if not, the container should be cleaned scrupulously. Tap water may be used for soaks because it is accepted as being free from pathogens.

- Unless the temperature of the soak is prescribed otherwise, a range of 40.5° to 43°C (105° to 109°F) is considered physiologically effective and comfortable for the client.
- The container holding the fluid should be positioned so that the part to be immersed is comfortable and the client is in good body alignment.
- During the treatment, which usually takes 15 to 20 minutes per soak, the temperature should be kept as constant as possible. This may be done by discarding some of the fluid every 5 minutes and replacing it or by adding solutions at a higher temperature while agitating the water. The client must remove the extremity from the soak while replacing or adding fluids.

Applying Cold

Dry Cold

Ice Bags Ice bags have essentially the same disadvantages as hot water bags, but they also are a relatively easy and inexpensive way to apply cold to an area. The following are recommendations for the use of an ice bag:

- Fill the bag with small pieces of ice to about two-thirds full. This makes the bag light in weight. Ice chips, rather than cubes, make it easier to mold the bag to a body part.
- Remove air from the ice bag in the same manner as removing air from a hot water bag.
- After securing the cap, test the ice bag for leaks and wipe off excess moisture.
- Place a cover on the ice bag to provide comfort and to absorb moisture that may accumulate on the outside of the bag.
- Apply an ice bag for 30 minutes and then remove it for about an hour before reapplying it. This technique prevents the effects of prolonged exposure to cold.

Cold Packs Commercially prepared ice bags are available in many health care agencies. These bags are sealed containers filled with a nontoxic substance. The bags are frozen in the freezing compartment of a refrigerator. An advantage of these bags is that the frozen solution remains pliable and can be easily molded to fit a body part. They are covered with a ribbed cotton sleeve so that the bag can be slipped onto an extremity. Or, the bag can simply be placed on a body part, such as the head. These bags cannot be reused.

Cooling Blankets A cooling blanket may be used to lower body temperature by placing the client on a special hypothermia blanket or pad. This apparatus has coils through which refrigerated solution is circulated. (It operates much

P R O C E D U R E 4 3 - 5

Applying Warm Sterile Compresses to an Open Wound

Equipment

Prescribed solution (warmed to
approximately 40° to 43°C (105° to
110°F)
Sterile container for solution
Sterile gauze dressings or
compresses

Sterile gloves
Clean disposable gloves
Waterproof pad
Dry bath towel
Bath blanket
Tape or ties

Aquathermia or external heating
device (optional)
Sterile bath thermometer
(if available, to check temperature
of solution)

Action	Rationale
1 Assess client for any circulatory impairment to area where compress is to be applied (numbness, tingling, impairment in temperature sensation, or cyanosis).	Circulatory impairment may interfere with client's ability to perceive heat and place him or her at risk of injury from the application of heat.
2 Check physician's order for warm compresses. Explain procedure to client.	An explanation encourages client cooperation and reduces apprehension.
3 Gather equipment.	This provides for organized approach to task.
4 Wash your hands.	Handwashing deters spread of microorganisms.
5 Close door or curtain. Use bath blanket as needed when exposing area for application of warm compresses. Position waterproof pad under client.	This provides for privacy and warmth.
6 Assist client to comfortable position that provides easy access to area.	This allows comfort and ease of application of compresses.
7 Place opened, cuffed plastic bag near working area.	Soiled dressings may be placed in disposal bag without contaminating outside surfaces of bag.
8 Prepare aquathermia pad or external heating device (optional).	External heating device allows compress to retain heat for longer interval.
9 Using sterile technique, open dressings and warmed solution. Pour solution into sterile container, and carefully drop gauze for compresses into sterile solution.	Sterile technique is used for warm moist compresses to an open wound.
10 Don clean disposable glove, and remove any dressing carefully. Discard dressing in disposable plastic bag. Pull off soiled glove inside out, and drop it in bag.	This prevents spread of microorganisms by contaminated dressings.
11 Assess wound healing or presence of infection.	Document condition of wound before application of compress.
12 Don sterile gloves (see Procedure 26-2).	Gloves maintain surgical asepsis.
13 Retrieve sterile compress from warmed solution, and squeeze moisture from it. Apply carefully, and gently mold around wound. Be alert for client's response to heat.	Excess moisture may contaminate surrounding area and is uncomfortable for client. Molding compress to skin promotes retention of warmth around wound site.
14 Cover the gauze compresses with dry bath towel, and secure in place if necessary.	Towel provides additional insulation.
15 Apply aquathermia pad or external heating device over towel (optional).	This controls temperature and extends therapeutic effect of compress.

(continued)

P R O C E D U R E   4 3 - 5 (continued)

Applying Warm Sterile Compresses to an Open Wound

Action	Rationale

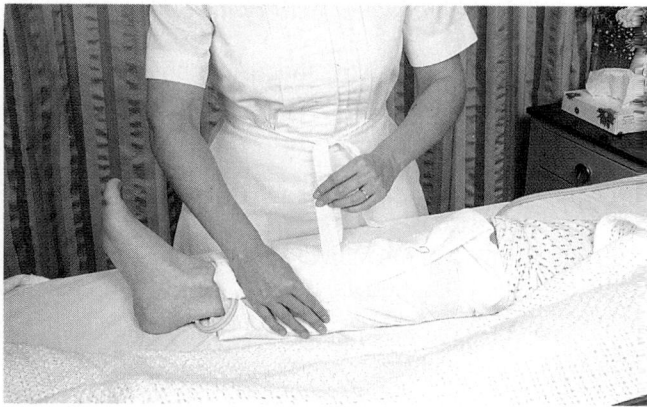

Action 15: Applying and securing pad in place. (Photo © Ken Kasper.)

Action	Rationale
16 Monitor condition of skin and client's response to warm compress at frequent intervals.	Impaired circulation may affect sensitivity to heat.
17 After 30 minutes (or time ordered by physician), remove warm compress. Carefully observe condition of skin around wound and client's response to application of heat.	Maximum therapeutic effects of heat occur within 20 to 30 minutes. Extended use of heat (beyond 45 minutes) results in tissue congestion and vasoconstriction. This *rebound phenomenon* results in increased risk to client of burns from application of heat.
18 Apply sterile dressing to wound (see Procedure 43-1).	Dressing protects wound from microorganisms in environment.
19 Dispose of equipment appropriately. Wash hands.	This deters spread of microorganisms.
20 Record clients' response and condition of wound and surrounding skin area.	This provides for accurate documentation of procedure.

like an Aqua K heating unit, except that the liquid is cooled instead of heated.) This method of reducing high body temperature may be used in place of a sponge bath.

Moist Cold

Cold Compresses   Moist, cold local applications are called **cold compresses**. They might be used for an injured eye, a headache, a tooth extraction, and, sometimes, for hemorrhoids. The texture and thickness of the material used depend on the area to which it is to be applied. For example, eye compresses could be prepared from surgical gauze compresses, which have a small amount of cotton filling. A washcloth makes an excellent compress for the head or the face.

The material used for the application is immersed in a clean basin appropriate for the size of the compress that contains pieces of ice and a small amount of water. The compress should be wrung thoroughly before it is applied to avoid dripping, which is uncomfortable for the client and may also wet the bed or clothing. The compresses should be changed frequently. The application should be contin-

ued for 20 minutes and repeated every 2 to 3 hours. Ice bags or commercial devices for keeping the compresses cold decrease the frequency with which the compresses must be changed.

Alcohol or Cold Sponge Bath   Alcohol or cold sponge baths are used to reduce body temperature. Plain water may be used, but alcohol added to water makes the temperature more easy to tolerate for most clients and removes heat from skin surfaces rapidly. Cold water often produces a strong initial reactionary effect, which elevates the temperature even further. This is observed when the client shivers and has gooseflesh.

The following techniques are recommended for administering an alcohol or cold-water sponge bath:

- Prepare a water and alcohol solution at about 29.5° to 32°C (85° to 89.6°F). If plain water is used, prepare it at a temperature of about 29.5°C (85°F), but add ice chips to bring the temperature down while bathing the client until the water temperature reaches about 18°C (64.4°F).

- Protect the client's bed with moisture-proof material.
- Prepare several ice bags. One ice bag is placed on the client's head to promote comfort. Others are placed in the groin and axillary areas, where blood vessels are close to the skin surface. The ice bags help to cool the client further.
- Drape the client properly to prevent shivering as various parts of the body are exposed for bathing.
- Sponge the face, neck, arms, and legs for 3 to 5 minutes and the back for 10 minutes. The anterior chest and abdomen usually are not sponged. Cover, but do not dry, each part as it is sponged. Evaporation of moisture on the skin helps to reduce body temperature.
- Move from one part of the body to another, and continue the bathing for 25 to 30 minutes. If the bath is short in duration, the body does not adjust to the

coolness. It then reacts to conserve heat, and the client's temperature may go even higher.
- Check the client's color and pulse rate during the bath. If the client becomes pale or cyanotic, or if the pulse rate increases or becomes irregular, discontinue the bath.
- Pat the client dry after the bath is completed. The friction of rubbing him or her dry may raise body temperature.
- Check the client's body temperature about 30 minutes after the bath to evaluate the effectiveness of the cool bath.

Evaluating

The effectiveness of the plan of care is evaluated based on the established client goals. If the goals are met, the plan was effective.

CASE STUDY

Mary Cupp, aged 35, has had abdominal surgery for removal of an ovarian tumor. Because the tumor was malignant, chemotherapy was initiated. After Mary was discharged from the hospital, her incision became red and swollen and she was having what she described as "thick, green, drainage." She was readmitted to the hospital for treatment of the infected wound. On admission, her vital signs were temperature, 102; pulse, 96; respirations, 22; blood pressure, 134/66. Her white blood cell count was 17,000. A physical assessment included the findings that the abdominal wound was not healed, with about half of the wound being open; that the area surrounding the

wound for 1 inch (2.5 cm) on all sides was red and edematous; and that the drainage was foul-smelling, copious, and purulent.

Nursing Diagnosis

Impaired Skin Integrity related to failure of abdominal wound healing as evidenced by open wound with purulent drainage, red and edematous wound edges, and elevated white blood cell count and temperature

NURSING CARE PLAN

for Mrs. Cupp

Nursing Diagnosis:	Impaired Skin Integrity related to failure of abdominal wound healing as evidenced by open wound with purulent drainage, red and edematous wound edges, and elevated white blood cell count and temperature
Long-Term Goal:	The client's abdominal wound will show progressive healing and absence of infection.
Goal:	By 1/6/93, the client will: • Demonstrate wound healing by (1) having decreased wound swelling and redness, (2) the surrounding skin will be less excoriated with no further breakdown, (3) body temperature will be normal, and (4) incisional pain will decrease

(continued)

NURSING CARE PLAN (continued)

for Mrs. Cupp

Nursing Actions
Change dressing every 4 hours using sterile technique. Irrigate wound with sterile saline and pack wound with saline-soaked 4 × 4s. Apply 8 × 10 sterile abdominal dressing over 4 × 4s.

Apply Montgomery straps over client's wound dressing.

Wear gown, gloves, and mask during dressing procedure. Use good handwashing technique before and after procedure.

Assess drainage for amount, color, odor, and consistency with each dressing change. Assess temperature every 4 hours.

Rationale
Sterile technique reduces potential infection of wound. Saline irrigation cleanses the wound and promotes healing which exudates would inhibit. An abdominal dressing over 4 × 4s protects the wound and promotes upward absorption of drainage. The soaked 4 × 4s prevent the dressing from clinging to dried wound drainage, which would further irritate wound with each dressing change.

Montgomery straps prevent skin damage and increase client's level of comfort by eliminating need for repeated removal of dressings and adhesives.

Using CDC guidelines for care of wounds with purulent drainage decreases chances of contamination.

Early detection of futher infection allows for prompt intervention.

Evaluative Statement
1/6/93 Goal met. Wound edges clean and pink. No further excoriation noted. Serous light yellow drainage on 4 × 4s. No sanguineous drainage noted. Temperature 99°F.

J. Weber, RN

Goal: By 1/6/93, the client will:
- Participate in self-care activities to promote wound healing and to prevent reinfection

Nursing Actions
Teach client the importance of proteins and vitamins in promoting wound healing. Identify those foods high in protein and vitamins for client and wife (protein—meat, eggs, fish, milk, leafy vegetables).

Rationale
A draining wound increases need for protein because exudate is high in protein. Protein replaces body mass lost during catabolism of cells from surgery and wound. This, in addition to bed rest, leads to a negative nitrogen balance. Increased calories are needed to restore weight, spare protein, and replace losses during surgery and stress periods. Stress and catabolism cause the early postoperative client to lose an increased amount of nitrogen and weight. Weight loss is common postoperatively, whereas an immediate weight gain postoperatively

Evaluative Statement
1/6/93 Goal partially met. Client choosing appropriate foods from menu, but lacks appetite. Eats half of each tray. Fails to eat much meat and other protein sources. Fluid intake adquate: 2000 to 2500 mL/day.

J. Weber, RN

(continued)

N U R S I N G   C A R E   P L A N *(continued)*

for Mrs. Cupp

Nursing Actions	Rationale	Evaluative Statement
	may indicate fluid retention. Vitamin A enhances wound healing and resistance to infection. Vitamin B_{12} promotes tissue synthesis; iron replaces that lost in blood loss; zinc promotes protein synthesis and wound healing. Vitamin C assists with synthesis of collagen, formation of capillaries, and resistance to infection. Vitamin K assists with synthesis of prothrombin (Eschleman, 1991).	
Encourage intake of 2000 mL of fluids per day.	Adequate hydration is necessary to replace losses through wound drainage and exudates and to maintain hydration.	
Teach client to splint abdomen and proper method of turning, coughing, and deep breathing every 2 hours. Assist client until she is able to do it by herself. Increase ambulation length each time as tolerated by client.	Activity stimulates appetite and sleep—both necessary for wound healing. Immobilization promotes a negative nitrogen balance and delays wound healing. Activity increases circulation to the wound and promotes healing by bringing increased leukocytes, oxygen, nutrients, antibodies, platelets, and erythrocytes to the damaged area. Increased circulation to the area also increases removal of toxins and debris.	

Goal:

By 1/6/93, the client will:
• Demonstrate safe and effective dressing change procedure

Nursing Actions	Rationale	Evaluative Statement
Teach client sterile procedure. Provide rationale for sterile dressing changes and avoidance of touching wound drainage. Demonstrate procedure and allow time for return demonstration.	Allowing the client to participate in self-care and promoting understanding of the procedure and purpose promote compliance and self-care.	1/6/93 Goal met. Client able to change abdominal dressing using sterile technique.

K E Y   P O I N T S

• The skin, as the largest organ of the body, provides protection, sensation, and fluid balance; it also facilitates communication and self-concept.
• A wound is a disruption in the normal integrity of the skin and tissues and may be described using various terms.

• Wounds heal more rapidly in a person who has a healthy physical status, proper nutrition, and intentional (surgical) trauma.

- Wounds heal by primary, secondary, or tertiary intention. Both the stress response and the inflammatory response influence tissue healing from the initial trauma through scar formation.
- Wound healing is affected by age, circulation and oxygenation, wound condition, and client wellness.
- Wound complications are infection, hemorrhage, dehiscence, and evisceration.
- Common psychological effects of wounds are pain, anxiety, fear, and altered self-concept.
- Wounds are assessed for appearance, skin sutures, drains, tubes, drainage, pain, and complications.
- Changing a dressing requires various supplies, may require bandages or binders, and is carried out using knowledge and skill.

- Heat and cold have local and systemic effects; both are used as therapeutic agents to treat traumatized body tissues.
- When assessing before the application of heat or cold, consideration is given to factors that influence tolerance, physical and mental status, the area to be treated, and the equipment to be used.
- Heat and cold may be applied in either dry or moist forms. Specific guidelines for performing procedures facilitate client safety and prevent tissue damage.

STUDY QUESTIONS

1. When a wound is accompanied by broken skin, it is labeled
   a. a closed wound
   b. an open wound
   c. an unintentional wound
   d. a contaminated wound
2. Which of the following surgical clients would be at greatest risk for a problem with wound healing?
   a. a healthy 10-year-old
   b. a 25-year-old with a surgical removal of the appendix
   c. a 50-year-old who exercises regularly
   d. a 75-year-old with a chronic illness
3. When changing the dressing on a flank wound, you note the drainage to be thin and light red. Which term would most accurately document this drainage?
   a. purulent
   b. serous
   c. sanguineous
   d. serosanguineous
4. A component of preparing for home care of a wound is to teach the symptoms of infection. Which of the following signs and symptoms should the client immediately report?
   a. crust formation across the incision line
   b. decreased drainage
   c. oral temperature of 101°F (38°C)
   d. mild incisional pain on exertion
5. The priority in caring for the client with a wound in an emergency situation is to:
   a. stop the bleeding
   b. apply ice as appropriate
   c. call 911
   d. assess airway patency
6. The tissue that forms across a wound during the proliferation phase of wound healing is:

   a. granulation tissue
   b. inflammatory tissue
   c. avascular tissue
   d. scar tissue
7. Mr. Jones has had a skin cancer removed from his left arm. The wound healed rapidly with minimal scarring. The wound healed by what process?
   a. tertiary intention
   b. secondary intention
   c. primary intention
   d. epithelial intention
8. Which of the following principles is used when determining that a dressing should be changed or reinforced?
   a. contamination moves through a moist medium
   b. aseptic procedures decrease the risk of infection
   c. blood on the dressing creates anxiety
   d. dry dressings are more comfortable
9. On the first day after thoracic surgery, Mr. Sol looks pale and has a low blood pressure and a rapid pulse rate. These are symptoms of what wound complication?
   a. infection
   b. hemorrhage
   c. dehiscence
   d. anxiety
10. Which of these basic turns would be most appropriate when applying a roller bandage to an elbow or a knee?
    a. circular turn
    b. spiral turn
    c. spica turn
    d. figure-of-eight turn
11. Systemic responses to the application of heat to large areas of the body are the result of vasodilation. What assessment finding would result in discontinuation of the treatment?

a. increased blood pressure
b. decreased blood pressure
c. decreased peripheral pulses
d. sweating

12. Which of the following treatments is an example of moist heat?
    a. heat cradle
    b. hot water bottle
    c. heat lamp
    d. sitz bath

13. Your neighbor has sprained her ankle and asks you how long she should leave on the ice bag. What would you tell her?
    a. for 30 minutes and then leave it off for 1 hour
    b. for 1 hour out of every 4
    c. for 2 hours and then leave it off for 2 hours
    d. as long as your leg hurts

14. Findings from which of the following assessments would indicate that an alcohol sponge bath should be stopped?
    a. pulse rate and skin color
    b. skin temperature
    c. amount of sweating
    d. amount of shivering

15. What statement would indicate that one of the client outcomes for the application of heat or cold has been met?
    a. "I feel so sleepy."
    b. "Why do I have all this drainage?"
    c. "My pain is much better."
    d. "My leg looks more swollen."

Answers With Rationale

1. The correct response is *b*. In an open wound, the skin is broken; it may be intentional or unintentional. A closed wound does not have broken skin, although soft tissue is damaged. A contaminated wound is the result of a break in surgical asepsis, accidental wounds, or contamination by bacteria.

2. The correct response is *d*. Physiologic alterations in elderly people result in diminished fibroplastic activity and circulation, and chronic illnesses impede the healing process. Children and healthy adults have less risk for problems.

3. The correct response is *d*. Purulent drainage is the result of infection and usually is thick and discolored. Serous drainage is clear and watery. Sanguineous drainage is primarily blood. Serosanguineous drainage is a mixture of serum and blood and is most common in surgical wounds.

4. The correct response is *c*. An elevated temperature is a systemic response to infection. The other responses are normal symptoms of a healing wound.

5. The correct response is *d*. The priority activity in any emergency situation is to assess for an open and intact airway.

6. The correct response is *a*. Granulation tissue forms across the wound during the proliferation phase of wound healing. The other responses are incorrect in describing the wound during this phase.

7. The correct response is *c*. Most surgical incisions and small sutured incisions heal by primary intention. Secondary intention healing takes place in large wounds when edges cannot be approximated. Tertiary intention healing occurs when there is an extended interval between the occurrence of the wound and suturing it.

8. The correct response is *a*. Wound contamination can occur as pathogens move through a moist medium. Therefore, a saturated dressing should be changed or reinforced. The other principles are accurate but do not answer the question.

9. The correct response is *b*. Hemorrhage is manifested by a falling blood pressure, a rapid pulse rate, and pallor.

10. The correct response is *d*. A figure-of-eight turn is used to apply roller bandages to joints. The other turns would slip off or be inappropriate.

11. The correct response is *b*. The application of heat to large areas of the body causes peripheral vasodilatation. As a result, the blood pressure would fall, possibly causing the client to become dizzy or faint. The nurse would discontinue the treatment if the blood pressure decreased.

12. The correct response is *c*. A sitz bath is an example of moist heat. The other responses are examples of dry heat.

13. The correct response is *a*. An ice bag should be applied for 30 minutes and then be removed for 1 hour. This prevents the effects of prolonged exposure to cold. The other responses are incorrect.

14. The correct response is *a*. Assessments of the client's pulse rate and skin color should be made at regular intervals during an alcohol sponge bath. If the client becomes pale or cyanotic, or if the pulse rate increases or becomes irregular, the sponge bath should be stopped.

15. The correct response is *c*. The reduction of pain is one of the desired outcomes of applications of heat or cold.

BIBLIOGRAPHY

Bale, S., & Harding, K. G. (1990). Using modern dressings to effect débridement. *Professional Nurse, 5,* 244, 246 248.

Carpenito, L. J. (1992). *Nursing diagnosis: Application to clinical practice* (4th ed.). Philadelphia: Lippincott.

Cerrato, P. L. (1988). What diet does for wound healing. *RN, 51*(6), 73–76.

Cooper, D. M. (1990a). Optimizing wound healing: A practice within nursing's domain. *Nursing Clinics of North America, 25*(1), 165–180.

Cooper, D. M. (1990b). Wound healing. *Nursing Clinics of North America, 25*(1), 163–164.

Cooper, D. M., & Schumann, D. (1979). Postsurgical nursing intervention as an adjunct to wound healing. *Nursing Clinics of North America, 14*(4), 713–725.

Cuzzell, J. Z., & Stotts, N. A. (1990). Wound care: Trial and error yields to knowledge. *American Journal of Nursing, 90*(10), 53–54.

Eschleman, M. M. (1991). *Introductory nutrition and diet therapy* (2nd ed.). Philadelphia: Lippincott.

Flynn, J. M., & Hackel, R. (1990). *Technological foundations in nursing.* East Norwalk, CT: Appleton & Lange.

Flynn, M. E., & Rovee, D. T. (1982). Promoting wound healing. *American Journal of Nursing, 82*(10), 1543–1558.

Fritz, C. (1982). Emergency! First aid for wounds. *Nursing, 10,* 68–75.

Gallaher, L. P., & Kreidler, M. (1987). *Maximizing human potential throughout the life cycle.* East Norwalk, CT: Appleton & Lange.

Gauthier, K. D., & LeMone, P. (1990). Trauma: The acute response. *AAOHN Journal, 38*(10), 475–481.

Guidelines for prevention of transmission of human immunodeficiency virus and hepatitis B virus to health-care and public-safety workers. (1989). *Morbidity and Mortality Weekly Report,* 5–6.

Hotter, A. N. (1982). Physiologic aspects and clinical implications of wound healing. *Heart and Lung, 11*(6), 522–540.

Huggins, B. (1990). Trauma physiology. *Nursing Clinics of North America, 25*(1), 1–10.

Jones, P. L., & Millman, A. (1990). Wound healing and the aged patient. *Nursing Clinics of North America, 25*(1), 263–277.

Lomas, C. (1988). From theory to practice . . . wound care. *Nursing Times, 84,* 63, 65–66.

McConnell, E. A. (1990). How to tape a dressing. *Nursing, 20*(6), 23.

Meehan, P. A., & Mayz, E. J. (1988). Nursing management of an open abdominal wound. *Critical Care Nurse, 8*(6), 29–30, 32–34.

Metheny, N. M. (1992). *Fluid and electrolyte balance: Nursing considerations* (2nd ed.). Philadelphia: Lippincott.

Morrison, M. J. (1989). Wound cleaning—which solution? *Professional Nurse, 4*(2), 220–222, 224–225.

Neuberger, G. B., & Reckling, J. B. (1985). A new look at wound care. *Nursing, 15*(2), 34–42.

Patrick, M. L., Woods, S. L., Craven, R. F., Rokosky, J. S., & Bruno, P. M. (1991). *Medical-surgical nursing: Pathophysiological concepts* (2nd ed.). Philadelphia: Lippincott.

Phipps, W., Long, B., Woods, N., & Cassmeyer, V. (1991). *Medical-surgical nursing: Concepts and clinical practice* (4th ed.). St. Louis: Mosby.

Rodeheaver, G., et al. (1982). Bacterial activity and toxicity of iodine-containing solutions in wounds. *Archives of Surgery, 117,* 181–186.

Smeltzer, S. C., & Bare, B. G. (1992). *Brunner and Suddarth's textbook of medical–surgical nursing* (7th ed.). Philadelphia: Lippincott.

Spencer, R. T., et al. (1989). *Clinical pharmacology and nursing management* (3rd ed.). Philadelphia: Lippincott.

Stotts, N. A. (1990). Seeing red and yellow and black. The three-color concept of wound care. *Nursing, 20*(2), 59–61.

Sutton, J. (1989). Accurate wound assessment. *Nursing Times, 85*(September 20–26), 68, 71.

Wieck, L., King, E. E., & Dyer, M. (1986). *Illustrated manual of nursing techniques* (3rd. ed.). Philadelphia: Lippincott.

Willey, T. (1992). Use a decision tree to choose wound dressings. *American Journal of Nursing, 92*(2), 43–46.

Wound-care update 91. (1991). *Nursing, 21*(4), 47–50.

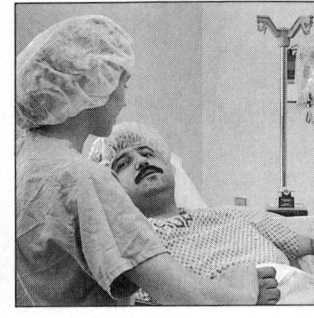

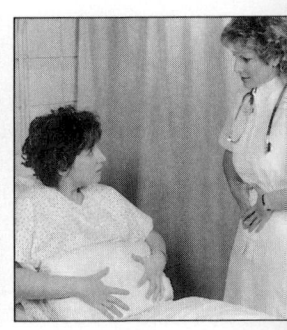

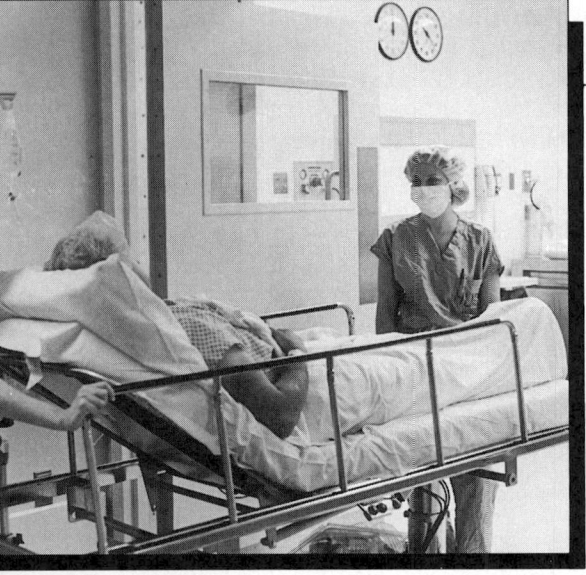

Perioperative Nursing

OBJECTIVES

After studying this chapter, the learner should be able to:

Define key terms used in the chapter.

Describe the surgical experience, including perioperative phases, categories of surgery, types of anesthesia, and informed consent.

Conduct a preoperative nursing history and physical assessment to identify client strengths as well as factors that increase surgical and postoperative complication risk.

Demonstrate preoperative exercises: deep breathing, coughing, and leg exercises.

Prepare a client physically and psychologically for surgery.

Describe the nurse's role in the intraoperative phase.

Identify assessments specific to the prevention of complications in the immediate postoperative phase.

Plan and implement interventions for postoperative care to prevent complications, promote a return to health, and facilitate coping with alterations.

Use the nursing process to knowledgeably develop an individualized plan of care for the surgical client during each phase of the perioperative period.

KEY TERMS

atelectasis
elective surgery
emergency surgery
general anesthesia
hemorrhage
hypovolemic shock
informed consent
intraoperative phase
paralytic ileus
perioperative nursing
perioperative period
pneumonia
postoperative phase
preoperative phase
pulmonary embolus
regional anesthesia
shock
thrombophlebitis

44

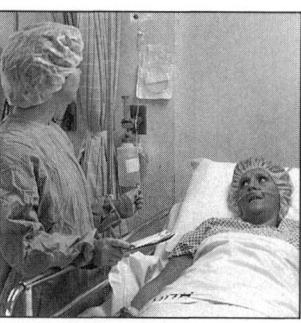

The medical treatment of a wide variety of illness and injuries often is some type of surgical intervention Surgery is an invasive method of treatment that may be planned or unplanned, major or minor, and that may involve any body part or system. Surgical procedures require physical and psychosocial adaptations and are stressors for both the client and the family, no matter what the extent. The client's recovery from a surgical procedure requires skillful and knowledgeable nursing care that is both collaborative and independent. All phases of the nursing process are used before, during, and after surgery to make assessments and provide interventions necessary to promote the recovery of health, prevent further injury or illness, and facilitate coping.

This chapter discusses nursing care appropriate to preparing the client for surgery, supporting the client during surgery, and assisting with recovery after surgery. The nurse's role during each stage is described, using the phases of the nursing process. Selected nursing diagnoses are included, and the application of the nursing process in the clinical setting is described at the end of the chapter in a case study and care plan for the surgical client.

The Surgical Experience

Regardless of the surgical intervention required, all clients progress through specific perioperative phases, have a defined surgical procedure, require anesthesia, and give their consent for surgery. This part of the chapter describes those components of the surgical experience to serve as a knowledge base for the application of the nursing process when giving nursing care to the client who is undergoing surgery.

Perioperative Period

The client who is having surgery progresses through several distinct phases, with the entire time frame labeled the **perioperative period**. **Perioperative nursing** is the name given to the wide variety of nursing activities carried out before, during, and after surgery. The three phases of the perioperative period are the **preoperative phase**, beginning with the decision that surgical intervention is necessary and lasting until the client is transferred to the operat-

ing room table; the **intraoperative phase**, extending from admission to the surgical department (or operating room) to transfer to the recovery area; and the **postoperative phase**, lasting from admission to the recovery area to the complete recovery from surgery. The nursing process is used during each phase to meet physical and psychosocial needs and facilitate the client's return to health. Each of these phases, with related client needs and nursing activities, are described in the remainder of the chapter.

Classification of Surgical Procedures

Surgical procedures usually are categorized by the major classifications of urgency, risk, and purpose. Table 44-1 lists each classification, with purposes and selected examples for each. The classifications are described below.

Based on Urgency Surgery may be classified as **elective surgery**, meaning that it is preplanned and based on the client's choice; *urgent surgery*, in which the surgery is necessary for the client's health but not an emergency; and **emergency surgery**, when surgery must be done immediately to preserve the client's life, body part, or body function.

Based on Degree of Risk Surgery is classified as *major* or *minor* based on the degree of risk for the client. Minor surgery may be done in a physician's office, in an outpatient clinic, in same-day surgery settings, or in the operating room of a hospital. This classification means that the surgical procedure usually is brief, carries a low risk, and results in few complications. In contrast, major surgery always requires hospitalization, usually is prolonged, has a higher degree of risk, involves major body organs or life-threatening situations, and has the potential of postoperative complications.

Based on Purpose Descriptors used to classify surgical procedures based on purpose include *diagnostic, ablative, palliative, reconstructive, transplant*, and *constructive*.

Combinations Surgical procedures may combine several classifications and labels (eg, a client who has been in an automobile accident and has severe trauma and bleeding may require major, reconstructive, emergency surgery). It is important to remember that no matter the defined degree of risk, any surgical procedure imposes physical and psychological stress and seldom is considered minor by the client.

Anesthesia

Anesthesia, depending on its classification as *general* or *regional*, produces such states as narcosis (loss of consciousness), analgesia, relaxation, and loss of reflexes. General anesthesia produces all of these responses, whereas regional anesthesia does not cause narcosis, but does result in analgesia and reflex loss. Anesthetic agents

TABLE 44-1

Classification of Surgical Procedures

Classification	Purpose	Examples
Based on Urgency		
Elective: Delay of surgery has no ill effects; can be scheduled in advance based on client's choice	• To remove or repair a body part • To restore function • To improve health • To improve self-concept	Tonsillectomy, hernia repair, cataract extraction and lens implant, hemorrhoidectomy, hip prosthesis, scar revision, face-lift, mammoplasty
Urgent: Usually done within 24–48 hours	• To remove or repair a body part • To preserve or restore health • To restore function • To prevent further tissue damage	Removal of gallbladder, coronary artery bypass, surgical removal of a malignant tumor, colon resection, amputation
Emergency: Done immediately	• To preserve life (plus purposes as listed above)	Control of hemorrhage, repair of trauma, perforated ulcer, intestinal obstruction, tracheostomy
Based on Degree of Risk		
Major: may be elective, urgent, or emergency	• To preserve life • To remove or repair a body part • To restore function • To improve or maintain health	Carotid endarterectomy, cholecystectomy, nephrectomy, colostomy, hysterectomy, radical mastectomy, amputation, trauma repair
Minor: Primarily elective	• To restore function • To remove skin lesions • To correct deformities	Teeth extraction, removal of warts, skin biopsy, dilatation and curettage, laparoscopy, cataract extraction, arthroscopy
Based on Purpose		
Diagnostic	• To make or confirm a diagnosis	Breast biopsy, laparoscopy, bronchoscopy, exploratory laparotomy
Ablative	• To remove a diseased body part	Appendectomy, subtotal thyroidectomy, partial gastrectomy, colon resection, amputation
Palliative	• To relieve or reduce intensity of an illness; is not curative	Colostomy, nerve root resection, debridement of necrotic tissue, balloon angioplasties, arthroscopy
Reconstructive	• To restore function to traumatized or malfunctioning tissue • To improve self-concept	Scar revision, plastic surgery, skin graft, internal fixation of a fracture, breast reconstruction
Transplant	• To replace organs or structures that are diseased or malfunctioning	Kidney, liver, cornea, heart, joints
Constructive	• To restore function in congenital anomalies	Cleft palate repair, closure of atrial-septal defect

are administered by a physician, an anesthesiologist (medical doctor), or a nurse anesthetist.

General Anesthesia

When a client is given drugs by inhalation, intravenous, rectal, or oral route to produce central nervous system depression, it is termed **general anesthesia**. The desired action of general anesthesia is loss of consciousness, relaxation of skeletal muscles, and reduction of reflex action. The choice of route and type of anesthesia is primarily made by the anesthesiologist after discussion with the client. Many factors influence the choice, including the type and length of surgery and the physical and psychological status of the client (Meeker & Rothrock, 1991). Inhalation anesthesia often is used because it has the advantage of rapid excretion and reversal of effects.

There are three phases of general anesthesia—induction, maintenance, and emergence. Induction begins with administration of the anesthetic agent and continues until the client is ready for the incision. Maintenance continues from this point until near the completion of the procedure. Emergence starts as the client begins to "emerge" from the anesthesia and usually ends when the client is ready to leave the operating room; the length of time depends on the depth and length of anesthesia (Meeker & Rothrock, 1991).

General anesthesia has both advantages and disadvantages. The advantages are that it can be used for clients of any age and for any surgical procedure, leaving the client unaware of physical trauma. There are, however, major risks of circulatory and respiratory depression.

Regional Anesthesia

Regional anesthesia occurs when an anesthetic agent is injected or applied topically near a nerve or nerve pathway, inhibiting the transmission of sensory stimuli to central nervous system receptors. The client receiving the regional anesthesia remains awake but loses sensation in a specific part of the body. In some instances, reflexes also may be lost. Regional anesthesia may be accomplished by surface anesthetic, local infiltration, nerve blocks, or subdural or epidural blocks. These are defined as follows:

- Surface (topical) anesthesia is used on mucous membranes, open skin surfaces, wounds, and burns. Cocaine, 4% to 10% solution, is the most commonly used agent; others are lidocaine (Xylocaine) and benzocaine.
- Local infiltration with an agent such as lidocaine or tetracaine 0.1% is used in minor surgical procedures such as skin biopsy and suturing small wounds.
- Nerve blocks are done by injecting a local anesthetic around a nerve trunk supplying the area of surgery, such as the jaw, face, and extremities.
- Subdural blocks are used to provide spinal anesthesia. The injection of a local anesthetic into the subarachnoid space (through a lumbar puncture) causes sensory, motor, and autonomic blockage and is used for surgery of the lower abdomen, perineum, and legs. Adverse effects of spinal anesthesia may include hypotension, headache, and urine retention.

Informed Consent

Informed consent is when a client voluntarily agrees to undergo a particular procedure or treatment (such as surgery) after having received the following information, which should be given to the client in understandable words:

- Description of the procedure or treatment
- Name and qualifications of the person performing the procedure or treatment
- Explanation of the risks involved, including potential for damage, disfigurement, or death
- That the client has the right to refuse treatment and that consent can be withdrawn

Informed consent protects the client, the physician, and the health care institution. The form that is signed is a legal document as well as an ethical imperative. The responsibility for securing informed consent from the client lies with the person who will perform the procedure; this usually is the physician. The nurse, signing as witness, signifies that the client signed the consent form and was alert and aware of the act. The client always has the right to refuse treatment.

Consent forms are not legal if the client is confused, unconscious, sedated, mentally incompetent, or considered a minor (specific guidelines for minors are written in states in the United States and in provinces in Canada). Consent may be given in those instances by a parent, spouse, next of kin, or legal guardian. In emergency situations, the physician may obtain consent over the telephone or by court order. More detailed information about informed consent can be found in Chapter 6. An example of an informed consent form is shown in Figure 44-1.

Preoperative Nursing Care

Clients who require surgical intervention and nursing care enter the health care setting in a wide variety of situations, ranging from essentially healthy people who have planned elective procedures to emergency admissions for treatment of trauma. Surgical clients may be any age and at any point on the health–illness continuum. It is the nurse's responsibility to identify factors that affect risk from a surgical procedure, assess physical and psychosocial needs of the client and family, and establish a plan of care, based on appropriate nursing diagnoses, that includes interventions to meet needs and facilitate recovery as the client progresses through the perioperative period.

Assessing

The importance of preoperative assessment cannot be overemphasized. Surgery is a major trauma to the body, and preoperative assessments identify factors that may place the client at greater risk for complications during and after surgery. Assessment of the surgical client includes a nursing history and physical assessment to establish baseline data, identify risk factors, and determine teaching and psychosocial needs of the client and the client's family.

Nursing History

The nursing history assesses risk factors and strengths in the client's physical and psychosocial status. Information significant to the surgical experience includes a health history, life-style habits, and coping patterns and support systems, including client perceptions of self and surgery.

Health History   Health history data that identify risk factors and individualized assessments are developmental level, medical history, medications, previous surgeries, and perceptions and knowledge of the surgery to be done.

Developmental Considerations   Infants and older adults are at a greater risk from surgery than are children and young and middle-aged adults. The infant has a lower total blood volume, making even a small loss of blood a serious consideration because of the risk of dehydration and the inability to respond to the need for increased oxygen during

PRESBYTERIAN–UNIVERSITY OF PENNSYLVANIA MEDICAL CENTER

CONSENT TO OPERATION AND/OR PROCEDURE OR TREATMENT, ADMINISTRATION
OF ANESTHETICS AND RENDERING OF OTHER MEDICAL SERVICE

Patient _____ Age _____

Date _____ Time _____

    1. I AUTHORIZE and DIRECT _____ M.D., with the
Associates and Assistants of his choice to perform upon—

_____

("Myself" or state name of patient)

The following operation and/or procedure or treatment _____

_____

_____

and if any unforeseen condition arises in the course of the operation calling in their judgment for other operations, diagnostic or therapeutic procedures including blood transfusions in addition to or different from those now contemplated, I further request and authorize them to do whatever is deemed advisable for my recovery, health and well-being.

    2. The nature, purpose, and possible risks and alternate methods of treatment have also been discussed and consequences of the proposed operation and/or procedure or treatment have been explained to me. I am aware that the practice of medicine and surgery is not an exact science and I acknowledge that no guarantee or assurance has been made to me as to the results.

    3. I consent to the administration of anesthesia and supportive measures by or under the direction of the Department of Anesthesiology of the Presbyterian–University of Pennsylvania Medical Center, and to the use of such anesthetics as the members of the Department deem advisable.

I have been advised of the alternative type of anesthesia, if any, and the possible consequences of the use of each type have been explained to me.

    4. I certify that I understand the above, acknowledge that the explanations referred to above have been made, and consent to the operation and/or procedure or treatment and the administration of anesthesia and supportive measures.

    5. I further understand that if I do not understand any aspect of this consent form that I may request and receive additional explanation and information.

    6. I agree that any tissue or other body parts removed will go to the Department of Pathology for pathological examination and photography and then be preserved or disposed of by that Department at their discretion unless otherwise stated.

SIGNATURE OF PATIENT _____

When patient is a minor or incompetent to give consent:
SIGNATURE of person authorized to consent for Patient:

_____

and Relationship to Patient _____

Witness to authenticity of signature _____

I have explained the procedure to the patient and/or nearest relative, along with possible risks, alternate methods of treatment and consequence of the procedure, and to the best of my knowledge the patient understands and comprehends and concurs with the performance of this procedure.

_____
          M.D.   Date

CONSENT TO OPERATION

F I G U R E   4 4 - 1

Example of an informed consent form.

surgery. The infant also has difficulty maintaining stable body temperature during surgery because the shivering reflex is not well developed, making potential hypothermia or hyperthermia more likely.

Physiologic changes associated with aging (described in Chapter 12) place the elderly client at risk for surgery. These changes, summarized in the accompanying display, decrease the older adult's ability to respond to the stress of surgery, alter the response to preoperative and postoperative medications and anesthesia, and prolong or alter wound healing processes. With an increasingly elderly population, assessment of physiologic changes is critical in providing knowledgeable, safe, holistic nursing care to the elderly surgical client.

Medical History The medical history provides information about past and current illnesses; pathologic changes associated with past and current illnesses increase surgical risk as well as the potential for postoperative complications. Preoperative assessments and documentation are necessary to provide a data base for individualized assessments and interventions in the intraoperative and postoperative phases of care. The following are selected examples and associated risks:

Cardiovascular diseases (thrombocytopenia, hemophilia, recent myocardial infarction or cardiac surgery, congestive heart failure, arrhythmias)—increase the potential for hemorrhage and hypovolemic shock, hypotension, venous stasis, thrombophlebitis, and overhydration with intravenous fluids.

Pulmonary disorders (pneumonia, bronchitis, asthma, chronic obstructive pulmonary diseases)—increase the possibility of respiratory depression from anesthesia as well as postoperative pneumonia, atelectasis, and alterations in acid–base balance.

Kidney and liver function alterations—influence the client's response to anesthesia, affect fluid and electrolyte as well as acid–base balance, alter the metabolism and excretion of drugs, and impair wound healing.

Metabolic disorders, especially diabetes mellitus—increase the potential for hypoglycemia or acidosis and impede wound healing.

Medications Use of drugs, whether prescribed or over-the-counter, can affect the client's reaction to and increase the risk from the stress of surgery and the effects of the

FOCUS ON THE OLDER ADULT

Physiologic Changes With Aging That Increase Surgical Risk

System	Change	Preoperative Nursing Interventions
Cardiovascular	• Decreased cardiac output, heart rate, and cardiac reserve • Decreased peripheral circulation • Increased vascular rigidity	• Establish baseline data of vital signs. • Assess peripheral pulses. • Teach leg exercises, turning, and ambulating. • Document normal activity levels and tolerance of fatigue.
Respiratory	• Reduced vital capacity • Diminished cough reflex • Decreased oxygenation of blood	• Establish baseline data of respiratory depth and rate. • Teach coughing and deep-breathing exercises. • Assess color of skin.
Neurologic	• Sensory deficit • Decreased reaction time	• Orient to surroundings. • Institute safety measures (eg, elevate side rails, use night light). • Allow additional time for questions and teaching.
Renal	• Decreased renal blood flow • Reduced bladder capacity	• Assess amount and times of voiding. • Monitor fluid and electrolyte status. • Institute intake and output.
Integument	• Decreased vascularity • Dry, inelastic	• Assess skin status. • Monitor fluid status. • Monitor nutritional status.

anesthetic agent. Medications usually are cancelled when a client goes to surgery, but it is important for the nurse to know the purposes and specific actions of drugs as well as physician's orders; specific medications may be given even when the client is going to surgery (eg, clients with heart or cardiovascular problems and those with diabetes mellitus).

Surgical risk is increased by drugs in the following categories:

Anticoagulants—may precipitate hemorrhage

Diuretics—may cause electrolyte imbalances, with resulting respiratory depression from anesthesia

Tranquilizers—may increase the hypotensive effect of anesthetic agents

Adrenal steroids—abrupt withdrawal may cause cardiovascular collapse in long-term users

Antibiotics—those in mycin group, when combined with certain muscle relaxants used during surgery, can cause respiratory paralysis.

Previous Surgery   Data about previous surgeries provide a knowledge base for meeting physical and psychological needs throughout the perioperative period.

Physical implications of previous surgeries are important to the intraoperative and postoperative phases (eg, previous heart or lung surgery may necessitate adaptations in anesthesia and in positioning during surgery). Complications after prior surgery, such as pneumonia, thrombophlebitis, or wound infection, provide data to support careful postoperative monitoring.

The client's past experiences with surgery also affect the plan of care established in the preoperative phase, especially if those experiences were negative. When the interview elicits negative feelings about the surgical experience, pain control, or nursing interventions carried out to prevent complications during previous surgeries, teaching and mutual goal setting are even more important.

Perceptions and Knowledge of Surgery   Included in the medical history review are the client's perceptions and knowledge of the surgical procedure to be performed. Questions asked or statements made by the client provide a base for meeting psychological and family needs when preparing the client for surgery.

Life-Style   The nursing history data about the client's lifestyle provide valuable information about surgical risk and postoperative recovery and rehabilitation. Areas especially important for the surgical client are nutrition, use of alcohol or nicotine, activities of daily living, and occupation.

Nutrition   Both malnutrition and obesity increase surgical risk. Surgery increases the body's need for nutrients, necessary for normal tissue healing and resistance to infection. The client who is malnourished is at higher risk for alterations in fluid and electrolyte balance, delay in wound healing, and wound infection. The obese client is at increased risk for pulmonary, cardiovascular, and gastrointestinal problems. Fatty tissue is more difficult to suture and has

less resistance to infection; postoperative complications of delayed wound healing, wound infection, and disruption in the integrity of the wound are more common (Smeltzer & Bare, 1992).

Use of Alcohol or Nicotine   Clients whose alcohol intake habitually is large require larger doses of anesthetic agents and postoperative analgesics, increasing the risk of drug-related complications. Clients who smoke are at higher risk for respiratory complications after surgery; pulmonary secretions are retained by all clients during anesthesia, but the smoker, who already has increased mucous secretions, has more difficulty clearing the respiratory passages after surgery. In addition, the tracheobronchial mucosa is chronically irritated in people who smoke; anesthesia further increases this irritation.

Activities of Daily Living   Exercise and rest and sleep habits are important considerations in preventing postoperative complications and facilitating recovery. A client with a well-established exercise program has improved cardiovascular, respiratory, metabolic, and musculoskeletal function, thereby lowering the risks of surgery. Rest and sleep are essential to physical and emotional adaptation and recovery from the stress of surgery. Information from the nursing history allows the nurse to individualize interventions to promote rest and sleep.

Occupation   Many surgical procedures require a delay in returning to a career or occupation or may necessitate a change in the way the client supports self and family. Knowledge of a client's usual work and concerns about returning to work prepare the nurse for necessary teaching and referrals.

Coping Patterns and Support Systems   Assessment of the client's psychologic, sociocultural, and spiritual dimensions is as important as the physical history and examination. Surgery is a major psychological stressor and affects coping patterns, support systems, and sociocultural needs.

Coping Patterns   A surgical procedure, no matter whether planned or unexpected, major or minor, causes anxiety and fear. The nursing history interview often is a time when the nurse can use cues from verbal and nonverbal communication of the client and family to identify fears and concerns and to plan nursing interventions to provide information and emotional support necessary to the successful recovery from surgery.

Surgery is an unknown experience over which a person has no control; the resulting anxiety may be expressed in many ways, such as anger, withdrawal, apathy, confrontation, questioning. Therapeutic communication skills are essential in establishing a trusting nurse–client relationship necessary to identify and resolve fear. The causes of fear in the preoperative phase include the following:

Fear of the unknown: The client has fears about the surgery itself, the anesthesia, the diagnosis, the future, financial and family responsibilities, response to pain, possible disfigurement or disability.

Fear of pain or death: Common fears are that the anesthesia will not "put me to sleep," that death will occur during surgery, or that the client will not be able to handle postoperative pain.

Fear of changes in body image and self-concept: Surgical procedures often leave the client with permanent changes in body structure, function, or appearance. Clients commonly fear alterations in physical attractiveness, social relationships, life-style, and sexuality.

The nurse should encourage the client to identify and verbalize fears; often simply talking about fears helps to diminish the magnitude that has built up. At the same time, incorrect knowledge can be identified and corrected, strengths can be identified, and teaching can be done. The reduction of fear is of major importance in preoperative preparation; emotional stress added to the physical stress of surgery increases surgical risk.

Support Systems Coping with stress can be facilitated through various support systems identified during the assessment phase of preoperative nursing care. As much as possible, family members or significant others should be part of the initial interview and should be included in discussions of fears and concerns. Family members should be encouraged to be part of the surgical experience, providing support before and after surgery.

By identifying spiritual beliefs in the nursing history, the nurse can support the client's spiritual needs through acceptance, participation in prayer, or referral to clergy or chaplain. Faith in a higher being provides support and helps to reduce fears.

The need for other support systems also can be identified in the initial interview (eg, the client having a colostomy or mastectomy may have many questions answered and anxieties reduced by a preoperative visit from a person who has had the same operation and adapted successfully).

The nursing history should elicit those ways in which a client provides self-support to reduce stress. These are discussed in Chapter 9 and range from listening to music to actively practicing relaxation techniques.

Sociocultural Needs A person's perceptions of and reactions to the surgical experience are influenced by sociocultural factors, including family health beliefs and practices, economic factors, and cultural background.

As discussed in Chapter 2, each person is influenced by family health beliefs and practices. If a client who requires surgery has grown up in a family that believes that surgical intervention is the last possible option in treating illness, he or she may refuse to have surgery or may be convinced that death will result. The resulting anxiety and physical condition make this particular client even more susceptible to surgical risk; a self-fulfilling prophecy has come true. Reactions to teaching, physical care, and pain also are influenced by family values (eg, the male client reared with the

belief that it is unmanly to acknowledge pain presents a stoic acceptance of pain and refuses needed medications postoperatively).

Economic factors influence the point on the health–illness continuum at which a person seeks medical care or has elective surgery. Cultural influences on the surgical experience also impact the client's responses and perceptions. Cultural backgrounds may require nursing interventions individualized to meet needs in such areas as language spoken, foods eaten, family interactions and participation, personal space, and health beliefs and practices (eg, a client from a cultural background that believes that bed rest is the most important treatment for illness or injury may have difficulty accepting the need for postoperative exercises and ambulation).

Preparing for Ambulatory Surgery

Surgical procedures performed in ambulatory (also referred to as outpatient or same-day) surgical settings are becoming more common as hospitals respond to government regulations formulated to reduce length of hospital stay as well as costs from third-party insurance companies. These surgical settings may be found as freestanding units, in hospitals, and in physicians' offices.

Many procedures that formerly required hospitalization are done routinely in ambulatory surgery and are in fact mandated by the federal government and the Health Care Financing Administration. Included are such procedures as cataract extraction, arthroscopy, hemorrhoidectomy, crushing of kidney stones and gallstones with sound waves, and gynecologic procedures.

By allowing the client to spend the night before surgery at home and to return to his or her own home to convalesce, much of the stress associated with surgery is eliminated. Clients who are elderly or chronically ill or who do not have support systems that are willing or able to provide the care needed after surgery may require additional teaching and home care.

Preoperative nursing assessments and teaching are key elements in providing care for the ambulatory surgical client (Fig. 44-2). Preoperative teaching often can be combined with preoperative screening tests, which usually are done 2 to 5 days before the scheduled surgery. Preoperative teaching should cover certain points:

- Instruct the client to do the following:
  - List medications routinely taken and ask the physician which should be taken or omitted the morning of surgery
  - Notify the surgeon's office if a cold or infection develops before surgery
  - List allergies and be sure the operating staff is aware of these
  - Remove nail polish and not wear makeup for the procedure
  - Leave all jewelry and valuables at home
  - Wear clothing that buttons in front; short-sleeved garments are better for surgery on the hands

PRE-ADMISSION TEACHING/TESTING
PERI-OPERATIVE ASSESSMENT

PLANNED SURGERY & DATE: _____

DATE OF VISIT: _____

SURGICAL HISTORY: _____

Lab Ordered:

Abnormal Lab work called to

Dr. _____ on _____ Initials _____

ANESTHESIA HISTORY: _____

X-ray

SYSTEMS REVIEW: **Allergy:** _____

Dental: _____

Abnormal X-ray called to

CONTACT LENS/IOL: _____

Dr. _____ cn _____ Initials _____

HEARING AID: _____

EKG

CARDIOVASCULAR

Rheumatic Fever: _____ Murmur: _____

Hypertension: _____ Infarction: _____

Date Last EKG: _____

Abnormal EKG work called to

Dr. _____ cn _____ Initials _____

RESPIRATORY

PRE-OP TEACHING GUIDELINES

Pneumonia: _____ TBC: _____

Asthma: _____ Recent URI: _____

Date Last CXR: _____

___ Pre-Op Injection   ___ Shave Prep

___ Transported to Holding Room   ___ Awake in Recovery Room

___ Visitors To Waiting Room   ___ Oxygen Face Tent

___ I.V. Fluids   ___ Deep Breaths & Cough

HEMATOLOGY

Bleeding Tendency: _____

___ Pneumatic Boots (Appr. Surg.) ___ Frequent Check BP & P

___ Leggins (Cysto or GYN)   ___ NPO after MN or Liq. Breakfast

GI

Recent Vomiting: _____ Diarrhea: _____

Jaundice: _____ Hepatitis: _____

___ Taken to O.R.   ___ Cannot Drive Self Home

___ Strap   ___ Jewelry, Make-up Left Home

___ BP Cuff, Monitor Pads   ___ Wear Loose Clothing

___ Bovie Pad   ___ Video _____

GYN

L.M.P.: _____ Para: _____

Gravida: _____

___ Hand-out/Packet _____

NOTES: _____

GU

UTI/Problems: _____

NEUROPSYCH

Syncope: _____ Epilepsy: _____

MUSCULOSKELETAL

Neck or

Arthritis: _____ Back Inj.: _____

R.O.M.: _____ Prothesis: _____

Skin Integrity: _____

RECOVERY ROOM FOLLOW UP: _____

METABOLIC

Diabetes: _____

Thyroid: _____

POST-OP FOLLOW-UP: _____

MEDICATIONS: _____

B/P _____ T. _____ P. _____ R. _____ WT. _____

HT. _____ **PHONE:** _____

Example of a same-day surgery assessment record.

- Have someone available for transportation home after recovery from anesthesia
- Give the client written instructions about limitations on eating or drinking before surgery, with a specific time to begin the limitations.
- Give the client written instructions about when and where to arrive for the procedure as well as the estimated time when the procedure will be performed.

Physical Assessment

Assessment of the client's current physical status done during the nursing examination provides data for interventions to decrease surgical risk and potential postoperative complications. Depending on the situation, the physical examination is done as described in Chapter 24. Table 44-2 summarizes assessments specific to the surgical client.

Screening Tests

Various screening tests done in the preoperative phase provide objective data of normal body function or, if abnormal, provide data for medical interventions to improve physical status and thus decrease potential surgical complications. The nurse's role is to ensure that the tests are

ordered and done, that the results are recorded in the client's record before surgery, and that abnormal findings are reported. Additionally, abnormal results provide data to support nursing diagnoses and collaborative problems. Usual screening tests include chest x-ray, electrocardiography, complete blood count, measurement of electrolyte levels, and urinalysis. These tests are discussed in Chapter 27; normal findings for laboratory tests are found in Appendix B. Significant abnormal findings are an elevated white blood cell count (presence of infection), decreased hematocrit and hemoglobin level (presence of bleeding, anemia), hyperkalemia or hypokalemia (increased risk of cardiac problems), elevated blood urea nitrogen or creatinine levels (possible renal failure), and abnormal urine constituents (indicating infection, fluid imbalances, renal failure).

Diagnosing

Nursing diagnoses for the client in the preoperative phase may be identified for various actual or potential problems, based on the analysis of subjective and objective data obtained from the nursing history and physical examination as well as information from other health team members and screening tests. Many diagnoses reflect assessment of potential risk and are made to provide interventions to

T A B L E   4 4 - 2

Preoperative Physical Assessments

Component	Assessment	Purpose
General survey	• Height • Weight • Vital signs	• Indicates nutritional status, especially obesity and malnutrition • Provides baseline data for intraoperative and postoperative phases • May indicate fluid and electrolyte imbalances or underlying infection
	• General appearance	• Reflects energy levels, physical and emotional status
Status of skin	• Oral cavity • Skin turgor • All skin surfaces, especially over bony prominences	• Indicates hydration levels • Significant in hydration status • Indicates potential for injury or pressure ulcers during and after surgery.
Respiratory status	• Respiratory depth, rate • Adventitious sounds on auscultation • Diameter and shape of thorax	• Any abnormalities found would indicate potential respiratory difficulties during surgery, or postoperative atelectasis or infection.
Cardiovascular status	• Apical pulse: character, rate, rhythm • Peripheral pulses • Presence of edema	• Provides baseline data for intraoperative and postoperative phases • Abnormal findings indicate potential complications intraoperatively and postoperatively, such as thrombophlebitis, emboli, congestive heart failure, arrhythmias
Abdominal status	• Size, shape, symmetry • Bowel sounds • Last bowel movement	• Provides baseline data for postoperative assessments
Neurologic status	• Level of consciousness • Mood • Motor and sensory function	• Provides baseline data for postoperative assessments • Especially important to postoperative assessment after spinal anesthesia

meet client needs during the intraoperative and postoperative phases. Nursing care throughout the perioperative period must be consistent and documented; the preoperative nursing diagnoses are the bases for consistent holistic care from admission through recovery.

Examples of nursing diagnoses appropriate to the preoperative period are as follows:

Anticipatory Grieving related to perceived loss of normal body image resulting from scheduled amputation of left leg after traumatic injury

Anxiety related to the effects of surgical procedure (on lumbar vertebrae for repair of ruptured intervertebral disk) on ability to function as primary wage earner and head of the family

Anxiety related to knowledge deficit about preoperative and postoperative routines and procedures

Fear related to surgery for treatment of cancer of the breast and unknown future

High Risk for Infection related to age (77), obesity, and abdominal incision to remove intestinal tumor

Ineffective Airway Clearance related to 25-year history of smoking and administration of anesthesia during surgery

Ineffective Individual Coping related to conflict between need for surgery and religious belief (member of Christian Scientist faith)

Planning: Client Goals

Preoperative nursing care is affected by the length of the preoperative phase. Clients who enter the hospital through the emergency department with the need for immediate surgery and those who have ambulatory surgery may not have time for comprehensive assessments and teaching. There has been a tremendous increase in the number of same-day surgeries, in which clients are admitted early the morning of surgery. In such cases, it is imperative for the nurse to use standardized preoperative plans and individualize the plans for the particular client and family. For the client having elective surgery (with admission the day before the procedure), expected client goals can be established. Goals are standard for all clients having surgery, but nursing interventions must be designed to meet priority needs of specific clients and situations.

Planning for the entire perioperative period is done in the preoperative phase and includes goals that have been mutually discussed and agreed on by the nurse, the client, and the family. Standards of care established by the Association of Operating Room Nurses (1989) address client knowledge, safety, physical status, and rehabilitation. More specific goals that would be appropriate are as follows. The client will:

- Be physically and emotionally prepared for surgery
- Demonstrate turning, coughing, and deep-breathing exercises
- Verbalize understanding of postoperative pain control

- Maintain fluid intake and nutritional balance to meet needs

To help the client meet these goals during the preoperative phase, the nurse must accomplish the following:
- Establish a data base and plan of care to meet client needs throughout the perioperative period
- Identify and meet client and family learning needs
- Identify physical and psychosocial risk factors
- Provide interventions to maximize physical and emotional safety and security

Implementing

Preoperative nursing interventions provide the client with the necessary physical and psychological preparation for surgery and the postoperative phase. This section of the chapter discusses implementing the plan of care to meet established client goals; Procedure 44-1 outlines the actions and rationales for preoperative client care.

Preparing the Client Psychologically

As discussed in the assessment section, surgery is almost always viewed as a life crisis and evokes anxiety and fear. Anxiety can be reduced and recovery can be facilitated by nursing actions that focus on therapeutic communications and client and family teaching.

Communicating   The nurse uses therapeutic communication skills and techniques, as described in Chapter 20, to establish a supportive and trusting nurse–client relationship and to facilitate psychological safety and security. Guidelines for the nurse in meeting psychological needs of the surgical client are as follows:
- Establish and maintain a therapeutic relationship, allowing the client to verbalize fears and concerns.
- Use active listening skills to identify and validate verbal and nonverbal responses indicative of anxiety and fear.
- Use touch, as appropriate, to demonstrate genuine empathy and caring.
- Be prepared to respond to common client questions about surgery:
  - Will I lose control of body functions while I'm having surgery?
  - How long will I be in the operating and recovery rooms?
  - Where will my family be?
  - Will I have pain when I wake up?
  - Will the anesthetic make me sick?
  - Will I need a blood transfusion?
  - How long will it be before I can eat?
  - What kind of scar will I have?
  - When will I be able to be sexually active?
  - When can I go back to work?

Remember that each client is a unique individual and will respond to the surgical experience in a unique way.

PROCEDURE 44-1

Preoperative Client Care

Action	Rationale
General	
1 Identify clients for whom surgery is a greater risk:	This allows for recognition of clients who may be prone to complications after surgery.
a Very young and elderly clients	
b Obese or malnourished clients	
c Clients with fluid and electrolyte imbalances	
d Clients in poor general health from chronic diseases and infectious processes	
e Clients taking certain medications (ie, anticoagulants, antibiotics, diuretics, depressants, steroids)	
f Clients who are extremely anxious	
2 Review nursing data base, history, and physical examination. Check that baseline data are recorded.	Review identifies clients who are surgical risks.
3 Check that diagnostic testing has been completed and results are available.	This check may influence type of surgery and anesthetic as well as timing of surgery or need for additional consultation.
4 Promote optimal nutritional and hydration status.	This promotes wound healing.
5 Identify learning needs of client. Conduct preoperative teaching regarding the following:	This minimizes surgical risk and allays anxiety by preparing clients for postoperative period.
a Coughing and deep-breathing exercises	
b Management of pain after surgery	
c Leg exercises and ambulation	
d Postoperative equipment and monitoring devices	

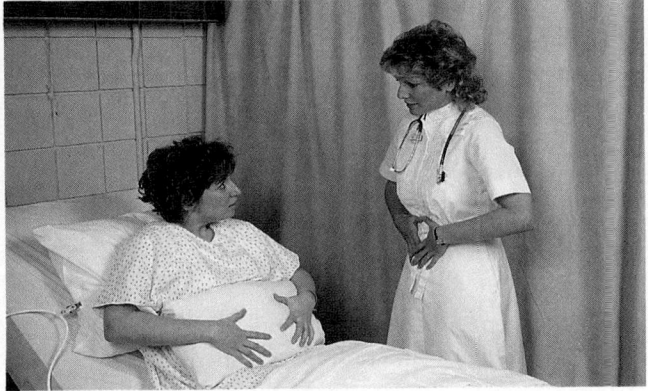

Action 5a: Teaching client to splint incision before coughing. (Photo © Ken Kasper.)

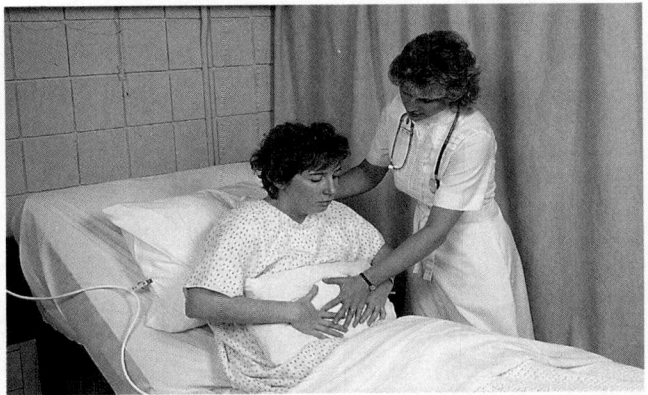

Action 5a: Teaching client to cough. (Photo © Ken Kasper.)

Action	Rationale
Day Before Surgery	
6 Provide emotional support. Answer questions realistically. Provide spiritual assistance if requested.	This allays client's misconceptions and fears.

(continued)

P R O C E D U R E 4 4 - 1 (continued)

Preoperative Client Care

Action	Rationale
7 Follow preoperative dietary restrictions.	This reduces risk of vomiting and aspiration during surgery. Anesthetic agents temporarily depress gastrointestinal function and processes.
8 Prepare for elimination needs during and after surgery.	Anesthetic agents and abdominal surgery interfere with normal elimination function. A urinary catheter inserted preoperatively minimizes risk of inadvertent trauma to bladder during surgery.
9 Shave and prepare the operative site if ordered by physician.	Prepping reduces number of microorganisms present on skin.
10 Attend to client's special hygiene needs (ie, use of antiseptic cleaning agents).	This decreases potential for infection.
11 Provide for adequate rest.	Rest minimizes stress before surgery.
Day of Surgery	
12 Check that proper identification band is on client.	Double-checking ensures identity of client.
13 Check that preoperative consent forms are signed and medical record is in order.	This fulfills legal requirement related to informed consent.
14 Check vital signs. Notify physician of any pertinent changes (ie, rise or drop in blood pressure, elevated temperature, cough, symptoms of infection).	This provides baseline data for comparison.
15 Provide hygiene and oral care. Remind client not to swallow water if NPO for surgery.	This promotes comfort.
16 Continue nutritional and hydration preparation.	This prepares client for operative procedure.
17 Remove cosmetics and prostheses (eg, contact lenses, false eyelashes, dentures, and so forth). Assess for loose teeth.	These interfere with assessment during surgery.
18 Have client empty bladder and bowel prior to surgery.	An empty bladder and bowel minimizes risk of injury or complications during and after surgery.
19 Place valuables in appropriate area. Hospital safe is most appropriate place for valuables. They should not be placed in narcotics drawer.	This ensures safety of valuables and personal possessions.
20 Attend to any special preoperative orders.	This prepares client for operative procedure.
21 Complete preoperative checklist and record of client's preoperative preparation.	This ensures accurate documentation.
22 Administer preoperative medication as ordered by physician.	Medication reduces anxiety, provides sedation, and diminishes salivary and bronchial secretions.

One note of caution: The nontherapeutic use of false reassurance must be avoided. In an attempt to allay anxiety and fear, the nurse may be tempted to reassure the client that he or she will be fine. These responses deny the client's emotional needs, shut off therapeutic communications, and may not be true.

Teaching Teaching postoperative activities is done in the preoperative phase and is the nurse's responsibility. Clients and families need to know about surgical events and sensations, how to manage pain, and how to perform the physical activities necessary to decrease postoperative complications and facilitate recovery. The teaching–learning process (see Chapter 21) is individualized to meet both specific and common client needs.

The timing of teaching is a significant consideration; teaching that is done too far in advance of surgery or when the client is anxious will be less effective. In today's health care delivery system, clients often enter the hospital the day before or the day of surgery, and teaching must be adapted to this schedule. Many institutions provide teaching sessions before admission so that the client is prepared for surgery. Whether done before or after admission, a preoperative teaching checklist gives nurses organized and comprehensive guidelines for instruction (see the accompanying display).

Nursing research has indicated that the success of preoperative teaching varies with the timing of the teaching, the individual client and his or her support systems, the type of surgery, and group versus individual sessions (Voss, 1986). Preoperative teaching has proved to be beneficial in decreasing postoperative complications and in positively influencing recovery.

Surgical Events and Sensations Clients and their families need to know when surgery is scheduled, about how long surgery and recovery room care will last, and what will be done before, during, and after surgery (procedures, medications, equipment). If the surgery is elective, a tour of the operating room suite is helpful in reducing anxiety and fear of the unknown (although especially helpful for children, this also is useful in teaching adult clients). An explanation of the surgical events includes a description of the various members of the health care team. An outline of surgical events is found in the display.

Clients also need to know what sensations they will be experiencing during the perioperative period. Although the sensations will differ depending on the type of surgery, teaching should include the following:
- Feelings experienced from preoperative medications, such as a dry mouth and drowsiness
- Sensations that normally occur after surgery and anesthesia, such as a sore throat from an endotracheal tube, a gradual return of feeling and movement after spinal anesthesia, and a lower tolerance of activity with increased fatigue
- Sensations experienced after surgery, such as incisional pain, intravenous catheters and fluids, tight dressings, dry mouth, and drowsiness

Pain Management Pain is a normal part of the surgical experience and an area of major concern for the client and family. The following are guidelines for teaching the client about pain control:
- Medications to relieve pain will be ordered by the physician and administered by the nurse.
- Pain medications usually are ordered on an as-needed (prn) basis, with a time restriction between doses (eg, every 3 to 4 hours). The client needs to ask for the medication and should do so before the pain is severe; if the medication does not control the pain, a different one can be ordered.
- Medications for pain usually are given by injection for the first few days (and as long as the client is NPO); with food intake and decreasing pain levels, oral medications can be used.

Sample Preoperative Teaching Checklist: Activities and Events

Preoperative phase
- Exercises and physical activities
    Deep-breathing exercises
    Coughing
    Incentive spirometry
    Turning
    Leg exercises
- Pain management
    Meaning of prn orders
    Timing for best effect
    Splinting incision
- Visit by anesthesiologist
- Physical preparation
    NPO
    Sleeping medication the night before
    Preoperative checklist (review items)
- Visitors and waiting room
- Transported to operating room by stretcher

Intraoperative phase
- Holding area
    Skin preparation
    Intravenous fluids
    Medications
- Operating room
    Operating room table
    Lights
    Restraints
    Sensations
    Staff

Postoperative phase
- Postanesthesia recovery area
    Frequent vital signs
    Dressings
    Intravenous lines
    Pain medications
    Family notification
    Sensations
    Staff
- Transfer to unit (on stretcher)
    Frequent vital signs
    Sensations
    Pain medications
    NPO, diet
    Exercises
    Ambulation
    Family visits

- There is little danger of addiction to pain medications when they are used in the postoperative management of pain.
- The use of relaxation techniques (such as deep breathing and guided imagery) facilitates the effects of pain medications.
- Pain medications allow the client to manage pain and increase his or her ability to carry out activities and exercises necessary to recovery.

Alternate methods of pain control also are used for relief of pain after surgery. Transcutaneous electrical nerve stimulation (TENS) is a nonpharmacologic technique that increases nerve fiber activity to close the gate to small nerve fibers; it also is believed to stimulate the release of endorphins, which are chemicals produced in the body that mediate pain perception. A TENS unit has electrodes that are placed on the skin along each side of the surgical incision. The client controls the electric current by pushing a button when feeling pain. A patient-controlled analgesia pump allows the client to administer his or her own analgesic. When the client pushes the control button on the pump, a preset dose of analgesic medication is administered automatically. The time intervals between doses and the amount of medication that can be used within a given period are programmed into the device. The client must be taught before surgery how to use both of these methods of pain control, and the nurse is responsible for assessing the effectiveness of the pain relief. Further discussion of pain control is found in Chapter 32.

Physical Activities   The most common causes of postoperative complications are cardiovascular and pulmonary alterations, including atelectasis, pneumonia, thrombophlebitis, and emboli. Physical activities to reduce the potential of these complications are taught in the preoperative period. The following sections describe deep (diaphragmatic) breathing, coughing, incentive spirometry, leg exercises, and turning in bed. The client should be able to verbalize the purpose and demonstrate the activities before going to surgery. (This section gives the rationale for the activities; postoperative complications are discussed later in the chapter.)

Deep Breathing   During surgery, the cough reflex is suppressed, mucous accumulates in the tracheobronchial passageways, and the lungs do not fully ventilate. After surgery, respirations often are less effective as a result of the anesthesia, pain medications, and pain from the incision (eg, clients who have thoracic or high abdominal incisions are especially prone to shallow breathing because of incisional pain with deeper respirations). As a result, alveoli do not inflate and may collapse and secretions are retained, increasing the potential for atelectasis and pulmonary infection.

Deep-breathing exercises hyperventilate the alveoli and prevent their recollapse, improve lung expansion and volume, help to expel anesthetic gases and mucus, and facilitate oxygenation of tissues.

The following are guidelines for teaching effective deep-breathing exercises:
- Place the client in semi-Fowler's position, with support for the neck and shoulders.
- Ask the client to place the hands over the rib cage, so he or she can feel the chest rise as the lungs expand.
- Ask the client to:
  - Exhale gently and completely.
  - Inhale through the nose gently and completely.
  - Hold his or her breath and mentally count to three.
  - Exhale as completely as possible through the mouth with lips pursed (as if whistling).
  - Repeat three times.
- This exercise should be done every 1 to 2 hours while the client is awake for the first 24 to 48 hours after surgery and as necessary thereafter, depending on risk factors and pulmonary status.

Coughing   Coughing facilitates the removal of retained mucus from the respiratory tract and usually is taught in conjunction with deep breathing. Coughing is painful; the client should be taught how to splint the incision (ie, to support the incision with a pillow or folded bath blanket, as shown in Procedure 44-1) and to use the period after pain medication has been administered to best advantage. The following are guidelines for teaching effective coughing:

- Place the client in a semi-Fowler's position, leaning forward.
- Provide a pillow or folded bath blanket to use in splinting the incision.
- Ask the client to:
  - Inhale and exhale deeply and slowly through the nose three times.
  - Take a deep breath and hold it for 3 seconds.
  - "Hack" out for three short breaths.
  - With mouth open, take a quick breath.
  - Cough deeply once or twice.
  - Take another deep breath.
- Repeat the exercise every 2 hours while awake.

Incentive Spirometry   An incentive spirometer (see the display Sample Preoperative Teaching Checklist: Activities and Events) often is ordered for clients having surgery, and the proper technique for using it should be practiced preoperatively. This device helps to increase lung volume and inflation of alveoli and facilitates venous return. The following points should be included in client teaching:
- Sit upright or elevate the head of the bed 45 degrees.
- Take two or three normal breaths and then insert the spirometer's mouthpiece into the mouth.
- Inhale through the mouth and hold the breath for 3 to 5 seconds.
- Exhale slowly and fully.
- Repeat the sequence 10 times during each waking hour for the first 5 days after surgery (except immediately before or after meals).

Leg Exercises   During surgery, venous blood return from the legs slows; some surgical positions also may decrease venous return. With circulatory stasis of the legs, thrombophlebitis and resultant emboli are potential complications. Leg exercises increase venous return through flexion and contraction of the quadriceps and gastrocnemius muscles. The following are guidelines for teaching the client leg exercises (Fig. 44-3):

- Alternately point toes toward the chin (dorsiflex) and toward the foot of the bed (plantar flex); then, make a circle with the toes.
- Flex and extend the knees, pressing them down toward the mattress on extension.
- Raise and lower each leg, keeping the leg straight.
- Repeat the exercises every 1 to 2 hours.

Leg exercises must be individualized to client needs, physical condition, physician preference, and agency protocol.

Turning in Bed   Turning in bed improves venous return, respiratory function, and gastrointestinal peristalsis. Although turning in bed sounds like a simple procedure, incisional pain makes it more difficult, and it should be practiced before surgery. To turn in bed, the client should raise one knee, reach across to grasp the side rail (on the side toward which he or she is turning), and roll over while pushing with the bent leg and pulling on the side rail. A small pillow is useful in splinting the incision while turning. The client should turn from side to side every 2 hours.

Preparing the Client Physically

The physical preparation of the client for surgery may vary, depending on the client's physical status and special needs, type of surgery to be done, and physician's orders. Certain independent and interdependent nursing interventions are appropriate for all surgical clients in the areas of hygiene and skin preparation, elimination, nutrition and fluids, and rest and sleep. The nurse also is responsible for the preparation and safety of the client on the day of surgery.

Hygiene and Skin Preparation   Intact skin is the body's first line of defense against microorganisms, and an alteration in skin integrity (such as the surgical incision) provides a potential source of infection. Therefore, the skin is prepared to minimize skin contamination and decrease the risk of postoperative wound infection.

The skin is cleaned by scrubbing the operative site one or more times with an antibacterial soap or solution to remove bacteria. This can be done by the client while taking a bath or shower. Ideally, a shower is taken the evening before or the morning of surgery. Shampooing the hair and cleaning the fingernails also help to reduce the number of organisms present.

The incisional area usually is shaved before surgery because hair serves as a reservoir for bacteria. This may be done by the nurse or by surgery personnel. Although shaving the skin was once done routinely the evening before surgery, it is now most often done immediately before the

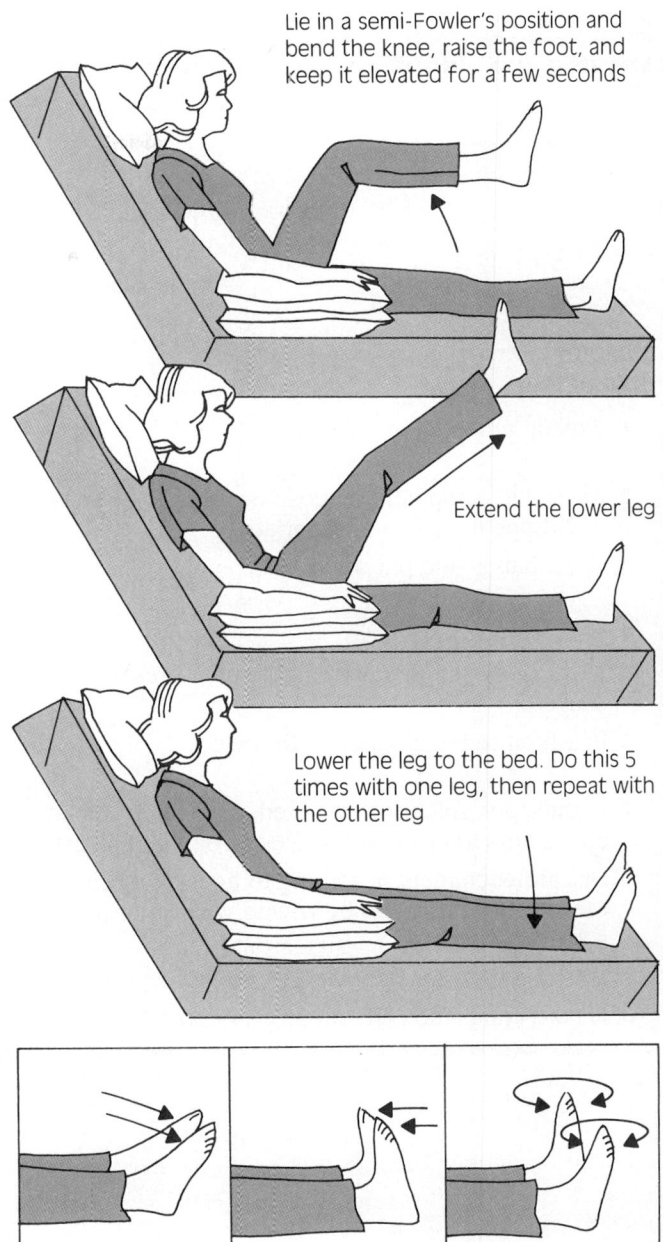

Lie in a semi-Fowler's position and bend the knee, raise the foot, and keep it elevated for a few seconds

Extend the lower leg

Lower the leg to the bed. Do this 5 times with one leg, then repeat with the other leg

A. Point the toes of both feet toward the foot of the bed. Relax both feet

B. Pull toes toward the chin. Relax both feet

C. Make circles with both ankles. First circle to the right, then to the left. Repeat 3 times, Relax feet

F I G U R E   4 4 - 3

Leg exercises to increase venous return.

operation, usually in the surgical holding area, based on findings that small cuts made by the razor serve as sites for bacterial growth; increased time for growth of bacteria raises the potential for infection. The procedure for shaving the skin of the preoperative client is outlined in Procedures 44-2 and 44-3. Presurgical shaving is not always done; *(Text continues on p. 1324)*

P R O C E D U R E   4 4 - 2

Shaving the Skin of the Preoperative Client (Dry Shave)

Equipment

Adequate lighting
Electric clippers
Scissors

Gloves
Antiseptic solution and applicator
  (if ordered)

Action	Rationale
1 Explain procedure to client.	Explanation facilitates cooperation and provides reassurance for client.
2 Assemble equipment. Expose the area to be shaved, and drape the client appropriately.	Having equipment ready saves time. Draping client provides for privacy.
3 Wash hands and put on gloves.	Handwashing deters the spread of microorganisms. Gloves are worn as part of universal precautions.
4 Shave with the clippers.	Shaving minimizes risk of abrasions on operative area.
5 Move drape and continue until entire area is shaved.	This provides for client's privacy.
6 Brush off remaining hair with towel.	This minimizes skin irritation and improves client's comfort.
7 If antiseptic solution is ordered, use cotton-tipped applicators to clean in crevices (groin, umbilicus).	This is additional protection against microorganisms that may accumulate in crevices.
8 Discard equipment according to agency policy. Clean electric clippers by wiping with antiseptic solution.	This protects against injury from razor blade.
9 Wash hands after removing gloves.	Handwashing deters the spread of microorganisms.
10 Record completion of skin preparation.	This provides documentation for procedure.

P R O C E D U R E   4 4 - 3

Shaving the Skin of the Preoperative Client (Wet Shave)

Equipment

Adequate lighting
Bath blanket
Gloves

Prep kit containing:
  Razor
  Sponge soaked with antiseptic
    soap
  Waterproof pad
  Basin
  Cotton-tipped applicator
  Washcloth

(continued)

PROCEDURE 44-3 *(continued)*

Shaving the Skin of the Preoperative Client (Wet Shave)

Equipment

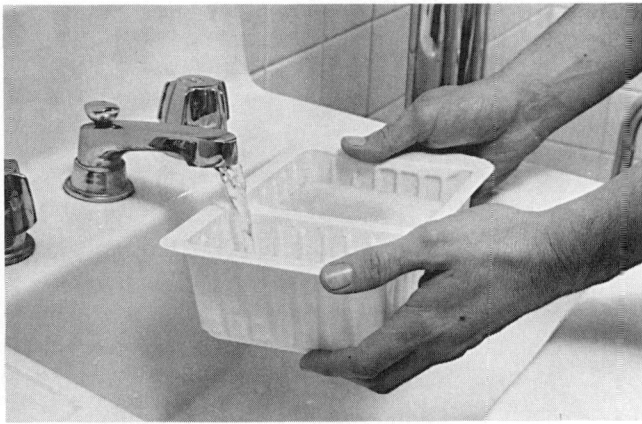

Wetting prepared prep kit.

Action	Rationale
1 Explain procedure to client.	Explanation facilitates cooperation and provides reassurance for client.
2 Assemble equipment. Expose the area to be shaved, and drape the client appropriately.	Having equipment ready saves time. Draping client provides for privacy.
3 Wash hands and put on gloves.	Handwashing deters the spread of microorganisms. Gloves are worn as part of universal precautions.
4 Place waterproof pad under area to be shaved.	Pad protects bed linens.
5 Apply soap solution to small areas of the skin, and work up a lather.	Soap emulsifies normal fatty substances on the skin and loosens dirt so that water can penetrate and soften the hair.
6 Shave with one hand while gently stretching the skin taut with the other hand. Hold the razor between a 30- and 45-degree angle, and take long gentle strokes in the direction of hair growth. Rinse hair and soap from razor as necessary.	Stretching the skin eliminates wrinkles and smooths the skin so that the nurse can accomplish a close shave. Gentle, long strokes with the razor held at a 30- to 45-degree angle help to prevent nicking and cutting the skin. Shaving in the direction of hair growth helps to minimize skin irritation.

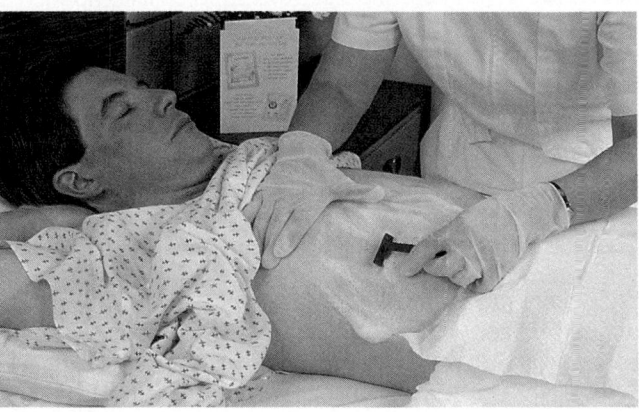

Action 6: Shaving area while gently stretching skin taut with other hand. (Photo © B. Proud.)

(continued)

P R O C E D U R E   4 4 - 3 *(continued)*

Shaving the Skin of the Preoperative Client (Wet Shave)

Action	Rationale
7 Continue moving drape until entire area is shaved. Replace razor if it becomes dull.	This provides for client's privacy. Sharp edge on razor reduces risk of injury.
8 Use washcloth and warm water to remove any excess soap and remaining hair. Dry carefully.	This minimizes irritation to skin.
9 Stoop so that the eyes are at the level of the shaven area to check for isolated hairs that may have been missed by razor.	Looking at the area with the eyes at the level of the skin helps in checking whether all hair has been removed.
10 Report any cuts in skin to physician or charge person.	Cuts in skin may be a potential source of infection.
11 Discard equipment according to agency policy. Clean electric clippers by wiping with antiseptic solution.	This protects against injury from razor blade.
12 Wash hands after removing gloves.	Handwashing deters the spread of microorganisms.
13 Record completion of skin preparation.	This provides documentation for procedure.

depilatory creams or hair clippers may be used to remove hair (and are recommended by the Centers for Disease Control). Agency protocol should be followed for timing, people responsible, and method.

Elimination   Emptying the bowel of feces is no longer a routine procedure before surgery, but the nurse should use preoperative assessments to determine the need for an order for bowel elimination. If the client has not had a bowel movement for several days or has had preoperative barium diagnostic tests, an enema helps to prevent postoperative constipation.

If the client is scheduled for surgery of the gastrointestinal tract, cleansing enemas usually are ordered. Peristalsis does not return for 24 to 48 hours after the bowel is handled, so preoperative cleansing helps to decrease postoperative constipation. An empty bowel also prevents contamination of the surgical area during surgery.

Insertion of an indwelling urinary catheter may be ordered before surgery, especially in clients having pelvic surgery, to prevent bladder distention or accidental injury. If the client does not have an indwelling catheter in place, she should void immediately before receiving preoperative medications to ensure an empty bladder during surgery.

Nutrition and Fluids   The diet order for the client having surgery depends on the type of surgery and type of anesthesia to be used. Clients having general anesthesia or major regional anesthesia are made NPO 8 to 12 hours before the surgery (often at midnight before next-morning surgery) to prevent aspiration of gastric contents if the client should vomit while anesthetized. The nurse explains the reason to the client, removes all food and fluids from the bedside, and

places a sign over the bed so that all health team members and visitors know about the restriction. If the client eats or drinks, the physician should be notified at once.

Clients need to be well nourished and hydrated before surgery to counterbalance fluid, blood, and electrolyte loss during surgery and to facilitate tissue healing after surgery. Preoperative assessments provide a base for physical preparation for surgery, including the need for supplemental nutrition, fluids, or electrolytes. The client who is undernourished may require parenteral nutrition (see Chapter 33) and intravenous electrolyte replacements. If the client's screening tests show a hemoglobin level of less than 10 g/dL and a hematocrit less than 33%, blood may be given preoperatively to maintain volume and increase oxygenation of tissue during surgery.

Rest and Sleep   Rest and sleep are important components in reducing stress before surgery and in healing and recovery after surgery. The nurse can facilitate rest and sleep in the immediate preoperative period by meeting psychological needs, carrying out teaching, providing a quiet environment, and administering the ordered bedtime sedative medication.

Physical Preparation: Day of Surgery

The preoperative checklist (Fig. 44-4) outlines the nurse's responsibilities on the day of surgery; these activities must be completed before the client is transported to surgery. Some of these activities have already been described (NPO, preoperative teaching, informed consent, skin preparation, screening tests, bladder elimination); other nursing responsibilities include the following:

Pre-Op Surgical Checklist

Nurse's Name: _____

O.R.		Comments or Lab Values	Nurses' Initials
	PRE OP HYPO ORDERED		
	NPO AFTER MIDNIGHT OR AS ORDERED		
	I.D. BAND ON PATIENT		
	PRE-OP TEACHING DONE		
	SURGICAL PERMIT SIGNED		
	INFORMED CONSENT SIGNED (IOL OR LASER CASES)		
	OPERATIVE AREA SHAVE PREPPED		
	HISTORY AND PHYSICAL DICTATED		
	CBC REPORT ON CHART	HGB.	
		HCT.	
	URINALYSIS REPORT ON CHART		
	PROFILE REPORT ON CHART IF ORDERED	K+	
	(NORMAL RANGE K+ 3.5 to 5)		
	BLOOD SCREENED _____ TYPED & X MATCHED	Exp. Date # of Units Set Up	
	PT AND PTT	PT PTT	
	CHEST X-RAY REPORT ON CHART		
	EKG		
	T _____ P _____ R _____ BP _____		
	DENTURES OR PARTIAL PLATE REMOVED		
	CONTACT LENSES OR GLASSES REMOVED		
	JEWELRY REMOVED OR SECURED		
	HAIR PINS. MAKE UP AND NAIL POLISH REMOVED		
	HEARING AID TO O.R. WITH PATIENT		
	BATHED		
	O.R. GOWN ON PATIENT		
	VOIDED OR CATHETERIZED AND FOLEY EMPTIED		
	PRE-OP ANTIBIOTIC GIVEN IF ORDERED		
	PRE-OP MEDICATION GIVEN		
	ALLERGIES		
	FAMILY O.R. WAITING ROOM		
	OLD CHART TO O.R.		
	X-RAY FILMS FROM FLOOR TO O.R.		

Floor Nurse Sending Patient to O.R.: _____ O.R. Nurse Receiving Patient: _____

Arrival Time: _____

COMMENTS:

FIGURE 44-4

Example of a preoperative checklist.

- Take and record vital signs to serve as baseline data for the intraoperative phase, and assess for and report any abnormal findings (such as an elevated temperature).
- Prepare the client physically for the intraoperative phase.

  Have the client remove all personal clothing and put on an operating room gown.

  Remove all hairpins or hairpieces. This prevents injury to the client during surgery as well as possible loss of hairpieces or wigs.

  Remove makeup and fingernail polish to allow intraoperative and postoperative assessment of skin and nailbeds for circulation and oxygenation of tissues.

  Remove all prostheses, such as dentures or partial plates, eyeglasses, contact lenses, and artificial limbs. Dentures may cause respiratory obstruction during anesthesia; other prostheses may be damaged or lost. Be sure items are stored safely while the client is in surgery.

  Remove jewelry to prevent loss or injury from swelling during or after surgery; if the client prefers not to remove a wedding band, it can be securely taped to the finger (in some types of surgery, leaving jewelry on is not allowed). When jewelry is removed, it should be given to a family member or locked in a safe place.

  Leave on a hearing aid, and be certain that operating and recovery room nurses know the client has one.

  Be sure that the client's identification bracelet is in place to ensure accurate identity.

  If the client has allergies, be sure they are noted according to institutional policy (eg, on the front of the client's record or on an allergy bracelet).

- To carry out any special procedures that are ordered, such as securing previous records, inserting a nasogastric tube, starting an intravenous line, applying antiembolic stockings, or giving medications.
- Give the preoperative medications that are ordered, either at a scheduled time or on call (the operating room will call and tell the nurse to give the medication). Commonly ordered medications are as follows:

  Sedatives and tranquilizers, such as pentobarbital (Nembutal), chlorpromazine (Thorazine), or diazepam (Valium), to alleviate anxiety and facilitate anesthesia induction

  Anticholinergics, such as atropine and glycopyrrolate (Robinul), to decrease pulmonary and oral secretions and to prevent laryngospasm

  Narcotic analgesics, such as morphine and meperidine hydrochloride (Demerol), to facilitate client sedation and relaxation and to decrease the amount of anesthetic agent needed

  Neuroleptanalgesic agents (Innovar) to cause a general state of calmness and sleepiness

  Histamine$_2$-receptor antihistaminics, such as cimetidine (Tagamet) and ranitidine (Zantac), to decrease gastric acidity and volume, so that if vomiting and aspiration occur during surgery, there is less danger of the client developing aspiration pneumonia

- Maintain client safety by elevating side rails, lowering the bed, and instructing the client to stay in bed.
- Meet the family (or other support person's) needs. The family may visit the morning of surgery and are told where the client will be taken after surgery (if a different location, such as the intensive care unit). The waiting area for the family is described, and the family is taken there after the client leaves for the operating room. The family also is told that the surgeon will come to the waiting room to tell them what happened in surgery.
- Document, through checklists and narrative charting, the nursing interventions carried out.
- Assist in moving the client from the bed to the operating room stretcher when it is time to transport the client to surgery, ensuring accurate identification.
- Prepare the client's bed and room for postoperative care.

  Make a surgical bed.

  Have necessary equipment and supplies in the room for postoperative care (equipment to measure vital signs, intravenous standard, and so forth).

Evaluating

Evaluation of the plan of care for the preoperative phase is based on the client goals. The plan is effective if the client is physically and emotionally prepared for surgery, can verbalize events and sensations of the perioperative period, and can demonstrate postoperative exercises and activities.

Intraoperative Nursing Care

The intraoperative phase begins with admission of the client to the surgical area and lasts until the client is transferred to the recovery area. Although the surgeon has the dominant role during this phase, the nurse has specific responsibilities and roles in collaboratively meeting client needs. The nursing process uses the preoperative data and plan as a base.

The type of surgery scheduled influences the assessments and interventions carried out by the nurse. For example, the nurse's role when caring for the client having outpatient or same-day surgery may be that of providing client care from admission through dismissal (same-day surgery is described later in this chapter), whereas the nurse's role for hospital-based surgery usually is specific to the phases (ie, one group of nurses provides care on the hospital unit preoperatively and postoperatively, another group practices operating room nursing, and still another group provides specific postanesthesia recovery room care). This section of the chapter discusses the role of the nurse specific to intraoperative care.

Assessing

The first room the client enters when he or she is transferred to the surgical area usually is the holding area. Nurses in surgical scrub dress identify the surgical client, assess the client's emotional and physical status, and verify the information on the preoperative checklist. They also may carry out ordered immediate preoperative care, including performing skin preparation, starting intravenous fluids (using a large-gauge intercatheter), and giving preoperative medications. The client's response to procedures is assessed and events of surgery are explained. When the operating room is prepared, a nurse from the operating room arrives to transport the client to the operating table

In the operating room, the client is positioned on the operating table, anesthetized, and draped. The operating room nurse assesses the client and reviews preoperative data, paying particular attention to factors that increase surgical risk. The nurse also assesses the client during positioning and monitors supplies used to maintain safety for the client.

Diagnosing

Client problems in the intraoperative period are primarily related to the position of the client during the procedure, the effects of the anesthesia, and the incision. Appropriate nursing diagnoses include the following:

> Impaired Skin Integrity related to 4-inch midline abdominal incision
> Fluid Volume Deficit related to loss of blood during surgery
> High Risk for Injury related to positioning, anesthesia, and environmental hazards

Collaborative problems might include the following (Carpenito, 1991):

> Potential complication: Hemorrhage
> Potential complication: Infection
> Potential complication: Neuromuscular damage

Planning: Client Goals

The planning phase of the nursing process focuses on preventing potential complications and client problems and on ensuring client safety.

Client goals for the intraoperative phase are as follows. The client will:

- Remain free of neuromuscular damage
- Maintain intact skin surfaces
- Have symmetric breathing patterns
- Be free of injury from burns, inaccurate count of supplies, and wound contamination

During the intraoperative phase, the nurse performs the following tasks:

- Assesses and monitors the client's physiologic response
- Positions the client to prevent injury or alterations in skin or in respiratory or neuromuscular function
- Maintains client's physical safety
- Maintains aseptic technique

Implementing

During surgery, nurses function either as scrub nurses or as circulating nurses. *Scrub nurses* assist the surgeon during the surgery and maintain surgical asepsis while draping and handling instruments and supplies. The *circulating nurse* assesses the client on admission to the operating room, helps to position the client on the operating table, helps with monitoring devices, gets additional supplies, and (at the end of the operation) counts the number of instruments, needles, and gauze sponges used during the operation to prevent the accidental loss of an item in the wound.

Positioning

The client is placed in a specific operative position after anesthesia has produced loss of consciousness and reflexes. The nurse must ensure client safety and comfort in positioning to prevent alterations in respiratory, vascular, and neuromuscular function. The potential of skin injury is avoided by lifting the client to a position, rather than rolling or pulling him or her, which can cause shearing force, in which two or more tissue layers slide on each other, stretching subcutaneous blood vessels, obstructing blood flow, and contributing to pressure ulcers (Groah, 1983).

Although the various operative positions are not included here, the nurse needs to know which position was used and significant nursing considerations for that position. Two examples are as follows:

> *Trendelenburg's position:* The downward displacement of the abdominal viscera decreases diaphragm movement and respiratory exchange; blood pools in the upper torso and blood pressure increases; hypotension can result with return to the supine position.
> *Lithotomy position:* The placement of legs in stirrups causes pooling of blood in the legs, increasing the potential of thrombophlebitis. Pressure also can damage the peroneal nerve, with resultant footdrop.

Draping

Drapes are used to establish a sterile field around the operative site, preventing the passage of microorganisms between sterile and nonsterile areas. The only area left exposed is the incision site. Plastic adhesive drapes may be used to form a complete seal over the skin; with these drapes, skin color is visible and the incision is made through the drape.

Documenting

Throughout surgery, the nurse documents item counts, monitored data, positioning, medications, dressings, and so forth, on the intraoperative record.

Transfer to the Postanesthesia Recovery Room

After the operation, the client is carefully moved from the operating table to a stretcher. This is an especially critical time; sudden or rough handling can cause severe hypotension or potentially lethal cardiac or respiratory arrest.

The client is then moved to the postanesthesia recovery (PAR) room, and relevant preoperative and postoperative assessments and interventions are communicated to the PAR nurses.

Evaluating

Evaluation of the effectiveness of the plan of care for the intraoperative phase is based on the established client goals. If goals are met, the plan was effective.

Postoperative Nursing Care

The postoperative phase can be divided into two stages—immediate care (usually provided in the PAR room) and ongoing postoperative care, lasting from return to the unit through convalescence. Nursing assessments and interventions are consistent with those in the preoperative and intraoperative phases and are carried out to maintain function, promote recovery, and facilitate coping with alterations in structure or function.

In this section, assessments and nursing interventions are combined in discussing the immediate postoperative care; the phases of the nursing process are used to describe ongoing postoperative care.

Immediate Postoperative Care

Nurses in the PAR room assess and evaluate postoperative clients, with emphasis on preventing complications from anesthesia or the surgery (Drain & Christoph, 1987). Assessments are continuous and ongoing, using preoperative and intraoperative data as the bases for comparison. The assessments made in the PAR room are respiratory status, cardiovascular status, central nervous system status, fluid status, wound status, and general condition. These assessments are made every 10 to 15 minutes initially. The average PAR room stay is about 2 hours.

Respiratory Status   Assessments of respiratory function are made by monitoring respiratory rate, rhythm, and depth and by observing skin color. Cardiovascular and neurologic assessments provide data about oxygenation. The following assessments indicate ineffective ventilation:

- Restlessness, apprehension
- Unequal chest expansion with use of accessory muscles
- Shallow, noisy respirations
- Cyanosis
- Rapid pulse rate

During the surgical procedure with general anesthesia, an artificial airway is inserted to maintain patent air passages. The airway is not removed until the laryngeal and pharyngeal reflexes return, allowing the client to control the tongue, cough, and swallow.

Respiratory obstruction is the most common PAR emergency. It may be due to secretion accumulation, obstruction by the tongue, laryngospasm (a sudden violent contraction of the vocal cords), or laryngeal edema. Assessments of respiratory obstruction include those previously outlined plus wheezing or crowing sounds with respiratory effort.

Positioning, administering oxygen, and suctioning may all be used to maintain a patent airway and tissue oxygenation.

Cardiovascular Status   Evaluation of cardiovascular function includes assessing blood pressure and pulses, skin color, respirations, and the wound.

Blood pressure findings are compared with baseline data from the preoperative period; hypotension may be the result of varied factors, including anesthetic agents, preoperative medications, position changes, blood loss, respiratory alterations, and peripheral blood pooling. Transient hypertension also can occur as a result of anesthetic effects, respiratory insufficiency, the surgical procedure, or the excitement phase of recovery from anesthesia. Low blood pressure can be increased by oxygen administration, deep breathing, leg exercises, verbal stimulation (to help expel anesthetic gases and facilitate increasing level of consciousness), and maintenance of accurate intravenous flow rates.

All pulses are assessed for bilateral equality, rhythm, rate, and character. Of special significance are assessments of abnormal function—arrhythmias, absence of pulses, and tachycardia. Tachycardia, an early symptom of shock, must be carefully evaluated. Other related assessments are cyanosis, edema, skin temperature, and urine output.

Central Nervous System Status   Anesthetics cause loss of consciousness and reflexes; the return of central nervous system function is assessed through response to stimuli and orientation. Reflexes return in reverse order, with the usual pattern being (1) unconsciousness, (2) response to touch and sounds, (3) drowsiness, (4) awake but not oriented, and (5) awake and oriented (McConnell, 1987). Nurses in the PAR room verbally reorient the client frequently by touching and calling him or her by name.

Fluid Status   Fluid imbalance may be the result of such factors as preoperative fluid restriction, fluid loss during surgery, wound drainage, or stress (with retention of sodium and water).

Assessments of fluid status include skin turgor, vital signs, urine output, wound drainage, and intravenous fluids; potential fluid volume deficit or excess is a risk. Assessments of intravenous fluids include the type of fluid ordered, the rate, the needle insertion site, and the tubing.

Wound Status The nurse in the PAR room assesses the wound dressing for amount, consistency, and color of drainage as well as for any tubes or drains and drainage by that route. It also is important to assess under the client for drainage.

Large amounts of bright red drainage combined with other abnormal physical status assessments (restlessness, pallor, cold moist skin, decreasing blood pressure, increasing pulse and respiratory rates) may indicate hemorrhage and hypovolemic shock. These symptoms should be reported immediately.

General Condition Other assessments and interventions are made to ensure physical and emotional comfort and safety. If the client is having pain and his or her condition has stabilized, pain medications are given (usually by the intravenous route). Most clients are cold and should be covered with blankets to keep them warm. Psychological comfort is provided by constant reorientation and reassurance that the surgery is over. Physical safety is maintained by careful assessments, proper positioning, and use of side rails and restraints.

The client is dismissed from the PAR room when physical status and level of consciousness are considered stable. The family is notified that the client is being transferred back to his or her room, and the PAR room nurse makes a verbal report to the unit nurse about the assessments and interventions during the intraoperative and immediate postoperative phases.

Ongoing Postoperative Care

Nurses use the nursing process during all phases of perioperative care, with the focus being the special and unique needs of each client in each phase. Ongoing postoperative care is planned to facilitate recovery from surgery and coping with alterations. The plan of care is based on individualized nursing diagnoses and includes promoting physical and psychological health, preventing complications, and teaching self-care when the client returns home. Procedure 44-4 outlines postoperative client care.

Assessing

The nurse on the unit assists PAR room personnel in transferring the client to the bed in his of her room and, using data from the preoperative and intraoperative phases, makes an initial assessment. A postoperative checklist or flow sheet (Fig. 44-5) may be used. The initial assessment

often is combined with the implementation of postoperative physician orders and includes the following:

Vital signs: Assess temperature, blood pressure, and pulse and respiratory rates. Note alterations from postoperative and PAR room data as well as symptoms of complications (as discussed under Immediate Postoperative Care).

Color and temperature of skin: Assess for warmth, pallor, cyanosis, diaphoresis.

Level of consciousness: Assess orientation to time, place, and person as well as reaction to stimuli and ability to move extremities.

Intravenous fluids: Assess type and amount of solution, flow rate, tubing, and infusion site.

Wound: Assess dressing and dependent areas for drainage (color, amount, consistency). Assess drains and tubes and be sure they are intact, patent, and properly connected to drainage systems.

Other tubes: Assess indwelling urinary catheter, gastrointestinal suction, and so forth, for drainage, patency, and amount of output. Be sure dependent drainage bags are hanging properly and suction drainage is attached and functioning. If oxygen is ordered, ensure placement of ordered application and flow rate.

Altered comfort level: Assess for pain (location, duration, intensity) and, if present, determine if analgesics were given in the PAR room. Assess for nausea and vomiting.

Position and safety: Place the client in an ordered position (eg, after spinal anesthesia, client may have to remain flat for a specified period), or if the client is not fully conscious, place him or her in the side-lying position. Elevate the side rails and place the bed in low position.

Comfort: Cover the client with a blanket, reorient him or her to the room as necessary, and allow family members to remain with the client after initial assessment is completed.

After assessment, document time of arrival and all assessments. Follow agency protocol for assessment routines: common time frames are every 15 minutes until stable, turning every 1 to 2 hours for the first 24 hours and every 4 hours thereafter.

Although the nurse can use agency protocol for guidelines in the immediate postoperative period, the individual nurse is responsible for adjusting the frequency and priorities of assessment to the specific needs of each client.

Diagnosing

Nursing diagnoses in the postoperative phase may be made for actual or potential altered responses or for collaborative problems to implement nursing actions necessary for monitoring and preventing postoperative complications. When making nursing diagnoses, the nurse uses assessment data and plans of care established before and during surgery and includes the family.

R E S E A R C H I N N U R S I N G Making a Difference

Perioperative Nursing Care

Nurses provide care to cl ents of all ages who require surgical treatment for injury or illness. Nursing assessments and interventions are critical factors in facilitating the client's return to health and are carried out to meet many client care needs. The nursing studies described here are examples of two areas of perioperative care that require nursing knowledge and skill: pain management and monitoring of vital signs.

Related Research

Davis, M. J., & Nomura, L. A. (1990). Vital signs of class I surgical patients. *Western Journal of Nursing Research, 12*(1), 28–37.

The authors of this study noted that hospital protocols for taking postoperative vital signs made no distinction between clients with different surgical procedures and different preoperative status. The vital signs of 250 class I clients (those with no existing organic, physiologic, biochemical, or psychiatric problems) were evaluated to see if the existing protocol was appropriate. Based on findings, the protocol for this class of surgical client was changed to a less frequent schedule, saving nurse time without increasing postoperative risk to the client.

Heidenreich, T., & Giuffre, M. (1990). Postoperative temperature measurement. *Nursing Research, 39*(3), 153–155.

The purpose of this study was to determine the validity of using the axillary site for postoperative temperature measurement. A sample of 11 men and 7 women, ranging in age from 53 to 86 years, directly admitted to the intensive care unit from the operating room with major surgical procedures were subjects for the study. Comparisons of rectal temperature, axillary temperature, and core body temperature were made. Findings from the study suggest that the best reflection of core body temperature is the rectal measurement, using a mercury thermometer for 5 minutes. An important finding was the relation between age and core body temperature, with the elderly client being more susceptible to hypothermia in the surgical setting.

Oberle, K., Wry, J., Paul, P., & Grace, M. (1990). Environment, anxiety, and postoperative pain. *Western Journal of Nursing Research, 12*(6), 745–753.

This study was conducted to explore relations between environment, anxiety, and postoperative pain. Two settings were used—an old and a new hospital—to examine the effect of physical and organizational factors on pain levels after surgery. Pain intensity after surgery, anxiety levels, and information about analgesic administration in the postoperative period were used as data from 290 clients. Findings from the study support the hypothesis that environment can affect anxiety levels, with a trend toward decreased anxiety in the new hospital. No relation was found between anxiety and pain. It is suggested that the tendency toward decreased anxiety be considered when building new facilities or modifying client care areas for the surgical client.

Daake, D. R., & Gueldner, S. H. (1989). Imagery instruction and the control of postsurgical pain. *Applied Nursing Research, 2*(3), 114–120.

This study examined the effectiveness of the use of the method of pleasant imagery for the control of pain in postoperative clients. Pleasant imagery is a learned technique in which clients mentally relive an enjoyable, relaxing experience to decrease pain intensity or to substitute a nonpainful sensation for pain during the postoperative period. A sample of clients who were taught this technique before surgery were compared with a sample who did not have this instruction. The results of the study strongly suggest that pleasant imagery can be effective in reducing the perception of postoperative pain. It is recommended that nurses routinely incorporate this technique in preoperative teaching plans.

Summary

These studies illustrate the importance of research into independent nursing interventions as part of collaborative problems in the surgical client. The studies described also reflect the holistic nature of nursing knowledge, with research conducted to explore established protocols, age-related nursing needs, environmental influences, and alternate methods of pain control. Nursing research will continue to provide the knowledge necessary to the caregiver role of the nurse in providing holistic and individualized care in the clinical setting.

Examples of postoperative nursing diagnoses include the following:

High Risk for Infection related to traumatic wound of right arm in farm vehicle accident

Pain related to right flank incision

Altered Family Processes related to loss of economic stability following surgical treatment for bone malignancy

Impaired Verbal Communication related to repair and wiring of fractured jaw

Impaired Skin Integrity related to incision on left anterior thorax

Impaired Physical Mobility related to inability to be independent in movement secondary to surgical repair of fractured right hip

(Text continues on p. 1334)

PROCEDURE   44-4

Postoperative Care When Client Returns to Room

Action	Rationale

Immediate

1 Place client in safe position on side with face down and neck slightly extended. Note level of consciousness.

This prevents aspiration of vomitus and airway obstruction.

2 Monitor and record vital signs frequently. Assessment order may vary, but usual frequency includes taking vital signs every 15 minutes the first hour, every 30 minutes the next 2 hours, every hour for 4 hours, and, finally, every 4 hours.

Comparison with baseline preoperative vital signs may indicate impending shock or hemorrhage.

3 Provide for warmth. Assess skin color and condition.

Depressed level of functioning results in fall in body temperature.

4 Check dressings for color, odor, and amount of drainage, and feel under client for bleeding.

Hemorrhage and shock are life-threatening complications of surgery.

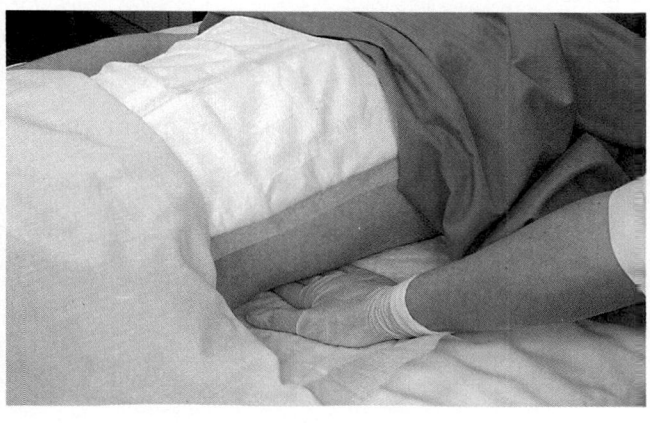

Action 4: Feeling under client for bleeding. (Photo © B. Proud.)

5 Verify that all tubes are patent and equipment is operative.

This ensures maintenance of vital functions.

6 Maintain intravenous infusion at correct rate.

This provides nutrition and prevents dehydration and electrolyte imbalances.

7 Provide for a safe environment. Keep bed in low position with side rails up. Have call bell within client's reach. Have No Smoking sign posted if client is receiving oxygen.

This prevents accidental injury.

8 Relieve pain by administering medications ordered by physician. Check record to verify if analgesic medication was administered in recovery room.

Analgesics are used for relief of postoperative pain.

9 Record assessments and interventions on chart.

This provides for accurate documentation.

(continued)

P R O C E D U R E 4 4 - 4 *(continued)*

Postoperative Care When Client Returns to Room

Action	Rationale
General	
10 Promote optimal respiratory function: a Coughing and deep breathing b Incentive spirometry c Early ambulation d Frequent position change e Administration of oxygen as ordered	Anesthetic agents may depress respiratory function. Clients who have existing respiratory or cardiovascular disease or abdominal or chest incisions or who are obese or elderly or in a poor state of nutrition are at greater risk of developing respiratory complications.
11 Maintain adequate circulation: a Maintenance of intravenous therapy b Early ambulation c Application of antiembolic stockings if ordered by physician d Leg and range-of-motion exercises if not contraindicated	Preventive measures can improve venous return and circulatory status.
12 Assess urinary elimination status: a Promote voiding by offering bedpan at regular intervals b Monitor catheter drainage if present c Measure intake and output	Anesthetic agents may temporarily depress bladder tone and response.
13 Promote optimal nutritional status and return of gastrointestinal function: a Assess for return of peristalsis b Assist with diet progression c Encourage fluid intake d Monitor intake e Medicate for nausea and vomiting as ordered by physician	Anesthetic agents depress peristalsis and normal functioning of gastrointestinal tract.

Action 13a: *Assessing for return of peristalsis. (Photo © B. Proud.)*

Action	Rationale
14 Promote wound healing: a Use surgical asepsis b Assess condition of wound c Assess any drainage	Alterations in nutritional, circulatory, and metabolic status may predispose clients to infection and delayed healing.
15 Provide for rest and comfort.	This shortens recovery period and facilitates return to normal function.
16 Provide emotional and spiritual support.	This facilitates individualized care and client's return to normal health.

POST-OP
PROGRESS FLOW RECORD

Name _____

M.R. # _____

DATE									
TIME									
BP									
PULSE									
RESPIRATIONS									
TEMPERATURE									
I.V.									
WOUND									
DRAIN (S)									
LOC									
PAIN									
NAUSEA									
FOLEY/ OTHER CATH OR VOIDING									
TURN, COUGH DEEP BREATHE									
MOVES ALL EXTREMITIES									
Initials									

Key _____   _____

_____   _____

640-044-830/0800751

FIGURE 44-5

Example of a postoperative progress record.

Appropriate collaborative problems for the client in the postoperative period include the following (Carpenito, 1991, p. 644):

Potential complication: Hemorrhage
Potential complication: Evisceration
Potential complication: Dehiscence
Potential complication: Urinary retention
Potential complication: Thrombophlebitis
Potential complication: Paralytic Ileus

Planning: Client Goals

The plan of care in the postoperative phase begins in the preoperative phase, when nursing activities to reduce stress and teach postoperative activities are carried out. From admission, the client and family are prepared for uneventful recovery and self-care on dismissal. Specific client goals are individualized, based on risk factors, surgical procedure, and unique needs. Examples of postoperative goals are as follows. The client will:

- Carry out leg exercises every 2 to 4 hours as taught
- Deep breathe and cough effectively every 2 hours as taught
- Verbalize decreasing levels of pain
- Have a balanced intake and output
- Regain normal bowel and bladder elimination
- Have a well-healed surgical incision
- Remain free of infection
- Verbalize any concerns about appearance of wound
- Verbalize and demonstrate self wound care

The aims of nursing are as follows:

- Assess and monitor client's physical and emotional status.
- Promote physical and psychological comfort and safety.
- Prevent complications.
- Facilitate coping with alterations in structure or function.
- Promote a return to health and maximize wellness.

Implementing

Many nursing activities implemented in the postoperative phase have been discussed in this chapter or are fully discussed in other chapters; therefore, this section focuses on the nursing interventions implemented to meet the client goals of the plan of care. Nursing care is presented in three broad areas—preventing complications, promoting a return to health, and facilitating coping with alterations.

Preventing Complications A wide variety of factors increase the risk of postoperative complications. These have been described in the preoperative and intraoperative sections of this chapter and include age, health habits, physical condition, medical history, psychological status, and surgical intervention (anesthesia, positioning, wound). Preoperative assessments and teaching are implemented to decrease the risk of postoperative complications; this section describes the implementation of those activities, focusing on preventing respiratory, cardiovascular, and wound complications.

Preventing Cardiovascular Complications Nursing interventions to prevent or monitor for cardiovascular complications are as follows:

- Assess and document vital signs as ordered and as the client's status dictates using preoperative assessments as a baseline.
- Provide covers as necessary to prevent chilling.
- Maintain fluid balance:
  - Maintain accurate intake and output.
  - Monitor rate and type of intravenous fluids.
  - Assess skin turgor and hydration of mucous membranes.
- Monitor amount, color, and consistency of wound drainage.
- Implement leg exercises and turning in bed every 2 hours.
- Assist with ambulation. Ambulation usually begins the evening of surgery and increases as tolerated; blood pressure and pulse and respiratory rates monitor tolerance.
- Apply and follow protocols for antiembolic stockings, if ordered.
- Give anticoagulant medications as ordered.
- Assess and record Homans' sign every 8 hours. Homans' sign is determined by asking the client to dorsiflex the foot and assessing for pain in the calf. If the client has pain with dorsiflexion, the Homans' sign is positive. When thrombophlebitis is present, pain results from the pressure of the muscles on the inflamed vein.
- Avoid positioning that will impede venous return (eg, do not raise the knee gatch or place pillows under the knees).

Specific cardiovascular complications are described in the following paragraphs.

Shock is the body's reaction to acute peripheral circulatory failure as the result of an alteration in circulatory control or to a loss of circulating fluid. The type of shock most commonly seen in the postoperative client is **hypovolemic shock**, which occurs with a decrease in blood volume. Common assessments of shock are hypotension; cold, clammy skin; a weak, thready, and rapid pulse; deep, rapid respirations; decreased urine output; thirst; apprehension; and restlessness. The primary purpose of care for the client in shock is to improve and maintain tissue perfusion by eliminating the cause of the shock. The following are recommended interventions in caring for the client in shock:

- Maintain airway.
- Place the client in a flat position with the legs elevated 45 degrees. (The Trendelenburg or "shock" position is no longer recommended because this position causes the diaphragm to ascend, reducing total lung volume and ventilation [Patrick, Woods, Craven, Rokosky, & Bruno, 1991].)

- Be prepared to assist with fluid administration as well as administration of whole blood or its components.
- Administer oxygen therapy as indicated.
- Place extra covering on the client to maintain warmth.
- Administer medications as ordered.
- Monitor vital signs and general condition continuously.
- Provide psychological support to the client and family.

Hemorrhage is an excessive blood loss, either internally or externally. Hemorrhage may lead to hypovolemic shock. It may occur from a slipped suture, a dislodged clot in the wound, or stress on the operative site; it also may be the result of pathophysiologic conditions or certain medications. Common assessments of hemorrhage are the early symptoms of restlessness, anxiety, and frank bleeding and the symptoms listed above for shock. The primary purposes of care for the client having a hemorrhage include stopping the bleeding and replacing blood volume. The following interventions are recommended when caring for the client who is hemorrhaging:

- Apply a pressure dressing to the bleeding site.
- Be prepared to have the client return to the operating room if bleeding cannot be stopped or is massive.
- Give nursing care as outlined for the client in shock.

Thrombophlebitis is an inflammation of a vein associated with thrombus (blood clot) formation. Thrombophlebitis is most commonly seen in the legs in the postoperative client. Common assessments of thrombophlebitis are pain and cramping in the calf or thigh of the involved extremity, redness and swelling in the affected area, elevated temperature, and positive Homans' sign (pain with dorsiflexion of the foot). Care for the client with thrombophlebitis includes preventing a clot from breaking loose and becoming an embolus that travels to the lungs, heart, or brain and preventing further clot formation. Interventions in caring for the client with thrombophlebitis are as follows:

- Administer anticoagulant medications as ordered.
- Maintain bed rest as ordered.
- Use high antiembolic stockings, and follow protocols for care.
- Elevate the affected leg to heart level.
- Do *not* massage or rub the legs.
- Give analgesics and use external heat applications as ordered.
- Measure bilateral calf or thigh circumference every shift.
- Provide emotional support to the client and family.

An *embolus* is a blood clot or other foreign substance that is dislodged and travels through the bloodstream until it lodges in another smaller vessel. In postoperative clients, the embolus often is part of a thrombus that breaks free from a vein wall. If the embolus lodges in the pulmonary vessels, it is called a **pulmonary embolus**. Common assessments of a pulmonary embolus include dyspnea, chest pain, cough, cyanosis, rapid respirations, tachycardia, and anxiety. The primary purposes of care are to stabilize cardiovascular and respiratory function and to prevent further emboli. The following are recommended interventions for the client with a pulmonary embolus:

- Contact the physician immediately if symptoms occur; pulmonary embolus is a life-threatening complication and immediate treatment is necessary.
- Maintain bed rest with the client in semi-Fowler's position.
- Maintain fluid balance; especially assess and maintain intravenous fluid rates to prevent overhydration.
- Administer oxygen therapy as appropriate.
- Administer anticoagulant medications as ordered.
- Administer prescribed analgesic medications for pain; use caution with narcotic analgesics, which depress respirations.
- Assess vital signs and general status frequently.
- Instruct client to avoid Valsalva's maneuver (forced exhalation against a closed glottis, such as straining to have a bowel movement) to prevent increased intrathoracic pressure and, possibly, increased emboli.
- Provide emotional support for client and family.

Preventing Respiratory Complications Nursing interventions to prevent or monitor for respiratory complications are as follows:

- Assess and monitor vital signs, using preoperative assessments as a baseline.
- Implement deep breathing, coughing, incentive spirometry, and turning in bed every 2 hours.
- Ambulate as ordered.
- Maintain hydration.
- Avoid positioning that decreases ventilation.
- Carefully monitor responses to narcotic analgesics.

Specific respiratory complications are described in the following paragraphs.

Pneumonia is an inflammation of the alveoli as the result of an infectious process or presence of foreign material, which can occur postoperatively as a result of aspiration, infection, depressed cough reflex, and increased secretions from anesthesia, dehydration, and immobilization. Assessments common to pneumonia are an elevated temperature, chills, cough productive of purulent or rusty sputum, crackles and wheezes, dyspnea, and chest pain. The purposes of care are to treat the underlying infection, maintain respiratory status, and prevent the spread of microorganisms. The following are recommended interventions in caring for the client with pneumonia:

- Promote full aeration of the lungs by positioning the client in semi-Fowler's or Fowler's position.
- Administer oxygen therapy as indicated.
- Maintain nutritional and fluid status.
- Administer antibiotic medications as ordered.
- Administer expectorants and analgesics as ordered.
- Implement deep-breathing and coughing exercises every 2 hours.
- Maintain personal hygiene, including frequent oral hygiene.
- Teach proper disposal of tissues and sputum.
- Ensure rest and comfort.
- Provide emotional support to client and family.

Atelectasis is the incomplete expansion or collapse of alveoli with retained mucus, involving a portion of the lung and resulting in poor gas exchange. Assessments of atelectasis are decreased lung sounds over affected areas, dyspnea, cyanosis, crackles, restlessness, and apprehension. The primary purposes of care for the client with atelectasis are to ensure oxygenation of tissues, prevent further atelectasis, and expand involved lung tissues. The following are recommended interventions in caring for the client with atelectasis:

- Position the client in semi-Fowler's position.
- Administer oxygen therapy as indicated.
- Implement deep breathing, coughing, and incentive spirometry every 2 hours.
- Implement leg exercises every 2 hours and ambulate as ordered.
- Maintain hydration.
- Administer analgesics for pain as ordered.
- Provide emotional support to client and family.

Preventing Wound Complications   Nursing interventions to prevent or monitor for wound complications are as follows:

- Assess vital signs, especially monitoring elevated temperature.
- Maintain hydration.
- Maintain nutritional status; encourage diet selection high in carbohydrates, proteins, calories, and vitamins.
- Use medical asepsis (handwashing) protocols.
- Follow Centers for Disease Control guidelines for wound care (see Chapter 43).
- Maintain aseptic technique in dressing changes and care of tubes or drains.

Specific wound complications are **dehiscence** (separation of the layers of a surgical wound) and **evisceration** (disruption of a wound with protrusion of body organs). Both complications are described in Chapter 43.

Promoting a Return to Health   Nurses provide interventions in ongoing postoperative care to promote the return of clients' physical and psychological functioning to as near a normal state as possible. The plan of care includes activities to meet elimination, fluid and electrolyte, nutrition, and rest and comfort needs.

Meeting Elimination Needs   Both urinary and bowel elimination can be altered by anesthesia, manipulation of organs during the surgical procedure, inactivity, and altered fluid and food intake during the perioperative period.

The return of normal *bowel elimination* is promoted by the following nursing interventions:

- Assess for the return of peristalsis.
  - Auscultate bowel sounds every 4 hours when client is awake.
  - Assess abdominal distention, especially if bowel sounds are not audible or are high-pitched (indicative of possible **paralytic ileus**, which is an absence of peristalsis).
  - Assess client's ability to pass flatus or stool.

- Assist with movement in bed and ambulation (to help relieve gas pains, a common postoperative discomfort).
- Encourage food and fluid intake when ordered, especially fruit juices and high-fiber foods.
- Maintain privacy when client is using the bedpan, commode, or bathroom.
- Administer colon tubes, suppositories, or enemas if ordered.

The return of normal *urinary elimination* is promoted by the following nursing interventions:

- Monitor intake and output.
- Assist with assumption of normal position to void.
  - Place client in upright sitting position when using bedpan.
  - Use bedside commode or assist client to bathroom, when able.
  - Help male clients stand upright to void.
- Assess for distention of the bladder (palpate above the symphysis pubis) if the client does not void within 8 hours after surgery or if the client voids frequently with amounts of less than 50 mL.
- Maintain ordered rate of intravenous fluids.
- Encourage PO fluids, when ordered.
- Provide privacy when the client is using the bedpan, commode, or bathroom.
- Carry out catheterization procedure, if ordered.

Meeting Fluid and Nutrition Needs   Fluid and nutrition needs can be met by the following nursing interventions:

- Monitor intake and output.
- Maintain intravenous fluids as ordered.
- Assess for dehydration and weight loss, if appropriate.
- Provide oral hygiene before meals and as needed.
- Monitor tolerance of ordered diet. (After surgery, diets usually progress from clear liquids to full liquids to soft to regular.)
- Maintain an environment conducive to good appetite (keep bedside articles clean and neat, eliminate odors).
- Encourage the client to sit up in bed or a chair for meals.
- Encourage family participation in meals.
- Remember that the presence of drains, gastric suction, fever, and intravenous therapy increases the risk of fluid and electrolyte imbalances in the surgical client.

Meeting Comfort and Rest Needs   After surgery, comfort needs often are a priority for the client. Alterations in comfort are the result of many factors, including nausea, vomiting, hiccups, thirst, and surgical pain. The following are nursing interventions to meet comfort and rest needs by providing relief for various disturbances:

Nausea and Vomiting
- Maintain a clean environment.
- Provide oral hygiene as needed.
- Avoid a large intake of food or fluids at one time, especially after being NPO.

- Maintain bowel elimination.
- Assess allergic response to antibiotics or analgesics.
- Administer ordered medications.

Thirst
- Provide oral hygiene as needed.
- Offer sips of water or ice chips when NPO (if allowed).

Hiccups
- Have the client do the following:
  - Take several swallows of water while holding his or her breath (if not NPO)
  - Rebreathe into a paper bag
  - Eat a teaspoon of granulated sugar
- Placing gentle pressure over the closed eyelids
- Administering ordered medications

Surgical Pain
- Assess for pain, and offering ordered analgesics every 3 to 4 hours during the first 24 to 36 hours after surgery.
- Reinforce preoperative teaching about pain management.
- Offer other comfort measures: position changes, back rubs, relaxation techniques.

Comfort and rest also are facilitated by providing personal hygiene, keeping the bed linens and environment clean, providing quiet during rest periods and at night, and allowing family members to remain with the client.

Facilitating Coping With Alterations

Surgical incisions often alter physical appearance and normal physiologic function, leading to actual or potential alterations in self-concept and body image and threatening psychological security. Changes in the way a person perceives himself can influence all of the human dimensions and areas of human functioning—self-esteem, relationships with others, sexual identity, spiritual beliefs, sociocultural values, and independent conduct of activities of daily living and work.

Many surgical clients have the same reaction to loss of a body part as to a death (crisis is discussed in Chapter 9; loss and grief are discussed in Chapter 13). The response and the adaptation made by the client are influenced by multiple factors, including age, values and beliefs, socio-cultural background, significance of the body part, visibility of the body part, time to prepare for the change, and support people available. The nurse must be aware and accepting of the client's needs and must establish interventions to meet needs in coping with change. The nursing process is used to implement interventions, beginning with the client's decision to have surgery and continuing through convalescence. Nursing activities to facilitate coping are as follows:

- Accept each client as a unique individual.
- Identify through verbal and nonverbal cues clients who are at risk for alterations in self-concept (risk is increased if the client has little support from others, a visible alteration, or an alteration that will seriously affect functional ability).
- Allow time for clients and families to verbalize feelings about the alteration, and do not assume that all clients will have problems.
- Support strengths and effective coping mechanisms.
- Allow the client to be part of goal-setting and decision-making throughout the surgical experience.
- Provide teaching and honest information to the client and family about all aspects of care.
- Work collaboratively with other members of the health team and provide referrals as necessary to meet physical, psychological, and spiritual needs.

Evaluating

As with any client, the plan of care for the surgical client is evaluated based on the established client goals. The plan has been effective if the client is discharged after surgery without complications, with a healing wound, and with knowledge and ability for self-care.

Evaluation of the client's postoperative status after same-day surgery is focused on ensuring that the client can safely be cared for at home. After surgery and recovery from the anesthetic, the client is asked to sit up and drink liquids. The client who is no longer drowsy or dizzy, has stable vital signs, and has voided is allowed to go home accompanied by a responsible adult. The client is not allowed to drive himself home. The usual length of time from completion of surgery to dismissal from the facility is 1 to 3 hours, providing established criteria have been met. Written and verbal instructions for home care are given to the client and family.

 C A S E   S T U D Y

Joe Lopez, aged 62, has been admitted to the hospital on 2/7/93 for surgical removal of the prostate gland on 2/8/93. He states that he has been having difficulty "passing his water" and the doctor has told him that his prostate is enlarged. The enlargement is not believed to be due to cancer. Mr. Lopez has no history of previous surgeries and has always been healthy. His wife and son accompanied him to the hospital. A physical assessment finds height, 5'8"; weight, 145 lb; temperature, 98.4; pulse, 88; respirations, 16; blood pressure, 134/86. Laboratory findings (done before admission) include normal potassium, complete blood count, electrocardiogram, chest x-ray, and urinalysis. Mr. Lopez asks many questions and states: "You know, I've never had surgery before—I'm a little nervous."

NURSING CARE PLAN

for Mr. Lopez

Nursing Diagnosis:	Anxiety related to knowledge deficit about perioperative surgical events
Long-Term Goal:	The client will be emotionally prepared for surgery.

Goal: On 2/7/93, the client will:
- Verbalize concerns related to surgery

Nursing Actions	**Rationale**	**Evaluative Statement**
Assess level of client's anxiety before initiating preoperative teaching.	Excessive fear and apprehension may trigger the adrenocortical stress reaction and produce changes in electrolyte metabolism, and necessitate postponing surgery (Metheney, 1991). Thus, emotional stress increases one's surgical risks. Creating an environment where the client is comfortable in expressing thoughts and concerns decreases psychological stress.	2/7/93 Goal met. Client continued to ask questions about surgery and expressed fear of postoperative pain and immobility. *J. Weber, RN*

Goal: By 2/8/93, the client will:
- Appear less anxious about surgery as evidenced by vital signs in her normal range: blood pressure 130/80; pulse, 80; respirations, 24; temperature 98.6; and the absence of crying

Nursing Actions	**Rationale**	**Evaluative Statement**
Encourage client and family questions to uncover unknown fears and concerns.	The family and significant others can convey anxiety if they lack understanding and are anxious. Moderate to severe anxiety also decreases one's readiness to learn.	2/8/93 Goal met. Vital signs: blood pressure, 136/80; pulse, 88; respirations, 24; temperature 98.4. No more episodes of tears. *J. Weber, RN*
Establish a therapeutic relationship with client by active listening and touch.	The family is an important support system to help client cope. Each person is influenced by family health beliefs and practices.	

Goal: By 2/8/93, the client will:
- Be able to explain purpose of surgery and surgical events to occur

Nursing Actions	**Rationale**	**Evaluative Statement**
Explain purpose of surgery and surgical events and postoperative events to occur to client and family.	It is necessary to identify the client's concerns and fears to provide correct information and emotional support. Because surgery is an unknown experience, a variety of fears (ie, death, pain, alteration in body image) may exist, and anxiety may be expressed in different ways. Simply talking about fears may reduce them.	2/8/93 Goal met. Client verbalized need for surgery and surgical events to occur. *J. Weber, RN*

(continued)

NURSING CARE PLAN *(continued)*

for Mr. Lopez

Assess the activities the client will engage in before surgery. This helps the nurse assess client's preoperative nutritional and physical status.

Goal: By 2/8/93, the client will:
• Visit with significant pastoral representative

Nursing Actions	**Rationale**	**Evaluative Statement**
Suggest to client to inform church pastor of impending surgery, or ask if the client would like to be visited by one of the hospital's pastoral care ministers.	A relationship with a higher being may provide client support by providing hope, meaning, and purpose in life during times of crisis.	2/8/93 Goal met. Client's pastor visited. Family at bedside and client lying comfortably in bed visiting with them. Client and family voice no further questions about surgery. *J. Weber, RN*

Long-Term Goal: Client will demonstrate understanding of nursing procedures and self-care activities necessary to prevent postoperative complications (infection, pneumonia, emboli, fluid and electrolyte imbalance).

Goal: On 2/7/93, the client will:
• Identify importance of proper nutrition, exercise, and rest before surgery

Nursing Actions	**Rationale**	**Evaluative Statement**
Inform client of the importance of proper nutrition, fluids, and exercise during preoperative teaching.	Correct information clarifies any erroneous beliefs and lets client know what to expect. Good nutrition prevents postoperative negative nitrogen balance. Decreased intake of protein and vitamin C delays wound healing and promotes infection. Activity stimulates appetite, circulation, and sleep, decreasing stress and promoting recovery.	2/7/93 Goal met. Client verbalized importance of proper nutrition, exercise, and rest before surgery. *J. Weber, RN*

Goal: By 2/8/93, the client will:
• Verbalize perioperative events of surgery

Nursing Actions	**Rationale**	**Evaluative Statement**
Inform client of surgery schedule, approximate length of surgery, and recovery room care. Offer agency booklet, "You and Your Surgery."	Correct information clarifies any erroneous beliefs and reduces anxiety by letting clients know what to expect.	2/8/93 Goal met. Client verbalized events of preoperative, intraoperative, and postoperative events of surgery. *J. Weber, RN*

Goal: By 2/8/93, the client will:
• Express understanding of postoperative pain control

(continued)

NURSING CARE PLAN (continued)

for Mr. Lopez

Nursing Actions
Request anesthesiologist visit by 2/8/93.

Explain nursing management of postoperative pain and the importance of communicating pain needs to the nurse.

Inform client of the cause of normal postanesthesia feelings of dry mouth, dizziness, sore throat, and fatigue.

Rationale
Fear is reduced when clients trust that their pain can and will be managed.

Clients on a prn analgesic regimen need to understand the importance of their communicating pain needs.

Knowledge facilitates control.

Evaluative Statement
2/8/93 Goal met. Client verbalized relief that pain would be managed.

J. Weber, RN

Goal: By 2/8/93, the client will:
• Correctly demonstrate how to turn, cough, deep breathe, exercise legs, and splint incision
• Verbalize understanding of purpose of indwelling (Foley) catheter and T-tube

Nursing Actions
Complete preoperative checklist by teaching client purpose of the following:
• Maintenance of NPO status and administration of preoperative medication

• Removal of jewelry, makeup, hairpieces
• Elevation of side rails
• Family waiting room

• Use of Foley catheter
• Use of T-tube

Demonstrate necessary postoperative exercises to client and explain how these activities prevent complications:
• Turning, coughing, and deep breathing

Rationale

Preoperative medications are given to alleviate anxiety, facilitate anesthesia induction, promote relaxation, and decrease pulmonary, oral, and gastric secretions.

These can interfere with surgery.

Raising side rails after administration of preoperative medications promotes patient safety.

A Foley catheter prevents bladder distention.

Turning promotes ventilation, venous return, and gastrointestinal peristalsis, all physiologic processes that are slowed during surgery. During surgery, cough reflex is suppressed, mucus accumulates, and lungs do not ventilate fully. Effective coughing removes retained mucus.

Evaluative Statement
2/8/93 Goal met. Client correctly demonstrated turning, coughing, deep breathing, leg exercises, incision splinting, and use of incentive spirometer; verbalized need for Foley and T-tube.

J. Weber, RN

(continued)

NURSING CARE PLAN *(continued)*

for Mr. Lopez

• Splinting of wound	Splinting aids in comfort and promotes lung expansion and oxygenation of tissues. This should be done once every 1 to 2 hours for 24 to 48 hours postoperatively.
• Leg exercises	During surgery, venous return slows and may promote circulatory stasis. Leg exercises increase venous return and prevent thrombophlebitis and emboli. These should be done every 1 to 2 hours when client is awake.
• Incentive spirometer usage	Using an incentive spirometer inflates alveoli and promotes venous return. This is done 10 times during waking hours for first 5 days postoperatively. Avoid doing this before and after meals.

KEY POINTS

- Surgery is a stressful time for the client and family, imposing physical and psychosocial alterations and adaptations.
- The time before, during, and after surgery is called the perioperative period; it is divided into preoperative, intraoperative, and postoperative phases.
- Surgical procedures are categorized by urgency, risk, and purpose.
- Anesthesia may be general or regional. General anesthesia is given to induce narcosis, loss of reflexes, and relaxation of skeletal muscles; regional anesthesia produces sensory loss but the client remains awake
- Clients agree to surgery by signing an informed consent form.
- Preoperative assessment identifies physical and psychosocial risk factors and strengths.
- Preoperative nursing interventions to prepare the client for the intraoperative and postoperative phases include therapeutic communications, preoperative teaching, and physical preparation.

- Intraoperative nursing roles are either as a scrub nurse or as a circulating nurse; each has specific client responsibilities.
- Immediate postoperative nursing care in the PAR area focuses on assessing and monitoring to prevent complications from anesthesia or surgery.
- Ongoing postoperative nursing care is planned to facilitate recovery from surgery and coping with alterations; both the client and the family are part of care.
- Ambulatory surgery is provided on an outpatient basis; preoperative assessment and teaching are critical elements in safe surgery and recovery.
- The nursing process is used throughout the perioperative period to provide knowledgeable, holistic, individualized client care.

STUDY QUESTIONS

1. Mrs. Ogg has surgery for treatment of a ruptured spleen as the result of an automobile accident. This type of surgery belongs in which of the following categories?

    a. minor, diagnostic
    b. minor, elective
    c. major, emergency
    d. major, palliative

2. A general anesthetic is given for specific purposes during a surgical procedure. Which one of the following purposes are *not* included?
   a. loss of consciousness
   b. relaxation of skeletal muscles
   c. reduction of reflex action
   d. localized loss of sensation

3. You have been asked to witness a client signature on an informed consent form for surgery. You would recognize that the document is valid for which one of these clients?
   a. a 92-year-old who is severely confused
   b. a 45-year-old who is oriented and alert
   c. a 10-year-old who is oriented and alert
   d. a 36-year-old who has had a narcotic

4. Although surgical clients may be taking any number of medications before surgery, which of the following categories of drugs would be most likely to increase surgical risk?
   a. anticoagulants
   b. antacids
   c. laxatives
   d. sedatives

5. The obese client who has surgery is at risk for which of the following postoperative complications?
   a. hunger
   b. impaired wound healing
   c. hemorrhage
   d. gas pains

6. Which of these teaching methods would be most effective in preoperative teaching for same-day surgery?
   a. lecture
   b. discussion
   c. audiovisuals
   d. handouts

7. Mr. Ying is scheduled for surgery. He says to you, "I am so frightened—what if I don't wake up?" What would be your best response?
   a. "You have a wonderful doctor."
   b. "Let's talk about how you are feeling."
   c. "Everyone wakes up from surgery!"
   d. "Don't worry, you will be just fine."

8. A patient-controlled analgesia pump allows the postoperative client to:
   a. be totally pain free
   b. take unlimited amounts of medication
   c. choose the type of pain medication
   d. administer his or her own analgesic

9. Mr. Moreno has had a surgical procedure that ne-cessitated a thoracic incision. You anticipate that he will have a higher risk for postoperative complications involving which body system?
   a. the respiratory system
   b. the circulatory system
   c. the digestive system
   d. the nervous system

10. While assessing a client in the PAR room, the nurse notes increased wound drainage, restlessness, a decreasing blood pressure, and an increase in the pulse rate. The most probable cause for these findings is:
    a. thrombophlebitis
    b. atelectasis
    c. infection
    d. hemorrhage

11. A positive Homans' sign is documented when the nurse assesses:
    a. pain in the calf with dorsiflexion of the foot
    b. increased respiratory rate with exertion
    c. decreased blood pressure after the first ambulation
    d. pain in the foot with flexion of the knee

12. Gas pains are a common postoperative discomfort. Which of the following nursing actions implemented in the plan of care would be most likely to relieve gas pains?
    a. cough and deep breathe every 2 hours
    b. maintain NPO status for 48 hours
    c. encourage frequent ambulation
    d. take vital signs every 4 hours

13. Which of the following surgical clients would be at a greater risk for alterations in body image?
    a. female, aged 19, large facial laceration
    b. female, aged 42, gallbladder surgery
    c. male, aged 14, fractured clavicle
    d. male, aged 52, hernia repair

14. The older adult often has reduced vital capacity as a normal physiologic change. Which nursing action would be most important for the postoperative care of the elderly surgical client specific to this change?
    a. Take and record vital signs every shift.
    b. Turn, cough, and deep breathe every 4 hours.
    c. Encourage increased intake of PO fluids.
    d. Assess bowel sounds daily.

15. The rationale for the use of leg exercises after surgery is that leg exercises:
    a. promote respiratory function
    b. maintain functional abilities
    c. provide diversional activities
    d. increase venous return

Answers With Rationale

1. The correct response is *c*. This surgery would involve a major body organ, has the potential of postoperative complications, requires hospitalization, and must be done immediately to preserve the client's life.

2. The correct response is *d*. Whereas *a*, *b*, and *c* are all purposes of a general anesthetic, a localized loss of sensation occurs with a regional anesthetic.

3. The correct response is *b*. A consent forms is not legal if the client signing the form is confused, sedated, or a minor.

4. The correct response is *a*. Anticoagulant drug therapy would increase the risk of hemorrhage during surgery. The other categories of drugs normally would not increase surgical risk.

5. The correct response is *b*. Fatty tissue is more difficult to suture, less resistant to infection, and more prone to delayed wound healing.

6. The correct response is *d*. Although all of the responses might be useful in teaching clients and families before ambulatory surgery, written instructions are most effective in providing information.

7. The correct response is *b*. This response allows the client to talk about feelings and fears and is therapeutic. The other responses give false reassurance.

8. The correct response is *d*. A patient-controlled analgesia pump does allow the client to administer his or her own analgesic. Use of this device does not allow the client to take unlimited amounts of medication, choose the type of pain medication, or be totally pain free.

9. The correct response is *a*. A thoracic incision makes it more painful for the client to take deep breaths or cough. Shallow respirations and ineffective coughing increase the risk for respiratory complications.

10. The correct response is *d*. Increased wound drainage, restlessness, decreasing blood pressure, and increasing pulse rate are assessment findings that indicate hemorrhage.

11. The correct response is *a*. Calf pain with dorsiflexion of the foot is a positive Homans' sign. This sign is positive when the client has thrombophlebitis.

12. The correct response is *c*. Frequent ambulation stimulates peristalsis and relieves gas pains. The other responses are incorrect in this situation.

13. The correct response is *a*. The reaction of the client to an accidental or intentional incision is influenced by age, time to prepare for the change, and visibility of the trauma. Large facial wounds increase the risk of an alteration in body image.

14. The correct response is *b*. Reduced vital capacity in elderly people increases the risk of respiratory complications, including pneumonia and atelectasis. Having the client turn, cough, and deep breathe every 4 hours maintains respiratory function and helps to prevent complications.

15. The correct response is *d*. Leg exercises in the postoperative period do increase venous return. As a result, the client has decreased risk of thrombophlebitis and emboli.

BIBLIOGRAPHY

Alverson, E. (1987). The preoperative interview: Its effect on perioperative nurses' empathy. *AORN Journal, 45*, 1162–1164.

Association of Operating Room Nurses. (1989). *Standards of nursing practice*. Denver: Author.

Carpenito, L. J. (1991). *Nursing care plans and documentation: Nursing diagnoses and collaborative problems*. Philadelphia: Lippincott.

Carpenito, L. J. (1992). *Nursing diagnoses: Application to clinical practice* (4th ed.). Philadelphia: Lippincott.

Caruso, C. C., Hadley, B. J., Shukla, R., Frame, P., & Khoury, J. (1992). Cooling effects and comfort of four cooling blanket temperatures in humans with fever. *Nursing Research, 41*(2), 68–72.

Daake, D. R., & Gueldner, S. H. (1989). Imagery instruction and the control of postsurgical pain. *Applied Nursing Research, 2*(3), 114–120.

Davis, M. J., & Nomura, L. A. (1990). Vital signs of class I surgical patients. *Western Journal of Nursing Research, 12*(1), 28–41.

Dickinson, S. P., & Bury, G. M. (1989). Pulmonary embolism. *Nursing, 19*(4), 34–42.

Drain, C., & Christoph, S. (1987). *The recovery room: A critical care approach to postanesthesia nursing* (2nd ed.). Philadelphia: Lippincott.

Frauline, K. E., & Borchardt, A. (1988). Guide to solving postanesthesia problems. *Nursing, 18*(5), 66–68.

Groath, L. (1990). *Operating room nursing: Perioperative practice* (2nd ed.). Norwalk, CT: Appleton & Lange.

Groath, L., & Howery, D. (1992). 25 predictions for perioperative nursing. *Nursing, 22*(1), 48–49.

Gruendemann, B. J. (1985). Dare to excel in ambulatory surgery. *AORN Journal, 41*(2), 330–331, 333, 337.

Heater, B. S., Olson, R. K., & Becker, A. M. (1990). Helping patients recover faster. *American Journal of Nursing, 90*(10), 19–20.

Heidenreich, T., & Giuffre, M. (1990). Postoperative temperature measurement. *Nursing Research, 39*(3), 153–155.

Lammers, P. (1986). Ambulatory surgery: Competition creates challenges. *AORN Journal, 44*(1), 87–94.

Jackson, M. F. (1988). High risk surgical patients. *Journal of Gerontological Nursing, 14*(1), 8–15.

McCormack, M. (1990). Managing hemorrhagic shock. *American Journal of Nursing, 90*(8), 22–29.

Meeker, M. H., & Rothrock, J. C. (1991). *Alexander's care of the patient in surgery* (9th ed.). St. Louis: Mosby.

Montanari, J. (1985). Documenting your postop assessment findings. *Nursing, 15*(8), 31–35.

Oberle, K., Wry, J., Paul, P., & Grace, M. (1990). Environment, anxiety, and postoperative pain. *Western Journal of Nursing Research, 12*(6), 745–757.

Patrick, M. L., Woods, S. L., Craven, R. F., Rokosky, J. S., & Bruno, P. M. (1991). *Medical–surgical nursing: Pa-*

thophysiological concepts (2nd ed.). Philadelphia: Lippincott.

Pope, K. E. (1990). Cost containment and the short-stay needs of surgical patients. *Nursing Management, 21*(3), 61–64.

Reeder, J. M. (1989). Ethical dilemmas in perioperative nursing practice. *Nursing Clinics of North America, 24,* 999–1007.

Rowland, M. A. (1990). Myths—and facts—about postop discomfort. *American Journal of Nursing, 90*(5), 60–64.

saltiel-Berzin, R. (1992). Managing a surgical patient who has diabetes. *Nursing, 22*(4), 34–42.

Smallwood, S. B. (1988). Preparing children for surgery. *AORN Journal, 47*(1), 177–185.

Smeltzer, S. C., & Bare, B. G. (1992). *Brunner and Suddarth's textbook of medical–surgical nursing* (7th ed.). Philadelphia: Lippincott.

Spearing, C., & Cornell, D. J. (1988). Incentive spirometry: Inspiring your patients to breathe deeply. *Nursing, 17*(9), 50–51.

Voss, S. J. (1986). Ambulatory surgery scheduling: Assuring a smooth patient flow. *AORN Journal, 43*(5), 1009–1012.

Wiseman, S. J. (1990). Patient advocacy: The essence of perioperative nursing in ambulatory care surgery. *AORN Journal, 51*(3), 754, 758–759.

Appendices

Equivalents

Metric Units

The metric system, developed by the French, uses the *meter* as the basic unit. The metric system is a decimal system, with prefixes that designate the various multiples or divisibles of 10. The most commonly used prefixes in medicine are

Milli, which means one one-thousandth (0.001)
Centi, which means one one-hundredth (0.01)
Kilo, which means one thousand (1000)

These prefixes may be affixed to any of the three basic units of measurements, which are

Meter (m), the unit of length
Gram (g), the unit of weight
Liter (L), the unit of volume
Therefore
1 millimeter (mm) = 0.001 m
1 milligram (mg) = 0.001 g
1 milliliter (mL) = 0.001 L
1 kilometer (km) = 1000 m
1 kilogram (kg) = 1000 g
1 kiloliter (kl) = 1000 L

Length
The meter (a little longer than a yard) and the kilometer (about 0.6 mile) seldom are used in medicine or nursing. The commonly used measure of length is 1 centimeter (cm) = 0.01 m = about 0.4 inch.

Volume
The most frequently used measures of volume are the *liter* and the *milliliter*. Some useful equivalents to know are
1000 milliliters (mL) = 1 liter (L)
1000 cubic centimeters (cc) = 1 liter (L)
1 milliliter (mL) = 1 cc

Weight
The gram designates the weight of 1 mL of distilled water to 4°C. The most frequently used units of weight are
1,000,000 micrograms (mcg or μg) = 1 gram (g)
1000 micrograms (mcg) = 1 milligram (mg)
1000 milligrams (mg) = 1 gram (g)
1000 grams (g) = 1 kilogram (kg) = 2.2 pounds (lb)

TABLE A-1

Metric and Household Equivalents	
Metric Unit	**Household Unit**
5 mL	1 tsp
15 mL	1 Tbs
180 mL	1 full teacup
240 mL	1 full glass

Metric Units and Their Household Equivalents

Household measurement is inaccurate, with wide variations in the size of teaspoons, teacups, and so forth. The generally accepted household measures are

  60 drops (gtt) = 1 teaspoon (tsp or t)
  3 tsp = 1 tablespoon (Tbs or T)
  12 Tbs = 1 teacup
  16 Tbs = 1 glass (or a standard measuring cup)

Apothecary Units

In the apothecary system
  The unit of weight is the *grain*.
  The unit of volume is the *minim*.
Of the many units of measure in the apothecary system, you should know the following units, abbreviations, and equivalents.

Weight

  60 grains (gr) = 1 dram (dr or ʒ)
  8 drams (dr or ʒ) = 1 ounce (oz or ℥)

Volume

  60 minims (min) = 1 fluid dram (fl dr or fʒ)
  8 fl dr = 1 fluid ounce (fl oz or f℥)
  16 fl oz = 1 pint (pt)
  2 pt = 1 quart (qt)
  4 qt = 1 gallon (gal)
In the apothecary system, when the symbol or abbreviation is used, the quantity is written in lowercase Roman numerals and follows the symbol. Arabic numerals are used, however, in preference to large Roman numerals. For example
  5 gr = gr v
  8 dr = ʒ viii
  The quantity one-half may be indicated by the symbol ss.
  1½ gr = gr iss
  7½ gr = gr viiss
Other fractional parts are expressed as common fractions, for example, gr 1/250, gr 1/10.
When pint, quart, and gallon are written, the quantity is expressed in Arabic numerals, (eg, 1½ pints or 7½ quarts).

Apothecary Units and Their Household Equivalents

  1 drop = 1 minim (m i)
  1 tsp = 1 dr (ʒ i)
  1 Tbs = ½ oz (℥ ss)
  2 Tbs = 1 oz (℥ i)
  1 teacup = 6 oz (℥ vi)
  1 glass or measuring cup = 8 oz (℥ viii)
  2 measuring cups = 1 pt

TABLE A-2

Most Commonly Used Approximate Equivalents*		
Metric	**Apothecary**	**Household**
0.06 g	gr i	
0.06 mL	min i	1 drop
1.0 g	gr xv	
1.0 mL	min xv	⅕ tsp
5 mL	(1 dr) ʒ i	1 tsp
15 mL	(½ oz) ʒ ss	1 Tbs
30 mL	(1 oz) ʒ i	2 Tbs
500 mL	(16 oz) ʒ 16	1 pt
1000 mL	(32 oz) ʒ 32	1 qt

*There are many discrepancies among these approximate equivalents. For example, 30 mL is the accepted equivalent for 1 oz (29.57 mL is the exact equivalent); however, multiplying 5 mL per dram by 8 (ʒ viii per ounce) results in an equivalent of 40 mL for 1 oz rather than the accepted equivalent of 30 mL = 1 oz.

Such discrepancies are inevitable when two systems are used whose equivalents are not exact. The discrepancies are within a 10% margin of error, which usually is acceptable in pharmacology.

TABLE A-3

Commonly Used Metric Units and Their Approximate Apothecary Equivalents		
Metric		**Apothecary**
1 g	1000 mg	gr xv
0.6 g	600 mg	gr x
0.5 g	500 mg	gr viiss
0.3 g	300 mg	gr v
0.2 g	200 mg	gr iii
0.1 g	100 mg	gr iss
0.06 g	60 mg	gr i
0.05 g	50 mg	gr ¾
0.03 g	30 mg	gr ½ or gr ss
0.02 g	20 mg	gr ⅓
0.015 g	15 mg	gr ¼
0.016 g	16 mg	gr ¼
0.010 g	10 mg	gr ⅙
0.008 g	8 mg	gr ⅛
0.006 g	6 mg	gr 1/10
0.005 g	5 mg	gr 1/12
0.003 g	3 mg	gr 1/20
0.002 g	2 mg	gr 1/30
0.001 g	1 mg	gr 1/60
	0.6 mg	gr 1/100
	0.5 mg	gr 1/120
	0.4 mg	gr 1/150
	0.3 mg	gr 1/200

APPENDIX B

Normal Adult Laboratory Values*

Commonly Used Abbreviations

kg = kilogram
g = gram
mg = milligram
μg = microgram
μμg = micromicrogram
ng = nanogram
mEq = milliequivalent
L = liter
dl = 100 milliliters
mL = milliliter
cu mm (mm³) = cubic millimeter
nM = nanomolar
mIU = milliInternational Unit
pg = picogram
mm = millimeter
μ = micron or micrometer
mm Hg = millimeters of mercury
mU = milliunit
μU = microunit
IU = International Unit

*Laboratory values may vary according to techniques used in different laboratories.

TABLE B-1

Hematologic Values—Reference Ranges		
Determination	**Conventional**	**SI**
Coagulation Factors		
Factor I (fibrinogen)	0.15–0.35 g/100 mL	4.0–10.0 μmol/L
Factor II (prothrombin)	60%–140%	0.60–1.40 μmol/L
Factor V (accelerator globulin)	60%–140%	0.60–1.40 μmol/L
Factors VII to X (proconvertin to Stuart factor)	70%–130%	0.70–1.30 μmol/L
Factor X (Stuart factor)	60%–140%	0.70–1.30 μmol/L
Factor VIII (antihemophilic globulin)	50%–200%	0.50–2.0 μmol/L
Factor IX (plasma thromboplastic cofactor)	60%–140%	0.60–1.40 μmol/L
Factor XI (plasma thromboplastic antecedent)	60%–140%	0.60–1.40 μmol/L
Factor XII (Hageman factor)	60%–140%	0.60–1.40 μmol/L
Coagulation Screening Tests		
Bleeding time (Simplate)	2–8 min	180–540 sec
Prothrombin time	9.5–12 sec	Less than 2 sec from control
Partial thromboplastin time (activated)	20–45 sec	25–37 sec
Whole blood clot lysis	No clot lysis in 24 hr	0/day
Fibrinolytic Studies		
Euglobin lysis	No lysis in 2 hr	0 (in 2 hr)
Thrombin time		Control +5 sec

(continued)

T A B L E B - 1 (*continued*)

Hematologic Values—Reference Ranges

Determination	Conventional	SI
Complete Blood Count		
Hematocrit	Male: 42%–50%	Male: 0.42–0.52
	Female: 40%–48%	Female: 0.37–0.48
Hemoglobin	Male: 13–18 g/dL	Male: 8.1–11.2 mmol/L
	Female: 12–16 g/dL	Female: 7.4–9.9 mmol/L
Leukocyte count	5000–10,000/mm^3	4.3–10.8 × 10^9/L
Erythrocyte count	4.2 million–5.9 million/mm^3	4.2–5.9 × 10^{12}/L
Mean corpuscular volume (MCV)	80–94 μm^3	80–94 fl
Mean corpuscular hemoglobin (MCH)	27–32 pg	1.7–2.0 fmol
Mean corpuscular hemoglobin concentration (MCHC)	33%–38%	19–22.8 mmol/L
Erythrocyte sedimentation rate (Zeta Centrifuge)	41%–54%	Male: 1–13 mm/h
		Female: 1–20 mm/h
Erythrocyte Enzymes		
Glucose-6-phosphate dehydrogenase	5–15 U/g Hb	5–15 U/g
Pyruvate kinase	13–17 U/g Hb	13–17 U/g
Ferritin (serum)	Females: 5–100 ng/mL	
	Males: 10–270 ng/mL	
Folic acid, RIA	4–16 ng/mL	
Haptoglobin	50–250 mg/dL	1.0 g–3.0 g/L
Hemoglobin Studies		
Electrophoresis for A$_2$ hemoglobin	1.5%–3.5%	0.015–0.035
Hemoglobin, met- and sulf-	0	0
Serum hemoglobin	2–3 mg/100 mL	1.2–1.9 μmol/L
Lupus erythematosus (LE) preparation		
Heparin as anticoagulant	0	0
Defibrinated blood	0	0
Muramidase	Serum, 3–7 μg/mL	3–7 mg/L
	Urine, 0–2 μg/mL	0–2 mg/L
Osmotic fragility of erythrocyte	Increased if hemolysis occurs in over 0.5% NaCl; decreased if hemolysis is incomplete in 0.3% NaCl	
Peroxide hemolysis	Less than 10%	<0.10
Platelet count	100,000–400,000/mm^3	150–350 × 10^9/L
Platelet Function Tests		
Clot retraction	50%–100%/2 hr	0.50–1.00/2 hr
Platelet aggregation	Full response to ADP, epi- nephrine and collagen	1.0
Platelet factor 3	33–57 sec	33–57 sec
Reticulocyte count	0.5%–1.5% red cells	0.005–0.15
Vitamin B$_{12}$	90–280 pg/mL (borderline: 70–90)	66–207 pmol/L (borderline: 52–66)

T A B L E   B - 2

Blood, Plasma or Serum Values—Reference Ranges

Determination	Conventional	SI
Acetoacetate plus acetone	0.3–2.0 mg/dL	3–20 mg/L
Aldolase	1.3–8.2 mU/mL	12–75 nmol sec⁻¹/L
Alpha amino nitrogen	3.0–5.5 mg/100 mL	2.1–3.9 mmol/L
Ammonia	80–110 μg/100 mL	47–65 μmol/L
Ascorbic acid	0.4–1.5 mg/100 mL	23–85 μmol/L
Bilirubin (van den Bergh test)	1 minute: 0.4 mg/100 mL	Up to 7 μmol/L
	Direct: 0.1–0.2 mg/dL	Up to 17 μmol/L
	Total: 1.0 mg/100 mL	
	Indirect: 0.1–1.0 mg/dL	
Blood volume	8.5%–9.0% of body weight in kg	80–85 mL/kg
	Toxic level: 17 mEq/L	
Bromsulphalein (BSP)	Less than 5% retention 45 min after 5 mg/kg IV	<0.05 L
Calcium	8.5–10.5 mg/100 mL	2.1–2.5 mmol/L
Carbon dioxide content	24 mEq–32 mEq/L	24–30 mmol/L
Carcinoembryonic antigen (CEA)	0.25 mg/mL	0–2.5 μg/L
Carotenoids	0.8–4.0 μg/mL	1.5–7.4 μmol/L
Ceruloplasmin	27–37 mg/100 mL	1.8–2.4 μmol/L
Chloride	95–105 mEq/L	100–106 mmol/L
Cholesterol	<200 mg/dL	
Cholinesterase (pseudocholinesterase)	0.5 pH U or more/hr	0.5 arb unit or more
	0.7 pH U or more/hr for packed cells	
Copper	Total: 100–200 μg/100 mL	16–31 μmol/L
Creatine phosphokinase (CPK)	Female: 50–250 mU/mL	0.08–0.58 μmol sec⁻¹/L
	Male: 50–325 mU/mL	
Creatinine	0.7–1.4 mg/100 mL	60–130 μmol/L
Ethanol	0.3%–0.4%, marked intoxication;	65–87 mmol/L
	0.4%–0.5%, alcoholic stupor;	87–109 mmol/L
	0.5% or over, alcoholic coma	>109 mmol/L
Glucose	Fasting: 60–110 mg/100 mL	3.9–5.6 mmol/L
Iron	65–170 μg/100 mL (higher in males)	9.0–26.9 μmol/L
Iron-binding capacity	250–410 μg/100 mL	44.8–73.4 μmol/L
Lactic acid	0.6–1.8 mEq/L	0.6–1.8 mmol/L
Lactic dehydrogenase isoenzymes	100–225 mU/mL	1.00–2.00 μmol sec⁻¹/L
Lead	50 μg/100 mL or less	Up to 2.4 μmol/L
Lipase	2 U/mL or less	Up to 2 arb units
Lipids, total	400–1000 mg/dL	3.10–5.69 mmol/L
Magnesium	0.33–2.4 mEq/L	0.8–1.3 mmol/L
5′ Nucleotidase	0.3–3.2 Bodansky U	30–290 nmol sec⁻¹/L
Osmolality	280–300 mOsm/kg water	285–295 mmol/kg
Oxygen saturation (arterial)	95%–100%	0.96–1.00 L
Pco_2	35–45 mm Hg	4.7–6.0 kPg
pH	7.35–7.45	Same
Po_2	95–100 mm Hg (dependent on age while breathing room air)	10.0–13.3 kPa
	Above 500 mm Hg while on 100% O_2	
Phenylalanine	0–2 mg/100 mL	0–120 μmol/L

(continued)

T A B L E   B - 2 (continued)

Blood, Plasma or Serum Values—Reference Ranges

Determination	Conventional	SI
Phosphorus (inorganic)	3.0–4.5 mg/100 mL	1.0–1.5 mmol/L
Potassium	3.8–5.0 mEq/L	3.5–5.0 mmol/L
Primidone (Mysoline)	Therapeutic level, 4–12 μg/mL	18–55 μmol/L
Protein, total	6.0–8.0 g/100 mL	60–84 g/L
Albumin	3.5–5.0 g/100 mL	33–50 g/L
Globulin	1.5–3.0 g/100 mL	23–35 g/L
Electrophoresis	% of total protein	% of total protein
Albumin	3.3–5.0 g/dL	0.52–0.68
Globulin		
Alpha$_1$	0.2–0.4 g/dL	0.042–0.072
Alpha$_2$	0.6–1.0 g/dL	0.068–0.12
Beta	0.6–1.2 g/dL	0.093–0.15
Gamma	0.7–1.5 g/dL	0.13–0.23
	0.3–0.7 mg/dL	0–0.11 mmol/L
Sodium	135–145 mEq/L	135–145 mmol/L
Sulfate	0.5–1.5 mg/100 mL	0.05–1.2 mmol/L
Transaminase (SGOT) (aspartate aminotransferase)	7–40 U/mL	0.08–0.32 μmol sec^{-1}/L
Urea nitrogen (BUN)	10–20 mg/100 mL	2.9–8.9 mmol/L
Uric acid	2.5–8.0 mg/100 mL	0.13–0.42 mmol/L
Vitamin A	50–220 μg/dL	0.5–2.1 μmol/L

T A B L E   B - 3

Urine Values—Reference Ranges

Determination	Conventional	SI
Acetone plus acetoacetate (quantitative)	0	0 mg/L
Alpha amino nitrogen	64–199 mg/day; not over 1.5% of total nitrogen	4.6–14.2 mmol/day
Amylase	35–260 U/mL	24–76 arb units
Calcium	150 mg/day or less	3.8 mmol/day or less
Catecholamines	Epinephrine, 10%–40%	<55 nmol/day
	Norepinephrine, 60%–90%	<590 nmol/day
Copper	20–70 μg/day	0–1.6 μmol/day
Coproporphyrin	50–300 μg/day	80–380 nmol/day
Creatine	0–200 mg/24 hr	<0.75 mmol/day
Cystine or cysteine	0	0
Follicle-stimulating hormone		
Follicular phase	5–20 IU/day	Same
Midcycle	15–60 IU/day	
Luteal phase	5–15 IU/day	
Menopausal	50–100 IU/day	
Men	5–25 IU/day	
Hemoglobin and myoglobin	0	
5-Hydroxyindole acetic acid	2–9 mg/day (women lower than men)	10–45 μmol/day

(continued)

Urine Values—Reference Ranges

Determination	Conventional			SI	
Phenolsulfonphthalein (PSP)	At least 25% excreted by 15 min; 40% by 30 min; 60% by 120 min			0.25 L	
Phosphorus (inorganic)	Varies with intake; average 1 g/day			32 mmol/day	
Porphobilinogen	0			0	
Protein, quantitative	<150 mg/24 hr			<0.15 g/day	
Steroids					

17-Ketosteroids (per day)	Age (yr)	Male (mg)	Female (mg)	Male (μmol/day)	Female (μmol/day)
	10	1–4	1–4	3–14	3–14
	20	6–21	4–16	21–73	14–56
	30	8–26	4–14	28–90	14–49
	50	5–18	3–9	17–62	10–31
	70	2–10	1–7	7–35	3–24

Determination	Conventional	SI
17-Hydroxysteroids	3–8 mg/day (women lower than men)	8–22 μmol/day as hydrocortisone
Sugar		
Quantitative glucose	0	0 mmol/L
Identification of reducing substances		
Fructose	0	0 mmol/L
Pentose	0	0 mmol/L
Titratable acidity	20–40 mEq/day	20–40 mmol/day
Urobilinogen	<0.25 mg/dL	To 1.0 arb unit
Uroporphyrin	Up to 50 μg in 24 hr	0 nmol/day
Vanilmandelic acid (VMA)	0.7–6.8 mg/24 hr	Up to 45 μmol/day

T A B L E   B - 4

Cerebrospinal Fluid Values—Reference Ranges

Determination	Conventional	SI
Bilirubin	0	0 μmol/L
Chloride	100–130 mEq/L	
Albumin	15.5–32.0 mg/dL	0.295 g/L ± 2 SD (0.11–0.48)
IgG	0–6.6 mg/dL	0.043 g/L ± 2 SD (0–0.086)
Glucose	50–75 mg/100 mL (30%–50% less than blood)	2.8–4.2 mmol/L
Pressure (initial)	70–180 mm H_2O	70–80 arb units
Protein		
Lumbar	15–45 mg/100 mL	0.15–0.45 g/L
Cisternal	15–25 mg/100 mL	0.15–0.25 g/L
Ventricular	5–15 mg/100 mL	0.05–0.15 g/L

T A B L E   B - 5

Special Endocrine Tests—Reference Ranges

Steroid Hormones

Aldosterone	Excretion: 5–19 μg/24 hr	14–53 nmol/day
Fasting, at rest, 210 mEq sodium diet	Supine: 48±29 pg/mL	133 ± 80 pmol/L
	Upright: (2h) 65±23 pg/mL	180 ± 64 pmol/L
Fasting, at rest, 110 mEq sodium diet	Supine: 107±45 pg/mL	279 ± 125 pmol/L
	Upright: (2h) 239±123 pg/mL	663 ± 341 pmol/L

(*continued*)

Special Endocrine Tests—Reference Ranges

Steroid Hormones

Fasting, at rest, 10 mEq sodium diet	Supine: 175±75 pg/mL	485 ± 208 pmol/L
	Upright: (2h) 532±228 pg/mL	1476 ± 632 pmol/L
Cortisol		
Fasting	8 AM: 5–25 μg/100 mL	0.14–0.69 μmol/L
At rest	8 PM: below 10 μg/100 mL	0–0.28 μmol/L
20 U ACTH	4-hour ACTH test: 30–45 μg/100 mL	0.83–1.24 μmol/L
Dexamethasone at midnight	Overnight suppression test: below 5 μg/100 mL	<0.14 nmol/L
	Excretion: 20–70 μg/24 hr	55–193 nmol/day
11-Deoxycortisol	Responsive: over 7.5 μg/100 mL (after metrapone)	>0.22 μmol/L
Testosterone	Adult male: 300–1100 ng/100 mL	10.4–38.1 nmol/L
	Adolescent male: over 100 ng/100 mL	>3.5 nmol/L
	Females: 25–90 ng/100 mL	0.87–3.12 nmol/L
Unbound testosterone	Adult male: 3.06–24.0 ng/100 mL	106–832 pmol/L
	Adult female: 0.09–1.28 ng/100 mL	3.1–44.4 pmol/L

Polypeptide Hormones

Adrenocorticotrophin (ACTH)	15–70 pg/mL	3.3–15.4 pmol/L
Calcitonin	Undetectable in normals	0
	>100 pg/mL in medullary carcinoma	>29.3 pmol/L
Growth hormone		
Fasting, at rest	Below 5 ng/mL	<233 pmol/L
After exercise	Children: over 10 ng/mL	>465 pmol/L
	Male: below 5 ng/mL	<233 pmol/L
	Female: up to 30 ng/mL	0–1395 pmol/L
After glucose	Male: below 5 ng/mL	<233 pmol/L
	Female: below 10 mg/mL	0–465 pmol/L
Insulin		
Fasting	6–26 μU/mL	43–187 pmol/L
During hypoglycemia	Below 20 μU/mL	<144 pmol/L
After glucose	Up to 150 μU/mL	0–1078 pmol/L
Luteinizing hormone	Male: 6–18 mU/mL	6–18 U/L
Preovulatory or postovulatory	Female: 5–22 mU/mL	5–22 U/L
Midcycle peak	30–250 mU/mL	30–250 U/L
Parathyroid hormone	<10 μl equiv/mL	<10 mL equiv/L
Prolactin	2–15 ng/mL	0.08–6.0 nmol/L
Renin activity		
Normal diet	Supine: 1.1 ± 0.8 ng/mL/hr	0.9±0.6 nmol/L/hr
	Upright: 1.9 ± 1.7 ng/mL/hr	1.5 ± 1.3 nmol/L/hr
Low-sodium diet	Supine: 2.7 ± 1.8 ng/mL/hr	2.1 ± 1.4 nmol/L/hr
	Upright: 6.6 ± 2.5 ng/mL/hr	5.1 ± 1.9 nmol/L/hr
High-sodium diet	Diuretics: 10.0 ± 3.7 ng/mL/hr	7.7 ± 2.9 nmol/L/hr

Thyroid Hormones

Thyroid-stimulating hormone (TSH)	0.5–3.5 μU/mL	0.5–3.5 mU/L
Thyroxine-binding globulin capacity	15–25 μg T_4/100 mL	193–322 mU/L
Total triiodothyronine by radioimmunoassay (T_3)	70–190 ng/100 mL	1.08–2.92 nmol/L
Total thyroxine (T_4) by RIA	4–12 μg/100 mL	52–154 nmol/L
T_3 resin uptake	25%–35%	0.25–0.35
Free thyroxine index ($FT_4$1)	1–4 ng/100 mL	12.8–51.2 pmol/L

APPENDIX C

U.S. Nutritional Tables

TABLE C-1

U.S. Recommended Daily Allowances

Category	Age (yr) or Condition	Weight† (kg)	Weight† (lb)	Height† (cm)	Height† (ln)	Protein (g)	Fat-Soluble Vitamins Vitamin A (µg RE)‡	Vitamin D (µg)§	Vitamin E (mg α-TE)¶	Vitamin K (µg)	Vitamin C (mg)
Infants	0.0–0.5	6	13	60	24	13	375	7.5	3	5	30
	0.5–1.0	9	20	71	28	14	375	10	4	10	35
Children	1–3	13	29	90	35	16	400	10	6	15	40
	4–6	20	44	112	44	24	500	10	7	20	45
	7–10	28	62	132	52	28	700	10	7	30	45
Males	11–14	45	99	157	62	45	1000	10	10	45	50
	15–18	66	145	176	69	59	1000	10	10	65	60
	19–24	72	160	177	70	58	1000	10	10	70	60
	25–50	79	174	176	70	63	1000	5	10	80	60
	51+	77	170	173	68	63	1000	5	10	80	60
Females	11–14	46	101	157	62	46	800	10	8	45	50
	15–18	55	120	163	64	44	800	10	8	55	60
	19–24	58	128	164	65	46	800	10	8	60	60
	25–50	63	138	163	64	50	800	5	8	65	60
	51+	65	143	160	63	50	800	5	8	65	60
Pregnant						60	800	10	10	65	70
lactating											
1st 6 mo						65	1300	10	12	65	95
2nd 6 mo						62	1200	10	11	65	90

* Designed for the maintenance of good nutrition of practically all healthy people in the United States. The allowances, expressed as average daily intakes over time are intended to provide for individual variations among most normal people as they live in the United States under usual environmental stresses. Diets should be based on a variety of common foods to provide other nutrients for which human requirements have been less well defined.

† Weights and heights of reference adults are actual medians for the U.S. population of the designated age, as reported by NHANES II. The use of these figures does not imply that the height-to-weight ratios are ideal.

‡ Retinol equivalents. 1 RE = 1 µg retinol or 6 µg beta-carotene.

§ As cholecalciferol. 10 µg cholecalciferol = 400 IU of vitamin D.

¶ α-Tocopherol equivalents. 1 mg d-α-tocopherol = 1 α-TE.

‖ 1 NE (niacin equivalent) is equal to 1 mg of niacin or 60 mg of dietary tryptophan.

(Food and Nutrition Board. [1989]. *National Research Council recommended dietary allowances* [10th ed.]. Washington, D.C.: National Academy Press.)

	Water-Soluble Vitamins					Minerals						
Thiamin (mg)	Ribo-flavin (mg)	Niacin (mg NE)‖	Vitamin B$_6$ (mg)	Folate (μg)	Vitamin B$_{12}$ (μc)	Cal-cium (mg)	Phos-phorus (mg)	Mag-nesium (mg)	Iron (mg)	Zinc (mg)	Iodine (μg)	Sele-nium (μg)
0.3	0.4	5	0.3	25	0.3	400	300	40	6	5	40	10
0.4	0.5	6	0.6	35	0.5	600	500	60	10	5	50	15
0.7	0.8	9	1.0	50	0.7	800	800	80	10	10	70	20
0.9	1.1	12	1.1	75	1.0	800	800	120	10	10	90	20
1.0	1.2	13	1.4	100	1.4	800	800	170	10	10	120	30
1.3	1.5	17	1.7	150	2.0	1200	1200	270	12	15	150	40
1.5	1.8	20	2.0	200	2.0	1200	1200	400	12	15	150	50
1.5	1.7	19	2.0	200	2.0	1200	1200	350	10	15	150	70
1.5	1.7	19	2.0	200	2.0	800	800	350	10	15	150	70
1.2	1.4	15	2.0	200	2.0	800	800	350	10	15	150	70
1.1	1.3	15	1.4	150	2.0	1200	1200	280	15	12	150	45
1.1	1.3	15	1.5	180	2.0	1200	1200	300	15	12	150	50
1.1	1.3	15	1.6	180	2.0	1200	1200	280	15	12	150	55
1.1	1.3	15	1.6	180	2.0	800	800	280	15	12	150	55
1.0	1.2	13	1.6	180	2.0	800	800	280	10	12	150	55
1.5	1.6	17	2.2	400	2.2	1200	1200	320	30	15	175	65
1.6	1.8	20	2.1	280	2.6	1200	1200	355	15	19	200	75
1.6	1.7	20	2.1	260	2.6	1200	1200	340	15	16	200	75

T A B L E   C - 2

U.S. Mean Heights and Weights and Recommended Energy Intake

Category	Age (yr) or condition	Weight (kg)	Weight (lb)	Height (cm)	Height (In)	REE* (kcal/day)	Multiples of REE	Average Energy Allowance (Kcal)† Per kg	Per day‡
Infants	0.0–0.5	6	13	60	24	320		108	650
	0.5–1.0	9	20	71	28	500		98	850
Children	1–3	13	29	90	35	740		102	1300
	4–6	20	44	112	44	950		90	1800
	7–10	28	62	132	52	1130		70	2000
Males	11–14	45	99	157	62	1440	1.70	55	2500
	15–18	66	145	176	69	1760	1.67	45	3000
	19–24	72	160	177	70	1780	1.67	40	2900
	25–50	79	174	176	70	1800	1.60	37	2900
	51+	77	170	173	68	1530	1.50	30	2300
Females	11–14	46	101	157	62	1310	1.67	47	2200
	15–18	55	120	163	64	1370	1.60	40	2200
	19–24	58	128	164	65	1350	1.60	38	2200
	25–50	63	138	163	64	1380	1.55	36	2200
	51+	65	143	160	63	1280	1.50	30	1900
Pregnant	1st trimester								+0
	2nd trimester								+300
	3rd trimester								+300
Lactating	1st 6 mo								+500
	2nd 6 mo								+500

*Calculation based on FAO equations then rounded.

†In the range of light to moderate activity, the coefficient of variation is ±20%.

‡Figure is rounded.

(Food and Nutrition Board. [1989]. *National Research Council recommended dietary allowances* [10th ed., p. 33]. Washington, D.C.: National Academy Press.)

APPENDIX D

Canadian Nutritional Tables

TABLE D-1

				Requirements*					
Average Energy Requirements*									
Age	Sex	Average Height (cm)†	Average Weight (kg)†	kcal/ kg†,‡	MJ/kg‡	kcal/day§	MJ/ day‖	kcal/ cm#	MJ/ cm‖
Months									
0–2	Both	55	4.5	120–100	0.50–0.42	500	2.0	9	0.04
3–5	Both	63	7.0	100–95	0.42–0.40	700	2.8	11	0.05
6–8	Both	69	8.5	95–97	0.40–0.41	800	3.4	11.5	0.05
9–11	Both	73	9.5	97–99	0.41	950	3.8	12.5	0.05
Years									
1	Both	82	11	101	0.42	1100	4.8	13.5	0.06
2–3	Both	95	14	94	0.39	1300	5.6	13.5	0.06
4–6	Both	107	18	100	0.42	1800	7.6	17	0.07
7–9	M	126	25	88	0.37	2200	9.2	17.5	0.07
	F	125	25	76	0.32	1900	8.0	15	0.06
10–12	M	141	34	73	0.30	2500	10.4	17.5	0.07
	F	143	36	61	0.25	2200	9.2	15.5	0.06
13–15	M	159	50	57	0.24	2800	12.0	17.5	0.07
	F	157	48	46	0.19	2200	9.2	14	0.06
16–18	M	172	62	51	0.21	3200	13.2	18.5	0.08
	F	160	53	40	0.17	2100	8.8	13	0.05
19–24	M	175	71	42	0.18	3000	12.4		
	F	160	58	36	0.15	2100	8.8		
25–49	M	172	74	36	0.15	2700	11.2		
	F	160	59	32	0.13	1900	8.0		
50–74	M	170	73	31	0.13	2300	9.6		
	F	158	63	29	0.12	1800	7.6		
75+	M	168	69	29	0.12	2000	8.4		
	F	155	64	23	0.10	1500	6.0		

* Requirements can be expected to vary within a range of ±30%.

† Figures rounded to the closest whole number when 10 or more and to the closest 0.5 when below 10.

‡ First and last figures are averages at the beginning and at the end of the 3-month period.

§ Figures rounded to the nearest 50 when below 1000 and to the nearest 100 when 1000 or more.

‖ Figures include 2 decimals if value is less than 1 and 1 decimal if 1 or more.

Figures rounded to the nearest 0.5.

(*Recommended nutrient intakes for Canadians.* [1983]. Ottawa: Bureau of Nutritional Sciences.)

T A B L E   D - 2

Canadian Recommended Nutrient Intake Based on Age and Body Weight Expressed as Daily Rates

Age	Sex	Weight (kg)	Protein (g)	Vitamin A (RE*)	Vitamin D (µg)	Vitamin E (mg)	Vitamin C (mg)	Folate (µg)	Vitamin B₁₂ (µg)	Calcium (mg)	Phosphorus (mg)	Magnesium (mg)	Iron (mg)	Iodine (µg)	Zinc (mg)
Months															
0–4	Both	6.0	12†	400	10	3	20	25	0.3	250‡	150	20	0.3§	30	2§
5–12	Both	9.0	12	400	10	3	20	40	0.4	400	200	32	7	40	3
Years															
1	Both	11	13	400	10	3	20	40	0.5	500	300	40	6	55	4
2–3	Both	14	16	400	5	4	20	50	0.6	550	350	50	6	65	4
4–6	Both	18	19	500	5	5	25	70	0.8	600	400	65	8	85	5
7–9	M	25	26	700	2.5	7	25	90	1.0	700	500	100	8	110	7
	F	25	26	700	2.5	6	25	90	1.0	700	500	100	8	95	7
10–12	M	34	34	800	2.5	8	25	120	1.0	900	700	130	8	125	9
	F	36	36	800	2.5	7	25	130	1.0	1100	800	135	8	110	9
13–15	M	50	49	900	2.5	9	30‖	175	1.0	1100	900	185	10	160	12
	F	48	46	800	2.5	7	30‖	170	1.0	1000	850	180	13	160	9
16–18	M	62	58	1000	2.5	10	40‖	220	1.0	900	1000	230	10	160	12
	F	53	47	800	2.5	7	30‖	190	1.0	700	850	200	12	160	9
19–24	M	71	61	1000	2.5	10	40‖	220	1.0	800	1000	240	9	160	12
	F	58	50	800	2.5	7	30‖	180	1.0	700	850	200	13	160	9
25–49	M	74	64	1000	2.5	9	40‖	230	1.0	800	1000	250	9	160	12
	F	59	51	800	2.5	6	30‖	185	1.0	700	850	200	13	160	9
50–74	M	73	63	1000	5	7	40‖	230	1.0	800	1000	250	9	160	12
	F	63	54	800	5	6	30‖	195	1.0	800	850	210	8	160	9
75+	M	69	59	1000	5	6	40‖	215	1.0	800	1000	230	9	160	12
	F	64	55	800	5	5	30‖	200	1.0	800	850	210	8	160	9
Pregnancy (additional)															
1st trimester			5	0	2.5	2	0	200	0.2	500	200	15	0	25	6
2nd trimester			15	0	2.5	2	10	200	0.2	500	200	45	5	25	6
3rd trimester			24	0	2.5	2	10	200	0.2	500	200	45	10	25	6
Lactation (additional)			20	400	2.5	3	25	100	0.2	500	200	65	0	50	6

* Retinol equivalents

† Protein is assumed to be from breast milk and must be adjusted for infant formula.

‡ Infant formula with high phosphorus should contain 375 mg calcium.

§ Breast milk is assumed to be the source of the mineral.

‖ Smokers should increase vitamin C by 50%.

(Minister of National Health and Welfare. [1990]. *Nutrition recommendations: Report of the Scientific Review Committee* [p. 204]. Ottawa: Author.)

Glossary

Abduction: lateral movement of the body part away from the midline of the body

Abrasion: wound that results from scraping or rubbing off skin or mucous membrane

Abscess: localized collection of pus

Absorption: process by which drugs are transferred from the site of entry into the body to the bloodstream

Abstinence: refraining from sexual activity, particularly sexual intercourse; a method of birth control

Accommodation: (1) ability to adjust the eye to see at various distances; (2) process by which intellectual acts are changed to handle increasingly complex information

Accreditation: process by which an educational program is evaluated and then recognized as having met certain predetermined standards of education

Acid: substance containing a hydrogen ion that can be liberated or released

Acidosis: condition characterized by a proportionate excess of hydrogen ions in the extracellular fluid, in which the pH falls below 7.35

Acne: skin condition due to inflammation and infection of sebaceous glands

Acquired immunodeficiency syndrome (AIDS): fatal condition in which the body's immune system is rendered ineffective as a result of infection by the retrovirus HIV

Active exercise: joint movement activated by the person

Active immunity: antibodies against harmful effects of microorganisms or toxins that are self-produced

Active transport: movement of ions or molecules across cell membranes, usually against a pressure gradient and with the expenditure of metabolic energy

Activities of daily living (ADLs): normal tasks of daily life

Acupressure: application of pressure or massage, or both, to usual acupuncture sites

Acupuncture: technique that uses long, thin needles to prick specific parts of the body to produce insensitivity to pain

Acute illness: rapidly occurring illness that runs its course, allowing the person to return to his or her previous level of functioning

Acute pain: episode of pain that lasts for seconds to less than 6 months

Adaptation: continuous change and adjustment of living things to other living things and to environmental conditions

Addictive: substance to which a person develops a psychological and physiologic dependency

Adduction: movement of a body part toward the midline of the body

Admitting: (1) act of entering something into a system; (2) department that enters a client into a health care facility

Adolescence: period of develop-

ment between childhood and adulthood, characterized by the onset of puberty

Adolescent: period from age 12 to 18 years

Adult day-care centers: centers providing day-care service (including recreation and nutrition) for older adults

Advance directive: written directive that allows people to state in advance what their choices for health care would be if certain circumstances should develop

Adventitious breath sounds: abnormal breath sound heard over the lungs

Advocacy: protection and support of another's rights

Aerobic bacteria: bacteria that require oxygen to live and grow

Aerobic exercise: exercise that promotes cardiovascular fitness; it increases blood flow, heart rate, and the metabolic demand for oxygen over a period of time

Affective learning: changes in attitudes, values, and feelings

Ageism: attitudes that stereotype the older adult on the basis of chronologic age

Agglutinin: antibody that causes a clumping of specific antigens

Agnostic: person who holds that nothing can be known about the existence of a god

Albuminuria: albumin in the urine; indication of kidney disease

Alkali: substance that can accept or trap a hydrogen ion; synonym for base

Alkalosis: condition, characterized by a proportionate lack of hydrogen ions in the extracellular fluid concentration, in which the pH exceeds 7.45

Alopecia: baldness

Alternative care: general term used to identify various methods of non-hospital health care, including residential housing, day-care, respite care, hospice, and extended-care facilities

Alveoli: small air sacs at the end of the terminal bronchioles that are the site of gas exchange

Alzheimer's disease: type of dementia in which discrete patches of brain tissue degenerate; this devastating disease eventually affects all body systems

Ambulatory care centers: health care settings, either hospital or community-based, that provide a wide variety of services (medical, surgical, mental health, drug related)

Ambulatory surgery: surgery performed on an outpatient basis, with admission and discharge the same day; also known as *same-day* or *outpatient surgery*

Amino acid: basic building blocks used to manufacture protein and the end products of protein digestion

Ampule: glass flask containing a single dose of medication for parenteral administration

Anaerobic bacteria: bacteria that can live without oxygen

Anaerobic exercise: exercise in which the supply of oxygen is less than the demand created by contracting muscles; oxygen debt results

Analgesic drug: pharmaceutical agent used to relieve pain

Anaphylactic reaction: severe reaction occurring immediately after exposure to a drug; characterized by respiratory distress and vascular collapse

Androgen: steroid hormone (eg, androsterone, testosterone) produced primarily by the testes in males but also produced to a lesser extent by the adrenal glands in both sexes and the ovaries in the female

Andropause: midlife decrease in androgen levels in men; men remain capable of reproduction

Anion: ion that carries a negative electric charge

Ankylosis: fixation or immobilization of a joint

Anorexia: lack or loss of appetite for food

Anorexia nervosa: eating disorder characterized by the denial of appetite and bizarre eating habits

Anoxia: absence of oxygen

Antagonistic effect: combined effect of two or more drugs that produces less than the effect of each drug alone

Anterior fontanelle: diamond-shaped membrane-covered space remaining *at* the junction of the frontal and parietal bone sutures in a fetus or infant

Anthropometric: measurements of the body and body parts

Antibacterial: agent that kills bacteria or suppresses their growth

Antibody: immunoglobin produced by the body in response to a specific antigen

Anticipatory guidance: identification of expected learning needs that commonly arise as a result of past or current health problems

Antigen: foreign material capable of inducing a specific immune response

Antipyretic: agent that reduces fever

Antiseptic: substance that inhibits the growth of bacteria

Anuria: technically, no urine voided; 24-hour urine output is less than 100 mL; synonyms are *complete kidney shutdown* and *renal failure*

Anxiety: vague sense of impending doom or apprehension precipitated by new and unknown experiences

Apical-radial pulse rate: rates counted simultaneously for 1 minute at the apex of the heart and at the radial artery

Apnea: absence of breathing

Approximate: to bring the two edges of a wound together (usu-

ally held together with suture materials)

Arousal: condition in which the cortical area of the brain receives and responds appropriately to stimuli

Arousal threshold: intensity of stimulus required to produce awakening

Arrhythmia: irregular pattern of heartbeats; synonym for *dysrhythmia*

Arterial blood gas analysis: examination of arterial blood to determine the pressure exerted by oxygen and carbon dioxide in the blood and the blood's pH

Ascites: accumulation of fluid in the peritoneal cavity

Asepsis: absence of disease-producing microorganisms; being free of infection

Assault: threat or an attempt to make bodily contact with another person without that person's permission

Assertiveness: ability to stand up for oneself and others using open, honest, and direct communication

Assessing: systematic and continuous collection, validation, and communication of client data

Assimilation: process by which a person interprets information to fit the current level of cognition

Asymmetry: lack of symmetry of parts or organs on opposite sides of the body

Atelectasis: incomplete expansion or collapse of the lungs

Atheist: person who denies the existence of a god

Atrioventricular node (AV node): tissue at the base of the atrial septum that normally picks up the electric current from the sinoatrial node

Atrophy: decrease in the size of a body structure

Attachment: active, affectionate, reciprocal relationship between two persons

Attitude: feeling or emotion, generally including a positive or negative judgment toward people, objects, or ideas

Auditory: pertaining to hearing

Auscultation: listening for sounds within the body

Authoritative knowledge: knowledge that comes from an expert and is accepted as truth based on a perceived level of expertise

Autocratic leadership: leadership style in which the leader assumes complete control over the decisions and activities of the group

Autonomy: self-determination; being independent and self-governing

Bandage: piece of gauze or other material used to cover a wound

Barium enema: x-ray visualization of the large intestine after the introduction of barium into the lower intestine

Basal metabolism: amount of energy required to carry out involuntary activities of the body at rest

Base: substance that can accept or trap a hydrogen ion; synonym for *alkali*

Base of support: foundation that provides stability for an object

Basic human needs: something essential to the health and survival of humans; common to all people

Battery: assault that is carried out

Bedsore: area of cellular necrosis caused by a lack of circulation to the involved area; synonym for *pressure* or *decubitus ulcer*

Beliefs: special class of intellectual attitudes based primarily on faith as opposed to fact

Beneficence: principle of doing good

Bereavement: state of grieving or going through the grief process

Bigeminal pulse: pulse rhythm in which every two pulsations is followed by a pause

Bilateral: pertaining to two sides of the body

Binder: type of bandage, usually designed to fit a large body area

Biomedical ethics: discipline that applies general ethical theories to the field of biomedicine

Biopsy: removal of a piece of tissue for microscopic examination

Biot's respirations: respirations of the same depth followed by a period of apnea

Bisexuality: having sexual feelings for people of both sexes

Blended family: two single-parent families joined together to form a new family unit

Blood pressure: force of blood against arterial walls

Blood transfusion: infusion of whole blood from a healthy person into a recipient

Body fluid: liquid part of the body consisting of both water and its solutes

Body image: how a person experiences his or her body

Body language: nonverbal communication

Body mechanics: efficient use of the body as a machine and as a means of locomotion

Body substance isolation (BSI): type of isolation that considers all body substances as potentially infective regardless of a person's diagnosis

Body water: liquid part of the body consisting of water only

Bolus: single injection of a concentrated solution administered intravenously

Bounding pulsation: pulse that reaches a higher level than normal and then quickly disappears

Bowel movement: emptying of the intestinal tract; synonym for *defecation*

Bowel training program: program that manipulates factors within a person's control (timing of defecation, exercise, diet) to produce a regular pattern of comfortable defecation without medication or enemas

Bradycardia: slow heart rate

Bradypnea: abnormally slow rate of breathing

Brief pain: pain that passes quickly; synonym for *transient pain*

Bronchodilator: medication that relaxes contractions of smooth muscles of the bronchioles

Bronchoscope: lighted, tubular instrument used for visual examination of the bronchi

Bronchoscopy: visual examination of the trachea and bronchi

Bronchovesicular: normal breath sounds heard over the mainstem bronchus

Bruit: unusual sound, usually abnormal, heard in auscultation

Buffer: substance that prevents body fluid from becoming overly acid or alkaline

Bulimia: eating disorder characterized by episodes of gorging followed by purging; often occurs in conjunction with anorexia nervosa

Burnout: behaviors exhibited as the result of prolonged occupational stress

Calorie: measure of heat, or energy; *kilocalorie*, commonly referred to as a calorie, defined as the amount of heat required to raise 1 kg of water 1°C

Capillarity: process by which a liquid at the point of contact with a solid rises; synonym for *capillary action*

Caput succedaneum: localized edema, congestion, and petechiae on the fetal and neonatal scalp, crossing suture lines

Cardiac output: volume of blood pumped from the left ventricle per minute

Cardinal signs: body temperature, pulse and respiratory rates, and blood pressure; synonym for *vital signs*

Cardiogenic shock: shock caused by a decrease in cardiac output

Caregiver burden: stress responses experienced during prolonged periods of home care by family caregivers

Caries: cavitation of the teeth

Carrier: person or animal that is without signs of illness but that has pathogens on or within the body that can be transferred to others

Cartilage: noninvasive connective tissue found in the joints as well as in the nose, ear, thorax, trachea, and larynx

Category-specific isolation sys-

tem: type of isolation system that groups infectious diseases that require similar infection control techniques together

Cathartic: medication that strongly increases gastrointestinal motility and promotes defecation

Catheter: tube for injecting or removing fluids

Cation: ion that carries a positive electric charge

Cellular fluid: fluid within the cell; synonym for *intracellular fluid*

Center of gravity: point at which the mass of an object is centered

Centers for Disease Control (CDC): U.S. government agency whose responsibilities include investigation, identification, prevention, and control of disease

Central venous catheter: venous access device usually introduced into the subclavian or internal jugular veins and passed to the superior vena cava just above the right atrium

Certification: process by which a person who has met certain criteria established by a non-governmental association is granted recognition

Cerumen: heavy, brown, waxy secretion in the external canal of the ear that is secreted by the ceruminous glands

Ceruminous gland: gland found in the external auditory canal that secretes a substance called *cerumen*

Change: process of transforming, altering, or modifying something

Change agent: person who purposefully and systematically implements change

Change of shift report: communication method used by nurses completing care for a client to transmit client information to nurses about to assume responsibility for continuing care; may be exchanged verbally in a meeting or audiotaped

Channel: a term used in communication theory to denote the medium selected to convey the message; the channel may

target any of the receiver's senses

Charting by exception: shorthand method for documenting client data that is based on well-defined standards of practice; only exceptions to these standards are documented in narrative notes

Chemical name: precise description of a drug's chemical composition

Cheyne-Stokes respirations: gradual increase and then gradual decrease in depth of respirations followed by a period of apnea

Child abuse: intentional, nonaccidental physical or mental abuse of a child by a parent or other caregiver

Chiropodist: one who treats foot disorders; synonym for *podiatrist*

Chiropody: health discipline that deals with the treatment of foot disorders; synonym for *podiatry*

Cholecystogram: x-ray examination of the gallbladder

Cholesterol: fat-like substance found only in animal tissues; it is important for cell membrane structure, a precursor of steroid hormones, and a constituent of bile; high serum cholesterol levels are a risk factor in the development of atherosclerosis

Chronic disorder: illness or condition for which there is no cure; it persists over an extended period (more than 6 months) and often affects one's ability to meet basic needs

Chronic illness: irreversible illness that causes permanent physical impairment and requires long-term health care

Chronic pain: episode of pain that lasts for 6 months or longer; may be intermittent or continuous

Chyme: semifluid state that food is in when it leaves the stomach

Circadian rhythm: rhythm that completes a full cycle every 24 hours; synonym for *diurnal rhythm*

Circadian synchronization: condition existing when a per-

son's sleep–wakefulness patterns follow his or her inner biologic clock

Circulating nurse: nurse working in the operating room who assesses the client, helps position the client for surgery, secures supplies, and maintains count of items used during surgery

Circumduction: moving the distal part of the limb to trace a complete circle while the proximal end of the bone remains fixed

Civil law: rule that regulates relationships among people; synonym for *private law*

Cleft lip: congenital fissure, or split, in lip

Cleft palate: congenital fissure, or split, in the roof of the mouth (ie, the palate)

Client: person requiring health care

Client goal: statement describing an expected client outcome

Closed wound: injury in which there is no break in the skin

Clubbing: rounding and swelling of nailbeds

Cognition: cerebral functioning; process of perceiving and understanding one's world

Cognitive learning: storing and recalling of new knowledge in the brain

Cohabitating family: people who choose to live together for various reasons; includes unmarried adults, communes, group marriages, and gay or lesbian relationships

Coitus: sexual activity in which the penis is placed in the vagina; synonym for *sexual intercourse*

Coitus interruptus: method of contraception; the penis is removed from the vagina before ejaculation

Cold: relative state meaning the absence of heat

Collaborative problem: actual or potential health problem that may occur from complications of disease, diagnostic studies, or the treatment regimen; the nurse works together with other members of the health care team toward its resolution

Colloid osmotic pressure: pressure exerted by plasma proteins on permeable membranes in the body; synonym for *oncotic pressure*

Colon: section of the large intestine from the cecum to the rectum

Colonization: harmless growth of microorganisms in or on the body

Colonoscopy: visual examination of the entire large intestine

Common law: law resulting from court decisions that is then followed when other cases involving similar circumstances and facts arise; common law is as binding as civil law

Communication: process of sharing information; process of generating and transmitting meanings

Compensation: substitution of what is perceived as a good for a perceived weakness

Competence: way a person performs the tasks or role expectations that are important to him or her

Complaint: legal statement of the plaintiff's claim; once filed, it initiates legal proceedings

Complete proteins: proteins that contain all the essential amino acids in sufficient quantities for protein synthesis to occur; also termed *high-biologic-value proteins*

Compliance: act of completing what is expected

Compress: several layers of moist, absorbent cloth or gauze folded to cover a small body area

Computerized nursing care plan: plan of client care developed by computer software programs that enable the nurse to call up screens listing causes, goals, and related nursing interventions for nursing diagnoses and medical diagnoses

Computed tomography (CT): scanning procedure that produces a cross-sectional image of a body part and reflects various tissue densities

Concept: abstract images that are formed as impressions from the environment and organized into symbols of reality

Conceptual framework model: set of concepts, along with the statements that arrange the concepts into an understandable pattern

Concurrent audit: evaluation of nursing care and client outcomes conducted while the client is receiving care; may use direct observation of nursing care, client interview, and chart review

Condom catheter: tube for draining urine; it connects a device applied externally to the penis to a collection bag

Conduction: transfer of heat to another object during direct contact

Confidentiality: respecting privileged information

Congenital anomaly: absence of, deformity in, or excess of body parts present at birth and resulting from faulty in utero development or chromosomal abnormality

Congenital syphilis: a sexually transmitted disease, acquired by an infant in utero from an infected mother; the disease is passed from mother to infant across the placenta

Congestion: presence of excessive fluids or secretions in an organ or body tissue

Constant fever: body temperature that remains consistently elevated and fluctuates less than 2°C (3.5°F); sometimes called a *continuing fever*

Constipation: passage of dry, hard, fecal material

Continuing care retirement community: self-contained retirement agencies that provide services to the elderly clients; designed to serve residents as their needs change with illness and increasing age

Continuity of care: coordination of services provided to clients before they enter a health care setting, during the time they are in the setting, and after they leave the setting

Continuous subcutaneous infusion (CSI): method for delivery of small doses of narcotics or opioids that is controlled by an infusion pump and absorbed from subcutaneous tissue

Continuum: graduated scale

Contraception: prevention of conception or pregnancy; also used to describe methods used for birth control

Contract: exchange of promises between two parties

Contractual agreement: pact made between two persons for the achievement of mutually set goals

Contracture: permanent contraction state of a muscle

Contralateral stimulation: stimulation to an area opposite the affected area

Contusion: wound in which the skin remains intact; often called a *bruise*

Convalescent period: stage of an infection that represents recovery from the infection

Convection: dissemination of heat by motion between areas of unequal density

Coping mechanism: patterns of behavior used to neutralize, deny, or counteract anxiety

Core temperature: temperature of internal areas of the body

Counseling: giving guidance, assisting with problem solving

Crackles: noncontinuous sounds that occur when air moves through airways that contain fluid; formerly called *rales*

Credentialing: general term that refers to ways in which professional competence is maintained

Crenation: process of losing fluid from a red blood cell, which eventually results in a shrunken, knobbed cell because of loss in intracellular water

Crime: offense against people or property; the act is considered to be against the government, referred to in a lawsuit as "the people," and the accused is prosecuted by the state

Crisis: (1) point at which body temperature drops rapidly to normal; (2) occurs when coping and defense mechanisms are no longer effective, resulting in high levels of anxiety, disorganized behavior, and the inability to function normally

Crisis intervention: five-step problem-solving technique to promote adaptation and improve future coping

Crisis intervention centers: centers that provide counseling or psychotherapy to reduce stress and facilitate coping in people in a life crisis

Criteria: specified behavior; for example, the measurable criteria in a client goal specifies how the client must perform the desired behavior

Crossmatching: act of determining the compatibility of two blood specimens

Cue: significant data that is helpful in making decisions

Cultural assimilation: process that occurs when a minority group, living as part of a dominant group within a culture, loses the cultural characteristics that made it different

Cultural care deprivation: a lack of culturally assistive, supportive, or facilitative acts in the health care setting

Cultural imposition: tendency of some to impose their beliefs, practices, and values on another culture because they believe that their ideas are superior to those of another person or group

Culture: sum total of human behavior or social characteristics peculiar to a specific group and passed from generation to generation or from one to another within the group

Culture shock: those feelings, usually negative, a person experiences when placed in a different culture

Cumulative effect: occurs when the body cannot metabolize a drug before additional doses are administered

Cunnilingus: kissing, sucking, and licking female genitalia, particularly the vulva, clitoris, and vaginal introitus

Cupping: manual percussion of lung areas to loosen pulmonary secretions

Cutaneous pain: superficial pain usually involving the skin or subcutaneous tissue

Cutaneous stimulation: pain relief methods that use stimulation of the skin by massage, application of heat or cold, vibration, and pressure

Cyanosis: bluish coloring of the skin and mucous membranes

Cystoscopy: direct visual examination of the bladder, ureteral orifices, and urethra with a cystoscope

Cytologic study: study of cells and fluids from the body

Dandruff: condition characterized by itching and flaking of the scalp

Dangling: position in which the person sits on the edge of the bed with the legs and feet over the side of the bed

Data: information

Data base: all the pertinent client information that enables a comprehensive and effective plan of care to be designed and implemented for the client

Data cluster: grouping of client data or cues that points to the existence of a client health problem

Day-care center: centers that provide care for infants, children, elderly people, and people with special health care needs

Death: termination of life and its related clinical signs

Débridement: cleaning away of infected and devitalized tissue from a wound

Decubitus ulcer: area of cellular necrosis caused by a lack of circulation to the involved area; synonym for *pressure ulcer* and *bedsore*

Deductive reasoning: thinking in which a general or broad idea is examined and then specific ideas or actions are considered

Defamation: wrongs of slander and libel; making derogatory remarks about one person to another

Defecation: emptying of the intestinal tract; synonym for *bowel movement*

Defendant: person accused of a tort or crime

Defense mechanisms: forms of self-deception; unconscious process the self uses to protect itself from anxiety or threats to self-esteem

Dehiscence: separation of the layers of a surgical wound; may be partial, superficial, or a complete disruption of the surgical wound

Dehydration: decreased water volume

Delta sleep: deep sleep, occurring during stage III and especially stage IV in NREM sleep

Dementia: organic impairment of intellectual functioning, gradually leading to interference with social or occupational functioning, memory, and often personality integration

Democratic leadership: leadership style characterized by a sense of equality between the leader and followers

Denial: refusal to acknowledge some truth; form of self-deception

Dentition: complement of natural teeth in place in the alveoli of the dental arch

Denver Development Screening Test (DDST): screening test for determining atypical developmental patterns in infants and children

Deontological: ethical system in which actions are right or wrong independent of the consequences they produce

Dependent intervention: nursing action carried out at the instruction or order of an authorized health care professional other than a nurse; synonym for *physician-initiated* or *physician-prescribed intervention*

Dependent variables: factors in a research study that alter in response to independent variables

Depilatory: agent that destroys hair shafts or mechanically removes hair

Depolarize: to destroy polarity

Deposition: legal testimonies; may be given by the plaintiff, defendants, fact witnesses, and expert witnesses

Dermis: underlying portion of the skin

Development: increase in the complexity of function and progression to skill advancement

Development theory: theory to describe the orderly and predictable process of the growth and development of humans, individualized by social, biologic, and environmental factors

Developmental crisis: predictable patterns of behavior and change occurring throughout the lifespan

Development delay: measure of development that lags behind the normal range for a given age

Developmental task: successful achievement of psychomotor, psychosocial, or cognitive skills at certain periods in life; failure to obtain the developmental task can lead to unhappiness and difficulty with later tasks

Diagnosis: analysis of client data to identify client strengths and health problems that independent nursing intervention can prevent or resolve

Diagnostic related groups (DRGs): classification of clients by major medical diagnosis for the purpose of standardizing health care costs (see *prospective payment*)

Diarrhea: passage of liquid and unformed stools

Diastolic pressure: least amount of pressure exerted on arterial walls, which occurs when the heart is at rest between ventricular contractions

Diffuse pain: pain that covers a large area

Diffusion: tendency of solutes to move freely throughout a sol-

vent from an area of higher concentration to an area of lower concentration until equilibrium is established

Diluent: liquid used to reconstitute powdered medications

Direct transfusion: infusion of blood while it is being taken from the donor

Disaccharides: double sugars composed of two monosaccharides; the most common disaccharides are sucrose (table sugar), lactose (milk sugar), and maltose (grain sugar)

Discharge planning: systematic process of preparing the client to leave the health care facility and for maintaining continuity of care

Discharge summary: description of where the client stands in relation to problems identified in the record at discharge; documents any special teaching or counseling the client received, including referrals

Discipline: specific and unique body of knowledge that uses existing and new knowledge to creatively solve problems and meet human needs within everchanging boundaries

Disease: pathologic change in the structure or function of the body or mind

Disease-specific isolation system: isolation system that lists each infectious disease separately along with the individual interventions and barriers that are necessary to prevent transmission of that specific pathogenic organism

Disinfectant: substance, usually intended for use on inanimate objects, that destroys pathogens but not spores

Disinfection: process by which pathogens but not spores are destroyed

Displacement substitution of more acceptable behavior for an unacceptable behavior

Distribution: movement of drugs by the circulatory system to the site of action

Diurnal enuresis: involuntary

urination that occurs during wakefulness

Documentation: written, legal record of all pertinent interventions with the client—assessments, diagnoses, plans, interventions, and evaluations

Dominant group: group within a culture that has the authority to control the value system and determine the rewards of the system; usually the largest group in a society

Donor: person who donates blood to be given to another person

Dorsal position: position in which the client lies flat on his or her back with legs together

Dorsal recumbent position: position in which the client is placed on his or her back close to the edge of the bed with the legs separated and knees flexed

Dorsiflexion: backward bending of the hand or foot

Down's syndrome: congenital conditions characterized by physical malformations and some degree of mental retardation; caused by a defect in chromosome 21; also called *trisomy 21 syndrome*

Dressing: protective covering placed over a wound

Drug: substance that modifies body functions when taken into the living organism; synonym for *medication*

Drug allergy: hypersensitivity caused by previous exposure to a medication; may occur immediately or be delayed; manifestations range from mild to severe

Drug tolerance: tendency of the body to become accustomed to a drug over time; larger doses are required to produce the desired effects

Dry cough: forceful expiratory effort; also known as *nonproductive cough*

Dull pain: gnawing discomfort less intense and acute than sharp pain

Durable Power of Attorney for Health Care: advance directive that appoints an agent a person trusts to make decisions about health care in the event of the appointing person's incapacity

Dynorphin: recently discovered opioid that appears to have potent analgesic activity

Dyspareunia: painful coitus that occurs most often in women and rarely in men

Dyspnea: difficult breathing

Dysrhythmia: irregular pattern of heartbeats; synonym for *arrhythmia*

Dysuria: difficulty in voiding; may or may not be associated with pain; a feeling of warm local irritation occurring during voiding is called *burning*

Ecchymosis: collection of blood in subcutaneous tissues that causes a purplish discoloration

Edema: accumulation of fluid in extracellular spaces

Ego integrity/despair: last stage of life according to Erikson, which begins around age 60. The stage is characterized as a time to review one's life and find wholeness and acceptance, or unresolved problems and missed opportunities

Ejaculation: expulsion of semen from the penis resulting from stimulation from sexual arousal

Elective surgery: surgery that is recommended but can be omitted or delayed without catastrophe

Electrocardiogram (ECG; EKG): graphic record produced by the electrocardiograph

Electrocardiograph: instrument that measures and records electric impulses of the heart

Electroencephalogram (EEG): graphic record produced by the electroencephalograph

Electroencephalograph: instrument that measures and records electric impulses of the brain

Electrolyte: substance capable of breaking into ions and developing an electric charge when dissolved in solution

Electromyograph (EMG): instrument that records muscle tone

Electronic infusion device: automatically regulates the amount of fluid infused intravenously at any one time and signals by way of an alarm system when air is in the tubing, flow is obstructed, or the solution level of the bottle or bag is getting lower

Electronic medical record: computer-generated medical record; may use any of several information software programs to store client data

Electrooculogram: recording of the electric current or potential produced by eye movements

Embolism: blocking of an artery by a blood clot or by other foreign matter brought to the site by the blood flow

Embolus: foreign body or air in the circulatory system; plural form is *emboli*

Emergency surgery: surgery that must be performed immediately to save the person's life or a body organ

Emollient: agent that soothes and softens the part of the body to which it is applied; usually applies to agents affecting the body surface

Empathy: intellectually identifying with the way another person feels

Empty nest syndrome: feeling of loss after all children have moved away from home

Endogenous: infection in which the causative organism comes from microbial life the person himself or herself harbors

Endorphins: morphine-like substances released by the body that appear to alter the perception of pain

Endoscope: flexible or rigid lighted tube that allows direct visual examination of various body cavities and organs

Endoscopic retrograde cholangio-pancreatography (ERCP): injection of a contrast medium through an endoscope for visualization of the pancreatic ducts and the hepatobiliary tree

Endoscopy: direct visualization of hollow organs of the body using an endoscope or flexible, lighted tube

Endotracheal tube: polyvinyl-chloride airway that is inserted through the nose or the mouth into the trachea using a laryngoscope as a guide

Endurance: ability to sustain movement or to perform an activity over time

Enema: introduction of solution into the lower intestinal tract

Enkephalins: opioids that are widespread throughout the brain and dorsal horn of the spinal cord and are believed to reduce pain sensation by inhibiting the release of substance P

Enteral nutrition: alternate form of feeding that involves passing a tube into the gastrointestinal tract to allow instillation of the appropriate formula

Enuresis: involuntary urination; most often used to refer to a child who involuntarily urinates during the night

Environment: condition of both internal and external physical factors affecting and influencing the growth and development of the person

Epidermis: a superficial portion of the skin

Epidural analgesia: means of providing pain relief with an opioid injection delivered by way of a catheter inserted in the midlumbar region into the epidural space

Erect position: position in which the client stands

Erectile failure: condition in which a man is unable to attain or maintain an erection to such an extent that he cannot have satisfactory coitus; synonym for *impotence*

Erection: condition that results when erectile tissue of the penis fills with blood as a result of stimulation

Erogenous zones: areas of the body that produce sexual desire and arousal when stimulated

Esophagogastroduodenoscopy: visual examination of the esophagus, stomach, and duodenum; also called *gastroscopy*

Essential hypertension: abnormally elevated blood pressure with no known cause; synonym for *primary hypertension*

Ethics: system dealing with standards of character and behavior related to what is right and wrong

Ethics committee: group of people whose chief functions include education, policy development, case review, and consultation pertinent to ethical issues

Ethics of caring: ethical system that advocates attending and relating to people in a way that prevents their being reduced to the moral status of objects

Ethnic group: minority groups that retain distinct customs, language, or social values as a result of a common heritage

Ethnicity: sense of identification that a cultural group collectively has; the sharing of common and unique cultural and social beliefs and behavior patterns, including language and dialect, religious practices, literature, folklore, music, political interests, food preferences, and employment patterns

Ethnocentrism: judgment of other people based on the standards and practices of one's own culture

Euphoria: unrealistic sense of well-being

Eupnea: normal respirations

Euthanasia: mercy killing; the deliberate termination of the life of a person

Evaluating: measurement of the extent to which the client has achieved the goals specified in the plan of care; factors that positively or negatively influence goal achievement are identified, and the plan of care is terminated or revised

Evaporation: conversion of liquid to a vapor

Evisceration: protrusion of viscera through an incisional area

Excretion: removal of a drug from the body

Excruciating pain: pain that could be described to range between 8 and 10 on a scale of 1 to 10; synonym for *severe pain*

Exhalation: act of breathing out; synonym is *expiration*

Exit from the reservoir: point of escape for organisms from a reservoir

Exogenous: infection in which the causative organism is acquired from outside the host

Expectorant: drug that facilitates the removal of respiratory secretions

Expert witness: nurse who explains to the judge and jury what happened based on the client's record and who offers an opinion as to whether the nursing care met acceptable standards of practice

Expiration: act of breathing out; synonym for *exhalation*

Expiratory reserve volume (ERV): additional amount of air that can be exhaled beyond tidal volume

Extended-care facility: type of care given after hospitalization of acute illness; includes residential care and intermediate or skilled nursing home care

Extended family: nuclear family and other related people

Extension: state of being in a straight line

External respiration: act of lung ventilation, oxygen absorption, and carbon dioxide elimination

External rotation: body part turning on its axis away from the midline of the body

Extracellular fluid (ECF): fluid outside the cells; includes intravascular and interstitial fluids

Extraneous variables: unknown factors that affect research outcomes

Exudate: fluid and cells that escape from blood vessels of wounds (drainage)

Fact witness: nurse who has knowledge of the actual incident prompting a legal case; bases testimony on firsthand knowledge of the incident not on assumptions

Failure to thrive (FTT): physical and developmental retardation of infants or children resulting from physical or emotional neglect

Faith: (1) spiritual dimensions of a person's life regardless of religious affiliation; (2) confident belief in something for which there is no proof or material evidence

False imprisonment: unjustifiable retention or prevention of the movement of another person without proper consent

Fasting state: abstinence from food and fluids

Fatty acids: structural components of fats

Feces: intestinal waste products

Feedback: verbal and nonverbal evidence that the message is received and understood

Fellatio: kissing, sucking, and licking the male genitalia, particularly the scrotum and penis

Felony: (1) crime punishable by imprisonment in a state or federal penitentiary for more than 1 year; (2) crime of greater offense than a misdemeanor

Fertilization: process in reproduction by which the male sperm unites with the female ovum

Fetishism: practice of arousing sexual desires with inanimate objects

Fever: elevation above the upper limit of normal body temperature; synonym for *pyrexia*

Fiber: all dietary plant material that is not digestible by gastrointestinal tract, enzymes, and secretions

Fidelity: keeping promises and commitments made to others

Fight-or-flight response: the body prepares itself against threat, to either resist (fight) or evade (flight) the danger

Filtration: passage of a fluid through a permeable membrane whose spaces do not allow certain solutes to pass; passage is from an area of higher pressure to one of lower pressure

Filtration pressure: difference between colloid osmotic pressure and blood hydrostatic pressure

Fingerprint: impression of an examiner's fingerprints on the skin made by applying pressure over the sternum

Fitness: degree of physical functioning characterized by physical strength, flexibility, endurance, and strong cardiovascular functioning

Flaccidity: decreased muscle tone; synonym for *hypotonicity*

Flatulence: excessive formation of gases in the gastrointestinal tract

Flatus: intestinal gas

Flexibility: ability to use a muscle through its entire range of motion

Flexion: state of being bent

Flowsheets: graphic record of abbreviated aspects of client's condition (eg, vital signs, routine aspects of care)

Fluid balance: state in which water and its solutes in the body are in normal proportions and concentrations and are in appropriate body compartments

Fluid imbalance: state in which water and its solutes in the body are in improper proportions and concentrations or are improperly located in body compartments

Fluid volume deficit: deficiency in the amount of both water and electrolytes in extracellular fluid; water and electrolyte proportions remain near normal

Fluid volume excess: excessive retention of water and sodium in extracellular fluid in near-normal proportions

Fluoroscopy: radiologic visualization of motion without its being recorded on film

Flushing: red appearance of the skin

Foley catheter: tube introduced through the urethra into the bladder for the purpose of withdrawing urine

Fomite: inanimate object other than food that can absorb and transmit infectious material

Food and Drug Administration (FDA): federal agency that has responsibility for enforcing federal regulations concerning the manufacture and distribution of food, drugs, and cosmetics to protect consumers against the sale of impure or dangerous substances

Footdrop: complication resulting from extended plantar flexion

Forced vital capacity (FVC): maximal amount of air that can be inhaled followed by a fast maximal forced exhalation with the greatest effort

Foreplay: activity engaged in before sexual intercourse to further stimulate sexual arousal

Formal teaching: planned teaching based on learner objectives

Fowler's position: semisitting position with the head of the bed raised 45 to 60 degrees

Fraud: willful and purposeful misrepresentation that could cause, or has caused, loss or harm to people or property

Fremitus: vibration of the chest wall that can be palpated during the physical examination

Frequency: increased incidence of voiding

Friction rub: crackling sounds heard in the chest cavity caused by inflamed pleura rubbing against the chest wall

Full stage of infection: stage of an infection characterized by the presence of specific signs and symptoms

Functional health: level of health defined by one's ability to carry out usual and desired daily activities

Functional incontinence: state in which a person experiences an involuntary, unpredictable passage of urine

Fungi: plant-like organisms (molds and yeasts) that also can cause infection.

Gastric gavage: introduction of nourishment into the stomach by mechanical means

Gastroenteritis: inflammation of the lining of the stomach and the intestine resulting from irritation, allergic reaction to foods, or emotional upset

Gate control theory: theory that explains that excitatory pain stimuli carried by small-diameter nerve fibers can be blocked by inhibiting signals carried by large-diameter nerve fibers

Gay: commonly used term that is synonymous with *homosexual*

General adaptation syndrome (GAS): biochemical model of stress describing the body's general response to stress

General anesthesia: anesthetic drugs that produce narcosis, relaxation of skeletal muscles, and reduced or absent reflex action

General systems theory: theory that explains how parts of whole things work together in systems, including relations between wholes and parts as they function, behave, and react

Generativity/self-absorption: middle adulthood stage of life according to Erikson that centers around ages 30 to 60, but also continues into older adulthood; stage is characterized by a desire to establish and guide the next generation or by a sense of stagnation and concentration on oneself

Generic name: name assigned by the manufacturer who first develops a drug; it is often derived from the chemical name

Gerontologic nursing: nursing specialty concerned with the care of both the well and the ill older adult

Gerontology: study of all aspects of the aging process and their consequences

Gingiva: tissue surrounding the teeth; gingivae (plural) are often called the *gums*

Gingivitis: inflammation of the gingivae or gums

Glycosuria: presence of sugar in the urine; if due to an unusually large intake of sugar or to marked emotional disturbances and is temporary, there is little cause for alarm

Goal: aim or end; expected outcome

Gonorrhea: highly contagious sexually transmitted bacterial infection of the genitourinary system caused by the organism *Neisseria gonorrhoeae*

Good Samaritan law: law that holds certain health practitioners blameless when undertaking to aid a person in an emergency

Gram-negative bacteria: bacteria with chemically more complex cell walls that can be decolorized by alcohol

Gram-positive bacteria: bacteria with a thick cell wall that resists decolorization (loss of color) and are stained violet

Granulation tissue: new tissue composed of fibroblasts and small blood vessels

Grief: emotional response to loss. *Dysfunctional grief:* distorted or abnormal grief response, including *inhibited grief* (suppression of grief reaction) and *unresolved grief* (lengthy or denied grief reaction). *Abbreviated grief:* short but genuine grief reaction. *Anticipatory grief:* grief reaction before actual loss.

Ground: conducting connection between a source of electricity and the earth

Group process: study of a group's characteristics and ways of functioning

Growth: increase in physical size of an organism or any of its structural organs

Gurgles: continuous musical sounds that are audible in expiration or inspiration, or both; formerly called *rhonchi*

Gustatory: pertaining to taste

Halitosis: offensive breath

Health: state of optimal functioning or well-being

Health-belief model: what people believe to be true about themselves in relation to health

Health maintenance organization (HMO): broad term encompassing various health care delivery systems that use group practice and provide an incentive to use a prepaid comprehensive health care system

Health problem: condition related to health requiring intervention if disease or illness is to be prevented or resolved and coping and wellness are to be promoted

Health risk appraisal: assessment of the total person, identifying both healthy and unhealthy practices

Heat: energy of the motion of molecules of a material

Heave: upward lift or rising of the chest, particularly of the precordial chest area

Helping relationship: interaction that sets the climate of movement of the participants toward common goals

Hematuria: blood in the urine; if present in large enough quantities, urine may be bright red or reddish brown

Hemiplegia: paralysis of half of the body

Hemolysis: process of freeing a red blood cell of its hemoglobin by destruction of the cell membrane

Hemoptysis: sputum containing blood

Hemorrhage: excessive blood loss due to the escape of blood from blood vessels

Hemorrhoids: abnormally distended rectal veins

Heparin lock: intravenous needle or catheter with an injection pad attached at the end

Herpes simplex II (genital herpes): highly contagious viral infection caused by the type 2 strain of the herpes simplex virus (HSV) and transmitted by direct person-to-person contact, particularly sexual

Hesitancy: delay or difficulty in initiating voiding

Heterosexuality: having sexual feelings for a person of the opposite sex

Hiccups: involuntary spasmodic contractions of the diaphragm; synonym for *singultus*

Hierarchy of needs: as defined by Maslow, certain needs are more basic than others; a person strives to at least minimally meet certain needs before attending to others

High-level wellness: functioning to one's maximum potential while maintaining balance and purposeful direction in the environment

Hirsutism: excessive growth of body hair

Holism: concept that views a person as more than the total sum of parts and shows concern and interest in all aspects of the person—physical, psychological, social, and spiritual

Holistic health care: health care that takes into account the whole person interacting in the environment

Holistic nursing care: care given with regard for all the components and human dimensions of a person ("the whole person")

Home health agency: agency, eligible to receive federal funds, that provides home-based care; may be independent, hospital operated, or health department managed

Home health care: that component of a continuum of comprehensive health care whereby health services are provided to individuals and families in their places of residency for the purpose of promoting, maintaining, or restoring health or maximizing the level of independence while minimizing the effects of disability and illness

Homeostasis: various physiologic and psychological mechanisms respond to changes in the internal and external environment to maintain a balanced state

Homeothermic: ability to regulate and maintain body temperature, regardless of environmental temperature

Homosexuality: having sexual feelings for a person of the same sex

Hospice care: provision of care and support to dying clients and their families through spiritual, emotional, and physical interventions

Host: animal or person on or within which microorganisms live

Hot—cold theory: theory that asserts that many diseases, foods, and herbs can be categorized as hot or cold; when there is an imbalance in the body, the proper foods must be taken to rebalance the body

Human dimension: physical, emotional, intellectual, environmental, sociocultural, and spiritual components of a person

Human sexuality: integration of the physical, mental, emotional, and social aspects of a person that denote maleness or femaleness

Humanism: concern and understanding of others that attests to the dignity and worth of all people

Hydration: union of a substance with water; term often is used as the opposite of dehydration, in which case it means that there is normal intracellular and extracellular water volume

Hydrolytic: substance capable of a reaction that takes up water

Hydrometer: instrument used to determine the specific gravity of urine

Hydrostatic pressure: force exerted by a fluid against the container wall

Hygiene: science dealing with the preservation of health and well-being

Hyperalimentation: intravenous infusion of solution that contains sufficient nutrients to support life and maintain normal growth and development; synonym for *total parenteral nutrition*

Hypercalcemia: excess of calcium in the extracellular fluid

Hyperextension: state of exaggerated extension

Hyperkalemia: excess of potassium in the extracellular fluid

Hypermagnesemia: excess of magnesium in the extracellular fluid

Hypernatremia: excess of sodium in the extracellular fluid

Hyperperistalsis: more than 34 bowel sounds per minute

Hyperphosphatemia: above normal serum concentration of inorganic phosphorus

Hyperpyrexia: high fever, above 41°C (105.8°F)

Hypersomnia: condition charac-

terized by excessive sleeping, especially daytime sleeping

Hypertension: blood pressure elevated above the upper limit of normal

Hypertonic: having a greater concentration than the solution with which it is being compared

Hyperventilation: condition in which there is more than the normal amount of air entering and leaving lungs

Hypervolemia: excess of plasma

Hypnosis: technique that produces a subconscious condition accomplished by suggestions made by a hypnotist

Hypnotic: pharmaceutical agent used to induce sleep

Hypocalcemia: insufficient amount of calcium in the extracellular fluid

Hypokalemia: insufficient amount of potassium in the extracellular fluid

Hypomagnesemia: insufficient amount of magnesium in the extracellular fluid

Hyponatremia: insufficient amount of sodium in the extracellular fluid

Hypophosphatemia: below normal serum concentration of inorganic phosphorus

Hypoproteinemia: insufficient amount of protein substances in the extracellular fluid

Hypospadias: developmental anomaly in male infants in which the urethral opening is on the underside of the penis or on the perineum

Hypotension: blood pressure below the lower limit of normal

Hypothermia: body temperature below the lower limit of normal

Hypotonic: having a lesser concentration than the solution with which it is being compared

Hypovolemia: deficiency of plasma

Hypovolemic shock: shock due to a decrease in blood volume

Hypoxemia: deficient oxygenation of blood

Hypoxia: inadequate amount of oxygen available to the cells

Iatrogenic disease: disease caused unintentionally by drug therapy

Iatrogenic infection: infection that occurs as a result of a treatment or diagnostic procedure

Ideal self: self a person would like to be or thinks he or she should be; includes aspirations, moral ideas, and values

Idiosyncratic reaction: unusual, unexpected response to a drug

Ileal conduit: urinary diversion in which the ureters are connected to the ileum with a stoma created on the abdominal wall

Illness: abnormal process in which any aspect of the person's functioning is altered (in comparison to the previous condition of health)

Imagery: pain relief modality that uses mind–body interaction; the imaging of the eradication of the source of the pain or its healing in a pleasurable environment

Immune response: specific reactions in the body as it responds to an invading foreign protein such as bacteria or, in some cases, the body's own proteins

Immunization: process of rendering a person immune or resistant to particular antigenic agents or bacteria

Immunoglobulin: animal protein found in body fluids with known antibody activity and characteristics

Impaction (fecal): collection in the rectum of hardened feces that cannot be passed

Implementing: carrying out the plan of care

Impotence: condition in which a man is unable to attain or maintain an erection to such an extent that he cannot have satisfactory sexual intercourse; synonym for *erectile failure*

Incentive spirometer: equipment to help maximize lung inflation

Incest: practicing sexual behavior between people who are so closely related that marriage between them is legally or culturally not allowed

Incident report: documentation that describes any injury or potential for injury suffered by a client in a health care agency

Incision: wound made with a sharp, cutting instrument

Incomplete proteins: proteins that lack or contain insufficient amounts of all the essential amino acids necessary for protein synthesis; also termed *low-biologic-value proteins*

Incontinence: inability to voluntarily control the discharge of urine or feces

Incubation period: stage of infection that includes the interval between the invasion of the body by the pathogen and the appearance of symptoms of infection

Independent intervention: (1) nursing action carried out at the instruction or order of a nurse; (2) actions within the legal scope of nursing's independent domain; synonym for *nurse-initiated* or *nurse-prescribed intervention*

Independent variables: factors in a research study that differ

Indirect transfusion: infusion of blood from a container in which the donor's blood was received

Individual supply: system of supplying a client's medications for a period of time

Inductive reasoning: pattern of reasoning that begins with specific findings from which general conclusions are drawn (specific to general)

Indwelling catheter: catheter that remains in place for continuous urine drainage; synonym for *Foley catheter*

Infancy: period from 1 month to 1 year of age

Infection: disease state resulting from pathogens in or on the body

Infiltration: escape of fluid into subcutaneous tissue

Inflammatory response: localized response of the body to injury or infection; protective mechanism that eliminates invading pathogens and allows for tissue repair to occur

Informal teaching: unplanned teaching sessions dealing with the client's immediate learning needs and concerns

Informed consent: knowledgeable, voluntary permission obtained from a client to perform a specific test or procedure

Inguinal hernia: abnormal protrusion of the intestine or omentum through a weak point in the abdominal wall or downward at an angle into the inguinal canal

Inhalation: (1) act of breathing in; synonym for *inspiration*; (2) administration of a drug in solution by way of the respiratory tract

Injection: introduction of medication into the body by a syringe attached to a needle

Inner canthus angle of the eye where the upper and lower lids meet

Inpatient: person who enters a health care setting for a stay ranging from 24 hours to many years

Insensible water loss: nonperceptible water lost from the body as moisture through the breath and by evaporation from the skin

Insomnia: difficulty in falling asleep, intermittent sleep, or early awakening from sleep

Inspection: purposeful and systematic observation

Inspiration: act of breathing in; synonym for *inhalation*

Inspiratory reserve volume (IRV): additional amount of air that can be inspired beyond the tidal volume

Instillation: pouring or dropping a liquid into a body cavity or onto a surface

Insulator: poor conductor of heat

Integument skin

Integumentary system: skin and its appendages (ie, hair, glands in the skin, and nails)

Intellectualization: defense mechanism that separates the emotion of an event from the facts because the emotion is too painful to be acknowledged

Intensive-level care: care warranting close observation, monitoring, or treatment requiring skilled care

Interdependent intervention: nursing action performed by the nurse in collaboration with other members of the health care team; synonym for *collaborative intervention*

Intermediate-level care: care warranting skilled services for a client in which an improvement in function is expected; synonym for *rehabilitative-level care*

Intermittent fever: body temperature that alternates between fever and normal or subnormal temperature

Intermittent pulse: normal pulse rhythm broken by periods of irregular rhythm

Internal respiration: act of using oxygen by body cells; synonym for *tissue respiration*

Internal rotation: body part turning on its axis toward the midline of the body

Interpersonal skills: elements required for positive relationships to exist between people

Interstitial fluid: fluid between the cells

Interview: planned communication for a specific purpose (eg, data collection)

Interviewing techniques: communication skills specifically designed to gather and validate information

Intracellular fluid (ICF): fluid within the cell; synonym for *cellular fluid*

Intractable pain: severe pain that is extremely resistant to relief measures

Intradermal injection: injection into the muscle tissue

Intraoperative phase: period lasting from admission to the operating room area to transfer to the postanesthesia recovery area after surgery is completed

Intravascular fluid: fluid within the vascular system; synonym for *plasma*

Intravenous infusion: injection of relatively large quantities of solution into a vein

Intravenous injection: injection into the vein

Intravenous pyelogram (IVP): x-ray examination of the kidneys and ureters after a contrast material is injected intravenously to determine the kidney's ability to excrete urine

Introjection: person internalizes some aspect of the external world and keeps it intact in his psyche

Intuitive problem solving: direct understanding of a situation based on a background of experience, knowledge, and skill that makes expert decision making possible

Inunction: rubbing substances into the skin

Invasion of privacy: action that invades the right of a person to be left alone

Ion: atom or molecule carrying an electric charge in solution

Ionization: process by which substances dissociate to form ions

Irrigation: flushing of a tube, canal, or area with solution

Ischemia: deficiency of blood in a particular area

Isokinetic exercise: exercise involving muscle contractions with resistance varying at a constant rate

Isolation: protective procedure designed to prevent the transmission of specific microorganisms; also called *protective aseptic techniques* and *barrier techniques*

Isometric exercise: exercise in which muscle tension occurs without a significant change in muscle length

Isotonic: (1) having about the same concentration as the solution with which it is being compared; (2) exercise in which muscles shorten (contract) and move

Jaundice: yellow appearance of the skin

Kardex nursing care plan: trade name for a care plan documentation system that encompasses (1) prescriptions for nursing care related to activities of daily living; (2) nursing diagnoses and related client goals and nursing orders; and (3) the nursing care related to diagnostic measures and the medical regimen.

Kegel exercises: repetitious contraction and relaxation of the pubococcygeal muscle to improve vaginal tone and urinary continence

Kinesthesia: awareness of positioning of body parts and body movement

Knee–chest position: position in which the client kneels with the body at a 90-degree angle to the hips

Korotkoff sounds: series of sounds that correspond to changes in blood flow through an artery as pressure is released

Kussmaul's respiration breathing: an extreme rate and depth of breathing

Laceration: wound caused by a blunt instrument or object that tears tissue

Laissez-faire leadership: leadership style in which the leader relinquishes all power to the group

Language: prescribed way of using words; a means to express thoughts and feelings

Lanugo: fine hair that covers the fetus and decreases as full gestation approaches

Laryngoscope: lighted, tubular instrument used for visual examination of the larynx

Laryngoscopy: visual examination of the larynx

Lateral: pertaining to the side

Law: rule of conduct established and enforced by the government of a society

Lawsuit: legal action in a court of law

Laxative: drug used to induce emptying of the intestinal tract

Lead: placement pattern of electrodes used in electrocardiography

Leadership: ability to direct or motivate others toward the achievement of predetermined goals

Learning: increasing one's knowledge; having one's behavior changed in a measurable way as a result of an experience

Learning readiness: client's willingness to engage in the teach-ing–learning process (emotional readiness) and experiential readiness to begin the challenge of learning

Lesbian: term used to describe a female homosexual

Liability: legal responsibility for one's acts (and failure to act); includes responsibility for financial restitution of harms resulting from negligent acts

Libel: untruthful, written statement about a person that subjects him or her to ridicule or contempt

Licensure: to be given a license to practice nursing in a state or province after successfully meeting requirements

Life review/reminiscence: universal phenomenon identified by Butler as a review of one's life through one's recollections

Ligaments: tough fibrous bands that bind joints together and connect bones and cartilage

Line of gravity: vertical line that passes through the center of gravity

Linguistic: speech designed to convey meaning

Lipid: group name for fatty substances, including fats, oils, waxes, and related compounds

Liter (L): metric standard of measurement for liquids; one liter contains 1000 milliliters

Literacy: ability to read and write

Lithotomy position: same as the dorsal recumbent position except the feet are placed in stirrups and the buttocks are at the edge of the examination table

Litigation: process of lawsuit

Liver biopsy: needle aspiration of a liver tissue specimen

Living will: advance directive specifying the medical care a person would want or refuse should he or she lack the capacity to consent to or refuse treatment himself or herself

Local adaptation syndrome (LAS): localized response of the body to stress, precipitated by trauma or pathology

Localized symptoms: symptoms that are limited or restricted to a discrete area

Long-term care facilities: nursing homes

Loss: inaccessibility or change in a valued person, object, or situation. *Actual loss:* loss tangible to both the person sustaining the loss and to others. *Perceived loss:* loss tangible only to the person sustaining it. *Physical loss:* loss of life, limb, an object, person, pet, or job. *Psychological loss:* loss that affects a person's self-image. *Anticipatory loss:* loss behaviors displayed before the actual loss occurs

Love and belonging needs: understanding and acceptance of others in giving and receiving love

Lozenge: small, solid medication intended to be held in the mouth until it dissolves

Lumbar puncture: insertion of a needle into the subarachnoid space; synonym for *spinal tap*

Lysis: gradual return of an elevated body temperature to normal

Macromineral: mineral that is needed by the body in amount greater than 100 mg/day

Macronutrient: essential nutrient that supplies energy and builds tissue, such as carbohydrate, fat, and protein

Macroshock: electric current passing through a relatively large area of a person

Magnetic resonance imaging (MRI): use of magnetism and radio waves to produce cross-sectional images of body tissues on a computer screen

Maintenance-level care: care warranting assistance with personal care and homemaker services for a client for whom there is no expected change of condition

Malnutrition: literally "bad nutrition"; may be related to dietary excesses or deficiencies, or may occur secondary to illness or treatments

Malpractice: act of negligence as applied to a professional person, such as a physician, nurse, or dentist

Management: process of directing others toward goal achievement

Manslaughter: second-degree murder

Many-tailed binder: type of bandage with multiple tails; synonym for *scultetus binder*

Masochism: practice of inflicting discomfort on oneself for sexual stimulation

Mastectomy: surgical excision of the breast, used as a treatment for breast cancer; surrounding tissue and lymph nodes may also be removed

Masturbation: self-stimulation for sexual satisfaction

Maturation: physical developmental changes influenced by genetic and environmental factors

Mechanism: patterns of action performed by different parts of the body to serve a common goal

Meconium: first stool of a neonate

Medicaid: Title XIX (Social Security Act, 1965) to make health care available to those people with less than the minimum income who do not qualify for Medicare

Medical asepsis: practices designed to reduce the number and transfer of pathogens; synonym for *clean technique*

Medical diagnosis: statement about a specific disease process using terminology from a well-developed classification system accepted by the medical profession

Medicare: Title XVIII (Social Security Act 1965) to provide a measure of health coverage to all Social Security recipients

Medication: substance that modifies body functions when taken into the living organisms; synonym for *drug*

Menarche: initiation of the menstrual cycle

Meniscus: curved surface at the top of a column of liquid in a tube

Menopause: decrease of cyclic hormonal production and cessation of menses in females, usually between ages 45 and 60 years

Menses: monthly menstrual period

Mentorship: relationship in which an experienced person (the mentor) advises and assists a less experienced person

Message: term used in communication theory to denote the actual physical product of the source or encoder (eg, a speech, interview, phone conversation, chart)

Metabolic acidosis: proportionate deficiency of bicarbonate ions in the extracellular fluid

Metabolic alkalosis: proportionate excess of bicarbonate ions in the extracellular fluid

Metabolism: (1) chemical changes in the body by which energy is provided; (2) breakdown of a drug to an inactive form; also referred to as *biotransformation*

Micromineral: mineral or tract element that is needed by the body in an amount less than 100 mg/day

Micronutrient: vitamin or mineral needed in much smaller amount to regulate and control body processes

Microshock: electric current passing through a relatively small area of a person, usually part of the heart

Micturition: process of emptying the bladder; urination; voiding

Midlife crisis: realization that the halfway point in life has been reached and youthful goals may not have been achieved

Mild pain: pain that could be described as being between 1 and 3 on a scale of 1 to 10; synonym for *slight pain*

Milia: tiny, pearly white bumps across the nose, cheeks, or forehead of an infant, caused by accumulation of sebum in the ducts of the sebaceous glands

Milliequivalent (mEq): unit of measurement to describe electrolyte chemical activity; one milliequivalent is equivalent to the activity of 1 milligram of hydrogen

Milliliter (mL): one thousandth of a liter

Minerals: inorganic elements found in nature

Minority group: group having

some physical or cultural characteristic that identifies the people within the group as different from the dominant culture

Misdemeanor: crime of lesser offense than a felony and punishable by fines, imprisonment (usually for less than 1 year) or both

Model: abstract outline or visual representation of a complex state or occurrence

Moderate pain: pain that could be described as being between 4 and 7 on a scale of 1 to 10; between pain that is described as mild or severe

Molding: shaping of the fetal head that occurs at birth to accommodate to the size and shape of the birth canal

Mongolian spot: smooth, brown to gray-blue nevus typically found in the sacral region in Asians, blacks, native (North) Americans, and some southern Europeans; usually disappears during early childhood

Monilian infection: infection by the parasitic fungus *Monilia (Candida)*; usually sexually transmitted

Monosaccharides: simple sugars containing one sugar molecule. Glucose (blood sugar) and fructose (fruit sugar) are the most common monosaccharides; monosaccharides also are the end products of carbohydrate digestion

Morality: judgment about justice in personal and social situations

Morals: like ethics, concerned with what constitutes right action; more informal and personal than the term ethics

Moratorium: identity state in which a person is considering various alternatives before making a commitment

Mourning: period during which a person learns to accept grief

Murder: illegal killing of another person. *First-degree murder:* murder with malice aforethought. *Second-degree murder:* murder without previous deliberation; also called *manslaughter*

Mutual aid self-help groups (MASH): member-organized and self-run help groups that offer emotional support and education to assist members in coping with personal and health problems

Myelination: production of myelin, a lipid substance that forms a sheath around the axon of certain nerve fibers

Narcolepsy: condition characterized by an uncontrolled desire to sleep

Narrative: descriptive record of the client's condition; includes client's response to interventions by health professionals and client's progress toward goal achievement

Nasal cannula: disposable, plastic device that delivers oxygen with two protruding prongs for insertion into the nostrils

Nasal speculum: instrument used for inspection of the internal nares

Nasogastric feeding: feeding a client through a tube inserted into the nares and down to the stomach

Necrosis: death of cells

Negativism: negative verbalizations and behaviors

Negligence: performing an act that a reasonably prudent person under similar circumstances would not do, or failing to perform an act that a reasonably prudent person under similar circumstances would do

Neonate: period from birth to 1 month of age

Neurologic hammer: instrument used to test reflexes

Neuromodulator: endogenous opioid chemical regulators that appear to have analgesic activity and alter pain perception

Nitrogen balance: comparison between nitrogen intake (protein eaten) and nitrogen output (protein excreted in the urine, feces, hair, nails, and skin)

Nits: lice eggs

Nociceptors: pain receptors

Nocturia: frequency of urination during the night

Nocturnal emission: ejaculation due to erotic dreams while sleeping; synonym for *wet dream*

Nocturnal enuresis: involuntary urination while a person is sleeping

Nocturnal myoclonus: condition characterized by marked muscle contraction that results in the jerking of one or both legs during sleep

Noncompliance: nonadherence to a therapeutic recommendation

Nonelectrolyte: molecules that remain intact and do not ionize

Nonmaleficence: principle of avoiding evil

Nonproductive cough: forceful expiratory effort without production of mucus; also called a *dry cough*

Nonverbal communication: exchange of information without the use of words

Normal flora: microorganisms that normally inhabit various body sites and are part of the body's natural defense system

Nosocomial infection: hospital-acquired infection

NREM: non–rapid eye movement that characterizes four stages of sleep

Nuclear family: family unit, family of marriage, parenthood, or procreation, and their immediate children

Nurse practice act: law established to regulate nursing practice

Nursing: profession focusing on the holistic person receiving health care services and providing a unique contribution to the prevention of illness and maintenance of health

Nursing actions: any action performed by a nurse to assist clients to meet health goals: promote wellness, prevent disease or illness, restore health, facilitate coping with altered functioning

Nursing audit: method of evaluating the outcomes of nursing care or the process by which these outcomes are achieved using a review of client records

Nursing care conference: formal

meeting of nurses to discuss some aspect of client's care

Nursing care plan: written guide to direct the efforts of the nursing team as they work with clients to meet health goals; specifies prioritized nursing diagnoses, client goals, and nursing orders

Nursing care rounds: procedure in which a group of nurses visit clients individually at bedside to gather information that helps to plan and evaluate nursing care

Nursing diagnosis: actual or potential health problem that independent nursing intervention can prevent or resolve. *Actual problem* is present. *Possible problem* may be present, but more data are needed to confirm or disconfirm the problem. *Potential problem* may occur; defining characteristics are present as risk factors

Nursing ethics: discipline that takes as its domain the ethical issues and analysis used by nurses to make ethical judgments

Nursing history: assessment of the client by interview to identify the client's health status, strengths, health problems, health risks, and need for nursing

Nursing order: prescribes the nursing care to be given to assist clients to meet health goals

Nursing process: five-step systematic method for giving client care; involves assessing, diagnosing, planning, implementing, and evaluating

Nursing theory: attempts to describe or explain the phenomenon (process, occurrence, or event) called nursing; includes the concepts of person, health, environment, and nursing

Nutrient: specific biochemical substance used by the body for growth, development, activity, reproduction, lactation, health maintenance, and recovery from illness or injury

Nutrition: study of the nutrients and how they are handled by the body, as well as the impact of human behavior and environment on the process of nourishment

Obesity: weight greater than 20% above ideal body weight

Object permanence: awareness that an object or person does not cease to exist when out of sight

Objective data: information perceptible to the senses; may be verified by another person

Objectivity: remaining neutral while applying research criteria

Observation: conscious and deliberate use of the five senses to gather data

Occult blood: blood present in such minute quantities that it cannot be detected with the unassisted eye

Official name: name by which a drug is identified in official publications

Old-old: term used to describe older adults over age 75; sometimes referred to as frail-old

Older adult: after middle age; refers to adults over age of 65

Olfactory: pertaining to smell

Oliguria: scanty or greatly diminished amount or urine voided in a given time; 24-hour urine output is 100 to 400 mL

Oncotic pressure: pressure exerted by plasma proteins on permeable membranes in the body; synonym for *colloid osmotic pressure*

Open wound: injury characterized by a break in the continuity of the skin so that there is exposure of underlying tissue to the atmosphere

Ophthalmoscope: lighted instrument used for examination of the interior eye

Opioid: more correct term for narcotic analgesics, since these drugs act by binding to opiate receptor sites in the central nervous system

Opportunist: bacteria that may potentially be harmful

Organism: a living being

Orgasm: apex of sexual activity in which rhythmic contractions of the genital organs and many other physiologic changes occur

Orgasmic dysfunction: condition in which a woman is unable to reach orgasm

Orthopedics: correction or prevention of disorders of the locomotion of the body

Orthopnea: type of dyspnea in which breathing is easier when the client sits or stands

Orthostatic hypotension: temporary fall in blood pressure associated with assuming an upright position; synonym for *postural hypotension*

Osmolality: property of a solution that describes the total number of dissolved particles in a solution; the concentration of solutes in a solvent

Osmoreceptors: special neurons that are sensitive to changes in osmotic pressure of surrounding fluids

Osmosis: passage of a solvent through a semipermeable membrane from an area of lesser concentration to an area of greater concentration until equilibrium is established

Osmotic pressure: drawing power for water or the attraction for water exerted by solute particles

Ossification: formation of or conversion into bone or a bony substance

Osteomalacia: softening of the bones, usually due to a deficiency or loss of calcium salts from the body

Osteoporosis: condition characterized by loss of calcium from bone tissue

Ostomy: general term referring to an artificial opening; usually used to refer to an opening created for the excretion of body wastes

Otoscope: lighted instrument used for examination of the external ear canal and the tympanic membrane (eardrum)

Outcome: end product of nursing care; client outcomes are measurable changes in client behavior or state of health

Outer canthus: lateral angle of the

eye where the upper and lower lids meet

Overhydration: above-normal amounts of water in extra-cellular spaces

Overweight: weight between 10% and 20% above ideal body weight

Ovulation: discharge of ovum from the female ovary at about the midpoint of each menstrual cycle

Ovum: female reproductive cell, often called an *egg*

Pack: moist cloths or dressings applied to a large body area

Pain: sensation of physical or mental suffering or hurt that usually causes distress or agony to the one experiencing it

Pain threshold: amount of stimulation required before a person experiences the sensation of pain

Pain tolerance: point beyond which a person is no longer willing to endure pain (ie, pain of greater duration or intensity)

Pallor: paleness of the skin

Palpation: method of examining by feeling a part with the fingers or hand

Palpitation: perception of one's own heartbeat

Paracentesis: withdrawal of fluid from a body cavity, usually from the abdominal cavity

Parainsomnia: patterns of waking behavior that appear during sleep (eg, sleep walking, sleep talking, nocturnal erections)

Parallax: apparent change of position of an object when observed from two different angles

Paralytic ileus: paralysis of intestinal peristalsis

Paraplegia: paralysis of the legs

Parenteral: outside of intestines or alimentary canal; popularly used to refer to injection routes

Parenteral nutrition: form of feeding that completely bypasses the gastrointestinal tract and meets the client's nutritional needs by way of nutrient-filled solutions administered intravenously

Paresthesia: numbness and tingling

Passive exercise: manual or mechanical means of moving the joints

Passive immunity: antibodies against harmful effects of micro-organisms or toxins are produced by other people or animals and passed on to a person; two common examples: a passive immunity is acquired by a fetus from its mother in utero or by an infant from its mother through breastfeeding

Pathogen: disease-producing microorganism

Patient-controlled analgesia (PCA): method of controlling pain that involves an infusion pump that holds a vial of an intravenous analgesic that the client controls and self-adminis-ters in small doses

Pediculicide: preparation for destroying lice

Pediculosis: infestation with lice

Perception: conscious process of organizing and interpreting data from the senses into meaningful information

Percussion: technique in physical examination that involves strik-ing the finger of one hand into the finger of the other hand to evaluate some organ

Percussion hammer: instrument with a rubber head used for tap-ping a body surface

Perfusion: passing of fluid through body tissue

Periodontitis: extensive inflamma-tion of the gums and alveolar tissues; synonym for *pyorrhea*

Perioperative nursing: wide vari-ety of nursing activities carried out before, during, and after surgery

Perioperative period: entire period from the decision to do or have surgery through recovery from surgery

Periorbital edema: edema or swelling around the orbit of the eye

Peripheral resistance: restraint to blood flow created by arteriole walls in a partial state of contraction

Peristalsis: involuntary, progres-sive wavelike movement of the

musculature of the gastrointesti-nal tract

Person: a living human being with all the characteristics that make up an individual personality

Personal hygiene: measures of personal cleaning and grooming that promote physical and psy-chological well-being

Personal space: external environ-ment surrounding a person that is regarded as being part of that person

Petechiae: small, purplish hemor-rhagic spots on the skin that do not blanch with applied pressure

pH: expression of hydrogen ion concentration and resulting acidity of a substance

Phagocytosis: engulfing of micro-organisms, foreign particles, or other cells by phagocytes

Phantom limb pain: sensation of pain without demonstrable physiologic or pathologic sub-stance; commonly observed after the amputation of a limb

Pharmacodynamics: study of drug activity at the cellular level

Pharmacokinetics: study of the movement of drug molecules in the body in relation to its absorption, distribution, metab-olism, and excretion

Pharmacology: study of actions of chemicals on living organisms

Pharmacopeia: official drug document

Philosophy: study of wisdom, of fundamental knowledge, and of the process used to develop and construct our own perception of life

Phlebitis: inflammation of a vein

Phlegm: thick, respiratory secretions

Physical assessment: systematic examination of the client for objective data to better define the client's condition and help the nurse in planning care; usu-ally performed in a head-to-toe format

Physiologic jaundice: yellowness of the skin, sclera, and mucous membranes due to excessive bilirubin in the blood of a neo-nate caused by immature liver function at birth; as the liver function matures, the jaundice disappears, usually within a few days

Physiologic needs: need for oxygen, food, water, temperature, elimination, sexuality, activity, and rest; these needs have the highest priority and are essential for survival

Piggyback infusion: intermittent intravenous administration of medications through a primary intravenous line with the additive container positioned higher than the primary intravenous solution

Placebo: Latin word meaning "I shall please"; an inactive substance that gives satisfaction to the person using it

Plaintiff: person or government bringing a lawsuit against another

Planned change: process of effecting change by purposeful and systematic efforts

Planning: establishment of client goals to prevent, reduce, or resolve the problems identified in the nursing diagnoses and determination of related nursing interventions

Plantar flexion: flexion of the foot so that the foot is in a dropped position

Plaque: transparent, adhesive coating on teeth consisting of mucin, carbohydrate, and bacteria

Plasma: liquid constituent of blood; synonym for *intravascular fluid*

Play: activities that allow the child to discover and begin to control the environment

Pleural friction rub: dry grating sound caused by inflammation of pleural surfaces

Pneumonia: inflammation or infection of the lungs

Podiatrist: one who treats foot disorders; synonym for *chiropodist*

Podiatry: health discipline that deals with the treatment of foot disorders; synonym for *chiropody*

Poikilothermic: maintenance of body temperature at or near the temperature of the environment

Polarity: presence of electrically charged particles

Polyp: tumor on a stem that bleeds easily and may become malignant

Polypharmacy: dispensing or use of multiple drugs for one or more health problems

Polypnea: fast respiratory rate; synonym for *tachypnea*

Polysaccharides: complex CHO compounds composed on ten or more glucose units; starch, dextrins, and cellulose are common polysaccharides

Polysomnography: sleep study consisting of an electroencephalographic recording of the stages of sleep and any episodes of apnea, continuous monitoring of arterial oxygen saturation, and an electrocardiographic recording to detect any cardiac dysrhythmias

Polyuria: excessive output of urine (diuresis)

Portal of entry: point at which organisms enter a host

Postanesthesia recovery (PAR) room: area to which clients are taken after surgery is completed for assessment of recovery from anesthesia and monitoring of potential complications

Posterior fontanelle: triangular membrane-covered space remaining at the junction of the occipital and parietal bone sutures in a fetus or an infant

Postoperative phase: period lasting from admission to the postanesthesia recovery area through recovery and convalescence

Postural hypotension: temporary fall in blood pressure associated with assuming an upright position; synonym for *orthostatic hypotension*

Power: ability to influence others to achieve a desired effect

Preceptorship: process by which an experienced person facilitates an orientee's introduction to new responsibilities by way of teaching and guidance

Precordium: anterior surface of the chest wall overlying the heart and its related structures

Preferred provider arrangement (PPA): any arrangement whereby clients are channeled to specific individual providers of health plans

Preferred provider organization (PPO): any arrangement whereby clients are channeled to specific organizations as providers of health plans

Prefilled cartridge: previously prepared single dose of medication inserted into a holder for injection

Preformed water: water in food

Pregnancy: condition resulting from union of a sperm and an egg; period from fertilization of the ovum to delivery of the neonate about 9½ lunar months in humans

Prelinguistic: sounds that precede speech in infancy

Premature beat: irregular rhythm in which a heartbeat occurs sooner than the pace at which previous ones were noted

Premature ejaculation: condition in which a man consistently reaches orgasm and ejaculation during sexual activity before or soon after coitus begins

Premenstrual (tension) syndrome (PMS): menstrual cycle–related distress; occurs a few days before the onset of menstruation

Preoperative phase: period lasting from the decision that surgery is necessary until the client is transferred to the operating room area

Presbycusis: age-related hearing loss in which there is decreased ability to distinguish higher frequencies

Presbyopia: condition of aging in which decreased elasticity of the eye lens hinders accommodation to close vision

Preschooler: period from ages 3 to 6 years

Prescription: used by physician to convey medication plans for a client

Pressure ulcer: area of cellular necrosis caused by a lack of circulation to the involved area; synonym for *bedsore* and *decubitus ulcer*

Primary hypertension: abnormally elevated blood pressure with no known cause; synonym for *essential hypertension*

Priority setting: process of ranking client problems in terms of the threat they pose to client well-being

Private law: rule that regulates relationships among people; synonym for *civil law*

Privileged communication: information that cannot be revealed in court by the person receiving it

Problem-oriented record (POR): documentation system organized according to the person's specific health problems; includes data base, problem list, plan of care, and progress notes

Process: series of actions, changes, or functions to bring about a result

Proctosigmoidoscopy: visual examination of the rectum, rectosigmoid junction, and lower sigmoid colon

Prodromal stage: stage of an infection when a person is most infectious; early signs and symptoms of disease are present but are vague and nonspecific

Productive cough: cough that produces respiratory tract secretions

Projection: a person attributes his own undesirable or unacceptable impulses to another person or object

Pronation: assumption of the prone position, such as when the patient is lying on his or her abdomen

Prone position: lying horizontal, with face downward and palms turned downward

Prospective payment: under this plan, clients are classified by major diagnostic related groups, with a rate or payment amount assigned prospectively to each group for reimbursement of health care providers

Proteinuria: albumin in the urine; indication of kidney disease

Protocol: written plan that details the nursing activities to be executed in specific situations

Protrusion: state or condition of being forward or projecting

Pseudomenstruation: slight, bloody, mucous discharge from the vagina of a female infant in response to maternal hormonal influences

Psychiatric hospital: institution that provides in-hospital mental health services for clients with acute or chronic alterations

Psychiatric nurse specialist: community health nurse with a specialty in psychiatric nursing

Psychogenic pain: pain for which no physical cause can be identified

Psychomotor learning: acquisition of physical skills

Psychosocial development: development governed by social, cultural, and emotional variables

Psychosomatic disorder: physiologic alterations and illness believed to be due to psychological influences

Puberty: period during which primary and secondary sexual characteristics develop and the capability of sexual reproduction is attained

Public health service: local, state, or national official agency that provides community services for the promotion of health and prevention of illness

Public law: rule that regulates relationships between people and their government

Pulmonary embolism: embolism carried to the lungs

Pulse: wave produced in the wall of an artery with each beat of the heart

Pulse deficit: difference between the apical and radial pulse rates

Pulse oximetry: noninvasive technique that measures the oxygen saturation (SaO_2) of arterial blood

Pulse pressure: difference between systolic and diastolic pressures

Puncture wound: injury caused by a pointed object that penetrates the skin; synonym for *stab wound*

Purkinje system: interlacing network in the heart that carries electric currents through the ventricles

Purulent: containing pus

Pyorrhea: extensive inflammation of the gums and alveolar tissues; synonym for *periodontitis*

Pyrexia: elevation above the upper limit of normal body temperature; synonym for *fever*

Pyuria: pus in the urine; urine appears cloudy

Quality assurance program: ongoing evaluation program designed and implemented to secure the excellence of health care; may involve an assessment of structure, process, and outcome standards

Quickening: first perceptible movement of the fetus in utero

Race: division of human beings based on distinct physical characteristics

Radiation: diffusion or dissemination of heat by electromagnetic waves

Radiography: examination by x-ray film

Radioisotope: radioactive chemical

Radiopaque: substance that x-rays cannot penetrate

Rales: abnormal lung sound described as crackling in nature

Range of motion: complete extent of movement of which a joint is normally capable

Rape: sexual violation of a person by someone who uses force, threats, and abuse

Rapport: feeling of mutual trust experienced by people in a satisfactory relationship

Rationalization: giving questionable behavior a logical or socially acceptable explanation; intellectual behavior justification

Reaction formation: giving a reason for behavior that is opposite from its true cause

Reactive hyperemia: body's flooding of an area with blood after the area has suffered from poor circulation for a period

Readiness: condition of possessing the ability to change

Reality orientation: method of care used to promote awareness of reality in confused or disoriented clients

Receiver (decoder): term used in communication theory that specifies the person or object to which the message is directed

Reception: process of receiving data about the internal or external environment through the senses

Receptor: specialized structures within a cell that interact with a drug

Recipient: person who receives another person's blood

Recommended dietary allowance (RDA): recommendations for average daily amounts of essential nutrients that healthy population groups should consume over time

Reconstitution: addition of fluid to a powdered drug to create a solution for administration

Record (medical record, chart): legal document consisting of a compilation of a person's health care information

Referred pain: pain in an area removed from that in which stimulation has its origin

Reflex: unconscious effecting of a particular automatic response mediated by the nervous system

Reflex incontinence: state in which a person experiences an involuntary loss of urine, occurring at somewhat predictable intervals when a specific bladder volume is reached

Reflex pain response: automatic response of the central nervous system to the stimulus of pain

Regional anesthesia: anesthetic drug is injected or applied topically to inhibit transmission of sensory stimuli

Registration: official listing of the names and qualifications of people who meet minimum requirements to practice in the occupation or profession of their choice

Regression: behavior that is more characteristic of an earlier age

Rehabilitation: process of restoring a person's highest level of possible wellness and returning that person's ability to live and work as normally as possible after a disabling illness or injury

Rehabilitation center: community center providing rehabilitation services

Rehabilitative-level care: care warranting skilled services for a client in whom an improvement of function is expected; synonym for *intermediate-level care*

Reinforcement: affirmation of clients who have mastered new knowledge, attitudes, or skills

Relapsing fever: body temperature that returns to normal for at least a day after which fever returns

Relationship: interaction of people over time

Relax: to become less rigid, slacken effort, and decrease tension

Religion: organized system of beliefs about a higher power; often includes set forms of worship, spiritual practices, and codes of conduct

REM: rapid eye movement that characterizes the dream state of sleep

Remittent fever: body temperature that fluctuates several degrees above normal but does not reach normal between fluctuations

Repolarization: process of restoring polarity

Report: oral, written, or computer-based communication of client data with the purpose of informing others

Repression: exclusion of an anxiety-producing event from conscious awareness

Reservoir: natural habitat for the growth and multiplication of microorganisms

Resident flora or bacteria: microorganisms that normally live on a person's skin

Residual urine: urine that remains in the bladder after the act of micturition

Residual volume (RV): air remaining in the lungs after maximal exhalation

Resonance: quality of the sound heard on percussion of a hollow structure such as the chest

Respiration: act of breathing and using oxygen in body cells

Respiratory acidosis: proportionate excess of carbonic acid in the extracellular fluid

Respiratory alkalosis: proportionate deficiency of carbonic acid in the extracellular fluid

Respiratory distress syndrome: condition of the neonate marked by dyspnea, cyanosis, expiratory grunt and intercostal retractions; usually caused by immaturity of lung function and occurs most frequently in premature infants

Respite care: care in which someone comes into the house for a few hours to relieve the caregiver; sometimes the client is sent to a nursing home for a short period to give the caregiver a rest

Respondeat superior: master–servant rule that states that an employer is legally liable for his or her employee's acts

Responsibility: obligation to perform some act for which one can be held accountable

Rest: condition in which the body is in a decreased state of activity with the consequent feeling of being refreshed

Restraint: device used to limit movement or immobilize a client

Retarded ejaculation: condition in which a man is unable to ejaculate into the vagina or has delayed intravaginal ejaculation

Retention: inability to void although urine is produced by the kidneys and enters the bladder; excessive storage of urine in the bladder

Retention sutures: sutures used to provide extra support in wounds in obese clients or in wounds with increased risk of dehiscence

Reticular activating system: network of neurons in the core of the brain stem with ascending and descending tracts to other areas of the brain that monitors and regulates incoming sensory stimuli and level of arousal

Retrograde pyelogram: x-ray examination of the kidney and ureters after a contrast material is injected into the renal pelvis through the ureter

Retrospective audit: evaluation of nursing care and client outcomes after the client has been discharged (may use post-discharge questionnaires, client interviews, or chart review)

Rh: an inherited antigen

Rhonchi: abnormal, continuous sound characterized by a sonorous, dry, coarse sound heard over the large airways; may clear with a cough; synonym for *gurgles*

Right: claim to a particular privilege

Risk factor: something that increases a person's chance for illness or injury

Risk management: process of identifying, analyzing, and treating risks to improve client care and reduce malpractice claims

Roentgen ray: high-energy electromagnetic wave capable of penetrating solid matter and acting on photographic film; synonym for *x-ray*

Role performance: ability to successfully execute societal expectations regarding role-specific behaviors

Rotation: turning on an axis

Sadism: practice of inflicting harm on another person for sexual stimulation

Sadomasochism (S & M): practice of using sadism and masochism simultaneously

Safety and security needs: person's need to be protected from actual or potential harm and to have freedom from fear

Sanguineous: containing or mixed with blood

Saturated fatty acids: primarily animal fats that have a solid consistency at room temperature

Scar: connective tissue that fills a wound area

Schemata: mental representation of familiar experiences or events

School-age: period from ages 6 to 12 years

School phobia: unrealistic fear of attending school, possibly reflecting severe, abnormal separation anxiety

Scientific knowledge: knowledge arrived at by applying scientific methods

Scientific method: systematic problem-solving process that involves (1) problem identification, (2) data collection, (3) hypothesis formulation, (4) plan of action, (5) hypothesis testing, (6) interpretation of results, and (7) evaluation resulting in conclusion or revision of the study

Scrub nurse: nurse who assists the surgeon during surgery, maintaining surgical asepsis while draping, handling instruments, and handling supplies

Scultetus binder: type of bandage with multiple tails; synonym for *many-tailed binder*

Sebaceous gland: gland found in the skin that secretes an oily substance called sebum

Sebum: fatty secretion of the sebaceous glands

Secondary hypertension: abnormally elevated blood pressure caused by known abnormality

Sedative hypnotic: pharmaceutical agent used to induce sleep

Self-actualization needs: need to reach one's potential through full development of one's unique capabilities; highest level need

Self-concept: mental image or picture of self; includes body image, subjective self, ideal self, and social self

Self-esteem: person's perception of his or her total being, including self-worth and body image

Self-esteem needs: need to feel good about oneself and to believe others hold one in high regard

Self-identity: conscious sense of who a person is and what it is that makes that person unique

Semantics: study of the meaning of words

Semen: seminal plasma containing sperm

Semi-Fowler's position: low, semi-sitting position with the head of the bed raised 15 to 30 degrees

Semipermeable membrane: selectively permeable membrane that allows water to pass through it but is either impermeable or selectively permeable to solutes

Sensoristasis: arousal state of the reticular activating system; general drive state

Sensory deficit: impaired functioning of one or more senses: visual, auditory, olfactory, gustatory, tactile, kinesthetic, visceral

Sensory deprivation: condition resulting from decreased sensory input or input that is monotonous, unpatterned, or meaningless

Sensory overload: condition resulting from excessive sensory input to which the brain is unable to meaningfully respond

Sensory/perceptual alteration: disturbance in the body's ability to receive or process data from its internal or external environment. NANDA-approved nursing diagnosis

Separation anxiety: condition that occurs when a child is afraid of being sent away from caregivers who are loved and provide security

Serous: resembling blood serum; clear and watery in appearance

Set point: level at which the hypothalamus attempts to maintain body temperature

Severe pain: pain that could be described as being between 8 and 10 on a scale of 1 to 10; synonym for *excruciating pain*

Sexual dysfunction: condition that prevents a person or couple from engaging in or obtaining satisfaction from sexual activity

Sexual harassment: unwelcome verbal or physical advance or sexually explicit statement (eg, leers, pats, grabs, jokes, requests for dates, and even rape) that interferes with one's ability to do one's job by making one feel humiliated, intimidated, or uncomfortable

Sexual intercourse: sexual activity in which the penis is placed in the vagina; synonym for *coitus*

Sexuality: degree to which a person exhibits and experiences maleness and femaleness physically, emotionally, and mentally

Sexually transmitted disease: pathologic condition spread by sexual activity and intimate genital contact

Sharp pain: quick, sticking, and intense discomfort

Shearing force: force created when layers of tissue move on one another

Shifting pain: discomfort that moves from one area to another

Shock: body's reaction to acute peripheral circulatory failure due to an abnormality of circulatory control or to a loss of circulating fluid

Significance: way a person believes that he or she is loved and approved of by the people who are important in his or her life

Sims' position (right and left): position in which the client is on his or her side with the top knee flexed sharply into the abdomen and the lower knee less sharply flexed

Single-parent family: family with only one parent, predominantly female

Singultus: involuntary spasmodic contractions of the diaphragm; synonym for *hiccups*

Sinoatrial node (SA node): tissue in the right atrium where the heartbeat originates; also called the *heart's pacemaker*

Situational crisis: change that results when a person faces an event or situation that causes a disruption in his life

Situational stress: changing events or situations that occur in day-to-day life

Sitz bath: special type of bath that applies heated water to the pelvic or rectal area

Skin sutures: used to approximate wound tissues and skin; may be silk, synthetic, wire, or metal staples

Skin tests: tests to determine antigen–ant body reaction

Slander: untruthful oral statement about a person that subjects him or her to ridicule or contempt

Sleep: state of altered consciousness throughout which varying degrees of stimuli preclude wakefulness

Sleep apnea: periods of no breathing during sleep that may last from 15 seconds to 2 minutes

Sleep cycle: passage through the four states of NREM sleep (I, II, III, IV), then reversal (IV, III, II), and finally instead of reentering stage I and awakening, entering REM sleep and returning to stage II

Sleep deprivation: condition resulting from decreased REM sleep, NREM sleep, or total sleep, characterized by progressive symptoms—irritableness or complete personality disintegration

Slight pain: pain that could be described as being between 1 and 3 on a scale of 1 to 10; synonym for *mild pain*

Smegma: thick secretion of sebaceous glands found under the labia minora and around the clitoris in the female and under the male prepuce

SOAP format: method of charting narrative progress notes; organizes data according to subjective information (S), objective information (O), assessment (A), and plan (P)

Social isolation: sense of aloneness because of decreasing relationships with others, resulting from attitudinal, geographic, financial, or illness-related factors

Social self: way a person believes that others see him or her

Socialization: integration of behavior patterns, attitudes, motivations, and values deemed important by a person's culture

Sodomy: term used to describe sexual activity of placing the penis into the rectum; synonym for *anal sex*

Soixante-neuf: French word meaning 69; refers to a couple engaging in cunnilingus and fellatio simultaneously while assuming a position resembling the number 69

Solute: substance dissolved in a solution

Solvent: liquid holding a substance in solution

Somatic pain: pain originating in structures in the body's external wall

Somnambulism: sleep walking

Sordes: accumulation of mucus and crust formation on the teeth and around the lips

Source (encoder): term used in communication theory to specify the one who prepares and sends a message to the receiver

Source-oriented record: documentation system in which each health care group records data on its own separate form

Spasticity: increased muscle tone

Specific dynamic action: caloric cost of digesting, absorbing, and metabolizing food; represents about 10% of total calorie intake

Speed shock: body's reaction to a rapid injection of a substance into the circulatory system

Sperm: male reproductive cell; synonym for *spermatozoan*

Spermatogenesis: development of mature sperm in the male testes

Spermicide: chemical agent used to destroy sperm

Sphincter: circular muscle that constricts a passage or closes a natural orifice

Sphygmomanometer: instrument used for the indirect measurement of blood pressure

Spina bifida: congenital anomaly in which there is a defective closure of the bony encasement of the spinal cord; the spinal cord and meninges may protrude through the defective closure

Spinal tap: insertion of a needle into the subarachnoid space; synonym for *lumbar puncture*

Spiritual distress: nursing diagnosis describing an alteration in spiritual health (eg, spiritual pain, alienation, anxiety, guilt, anger, loss, despair)

Spiritual need: lack of anything necessary for spiritual health

(eg, meaning and purpose, love and relatedness, forgiveness)

Spirituality: anything that pertains to a person's relationship with a nonmaterial life force or higher power

Spirometer: instrument used to measure lung capacities and volumes; one type is used to encourage deep breathing (incentive spirometry)

Spooning: nail having a concave outer surface

Stab wound: injury caused by a pointed object that penetrates the skin; synonym for *puncture wound*

Standard: acceptable, expected, level of performance established by authority, custom, or consent

Standard of care: description of conduct that illustrates what a reasonably prudent person would have done or would not have done under similar circumstances

Standardized care plan: prepared plan of care that identifies the nursing diagnoses, client goals, and related nursing orders common to a specific population (eg, normal neonates) or problem

Standards of nursing: optimal levels of nursing care used for comparison of actual performance

Standing order: document that details the nursing care to be implemented in specific nursing situations, frequently when a physician is not present; may expand scope of nursing responsibilities

Stare decisis: Latin phrase meaning "Let the decision stand"; basis for common law

Step-family: family in which children live with one birth parent and one non–birth parent

Stereotyping: assigning characteristics to a group of people without considering specific individuality

Sterilization: (1) the process by which all microorganisms, including spores, are destroyed; (2) surgical procedure performed to render a person infertile

Stertorous breathing: noisy respirations

Stethoscope: instrument used in auscultation to convey to the ear sounds produced in the body

Stimulus: agent, act, or other influence capable of initiating a response by the nervous system

Stock supply: system of supplying large quantities of medication on a nursing unit

Stoma: artificial opening for waste excretion located on the body surface

Stool: excreted feces

Strength (muscle): ability of the muscle to move actively against resistance

Stress: condition in which the human system responds to change in its normal balanced state

Stress incontinence: state in which the person experiences a loss of urine of less than 50 mL that occurs with increased abdominal pressure

Stressor: anything causing a person to experience stress; change in the balanced state

Stretching exercises: exercises that allow muscles and joints to be stretched gently through their full range of motion and that promote flexibility

Striae: (1) elevated or depressed line or band surrounding tissue; (2) difference in color and texture

Stridor: harsh, high-pitched sound usually heard on inspiration when upper airways become narrowed

Stroke volume: quantity of blood forced out of the left ventricle with each contraction

Subconjunctival hemorrhage: bleeding under the conjunctiva into the sclera of the eyeball as a result of increased vascular tension

Subculture: group of people with different interests or goals than the primary culture

Subcutaneous injection: injection into the subcutaneous tissue that lies between the epidermis and the muscle

Subjective data (symptoms, covert data): information perceived only by the affected person

Subjective self: how one sees oneself; who one thinks one is

Sublimation: conscious expression of an unacceptable impulse or feeling in a more acceptable way

Sublingual: area in the mouth under the tongue

Sudden infant death syndrome (SIDS): sudden death of any infant or young child without demonstrated cause

Suffocation: stoppage of breathing or the lack of air reaching the lungs; synonym for *asphyxiation*

Sundowning syndrome: describes a phenomenon when a person habitually becomes confused or disoriented with darkness

Supination: assumption of the supine position, such as when the client is lying on his or her back

Supine position: position in which the client lies flat on his or her back with legs together (dorsal position)

Suppository: oval- or cone-shaped substance that is inserted into a body cavity and that melts at body temperature

Suppressant: drug that depresses a body function

Suppression: person consciously turns his or her attention away from a perceived threat

Suprapubic catheter: catheter inserted into the bladder through a small abdominal incision above the pubic area

Surgical asepsis: practices that render and keep objects and areas free from microorganisms; synonym for *sterile technique*

Surgical risk: classification of surgery as major or minor; major surgery has the potential for significant client risk and postoperative complications

Susceptibility: degree of resistance of a host to a pathogen

Suture: line of union between adjoining bones of the skull

Symmetry: correspondence in shape, size, and relative position of parts on opposite sides of the body

Sympathomimetic agent: drug that produces effects that mimic the action of the sympathetic nervous system

Symptom: abnormality indicative of illness as experienced by the client; synonym for *subjective data*

Synergistic effect: combined effect of two or more drugs is greater than the effect of each drug alone

Synovial joint: freely movable joint in which there is a space between the articulating bones

Syphilis: sexually transmitted disease caused by the bacterium *Treponema pallidum*

Systemic symptoms: symptoms manifested throughout the entire body

Systolic pressure: highest point of pressure on arterial walls when the ventricles contract

Tachycardia: rapid heart rate

Tachypnea: abnormally rapid rate of breathing

Tactile: pertaining to touch

Tandem infusion: intermittent intravenous administration of medications through a primary intravenous line with the additive container positioned at the same level as the primary intravenous solution

Target heart range: between 70% and 85% of the maximum heart rate (ie, the greatest number of beats per minute of which the heart is capable)

Tartar: hard deposit on the teeth near the gum line formed by plaque buildup and dead bacteria

Teaching: planned method or series of methods used to help someone learn

Temperament: person's style of approaching people, situations, or events

Temperature: refers to the hotness or coldness of a substance

Tendons: strong, flexible, inelastic fibrous bands that attach muscle to bone

Terminal illness: illness from which there is no reasonable expectation of recovery or cure

Theory: statement that explains or characterizes a process, an occurrence, or an event based on observed facts but lacking absolute or direct proof

Therapeutic touch: unblocking, or "unruffling," of congested areas of energy in the body and redirecting the energy for the promotion of comfort, relaxation, healing, and sense of well-being

Third-space fluid shift: distributional shift and trapping of body fluids into body spaces such as the pleural, peritoneal, or pericardial, or into the interstitial space (plasma-to-interstitial shift)

Thoracentesis: aspiration of fluid or air from the pleural space

Thrill: abnormal tremor accompanying a vascular or cardiac murmur felt on palpation

Thrombophlebitis: inflammation in a vein associated with thrombus formation

Thrombus: blood clot; plural is *thrombi*

Tidal volume (TV): amount of air inspired and expired in a normal respiration

Tissue respiration: act of using oxygen by body cells; synonym for *internal respiration*

Toddler: period from ages 1 to 3 years

Tonus: normal, partially steady state of muscle contraction

Topical: application of a substance directly to a body site

Tort: wrong committed by a person against another person or his property

Total body water (TBW): total amount of water in the body, expressed as a percentage of body weight. The term *total body fluid* also is used; fluids usually are considered to include water and electrolytes

Total incontinence: state in which a person experiences a continuous and unpredictable loss of urine

Total lung capacity (TLC): amount of air equal to the tidal volume plus the residual volume

Total parenteral nutrition (TPN): feeding a nutritionally complete hypertonic solution through a major central vein; synonym for *hyperalimentation*

Trace elements: minerals found in the body in quantities less than 5 g and needed in only small amounts (18 mg or less)

Tracheostomy tube: curved tube inserted into an artificial opening made into the trachea that comes with varied angles and in multiple sizes

Trade name: drug name selected and trademarked by the company selling the drug to market the drug; also called *brand name* or *proprietary name*

Traditional family: composed of a husband, wife, and their children, who live together in one house

Traditional knowledge: knowledge passed down from generation to generation

Tranquilizer: pharmaceutical agent used primarily to reduce anxiety

Transducer: instrument that converts energy from one form to another

Transient flora or bacteria: microorganisms picked up on the skin as a result of normal activities that can be easily removed

Transient pain: pain that passes quickly; synonym for *brief pain*

Transsexuality: condition in which the person feels trapped within a body of the wrong sex

Transvestism: practice of arousing sexual desire by wearing clothing of the opposite sex

Transcultural nursing: providing nursing care that is planned and implemented in a way that is sensitive to the needs of individuals, families, and groups representing the diverse cultural populations within our society

Trauma: injury

Tremor: involuntary muscular movements

Trendelenburg's position: elevating the feet and legs while keeping the trunk flat on the bed; the head may rest on a small pillow

Trial: hearing of evidence in a legal case before a judge (and jury) with the intent of reaching a decision or verdict

Trichomonal infection: sexually transmitted disease caused by the parasitic protozoa *Trichomonas vaginalis*

Triglycerides: predominant form of fat in food and the major storage form of fat in the body; composed of one glyceride molecule and three fatty acids

Trimester: one of the three periods of about 3 months into which pregnancy is divided

Tuning fork: instrument that sets up vibrations; used primarily for testing hearing

Turgor: tension of a cell determined by its hydration

Tympany: drumlike sound on percussion resulting from the presence of air or gas

Typing: determining a person's blood type

Ultrasonography: use of ultrasound to produce an image or photograph of an organ or tissue

Ultrasound waves: extremely high-frequency and inaudible sound waves

Unilateral: affecting or occurring on one side only

Unit dose: separate packaging and labeling of individual drug doses

United States Dietary Guidelines: general recommendations for choosing a healthy diet made by the U.S. Department of Agriculture and the U.S. Department of Health and Human Services

Universal precautions: isolation system that considers blood, body fluids containing blood, semen, and vaginal secretions of all clients as potentially infective

Unsaturated fatty acids: primarily vegetable fats that are liquid at room temperature and referred to as oils

Upper GI series: x-ray film visualization of the esophagus, stomach, and duodenum

Urge incontinence: state in which a person experiences involuntary passage of urine that occurs soon after a strong sense of urgency to void

Urgency: strong desire to void

Urinalysis: laboratory examination of a urine specimen

Urination: process of emptying the bladder; micturition; voiding

Urinometer: instrument used to measure the specific gravity of urine

Utilitarianism: ethical theory that states that those acts that produce the greatest overall balance of good for the greatest number of people are right

Vaginal speculum: two-bladed instrument used to examine the vaginal canal and cervix

Vaginismus: condition in which the muscles of the vagina contract tightly to prevent penile penetration

Validation: act of confirming or verifying

Valsalva's maneuver: forcible exhalation against a closed glottis, resulting in increased intrathoracic pressure

Value system: organization of values ranked along a continuum of importance

Values: set of beliefs that are meaningful in life and that influence relationships with others

Variables: factors in a research study

Varicosity: swollen, twisted vein

Vector: nonhuman carrier, usually an arthropod, that transfers pathogens from one host to another

Vehicle: means for transmitting organisms

Ventilation: exchange of gases

Veracity: truth telling

Verbal communication: exchange of information using words

Verdict: decision reached by a jury in a legal proceeding

Vernix caseosa: cheeselike substance made of sebum and epithelial cells; acts in utero as a protective covering for the skin of the fetus

Vesicular: pertaining to vesicles or small blisters

Vesicular breathing: normal sound of respirations heard on auscultation over peripheral lung areas

Vial: glass bottle with self-sealing stopper through which medication is removed; may be single or multiple dose

Vibration: rhythmic contraction and relaxation of the arms and shoulders while holding the hands flat on the client's chest wall

Virginity: state of a person who has never engaged in sexual activity, particularly sexual intercourse

Virtue: attainment of moral–ethical standards

Virulence: ability to produce disease

Virus: smallest of all microorganisms that can be seen only by using an electron microscope

Visceral: pertaining to inner organs

Visceral pain: pain originating in the internal organs in the thorax, cranium, or abdomen

Visual: pertaining to sight

Visual recognition memory: remembering what occurs as a result of a visual stimulus

Vital capacity (VC): maximal amount of air that can be exhaled after maximal inhalation

Vital signs: body temperature, pulse and respiratory rates, and blood pressure; synonym for *cardinal signs*

Vitamins: organic substances needed by the body in small amounts to help regulate body processes; are susceptible to oxidation and destruction

Voiding: process of emptying the bladder; also called *micturition* or *urination*

Voluntary agency: nonprofit organizations that provide health care for communities; usually dealing with a particular segment or aspect

Waiver: legal provision that gives up a right or claim

Wellness: state of human functioning in which a person achieves maximum attainable function and quality of life

Wellness diagnosis: clinical judgment about an individual, family, or community in transition from a specific level of wellness to a higher level of wellness

Wheeze: high-pitched continuous sound that occurs during expiration or inspiration as a result of narrowed air passages

Widowhood: status change resulting from the death of a husband or wife

Wound: injury that results in a disruption in the normal continuity of a body structure

X-ray: high-energy electromagnetic wave capable of penetrating solid matter and acting on photographic film; synonym for *roentgen ray*

Yin–yang: energy forces in Chinese teaching that must be in balance for good health; expression of strong emotions results in disharmony and imbalance between these forces

Z-track: zigzag technique used to administer irritating medications intramuscularly

Photo Credits

Cover Photos

Front and back cover photos: Gates Rhodes, courtesy of the School of Nursing, University of Pennsylvania

Spine photo: courtesy of Lippincott Learning Systems

Unit and Chapter Opener Photos

Denise Angelini, courtesy of the School of Nursing, University of Pennsylvania: Unit II; Chapters 8, 12, 17, 25, 32, and 44

Jane Barry: Chapter 38

J. Barstys/H. Armstrong Roberts: Chapter 13

William Boehm: Chapter 11

Robert Coldwell, courtesy of Community Home Health Services of Philadelphia: Chapter 28

Denise Gilfillan: Unit III

© Ken Kasper: Chapters 15 and 42

Lippincott Learning Systems: Unit VI; Chapters 23, 26, 31, 35, and 43

Eugene Mopsik/H. Armstrong Roberts: Chapter 30

Robert Neroni, courtesy of Thomas Jefferson University: Chapter 5

© B. Proud: Unit I; Chapters 6, 29, 34, and 36

Gates Rhodes, courtesy of the School of Nursing, University of Pennsylvania: Units IV, V, VII, VIII; Chapters 1, 2, 3, 4, 7, 9, 10, 14, 16, 18, 19, 20, 21, 22, 24, 27, 33, 37, and 41

H. Armstrong Roberts: Unit IX

Don Walker, courtesy of Thomas Jefferson University: Chapter 40

J. Whitmer/H. Armstrong Roberts: Chapter 39

Index

Numbers followed by *f* indicate a figure; *t* following a page number indicates tabular material.